SURGERY

A PROBLEM-SOLVING APPROACH

SECOND EDITION

EDITED BY

JOHN H. DAVIS, M.D.
Professor, Department of Surgery
University of Vermont College of Medicine
Burlington, Vermont

GEORGE F. SHELDON, M.D.
Professor and Chairman
Department of Surgery
The University of North Carolina
Chapel Hill, North Carolina

WILLIAM R. DRUCKER, M.D.
Professor, Department of Surgery
Uniformed Services University of the Health Sciences
School of Medicine
Bethesda, Maryland

ROGER S. FOSTER Jr., M.D.
Wadley Glenn Professor of Surgery
Emory University
Chief, Surgical Services
Crawford Long Hospital of Emory University
Atlanta, Georgia

RICHARD L. GAMELLI, M.D.
Professor of Surgery and Pediatrics
Loyola University School of Medicine
Director, Shock-Trauma Institute
Chief, Burn Center
Department of Surgery
Loyola University Medical Center
Maywood, Illinois

DONALD S. GANN, M.D.
Professor and Associate Chairman
Department of Surgery
The University of Maryland School of Medicine
Baltimore, Maryland

ERNEST E. MOORE, M.D.
Chief, Department of Surgery
Denver General Hospital
Professor and Vice-Chairman of Surgery
University of Colorado Health Sciences Center
Denver, Colorado

BASIL A. PRUITT Jr., M.D.
Commander and Director
U.S. Army Institute of Surgical Research
Fort Sam Houston, Texas

With 1400 illustrations

Mosby

St. Louis Baltimore Berlin Boston Carlsbad Chicago London Madrid
Naples New York Philadelphia Sydney Tokyo Toronto

Mosby
Dedicated to Publishing Excellence

Editor: Susie H. Baxter
Developmental Editor: Ellen Baker Geisel
Project Manager: Mark Spann
Production Editor: Melissa Martin
Designer: David Zielinski
Manufacturing Supervisors: Kathy Grone and Karen Lewis

SECOND EDITION

Printed in the United States of America
Composition by Graphic World
Printing/binding by Maple-Vail Book Manufacturing Group

Mosby–Year Book, Inc.
11830 Westline Industrial Drive
St. Louis, Missouri 63146

International Standard Book Number 0-8016-7169-8

95 96 97 98 99 / 9 8 7 6 5 4 3 2

CONTRIBUTORS

Paul S. Auerbach, M.D., M.S.
Professor and Chief
Division of Emergency Medicine
Department of Surgery
Stanford University Hospital
Stanford, California
Chapter 18: Environmental Injuries

George M. Babikian, M.D.
Assistant Clinical Professor of Orthopedics
University of Vermont College of Medicine
Maine Medical Center
Portland, Maine
Chapter 19: Musculoskeletal Injuries and Fractures

W. Henry Barber, M.D., D. Phil.
Professor of Surgery
Surgical Director of Renal Transplantation
Department of Surgery
University of Mississippi Medical Center
Jackson, Mississippi
Chapter 21: Organ Transplantation

A. Griswold Bevin, M.D.
Professor of Plastic Surgery
Director, The Hand Rehabilitation Center
Department of Surgery
Division of Plastic and Reconstructive Surgery
The University of North Carolina at Chapel Hill
School of Medicine
Chapel Hill, North Carolina
Chapter 51: Hand

John Bostwick III, M.D.
Professor and Chairman
Division of Plastic Surgery
Emory University School of Medicine
Atlanta, Georgia
Chapter 45: Breast

Kenneth W. Burchard, M.D.
Associate Professor
Department of Surgery
Dartmouth-Hitchcock Medical Center
Lebanon, New Hampshire
Chapter 2: Assessment of the Surgical Patient: Temperature Alteration

William F. Chandler, M.D.
Professor
Section of Neurosurgery
University of Michigan
Ann Arbor, Michigan
Chapter 26: Central Nervous System

Rachel L. Chin, M.D.
Resident Physician
Division of Emergency Medicine
Department of Surgery
Stanford University Hospital
Stanford, California
Chapter 18: Environmental Injuries

Raphael S. Chung, M.D.
Staff Surgeon
Department of Surgery
Cleveland Clinic Foundation
Cleveland, Ohio
Chapter 35: Biliary System

William G. Cioffi Jr., M.D.
Chief, Burn Study Branch
United States Army Institute of Surgical Research
Fort Sam Houston
Clinical Associate Professor of Surgery
University of Texas at San Antonio
San Antonio, Texas
Chapter 5: Circulation and Shock
Chapter 17: Thermal Injuries

Orlo H. Clark, M.D.
Professor and Vice Chair, Department of Surgery
University of California, San Francisco
Chief of Surgery, UCSF—Mount Zion
Staff Surgeon, Surgical Services
Veterans Administration Medical Center
San Francisco, California
Chapter 47: Parathyroid Glands

Laurence H. Coffin, M.D.
Professor of Surgery
University of Vermont College of Medicine
Burlington, Vermont
Chapter 41: Heart: Acquired Disease

John H. Davis, M.D.
Professor of Surgery
University of Vermont College of Medicine
Burlington, Vermont
Chapter 1: Surgery: Past, Present, and Future
Chapter 2: Assessment of the Surgical Patient: Problem-Solving Approach
Chapter 42: Aorta and Peripheral Arteries
Chapter 43: Veins and Lymphatics

Mark H. Deierhoi, M.D.
Associate Professor of Surgery and Pathology
University of Alabama Medical Center
University Hospital
Birmingham, Alabama
Chapter 21: Organ Transplantation

Edwin A. Deitch, M.D.
Professor and Chairman of Surgery
University of Medicine and Dentistry New Jersey
New Jersey Medical School
Newark, New Jersey
Chapter 16: Multiple Organ Failure

Arnold Diethelm, M.D.
Professor and Chairman
Department of Surgery
University of Alabama School of Medicine
Birmingham, Alabama
Chapter 21: Organ Transplantation

Lisa Susan Dresner, M.D.
Assistant Professor of Surgery
State University of New York
Health Science Center at Brooklyn
Attending Surgeon
King's County Hospital Center
Brooklyn, New York
Chapter 31: Small Intestine

David J. Dries, M.S.E., M.D.
Associate Professor of Surgery
Stritch School of Medicine
Assistant Director
Shock-Trauma Institute
Loyola University Medical Center
Maywood, Illinois
Chapter 4: Respiratory Function

Robert P. Drucker, M.D.
Pediatric Clerkship Director
Duke University School of Medicine
Associate Professor
Department of Pediatrics
Duke University Medical Center
Durham, North Carolina
Chapter 3: Body Fluids and Fluid Therapy

William R. Drucker, M.D.
Professor of Surgery
Uniformed Services University of the Health Sciences
Bethesda, Maryland
Chapter 1: Surgery: Past, Present, and Future
Chapter 3: Body Fluids and Fluid Therapy

Quan-Yang Duh, M.D.
Assistant Professor in Residence
Department of Surgery
University of California, San Francisco
Assistant Chief, Surgical Services
Veterans Administration Medical Center
San Francisco, California
Chapter 47: Parathyroid Glands

Samir M. Fakhry, M.D.
Assistant Professor of Surgery
University of North Carolina School of Medicine
Director of Surgical ICU
University of North Carolina Hospitals
Chapel Hill, North Carolina
Chapter 6: Bleeding, Coagulation, and Blood Component Replacement Therapy

Josef E. Fischer, M.D.
Christian R. Holmes Professor and Chairman
Department of Surgery
University of Cincinnati College of Medicine
Surgeon-in-Chief
University Hospital and Christian R. Holmes Division
University of Cincinnati Medical Center
Cincinnati, Ohio
Chapter 34: Liver and Portal Venous System

John L. Flowers, M.D.
Assistant Professor of Surgery
Director, Center for Advances in Videoscopic Surgery
The University of Maryland School of Medicine
Baltimore, Maryland
Chapter 30: Stomach

Andrew H. Foster, M.D.
Assistant Professor of Surgery
Director, Surgical Electrophysiology
Division of Thoracic and Cardiovascular Surgery
The University of Maryland School of Medicine
Baltimore, Maryland
Chapter 8: The Biologic Response to Injury

Roger S. Foster Jr., M.D.
Wadley Glenn Professor of Surgery
Emory University
Chief, Surgical Services
Crawford Long Hospital of Emory University
Atlanta, Georgia
Chapter 2: Assessment of the Surgical Patient: Problem-Solving Approach
Chapter 12: Principles of Cancer Biology and Cancer Treatment
Chapter 20: Skin and Soft Tissue
Chapter 45: Breast
Chapter 46: Thyroid Gland

Wesley C. Fowler Jr., M.D.
Palumbo Professor and Associate Chairman
University of North Carolina School of Medicine
Ob/Gyn Director, Division of Gynecologic Oncology
University of North Carolina Hospitals
Chapel Hill, North Carolina
Chapter 39: Gynecologic System

Douglas L. Fraker, M.D.
Senior Investigator
Head, Surgical Metabolism Section
Surgery Branch
National Cancer Institute
Bethesda, Maryland
Chapter 50: Endocrine Pancreas

Richard L. Gamelli, M.D.
Professor of Surgery
Loyola University School of Medicine
Director, Shock-Trauma Institute
Chief, Burn Unit
Department of Surgery
Loyola University Medical Center
Maywood, Illinois
Chapter 2: Assessment of the Surgical Patient: Problem-Solving Approach
Chapter 5: Circulation and Shock
Chapter 7: Renal Function and Acute Renal Failure
Chapter 9: Nutritional Support: Parenteral Alimentation

Donald S. Gann, M.D.
Professor and Associate Chairman
Department of Surgery
The University of Maryland School of Medicine
Baltimore, Maryland
Chapter 8: The Biologic Response to Injury
Chapter 48: Adrenal Gland

Cleon W. Goodwin, M.D.
Director, Burn Center
New York Hospital
Johnson and Johnson Associate Professor
Cornell University Medical College
New York, New York
Chapter 10: Management of Surgical Infection: Pathogenesis, Diagnosis, and Treatment
Chapter 17: Thermal Injuries

Philip H. Gordon, M.D., F.R.C.S.(C.)
Professor of Surgery and Oncology
McGill University
Director, Colon and Rectal Surgery
Sir Mortimer B. Davis—Jewish General Hospital
Montreal, Quebec, Canada
Chapter 33: Colon, Rectum, and Anus

Scott M. Graham, M.D.
Assistant Professor of Surgery
Director, Surgical Endoscopy
The University of Maryland School of Medicine
Baltimore, Maryland
Chapter 30: Stomach

A. Gerson Greenburg, M.D., Ph.D.
Professor of Surgery
Brown University School of Medicine
Surgeon-in-Chief
Miriam Hospital
Providence, Rhode Island
Chapter 37: Abdominal Wall and Hernia

Carl E. Haisch, M.D.
Associate Professor of Surgery
East Carolina University School of Medicine
Director of Surgical Immunology and Transplantation
Attending in Transplantation, Trauma, and General Surgery
Pitt County Memorial Hospital
Greenville, North Carolina
Chapter 13: Molecular Biology for Surgeons
Chapter 22: Chronic Vascular and Peritoneal Access

Douglas W. Hanto, M.D., Ph.D.
Associate Professor of Surgery
Division of Transplantation
University of Cincinnati College of Medicine
Cincinnati, Ohio
Chapter 34: Liver and Portal Venous System

James C. Hebert, M.D.
Professor of Surgery
University of Vermont
Program Director, General Surgery
Medical Center Hospital of Vermont
Burlington, Vermont
Chapter 44: Spleen and Lymph Nodes

Nicholas H. Heintz, Ph.D.
Associate Professor of Pathology
University of Vermont College of Medicine
Burlington, Vermont
Chapter 13: Molecular Biology for Surgeons

Robert E. Hermann, M.D.
Senior Surgeon, Past Chairman
Department of General Surgery
Cleveland Clinic Foundation
Cleveland, Ohio
Chapter 35: Biliary System

Julian T. Hoff, M.D.
Professor of Surgery
Head, Section of Neurosurgery
University of Michigan School of Medicine
Ann Arbor, Michigan
Chapter 26: Central Nervous System

Olivier Huber, M.D.
Medecin-adjoint
Department of Digestive Surgery
University Hospital of Geneva
Geneva, Switzerland
Chapter 29: Esophagus

Sally A. Huber, M.D.
Associate Professor of Pathology
University of Vermont College of Medicine
Burlington, Vermont
Chapter 13: Molecular Biology for Surgeons

John G. Hunter, M.D.
Associate Professor of Surgery
Emory University School of Medicine
Chief, GI Division
Department of Surgery
Emory University Hospital
Atlanta, Georgia
Chapter 32: Appendix

Anthony L. Imbembo, M.D.
Professor and Chairman
Department of Surgery
The University of Maryland School of Medicine
Surgeon-in-Chief
University of Maryland Hospital
Baltimore, Maryland
Chapter 30: Stomach

Krista L. Kaups, M.D.
Assistant Professor of Surgery
University of Vermont College of Medicine
Co-Director, Surgical Intensive Care Unit
Medical Center Hospital of Vermont
Burlington, Vermont
Chapter 14: Critical Care

Blair A. Keagy, M.D.
Professor of Surgery
University of North Carolina School of Medicine
University of North Carolina Hospitals
Chapel Hill, North Carolina
Chapter 25: Critical Evaluation of Data

Roger G. Keith, M.D., F.R.C.S., F.R.C.S.(C.)
Professor and Chairman
Department of Surgery
University of Saskatchewan
Saskatoon, Saskatchewan, Canada
Chapter 36: Pancreas

Mark J. Koruda, M.D.
Associate Professor of Surgery
University of North Carolina School of Medicine
Chief, Gastrointestinal Surgery
University of North Carolina Hospitals
Chapel Hill, North Carolina
Chapter 9: Nutritional Support: Enteral Alimentation

Thomas J. Krizek, M.D.
Professor and Vice Chairman
Department of Surgery
Director, Division of Plastic Surgery
The University of South Florida
Tampa, Florida
Chapter 20: Skin and Soft Tissue

Bruce J. Leavitt, M.D.
Associate Professor of Surgery
Division of Thoracic and Cardiac Surgery
Department of Surgery
University of Vermont College of Medicine
Burlington, Vermont
Chapter 41: Heart: Acquired Disease

Frank R. Lewis Jr., M.D.
Professor of Surgery
Case Western Reserve University
Chairman, Department of Surgery
Henry Ford Hospital
Detroit, Michigan
Chapter 32: Appendix

Patricia A. Lodge, Ph.D.
Post-Doctoral Fellow
Department of Neurology
Vanderbilt University School of Medicine
Nashville, Tennessee
Chapter 13: Molecular Biology for Surgeons

Solange D. MacArthur, M.D.
Assistant Professor of Surgery
State University of New York
Attending Physician
Department of Surgery
King's County Hospital Center
Brooklyn, New York
Chapter 31: Small Intestine

Daniel Marelli, M.D., M.Sc., F.R.C.S.(C.)
Chief Resident in Cardiothoracic Surgery
McGill University Faculty of Medicine
The Montreal General Hospital
Montreal, Quebec, Canada
Chapter 28: Lungs, Chest Wall, Mediastinum, Pleura, and Diaphragm

Stephen J. Mathes, M.D.
Professor of Surgery
University of California at San Francisco
Head, Division of Plastic and Reconstructive Surgery
San Francisco, California
Chapter 11: Wound Healing

Jack W. McAninch, M.D.
Professor of Urology
University of California at San Francisco
Chief of Urology
San Francisco General Hospital
San Francisco, California
Chapter 38: Genitourinary Disorders

Brent R.W. Moelleken, M.D.
Chief Resident
Department of Plastic and Reconstructive Surgery
University of California at San Francisco
San Francisco, California
Chapter 11: Wound Healing

Ernest Eugene Moore, M.D.
Chief, Department of Surgery
Denver General Hospital
Professor and Vice-Chairman of Surgery
University of Colorado Health Sciences Center
Denver, Colorado
Chapter 15: Early Care of Multisystem Trauma

Frederick A. Moore, M.D.
Chief, Surgical Critical Care
Denver General Hospital
Associate Professor of Surgery
University of Colorado Health Sciences Center
Denver, Colorado
Chapter 15: Early Care of Multisystem Trauma

David S. Mulder, M.D., M.Sc., F.R.C.S.(C.)
Professor and Chairman
Department of Surgery
McGill University Faculty of Medicine
Surgeon-in-Chief
The Montreal General Hospital
Montreal, Quebec, Canada
Chapter 28: Lungs, Chest Wall, Mediastinum, Pleura, and Diaphragm

Dao M. Nguyen, M.D., M.Sc., F.R.C.S.(C.)
Chief Resident in Cardiothoracic Surgery
McGill University Faculty of Medicine
Montreal, Quebec, Canada
Chapter 28: Lungs, Chest Wall, Mediastinum, Pleura, and Diaphragm

Santhat Nivatvongs, M.D.
Professor of Surgery
Mayo Medical School
Consultant in Colon and Rectal Surgery
Mayo Clinic
Rochester, Minnesota
Chapter 33: Colon, Rectum, and Anus

Jeffrey A. Norton, M.D.
Professor of Surgery
Washington University School of Medicine
Chief of Endocrine and Oncologic Surgery
Barnes Hospital
St. Louis, Missouri
Chapter 50: Endocrine Pancreas

Nelson Oyesiku, M.D.
Assistant Professor
Department of Neurosurgery
Emory University School of Medicine
Attending Neurosurgeon
Emory University Hospital
Atlanta, Georgia
Chapter 49: Pituitary Gland

George J. Palmer, M.D.
University of North Carolina at Chapel Hill
Chapel Hill, North Carolina
Chapter 25: Critical Evaluation of Data

Thomas P. Paxton, M.D.
Trauma Research Fellow
Department of Surgery
Loyola University Medical Center
Loyola University Shock-Trauma Institute
Maywood, Illinois
General Surgery Resident
University of Health Sciences
The Chicago Medical School at Mount Sinai Hospital Medical Center
Chicago, Illinois
Chapter 9: Nutritional Support: Parenteral Alimentation

Carlos A. Pellegrini, M.D.
Professor and Chairman
Department of Surgery
University of Washington School of Medicine
Seattle, Washington
Chapter 29: Esophagus

Jack Pickleman, M.D.
Professor of Surgery
Chief, Division of General Surgery
Loyola University Stritch School of Medicine
Maywood, Illinois
Chapter 2: Assessment of the Surgical Patient: Abdominal Pain

David B. Pilcher, M.D.
Professor of Surgery
Department of Surgery
University of Vermont College of Medicine
Burlington, Vermont
Chapter 42: Aorta and Peripheral Arteries

Steven C. Poplawski, M.D.
Assistant Professor of Surgery
Director, Liver Transplantation
University of Alabama Medical Center
Birmingham, Alabama
Chapter 21: Organ Transplantation

Basil A. Pruitt Jr., M.D.
Commander and Director
U.S. Army Institute of Surgical Research
Fort Sam Houston, Texas
Chapter 10: Management of Surgical Infection: Pathogenesis, Diagnosis, and Treatment
Chapter 17: Thermal Injuries

Chen Feng Qi, M.D., Ph.D.
Research Associate
Division of Surgical Immunology and Transplantation
East Carolina University
Greenville, North Carolina
Chapter 13: Molecular Biology for Surgeons

Robert A. Read, M.D., Ph.D.
Assistant Professor of Surgery
University of Colorado Health Sciences Center
Director of Surgical Education
Denver General Hospital
Denver, Colorado
Chapter 15: Early Care of Multisystem Trauma

Michael A. Ricci, M.D.
Assistant Professor of Surgery
University of Vermont College of Medicine
Burlington, Vermont
Chapter 43: Veins and Lymphatics

Frederick B. Rogers, M.D.
Assistant Professor of Surgery
University of Vermont College of Medicine
Director of Trauma Services
Medical Center Hospital of Vermont
Burlington, Vermont
Chapter 14: Critical Care

Robert Rutledge, M.D.
Associate Professor
Division of General Surgery
University of North Carolina Hospital
University of North Carolina School of Medicine
Chapel Hill, North Carolina
Chapter 6: Bleeding, Coagulation, and Blood Component Replacement Therapy

Steven R. Shackford, M.D.
Professor and Chairman
Department of Surgery
University of Vermont College of Medicine
Surgeon-in-Chief
Medical Center Hospital of Vermont
Burlington, Vermont
Chapter 14: Critical Care

George F. Sheldon, M.D.
Professor and Chairman
Department of Surgery
University of North Carolina
Chapel Hill, North Carolina
Chapter 1: Surgery: Past, Present, and Future
Chapter 6: Bleeding, Coagulation, and Blood Component Replacement Therapy

Geoffrey Silver, M.D.
Instructor of Surgery
Harvard Medical School
Associate Director, Emergency Unit
Department of Surgery
Division of Trauma and Critical Care
Boston, Massachusetts
Chapter 7: Renal Function and Acute Renal Failure

Rebecca Smith-Coggins, M.D.
Assistant Professor of Surgery and Emergency Medicine
Emergency Medicine Residency Director
Stanford University School of Medicine
Stanford University Hospital
Stanford, California
Chapter 18: Environmental Injuries

Robert A. Sofferman, M.D.
Professor of Surgery
Division of Otolaryngology
University of Vermont College of Medicine
Chairman, Division of Otolaryngology
Otology, Neurology, Head and Neck Surgery
University of Vermont Health Center
Burlington, Vermont
Chapter 27: Head and Neck

David H. Stern, M.D.
Associate Professor of Anesthesiology
University of Rochester School of Medicine and Dentistry
Attending Anesthesiologist
Strong Memorial Hospital
Rochester, New York
Chapter 24: Perioperative Anesthesia

George T. Tindall, M.D.
Professor and Chairman
Department of Neurosurgery
Emory University School of Medicine
Atlanta, Georgia
Chapter 49: Pituitary Gland

Linda Van Le, M.D.
Assistant Professor
Division of Gynecologic Oncology
Department of Obstetrics and Gynecology
University of North Carolina School of Medicine
Chapel Hill, North Carolina
Chapter 39: Gynecologic System

David P. Vogt, M.D.
Department of General Surgery
Cleveland Clinic Foundation
Cleveland, Ohio
Chapter 35: Biliary System

Daniel von Allmen, M.D.
Fellow, Division of Pediatric Surgery
Department of Surgery
University of Cincinnati College of Medicine
Children's Hospital Medical Center
Cincinnati, Ohio
Chapter 23: Pediatric Surgery

Richard B. Wait, M.D., Ph.D.
Professor and Chairman
Department of Surgery
SUNY-Health Science Center at Brooklyn
Downstate Medical Center
Brooklyn, New York
Chapter 31: Small Intestine

Raymond R. White, M.D.
Assistant Clinical Professor of Orthopedics
University of Vermont College of Medicine
Maine Medical Center
Portland, Maine
Chapter 19: Musculoskeletal Injuries and Fractures

William R. Wilson Jr., M.D.
Assistant Professor of Surgery and Pediatrics
Chief, Division of Pediatric Cardiac Surgery
Medical College of Ohio
Toledo, Ohio
Chapter 40: Heart: Congenital Disease

Moritz M. Ziegler, M.D.
Professor of Surgery and Pediatrics
University of Cincinnati College of Medicine
Director, Division of Pediatric Surgery
Surgeon-in-Chief
Children's Hospital Medical Center
Cincinnati, Ohio
Chapter 23: Pediatric Surgery

PREFACE

A textbook should serve as the first source of information about disease pathogenesis and its clinical manifestations. It should supply fundamental information that allows the student, resident, or practitioner to develop a base of knowledge about a condition. However, no textbook is so complete that it can cover everything, nor is any so exhaustive that it can provide a thorough understanding of all problems. Thus the book should include, as does this text, citations of current publications that allow the physician to seek more detailed information.

In organizing this new edition of our textbook, we have given high priority to the needs of residents and students, but we have also paid special attention to the recertification review needs of the surgical practitioner.

When the first edition of this book, *Clinical Surgery,* was being prepared, some of the available surgical texts met the criteria mentioned previously. Then why another one? As stated in the Preface to the first edition, the book was written after a survey of medical students, residents, and practicing surgeons documented a need for a surgical textbook with a problem-solving approach, a textbook organized in a manner that parallels the process by which surgery is actually practiced. An editorial board reviewed the results of the demographic survey, established discrete educational goals for the book, defined the needs of practicing surgeons, and determined the organization and content of the first edition.

This new edition, appropriately titled *Surgery: A Problem-Solving Approach,* has given us the opportunity to refine both content and organization. In order to update the text by including new developments that have changed surgical care, the book has been virtually rewritten. Many new authors have contributed chapters, and those who wrote for the first edition have revised their material extensively. Some sections and chapters have been combined to present the material more concisely and practically. For example, the chapter Assessment of the Surgical Patient includes discussions of the problem-solving approach in patient care, abdominal pain, and temperature changes. Body fluids and fluid therapy have been combined into a single chapter, as have bleeding, coagulation, and blood component replacement therapy. Icons and boldface subheadings have been added to make the material more accessible.

At the beginning of each chapter is a chart, diagram, or anatomic plate highlighting a particular aspect of the area under consideration. The introductory chapter provides an overview of the events and developments that have given us our surgical heritage and discusses how current changes in health care may affect the future of our specialty.

Part One is organized around biologic phenomena in surgery and reviews the basic science that influences the management of surgical problems. This section includes a new chapter, Molecular Biology for Surgeons, which summarizes what currently is one of the most active areas of research. Another important chapter, The Biologic Response to Injury, describes in detail the pathophysiologic changes elicited by injury and discusses subsequent therapeutic measures.

Because surgeons are caring for an ever-increasing number of critically ill and injured patients, we have devoted Part Two to these areas: Critical Care, Early Care of Multisystem Trauma, Multiple Organ Failure, Thermal Injuries, Environmental Injuries, and Musculoskeletal Injuries and Fractures. Although some historically prominent surgical diseases now can be prevented or treated by other means, the complexity of intensive care has increased and the number of critically ill surgical patients continues to rise. Excellent emergency medical services across the country are delivering more severely injured patients to the hospital than ever before, and more of those patients are surviving their initial injuries and surgical interventions. Treatment of critically ill or injured patients requires swift decision making, which in turn requires a knowledge of the problems commonly encountered and the treatment options available.

Part Three covers some special areas that typically are not part of a general surgeon's everyday practice but that nonetheless are germane. Surgeons must be knowledgeable in these areas for two reasons: (1) when no specialist is available, they must know how to manage patients with problems that ordinarily are the purview of a surgical specialist; and (2) they must know what assistance their specialist colleagues can provide. For example, most surgeons will never perform an organ transplantation, yet any surgeon may be called upon to care for a patient awaiting transplantation or to help a deceased patient's grieving family make a decision about organ donation.

Part Four covers diseases that are specific to organs and systems. Although discussing all diseases in a single text is nearly impossible (and multivolume encyclopedias of surgery are available), the principles of management are similar for broad categories of surgical diseases. Therefore we have organized these chapters using a problem-solving format. Each chapter provides thorough and expert coverage of a particular organ and its diseases, as well as sufficient background in basic science (e.g., embryology, anatomy, biochemistry, pathology) to enable the surgeon to understand the relevant pathophysiology, to select appropriate diagnostic procedures, and to evaluate the treatment options. In order to be inclusive yet avoid the need to present uncommon diseases in detail, we have concluded each chapter in Part Four with a review table. Thus the reader can quickly identify similar disease processes, applicable diagnostic tests, and appropriate therapeutic approaches.

All members of the editorial board greatly appreciate the reviewers' critiques, which were useful in updating and reorganizing this text, and the secretarial assistance given each editor, which kept the revision program on track.

We hope that this book facilitates the learning process for all its readers and thereby improves patient care—the goal of every surgeon and of all physicians.

The Editors

DEDICATION

The editors dedicate this textbook to the many physicians and surgeons who gave of their time and energy in providing our education. They gave many nights and weekends and missed social events or precious time with their families to provide our education and help us through difficult times. Some are no longer with us, and many have retired from active practice; however, none is forgotten. We wish to express our gratitude for their efforts.

Special thanks go to our wives and families, who also gave up many nights and weekends as we labored to produce this textbook. Without their help and understanding, we could not have accomplished our goal.

John H. Davis, M.D.
George F. Sheldon, M.D.
William R. Drucker, M.D.
Roger S. Foster Jr., M.D.
Richard L. Gamelli, M.D.
Donald S. Gann, M.D.
Ernest E. Moore, M.D.
Basil A. Pruitt Jr., M.D.

CONTENTS

VOLUME I
CONCEPTS AND PROCESSES

PART ONE
BIOLOGIC PHENOMENA IN SURGERY

PART TWO

MANAGEMENT OF CRITICALLY ILL OR INJURED PATIENTS

PART THREE

SPECIAL AREAS

VOLUME II
CLINICAL PRACTICE

PART FOUR

DISEASES OF THE ORGANS AND SYSTEMS

CHAPTER

1

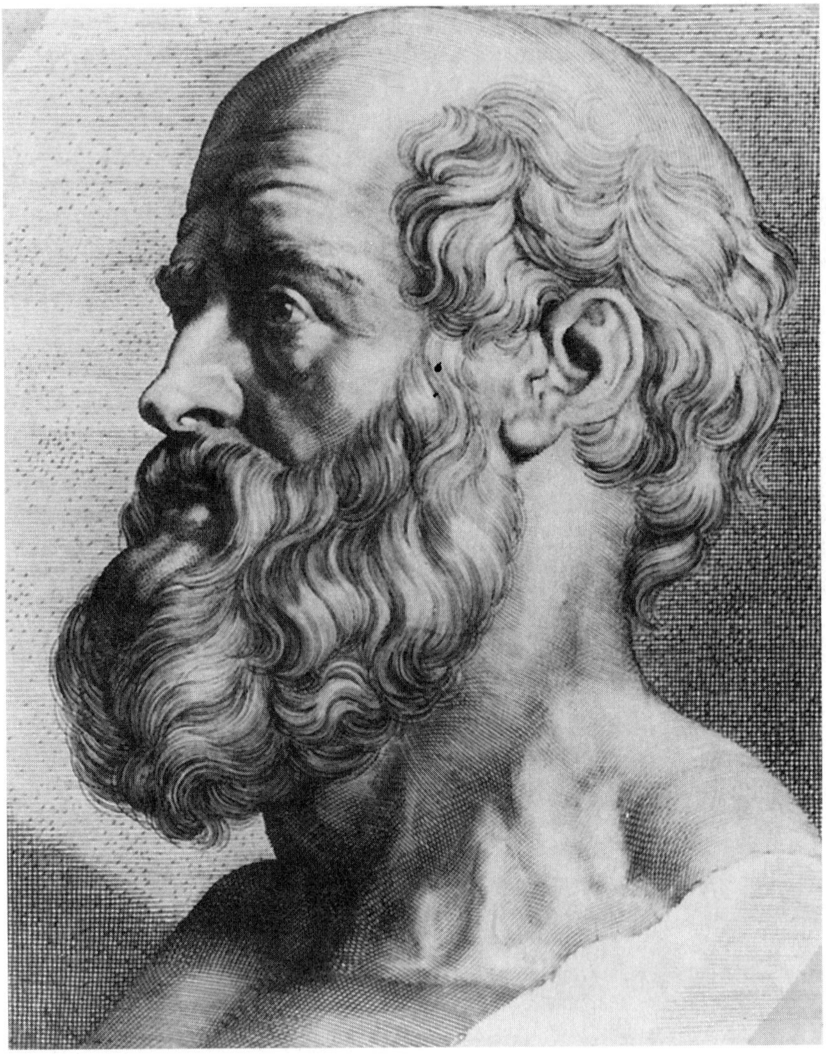

SURGERY: PAST, PRESENT, AND FUTURE

John H. Davis • William R. Drucker • George F. Sheldon

HISTORICAL PERSPECTIVE

Although surgery has been practiced since about 4000 BC, it was a crude and unscientific trade limited to a few operations without anesthesia or asepsis. Surgery became accepted as an academic discipline only after anatomy was developed as a science fundamental to medicine. Thus surgery rode into the academic arena on the back of anatomy; most of the early professors of surgery were appointed with the dual responsibilities of professor of surgery and anatomy and midwifery (obstetrics).

In 1805, at the University of Pennsylvania (the first medical school in the United States), the Edinburgh administrative arrangement of a combined department of surgery, anatomy, and midwifery was dissolved into component parts. Philip Syng Physick (1768-1837) became the first professor and chair of surgery in the oldest medical school in the United States.

Surgery, as we know it today, began in 1846, when the first successful operation under anesthesia was performed in the Ether Dome of the Massachusetts General Hospital on October 16, 1846. John Collins Warren agreed to try sulphuric ether as an anesthetic, at the suggestion of W.T.G. Morton, a dentist who was studying medicine. Morton had become convinced of the anesthetic properties of ether and urged Warren to try it. Although skeptical of its usefulness, Warren removed a tumor of the neck using ether anesthesia and turned to his audience at the completion of the procedure and exclaimed, "Gentlemen this is no humbug."

In March 1842, Crawford W. Long of Danielsville, Georgia, used ether anesthesia to remove a small tumor on the back of a patient's neck. He subsequently used ether in other operations, but he never published his results so that Morton has been credited with the discovery of anesthesia.

During this same period antiseptic surgery came into being. Two physicians made remarkable observations concerning infection and its etiology. The first, Oliver Wendell Holmes (1809-1894), recognized that the surgeon's dirty hands might cause an infection and published an article in the *New England Journal of Medicine* (1843), "On the Contagiousness of Puerperal Fever." This article met strong opposition from the leading American obstetricians, and Holmes was severely criticized.

In Vienna, Ignatz Semmelweis (1818-1865) came to the same conclusion 10 years later. He observed that mortality was highest in clinics in which students and physicians entered the obstetric ward directly from the dissecting room. He insisted that all hands be washed before any examination of the pregnant female and that the floors be scrubbed with calcium chloride. The mortality rate dropped immediately and significantly, but Semmelweis was so ridiculed by his contemporaries that he died in an insane asylum a few years later.

Pasteur's discovery of the role of microbes as a cause of disease in anthrax opened the way for surgeons to study the possibility that microbes were the cause of infection and the high mortality that followed surgical procedures. Pasteur's work did not fall on deaf ears. Joseph Lister, (1827-1912) a Scottish surgeon, had a great interest in microscopic anatomy and physiology and was pursuing studies on the pathogenesis of inflammation and intravascular coagulation. In 1860, he became the Professor of Surgery at Glasgow and turned his attention to the frightful mortality that occurred after amputations and compound fractures. Mortality rates often would reach 45% in hospitals throughout the United Kingdom as well as the rest of the world. Having heard of Pasteur's discoveries, Lister began to study the possibility of sterilizing the operative field to prevent the emergence of pathogenic bacteria. He reasoned that if he could destroy the bacteria, wound infection would not occur and the mortality rate would drop. He tried various antiseptic solutions, but eventually settled on carbolic acid spray and developed a method for spraying not only the wound but the entire room. He noted a striking drop in wound infection and mortality in compound fractures and amputations. The word spread quickly and Listerism, as it was known, slowly began to be adopted throughout the world. However, great opposition to Listerism continued to rage for many years with some of the greats of medicine disbelieving that anything invisible to the eye could possibly cause disease.

Many scoffed at Lister's discovery, and thought that bacteria were scientific playthings with no real effect on human disease. German surgeons, especially Bilroth, of Vienna, accepted Lister's investigations so that German surgery advanced while surgery in Europe, Great Britain, and the United States stood still. Over time, however, more and more physicians tried the carbolic acid spray and obtained results similar to those of Lister. Eventually antisepsis, as it was called, became the watchword of surgery. Asepsis was developed by Bergmann in Germany and eventually replaced antisepsis as the method of preventing bacterial contamination in operating rooms and in wounds.

During the latter half of the nineteenth century, many new operations were developed and all body cavities became open to the surgeon because of the availability of anesthesia and antisepsis.

The publication of *Cellular Pathology* in 1858 by Rudolph Virchow had an enormous impact on medicine by demonstrating that organs were made up of cells and that cellular dysfunction caused disease. Although Virchow gave credit for the discovery of cellular pathology to Morgagni, some 100 years earlier, it was Virchow who popularized and promoted the concept of cellular pathology. Before this time disease was thought to arise from the miasmas that arose from a variety of sources including the cold, dark earth. Virchow demonstrated that all organs were made up of individual cells, some identical and some different, depending on the organ or tissue they made up. At the same time all had some common elements such as a nucleus and a nucleolus. Disease caused changes in the cellular structure, which could be observed under the microscope. It thus became possible to classify some of these cellular changes into diseases such as inflammation, degenerative changes, and tumors.

William S. Halsted, Professor of Surgery at the new School of Medicine at The Johns Hopkins University, changed American surgery in many ways. Halsted had spent a great deal of time studying the methods of European surgeons, where he was most impressed by the German system of residency training that he observed in Langenbeck's clinic. After The Johns Hopkins Hospital opened its doors in 1889, Halsted was named surgeon-in-chief in 1892. He immediately set about developing a residency system similar to the one he had observed in the German clinics. We must remember there were no other residencies in this country at that time. The Halsted system became the model for surgical residencies throughout the United States and profoundly influenced the training of young surgeons.

The principles of the residency training program were as follows:

1. The resident lived in the hospital, thus allowing the young physician to observe the patient over time.
2. The responsibility for the management of the patient was delegated to the "in-house physician" based on his continuous observation of the patient.
3. Progression of the resident's responsibility was determined by the chief of the clinic.
4. The resident received a broad exposure to all types of surgery performed at the hospital. Thus the hospital provided an educational environment organized and directed by able surgeons dedicated to educating highly qualified young surgeons who would be the future teachers of surgery.

Considered the father of scientific surgery in this country, Halsted was a painstaking experimenter who not only trained 17 chief residents in clinical surgery but also made them into active investigators. The German system demanded that the chief of surgery be an excellent clinical surgeon and a good teacher and have at his disposal a laboratory where he was expected to advance the science of surgery by independent investigation. Most of Halsted's residents became professors of surgery when he finally allowed them to complete the residency, which often required 8 or 10 years, since there were no guidelines for the length of a residency.

Halsted's early study in Austria and Germany gave him basic scientific knowledge that was not yet flourishing in the United States. He witnessed the application of this science to surgery in the great European clinics and became acquainted with Lister's principles of antiseptic surgery. Halsted was a meticulous operator who took great care with tissues. He made many contributions to the surgery of breast tumors, including the radical mastectomy, which was the treatment of choice until recent years. He also developed operations for inguinal hernia, biliary and thyroid disease, and aneurysm. Some of his initial research also had a bearing on immunology and transplantation.

Thus at the turn of the century scientific surgery was

slowly being introduced, particularly at The Johns Hopkins School of Medicine, as was the idea of graduate training in surgery. However, most physicians were graduating from 2-year proprietary medical schools with little or no clinical experience (recall that it was Osler who first put the students on the wards to gain practical clinical experience at The Johns Hopkins Hospital). Surgery was taught almost exclusively by lecture, with some practical demonstrations on cadavers. It was not easy to observe an operation, because they were not very common, in contrast to the busy German clinics. Reflecting the tardy acceptance of antisepsis and asepsis, Rudolph Matas reported in 1890 that of the 6083 admissions to Charity Hospital in New Orleans in 1 year, only 290 patients had what he would classify as a major operation.

TABLE 1-1 MAJOR FACTORS IN STUDENTS' CAREER DECISIONS

FACTOR	STUDENTS RESPONDING (%)
Required clerkship	73
Gratification from the type of practice	71
Lifestyle of specialty	50
Medical school electives	48
Role model	40
Psychologic needs in the field	22
Length of residency training	14
Financial rewards of specialty	12
Family background	12
Research	9
Other	14

From *Bull Am Coll Sur* 68:5, 1983.
Students instructed to choose as many responses as appropriate.

MEDICAL EDUCATION: A UNIVERSITY RESPONSIBILITY

While surgery was advancing after the development of cellular pathology and anesthesia, medical education remained unscientific and of a trade-school character. Proprietary schools were abundant, with few or no standards, and often consisted of two courses of lectures of identical material given in two consecutive years. The lectures did not start until after the completion of the harvest and were completed in time for spring planting. The students paid a fee to the instructor for the course and, after completion of the course material, were permitted to practice medicine. Many of these proprietary schools were worthless in their content but lucrative to those who ran them.

Reflecting concern about the proliferation of proprietary medical schools, Abraham Flexner was commissioned by the Carnegie Foundation to review and evaluate American medical schools and report his findings. The Flexner report, published in 1910, recommended that most of the approximately 160 medical schools be closed. Only Harvard, Western Reserve, and Johns Hopkins were in compliance with his recommendations. After the Flexner report, only 88 medical schools remained open.

In 1908 only 11 medical schools required more than 2 years of college before matriculating in medicine. In addition, very few schools had a working relationship with a parent university and with a hospital, both of which Flexner thought were necessary for a good educational program. It was becoming obvious that surgery should be taught as a graduate field; nevertheless, because licensing after graduation from medical school included the right to carry out surgical procedures, it was important for surgery to be taught in medical school.

A student planning a career in surgery clears a significant number of hurdles by preparing for and attaining admission to medical school. Some students contemplate a career in surgery because of an attraction to the field or identification with a role model, perhaps before college. However, most students choose a specialty during their clinical years in medical school and are most influenced by contact in the last 2 years of medical school, during clinical rotations (Table 1-1). Approximately 71% of students who decide to become surgeons do so because of identification with role models or because of the stimulation they receive as students while participating in the care of surgical patients.

Thus medical education was undergoing tremendous change during the first half of the twentieth century. The medical curriculum became 4 years in length and, in general, 4 years of college preparatory work was required for admission to medical school. Most schools developed a program of 2 years of basic science study, including laboratory work, and then 2 years of clinical work in the hospital. The rapid increase in our basic science knowledge required increasing the number of teachers in the basic sciences and significantly increasing the sophistication of their laboratories and the physical space for this expansion. There was also an increased need for clinical teachers as medicine became more complex. To meet this need, the number of full-time clinicians increased and the cost for modern medical education increased dramatically.

MEDICAL LICENSURE AND QUALIFYING EXAMINATIONS

All graduates from medical school must obtain licensure to practice medicine. Licensure by states developed in response to the chaotic credentialing practices of the eighteenth and nineteenth centuries. Texas was the first state to have a licensing board, but by 1900, 36 states had some requirements for medical practice. In 1902, the *Journal of the American Medical Association* published an editorial suggesting that reciprocity based on a board examination was an idea that had come of age; the possibility of a national board to administer medical examinations was suggested.

In 1915, William Rodman, President of the AMA, announced formation of the National Board of Medical Examiners (NBME), under Dr. Walter Biering's leadership. During its first 5 years of existence, only 32 applicants were interviewed and 16 examined; however, 3325 applicants representing eight states eventually took the test, with an 83% pass rate. By 1922, with the aid of a Carnegie Foundation Fund grant, parts one and two of the examination were developed. Between 1920 and 1950, a three-part examination evolved. Another milestone was passed in 1950, when Dr. John Hubbard developed a multiple-choice concept with psychometric evaluations. The NBME has grown rapidly since 1950, and the NBME examination is now accepted as a route to licensure in all but three states. Seventy-five percent of the 127 medical schools require at least part one of the NBME examination and 70% require part two. In all licensing jurisdictions but one, diplomats of the NBME were required to pass an examination by the jurisdiction in which they sought licensure.

The NBME also provides examination services to other agencies, including in-training, certification, and self-assessment examinations. The Educational Commission for Foreign Medical Graduates (ECFMG) also functions under the auspices of the NBME testing commission. The ECFMG, which began testing in 1957, has examined over 37,000 applicants, with a 68% pass rate.

The Federation of State Medical Boards was founded in 1912 to improve medical licensure in the United States and was one of the founders of the NBME. Currently, the Federation Licensing Examination (FLEX), which in 1973 was administered to 2000 physicians, is somewhat controversial. However, by 1974 all but two states used FLEX as an alternative route to licensure to the three parts of the NBME examination.

In 1976, the Health Professions Assistance Act was passed. This legislation requires that a person pass parts one and two of the NBME examination to practice medicine in the United States. As a result of this legislation, some legal redefinition by the NBME was necessary. A Visa Qualifying Examination (VQE) became an additional method for foreign nationals to enter training in the United States.

A new examination, the USMLE (United States Medical Licensure Examination) has now supplanted the NBME and FLEX. As it is a product of the National Board, it retains many characteristics of the national board examination.

GRADUATE MEDICAL EDUCATION (RESIDENCY)

Initially, a surgeon did all operations, particularly when there were few of them. As surgery became more successful and more and more surgical procedures were developed, fragmentation (specialization) began to evolve. At first there were no training programs, but individual surgeons began to limit their activities to one anatomic region, such as the abdomen, the head and neck, or the chest, or to a type of surgery, such as vascular or cancer surgery, and the specialties developed.

The transformation of the Halsted concept of Graduate Medical Education (GME) from an organized university hospital–based system intended to produce teachers and upgrade the practice of surgery to multispecialty, heterogenous programs with widely divergent goals, standards, and control resulted in the second major challenge to medical education in this century. The first challenge, the plethora of proprietary schools with minimum standards for education, had been resolved by the combined efforts of medical schools, medical societies, and the persuasive effect of the Flexner Survey of the existing state of medical schools at the turn of the century. The second challenge was to establish workable controls for GME.

Regulation

As residency programs in all specialties became a reality, the need for some kind of standardization was evident. For instance, programs varied in the length of the residency as well as the content of the program. In some programs there was a large clinical (operative) experience and in other programs there was very little. In 1927, the AMAs Council on Medical Education and Hospitals published a list of hospitals that had approved graduate medical education programs. By 1928 the AMA house of delegates approved basic standards for residency programs titled "Essentials of Approved Residencies and Fellowships," which have continued in some form to the present.

The American Board of Surgery was established in 1937. The board set the length of residency training, established the content of training in broad terms, and examined the candidates at the completion of their training with both a written and oral examination in an attempt to determine competency (the residency review committees did not yet exist). Standards for approved surgical education programs were published, entitled "Fundamental Requirements for Graduate Training in Surgery."

The surgeons not only initiated residency education but were the first specialty to develop a unified committee for overseeing graduate education. This was accomplished by the creation in 1950 of a joint conference committee on graduate training in surgery, with equal representatives from the three constituents most thoroughly involved in graduate education, The American Board of Medical Specialties (ABMS), The American College of Surgeons (ACS), and The Council on Medical Education of the AMA. This committee formed a new pattern for the regulation of specialists and left the specialty boards free to concentrate on basic standards and examination techniques. The committee was later named the Residency Review Committee, under the Accreditation Council for Graduate Medical Education, and 11 other specialties established similar tripartite conference committees within the next decade.

The specialty of internal medicine developed in a similar fashion, with a committee sponsored by the American College of Physicians, the AMA, and the American Board of Internal Medicine. The conference committees appointed by sponsors recommend the educational standards, with final decision for accreditation developed through the staffing of the AMA. In 1953 the two committees embraced the idea of establishing residency review committees, an idea proposed a year earlier by the Council on Medical Education. By 1956 all but three specialty boards had established residency review committees. Currently, 32 societies and organizations sponsor residency review committees, which remain heavily financed and staffed by the AMA. At its inception, the Residency Review Committee had a limited function that involved accrediting positions and programs more than developing broad educational policies. Instead of working to unify the GME, the review committee fragmented it further by making the existing fragmentation more efficient. Lacking university direction or control, the residency program predominantly became truly a training program rather than an academic educational program by relying on the methods of apprenticeship and associateship. The focus of most programs was on the hospital rather than on the university.

The residency review committee for surgery has become an important tool in improving the quality of graduate medical education. The most common reasons for an adverse action from any residency review committee are insufficient mix of operations, lack of a scholarly environment, and insufficient experience in certain areas such as the emergency room or intensive care unit.

In the 1960s, the Millis report, entitled "A Rational Public Policy for Medical Education and its Financing," was published under the close scrutiny of the federal government. This report resulted in the formation of the Liaison Committee of Graduate Medical Education (LCGME) in 1972. A coordinating council on medical education was also formed to approve and further develop this process.

These activities gradually expanded. Although only 388 hospitals with 7500 physicians participated in the process in 1930, by 1980 over 1000 hospitals and 75,000 physicians were under the purview of this organization. The *Manual of Structures and Functions* was developed to stabilize the process, and continued evolution resulted in the formation of the ACGME (Accreditation Council on Graduate Medical Education) as a successor to the LCGME (see box on p. 6). Maturing of this process has resulted in specialty societies, placing members of the residency review committees under the overall purview of the ACGME, which delegates its authority to the residency review committees. The residency review committee for each surgical specialty is composed of representatives from the ACS, the ABMS, and the AMA.

Role of Universities

In time, medical schools could no longer ignore the expansion of residency programs coupled with the rapid growth of specialties. Some period of GME became the *de facto* gateway to specialty practice and an integral part of the complete education of most physicians. The influence of new information and technology on the expansion of GME created a self-perpetuating process. As the university-based residency programs drew on their German educational heritage to emphasize the integral role of investigative work in residency education, the residency programs became an important source for the growth of science and technology.

This goal was fostered and accelerated by the National Institute of Health (NIH), established during the internecine period in 1930. The NIH became the instrument of choice for federal support of biomedical research through passage of an omnibus medical research act in 1950. New disease-oriented institutes began to develop, and the NIH became pluralistic. Research flowed within NIH and through extramural support awarded largely to universities. The result in growth and special areas of research led to an obvious need for university sponsorship of residency programs to convey the new technology information into programs for the graduate education of physicians.

While retaining their base primarily in hospitals, the programs of GME for physicians have become a major responsibility for medical schools over the last two decades. Debates still continue over the concept of "corporate" responsibility in regard to the extent to which medical schools should assume responsibility for the conduct of the residency programs. But the faculty for the graduate programs has become largely congruent with the faculty responsible for the undergraduate phase of medical education. By 1979, 93% of graduating medical students have plans to continue with a residency program leading to board certification and a specialty.

Over 95% of these residents were in programs associated with the medical school.

The independent specialty certifying boards retained responsibility for the organization and assessment of programs of GME. This programmatic, fragmented focus has continued to cause an undesirable degree of separation between residency programs and their sponsoring universities and hospitals. One formal step toward unification occurred after the publication in 1965 of the Coggeshall Report sponsored by the AAMC (Association of American Medical Colleges) and the report of the Citizens (Millis) Commission on Graduate Medical Education the following year. These reports put the final touch to the decline of independent internships by placing the internship as the first year in a graded program of university-sponsored GME. However, the recommendation of the Millis Commission to establish a commission on GME with responsibility for the development of comprehensive policies was not carried out. Clearly, the establishment of such a commission would have a significant impact on the several organizations involved with GME: the suggested changes were similar to the changes that occurred almost 50 years earlier when state licensing boards relinquished formal control over the undergraduate curriculum.

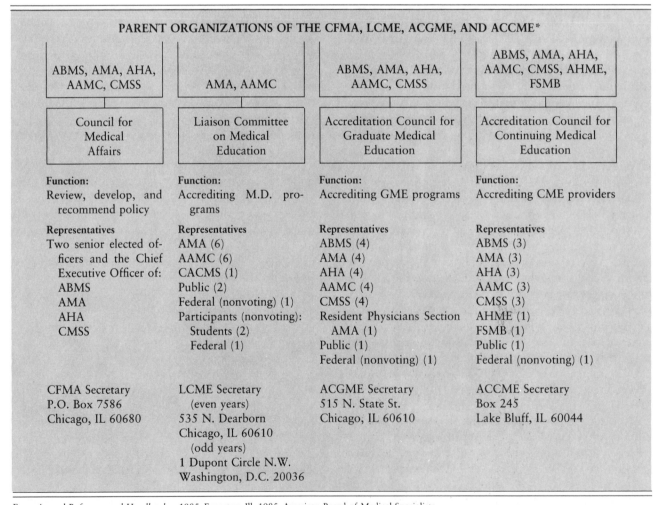

PARENT ORGANIZATIONS OF THE CFMA, LCME, ACGME, AND ACCME*

ABMS, AMA, AHA, AAMC, CMSS	AMA, AAMC	ABMS, AMA, AHA, AAMC, CMSS	ABMS, AMA, AHA, AAMC, CMSS, AHME, FSMB
Council for Medical Affairs	Liaison Committee on Medical Education	Accreditation Council for Graduate Medical Education	Accreditation Council for Continuing Medical Education
Function: Review, develop, and recommend policy	**Function:** Accrediting M.D. programs	**Function:** Accrediting GME programs	**Function:** Accrediting CME providers
Representatives Two senior elected officers and the Chief Executive Officer of: ABMS, AMA, AHA, CMSS	**Representatives** AMA (6), AAMC (6), CACMS (1), Public (2), Federal (nonvoting) (1), Participants (nonvoting): Students (2), Federal (1)	**Representatives** ABMS (4), AMA (4), AHA (4), AAMC (4), CMSS (4), Resident Physicians Section AMA (1), Public (1), Federal (nonvoting) (1)	**Representatives** ABMS (3), AMA (3), AHA (3), AAMC (3), CMSS (3), AHME (1), FSMB (1), Public (1), Federal (nonvoting) (1)
CFMA Secretary, P.O. Box 7586, Chicago, IL 60680	LCME Secretary (even years) 535 N. Dearborn, Chicago, IL 60610 (odd years) 1 Dupont Circle N.W. Washington, D.C. 20036	ACGME Secretary, 515 N. State St., Chicago, IL 60610	ACCME Secretary, Box 245, Lake Bluff, IL 60044

From *Annual Reference and Handbook—1985,* Evanston, Ill, 1985, American Board of Medical Specialists.

AAMC, Association of American Medical Colleges; *ABMS,* American Board of Medical Specialities; *AHA,* American Hospital Association; *AHME,* Association for Hospital Medical Education; *AMA,* American Medical Association; *CACMS,* Committee on Accreditation of Canadian Medical Schools; *CMSS,* Council of Medical Specialty Societies; *FSMB,* Federation of State Medical Boards; *CFMA,* Council for Medical Affairs; *LCME,* Liaison Committee on Medical Education; *ACGME,* Accreditation Council for Graduate Medical Education; *ACCME,* Accreditation Council for Continuing Medical Education.

*Parent organizations establish policy.

Related Issues

Residency Positions

The Association of American Medical Colleges (AAMC) has clearly stated the overreaching concerns referable to all GME. All graduates of accredited medical schools in the United States must have an opportunity to complete their formal education in a quality graduate (residency) program, and stable funding should exist for these programs. The medical academic community voices the additional concern about continuing adequate support for research because of its intrinsic usefulness and as a key component in programs of undergraduate and graduate medical education. Between 1950 and 1975 when the number of physicians in the United States increased by 79%, the number of internship positions increased by 10%. During that same period, the number of graduates of training programs increased by 120%, and the number of residencies available increased by 200%.

A so-called "Jaws" phenomenon appears to be evolving in that the number of graduates of medical schools seeking positions in surgery is now about equal to the number of available residency positions (Figure 1-1). The number of positions available in General Surgery is about 1040, and about equal to the number of applicants. The most competitive programs (the 4 "Os") are ophthalmology, obstetrics–gynecology, otolarnygology, and orthopedics. The primary cause of this phenomenon is the decrease of the total number of training programs, from 723 to 271. The enlarged pool of graduates and the static or decreasing number of residency positions create a potential unavailability of training in the specialty of a student's choice.

Another factor contributing to this phenomenon is the number of foreign medical graduates taking graduate education positions in the United States. In 1982 NRMP showed a narrowing gap between graduate medical education positions and the number of US graduates. For example in 1984, US medical schools graduated 16,800 students. Because foreign medical graduates held 23% of the graduate medical education positions (approximately 1500), the ratio of US graduates to graduate medical education positions was 0.99. In general surgery the positions available for training did increase from 3977 in 1951 to a peak of 8305 in 1983 and 1984. The increase in positions occurred at a time when program consolidation was also occurring. For example, the total number of programs increased from 503 in 1951 and 1952 to 723 in 1959 and 1960. However, the peak of 723 declined to 271 by 1993. One underemphasized point about the complex manpower figures is that chief surgical resident positions, which represent the potential manpower pool, have actually decreased from approximately 1100 to 950 positions.

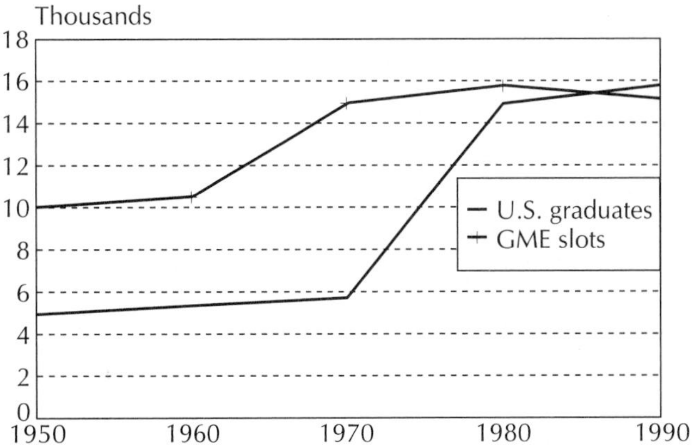

FIGURE 1-1 Medical school graduates and GME training positions.

Although the direction of GME in the United States continues to be fragmented, the academic medical centers have become the hub for virtually all programs of residency education. GME has become as important as undergraduate medical education in the preparation of physicians. Continued failure to achieve a functional coordination of the planning and conduct of the programs of graduate education currently sponsored by 50 to 60 specialties has raised the possibility of government intervention to achieve this objective. The government's interest in resolving this issue is indicated by the Budget Reconciliation Bill passed by Congress in the spring of 1986 which provided for a National Advisory Committee for Graduate Medical Education. Whether this committee acts to move GME more fully under the aegis of medical schools to promote more integration between the undergraduate and graduate medical programs of medical education and coordinate more directly the programs of GME remains to be seen. In the absence of a direct link between the funding of graduate education and the processes by which residency programs are accredited and physicians are certified, the basic question regarding the extent to which medical schools should accept responsibility for the design, conduct, and quality of GME will be asked.

Until some move is made, the surgical residency program in concert with all other programs in GME probably will continue to be based in hospitals, most of which today are strongly tied to a university. Specialty boards will continue to provide the examination for certification, and they will specify the duration, as well as strongly influence the content of the programs. The Residency Review Committee, answerable to the Accreditation Council for Graduate Medical Education, will retain responsibility for accrediting residency programs. All trends indicate that medical schools will continue to serve in the dual capacity of instructing medical students and residents. The academic medical centers will continue to provide the basis for biologic and clinical research, although it is probable that the scope of investigation, however it is financed, will be broadened to include a more widespread commitment to studies of social and economic issues that relate to medical care.

In 1986 the Council on Graduate Medical Education (COGME) was created by legislation charged with manpower and other issues. Current health reform legislation will centralize GME financing and numbers. Health care reform through the development of more primary care physicians at the expense of the specialists is current popular dogma.

Specialization beyond General Surgery

A relatively recent phenomenon in the education of surgeons has been training beyond the 5 years of general surgery. Today approximately 60% of all residents completing programs in general surgery take additional training for certificates of added qualifications or move into other programs that involve further specialization. Some programs require a physician to be certified in general surgery before becoming a candidate for further training in other specialties (Table 1-2). The first example of this phenomenon was the formation of the American Board of Thoracic Surgery in 1948. This Board requires preliminary training in general surgery and then 2 years of cardiothoracic surgery before a physician can become a specialist in cardiothoracic surgery. A physician who completes such a training program then has specialty certification in both general and thoracic surgery. Pediatric surgery has a comparable requirement. The American Board of Medical Specialties (ABMS) has approved additional Certificates of Added Qualifications in Critical Care Medicine, Hand Surgery, and Vascular Surgery. This increase in specialty certification will probably continue and the mechanism will be Certification of "Added Qualification." Currently, approximately 65% of residents completing training in General Surgery specialize beyond first certification.

Board Certification

The culmination of residency education is the specialty certification board examination given under the regulation of the American Board of Medical Specialists. Currently, 24 boards participate in this conglomerate organization, which was founded in 1933. However, some boards have been in existence for a longer time: For example the Ophthalmology Board was founded in

TABLE 1-2 REQUIREMENTS FOR SPECIALTY BOARD CERTIFICATION

	GME YEARS REQUIRED TO CERTIFICATION			
AMERICAN BOARD OF	PRELIMINARY TRAINING REQUIREMENTS	SPECIAL RESIDENCY REQUIREMENT	(MINIMUM)*	REQUIRED
Allergy/Immunology	3	2	5	No
Anesthesiology	1	3	4	Yes
Colo/Rectal Surgery	5	1	6	Yes
Dermatology	1	3	4	Yes
Emergency Medicine	1	2	3	Yes
Family Practice		3	3	Yes
Internal Medicine		3	3	No
Neurosurgery	1	5	8	Yes
Nuclear Medicine	2	2	4	No
Ob./Gyn.		4	6	Yes
Ophthalmology	1	3	4	Yes
Orthopedic Surgery		5	7	Yes
Otolaryngology	1	3	5	Yes
Pathology		4	4	Yes
Pediatrics		3	3	No
Physical Medicine/Rehabilitation	1	3	4	No
Plastic Surgery	3	2	5	No
Preventive Medicine	3	1	4	Yes
Psychiatry/Neurology		4	4	Yes
Radiology		4	4	No
Surgery		5	5	Yes
Thoracic Surgery	5	2	7	No
Urology	2	3	6	Yes

From *Annual Report and Reference Handbook—1985,* Evanston, Ill, 1985, American Board of Medical Specialists.

*Total may be greater than sum of preliminary training requirements due to practical experience requirements or to other creditable experience.

1917. During one period of the development of board certification, "affiliate" boards were formed, which in many cases eventually became independent certifying agencies, as was the case with thoracic surgery. Today the affiliate board concept has been superseded by joint boards, such as the American Board of Emergency Medicine, which is composed of boards for Emergency Medicine, Surgery, and Internal Medicine and recently has become an independent board.

In 1937 the American Board of Surgery was founded to provide an examination for general surgeons and other members of the surgical community. Subsequent founding of boards for many surgical specialties represented the development of new surgical techniques in areas of progress. In 1975 pediatric surgery was granted a special certificate, and 128 surgeons were examined. In 1983 General-Vascular Surgery was added as an additional area of certification of special competence. The Special Competence Certificate has been superseded by a Certificate of Added Qualification.

The trend to increase credentialing is gaining momentum. The American Board of Surgery, the American Board of Plastic Surgery, and the American Board of Orthopaedic Surgery now offer certification in surgery of the hand. Certification in Surgical Oncology, Critical Care Medicine, and other areas may soon follow. The American Board of Surgery, in an effort to halt fragmentation, declared a moratorium on additional certificates in 1989.

Currently, approximately 60% of graduates of General Surgery training programs take additional training in one of the fields that require general surgery board examinations for admission into a training program. The various boards are charged with examining and certifying as specialists those physicians who have completed approved training programs in surgery and the specialties of surgery. The involvement of the various boards in the program is limited to participation in and representation on the residency review committees, making the process somewhat less centralized than it is in Canada and England.

A physician entering graduate training in surgery should become familiar with the program requirements of his specialty as soon as possible. Different training programs vary slightly in the number of years of training required and the opportunities available. However, programs in surgery differ from those in other specialties, such as internal medicine and pediatrics, in several fundamental ways. Programs in surgery require the resident to perform a number of operations in a variety of characteristic areas to pass the credentials committee of the respective board. In addition, all fields require a period of chief residency in which the resident must fulfill defined responsibilities to qualify for the board examination. Junior residency does not qualify a person for examination.

Although the examination process in surgery varies somewhat among the surgical specialties, they all share certain general characteristics. The resident's program director submits a certified number of operative procedures to the credentials committee of the respective board. If then accepted for examination, the applicant must usually pass a qualifying examination (written). Once the applicant successfully completes that examination, that person is admitted to a certifying examination (usually an oral examination). Most boards allow several opportunities (up to three) to take the examination to become a certified specialist. Some boards require an additional year of training if the applicant has not passed the examination by the third attempt. Some boards require a period of practice before qualifying for the credentials committee.

Economic Influences

Today's students are completing their medical education often in debt for $60,000 to $80,000. Congress provided financial support for medical education through Medicare legislation by making money available to hospitals to pay for direct and indirect costs of medical education. Patient revenues absorbed the higher cost of maintaining teaching hospitals. However, the cost of and commitment to this program are now being questioned because of the increasing public perception that there are too many physicians, particularly too many specialists already trained.

In 1984 the federally sponsored Medicare program spent $1 billion directly for medical education. The current administration's budget proposes to freeze these payments and halve the indirect subsidy for medical education, thereby netting a savings of 30% from the estimated total of $2.3 billion spent on medical education. In the drive of the government to bring the cost of health care under control, the ensuing debates over the related issues of the number of residents, specialty choice, and geographic distribution of physicians, and the need for greater accountability for the allocation of public funds in support of GME will have a profound effect on teaching hospitals.

At present, the reality of a more tightly fisted government and the broad concern over the size of the physician population virtually preclude programs in the United States from accepting positions from other countries. However, it is unlikely that the talents and imaginations of surgical educators will be unable to develop responsible means to continue the time-honored tradition for leading surgical centers to educate surgeons from abroad while at the same time providing the quality residency education required for the surgeons of tomorrow in the United States. The threat of reduced support for biomedical research, concomitant with a diminishing role for acute care hospitals on the increasingly pernicious influence of malpractice litigation on educational programs, will only compound difficulties that academic medical centers can expect to face in the near future.

Changing Health Provider Plans

A broader based change that already has begun to influence the graduate programs of medical education is the accelerating movement to a highly competitive health care system. Driven by a concern about the escalating cost of medical care, corporate America has prompted the private insurance industry to develop mechanisms to control pricing. Industry and government have joined forces to stimulate the development of restricted provider health plans such as health maintenance organizations (HMOs) and preferred provider organizations (PPOs). Although many students envision a career as a private solo office practitioner based on role models from their youth, fewer and fewer of them achieve that goal.

Specialty groups, clinics, and HMOs, have grown considerably in the past few years, as has the number of people served by HMOs. Presently more than 575 HMOs serve more than 33,092,954 people, representing an 18% increase since 1983 and 1984. PPOs are also increasing rapidly. Both HMOs and PPOs are expected to grow so rapidly that by 1995 the vast majority of the population will be in some type of restricted provider health plan. Traditional fee-for-service medicine probably will no longer be used, replaced by systems designed to control use, ensure quality, and restrain pricing. These plans specifically omit provision for the cross-subsidy of residency education that currently receives at least 80% of its financial support from insurance payments for patient care. In the shift of third-party payers to limit their financial liability to direct coverage for the medical care of subscribers, the other casualties will be financing the care of indigent patients and regional standby services.

The interaction of societal and economic pressures with advances in surgical technology and information will foster innovative responses from surgical educators. Certainly the practices and policies of GME will be reexamined in response to societal and economic pressures. In addressing these global issues, the graduate programs in medical education have an unparalleled opportunity to overcome the problems of the past while planning for the continuing evolution of residency education that started with Halsted almost a century ago.

Medical Manpower

According to the AMA, 600,789 physicians were practicing in the United States and its possessions in 1989. That number included 68,986 residents in all years of training and 118,789 physicians in the surgical specialties including obstetrics and gynecology (Table 1-3).

Many studies of physician and surgeon manpower have been conducted. Two of these reports predicted an excess supply of physicians in 1990. Interest in this alleged excess grows primarily from health care cost information and from the belief that physicians are responsible for much of the cost of health care.

TABLE 1-3 HEALTH MANPOWER

SPECIALTY	NUMBER	PERCENTAGE
Primary care	207,325	34.5
Surgery	135,125	22.5
Residency	82,103	13.7
Other	176,236	29.3
TOTAL	600,789	100

From American Medical Association: *Physician characteristics and distribution in the US*, 1990.

In 1958, the BANE Committee reported on physician manpower and their report suggested that there was an inadequate number of physicians. Their report recommended the following:

1. A 50% increase in the number of graduates of medicine and osteopathy by 1975.
2. Establishment of a consultant group to study educational needs in the health professions.
3. Development and implementation by professional organizations of active programs for recruitment of qualified students into medicine.
4. Establishment of new medical schools.

Directly or indirectly, the recommendations of the BANE report were accepted into public policy and incorporated into many aspects of the Medicare legislation of 1965.

In 1975 the American College of Surgeons and the American Surgical Association published a report titled "Studies on Surgical Services for the United States" (SOSSUS). The federal government and other co-sponsors participated in this study, which covered the period from 1970 to 1975 and involved 10 committees of surgeons that developed assessments of fitness, performance, and confidence of surgeons. The SOSSUS study recommended among other things that a surgical residency output of 1600 to 2000 surgeons per year would be an adequate goal (currently about 3000 surgeons complete training annually).

Perhaps the most influential of all the health personnel studies was the Graduate Medical Education National Advisory Committee (GMENAC), chartered in 1976 by the Secretary of the Department of Health and Human Services (HHS), formerly the Department of Health Education Welfare (HEW). The committee, composed of 19 members from the private sector and three federal government representatives, issued a report in September, 1980. The report identified seven major personnel problems and made 107 recommendations directed specifically at physicians. The most influential observation was that by 1990 the surplus of physicians would exceed 70,000. The report projected that graduates of foreign medical schools entering the United States would account for 40,000 to 50,000 of these surplus physicians. The report also concluded that substantial geographic and specialty imbalances would occur and attempted to identify other problems, such as the cost of medical education and the role of medical schools and physician choice of specialty. The report highly favored recommendations for increasing the number of primary care physicians. Although the GMENAC study projected excess physicians in some fields, it did not recommend limiting these specialties.

A report by the Bureau of Resources and Services criticized the methods of the GMENAC report and projected a smaller increase (59%) of physicians by 1990. This study concluded that the GMENAC model overpredicted the growth in subspecialties and that considerable difficulties exist in projecting physician supply using growth patterns related to the general population.

Increased changes in health care delivery patterns complicated the personnel issue. However, approximately 50 medical schools diminished their enrollment during 1984 in response to predictions of future physician oversupply.

The various personnel surveys have not given adequate attention to the output of residencies. These surveys globally group residents and fail to consider that beginning residents in surgery frequently enter other specialties. Moreover, the studies discussed earlier failed to consider that in surgical fields the number of residents trained has been relatively constant for 15 years and constitutes fewer than 3000 certified specialists in nine fields of surgery. That number is only slightly higher than the initial 1975 SOSSUS recommendation.

The studies also failed to consider the length of training in surgery, which means that persons who are currently in the educational system will not move into practice for several years. Nor do such studies consider the varying practice patterns for surgeons. At different points in a person's career, a surgeon may not actually perform some operations falling within the broad definition of their specialty. For example some general surgeons have an extensive practice in vascular surgery and thoracic surgery, whereas others do not, a fact dictated by hospital privileges, practice patterns, and training. In addition, the cost of malpractice insurance and the overhead expenses of a practice are so great that today many surgeons are leaving practice at an earlier date, thereby reducing the number of available physicians.

SELECTION OF A RESIDENCY PROGRAM

Selection of a residency is the most important decision that a graduate physician can make because it affects an entire career and productivity. Quality of the residency taken is more important to the physician than the medical school and undergraduate educational experiences because residencies are longer than the period of medical school or undergraduate education. Figure 1-2 lists the choices of 1993 graduates.

Before committing to a residency program, the student is wise to consider several points. To see if programs

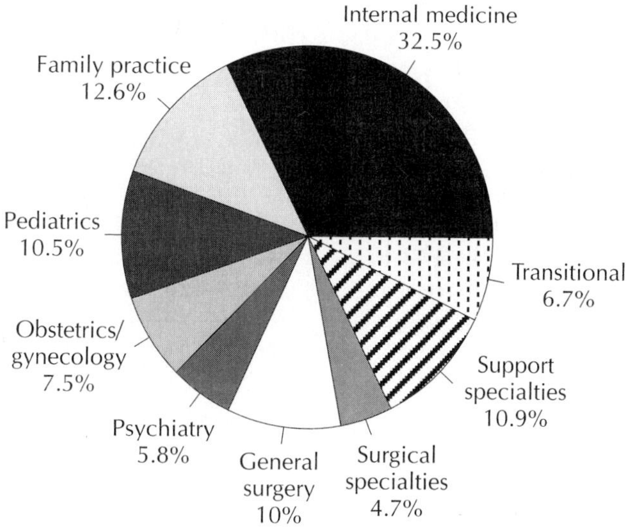

FIGURE 1-2 National Resident Matching Program, 1993. First graduate year choices of 16,896 graduates.

comply with requirements, applicants to training programs should consult the *Directory of Approved Residency Programs* and review the essentials as well as special requirements for graduate medical education as they interview at each institution. Other important information concerns the general tone of the educational program as demonstrated by residents' satisfaction with their training experience, performance on the American Board of Surgery examination, and faculty interest in the residency programs. In addition, with the changing climate in medicine, some university hospitals are affiliating with other institutions to provide a more diverse educational experience.

Among the requirements of graduate medical education are time and commitment, which predictably affect lifestyle. Students in the 20- to 25-year-old age group, which encompasses most recent graduates of medical school, are often raising families and are not living independently at a time of great change in their personal lives.

One of the characteristics of surgical residency programs is the large amount of time demanded, generally acknowledged to exceed that of other specialties. In 1977 Chao and Curran documented activities of residents and fellows. This study, commissioned by the National Institute of Medicine, shows weekly hourly commitments required of residents to fulfill their service and meet their educational needs. The mean time required was 63 hours weekly, of which 19 hours involve joint teaching duties; 15 hours were devoted to nonpatient care pursuits; 10 hours involved formalized learning; and 5 hours were devoted to research, teaching, and administration. A related and unresolved dilemma of medical education is the transition from the student to the student practitioner and the proper mix of time for these activities. The proper mix of activities can never be precisely determined; learning rates and patient demands vary among residents and institutions.

Surgical training usually requires a 70-hour week. Current salaries for residents vary from approximately $15,000 annually for a starting graduate position to $30,000 by the end of training, with some regional and local variations. The large contribution of federal dollars to training programs has recently been challenged; any reduction in federal financial support will have a predictable and significant adverse effect on graduate medical education.

Despite the changes in health care systems, two recommendations regarding graduate medical education are pertinent. Students should avail themselves of counseling early in their clinical years as they prepare for graduate training in medical education, and advisors and counselors should help them compete realistically for training programs in surgery consistent with their career goals.

TABLE 1-4 SPECIALTY CERTIFICATES ISSUED 1980 TO 1990

AREA	NO. OF CERTIFICATES
Surgery	9,445
Obstetrics and gynecology	10,345
Radiology	9,633
Primary care	
Pediatrics	21,105
Internal medicine	48,356
Family practice	22,894
Total primary care	92,355 (49%)

TABLE 1-5 SURGICAL RESIDENTS BY SPECIALTY: 1982/83 TO 1991/92

SPECIALTY	82/83	86/87	91/92
General surgery	8,683	8,118	7,696
Orthopedic surgery	2,575	2,721	2,793
Otorhinolaryngology	1,025	1,105	1,186
Urology	977	940	977
Neurological surgery	604	692	717
Plastic surgery	424	410	448
Thoracic surgery	294	297	316
Colon and rectal surgery	50	48	50
Pediatric surgery	30	30	41
Vascular surgery	....*	74	93
SUBTOTAL	14,662	14,435	14,317
Obstetrics/Gynecology	4,918†	4,616†	4,781
Ophthalmology	1,553‡	1,549‡	1,574
TOTAL	21,133	20,600	20,672

*Vascular surgery programs not accredited until 1984/85.
†Counts from the Council on Resident Education in Obstetrics and Gynecology's Resident Data Bank, Washington, DC (1989).
‡Counts from the American Medical Association: *Directory of residency training programs,* Chicago, 1985, 1987, The Association.
From American College of Surgeons: *Longitudinal Study of Surgical Residents, 1991-1992.*

TABLE 1-6 SURGICAL SPECIALTY CERTIFICATION OF GRADUATING MEDICAL STUDENTS, 1985 TO 1992*

SPECIALTY CERTIFICATION LIST	1985	1988	1989	1992
General surgery	6.2	5.6	5.3	2.1
Surgical subspecialties	0.6	0.7	0.8	3.7
Colon and rectal surgery	0.0	0.1	0.2	0.3
Neurological surgery and critical care medicine	1.0	1.2	1.0	1.0
Orthopaedic and hand surgery	5.7	5.4	5.1	5.3
Otolaryngology	2.4	2.3	2.3	2.4
Plastic and hand surgery	1.4	1.3	1.4	1.5
Thoracic surgery	0.9	0.9	0.8	1.2
Urology	2.0	1.6	1.6	1.9

*Numbers shown are percentages.
Modified and selected from Kassebaum DG, Szenas PL: Specialty preferences of graduating medical students: 1992 update, *Acad Med* 802, 1992.

TABLE 1-7 NONSURGICAL SPECIALTY CERTIFICATION OF GRADUATING MEDICAL STUDENTS, 1985 TO 1992*

SPECIALTY CERTIFICATION LIST	1985	1988	1989	1992
Family practice	13.3	11.3	11.8	9.0
Family practice subspecialties	....	....	....	1.9
General internal medicine	10.7	8.1	6.0	3.2
Internal medicine subspecialties	10.6	11.7	13.5	16.4
Obstetrics/Gynecology	5.4	5.3	4.6	2.7
Ob/Gyn subspecialties	1.6	1.8	2.1	4.1
Ophthalmology	3.6	3.5	3.4	3.4
General pediatrics	5.8	5.3	4.9	2.4
Pediatric subspecialties	2.3	2.9	3.1	5.3
Psychiatry	4.2	4.6	4.1	1.6
Radiology	0.2	0.5	0.2	0.5
Radiology subspecialties	5.5	6.4	6.2	6.7

*Numbers shown are percentages.
Modified and selected from Kassebaum DG, Szenas PL: Specialty preferences of graduating medical students: 1992 update, *Acad Med,* 802, 1992.

A student seeking training in surgery usually consults the *Directory of Approved Residency Programs* published annually by the AMA. The publication contains a list of approved graduate medical education programs, including the geographic and other information a prospective surgery resident needs.

Currently, 6900 accredited residency programs, including 581 specialty programs in internal medicine and pediatrics, come under the accreditation process. In 1991 these programs offered 86,000 resident positions, of which 1724 were unfilled. In the same year 86,217 residents were enrolled in accredited educational programs. These included 60,044 US Liaison Committee on Medical Education (LCME) graduates, 406 Canadian LCME graduates, 1150 osteopathic graduates, and 13,525 foreign medical graduates. Of the foreign medical graduates, 7381 were US citizens and 6065 were foreign nationals.

Although currently there are more residency positions than candidates, particularly when one excludes foreign nationals, the attraction and availability of different specialties are not universal. For example, the 1985 National Resident Matching Program (NRMP), conducted through the Council of Medical Specialty Societies (CMSS), has a ratio of 1.2 for residency positions per applicant. However, less than 70% of available positions were filled in family practice, pediatrics, psychiatry, and pathology. In internal medicine 70% to 80% of available positions were filled and 80% to 90% of available positions in general surgical, the surgical specialties, and obstetrics/gynecology residencies were filled. In specialties with a relatively small number of positions, such as neurosurgery, urology, ophthalmology, and otolaryngology, insufficient positions were available to accommodate the applicants. In fact, 41.5% of US seniors whose first choice was a specialty of surgery failed to match in the NRMP in 1984. Table 1-4 lists the number of specialty certificates issued between 1980 and 1990. Table 1-5 indicates the number of surgical residents by specialty, and Table 1-6 indicates the percentage of students graduating between 1985 and 1992 who received certification in surgery. Table 1-7 gives the percentage of students who were certified in nonsurgical specialties in the same years (1985 to 1990).

The result in competition for physicians in specialties has led the national crediting bodies to consider the possibility of a second match. Such a match would occur after 2 years of preliminary surgical training. An additional phenomenon has been the change of specialties outside the match because of career changes. In fact about 25% of persons entering a basic surgical field will branch into a specialty after 1 or 2 years. In addition, approximately two thirds of all finishing residents of general surgery will take specialized training beyond the 5-year core program in general surgery.

The patterns of medical and surgical practice have changed dramatically in the past 10 years and will continue to do so in the near future.

GLOSSARY

board certified The term *board certified* applies to those physicians who have successfully passed the national examination given by a particular specialty board

board eligible When a resident has successfully completed an accredited residency program and has met requirements specified by a particular specialty board, the physician is considered board eligible

graduate education The years of training between undergraduate medical education and continuing medical education; includes both residency and fellowship training

fellowship A period of training that follows residency during which the physician may further subspecialize and/or continue research in a specific area

internship The first year of residency training, generally required for state licensure; now referred to as postgraduate year No. 1 (PGY No. 1)

residency A period of training that provides the medical school graduate with clinical practice experience in a specialty or subspecialty area; the residency period is designed to (1) give the physician proficiency in a field of practice including the acquisition of special skills and techniques and (2) give the physician sufficient education for continued development; the term *resident* or *resident physician* identifies a person engaged in residency training; the duration of a residency varies from specialty to specialty and usually coincides with the period of training required for board certification.

specialty There are 23 specialty areas that describe the different practices of medicine. Table 1-2 lists 19 of these areas.

specialty society Professional specialty societies are independent groups of practicing physicians with common specialty training; these societies range from small associations of program directors in graduate medical education and medical school department chairmen to large specialty colleges and academies; the Council of Medical Specialty Societies (CMSS) has 24 major colleges and academies as members

subspecialty Within the 23 medical specialties, there are 31 subspecialty areas; for example, within the specialty of internal medicine, there are 10 subspecialty areas of practice: cardiovascular disease, critical care medicine, endocrinology and metabolism, gastroenterology, hematology, infectious disease, medical oncology, nephrology, pulmonary disease, rheumatology

Terminology of Accreditation Process

Accreditation Council for Graduate Medical Education (ACGME) The ACGME is the successor to the LCGME and remains an independent autonomous body that has responsibility for accrediting and reviewing programs in graduate medical education

Council on Medical Education (CME) Established in 1927 by the American Medical Association to review and approve graduate medical education; in 1928 the CME developed standards for residency programs entitled "Essentials of Approved Residencies and Fellowships"

Liaison Committee on Graduate Medical Education (LCGME) Established in 1972 by the American Medical Association, American Hospital Association, Council of Medical Specialty Societies, American Board of Medical Specialties, and Association of American Medical Colleges, the LCGME was the successor entity to the Council on Medical Education and assumed responsibility for accreditation of graduate medical education programs; the LCGME improved the accreditation process and made significant progress toward more consistent quality of graduate programs across the nation

Residency Review Committees (RRCs) RRCs were established in the early 1950s by the Council on Medical Education of the American Medical Association in cooperation with specialty boards and some specialty colleges; RRCs recommend minimum requirements for residency programs and review programs to determine if they meet these established requirements

■ From *The Commonwealth Fund Task Force on Academic Health Centers,* New York, 1985, Harkness House.

SUGGESTED READINGS

Annual Report and Reference Handbook—1985, Evanston, Ill, 1985, American Board of Medical Specialties.

Association of American Medical Colleges: External examinations for the evaluation of medical education achievement and for licensure, *J Med Educ* 1981.

Barker HG: *The structure and support of contemporary residency programs in surgery,* Springfield, Ill, 1971, Charles C Thomas.

Bernard C: *An introduction to the study of experimental medicine,* New York, 1927, MacMillan. (Translated by Henry Copley Greene.)

Billroth T: *General surgical pathology and therapeutics, classics of surgery library,* Birmingham, 1984, LB Adams, Jr.

Blendon RJ, Alteman DE: Special report: public attitudes about health care costs, *N Engl J Med* 311:613, 1984.

Bowers JZ, Purcell EF: *Advances in American medicine: essays at the bicentennial,* New York, 1976, Josiah Massey Foundation.

Carter BN: The fruition of Halsted's concept of surgical training, *Surgery* 32:518, 1935.

Chao W, Curran E: A description of house officer effort by activity category, specialty and type of hospital, *Clin Chim Acta* 78(1):79, 1977.

Drucker WR: Problems and solutions for graduate surgical education in Canada. In Barber HG, editor: *The structure and support of contemporary residency programs in surgery.* Transactions of the 31st Annual Meeting of the Allen O. Whipple Surgical Society, Springfield, Ill, 1971, Charles C Thomas.

Eighty-third annual report on medical education in the United States (1982-1983), *JAMA* 250:1501, 1983.

Executive Services Department: *Longitudinal study of surgical residents, 1984/85,* Chicago, 1986, American College of Surgeons.

Final report of the Commission on Medical Education, New York, 1932, Office of the Director of Study.

Fishman AP, Richards DW: Circulation of the blood. In *Man and ideas,* New York, 1964, Oxford University Press.

Flexner A: *Medical education in the United States and Canada,* New York, 1910, The Carnegie Foundation.

Flexner A: *Medical education: a comparative study,* New York, 1925, MacMillan.

Garrison FH: *An introduction to the history of medicine,* Philadelphia, 1919, WB Saunders.

Halsted WS: *Surgical papers,* Baltimore, 1928, The Johns Hopkins Press.

Halsted WS: The training of a surgeon, *Bull Johns Hopkins Hospital* 15:267, 1904.

Heuer GJ: Graduate teaching of surgery in university clinics, *Ann Surg* 102:507, 1935.

Hubbard JP: *Measuring medical education: the tests and the experience of the National Board of Medical Examiners,* Philadelphia, 1978, Lea & Febiger.

Inglehart JK: Difficult times ahead for graduate medical education, *N Engl J Med* 312:1400, 1985.

King IS: Medical education: the decade of massive change, *JAMA* 251:219, 1984.

Lloyd JS, editor: *Residency director's role in specialty certification,* Chicago, 1985, American Board of Medical Specialties.

Lyons AS, Petrucelli RJ: *Medicine: an illustrated history,* New York 1978, Harry N Abrams.

MacKenzie WC: Interest and concern of the Royal College of Surgeons in residency programs, *Can Med Assoc J* 95:697, 1966.

Major RH: *Classic descriptions of disease,* Springfield, Ill, 1945, Charles C Thomas.

Medical education: institutions, characteristics, and programs, Washington, DC, 1933, Association of American Medical Colleges.

Medical school admission requirements, 1983-84, Washington, DC, 1985, Association of American Medical Colleges.

Mettler CC, Mettler FA: *History of medicine,* Philadelphia, 1947, The Blakiston Co.

Moore FD: Surgery. In Bowers JZ, Purcell EF, editors: *Advances in American medicine: essays at the Bicentennial,* vol 2, New York, 1976, The Josiah Massey, Jr. Foundation, in cooperation with the National Library of Medicine.

Morton JH, Aufses AH Jr, Beilgh TJ: An assessment of surgical training, *Am Coll Surg Bull,* 20, 1981.

Nuland SB: *The origins of anesthesia, classics of medicine library,* Birmingham, 1983, LB Adams, Jr.

Numbers RL, editor: *The education of American physicians,* Los Angeles, 1980, University of California Press.

Personnel needs and training for biomedical research and behavioral research, Washington, DC, 1983, National Academy Press.

Projections of physician supply in the U.S.—March, 1985, Washington, DC, 1985, US Department of Health and Human Services, Public Health Service, Health Resources and Services Administration.

Report of the New York State Commission on Graduate Medical Education, New York, 1986, State of New York Department of Health.

Rutkow IM: *Surgery: an illustrated history,* St Louis, 1994, Mosby.

Sawyers, JL: Graduate surgical education, *Am Surg* 47:1, 1981.

Sheldon GF: 1984 A.A.S.T. presidential address: medical education and the trauma surgeon—the role of the A.A.S.T., *J Trauma* 25(8):727, 1985.

Starr P: *The social transformation of American medicine,* New York, 1982, Basic Books.

Stevens R: *American medicine and the public interest,* New Haven, Conn, 1971, Yale University Press.

Swanson AG: The evolution of graduate medical education, *J Med Educ* (suppl) 55:1039, 1981.

Task Force on Academic Health Centers: *Prescription for change, the commonwealth fund, report of the Task Force on Academic Health Centers,* New York, 1985, Harkness House.

Undergraduate education in surgery, *Am Coll Surg Bull* 68(5): 1983.

Virchow R: *Cellular pathology,* London, 1860, John Churchill. (Translated by Frank Chance.)

Wangensteen OH, Wangensteen SD: *The rise of surgery: from empiric craft to scientific discipline,* Minneapolis, 1978, University of Minnesota Press.

Welch WH: *Papers and addresses,* vol 3, Baltimore, 1920, The Johns Hopkins University Press.

Zimmerman LM, Veith I: *Great ideas in the history of surgery,* Baltimore, 1961, Williams & Wilkins.

Zuidema GE: The status of surgical manpower, *Am Coll Surg Bull* 29:2, 1984.

Zuidema GE, Moore FD: *Surgery in the United States,* Chicago, 1975, The American College of Surgeons and The American Surgical Association.

Part One, which covers biologic phenomena in surgery, is exciting to the editors; we trust the reader will find it equally so. These chapters present biology written by surgeons for their colleagues. As practicing surgeons, we must often make decisions without the amount of precise data we would like. In science we usually have more exact and complete data, but scientific knowledge and understanding are constantly changing. Therefore we must build on the old science, replace the outmoded, add what appears to be reasonable according to available data, and incorporate the new scientific information into our practices. No surgeon has seen every disease, nor do patients always manifest the classic picture of a particular disorder. Thus surgeons who carry an understanding of human biologic phenomena into daily practice are better able to assess the problems they face and to institute proper therapy, even if they have neither seen nor heard of the specific disease. Surgery is not simply a learned mechanical skill, nor is medicine a mnemonic system of signs and symptoms. Rather, the sound practice of medicine and surgery is a science, requiring a thorough and working knowledge of biologic phenomena.

PART ONE

BIOLOGIC PHENOMENA IN SURGERY

CHAPTER 2

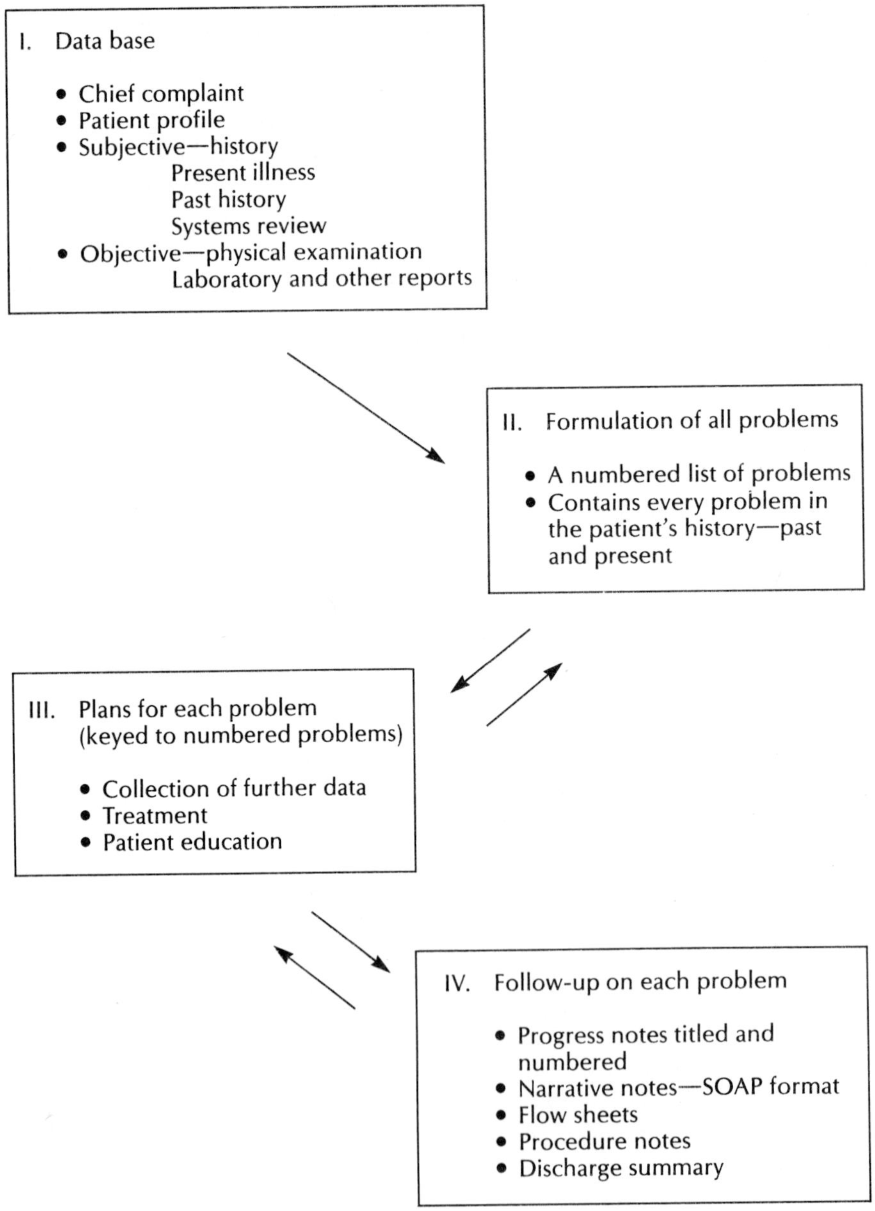
I. Data base
• Chief complaint
• Patient profile
• Subjective—history
Present illness
Past history
Systems review
• Objective—physical examination
Laboratory and other reports
II. Formulation of all problems
• A numbered list of problems
• Contains every problem in the patient's history—past and present
III. Plans for each problem (keyed to numbered problems)
• Collection of further data
• Treatment
• Patient education
IV. Follow-up on each problem
• Progress notes titled and numbered
• Narrative notes—SOAP format
• Flow sheets
• Procedure notes
• Discharge summary

ASSESSMENT OF THE SURGICAL PATIENT

John H. Davis • Roger S. Foster Jr. • Richard L. Gamelli
Jack Pickleman • Kenneth W. Burchard

This chapter provides both a systematic approach to data gathering and critical thinking in surgery and a guide to understanding the overall organization of this text. The major emphasis is on the process of critical thinking and decision making in surgery. Appropriate decisions in patient management require an organized approach to collection of information and a systematic approach to assessment of that information. Clinical surgery shares with other fields of medicine many of the data-gathering and decision-making processes. Surgery is distinct from other fields in its use of highly developed surgical skills for patient treatment and in the speed with which some management decisions must be made. From data collection to formulation of a treatment plan, this chapter describes a systematic approach to the care of the surgical patient that we believe leads to better patient care. The approach described in this chapter is an adaptation of the problem-solving approach to clinical thinking and record keeping developed by Dr. Lawrence Weed.[3]

PROBLEM-SOLVING APPROACH

Identifying Problems

Identifying and enumerating a patient's problems is quite different from establishing a final diagnosis. The final diagnosis may be the ultimate definition of the patient's problem, but before reaching the final diagnosis, the surgeon identifies problems with an increasing degree of diagnostic sophistication. For example, a patient with a gallstone impacted in the distal common duct does not first come to the clinician with a well-defined problem. The presenting problem may be "jaundice," which is not a disease but an objective finding. Initial evaluation of the patient may establish that the patient has an obstructive type of jaundice, and the problem definition is refined to "obstructive jaundice." Further diagnostic evaluation that demonstrates the presence of a stone would lead to a final definition of the problem as "common duct stone." The chapters in this text reflect these increasingly specific levels of problem identification.

It is essential that the surgeon take care not to define the problem with more specificity than the available data warrant. Labeling a problem prematurely with a specific diagnosis may lead to failure to consider reasonable alternative diagnoses. Only when a problem has been defined with a reasonable certainty is it appropriate to proceed with a working diagnosis that may have treatment implications. Even when the problem has been sufficiently defined so that a working diagnosis is established, the surgeon must approach all diagnostic labels with an element of skepticism. Working diagnoses are hypotheses to explain the patient's signs, symptoms, and laboratory findings. The surgeon must be alert to subsequent observations that are not consistent with the working diagnosis.

■ Problem-Solving Approach section contributed by John H. Davis, Roger S. Foster Jr., and Richard L. Gamelli.

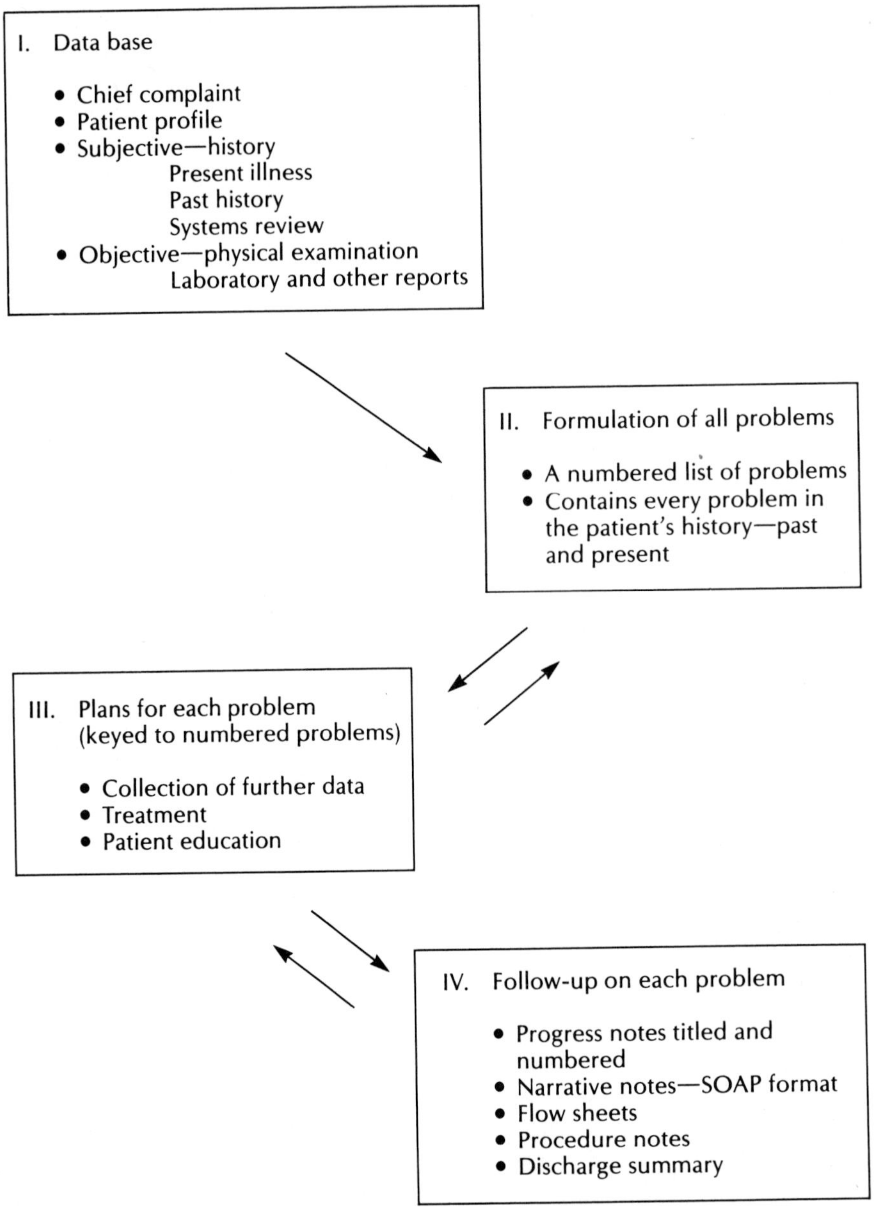

FIGURE 2-1 A schematic display of the problem-oriented medical record. As data and the patient's course dictate, the formulation of problems is modified, the problem list updated, the plans made current, and the outcome noted in subsequent progress notes; hence the bidirectional arrows. The care of patients is a constant integrative process that frequently requires reassessment and reformulation of plans.

Structuring the Problem-Solving Approach

Defining the patient's problems with increasing degrees of sophistication is accomplished through the traditional research techniques of data acquisition and analysis. The problem-solving approach is shown diagrammatically in Figure 2-1. Data obtained from taking the patient's history are *subjective* data. Subjective data include the patient's profile, history of the current illness, any past history or family history potentially related to the problem, the patient's interpretation or understanding of the problem, and any previous treatment or surgical procedures. Also included are negative aspects of the history that may be pertinent to the problem.

Objective data include the physiologic data (e.g., weight, height, temperature, pulse, and blood pressure), the physical examination data, and data from any previously obtained laboratory tests or other diagnostic studies.

Based on the surgeon's assessment of the subjective and objective data, an initial problem list is formulated. Using this problem list, an *initial plan* is made for each problem. This plan generally has three separate subcomponents: (1) diagnostic plans; (2) therapeutic plans; and (3) patient education plans (often this may also be parent, spouse, or partner education).

The mnemonic for organization of the medical record in the problem-oriented format is SOAP. For example:

Problem 1
- Subjective:
- Objective:
- Assessment:
- Plans:

If the patient is believed to have more than one problem, each problem is separately identified and categorized in a similar fashion:

Problem 2
- Subjective:
- Objective:
- Assessment:
- Plans:

The advantage of the problem-solving approach is its organization of clinical thinking. The list of problems serves as an index to alert the surgeon to other issues that may confound the management of a specific surgical problem. The problem list occasionally may provide clues that allow several problems to be redefined under the heading of a single problem. For example, the initial problem list might read:

Problem 1 Weight loss
Problem 2 Diarrhea
Problem 3 History of duodenal ulcer
- a. Closure of perforation 5 years previously (1989)
- b. Vagotomy and pyloroplasty 4 years previously (1990)
- c. Distal gastrectomy and Billroth II anastomosis for recurrent duodenal ulcer 2 years previously (1992)

Problem 4 Anemia
Problem 5 Intermittent abdominal pain

A diagnostic workup establishes that problems 1 through 5 appear to be related to a marginal ulcer and hypergastrinemia. The problem can now be redefined as:

Problem 1 Hypergastrinemia with complications
- a. Post closure of duodenal perforation (1989)
- b. Vagotomy and pyloroplasty (1990)
- c. Distal gastrectomy and Billroth II anastomosis (1993)
- d. Marginal ulcer and anemia secondary to bleeding
- e. Current therapy with H_2-receptor blocking agent

Further diagnostic evaluation and treatment might refine the problem title to:

Problem 1 Zollinger-Ellison syndrome resolved
- a. Resection of solitary islet cell tumor of the pancreas (1994)
- b. Post closure of duodenal perforation (1989)
- c. Vagotomy and pyloroplasty (1990)
- d. Distal gastrectomy and Billroth II anastomosis (1993)

Process of Clinical Assessment

The process of clinical assessment, or the evaluation of the patient and the patient's course, is a critical part of patient management that must precede and accompany any surgical or nonsurgical intervention. It is competence in the evaluative process that distinguishes the surgeon as a professional from an operating technician. Good surgical care depends first on a fundamental knowledge of anatomy, physiology, pathology, available diagnostic technology, and therapeutic technology; second, on an organized system for assessing the patient; and third, on competence in surgical skills. The process of assessment is the critical link between knowledge and performance.

The decision tree in Figure 2-1 and the faceplate of the chapter diagram the assessment process. As the bidirectional arrows imply, the assessment process recycles as more data become available or as the patient's progress or response to treatment is evaluated.

Initial Assessment

After a patient's problem or problems have been identified, the next steps in initial assessment are localizing the problem, determining the type of pathologic process, and determining the urgency of intervention.

Identification

Identification in the assessment process involves determining whether the patient has a problem. Are there symptoms? Does the physical examination reveal any abnormalities? Are abnormalities seen on laboratory test results or in other diagnostic procedures? The initial assessment should focus on the most specific problems.

Localizing the Problem

Localization in the assessment process is the anatomic localization. Does the problem involve a single organ? Multiple organs? Which organ or organs? Is it a systemic process? For example, in a patient experiencing intermittent severe abdominal pain (colic), the surgeon attempts to determine which organ is responsible: the colon? the appendix? the gallbladder? the small bowel? the ureter?

Determining the Pathologic Process

In determining the type of pathologic process in the assessment, the surgeon considers the basic categories of disease: Is it congenital, degenerative, traumatic, inflammatory, toxic, metabolic, or neoplastic?

Determining the Urgency of Intervention

The immediate need for intervention is determined primarily by the presenting problem. Fortunately, many problems do not require immediate diagnostic or therapeutic intervention. The few that do require action on the surgeon's part to maintain the patient's life. Examples of the need for immediate intervention are described below.

SUDDEN LOSS OF AIRWAY PATENCY. The problem is the patient is unable to breathe; this might be caused by an obstruction, such as a bolus of food that was aspirated and caught in the airway. It may also be caused by aspirated blood or vomitus following a motor vehicle accident in which the patient suffered severe facial injuries, with multiple fractures or major hemorrhage or both in and around the mouth.

INABILITY TO VENTILATE THE LUNGS PROPERLY. The problem may be a crushed chest (e.g., following a motor vehicle accident) involving both a flail segment and inability to adequately oxygenate the blood circulating through the lung. The problem could also be severe pneumonia in which the lung is so congested from infection that adequate gas exchange is impossible. Another possibility is muscular paralysis that renders the patient unable to expand and contract the chest normally. Regardless of the underlying pathologic process, the problem remains the patient's inability to breathe, and the need for intervention is immediate.

CARDIOVASCULAR COLLAPSE. The patient has inadequate circulation, which might be caused by failure of the heart (such as is seen with an acute myocardial infarction) or might result from a severe arrhythmia in which the heart is unable to effectively pump the blood (such as is seen with ventricular fibrillation). Cardiovascular collapse also might be caused by severe dehydration in which there is an inadequate volume of fluid in the circulation for the heart to pump. Regardless of the pathologic mechanism, the problem remains cardiovascular collapse, and the need for intervention is immediate.

MAJOR HEMORRHAGE (EXSANGUINATION). Exsanguination may result from internal or external bleeding. The problem arises because the loss of blood volume is such that an effective cardiac output is impossible, and the blood pressure falls. This loss could be caused by major hemorrhage from a duodenal ulcer or from numerous other sites of internal bleeding (such as occurs with a ruptured abdominal aortic aneurysm), or it could be caused by external hemorrhage from a gunshot wound. The pathologic process may be unknown at the time the patient is initially seen, but the problem remains major hemorrhage and shock.

RAPIDLY DETERIORATING NEUROLOGIC STATUS. Rapid deterioration in neurologic status may be seen in a patient who has been in an accident and sustained a head injury, but who was awake at the scene. On entering the emergency department, however, the patient begins to demonstrate a deteriorating neurologic status. The underlying pathologic process might be something such as an epidural hematoma, but the initial problem remains a deteriorating neurologic status.

In these emergency conditions, the problem list necessarily must be short and should consist only of the problem for which the physician is treating the patient, as mentioned above; the second problem should be listed as an inadequate data base. Under these circumstances there is no time to obtain a complete history, to discover other problems that the patient may have, or to spend any time defining such problems. Therefore an incomplete data base is problem no. 2, which alerts the physician that at a later time, once the patient's condition has been stabilized and treatment is under way, further evaluation of the patient is needed. Early in the management of emergency patients, the physician keeps the organizational approach in mind and records it after the patient's condition is initially stabilized.

Another group of problems requires urgent diagnostic or therapeutic intervention, or both, usually within 6 to 12 hours of onset. Examples of these problems are given below.

SEVERE ABDOMINAL PAIN. Abdominal pain that comes on suddenly in a patient who has been relatively well usually occurs secondary to a process that will require surgical intervention. Such pain may occur with a perforated viscus, which can lead to acute peritonitis. The pain might be quite well localized as is seen with torsion of a testicle. It might last for several hours, as is seen with an ischemic leg after an embolus develops.

SEVERE FEBRILE EPISODE. A severe febrile episode is the sudden onset of high fever, ranging from 40° to 41.1° C (104° to 106° F), in an adult who was previously well. This usually heralds serious illness; a fever workup must be undertaken immediately, and steps must be taken to lower the body temperature. This immediate action generally does not apply to children, because they can develop a very high fever with a relatively minor illness and seem to tolerate it quite well.

NEW OR RAPID ONSET OF DYSFUNCTION

Depression of mental status. Depressed mental status is an urgent situation that may be seen in patients who are taking drugs, particularly those who are using drugs for other than medical purposes. It also may be seen after a mild head injury in which the patient appears to have no symptoms for a period of time and then gradually shows a depression of mental status, suggesting that a subdural hematoma may be present.

Paralysis or paresis. Paralysis or paresis can be seen

in a patient who has had a transient ischemic attack that causes temporary cerebral ischemia, usually secondary to stenosis of the carotid artery. It can also be seen in patients who have a completed stroke.

Complete urinary retention. The problem of complete urinary retention is acute and painful. It can be seen in patients who may or may not have been having urinary difficulties over a period of time but who suddenly can no longer void any urine. No matter how hard they try, they are completely obstructed; the bladder distends, and the pain and cramping are relatively severe.

Total obstipation. Many people have difficulty moving their bowels, but an urgent problem arises when they are unable to pass anything at all through the rectum for several days. This condition usually is accompanied by cramping abdominal pain and frequently distention. The problem is complete obstipation, although the underlying pathologic process may vary, from a malignant tumor causing obstruction to certain types of inflammation or a volvulus of the colon.

Localized circulatory ischemia. The most common scenario for localized circulatory ischemia is the patient who has had some ischemic signs in an extremity, usually the leg, and who then has a sudden, final occlusion of the circulatory process. The leg becomes cold, white, and quite painful. In this situation it is urgent that circulation be restored within a matter of hours, or tissue may be lost. A similar situation can be seen in a patient with a cardiac arrhythmia, either chronic or acute, that throws an embolism into one of the distal arteries, causing immediate ischemia. A similar problem can be seen on the venous side of the circulation in a patient who has developed deep venous thrombosis, frequently in the postoperative period. The sudden onset of chest pain, hemoptysis, and difficulty breathing suggests a pulmonary embolus. The urgency of this condition is determined by the size of the embolus, which may convert an urgent situation into an emergency.

Alterations in breathing. Some rates of breathing may be too rapid for the patient to sustain for a long period without complete exhaustion. Rapid breathing may be seen in adult respiratory distress syndrome (ARDS), in which pulmonary gas exchange is compromised, and the patient attempts to maintain oxygenation by breathing more quickly. Because only a few hours of this type of breathing will totally exhaust the patient, urgent intervention is required. Respirations may also be too slow to maintain adequate ventilation; this is often caused by drug overdose.

Pernicious nausea and vomiting. Nausea and vomiting accompany many diseases but usually are not severe enough to require urgent intervention. However, patients who develop complete pyloric obstruction may begin to vomit fairly large quantities in an explosive manner every few minutes. They sometimes fill many basins with material, creating not only rapid dehydration but also hypochloremic hypokalemic alkalosis. They require urgent decompression of the stomach and supportive fluid therapy until the underlying problem can be defined and treated.

PULSATILE EXPANDING MASS. Pain usually accompanies a pulsatile expanding mass; otherwise the patient might not have sought medical attention. Pain in the abdomen or lower back accompanied by a pulsatile mass in the abdomen suggests impending rupture of an abdominal aortic aneurysm.

Initial assessment of the above problems should include both a preliminary hypothesis as to the problem or the general type of problem and a determination of the urgency of the problem. The findings on physical examination and/or any imaging studies usually contribute to anatomic localization of the problem. Generalized symptoms such as fatigue, chills, sweating, and anorexia, as well as physiologic data such as temperature and pulse rate, generally provide the initial clues to the type of pathologic process. The duration of symptoms, their severity, and the rapidity with which they change are the major clues to the urgency of intervention.

Hypothesis Formation and Testing

Diagnostic hypotheses come from the surgeon's knowledge and experience (pattern recognition), as well as from logical deductions based on analysis of the data. The initial hypotheses are constantly tested. Sometimes testing of hypotheses involves returning to the patient for further history (subjective data) or clarification of details. Sometimes portions of the physical examination are repeated. Frequently laboratory tests and diagnostic imaging procedures are obtained either to further support or to eliminate the diagnostic hypotheses. Initial hypotheses that fail to explain the findings are discarded. The remaining possibilities are then weighed as to their importance.

Weighing Initial Diagnostic Hypotheses

Several criteria are used to weigh the initial diagnostic hypotheses. One important criterion is the probability of a diagnosis based on its frequency in a patient of the given age, gender, and circumstances. Reasonable hypotheses about diagnoses involving potentially life-threatening conditions are given important weight for additional evaluation that will either exclude or further support them. Hypotheses about conditions that are potentially treatable also are weighed more heavily than diagnostic hypotheses of conditions that have no effective treatment. Further definition of nontreatable conditions may have research implications or may on occasion be important in establishing a prognosis; except for these two reasons, however, further testing is inappropriate. For humanitarian as well as cost-containment reasons, the clinical dictum is that a test should not be ordered if the information will not be used in the patient's care.

Working Diagnosis

At the completion of the diagnostic evaluation, the surgeon should arrive at a working diagnosis or formulation of the problem. In the real world of the clinical practice of surgery, one frequently does not arrive at a working diagnosis that is absolutely certain. The surgeon must settle for a working diagnosis that is either most probable or most important to exclude. After establishing the working diagnosis, the next step frequently is therapeutic intervention, which can lead to correction of the patient's problem and correction or refinement of the working diagnosis.

Efficiencies and Pitfalls in the Assessment Process

An experienced surgeon very quickly begins to formulate and discard hypotheses about a patient's problem. Whereas a beginner may collect comprehensive history and physical examination data before beginning the assessment, an experienced surgeon frequently arrives at a diagnosis quickly through a series of highly relevant and specific questions and a limited physical examination to test various initial hypotheses. The diagnostic efficiency of a mature clinician is a goal to be sought. However, some pitfalls must be avoided. A premature final diagnosis may trap the unwary into failing to obtain necessary subjective or objective data, leading to an incorrect diagnosis. Overly direct or leading questions may cause the patient to give answers that he believes the clinician wants, or they may close off the patient from volunteering an important detail. Moreover, additional problems may exist that are important to the patient's overall health, and these should not be overlooked.

Systems exist both to maintain efficiency and to help prevent oversight. These systems include systematic questionnaires that the patient fills out, checklists for the clinician to ensure that relevant data or steps are not missed, and efficient use of ancillary personnel, to whom are delegated standardized tasks of data collection and recording. Depending on the training of the ancillary personnel, they may obtain and record the standard vital signs or they may conduct routine parts of the physical examination.

The Medical Record

Proper organization of the medical record can contribute in a major way to both the quality and efficiency of patient care. A good record improves and speeds communication between physicians and other health care workers. A good record also helps coordinate care when it is provided by many different physicians, documents the progression of the patient's problem or problems, and clarifies the process of clinical thinking.

Just as an index, section headings, tables, and graphs contribute to the organization of a scientific paper or textbook, so do they in a medical record. Consistency and order are imperative. The basic components of a complete problem-oriented medical record are illustrated in Figure 2-1.

Data Base

The data base should be a defined data base that screens for abnormalities that are important and appropriate for the age and demographic characteristics of the patient population. The data base traditionally includes the chief complaint, patient profile, review of systems, physical examination, and laboratory data. Data recording is more efficient if checklists are used for reviewing systems and recording physical examination data. Under numbered headings related to the patient's specific problems, the record should have subheadings for the subjective information (history), the objective information (physical examination and any available laboratory tests or imaging studies), the initial assessment, and the initial plans. Although the problem list is constructed after the history and physical examination are completed and therefore is shown second in Figure 2-1, the record should be assembled so that the problem list is the first page of the medical record and thus serves as an index to it. The problem list (Figure 2-2) is modified as new problems are identified and as active problems are further clarified or resolved.

The subjective items in the patient's history should be grouped together under "history" or "subjective data." Generally the history should be recorded in chronologic order, but for long, complex histories it may be more appropriate to first describe the current episode and then to summarize the patient's past history associated with the problem. All subjective data, both positive and negative, is recorded under the problem that contributes to the assessment. The important information is recorded concisely; excessive detail may deter others from reading the record.

Objective data pertinent to the problem should also be recorded concisely and objectively. Subjective information from the history should not be intermingled. Long lists of relatively minor negative findings should not be recorded under the problem heading; these are frequently best handled by a standardized checklist format. Details should be recorded objectively and precisely. Abbreviations should not be used unless they are universally accepted. Measurements should be made and recorded using the metric system. Measurements in fingers, hands, and stones were replaced long ago with more standard units. Measurements in eggs, fruits, and vegetables are even worse.

Often, data from repetitive observations or labora-

Master problem list

Name: White female

Date of birth: 07-02-52

Medical record no. xxx-xx-xxx

Date onset noted	Active problems (number 1,2,3, etc.)	Date resolved	Inactive/resolved problems
1966	#1	 1976 1974 1970	Membranous nephropathy a. Renal biopsy 1968 b. Immunosuppressive therapy 1. 1970 azathioprine 2. 1970 prednisone c. Psychotic reaction due to prednisone
1970	#2	1982	Chronic renal failure with complications a. 1970 anemia b. 1970 easy bruisability c. 1970 cramping of extremities d. 1976 anorexia and nausea
1973	#3	1973	Tubal ligation
1975	#4 Degenerative disc disease L4-5 without nerve involvement		
6/9/78	#5	1/3/82 2/29/84	Hemodialysis a. Saphenous fistula L thigh removed
1/3/82	#6 Cadaver renal transplant	1/82	a. Acute rejection episode treated with ATG
		1982	b. Herpes simplex stomatitis
	c. Azathioprine, prednisone immunosuppression		
1985	#7 Hypercholesterolemia		
1985	#8 Hypertension		

FIGURE 2-2 Example of a master problem list that is placed at the front of the patient's record. The master problem list provides a concise overview of the patient's medical problems and serves as an index to the content of the medical record.

tory studies are best followed on a flow sheet or a graph. Judgment should be used here, just as it would be in a scientific paper. The initial plans are organized by problem and grouped into three subcomponents:

1. Diagnostic

1.1 Diagnostic workup: the plans for ruling out or confirming the various diagnostic possibilities arising from the initial assessment.

1.2 Parameters to be followed to determine the course of the disease, response to therapy, and possible side effects of treatment (e.g., frequency of vital signs, repeat laboratory studies, or repeat physical examination).

2. Therapeutic

The statement here should include planned procedures and medications, as well as a precise statement of the goals. Contingency plans in the event the initial therapeutic plan fails should be indicated.

3. Patient education

This is the information to be provided to the patient and family or partner.

Progress Notes (SOAP)

Progress notes are numbered and titled to correspond to a specific problem. Each progress note contains the four SOAP subcomponents: subjective and objective data, assessment, and plans (diagnostic and therapeutic). It is important to number and title each progress note, including the date and time, so that there is no misunderstanding the physician's thinking and when it took place. A patient may have five problems on his problem list, but on a specific day, progress notes may be written on only three of them (e.g., problems 1, 2, and 5). Because no progress has occurred in problems 3 and 4, no note is necessary. These may be stationary problems; for example, problem 3 may be low back pain caused by osteoarthritis, in which no new therapy is contemplated and the patient's condition is unchanged. Problem 4 may be cataracts (mild), for which no therapy is planned in the immediate future.

Under each of the numbered and titled progress notes, the SOAP format is used. Recording by problem the subjective and objective changes that have occurred tells the reader immediately what is happening. The assessment demonstrates the clarity of the physician's thinking about the problem, and the plans tell clearly what is to be done based on the assessment. If an imaging study is to be ordered, it tells the reader it is specific for this problem and how it will alter the assessment or lead to a therapeutic intervention. In an unstructured record, a jumble of imaging studies may be ordered, and the reader is confused as to why they were. The shotgun approach—"get every test and hope something turns up"—is not only dangerous but also very expensive. The structured problem progress notes explain why the test is being ordered and how it will affect diagnosis and therapy.

Flow Sheets

Narrative notes are inadequate for recording certain types of data. When several variables are being followed sequentially over time, the patterns of change become much more evident when the variables are organized in graphic or tabular form. The data placed on a flow sheet can include vital signs, physical findings, fluid intake and output, laboratory values, and medications (Figure 2-3). For patients with rapidly changing problems (e.g., trauma patients, patients in intensive care units, and patients undergoing cardiac resuscitation), the most valuable and sometimes the sole "progress note" is a well-constructed flow sheet. Choosing the parameters to be followed and the frequency with which they are to be followed requires judgment. The parameters to be followed should be the key indicators that would trigger a therapeutic intervention. The point of the flow sheet is to allow the pattern of changes in the important variables to emerge. Compulsive cluttering of the flow sheet with trivial details is almost as bad as omitting a critical parameter. The intervals at which the data should be obtained and recorded depend on how fast the patient's condition is changing and how fast a change in treatment might be required.

The common flow sheets on a surgical service are the vital sign sheets for respiration, blood pressure, pulse, and temperature; the anesthesia records; and the fluid balance records. Flow sheets are critical to the management of trauma patients, burn patients, patients with gastrointestinal hemorrhage, patients in intensive care units, patients receiving total parenteral nutrition, and organ transplant patients. The value of using flow sheets to follow long-term problems in outpatients should not be overlooked. Whenever a patient's problem is complex or whenever several variables are involved, the clinician should consider using a flow sheet to clarify patterns of change and to improve the likelihood that intelligent decisions will be made.

Operation Notes

Each patient undergoing surgery should have a preoperative progress note written that clearly spells out the reason for the surgery and succinctly reviews the pertinent preoperative data. Such a review should clarify the rationale for the surgery and ensure that the patient is appropriately prepared and evaluated for the planned procedure.

On the day of surgery, a brief operative note should be recorded in the written medical record. This note should include the following:

1. Preoperative diagnosis (problem that is the indication for surgery)
2. Postoperative diagnosis
3. Procedure
4. Surgeon and assistants
5. Findings at surgery
6. Complications
7. Tissues removed
8. Drains placed
9. Estimated blood loss
10. Patient's condition on leaving the operating room
11. Anesthesia used

In more complex cases, it is also beneficial for the surgeon to sketch the surgical result. This has proved valuable in our experience with complex vascular reconstructive cases and also when gastrointestinal surgery must be repeated.

In addition to the brief operative note, most surgeons dictate a formal operative note for typing later. This note includes the patient's name, date of birth, and medical record number, the date of the procedure, the surgeon and assistants, the preoperative diagnosis, the postoperative diagnosis, the procedure performed, the indications for the surgery, the findings at the time of surgery, a narrative description of the surgical procedure that gives the details of the operation, the materials used

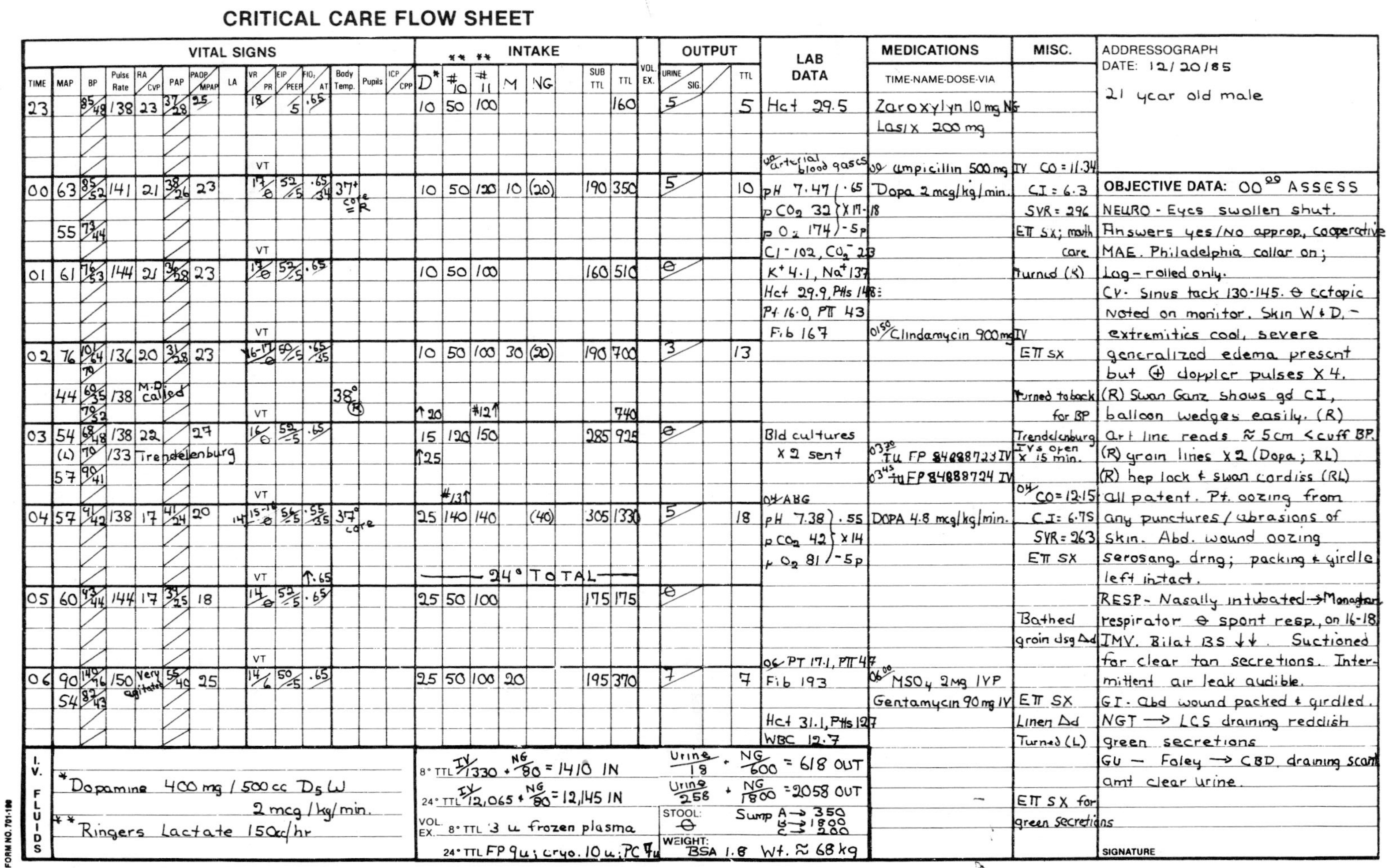

FIGURE 2-3 Flow sheet covering 8 hours in the care of a 21-year-old male who had been injured in a motor vehicle accident and had been trapped in the vehicle for 2 hours. The patient sustained a cerebral contusion, a cardiac contusion, a traction injury to the right upper extremity, and a degloving avulsion injury to the abdomen with mesenteric tear and colon perforation. Complications that developed included acute renal failure, adult respiratory distress syndrome, and a consumptive coagulopathy. The meanings of the column abbreviations are: *MAP*, mean arterial pressure; *BP*, blood pressure; *RA*, right atrial pressure; *CVP*, central venous pressure; *PAP*, pulmonary artery pressure; *PAOP*, pulmonary artery obstructive pressure; *MPAP*, mean pulmonary artery pressure; *LA*, left atrial pressure; *VR*, ventilator rate; *PR*, patient-initiated respiratory rate; *EIP*, end inspiratory pressure or delta P; *PEEP*, positive end-expiratory pressure; FiO_2, fractional inspired oxygen concentration; *AT*, airway temperature; *VT*, tidal volume; *ICP*, intracranial pressure; *CPP*, cerebral perfusion pressure; *Sub TTL*, subtotal; *TTL*, total; *Vol ex*, volume expanders; *SG*, specific gravity; *Misc*, miscellaneous.

or implanted, complications, blood loss, fluid replacement, specimens sent to the laboratory, and the patient's condition on leaving the operating room.

Discharge Summaries

The discharge summary should also be written in a problem-oriented form, and the problem sheet should be the top page of the discharge summary. Serving as an index, the problem sheet tells the physician reviewing the record exactly what the patient's problems have been in the past or are currently. The discharge note should then contain a summary of each numbered and titled problem with the minimum amount of verbiage necessary to clearly state the data base and the status of each problem at the time of discharge. Long-winded narrative summaries, which usually make up a discharge note, often are impossible to evaluate as to what has happened to the patient, what treatment is currently going on, and what the plans for the future may be. Written in the problem-oriented format, the discharge note should be perfectly clear as to where the diagnosis and treatment of each problem stand at a particular time; this enables the referring physician to make decisions on gathering more data or to change or stop the treatment regimen. The surgeon, who is so dependent on referrals, thus informs the referring colleague of exactly what took place during the hospitalization and what the status of each problem was at the time of discharge. The referring physician then has no doubt about what elements require follow up, what additional studies may be helpful over time, and what changes in therapeutic intervention may be needed during the patient's course. A flow sheet that accompanies the discharge summary is extremely important in many cases involving complex, ongoing problems.

Auditing Care of the Surgical Patient

Problem-Oriented Record in Auditing

A particular advantage of the problem-oriented record is that it allows an organized audit of medical care. The problem-oriented record forces the physician into clarity of thinking by relating each of the pieces of the data base to a specific problem and allows the plans for diagnosis and therapy to be clearly delineated. Because every test ordered and every procedure done must be related to a specific problem, the thinking of the physician writing the record becomes well defined. Organization of the records becomes the tool for teaching and learning by the physician as the record is audited later by a teacher, by the physician himself, or by peer review.

Medical education all too frequently forces a student into learning facts and making lists and tables to try to remember even more facts. The "A" student is often the one who can remember the most facts, and many teachers are guilty of teaching by showing how many facts they know. The real effort at teaching should be to see if the student or the teacher is thorough and reliable, has a sound analytic sense, and is efficient. By examining the problem-oriented record, these characteristics can be delineated. To do this, it may be necessary to periodically spot-check certain aspects of the patient's subjective and objective data to determine the treating physician's thoroughness and reliability. The formulation of the problems from the data base provides clear evidence of the analytic sense of the physician and is of major importance in patient care. Efficiency can be somewhat harder to determine, because it is related to time and function. It is difficult to tell from auditing the record whether it took an hour, a day, or a week to complete the workup, and efficiency can only be determined by indirect means. However, an aspect of efficiency is using various tests and diagnostic imaging techniques in a manner that is properly sequenced and that results in no extra time in the hospital for the patient. Too often a record shows that several tests were ordered, no thought was given to sequence, and a particular test was cancelled because another test interfered (e.g., a barium swallow examination was given before a barium enema, thus impairing a satisfactory examination by enema).

Thoroughness is also an important aspect of good medical practice. In reviewing the record, one can quickly see whether the data base contains things such as a patient profile that has been carefully done or if the system's review is complete. For example, if the patient profile reveals that a patient with peripheral vascular disease does not do any walking and has not been out of the house for months or years because of other problems, then revascularization of his legs to allow him to walk great distances is rather foolish.

Reliability is equally as important as thoroughness. Periodic spot-checks of the data base can rapidly determine the reliability of the physician who performed the test. For example, is what is written reproducible and accurate? If the material presented is not reliable, then it is important to find out whether the physician is simply careless; lacks skills in hearing, seeing, and palpating; or is dishonest. It is also possible that the physician does not relate well to patients and therefore does not obtain the proper data. If a teacher is doing the auditing, he or she should not obtain the data for the student but should stand by the student and force him to perform properly and then stay with him until the performance has been mastered. Too often this is ignored by the teacher, who is simply disgusted with what he or she has found and walks away, leaving the student to learn by himself or never to learn at all.

Finally, a sound analytic sense is perhaps the most important asset to the good practice of medicine. The data base, or at least pieces of it, can be obtained by people other than physicians, but it requires the educational background of the physician the analyze the data base and develop the problem list. Problems should always be formulated at the highest level of understanding. An audit that shows four or five problems that a more experienced physician would quickly group under one problem states very clearly the level of understanding of the physician who wrote the record. This finding simply tells the auditor that the physician needs more experience and is doing little or no reading on the subject. Any standard textbook, such as this one, would allow the student to combine the various items listed as separate problems and group them under one problem. Instead of trying to memorize patterns of disease and groups of symptoms, the student should be sent to his textbooks or the library or, in today's world, perhaps to a computer to find the answers about the multiple symptoms he has grouped as separate problems. When trained in this way, the disciplined mind will almost always remember such patterns in the future, and they will not have to be looked up each time. This method is far different from giving the student a list of diseases or syndromes and expecting him to memorize them and retain that information for something that he might not see for months or years.

Once these disciplines have been developed in the young physician, they set a lifelong pattern for writing clear records and properly using sources of knowledge such as textbooks, libraries, and computers. The patient cannot expect every physician to know all the answers to all problems. However, the patient has a right to expect the physician to be thorough and reliable, to have a sound analytic sense, and to use the patient's time and money efficiently.

ABDOMINAL PAIN

The word "pain" derives from the Latin word *poena*, meaning punishment. Managing patients with acute and chronic pain syndromes plays a prominent role in the practice of most physicians. Unfortunately, the treatment results often are compromised by the physician's unfamiliarity with the general concepts of pain perception and management and the more specific pain syndromes that should suggest specific diagnostic steps and treatment. This section discusses specific clinical approaches to patients with postoperative pain and abdominal pain resulting from acute surgical illness. The body of literature dealing with the appreciation of pain is vast, and clearly our current knowledge is rudimentary.

▪Abdominal Pain section contributed by Jack Pickleman.

Innervation of the Abdomen

The efferent innervation of the abdomen is via the autonomic nervous system (ANS), which is functionally divided into two parts, depending on the neurotransmitter released by the postganglionic fibers. The sympathetic nervous system (SNS) releases catecholamines such as norepinephrine, and the parasympathetic nervous system (PNS) releases acetylcholine. These two systems innervate the same intra-abdominal structures but in general have opposing effects (e.g., the SNS decreases motility and visceral blood flow and increases sphincter contraction, whereas the PNS opposes each of these actions). Parasympathetic fibers originate from the vagus nerves and the sacral nerve roots as the pelvic splanchnic nerves. The SNS arises only from the thoracic spinal cord. Afferent nerves from the abdominal viscera are distinct from the ANS.

Pain Receptors

Specific pain receptors are located in the abdominal viscera, mesentery, blood vessels, and parietal peritoneum. Fibers from the viscera travel to the spinal cord, closely following the ANS splanchnic nerves. Afferents from the parietal peritoneum reach the cord by way of segmental spinal nerves. All these visceral and parietal afferents enter the posterior spinal cord and may converge onto the same secondary fibers, because the number of primary afferents from the gut and skin far exceeds the number of secondary neurons.

When visceral pain fibers are stimulated, pain signals pass through some of these shared neurons, and the person feels that the sensation actually originates from the skin. This explains the phenomenon of *referred pain*, which is pain perceived at a point distant from the source of actual stimulation. For instance, diaphragmatic pain afferents follow the phrenic nerve (C3-5) to the spinal cord and converge with secondary fibers, receiving cutaneous afferents from the shoulder. This explains why a patient with diaphragmatic inflammation may complain of unilateral shoulder pain. Referred epigastric pain is associated with viscera whose afferents enter T5-8; these include the stomach, the duodenum, and the entire pancreaticobiliary system. This explains why biliary colic can "radiate" to the right scapula. Referred periumbilical pain is associated with viscera whose afferents enter T9 and T10, including the small bowel, appendix, and ovaries. Referred hypogastric pain is associated with viscera whose afferents enter T11 and T12, such as the colon, rectum, bladder, and uterus. Thus ureteral colic may yield pain in the flank that radiates to the ipsilateral testicle and thigh.[7,11] Some primary pain afferents do not synapse with ascending lateral spinothalamic tract fibers, but rather join with ANS afferents within the spinal cord. Other fibers from the spinothalamic tracts may give off collaterals in the brain stem that go to the hypothalamus, limbic system, and frontal cortex; these centers may in turn stimulate the ANS. These pathways explain why visceral reflexes frequently accompany abdominal pain. Severe visceral or somatic pain may lead to a secondary ANS outpouring, with diaphoresis, changes in pulse and blood pressure, and nausea and vomiting.

The gastrointestinal (GI) tract contains numerous pain receptors that for simplicity's sake may be subdivided; however, the actual anatomic paths may be similar. Mucosal receptors lie in or just below the GI tract epithelium and may respond to various chemical and mechanical stimuli. Acid and alkaline solutions and nonisotonic solutions may stimulate these receptors. Therefore these receptors serve as sensors of the texture, acidity, and osmolality of GI tract contents.

A second kind of GI pain receptor is the tension receptor of visceral muscle layers. This receptor discharges during both gut contraction and passive distention of the lumen and may be viewed as a sensor of the degree of filling of a viscus and of the effectiveness of a contraction of the viscus in propelling bowel contents. Serosal receptors under the serosa or in the adjacent mesentery are mechanical receptors and may monitor visceral fullness.[9]

Hence visceral pain sensations can be produced by four conditions: (1) irritation of the mucosa or serosa; (2) traction on the mesentery; (3) distention of a viscus; and (4) forceful contraction of a viscus. The vagueness of visceral pain is attributed to the convergence of visceral afferent input into the central nervous system (CNS). In an apparent attempt at economy, each receptor type is activated by a variety of visceral stimuli, leading to confusion in perception of each form of stimulation. However, somatic abdominal pain is transmitted by those fibers whose receptors lie in the parietal peritoneum, the root of the mesentery, and the abdominal wall. When such nerves are stimulated, the patient complains of a sharper, well-localized pain, often aggravated by deep breathing, coughing, movement, or palpation.

Causes of Pain

Because numerous disorders can cause abdominal pain, it is fruitless to attempt to memorize salient points for each disease. Instead, the physician should take a general approach to a patient with abdominal pain, recognizing the virtually endless list of both intra-abdominal and extra-abdominal processes that may cause pain and the unique characteristics of visceral and somatic pain. A list of the more common intraperitoneal causes of abdominal pain is given in the left-hand box on p. 31, and a list of predominantly nonsurgical problems that may mimic acute surgical conditions is presented in the right-hand box on p. 31.

Approach to the Patient with Acute Abdominal Pain

One of the most common problems a general surgeon confronts is a patient with acute or chronic abdominal pain. If the surgeon takes a reasoned, orderly approach to the history, physical examination, and interpretation of laboratory tests and radiographs, most patients can be accurately assessed and treated. Failure to approach these cases logically may lead to three outcomes, all adverse: (1) failure to operate on a patient with a genuine surgical condition; (2) an ill-timed operation, performed either too soon, before volume resuscitation is complete, or too late, after peritonitis and sepsis have become established; and (3) an operation performed through a poorly chosen incision because of either initial misdiagnosis or failure to consider other reasonable diagnoses. Common intra-abdominal and extra-abdominal causes of pain are presented in the boxes on p. 31.

History

It is best to let the patient give his entire current history before asking specific questions. With patience, the whole story may be revealed with minimum input from the examiner. The past medical history and information concerning associated illnesses such as cardiovascular disease, hypertension, diabetes, and bleeding disorders should be elicited. A history of previous similar symptoms should be specifically sought, as should the presence of any prodromal symptoms.

The exact sequence of symptoms is critical. For instance, a patient with appendicitis may have both nausea and abdominal pain at the time of presentation, but the former symptom rarely precedes the latter. The examiner should ascertain whether the pain began gradually or suddenly and whether the maximum pain occurred immediately. The examiner should also ask the patient which actions bring on the pain or alleviate it.

The location and changes in location of the pain are obviously important, but when questioning the patient, the examiner should remember that early visceral pain is sensed vaguely and parallels the embryologic origin of the affected organ; that is, pain in organs derived from the foregut is perceived as epigastric pain; pain in organs derived from the midgut manifests as periumbilical pain; and pain in organs derived from the hindgut is felt as lower abdominal pain. Somatic pain is accurately perceived in the area of parietal peritoneal involvement.

The character of the pain should be determined. Colic is intermittent and crampy and occurs in waves associated with obstruction of the biliary, urinary, or intestinal tract. The pain of acute cholecystitis may be described as upper abdominal pain or chest pressure, sometimes mimicking a myocardial infarction. The severity of the pain is obviously a reflection not only of the

INTRA-ABDOMINAL CAUSES OF ACUTE PAIN

Inflammation
Peritonitis
- Primary
- Perforated viscus (stomach, small intestine, or colon)

Hepatitis
Cholecystitis
Pancreatitis
Regional enteritis
Colitis (ischemic, ulcerative, Crohn's, amebic)
Appendicitis
Diverticulitis
Intra-abdominal abscess

Mechanical Obstruction
Small-bowel obstruction
Large-bowel obstruction
Biliary colic
Renal colic

Hemorrhage
Intraperitoneal bleeding
- Ruptured liver
- Ruptured spleen
- Ruptured abdominal aortic aneurysm

Ischemia
Mesenteric occlusion
Omental infarction

Gynecologic Factors
Ovarian cyst (rupture, twisting)
Degenerated fibroid
Ectopic pregnancy
Endometriosis
Pelvic inflammatory disease

Urinary Tract
Nephritis
Pyelitis
Perinephric abscess
Prostatitis

pathologic process but also of the patient's pain threshold and emotional response. Colicky pain or ischemic pain of the intestines generally is perceived as more severe than inflammatory pain; likewise, chemical peritonitis secondary to a perforated duodenal ulcer often is more severe than fecal peritonitis from a ruptured appendix or colonic diverticulitis.

If vomiting is a symptom, it is important to note the frequency and character of the vomitus; likewise, the patient should be asked about recent passage of urine, stool, or flatus. In girls and women, an exact menstrual history must be obtained, because this may be the only clue to gynecologic pathologic process, such as ectopic pregnancy.

EXTRA-ABDOMINAL CAUSES OF ACUTE PAIN

Cardiopulmonary
Myocardial infarction
Pneumonia
Empyema

Neurogenic
Spinal cord tumor
Spinal nerve root compression
Herpes zoster
Abdominal epilepsy

Metabolic
Uremia
Diabetic ketoacidosis
Porphyria
Adrenal insufficiency

Toxic
Insect bites
Venoms
Drugs
Lead poisoning

Miscellaneous
Rectus sheath hematoma
Sickle cell crisis

Physical Examination

Examination of the abdomen should begin with auscultation for bowel sounds. Although many acute abdominal conditions may lead to a partial ileus with decreased sounds, patients with bowel obstruction have hyperactive sounds that point to the diagnosis. After auscultation, all quadrants of the abdomen should be gently palpated. Nothing is less productive than a hurried trial of initial deep palpation, yielding pain and guarding, so that any subsequent examinations are compromised by the patient's inability to relax and cooperate. Evidence of peritoneal irritation is manifested even on gentle palpation, but after this, deeper palpation should be attempted; this will also define the presence of localized or generalized peritonitis and identify any masses present. Evidence of peritoneal irritation should be sought next. The usual method of deep palpation followed by rapid release (rebound tenderness) should be discouraged, because it causes pain even in patients without peritonitis and it is not a reproducible test. A far more accurate test is gentle shaking of the patient's torso back and forth laterally by holding the hips. This causes inflamed peritoneal surfaces to rub on one another, yielding specific somatic pain. A rectal or pelvic examination completes the assessment and should never be omitted.[6]

Laboratory Tests and Diagnosis

Laboratory tests may provide helpful information. A complete blood count, urinalysis, serum amylase test and, in women, a beta-subunit human chorionic gonadotropin (HCG) test should be performed, along with other studies as specifically indicated. The serum amylase test is nonspecific; the serum amylase level is elevated in a small percentage of nearly all acute abdominal conditions. Therefore, although elevation of this enzyme remains the cornerstone of the diagnosis of acute pancreatitis, elevations must be interpreted cautiously. In straightforward presentations, patients with entities such as acute appendicitis or cholecystitis should not receive abdominal radiographs, because these are wasteful and only rarely yield clinically significant information. However, if other conditions are suspected or in obscure situations, four radiographic views of the abdomen are mandatory. Likewise, abdominal paracentesis has no role in the assessment of patients with acute abdominal pain, except for patients with ascites from any cause who have acute abdominal pain. In this case, an elevated white blood cell count in the peritoneal fluid may be the only indication of an infectious process in the peritoneal cavity.

Depending on the urgency of the clinical situation, additional tests may be required to secure a diagnosis. The box at right lists tests that may be useful in evaluating a patient with abdominal pain. Some general rules concerning their use should be noted:

1. No test should be performed unless its result will alter the need for additional tests or treatment. For example, in a patient with the clinical diagnosis of acute appendicitis, if an abdominal radiographic examination is performed and discloses or fails to disclose an appendiceal fecalith, the patient still requires surgery. Therefore this test is not indicated.
2. Tests should not duplicate results already obtained. For example, a patient with jaundice who has a pancreatic mass defined by abdominal ultrasound does not also require an abdominal computed tomography (CT) scan to delineate the same mass.
3. The "Mount Everest syndrome" should be avoided. This involves performing a test just because the facilities to do it are available. For example, if a patient is jaundiced and gallstones have been demonstrated on abdominal ultrasound, performing a percutaneous transhepatic cholangiogram will demonstrate the common duct stones but will not alter the need for surgery.
4. When the physician is choosing between various tests, a balance should be sought, including considerations of cost, diagnostic yield and relative accuracy, and potential morbidity. For example, if a patient has painless jaundice, and carcinoma of the pancreas is suspected, an upper gastrointestinal (GI) radiograph, although inexpensive and safe, is unlikely to help make the diagnosis. Something more expensive (abdominal CT scan) or more invasive (endoscopic retrograde cholangiopancreatography [ERCP]) is required.

LABORATORY TESTS

Blood Tests
Complete blood count
Liver function tests
- Albumin
- Prothrombin time
- Serum glutamic-oxaloacetic transaminase (SGOT)
- Serum glutamic-pyruvic transaminase (SGPT)
- Alkaline phosphatase
- Bilirubin

Amylase
Culture and sensitivity

Urine Tests
Urinalysis
Culture and sensitivity
Amylase
Human chorionic gonadotropin (HCG)

Imaging
Four views of the abdomen
- Supine abdomen
- Upright abdomen
- Left lateral decubitus
- Upright chest

Upper GI
Barium enema
Oral cholecystogram
Intravenous pyelogram (IVP)
Abdominal ultrasound
Abdominal computed tomography (CT) scan
Percutaneous transhepatic cholangiogram (PTC)
Endoscopic retrograde cholangiopancreatography (ERCP)

Nuclear Medicine Tests
Liver/spleen scan
Biliary excretion scan (BIDA, HIDA, PIPIDA)
Gallium scan

Miscellaneous Tests
Abdominal paracentesis
Laparoscopy

The specific diagnostic workup of patients suspected to have one of the conditions listed in Chapter 36 is beyond the scope of this chapter. However a careful clinical evaluation followed by the approach just outlined should lead to a quickly made, inexpensive, and accurate diagnosis in most cases.

The treatment of acute abdominal pain is based on the fact that the pain is a symptom and not a diagnosis.

Appropriate treatment is control of the underlying process. To treat abdominal pain with analgesics without diagnosing and resolving the primary intra-abdominal pathologic condition may be a disservice to the patient.

Managing Postoperative Abdominal Pain

Studies have shown that many patients may fear an operation more for the potential pain than for the risks involved. The relief of pain, of utmost concern to the patient, is poorly handled on most surgical services, and numerous studies have documented inadequate pain relief for most postoperative patients. This phenomenon is hard to understand, because it is generally agreed that even the most severe pain can be managed well by appropriate use of narcotics. Excessive postoperative pain may result in a decrease in ambulation, pulmonary toilet, and other activities important to the patient's recovery.

What are the reasons for this suboptimal use of pain medications? One is the somewhat irrational fear of side effects, including respiratory depression, drowsiness, urinary retention, and constipation. In reality, far fewer than 1% of all postoperative patients who receive narcotics develop any symptoms of respiratory depression; thus this problem is obviously of minor import. If respiratory depression does occur, a rapidly effective antidote (naloxone) is available. The fear of turning a previously functional patient into a drug addict is another concern that is constantly reiterated. Actually, it is extremely rare for such a progression to take place (affecting less than 1 patient in 1000, according to some studies).[4] No study yet has shown that adequate hospital pain relief leads to addiction; if physical dependency occurs, withdrawal is easily accomplished once the pain is no longer present. Despite this, pain medications continue to be given sparingly, much to the chagrin of most patients.[4]

Usual analgesic orders specify a dose range to be given at prescribed intervals on an as-needed basis. This places the burden on the patient, who may not wish to be a nuisance to the staff or who may make frequent demands, leading to the conclusion that he is emotionally labile or neurotic. Nurses share the strange belief that addiction is a potential sequela of narcotic administration and are therefore likely to pressure patients to "tough it out" and wait as long as possible before the next dose.

A number of facts concerning narcotic use and postoperative pain relief should be understood by all physicians. First, many physicians believe the duration of action for all narcotics is the same. In fact, the equianalgesic peak effect of meperidine (Demerol) is only 3 hours; therefore if administration every 6 hours is prescribed, the patient may receive no effective analgesia as much as half the time. The same is true for morphine. Alternately, levorphanol (Levo-Dromoran) has a longer half-life; if it is ordered every 3 hours, serum levels may be excessive, leading to side effects.

Second, it is important to consider the route of administration. Intravenous administration produces a rapid peak effect but no sustained relief; therefore intramuscular administration is the preferred route for postoperative patients who are not receiving oral intake. The site of intramuscular injection is important. Using the deltoid muscle, because of greater blood flow and less adipose tissue, leads to better pain relief than using the gluteal site, especially if the patient is female, obese, or elderly with increased fat in the latter region.

Third, oral administration of analgesics should begin as soon as possible. This obviously eases some of the burden on the patient and nursing staff and can provide sustained pain relief. However, because most narcotics are rapidly metabolized in the liver, dosages of these drugs must be significantly increased if equianalgesic doses are to be provided. For instance, 400 mg of oral meperidine gives roughly the same analgesic effect as 100 mg given intramuscularly. Hydromorphone (Dilaudid), methadone (Dolophine), and levorphanol (Levo-Dromoran) are the preferred narcotics for oral use.

Finally, all narcotics are equally effective in relieving pain when given in equianalgesic doses. Therefore merely changing a drug because of inadequate pain relief without increasing the effective dose makes no sense.[10]

Recognizing the mechanism of action of narcotics can lead to more rational use of these drugs. The primary action of opioids is to increase the tolerance of perceived pain; patients are still aware of the pain, but the experience is not as disturbing. This change in pain perception is most effective before the pain recurs or reaches severe intensity. Thus the patient should not be encouraged to endure the pain and wait longer; instead, the dose and frequency should be increased to maintain sufficient plasma levels at all times. One recent attempt to optimize patient analgesia makes use of a patient-controlled mechanical device that delivers small doses of intravenous narcotics via a switch controlled by the patient. Most studies involving this apparatus have noted increased pain relief and a decreased total dose of narcotic used. Expense is clearly a drawback, but if a value is put on nursing time, this device may yet prove cost effective.[5]

Delivery of Optimal Postoperative Pain Control

How is it possible to bring about optimal postoperative pain control in a hospital setting? First, the as-needed routine should be abolished as unduly punishing and inconsistent with the fact that it requires less narcotic to prevent pain than to treat it. Similarly, a fixed drug administration schedule is not practical because of the wide differences in analgesic requirements, which would lead to both overtreatment and undertreatment.

We suggest that an as-needed order be written that specifies a range of narcotic doses. The patient could then be asked at 2-hour intervals whether he requires any analgesic and whether he needs a relatively small or large dose. With this regimen it is likely that less total narcotic would be administered; pain control would be optimized; and the patient would never have to suffer needlessly while waiting for the next dose. Clearly such an approach would meet with initial resistance from nurses, hospital staff, and attending physicians, to whom many of these concepts are foreign. But with increased awareness of the mechanisms of pain and the pharmacology of analgesic drugs, a more rational and effective approach to postoperative pain is possible.

TEMPERATURE ALTERATION

As an isolated clinical problem, temperature change usually is not the primary reason for initial surgical evaluation or treatment. For instance, fever alone leads to surgical diagnostic-therapeutic interventions only rarely, such as with fever of unknown origin. However, even in this circumstance surgical exploration is recommended only after exhaustive investigation strongly suggests that the disease process is located in the abdomen.*

After surgery, temperature changes, particularly fever, are common and often are the major clinical indication of a postoperative complication. For this reason expertise in temperature evaluation is critical to good surgical practice. In this setting a temperature change may lead to surgical intervention as a diagnostic or therapeutic procedure.

This chapter reviews the physiology of temperature changes and presents a schema for assessing these changes, particularly fever, in the postoperative period.

Physiology of Temperature Regulation

Modern Concepts

The modern understanding of temperature regulation dates primarily from the demonstration of endogenous pyrogen by Bennett and Beeson in 1948.[14,100,113] Significant progress has been made in characterizing endogenous pyrogen and its effects on the hypothalamus.

Temperature is regulated by a cluster of thermoregulatory neurons near the floor of the third ventricle in the preoptic area of the hypothalamus. The thermoregulatory center establishes the *set point* for body temperature. Normally this set point allows for a diurnal variation in temperature, with a peak at about 6 PM. The time and magnitude of the peak are constant findings in each person. Ninety-eight percent of normal people have a temperature range of 36.2° to 37.5° C (97° to 99.9° F).[24,40,92]

Body temperature depends on the difference between heat production and heat loss. Normally, approximately 2400 kcal of heat is produced per day. Heat production is increased by exercise, shivering, catecholamines, and thyroxin. Heat is a product of metabolism, primarily in skeletal muscle and the liver. When increased heat production is required, skeletal muscle responds, producing shivering.[92]

Heat loss occurs through four mechanisms. The first, radiation, is dependent on the temperature difference between the skin and surroundings. Under normal circumstances about 60% of heat loss is due to radiation. The second mechanism is evaporative loss, which occurs secondary to insensible perspiration. Normally approximately 25% of heat loss is due to this mechanism. Through increased perspiration, evaporation is the mechanism most responsive to a need for acute heat loss. The third mechanism, convection, results in heat loss as air passes over a surface, the method by which a fan helps cool the body. The fourth mechanism, conduction, results in heat loss through direct contact with a cooler object, such as being immersed in cold water or being placed on a cooling blanket.[92]

The causes of temperature change may be grouped into three broad categories: (1) disruption of hypothalamic function, (2) excessive exposure to environmental cold or heat, and (3) resetting of the hypothalamic set point.

Hypothalamic dysfunction may be caused by direct trauma to the hypothalamus, such as hemorrhage or compression. This usually results in elevated body temperature and is seen most frequently after head trauma or neurosurgical procedures.[80,92]

General anesthesia may also cause hypothalamic dysfunction. When anesthesia is accompanied by muscular paralysis, inhalation of cool gases, administration of room-temperature intravenous fluids or cool blood, evaporative loss with an open thoracic or abdominal cavity, and irrigation of pleural or peritoneal surfaces with room-temperature solutions, hypothermia frequently follows.[92,105]

Excessive environmental exposure is the mechanism of fever in heatstroke, in which heat loss mechanisms are unable to produce adequate body cooling.[92]

Temperature change in surgical patients most commonly results from resetting of the hypothalamic thermoregulatory set point to a higher level, frequently as a result of production of endogenous pyrogen.[92] As mentioned previously, endotoxin is the exogenous pyrogen responsible for fever from some bacterial injections. After approximately 90 minutes, endotoxin injection in humans results in increased oxygen consumption, which precedes elevation in body temperature. In contrast, en-

*References 45, 54, 63, 67, and 94.

■Temperature Alteration section contributed by Kenneth W. Burchard.

dogenous pyrogen produces fever almost immediately when injected into the carotid artery in experimental animals.[41] Endogenous pyrogen is a similar, if not the same, molecule as lymphocyte-activating factor (interleukin-1), which has been shown to be a factor in host defense.[41,93] Although demonstrated previously only in animal models, interleukin-1-leukocyte pyrogen recently has been demonstrated in humans during fever.[23]

Endogenous pyrogen (interleukin-1) is released in humans from neutrophils, monocytes, eosinophils, tissue from patients with Hodgkin's disease, Kupffer's cells, splenic sinusoidal cells, alveolar macrophages, and cells lining the peritoneum. Substances that cause human leukocytes to release endogenous pyrogen are bacteria, yeast, endotoxin, and etiocholanolone (a steroid). The release of endogenous pyrogen requires the synthesis of new messenger ribonucleic acid (mRNA) and protein. Endogenous pyrogen is a small protein with an approximate molecular weight of 15,000 daltons and is not species specific.*

Endogenous pyrogen may affect the thermoregulatory center set point by acting through other molecules. In primates, serotonin produces an increase in the thermoregulatory set point, and norepinephrine produces a decrease. Prostaglandins of the E series have been shown to cause fever when injected into the hypothalamus of cats and rabbits.[41,46,82]

Endogenous pyrogen has been shown to induce the synthesis of prostaglandins in the hypothalamus. Prostaglandin may be the central transmitter that initiates fever. It is interesting that antipyretics such as salicylates and acetaminophen interfere with the synthesis of prostaglandins. Cyclic adenosine monophosphate (cAMP) also has been shown to cause fever when injected into the hypothalamus. Endogenous pyrogens may stimulate the synthesis of prostaglandins, which subsequently increases cAMP to reset the thermoregulatory center. Antipyretics do not affect fever induced by prostaglandins or cAMP.†

Treating Elevated Temperature

The therapy for elevated body temperature begins with enhancing heat loss. Lowering the room temperature increases radiation loss. Applying volatile solutions to the skin, such as a tepid mixture of water and alcohol, increases evaporative loss. Convection may be increased by increasing air movement. Conductive heat loss may be increased by placing the patient in contact with a cool object, such as a cooling blanket. For patients using a respirator, cooling the temperature of inhaled gases is an effective way of reducing body temperature.[92] The second major therapeutic maneuver is to reset the thermoregulatory center. This is done by administering salicylates or acetaminophen, which interfere with prostaglandin synthesis.[78]

*References 14, 24, 31, 40, and 59.

†References 24, 33, 41, 46, and 82.

Treating Lowered Temperature

The therapy for lowered body temperature begins with reducing heat loss. Raising the room temperature and covering the patient with blankets reduces evaporative heat loss. Heat may be transmitted to the patient by warming blankets and by warming intravenous solutions and inhaled gases to body temperature. Patients who have hypothermia and severe vasoconstriction may develop hypertension despite significant hypovolemia. As rewarming takes place, subsequent vasodilatation may result in precipitous hypotension. Therefore intravascular volume resuscitation of patients with hypovolemia and hypothermia must be pursued as aggressively as rewarming.

Measuring Temperature

Several studies have evaluated temperature measurement in humans with normothermia. Rectal temperature has been found to be significantly greater than temperatures measured in the esophagus, the right side of the heart, and the oral cavity. This difference may be accentuated in febrile states, in which the rectal temperature may be as much as 0.2° C (1.4° F) higher than that of the right side of the heart.[43,84] However, for routine clinical evaluation, rectal temperature remains the most practical determinant of core body temperature.

Assessment of Postoperative Temperature Changes

Because temperature change, particularly fever, is a common postoperative problem, it is often the initial stimulus for careful assessment of the patient. This section describes a method of assessing primarily postoperative fever at various times after surgery. A method of evaluating postoperative hypothermia is presented later. In Figures 2-4 to 2-10, temperature change is the entry point in surgical decision making. Before physicians examine a patient after surgery, they and other medical personnel have certain preconceived notions about the most common causes of temperature change at that time. In Figures 2-4 through 2-10, these are listed under Most Common Cause. For instance, even a beginning surgical clerk should understand that fever after a cholecystectomy would not likely be caused by meningitis. A history and physical examination are done that allow the clinician to determine the most likely cause or causes. Laboratory tests are then used to confirm or refute a diagnosis or diagnoses, and appropriate therapy follows. This process avoids the expensive, "shotgun" method of approaching postoperative temperature change.[49]

The following text provides information about the most common causes of temperature elevation and

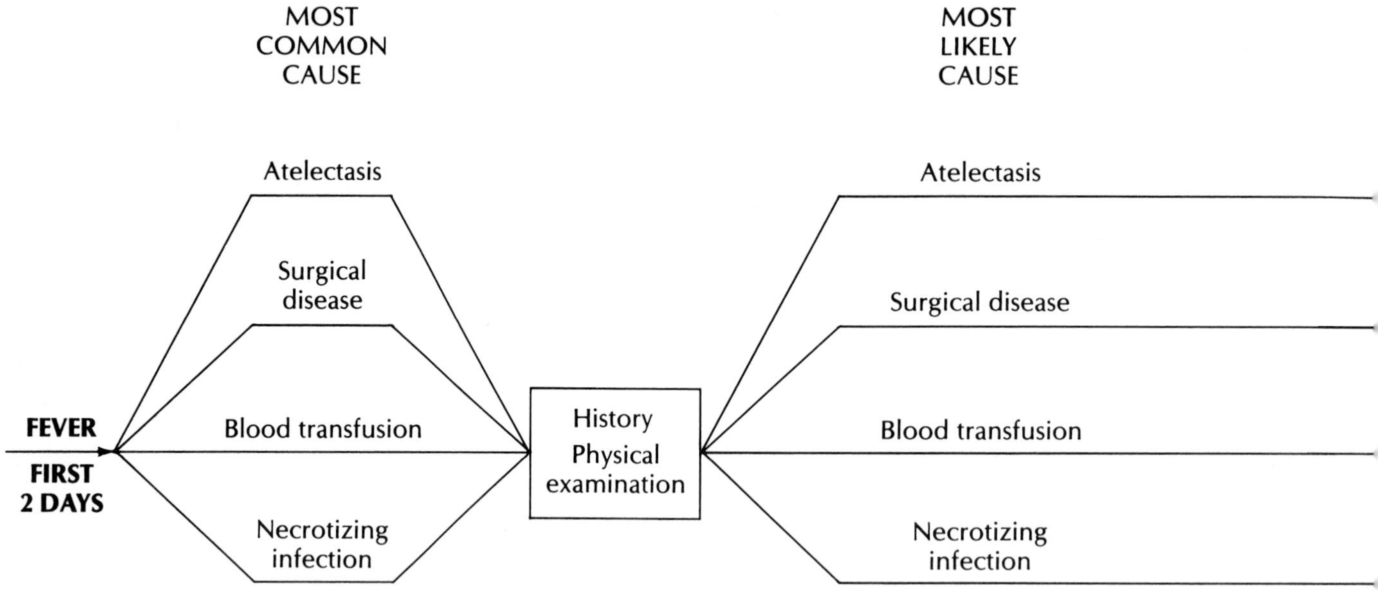

FIGURE 2-4 Evaluation of temperature changes during or immediately after surgery. *ICP,* Intracranial pressure; *CXR,* chest radiograph; *ABG,* arterial blood gases; *Hgb,* hemoglobin level; K^+, potassium level; *CPK,* creatine phosphokinase.

depression during the various time periods after surgery. Because some causes may overlap during the various time periods, the most detailed discussion is presented when the particular cause is most likely to be the origin of postoperative temperature elevation. The textual material and algorithms are designed to promote a sequential, logical approach to evaluation of postoperative temperature changes.

Fever during or Immediately after Surgery

Fever during surgery or in the immediate postoperative period (Figure 2-4) most commonly occurs secondary to the surgical disease itself or to atelectasis, blood transfusion, or malignant hyperthermia.

SURGICAL DISEASE. When a patient is operated on for a disease that is accompanied by bacteria, such as perforated diverticulitis or drainage of an intra-abdominal abscess, the remaining pyrogens may produce an elevated temperature both during surgery and shortly thereafter. This is particularly true if a large infected cavity has been manipulated, with subsequent transient bacteremias or transient release of pyrogen into the circulation. Otherwise, operations that do not involve microbiologic organisms are unlikely to produce an elevated temperature, except for neurosurgical procedures in which hypothalamic dysfunction may develop.[92]

Knowledge of the patient's condition before surgery (particularly if the patient were suffering from severe sepsis) or knowledge of infection at the time of surgery would provide the historical information supporting the diagnosis of surgical disease as a determinant of fever during surgery or in the immediate postoperative period. Knowledge of the nature of a neurosurgical procedure that might interfere with hypothalamic function would also support the role of surgical disease and procedure as contributing to temperature elevation.

Physical findings that would support the diagnosis of continuing infection in the immediate postoperative period include hypotension, tachycardia, obtunded mental status, and vasoconstriction. With lesser degrees of sepsis, mild hypotension with warm extremities would be most consistent with continuing infection. With CNS surgery, physical findings demonstrating global or focal neurologic dysfunction would support the possibility of hypothalamic dysfunction.

The laboratory test that would support the likelihood of significant ongoing infection is Gram's stain confirmation of the presence of bacteria or fungi at surgery. The diagnosis of hypothalamic dysfunction with hyperthermia after CNS surgery would be supported by a finding of increased intracranial pressure or by laboratory tests confirming the diagnosis of diabetes insipidus—a large urine volume with low osmolarity and a rising serum osmolarity.[16,76] In addition, a computed tomography (CT) scan of the head might demonstrate a significant intracranial pathologic process.

At this point the therapy for elevated temperature caused by an infection, presuming adequate surgical drainage, comprises resuscitation and antibiotics. However, if evidence of severe septic shock persists (i.e., hy-

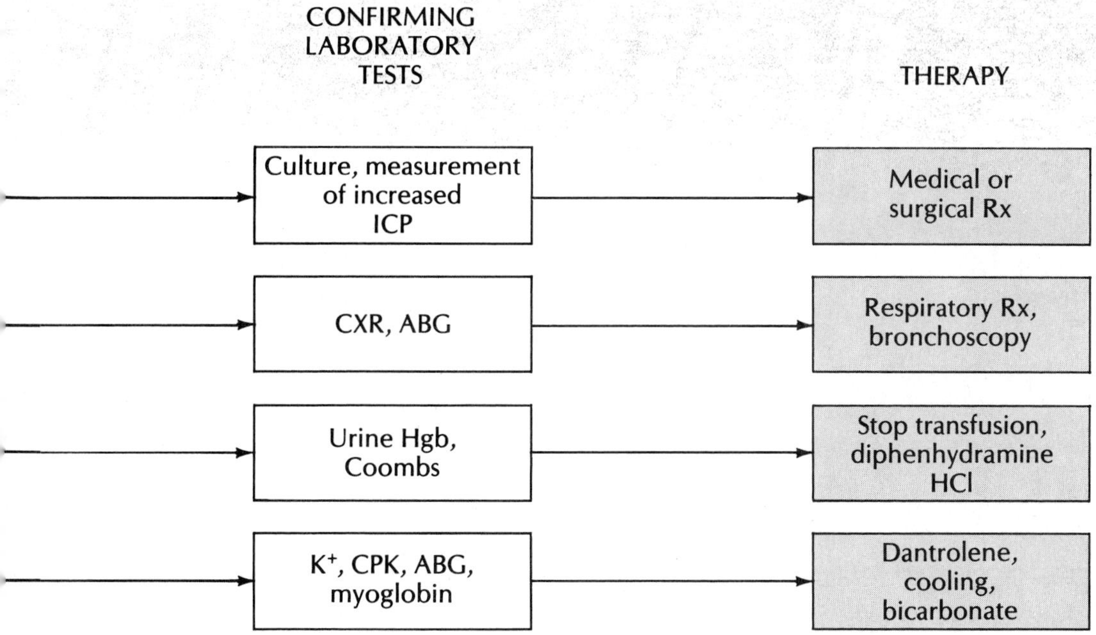

potension, tachycardia, vasoconstriction, mental confusion, acidosis, or oliguria), the possibility of inadequate surgical intervention must be considered. Proper therapy in this context might require further surgery. After CNS surgery, unless a CT scan shows evidence of a surgically correctable problem, the usual therapy is to reduce intracranial pressure, through such measures as hyperventilation to a partial pressure of carbon dioxide (P_{CO_2}) of approximately 25 mm Hg and administration of an osmotic diuretic such as mannitol.[58,80]

ATELECTASIS. Atelectasis usually does not cause the temperature to rise during or immediately after surgery. However, atelectasis usually begins during surgery and must be considered. This is particularly true for a collapsed major section of lung resulting from intubation of the right or left main bronchus. A history of general anesthesia with endotracheal intubation is enough to raise the suspicion of atelectasis. With major atelectasis, physical examination would demonstrate diminished breath sounds in the atelectatic area, along with tracheal deviation toward the atelectatic area. The confirming laboratory test is a chest radiograph. Therapy involves moving the endotracheal tube into the trachea and may require bronchoscopy. Atelectasis in the period 24 to 48 hours after surgery is discussed further in the section Fever During the First 2 Days After Surgery.

BLOOD TRANSFUSION. Febrile reactions to blood transfusions most commonly occur secondary to antibodies against transfused leukocytes. When awake, the patient usually feels cold approximately 30 minutes after the blood transfusion is started, and elevated temperature appears 30 to 60 minutes later. This temperature elevation usually does not indicate red cell incompatibility. In rare cases bacterial pyrogens in the blood transfusion may cause fever.[83]

A history of temperature elevation developing during a blood transfusion or shortly thereafter without other history or physical evidence would support the suspicion of blood transfusion as the cause. The usual febrile reactions to blood transfusions do not cause abnormalities in laboratory test results. Only red cell incompatibility would be expected to produce an elevation in urine hemoglobin or a positive result on the Coombs' test. The treatment for fever from a blood transfusion is to stop the transfusion and administer aspirin.[83]

MALIGNANT HYPERTHERMIA. Malignant hyperthermia is a rare phenomenon with an incidence of 1 in 15,000 administrations of a general anesthetic in children and 1 in 50,000 to 100,000 in adults. It is more commonly associated with administration of halogenated inhalation anesthetics and the depolarizing muscle relaxant succinylcholine. There appears to be a genetic susceptibility.[85] With malignant hyperthermia, physical examination reveals severe hyperthermia, tachycardia, arrhythmias, and muscle rigidity. Laboratory test results show severe metabolic acidosis and elevated levels of serum potassium, urine myoglobin, and serum creatine phosphokinase (CPK). Metabolic acidosis and hyperkalemia associated with muscle rigidity and hyperthermia should lead to therapy. Malignant hyperthermia is

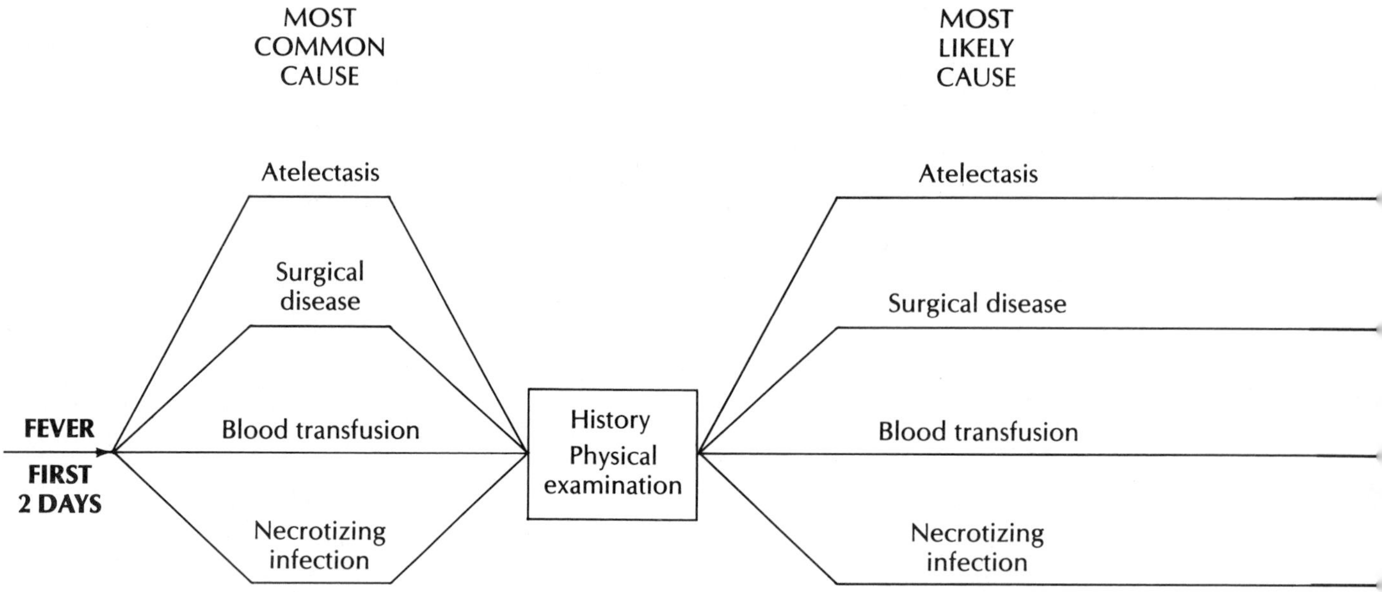

FIGURE 2-5 Evaluation of temperature changes during first 2 days after surgery. *CXR,* Chest radiograph; *ABG,* arterial blood gases; *ICP,* intracranial pressure.

best treated with dantrolene, a skeletal muscle relaxant. In addition, aggressive body cooling, with instillation of cold solutions in the abdominal cavity or using a cooling blanket, is recommended. Anesthetics must be stopped. Bicarbonate is used to treat severe metabolic acidosis. Arrhythmias are treated with standard medications. Brisk diuresis should be induced using volume loading and osmotic diuretics to prevent damage from myoglobin.[70,85]

Fever during the First 2 Days after Surgery

During the first 2 days after surgery (Figure 2-5), the most common causes of fever are atelectasis, blood transfusion, necrotizing infections, and continuation of the surgical disease.

ATELECTASIS. Atelectasis is the most common cause of fever in the first 2 days after surgery.[19,21,77,110] Although intubation of a main bronchus may result in major lobar collapse or collapse of the entire lung, the most common cause of atelectasis is hypoventilation both during surgery and in the immediate postoperative period. After surgery, hypoventilation occurs secondary to splinting from pain and the use of narcotic analgesics. Significant atelectasis is most likely to follow thoracic or upper abdominal incisions and is most common in patients with poor pulmonary mechanics before surgery.[19,77,101]

The cause of atelectasis-induced fever is uncertain. In 1963 bacteria were considered the most likely cause.[73] However, currently the cause is not well defined. It is interesting that interleukin-1, an endogenous pyrogen, has been shown to be produced by alveolar macrophages.[41,71] One might speculate that atelectasis leads to production of interleukin-1 by aleveolar macrophages.

A history of having undergone an operation under general anesthesia, particularly with a thoracic or abdominal incision, should alert the clinician to the possibility of atelectasis as a cause of fever. On physical examination, minor atelectasis commonly produces rales at the lung bases. However, significant atelectasis manifests physical findings consistent with consolidation—dullness to percussion, tubulovesicular or tubular breath sounds, and egophony.[77] Although physical findings consistent with consolidation might be considered evidence of pneumonia, without a significant episode of aspiration, it would be unusual for a surgical patient to develop pneumonitis as a cause of consolidation in the first 2 days after surgery.

Atelectasis most commonly is diagnosed by history and physical examination, and no further investigation is warranted. When confirmation is needed, a chest radiograph may reveal various degrees of atelectasis, from segmental to complete collapse of a lobe or lung.[48,77] Atelectasis produces an increase in intrapulmonary shunt and thereby a decrease in the partial pressure of oxygen (PO_2), which may be confirmed by blood gas studies.[77,100]

Because atelectasis most commonly results from hypoventilation, the most effective therapy for atelectasis is physiologic expansion of the lung with negative pressure and incentive spirometry.[20,77] In some cases more aggressive respiratory therapy with suctioning, chest percussion, or bronchoscopy may be required. Only

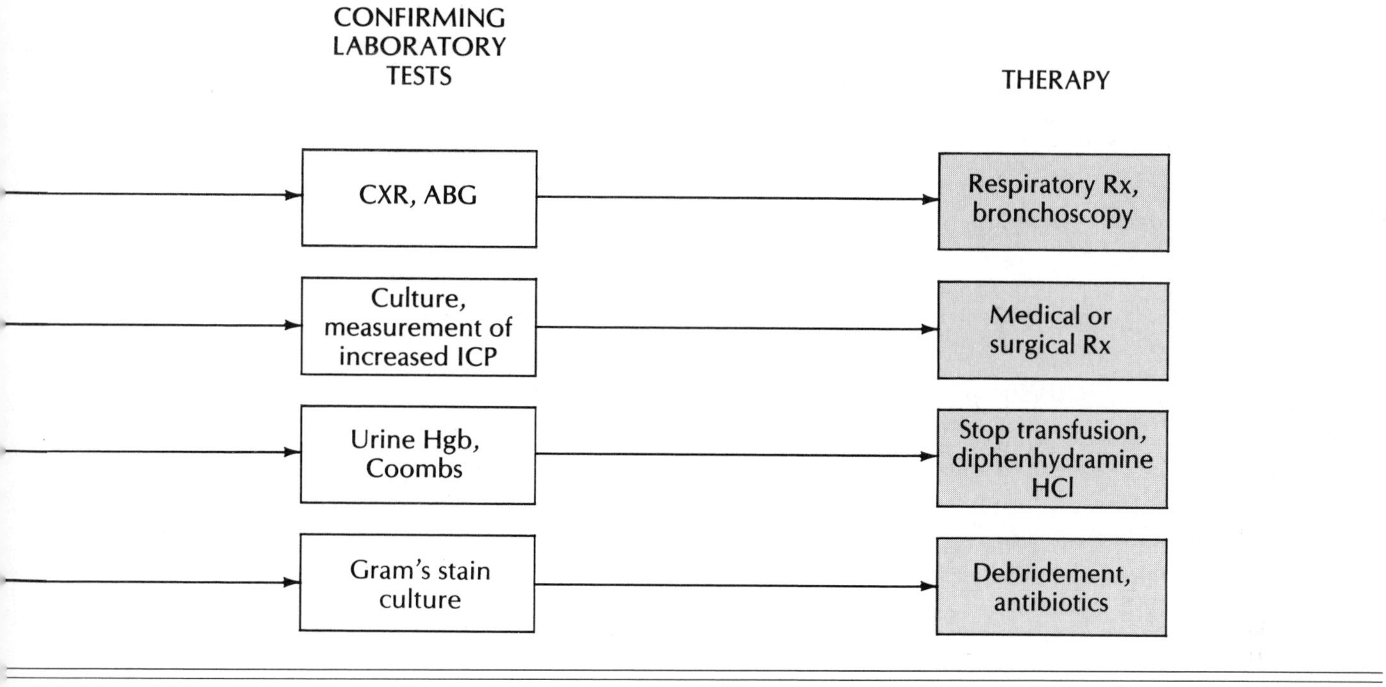

rarely are endotracheal intubation and ventilator support required as primary treatment for atelectasis.[77]

NECROTIZING WOUND INFECTIONS. Although it is rare, necrotizing wound infections may declare themselves within the first 2 days after surgery. The elevated temperatures associated with atelectasis and blood transfusion are not commonly associated with marked clinical toxicity, as evidenced by sustained tachycardia, marked respiratory distress, and obtunded mental status. On the other hand, necrotizing wound infection that develops secondary to virulent bacterial invasion produces severe toxicity. Necrotizing wound infections most commonly occur after operations on the gastrointestinal tract. Although classically described with clostridial organisms, nonclostridial polymicrobial synergism may result in a similar picture.[60,68,99]

Physical examination will reveal evidence of severe clinical toxicity, with tachycardia, tachypnea, and possibly hypotension and obtunded mental status. The classic signs of necrotizing wound infection are edematous wounds with bronze, gray, or purple discoloration that may exude a brown, watery fluid and may demonstrate hemorrhagic bullae or palpable crepitus. These classic physical findings may be preceded by severe pain in the wound, associated with mental depression and shiny skin.[60,68,99]

Laboratory confirmation of the organisms in a necrotizing wound infection may be obtained from aspiration of fluid from a bulla or culture of the necrotized tissue. Gram's staining should be done immediately to determine if gram-positive rods consistent with clostridia are present. Such necrotizing infections require aggressive surgical intervention (debridement of all destroyed tissue) along with the antibiotic therapy appropriate for the organisms seen on the Gram's stain.[60,68,99]

OTHER CAUSES. Fever during the first 2 days after surgery may also be caused by surgical disease or blood transfusion. These causes are discussed in the preceding section, Fever During or Immediately After Surgery.

Fever 2 to 4 Days after Surgery

Postoperative fever on days 2 to 4 (Figure 2-6) is associated with diseases representing complications that frequently occur in areas distant from the surgical site. In addition to the causes already discussed, at this point urinary tract infection, intravenous line infection, pneumonia, leg vein phlebitis, and pulmonary embolism must be considered.

URINARY TRACT INFECTION. Because bladder catheterization is used so often, urinary tract infection is the most common nosocomial infection, and it must be considered in any patient with a catheter in place for several days after surgery.[47,49,72,73] Urinary tract infection is suspected when urinalysis demonstrates white cells or bacteria and is confirmed by a positive urine culture. Usually a urine culture is considered positive when 10^5/ml or more organisms are present in the urine. Recently, however, patients with indwelling catheters were shown to have progressed from fewer than 10^5/ml to more than 10^5/ml, suggesting that sometimes a concentration of bacteria below 10^5/ml must be considered significant.[107] Therapy involves administering specific antibiotics and,

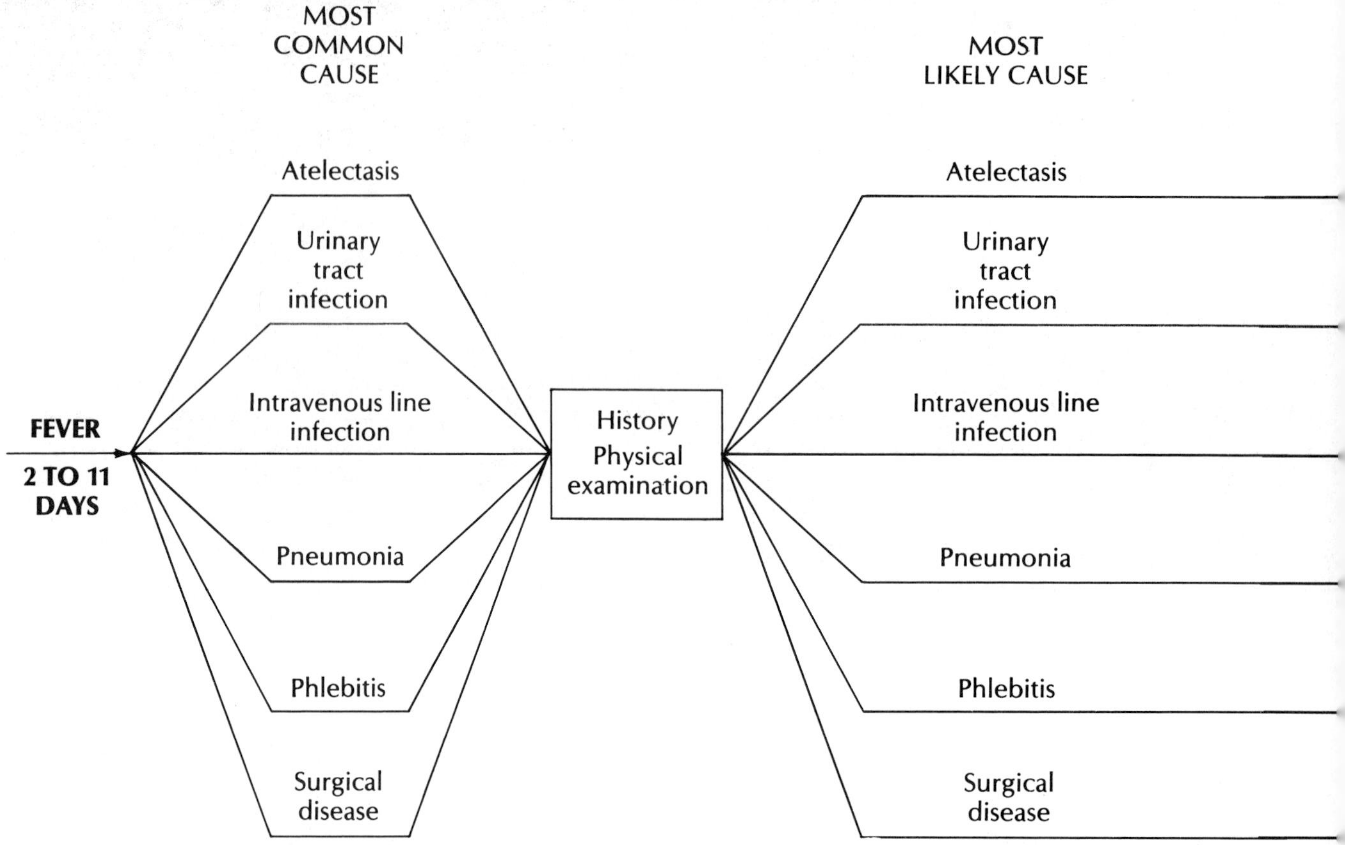

FIGURE 2-6 Evaluation of temperature changes 2 to 4 days after surgery. *CXR,* Chest radiograph; *ABG,* arterial blood gases; *C & S,* culture and sensitivity; *Tip,* catheter tip; *CT,* computed tomography.

when possible, removing the indwelling catheter.

INTRAVENOUS LINE INFECTION. Intravenous line infection, nonseptic phlebitis, and septic phlebitis are common sequelae of catheter use. Catheter colonization has been documented in as many as 34% of patients overall and in 54% for both peripheral and central venous lines if catheters are left in place for 4 days or longer.* Infection of a central venous catheter may occur with both monitoring devices and total parenteral nutrition (TPN) lines. When suspected as a source of infection, the central catheter should be removed and cultured by a semiquantitative technique.[79,103,104]

With both septic and nonseptic peripheral catheter-induced phlebitis, physical examination may reveal tenderness, a clot in the vein proximal to the insertion site, and erythema and edema surrounding the insertion site. With central venous catheters, septic and nonseptic phlebitis may start with edema of the arm, extending to the shoulder. When thrombosis involves a subclavian vein, coexistent thrombosis of the external jugular vein or internal jugular vein may be evident clinically.

*References 12, 15, 25, 27, 79, 103, and 104.

The diagnosis of septic peripheral phlebitis is confirmed by demonstrating organisms in the clot (through Gram's stain or culture). Peripheral nonseptic phlebitis is treated by removing the catheter, elevating the extremity, and applying heat. Septic peripheral phlebitis is treated by removing the catheter, elevating the limb, applying heat, administering antibiotics, and frequently by excising the clotted segment of vein.[15] Central venous line phlebitis requires removal of the catheter and systemic heparinization. Streptokinase therapy is contraindicated at this point after surgery. Septic central vein thrombophlebitis is diagnosed when the physical findings of central vein phlebitis are associated with positive blood culture results that are commonly repetitively positive for the same organism. This is most often successfully treated by removing the catheter and using a combination of heparin and antibiotics.[57] Thrombectomy of a central vein is rarely required, even with infected thrombophlebitis.[112]

PNEUMONIA. Pneumonia is a common nosocomial infection.[44,107] Important risk factors are pulmonary edema, malnutrition, smoking, long operations, and a long preoperative hospital stay.[50] During the first few

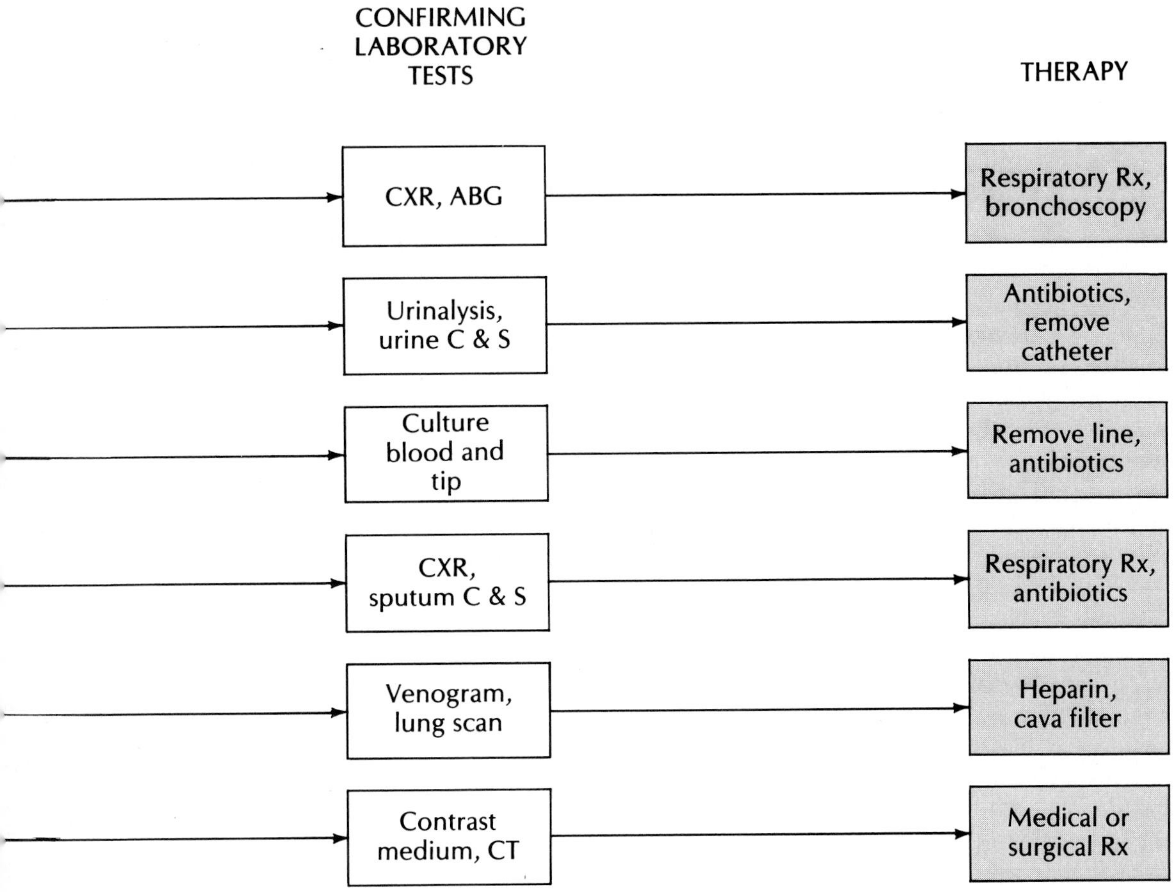

days after surgery, the nasopharynx or tracheobronchial tree becomes colonized with hospital organisms.[77,109] Subsequent pneumonias most commonly occur secondary to staphylococcal or gram-negative bacterial infection. The diagnosis of pneumonia primarily depends on findings of elevated temperature, a physical examination consistent with consolidation, an elevated white blood count, a chest radiograph that demonstrates a new infiltrate, and sputum that demonstrates organisms and white cells on Gram's stain with pathogens on culture.[77] A positive blood culture result with the same organism cultured from the sputum strongly supports the diagnosis of pneumonia.[109] Therapy involves administering antibiotics and chest physiotherapy. If significant problems with raising tracheobronchial secretions persist, bronchoscopy may be required. In rare cases a diagnosis of pneumonia can be made on the basis of an elevated temperature and purulent sputum, without a new infiltrate shown on chest radiograph.[109]

One commonly overlooked area on chest radiographs is the left lower lung field, where atelectasis or infiltrate may not be readily apparent. This is particularly true with the anteroposterior chest radiographs obtained in intensive care units. A pathologic condition in this area may be evident only as the "silhouette sign" or "ivory heart sign," which results in loss of the medial aspect of the left side of the diaphragm and a denser than normal heart shadow on the left side.[48] Left pleural effusion is also in the differential diagnosis of the ivory heart sign. A lateral decubitus chest radiograph will determine if the ivory heart sign has developed secondary to the presence of pleural fluid. If this is not the case, bronchoscopy, with attention directed to the left lower bronchi, should result in re-expansion of atelectasis. If this does not resolve the ivory heart sign, pneumonia in the left lower lung field may be presumed.

PHLEBITIS AND PULMONARY EMBOLISM. Deep vein thrombosis that is not associated with intravenous line catheterization occurs most commonly in the lower extremities. The pathogenesis of deep vein thrombosis is concisely described by Virchow's triad of trauma, stasis, and a hypercoagulable state.[95] Trauma refers to trauma directly to the vein in question. Stasis is diminished blood flow, and hypercoagulable state is any process that makes blood more likely to clot. After surgery not performed on the lower extremities, deep vein thrombosis occurs secondary to stasis and the hypercoagulable state. Stasis occurs from immobility of the lower extremities in the operating room and is aggravated by conditions associated with diminished cardiac output, such as hypovolemia or congestive heart failure. Hypercoagulability follows any injury, including surgical trauma. The risk of deep vein thrombosis is increased with obesity, cancer, age over 40 years, cardiac or peripheral vascular disease, and a history of deep vein thrombosis.[30,95]

Although clots may develop in veins in the extremities during surgery, the clinical evidence of deep vein thrombosis usually does not declare itself until several days later, as either deep vein thrombosis or pulmonary embolism. Physical findings consistent with deep vein thrombosis in a lower extremity are tenderness in the calf, edema of one leg more than the other (usually extending from the ankle cephalad), and pain on movement of the calf. Warmth and erythema may be present, but these are more likely with superficial vein thrombosis.

With pulmonary embolism, physical examination usually reveals tachycardia and tachypnea and, more rarely, a pleural friction rub, chest splinting, and a gallop rhythm.[86]

Most often deep vein thrombosis and pulmonary embolism cannot be diagnosed simply by physical examination. The diagnosis usually requires a high index of suspicion and confirming laboratory tests. For deep vein thrombosis, plethysmography is most useful when the examination result is normal, since the false negative rate is low.[26,75] However, because plethysmography has a high false positive rate, duplex ultrasound scanning usually is indicated before therapy is begun to prove the diagnosis of deep vein thrombosis. With pulmonary embolism, a significant drop in blood Po_2 and Pco_2 is consistent with the diagnosis. A chest radiograph may reveal no abnormality, segmental atelectasis, pleural effusion, or wedge-shaped defect in the periphery consistent with an infarcted segment. The likelihood of pulmonary embolism is confirmed by a positive ventilation/perfusion lung scan and, when equivocal, pulmonary angiography.[55,98]

The initial therapy for deep vein thrombosis or pulmonary embolism in the postoperative period is heparinization. Streptokinase is contraindicated.[22] Only rarely is interruption of the vena cava with ligation, a clip, or an umbrella indicated.[26,42,56] Still more rarely is pulmonary embolectomy indicated.[81,98]

OTHER CAUSES. Atelectasis and continuing surgical disease are possible causes of fever during this period. These are reviewed in the section on Fever During or Immediately After Surgery.

Fever 5 to 10 Days after Surgery

Fever that occurs 5 to 10 days after surgery is the most difficult to evaluate, because the greatest number of potential causes are present at this time (Figure 2-7). Infections from the hospital environment or the patient's own flora are most prevalent.

WOUND INFECTION. Wound infection most commonly results from contamination of the wound with the patient's own flora at the time of surgery.[37,88,111] These may be skin organisms, or infection may occur secondary to contamination from organisms present in the tissue undergoing operation (e.g., colonic bacteria during colonic resections). Although bacteria contaminated the wound at the time of the procedure, several days must pass before bacterial growth produces a clinically evident infection. Wound infection is most likely to occur when the operation has encompassed a contaminated field with frank infection or spillage of intestinal contents.* Closing the subcutaneous tissue after an operation in a contaminated field establishes a greater probability of wound infection developing.[37] Wound infections are also more likely to occur in patients who have depressed immunocompetence from shock, malnutrition, malignancy, prior sepsis, or severe injury.[89]

During this period all wounds, not just abdominal wounds, require inspection for erythema, tenderness, edema, and warmth. When a wound infection is suspected, partly opening the wound and probing it to examine the contents may prove diagnostic. If purulent material is encountered, the wound must be opened completely for drainage. Antibiotic therapy may be necessary if the patient appears to be suffering significantly from sepsis and if there is surrounding cellulitis extending away from the edges of the wound. Otherwise, simply opening the wound usually is adequate therapy.

WOUND DEHISCENCE. All wounds are weakest approximately 5 to 7 days after injury.[66] Therefore wound dehiscence usually declares itself during this period. This is true for any wound, including intestinal anastomoses, in which the wound dehiscence produces an anastomotic leak (see below). Malnutrition, previous or ongoing sepsis, cancer, diabetes, steroid use, and wound infection all increase the risk of wound dehiscence.[66] Wound dehiscence declares itself most commonly with serous fluid, representing intra-abdominal or intrapleural contents, emanating from the wound.

A wound dehiscence must be differentiated from a seroma, in which serous fluid has accumulated only in the wound proper and has not been leaking from an enclosed serosal surface. This is done by partially opening the wound and palpating the fascial closure. With a dehiscence the fascial closure is disrupted; with a seroma the fascial closure remains intact.

*References 35, 37, 88, 108, and 111.

When possible, the best treatment for dehiscence is reclosure of the wound. Occasionally a patient is too ill to undergo this procedure. In these cases simply packing the wound is the correct therapy; the resulting hernia is repaired later.

ANASTOMOTIC LEAK. The same risk factors that pertain to wounds likely to dehisce apply to anastomoses that are likely to break down.[65,66] Gastrointestinal tract anastomoses are much more likely to dehisce than bronchial or vascular anastomoses. Within the gastrointestinal tract, colonic anastomoses are more likely to break down than are small bowel or stomach anastomoses.[65,66]

Fever may be the first manifestation of an anastomotic leak. Physical examination may reveal tenderness, edema, erythema, and warmth. Abdominal examination may reveal physical findings consistent with peritonitis. An anastomotic dehiscence usually is confirmed by contrast instillation in the areas suspected of leaking. With a gastrointestinal anastomotic leak, demonstration of intestinal contents from a drain or through a wound is diagnostic. Treatment of an anastomotic leak is based on the principles of (1) controlling sepsis, (2) relieving a distal obstruction, and (3) decompressing flow proximal to the leak. A gastrointestinal anastomotic leak may require surgical diversion.

INTRA-ABDOMINAL ABSCESS. An intra-abdominal abscess without an associated anastomotic leak may develop during this period. Intra-abdominal abscesses most commonly follow operations associated with contamination of the abdominal cavity.[86] Intra-abdominal abscesses are most likely to develop in patients suffering significant immunoincompetence (e.g., cancer, malnutrition, previous sepsis, trauma, chemotherapy, diabetes, and human immunodeficiency virus [HIV] infection or acquired immunodeficiency syndrome [AIDS]). An intra-abdominal abscess should be considered a possible cause of fever in any patient who has undergone a major intra-abdominal procedure. Physical examination may reveal localized tenderness in the abdomen with physical findings consistent with peritonitis. In addition, edema or erythema may localize to an area where an intra-abdominal abscess has formed. In women, a pelvic examination may reveal bulging tenderness in the cul-de-sac consistent with a pelvic abscess. In men, a rectal examination may reveal a similar finding. Several diagnostic studies can confirm the presence of an intra-abdominal abscess—plain radiographs of the abdomen that reveal pockets of gas outside the intestinal lumen; a gallium scan; indium-labeled leukocytes; or an ultrasound or CT scan of the abdomen that shows a fluid collection.* Of these, the CT scan has proved to be the most useful.[38,62,69] The treatment for an intra-abdominal abscess is drainage, which may require further surgical intervention. Recently, however, percutaneous drainage of intra-abdominal abscesses has become a widely used technique and has shown excellent results.[53,61]

MENINGITIS. Meningitis is an unusual infectious complication in the postoperative period. Only patients who have a communication of cerebrospinal fluid (CSF) with the external environment (e.g., patients suffering basilar skull fractures with rhinorrhea or CSF leakage from an ear) are at risk for meningitis. The findings of a physical examination would be consistent with evidence of a basilar skull fracture and possibly nuchal rigidity. Because changes in mental status are common to all cases of sepsis, finding a patient to be more somnolent offers no particular support of meningitis as a diagnosis. Laboratory confirmation of meningitis is based on culture of cerebrospinal fluid. The treatment is antibiotic therapy.

ACALCULOUS CHOLECYSTITIS. Particularly in injured males, even with minimal trauma, acalculous cholecystitis should be considered a cause of postoperative fever.[52,61,72] With this disorder, fever commonly is associated with tenderness in the right upper quadrant and occasionally a palpable gallbladder. The patient may develop jaundice. Laboratory tests that confirm a diagnosis of acalculous cholecystitis are ultrasonography showing an edematous gallbladder wall with sludge in the gallbladder and a DISIDA scan demonstrating nonvisualization of the gallbladder.[39] However, false positive results from DISIDA scans are common in critically ill surgical patients with either other intra-abdominal disorders or sepsis from other foci that may be depressing liver function. In particular, an acutely congested liver, acute pancreatitis, and/or a perforated duodenal ulcer may cause a false positive result. The best diagnostic test is visualization of the gallbladder. This does not necessarily require a major surgical procedure using general anesthesia; it may be accomplished with a transverse subcostal incision using local anesthesia. If the gallbladder appears normal, acalculous cholecystitis is not the disease, and the incision can be closed using local anesthesia. If the gallbladder is obviously inflamed or if omentum surrounds the gallbladder, general anesthesia with a standard approach to the gallbladder may then follow. The treatment of choice for acalculous cholecystitis is cholecystectomy. In some cases cholecystostomy is adequate therapy.[52,64,87]

A new diagnostic approach being tried in several centers is the use of laparoscopy to determine if the gallbladder is inflamed and thus the cause of the problem.

EMPYEMA. After the development of pneumonia and, in particular, after insertion of a chest tube for hemothorax, empyema may emerge as a major determinant of elevated temperature during this period.[32] The usual chest radiograph may not adequately define an area of pleural fluid collection. Thoracentesis under these cir-

*References 31, 34, 38, 62, and 114.

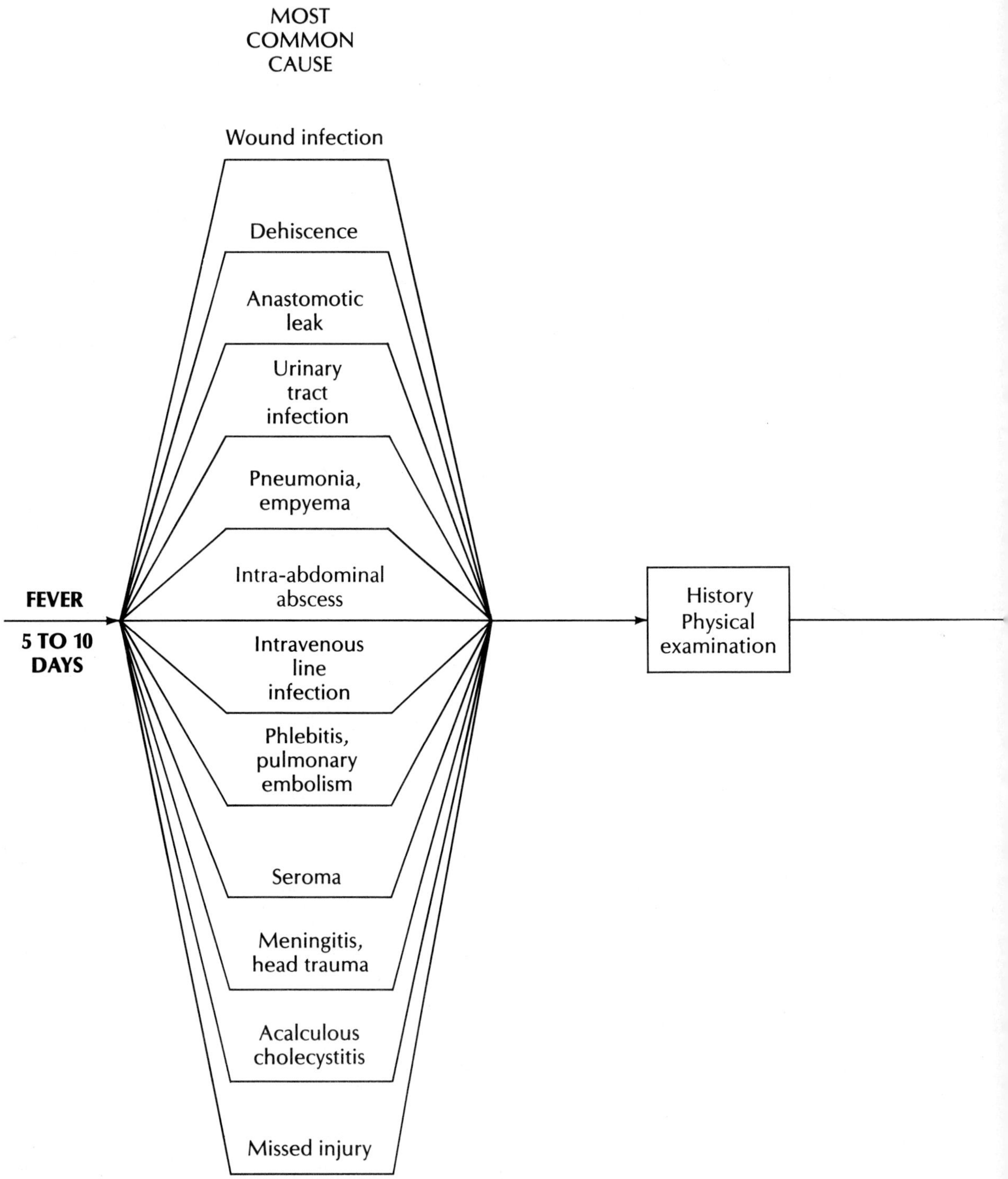

FIGURE 2-7 Evaluation of temperature changes 5 to 10 days after surgery. *CT,* Computed tomography; *C & S,* culture and sensitivity; *CXR,* chest radiograph; *LP,* lumbar puncture.

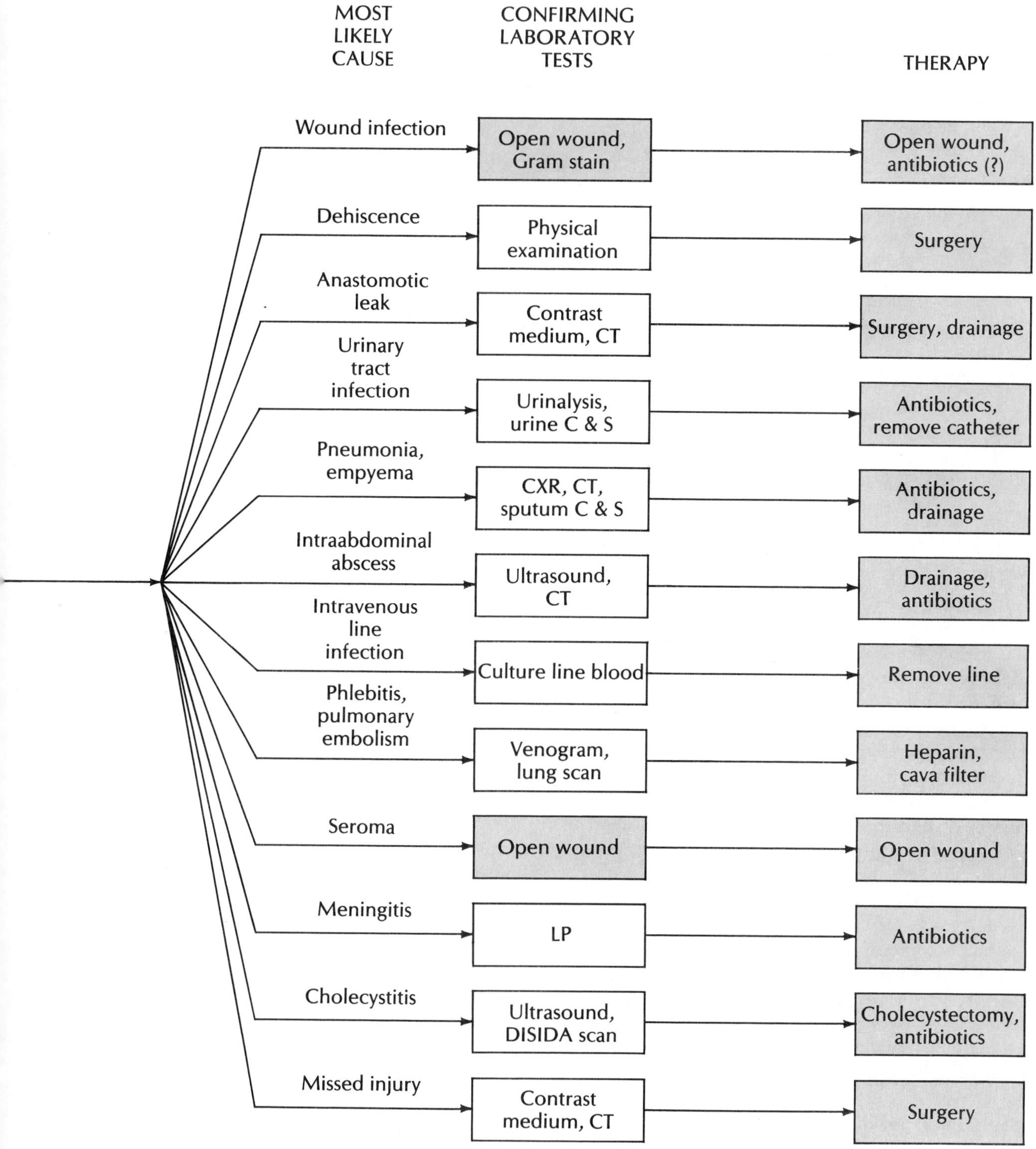
MOST LIKELY CAUSE
CONFIRMING LABORATORY TESTS
THERAPY
Wound infection
Open wound, Gram stain
Open wound, antibiotics (?)
Dehiscence
Physical examination
Surgery
Anastomotic leak
Contrast medium, CT
Surgery, drainage
Urinary tract infection
Urinalysis, urine C & S
Antibiotics, remove catheter
Pneumonia, empyema
CXR, CT, sputum C & S
Antibiotics, drainage
Intraabdominal abscess
Ultrasound, CT
Drainage, antibiotics
Intravenous line infection
Culture line blood
Remove line
Phlebitis, pulmonary embolism
Venogram, lung scan
Heparin, cava filter
Seroma
Open wound
Open wound
Meningitis
LP
Antibiotics
Cholecystitis
Ultrasound, DISIDA scan
Cholecystectomy, antibiotics
Missed injury
Contrast medium, CT
Surgery

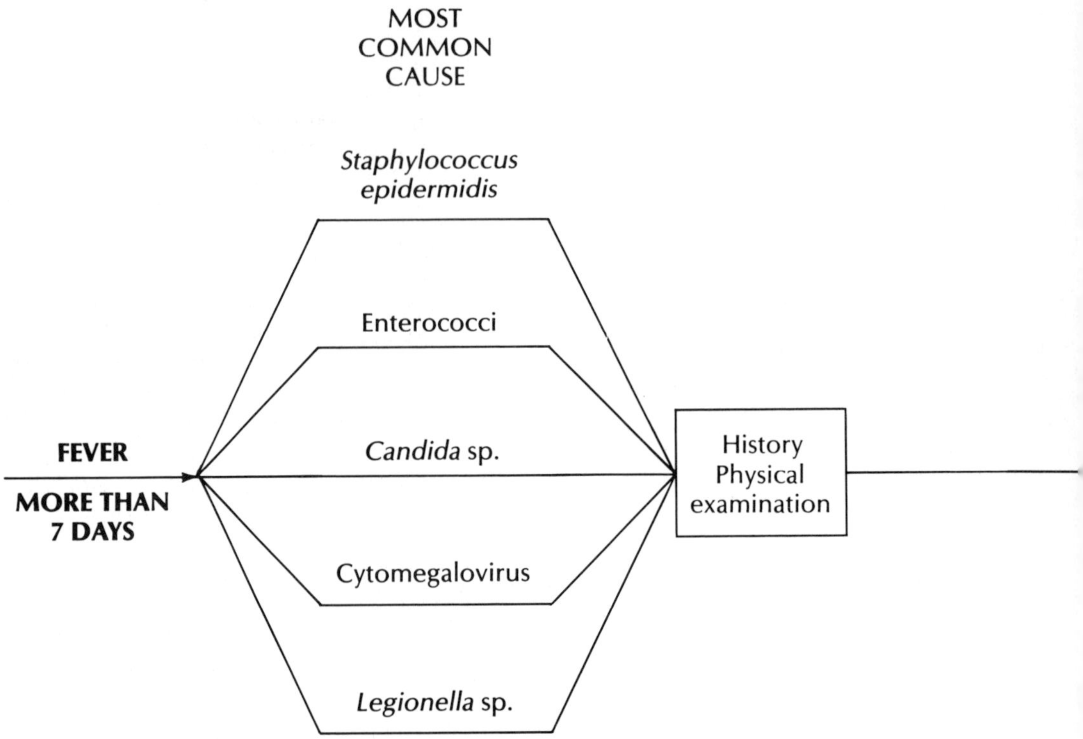

FIGURE 2-8 Evaluation of temperature changes more than 7 days after surgery ("unusual" organism sepsis). *C & S*, Culture and sensitivity.

cumstances may fail to sample a loculated area of pleural fluid. Ultrasonography or computed tomographic scanning may be required to locate pleural fluid collections accurately during this period and to rule out empyema. In addition, a computed tomographic scan of the chest may reveal a lung abscess or other areas of pleural fluid collection that were not suspected by the plain chest radiograph.[91] The initial treatment for empyema is chest tube drainage. If this procedure proves inadequate, partial rib resection and aggressive opening of the empyemic cavity is required.[97]

MISSED INJURY. After observation or exploration for trauma has been completed, a subtle injury to an abdominal or a thoracic organ, particularly the esophagus or pancreas, may be missed during the initial evaluation. Such a missed injury may declare itself as a fever during this period. The diagnosis of a missed injury is based primarily on a high index of suspicion stemming from the mechanism of the initial trauma. A variety of diagnostic studies, including instillation of contrast material, ultrasonography, and CT scanning, may be required to establish the cause of a septic focus. Most often this initially is diagnosed as an intra-abdominal abscess or empyema, and a subsequent pancreatic, esophageal, or other intestinal fistula is recognized after the abscess is drained. The treatment for missed injury is drainage of purulent collections, drainage of any fistulae, and possibly surgery to control fistulous drainage or to repair the fistula.

OTHER CAUSES. The other causes of fever mentioned in the above text have been covered in previous sections.

Fever More Than 7 Days after Surgery—Unusual Organism Sepsis

Once critically ill surgical patients have spent 7 days or longer in the hospital, a combination of several factors predisposes them to infection with organisms that in the past have been considered of low virulence. These factors are (1) gastrointestinal surgery; (2) older age; (3) previous bacterial sepsis; (4) antibiotic therapy; (5) presence of a central venous catheter; (6) respiratory therapy; and (7) total parenteral nutrition. If fever develops more than 7 days after surgery in patients with these risk factors, infection with one of the organisms described below should be considered high on the list of possibilities (Figure 2-8).

FUNGAL SEPSIS. Fungi (particularly *Candida*) are organisms found primarily in the gastrointestinal tract in most people. The risk factors described earlier allow for fungal colonization of many sites, particularly the skin, gastrointestinal tract, and urinary tract. Subsequent invasion occurs, with a clinical picture similar to that of

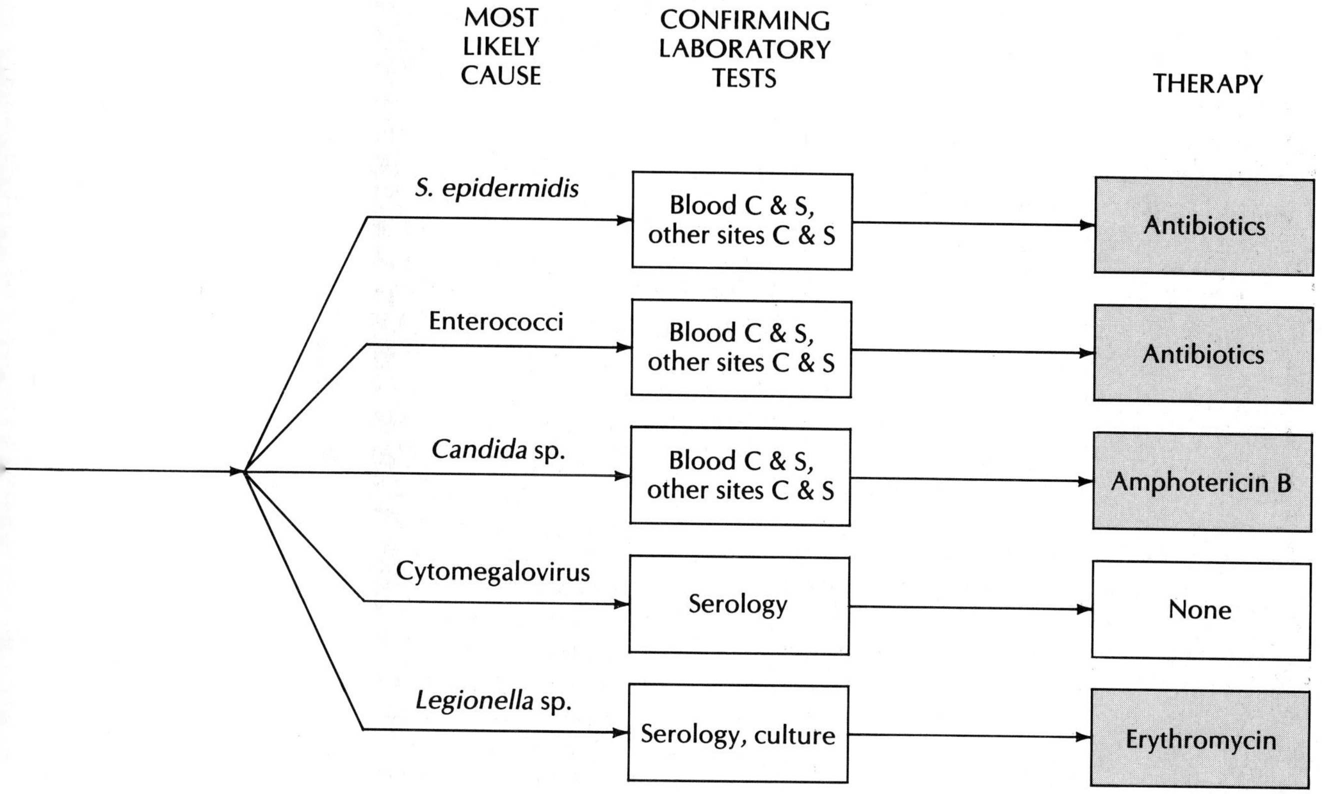

bacterial sepsis. Mortality with fungal sepsis is approximately 40%. The diagnostic criteria for disseminated fungal sepsis have been well described (see box). Once a diagnosis of likely or proven fungal dissemination is made, the treatment of choice is therapy with amphotericin B.[28,106]

STAPHYLOCOCCUS EPIDERMIDIS SEPSIS. *Staphylococcus epidermidis* is emerging as an organism that is frequently cultured from the bloodstream of critically ill surgical patients.[29] The risk factors for developing *S. epidermidis* sepsis are similar to those described for fungal infection. In fact, *S. epidermidis* is sometimes seen in patients who have fungal sepsis.[28] The diagnostic criteria for invasive *S. epidermidis* infection have also been described (see box). Invasive *S. epidermidis* requires specific antibiotic therapy.

ENTEROCOCCAL INFECTION. *Enterococcus* is a ubiquitous organism in the gastrointestinal tract of humans. Similar to the *Candida* organism, it becomes prevalent after gastrointestinal procedures and antibiotics that in general kill enteric pathogens other than the enterococci. Although well described as a pathogen in meningitis and endocarditis, the role of enterococci in determining mortality in surgical patients is a difficult subject. Several investigations have failed to prove that the *Enterococcus* organism per se is a major determinant of mortality.[17,51]

DIAGNOSIS OF DISSEMINATED FUNGAL SEPSIS

Definitive Diagnosis

Culture of organism from tissue
Endophthalmitis
Burn wound invasion
Positive peritoneal fluid culture

Likely Dissemination

Two positive blood cultures at least 24 hours apart (without central venous catheter)
Two positive blood cultures, the second of which was obtained more than 24 hours after removal of a colonized catheter
Three or more colonized sites: leg, urine, sputum, or wound

DIAGNOSIS OF INVASIVE *STAPHYLOCOCCUS EPIDERMIDIS* SEPSIS

Definitive Diagnosis

Positive blood culture with culture from a tissue or cavity

Likely Invasion

Repeatedly positive blood cultures
Other foci of *S. epidermidis* (e.g., urine or wounds)
Marked antibiotic resistance

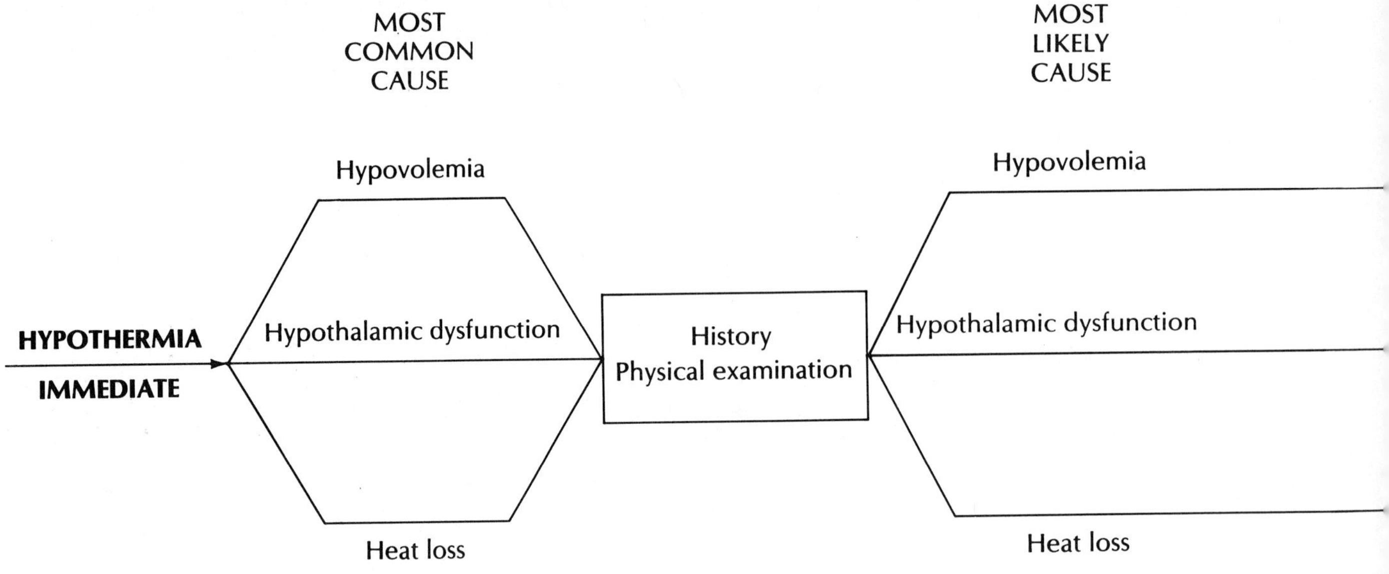

FIGURE 2-9 Evaluation of hypothermia during or immediately after surgery. *CVP*, Central venous pressure.

However, the consensus is that enterococci in the bloodstream require specific antienterococcal therapy. Of interest is the propensity for *Enterococcus* organisms to invade along with gram-negative organisms, commonly with both organisms located in a site that usually would be considered of low invasive potential (e.g., an open wound or a drain site). The possibility has been raised that enterococci and gram-negative organisms may act synergistically to invade such areas.[17]

SERRATIA **INFECTION.** *Serratia marcescens* infection is emerging as a major cause of morbidity in patients after surgery, especially those hospitalized in intensive care units. As with fungi and *S. epidermidis, Serratia* organisms were thought to be innocuous but now have become virulent in patients with the risk factors described previously. The major portals of entry for *Serratia* organisms are the urinary and respiratory tracts. *Serratia* organisms also have been noted to cause postoperative wound infections. Culture of *Serratia* organisms from sputum with other clinical evidence of pneumonia, positive blood cultures, significant urine cultures, or wound infections with *Serratia* organisms all require systemic antibiotic therapy based on the sensitivity of the organism. In general, gentamycin has emerged as the main therapy.[115]

CYTOMEGALOVIRUS INFECTION. Cytomegalovirus (CMV) infections are seen predominantly in immunosuppressed patients.[89,90] Physical examination may reveal a maculopapular rash and hepatosplenomegaly. Cytomegalovirus infection is confirmed by immunologic tests. Therapy of active CMV infection involves reducing any immunosuppressive treatment or treating the infection with antiviral drugs, or both.

LEGIONELLA **INFECTION.** *Legionella* infection also occurs in critically ill, immunocompromised surgical patients. It begins primarily as a pneumonia that may be interstitial, simulating pulmonary edema.[18] *Legionella* infection is confirmed by serologic tests and cultures of sputum. Currently erythromycin is the treatment of choice for *Legionella* infection.[19]

Hypothermia during or Immediately after Surgery

As mentioned in the section Physiology of Temperature Regulation, several events can occur with general anesthesia and major surgery that predispose a patient to hypothermia during surgery and in the immediate postoperative period. Anesthetic inhibition of thermoregulatory center function, inhalation of cool anesthetic gases, administration of room temperature intravenous fluids and cool blood, evaporative loss with an open thoracic or abdominal cavity, and irrigation of pleural or peritoneal surfaces with room temperature solutions all may cause hypothermia. Intraoperative and postoperative hypothermia are common in patients undergoing major surgery, particularly those requiring management in the intensive care unit after surgery. In a recent study of 100 such patients, 77% developed a temperature below 36° C (97° F) during surgery, and about 50% had hypothermia at the end of the surgery. Hypothermia was associated with a greater fluid requirement during the operation and a longer period of surgery. In surgical patients, hypothermia may continue

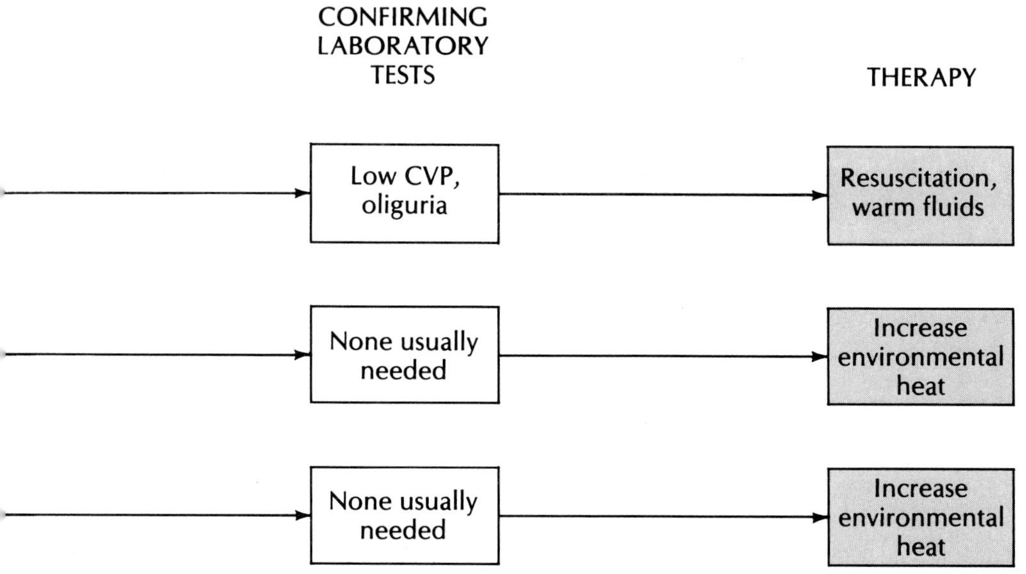

to be a problem until 2 hours after surgery (approximately 40%), but by 4 hours after surgery 80% of the patients should be normothermic. At this point persistent hypothermia is associated with an increased risk of mortality.[107]

The most common causes of persistent hypothermia several hours after surgery are (1) hypovolemia, (2) hypothalamic dysfunction, and (3) environmental heat loss (Figure 2-9).

HYPOVOLEMIA. Hypovolemia that requires continuing administration of room temperature or cooler intravenous fluids or blood may result in persistent hypothermia. If bleeding is the major cause of hypovolemia, treating a bleeding focus or associated coagulopathy will diminish the requirement for infusion of cool fluids. All inhaled gases and all fluids administered to such a patient should be warmed to body temperature if possible. Inability to reverse hypotension in a patient with hypothermia and hypovolemia within the first 4 hours after surgery is a poor prognostic indicator.[105] Therefore every effort should be made to reverse the cause of persistent hypovolemia, restore perfusion, and elevate body temperature.

HYPOTHALAMIC DYSFUNCTION. As stated earlier, anesthesia may cause hypothalamic dysfunction that allows hypothermia to develop. Neurosurgical diseases that cause hypothalamic injury usually result in hyperthermia, but they may result in hypothermia. The history and the findings from a physical examination will be consistent with neurologic dysfunction as described in the previous discussion of hypothalamic dysfunction on page 34. Treatment consists of general measures to increase body temperature and therapy for the neurosurgical disease.

ENVIRONMENTAL HEAT LOSS. Placing a patient who has undergone surgery in a cool, air-conditioned recovery area without blankets and allowing him to breathe room temperature gases sets the stage for significant environmental heat loss. Large, open wounds that may have moist dressings also cause significant heat loss. The history and the findings from a physical examination should reveal the nature of the surgical procedure and exposure of the patient to environmental heat loss. Therapy consists of general measures to reduce heat loss, as previously described, with particular attention to covering the patient with a large forced-air-heated "air blanket" and warming inhaled gases.

Hypothermia Several Days after Surgery

The most common causes of hypothermia several days after surgery are systemic sepsis and evaporative water loss (Figure 2-10). As described earlier, infection most commonly raises the temperature after surgery. Occasionally, however, particularly in severe gram-negative sepsis, a patient with an infection will demonstrate hypothermia rather than hyperthermia.[102] However, other accompaniments of sepsis may be present, such as a shift of white blood cells to immature polymorphonuclear leukocytes, glucose intolerance, depressed mentation, tachycardia, and tachypnea. A systematic search for an infected focus must be begun in a fashion similar to that described for an elevated temperature. Measures

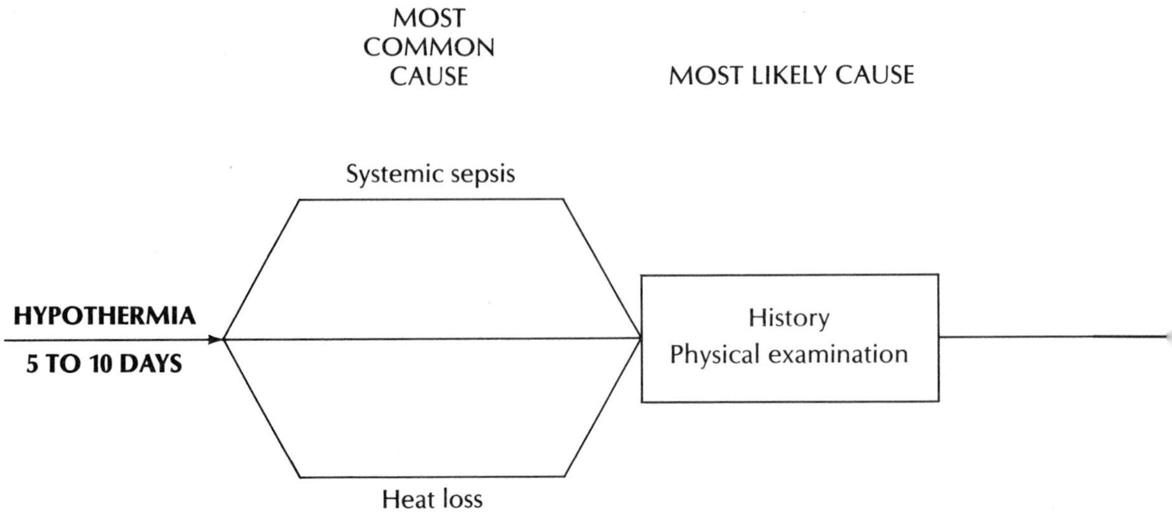

FIGURE 2-10 Evaluation of hypothermia several days after surgery. *WBC,* White blood cells.

to elevate body temperature should be carried out as described previously until the source of sepsis is treated.

Persistent environmental heat loss leading to hypothermia several days after surgery or injury most commonly occurs in patients with significant loss of skin function, particularly burn patients. At this point hypothermia primarily occurs secondary to heat loss from evaporation of water from the burn wound. However, it is at just this time that burn wound sepsis may be declaring itself, and the clinician should not presume that the hypothermia is only secondary to heat loss from water evaporation. The prime therapy for reducing or eliminating hypothermia on this basis is to provide skin grafts. However, temporizing measures, such as increasing the room temperature, covering the patient with burn dressings, and administering warm intravenous fluids and inhaled gases, may help ameliorate the hypothermia.

REFERENCES

Problem-Oriented Approach

1 Abrams JS, Davis JH: Advantages of the problem-oriented medical record in the care of the severely injured patient, *J Trauma* 14:361, 1974.

2 Hurst JW, Walker HK: *The problem-oriented system,* New York, 1972, Medcom.

3 Weed LL: *Medical records, medical education and patient care,* Cleveland, 1969, Case Western Reserve University Press.

Abdominal Pain

4 Angell M: The quality of mercy, *N Engl J Med* 306:98, 1982.

5 Bennett RL, Batenhorst RL, Bivins, BA et al: Patient-controlled analgesia, *Ann Surg* 195:700, 1982.

6 Diethelm AG: The acute abdomen. In Sabiston DC, editor: *Davis-Christopher textbook of surgery,* ed 13, Philadelphia, 1986, Saunders.

7 Fitts WT, Gadzik JP: The acute abdomen. In Hardy JD, editor: *Rhoads' textbook of surgery,* ed 5, Philadelphia, 1977, JB Lippincott.

8 Guyton AC: *Textbook of medical physiology,* Philadelphia, 1981, WB Saunders.

9 Leek BF: Abdominal and pelvic visceral receptors, *Br Med Bull* 33:163, 1977.

10 Perry SW, Rogers W: Classical management of postop pain with narcotics, *Infect Surg* 115, 1984.

11 Silen W: Abdominal pain. In Petersdorf RG et al: *Harrison's principles of internal medicine,* ed 10, New York, 1983, McGraw-Hill.

Temperature Alteration

12 Altemeier WA, McDonough JJ, Fullen WD: Third day surgical fever, *Arch Surg* 103:158, 1971.

13 Atkins E, Bodel P: Clinical fever: its history, manifestations, and pathogenesis, *Fed Proc* 38(1):57, 1979.

14 Atkins E, Bodel P, Frances L: Release of an endogenous pyrogen in vitro from rabbit mononuclear cells, *J Exp Med* 126:357, 1968.

15 Baker CC, Petersen SR, Sheldon GF: Septic phlebitis: a neglected disease, *Am J Surg* 138:97, 1979.

16 Balestrieri FJ, Chernow B, Rainey TG: Postcraniotomy diabetes insipidus: who's at risk? *Crit Care Med* 10(2):108, 1982.

17 Barrall DT, Kenney PR, Slotman GJ et al: Enterococcal bacteremia in surgical patients, *Arch Surg* 120:57, 1985.

18 Bartlett JG: New developments in infectious diseases for the critical care physician, *Crit Care Med* 11(7):563, 1983.

19 Bartlett RH: Pulmonary pathophysiology in surgical patients, *Surg Clin North Am* 60(6):1323, 1980.

20 Bartlett RH, Brennan ML, Gazzaniga AB, et al: Studies on the pathogenesis and prevention of postoperative pulmonary complications, *Surg Gynecol Obstet* 137:925, 1973.

21 Becker A, Barak S, Braum E et al: The treatment of postoperative pulmonary atelectasis with intermittent positive pressure breathing, *Surg Gynecol Obstet* 111:517, 1960.

22 Bell WR, Meek AG: Guidelines for the use of thrombolytic agents, *N Engl J Med* 301(23):1266, 1979.

23 Bendtzen K, Baek L, Berild D et al: Demonstration of circulating leukocytic pyrogen/interleukin-1 during fever, *N Engl J Med* 310(9):596, 1984.

24 Bernheim HA, Block LH, Atkins E: Fever: pathogenesis, pathophysiology, and purpose, *Ann Intern Med* 91:261, 1979.

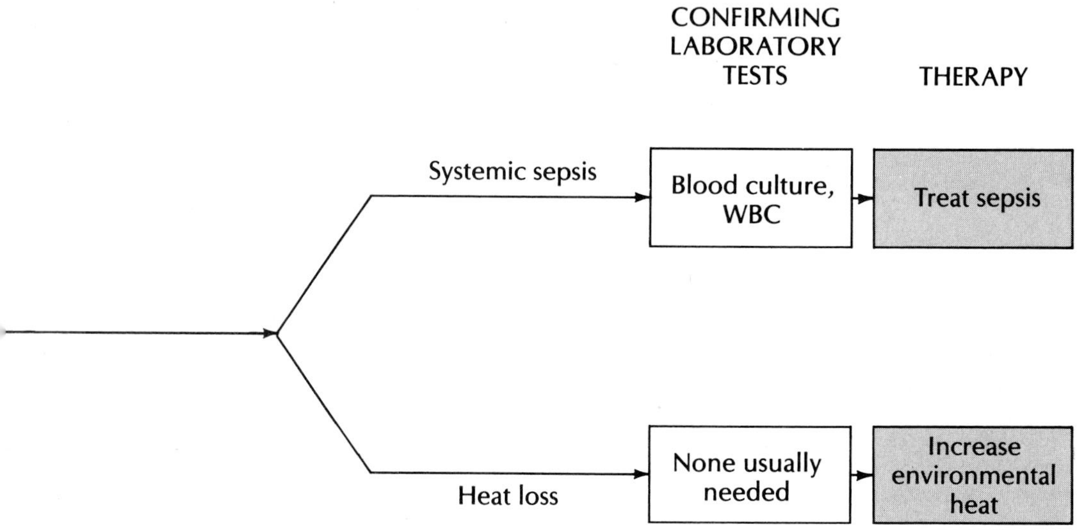

25 Bjornson HS, Colley R, Bower RH et al: Association between microorganism growth at the catheter insertion site and colonization of the catheter in patients receiving total parenteral nutrition, *Surgery* 92(4):720, 1982.
26 Blumenberg RM, Gelfand ML: Long-term follow-up of vena caval clips and umbrellas, *Am J Surg* 134:205, 1977.
27 Bozzetti F, Terno G, Camerini E et al: Pathogenesis and predictability of central venous catheter sepsis, *Surgery* 91(4):383, 1982.
28 Burchard KW, Minor LB, Slotman GJ et al: Fungal sepsis in surgical patients, *Arch Surg* 118:217, 1983.
29 Burchard KW, Minor LB, Slotman GJ et al: *Staphylococcus epidermidis* sepsis in surgical patients, *Arch Surg* 119:96, 1984.
30 Cade FJ: High risk of the critically ill for venous thromboembolism, *Crit Care Med* 10(7):448, 1982.
31 Caffee HH, Watts G, Mena I: Gallium-67 citrate scanning in the diagnosis of intra-abdominal abscess, *Am J Surg* 133:665, 1977.
32 Caplan ES, Hoyt NJ, Rodriguez A et al: Empyema occurring in the multiply traumatized patient, *J Trauma* 24(9):785, 1984.
33 Clark WG, Moyer SG: The effects of acetaminophen and sodium salicylate on the release and activity of leukocytic pyrogen in the cat, *J Pharmacol Exp Ther* 181(1):183, 1972.
34 Coleman RE, Black RE, Welch DM et al: Indium-111–labeled leukocytes in the evaluation of suspected abdominal abscesses, *Am J Surg* 139:99, 1980.
35 Coles B, Van Heerden JA, Keys TF et al: Incidence of wound infection for common general surgical procedures, *Surg Gynecol Obstet* 154:557, 1982.
36 Collins GJ, Rich NM, Andersen CA et al: Phleborrheographic diagnosis of venous obstruction, *Ann Surg* 189(1):25, 1979.
37 Cruse PJE, Foord R: The epidemiology of wound infection, *Surg Clin North Am* 60(1):27, 1980.
38 Daffner RH, Halber MD, Morgan CL et al: Computer tomography in the diagnosis of intra-abdominal abscesses, *Ann Surg* 189(1):29, 1979.
39 Deitch EA, Engel JM: Acute acalculous cholecystitis, *Am J Surg* 142:290, 1981.
40 Dinarello CA, Wolff SM: Pathogenesis of fever in man, *N Engl J Med* 298(11):607, 1978.
41 Dinarello CA, Wolff SM: Molecular basis of fever in humans, *Am J Med* 72:799, 1982.
42 Donaldson MC, Wirthlin LS, Donaldson GA: Thirty years' experience with surgical interruption of the inferior vena cava for prevention of pulmonary embolism, *Ann Surg* 191(3):367, 1980.
43 Eichna LW, Berger AR, Rader B et al: Comparison of intracardiac and intravascular temperatures with rectal temperatures in man, *J Clin Invest* 30:353, 1951.
44 Eickhoff TC: Pulmonary infections in surgical patients, *Surg Clin North Am* 60(1):175, 1980.
45 Espositio AL, Gleckman RA: A diagnostic approach to the adult with fever of unknown origin, *Arch Intern Med* 139:575, 1979.
46 Feldberg W, Saxena PN: Fever produced by prostaglandin E_1, *J Physiol* 217:547, 1971.
47 Fowler JE: Nosocomial catheter-associated urinary tract infection, *Infect Surg* 43, 1983.
48 Fraser RG, Pare JAP: *Diagnosis of disease of the chest,* Philadelphia, 1977, WB Saunders.
49 Freischlag J, Busuttil RW: The value of postoperative fever evaluation, *Surgery* 94(2):358, 1983.
50 Garibaldi RA, Britt MR, Coleman ML et al: Risk factors for postoperative pneumonia, *Am J Med* 70:677, 1981.
51 Garrison RN, Fry DE, Berberich S et al: Enterococcal bacteremia: clinical implications and determinants of death, *Ann Surg* 196(1):43, 1982.
52 Gately JF, Thomas EJ: Acute cholecystitis occurring as a complication of other diseases, *Arch Surg* 118:1137, 1983.
53 Gerzof SG, Robbins AH, Johnson WC et al: Percutaneous catheter drainage of abdominal abscesses: a five-year experience, *N Engl J Med* 305(12):653, 1981.
54 Gleckman R: Fever of unknown origin: the value of abdominal exploration, *Postgrad Med* 62(1):191, 1977.
55 Goodall RJR, Greenfield LJ: Clinical correlations in the diagnosis of pulmonary embolism, *Ann Surg* 191(2):219, 1980.
56 Greenfield LJ, Zocco J, Wilk J et al: Clinical experience with the Kim-Ray Greenfield vena caval filter, *Ann Surg* 185(6):692, 1977.
57 Griffith GL, Maull KI, Sachatello CR: Septic pulmonary embolization, *Surg Gynecol Obstet* 144:105, 1977.

58 Gurdjian ES, Gurdjian ES: Acute head injuries, *Surg Gynecol Obstet* 146:805, 1978.
59 Hahn HH, Char DC, Postel WB et al: Studies on the pathogenesis of fever, *J Exp Med* 126:385, 1967.
60 Hart GB, Lamb RC, Strauus MB: Gas gangrene. I.A. Collective review, *J Trauma* 23(11):991, 1983.
61 Herlin P, Ericsson M, Holmin T et al: Acute acalculous cholecystitis following trauma, *Br J Surg* 69:475, 1982.
62 Herman CM: Detection and management of intra-abdominal abscess, *Infect Surg* 737, 1983.
63 Howard PH, Hardin WJ: The role of surgery in fever of unknown origin, *Surg Clin North Am* 52(2):397, 1972.
64 Howard RJ: Acute acalculous cholecystitis, *Am J Surg* 141:194, 1981.
65 Hunt TK: *Fundamentals of wound management in surgery,* South Plainfield, NJ, 1976, Chirurgecom.
66 Hunt TK, editor: *Wound healing and wound infection,* New York, 1980, Appleton-Century-Crofts.
67 Jacoby GA, Swartz MN: Fever of undetermined origin, *N Engl J Med* 289(26):1407, 1973.
68 Janevicius RV, Hann SE, Batt MD: Necrotizing fasciitis, *Surg Gynecol Obstet* 154:97, 1982.
69 Koehler PR, Knochel JQ: Computed tomography in the evaluation of abdominal abscesses, *Am J Surg* 14:675, 1980.
70 Kolb ME, Horne ML, Martz R: Dantrolene in human malignant hyperthermia, *Anesthesiology* 56:254, 1982.
71 Koretzky GA, Elias JA, Kay SL et al: Spontaneous production of interleukin-1 by human alveolar macrophages, *Clin Immunol Immunopathol* 29:443, 1983.
72 Krieger JN, Kaiser DL, Wenzel RP: Nosocomial urinary tract infections cause wound infections postoperatively in surgical patients, *Surg Gynecol Obstet* 156:313, 1983.
73 Kunin CM: Urinary tract infections, *Surg Clin North Am* 60(1):223, 1980.
74 Lansing AM, Jamieson WG: Mechanisms of fever in pulmonary atelectasis, *Arch Surg* 87:184, 1963.
75 Lepore TJ, Savran J, Van De Water J et al: Screening for lower extremity deep venous thrombosis, *Am J Surg* 135:529, 1978.
76 Levitt MA, Fleischer AS, Meislin HW: Acute post-traumatic diabetes insipidus: treatment with continuous intravenous vasopressin, *J Trauma* 24(6):532, 1984.
77 Lewis FR: Management of atelectasis and pneumonia, *Surg Clin North Am* 60(6):1391, 1980.
78 Lovejoy FH: Aspirin and acetaminophen: a comparative view of their antipyretic and analgesic activity, *Pediatrics* 62 (suppl):904, 1978.
79 Maki DG, Weise CE, Sarafin HW: A semiquantitative culture method for identifying intravenous catheter–related infection, *N Engl J Med* 296(23):1305, 1977.
80 Marsh ML, Marshall LF, Shapiro HM: Neurosurgical intensive care, *Anesthesiology* 47(2):149, 1977.
81 Mattox KL, Feldtman RW, Beall AC et al: Pulmonary embolectomy for acute massive pulmonary embolism, *Ann Surg* 195(6):726, 1982.
82 Milton AS, Wendlandt S: Effects on body temperature of prostaglandins of the A, E, and F series on injection into the third ventricle of unanesthetized cats and rabbits, *J Physiol* 218:325, 1971.
83 Mollison PL: *Blood transfusion in clinical medicine,* St Louis, 1983, Mosby.
84 Molnar GW, Read RC: Studies during open-heart surgery on the special characteristics of rectal temperature, *J Appl Physiol* 36(3):333, 1974.
85 Nelson TE, Flewellen EH: The malignant hyperthermia syndrome, *N Engl J Med* 309:416, 1983.
86 Nichols RL: Infections following gastrointestinal surgery: intra-abdominal abscess, *Surg Clin North Am* 60(1):197, 1980.
87 Orlando R, Gleason E, Drezner AD: Acute acalculous cholecystitis in the critically ill patient, *Am J Surg* 145:472, 1983.
88 Owens ML: Epidemiology of surgical wound infections, *Infect Surg* 833, 1983.
89 Pas RF: Cytomegalovirus in the surgical patient, *Infect Surg* 571, 1983.
90 Pass RF, Whitley RJ, Diethelm AG et al: Cytomegalovirus infection in patients with renal transplants: potentiation by antithymocyte globulin and an incompatible graft, *J Infect Dis* 142:9, 1980.
91 Roddy LH, Unger KM, Miller WC: Thoracic computer tomography in the critically ill patient, *Crit Care Med* 9(7):515, 1981.
92 Roe CF: Surgical aspects of fever, *Curr Probl Surg* 11:3, 1968.
93 Rosenwasser LJ, Dinarello CA: Ability of human leukocytic pyrogen to enhance phytohemagglutinin-induced murine thymocyte proliferation, *Cell Immunol* 63:134, 1981.
94 Rothman DL, Schwartz SI, Adams JT: Diagnostic laparotomy for fever or abdominal pain of unknown origin, *Am J Surg* 133:273, 1977.
95 Russell JC: Prophylaxis of postoperative deep vein thrombosis and pulmonary embolism, *Surg Gynecol Obstet* 157:80, 1983.
96 Sabiston DC: Pathophysiology, diagnosis, and management of pulmonary embolism, *Am J Surg* 138:384, 1979.
97 Sabiston DC, Spencer FC: *Gibbon's surgery of the chest,* Philadelphia, 1976, WB Saunders.
98 Sasahara AA, Sonneblick EH, Lesch M, editors: *Pulmonary emboli,* New York, 1975, Grune & Stratton.
99 Serota AI, Finegold SM: Necrotizing soft tissue infections following abdominal surgery, *Infect Surg* 50, 1982.
100 Sigal SL: Fever theory in the seventeenth century: building toward a comprehensive physiology, *Yale J Biol Med* 51:571, 1978.
101 Siler JN, Rosenberg H, Mull TD et al: Hypoxemia after upper abdominal surgery: comparison of venous admixture and ventilation/perfusion inequality components, using a digital computer, *Ann Surg* 179(2):149, 1974.
102 Simmons RL, Howard RJ, editors: *Surgical infectious diseases,* East Norwalk, Conn, 1982, Appleton-Century-Crofts.
103 Singh S, Nelson N, Acosta I et al: Catheter colonization and bacteremia with pulmonary and arterial catheters, *Crit Care Med* 10(11):736, 1982.
104 Sise MJ, Hollingsworth P, Brimm JE et al: Complications of the flow-directed pulmonary artery catheter: a prospective analysis in 219 patients, *Crit Care Med* 9(4):315, 1981.
105 Slotman GJ, Jed EH, Burchard KW: Adverse effects of hypothermia in postoperative patients, *Am J Surg* 149:495, 1985.
106 Solomkin JS, Flohr A, Simmons RL: *Candida* infections in surgical patients: dose requirements and toxicity of amphotericin B, *Ann Surg* 195(2):177, 1982.
107 Stark RP, Maki DG: Bacteriuria in the catheterized patient: what quantitative level of bacteriuria is relevant? *N Engl J Med* 311:560, 1984.
108 Stone HH, Hester TR: Incisional and peritoneal infection after emergency celiotomy, *Ann Surg* 177(6):669, 1973.
109 Talbot GH: Nosocomial pneumonia in the surgical patient, *Infect Surg* 557, 1984.
110 Thoren L: Postoperative pulmonary complications: observations on their prevention by means of physiotherapy, *Acta Chir Scand* 107:193, 1954.
111 Wenzel RP, Hunting KJ, Osterman CA: Postoperative wound infection rates, *Surg Gynecol Obstet* 144:749, 1977.
112 Winn RE, Tuttle KL, Gilbert DN: Surgical approach to extensive suppurative thrombophlebitis of the central veins of the chest, *J Thorac Cardiovasc Surg* 81:564, 1981.
113 Wood WB: The Shattuck lecture: studies on the cause of fever, *N Engl J Med* 258(21):1023, 1958.
114 Wright HK, Dunn E, MacArthur JD et al: Specific but limited roles of new imaging techniques in decision making about intra-abdominal abscesses, *Am J Surg* 143:456, 1982.
115 Yu VL: *Serratia* infection in the surgical patient, *Infect Surg* 127, 1984.

CHAPTER

3

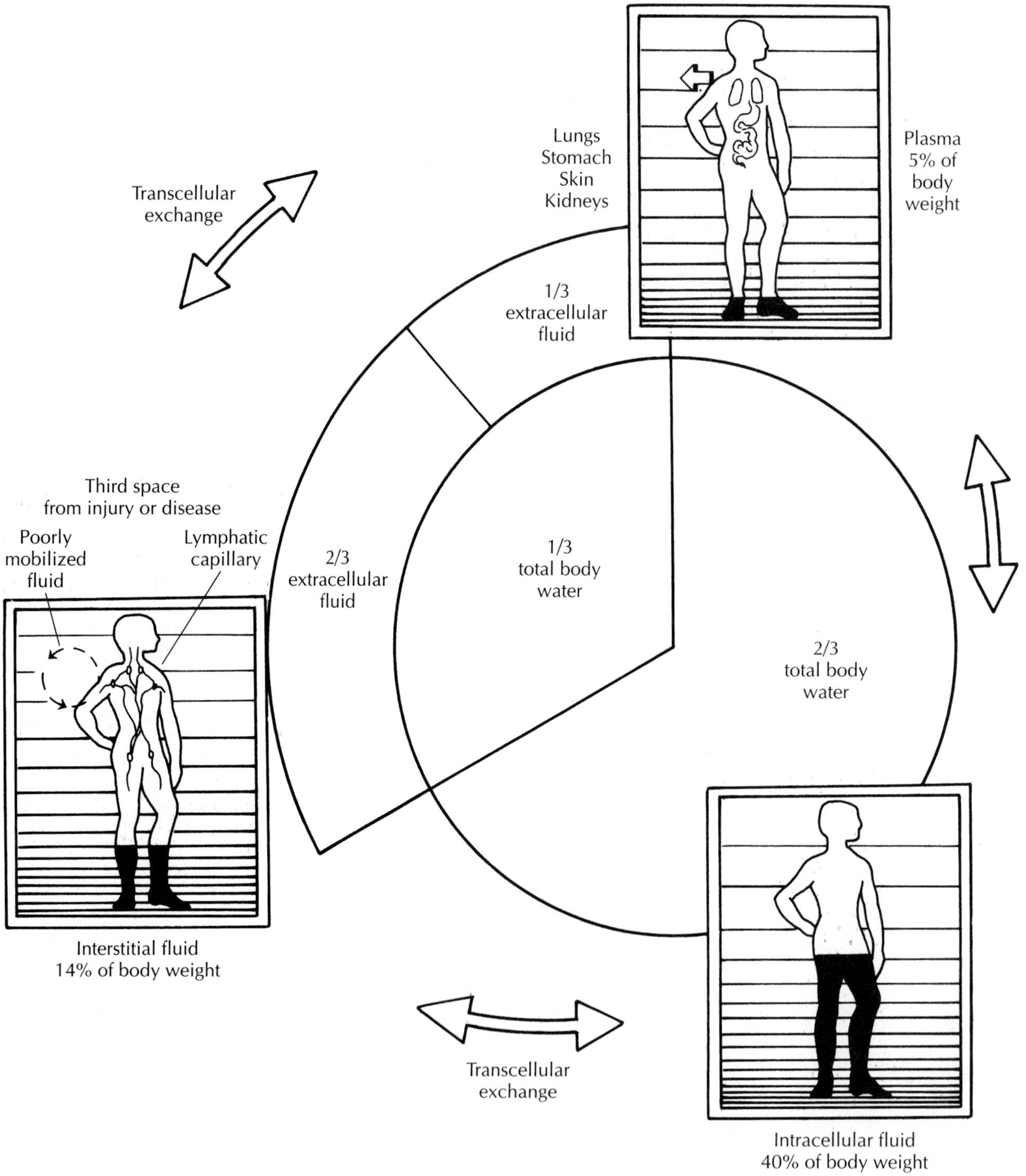
Transcellular exchange
Lungs
Stomach
Skin
Kidneys
Plasma 5% of body weight
1/3 extracellular fluid
Third space from injury or disease
Poorly mobilized fluid
Lymphatic capillary
2/3 extracellular fluid
1/3 total body water
2/3 total body water
Interstitial fluid 14% of body weight
Transcellular exchange
Intracellular fluid 40% of body weight

BODY FLUIDS AND FLUID THERAPY

Robert P. Drucker • William R. Drucker

> The biological sanctities of this solution of several simple salts is very impressive. Apparently, it not only permitted the inception of the experiment which we call life, but remains its inviolable basis.
>
> James L. Gamble, 1946

BODY FLUID

Fluid constitutes the transport system that nourishes, informs, and protects all tissues of the body. Pumped through conduits of widely divergent size, fluid flows across extracellular open spaces and enters the confines of cellular envelopes obedient to laws of physics and chemistry. Within the cell it serves as a medium for metabolic processes. Outside the cell it functions as the vehicle for delivery of substrates required for the production of energy and of the oxygen needed to metabolize these substrates effectively. It protects the cellular machinery by removing the products of metabolism, principally urea, carbon dioxide (CO_2), and heat, for dissipation into the environment surrounding the body. Simultaneously, it facilitates the neural integration of body functions by transporting hormones to receptor sites, thereby providing the principal line of communication between cells.

The conventional division of body fluid into several compartments or phases belies the reality of a system without rigid boundaries (Figure 3-1). Because the volumes of these compartments were determined by isotopic dilutions, the results reflect the behavior of these isotopes and obscure recognition of the continual movement of water and certain ions across isotopically defined boundaries.

The Milieu Intérieur and Homeostasis

> The stability of the milieu intérieur is the primary condition for freedom and independence of existence; the mechanism which allows of this is that which ensures in the milieu interieur the maintenance of all the conditions necessary to the life of the elements.
>
> Claude Bernard, 1878

> This theory of the constancy of the milieu intérieur was an induction from relatively few facts, but the discoveries of the last fifty years and the introduction of physico-chemical methods into physiology have proved that it is well founded.
>
> Lawrence Henderson, 1913

The concept of a constant internal environment, first clearly enunciated by the great French physiologist, Claude Bernard, drew heavily on the observations and deductions of Charles Darwin regarding the survival of the fittest in each species.[22] Although it was not artic-

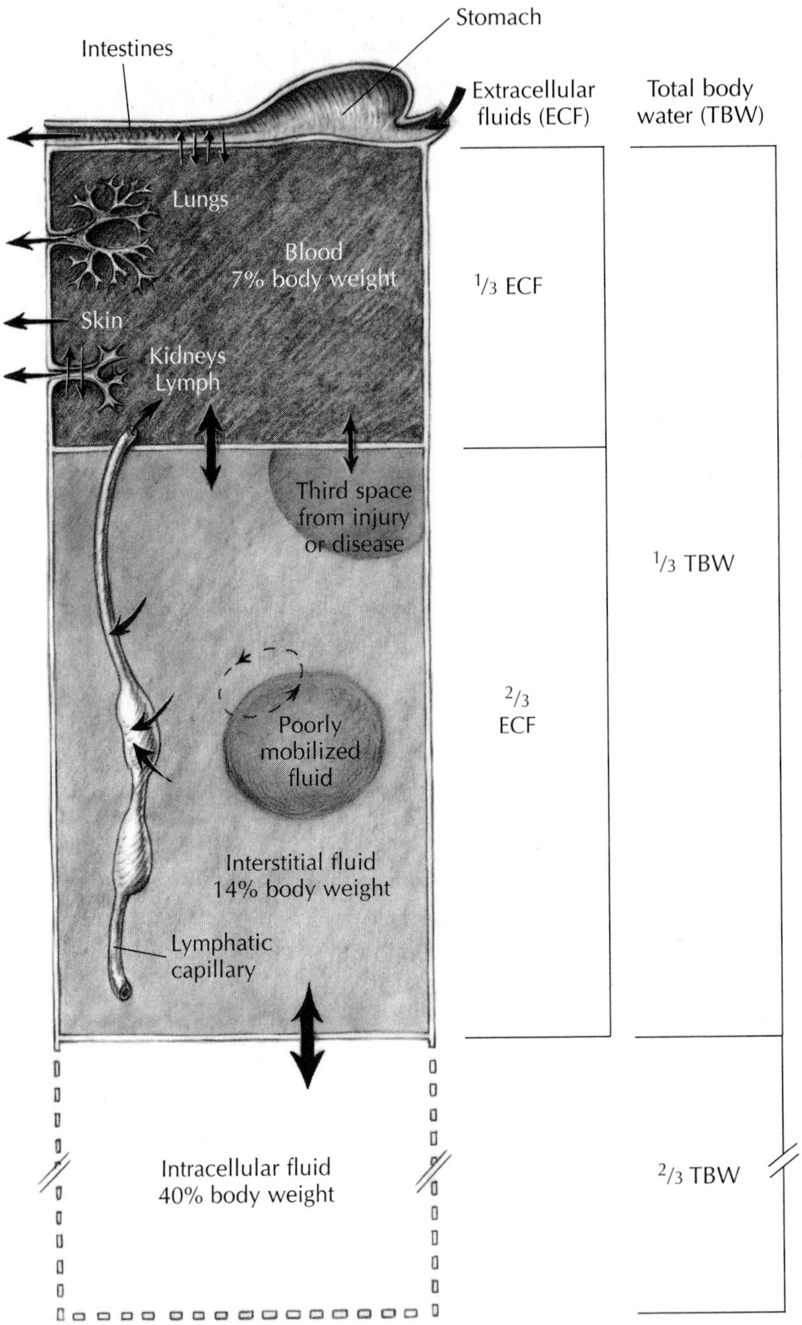

FIGURE 3-1 Exchange of fluid across compartments.

ulated clearly, the idea that an internal sea of salt water is essential for human existence was applied by Latta and O'Shaunessey 50 years earlier when they treated cholera victims by administration of salt solutions.[62,85] However, it was Bernard, writing just after the United States dissolved into the bitter Civil War, who recognized that higher animals lived in two very different environments: a milieu exterieur in which the body resides and "a milieu intérieur" in which the tissue elements live. As he stated, "The circulation of the blood forms a true organic environment, intermediary between the external environment in which the individual as a whole lives and the molecules of the living cells which would otherwise not come into direct relationship with the external environment."[15] Theodor Schwann, working in the laboratory of Johannes Miller in 1839, had introduced the concept of the cell as the basic unit of tissue structure.[21] Based on earlier studies of the chemistry of blood and tissues, Bernard conceived of a sea with approximately constant content of water and salt and organic matter bathing all cells to provide the environment necessary for their survival. Another 50 years passed before the concept was clearly elucidated that the constancy of this milieu intérieur is protected by multiple intrinsic mechanisms. The success in preserving vital physiologic processes during adversity was termed *homeostasis* by Walter Cannon, the professor of physiology at Harvard.[17]

> The coordinated physiological processes which maintain most of the steady states in the organism are so complex and so peculiar to living beings—involving as they may, the brain and nerves, the heart, lungs, kidneys and spleen, all working cooperatively—that I have suggested a special designation for these states, *homeostasis*.
>
> Walter Cannon, 1939

Physiologic thinking subsequently has been led by the concept that fitness for survival is directly related to the capacity of an organism to maintain homeostasis. No area in biology has benefited more demonstrably from direct application of this concept than has the study of mechanisms supporting homeostasis of the milieu intérieur; the extracellular fluid (ECF) aided by the circulation is the true milieu of life because it bathes the cells of the body.

Circulation of Body Fluids

Within the body, fluids are in a state of dynamic equilibrium; any deviation from the norm is corrected rapidly by internal adjustments mediated by the neural, endocrine, and circulatory systems.[26,102,112] The burden of maintaining constancy of body fluids falls on the kidney and the extrarenal control mechanisms that affect kidney function. The adjustments are accompanied by an appropriate increase or decrease in renal excretion of water. Overall, the volume of fluid in the body is controlled to maintain an optimal circulation. Volume regulation per se has no intrinsic value, but in terms of providing a circulation adapted to the changing demands of the organism, the regulation of circulatory volume assumes the primary homeostatic priority.[16,92]

Any condition that interferes with the circulatory volume promotes a prompt alteration to protect the existing blood volume without regard to other priorities for homeostasis. Also, when the circulatory volume is depleted, the kidney cannot regulate disturbances in osmolality by excretion of the relative excess of water, or alternatively, of sodium. Thus regulation to preserve normovolemia must dominate osmoregulation. However, the osmoreceptor is exquisitely sensitive. When the intrinsic defense mechanisms are forced to make a choice among regulation of circulatory volume, solute content, and composition of body fluids, the defense of circulatory volume always wins. Once this essential fact is understood, many of the apparent enigmas of electrolyte and fluid balance become comprehensible.[30,94]

The stimuli for volume regulation are linked with changes in flow and pressure in the heart arterial system.[16] Clearly, an understanding of fluid and electrolyte balance requires a firm appreciation of the anatomy, function, and regulation of the circulatory system, which distributes blood and its essential substrates to the tissues and removes the by-products of metabolism.

Acting together, the endocrine, nervous, and circulatory systems constitute the principal coordinating and integrating mechanism in the body. A study of fluid physiology goes a step beyond control of the fluid that passes through the circulatory system to consider the circulation of the fluid across the barrier and membranes that separate the vascular and perivascular spaces from the environment external to the body and from the internal environment of the interstitial fluid and the cell. Because life as we know it is cellular, the primary concern for fluid physiology relates to the mechanisms that support a constant internal environment in the presence of losses and gains of fluids and electrolytes and disturbances of cellular function by disease.

Compartments

A century ago, Carl Voit, professor of physiology at the University of Munich and a former student of Liebig, advanced the concept that not only the milieu intérieur but also the total water content of the body retains a constant relationship to body weight.[117] When allowance was made for fat, about 70% to 75% of the lean body mass was estimated to be water. Pace and Rathbun,[86] using the specific-gravity technique that had been developed by the US Navy physiologist Albert Behnke for measuring proportion of fat in the body, confirmed and extended his studies of water content to demonstrate in guinea pigs that nitrogen, as well as water contents of the body, are remarkably constant. However, Moultin,[77] confirming earlier studies of the human fetus, found that the amount of water as a percentage of lean body mass decreases after birth until chemical maturity is reached, while a reciprocal change occurs in the amount of nitrogen.

Harrison and colleagues,[50] the harbingers of clinicians dedicated to the study of fundamental biologic problems, drew on these results in their investigations that led to the concept that the high water content of the fetus is a result of the relatively high extracellular phase. They found that with growth of the fetus, the increasing cellular mass retains a constant cellular composition, including the concentration of potassium, whereas the amount of extracellular fluid decreases and fat increases relative to total body weight. Extending these studies by using chloride (Cl^-) as an index of extracellular fluid volume, they calculated that the distribution of fluid between extracellular and intracellular phases also attains a relatively constant balance in healthy animals after birth. These fundamental studies, confirmed by others using many different substances thought to be distributed only in ECF, constitute the basis for our current concept: the water content of each tissue is divided into two main compartments—intracellular and extracellular. Although the distribution varies widely among tissues, it is reasonably constant for any one tissue (see Figure 3-1).

Extracellular Fluid

ECF is readily defined as all body water external to cells. Based on the pioneering studies of ECF volume, today we think that approximately two thirds of body water is contained in cells. Of the fluid remaining in the extracellular spaces, one third is within the vascular system and two thirds reside in the interstitial spaces located between the vascular system and the cells of tissues (see Figure 3-1). Based on more modern techniques using heavy water (D_2O), Schloerb and colleagues[100] calculated total body water to be only 60% of body weight in men and closer to 50% in women because of the slightly greater amount of anhydrous adipose tissue normally present in women.

Interstitial volume, which cannot be measured directly, is calculated as the difference between total ECF and intravascular volume. As an example for clinical purposes, one can readily estimate that a healthy 70 kg man has about 42 L of total body water. Two thirds of this fluid, or 28 L, resides within cells, whereas 14 L is in the extracellular "compartment." Slightly less than 5 L constitutes the plasma volume, and the residue of the 14 L of ECF is moving through the interstitial spaces. ECF fluid external to the circulating blood, termed *interstitial fluid,* moves in several directions. Not only is there a continuous rapid exchange between plasma and interstitial fluid across the capillaries and a rapid flux of fluid into and out of cells—"fast extracellular fluid"—there also is a large exchange of isotonic fluid across the bowel wall, which probably exceeds in daily volume the entire ECF volume.[30] Less rapid exchanges of fluid occur with the cerebrospinal fluid and the pleural and peritoneal spaces—*transcellular fluid.* An appreciable quantity of interstitial fluid returns to the plasma via the lymphatics.

Isotopic studies also indicate that a small amount of interstitial fluid is relatively immobile, such as fluid within synovial spaces, matrices of bone, and cartilage (see Figure 3-1). In certain disorders these small "satellite" circulations may become a serious threat to fluid balance. For instance, impaired return or increased loss of fluid from the capillaries, as in intestinal obstruction, peritonitis, or blunt trauma, may lead to sequestration in a "third space" (i.e., gut, pleura, peritoneum, or swollen, injured cells, with corresponding reduction in *effective* circulating volume).[30,48,61,106]

Transcapillary Fluid Exchange: Starling Forces

The anatomy of the ECF clearly divides it into two separate compartments, the plasma and interstitial fluid, with generally similar composition of electrolytes. Almost a century has passed since the brilliant English physiologist, Sir Ernest Starling, developed the hypothesis governing the exchange of solutes and water between these components of extracellular fluid. Experience has validated the concept that the differential between the forces of osmotic and hydrostatic pressure within the capillary and in the interstitial fluid are primarily responsible for both the filtration and reabsorption of solutes and water across the capillary. Today, however, it is clear that many other factors also influence this exchange.

Although a detailed consideration of the Starling forces is beyond the scope of this chapter, it is important to emphasize that capillary exchange is a more complex process than indicated by the original Starling equation. For instance, there is a difference in osmotic pressure between the two solutions, separated by the capillary membrane, to which the impermeable solute particles and the asymmetrically distributed diffusible ions contribute. This effect described by F.G. Donnan in 1924 has subsequently been amplified to embrace an osmotic reflection coefficient (of Staverman), which varies with the anatomic configuration of the capillary in different locations. This quantitative measure of the difference between the theoretical and actual values of osmotic pressure is also influenced by drugs, hormones, and circulating metabolic products. A filtration coefficient has been derived to emphasize the differences that can occur in transcapillary exchange between different organs and regions of the body (see box).

Today, as a consequence of the intense interest by electron microscopists in this important aspect of body fluid physiology, a consensus has developed about capillary and lymphatic ultrastructure.[18] A broad spectrum of substances are transported across different capillary walls, ranging from water and a few monosaccharides and amino acids crossing the "tight" endothelium of the central nervous system to the very "leaky" hepatic sinusoids, which permit the passage of chylomicrons up to 200 nm in diameter. The endothelial permeability is specific for each tissue. In addition to leaks via the clefts between adjacent cells for passage of ions and water, several other endothelial pathways are characteristic for individual capillary beds through which fluid, small solutes, and proteins are transported passively.[122]

Many control systems serve the primary goal of maintaining cardiac output and blood pressure. It is clear, however, that in meeting this task they have a significant

STARLING STAVERMAN EQUATION

$$J_v = K_f(P_c - P_i) - \sigma(\pi_c - \pi_i)$$

J_v is the net water flux across capillary walls; filtration has a positive value, and reabsorption has a negative value.

σ is Staverman's osmotic reflection coefficient, which varies among capillary beds with differing structural and functional characteristics. This value can be changed by drugs, hormones, or endogenous metabolites that alter the permeability of capillaries for macromolecules.

K_f is the filtration coefficient, which, like σ, may vary among different capillary beds. It can be modified by many physiologic changes: arterial and venous blood pressure, arterial tone, activity of precapillary sphincters, and interstitial fluid pressure.

Adapted from Seldin DW, Giebison G, editors: *The regulation of sodium and chloride balance*, New York, 1990, Raven Press.

influence on Starling forces and thereby on the distribution of ECF. A key element in appreciating the influences of neurohumoral agents on the distribution of ECF is that the capillary, the site of fluid exchange between plasma and interstitial fluid, is not directly innervated. Thus the major influences are through alterations in vascular constriction, dilatation, and permeability or through interaction with other hormones. For example, significant influence on transcapillary fluid exchange have been found for hormones serving the autonomic nervous system, vasoconstrictor peptides, bradykinin, histamine, arginine vasopressin (ADH), ecinosoids, and the atrial natriuretic factor.

Lymph

In the course of his studies on the coagulation of blood, Hewson (1739-1774) extended his search to include fluid in the serous cavities and in the lymphatic vessels.[49] The finding that these fluids circulated like blood ultimately led to his concept of the formation of tissue fluid. Many scholars think that this concept ranks close to the discovery of the circulation for its importance in physiology.[21] Hewson considered that the fluids in the serous cavities, interstitial spaces, and lymph vessels were all derived from blood. He postulated that pores exist in the capillary walls to provide the requisite semipermeability for escape of fluid. Writing just before the American Revolution and two centuries before the structure of capillaries and lymphatics were clarified by electron microscopy, this insightful man made his many contributions to science before the age of 35 years when he died from an infection contracted during a dissection. Obviously, his concept of fluid exchange in the peripheral tissues was a necessary prelude to the development a century later of Bernard's concept of the milieu intérieur.

It is now clear that more fluid is filtered out of the capillaries than is reabsorbed; the volume difference is returned to the circulation through the lymphatic channels. This system is a dynamic part of the circulation of extracellular fluid. Within a 24-hour period the volume of fluid transported through the lymphatics is almost equivalent to the total plasma volume, slightly in excess of 4.5% of body weight. About one quarter to one half of the total quantity of circulating plasma protein is returned to the plasma by daily lymph flow.

The interstitial fluid destined for lymphatic return is led passively through minute interstitial channels that link the blood capillaries and lymphatics. The ultrastructure of these channels, beautifully described by Casley-Smith,[18] constitutes a continuous network throughout all capillary beds, being organized in a loosely connected, semirandom manner. The fine structure of lymphatic capillaries resembles the blood capillaries as a tube, albeit with marked irregularities of lumen; they have a continuous linking of endothelial cells.[18]

William Hunter, speaking from his profound knowledge of gross anatomy, had declared unequivocally shortly before the American Revolution that lymphatic vessels function as "the absorbing vessels" all over the body.[46] A century and a half later in the 1920s and 1930s, Cecil Drinker and his colleagues at Harvard used tiny glass tubes to cannulate lymphatic vessels for physiologic studies.[27] These studies provided support for the concept of fluid return to the venous blood via the lymphatic (absorbing) vessels. The mechanism for fluid entry into the lymphatics is thought to involve a phasic pressure gradient that is positive for inward flow of fluid for at least part of the contractile cycle of the lymph capillary.[27]

Interstitial fluid has at least three routes to enter the lumen of the ("closed") lymphatic capillaries: direct transport across the endothelial cells as free fluid, transport through vesicles, or transport via intercellular junctions. When the interstitial fluid load increases or after injury, the path between cells assumes greater significance and allows more fluid and larger molecules to enter the various channels.

Within the lymphatic system the central movement of fluid is influenced by many intrinsic and extrinsic forces. Of particular importance for the concepts of fluid physiology was the demonstration by Pullinger and Florey[91] (the latter perhaps better known for his work with penicillin) of anchoring fibers that exert a centrifugal pull on the lymph capillary. These fibers maintain patency of the lymph capillary when interstitial pressure is increased by an increase of fluid in the space. Thus return of lymph to the circulation is increased rather than obstructed when the interstitial pressure rises to positive values.[46] This return of lymph is a protection against the development of edema. Because of the anchoring fibers, lymph can flow effectively through the interstitium over a pressure range from the usual negative value of −7 mm Hg until the pressure reaches +2 mm Hg.

A competent system of valves necessary for a unidirectional flow of lymph was described initially by Rudbeck, professor of anatomy in Uppsala, in 1653, the same year that Bartholin in Copenhagen named the lymphatic system.[12,105] Contractility of the vessel supplemented by muscle activity, transmitted pulsations from closely adjacent blood vessels, respiratory movement plus the cyclic and opposite variation between intrathoracic and abdominal pressure, and changes in posture all contribute to the forward flow of lymph. Physical activity further increases the influence of extrinsic factors on this flow. The ultimate return of lymph to the venous system probably involves multiple communications, which become functional in disease or when lymphatic pressure rises. These "potential" channels and the well-recognized channels communicating between the renal and lymphatic vessels are supplemental to the large right lymphatic and large left thoracic (lymph) ducts that enter the subclavian veins. It is unlikely that a significant volume of lymph returns to the blood via lymph nodes.

The dynamics of peripheral fluid exchange are so rapid that the daily volume probably is greatly in excess of the 16 to 18 L of fluid reabsorbed into the circulation through the capillaries and the 2 to 4 L returned via the lymphatics, which was originally estimated by Landis and Pappenheimer.[61] In addition to its important role in the immune system, this circulation of lymph supports the homeostasis of transcapillary fluid exchange. The interstitial fluid and lymph flow probably function to a limited extent as a buffer for the circulatory system. It is clear that the lymphatics not only assist in the ordinary return of fluid to the venous system, but also they help to protect against the formation of edema with fluid overload. Furthermore, the lymphatic circulation may be viewed as being qualitatively important in supporting capillary exchange in restoration of circulatory volume after blood loss.[18,19,46,61] However, the volume receptors that regulate the renal excretion of salt and water are located within the vascular tree, not in the interstitial space.

Perhaps the primary function of lymph is to support the integrity of both interstitial and intravascular colloid osmotic pressures as Starling forces. For example, if the lymphatic system fails to maintain a low concentration of interstitial protein, the gradient of protein oncotic pressure between interstitium and plasma cannot be maintained. Consequently, the countercurrent mechanism of the kidneys fails, which is reflected by the kidneys' inability to concentrate urine when lymph drainage is blocked.[46] In this manner lymph has a vital role in support of hemostasis of circulatory volume.

Cells

Two thirds of body water is contained within cells, but only under extreme circumstances of hypovolemia may this fluid become available to defend circulatory volume. Cells are not directed to support the homeostasis of extracellular fluid; rather, the ultimate purpose of extracellular fluid is to nourish and protect the cells and to remove the waste products of their metabolism. Cellular metabolism is directed to the production and use of energy—life. Although cellular volume responds to alterations in the extracellular osmotic concentration, cells are equipped to protect their volume and thereby support a stable intracellular environment for metabolic activity. It is the extracellular fluid aided by the circulation that is the true milieu of life because it bathes the cells of the body.

Composition of Body Fluids

An appreciation of the influence of solutes on the exchange of fluids between compartments had been developing since Hewson's studies with the red globules of blood in the 1770s[49] and the pioneering scientific measurement of osmosis by Dutrochet in Paris and Thomas Graham in London in the early 1800s.[32,47] About this time Michael Faraday made his fundamental contribution to our concepts of fluid exchanges throughout the body by discovering that an electric current passed through a solution of hydrochloric acid (HCl) separated molecules into negatively and positively charged particles.[34] Free chloride with a negative charge (Cl^-) moved to the point of entry of the current, the anode, and free hydrogen with a positive charge (H^+) moved to the point of exit, the cathode. He termed a solute that could dissociate to conduct electricity an *electrolyte* and named the electrically charged atoms *ions.* Anions carried a negative charge to the anode, whereas cations carried a positive charge to the cathode. Applying these results to the study of plasmolysis in plants, he found that equimolar solutions of dissimilar solutes did not necessarily provide the same osmotic pressure. A molar solution of electrolytes such as sodium chloride (NaCl) produced twice the osmotic pressure of a molar solution of sucrose or mannitol.

The significance of Faraday's studies for movement of biologic fluids was not fully appreciated until 50 years later when Svante Arrhenius[9] at the Physical Chemistry Institute of Uppsala University published his theory of electrolytic dissociation in 1887. He explained the anomalous osmotic pressures Faraday had found for solutions of electrolytes with the hypothesis that passage of an electric current is not required for the ions to dissociate in the solution. His concept of the spontaneous dissociation of electrolytes in water was firmly established after he demonstrated that passage of an electric current did not alter the osmotic pressure of a solution of an electrolyte.[21]

Discovery that each element of a dissociated molecule had an osmotic force equivalent to the nondissociated parent molecule provided the necessary foundation for studies that led to the current concept that cellular volume is directly related to the osmotic pressure of its surrounding fluids. It also led to the monumental work of another clinical scientist, James Gamble, Professor of Pediatrics, who stimulated two generations of students by the originality of his studies and the clarity of his instruction.[42] Working with Ross and Tisdall at Harvard, he applied the Arrhenius theory of electrolytic dissociation to functional concepts of the chemical structure of body fluids.[43] The basis of his teaching was the concept that the chemical structure of ECF is determined by ions, each of which is controlled separately. To preserve electric neutrality, the concentration of cations must be balanced by the total concentration of anions. Because the salts of sodium constitute more than 95% of the solutes in ECF, it became apparent that the concentration of the sodium ion should play a critical role in fluid balance. Gamble reasoned that intracellular fluid (ICF), which could not be measured directly, should have an equivalent concentration of osmotically active cations and anions to preserve osmotic neutrality across the semipermeable cellular membrane. The finding of a slightly greater number of ions within muscle cells than in plasma was interpreted as a reflection of more polyvalent intracellular anions that protected electric equivalence without disturbing the molecular concentration. The cell also contains nondissociable proteinates of magnesium.[42]

The excitement that began in this era for discovery of fundamental concepts of body fluids is reflected by the multidisciplinary talents that became engaged in these studies. Working independently, Wallace Fenn, a physiologist; Baird Hastings, a biochemist; and H.E. Harrison, a pediatrician, used calculated corrections for the component of ECF in their measurement of electrolytes in muscle tissue.[36,50,52] Their results uniformly supported Gamble's estimation that the distribution of the concentration of base between muscle cells and ECF is very similar to its distribution between erythrocytes and plasma. Gamble had found that the acidosis of fasting resulted from a loss of sodium (Na^+) and potassium (K^+) ("fixed base") in the urine with a corresponding loss of body water.[43] This volumetric agreement in loss of salt and water suggested that the concentration of total fixed base was the same in the ICF and ECF compartments, with water being capable of diffusing freely across the cell membranes that separate the compartments.

These observations made it possible to assume the following:

1. There are no absolute barriers to the movement of water between compartments. Consequently, there is osmotic equilibrium among all phases of body fluids including plasma, interstitial, and intracellular spaces.
2. In contrast to inorganic ions and small molecules, the large protein molecules do not move across the capillary wall of most tissues. This lack of movement results in a slight disequilibrium in the distribution of the small inorganic ions according to the forces of the Gibbs-Donnan equation.
3. Cellular and extracellular water have similar properties (osmolality), but they differ markedly in the composition of their constituent solutes. In particular, sodium and chloride are considered to be largely absent from the ICF, whereas most potassium is contained within cells.

Hastings and Eichelberger[53] used these assumptions to make their calculations of the content and distribution of water among the compartments in muscle. They also found that an intravenous injection of a large volume of isotonic saline solution, which did not alter the acid-base balance, increased the volume of ECF in muscles without changing the size of muscle cells. This in vivo study provided confirmation of the concept that cell volume remains constant if the osmotic pressure of the ECF is not altered. The results added further evidence to support Gamble's concept of isosmolarity of all phases of body fluids.[42]

DEFENSE OF HOMEOSTASIS

Because life as we know it is cellular, the primary concern for fluid physiology relates to the mechanisms that support a constant internal environment in the presence of stress. The literature on this subject is so vast that in the interest of presenting a relatively concise orientation to current concepts, no attempt is made to credit many brilliant investigators who have contributed to our understanding of body fluids.

It is clear that the migration of living creatures from brackish water to dry land required a means of obtaining and conserving water. Perhaps surprisingly, the reptile was the first terrestrial vertebrate to obtain water by drinking it and absorbing it through the alimentary canal.[10] This section considers the mechanisms that control the fluid that is absorbed.

The Kidney

Man is provided with distinct mechanisms for the regulation of the amount as well as the composition of body fluids.

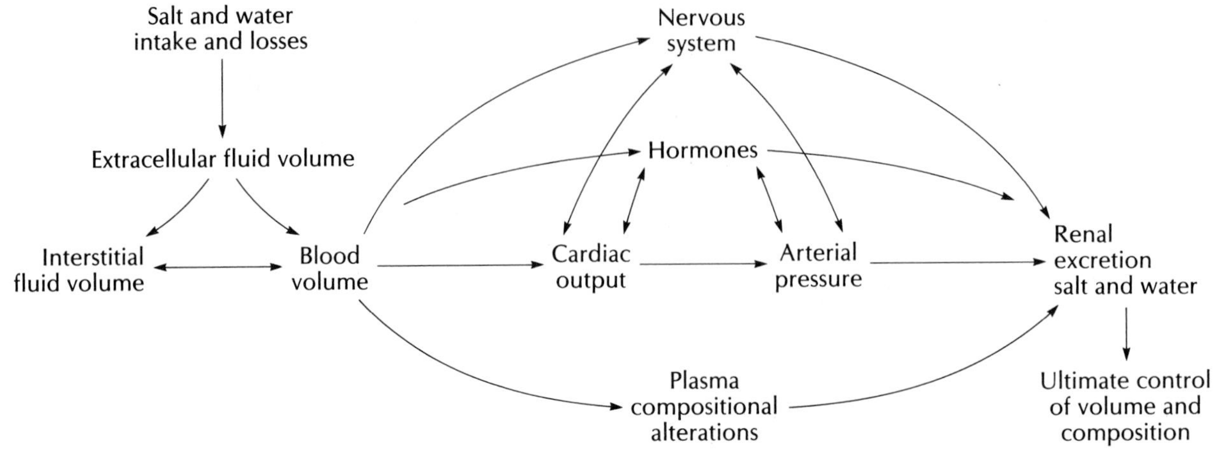

FIGURE 3-2 Systems controlling extracellular fluid volume. (Modified from Navar LG: Renal regulation of body fluid balance. In Staub NC, Taylor AE, editors: *Edema,* New York, 1984, Raven Press.)

> Thirst and appetite under the regulation of the central nervous system and the kidneys under the influence of circulatory, hormonal, and possibly neurogenic factors, subserve this office.
>
> Maurice Strauss, 1958

Because the composition of the milieu intérieur is determined not so much by what is randomly taken in, but rather by what is retained and what is excreted, the kidney is properly viewed as the prime organ for maintaining the constancy of the internal environment.[112] The kidney not only regulates the quantity of water, ions, and many solutes in the body in response to wide variations of intake and loss, but also is the ultimate arbiter of acid-base balances. It secretes two important hormones, erythropoietin and renin, as well as dihydroxycholecalciferol, the final and active metabolite of vitamin D. It also contributes to the production of prostaglandins.

The capacity of the kidney to respond rapidly and in an appropriate manner to deviations in the volume, solute content, and composition of body fluids is determined by changes in the glomerular filtration rate (GFR) or tubular resorption. These renal mechanisms respond to at least four groups of extrarenal signals: (1) hemodynamic factors such as perfusion pressure and renal blood flow; (2) neural activity directly to the kidney or indirectly to other systems influencing renal function; (3) alterations in the composition of the blood involving solute, specific ions, or the hematocrit (Hct); and (4) hormones[81] (Figure 3-2).

There are two fundamental seemingly paradoxical concepts regarding the critical role of the kidney to control extracellular fluid volume and tonicity. The excretion or retention of water is regulated to maintain a normal concentration of salt in body fluids, and the amount of salt in these fluids is regulated to protect the appropriate proportion of water in the body. Thus the volume of ECF depends on regulation of the quantity of total body sodium.[102] This reflects the virtual confinement of sodium and its attendant anions to the extracellular spaces. These ions, being the principal osmotic components of ECF, determine its volume. In determining ECF volume, sodium regulates circulatory volume. The kidney has a key role—it adjusts the excretion of sodium in response to volume stimuli to protect the homeostasis of extracellular volume, with its component, the circulatory volume.

In addition, the concentration of sodium (osmolality) in ECF is determined by water balance. The mechanisms to maintain isosmolality involve ADH, thirst, and renal concentration or dilution of urine. Acting in concert, these three mechanisms change the volume of water in which the body solutes are dispersed within and outside the cell. The stimulus to these mechanisms is the level of plasma osmolality. As illustrated in Figure 3-3, starting at 280 mOsm/kg there is a linear relationship between the rise in plasma osmolality and levels of ADH in the plasma. Thirst is stimulated to help defend plasma osmolality after the plasma level rises above 290 mOsm/kg. Because the defense of extracellular tonicity is so precise, it is reasonable to conclude that the quantity of sodium rather than its concentration determines the volume of ECF. This important concept explains why either hypernatremia or hyponatremia can occur with increased, decreased, or no change in volume of ECF. That is, osmolality of the ECF is not a reliable index of ECF volume. Clinical assessment remains the best guide to alterations in the volume of ECF.

Although more detailed discussion of renal physiology is beyond the intent of this chapter, no discussion of fluid physiology could be considered adequate with-

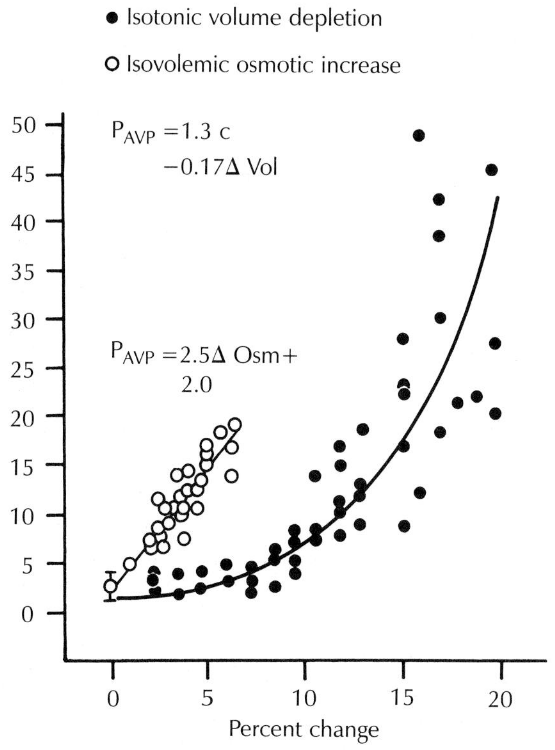

FIGURE 3-3 Relationship of plasma AVP to percentage of change in plasma osmolality *(open circles)* and to volume depletion *(solid circles)*. (From Dunn FL, Brennan TJ, Nelson AE et al: *J Clin Invest* 52:3213, 1973, The American Society for Clinical Investigation.)

out at least noting the fundamental contributions to this subject resulting from: (1) the micropuncture technique for study of glomerular and tubular fluid developed by Robert Chambers, A.N. Richards, and Joseph Wearn; (2) the quantitative studies using clearance methods in normal and diseased kidneys conducted by P.B. Rehberg, Homer Smith, and James Shannon; and (3) the conceptual stimuli of A.R. Cushney (1866-1926), the father of the modern view of renal physiology.[106]

Control of Cellular Water

Today, it is clear that one of the fundamental properties of cells is their capacity to regulate their volume.[69] For many years it was thought that cells behave like perfect osmometers, with cell water acting like a solvent. Approximately 70% to 75% of total cellular weight is water, which under normal physiologic circumstances remains constant in volume. Because the characteristics of the cellular envelope endow it with free permeability for water, maintenance of a constant cellular volume must require that either the activities of water (total concentration of solutes) are the same on both sides of the cell or metabolic energy is expended to create and maintain a difference in water activity across the plasma membrane. The consensus among most students of this problem is that cellular and extracellular water have similar osmolalities. Consequently, as long as the cellular content of solute remains constant, cellular volume is regulated by the osmolality of ECF (Figure 3-4). Ordinarily, this regulation is very precise and involves primarily thirst and ADH mechanisms (Figure 3-5). In health, the ECF osmolality varies no more than 1% from 287 mOsm/kg H_2O.[69,94,95]

However, maintenance of a normal steady-state content of cellular osmoles is a continuous energy-dependent process as indicated by the weight gain Krebs observed when tissue slices were placed in an isotonic medium under anaerobic conditions.[108] Some of the energy is consumed by preserving the integrity of large organic molecules. If cellular metabolism is impaired, these molecules are degraded rapidly into numerous smaller molecules, which, if they remain within the cell, cause a rapid increase in cellular osmolality.[70] The "cloudy swelling" of injured tissue can be explained in part on this basis. Contrary to this view, Mudge[78] found that swelling is caused by solutes entering the cell with a relatively greater increase of sodium than loss of potassium.

Unquestionably, cellular energy is required to maintain osmotic equilibrium across the cell membrane. It may be used to preserve the asymmetric distribution of the "bases" or "alkali" ions, K^+ and Na^+, between the cells rich in K^+ and ECF in which Na^+ is the dominant cation. The large cellular organic molecules that do not cross the plasma membrane create an osmotic force to draw ECF into the cell despite similar osmolality on both sides of the membrane. Furthermore, the intracellular organic macromolecules, by possessing an electric charge, attract "counterions" to preserve electroneutrality (Donnan excess), which adds to the osmotic force of these impermeable proteins. To offset this force, according to a theory proposed independently by Leaf and Wilson, two investigators at Harvard, there may be a "pump leak" in the cell membrane.[64,121]

This viable concept considers that Na^+, which easily gains entrance into the cell, is actively transported back to the surrounding interstitial fluid against both an electric and a chemical concentration gradient (see Figure 3-4). Lacking the coupling of this movement to an energy dissipating internal flux of another ion of solute or water, the outward movement of Na^+ must be coupled to energy metabolism. Through this mechanism, which makes the cellular membrane effectively impermeable to sodium, an extracellular osmotic pressure is created that offsets the swelling force of the nonpermeable cellular colloid solutes and their associated counterions. Diffusible anions, such as chloride, are largely excluded from the cell because of the electronegativity of ICFs.

According to this concept, under normal physiologic

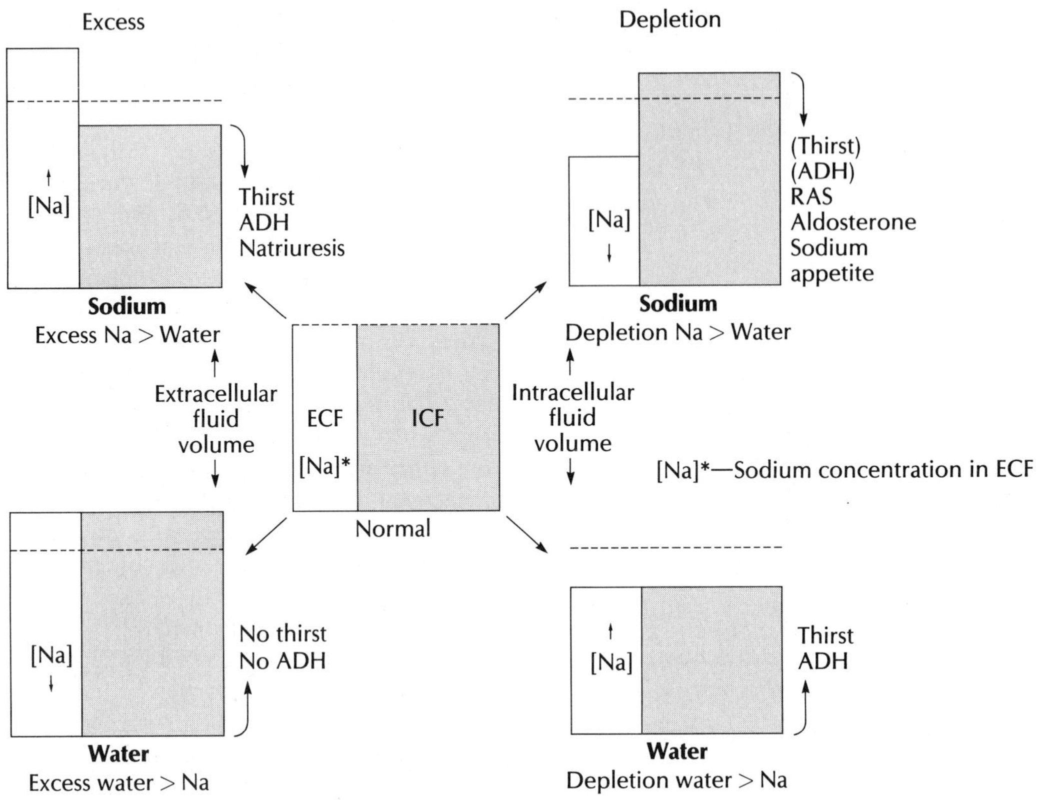

FIGURE 3-4 Changes in body fluid distribution and extracellular Na^+ during positive and negative sodium and H_2O balance. *ADH,* Antidiuretic hormone; *RAS,* renin-angiotensin system. (Modified from Andersson B, Leksell LG, Rundgren M: Regulation of body fluids: intake and output. In Staub NC, Taylor AE, editors: *Edema,* New York, 1984, Raven Press.)

conditions the total osmolality of fluid in metabolizing cells is the same as in the ECF. Also, there is no difference in the hydrostatic pressure between cells and the fluid that surrounds them (see Figure 3-4).

Controversy persists, however, about the mechanisms responsible for the cellular exclusion of sodium. The concept of a sodium-potassium pump that uses the cardiac glycoside-sensitive enzyme, Na^+, K^+-ATPase, is still favored. Inhibition of tissue metabolism, which can be accomplished simply by cooling, causes a net gain of intracellular solute with cellular swelling. The process is reversed by rewarming the tissue. There is now some evidence, however, at least in renal tissue, for a second sodium pump that also depends on metabolic energy but is insensitive to cardiac glycosides. Furthermore, ultrastructural studies of liver tissue have added a third possibility of cellular organelles, which may account for ouabain-resistant regulation of cellular volume. In all instances, exclusion of sodium is central to the regulation of a constant and normal cellular volume.

It is also clear that extrusion of sodium is not an absolute process because the cellular sodium concentration varies in accord with the extracellular concentration of sodium and the pH of the interstitium. This mechanism serves homeostasis by helping to modulate changes in cellular volume in response to pathologic alterations in the osmolality of ECF. For instance, when extracellular hyperosmolality develops, the influx of sodium is increased. In the new steady state, the cell has a higher than usual solute content and experiences a smaller decrease in volume than expected from the increase in extracellular osmolality (see Figure 3-4). An opposite sequence occurs in the presence of hypoosmolality in the ECF.

Control of Osmolality of Body Fluids

Perhaps the first recorded interest in a balance between the intake and output of fluids is credited to the writings of Celsius in the first century AD.[107] In his book *De Medicina,* he recommended measurement of fluid intake and urine excretion as indices of good health. It was not until after the Dark Ages that a graduate from the School of Medicine at Padua, Sanctorius, who was also a friend of Galileo, professor of physics, suggested that an "invisible perspiration" accounted for the usually smaller output than intake of fluid.[72] As one of the instigators of physical measurements in studies of biologic problems (owing to his association with Galileo), Sanctorius con-

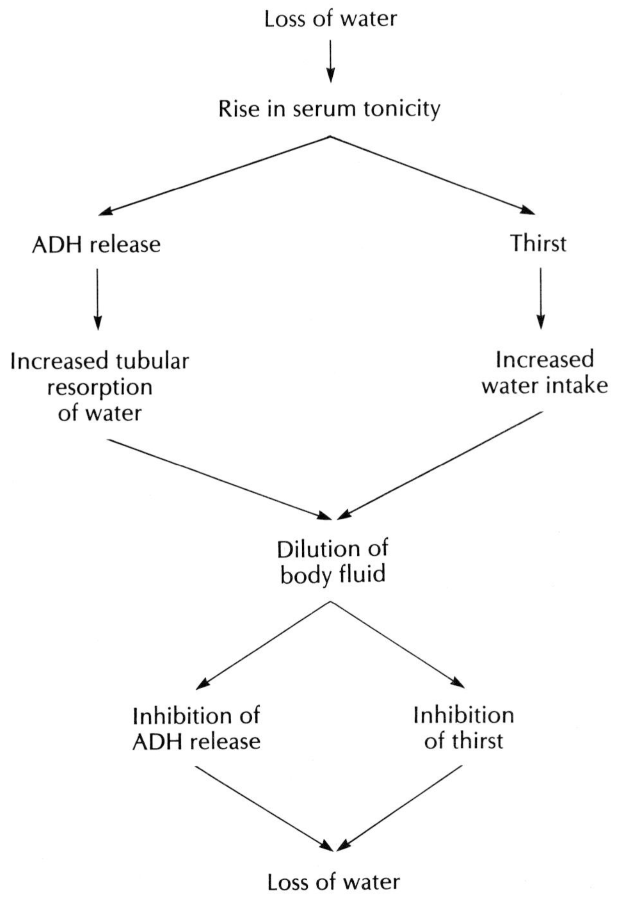

FIGURE 3-5 Regulation of concentration of body fluids. (From Leaf A, Cotran RS, editors: *Renal physiology*, ed 3, New York, 1985, Oxford University Press.)

structed a huge scale to record the fluctuations of body weight during meals, work, and sleep. Not only did he lay the foundation for the quantitative study of metabolism and water balance, he also set an example for succeeding generations by using himself as an experimental subject. His clear description and remarkably accurate quantitation of insensible perspiration were not properly understood until Lavoisier discovered oxygen just before the French Revolution and Liebig deduced early in the nineteenth century that water must be produced within the body by the combustion of foodstuffs.[63,67] Insensible perspiration through the lungs was recognized as containing CO_2, as well as water. At the beginning of the present century after Magnus-Levy found that ordinary combustion of food provides about 300 ml of water internally per day, the quantitative indices became available to conduct metabolic studies with more precise information about fluid balance.[71]

Throughout the nineteenth century, evidence accumulated to support the observation that the concentration of sodium in the serum remains within a very narrow range during health. The significance of this constancy and the mechanisms that support it, however, were not determined until biologic scientists turned their attention to the new field of endocrinology during the early part of the present century. It is true that Nothnagel suggested a century ago that water intake is regulated by a center located in the brain.[82] In addition, just before the end of the nineteenth century, the British physiologists Oliver and Schafer[84] discovered that extracts of the pituitary gland cause a rise in blood pressure when injected intravenously. Continuing his studies with Magnus and later with Herring, Schafer concluded in his Croonian lecture given in 1909 that the infundibular part of the pituitary gland secretes "a substance" into the blood that influences the secretion of urine through an indirect effect on the vascular system and a direct effect on renal epithelium.[98]

Almost 40 years later, Verney,[116] in his 1947 Croonian lecture to the Royal Society, reviewed his studies demonstrating conclusively that cerebral sensors participate in the regulation of ADH secretion. These sensors are stimulated when the carotid blood osmolality is raised with sodium salts or other cell-dehydrating substances. Verney postulated that ADH release is regulated by sensors located in the carotid artery, which are excited primarily by diminution of their own volume. However, the sensors have a certain degree of constant activity in euhydrated persons, which explains basal ADH secretion that is turned off by excessive intake of water.

It is now evident that when a supply of fresh water is unlimited, humans satisfy the need to maintain water balance by habitual or nonthirst-motivated drinking. However, to protect the homeostasis of body fluids, there are two backup systems involving an efficient thirst mechanism and secretion of ADH from the neurohypophysis. The two stimuli that usually activate these defense systems are a deficit of water without corresponding loss of sodium or an excessive intake of sodium, which causes an osmotic shift of water out of the cells into the ECF (see Figure 3-4). The common denominator of both stimuli is cellular dehydration and hyperosmolality of body fluids reflected by an increased tonicity in the serum (rise in concentration of serum Na^{+}*). These mechanisms of osmotic regulation by water intake through thirst and water conservation through ADH release are the chief guardians of the homeostasis of serum sodium concentration[6] (see Figure 3-5). Because osmoequilibrium exists across all fluid compartments, the serum sodium concentration reflects total body fluid osmolality and the relative distribution of water between the ICF and ECF compartments.

The efficiency of this thirst neurohypophyseal-renal

*In the absence of hyperglycemia or hyperlipidemia, *the serum concentration of sodium can be used as an index of total serum osmolality* because the salts of sodium comprise more than 90% of osmotically active solutes in the serum.

axis in maintaining the constancy of total solute activity of serum is reflected by the relatively narrow range of serum sodium concentration found in normal persons. The serum sodium concentration stays within the values of 136 and 143 mEq/L (or mOsm/L) in health despite often large individual variations in intake of salt and water. A rise of only 1% or 2% in osmotically effective total serum solute concentration elicits maximum release of ADH. A similar sensitivity exists in response to dilution of body fluids; a 2% increase in total body water is sufficient to suppress ADH output below detectable levels.[65]

The effectiveness of ADH is determined to a great extent by its capacity to dilute or concentrate the urine by a factor of four with reference to plasma. It acts to increase the permeability of the distal renal tubule and collecting duct to water. The duct is embedded in the hypertonic interstitium of the renal medulla. As a result, water leaves the duct to flow down a concentration gradient to the point at which the concentration of urine in the collecting duct becomes approximately equal to that of the surrounding medulla.

Conversely, in the absence of this hormone, the collecting duct becomes impermeable. This impermeability results in the escape of a hypotonic distal tubular fluid through the collecting system, which results in a water diuresis. Thus urine concentration can vary between 80 and 1300 mmole/kg, whereas the plasma osmolality remains very close to the range of 300 mmole/kg.[31]

The sensation of thirst provides the necessary backup mechanism to support this finely tuned and sensitive ADH control of water balance.[38,39] If there were not some means to signal the need for water intake, a continuing external loss of water would cause a progressive increase in total solute concentration in body fluids. Osmoregulatory thirst comes into action only when habitual drinking and the water in food plus maximum ADH effect do not maintain the serum concentration of sodium below a certain level (see Figure 3-5).

Control of Circulatory Volume

In addition to the stimulus of cellular dehydration and hyperosmolality, thirst is elicited by a second and quite distinct stimulus. An acute reduction of ECF volume also stimulates both thirst and ADH release and does so through receptors anatomically separate from the enteroreceptors responsible for mediating the osmotic regulation of water balance. However, there must be a pronounced reduction of ECF volume before the sensation of thirst and the secretion of ADH are stimulated. When hypovolemia stimulates thirst and ADH release, the afferent side of the reflux arc is mediated by stretch receptors in the low-pressure capacitance vessels near the heart and in the atria that activate vagal impulses in conjunction with the arterial baroreceptors that activate the renal renin-angiotensin system.[38,39,92,93] When this does occur, volume regulation takes precedence over osmotic control[6,115] (see Figures 3-2 and 3-4).

Ordinarily, the ECF volume receptors have minimum activity in day-to-day control of fluid balance.[65] Responsibility rests with the osmotic receptors to preserve the fine control of total serum osmolality and thereby protect ICF volume. For practical purposes, this is reflected by the serum concentration of Na^+ because as long as the cellular content of solute remains constant, cellular volume is regulated by the osmolality of ECF. This regulation is accomplished by small adjustments in volume intake and output. Thirst is rarely manifest as a symptom of hypovolemia other than as an emotional response. A loss of 10% to 20% of blood volume is probably required before the mechanisms eliciting thirst and release of ADH are stimulated by hypovolemia.[6,93,94]

The rise in serum osmolality that occurs after blood loss may have physiologic significance beyond a possible direct effect on mobilizing cell water to help refill plasma volume because hypovolemia induces a reset of the osmoreceptors. During hypovolemia the osmotic threshold for liberation of ADH is lowered, and release of ADH increases in response to superthreshold levels of plasma osmolality; that is, the plasma ADH response to a given change in osmolality is increased if there is a coincident decrease in ECF volume. This change suggests afferent input from the ECF receptors (left atrial stretch receptors) to the cells of the supraoptic nucleus and/or osmoreceptors (ICF volume receptors).[92] Opposite effects have been observed with the expansion of blood volume.[94]

The ADH-thirst system regulates total body fluid osmolality, not merely plasma or ECF osmolality, because no osmotic gradient is tolerated in the body except the renal medulla and perhaps certain serous glands. Thus by maintaining constant total body osmolality, the ADH-thirst mechanism defends the ratio of total body water to total exchangeable solute. As a result, the system indirectly maintains body water constancy, and the fluid volume in each compartment remains constant as long as a person is in electrolyte balance.

It is clear that a system oriented only to osmotic regulation will not maintain constancy of volume when solute is being gained or lost from the body. Lacking other control mechanisms, the body would either swell up or shrink isosmotically over a wide range determined only by the vicissitudes of appetite and thirst. Thus continued study of the sodium-regulatory mechanisms was directed by an appreciation that the volume of ECF must be determined by a balance between intake and output of this critical solute because its concentration as the dominant cation solute (balanced by an equivalent number of univalent anion solutes) was maintained with such constancy.

Historically, Thomas Addison, physician at Guy's Hospital, should be credited for stimulating the studies of internal secretion that led to discovery of the mechanisms of control of solute content in the ECF and thus indirectly of controlling the volume of fluid in the body.[2] In 1855 he drew attention to a remarkable group of symptoms in patients with disease of the previously unrecognized small glands situated above the kidneys. Many studies followed on the relation between the presumed adrenocortical hormone and the electrolyte disturbances found with adrenal insufficiency.*

By 1923 during his studies of the role of electrolytes in fluid physiology, Gamble had observed that patients with Addison's disease develop a fall in sodium level and a rise in potassium level in the serum.[43] The clinical observations of hypotension combined with hemoconcentration signifying a depleted volume led clinical investigators to make the obvious comparison between patients with Addison's disease and patients suffering from cholera. One century earlier O'Shaughnessy and Latta had reported success in treatment of dehydrated patients with cholera by infusion of saline solution.[62,85]

Thus the main treatment of Addison's disease became the administration of salt and water. Groups led by Harrop and Strauss in Boston, Swingle in Philadelphia, Loeb in New York, and Levy in Britain found that extracts of the adrenal gland also were successful in preventing the lethal dehydration of adrenal insufficiency.[51,66,68,114] Loeb and Atchley, on finding large losses of sodium in the urine, suggested "that the adrenal glands exert a regulatory effect upon the Na metabolism analogous to that of the parathyroid gland upon Ca and PO_4 metabolism."[68] Reflecting the prevailing concepts, they also suggested that the adrenal glands might be able to control the *concentration* (rather than quantity) of sodium in the blood and tissue fluids. Invited to participate in the final series of Harvey lectures before the United States entered World War II, Loeb provided a clear exposition of concepts that unequivocally tied an adrenal hormone into mechanisms regulating body hydration: a decrease in circulating "products of adrenocortical tissues" leads to dehydration, shock, and death.[68] This course of events, which involves the kidney, can be curtailed either by administration of large quantities of sodium salts and water or by large amounts of adrenocortical extract with some supplementary salt and water.

Perhaps less recognized at that time was the simultaneous work being conducted on the influence of adrenocortical extracts on the internal movement of water. After his discovery of insulin, Banting turned his attention to the adrenal gland as another organ of internal secretion. His studies in Canada, independent of similar work by Rogoff and Stewart in Cleveland, demonstrated clearly that adrenal-deficient animals lose plasma volume somewhere within the body.[11,96] Gaudino and Levitt[45] found that cells gained fluid during adrenal insufficiency. Later, work by Marks, the lifelong studies by Swingle, and most recently the work by Pirkle and Gann have demonstrated that increased adrenocortical steroids are required to prevent the movement of fluids into cells in adrenalectomized animals. They are also required to foster the refill of plasma volume following a major hemorrhage.* In view of recent findings that mild dehydration impairs the refill of plasma volume after hemorrhage, the beneficial role of adrenocortical steroids in this process observed in the adrenal-deficient animals may be to mobilize cellular fluid.[19,111]

Confusion over the relative influence of the several active adrenocortical compounds on physiologic processes was finally settled by the postwar development of partition chromatography and other new laboratory techniques. Simpson and Tait[104] identified aldosterone in 1952 and shortly thereafter isolated it as the primary salt-retaining hormone secreted by the adrenal gland. Ensuing studies were addressed to the mechanism of aldosterone action and the control of its secretion. However, it quickly became apparent that there is a multiplicity of interrelationship of sodium-retentive forces, none of which had a predominant role equivalent to the influence of ADH in the control of water loss. Thus several adrenocortical steroids, in addition to aldosterone, are involved in the regulation of fluid balance. Unquestionably, aldosterone is the most potent mineralocorticoid secreted from the adrenal; but cortisol, deoxycorticosterone, and corticosterone are all required for the smooth control of body fluids.[93] In addition, numerous other mechanisms have been proposed to assist with the control of sodium excretion; they are closely linked and usually act in harmony.

The net result of these and many other ingenious studies is the current concept of an "effective intravascular volume," which although hard to measure is sensed by volume-regulating mechanisms. Although it is not certain what change in intravascular volume is monitored, there are at least two groups of pressor or stretch receptors (see Figure 3-2). The first lines of defense against changes in circulatory volume are the mechanoreceptors located in the great veins of the thorax and in the atrial and ventricular walls. These low-capacitance vessels located near the heart send continuous signals via the vagus nerve to the brain regarding the "effective" intravascular volume. Capable of stretching at low pressure, these vessels are admirably suited to buffer alterations in circulatory volume to sustain cardiac output and arterial blood pressure. The physiologic backup for sensing more pronounced changes in volume is accomplished by the aortic and carotid baroreceptor network,

*References 20, 29, 51, 66, 68, 93, and 114.

*References 3, 29, 73, 90, 113, and 114.

which transmits a continuous sensory signal centrally over the sympathetic nerve. Both groups of volume receptors are sensitive to some parameter of intravascular volume, but they do not modulate the excretion or conservation of sodium in response to changes in the serum concentration of this ion.

Changes in the effective volume of circulating blood induce appropriate volume-regulatory changes of renal sodium excretion by cardiovascular reflexes and by activation of the renin-angiotensin system (see Figure 3-2). As noted earlier these mechanisms are also called on as reserve expedients to control water balance when very large deficits develop in the ECF volume. Ordinarily, however, control of water balance is achieved by the sensitive osmoreceptors.[65,81,93] It is likely that equally important mechanisms for modulating sodium excretion are provided by the awesome and complex constellation of intrinsic renal factors. These mechanisms control the relationship between GFR and tubular reabsorption of sodium.[115] Ordinarily, GFR remains stable while fine adjustments in sodium content in ECF are made by alterations in tubular reabsorption rates (see Figure 3-2).

The primary mechanism activated by the volume receptors to control the excretion of sodium is thought to be the renin-angiotensin system. Probably all of the renin that reaches the circulation originates in the kidney from the juxtaglomerular apparatus. It is stored, synthesized, and released from this site. This area probably should be regarded as part of the baroreceptor system because of its behavior in support of cardiovascular and fluid homeostasis.[93] Certainly, it is innervated by adrenergic neurons, and the release of its self-generated hormone is determined in part by the stretch receptors located in its afferent arterioles.

In addition to the stretch receptors, Davis has defined at least two other principal mechanisms governing the release of renin: increased sympathetic nerve activity and stimulation of the renal macula densa by changes in the composition of fluids in the proximal part of the distal tubule.[23] These stimuli are manifested clinically when the kidneys, acting like baroreceptors, respond to the decreased perfusion pressure of hypotension by releasing renin. Increased sympathetic activity induced by volume reduction in other parts of the body also induces an increased renal output of renin.

The renin released from the juxtaglomerular apparatus cleaves a circulating protein substrate, angiotensinogen, which is synthesized by the liver to release angiotensin I. Primarily in the lungs and to a lesser extent in the kidney, angiotensin I is converted rapidly to angiotensin II, which is the physiologically active component of the renin-angiotensin system. Angiotensin II in turn is degradated within a minute. During its brief role it probably exerts a positive feedback to foster the hepatic output of angiotensinogen.

A broad spectrum of physiologic alterations is produced by angiotensin II, including cardiovascular, endocrine, and metabolic effects. However, none are more important than its interrelated influences on blood pressure and fluid and electrolyte balance. Its action as a potent pressor agent is a result of direct constriction of vascular smooth muscle. However, it also has a central pressor effect modulated by the sympathetic nervous system. In the kidney, angiotensin II alters sodium excretion by its effect on hemodynamics, and it exerts a "short loop" negative feedback to inhibit the secretion of its parent renin. It may act on efferent arterioles to control glomerulus-tubular balance and thus single nephron sodium excretion. The influence of renin on body fluid balance through control of water intake and vasopressin secretion probably should be regarded as a reserve expedient to help control water balance in the presence of large deficits of ECF volume. However, there is no doubt that the renin-angiotensin system is a critical component in the regulation of sodium balance through its influence on the biosynthesis of the adrenocortical hormone aldosterone.[93]

The increased adrenal output of aldosterone under the stimulus of angiotensin II results from newly formed hormone by catalyzing the hydroxylation of desoxycorticosterone rather than release from preformed storage.[93] The output of aldosterone is quite independent of the secretion of glucocorticoids and originates from a separate anatomic site, the zona glomerulosa in the outer layer of the cortex. Nevertheless, as demonstrated initially by Banting, Rogoff, and Stewart, the glucocorticoids originating from the inner part of the adrenal cortex also are required for regulation of fluid balance.[11,93,96] In addition to angiotensin II, the secretion of aldosterone and the glucocorticoids is stimulated by adrenocorticotropic hormone (ACTH), particularly during emotional or physical stress, hemorrhage, or changes in posture.[93] Potassium promotes the secretion of aldosterone. Because deviation in the serum concentration of sodium greater than 10 to 20 mEq/L is required to increase the adrenal secretion of aldosterone, it is unlikely that sodium has a fundamental influence.

Aldosterone exerts its vital modulation of sodium balance by stimulating the active transport of sodium out of the fluid in the distal tubule and collecting duct. It also increases the secretion of potassium in sweat, salivary juice, and intestinal fluids and the urinary excretion of hydrogen and potassium.

The current concept of mechanisms supporting the homeostasis of body fluids involves the action of several hormones integrated by the circulatory and nervous systems. Although renin-angiotensin system, aldosterone, and vasopressin are key factors in maintaining this regulation, other hormones including several other corticosteroids, the sex hormones, estrogen and progesterone, the thyroid and parathyroid hormones, and a "na-

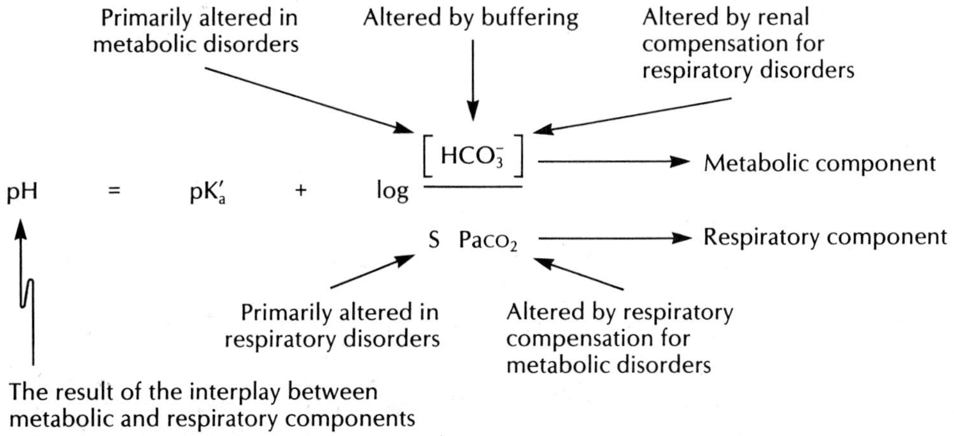

FIGURE 3-6 Challenges and defense of the bicarbonate/carbonic acid buffer system. (Modified from Kaehny WD. In Schrier RW, editor: *Renal and electrolyte disorders,* ed 4, Boston, 1992, Little, Brown.)

triuretic" hormone are required for optimal control of salt and water balance.

Control of Acid-Base Balance

In addition to control of volume and osmolality of body fluids, there is an exquisite system for maintaining the quantity and the close balance between the acids and bases in body fluids. The order of homeostatic priorities is clear: defense of the acid-base balance is subservient when tested by markedly adverse clinical circumstances to the protection of volume and osmolality. The defense of volume is the overriding mission of homeostatic mechanisms. Nevertheless, the H^+ activity of body fluids is a jealously guarded constituent of body composition.* This defense is an impressive task when one considers that 20,000 mmole carbonic acid and approximately 80 mmole of nonvolatile acids (50 to 100 mEq of H^+) are added to the body fluids daily[65]; approximately 2 lb of carbonic acid resulting from oxidation of food substances must be carried out of the body daily without disturbing appreciably the reaction of body fluids.[43]

In terms of the more conventional expressions of H^+ concentration as the negative logarithm to the base 10, these values represent a pH of 7.0 to 7.6 as a range compatible with life. Ordinarily, the pH of ECF is maintained with a much narrower range, between 7.35 and 7.45 (45 to 35 nmole/L). Although it is not possible to measure precisely the pH within cells, there is a reasonable consensus from studies that it is lower than the pH in ECFs and is in the range of pH 6.9. Each cell has a number of different options intimately involved with metabolic processes that may be used to maintain the acid-base status required for its survival. Within individual cells, it is probable that the pH varies among the organelles in cytoplasm and adds thereby to the complexity of control of body fluid pH.

The H^+ concentration is determined by a disassociation constant and the concentration ratio of free buffer anion to unassociated acid. The mathematic formulation of this relationship by Henderson in 1909 was transferred to a negative logarithmic expression by Hasselbalch 7 years later.[55,58] The resultant, and now familiar, Henderson-Hasselbalch equation:

$$pH = pK + \frac{[A^-]}{[HA]}$$

may be rewritten in terms of the major buffer system in the ECF (H_2CO_3 − $NaHCO_3$) as:

$$pH = 6.1 + \log \frac{HCO^-_3}{H_2CO_3}.$$

This equation provides the basis for chemical quantitation of clinical acid-base disturbances and makes abundantly clear that the physiologic defenses need only to reestablish the ratio between the concentrations of HCO^-_3 and H_2CO_3 rather than restore their absolute values to protect the pH of body fluids[43,58,59] (Figure 3-6).

Acid-base balance is challenged by two types of disorders, metabolic and respiratory, which work to alter the pH of body fluids. Homeostasis is defended by mechanisms that attempt to return the pH to its normal range. The metabolic challenges act by raising or lowering the serum concentration of bicarbonate, the numerator or "base" component of the Henderson-Hasselbalch equation. Respiratory alterations of pH are produced by excessive retention or excretion of $PaCO_2$, the denominator or "acid" component of this equation. Because H_2CO_3 varies directly with CO_2 ($CO_2 + H_2O \rightleftharpoons H_2CO_3$ through the action of carbonic anhydrase), a convenient

*H^+ represents the hydrogen ion concentration in nmole/L; HCO_3 represents bicarbonate concentration in mmole/L; $PaCO_2$ is the partial pressure of CO_2 in arterial blood, or arterial gas tension.

way to think of the equilibrium is that the pH varies directly with bicarbonate and inversely with CO_2 $\left(pH \propto \frac{HCO^-_3}{H_2CO_3}\right)$.

Defense of pH is provided by a three-tiered system: buffers, compensation, and correction. Buffers work as pairs including a weak acid and the salt of a strong alkali with the weak acid. For example, the three primary buffers of ECF are: $H_2CO_3 - NaHCO_3$, H protein – Na protein, and $NaH_2PO_4 - Na_2HPO_4$. These buffers can take up or release H^+ instantly in response to the addition of a strong acid (H^+ donor) or base (H^+ acceptor) in a way that minimizes but does not abolish the changes in pH. Because more detailed considerations of the chemistry of acids and bases and buffers are available in all standard textbooks of renal physiology, it is sufficient for our purposes to note that all buffer pairs in the ECF are in equilibrium with each other as are the buffer pairs in the ICF.[58,65]

Compensation is the second line of acid-base defense. Although slower in onset than buffering, the process is more effective. The primary buffer in the ECF ($H_2CO_3 - NaHCO_3$) is particularly suited to function in this matter because one component, H_2CO_3, is directly and rapidly regulated by pulmonary ventilation. Consequently, metabolic disorders with loss or gain of HCO^-_3 are quickly compensated by the lungs to lower or raise $PaCO_2$. However, when respiratory disorders are responsible for the challenges to acid-base balance, the kidney must act to preserve the 20:1 HCO^-_3/H_2CO_3 ratio. This adaptation requires 4 to 6 days to become totally effective in most instances.[88] Thus the second line of defense supporting the primary carbonic acid-bicarbonate buffer system depends on the independent and complementary function of two different organ systems: control of the concentration of H_2CO_3 by the lungs and of HCO^-_3 by the kidneys.

The third and definitive line of defense of acid-base homeostasis requires the cure or modification of the disease process to the extent that the lungs can correct the respiratory component and the kidneys can correct the metabolic component of the alteration. The disorders most commonly encountered that cause alterations in acid-base balance are hypoperfusion of tissues and renal failure in metabolic acidosis, liver failure in metabolic alkalosis, and hypoventilation or hyperventilation in respiratory acidosis and alkalosis, respectively. Clearly, when the primary disorder is pulmonary or renal, the third line of defense is compromised (see Figure 3-6).

FLUID AND ELECTROLYTE MANAGEMENT

The management of fluids and electrolytes is a major component of the overall care of the surgical patient.[74] This section focuses on general principles of basic fluid management and correction of fluid and electrolyte abnormalities. An essential portion of this management is a thorough knowledge of the normal body mechanisms for maintaining homeostasis, which are detailed in the preceding sections. The formulae given here are only guidelines and are better replaced by a good understanding of the principles involved. Every patient is different, and repeated clinical assessments are necessary.

Basic Fluid Management

The goal of any fluid and electrolyte management is to maintain normal volume and composition of body fluid. The easiest and safest way to accomplish this goal in a healthy individual is to provide a balanced diet and free access to water, allowing the body to make the appropriate adjustments. However, when it becomes necessary to limit oral intake or when there are alterations in the normal homeostatic mechanisms, it is important to balance input and output of all fluids and electrolytes. The key to all estimates of fluid administration is a reliable baseline weight for the patient.

Fluid Volume and Composition

Water

An average adult ingests 1,500 to 2,000 ml of water daily. Most is in the form of liquids, but solid foods also contain a high water content. In addition, there are two endogenous sources of water. The first is the water of oxidation, produced during the oxidation of carbohydrate, fat, and protein; the second is preformed water, or water of solution, which is the intracellular water released by the disruption of cells during catabolic states or as a result of injury. These endogenous sources are usually minimal and therefore do not play a major role in the calculations of daily fluid requirements. However, they may become critical in some disease states such as renal failure or major trauma.

There are four normal routes for the loss of water. The most readily apparent is the urine, which is the only loss mechanism that varies with the volume and composition of body fluid. The second is insensible water loss through the skin (75%) and the lungs (25%), which changes with alterations in the metabolic rate, respiratory rate, and body temperature. The third route of water elimination is through sweating, where the volume lost can vary greatly (up to 4000 ml/hr). For the afebrile patient in the controlled, air-conditioned environment in modern hospitals, these losses are minimal. The fourth route of water loss, the stool, normally accounts for only 0 to 250 ml of water daily. This can increase markedly in severe diarrhea.

The daily water requirement is the sum of the amount of water necessary to excrete the daily solute load plus the amount of insensible losses minus the fluid received, either exogenously or endogenously. The amount of water to excrete the solute load depends on both the quantity of solute to be removed and the concentrating ability of the kidney. Under normal circumstances, an adult generates approximately 600 mOsm of solute daily. If the kidney is capable of concentrating urine to a maximum of 1200 mOsm/kg of water, 500 ml of urine would have to be excreted. If the kidney is incapable of maximal concentration (e.g., during renal failure) or the amount of solute increases greatly (e.g., as a result of catabolism), a larger volume of water is needed.[14]

The kidneys also have a remarkable ability to dilute urine to as low as 50 to 100 mOsm/kg of water. Therefore under normal circumstances, the kidney can excrete as much as 6 to 12 L of water daily and maintain normal body osmolality.

Holliday and Segar[56] found that solute excretion ranged from 10 mOsm/100 kcal/day in infants receiving glucose and water to 40 mOsm/100 kcal/day in infants receiving cow's milk. Parenteral fluid should provide a solute load somewhere between these extremes, some of which will be derived from metabolism and some from exogenously administered electrolytes. Sufficient water should be available to minimize the need for the kidney to concentrate or dilute the urine. A useful estimate is 25 mOsm/100 kcal/day, requiring about 55 ml of water/100 kcal/day.

An estimate of the metabolic rate is the most accurate guide to insensible water loss. Holliday and Segar[56] assumed that hospitalized infants expend the same number of calories as infants at home because activity levels are comparable. However, adults are much less active when hospitalized, expending approximately half the number of calories during the hospital stay. The caloric expenditure of children is somewhere between these two extremes. Based on these assumptions, the estimated caloric expenditure can be calculated as follows:

For the first 10 kg of body weight	100 kcal/kg
For the next 10 kg of body weight	50 kcal/kg
For each additional kilogram	20 kcal/kg

For a 25-kg person, this calculation would be:

$$10 \text{ kg} \times 100 \text{ kcal/kg} +$$
$$10 \text{ kg} \times 50 \text{ kcal/kg} +$$
$$5 \text{ kg} \times 20 \text{ kcal/kg} = 1{,}600 \text{ kcal}$$

The insensible water loss can then be calculated using a rate of 45 ml of water lost for each 100 kcal metabolized. For the child in the preceding example, the estimate would be 720 ml per day (1600 kcal/100 kcal × 45 ml). Elevated body temperature raises the insensible losses. This rise can be estimated by increasing the previous estimate by 10% for each degree of fever greater than 37°C (98.6°F) (use 7% if the Fahrenheit scale is used).[55] If the child in this example had a temperature of 40°C (104°F), the estimated loss would be:

$$720 \text{ ml} + 10\% \times (40°\text{C} - 37°\text{C}) \times 720 \text{ ml} = 936 \text{ ml}$$

If the water required for excretion of the solute load, 55 ml/100 kcal, is added, the total 24-hour water requirement is 100 ml/100 kcal or, using the preceding equations:

For the first 10 kg of body weight	100 ml/kg
For the next 10 kg of body weight	50 ml/kg
For each additional kilogram	20 ml/kg

At best, these guidelines are only an approximation and are based on many assumptions including normal renal function, normal metabolic rate, and no other fluid losses. Frequent reassessment of the patient is required any time parenteral therapy is being administered. The patient's weight is the best guide to the adequacy of water administration.

Sodium

A normal adult ingests 3 to 5 g of salt daily, providing 50 to 90 mEq of Na^+ in the form of NaCl. The normal kidney excretes the excess salt. When a sodium-free diet is initiated, the kidneys are able to reduce excretion to less than 1 mEq/day, although a mild sodium deficit usually develops during the process. These extremes demonstrate the range of the kidney's ability to adjust to sodium intake, providing flexibility in the amount of sodium administered during parenteral therapy. Usually, about 70 mEq of Na^+ should be provided daily to compensate for losses in sweat and stool and to minimize the load on the kidneys.

Potassium

Potassium excretion cannot be reduced as much as sodium, but can decrease to 10 mEq/day. Normal kidneys are capable of excreting 700 mEq of potassium daily, although it takes several days to adjust to either extreme. It is necessary therefore to provide at least 20 mEq of potassium daily to allow for obligatory renal losses. Usually 40 to 60 mEq/day is preferred, once it is known that renal function is adequate.

Miscellaneous

Protein catabolism complicates fluid and electrolyte management through release of water and electrolytes. Therefore it is advisable to provide carbohydrate to decrease the amount of protein catabolism, especially in patients with renal failure. Usually 100 to 150 g/day is adequate.[41] If parenteral therapy is maintained longer than 1 week, it may be necessary to supplement calcium, magnesium, phosphorus, vitamins, and protein as well.

Routine Management

Many fluids for intravenous administration are commercially available. The remarkable ability of the kidney to adapt to the composition of administered fluids in order to maintain a constant environment allows most of these solutions to be used with minimal adjustments. A commonly used daily fluid plan for an adult with no underlying disturbances is D5 1/4NS with 20 mEq of KCl added per liter, administered at a rate of 100 ml/hr.

Postoperative Fluid Management

Fluid management is much more difficult after surgery; "routine" care has gone through many changes.[74] The many stresses of surgery are potent stimuli of ADH.[54,75,76] The patient is unable to excrete excess free water, so it is necessary to decrease the amount of free water administered. The ADH response may last from one to several days after surgery.

In addition, the postoperative patient frequently receives only enough intravenous glucose to minimize the negative nitrogen balance, and so has a low daily solute output, which further decreases the amount of free water that can be handled by the kidney. The amount of fluid to replace urinary loss is, therefore, restricted to a much narrower range. A useful approximation for a postoperative adult is 1 L daily. If an increased urine volume is needed, additional solute administration, usually in the form of NaCl, may be required. The kidney will excrete the solute with the added water.

Insensible losses are approximately the same after surgery as they were before, if there are no other changes. However, the insensible losses are increased if fever develops postoperatively.

Monitoring the patient's weight preoperatively and postoperatively is the best guide to the appropriate volume of fluid to administer. It must be remembered that an adult in the postoperative catabolic period who does not receive the preoperative equivalent of calories and protein should be expected to lose 0.1 kg to 0.2 kg (0.25 to 0.5 lb) of real body weight per day. If the weight remains constant, it may indicate the administration of excess fluid.

Weight can be helpful in determining if the patient received too much or too little fluid during surgery. The volume-overloaded patient is expected to excrete the excess fluid over the first few postoperative days as the ADH response diminishes. A fluid plan that attempts to replace all of the urinary losses will only perpetuate the problem of fluid excess.

It is unnecessary and potentially dangerous to administer any potassium during the first postoperative day. Some degree of renal compromise often develops due to surgery. Until compromise can be determined for a specific patient, it is prudent to avoid potassium. If there is no renal damage, the kidneys tend to excrete large quantities of potassium in postoperative patients. For these patients, supplementation of 60 to 100 mEq daily is often required.

CORRECTION OF IMBALANCES

The preoperative or postoperative patient may have abnormalities of body fluid in volume, osmolality, or composition. Understanding and correction, if possible, of underlying etiologies are imperative to optimum management. The following guidelines are only approximations. Nothing can replace close patient observation with frequent reassessment of the clinical status plus fluid output and administration.

Volume Abnormalities

Volume Excess

Excess body water occurs primarily in three situations: renal failure, congestive heart failure, and advanced liver disease. Management of these disorders is beyond the scope of this chapter, but alterations in fluid to be administered must be made to accommodate the decreased fluid output.

A common cause of volume excess in the postoperative patient is the over-vigorous administration of hypotonic fluids.[28] Many of the stresses associated with surgery, including anxiety, anesthesia, sedatives, narcotics, and pain, can stimulate the secretion of ADH.[54,75,76] This leads to retention of water, producing a urine osmolality greater than would be expected for the low plasma osmolality. Total body water (TBW) is increased, which leads to an increased secretion of sodium (see Figure 3-2), aggravating the hyponatremia.

Excess administration of isotonic salt solutions can expand the ECF space. The kidney's ability to excrete sodium is overwhelmed after a few days, leading to a pronounced volume overload.

Management of volume excess is directed toward the underlying pathologic process in the cases of organ impairment. For the postoperative patient or other patient with "inappropriate" ADH secretion, prevention is the key to therapy. Further therapy is discussed in the section on hyponatremia.

Volume Deficit

The two different types of dehydration, total body dehydration and extracellular dehydration, are considered in these sections. Hypovolemia caused by blood loss is not discussed here.

Total Body Dehydration (Primarily Water Loss)

Total body dehydration is seen uncommonly in surgical patients because most fluid disorders involve the loss of salt as well as water. When total body dehydration does occur, it usually happens in an unconscious patient who cannot express the severe sensation of thirst, a cardinal symptom of intracellular dehydration. Dehydration is most likely to occur in patients with a head injury, after a neurosurgical procedure that has produced diabetes insipidus, or as a consequence of an osmotic diuresis. Clinical signs of circulatory volume depletion are lacking, even with volume deficits equivalent to 10% of TBW because in total body ("pure") dehydration, the water loss is shared by all body fluid compartments. This sharing contrasts to the hypovolemia produced by the loss of salt and water (extracellular dehydration), which rapidly induces clinical signs of increased sympathetic activity. Blood pressure is well maintained with total body dehydration. However, because of the loss of water in excess of salt, the concentration of all body solutes begins to increase. In time, the circulatory volume becomes sufficiently reduced to induce renal conservation of sodium despite the increased plasma concentration of this solute (hyperosmolality), which ordinarily induces naturesis. This "dehydration reaction," described so clearly by Peters,[87] is applied to reabsorption of Na^+ by the kidneys to conserve water (volume). This reaction is an excellent example of the ordering of homeostatic priorities. Circulatory volume is defended at the expense of osmolality. The concentration of plasma proteins and Hct also is increased by depletion of total body water, and blood urea nitrogen (BUN) rises, reflecting prerenal azotemia.

Obviously, therapy for pure dehydration is administration of water; not so obviously, these patients also benefit from adding some salt to the water. Because many of these patients are obtunded or otherwise incapable of taking oral fluids, therapy is usually given intravenously. However, one must be careful not to reduce too rapidly the hyperosmolality produced by the relative lack of body water (see Hypernatremia).

Extracellular Dehydration (Desalting Dehydration, or Simple Volume Depletion)

For the surgical patient, the three primary causes of large losses of fluid volume are (1) hemorrhage; (2) gastrointestinal disorders; and (3) sequestration of fluid in various areas of the body (third space) associated with disorders such as intestinal obstruction, trauma, infection, and burns. From a therapeutic standpoint, the common denominator of the several disorders causing extracellular volume depletion in surgical patients is a loss of isotonic fluid.

Clinical manifestations are the guide to the diagnosis of volume depletion (Figure 3-7). Although body weight is a helpful measurement for evaluating external fluid loss, it is of no use for monitoring third-space changes. The rapidity of onset of symptoms depends on the character of the fluid lost. Changes of a reduced circulatory volume are seen more quickly when salt and water losses approximate ECF than when water alone is lost. The box on page 74 lists key features in the history, symptoms, physical signs, and laboratory findings. If the depletion is severe, central venous pressure monitoring is useful to help guide the rate of fluid administration to avoid acute pulmonary edema and congestive failure.

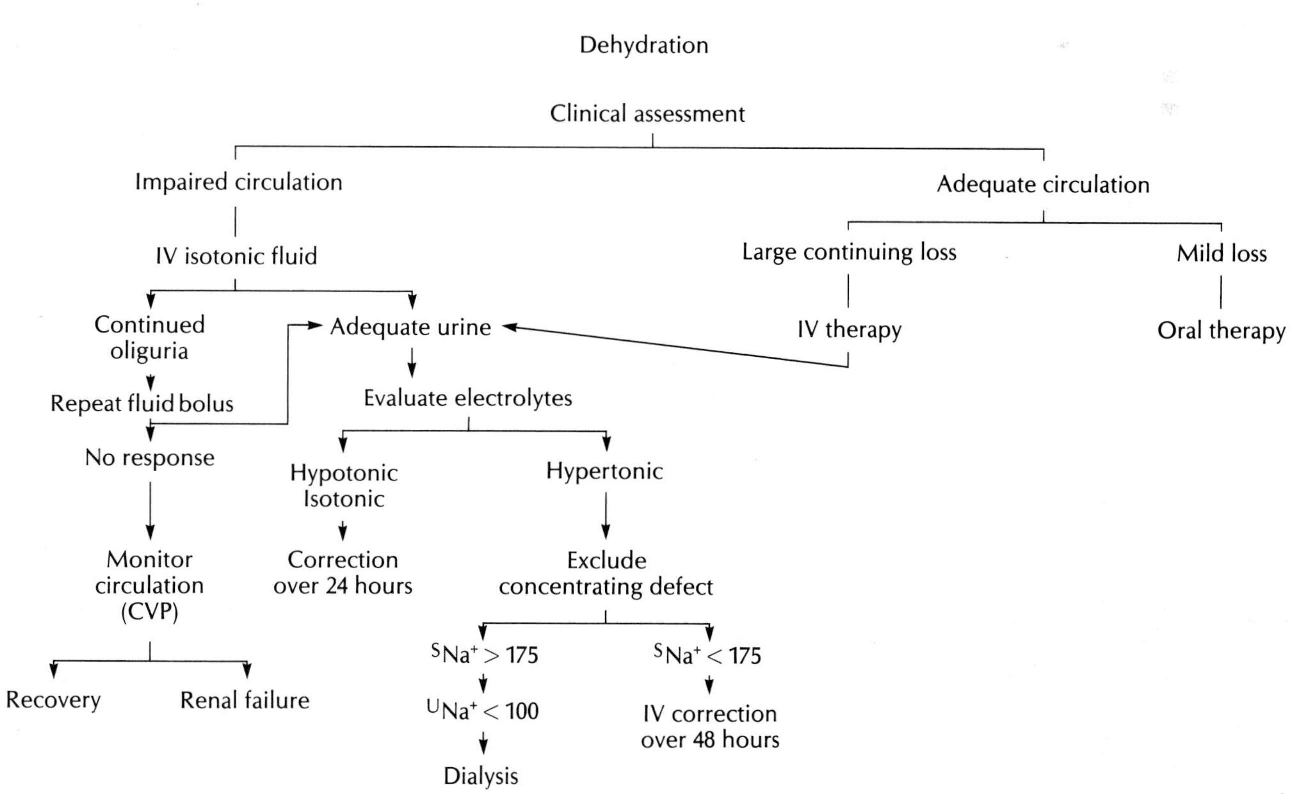

FIGURE 3-7 Dehydration.

FEATURES OF EXTRACELLULAR FLUID DEPLETION

History
Volume loss (stool, vomitus, blood)
Insufficient water and salt intake
Drug therapy
Preexisting renal disease

Symptoms
Thirst
Weakness
Anorexia
Apathy
Orthostatic dizziness or syncope

Physical Signs
Weight loss
Dry mucous membranes
Loss of tears
Decreased skin turgor
Decreased intraocular pressure
Orthostatic changes in blood pressure and pulse
Tachycardia
Prolonged capillary refill time

Laboratory Findings
Increased U_{osm} and specific gravity
Decreased urine volume
BUN increase disproportionate to creatinine
Increased hematocrit
Increased protein concentration

To a great extent these clinical signs are manifestations of the increased activity of the sympathetic nervous system, which is induced to defend homeostasis of circulatory volume. In an oliguric patient the laboratory data usually reveal an elevated urine specific-gravity level with rise in BUN, plasma creatinine, and Hct. Conversely, the Hct falls rapidly within 1 to 2 hours following any significant hemorrhage in a well-hydrated patient. Measurement of the concentration of sodium in the urine can facilitate the distinction between an extrarenal cause for fluid loss, "prerenal azotemia," and renal losses of sodium from intrinsic kidney disease. The homeostatic mechanisms protecting circulatory volume restrict renal sodium excretion to less than 5 mEq/L when extrarenal fluid losses are present (upper limit 20 mEq/L with prerenal azotemia), whereas the loss of sodium in the urine rises above 20 mEq/L when renal (or adrenal) problems are responsible for the loss of salt and water. A more precise assessment is the fractional excretion of sodium (FeNa):

$$\begin{aligned}(\text{FeNa}) &= \text{Sodium excreted} \div \text{Sodium filtered} \times 100\\ &= \frac{\text{Urine sodium}}{\text{Plasma sodium}} \div \frac{\text{Urine creatinine}}{\text{Plasma creatinine}} \times 100\\ &= \frac{\text{Urine sodium}}{\text{Plasma sodium}} \times \frac{\text{Plasma creatinine}}{\text{Urine creatinine}} \times 100\end{aligned}$$

This calculation is applicable only if the patient is oliguric. A value <1 is consistent with prerenal causes, and a value >3 indicates intrinsic renal disease. Another means of assessment is a comparison of urine to plasma osmolality. Uosm ÷ Posm >1.1 indicates prerenal causes, whereas lower levels usually indicate intrinsic disease or obstruction. Urine osmolality can be approximated by the specific gravity of the urine:

$$\text{Uosm} = (\text{specific gravity} - 1.000) \times 40{,}000$$

The degree to which ICF volume participates in defense of circulatory volume depends on (1) duration and extent of depletion and (2) whether there is a rise in plasma osmolality that pulls fluid out of the cells. Through mechanisms as yet poorly understood, ICF volume, in time, probably does help defend against acute isotonic losses of ECF greater than 10% to 15%.[44] The concentration of serum sodium is totally worthless as a test for determining volume loss because it may be reduced, normal, or elevated in dehydrated patients. The serum concentration reflects only a ratio: the number of milliequivalents of sodium per liter of serum. At issue is the deficiency in volume. Thus with isotonic losses, one should not expect to find a change in serum sodium levels. In these patients a change in serum sodium level results from either iatrogenic causes or movement of water from the cells to protect the circulation when volume loss has been large. Administration of potassium can cause a rise in serum sodium level. The problems associated with hyponatremia and hypernatremia are considered next.

The most common source of external fluid loss in a surgical patient is through the gastrointestinal tract. The key to therapy is the administration of a solution that approximates the fluid and electrolytes lost. Table 3-1 provides an estimation of electrolyte loss from different segments of the gastrointestinal tract. In addition to the estimated deficit, ongoing losses must be replaced.

The third space includes losses into the peritoneum, bowel wall, pericardium, and joint spaces. In the postoperative patient, the composition of this fluid approximates extracellular fluid. These losses can be very large. The peritoneum itself has a surface area of about 1 m^2. Several liters of fluid can be sequestered with only a slight change in the thickness of the peritoneum. Additionally, the bowel wall can hold large volumes of fluid. Technically, these fluids remain part of the ECF volume, but they no longer freely communicate with the ECF compartment. When fluid therapy is initiated to replenish third-space losses, a suitable choice is a solution that approximates ECF, such as lactated Ringer's solution. The volume to be infused can only be estimated for third-space losses, making frequent reevaluation mandatory. Unlike an external loss, the sequestered fluid will eventually return to the circulation.

TABLE 3-1 BODY FLUID COMPOSITION

SOURCE	Na^+ mEq/L	K^+ mEq/L	Cl^- mEq/L	HCO_3^- mEq/L	FLUID VOLUME ml/24 hr
Saliva	10	30	70	30	1500
Stomach	50	10-15	150	0	1500
Duodenum	140	5	80	0	100-2000
Pancreas	140	5	50-100	100	1000
Bile	130	5	100	40	600
Ileal	130	15-20	120	25-80	3000
Colon	60	30	40	0	0-250
Diarrhea	50	35	40	50	Variable
Sweat	50	5	55	0	Variable
Blood	140	4-5	100	25	---
Urine	0-100*	20-100*	70-200*	0	1500*

*Varies considerably with intake.

A useful guide to the functional ECF is the urine output. The hourly volume should be 1 to 2 ml/kg in a child, or 30 to 50 ml in an adult. However, reliance on this finding alone should be avoided. The kidneys may have been insulted by the volume deficit or by surgery and may not respond appropriately to the increased volume during therapy. Excess administration of glucose or an osmotic agent such as radiologic dyes may result in an osmotic diuresis, giving a false sense of security. A large fluid bolus of isotonic fluid can also increase the urine flow temporarily until the fluid has been redistributed.

Treatment of hypovolemia is based largely on clinical judgment. Although the rise in Hct is a good indicator of the extent of a volume deficit caused by combined water and salt losses (extracellular dehydration), the fall in Hct is at best an imprecise guide for the treatment of blood loss.[19,29] In addition, the change in Hct is useful for estimating the volume loss in pure dehydration if one takes into account that, in this circumstance, the change in Hct reflects loss of total body water rather than loss confined to the ECF. Usually, serial measurements of Hct combined with observations of urine output, blood pressure, and the clinical response to infusion of fluids are sufficient to provide dependable guides for the rate and volume of fluid therapy.

The most valuable guide to therapy for dehydration, with the exception of third-space losses, is careful monitoring of the patient's weight. This monitoring prevents excessive administration of fluid while discouraging overly cautious management.

When the extent of fluid loss requires the rapid infusion of fluid or when the patient has a precarious cardiovascular compensation, the use of a catheter to monitor the central venous pressure or insertion of a Swan-Ganz catheter to monitor the pulmonary capillary wedge pressure as an index of left atrial pressure provides more precise quantitation of the cardiovascular response to fluid infusion. Although often forgotten, crystalloid fluids can be infused, even to a patient with borderline cardiac compensation, at the rate of 15 ml/kg/hr without precipitating acute pulmonary edema, provided there is a need for additional fluid. Measurement of the concentration of electrolytes in plasma is not a substitute for clinical judgment supported by hemodynamic monitoring during the restoration of fluid volume. However, these laboratory values are critically important to assess the appropriate solute content and composition of the fluids used in this therapy.

The four basic principles of therapy for acute volume depletion are soundly based on the physiologic mechanisms that support body fluid homeostasis.

1. All losses incurred by hemorrhage, gastrointestinal disorders, and sequestered fluid are detrimental. Therefore all of these losses must be replaced.
2. Because these losses almost invariably are isotonic, they produce acute depletion of ECF (most importantly intravascular volume) with scant mobilization of intracellular water to replace the deficit. Consequently, replacement fluids except for allowing for insensible losses, should reflect the solute content and composition of the fluid that is lost (see Table 3-1). Coexisting alterations in plasma solute content and composition will be "fine-tuned" by body mechanisms supporting homeostasis after an adequate circulatory volume and a reasonable composition of solutes have been restored. Colloids other than blood are rarely needed during the initial 24 hours of therapy for an acute depletion of ECF or blood volume. A possible exception is the use of fresh-frozen plasma to manage disseminated intravascular coagulopathy.
3. Fluid losses frequently involve loss of fixed acid or base. Although the body cannot replace these losses, it can compensate partially for them. The

extent to which the kidney can correct acid-base imbalances cannot be overemphasized if only it is given the fluid volume and electrolytes (including potassium) with which to work. Therapy must be oriented initially toward volume replacement, even in the face of acid-base (composition) alterations.

4. An important adjunct to restoration of an adequate fluid volume is provision of sufficient calories to prevent or minimize the undesirable sequelae of starvation acidosis, loss of potassium, and loss of nitrogen. Gamble's classic studies demonstrated that a minimum of 100 g of carbohydrate/day will approach these objectives, as well as foster renal conservation of sodium.[41,43]

Osmolality Abnormalities

Hyponatremia

It is important to reemphasize that measurement of the serum sodium concentration may give an approximation to the osmolality of TBW, but yields no information about the total body sodium content. However, use of the serum concentration of sodium is a valid guide to total body osmolality with two exceptions: (1) Hyperlipidemia or extreme hyperproteinemia causes a spurious hypoosmolality because the lipid or protein occupies a disproportionate space in the sample of serum analyzed for its electrolyte content, and (2) hyperglycemia acting as an osmotic agent draws cellular fluid into extracellular spaces and thereby dilutes the serum concentration of sodium. There is a decrease of 1.6 mEq/L for each rise of 100 mg/100 ml of glucose. Total body fluid osmolality can be approximated of the basis of the serum concentration of sodium with correction for the contribution of glucose and urea in the serum by the formula:

$$2 \times (Na^+ + K^+) + \frac{\text{Glucose mg/100 ml}}{18} + \frac{\text{BUN mg/100 ml}}{2.8}$$

Although hyponatremia reflects hypoosmolality, hyponatremia is not equivalent to total body sodium depletion, nor does it provide information about the volume of plasma or TBW. Hyponatremia can occur with expanded, normal, or depleted body fluids. Ordinarily, a fall in osmolality induces a prompt diuresis by inhibition of ADH. Thus when plasma sodium falls, it reflects one or more of the following: (1) secretion of ADH in defense of plasma volume, which has superseded the role of ADH in protecting osmolality; (2) advanced disease of the liver, kidney, or heart with retention of water in excess of sodium; (3) the syndrome of inappropriate secretion of ADH (SIADH); or (4) in rare clinical situations, the osmoreceptors become "reset" to control serum sodium at a lower level. This "reset" may occur after prolonged or marked hypovolemic shock, or it may be part of the mechanism responsible for the edema associated with cardiac, renal, or hepatic dysfunction.

Treatment of hyponatremia must be individualized to each patient. It remains an area of significant controversy.[13,109,110] Prompt correction of hyponatremia is necessary only if the patient is symptomatic due to the abnormality. Young children and the elderly are more likely to be symptomatic. Most patients with seizures or coma secondary to hyponatremia have serum sodium levels less than 120 mEq/L, but the rate at which the serum concentration falls is more important than the absolute level. Acute decreases have been associated with a 50% mortality rate, whereas chronic development of hyponatremia is associated with very low mortality and few symptoms.[101]

The most common cause of hyponatremia in the surgical patient is the administration of inappropriate or excess fluids. For example, too much free water may be ingested or infused during the time of increased ADH production, that is, postoperatively, or replacement fluids that are hypotonic compared to the losses may be used.

In the asymptomatic patient with volume excess, attempts to provide correction by the administration of isotonic or hypertonic solutions will fail. These solutions only increase the already expanded ECF, stimulating natriuresis. Correction is achieved by restricting free water to replace only insensible losses (45 ml/100 kcal) and not replacing the urine volume. As negative water balance is achieved, the ECF decreases and natriuresis diminishes. The final result is an increased serum sodium.

In the symptomatic patient with marked hyponatremia and volume excess, it is necessary to raise the serum sodium concentration more quickly than can be achieved by fluid restriction alone. This process can be accomplished by stimulating the excretion of fluid using a potent loop diuretic such as furosemide or ethacrynic acid to establish negative water balance. The sodium and potassium lost in the urine are replaced using an isotonic or rarely a hypertonic saline solution. Fluid is replaced not to provide extra sodium, but only to replenish the urinary losses. The desired negative water balance can be approximated (the TBW fraction is about 60% for males and about 50% for females):

$$\text{Weight} \times \text{TBW fraction} = \text{TBW}$$

$$\frac{\text{Actual serum sodium concentration}}{\text{Desired serum sodium concentration}} \times \text{TBW} =$$

$$\text{TBW} - \text{Desired body water} = \text{Negative water balance}$$

Example: A stuporous 70 kg 55-year-old man with a serum sodium of 115 mEq/L:

$$70 \text{ kg} \times .60 = 42 \text{ L (TBW)}$$

$$\frac{115 \text{ mEq/L}}{135 \text{ mEq/L}} \times 42\text{L} = 35.8\text{L}$$

$$42\text{L} - 35.8\text{L} = 6.2\text{L}$$

The plan should be to remove 6.2 L of fluid over at least 6 to 8 hours by administering intravenous furosemide. Hourly measurements of urine volume and concentrations of sodium and potassium are necessary so that the electrolytes can be replaced. These calculations are at best only an approximation, and frequent reassessment of the patient is critical.

One objection to the preceding calculation is the realization that sodium is not distributed equally through the TBW but is mainly extracellular. However, as sodium is lost from the ECF compartment, the ICF compartment becomes relatively hypertonic and water moves into cells. This raises the apparent ECF concentration of sodium from what would be seen if only ECF water was lost. The net effect is the functional appearance that sodium is distributed throughout the TBW.[24]

Hyponatremia in a patient with a volume deficit is seen when fluid losses are only partially replaced and a hypotonic fluid is used. In the asymptomatic patient, the deficit can be corrected gradually using isotonic saline. In the symptomatic patient, it is helpful to approximate the sodium deficit:

$$\text{Weight} \times \text{TBW fraction} = \text{TBW}$$
$$135\ \text{mEq/L} - \text{Observed serum sodium} = \text{Cation deficit/L TBW}$$
$$\text{Cation deficit (mEq/L)} \times \text{TBW} = \text{Cation to be added}$$

Example: a lethargic 70 kg man with orthostatic hypotension has a serum sodium of 115 mEq/L:

$$70\ \text{kg} \times 0.60 = 42\text{L}$$
$$135\ \text{mEq/L} - 115\ \text{mEq/L} = 20\ \text{mEq/L cation deficit}$$
$$20\ \text{mEq/L} \times 42\text{L} = 840\ \text{mEq}$$

This is the maximum amount of cation needed. Half this amount should be given over the first 24 hours. If urgent therapy is required, part of this deficit can be corrected by the cautious administration of 3% NaCl.[8]

Another potential cause of hyponatremia in the volume-depleted patient is the excessive use of diuretics. Loop diuretics and thiazides decrease sodium reabsorption in the water-impermeable portions of the ascending loop of Henle. Most diuretics also waste potassium. As intracellular potassium concentrations fall, there may be shifts of sodium into cells. Replacement of potassium in these patients may increase the serum sodium concentration. These patients frequently show no signs of volume depletion.[37]

Hypernatremia

The only information that an elevated serum sodium provides is the presence of a deficiency in TBW relative to solute content.[28,59,102] For the surgeon, the situations most commonly encountered with hypertonic body fluids result from (1) the acute onset of diabetes insipidus in a postoperative neurosurgical patient or following a head injury (fever increases further the insensible water loss, thereby causing an even greater deficit of total body water); (2) the excessive administration of solutes without sufficient water; (3) the "dehydration reaction" in which a marked deficiency in circulatory volume occurs in association with a defect in total body water; and (4) the overuse of osmotic diuretics. It is important to remember that hypernatremia can be produced by intrinsic renal disease and by an excess of salt-retaining hormones. Common to all of these disorders is the failure of the patient to manifest or to be capable of responding to the strong stimulus of thirst that develops from hypertonicity. Many of these patients are either comatose or restrained in a manner that prevents easy access to water.

The risks of hypernatremic dehydration are greater than those of hyponatremic dehydration, due to compromise of the intravascular fluid. It has been associated with a significant mortality, both in infants and elderly persons.[8] Fortunately, hypernatremia is less common than hyponatremia, due probably more to the powerful thirst mechanism secondary to hypertonicity than to differences in the frequencies of renal dilution or renal concentration defects.[5,38]

Extrarenal sources for water loss in excess of sodium loss are the skin, respiratory tract, and gastrointestinal tract. A high environmental temperature as well as a febrile patient or one in a hypermetabolic state can lead to considerable water loss.

Acute management of the symptomatic patient with hypernatremic dehydration is to provide free water. The amount of free water can be approximated as follows:

$$\text{Normal weight} \times \text{TBW fraction} = \text{Normal TBW}$$
$$\frac{\text{Normal serum sodium concentration}}{\text{Measured serum concentration}} \times \text{TBW} = \text{Current TBW}$$
$$\text{Normal TBW} - \text{Current TBW} = \text{Water deficit}$$

Example: A comatose 70 kg woman with a serum sodium of 155 mEq/L:

$$70\ \text{kg} \times 0.50 = 35\text{L}$$
$$\frac{140\ \text{mEq/L}}{155\ \text{mEq/L}} \times 35\text{L} = 31.6\text{L}$$
$$35\text{L} - 31.6\text{L} = 3.4\text{L of water to be replaced}$$

Therefore 3.4 L of free water should correct the deficit. Some sodium also should be given because invariably there has been sodium loss as well. While waiting for initial laboratory studies to differentiate between hypernatremic, hyponatremic, or isotonic dehydration, one can safely use 0.9% saline (normal saline). This fluid is still hypotonic relative to the serum sodium in the hypernatremic patient. Once the diagnosis of hypernatremia is made, 5% dextrose in water can be administered cautiously until symptoms have resolved. It is then safer to change to a solution with one-fourth strength or one-half strength NaCl or lactated Ringer's solution.

The rate of correction depends on the rate of onset of hypernatremia. The faster the onset, the more rapid a safe correction can be made. In the acute situation, replacement can occur over a few hours, giving about half of the deficit during the first 12 hours. If the hypernatremia has been present for 7 days or more, brain cells have had a chance to accumulate idiogenic osmoles to maintain normal brain volume.[35] Vigorous water administration causes brain swelling, potentially resulting in death.[8] Correction must be slow; the deficit should be replaced over at least 48 hours.

When daily maintenance fluid requirements are calculated, it is important to realize that these patients may have a marked release of ADH, which decreases the normal urine volume. Therefore the allowance for daily urine volume should also be decreased.

Hypernatremia can also be caused by the excess administration of salt without water, such as the ingestion of salt tablets without water, or the vigorous administration of isotonic fluids to replace free water losses. Despite the kidney's remarkable ability to eliminate excess sodium, the mechanism can be overwhelmed. In these situations, furosemide should be used to increase salt excretion. If renal failure is present, dialysis is required.

Composition Abnormalities

Potassium

Potassium (K^+), the major determinant of intracellular solute, is involved in many metabolic processes. The transcellular movement of this important ion is influenced greatly by the acid-base balance of body fluids. Acidosis promotes the loss of potassium from its high intracellular concentration (150 mEq/L) into a low extracellular concentration (3.5 to 5.0 mEq/L). Alkalosis causes K^+ to move in the opposite direction, into cells, against a concentration gradient. In both instances, K^+ is exchanged for Na^+.

Hypokalemia

Low serum potassium can be related to an alteration in the intracellular/extracellular distribution of potassium, total body potassium depletion, or a combination of these. The most common cause of altered distribution is alkalosis, leading to an increased intracellular potassium concentration. Changes in distribution are also seen during the administration of glucose and/or insulin.

The usual causes for K^+ depletion in surgical patients are disorders of the gastrointestinal tract and renal losses under the influence of diuretics, mineral corticoids, or intrinsic renal disease. The diagnosis of hypokalemia is confirmed by neuromuscular abnormalities, in particular, weakness; electrocardiogram (ECG) changes of flattening and inversion of the T wave; and a low level of K^+ in the serum. The urine loss of K^+ may reach 20 to 25 mEq/L in compensation for H^+ with upper gastrointestinal vomiting disorders, but the loss exceeds these values when renal abnormalities are responsible. Aldosterone causes K^+ loss in the urine as Na^+ is retained. Loop diuretics induce an increased presentation of Na^+ to the sites of exchange with K^+ in the kidney. Probably the most rapid loss of K^+ occurs with diarrhea because the concentration of potassium may reach 40 to 60 mEq/L in liquid stool. Potassium depletion is rarely found without an associated deficit of water, sodium, and chloride, which should also be replaced. Acting through incompletely understood mechanisms, hypokalemia impairs renal concentrating abilities.

The therapy for true potassium deficit is the administration of potassium and the correction of the underlying problem if possible. Potassium should be given only when urine flow is adequate. Even a small amount of potassium given to an anuric patient can be fatal. Oral therapy is the preferred route of administration of potassium for several reasons. First, intravenous administration is painful and is often associated with phlebitis. Next, the excitability of the heart muscle is related to the extracellular concentration of potassium. The infusion of a bolus of potassium will give a temporarily high serum concentration until equilibration with the ICF can take place, leading to a higher risk of arrhythmias. Unfortunately, many of the patients with hypokalemia, especially those with gastrointestinal losses, are unable to take oral supplementation. In these situations, cautious intravenous administration of potassium is required.

There is no reliable formula for calculating the amount of potassium required because the serum level represents such a small fraction of the total body potassium. A rough guideline is that a decrease in serum potassium by 1 mEq/L indicates a total body deficit of about 80 mEq in an adult. A decrease of 2 mEq/L approximates a 200 mEq deficit and a 3 mEq/L drop suggests a 400 to 500 mEq deficit. Monitoring serum potassium levels during therapy is mandatory. Oral potassium replacement is usually provided in doses from 40 to 60 mEq/day, depending on the estimated deficit. If intravenous therapy is required, no more than 10 mEq of potassium should be given in an hour, except in rare circumstances. Infusion rates above this level can lead rapidly to hyperkalemia. The concentration of potassium in the solution should not exceed 40 mEq/L if given through a peripheral vein; higher concentrations are painful.

Hyperkalemia

Increased serum potassium levels are associated with changes in intracellular/extracellular distribution or result from a true body excess of potassium. Potassium redistribution is associated with acidosis, which promotes the movement of potassium from the ICF to the ECF. Correction will relieve the hyperkalemia without

TABLE 3-2 ACUTE, TEMPORARY MANAGEMENT OF HYPERKALEMIA

DRUG	AMOUNT	ONSET OF ACTION	DURATION OF ACTION
$NaHCO_3$	50-100 mEq over 15-20 minutes	15 minutes to hours	1-2 hr
Glucose and insulin	25 g/10 units over 5 minutes	30 minutes	2-3 hr
Calcium gluconate*	5-10 ml of 10% solution over 2 minutes; may repeat after 5 minutes	<5 minutes	1 hr

*See text.

the need for further management, as there is no change in the total body potassium.

Total body excess is rarely seen without alterations in renal function because the kidneys have a tremendous capacity for excreting potassium.[60] However, minor renal changes coupled with an increased potassium load can lead to significant hyperkalemia. Examples of endogenous potassium loads include major surgery, crush injuries, hemolysis, and gastrointestinal bleeding. Exogenous sources, such as foods high in potassium, blood transfusions, and high doses of penicillin (1.7 mEq of potassium/1 million U) also need to be considered.

The most serious manifestations of hyperkalemia are cardiac related. Arrhythmias are frequent at serum potassium levels over 8.0 mEq/L, but uncommon at levels under 6.5 mEq/L. The rate of rise in the serum potassium level is of major importance. If the rate of rise is slow; complications may not be seen until levels reach 8.0 mEq/L. However, if the rate of rise is rapid, serious changes in cardiac rhythm may be seen at levels of 6.5 to 7.0 mEq/L. ECG monitoring is an essential component of therapy, but cannot be relied on as the only way to predict hyperkalemia.[123]

Table 3-2 lists some of the acute, temporary guides to the management of hyperkalemia. The goal of treatment is to move potassium into cells, to counteract the cardiac toxicity, and to remove excessive potassium from the body.[60] Sodium bicarbonate is given to raise the pH, thereby driving the potassium into cells. An ampule of sodium bicarbonate contains either 44.5 or 50 mEq. One ampule should be infused over a 5-minute period. A second ampule can be given 10 to 15 minutes later. In children, the dose is 3 mEq/kg. The use of sodium bicarbonate may be limited in situations of significant volume overload or hypernatremia.

The administration of glucose to a normal person will stimulate the endogenous release of insulin, and potassium will be shifted into cells. This endogenous release is less reliable in the acutely ill patient, and the concomitant administration of insulin is advisable. The usual regimen is to give 1 ml/kg of a 50% dextrose solution up to 50 ml accompanied by insulin at a dose of 1 unit/kg up to 10 units. Alternatively, 200 ml of a 10% to 20% glucose solution containing 10 to 20 units of insulin may be given intravenously over the first 30 minutes.

Calcium has no effect on the serum potassium concentration. Its usefulness lies in its direct antagonism of the membrane-depolarizing effect of hyperkalemia. Calcium must be infused extremely carefully, if at all, in patients receiving digitalis, as it may induce arrhythmias. A volume equal to 0.5 ml/kg of a 10% calcium gluconate solution should be infused over 2 to 4 minutes and can be repeated after 5 minutes if ECG abnormalities persist.

A newer method to promote the movement of potassium from the ECF to the ICF is the use of beta agonists.[4,79] These drugs have been used in aerosolized form or administered intravenously. The decrease of serum K^+ is seen within 30 minutes following administration and is sustained for at least 2 hours.

None of these steps is definitive but should provide temporary stabilization while corrective measures are initiated. The key is the removal of potassium through the urine, cation-exchange resins, or dialysis. In mild hyperkalemia unassociated with significant volume depletion or following replacement of any deficits, diuretics can help increase potassium excretion. Potassium-sparing diuretics are obviously contraindicated.

Cation-exchange resins, such as sodium polystyrene sulfonate (Kayexalate), reduce potassium levels more slowly than any of the previous methods. However, the reduction is definitive because the potassium is removed from the body.[40,60,99] Approximately 1 mEq of potassium is removed for each gram of Kayexalate. Kayexalate can be given orally or rectally, and occasionally by both routes. It is more effective given orally because it stays in the gastrointestinal tract longer. However, its action is not seen as readily as during rectal administration because the greatest amount of sodium-potassium exchange is in the colon. The usual dose is 1 g/kg up to 25 to 50 g. Kayexalate is a constipating agent, so it is usually given in a 20% solution of sorbitol, which acts as an osmotic agent. This unpalatable solution can be mixed with food or given through a stomach tube every 3 to 4 hours up to four to five doses in a single day as needed.

If it cannot be tolerated orally, Kayexalate can also be given as a retention enema, mixed with sorbitol. To be effective, the enema must be retained for at least 30 to 60 minutes.

It must be remembered that Kayexalate is a cation *exchange* resin. For each 1 mEq of potassium removed, 1.3 to 1.7 mEq of sodium is replaced. This situation is potentially dangerous in a volume-overloaded patient.

TABLE 3-3 ACID-BASE DISTURBANCES

DISORDER	PRIMARY CHANGE	SECONDARY RESPONSE	NET EFFECT	APPROXIMATE RELATIONSHIP
Metabolic acidosis	↓ $[HCO_3^-]$	↓ P_{CO_2}	↓ pH	Change in P_{CO_2} = 1.0 to 1.5 × change in $[HCO_3^-]$
Metabolic alkalosis	↑ $[HCO_3^-]$	↑ P_{CO_2}	↑ pH	Change in P_{CO_2} = 0.5 to 1.0 × change in $[HCO_3^-]$
Respiratory acidosis	↑ P_{CO_2}	↑ $[HCO_3^-]$	↓ pH	Acute: change in $[HCO_3^-]$ = 0.1 × change in P_{CO_2}, but usually <30 mEq/L Chronic: change in $[HCO_3^-]$ = 0.35 – 0.5 × change in P_{CO_2}
Respiratory alkalosis	↓ P_{CO_2}	↓ $[HCO_3^-]$	↑ pH	Acute: change in $[HCO_3^-]$ = 0.25 × change in P_{CO_2}, but usually >18 mEq/L Chronic: change in $[HCO_3^-]$ = 0.25 – 0.5 × change in P_{CO_2}, usually >14 mEq/L

Dialysis is the ultimate mode of potassium removal but should be reserved for those patients in whom other measures have failed or for whom dialysis is required for other reasons.

Acid-Base Disorders

Body pH is maintained within a very narrow range by means of a complex buffer system and the excretion of excess acid or base through the kidneys and lungs. Key to the management of any acid-base disturbance is the determination of the underlying disorder. An arterial blood gas is the best initial test. Table 3-3 is a guide to the changes in pH, P_{CO_2}, and bicarbonate during the four basic types of acid-base disturbance. Any compensatory changes in bicarbonate or P_{CO_2} inconsistent with the expected changes shown in the table should raise the possibility of a mixed acid-base disturbance.

A single component of the blood gas by itself is not meaningful. For instance, the serum bicarbonate level can be low in metabolic acidosis or respiratory alkalosis. Administration of bicarbonate in the latter case is actually fighting against the compensatory mechanism and could be detrimental to the patient. Knowledge of the pH and the P_{CO_2} provides the additional information necessary to distinguish between the two. Correction of the underlying problem is the most important part of management.

Metabolic Acidosis

The leading causes of metabolic acidosis in surgical patients are (1) accumulation of nonvolatile acids and the end products from anaerobic metabolism from hypoperfusion of tissues, reduced arterial oxygen saturation, or ketoacids produced by starvation or diabetes mellitus; (2) excessive loss of alkaline gastrointestinal fluids; and (3) decreased acid excretion by the kidney as a result of either an associated reduction of circulatory volume or intrinsic renal failure. As noted earlier, when the H^+ rises in body fluids, HCO_3^- falls through immediate action of the HCO_3^-/H_2CO_3 buffer system; quickly thereafter respiration is stimulated to produce a compensatory reduction of the carbonic acid content of plasma to maintain the 20:1 ratio of the buffer system required for protection of the pH of body fluids.

Treatment directed exclusively to correct an abnormality in acid-base balance without attention to the underlying cause of the abnormality fails to recognize the hierarchic ordering of homeostatic priorities. As a result, single-minded devotion to correcting pH may be unnecessary, ineffectual, or actually detrimental. When the metabolic acidosis is caused by low flow, diarrhea, or loss of alkaline gastrointestinal secretions, restoration of an inadequate circulatory volume is mandatory. Return of renal perfusion usually allows the kidney to correct the acid-base abnormality. It is rarely necessary to use intravenous sodium bicarbonate to supplement volume therapy of acute metabolic acidosis.

Calculation of the anion gap can provide a clue to the cause of the acid-base imbalance. Subtraction of the sum of serum Cl^- and HCO_3^- concentration from the serum Na^+ concentration is a simple, convenient expression of the anion gap. Normally, this level is in the range of 4 to 12 mEq/L (or, because these are monovalent ions, the gap can be expressed as milliosmoles). Some laboratories add the serum concentration of K^+ to serum Na^+ in calculating the anion gap; the range of normal values is 9 to 17 mEq/L with this calculation. When the metabolic acidosis is caused by a loss of HCO_3^- by diarrhea or upper intestinal fluid loss, the anion gap is not increased because there is an equivalent loss of sodium. An elevated anion gap is usually associated with the accumulation of organic acids, such as in lactic acidosis, diabetic acidosis, salicylate toxicity, or intoxication with paraldehyde, methanol, or ethylene glycol. In these conditions the HCO_3^- is removed to "make room" for the acids. An increased respiratory loss of CO_2 compensates, in turn, to maintain the 20:1 ratio of the bicarbonate buffer system that protects pH. Normal anion gaps in metabolic acidosis are due to the loss of bicarbonate and a resulting increased chloride level, or the addition of chloride-containing acids (e.g., NH_4Cl, HCl, or $CaCl_2$).[33,80,83]

Treatment of metabolic acidosis must focus on the correction of the underlying disorder, and bicarbonate should be given only when absolutely necessary. If the serum bicarbonate level is only moderately low (greater than 15 mEq/L) and if the cause of the acidosis can be treated, bicarbonate replacement may not be necessary. The kidneys can make the appropriate adjustments over a few days.

A frequent situation in a surgical patient is lactic acidosis secondary to hypoperfusion. Administration of bicarbonate without correcting the volume depletion is futile. However, restoration of adequate volume without administration of bicarbonate can usually correct the acidosis. It is commonly thought that Ringer's lactate solution should be avoided in this situation because it will add to the acid load already present. However, the sodium lactate is not lactic acid, but a metabolic precursor of bicarbonate. As the ECF volume is increased and circulation to the liver is restored, anaerobic metabolism ceases and the lactate can be metabolized to bicarbonate, with correction of the acidosis.

If the bicarbonate level is markedly depressed (e.g., less than 10 mEq/L), intravenous bicarbonate may be necessary. A very rough approximation of the amount needed can be made:

Body weight × 0.4
× (desired bicarbonate − actual bicarbonate)
= Bicarbonate deficit

This calculation is based on an approximate volume of distribution for bicarbonate of about 40% of body weight during times of marked acidosis. The desired bicarbonate level used in the formula should be about 15 to 18 mEq/L to avoid overcorrection. About half of the deficit should be given over the first 12 hours while the blood gases and electrolytes are monitored.

Bicarbonate administration is hazardous. It may be contraindicated in the volume-overloaded patient who cannot tolerate the osmolarity or sodium load in sodium bicarbonate. It is also essential to monitor potassium levels carefully because potassium will be driven into cells. Symptomatic hypokalemia can occur if any potassium losses are not replaced simultaneously. Furthermore, as the circulatory volume is restored, the accumulated lactic acid and ketone bodies are metabolized to bicarbonate and thereby add endogenous assistance to correction of the acid-base imbalance. Other possible detrimental effects of bicarbonate include venous hypercapnia, decrease in intracellular pH, cerebrospinal fluid acidosis, tissue hypoxia, and circulatory congestion.[7] Therefore several other agents have been developed for the treatment of anaerobic lactic acidosis. These include Tris buffer (2-amino-2-hydroxymethyl-1, 3-propanediol) (THAM), Carbicarb, and dichloroacetate.[7]

CAUSES OF METABOLIC ALKALOSIS

Sodium Chloride Responsive
Gastric chloride loss (gastric suction, prolonged vomiting)
Diuretics*
Chloride restriction
Abrupt relief of hypercapnia

Sodium Chloride Resistant
Hyperaldosteronism
Bartter's syndrome
Cushing's syndrome
Severe potassium depletion
Excessive licorice ingestion

*See text.

Metabolic Alkalosis

Metabolic alkalosis is a result of the loss of acids or the gain of bicarbonate. There is a rise in mortality when a pH of 7.55 is exceeded, and a pH of 7.65 to 7.70 has been associated with an overall mortality of 80%.[120] It is difficult to administer enough bicarbonate to cause metabolic alkalosis because the kidneys have a striking ability to eliminate excess bicarbonate. One exception, however, occurs after excessive use of bicarbonate during resuscitation for a cardiac arrest. A surplus of bicarbonate also exists in a patient who has had chronic hypercapnia that is abruptly corrected by ventilation. The patient is then left with a relative abundance of alkali, which will be excreted gradually.

For the purposes of management, it is easier to classify conditions into two subgroups, depending on their responsiveness to NaCl (see accompanying box).

A common cause of metabolic alkalosis in a surgical patient is the removal of gastric hydrochloric acid by nasogastric suction or during prolonged vomiting. Administration of hydrochloric acid to balance the gastric losses will not correct the situation. The early loss of chloride from the stomach results in an imbalance in the sodium/chloride ratio. Sodium loss in the kidney is accompanied by bicarbonate loss because the serum chloride concentration is low. This mechanism provides a partial compensation for the acidosis. As gastric losses continue, the ECF becomes compromised, leading to an outpouring of aldosterone.

In its attempts to conserve volume, the kidney reabsorbs sodium, excreting K^+ and H^+ instead. Initially, K^+ is excreted, but when the serum potassium level drops low enough, H^+ is excreted instead. This renal loss of H^+ gives an acid urine and accounts for the "paradoxical aciduria." This condition is usually found in children who have prolonged vomiting caused by pyloric stenosis or in adults with "subtraction alkalosis." In this situation, the kidneys excrete K^+ and H^+ to conserve sodium after circulatory volume has become threatened. As the K^+ deficiency becomes pronounced, the production of NH_4^+ is augmented, which leads to a greater renal loss of H^+. The urine pH is usually near 7.0 in these patients despite the substantial metabolic alkalosis in their body fluids. Although the mechanisms are not fully understood, it seems likely that the K^+ deficiency causes a shift of H^+ into cells. In the renal epithelial cells, the change in ratio of these two ions promotes the secretion of H^+, while HCO_3^- reabsorption is inhibited by maintenance of a high threshold.

Therefore management depends on the replacement of volume, chloride, sodium, and potassium. An appropriate choice for a fluid to correct these deficits is isotonic saline with 40 to 60 mEq/L of potassium chloride. The preferred course of action is to try to prevent the development of any deficits. Gastric losses can be replaced with a specific mixture designed to approximate gastric fluid (see Table 3-1). However, 0.5 N saline with 20 mEq/L of potassium chloride is also an adequate solution. This fluid should be given at a rate that approximates the rate of gastric losses. In addition, normal maintenance fluids are given.

Most diuretics can cause a metabolic alkalosis and probably account for more patients with this acid-base abnormality than any other cause. Potassium-sparing and carbonic-anhydrase inhibitors are exceptions and can actually lead to metabolic acidosis. The other diuretics lead to a greater urinary excretion of chloride than bicarbonate. Therefore bicarbonate is transported with sodium, as outlined earlier. A potassium deficit is almost always present in metabolic alkalosis, requiring the replacement of potassium chloride once adequate urine flow has been ensured.

Rarely, in severe metabolic alkalosis (pH greater than 7.6 and serum HCO_3^- greater than 40 to 45 mEq/L), infusion of an acid solution may be necessary. A 0.1N to 0.2N solution of hydrochloric acid given through a central line is the therapy of choice.[1,119] The chloride deficit can be approximated using 40% of body weight for the apparent volume of distribution of chloride during alkalosis:

Body weight × 0.4 × (normal serum chloride − measure serum chloride) = chloride deficit

Half this amount can be given over the first 2 to 4 hours and the rest over the next 24 hours. Arterial blood gases and serum electrolytes should be monitored closely (every 4 to 6 hours).

Management of the sodium chloride-resistant forms of metabolic alkalosis depends on the treatment of the underlying disorder.

Respiratory Acidosis and Respiratory Alkalosis

Because the pulmonary control of CO_2 excretion constitutes the first line of defense of the pH of body fluids, any acute pulmonary disorder promptly induces a serious threat to homeostasis of pH. The only compensation the body can make beyond the limited modulation afforded by tissue buffers depends on renal alteration in the excretion of HCO_3^- and acid. This compensation requires time. For instance, in respiratory acidosis the kidneys do respond within 5 to 7 days by excretion of acid and reabsorption of HCO_3 to minimize the degree of acidemia.

Respiratory alkalosis caused by a decrease in arterial P_{CO_2} may be caused by a large number of disorders that produce hyperventilation. The characteristic clinical picture includes numbness, tingling, light-headedness, and even tetany, which can be induced by voluntary hyperventilation. The body buffers and renal compensatory mechanisms are not sufficiently prompt to prevent these changes induced by a sudden respiratory loss of carbonic acid. In time, the kidney reduces reabsorption of bicarbonate to bring the plasma level of bicarbonate closer to the required ration with P_{CO_2}.

In both respiratory acidosis and alkalosis, the only appropriate therapy is directed to correct the underlying respiratory disorder. Giving bicarbonate to a patient with respiratory acidosis is dangerous because the respiratory drive from an elevated H^+ concentration may be reduced. These disorders are properly treated by discovery of the underlying respiratory problem and dealing directly with this alteration.

Mixed Disorders

Unfortunately, patients do not always fall into one of the four standard categories of acid-base disorders; sometimes they exhibit components of two and sometimes three of them. A careful history and physical examination and determination of electrolytes and arterial blood gas are necessary to make a diagnosis.[59,80]

A frequent example of a mixed disorder is the patient with severe gastroenteritis, with prolonged vomiting and diarrhea. The diarrhea causes a metabolic acidosis as a result of the loss of bicarbonate through the stool. The serum chloride level is elevated because chloride is reabsorbed preferentially with sodium as a result of the lack of bicarbonate. However, vomiting causes a hypochloremic metabolic alkalosis as outlined earlier. Management of this mixed disorder is through the administration of fluids. The composition of the fluids depends on the relative contribution of each disorder. For example, if an aspiration pneumonia complicates the situation, it is not unusual to find components of a respiratory acidosis as well.

Clinical Examples

Following are some of the more commonly encountered surgical problems with fluid and electrolyte abnormalities. In reviewing these problems, it is worth emphasizing that patients rarely have a single abnormality but combine several. The general principles for each disorder still apply but may require modification, depending on other changes.

Upper Gastrointestinal Tract Losses

The metabolic alkalosis, hypokalemia, and sodium deficit associated with prolonged loss of gastric contents have been described. Obstruction of the jejunum leads to the loss of gastric, biliary, duodenal, pancreatic, and other jejunal secretions. Ileal obstruction initially shows fluid loss from the circulation into three "third spaces": the lumen of the bowel, the bowel wall, and the peritoneal cavity. Eventually, the entire bowel proximal to the obstruction loses its ability to handle fluids and electrolytes.[103] Large volumes of fluid can be lost quickly, leading to a depleted ECF space and ultimately causing hypovolemic shock. The electrolytes lost depend on the contribution of each of the secretions shown in Table 3-1 and should be replaced accordingly. In general, there is a need for sodium, chloride, potassium, and bicarbonate. A useful solution for small-bowel losses is lactated Ringer's solution with 15 mEq/L of potassium chloride.

Fully correcting the abnormalities is impossible until the obstruction has been relieved. Decompression of the GI tract with a nasogastric tube gains time, but preoperative restoration of fluid volume is essential. The rapidity with which the patient undergoes surgery depends on the clinical condition. If there is a closed loop obstruction with the risk of strangulation or perforation, urgent surgery is required with rapid fluid and electrolyte correction. In other patients, fluid and electrolyte balance can be optimized before surgery.

Lower Gastrointestinal Tract Losses

About 8 to 9 L of fluid enter the jejunum daily, mainly from endogenous secretions such as saliva and gastric juices (see Table 3-1). However, only about 0.6 L enters the colon where an additional 500 ml are reabsorbed. Therefore obstruction of the colon does not cause any major abnormalities until the obstruction has been present for a substantial period of time. Early losses are minimal and can usually be replaced with saline.

Diarrhea, if severe, can cause a marked depletion in the ECF.[30,42] Rapid transit of normal gastrointestinal secretions leads to a loss of sodium, potassium, and bicarbonate in excess of chloride. This loss results in a hyperchloremic acidosis and is one of the most common causes of metabolic acidosis with a normal anion gap. Treatment depends on the replacement of sodium, potassium, bicarbonate, and some chloride despite the elevated serum chloride levels. If the electrolyte abnormalities are not severe, oral therapy is usually adequate and appropriate.

Establishing the value of oral therapy has been a major goal of the World Health Organization (WHO), but its value has been recognized only recently in developed nations. The fluid recommended by the WHO consists of 90 mEq/L of sodium, 20 mEq/L of potassium, 80 mEq/L of chloride, 30 mEq/L of bicarbonate, and 111 mmole/L of glucose.[89] Opponents of this fluid argue that the sodium content is too high because it was chosen as a replacement for diarrhea caused by cholera, a rare problem in developed countries. Fluids using a lower sodium concentration have been used successfully.[57,97]

If oral replacement is not possible, the intravenous administration of 0.5N saline with 40 mEq/L of potassium chloride and 25 mEq/L of sodium bicarbonate can be used to approximate diarrheal losses. Electrolytes should be monitored with appropriate corrections as needed.

Fistulas

Fistulas may occur at any level of the gastrointestinal tract and can present a major challenge to fluid and electrolyte management. A fistula that drains completely outside the body, where the daily volume and electrolyte loss can be measured, is the easiest kind to handle. The best example of this situation is the surgically created ileostomy. Daily losses from the ileostomy in excess of normal stool losses need to be replaced to prevent any abnormalities.

Unfortunately, most fistulas present more of a problem. Even knowledge of the normal electrolyte concentrations and volumes of various gastrointestinal secretions is of little help. A fistula frequently diverts only part of the intestinal contents.

If the diversion is to an area that cannot be measured, as with a bilicolic fistula, determining the appropriate fluid volume is more difficult. Table 3-1 lists the electrolyte concentrations and volumes for each secretion, but intestinal contents are actually a combination of these in varying amounts. Fluid and electrolyte disorders are seen primarily with pancreatic, duodenal stump, ileal, bilicolic, and gastrojejunal anastomotic fistulas.[118]

Duodenal stump fistulas, following Billroth II-type gastrectomies, are high in bile and pancreatic secretions. One patient had a daily drainage of 1 to 4 L/day of a fluid with a sodium content of 121 mEq/L and a chloride of 54 mEq/L. The bicarbonate loss can be estimated at 67 mEq/L. As expected from these measurements, the patient developed a severe volume depletion and metabolic acidosis.[25]

Some guidelines can be helpful. Although bile and pancreatic secretions are alkaline, the contents in the upper jejunum are acidic and have a high sodium content. As the fluid moves through the gastrointestinal tract, there is a gradual exchange of K^+ for Na^+ and of HCO_3^- from the blood for intestinal Cl^-. Simultaneously, water is absorbed; when the contents reach the ileum, they are alkaline, with a high K^+ content and decreased volume. Therefore high fistulas usually cause a loss of sodium and give a metabolic alkalosis. Low fistulas lead to a metabolic acidosis and hypokalemia. These are only guidelines. A high fistula that is rich in bile and pancreatic secretions, as in the duodenal stump fistula discussed earlier, causes hyponatremia and metabolic acidosis.

Therapy depends on the fluid lost through the fistula. If possible, a sample of this fluid should be analyzed for electrolyte content to aid in fluid replacement. Weighing the patient daily provides a measure of the adequacy of volume replacement.

Peritonitis

Any disorder leading to peritonitis, such as perforation of the GI tract, pancreatitis, or a penetrating wound of the abdomen, causes an isotonic desalting dehydration.[28] The volume of fluid lost varies greatly with the specific cause, but it may reach a lethal level within a few hours. Fluid is sequestered ("third space") not only within the inflamed ("burned") peritoneal cavity, but it may also accumulate as edema in the bowel wall and within the paralyzed bowel lumen. Treatment of the volume deficit is straightforward: decompression of the GI tract with a nasogastric tube, rapid infusion of lactated Ringer's solution guided by the physiologic status of the patient, and urgent correction of the disorder causing the peritoneal "burn." Supplemental potassium (15 to 30 mEq/L) and glucose (100 g within 24 hours) are advantageous.

REFERENCES

1 Abouna GM, Veazey PR, Terry DB: Intravenous infusion of hydrochloric acid for treatment of severe metabolic alkalosis, *Surgery* 75:194, 1974.

2 Addison T: *The constitutional and local effects of diseases of the suprarenal capsules,* London, 1885, Highley.

3 Adolph EF, Gerbasi MJ, Lepore MJ: The rate of entrance fluid into the blood in hemorrhage, *Am J Physiol* 104:502, 1933.

4 Allon M, Dunlay R, Copkney C: Nebulized albuterol for acute hyperkalemia in patients on hemodialysis, *Ann Intern Med* 110:426, 1989.

5 Andersson B: Regulation of water intake, *Physiol Rev* 58:582, 1972.

6 Andersson B, Leksell LG, Rundgren M: Regulation of body fluids: intake and output. In Staub NC, Taylor AE, editors: *Edema,* New York, 1984, Raven Press.

7 Arieff AI: Indications for use of bicarbonate in patients with metabolic acidosis, *Br J Anaesth* 67:165, 1991.

8 Arieff AI, Guisado R: Effects on the central nervous system of hypernatremic and hyponatremic states, *Kidney Int* 10:104, 1976.

9 Arrhenius S: Über der Dissociation der im Wasser Gelösten Stoffe, *Z Physikal Chem* 1:631, 1887.

10 Baldwin EJ: *An introduction to comparative biochemistry,* Cambridge, England, 1948, Cambridge University Press.

11 Banting FG, Gairns S: Suprarenal insufficiency, *Am J Physiol* 77:100, 1926.

12 Bartholin T: *Vasa lymphatica, nuper hafniae in animantibus inventa, et hepatis exequiae,* Paris, 1653, DuPuis.

13 Berl T: Treating hyponatremia: damned if we do and damned if we don't, *Kidney Int* 37:1006, 1990.

14 Berl T, Schrier RW: Disorders of water metabolism. In Schrier RW, editor: *Renal and electrolyte disorders,* ed 4, Boston, 1992, Little, Brown.

15 Bernard C: *Lecons sur les phenomenes de la vie,* Paris, 1878, Bailliere.

16 Borst JGG, DeVies LA, VanLeeuwen AM et al: The maintenance of circulatory stability at the expense of volume and electrolyte stability. In Steward CP, Strengers T, editors: *Water and electrolyte metabolism,* Amsterdam, 1960, Elsevier.

17 Cannon WB: *The wisdom of the body,* New York, 1939, WW Norton.

18 Casley-Smith JR: The fine structure of tissues and tissue channels. In Hargens AR, editor: *Tissue fluid pressure and composition,* Baltimore, 1981, Williams and Wilkins.

19 Chadwick CDJ, Pearce FJ, Drucker WR: Influences of fasting and water intake on plasma refill during hemorrhagic shock, *J Trauma* 25:608, 1985.

20 Clark RG: Fluid, electrolyte and nutritional support. In Taylor S, Chisholm GD, O'Higgins N, Shields R, editors: *Surgical management,* London, 1984, William Heinemann Medical Books.

21 Courtice FC: The development of concepts of fluid balance. In Staub NC, Taylor AE, editors: *Edema,* New York, 1984, Raven Press.

22 Darwin C: *On the origin of the species by means of natural selection, or the preservation of favoured races in the struggle for life,* London, 1859, John Murray.

23 Davis JO, Freeman RH: Mechanisms regulating renin release, *Physiol* 56:1, 1976.

24 Dell RB: Pathophysiology of dehydration. In Winters RW, editor: *The body fluids in pediatrics,* Boston, 1973, Little, Brown.

25 Denton DA: Renal regulation of the extracellular fluid: I. A study of homeostasis in a patient with a duodenal fistula, *Med J Aust* 2:521, 1949.

26 DeVies LA, Tenholt SP, VanDaatselaar JJ et al: Characteristic renal excretion patterns in response to physiological, pathological and pharmacological stimuli. In Steward CP, Strengers T, editors: *Water and electrolyte metabolism,* Amsterdam, 1960, Elsevier.

27 Drinker CK: Extravascular protein and the lymphatic system, *Ann NY Acad Sci* 46:807, 1947.

28 Drucker RP, Drucker WR: Fluid and electrolyte therapy. In Cameron JL, editor: *Current surgical therapy,* ed 3, Toronto, 1989, BC Decker.

29 Drucker WR: Water and salt metabolism. In Schumer W, Nyhus LM, editors: *Corticosteroids in the treatment of shock,* Urbana, 1970, University of Illinois Press.

30 Drucker WR, Wright HK: Physiology and pathophysiology of gastrointestinal fluids. In Ellison EH, Julian OC, Thal AP, Wangensteen DH, editors: *Current problems in surgery,* Chicago, 1964, Mosby.

31 Dudley HAF: Body water and electrolytes. In Burnett W, editor: *Clinical science for surgeons,* London, 1981, Butterworths.

32 Dutrochet M: Nouvelles observations sur l'endosmose et l'exosmose, et sur la cause de ce double phenomene, *Ann Chim Phys* 35:393, 1827.

33 Emmett M, Narins RG: Clinical use of the anion gap, *Medicine* 56:38, 1977.

34 Faraday M: Experimental researches in electricity—seventh series: on electrochemical decomposition, *Philos Trans R Soc* 124:77, 1834.

35 Feig PU, McCurdy DK: The hypertonic state, *N Engl J Med* 297:1444, 1977.

36 Fenn WO: Electrolytes in muscle, *Physiol Rev* 16:450, 1936.

37 Fichman MP, Vorherr H, Kleeman CR et al: Diuretic-induced hyponatremia, *Ann Intern Med* 75:853, 1971.

38 Fitzsimmons JT: Thirst, *Physiol Rev* 52:468, 1972.

39 Fitzsimmons JT: The physiological basis of thirst, *Kidney Int* 10:3, 1976.

40 Flinn RB, Merrill JP, Welzant WR: Treatment of the oliguric patient with a new sodium-exchange resin and sorbitol, *N Engl J Med* 264:111, 1961.

41 Gamble JL: Physiological information gained from studies on the life raft ration, *Harvey Lect* 42:247, 1946.

42 Gamble JL: *Chemical anatomy, physiology and pathology of extracellular fluid,* Cambridge, 1957, Harvard University Press.

43 Gamble JL, Ross GS, Tisdall FF: The metabolism of fixed base during fasting, *J Biol Chem* 57:633, 1923.

44 Gann DS, Wright HK: Augmentation of sodium excretion in postoperative patients by expansion of the extracellular fluid volume, *Surg Gynecol Obstet* 118:1024, 1964.

45 Gaudino M, Levitt MF: Influences of the adrenal cortex on body water distribution and renal function, *J Clin Invest* 28:1487, 1949.

46 Gnepp DR: Lymphatics. In Staub NC, Taylor AE, editors: *Edema,* New York, 1984, Raven Press.

47 Graham T: Liquid diffusion applied to analysis, *Philos Trans R Soc Lond* 151:183, 1861.

48 Granger HJ, Laine GA, Barnes GE et al: Dynamics and control of transmicrovascular fluid exchange. In Staub NC, Taylor AE, editors: *Edema,* New York, 1984, Raven Press.

49 Gulliver G: *The works of William Hewson,* F.R.S. London, 1846, The Syndenham Society.

50 Harrison HE, Darrow DC, Yannet H: The total electrolyte content of animals and its probable relation to the distribution of body water, *J Biol Chem* 113:515, 1936.

51 Harrop GA, Nicholson WM, Strauss MB: Studies on the suprarenal cortex. V. The influence of the corticol hormone upon the excretion of water and electrolytes in the supradrenalectomized dog, *J Exp Med* 64:233, 1936.

52 Hastings AB: The electrolytes of tissues and body fluids, *Harvey Lect* 36:91, 1940.

53 Hastings AB, Eichelberger L: Exchange of salt and water between muscle and blood, *J Biol Chem* 117:73, 1937.

54 Hayes MA: Water and electrolyte therapy after operation, *N Engl J Med* 278:1054, 1968.

55 Henderson LJ: *The fitness of the environment,* New York, 1913, MacMillan.

56 Holliday M, Segar WE: The maintenance need for water in parenteral fluid therapy, *Pediatrics* 19:823, 1957.

57 Hunt JB, Elliott EJ, Fairclough PD et al: Water and solute absorption from hypotonic glucose—electrolyte solutions in human jejunum, *Gut* 33:479, 1992.

58 Kaehny WD: Pathogenesis and management of respiratory and mixed acid-base disorders. In Schrier RW, editor: *Renal and electrolyte disorders,* Boston, 1992, Little, Brown.

59 Krieger JW, Sherrard DJ, editors: *Practical fluids and electrolytes,* Norwalk, 1991, Appleton and Lange.

60 Kunis CL, Lowenstein J: The emergency treatment of hyperkalemia, *Med Clin North Am* 65:165, 1981.

61 Landis EM, Pappenheimer JR: Exchange of substances through the capillary walls. In Hamilton WF, editor: *Handbook of physiology,* Washington, DC, 1963, American Physiology Society.

62 Latta RW: Case of malignant cholera in which 480 ounces of fluid were injected into the veins with success, *Lancet* 2:688, 1831.

63 Lavoisier AL, Seguin A: Premier memoire sur la chaleur. In his Oeuvres, Tome, II. *Memories de chimie et de physique,* Paris, 1862, Paris Imprimerie Imperiale.

64 Leaf A: On the mechanism of fluid exchange of tissue in vitro, *Biochem J* 62:241, 1956.

65 Leaf A, Cotran RS: *Renal physiology,* Oxford, 1985, Oxford University Press.

66 Levy-Simpson S: The use of synthetic desoxycorticosterone acetate in Addison's disease, *Lancet* 2:557, 1938.

67 Liebig J: *Familiar letters on chemistry,* London, 1845, Taylor and Walton.

68 Loeb RF: The adrenal cortex and electrolyte behaviour, *Harvey Lect* 37:100, 1941.

69 Macknight ADC: Cellular volume under physiological conditions. In Staub NC, Taylor AE, editors: *Edema,* New York, 1984, Raven Press.

70 Macknight ADC: Cellular response to injury. In Staub NC, Taylor AE, editors: *Edema,* New York, 1984, Raven Press.

71 Magnus-Levy A: The physiology of metabolism. In VonNoorden C, Keenan WT, editors: *Metabolism and practical medicine,* Chicago, 1907, WT Kenner.

72 Major RH: Santorio Santorio, *Ann Med Hist* 10:369, 1938.

73 Marks LJ, King DW, Kingsbury PF et al: Physiologic role of the adrenal cortex in the maintenance of plasma volume following hemorrhage or surgical operation, *Surgery* 58:510, 1965.

74 Mengoli LR: Excerpts from the history of postoperative fluid therapy, *Am J Surg* 121:311, 1971.

75 Miller M, Moses A: Drug-induced states of impaired water excretion, *Kidney Int* 10:96, 1976.

76 Moran WH, Miltenberger FW, Shuayb WA, Zimmerman B: The relationship of antidiuretic hormone secretion to surgical stress, *Surgery* 56:99, 1961.

77 Moulton CR: Age and chemical development in mammals, *J Biol Chem* 57:79, 1923.

78 Mudge GH: Electrolyte and water metabolism of rabbit kidney slices: effect or metabolic inhibitors, *Am J Physiol* 167:206, 1951.

79 Murdoch IA, Dos Anjos R, Haycock GB: Treatment of hyperkalemia with intravenous salbutamol, *Arch Dis Child* 66:527, 1991.

80 Narins RG, Emmett M: Simple and mixed acid-base disorders: a practical approach, *Medicine* 59:161, 1980.

81 Navar LG: Renal regulation of body fluid balance. In Staub NC, Taylor AE, editors: *Edema,* New York, 1984, Raven Press.

82 Nothnagel H: Durst und Polydipsie, *Virchows Arch (Pathol Anat Physiol)* 86:435, 1881.

83 Oh MS, Carroll HJ: The anion gap, *N Engl J Med* 297:814, 1977.

84 Oliver G, Schafer EA: On the physiological action of extracts of pituitary body and certain other glandular organs, *J Physiol* (Lond) 18:277, 1895.

85 O'Shaughnessy WB: Experiments on the blood in cholera, *Lancet* 1:490, 1831.

86 Pace N, Rathbun EN: Studies on body composition. III. The body water and chemically combined nitrogen content in relation to fat content, *J Biol Chem* 158:685, 1945.

87 Peters JP: The significance of serum sodium, *McGill Med J* 18:130, 1949.

88 Pierce NF, Fedson DS, Brigham KL et al: The ventilatory response to acute base deficit in humans: time course during development and correction of metabolic acidosis, *Ann Intern Med* 72:633, 1970.

89 Pierce NF, Hirschorn N: Oral fluid—a simple weapon against dehydration in diarrhea: how it works and how to use it, *WHO Chron* 31:87, 1977.

90 Pirkle JC, Gann DS: Restitution of blood volume after hemorrhage: role of the adrenal cortex, *Am J Physiol* 230:1683, 1976.

91 Pullinger BD, Florey HW: Some observations on the structure and functions of lymphatics: their behavior in local edema, *Br J Exp Pathol* 16:49, 1935.

92 Ramsay DJ: Asymmetric control of vasopressin in the dog, *Am J Physiol* 243:E287, 1982.

93 Reid IA: Endocrine regulation of body fluid balance. In Staub NC, Taylor AE, editors: *Edema,* New York, 1984, Raven Press.

94 Robertson GL, Athar S: The interaction of blood osmolality and blood volume in regulating vasopressin secretion in man, *J Clin Endocrinol Metab* 42:613, 1976.

95 Robinson JR: *A prelude to physiology,* Oxford, 1975, Blackwell.

96 Rogoff JM, Stewart GN: Studies on adrenal insufficiency, *Am J Physiol* 84:649, 1928.

97 Santosham M, Daum RS, Dillman L et al: Oral rehydration therapy of infantile diarrhea, *N Engl J Med* 306:1070, 1982.

98 Schafer EA: Croonian lecture: the function of the pituitary body, *Proc R Soc Lond (Biol)* 81:442, 1909.

99 Scherr L, Ogden DA, Mead AW et al: Management of hyperkalemia with a cation-exchange resin, *N Engl J Med* 264:115, 1961.

100 Schloerb PR, Friis-Hansen BJ, Edelman IS et al: The measurement of total body water in the human subject by deuterium oxide dilution, *J Clin Invest* 29:1296, 1950.

101 Schrier RW, editor: *Renal and electrolyte disorders,* ed 4, Boston, 1992, Little, Brown.

102 Seldin DW, Giebison G, editors: *The regulation of sodium and chloride balance,* New York, 1990, Raven.

103 Shields R: The absorption and secretion of fluid and electrolytes by the obstructed bowel, *Br J Surg* 52:774, 1965.

104 Simpson SA, Tait JF: Recent progress in methods of isolation, chemistry and physiology of aldosterone, *Rec Prog Horm Res* 11:183, 1955.

105 Skavlem JH: The scientific life of Thomas Bartholin, *Ann Med Hist* 3:67, 1921.

106 Smith HG: Renal physiology. In Fishman AP, Richards DW, editors: *Circulation of the blood: men and ideas,* New York, 1964, Oxford University Press.

107 Spencer WG: *Celsus: de medicina with an English translator,* London, Loeb, Library, 1935, Heinemann.

108 Stern JR, Eggleston LV, Hems R et al: Accumulation of glutamic acid in isolated brain tissue, *Biochem J* 44:410, 1949.

109 Sterns RH: The management of hyponatremic emergencies, *Crit Care Clin* 7:127, 1991.

110 Sterns RH: Severe hyponatremia: the case for conservative management, *Crit Care Med* 20:534, 1992.

111 Stewart JD, Rourke GM: Intracellular fluid loss in hemorrhage, *J Clin Invest* 14:697, 1936.

112 Strauss MB: *Body water in man. The acquisition and maintenance of the body fluids,* Boston, 1957, Little, Brown.

113 Swingle WW, DaVango JP, Crossfield HC et al: Glucocorticoids and maintenance of blood pressure and plasma volume of adrenalectomized dogs subjected to stress, *Proc Exp Biol Med* 100:617, 1959.

114 Swingle WW, Parkins WM, Taylor AR et al: The influence of adrenal cortical hormone upon electrolyte and fluid distribution in adrenalectomized dogs maintained on a sodium and chloride free diet, *Am J Physiol* 119:684, 1937.

115 Valtin H: *Renal dysfunction: mechanisms involved in fluid and solute balance,* Boston, 1979, Little, Brown.

116 Verney EB: Croonian lecture: the antidiuretic hormone an the factors which determine its release, *Proc Roy Soc Lond (Biol)* 135:25, 1947.

117 Voit C: Physiologic des stoffwechels und der ernahrung. In Hermann L, editor: *Handbuch/der Physiologie,* vol 6 (part I), Leipzig, 1881, Vogel.

118 Weinberg J: Fluid and electrolyte disorders and gastrointestinal diseases. In Kokko JP, Tannen RL, editors: *Fluids and electrolytes,* Philadelphia, 1986, WB Saunders.

119 Williams DB, Lyons JH: Treatment of severe metabolic alkalosis with intravenous infusion of hydrochloric acid, *Surg Gynecol Obstet* 150:315, 1980.

120 Wilson RF, Gibson D, Percinel AK et al: Severe alkalosis in critically ill surgical patients, *Arch Surg* 105:197, 1972.

121 Wilson TH: Ionic permeability and osmotic swelling of cells, *Science* 120:104, 1954.

122 Wissig SL, Charonis AS: Capillary ultrastructure. In Staub NC, Taylor AE, editors: *Edema,* New York, 1984, Raven Press.

123 Wrenn KD, Slovis CM, Slovis BS: The ability of physicians to predict hyperkalemia from the ECG, *Ann Emerg Med* 20:1229, 1991.

CHAPTER

4

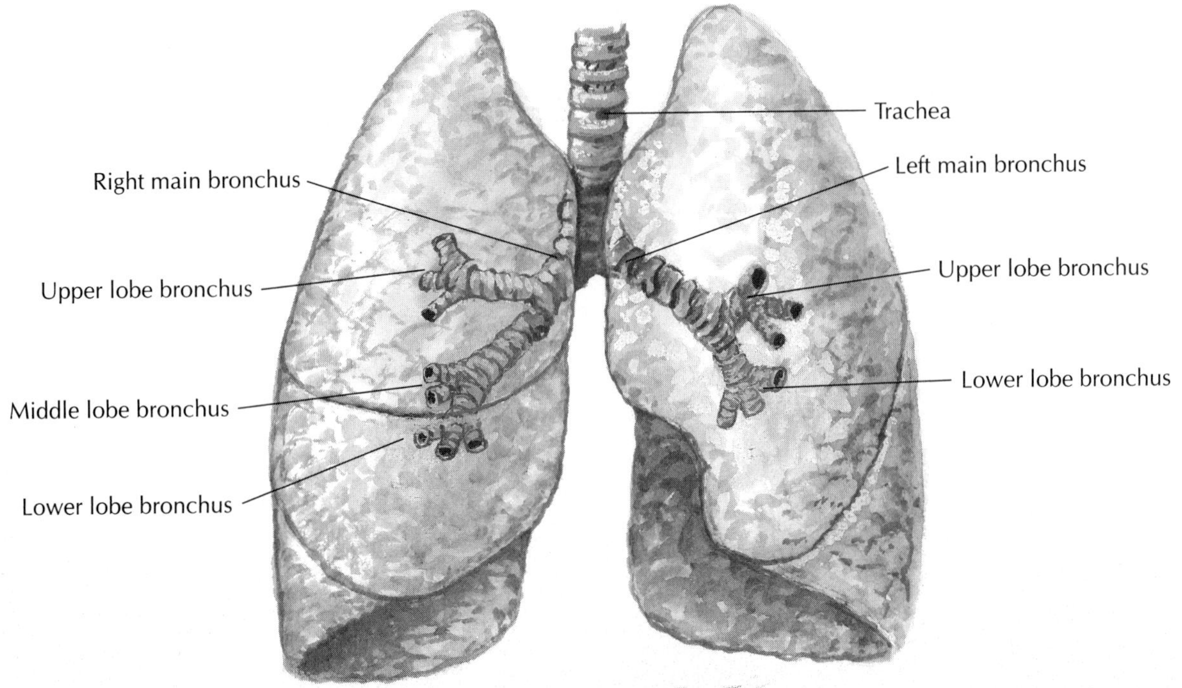
Trachea
Right main bronchus
Left main bronchus
Upper lobe bronchus
Upper lobe bronchus
Lower lobe bronchus
Middle lobe bronchus
Lower lobe bronchus

After Schlossberg

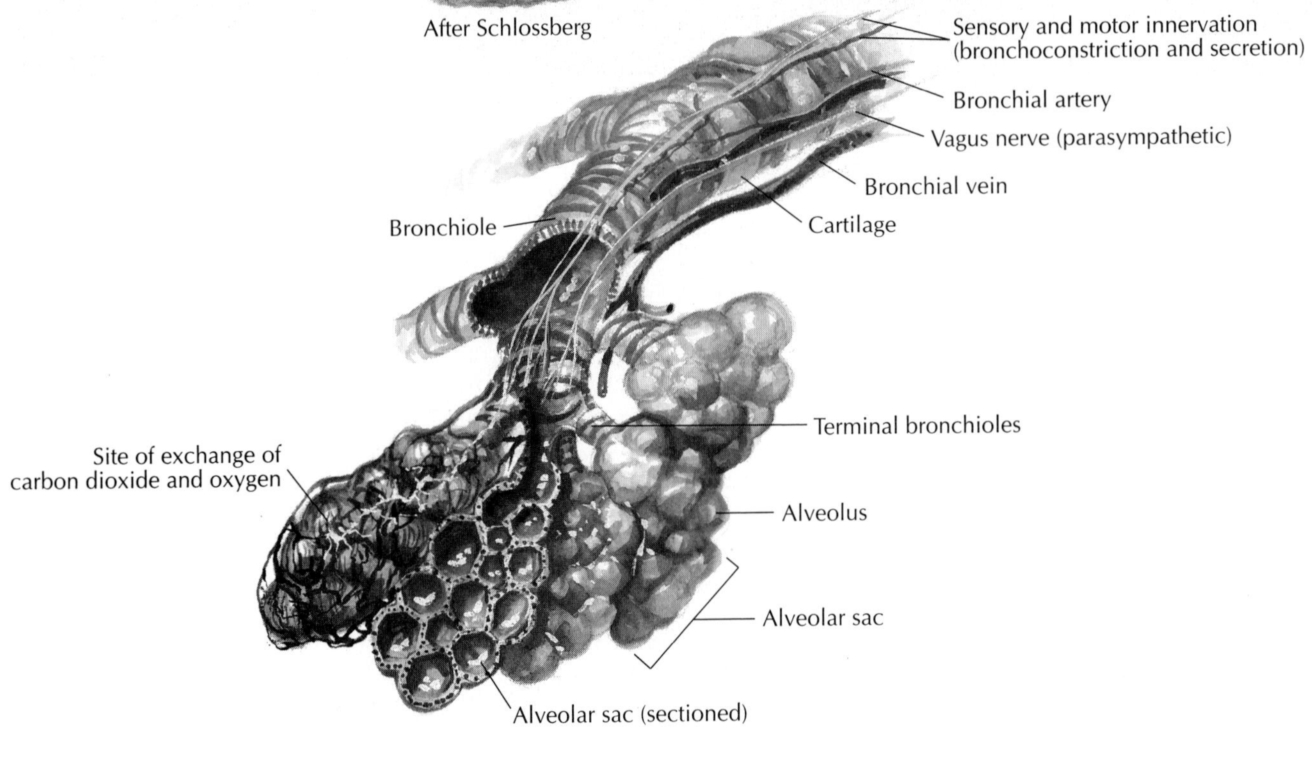
Sensory and motor innervation
(bronchoconstriction and secretion)
Bronchial artery
Vagus nerve (parasympathetic)
Bronchial vein
Bronchiole
Cartilage
Terminal bronchioles
Site of exchange of
carbon dioxide and oxygen
Alveolus
Alveolar sac
Alveolar sac (sectioned)

RESPIRATORY FUNCTION

David J. Dries

RELATED MATERIAL APPEARS IN CHAPTERS 5, 14, 15, AND 16

ANATOMIC AND PHYSIOLOGIC CONSIDERATIONS

Airways[48,74,78]

The upper airway extends from the nose through the cervical trachea. This area includes the nose, mouth, pharynx, larynx, and upper trachea. The nose moistens air and removes inhaled particular matter via a vascular mucous membrane with ciliated columnar epithelium. Air passing through the nose is completely humidified and warmed to body temperature by the time it reaches the tracheal bifurcation. Breathing through the mouth or an endotracheal tube may circumvent this mechanism, causing drying and irritation to the upper airway (Figure 4-1).

Anatomically, the pharynx is divided into the nasal pharynx, oral pharynx, and laryngopharynx. The pharynx is the common upper channel for both the respiratory and digestive tracts. From a position above the soft palate, the nasal pharynx separates the oral and nasal cavities during the act of swallowing. The oral pharynx reaches from the soft palate to the superior aspect of the epiglottis covering and protecting the upper opening of the larynx during deglutition. Posterior and lateral to the larynx is the hypopharynx. This structure extends from the lateral aspect of the epiglottis to the lower border of the cricoid where it becomes the esophagus. Pyriform sinuses are the lateral portions of the hypopharynx; foreign bodies are frequently caught here if they fail to enter the larynx or esophagus. One of the major functions of the larynx is prevention of entry of food and swallowed foreign particles into the trachea. Upward movement of the larynx and downward motion of the flaplike epiglottis accomplish this task.

The larynx extends from the epiglottis to the cricoid cartilage at the level of C6 where the trachea is reached. Vocal cord opposition allows the patient to increase intrathoracic pressure before coughing, with irritation of the larynx or tracheobronchial tree. Sounds are created by vibration and vocal cord movement. Higher tones are created by thinner, shorter, and tighter vocal cords. Notably, whispering does not require normal vocal cords and can be accomplished in the presence of severe inflammation. Prolonged tracheal intubation may damage vocal cords and result in speechlessness. Intubation for as short as several days may result in hoarse-

■ Portions of this chapter reprinted from Dries DJ: Perioperative mechanical ventilatory support, *Probl Crit Care* 5:565, 1991; and Dries DJ, Mathru M: Cardiovascular performance in embolism, *Anesthesiol Clin North Am* 10:755, 1992.

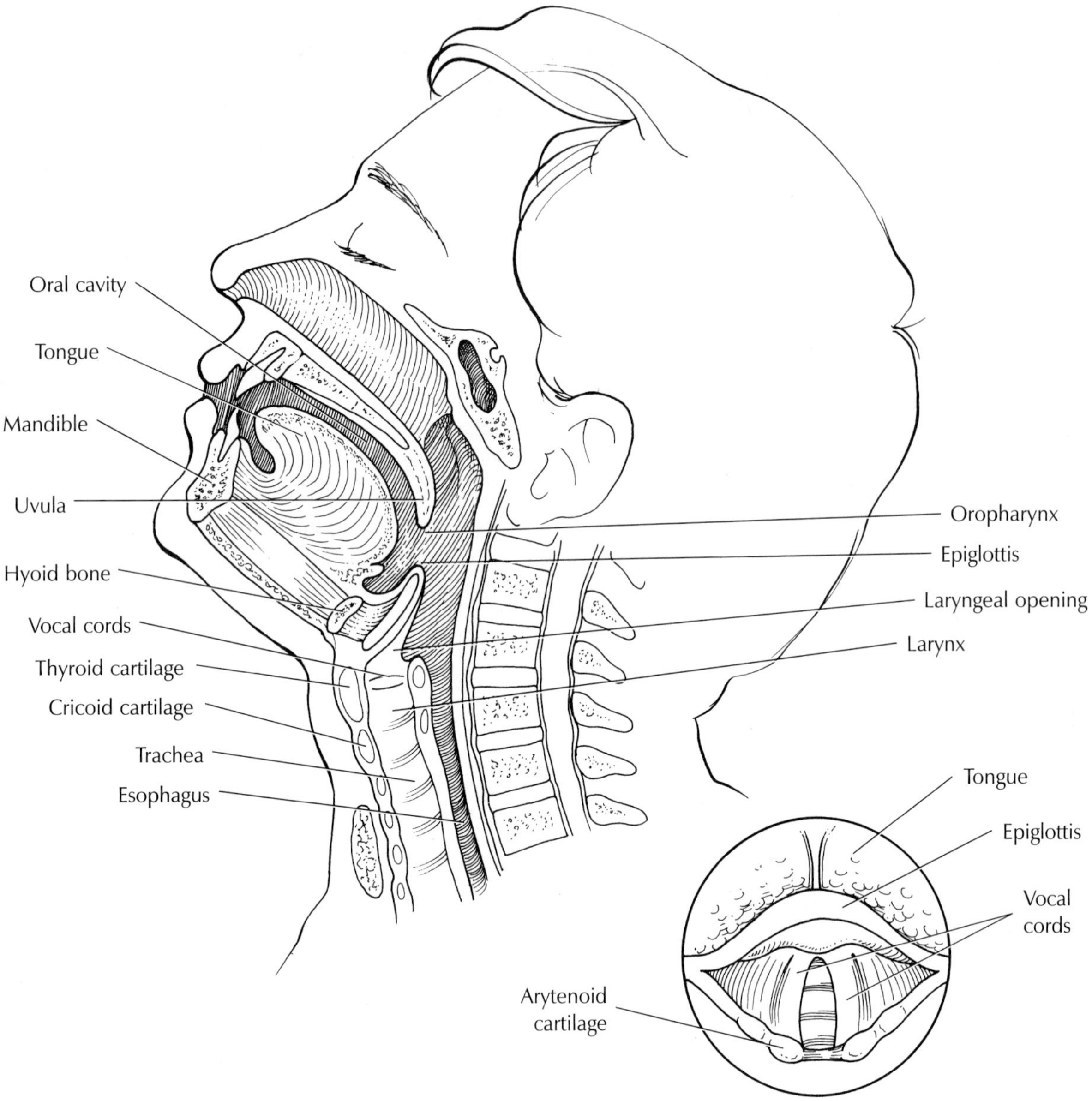

FIGURE 4-1 Anatomic landmarks of the head and neck. (Redrawn from Hines D, Bone RC: *J Crit Illness* 1:60, 1986.)

ness lasting for weeks or more serious upper airway injury.

In adults, the trachea is 10 to 12 cm long and is lined with a mucous membrane made up of pseudostratified, ciliated columnar epithelial cells interspersed with goblet cells. Cilia function to move mucoid secretions upward along the trachea to the opening of the larynx. Mucus ciliary clearance along with coughing removes most debris and inhaled particulate material, otherwise accumulating in the lungs. Remarkably, the cilia are so sensitive that use of one cigarette can cause paralysis for 20 to 30 minutes. Repeated smoking may replace this columnar epithelium with squamous epithelium. The trachea bifurcates into right and left mainstem bronchi at the fifth thoracic vertebra. In adults, the average trachea diameter is 16 mm, and respiratory stridor is not common until the lumen is 70% to 80% obstructed.

The right mainstem bronchus is shorter and placed more vertically than the left. In this position it is more directly in line with the trachea. Inhaled foreign bodies and aspirated oral secretions, thus, tend to go down the right mainstem bronchus, along with endotracheal tubes inserted below the level of the carina. The strength of the trachea lies in 16 to 20 cartilages presenting as incomplete rings spanning the anterior two thirds of the circumference of the trachea. At its posterior aspect, the trachea includes a fibrous and elastic tissue membrane with smooth muscle fibers. Endotracheal or tracheostomy tube balloons, if inflated above capillary pressure (30 torr), can inflict pressure necrosis on mobile tracheal cartilages. The fibrous tissue formed in the healing process may retract and narrow the tracheal lumen.

Lungs

The right lung normally consists of three lobes (upper, middle, and lower) and the left lung consists of two lobes (upper and lower). The right lung in the normal adult man is slightly larger, weighing 600 to 650 g, and is responsible for approximately 55% of total ventilation. The left lung is smaller, weighing 525 to 575 g, and accounts for the remaining 45% of total ventilation. The amount of blood or fluid present in the lung may dramatically affect the weight of this structure. Patients with severe congestive heart failure or acute respiratory failure may have lungs weighing in excess of 1000 g.

Lobar or secondary bronchi divide into two to five segmental bronchi. Normally ten pulmonary segments exist on the right and eight on the left. If bronchi are traced away from the pulmonary hilum, they are noted to branch and shrink. Bronchioles less than 1 mm in diameter have no cartilaginous rings and collapse readily with expiration. Terminal bronchioles are the smallest airways without alveoli. In first-order bronchioles, alveoli come directly off their sides and are referred to as respiratory bronchioles. The acinus consists of a first-order bronchiole that branches into succeeding smaller respiratory bronchioles, each with alveoli in their walls. Third-order respiratory bronchioles are followed by alveolar ducts, which are entirely alveolate. Alveolar ducts connect to an atrium, the entry point to main alveolar sacs.

The respiratory bronchioles and alveoli comprise the respiratory zone, that portion of the lung available for gas exchange. This volume is approximately 3000 ml in the normal adult. With each breath, a tidal volume of approximately 500 ml moves through the conducting zone composed of dead space to the respiratory zone, where the blood-gas interface occurs. A relatively small amount (12% or 350 of the 3000 ml) of gas in the respiratory zone is exchanged with each breath.

As each individual airway branches, the radius decreases. However, the total number of airways increases to a greater extent culminating in an increase in total airway cross-sectional area with each airway branch point. Overall resistance to gas flow is thus highest in the larger airways and decreases as total airway cross-sectional area increases. In the smaller airways, gas flow velocity decreases as gas flows through a larger cross-sectional area. Higher flow rates in large airways may cause turbulence, whereas in smaller airways, velocity slows and flow may become more laminar.

Bronchioles containing cartilage have the same gross appearance as the trachea. Distal bronchioles have fewer goblet cells and an increased number of special cuboidal cells. Longitudinal bands of elastin in bronchioles are important in elastic recoil of the lung. In the submucosal layer, helical tracts of muscular fibers run in opposite directions. Stimulation of this pattern of crossing muscles by hypoxemia, histamine, or serotonin may cause constriction.

The normal lung contains 200 to 600 million alveoli. The total alveolar surface area relates directly to body length and reaches 40 to 100 m^2 in the average adult. This area decreases by approximately 5% per decade after young adulthood. Alveolar epithelium comprises two cell types attached to a basement membrane. The most common cell type is the thin type I alveolar epithelial cell. The function of these cells appears to be passive exchange of gas. These cells are differentiated and cannot replicate when damaged. Interstitial connective tissue separates the basement membrane to which the type I alveolar cells adhere from the capillary. The diffusion barrier to alveolar gas normally consists of the alveolar cell wall, the basement membrane, the previously noted interstitial connective tissue, and the capillary cell wall. At its thinnest portion, the alveolar capillary membrane is usually 0.2 μM wide. The average thickness is up to 6 μM.

There are fewer type II alveolar cells, which are cuboidal with prominent organelles. These cells are commonly found at the junction of the alveolar septa and are covered with microvilli. Surfactant is produced in the cytoplasmic bodies and microsomes of these cells. Type II cells multiply to fill gaps created by injury to type I cells.

The third cell type in the alveolus is the macrophage. These cells migrate from capillaries to remove particles and foreign material in alveoli. They may then migrate into lymphatics or into the proximal bronchioles where they are removed by mucociliary clearance.

The pulmonary capillary endothelial cells are the final cell type forming the alveolar capillary membrane. These cells produce and degrade prostaglandins, among other vasoactive substances, and convert angiotensin I to angiotensin II. Joined by loose intercellular junctions, capillary endothelial cells are relatively permeable and may synthesize mediators responsible for local regulation of ventilation and perfusion relationships.

Pulmonary Vascular Bed

Right and left pulmonary arteries and their branches bring venous blood from the right ventricle to the pulmonary capillaries where gas exchange is accomplished within the alveoli. Bronchial arteries carry arterial blood

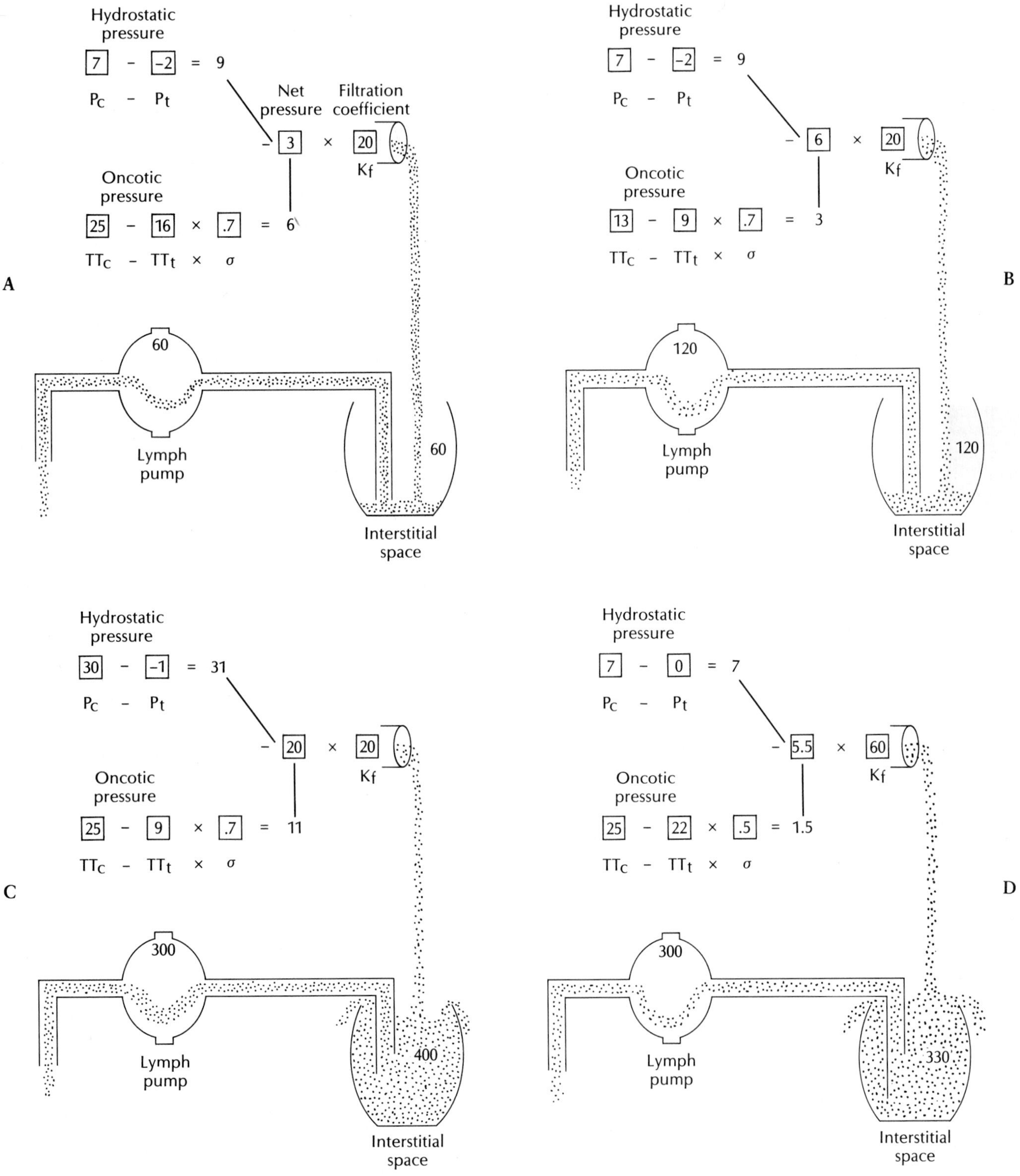

FIGURE 4-2 For legend see opposite page.

to supporting tissues of the lung, particularly bronchi. In general, one bronchial artery is noted on the right and two on the left; their branches follow the bronchial tree as far as the respiratory bronchioles. Superior and inferior pulmonary veins carry oxygenated blood from the pulmonary capillaries to the left atrium. Bronchial venous drainage may go to the azygous and hemiazygous venous systems or directly into the pulmonary veins. Bronchial venous blood entering the pulmonary veins causes desaturation, accounting for part of the normal physiologic shunt, which is 3% to 5% of the cardiac output.

Pulmonary arteries and veins divide and progressively shrink until they form capillaries in the alveolar capillary membranes. Pulmonary capillaries are found in the alveolar matrix. Two types of capillaries are noted. The first passes through corner junctions where adjacent alveolar lines merge. These junctional capillaries do not appear to participate in gas exchange, but contribute to pulmonary fluid homeostasis while other capillaries run in the alveolar septa, separating adjacent air spaces, and contribute directly to gas exchange (Figure 4-2). Collagen fibers suspend each side of septal capillaries. Increase in lung volume with inspiration creates traction on suspensory fibers, causing septal capillaries to bulge outward into the air space on a particular side of the alveolar septa. With half of the capillaries in any septa protruding into adjacent air space, the area of alveolar capillary contact is increased. Septal capillaries are thin where they bulge into alveoli and thick on the side remaining at the septum. The thick portion of these capillaries is predominantly concerned with fluid and protein transfer between blood and the pulmonary interstitium. The thin portion is devoted primarily to gas exchange. The interstitial space between alveoli and capillaries is generally thin, but thickens around larger arteries and veins. Initial accumulation of interstitial fluid occurs in the perivascular interstitial space.

Respiration[48,59,74,78]

Seventy percent of minute ventilation is normally due to the function of the diaphragm. Diaphragmatic muscle contraction during inspiration draws down a central tendon with increase in the volume of the thoracic cavity. At the same time, relaxation of abdominal muscles occurs, allowing the upper abdomen to protrude anteriorly. Costal fibers of the diaphragm help to elevate the six lower ribs, increasing the transverse diameter of the chest. Normally bowl shaped at rest, the diaphragm descends and flattens with inspiration to assume a saucer shape. With obstructive lung disease, diaphragmatic flattening occurs, leaving this structure saucer shaped following expiration. In this configuration, diaphragm function may be severely limited.

With quiet respiration, the diaphragm rises to its resting position at the sixth intercostal space anteriorly. With forced expiration, contraction of abdominal wall muscles increases intraabdominal pressure and can lead to diaphragmatic rise as high as the third or fourth intercostal space at the anterior aspect. Each hemidiaphragm is supplied by a branch of the phrenic nerve originating from the third to fifth cervical nerve roots. Intercostal muscles are innervated by corresponding intercostal nerves. An injury to the spinal cord at the level of C-6 will paralyze lower intercostal muscles, leaving the diaphragm intact. Diaphragmatic paralysis with injury creates paradoxical motion during breathing; in other words, the diaphragm moves upward with inspiration and downward with expiration.

Resting ventilation may be accomplished easily by one hemidiaphragm or intercostal muscles alone. With an increase in respiratory requirements or the work of breathing, ventilatory insufficiency may rapidly present if effectiveness of diaphragmatic contraction is altered by loss of coordination with intercostal contraction, changes in diaphragmatic position at end-expiration, increased pulmonary compliance, and abnormally increased intraabdominal pressure. A variety of disorders including neuromuscular disease, phrenic nerve injury, malnutrition, and metabolic disorders, may reduce diaphragmatic strength, compromising ventilatory reserve and limiting the ability to wean the patient from mechanical ventilatory support. During quiet tidal ventilation, the vertical chest cavity dimension increases from 1 to 4 cm. This change may exceed 8 cm during maximal inspiration. External intercostal muscle contraction pulls

FIGURE 4-2 The Starling relationship. Each part of the figure shows the net hydrostatic pressure: the hydrostatic pressure in the capillaries *(P_c)* minus the hydrostatic pressure in the tissue *(P_t)*. The oncotic pressure in the serum *(TT_c)* minus tissue oncotic pressure *(TT_t)* is then multiplied by the reflectance coefficient (σ) (the discount for permeability of protein through the capillary membrane). The net filtration pressure is the difference between these two. The filtration coefficient, with dimensions of ml/mm Hg/min (K_f), is multiplied by the net filtration force to give the amount filtered from the capillary into the interstitium. This filtered fluid is returned to the circulation by the lymphatic pump. **A,** Normal values for the lung. **B,** Results of hemodilution of lung fluid exchange. **C,** The effect of rise in capillary pressure filtration exceeds the capacity of the lymphatic pump, and interstitial edema results. **D,** With acute respiratory distress syndrome, the capillary is damaged and leaks. The protein reflectance (σ) falls. As a result, interstitial protein rises, and the effect of the oncotic pressure difference is discounted. The filtration fraction *(K_f)* rises, and although the fluid filtration force is only modestly elevated, for each 1 mm Hg net filtration force, the amount of fluid filtered is tripled. The result is an overwhelmed lymphatic pump and pulmonary edema.

the ribs upward and outward, increasing anteroposterior chest dimensions. Accessory muscles of inspiration (scalene, sternocleidomastoid, vertebral column extensors, anterolateral abdominal muscles, pectoralis muscles) may also increase chest wall expansion.

The muscles of the chest wall articulate with the ribs. The first rib is attached to the sternum and moves minimally with inspiration and expiration. The vertebral-sternal ribs (2 through 7) move about two axes simultaneously. One axis produces an increase in anteroposterior diameter of the chest using a pump handle motion. These ribs also move in a bucket handle fashion about the larger axis from their angles to the sternum, producing an increase primarily in transverse chest diameter. Ribs 8 through 10, also known as the vertebral chondral ribs, move only in a bucket-handle fashion with an increase in the transverse diameter of the chest. With diaphragmatic descent, these ribs move laterally, providing increased intraabdominal space for viscera displaced by diaphragmatic movement. Ribs 11 and 12 have no sternal or chondral attachments at the ventral ends and are thus called floating ribs.

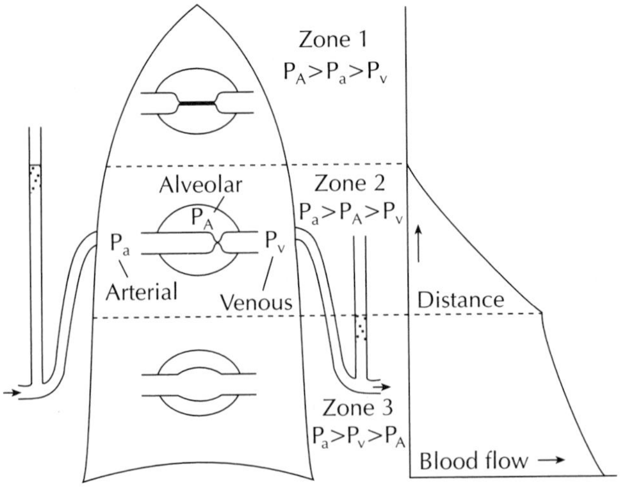

FIGURE 4-3 Model to explain the uneven distribution of blood flow in the lung based on the pressures affecting the capillaries. (From West JB, Dollery CT, Naimark A: *J Appl Physiol* 19:713, 1964.)

Pulmonary Microcirculation

Perfusion pressure and vascular resistance determine blood flow distribution within the pulmonary circulation. Flow through the pulmonary vascular bed varies with pressure gradient and inversely with resistance. For example, pulmonary arterial pressure is determined by preejection right ventricular diastolic pressure, right ventricular contractility, stroke volume, and large vessel compliance in the pulmonary vascular bed. Heart rate also affects diastolic blood pressure through the diastolic time interval. Pressures in the pulmonary vascular bed are lower than those in systemic vessels, largely due to increased pulmonary artery wall compliance and low pulmonary vascular resistance.

Due in part to the characteristics of the pulmonary vascular bed described earlier, gravity exerts a significant influence on intravascular pressure.[74,78] Arteries located below the level of the heart sustain an increase in vascular pressure equivalent to the weight of the fluid column between the right atrium and the artery. Arteries located above the heart experience a corresponding decrease in intravascular pressure due to the opposition of gravitational force to upward blood flow. Most pressure reduction occurs by the time blood passes the small muscular arterioles. Postarteriolar flow is determined by capillary resistance, alveolar pressure, and pulmonary venous pressure. The distensibility and collapsibility of the small pulmonary vessels make the pulmonary capillary resistance a more significant factor in determining blood flow distribution than systemic capillary resistance.

In relating the interaction between alveolar pressure and microvascular blood flow, three types or zones of interaction have been described (Figure 4-3). In the most superior or apical zone, alveolar pressure is greater than pulmonary artery pressure, collapsing septal capillaries and precluding blood flow.

Zone I capillary blood flow occurs through capillaries located at the triple points described previously. With spontaneous ambient ventilation, zone I exists in the most nondependent lung tissue, and maximum alveolar pressure is normally 2 to 4 cm of water.

Zone II is that region in which alveolar pressure is less than pulmonary artery pressure but greater than pulmonary venous pressure. Capillary flow in zone II is intermittent, decreasing in septal vessels when microvascular pressure falls below alveolar pressure during expiration or diastole.

In Zone III, pulmonary artery and pulmonary venous pressure exceed alveolar pressure and blood flow occurs throughout the cardiac cycle. Most healthy lung tissue falls within zone III unless alveolar pressure is elevated significantly above atmospheric pressure.[75] Described in terms of ventilation perfusion mismatch, Zone I represents dead space or ventilation (V) without perfusion (Q), Zone II contains high V/Q units (ventilation in excess of perfusion), and Zone III contains well-matched V/Q units.

Cross-sectional area and resistance of the capillaries are affected by pulmonary venous pressure as well as pleural and alveolar pressure and lung volume.[48] The effects of lung volume on septal and junctional capillary

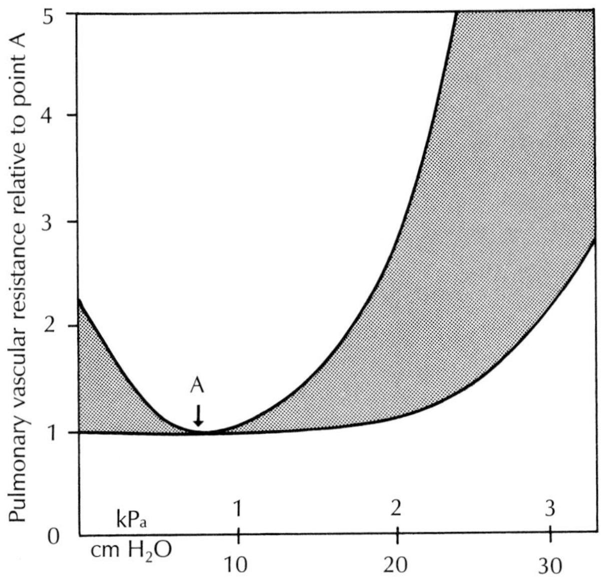

FIGURE 4-4 Representation of pooled experimental data on the change in pulmonary vascular resistance with lung inflation. It is evident that pulmonary vascular resistance is minimal at point A, which corresponds to functional residual capacity (FRC). From that point, with either decreasing or increasing lung inflation, pulmonary vascular resistance increases. (Redrawn from Nunn JF: *Applied respiratory physiology,* London, 1977, Butterworths.)

resistance are complex. Microvascular resistance is minimal at normal functional residual capacity and increases with changes in lung volume above or below functional residual capacity (Figure 4-4). Changes in microvascular resistance due to expansion or collapse of lung segments may divert flow to better expanded regions, thus improving ventilation and perfusion match. Negative alveolar pressure during inspiration may increase cross-sectional area, whereas extremes of negative or positive alveolar pressure can cause marked changes in regional blood flow distribution. Pulmonary artery pressure also affects regional blood flow. Pressure reduction decreases perfusion, particularly to nondependent lung regions. A decrease in pulmonary artery pressure blunts the impact of resistance changes among pulmonary vascular beds. Increased pulmonary artery pressure directs flow to nondependent areas and incorporates previously underperfused beds with higher vascular resistance. This effect increases flow through physiologic and pathologic right-to-left shunts.

Hypoxic pulmonary vasoconstriction (HPV) causes localized contraction of arterioles in the size range of 200 to 300 μm in diameter. This effect includes increased vascular resistance and diversion of blood to better oxygenated air spaces in response to regional reduction in alveolar oxygenation. Global constriction in response to hypoxemia includes increased pulmonary artery pressure and redistribution of blood flow to the nondependent regions of the lung with recruitment of poorly perfused capillaries and increasing surface area available for gas exchange. Among factors affecting HPV are inflammatory mediators, drugs, and shifts in pulmonary artery pressure. Use of vasodilators, particularly nitrates, may precipitate hypoxia through compromise of HPV. Sympathetic nervous system activity and circulating catecholamines may also change resistance to flow in the pulmonary vascular bed. In general, alpha-adrenergic stimulation causes vasoconstriction, whereas beta-adrenergic stimulation is associated with vasodilation. Mediators including angiotensin, histamine, acetylcholine, bradykinin, serotonin, and vasopressin, along with various neuropeptides, stimulate vasoconstriction or vasodilation, depending on resting vascular tone.

Between the pulmonary capillaries and the left atrium, vascular resistance is generally small. However, small veins and pulmonary venules display sympathetic nervous system innervation and may constrict in response to central nervous system sympathetic outflow. This effect reduces flow in upstream capillaries and arterioles. In the setting of head injury, hypoxemia, or other central nervous system pathology, large increases in postcapillary resistance and accelerated fluid egress into the pulmonary interstitium are noted to cause neurogenic pulmonary edema.[17]

Gas transfer between blood and the alveoli occurs by passive molecular diffusion down partial pressure gradients.[74] The diffusion distance across thin septal capillaries in small, allowing rapid transfer of gas molecules. A rapid flux of oxygen and carbon monoxide molecules along partial pressure gradients follows exposure of pulmonary arterial blood to alveolar gas. A new partial pressure equilibrium is reached rapidly. Oxygen molecules diffuse from a relatively high partial pressure in alveolar gas to lower partial pressure regions in the pulmonary arterial blood. In general, equilibration with alveolar oxygen is usually achieved before blood traverses one-third the length of an exchange capillary. Carbon dioxide molecules diffuse in the opposite direction along a gradient from the pulmonary arterial blood to alveolar gas. Due to increased water solubility, carbon dioxide exchanges even more readily across biologic barriers than does oxygen. Equilibration for carbon dioxide is almost instantaneous and is essentially unaffected by conditions impeding oxygen transfer. The partial pressures of nitrogen and other inert gasses are almost equal in alveoli and pulmonary blood unless the inspired gas concentration changes and a diffusion gradient is thus established.

Control of Respiration

Respiratory control begins with proprioceptors in the chest wall and lungs as well as chemoreceptors in the carotid bodies and medulla.[43,77] A fall in the pH, Pa_{O_2}, or P_{CO_2} may stimulate the respiratory drive. Changes in pH and P_{CO_2} affect the respiratory center, whereas Pa_{O_2} affects the carotid bodies. With a fall in pH, the respiratory center stimulates hyperventilation with a fall in P_{CO_2}. Hypoxia, as seen by a fall in P_{O_2}, stimulates the carotid bodies and respiratory center to hyperventilation. With hyperventilation, pH rises and P_{CO_2} falls, reducing the stimulus secondary to a low P_{O_2}.

Mechanical input to respiratory function comes from irritant, stretch, and juxtacapillary or J receptors. Stimulation of these receptors produces cough and hyperventilation. Juxtacapillary receptors and capillary receptors respond to factors, such as edema, which produce pulmonary stiffening. Rate and tidal volume fall with stimulation of mechanical receptors. With increased metabolic stress, oxygen demand and carbon dioxide production increase along with minute ventilation as Pa_{O_2}, Pa_{CO_2}, and arterial blood pH (pHa) remain unchanged. The most common stimuli to hyperventilation are hypoxemia and metabolic acidoses, which may also result secondarily from anaerobic metabolism driven by peripheral hypoxemia. A common example of respiratory control receptor interaction is the impact of increased inspired oxygen concentrations given to patients with chronic obstructive pulmonary disease. Removal of a hypoxemic stimulus in these patients, particularly those with mild to moderate carbon dioxide retention, eliminates drive from the aortic and carotid body chemoreceptors to maintain the ventilatory drive. Minute ventilation decreases and P_{CO_2} rises acutely. Thus in this situation it is critical to provide only the minimal oxygen concentration required to maintain respiratory control system function.

Gas Exchange

Atmospheric air is in large part nitrogen (79%) and oxygen (20.9%). Where gases are equilibrated with a liquid, as may occur in the lung, the partial pressure of gas in the liquid is the same as in the gas phase. Solubility of a gas in a liquid and the partial pressure of a particular gas dictate the portion of a gas dissolved in a liquid at the gas-liquid interface. Oxygen is relatively insoluble in serum. At normal oxygen tension in arterial blood, approximately 100 mm Hg, only 0.3 ml of oxygen is dissolved in each 100 ml of serum (Figure 4-5, *A*).

Hemoglobin is the biologic answer to limitations in the serum transfer of oxygen.[74] Again, hemoglobin saturation with oxygen depends on the partial pressure of oxygen in the blood. In contrast to the linear relationship of dissolved oxygen in serum, hemoglobin quickly absorbs oxygen at a P_{O_2} greater than 65 mm Hg and releases oxygen at a P_{O_2} less than 65 mm Hg. If fully saturated, blood may carry 1.34 ml of oxygen per gram of available hemoglobin. Thus with a hemoglobin of 15 g, each deciliter of blood carries approximately 20 ml of oxygen: 20 ml in hemoglobin and 0.3 ml dissolved in serum. As can be seen from the oxyhemoglobin desaturation curve, little oxygen is added to the blood above the P_{O_2} of 90 mm Hg, whereas desaturation occurs rapidly below a P_{O_2} of 65 mm Hg.

In contrast to the relatively complicated interaction between P_{O_2} and arterial oxygen content, over the physiologic range, P_{CO_2} and CO_2 content are nearly linearly related. As P_{CO_2} increases, a comparable change in milliliters of carbon dioxide dissolved in blood occurs. Blood acidity also changes as carbonic anhydrase hydrates carbon dioxide, producing or removing carbonic acid (H_2CO_3) (Figure 4-5, *B*).

Changes in ventilation cause inversely proportional changes in alveolar and arterial carbon dioxide tension. On the contrary, hyperventilation increasing alveolar oxygen tension greater than 100 mm Hg does not change oxygen content in the blood, as hemoglobin has already been fully saturated. Hyperventilation does alter carbon dioxide content inasmuch as carbon dioxide dissociation is a linear relationship. Hyperventilation may decrease the arterial P_{CO_2} below the normal level of 40 mm Hg while hypoventilation increases P_{CO_2}. Hypoventilation lowers P_{O_2}, but affects oxygen content of the blood little until arterial oxygen tension falls below 70 mm Hg, where hemoglobin desaturation begins to occur rapidly. Thus hyperventilation results in a fall in P_{CO_2}, whereas hypoventilation causes a rise in P_{CO_2} and little change in P_{O_2}. The previously discussed physical proprieties of oxygen, carbon dioxide, and hemoglobin make P_{CO_2} changes proportional to variation in ventilation. An increase in P_{CO_2} coincides with inadequate ventilation, whereas a decrease in P_{CO_2} is associated with hyperventilation. Changes in P_{O_2} may have many causes, including variation in inspired oxygen tension, variation in ventilation and perfusion relationships, and change in position of the oxygen-hemoglobin dissociation curve. P_{O_2}, therefore, is not an indicator of adequacy of ventilation.

Right Ventricular Anatomy and Physiology

A growing body of clinical and experimental evidence suggests that optimum manipulation of the cardiopulmonary system entails recognition that the lungs are more than a series of intertwined airways; a critical and sensitive link between the airways and vascular bed is involved. The circulation of the pulmonary vascular bed is unique and different in many ways from the systemic circulation. Right ventricular anatomy and function are profoundly different from those of the left. Principles of right ventricular resuscitation and care in right ventric-

A

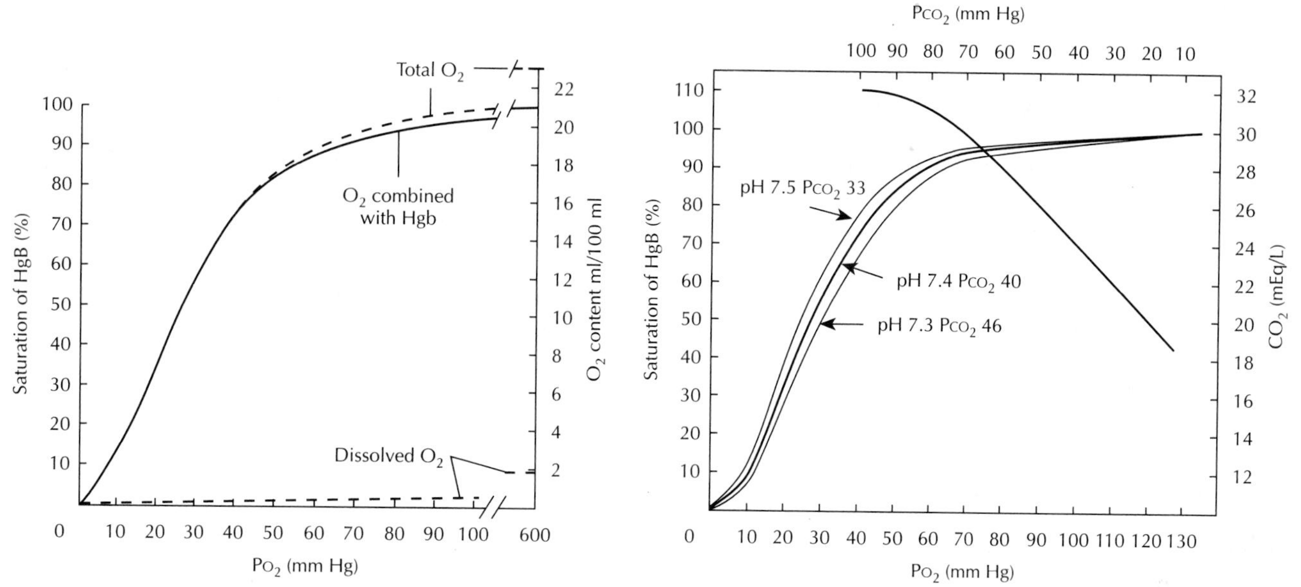

B

FIGURE 4-5 **A,** Dissociation curve *(solid line)* for pH 7.4, Pco_2 40 mm Hg, and 37° C. The total blood O_2 content is also shown for a hemoglobin concentration of 15 g/100 ml of blood. (Redrawn from Peters RM: *Am J Surg* 138:368, 1979.) **B,** Dissociation curves for oxygen and carbon dioxide in whole blood. The vertical axis on the left represents oxygen content and saturation, and on the right, carbon dioxide (CO_2) content. The horizontal axis on the bottom represents partial pressure of oxygen (Po_2), and on the top, partial pressure of carbon dioxide (Pco_2). Note that at 65 mm Hg, the oxyhemoglobin dissociation curve begins to flatten out, and above 90 mm Hg very little oxygen is added by increasing the partial pressure of oxygen. As Po_2 falls below 65 mm Hg, oxygen saturation decreases very fast. The CO_2 dissociation curve is straight over almost the complete range of $Paco_2$ seen clinically.

ular failure may change as therapeutic alternatives differ in the setting of right versus left ventricular failure.

During the last two decades interest in the right ventricle has renewed. This thin-walled chamber has long been obscured by its more muscular neighbor on the left side. The renewed interest in the right ventricle comes from an evolving awareness that dysfunction of this chamber plays a critical role in several frequently encountered, clinically important cardiopulmonary disorders. In an adult, the normal right ventricle is crescent-shaped with compliant walls. Because of a large surface-to-volume relationship, the right ventricle propels large amounts of blood into the pulmonary artery with minimal myocardial fiber shortening. The right ventricle is unable to generate high intracavitary pressures. Normally, the right ventricle functions as a low-pressure volume conduit, ejecting venous blood into the high compliance, low resistance pulmonary vascular bed.[76]

The left ventricle has less compliant walls than the right ventricle and a much smaller surface area/volume ratio. This chamber generates high pressures through the contraction and relaxation of circumferential muscle bundles. The left ventricle sustains stroke volume in the presence of elevated systemic arterial pressures, but is less suited than the right ventricle to handle increases in volume. The systolic performance of both ventricles is determined by the same three factors: preload, afterload, and contractility.[40,62] End-diastolic pressure represents the ventricular preload, whereas afterload is the resistance seen by the ventricle during contraction. Arterial pressure and vascular resistance are the commonly used indices of afterload. However, ventricular wall tension related to the product of chamber diameter and ventricular pressure is a more precise estimate of afterload. Augmentation of diastolic volume increases both preload and afterload. The vigor of muscle shortening that occurs at any given preload and afterload is called myocardial contractility. The Frank-Starling relationship provides a framework for assessing left and right ventricular performance.[62] Ventricular function curves relate systolic pump function to preload and contractility.

Qualitative differences exist between the left and right ventricles. For instance, the right ventricle is unable to maintain its ejection fraction when faced with an elevated afterload. Thus augmenting preload is necessary to preserve the stroke volume of the right heart in the presence of pressure stress. This volume compensation is less important when the normal left ventricle is confronted by afterload elevation, probably as a result of the increased contractile reserve of this chamber.[40]

The free wall of the right ventricle is perfused almost entirely by the right coronary artery.[24] The interventricular septum is supplied by both the left anterior descending coronary artery and the right coronary artery. As noted by Matthay and associates,[40] the total blood flow to the left ventricle is considerably greater than that to the right. The flow of blood per gram of tissue in the right ventricle is only about two-thirds that perfusing the left ventricle, and the right ventricle contains less muscle. The left ventricle also extracts more oxygen per gram of tissue than the right. In contrast to the left ventricle, blood flow to the myocardium of the right ventricle is distributed more evenly throughout the cardiac cycle, presumably as a result of the high pressures developed by the left ventricle during systole; thus perfusion occurs primarily during diastole. The driving pressure for perfusion of the right ventricle is aortic pressure minus right ventricular pressure. Systemic hypotension in association with left ventricular failure, therefore, results in right ventricular ischemia and abnormal contraction. In addition, an increase in right ventricular pressure, caused by increased afterload, may also reduce right coronary blood flow. This, in turn, limits the ability of the right ventricle to respond to increased pressure demands.[40]

Matthay and associates describe the response of the right ventricle to stress as a vicious cycle leading to circulatory collapse if the insult is sufficiently severe.[40] Right coronary blood flow increases to meet mild or moderate pressure loading of the right ventricle, despite the decrease in driving pressure, because the vessel dilation and resistance to flow decreases. Augmentation in preload also maintains right ventricular systolic function. However, this adaptation is limited because increasing right ventricular volume is associated with increased wall tension (and oxygen demand), decreased left ventricular compliance, and tricuspid regurgitation. These factors may decrease aortic pressure and cardiac output, reducing right coronary perfusion pressure while increasing the demand for oxygen by the myocardium. When right coronary vasodilatory reserve is exhausted, myocardial ischemia results and right ventricular systolic function is lost.[31,72] At this point, unless the right ventricle is resuscitated, circulatory collapse will follow (Figures 4-6 and 4-7).

Wiedemann and Matthay[76] define right ventricular failure as the point at which the systolic function of this chamber is inadequate to maintain adequate circulation. In face of even moderate pressure stress, right ventricular preload increases and ejection fraction decreases. Pe-

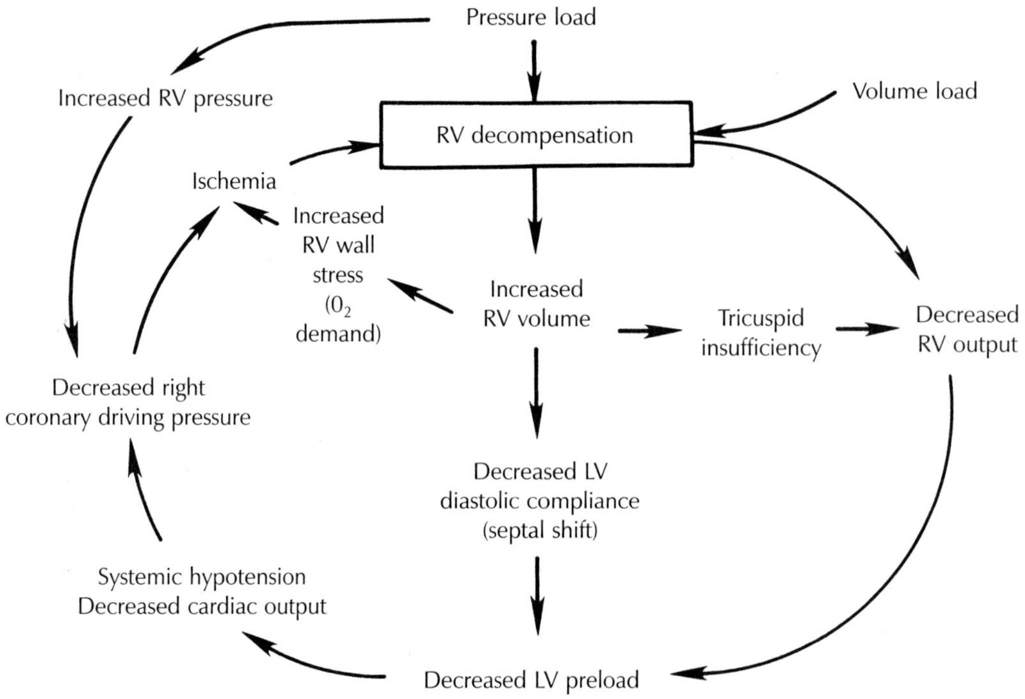

FIGURE 4-6 The pathophysiology of acute right ventricular failure (the "vicious circle") is schematically depicted. (Redrawn from Wiedemann HP, Matthay RA: *Crit Care Clin* 1:631, 1985.)

ripheral edema may be a manifestation of the increased mean right ventricular pressure with resultant elevation of right atrial pressure. Under these circumstances, right ventricular contractile function may still be normal. The variety of clinical manifestations of right heart stress (which has been discussed earlier) is determined by the interaction between the cause of the dysfunction and the intravascular volume status. Invasive hemodynamic monitoring may be misleading in this setting. Right ventricular decompensation in a previously normal chamber may not be associated with a high right atrial pressure despite a large ventricular volume, primarily because of the high compliance of the normal right ventricle. On the other hand, a chronically hypertrophied right ventricle may exhibit high diastolic pressures while normal circulation is maintained. In addition, due to the phenomenon of ventricular interdependence, left ventricular dysfunction, as suggested by a high wedge pressure in the absence of left ventricular disease, may be a manifestation of right ventricular failure (Figure 4-8).

Right Ventricular Resuscitation

If right ventricular outflow is diminished as a result of increased right ventricular afterload or depressed contractility, cardiac output can be restored by volume expansion. This has been shown in several situations, including acute respiratory distress syndrome (ARDS), right ventricular infarction, and acute pulmonary artery constriction.[31,68] Factors contributing to this improvement can be seen in the relationship between cardiac output and venous return. An augmented venous volume causes a rightward shift in the venous return curve, thus compensating for diminished cardiac output. It should be noted, however, that systemic mean pressure rises

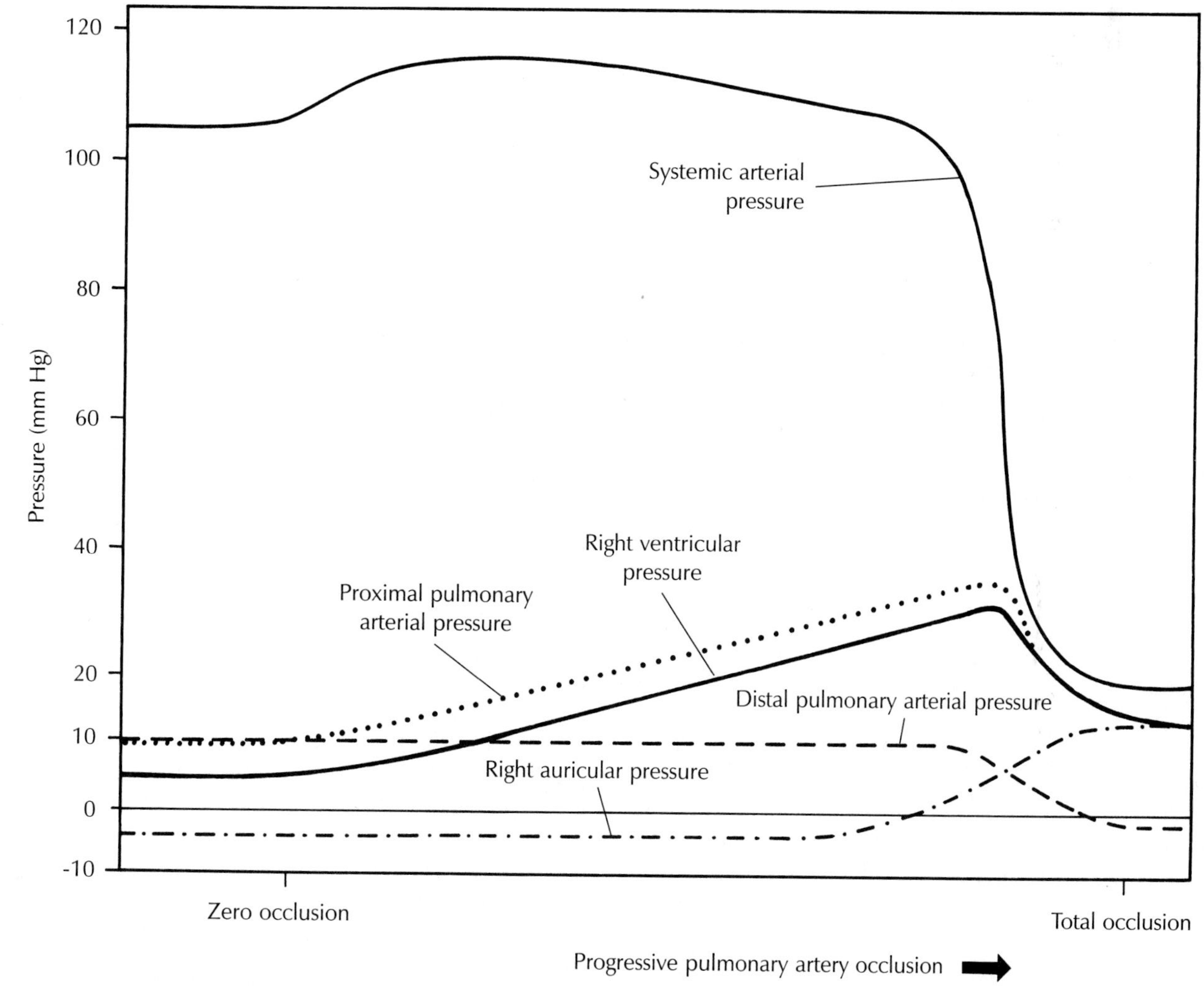

FIGURE 4-7 Mean pressures observed as the main pulmonary artery of a dog was progressively constricted for 4 to 5 minutes. The right ventricle was unable to generate a pulmonary artery pressure greater than 40 mm Hg, and circulatory collapse suddenly occurred. (Redrawn from Guyton AC, Lindsey AW, Gilluly JJ: *Circ Res* 2:326, 1954.)

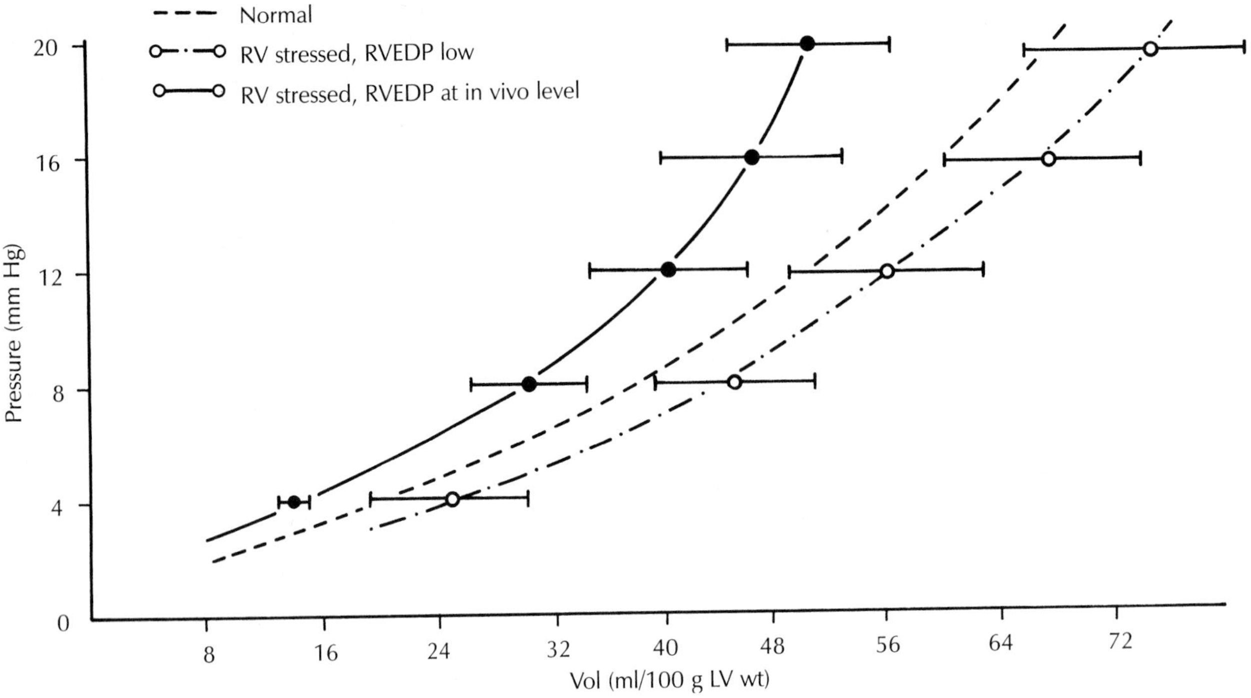

FIGURE 4-8 The left ventricular *(LV)* diastolic volume-pressure curve is shown in three groups of dogs: normal; dogs with right ventricular pressure stress, in which right ventricular end-diastolic pressure (*RVEDP*) is kept at the low levels found in normal animals; and dogs with right ventricular pressure stress in which the RVEDP is allowed to reach higher levels. This illustrates ventricular interdependence whereby right ventricular stress decreases left ventricular compliance. (Redrawn from Kelly DT, Spotnitz HM, Beiser GD et al: *Circulation* 44:403, 1971.)

with venous volume expansion, favoring the development of peripheral edema, and cardiac output may fall if the clinician administers a diuretic in an attempt to reduce or eliminate edema. Thus it may be necessary to accept peripheral edema to maintain cardiac output in patients with compromise of right ventricular function.[69]

The ability of increased right ventricular preload to maintain cardiac output is clearly limited. A decrease in left ventricular diastolic filling and tricuspid regurgitation may develop following volume loading to optimize right ventricular function. In addition, an increase in circulatory volume may cause a rise in wall tension and increased oxygen demand even though the compliance of the right ventricle is high. Right coronary perfusion pressure is also reduced by the high systolic pressure generation required to overcome increased right ventricular outflow resistance. In patients with ARDS, volume loading may be associated with worsening pulmonary edema if the right ventricular volume is raised to the degree that left ventricular compliance is reduced and pulmonary capillary wedge pressure is elevated. The point beyond which further volume loading is detrimental to right ventricular function is indicated by a precipitous rise in left or right-sided filling pressures without a concomitant increase in cardiac output.[54]

Maintenance of aortic pressure is critical to continued adequate right coronary artery perfusion and avoidance of myocardial ischemia with the onset of acute right ventricular failure. Thus therapy of acute right ventricular failure may at times include intraaortic balloon counterpulsation, aortic banding, and/or phenylephrine or noradrenaline infusion. Although right ventricular performance may be directly improved by pressors, the common mechanism in each of these therapies is an augmentation of aortic pressure.

A practical means of rapidly lowering afterload stress in acute right ventricular failure is oxygen therapy. As hypoxic pulmonary vasoconstriction contributes to elevated pulmonary vascular resistance in many patients with chronic obstructive pulmonary disease (COPD), ARDS, pulmonary thromboembolism, and interstitial lung disease, supplemental oxygen may lower pulmonary vascular resistance and pulmonary artery pressures when these disorders are associated with hypoxemia.

Right ventricular ejection fraction may also be increased by oxygen therapy.

Therapy of pulmonary arterial hypertension with vasodilators has produced conflicting and confusing results. A beneficial hemodynamic response to these agents has not been clearly defined, partly because pharmacologic agents may have several sites of action, in some cases altering ventricular contractility and preload. Other agents, such as selective beta-2 adrenergic agents, may decrease air flow obstruction and reduce pulmonary vascular resistance by this effect as well as by direct pulmonary vasodilation. However, some vasodilator agents may produce a decrease in arterial oxygen tension by increasing physiologic shunting and ventilation-perfusion mismatch within the lung. The risk in administering pharmacologic vasodilators to reduce primary right ventricular afterload is the potential for adverse effects on the systemic circulation. Patients with fixed low cardiac output due to right ventricular decompensation may be further compromised by systemic vasodilation associated with hypotension and the resultant loss of right coronary artery perfusion pressure. This may be the mechanism of death reported after administration of hydralazine or diazoxide to patients with severe pulmonary artery hypertension. The underlying disease process may also affect the results of vasodilator therapy in the pulmonary circulation.[50,60]

The final means of right ventricular resuscitation is augmentation of contractility with adrenergic agents including dobutamine, dopamine, norepinephrine, and isoproterenol. All of these drugs increase right ventricular contractility. Inotropic agents may produce minimum improvement of right ventricular performance if afterload is normal due to the normally steep slope of the right ventricular systolic function curve. The value of catecholamines in treating acute right heart failure secondary to increased pulmonary vascular resistance is suggested by Prewitt and associates.[53,54] These studies, limited to anesthetized and ventilated dogs, suggest that as pulmonary vascular resistance is gradually raised by glass bead embolization, right ventricular afterload increases, and cardiac output fails. Volume expansion is successful in improving cardiac performance in the early stages, but after a certain point cardiac output deteriorates with further volume administration. Right ventricular performance and cardiac output may be improved with administration of dopamine or norepinephrine.[53] Other agents, including albuterol, terbutaline, and theophylline, may also improve right ventricular contractility. Few data support a consistent pattern for use of these drugs.

Right ventricular contractility is increased by digitalis and other cardiac glycosides. However, it is difficult to say whether these agents should be used, because digitalis may exhibit adverse effects on right ventricular function as a result of pulmonary vasoconstriction. In addition, cardiac glycosides may cause a shift in the venous return curve to the left and thus adversely affect cardiac output.[69] Several authors suggest that unless coexisting left ventricular dysfunction is present, digitalis does not appear to relieve right ventricular dysfunction. Digitalis augments right heart function in the presence of left ventricular failure by reducing pulmonary venous pressure and right ventricular afterload. In the absence of left heart disease, no overall improvement and possible deterioration in right ventricular function may result from digitalis administration.

Pulmonary Vascular Assessment

As noted by Prewitt,[53,54] right ventricular afterload increases with alteration in the pulmonary vascular bed; however, despite the importance of these changes, the pathophysiology of acute pulmonary hypertension has only recently been elucidated.[21] Conventional pulmonary vascular resistance, calculated as pulmonary artery pressure minus left ventricular filling pressure divided by cardiac output, is assumed to reflect the flow resistance of the pulmonary vascular bed. Changes in pulmonary vascular resistance are thought to reflect changes in effective vascular caliber. A single pressure-flow coordinate is used to describe the vascular resistance; the assumption is made that the effective pulmonary vascular outflow pressure in zone III is equal to the left ventricular filling pressure.[75]

Recent work by several authors, using multicoordinate pulmonary vascular flow plots to investigate physiology and pathophysiology, has evaluated the pulmonary circulation. A linear relationship has been reported between incremental resistance and flow in the pulmonary vascular bed. This incremental resistance, however, must be distinguished from traditional pulmonary vascular resistance, because the extrapolated pressure intercept in these studies may exceed left ventricular filling pressure in zone III and alveolar pressure in zone II. Thus in the presence of pulmonary hypertension, the actual level of pulmonary artery pressure may result from an increase in the extrapolated pressure intercept, an increase in vascular resistance, or a combination of these factors. Vasoactive compounds may alter pulmonary hemodynamics by their effects on these factors together or individually.

To express this relationship graphically, a plot of upstream pressure (mean pulmonary artery pressure) against cardiac output, assuming a linear correspondence, should yield a straight line, with the extrapolated pressure axis intercept reflecting the relevant downstream pressure. In isolated lobe experiments, this pressure-flow relationship has been described using determinations of pressure-flow coordinates at several levels of cardiac output. These studies reveal that the extrapolated pressure intercept of the linear segment exceeded the apparent downstream pressure. Ducas and Prewitt[21] suggest that extrapolated pressure intercepts obtained from this animal work represent the mean closing pressure of the pulmonary vasculature and thus optimally represent the operative downstream pressure. The slope of the linear segment of the pressure flow plots obtained represents the incremental pulmonary vascular resistance. The derived closing pressure and the incremental resistance, rather than the classic pulmonary vascular resistance, may vary in the setting of pulmonary hypertension, such as that following pulmonary thromboembolism. Although pulmonary vascular resistance, as traditionally calculated, may change with a given intervention, incremental vascular resistance, as defined by the pressure-flow relationships described earlier, may not be affected. Data obtained from numerous animal experiments reveal that the incorrect assumption in the classic evaluation of pulmonary vascular resistance is that the appropriate downstream pressure in this relationship is the left ventricular end-diastolic pressure.[21]

RESPIRATORY FUNCTION TESTING

Measurement of pulmonary function during the preoperative period is a guide to surgical risk and may uncover an abnormality requiring therapy to improve lung function and forestall postoperative pulmonary complications. Spirometric, cardiovascular, and gas exchange assessments are available to facilitate evaluation of risk for pulmonary complications with various surgical procedures.

The most common spirometric measurements include forced vital capacity (FVC), forced expiratory volume in 1 second (FEV_1), maximal voluntary ventilation, and static lung volumes (Figure 4-9 and Tables 4-1 and 4-2). FVC is easily measured and highly reproducible. Data are available that allow comparison of a patient with control subjects of comparable height, weight, and age. Decreased FVC suggests restrictive ventilatory defects or a severe obstructive defect with hyperinflation. If FVC is less than 50% of the predicted value or less than 1.75 to 2 L in a normal adult, a higher risk of postoperative pulmonary complications is noted. Whereas FVC is an index of restrictive ventilatory defect, FEV_1 is a more direct measurement of airflow obstruction.[70] The hallmark of obstructive lung disease is an abnormal ratio of FVC/FEV_1. A FEV_1 of less than 800 ml warrants exclusion of patients from any type of thoracic resection. If FEV_1 reaches 2 L, patients are considered to have a moderate obstructive ventilatory defect. When FEV_1 exceeds 2 L, the mortality rate is approximately 10%. Maximal voluntary ventilation (MVV) evaluates obstructive and restrictive physiology and depends on the ability of the patient to cooperate and perform the task.

TABLE 4-1 LUNG VOLUME CHANGES WITH AGE AND ARDS*

	20 YEARS	70 YEARS	ARDS
Inspiratory reserve volume	2.5	1.2	0.3
Tidal volume	0.5	0.4	0.4
Expiratory reserve volume	1.8	0.8	0.3
Residual volume	1.2	1.8	1.5

*All values expressed in liters
From Wilson RF: *Critical care manual: applied physiology and principles of therapy,* Philadelphia, 1992, FA Davis.

TABLE 4-2 LUNG CAPACITY CHANGES WITH AGE AND ARDS*

	20 YEARS	70 YEARS	ARDS
Total lung capacity (TLC)	6.0	4.2	2.5
Vital capacity (VC)	4.8	2.4	1.0
Inspiratory capacity (IC)	3.0	1.6	0.7
Functional residual capacity (FRC)	3.0	2.6	1.8

*All values expressed in liters
From Wilson RF: *Critical care manual: applied physiology and principles of therapy,* Philadelphia, 1992, FA Davis.

Though not specific to a specific type of pulmonary function, MVV gives effective global assessment of patient pulmonary status and includes factors such as restriction, pain, general debilitation, and altered mental status, which may not be apparent on other types of pulmonary function testing. Other spirometric flow evaluations, including maximal mid-expiratory flow or the forced expiratory flow between 25% and 75% of exhaled volume ($FEV_{25-75\%}$), are thought to be sensitive indicators of small airway dysfunction. Midflow measurements are always abnormal in patients with COPD, and values less than predicted indicate a higher risk of postoperative pulmonary complications after thoracotomy or abdominal surgery.[3]

Patients with abnormal spirometric measurements may have coexisting changes in lung volumes or ratios between various lung volumes. Increase in the residual volume/total lung capacity ratio and/or functional residual capacity to total lung capacity indicate hyperinflation and gas trapping. However, lung volumes and flow measurements should be obtained before and after bronchodilator therapy. Improvement with bronchodilator therapy is considered a good prognostic sign in patients undergoing thoracic or abdominal surgery.

Additional information regarding patient tolerance of procedures entailing pulmonary compromise may be obtained from exercise testing. Spirometric testing and oxy-

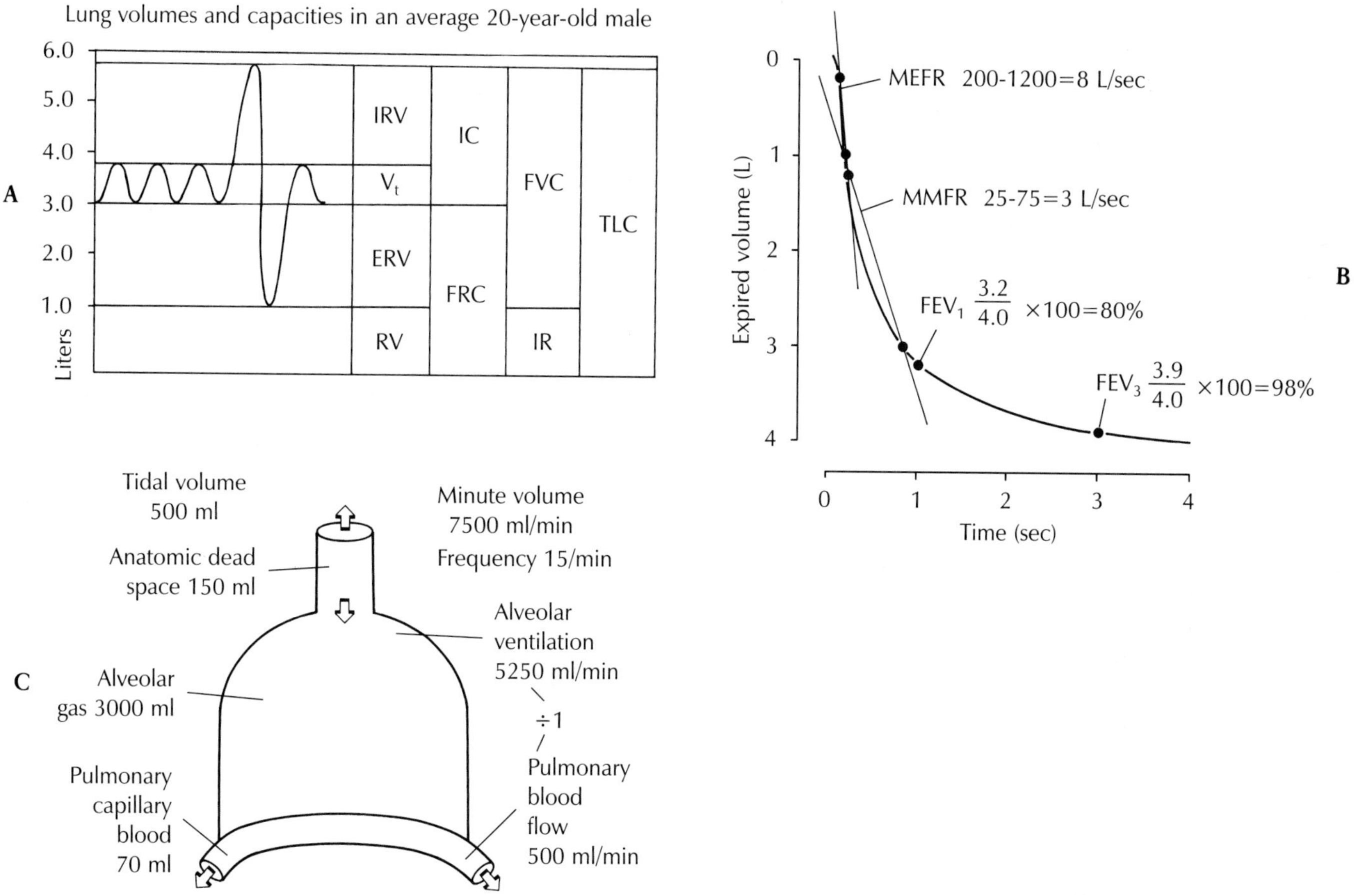

FIGURE 4-9 **A,** Spirometry in a normal patient. Normally, at least 75% of the forced expiratory volume should be exhaled during the first second. The maximum midexpiratory flow rate (MMFR), from 25% to 75% of the forced expiratory volume, should be about 4.0 L/second or about 240 L/min. Expiratory reserve volume (ERV) is the amount of air that can be exhaled after a normal exhalation; inspiratory reserve volume (IRV) is the amount of air that can be inhaled after an inspiration of a normal tidal volume; functional residual capacity (FRC), also called resting lung volume, consists of the EFV plus the RV and is the amount of air still present in the lungs after a normal exhalation; inspiratory capacity (IC) consists of V plus IRV and is the amount of air that can be inhaled after a normal exhalation. (Redrawn from Wilson RF: *Critical care manual: applied physiology and principles of anatomy,* Philadelphia, 1992, FA Davis.) **B,** Schematic representation of a normal forced vital capacity (FVC) maneuver (expired volume against time, *heavy line*) and the derivation of several variables commonly used to evaluate airway obstruction. (Redrawn from Smith TH, Thier SO: *Pathophysiology,* Philadelphia, 1985, WB Saunders.) **C,** Diagram of a lung showing typical volumes and flows. There is considerable variation among these values. (Redrawn from West JB: *Ventilation/blood flow and gas exchange,* Oxford, 1970, Blackwell.)

gen consumption with exercise have been evaluated and compared to morbidity and mortality data in patients undergoing various operative procedures. For example, maximal oxygen consumption may be expressed in milliliters per kilogram per minute. When it is less than 15 ml/kg/min, perioperative complications are frequent, but with oxygen consumption exceeding 20 ml/kg/min, patients generally tolerate surgery without problems.

Exercise testing provides a stress factor to highlight signs of impending cardiopulmonary failure. Other physiologic measures during exercise are also valuable. Elevated pulmonary artery pressure at rest or during exercise is indicative of poor prognosis. Mean pulmonary artery pressure greater than 30 mm Hg is associated with elevated right ventricular pressure and cor pulmonale. Other studies suggest that significant elevation of pulmonary artery pressure at rest or during exercise indicates inability to survive pulmonary resection.

In patients undergoing abdominal surgery, postoperative pulmonary complications occur even in the presence of normal lungs. The overall incidence of pulmonary complications is reported at 6% to 8% in postoperative patients. The key factors determining these complications are site of incision, preexisting lung disease, and smoking history. For nonabdominal surgery, the risk of subsequent pulmonary complications is less than 1%. As the incision site nears the diaphragm, the incidence of complications rises to 20% for an upper abdominal incision. The incidence of complications doubles for smokers and quadruples if smokers have COPD.[56]

To assess risks in patients undergoing upper abdominal surgery, the best tests appear to be simple spirometric testing and arterial blood gas analysis. Obstructive and restrictive disease can be detected with FVC, FEV_1, FEV_1/FVC, and $FEV_{25\text{-}75\%}$. Increased risk is suggested by an FEV_1 less than 2 L or less than 50% of predicted value. An FVC, FEV_1/FVC, or $FEV_{25\text{-}75\%}$ less than 50% of predicted value also suggests increased risk. High risk as reviewed by Boysen and associates[3,4] includes patients with FEV_1 less than 1 L, FVC less than 1.5 L or 20 ml/kg, and FEV_1/FVC below 35% of predicted value. Maximal voluntary ventilation below 50% of predicted value or less than 50 L/minute, $FEV_{25\text{-}75\%}$ less than 1 L/second, and carbon dioxide retention on arterial blood gas testing also suggest patients at high risk. Obtaining these data is relatively easy and inexpensive compared with other forms of testing. Spirometric evaluation is suggested for patients scheduled for thoracotomy or upper abdominal surgery with documented history of previous lung disease, smoking, or cough. Patients older than 70 years or the morbidly obese may warrant additional testing.

Relatively healthy subjects only require instruction in deep breathing preoperatively and postoperatively, which can be encouraged with the use of a device such as a disposable incentive spirometer. It has been repeatedly shown that patients with lung disease can achieve a threefold reduction in postoperative pulmonary complications by means of aggressive preparation such as deep-breathing maneuvers, chest physiotherapy, bronchodilators, and antibiotics. Preoperative education in the importance of deep breathing, coughing, and the use of incentive spirometry is likely to be more effective than attempting to teach these principles at a time when a patient has postoperative pain or is receiving analgesia. Bronchospasm should be minimized before surgery. It is useful to monitor pulmonary function during the preoperative period, as those who improve their pulmonary function have a better prognosis than those who do not.

In patients undergoing thoracotomy and pulmonary resection, postoperative pulmonary function must be assessed with consideration of the reduced lung mass available in the postoperative period. Boysen and associates[3,4] reviewed the indicators of high risk from pulmonary function data in patients undergoing pulmonary resection including pneumonectomy. Optimal indicators of high risk from pulmonary function data appear to be FEV_1 and MVV. To predict postoperative FEV_1 in patients undergoing pulmonary resection, the preoperative value for this term can be multiplied by the percent perfusion of uninvolved pulmonary tissue as obtained from a xenon perfusion scan. Routine pulmonary function studies combined with perfusion lung scanning may eliminate the need for more invasive testing, including balloon occlusion of the pulmonary artery, to determine tolerance of pulmonary resections.

Based on the experience of Boysen and associates,[4] a predicted postoperative FEV_1 greater than 800 to 1000 ml is required to justify pulmonary resection. Patients failing to meet this criterion require additional testing such as unilateral pulmonary artery balloon occlusion to assess changes in pulmonary artery pressure and right ventricular response before qualifying for pulmonary resection. In patients not requiring pneumonectomy, prediction of postoperative FEV_1 may be extended to resections less than a total lung by multiplying the predicted postoperative FEV_1 (obtained by spirometry and perfusion scanning) by the number of pulmonary segments remaining over the total number of pulmonary segments in the involved lung, assuming ten pulmonary segments on the right and eight on the left.

Operative Changes in Pulmonary Function

Among effects related to anesthetic administration are changes in lung volume, gas exchange, respiratory drive, and airway protection. General anesthesia causes a decrease in FRC of 15% to 25% in comparison with the supine awake state. These effects are seen in the shape and motion of the chest wall and diaphragm. A cephalad shift in the dependent portion of the diaphragm contributes to the decrease in FRC and the development of atelectasis, which has been noted within minutes after induction of anesthesia.

Anesthesia may cause an increase in intrapulmonary shunt, with distribution of perfusion to areas of low ventilation and increasing ventilation to areas of reduced perfusion. Normally, these alterations do not pose a significant threat, as they may be overcome by increasing the concentration of oxygen in the inspired gas. Inhalation anesthetics may also depress hypoxic pulmonary vasoconstriction through direct impact on the pulmonary vascular bed and secondarily through changes in cardiac performance.[48]

Normal response to hypoxia and hypercapnia is blunted by anesthetic agents, particularly with halogenated anesthetic agents and intravenous narcotics. Thus weaning patients from mechanical ventilation may be delayed because of residual effects of various anesthetic agents. This effect is particularly important in elderly patients receiving narcotics.[57]

General anesthesia predisposes to upper airway obstruction by allowing the tongue to fall against the posterior pharyngeal wall with loss of hypoglossal nerve function. Other anesthetic effects include reduction in defense mechanisms promoting bronchial hygiene, including swallowing and clearance of mucus and foreign particles. After operation, secretions may not be cleared and may pool in atelectatic lung segments. Prolonged immobilization, presence of an endotracheal tube, and ineffective cough aggravate this effect. Endotracheal intubation may also stimulate bronchospasm in patients with reactive airway disorders. In these persons, typified by asthmatics, halothane and ketamine are thought to be optimal anesthetic agents.

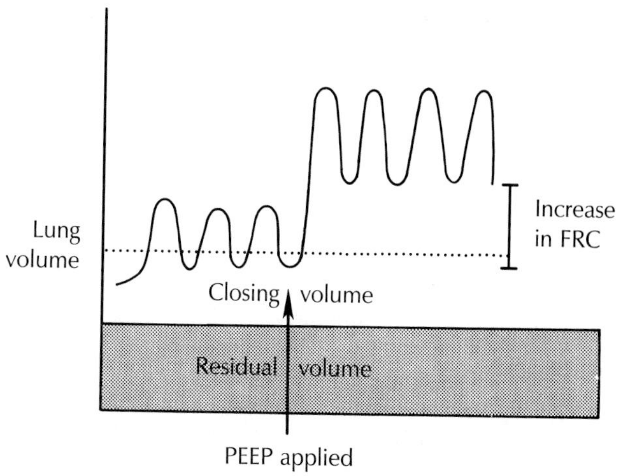

FIGURE 4-10 Impact of pressure ventilation on pulmonary volume in acute respiratory failure. (Redrawn from Dries DJ: *Probl Crit Care* 5(4):575, 1991.)

Postoperative Pulmonary Function

Common postoperative pulmonary complications include atelectasis and hypoxemia. Atelectasis ranges from radiologically invisible microatelectasis to radiologically apparent collapse of segments, lobes, or a complete lung. Microatelectasis is probably common, and macroatelectasis occurs in approximately 60% of patients undergoing various operative procedures. Atelectasis may cause cough, sputum production, fever, and leukocytosis. Fever and leukocytosis may be present secondary to bacterial growth in obstructive airways. As these symptoms resolve without antibiotic administration, this syndrome is not a form of pneumonia.[49]

Factors important in causing atelectasis include retention of secretions, altered pattern of breathing, and changes in small airway function. Mucus plugs that obstruct large airways cause absorption of alveolar gas by mixed venous blood leading to airway collapse unless collateral channels permit the entrance of fresh gas. In addition, the respiratory pattern changes after surgery with reduction in tidal volume by 20% and respiratory rate increase of approximately 25%. This change in breathing pattern results in decreased pulmonary compliance and closure of small airways. Small airway function also changes in the postoperative period. Closing volume, the lung volume at which small airways close, is normally less than expiratory reserve volume, allowing small airways to remain patent throughout the respiratory cycle. Postoperatively, expiratory reserve volume is reduced and becomes smaller than closing volume, leading to closure of small airways during the end-expiration phase of tidal breathing. In cigarette smokers or patients with COPD, this problem is magnified because the closing volume is already increased compared with normal. These individuals, along with the elderly, are particularly vulnerable to the development of atelectasis (Figure 4-10).

The treatment of atelectasis in the postoperative period is difficult to evaluate, in part because much of the atelectasis that occurs is clinically inconsequential and requires no special therapy. In contrast, atelectasis may pose a definite threat to patients with underlying pulmonary disorders or those undergoing thoracic or upper abdominal surgery. These patients should be treated before operation and through the perioperative period with measures intended to promote lung expansion. Postoperative pulmonary complications for high-risk patients may be reduced to the same degree as for low-risk patients with the use of a program including vigorous bronchial hygiene. Other modalities available to prevent atelectases, including spirometry, deep-breathing exercises, intermittent positive pressure breathing, and continuous positive airway pressure, have been studied in the perioperative period. In motivated patients, frequency of pulmonary complications is reduced and hospital stay was shortest with use of spirometry.[12] Due to ease of administration, spirometry is probably the pulmonary prophylactic of choice and may be performed as frequently as 10 times per hour while the patient is awake. Chest physiotherapy may also be beneficial in the setting of significant atelectasis.

Hypoxemia is a common finding in the early postoperative period. The mechanism of postoperative hypoxemia appears related to diffuse atelectasis, associated with the altered pattern of breathing described earlier and abnormal distribution of ventilation associated with anesthetics and operatively induced changes. The supine posture causes a 30% decrease in FRC compared with the upright position. In addition, anesthesia and muscle paralysis cause a reduction in lung and chest wall com-

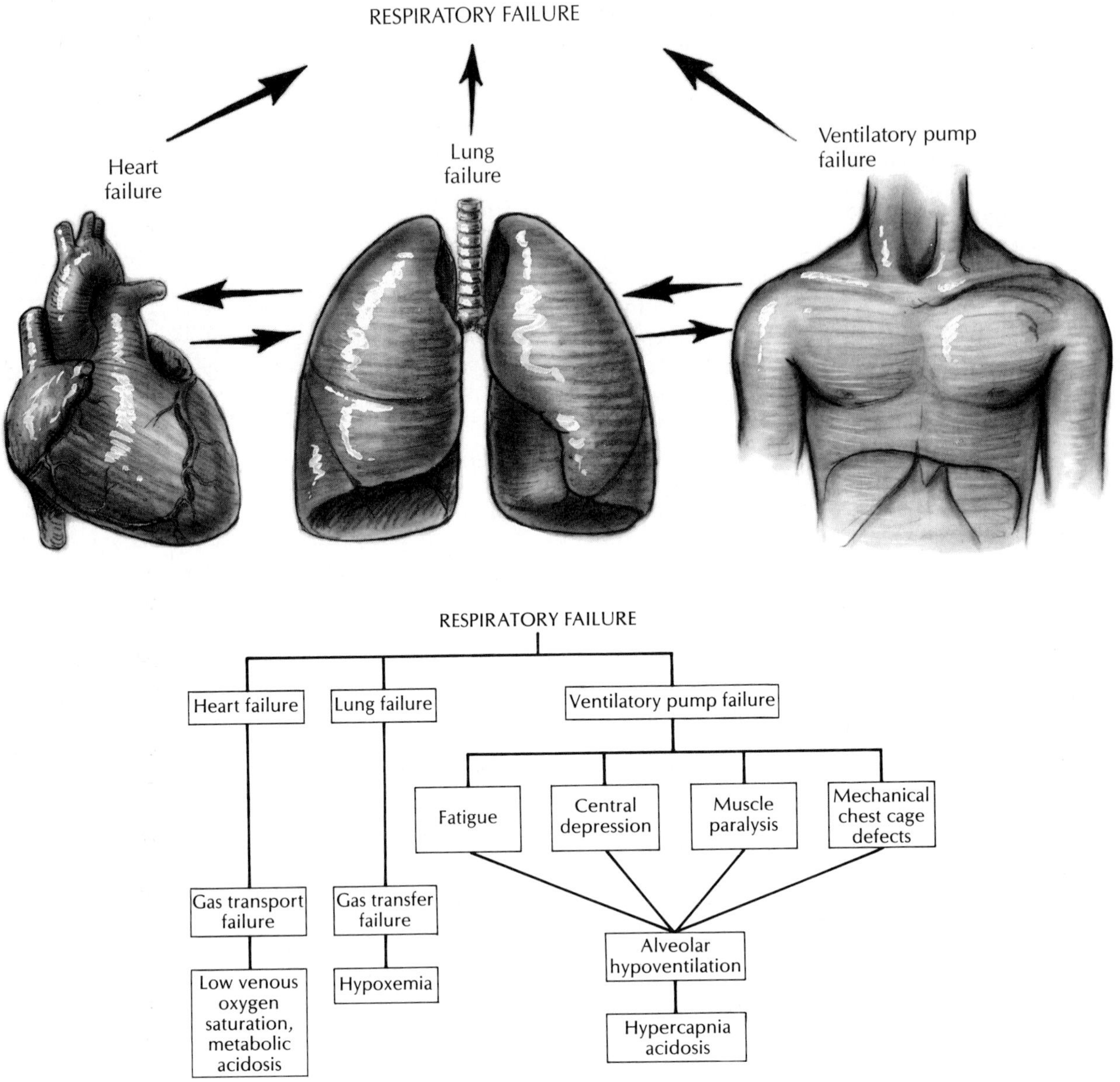

FIGURE 4-11 Proper respiratory function depends on the coordinated functioning of the heart, lungs, and ventilatory pump. Dysfunction in one part can cause deterioration in function in one or both other parts.

pliance and a change in diaphragmatic motion. During normal breathing, diaphragmatic excursion is greatest in the dependent areas of the lung. With general anesthesia, a further reduction in FRC occurs, although the ventilation of dependent lung zones remains dominant during spontaneous breathing. When muscle relaxation and mechanical ventilation are added to general anesthesia, lung inflation shifts to nondependent regions, where forces opposing inflation are reduced. This results in mismatched ventilation and perfusion as blood continues to flow preferentially to dependent lung regions. In most cases, the abnormalities in respiratory function described earlier improve over the initial days after operation, and a temporary increase in delivered fraction of oxygen concentration to the patient is all that is required to maintain adequate oxygen delivery while appropriate respiratory care is used (Figure 4-11).

PERIOPERATIVE MECHANICAL VENTILATORY SUPPORT

The majority of patients undergoing surgical procedures, in whom mechanical ventilatory support is used, are weaned and extubated based on clinical criteria with limited invasive measurements by the anesthesiologist in the postanesthesia care unit. A much smaller group of patients, due either to the complexity of operative procedure or to limitations of underlying medical problems, receive mechanical ventilation support in the initial postoperative period. These patients and others who fail initial ventilator weaning due to respiratory failure confront the clinician with decisions regarding ventilator type, mode of ventilation, inspired oxygen fraction, tidal volume, rate, use of positive end-expiratory pressure (PEEP), and decisions regarding waveform and flow rate. A wide array of possible therapeutic combinations is available. At times, the choices appear arbitrary because some of the literature regarding mechanical ventilatory support is anecdotal. This section describes the use of mechanical ventilatory support and some of the commonly available modes of mechanical ventilation. The physiologic implications and limitations of mechanical ventilation are also reviewed briefly.

TABLE 4-3 INDICATIONS FOR MECHANICAL VENTILATION CRITICAL VALUES*

MEASUREMENT	CRITICAL VALUE
Respiratory Mechanics	
Respiratory rate	>30 breaths/minute
Negative inspiratory force	<−20 mm Hg
Vital capacity	<7-10 ml/kg
Minute ventilation	<3 or >20 L/m
Gas Exchange	
Po_2 (with supplementary oxygen)	<55 mm Hg
Pco_2 (acutely)	>50 mm Hg
$P(A\text{-}a)Do_2$: (with 100% oxygen) (alveolar/arterial gradient)	>450 mm Hg

* Must be assessed in light of coincident medical problems and examination findings, such as altered mental status and use of accessory muscles for respiration.

Modified from Grum CM, Chauncey JB: *Clin Chest Med* 9:37, 1988.

Intubation

A critical initial decision is if and when to perform tracheal intubation and begin assistance with mechanical ventilation (Table 4-3). Benefits gained from intubation and mechanical ventilation include improved gas exchange, reduced work of breathing, and protection of airway patency. Unwarranted delay risks complications associated with hypoxemia, respiratory acidosis, or emergency attempts to secure the airway. Inappropriate initiation of mechanical ventilatory support exposes patients to the hazards of mechanical ventilation and mechanical airway control.[30,65]

By definition, respiratory insufficiency involves abnormal alveolar gas exchange with impaired oxygen transport or inadequate ventilation. Hypoxemia, and not hypercapnia, is the true threat to the patient in this situation. With apnea, life-threatening hypoxemia develops within minutes, as our usable oxygen stores are minimal. In the short term, an arterial oxygen tension $\leq$ 40 mm Hg is frequently associated with tissue hypoxia, metabolic acidosis, and vital organ failure. Thus a $Pao_2 \leq 55$ to 60 mm Hg, despite supplemental oxygen support, is almost always an indication to begin mechanical ventilation.

Hypercapnia requires more judgment when deciding between intubation and initiation of mechanical ventilatory support. Hypercapnia may represent a primary disturbance in alveolar ventilation or compensation for externally imposed metabolic alkalosis. Although primary hypercapnia may lead to acidosis and mental status changes, these effects are rarely life threatening.

Acidemia is frequently present with acute hypercapnia and may signify failing spontaneous ventilation. Acidemia is also common, however, with severe chronic hypercapnia because the bicarbonate store is generally inadequate to normalize arterial pH when the arterial CO_2 tension ($Paco_2$) is $\geq$ 40 to 70 mm Hg. It should also be noted that a $Paco_2 \geq 70$ to 80 mm Hg is associated with a nonlinear CO_2 content-$PaCO_2$ relationship and is tied to the balance between serum bicarbonate and carbon dioxide content, not $Paco_2$.[47]

Progressive hypercapnia and acidosis are important indicators of impending central nervous system depression, additional alveolar hypoventilation, apnea, and hypoxemia. Hypercapnia with acidemia is a signal that the patient is unable to effectively remove carbon dioxide, whatever the reason. Further deterioration is likely to be rapid and important, as little additional ventilatory reserve is present. Hypercapnia without acidemia or central nervous system depression is rarely a sufficient reason to initiate or maintain mechanical ventilatory support. Without acidemia, mental status changes may not be due to hypercapnia alone.

Few patients with hypercapnia develop CO_2 narcosis if hypoxemia is controlled with oxygen therapy. Occasionally, CO_2 narcosis seems to follow the use of even low flow oxygen. Oxygen administration in this setting may be carefully controlled using the venti-mask in which an upper limit is set for the fraction of inspired oxygen. Oxygen therapy can be titrated with finger pulse oximetry to achieve arterial saturation $\geq$ 85% to 90%, allowing additional safety in the administration of oxygen therapy. When this degree of oxygen saturation cannot be achieved without hypercapnia and respiratory acidosis, intubation and mechanical ventilation must be considered.

The often mentioned association between supplemental oxygen administration and worsening hypercarbia in the patient with COPD has been inappropriately extended to other hypoxemic patients with hypocarbia, needlessly prolonging hypoxemia as the fraction of inspired oxygen is slowly increased to achieve desired blood gas results. Unless COPD is evident from the history or physical examination, high fractions of inspired oxygen should be administered immediately to dyspneic or cyanotic patients. Finger oximetry may quickly establish whether adequate oxygenation can be achieved. If it cannot, intubation with mechanical ventilation and positive airway pressure are required.[65]

Mechanical ventilatory assistance should be initiated if the work required to maintain adequate gas exchange is greater than that which can be sustained indefinitely, even if gas exchange is still satisfactory. The work of breathing ordinarily requires less than 3% of the body's total oxygen consumption. With acute respiratory failure, or failure in weaning, ventilatory work may increase in excess of half of the body oxygen consumption. It is frequently difficult to accurately identify excessive respiratory work. Clinical indications include tachycardia, diaphoresis, accessary muscle use, patient distress, a widened paradoxical pulse, and an elevated respiratory rate. Even then, intubation may not be required if an episode of bronchospasm or heart failure can be rapidly reversed.

Even if gas exchange and respiratory work are normal, tracheal intubation is indicated if the airway cannot be kept clear of secretions or the lungs protected from aspiration. A frequent setting is the presence of a depressed state of consciousness or facial or neck trauma. Infection or infiltrative diseases of the upper airway may also contribute. Clues to this condition include coarse rhonchi over central airways or ineffective cough in the presence of tracheal suctioning.

Decisions regarding intubation and mechanical ventilatory assistance are based on clinical evidence. Early elective intubation is most often the wise course, even if CO_2 retention occurs without central nervous system depression or hypoxemia is marginally corrected with high concentrations of supplemental oxygen, particularly if the underlying disease process is unknown or unlikely to improve rapidly. If one delays intubation, improvement should be expected shortly after the initiation of nonintubation therapy. If improvement is not observed, immediate intubation is almost always required. Respiratory failure is sometimes the inevitable complication of heroic treatment for otherwise incurable illness. Medical staff and family are often reluctant to discontinue mechanical ventilatory support once it is initiated. Decisions regarding the initiation of mechanical ventilatory support with intubation should be made, therefore, with forethought regarding implications for patient comfort and inevitable decisions about supporting other organ system failure.

Initiating Mechanical Ventilation

Indications for mechanical ventilation overlap, but are not identical to those entailed in intubation for control of the airway. Mechanical ventilation is used to sustain ventilation when patient effort is inadequate or to gain control of a critically ill patient's ventilation, particularly during collapse of other organ systems. In the perioperative period, mechanical ventilation is used electively to support patients in the initial time of recovery from operative and anesthetic insults. A set of empiric criteria for determining the need for mechanical ventilation is presented in Table 4-3. It should be noted that clinical judgment and the trend of these values are more important than absolute numbers. Increasing severity of illness should always incline one to consider support with mechanical ventilation. Examples of illness where mechanical ventilation should be considered as the pathophysiologic process progresses are septic shock, development of ARDS, and the possibility of apnea. Early mechanical ventilation in the setting of respiratory failure may minimize further complications and irreversible injury by preserving lung volumes and preventing atelectasis.

Initial Ventilator Settings

A standard approach to initial ventilator settings is useful, particularly in a teaching hospital. Table 4-4 includes a set of widely accepted initial ventilator settings. The ventilator modes, or methods by which the machine provides each tidal volume, include control, assist-control, and intermittent mandatory ventilation (IMV) modes. The control mode is used only when the patient is not breathing spontaneously. In the assist-control mode, each mechanical breath is assisted or triggered if initiated by the patient during the designated cycle time. Otherwise, the ventilator provides a nontriggered or control breath. To initiate an assisted breath, the patient must lower airway pressure by a preset amount, which is usually 1 to 3 cm H_2O. Most authors refer to this value as trigger sensitivity. In the IMV mode, the patient receives a predetermined number of ventilator-generated tidal volumes each minute. Breaths from the ventilator either can be synchronized with patient effort or independent of patient respiration. Additional ventilation is made by spontaneous patient effort with tidal volumes in proportion to that effort.

Assist-control or IMV can be successfully used to initiate ventilatory support. An advantage of the assist-control mode is that the patient can increase minute ventilation simply by triggering additional mechanical breaths above the set back-up rate. During IMV, a similar increase in minute ventilation may require greater patient effort. Although practitioners in respiratory care units consider assist-control to be the preferred initial ventilation mode, in patients during the perioperative period where acute respiratory failure is unlikely, IMV at sufficiently high rates can be used with equally satisfactory results.[26,30,65] In the acute situation, the preferred mode of initiating ventilation uses a volume-cy-

TABLE 4-4 INITIAL VENTILATOR SETTINGS

Mode	IMV/SIMV*
Tidal volume	10-15 ml/kg
Backup rate	12 breaths/minute
Oxygen concentration	100%
Flow rate	40 L/minute
Inspiratory : expiratory time ratio	1:3

*Intermittent mandatory ventilation/synchronized intermittent mandatory ventilation

cled ventilator. The presence of unexpected changes in respiratory compliance or resistance in the acute situation may render pressure-cycled ventilation inadequate.

A high initial fraction of inspired oxygen is often recommended, because in many critically ill patients, a high degree of ventilation-perfusion mismatch is present with varying degrees of shunt. As adequate oxygenation is documented, preferably within 20 minutes with an arterial blood gas, the fraction of inspired oxygen can be rapidly reduced to prevent the toxic effects of oxygen therapy. In critically ill patients, the first arterial blood gas determination following operation is appropriate within minutes of arrival in the intensive care unit. While this time period is inadequate for total equilibration of arterial oxygen in patients with underlying lung disease (up to 25 minutes), an early blood gas measurement is useful to assess ventilation and gives an initial indication of the final arterial partial pressure of oxygen.[30,67]

Continuous monitoring with the finger oximeter precedes and complements the arterial blood gas measurement. A subsequent arterial blood specimen may be obtained at the 30-minute time point. By this time, oxygen transport equilibration should have occurred. An oxygen tension of 60 mm Hg or greater allows the oxygen saturation of the hemoglobin to remain in the flat portion of the oxygen/hemoglobin dissociation curve in most clinical situations. Until technology to reliably assess oxygenation at the tissue level becomes available, this guideline is widely accepted to determine oxygen therapy.

After assuring adequate oxygenation, the second priority is provision of adequate carbon dioxide elimination. Ventilation is generally proportional to the partial pressure of carbon dioxide in blood, which is usually between 35 and 45 mm Hg. Schuster[65] reviewed the relationship of minute ventilation, tidal volume, dead space, and CO_2 production. To summarize some of the factors requiring consideration:

$$Pa{CO_2} = (0.863)\ V{CO_2}/(V_E)\ (1 - (V_D/V_T)$$

In this relation minute ventilation (V_E), tidal volume (V_T), dead space (V_D), and CO_2 production ($V{CO_2}$) are related to the partial pressure of carbon dioxide in arterial blood ($Pa{CO_2}$). Assuming a dead space tidal ventilation volume ratio of approximately 0.6 with normal CO_2 production (180 ml/min) should yield a minute ventilation (tidal volume × rate) of 10 L/minute to achieve a partial pressure of carbon dioxide of 40 mm Hg in arterial blood. Generally, a tidal volume of 10 to 15 ml/kg is used in the average adult.

A flow rate of approximately 40 L/minute in the ventilator system generally allows an inspiratory to expiratory time ratio of 1:3. Higher flow rates may be required in patients with high inspiratory demands. Although high flow rates may decrease the inspiratory work of breathing, they may be associated with increased airway pressure. Alternatively, lower flow rates may decrease airway pressure but also reduce the expiratory time available. Decreased airway pressure may be useful when high pressures threaten venous return and cardiac output or if the risk of barotrauma is high.

Modes of Ventilation

Assist-Control

Originally, all ventilators delivered ventilation in a controlled fashion. In other words, a preset volume or pressure was delivered at a preset rate. Assist-control ventilation was developed to allow patient interaction with the ventilator, which resulted in reduction in discomfort related to the preset pattern of ventilation associated with a full control mode. The assist-control mode of ventilation allows the patient to trigger the ventilator with an inspiratory effort while assuring that a specified back-up rate is provided by the ventilator. The pressure or volume of each inspired breath is determined by the physician, and the frequency is set by the patient or the back-up rate if the patient makes no inspiratory efforts. Assist-control ventilation allows the patient to increase minute ventilation by simply increasing the frequency of respiratory efforts. In patients who are weak or debilitated or who have high metabolic demands due to underlying medical problems, ventilation can be increased with minimal metabolic cost to the patient.[39]

Intermittent Mandatory Ventilation

Downs and Klein[19] introduced intermittent mandatory ventilation approximately 15 years ago. This ventilatory mode was designed as a weaning tool and differs from assist-control in that machine response to a patient's inspiratory effort is limited to providing a predetermined number of breaths, which may be delivered in synchrony with the patient's own respiratory efforts. Additional breaths obtained during ventilation in the IMV or synchronization of the IMV mode SIMV mode are completely dependent on patient effort. SIMV is useful in preventing the patient from getting a double tidal volume, which could occur if a mandatory machine breath was delivered with a spontaneous breath. IMV/

SIMV is the most frequently used ventilatory mode in intensive care units. Potential benefits include decrease in weaning time, reduction in mean airway pressure, and reduction of adverse cardiovascular effects from PEEP. These benefits, however, are poorly documented in prospective studies.[73] IMV may not be the ventilatory method of choice during rapid changes in acid-base status or during times when respiratory muscle work needs to be minimized, such as respiratory muscle fatigue or cardiogenic shock.

Pressure Support Ventilation

Pressure support ventilation (PSV) is an augmentation of spontaneous respiratory efforts by a clinician-set amount of positive airway pressure. Pressure administration is maintained as long as a minimal inspiratory effort occurs. The patient has substantial control over duration and volume of inspiratory effort. Pressure support differs from continuous positive airway pressure in that pressure is applied only during inspiration. It is also different from older forms of intermittent positive pressure breathing in that pressure is maintained as a plateau as long as patient effort persists. Low levels of pressure support ventilation (5 to 10 cm H_2O) can reduce pressure work required for spontaneous air flow through an endotracheal tube. This support may improve comfort and optimize workload in patients requiring endotracheal tube placement for airway control without ventilatory support. This form of ventilation may also be used to complement spontaneous breaths during IMV/SIMV. Higher levels of pressure support can be used to augment patient respiratory efforts and thereby produce tidal volumes equivalent to those supplied by conventional mechanical ventilation. When this occurs, patient muscle work is eliminated and patient-ventilator synchrony is improved. Pressure support is thought to provide a more physiologic workload to ventilatory muscles than IMV/SIMV. In addition, because patient control over flow and volume of each breath is considerable, patient-ventilator synchrony improves along with patient comfort. A theoretical disadvantage to pressure support ventilation is that no minimal minute ventilation is guaranteed. In addition, cardiac filling can be compromised with pressure support ventilation, just as it can with intermittent positive pressure ventilation and other ventilatory modes.[63]

In pressure support ventilation the degree of ventilatory assistance is proportional to the preset pressure level. Maximum muscle unloading occurs at the maximum inspiratory pressure support level, defined as providing a tidal volume of 10 to 12 ml/kg. Theoretically, a pressure support level above this tidal volume range is unnecessary. Transition from partial to maximum respiratory unloading can be detected from changes in the breathing pattern. Maximum unloading of inspiratory muscles is characterized by an increase in tidal volume and a decrease in respiratory rate.

Several studies have suggested an advantage for pressure support ventilation over demand flow or continuous flow positive airway pressure in terms of decreasing oxygen consumption of respiratory muscles and diaphragmatic pressure time product in postsurgical patients. In addition to providing relief for respiratory work imposed by endotracheal tube size–airway size differential, low levels of pressure support ventilation are adequate to compensate for the work of breathing required to open demand valves in mechanical ventilatory systems.

Limited studies suggest the applicability of pressure support ventilation in weaning postoperative patients from mechanical ventilatory support.[63] Pressure support appears to provide a degree of ventilation similar to standard positive pressure ventilation. In selected patients, pressure support is adequate as a primary means of ventilatory support. However, in patients with unstable respiratory drive or changeable respiratory system impedance, pressure support ventilation is not advisable unless backed by volume cycled breaths at a frequency sufficient to meet overall ventilatory demand. Positive inspiratory pressure may also persist in the presence of circuit leak. A small breathing circuit leak may produce a continued demand, causing continuous positive airway pressure equal to the preset pressure support level because the expiratory criterion is not met. Many ventilators have secondary breath termination criteria to reduce this hazard. The patient may also fail to trigger the pressure-limited breath during pressure support ventilation when continuous in-line nebulizers are applied with flow rates that exceed patient mean flow rate. High nebulizer flow rates cause difficulty in triggering the pressure-limited breath, resulting in alveolar hypoventilation. In addition, bias flow would be sensed by the ventilator as the patient minute ventilation, preventing activation of a ventilator apnea alarm.

Pressure support has gained wide clinical application. However, guidelines for the application of pressure support ventilation during weaning have yet to be adequately formulated. No randomized prospective studies have evaluated the efficacy of pressure support ventilation in comparison to either SIMV or T-piece weaning on the duration and outcome of weaning from mechanical ventilatory support. Pressure support has the potential to be a primary means of ventilatory support. However, backup ventilation is required to meet patients' ventilatory demand in the event that pressure support fails.

High-Frequency Ventilation

Mechanical ventilation using higher than normal respiratory frequencies is defined as high-frequency ventilation (HFV). Generally, this is assumed to be greater than one breath per second. In a recent review, MacIntyre[37] described two basic types of high frequency ventilation with fundamentally different concepts of gas transport: (1) HFV using tidal breaths larger than anatomic dead space (V_D) operating under convective flow principles and (2) high-frequency ventilation using tidal breaths smaller than V_D operating under nonconvective flow principles. High-frequency ventilation using convective flow is generally given only with rates less than 300 bpm. As smaller tidal volume can be given at higher rates, high frequency ventilation using nonconvective flow principles can be administered at rates up to 50 breaths per second (50 Hz).

Convective flow high-frequency ventilation can be supplied by conventional positive pressure ventilators at rates up to 150 bpm. Valve response characteristics in these devices, however, prevent tidal volume from exceeding 200 to 300 ml at these high rates. Jet ventilators use pulses of gas injected through narrow cannulae into the endotracheal tube or trachea to deliver tidal breaths. The volume of these pulses may be increased by entraining additional gas from the adjacent endotracheal tube. Exhalation is passive, and no exhalation valve is required in the ventilator circuit. It is thought that these characteristics allow jet ventilators to supply large minute volumes without excessive air trapping. Reduced peak pressures and faster respiratory rates can alter ventilation and perfusion distribution and improve gas exchange in patients with large pulmonary air leaks.[8,9] Thus high-frequency ventilation is an acceptable mode of therapy in patients with bronchopleural fistula.

Other proposed benefits of high frequency ventilation include reduction in vascular pressure swings related to intracranial pressure and improvement in stroke volume in patients with cardiac dysfunction when high-frequency ventilation is synchronized with systole.[51] Finally, high-frequency ventilation allows airway surgical procedures to be performed with ventilatory support using low airway pressures. This effect has been demonstrated with laryngoscopy and bronchoscopy. Reduction in thoracic abdominal motion during anesthesia with high-frequency ventilation has reduced stone motion and facilitated extracorporeal shock wave lithotripsy. More common forms of adult respiratory failure do not appear to be ventilated or oxygenated better with the use of convective high-frequency ventilation at comparable airway pressures.

Nonconvective high-frequency ventilation has been provided with jet and oscillator devices. Jet devices function as described earlier, and oscillator devices put sinusoidal oscillations on the airways while gas is provided by bias flow. Airway pressure is manipulated by the inflow of fresh gas and vacuum control on the exhalation tubing. This mode of ventilation has produced effective oxygen and carbon dioxide transport. The physiology of this mode of ventilation has not been adequately determined.[20] PEEP and mean airway pressures can be reduced further with nonconvective high-frequency ventilation than other forms of mechanical ventilation. While this type of ventilation may reduce complications associated with high airway pressures, theoretically, at lung resonant frequencies, high alveolar pressures can develop despite low central airway pressures. Clinical data supporting use of all forms of high-frequency ventilation are still being obtained.

Positive End-Expiratory Pressure and Continuous Positive Airway Pressure (PEEP, CPAP)

PEEP and CPAP are pressure modalities designed to maintain airway patency in association with mechanical or spontaneous ventilation by providing a baseline level of continuous positive pressure, either in specific association with mechanical breaths or throughout the respiratory cycle of spontaneous respiration. These terms are often used interchangeably and incorrectly. PEEP is a fixed level of pressure applied at end expiration, whereas CPAP (more commonly applied) is a fixed pressure level given on a continuous basis. PEEP/CPAP is a useful method for increasing arterial oxygen tension and allowing reduction in oxygen administration. Functional residual capacity is increased, and the available alveolar surface area is also augmented with improved ventilation perfusion relationships and ultimately arterial oxygen tension. PEEP/CPAP may decrease the work of respiration in asthmatics and patients with chronic obstructive pulmonary disease who experience a form of spontaneous PEEP as a part of their disease process. PEEP/CPAP has not been demonstrated effective in the prevention of ARDS or atelectasis. Adverse effects attributed to PEEP include an increase in barotrauma related to positive pressure ventilation, depression of cardiac output, increased intracranial pressure, and contribution to inaccuracy in pulmonary artery pressure monitoring.[23,52]

No formula can predict the levels of PEEP/CPAP that will maximally benefit the patient. When patients require the administration of toxic oxygen concentrations to maintain adequate arterial oxygen saturation, an appropriate level of PEEP may be associated with improved tissue oxygen delivery. PEEP, therefore, may be increased to decrease oxygen administration as long as tissue oxygen delivery does not fall to undesirable levels. Monitoring with pulmonary artery catheter placement is probably appropriate in the acute application of PEEP or CPAP in excess of 10 cm H_2O. Significant changes in oxygen transport or other hemodynamic parameters require reevaluation of the level of PEEP or CPAP. In treating patients with PEEP, the hemoglobin should be kept in an optimal range through transfusion of packed red blood cells, and hypovolemia should be avoided.

Inotropic drugs may be required to augment the cardiac output and improve oxygen transport. In addition, there is no evidence to support the direct therapeutic benefit to the lungs with PEEP administration, although intracranial pressure and barotrauma can be increased with its use. PEEP should be used in situations in which improved arterial oxygen tension or exposure to potentially harmful levels of oxygen are demanded.

Inverse Ratio Ventilation

Inverse ratio ventilation is used in patients with diffuse lung disease and hypoxemia, which is refractory to standard PEEP/CPAP therapy. In this mode of ventilatory support, the inspiratory to expiratory time ratio is greater than 1:1 ($I{:}E \geq 1{:}1$). The rationale for inverse ratio ventilation is that longer duration of inspiratory positive pressure will open less compliant alveolar units with long-time constants, and shorter expiratory times will not allow these alveoli to collapse again.[37] Inverse ratio ventilation can raise mean airway pressures without a concomitant increase in PEEP pressure. However, inverse ratio ventilation is often uncomfortable and may require sedation or paralysis of the patient. In addition, hypotension has been noted due to decreased cardiac output, which is a function of increased mean airway pressure.

When used with the pressure control mode of ventilation, preset variables in patients treated with inverse ratio ventilation are peak airway pressure, ratio of inspiratory/expiratory time, respiratory rate, and the applied PEEP. Peak inspiratory flow rate and flow waveform are usually preset in the machines now available. Frequently, preset peak airway pressure is lower than with conventional positive pressure ventilation, but mean airway pressure is increased because of the increased filling time. Tidal volume is determined by the respiratory system mechanics of the patient. As the ratio of inspiratory to expiratory time increases and respiratory rate is also increased, the duration of expiratory time is decreased. This may be associated with production of intrinsic PEEP. Increase in intrinsic PEEP may result in smaller tidal volumes with a given pulmonary airway pressure pattern. Despite this limitation, P_{CO_2} can be maintained satisfactorily in most cases with the use of inverse ratio ventilation.

The chief benefit seen with inverse ratio ventilation is improved oxygenation. Improved oxygenation is thought to be related to increases in both mean airway pressure and intrinsic PEEP or end-expiratory lung volume. There are no established guidelines regarding the appropriate level of airway pressure when switching patients from more conventional modes of ventilation to inverse ratio ventilation. In addition, no controlled study to date has established reduced mortality or morbidity with inverse ratio ventilation in comparison with conventional positive pressure ventilation modes. Most of the uncontrolled studies of inverse ratio ventilation in adults have reported improved oxygenation.

Mandatory Minute Volume

Mandatory minute volume ventilation was introduced in 1977 by Hewlett and associates.[32] The intent of this ventilatory mode is facilitation of weaning from mechanical ventilatory support. This closed loop ventilation mode allows the patient to breathe spontaneously. The ventilator is set to provide a guaranteed minute ventilation volume if the spontaneous ventilation on the part of the patient drops below a preset level. If this drop occurs, a feedback mechanism is actuated and the machine delivers pressurized breaths of fixed volume until the desired minute volume of ventilation is obtained. Thus the level of machine support may vary between total ventilatory support and complete patient independence.[55] As the patient's spontaneous ventilation increases, machine support decreases and vice versa. In the mandatory minute volume mode, the ventilator does not provide any assistance until patient minute ventilation falls below the preset level. The ventilator assists only to the point of restoring the preset minute ventilation.

In the mandatory minute volume ventilation mode, the quality of spontaneous minute volume is not evaluated. Minute volume induced by less efficient rapid shallow breathing is not distinguished from minute volume induced by slow deep breathing, as long as the total minute ventilation of both breathing patterns is comparable. Rapid shallow breathing may be inadequate to wean the patient from mechanical ventilatory support and to actuate the ventilatory support mechanism, leading to the possibility of significant alveolar hypoventilation.[63] A recent innovation in this method has been the incorporation of pressure support ventilation in addition to mandatory minute volume ventilation. The use of pressure support was thought to ensure adequate tidal volume in patients with rapid shallow breathing, and the mandatory minute volume made would provide backup for pressure support in patients with unstable respiratory drive. Laboratory evaluation suggests that this combination of ventilatory modes improves treatment of alveolar hypoventilation in comparison to the use of pressure support ventilation alone.

Since its introduction, mandatory minute volume ventilation has gained limited clinical acceptance, as the advantages posed over more commonly used weaning modalities have not been established. This mode of ventilation has been incorporated in some commercially available ventilators that can provide both mandatory minute volume ventilation and pressure support ventilation. In this setting, efficacy, as seen in gas exchange, safety, morbidity, and mortality in comparison to conventional positive pressure ventilation modes, has yet to be established.

Other Ventilator Modes

In patients with severe unilateral lung disease, two ventilators may be used to ventilate the lungs independently through a double-lumen endotracheal tube. This mode of ventilation is termed independent lung ventilation.[33,65] With conventional ventilation, most minute ventilation and positive airway pressure are delivered to a more compliant lung, resulting in significant ventilation/perfusion mismatch. Independent lung ventilation allows the physician to determine tidal volume, fraction of inspired oxygen, and CPAP for each lung independently without synchronization. Hyperventilation, hyperexpansion, and potential barotrauma to the normal lung are reduced. Neuromuscular paralysis and sedation are often required. This technique is rarely necessary to achieve adequate gas exchange.

PHYSIOLOGY OF MECHANICAL VENTILATION

With the institution of mechanical ventilation, changes occur that alter both ventilatory mechanics and gas exchange. The most obvious change is the difference between respiratory muscle role in spontaneous breathing and with mechanical ventilation. During spontaneous breathing, respiratory muscles produce air flow by reducing intrathoracic and particularly pleural, alveolar, and airway pressures. During mechanical ventilation, air is forced into the lungs by application of positive pressure; and airway, alveolar, and pleural pressure are increased throughout inspiration (Figure 4-12). The impact of positive pressure ventilation on the mechanics of ventilation, with particular regard to the relationship between airway resistance and lung volume, is poorly understood. With increased inspiratory flow, associated with mechanical ventilation, ventilation becomes more uniform throughout the lungs, allowing ventilation-perfusion imbalance to increase.[36] Mechanical ventilation has also been associated with an increase in physiologic dead space in patients with normal lungs. Gas exchange may be enhanced in patients with significant underlying pulmonary disease.

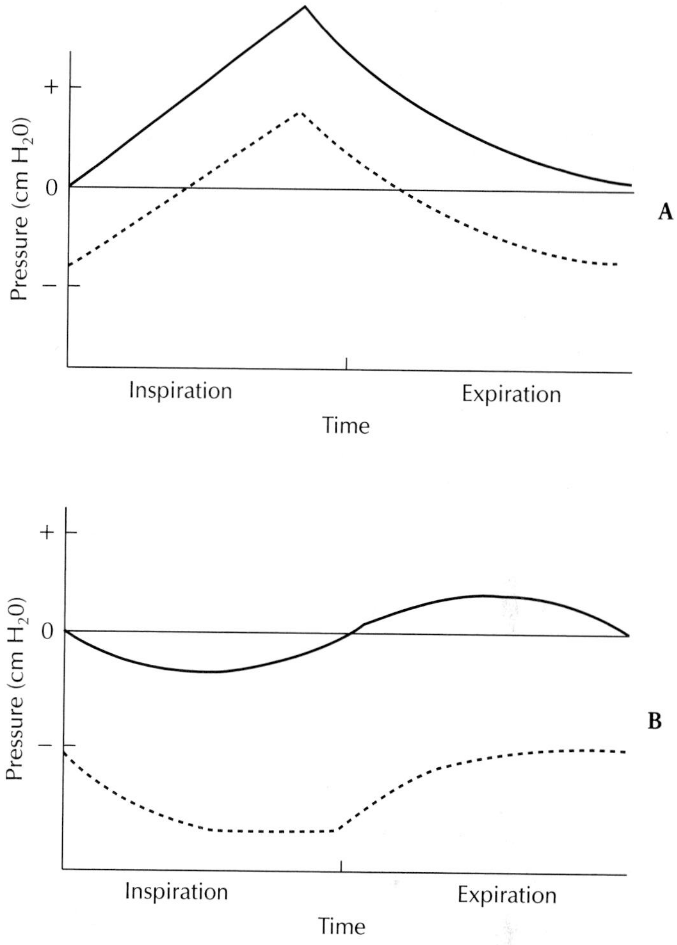

FIGURE 4-12 Effect of mechanical ventilation (**A**) on airway pressure *(solid line)* and pleural pressure *(dashed line)* in comparison to spontaneous ventilation (**B**). (From Kreit JW, Eschenbacher WL: *Clin Chest Med* 9:11, 1988.)

Another change associated with the institution of mechanical ventilation is placement of a mechanical airway, the endotracheal tube, having nonlinear pressure and flow characteristics with resistance increasing progressively as the flow increases. Pressure loss across the endotracheal tube depends primarily on the internal diameter. As tube size decreases, resistance increases dramatically (Figure 4-13). It has also been demonstrated that endotracheal tubes have a much higher resistance than the normal upper airway and that this difference in resistance may increase significantly as the gas flow rate is increased. The endotracheal tube may also elevate airway resistance by triggering bronchial constriction. This response may be triggered by receptor stimulation at the level of the larynx and trachea. Anatomic dead space is also affected by the placement of the endotracheal tube. If the upper airway volume is assumed to be approximately 0.5 ml per pound, endotracheal intubation should result in a decrease in anatomic dead space in most patients. In fact, 26-cm endotracheal tubes and connectors have volumes ranging from 39 to 45 ml as internal diameter increases from 7 to 9 mm. The clinical significance of this difference is unclear.

Mechanical ventilation is associated with a change in patient position from upright to supine. In the supine position, abdominal contents force the dome of the diaphragm in a cephalad direction and functional residual capacity is decreased. Thus airway and respiratory system resistance may increase. In addition, the pressure/

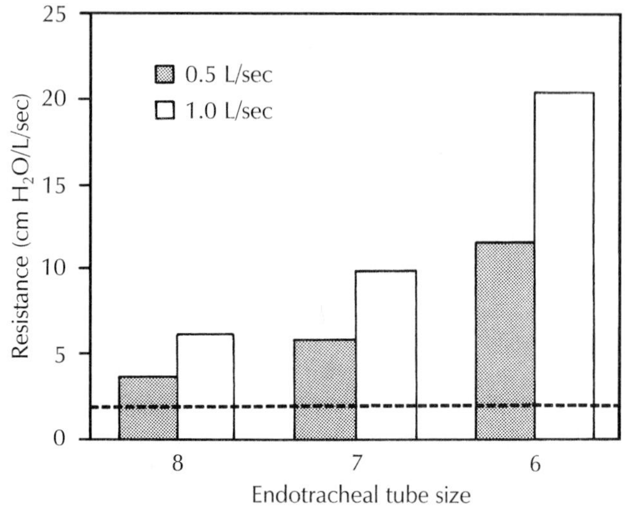

FIGURE 4-13 Resistances posed by endotracheal tubes of different diameters at airflow rates of 0.5 and 1.0 L/sec. The normal airway resistance of less than 2 cm H_2O/L/sec is indicated by the stippled line. (Based on data from Demers RR. Redrawn from Taylor RW, Shoemaker WC: *Critical care: state of the art* 12:394, 1991.)

volume relationship of the respiratory system becomes flatter in the supine position. Functional residual capacity may fall below the critical closing volume, contributing to the need for greater pressure to expand the lungs to a desired volume. Respiratory system compliance also decreases. When subjects move from the upright to supine position, ventilation and perfusion change depending on the comparison of functional residual capacity and critical closing volume. If functional residual capacity exceeds closing volume in the upright and supine positions, physiologic dead space decreases when the patient is supine. If, however, functional residual capacity falls below closing volume when the patient changes from the upright to the supine position, physiologic dead space increases. In patients with acute respiratory insufficiency, functional residual capacity is reduced below normal. These patients, therefore, will suffer additional gas exchange abnormality when they assume the supine position.[14,28,35,45]

Heart-Lung Interaction

Right ventricular preload is controlled by venous return to the right atrium, which is governed by a pressure gradient that develops between systemic venous pressure and right atrial pressure. The gradient for venous filling of the right side of the heart is in effect an extrathoracic-to-intrathoracic pressure gradient. During spontaneous inspiration, decreases in intrathoracic pressure produce a net increase in the pressure gradient to increase right ventricular filling and right ventricular ouput.[13] In 1948, Cournand and associates[13] noted that cyclic elevations of intrapleural pressure associated with mechanical lung inflation corresponded to phasic changes with decreased right ventricular stroke output. Subsequent studies revealed that right and left ventricular volumes when plotted against time during mechanical lung inflation changed so that right ventricular volume decreased and was minimal at peak inspiration. As intrathoracic pressure returned to baseline during exhalation from a mechanical breath, right ventricular volume increased. Reciprocal changes, though less in magnitude, occurred in the left ventricle. Thus a potential for control of right ventricular inflow as well as left ventricular performance exists with the application of positive intrapleural pressure associated with mechanical ventilation.[61]

Changes in lung volume imposed by mechanical lung inflation may also affect right ventricular outflow impedance by changing pulmonary vascular resistance. Given the low pressure-generating capacity of the right ventricle, one can appreciate the potential impact of positive pressure ventilation, not only on right ventricular output performance, but also on the input provided to the left ventricle. Subsequent studies using technology to evaluate the right ventricular ejection fraction demonstrated that continuous positive-pressure ventilation with large tidal volumes resulted in decreased right ventricular ejection fraction. Right ventricular ejection fraction increased as the level of spontaneous ventilation was allowed to increase as patients were weaned from continuous mechanical ventilation to a blend of spontaneous and mechanical breaths.

PEEP and CPAP continue to be studied with regard to effect on right ventricular performance. PEEP has been found to increase echocardiographically derived right ventricular area with increasing right atrial transmural pressure. As higher levels of PEEP/CPAP are used, right ventricular pressure overload appears to compromise the right ventricle with increasing right ventricular deformity and decreased left ventricular compliance imposed by the intervening interventricular septum.[10,34] At low levels, PEEP/CPAP appears to control right ventricular input, whereas higher pressure levels cause changes mainly at the level of right ventricular output impedance.

Mechanical ventilation also has complex effects on left ventricular function, including changes in preload, chamber compliance, afterload, and inotropic state. Left ventricular preload is in part mediated by changes in the right ventricle and pulmonary vascular bed imposed by mechanical ventilation. As right ventricular output impedance increases, the right ventricle fails as a pressure generator and left ventricular filling may be reduced. In addition, right ventricular failure is characteristically accompanied by right ventricular dilation. This tends to displace the interventricular septum toward the left, decreasing left ventricular compliance and filling secondary to increased right ventricular volume. This and similar observations form the basis for the concept of ventricular interaction. In addition to acting in series, both ventricles act in parallel and, by means of the interventricular septum and pericardium, influence each other in both systole and diastole.[2]

With specific regard to mechanical ventilation, the physiologic effects differ from those of spontaneous inspiration. Right ventricular output decreases during mechanical lung inflation as opposed to spontaneous inspiration where right heart output may increase due to improved venous return. When this decrease in right ventricular output is transferred to the left side of the heart, left ventricular stroke output decreases, in either late inspiration or early expiration.[64] If elevated pleural pressures are sustained (for example, by CPAP or PEEP), the predominant effect of mechanical ventilation on left ventricular preload is to decrease left ventricular preload significantly.

In contrast to spontaneous ventilation where negative intrathoracic pressure tends to increase left ventricular afterload, mechanical lung inflation is expected to decrease left ventricular afterload.[7] This observation has been supported in patients with ventricular fibrillation and cardiogenic shock; however, widespread support for this concept in patients with normal ventricular function has not been forthcoming.

Left ventricular contractility is mediated by neural, humoral, and mechanical factors in the presence of positive-pressure ventilation. Vagal reflexes activated by lung inflation may have negative chronotropic, inotropic, and vasodilatory effects.[11] In addition, humoral factors released during lung expansion have been identified in cross-circulation experiments mediating the decline in ventricular contractile function during the imposition of PEEP in intact animal experiments.[22] Mechanical factors may also decrease left ventricular pumping function.

Ventricular interaction may affect systolic as well as diastolic function. Geometric studies of changes occurring with spontaneous respiration and with PEEP suggest compromise of left ventricular systolic function.[58] These effects may be more pronounced in patients with preexisting wall motion abnormalities. PEEP or CPAP may also decrease myocardial blood flow, altering perfusion of the left ventricle and subjecting the ventricle to ischemia.

PROTOCOL FOR WEANING THE POST OPEN-HEART SURGERY PATIENT FROM VOLUME VENTILATION:

1. Place patient on ventilator with the following settings (usually selected by anesthesia):
   A. Mode: SIMV with 5 cm pressure support
   B. FIO_2 100%
   C. PEEP + 5 cm H_2O
   D. TV 10 ml/kg. Exceptions: bullous lung disease, present or past lung resection
   E. Ventilator rate 10
2. Wean FIO_2 in the decrements 100%-80%-60%-50%-40%, as long as PaO_2 > 70 mm Hg and pulse oximetry shows O_2 saturation over 92%.
3. At 0200 or thereabouts, after sedation has been discontinued, reduce SIMV rate in decrements of two breaths/min every 1-2 hours until SIMV rate of 6 breaths/min has been reached, keeping pH between 7.35 and 7.45. Take blood pressure and heart rate and follow O_2 saturation.
4. At 0600 or thereabouts, measure and record *spontaneous ventilation* (ventilator detached):
   A. Tidal volume
   B. Respiratory rate
   C. Negative inspiratory force
5. Calculate *rapid shallow breathing index* (RSBI). This is the respiratory rate breaths/min/tidal volume (liters). The RSBI is normally under 80. Generally, the respiratory rate should be under 30 breaths/min.
6. If values are acceptable (RSBI<80; NIF >-30cm) place patient on CPAP of 5 cm H_2O NIF +5, FIO_2 of 40%.
   If RSBI is between 80 and 100, do not put on CPAP, but await the decision of a physician. An RSBI over 100 indicates patient is not ready for CPAP.
7. Measure heart rate, respiratory rate, and blood pressure every 15 minutes for 30 to 60 minutes.
8. If the following criteria are met, patient can be extubated:
   A. Respiratory rate <30 breaths/min
   B. Pulse increase under 20 breaths/min
   C. Systolic pressure stable (no change over 20 mm Hg)
   D. O_2 saturation >90%
   E. Patient not distressed
9. If these criteria are *not* met, resume full ventilatory support.

Weaning from Mechanical Ventilation

As the patient recovers from the stress of surgery and anesthesia, mechanical ventilatory support is generally no longer required. In most patients, weaning per se is not needed. One can simply confirm adequacy of gas exchange during a short period of spontaneous breathing without respiratory compromise before completely removing ventilator support and the endotracheal tube.

Weaning is the gradual withdrawal of mechanical ventilatory support (see the box above). It is applied to those patients in whom recovery from previous insults is incomplete and in whom respiratory demand may be only partially reduced. A weaning plan may need to provide improvement in respiratory muscle strength and endurance.[65] The approach typically involved is standard to exercise physiology and includes periods of high intensity work followed by adequate rest in between these periods of increased activity. This strategy is most consistent with periods of T-tube weaning in which spontaneous breathing through the endotracheal tube is interposed between periods of mechanical ventilatory support.

Ultimate decisions regarding weaning and its efficacy are clinical. An experienced physician may be able to predict success or failure during weaning attempts. In an attempt to qualify and predict more accurately the success of weaning, a variety of indices, such as vital capacity, negative inspiratory pressure, minute ventilation, and tidal volume, have been proposed as predictors of weaning outcome. Unfortunately, the power of these studies to accurately predict outcome and weaning has been poor.[25,46,71] Tobin and Yang[71] suggest several factors that may affect the value of weaning indices from mechanical ventilation support. Differences among patient groups studied may be significant. In addition, techniques of measurement and the lack of consistent criteria to define successful weaning pose problems. These authors found that rapid shallow breathing as reflected by the ratio of respiratory frequency to tidal volume was the optimum predictor of weaning trial failure, whereas its absence was the most accurate predictor of success in weaning patients from mechanical ventilatory support.[71] It should be noted that the study of Tobin and Yang was limited to medical patients where weaning outcome is generally more difficult to predict than in the surgical perioperative population. Nonetheless, it is valuable to note the importance of rapid shallow breathing as a predictor of failure in weaning trials, particularly when mechanical ventilation has been in place for a long time.

It is also important that weaning not interfere with recovery. As ventilatory support is reduced, signs of respiratory fatigue must be sought carefully. Spontaneous breathing requires work, and ventilatory support must be adjusted so that patient effort does not exceed the patient capacity to meet the work required. Pressure support ventilation may play a significant part in reducing ventilator-imposed respiratory work in patients during weaning trials. Unassisted breathing during weaning trials is also clearly associated with increased work when a narrow endotracheal tube is in place. The most common method for assessing respiratory work is clinical observation for signs of distress or fatigue. Early signs of increasing respiratory work include rapid breathing occasionally followed by uncoordinated inspiratory activity—either respiratory alternans (alternating rib cage and abdominal breathing) or paradoxical abdominal motion (inward movement of the abdomen during inspiration).

The specific weaning technique used is frequently less important than the care with which it is applied. Different aspects of mechanical ventilation, i.e., oxygenation, ventilation, work of breathing, and airway patency, must be evaluated and support drawn separately as appropriate. For example, if oxygenation failure is the major indication for continuing mechanical ventilation, PEEP or CPAP and FIO_2 should be titrated until the patient can sustain a $PaO_2 \geq 60$ mm Hg with an FIO_2 at 0.50 or less and 5 cm H_2O or less of PEEP or CPAP. During weaning of mechanical ventilation, PEEP is typically reduced in 2 to 3 cm H_2O increments every 8 to 12 hours, assuming adequate oxygenation during that period. Although PEEP, fraction of inspired oxygen, and ventilator rate may be lowered in tandem, their separate effects on arterial blood gases and patient response to mechanical ventilation should be appreciated. Once the PEEP level is reduced to 5 cm H_2O or less, and the FIO_2 is 0.50 or less, further weaning can usually be rapid if the duration of ventilator support has been brief. Extubation may be considered after a trial of 1 to 2 hours of unassisted ventilation (see accompanying box) (Table 4-5).

WEANING PRIORITIES

1. $FIO_2 \leq 50\%$
2. PEEP/CPAP ≤ 5 cm H_2O
3. Rate (SIMV/IMV) ≤ 4 breaths/min
4. Pressure support level ≤ 5 cm H_2O
5. Assess for extubation
   a. Acute problems resolved/stable
   b. Mental status/airway control
   c. Secretion control

Modified from Dries D: *Probl Crit Care* 5(4):579, 1991.

Approaches to weaning include the T-tube technique in which periods of unassisted spontaneous breathing through a T tube or tracheostomy circuit are interposed between periods of mechanical ventilatory support. It is suggested that the patient rest completely when returned to ventilatory assistance. Short daytime weaning periods are used initially and are progressively increased in duration and/or frequency.

IMV is another commonly used technique for weaning patients from the ventilator. A transition from full ventilatory support to spontaneous breathing is made by gradually decreasing the ventilator rate, thus allowing the patient to provide necessary respiration. Pressure support ventilation is sometimes combined in this effort to reduce the work of breathing associated by the ventilator circuit and endotracheal tube. The ventilator rate can be decreased at a slow or rapid rate depending on the clinical assessment of patient respiratory status. Respiratory rate and tidal volume can be readily checked

TABLE 4-5 CRITERIA FOR WEANING

PARAMETER	NORMAL	ACCEPTABLE
Po_2 (torr)	>80 (FIo_2 .21)	70-80 (FIo_2 0.4-0.6)
Alveolar-arterial O_2 gradient (torr)	<100 (FIo_2 1.0)	<300-450 (FIo_2 1.0)
Pco_2 (torr)	35-45	30-55
Vital capacity (ml/kg)	70	10-20
Inspiratory force (cm H_2O)	50-100	20-30
Minute ventilation (1/min)	4-5	<10 (double on command)

Modified from Dries DJ: *Probl Crit Care* 5(4):580, 1991.

to assess the progress of the weaning trial. Weaning parameters along with normal values are given to permit comparison between patients with acceptable weaning parameters and normals. One should be mindful that the discrepancy can be impressive. Hemodynamic function profiles, with particular reference to the intrapulmonary shunt equation, may be valuable aids in determining weaning propriety. Marginal cardiac performance suggests cautious weaning at best, whereas elevated shunt is predictive of poor outcome in weaning from PEEP or CPAP.

In patients where chronic respiratory muscle weakness limits successful weaning, pressure support ventilation may be used independent of intermittent mandatory ventilation. Again, respiratory rate and tidal volume are monitored carefully in patients who receive weaning trials using pressure support. All patients who receive prolonged weaning trials require psychologic support, adequate sleep, nutrition, and physical and occupational therapy. Causes of failure include inadequately treated respiratory infection, bronchospasm, or cardiac failure.

Extubation is attempted when adequate gas exchange during spontaneous breathing at an acceptable level of respiratory work and supplemental oxygen are present. Airway control by mechanical means should no longer be necessary. Reintubation may be necessary if secretions cannot be adequately cleared, muscle fatigue or weakness supervenes, acute airway obstruction develops, or other organ system problems impose an unfavorable balance in a poorly compensated patient. In this setting, we frequently perform tracheostomy to facilitate airway management and ventilatory support after failed extubation. Upper airway obstruction may present as inspiratory wheezing or stridor within 24 hours of extubation. It is usually caused by glottic edema and may be treated with inhaled racemic epinephrine in the acute setting.

If the response is not rapid, reintubation is frequently necessary. In this case, the endotracheal tube is typically left in place for 2 to 3 days to allow edema to resolve before extubation is attempted. Recurrent problems of this type frequently entail tracheostomy.

Complications

A common problem presented to the manager of mechanical ventilatory support is the patient who is decompensating and fighting the ventilator. Patients in acute distress should be removed from the ventilator and bagged with 100% oxygen. Easy manual ventilation with patient improvement suggests a ventilator problem. Manual bagging, however, also results in an increased tidal volume, which may coincide with patient improvement. For example, patients with decreased lung compliance may have dyspnea despite adequate gas exchange, which coincides with receptor activation in the lungs due to increased interstitial fluid. The increased tidal volume of manual bagging corrects this feeling. Adding dead space to the ventilator system may prevent hyperventilation and hypocarbia.[18]

Difficulty with bagging after the ventilator is disconnected indicates a problem with the endotracheal tube or the lung chest-wall complex. Endotracheal tube narrowing secondary to secretion accumulation or tube malposition may be present. Physical examination, chest radiograph, and blood-gas determination should be performed rapidly. A suction catheter may be passed to check for endotracheal tube narrowing or blockage. Tube markings may assist assessment of tube position. Tube replacement may be necessary if the etiology of the problem is not rapidly apparent. Pneumothorax is suggested by endotracheal tube patency and physical examination. In the absence of pneumothorax, a clear endotracheal tube and respiratory distress may correspond with increased oxygen demand or impaired oxygen delivery, as may occur in heart failure, acute pulmonary injury, pulmonary emboli, or aspiration syndromes.

Grum and Chauncey[30] reviewed common ventilator problems. Calculation of static and dynamic compliance may be useful to identify the cause of acute distress and provide trends to look for in patient assessment. Static compliance is obtained by dividing the tidal volume by the static pressure obtained by occluding the exhalation port just before exhalation. Dynamic compliance is obtained by dividing tidal volume by peak inspiratory pressure (Table 4-6).

Although a review of the cellular mechanisms related to oxygen toxicity is beyond the scope of this manuscript, several comments are in order. Potential adverse effects of oxygen exposure where high tensions are involved can be divided into two broad groups: (1) alterations of normal physiology and (2) oxygen-induced tissue damage.[6,27] Physiologic changes involve extrapulmonary effects including suppression of erythropoiesis,

TABLE 4-6 COMMON VENTILATOR DILEMMAS

OBSERVED PROBLEM	INVESTIGATE
Low static and dynamic compliance (high plateau and peak pressure)	Pulmonary edema, consolidation, atelectasis, mainstem bronchus intubation, tension pneumothorax, chest wall constriction
Low dynamic compliance and normal static compliance (increased difference between peak and static pressure = resistance)	Bronchospasm Increased secretions Obstructed inspiratory circuit (check endotracheal tube)
Spontaneous positive end-expiratory pressure (auto-PEEP)	Obstructed expiratory circuit (for example, H_2O in tubing) Insufficient flow rate/expiratory time
Increased respiratory rate	Change in clinical status (for example, desaturation, bronchospasm, secretions, pulmonary embolism, sepsis) Low tidal volume Insufficient flow rate
Low exhaled volumes	Leak from circuit Cuff Leak Insufficient delivery/low flow rate Bronchopleural fistula Inaccurate measurement of exhalation
Increased exhaled volumes ("stacking breaths")	Hypersensitivity of demand valve High minute ventilation Insufficient flow rate Low I:E ratio
No spontaneous breaths	Backup rate too high, causing relative respiratory alkalosis Sedation Central nervous system lesion

Modified from Grum CM, Chauncey JB: *Clin Chest Med* 9:37, 1988.

depression of cardiac output, and systemic vasoconstriction. Physiologic effects in the pulmonary bed include ventilation depression, vasodilation of the pulmonary vasculature, and absorption atelectasis. Absorption atelectasis is usually not a major problem during oxygen administration in the absence of coexisting disease. High inspired oxygen concentrations, however, produce a washout of pulmonary nitrogen, which normally functions as a physiologic alveolar stent. Subsequently, the increased oxygen load in the alveolus is absorbed, leaving the alveolus devoid of gas with a tendency to collapse. Absorption atelectasis can both reduce the vital capacity and increase the shunting of blood through the lung. Surfactant formation is also decreased early after hyperoxic exposure.

In addition to decreased surfactant production, a protein-rich alveolar edema may be formed in the presence of excessive oxygen administration. Alveolar hemorrhage can occur with decreasing neutrophil and capillary endothelial cell counts and an increased monocyte population. Chronic changes associated with oxygen toxicity include increase in type II epithelial cells and surfactant production. These changes are associated with hyaline membrane formation and increased infiltration by fibroblasts.

When volunteers are exposed to 100% oxygen, systemic symptoms including malaise, nausea, and transient paraesthesia may occur. Tolerance in excess of 3 days is unusual. In injured patients, prolonged exposure to 100% oxygen has been associated with increased intrapulmonary shunts, dead space to tidal volume ratios, and lung weights. Radiographs obtained of these patients gave evidence of multilobar consolidation within 40 hours of ventilation with 100% oxygen.[1] At less than 100% oxygen, tolerance is much greater. Normal volunteers can withstand 55% oxygen for 1 week, with minimal discomfort or 35% oxygen for up to a month without symptoms of pulmonary function loss. Unfortunately, most of the data related to oxygen toxicity was not obtained in ventilator-dependent patients.

Ventilator-related barotrauma probably occurs in 3% to 7% of all patients requiring mechanical ventilation, though the reported range is 0.5% to 15% in the adult population.[5] All patients treated with mechanical ventilation are at risk. Factors associated with the development of barotrauma include high airway pressures, frequent positive pressure breaths, pulmonary or systemic infection, ARDS, diffuse pulmonary injury, and hypovolemia. Initial work on the mechanism of pulmonary barotrauma came in the late 1800s. Later studies in various animal models demonstrated that alveolar overinflation with positive-pressure ventilation produced extraalveolar air resulting from alveolar rupture, which tracked along alveoli and pulmonary vascular sheaths to the mediastinum. From this location, air can pass by way of the mediastinal pleura into the pleural space to cause pneumothorax or into other areas to produce subcutaneous emphysema, pneumopericardium, and pneumoretroperitoneum. Additional risk factors in the perioperative patient include thoracic trauma, central venous catheter placement, cardiopulmonary resuscitation, previous thoracotomy, and other surgical procedures. On rare occasions, pulmonary barotrauma may cause the development of tension pneumothorax, tension pneumomediastinum, tension pneumopericardium, and occasionally tension subcutaneous emphysema.

Barotrauma may compromise mechanical ventilation. Tracheal obstruction and intracranial pressure increase may also be associated with massive subcutaneous emphysema, and air embolism is a remote possibility. Common precautions thought to decrease the incidence of pulmonary barotrauma include reduction of the number of mechanical breaths, and careful control of peak inspiratory pressures by use of flow rates, sedation, and muscle relaxants as necessary. Intravascular volumes should be maintained and alternative means of ventilation used as needed. It is important to emphasize, however, that respiratory death should not occur due to avoidance of high PEEP or CPAP levels out of fear for pulmonary barotrauma.

COMMON CARDIOPULMONARY PROBLEMS

Pulmonary Embolism

The initial hemodynamic result of pulmonary embolism is acute reduction in the area of the pulmonary vascular bed. With acute reduction in the patent pulmonary vascular bed, pulmonary artery pressure (PAP) increases and right ventricular work must also increase to compensate. Normal pulmonary vascular reserve is such that 50% of the cross-sectional area must be lost before sustained pulmonary hypertension will be seen at normal levels of cardiac output.

McIntyre and Sasahara[41,42] evaluated angiographic and hemodynamic findings in patients with pulmonary thromboembolism who had no preexisting cardiopulmonary disease. The correlation obtained by these investigators between mean PAP and mean pulmonary vascular obstruction suggested that a PAP of 22 mm Hg corresponded to a 30% obstruction of the pulmonary vascular bed, and a pulmonary artery pressure of 36 mm Hg corresponded with a 50% occlusion. There was no correlation between angiographic findings, cardiac output, or pulmonary artery pressure in patients with chronic cardiopulmonary disease. In some patients with small pulmonary thromboemboli, cardiac index was severely depressed. The combination of pulmonary capillary wedge pressure and PAP was not a reliable indicator of the magnitude of pulmonary embolism in patients with preexisting congestive cardiac failure and superimposed pulmonary thromboembolism.[16]

In addition to the direct effect of vascular occlusion by thromboemboli as a cause of pulmonary hypertension, indirect evidence supports mediator-induced vasoconstriction.[16] For instance, as noted earlier, mean PAP increased to an average of 35 mm Hg when 50% of the pulmonary vascular bed was occluded by emboli, whereas this value increased from an average of 17 to only 23 mm Hg with unilateral pulmonary occlusion in healthy volunteers. Microemboli induced more mediator release, pulmonary permeability changes, and reflex effects than larger obstructing emboli in a variety of animal studies. The clinical relevance of this animal work must be viewed with some skepticism, as pulmonary hypertension created by microemboli may be more amenable to vasodilation and manipulation of mediators than larger, more clinically significant pulmonary emboli. In addition, anesthetic and other drugs given in animal studies may affect the response of the sympathetic nervous system and thus provide misleading information.

A canine study investigated the effects of pulmonary thromboembolism and norepinephrine on the previously described pulmonary pressure and flow characteristics.[21] Multiple parameters, including PAP and cardiac output, were obtained by opening systemic arterial-venous fistulae fitted with variable resistors. Embolization in this study produced significant pulmonary hypertension, with a threefold increase in pulmonary artery pressure and a fourfold increase in calculated pulmonary vascular resistance. When the pulmonary vascular pressure-flow data were plotted, however, these authors noted only a small increase in the overall mean incremental resistance (slope of the curve relating PAP to cardiac output). The increase in incremental resistance was much less than that suggested by the traditionally calculated pulmonary vascular resistance. Instead, there was a marked upward shift in the extrapolated pressure intercept, suggesting that the predominant mechanism of the increase in pulmonary artery pressure in this model was an elevation of the mean pulmonary vascular closing pressure, not a change in vascular resistance.

In a second arm of this study, norepinephrine was administered and the pulmonary artery pressure and cardiac output measurements were repeated. Before and after embolization, norepinephrine caused a significant increase in cardiac output and decreased the traditionally calculated pulmonary vascular resistance. When pulmonary vascular pressure-flow curves were calculated, however, norepinephrine did not in fact alter the slope of the curve (incremental resistance). Thus, the utility of norepinephrine therapy in pulmonary thromboembolism rests on reversal of the shock state by its beneficial pressor effects, whereas its inotropic effects improve right ventricular function. These positive changes are not associated with any pulmonary vascular effects. Any increase in pulmonary artery pressure with norepinephrine therapy is thought to be due to the change in right ventricular outflow.

Hydralazine has also been noted to have a beneficial hemodynamic impact in clinical and canine studies of pulmonary hypertension. Increased cardiac output without a change in PAP suggests that hydralazine has a specific pulmonary vasoactive property.[21] Pulmonary vascular pressure-flow relationships were determined before and after pulmonary embolization and hydralazine therapy. The effect of hydralazine was not to reduce pulmonary vascular resistance, but to induce a parallel downward shift in the pressure-flow curves, again consistent with a decrease in the pulmonary vascular closing pressure rather than reduction in incremental vascular resistance.

Thus an increase in vascular closing pressure, rather than a change in incremental resistance, is the principal mechanism explaining the increase in right ventricular afterload following pulmonary thromboembolism. Treatment intended to reduce right ventricular afterload may act by reduction in closing pressure or incremental resistance or both. These factors must be weighed along with other therapeutic considerations in hemodynamic manipulation designed to augment right ventricular performance after pulmonary thromboembolism.

In patients with pulmonary thromboembolism who have a marked diminution in cardiac output and blood pressure complicating an increase in right ventricular afterload, initial therapy should ensure appropriate right coronary perfusion pressure.[53] Norepinephrine, a drug with inotropic and pressor effects, is an excellent agent for short-term maintenance of hemodynamic stability. If a moderate decrease in cardiac output complicates the increased afterload, dobutamine or possibly isoproterenol may be used to increase right ventricular output. However, these agents may decrease systemic vascular resistance and systemic blood pressure; thus right ventricular coronary perfusion pressure as inferred from arterial pressure, pulmonary artery pressure, and central venous pressure must be carefully monitored. In these critically ill patients, end points of therapy should be guided by invasive hemodynamic monitoring.

In the canine studies reviewed earlier, data suggest that changes in incremental resistance and effective outflow pressure are responsible for the increase in PAP seen with thromboembolism. Thus vasoactive drugs may improve hemodynamics in the pulmonary vascular bed and decrease right ventricular afterload by reduction in either or both of these parameters. Norepinephrine and hydralazine may be effective for this purpose.

Adult Respiratory Distress Syndrome

After nearly two decades of work in support of patients with respiratory failure, recent reviews report mortality statistics ranging between 20% and 60% in patients with ARDS and as much as 90% in patients with both sepsis and ARDS. Supportive measures, including various forms of PEEP and extracorporeal membrane oxygenation, have improved arterial oxygenation, but had no apparent effect on reducing mortality related to this problem. In fact, Montgomery and associates[44] suggest that patients with ARDS do not die from respiratory failure, but rather from other causes. In this report, irreversible respiratory failure was associated with only 16% of deaths in patients with ARDS. Irreversible respiratory failure typically occurred in the setting of ongoing uncontrolled sepsis. Early deaths (defined as less than 72 hours) were generally the result of underlying illness or injury. Deaths occurring longer than 72 hours after trauma or illness culminating in ARDS were related to the sepsis syndrome.[44]

ARDS predisposed patients who survived the presenting illness or injury to lung infection. Possible mechanisms for lung infection with ARDS include secondary infection of necrotic or edematous lung tissue or infection transmitted by lung tissue injured during support of patients with respiratory compromise. ARDS was defined in this setting as a clinical condition comprising (1) PO_2/FIO_2 ratio less than 150 to 200, (2) diffuse radiographic infiltrates on plain chest radiograph involving all lung fields, (3) pulmonary artery wedge pressure less than 18 mm Hg, and (4) no other cause explaining 1 through 3.

In ARDS, one of the inciting events is alteration in permeability of the pulmonary vascular endothelium with development of interstitial and alveolar edema. A variety of mediators induce edematous thickening of alveolar capillary membranes and interstitium, which impairs pulmonary expansion. If this process is allowed to persist and progress, irreversible pulmonary fibrosis may result.

Although one of the defining characteristics of ARDS is diffuse lung injury on an anteroposterior chest radiograph, there does not appear to be homogenous distribution of gas exchange abnormality and mechanical alteration in pulmonary function.[38] Gattinoni and associates[29] demonstrate with CT scans heterogeneity in roentgenographic density changes in lung injury. Patients with ARDS are characterized by areas of normally aerated tissue, as well as areas appearing poorly aerated and consolidated. Recent studies suggest that in patients with severe ARDS, one third to one half of pulmonary tissue participates in tidal gas exchange. Often, there is a striking gravitational distribution of infiltrates, which may be reduced by the administration of PEEP. Areas of consolidation appear more extensive in dependent portions of the lung, and positional changes of the patient may alter this distribution, suggesting that at least a portion of the nonaerated lung may be recruitable.

Using inert gas techniques, Danzker[15] suggested that alteration of pulmonary function occurs in a nonhomogeneous pattern in patients with ARDS. Although the proportion of venous admixture corresponds to nonaerated lung, a significant fraction of lung units appear to have normal ventilation/perfusion ratios despite overall increase in shunt and pulmonary dead space. Evaluation of pressure/volume relationships in lungs of patients with ARDS suggests collapse and reopening of airways and alveoli during the phases of the respiratory cycle. These findings are consistent with changes of surface characteristics of the alveoli secondary to fluid accumulation or depletion of surfactant activity. Higher transpulmonary inflation pressure is required to treat these mechanical changes, which have been tied to the change in compliance characteristics previously reported with ARDS.

As summarized by Marcy and Marini,[38] CT scans, gas exchange assessment, and thoracic mechanics indicate that acute lung injury affects lung function in a nonhomogeneous distribution. For any transpulmonary pressure, there is a decrease in the absolute volume of aerated lung tissue. While some lung units are not aerated due to edema or atelectasis, other lung units are normally aerated and have normal compliance and ventilation/perfusion relationships. Thus the functioning lung in ARDS is not so much stiff as it is small. The mechanical ventilator must apply high pressures to the airway to deliver a tidal volume of smaller size (less than 10 ml/kg) into these small lungs. Higher applied ventilatory pressures place normally compliant alveoli at risk for inappropriate distention or rupture (Figure 4-14).

The dynamic pulmonary compliance curve of a 75-kg man with ARDS looks like that of a normal child.[66] In ARDS, as fibrosis follows edema, the elastic proprieties of pulmonary parenchyma are diminished such that progressively greater pressure is required to achieve inflation with a given tidal volume. Compliance in ARDS is decreased because of lung size primarily and fibrosis secondarily. Studies using animal models suggest that peak airway pressures greater than 40 to 50 cm H_2O irrevocably injure normal alveoli. At pressures greater than 40 cm H_2O there is no significant increase in alveolar inflation, but overdistension of already inflated alveoli may occur. It is common to think of the less compliant lung as stiff because increased alveolar and interstitial fluid makes inflation more difficult. It is more appropriate to recognize that ARDS represents a reduction in the effective functioning alveolar mass and consider the diseased lung as small rather than stiff.

The conventional approach to mechanical ventilation in the adult population is volume regulated. Delivery of a predetermined tidal volume is emphasized, and each breath is delivered in full, regardless of the airway pressure required to provide it. As pulmonary compliance is reduced, increased airway pressure results, which is applied directly to the reduced healthy alveolar mass. As previously noted, with airway pressure exceeding 40 cm H_2O, alveolar damage may occur. Therefore tidal volume should be adjusted to achieve inflation but to avoid overdistension of the remaining functioning alveolar units.

Care of the patient with ARDS frequently entails a transition from volume to pressure regulated ventilation. With the latter mode of ventilatory support, gas flows until a given pressure is reached or until a fixed time interval has elapsed in each respiratory cycle. Tidal volume generated is a variable reflecting underlying pulmonary compliance, and it increases as lung injury resolves.

The first priority in the management of the patient with ARDS must be reversal of hypoxemia. Initially, high fractions of inspired oxygen (greater than 50%) may be needed to maintain an acceptable level of arterial oxygen tension. When possible, inspired oxygen fraction should be reduced to less than 40% to reduce the risk of oxygen toxicity and absorption-driven atelectasis. The most effective supportive therapy for ARDS is continuous positive airway pressure or PEEP. This therapy improves reduced functional residual capacity and reverses hypoxemia associated with ARDS. Relief of hypoxemia allows downward titration of the inspired oxygen fraction to non-toxic levels.

The optimum use of PEEP remains controversial. In general, PEEP is increased gradually, with measurements made to identify the deleterious effects on cardiac output, oxygen transport, and/or organ function. Hemodynamic monitoring and augmentation of cardiac output with volume infusion or inotropic agents have been advocated to support the patient requiring increased levels of PEEP therapy. Initial titration of PEEP may occur in increments of 2 to 3 cm H_2O with frequent reassessment of arterial oxygen tension, intrapulmonary shunt fraction, and oxygen transport. A therapeutic end point is the level of PEEP that allows reduction of the fraction of inspired oxygen to a non-toxic level while adequate arterial oxygen tension and oxygen transport are sustained. Reduction in cardiac output by positive pressure ventilation and PEEP therapy may be effectively reversed by volume expansion. If adequate hemodynamic performance is obtained, judicious diuresis may decrease lung water and improve oxygenation. Excessive diuresis, however, when coupled with positive pressure ventilation and PEEP, may reduce preload, cardiac performance, and oxygen transport.

It is appropriate to consider a relatively new ventilatory mode such as inverse ratio ventilation only when conventional ventilatory modes are unable to provide adequate oxygenation without the administration of excessive amounts of PEEP, toxic levels of inspired oxygen, or high airway pressures. Therapies such as switching to pressure-limited ventilation with prolongation of the inspiratory to expiratory time (I:E) ratio must be seen as a continuum aimed at raising the mean airway pressure to the minimum effective level needed to optimize oxygenation and gas exchange. Gas exchange, hemodynamics, minute ventilation, and airway pressure must be frequently monitored when increased airway pressure ventilation is instituted. Routine use of pulmonary artery catheters is advocated.

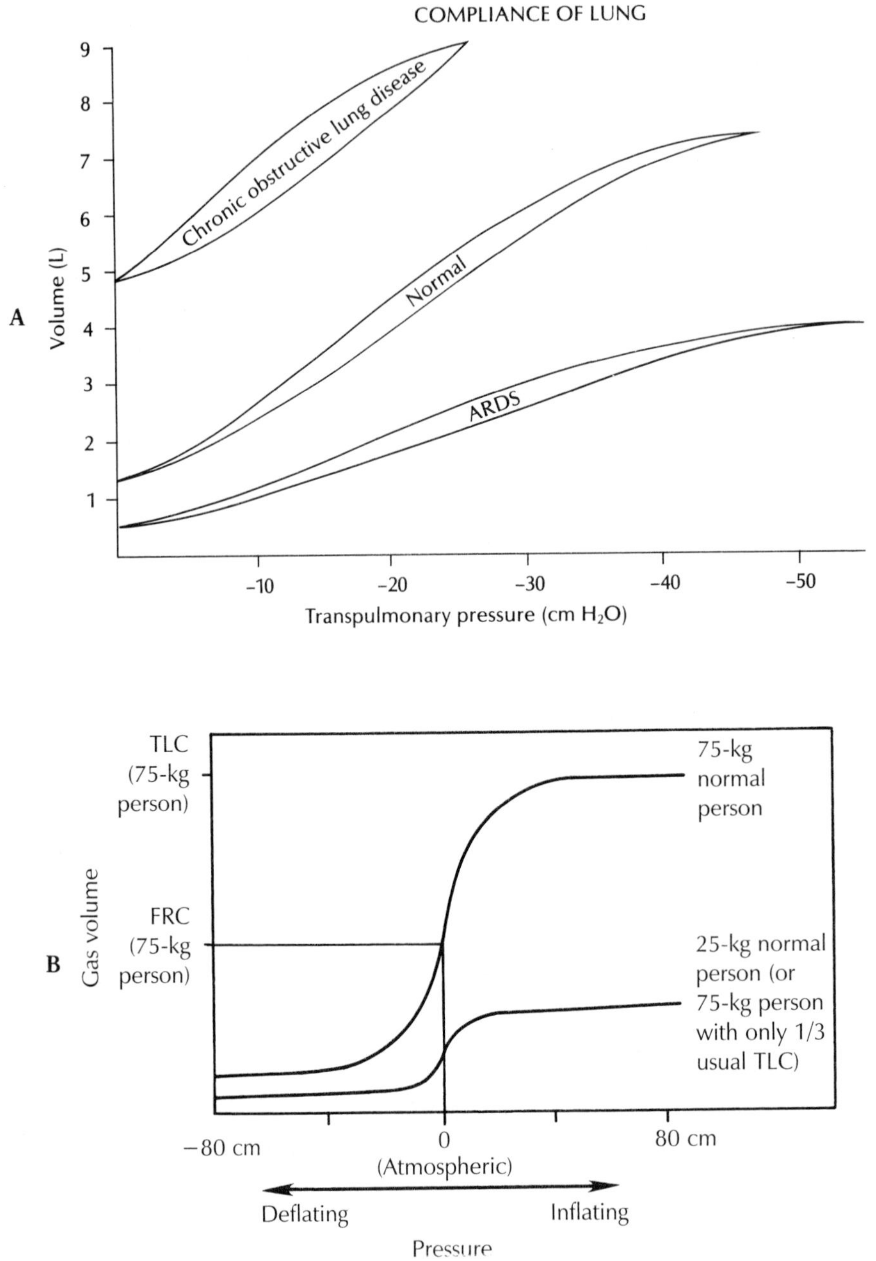

FIGURE 4-14 **A,** The three curves show the relation between transpulmonary pressure *(horizontal axis)* and change in lung volume *(vertical axis)*. The pressure per unit of volume change is higher during inspiration than during expiration. The S shape of the curves results because the range of linear elasticity of the lungs is limited. At low volumes extra pressure is needed to open closed alveoli; at high volumes the fibrous network of the lung limits further expansion. Patients with chronic obstructive pulmonary disease (COPD) have lungs with poor elastic recoil and increased end-expiratory volume. Patients with acute respiratory distress syndrome (ARDS) have lungs that have lowered end-expiratory volume. **B,** Volume/pressure (compliance) relationships. *TLC,* Total lung capacity; *FRC,* functional residual capacity. (Redrawn from Shapiro MB, Bartlett RH: *Arch Surg* 127:485, 1992.)

Volume-cycled ventilation is used by some workers to prolong the inspiratory to expiratory time ratio as initial therapy for hypoxemia in ARDS when conventional ventilation fails.[38] Pressure-controlled ventilation is an alternative method offering tighter control of airway pressure and possibly reducing the sedation required by patients. Use of pressure rather than volume control methods of ventilation, however, requires careful attention to minute ventilation to avoid progressive respiratory acidosis. As signs of improving oxygen exchange appear, the inspiratory time is reduced by decreasing the length of the inspiratory phase or changing the machine-set I:E ratio. This process continues as tolerated until conventional ventilation may be resumed.

Optimum ventilation in ARDS must be tailored to the needs of each patient. Evidence exists to support an approach preventing peak alveolar pressure from exceeding 35 to 40 cm H_2O and maintaining end-expiratory alveolar pressures above 7 to 10 cm H_2O. Within these limits, tidal volume, respiratory frequency, and inspiratory duration may be adjusted to obtain appropriate levels of ventilation and oxygen transport. Although the use of new ventilatory modes such as inverse ratio ventilation is attractive in patients with ARDS, no controlled clinical evaluation has been made to justify this therapy. Until additional clinical experience accrues, these methods must be considered unproven and applied cautiously with sensitivity to their potential benefits and hazards.

REFERENCES

1 Barber RE, Lee J, Hamilton WK: Oxygen toxicity in man, *N Engl J Med* 283:1478, 1970

2 Bove AA, Santamore WP: Ventricular interdependence, *Prog Cardiovasc Dis* 23:365, 1981.

3 Boysen PG: Preoperative pulmonary function testing. In Civetta JM, Taylor RW, Kirby RR, editors: *Critical care,* ed 2, Philadelphia, 1992, JB Lippincott.

4 Boysen PG, Block AJ, Olsen GN et al: Prospective evaluation for pneumonectomy using the 99m technician quantitative perfusion lung scan, *Chest* 72:422, 1977.

5 Brown DL, Kirby RR: Pulmonary barotrauma. In Civetta JM, Taylor RW, Kirby RR, editors: *Critical care,* ed 2, Philadelphia, 1992, JB Lippincott.

6 Bryan CL, Jenkinson SG: Oxygen toxicity, *Clin Chest Med* 9:141, 1988.

7 Buda AJ, Pinsky MR, Ingels NB et al: Effect of intrathoracic pressure on left ventricular performance, *N Engl J Med* 301:453, 1979.

8 Carlon GC, Howland WS, Ray C et al: Clinical experience with high frequency jet ventilation: a prospective randomized evaluation, *Chest* 84:551, 1983.

9 Carlon GC, Kahn RC, Howland WS et al: Clinical experience with high frequency jet ventilation, *Crit Care Med* 9:1, 1991.

10 Cassidy SS, Eschenbacher WL, Robertson CH et al: Cardiovascular effects of positive-pressure ventilation in normal subjects, *J Appl Physiol* 447:453, 1979.

11 Cassidy SS, Eschenbacher WL, Johnson RL et al: Reflex cardiovascular depression during unilateral lung hyper-inflation in the dog, *J Clin Invest* 64:620, 1979.

12 Celli BR, Rodriquez KS, Snider GL: A controlled trial of intermittent positive pressure breathing: incentive spirometry and deep breathing exercises in preventing pulmonary complications after abdominal surgery, *Am Rev Respir Dis* 130:12, 1984.

13 Cournand A, Motley HL, Werko L et al: Physiological studies of the effects of intermittent positive pressure breathing on cardiac output in man, *Am J Physiol* 152:162, 1948.

14 Craig DB, Wahba WM, Don HF et al: "Closing volume" in its relationship to gas exchange in seated and supine positions, *J Appl Physiol* 31:717, 1971.

15 Danzker D: Gas exchange in the adult respiratory distress syndrome, *Clin Chest Med* 3:57, 1982.

16 Dehring DJ, Arens JF: Pulmonary thromboembolism: disease recognition and patient management, *Anesthesiology* 73:146, 1990.

17 Demling R, Riessen R: Pulmonary dysfunction after cerebral injury, *Crit Care Med* 18:768, 1990.

18 Demling RH, Wilson RF: *Decision making in surgical critical care,* Philadelphia, 1988, BC Decker.

19 Downs JB, Klein EF Jr, Desautels D et al: Intermittent mandatory ventilation: a new approach to weaning patients from mechanical ventilators, *Chest* 64:331, 1973.

20 Drazen JM, Kamm RD, Slutsky AS: High frequency ventilation, *Physiol Rev* 64:505, 1984.

21 Ducas J, Prewitt RM: Pathophysiology and therapy of right ventricular dysfunction due to pulmonary embolism. In Brest AN, Fisk RL, editors: *Cardiovascular clinics: the right heart,* Philadelphia, 1987, FA Davis.

22 Dunham B, Grindlinger G, Utsunomiya T et al: Role of prostaglandins in positive end-expiratory pressure-induced negative inotropism, *Am J Physiol* 241:H783, 1981.

23 Elliot CG, Zimmerman GA, Clemmer TD: Complications of pulmonary artery catheterization in the care of critically ill patients: a prospective study, *Chest* 76:647, 1979.

24 Ferlinz J: Right ventricular function in adult cardiovascular disease, *Prog Cardiovasc Dis* 25:226, 1982.

25 Fiastro JF, Habib MP, Shon BY et al: Comparison of standard weaning parameters and the mechanical work of breathing in mechanically ventilated patients, *Chest* 94:232, 1988.

26 Field S, Kelly SM, Macklem PT: The oxygen cost of breathing in patients with cardiorespiratory disease, *Am Rev Respir Dis* 126:9, 1982.

27 Fisher AB: Oxygen therapy: side effects and toxicity, *Am Rev Respir Dis* 122:61, 1980.

28 Gal TJ: Pulmonary mechanics in normal subjects following endotracheal intubation, *Anesthesiology* 52:27, 1980.

29 Gattinoni L, Pesenti A, Avalli L et al: Relationships between lung computed tomographic density, gas exchange, and PEEP in acute respiratory failure, *Anesthesiology* 69:824, 1988.

30 Grum CM, Chauncey JB: Conventional mechanical ventilation, *Clin Chest Med* 9:37, 1988.

31 Guyton AC, Lindsey AW, Gilluly JJ: The limits of right ventricular compensation following acute increases in pulmonary circulatory resistance, *Circ Res* 2:326, 1954.

32 Hewlett AM, Platt AS, Terry VG: Mandatory minute volume, *Anesthesia* 32:163, 1977.

33 Hillman KM, Barber JD: Asynchronous independent lung ventilation, *Crit Care Med* 8:390, 1980.

34 Jardin F, Farcot J, Boisante L et al: Influence of positive end-expiratory pressure on left ventricular performance, *N Engl J Med* 304:387, 1981.

35 Kaneko K, Milic-Emili J, Dolovich MB et al: Regional distribution of ventilation and perfusion as a function of body position, *J Appl Physiol* 21:767, 1966.

36 Kreit JW, Eschenbacher WL: The physiology of spontaneous and mechanical ventilation, *Clin Chest Med* 9:11, 1988.

37 MacIntyre NR: New forms of mechanical ventilation in the adult, *Clin Chest Med* 9:47, 1988.
38 Marcy TW, Marini JJ: Inverse ratio ventilation in ARDS: rationale and implementation, *Chest* 100:494, 1991.
39 Marini JJ, Capps JS, Culver BH: The inspiratory work of breathing during assisted mechanical ventilation, *Chest* 87:612, 1985.
40 Matthay RA, Biondi JW, Schulman DS et al: Acute right heart failure—pathogenesis, diagnosis, and therapy, *Appl Cardiopulmonary Pathophysiol* 2:59, 1988.
41 McIntyre KM, Sasahara AA: Determinants of right ventricular function and hemodynamics after pulmonary embolism, *Chest* 65:534, 1974.
42 McIntyre KM, Sasahara AA: The hemodynamic response to pulmonary embolism in patients without prior cardiopulmonary disease, *Am J Cardiol* 28:288, 1971.
43 Mitchell RA, Berger AJ: Neural regulation of respiration, *Am Rev Respir Dis* 11:206, 1975.
44 Montgomery AB, Stager MA, Carrico CJ et al: Causes of mortality in patients with the adult respiratory distress syndrome, *Am Rev Respir Dis* 132:485, 1985.
45 Moreno F, Lyons HA: Effect of body posture on lung volumes, *J Appl Physiol* 16:27, 1961.
46 Morganroth ML, Morganroth JL, Nett LM et al: Criteria for weaning from prolonged mechanical ventilation, *Arch Intern Med* 144:1012, 1984.
47 Narins RG, Emmett M: Simple and mixed acid-base disorders: a practical approach, *Medicine* (Baltimore) 59:161, 1980.
48 Nunn JF: *Applied respiratory physiology,* ed 3, London, 1987, Butterworth.
49 Otto CW: Respiratory morbidity and mortality, *Int Anesthesiol Clin* 18:85, 1980.
50 Packer M: Vasodilator therapy for primary pulmonary hypertension, *Ann Intern Med* 103:258, 1985.
51 Pinsky MR, Marquez J, Martin D et al: Ventricular assist by cardiac cycle specific increases in intrathoracic pressure, *Chest* 91:709, 1987.
52 Potkin RT, Hudson LD, Weaver LV et al: Effect of positive end-expiratory pressure on right and left ventricular function in patients with the adult respiratory distress syndrome, *Am Rev Respir Dis* 135:307, 1987.
53 Prewitt RM: Hemodynamic management in pulmonary embolism and acute hypoxemic respiratory failure, *Crit Care Med* 18:S61, 1990.
54 Prewitt RM, Matthay MA, Ghignone M: Hemodynamic management in the adult respiratory distress syndrome, *Clin Chest Med* 4:251, 1983.
55 Ravenscroft RJ: Simple mandatory minute volume, *Anesthesia* 33:246, 1978.
56 Razma E, Jubran A: Pulmonary complications in the perioperative period, *Probl Crit Care* 5:586, 1991.
57 Rehder K, Sessler AD, Marsh HM: General anesthesia and the lung, *Am Rev Respir Dis* 112:541, 1975.

58 Robotham JL: Cardiovascular disturbances in chronic respiratory insufficiency, *Am J Cardiol* 47:941, 1981.
59 Roussos C, Macklen PT: The respiratory muscles, *N Engl J Med* 307:786, 1982.
60 Rubin LJ: Cardiovascular effects of vasodilator therapy for pulmonary artery hypertension, *Clin Chest Med* 4:309, 1983.
61 Santamore WP, Bove AA, Heckman JL: Cardiovascular changes from expiration to inspiration during IPPV, *Am J Physiol* 245:H307, 1983.
62 Sarnoff SJ, Berglund E: Ventricular function. I. Starling's law of the heart studied by means of simultaneous right and left ventricular function curves in the dog, *Circulation* 9:706, 1954.
63 Sassoon CSH: Positive pressure ventilation: alternate modes, *Chest* 100:1421, 1991.
64 Scharf SM, Brown R, Saunders N et al: Hemodynamic effects of positive-pressure inflation, *J Appl Physiol* 49:124, 1980.
65 Schuster DP: A physiologic approach to initiating, maintaining and withdrawing mechanical ventilatory support during acute respiratory failure, *Am J Med* 88:268, 1990.
66 Shapiro MB, Bartlett RH: Pulmonary compliance and mechanical ventilation, *Arch Surg* 127:485, 1992.
67 Sherter CB, Jabbour SM, Kovnat DM et al: Prolonged rate of decay of arterial PO_2 following oxygen breathing in chronic airways obstruction, *Chest* 67:259, 1975.
68 Sibbald WJ, Driedger AA, Myers ML et al: Biventricular function in the adult respiratory distress syndrome: hemodynamic and radionuclide assessment, with special emphasis on right ventricular function, *Chest* 84:126, 1983.
69 Sylvester JT, Goldberg HS, Permutt S: The role of the vasculature in the regulation of cardiac output, *Clin Chest Med* 4:111, 1983.
70 Tisi GM: Preoperative evaluation of pulmonary function, *Am Rev Respir Dis* 119:293, 1979.
71 Tobin MJ, Yang KL: A prospective study of indices predicting the outcome of trials of weaning from mechanical ventilation, *N Engl J Med* 324:1445, 1991.
72 Vlahakes GJ, Turley K, Hoffman JI: The pathophysiology of failure in acute right ventricular hypertension: hemodynamic and biochemical correlations, *Circulation* 63:87, 1981.
73 Weisman IM, Rinaldo JE, Rogers RM et al: Intermittent mandatory ventilation, *Am Rev Respir Dis* 127:641, 1983.
74 West JB: *Ventilation/blood flow and gas exchange,* Oxford, 1970, Blackwell.
75 West JB, Dollery CT, Naimark A: Distribution of bloodflow in isolated lung: relation to vascular and alveolar pressures, *J Appl Physiol* 19:713, 1964.
76 Wiedemann HP, Matthay RA: Acute right heart failure, *Crit Care Clin* 1:631, 1985.
77 Whipp BJ: Ventilatory control during exercise in humans, *Annu Rev Physiol* 45:393, 1983.
78 Wilson RF: Pulmonary physiology. In *Critical care manual: applied physiology and principles of therapy,* Philadelphia, 1992, FA Davis.

CHAPTER

5

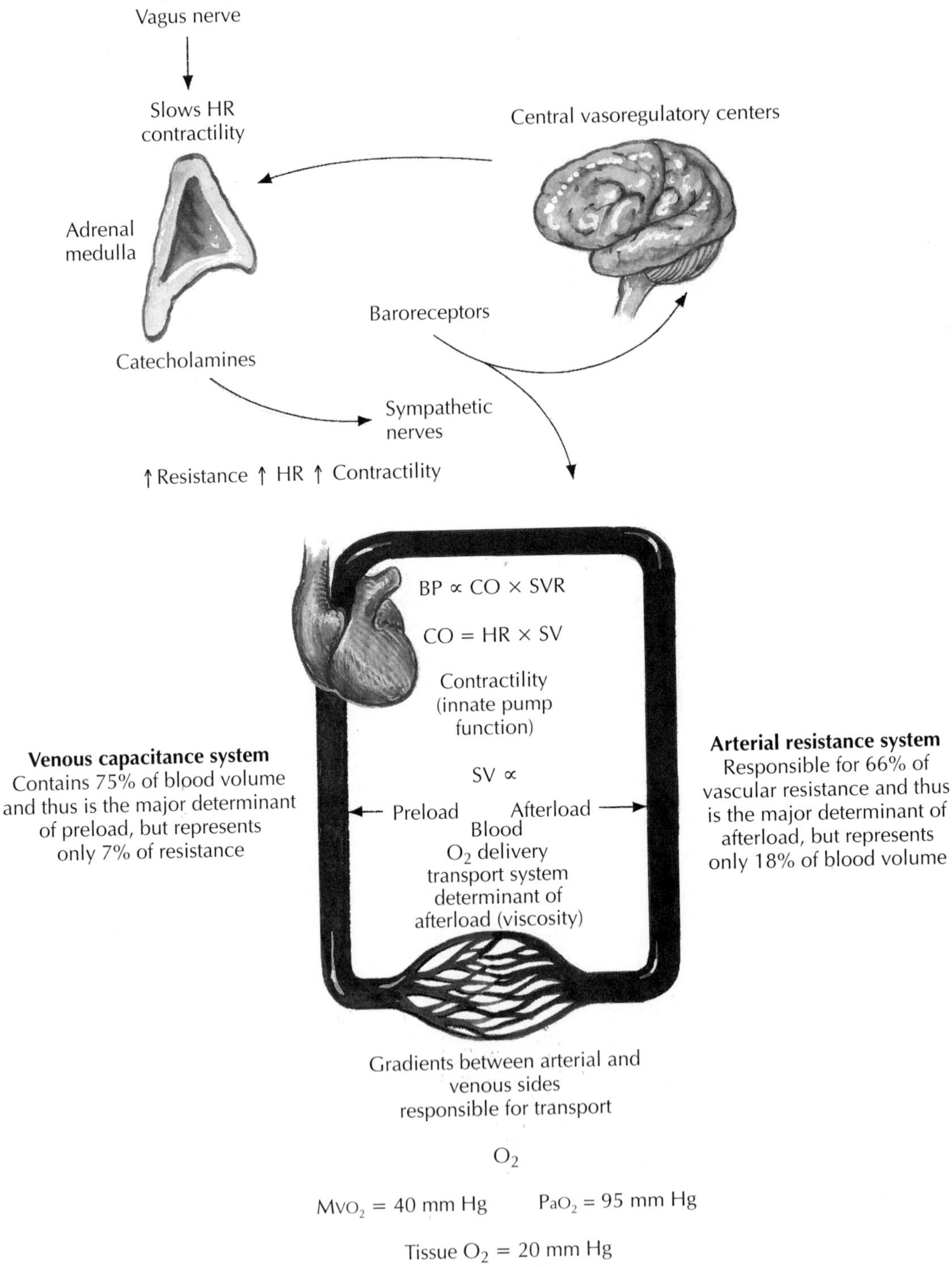

Vagus nerve
Slows HR
contractility
Central vasoregulatory centers
Adrenal
medulla
Baroreceptors
Catecholamines
Sympathetic
nerves
↑ Resistance ↑ HR ↑ Contractility
BP ∝ CO × SVR
CO = HR × SV
Contractility
(innate pump
function)
SV ∝
Preload
Afterload
Blood
O2 delivery
transport system
determinant of
afterload (viscosity)
Venous capacitance system
Contains 75% of blood volume
and thus is the major determinant
of preload, but represents
only 7% of resistance
Arterial resistance system
Responsible for 66% of
vascular resistance and thus
is the major determinant of
afterload, but represents
only 18% of blood volume
Gradients between arterial and
venous sides
responsible for transport
O2
MvO2 = 40 mm Hg
PaO2 = 95 mm Hg
Tissue O2 = 20 mm Hg

CIRCULATION AND SHOCK

William G. Cioffi Jr. • Richard L. Gamelli

> "Shock: manifestation of the rude unhinging of the machinery of life."
>
> Gross, 1872

Evaluation of a patient in shock involves a series of sequential analyses to determine the cause and to plan a rational treatment protocol. Although many conditions can result in shock, MacLean's definition of shock, "inadequate blood flow to vital organs or the inability of the body cell mass to metabolize nutrients normally,"[83] aptly describes the common endpoint of inadequate perfusion.

Decreased blood pressure is the most useful clinical marker, providing evidence of decreased perfusion of vital organs. However, blood pressure and blood flow may not be directly correlated. In 1917 Archibald and McLean stated, "While low blood pressure is one of the most constant signs of shock, it is not the essential thing, let alone the cause of it."[5] Thus although most patients in shock are hypotensive, not all hypotensive patients are in shock.

Regional perfusion (i.e., the volume flow of blood to a specific organ) depends not only on blood pressure but also on the caliber of the resistance vessels. A decrease in the vessels' size, causing increased resistance and subsequently increased blood pressure, may actually decrease flow, or perfusion. To evaluate a patient suspected of being in shock and to treat that patient appropriately, the physician must first thoroughly understand basic cardiovascular dynamics.

CIRCULATION DYNAMICS

The cardiovascular system is a transport system in which a pump (the heart) propels a medium (blood) in a closed circuit through elastic tubes (vessels). The system perfuses the cells of each organ system, providing oxygen and nutrients and removing the end products of cellular metabolism. The critical functions of the cardiovascular system are maintaining the constancy of the internal milieu and providing a primary defense against pathogenic organisms. The system's ability to perform these tasks is directly related to the integrity of each of many parts, which must function in a coordinated and integrated fashion. Complex control mechanisms regulate the activities and integrate the functions of each component of the circulatory system.

Cardiac Output

Preload

The heart is capable of changing its output over an extremely wide range. Resting cardiac output, approximately 5 L/min, can be increased up to five times by increasing the stroke volume or heart rate. Stroke volume can be increased by increasing preload or by altering the contractile state of the myocardium. *Preload* refers to the ventricular end-diastolic volume, which is related to the stretch and, ultimately, tension placed on myocardial fibers before contraction. *Contractility* is the inherent capacity of the myocardium to function as a pump. While studying cardiac muscle kinetics in isolated muscle preparations, Otto Frank[48] and Ernest Starling[136] advanced the concepts of preload and contractility as they relate to myocardial performance. In describing preload Starling stated that "the energy of contraction is proportional to the initial length of the cardiac muscle fiber."[58] Increasing the length of individual fibers before contraction (i.e., increasing preload) increases the resting tension, resulting in an increased velocity of contraction for those fibers. Increasing the length of individual muscle fibers before contraction allows the fibers to contract at a faster velocity until they shorten to the same specific end contraction length, assuming other variables to be constant. Increasing precontraction length yields an increased distance of contraction. Thus when precontraction stretch is greater (i.e., augmented preload), contraction is greater. These changes occur without altering the inherent contractile properties or contractility of the muscle. Figure 5-1 contains both length-tension curves and force-velocity curves for various fiber lengths (i.e., preloads). The maximum velocity of contraction (V_{max}) at which fibers may shorten, or contractility, was not altered by precontraction stretch in these preparations.

Sarnoff and Mitchell[112,114] expanded Starling's theory and introduced the concept of ventricular function curves. In an intact normal ventricle, the volume of blood that fills the ventricle during diastole determines the initial length of the muscle fibers before contraction. Increasing preload by volume loading increases stroke volume at the expense of increased cardiac work. The increase in stroke volume can be explained by extending individual cardiac fiber physiology to the intact ventricle. A greater end-diastolic ventricular volume results in a greater stretch of muscle fibers that contract to their

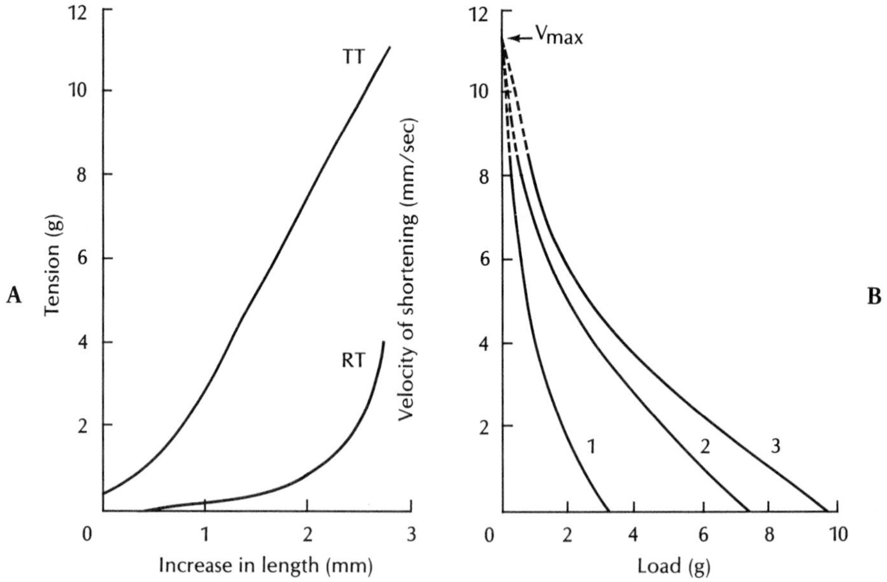

FIGURE 5-1 Length-tension velocity of shortening relationships in isolated papillary muscle of the cat heart. **A,** Under isometric conditions both resting tension *(RT)* and total developed tension *(TT)* increase with increasing muscle length. **B,** Force-velocity (or tension-velocity) curves for three different initial muscle lengths *(1, 2,* and *3).* Velocity of shortening of contractile elements falls as tension (load) increases in all three instances. Load, P_0, at which no shortening occurs (i.e., point where curves intercept abscissa, indicating velocity equals 0) becomes greater as initial length is increased, but maximum velocity (V_{max}), determined by extrapolating curves to intercept ordinate (load = 0), is virtually the same for all three initial lengths. (Redrawn from Sonnenblick EH: *Fed Proc* 21:975, 1962.)

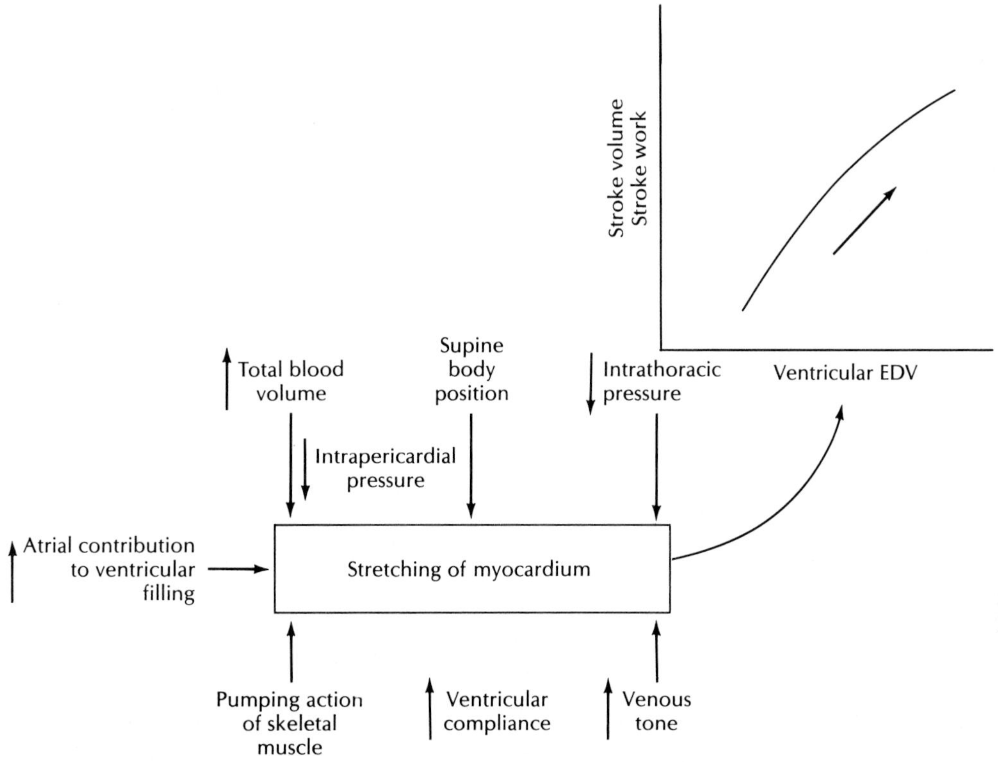

FIGURE 5-2 Relationship between ventricular end-diastolic volume *(EDV)* and ventricular performance (Frank-Starling curve), with a summary of the major factors affecting EDV. (Modified from Braunwald E, Ross S, Sonnenblick EH: *Mechanisms of contraction of the normal and failing heart,* Boston, 1967, Little, Brown.)

initial length, yielding an ejection of the extra blood (Figure 5-2).

A point often debated in the literature is whether at high end-diastolic volumes, preload and cardiac output become inversely correlated (i.e., decreasing myocardial performance despite increasing preload). Theoretically, the contractile elements of individual cardiac muscle fibers may become overstretched, resulting in poor interdigitation and decreased function. However, in an intact ventricle this does not appear to occur to any significant extent.[92] More likely, increasing diastolic volume, causing increased diastolic pressure, results in subendocardial ischemia, which then impairs function.

Afterload

Another important determinant of cardiac output is the resistance the ventricle must overcome during isovolumetric contraction to open the aortic valve and begin ejection of blood. This force is called *aortic impedance,* or *afterload.* In an intact ventricle, aortic impedance is governed by factors that determine the pressure/flow relationship in the aorta, such as the compliance of the aorta and the inertia and viscosity of the blood, as well as by mechanical factors, such as the size of the valve orifice. The inertia of the blood depends on the force at which it is expelled and the resistance of the vascular system.

Clinically, systemic vascular resistance (SVR) is used to assess afterload. In individual muscle preparations, increases in afterload decrease the velocity of contraction (Figure 5-3). In an intact heart, increasing afterload increases the resistance the ventricle must overcome to begin ejection; ejection velocity also decreases. Because systolic time is governed by the electromechanical properties of the muscle and is relatively constant, increased afterload results in less time for actual ejection. Acute increases in afterload decrease stroke volume. However, this decrease in stroke volume yields an increase in preload secondary to the unejected blood. Augmentation in preload then restores the stroke volume to normal. This occurs at the expense of increased work and oxygen (O_2) consumption. This feedback mechanism has limits, and eventually increases in afterload effect a decrease in stroke volume while still increasing ventricular work and O_2 consumption. Conversely, a decrease in afterload allows the ventricle to eject more blood while not in-

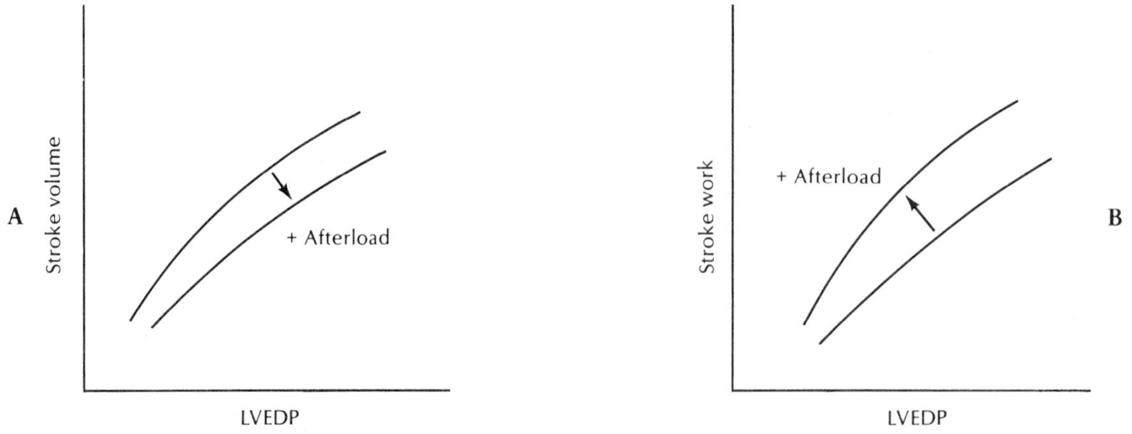

FIGURE 5-3 In the intact ventricle, with no increase in contractile state, elevation of blood pressure would tend to diminish stroke volume relative to left ventricular end-diastolic pressure *(LVEDP)* (**A**), but stroke work and power would be augmented (**B**).

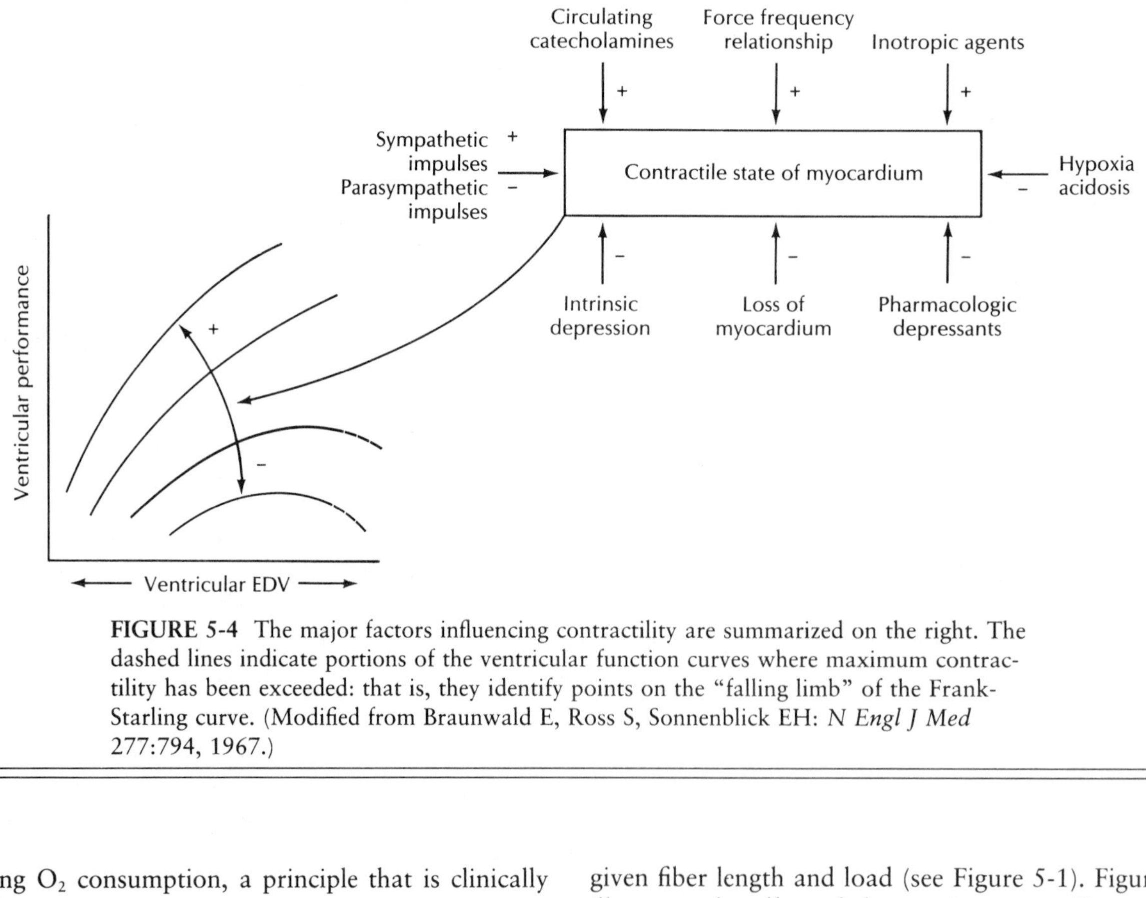

FIGURE 5-4 The major factors influencing contractility are summarized on the right. The dashed lines indicate portions of the ventricular function curves where maximum contractility has been exceeded: that is, they identify points on the "falling limb" of the Frank-Starling curve. (Modified from Braunwald E, Ross S, Sonnenblick EH: *N Engl J Med* 277:794, 1967.)

creasing O_2 consumption, a principle that is clinically useful.

Contractility

Because there is no precise, workable definition of contractility, the concept is best depicted by ventricular function curves. In general, contractility is the maximum velocity that contractile elements can shorten for any given fiber length and load (see Figure 5-1). Figure 5-4 illustrates the effect of changes in contractility on ventricular function. An increase in contractility shifts the function curve upward and to the left, resulting in increased cardiac performance at the same preload. Alterations in preload and contractility increase cardiac output at the expense of increasing cardiac work and O_2 consumption. Faster heart rates increase cardiac output not only by increasing ejections per minute, but also by altering contractility by increasing the intracellular calcium flux between the cytosol and sarcoplasmic reticulum.[16]

Autonomic Innervation

Autonomic innervation by the sympathetic and parasympathetic nervous systems partially regulates cardiac function by effecting either positive or negative chronotropic or inotropic activity. Parasympathetic intervention by the vagus nerve is mediated by the neurotransmitter acetylcholine. The right vagus sends fibers to the right atrium and the SA node and the left vagus to the AV node. The right vagus decreases the SA node pacemaker rate and thus decreases the heart rate. The left vagus acts to retard AV nodal conduction and increases the refractory period of the AV node but has little effect on the ventricular myocardium. Atropine blocks the cardiac vagal effects. Sympathetic control of the heart is mediated by the adrenal glands, which secrete catecholamines into the circulation, and by the cardiac nerves, which originate from the upper thoracic and lower cervical sympathetic chains. The sympathetic system, with its catecholamine neurotransmitters, acts through a series of alpha- and beta-receptors. The heart contains specific beta-receptors, designated beta$_1$, which are also found in the liver. Stimulation of cardiac beta-receptors by catecholamines increases heart rate, AV nodal conduction velocity, and myocardial contractility, actions that increase cardiac output. The influence of the autonomic system is a balance of the parasympathetic and sympathetic tone, and at various times one may predominate over the other.

Energetics

The energy the heart requires for its mechanical work comes primarily from oxidative decomposition of nutrients. The organ has a limited capacity for anaerobic metabolism. At rest the heart accounts for approximately 10% of the body's basal O_2 consumption, which may be increased up to fourfold during strenuous exercise. The percentage of delivered oxygen extracted by the heart is greater than that of any other organ system; approximately 75% of the oxygen delivered via the coronary circulation is extracted.[110] The efficiency of the heart, or the fraction of total energy expenditure that is converted to mechanical work, depends on prevailing conditions and varies between 15% and 40%.[19] The heart is considerably less efficient when working against high pressure or afterload than when ejecting against low pressure or afterload.

Cardiac muscle consumes a different mix of nutrients than skeletal muscle, using equal quantities of fatty acids, glucose, and lactate as energy substrates in the nonexercising state. The proportions of the individual substrates consumed are primarily determined by their supply. Extreme exercise results in a shift of substrate usage; free fatty acid and glucose usage decreases by 30%, and lactate usage doubles.[69]

Because the heart is extremely adaptable in its substrate usage, the chief danger of coronary insufficiency lies not in substrate shortage but rather in oxygen insufficiency. The heart's oxygen requirements depend on four variables: intramyocardial wall tension, heart rate, myocardial contractility, and afterload. Intramyocardial wall tension is directly proportional to intraventricular pressure, which is related to the radius of the ventricle and thus volume, or preload. Laplace's law describes this relationship: $T = PR/2h$, where T is tension, P is pressure, R is radius, and h is wall thickness. Thus the greater the preload, the more dilated the ventricle and the higher the tension. The O_2 consumption of the heart is not directly related to the mechanical work the heart performs; rather, it is directly related to the pressure developed by the ventricle and heart rate.[67,113] Drugs that affect the rate of left ventricular pressure development (i.e., inotropes) greatly increase O_2 consumption.[131] Oxygen consumption is approximately proportional to the square root of the heart rate.[116] When cardiac output is increased by only increasing stroke volume (through changes in preload, not through changes in contractility) while maintaining a constant heart rate, myocardial O_2 consumption is only slightly increased.

BLOOD

In an average adult, blood accounts for approximately 6% to 8% of total body weight, or a volume of 4 to 6 L. The red cell mass, which accounts for 40% to 45% of the blood volume, is responsible for the most critical function of blood—O_2 delivery. Oxygen transport to tissues depends primarily on four factors: hemoglobin (Hb) concentration, O_2 saturation of arterial Hb (SaO_2), cardiac output, and the affinity of Hb for O_2. The Hb content of blood is usually about 15 g/dl. The amount of O_2 bound to Hb and the amount dissolved in plasma determine the arterial O_2 content. The quantity of bound O_2 is determined by the following equation:

$$HbO_2 = Hb \times 1.36 \times SaO_2$$

where 1.36 is the mean volume of O_2 that can be bound to 1 g of Hb when SaO_2 equals 1.0. The amount of dissolved O_2 in plasma is defined as:

$$DO_2 = PaO_2 \times 0.003$$

where PaO_2 is the arterial partial pressure of O_2 and 0.003 is the solubility constant of O_2 in plasma.

Normally, Hb is 15 g/dl, SaO_2 is 97%, and PaO_2 = 80. Thus the arterial O_2 content (CaO_2) is:

$$(15 \times 1.36 \times 0.97) + (80 \times 0.003) = HbO_2 + DO_2$$
$$= 20 \text{ ml } O_2/\text{dl}$$

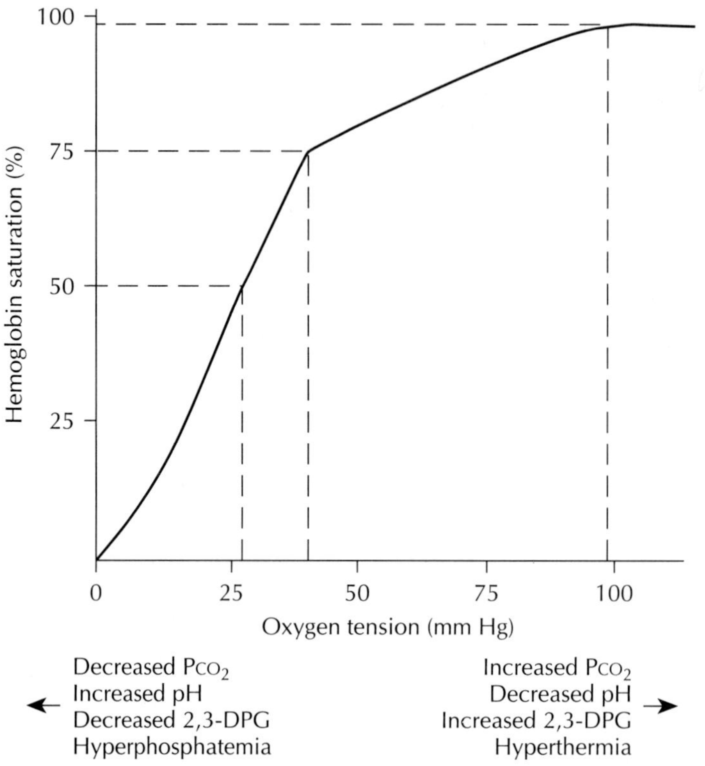

FIGURE 5-5 Important points on the curve are PO_2 at half saturation (26 mm Hg), 75% saturation (40 mm Hg), and 97% saturation (99 mm Hg). The heavy line represents the normal working range between arterial and mixed venous blood. Situations resulting in shifts of the curve are also illustrated.

At an average cardiac output of 5 L/min, O_2 delivery, or CaO_2, is 1000 ml/min. Because normal resting O_2 consumption is only 250 ml/min, an excess of 750 ml/min of O_2 is supplied to the tissues. Thus the venous O_2 content (CvO_2) is 15 ml O_2/dl, and a normal arterial venous O_2 difference is 5.

The affinity of Hb for O_2 is determined by such things as pH, temperature, and the partial pressure of O_2 (PO_2) and carbon dioxide (PCO_2). The Hb molecule is a tetramer capable of carrying four molecules of oxygen. The affinity of Hb for O_2 increases with each successive O_2 molecule bound. Thus a fully saturated Hb molecule binds O_2 tighter and easier than does Hb bound with two O_2 molecules. This arrangement explains why the binding of O_2 to Hb is not a linear relationship and why the oxyhemoglobin dissociation curve is sigmoid (Figure 5-5). At high O_2 concentrations, such as are found in the pulmonary circuit, O_2 binds more easily to Hb, allowing for maximum loading. This corresponds to the flat upper portion of the curve. At the tissue level, where PO_2 is lower, O_2 more easily dissociates from Hb, allowing for maximum unloading. This corresponds to the steep portion of the curve.

The partial pressure gradient of oxygen between the capillaries and cells is the primary determinant of the amount of O_2 that diffuses into the cells. The end-capillary PO_2, or the venous partial pressure of O_2 (PVO_2) for that capillary bed, is a function of arterial PO_2, blood flow, and degree of O_2 extraction. Because O_2 demand and the ability of tissues to extract O_2 vary in different tissue beds, normal values of PVO_2 also vary, depending on the organ in question (Figure 5-6). In general, tissues tolerate PVO_2 levels of 28 mm Hg. Because skeletal muscles can function anaerobically for periods of time without untoward consequences, exercising muscle may tolerate a PVO_2 level as low as 20 mm Hg. The average PVO_2 for the entire body is approximately 40 mm Hg. Assuming a normal oxyhemoglobin dissociation curve, this would correspond to an Hb saturation of 75%, which means that a considerable portion of the O_2 has not been extracted. Increasing extraction caused by increased demand yields a lower PVO_2. Decreasing PVO_2 values reflect decreased tissue O_2 levels, because tissue O_2 levels depend on O_2 delivery. The degree to which tissue O_2 may decrease before cellular dysfunction occurs is finite (Figure 5-7).

Shifts in the oxyhemoglobin dissociation curve may alter the amount of O_2 available to the tissues. Right-

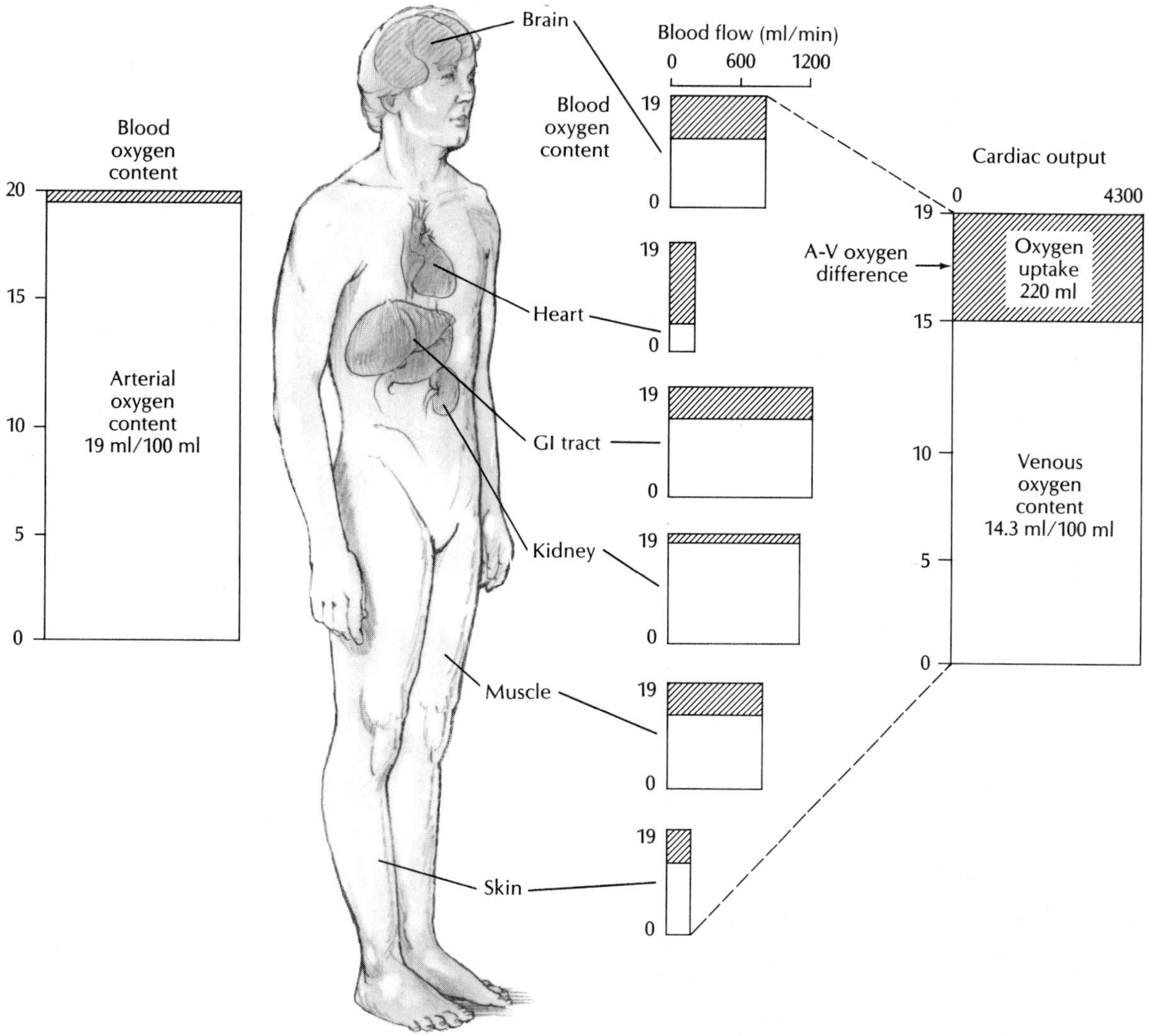

FIGURE 5-6 The blood flow through some tissues is voluminous relative to the oxygen requirements (kidney and skin). In contrast, the myocardium extracts most of the oxygen from the blood. The arteriovenous (A-V) oxygen differences represent the relationship between blood flow and oxygen use in various tissues. (Redrawn from Rushmer RF: *Cardiovascular dynamics,* ed 3, Philadelphia, 1970, WB Saunders.)

ward shifts of the curve caused by hypercapnia, acidosis, increasing levels of 2,3-diphosphoglycerate, and increasing temperature are associated with O_2 being less tightly bound to Hb molecules. Alkalosis and hyperphosphatemia cause the curve to shift left and can cause O_2 to be bound more tightly (see Figure 5-5). Rightward shifts facilitate O_2 unloading at the tissue level, because more O_2 is unloaded at the same PO_2. Leftward shifts retard O_2 unloading. Profound alkalosis may be detrimental, because with a leftward shift of the curve, a lower PO_2 is required for O_2 release. In the pulmonary circuit the curve normally is shifted to the left, resulting in increased Hb saturation. At the tissue level the curve shifts to the right, facilitating O_2 unloading. This phenomenon, called the *Bohr effect,* is thought to occur secondary to the differences in pH and partial pressure of carbon dioxide between the lungs and tissues.[11,71] A term commonly used to describe the oxyhemoglobin dissociation curve is the P_{50} value. This is the partial pressure of oxygen at which the SaO_2 is 50%. Rightward shifts of the curve increase the P_{50}, and leftward shifts decrease it.

The red cell mass of blood significantly contributes to the viscosity of blood, which plays a major role in determining vascular resistance. Viscosity varies little between a hematocrit of 0% and 40% but rapidly in-

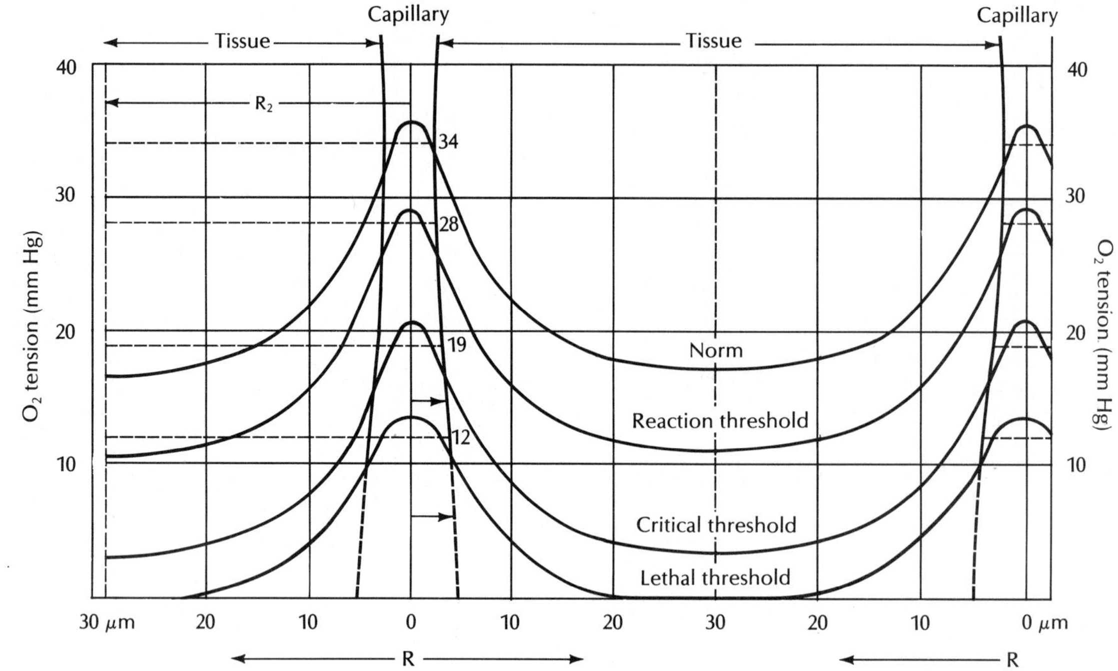

FIGURE 5-7 Oxygen concentration in the vicinity of capillaries under conditions of progressively greater hypoxemia. Also indicated are the levels at which tissue reaction and ultimately dysfunction may occur. (Redrawn from Thews G: Gaseous diffusion in the lungs and tissues. In Reeve EB, Guyton AC, editors: *Physical basis of circulatory support,* Philadelphia, 1967, WB Saunders.)

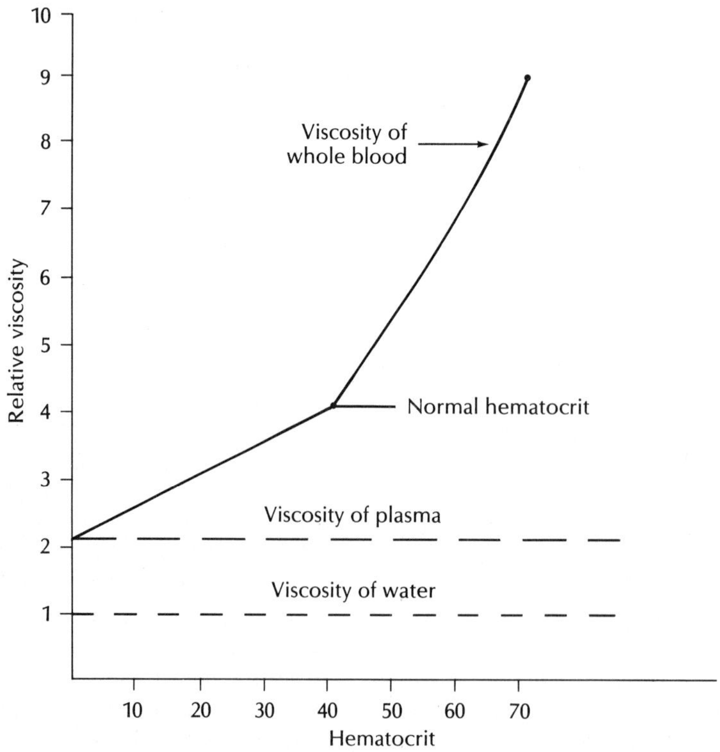

FIGURE 5-8 Relative viscosity of the blood as a function of hematocrit.

creases as hematocrit increases past this level (Figure 5-8). Although increasing hematocrit may yield an increased O_2-carrying capacity, it also may result in a decrease in cardiac output secondary to increased vascular resistance, with the net effect of decreased O_2 delivery.

VESSELS

Functional Organization

Functionally six classes of vessels make up the circulatory system: (1) elastic vessels; (2) resistance vessels; (3) sphincter vessels; (4) exchange vessels; (5) capacitance vessels; and (6) shunt vessels (Figure 5-9).

The walls of elastic vessels, such as the aorta, contain a high proportion of elastic fibers. A major function of elastic vessels is to convert the pulsatile systolic inflow of blood to a smoother outflow in the more distal arteries. When each stroke volume is ejected into the aorta, the vessel's elasticity allows it to be stretched so that blood is stored in that region of the vessel. The elastic recoil allows return to the vessel's original dimension, resulting in movement of blood into the next segment, where it is stored (Figure 5-10). This process, the compression chamber effect, is repeated in a continual manner along the elastic arteries, resulting in a forward flow of blood.[116]

Resistance vessels are primarily small-lumen, thick-walled vessels with a large proportion of smooth muscle in their walls. Smooth muscle reactivity within resistance vessels is the decisive factor in the regulation of flow into each vascular bed and thus in the distribution of cardiac output throughout the overall circulation.

The terminal segments of precapillary arterioles, the sphincter vessels, determine the actual number of open capillary beds and thus the size of the capillary exchange surface.

The actual exchange vessels, or capillaries, are essentially noncontractile, with diameters that change passively as a result of both tissue and blood pressure changes. The functional surface area of capillaries is approximately 60 m^2 in the systemic circulation and 40 m^2 in the pulmonary circuit.

The capacitance vessels, or veins, are easily distended, extremely compliant vessels that serve as blood reservoirs. The venous vessels of the liver, the large veins of the splanchnic region, and the veins of the subpapillary plexus of the skin can hold an additional 1 L of blood above their minimum volume.

The shunt vessels function as arterial venous anastomoses that bypass capillary flow. The opening of these vessels may reduce or entirely interrupt capillary blood flow.

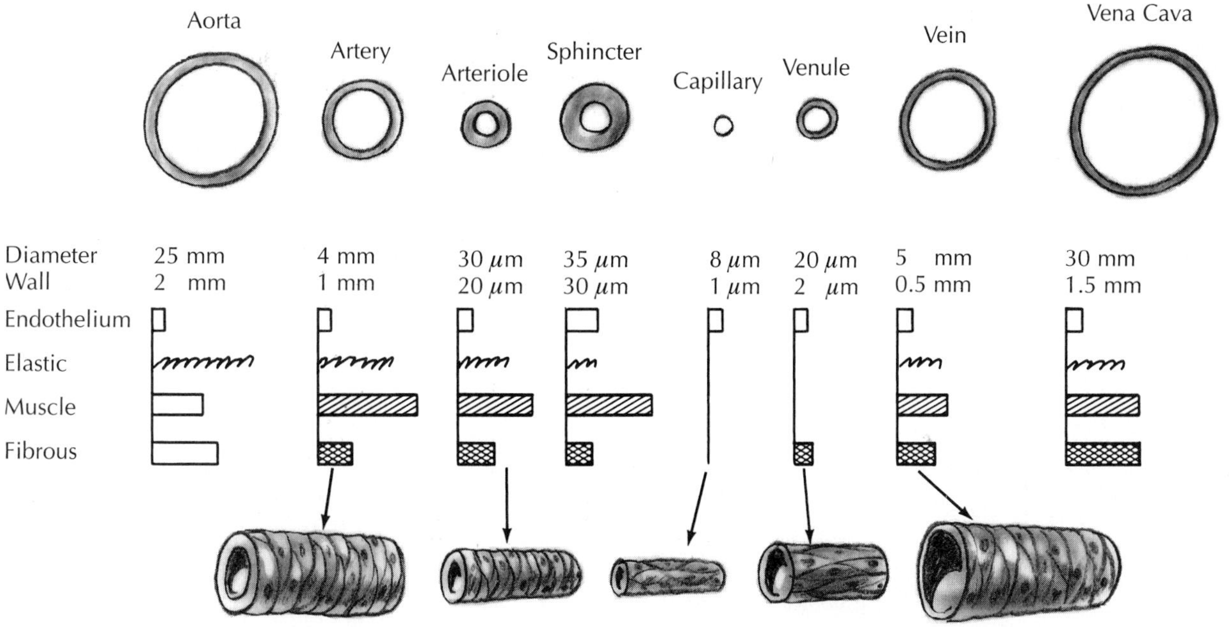

FIGURE 5-9 The relative amount of elastic tissue and fibrous tissue is greatest in the aorta and least in small branches of the arterial tree. Smaller vessels have more prominent smooth muscle in the media. Capillaries consist only of endothelial tubes. The walls of the veins are much like the arterial walls but are thinner in relation to their caliber. Not pictured are the shunt vessels, which are similar to sphincter vessels. (Redrawn from Rushmer RF: *Cardiovascular dynamics*, ed 3, Philadelphia, 1970, WB Saunders.)

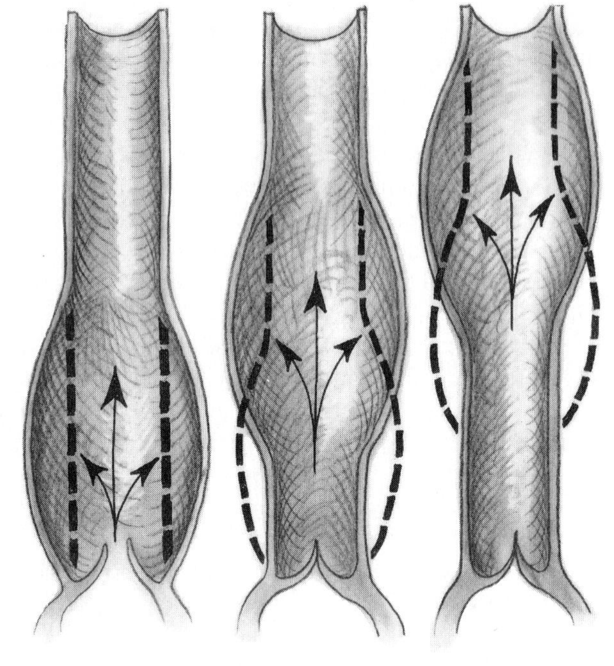

FIGURE 5-10 The initial systolic stretching of the aorta next to the heart so that blood is stored in this region *(left)* is followed by a return to the original dimensions here and stretching and storage of blood in the next segment *(middle)*; this process is repeated in a continual progression along the elastic arteries *(right)*.

Distribution of Volume Versus Resistance

Vascular resistance is the sum of the resistances of all vascular beds in the body. The aorta and other large vessels contribute 20%, the terminal resistance vessels 50%, the capillaries 23%, and the veins and venules 7% of the total vascular resistance. The overall resistance of the systemic circulation in concert with total volume flow determines the blood pressure at any given moment. Eighty-four percent of the blood volume is found in the systemic circulation, whereas only 9% is found in the pulmonary system and 7% in the heart. In the systemic circulation the arteries contain approximately 18% of the total volume, the capillaries only 7%, and the veins and venules 75% (Figure 5-11).

Arterial System

Flow

Aortic flow occurs only during the ejection period of systole. Flow peaks at the end of the first third of the ejection time and has returned to zero by the end of the ejection period. From the onset of the relaxation period to the closure of the aortic valves, a brief period of retrograde flow into the ventricle occurs. During diastole, blood stands still in the ascending aorta until the next ejection. Under resting conditions peak velocities in the human aorta reach 140 cm/sec, with an average velocity of 70 cm/sec. Some antegrade diastolic flow develops in the descending aorta and distal arteries, but at rest retrograde flow can be demonstrated as far distal as the femoral and brachial vessels. Not until the blood reaches the terminal arteries and arterioles does a progression from pulsatile to more continuous flow develop (Figure 5-12).

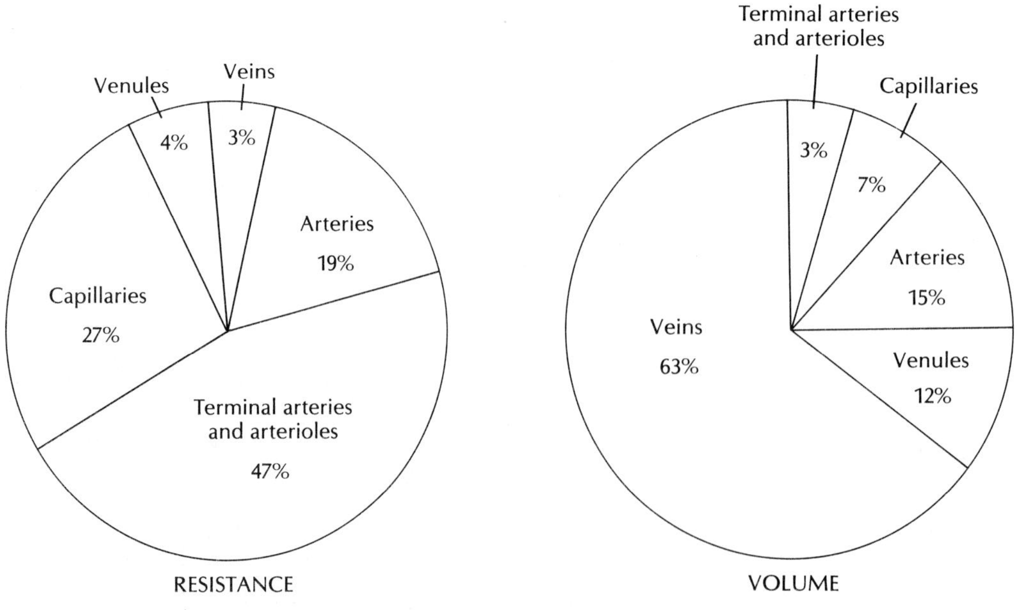

FIGURE 5-11 Distribution of vascular resistance and blood volume.

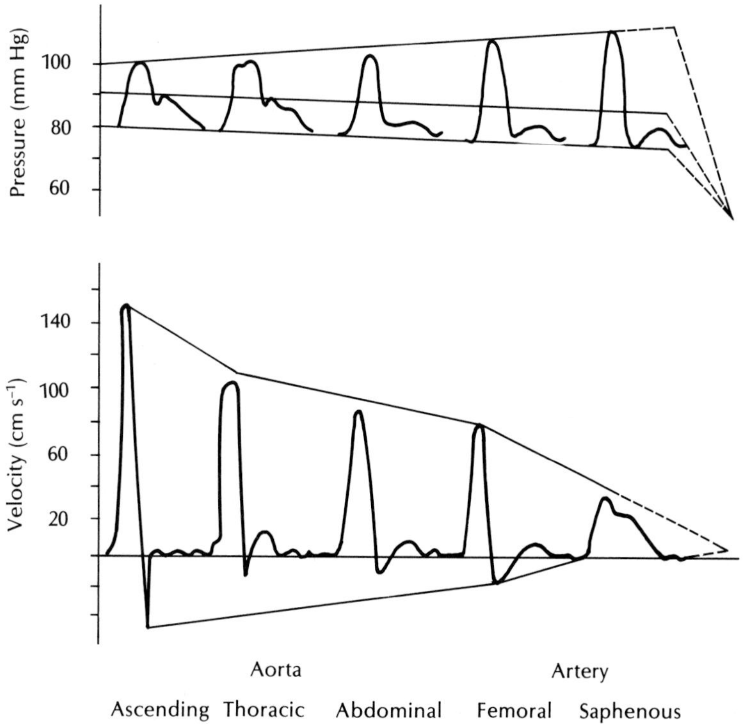

FIGURE 5-12 Changes in pressure and flow pulses in the aorta and leg arteries. Note the development of an anterograde flow component during diastole and the rise in systolic pressure at increasing distances from the heart. (Redrawn from McDonald DA: *Blood flow in arteries,* ed 2, London, 1974, Arnold.)

REGIONAL CHARACTERISTICS

Local regulation. The volume flow ($\dot{V}$) of blood through vessels is directly related to the pressure gradient (P) between segments and inversely related to the resistance (R) in that segment:

$\dot{V} = P/R$

The pressure gradient depends on the driving force of the heart. Resistance to flow depends on the geometry of the vessel and the viscosity of the blood as described by

R = 8 Lv/r4

where L is the length of the tube, v the viscosity, and r the radius of the vessel. Simply, mechanical resistance is proportional to the length/cross-sectional area ratio. An increase in vessel diameter causes a decrease in resistance and an increase in flow. If the radius of the vessels is increased twofold, the resistance to flow drops to 6% of the original value. To increase flow twofold, the vessels' radius must increase by only 20%. These relationships were described under conditions of streamlined flow in nondistensible tubes with Newtonian fluids at a constant temperature. This hardly describes the vascular system, but in general the principles hold true. (More detailed analyses of circulatory hemodynamics that allow for the differences in the vascular system have been performed.[22,52,82]) Despite this inconsistency, the decisive mechanism for regulation of flow relates to the vessel's cross-sectional area, because a relatively small change in the radius effects a large change in resistance.

Distribution of blood flow to each organ system primarily depends on the resistance to flow in the vascular beds. Table 5-1 shows the distribution of a normal cardiac output of approximately 5 to 6 L, representing the system at rest. However, at various times of stress vascular resistance can drastically alter regional flows.

Many substances involved in cellular metabolism have a direct effect on the state of contraction of the vascular musculature in various organ beds. These processes constitute the metabolic autoregulation of peripheral blood flow. *Autoregulation* is the ability of an isolated organ to maintain a constant blood flow in the face of variable perfusion pressure. Autoregulation is a feature of the vascular system and not a reflection of reflex control, since it occurs in the denervated organ.[135] The exact mechanism of autoregulation is unknown.[66] The vessels of the brain best demonstrate this type of response. Hypoxia causes vasodilatation and associated changes in regional blood flow. Local increases in carbon

TABLE 5-1 DISTRIBUTION OF CARDIAC OUTPUT

	CARDIAC OUTPUT (%)	ML/MIN
Brain	13	750
Coronary vessels	4	250
Muscles	21	1200
Splanchnic region	24	1400
Kidneys	19	1100
Skin	9	500
Other organs	10	600
Total systemic circulation	100	5800

dioxide or hydrogen concentration may also cause vasodilatation. Other metabolites such as lactate, produced in greater amounts during exercise, especially in the muscle beds, also exert a dilator action.

Myogenic autoregulation, or the *Baylis effect,* is the ability of vascular smooth muscle to contract in response to pressure increases, thereby yielding little or no increase in volume flow.[13] In vascular beds such as the kidney, this stabilizes the blood supply over a range of pressures from 120 to 200 mm Hg.[44,115]

However, autoregulation does not totally explain the extreme changes in perfusion seen at various times. Neurovasomotor mechanisms, mediated by the autonomic nervous system, control a large portion of regional blood flow. The sympathetic fibers are predominantly involved, although the parasympathetic fibers act in some responses. All blood vessels except capillaries are innervated. The density of this innervation varies widely in different organs and different parts of the vascular system. Small arteries and arterioles of the skin, skeletal musculature, kidneys, and splanchnic region receive a dense innervation of sympathetic fibers, whereas the innervation of those in the brain and heart is relatively sparse.

Norepinephrine, which stimulates the receptors that cause vasoconstriction, usually mediates neuromuscular transmission. The degree of vascular smooth muscle contraction depends on the frequency of the efferent impulses in these nerves. Increases in impulse frequency produce vasoconstriction and decrease vasodilatation. The basal tone that prevails when the vasoconstrictor fibers are silent limits the amount of vasodilatation. A sympathetic cholinergic vasodilator system has been described in skeletal muscle.[54] Its importance is unknown, but it acts via acetylcholine, which binds to gamma-receptor. Chemicals and hormones also act directly on the vessels to produce vasoconstriction and dilatation. Both hypoxemia and acidosis have been shown to produce marked vasodilatation. The circulating catecholamines, epinephrine or norepinephrine, are released continuously in small quantities from the adrenal medulla and have a considerable effect on vascular smooth muscle. The presence of alpha- and beta-adrenergic receptors explains differential responses of the vessel musculature to these catecholamines.[3] Engagement of alpha-receptors elicits vasoconstriction, and beta-receptors elicit vasodilatation. Epinephrine acts on both alpha- and beta-receptors, whereas norepinephrine acts predominantly on alpha-receptors. In low concentrations epinephrine stimulates predominantly beta-receptors, thus causing vasodilatation. In higher doses the vasoconstrictive response predominates. Almost all blood vessels have alpha- and beta-receptors; however, they differ in proportion and absolute numbers in different parts of the circulatory system. The vessels of the brain and heart are the most sparsely innervated by sympathetic nerves and have the lowest concentration of receptors, whereas the skin, liver, and mesenteric vascular beds are most densely innervated and have the greatest number of receptors. When levels of circulating catecholamines are high, as in hypotension, they increase blood pressure by causing vasoconstriction. Increasing vasoconstriction decreases blood flow to regional beds, especially those with rich innervation and large numbers of receptors. However, the brain and heart are relatively spared and maintain a near-normal flow. Because the veins are also innervated by sympathetic nerves and have sympathetic receptors, stimulation can cause venoconstriction, increasing the blood return to the heart. Maximum sympathetic discharge, causing vasoconstriction, may increase blood return to the heart by 2½-fold. Conversely, stimulation of beta-receptors or other vasodilatory receptors can cause marked venodilatation. Thus a combination of all these factors can alter regional blood flow, depending on the needs of the individual organ system and the ability of the vascular system to meet these demands.

Venous System

Pressures and Flow

Flow within the venous system is continuous and nonpulsatile. The pressure drop within the venous system is relatively sharp, with pressure of 15 to 20 mm Hg near the capillaries, 15 mm Hg in the small veins, 5 to 6 mm Hg in the extrathoracic veins, and 2 to 4 mm Hg in the intrathoracic veins and right atrium. This pressure gradient, plus the residual arterial pressure, provides the basic driving force for venous flow. The venous circuit does demonstrate reflex vasoconstriction secondary to stimuli such as asphyxia and hypovolemia. The central venous pressure, which refers to the right atrial pressure, determines the amount of blood return to the right ventricle.

A major impedance to venous flow is gravity or hydrostatic pressure. Three mechanisms facilitate venous flow: the muscle pump, the respiratory pump, and the heart's suction effects. The pumping action of skeletal

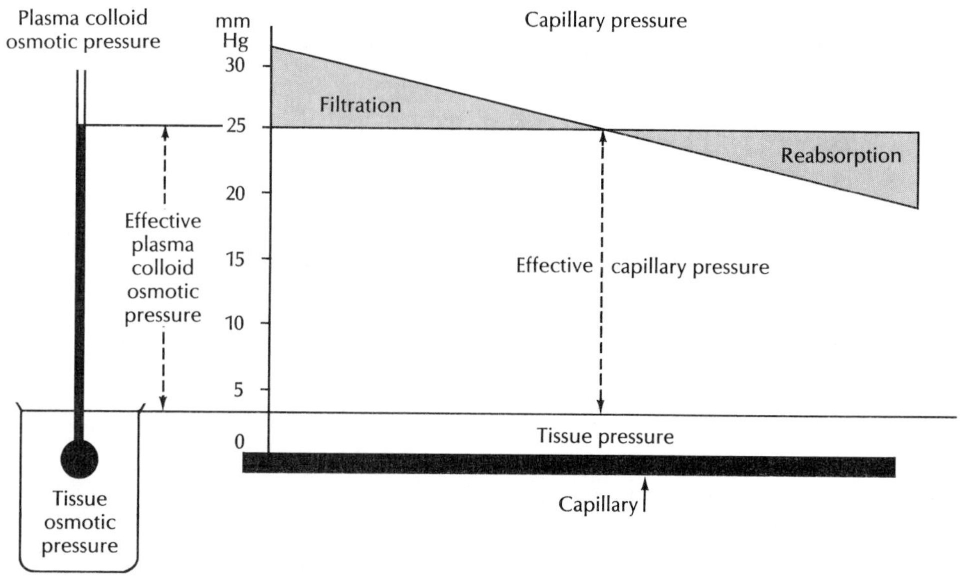

FIGURE 5-13 The difference in protein concentration in tissues and in the plasma determines the effective colloid osmotic pressure of the plasma. The effective capillary pressure is the difference between capillary pressure and tissue pressure. The pressure gradient in capillaries under a specific set of conditions may produce filtration at the arteriolar end of the capillary and reabsorption in the venular end of the capillary with no net fluid exchange. Such complete fluid balance is the exception rather than the rule. (Redrawn from Rushmer RF: *Cardiovascular dynamics,* ed 3, Philadelphia, 1970, WB Saunders.)

muscle, resulting from compression of the veins by muscle contraction, helps propel blood in an antegrade fashion; that is, as muscles contract, venous flow is augmented. Retrograde flow is prevented in the extremities by the venous valves. The respiratory pump is active during inspiration when the intrathoracic pressure drops from 15 mm Hg to zero. This pressure drop causes greater dilatation in the intrathoracic vessels and results in decreased resistance to flow while simultaneously exerting an effective suction on the adjacent vessels. Finally, the downward displacement of the tricuspid valve plane during ejection yields lower pressure in the atrium and adjacent parts of the vena cava, resulting in a suction effect.

Microcirculation

The total effective capillary exchange area is approximately 1000 m^2 and is distributed among approximately 40 billion capillaries. Under resting conditions blood is actually flowing through only one fourth of the capillaries, with a cross-sectional area of approximately 2500 cm^2.[45] Flow through individual capillary beds depends on three factors: the regional blood flow to that organ system, the state of the precapillary sphincters present at each capillary bed, and the arterial venous anastomoses, or shunt vessels, that provide direct communication between small arteries and veins bypassing the capillary system. Exchange between the blood and the interstitial fluid occurs by two methods. The first is by diffusion, in which the exchange of fluid and materials passes between the blood and the interstitial space, dependent on the relative concentrations of the materials in each space. The rate of diffusion of water from the entire capillary surface of the body is approximately 60 L/min or 85,000 L/day. The second mechanism of exchange is filtration and reabsorption, which is explained by Starling's theory (Figure 5-13).[136]

A dynamic equilibrium prevails between the amount of fluid filtered out of the capillaries at their arterial end and the amount reabsorbed at the venous end. The capillary hydrostatic pressure, the interstitial fluid pressure, the colloid osmotic pressure of the plasma and interstitial fluid determine the amount of filtration and reabsorption in the capillaries. Changes in these pressures can result in a relatively rapid volume shift between the intravascular and interstitial space, affecting hemodynamics.

INTEGRATION

Blood Pressure Maintenance

In clinical practice it is nearly impossible to measure regional blood flow and tissue perfusion. Blood pressure measurements usually are used, but these are crude assessments of body blood flow because, as previously shown, flow depends on more than just pressure. Although blood pressure depends on several factors, the generation of blood pressure can be fundamentally explained as:

BP = Cardiac output (CO) × Peripheral vascular resistance (PVR)

Maintenance of blood pressure depends not only on the heart's ability to pump blood at a sufficient rate and volume but also on the ability of the vasoregulatory mechanism to maintain vasomotor tone. Because cardiac output is a function of heart rate (HR) and stroke volume (SV), the above equation can be further modified to:

BP = HR × SV × PVR

Changes in each component of the equation may cause changes in blood pressure.

Regulatory Mechanisms

Maintaining perfusion depends on the body's regulatory mechanisms, which affect heart rate, cardiac performance, and peripheral vascular resistance. A variety of receptors continuously monitor the functional aspect of the circulation. The afferent impulses from these receptors are centrally transmitted to the vasomotor center in the medulla. The resulting response can be categorized as one of three types, depending on the time of onset: (1) short-term, or acute, control mechanisms; (2) intermediate-term control mechanisms; or (3) long-term control mechanisms.

Short-Term Control Mechanisms

Short-term, or acute, control mechanisms are mostly vasomotor adjustments enacted by baroreceptors, chemoreceptors, and ischemic reflexes that require only minutes to take effect.

BARORECEPTORS. The major baroreceptors are located in the carotid sinus, the aortic arch, and the cardiac atria. The carotid sinus is an isolated area at the carotid bifurcation that has a thinner, more elastic medium innervated by the carotid sinus nerve, a branch of the glossopharyngeal nerve. The aortic arch baroreceptor is anatomically similar and is innervated by a branch of the vagus nerve, as are the atrial stretch receptors. The arterial baroreceptors monitor blood pressure as assessed by vessel wall stretching. Impulses are continuously generated at a pressure-dependent rate, with increased blood pressure increasing the number of impulses. Heightened stretch receptor activity decreases sympathetic tone and enhances parasympathetic response. The cardiac stretch receptors in the atrium are sensitive to changes in intravascular volumes. The function of these receptors is less understood. Two types have been reported: receptors that are discharged during atrial systole and beta-receptors that are discharged during diastole. In 1914 Bainbridge[8] described a reflex in which rapid infusion of a large volume of fluid caused a reflex tachycardia. It has been postulated that increasing volume causes a reflex stimulation of the beta-receptors. This response results in an increase in sympathetic cardiac tone, causing a faster heart rate to help eject the larger volume of blood. Engagement of the Bainbridge reflex requires a low baseline heart rate, and many have questioned its clinical significance. Atrial stretch receptors also help regulate secretion of hypothalamic antidiuretic hormone through an increase in atrial pressure, which causes a decrease in antidiuretic hormone secretion. These same receptors are thought to regulate secretion of a group of peptides known as *atrial natriuretic peptides* (ANP). Increased atrial stretch and tachycardia augment release of ANP, producing a renal natriuretic effect.

CHEMORECEPTORS. The major chemoreceptors, the carotid and aortic bodies, respond to changes in arterial PO_2 and PCO_2. They consist of highly vascularized groups of so-called glomus cells. The afferent impulses, increased by a decrease in flow or in PO_2, stimulate both the respiratory and circulatory centers of the medulla, causing vasoconstriction, a decrease in heart rate, and an increase in respiratory rate.

ISCHEMIC REFLEX. The ischemic reflex is regulated by cerebral blood flow; thus decreases in flow cause stimulation of the autonomic medullary center, resulting in general vasoconstriction mediated by the sympathetic nervous system.

Intermediate-Term Control Mechanisms

TRANSCAPILLARY VOLUME SHIFT. Increases in arterial pressure produce a rise in effective capillary pressure, which increases filtration into the interstitial space, reducing intravascular volume. A decrease in pressure (and usually blood volume) results in the converse, yielding increased capillary resorption of fluid from the interstitial space, which results in increased vascular volume.[45,58] Lister and colleagues[78] have measured the refilling that occurs secondary to the Starling forces at 50 to 120 ml/hr, but other researchers have reported values as high as 1 L/hr. Prolonged hypovolemia will cause this mechanism to fail because constriction of postcapillary sphincters persists while precapillary sphincters relax.[91] Intracellular fluid also plays a role by contributing water to the interstitial space as a result of contracted volume. The shifts from the intracellular space take longer to become effective than do the simple transcapillary volume shifts, but the former are responsible for intravascular volume repletion when hypertonic saline is used for resuscitation.

RENIN-ANGIOTENSIN SYSTEM. Decreased renal perfusion in any form, whether caused by generalized hypotension, vasoconstriction, or flow-limiting lesions of the renal vessels, can cause an increased release of renin. The mechanism by which decreased renal perfusion stimulates renin release is poorly understood. The juxtaglomerular cells of the kidney synthesize and store the enzyme renin. When released, renin splits angiotensinogen, an alpha-globulin formed in the liver, producing angiotensin I, which is then converted in the lungs and kidneys to angiotensin II. The most important effect of angiotensin II is that it serves as a strong stimulus for aldosterone release. In addition, it activates the central sympathetic nervous system and is a potent vasoconstrictor. The systemic vasoconstrictor effect is probably insignificant because of the extremely low physiologic concentrations normally encountered, although regional effects may be of greater magnitude. In addition, the plasma half-life of angiotensin II is only 4 to 6 minutes. It plays a less important role as a weak inotrope.

Long-Term Control Mechanisms

The long-term control mechanisms of blood pressure predominantly involve the kidney. Renal response is intimately related to both vasopressin and aldosterone. Vasopressin, or antidiuretic hormone, may cause vasoconstriction, but its main effect is to control the reabsorption of water in the distal tubule of the kidney. Increases in blood volume activate the atrial receptors that inhibit vasopressin release from the posterior pituitary, causing the kidney to excrete more fluid. The release of aldosterone, produced and stored in the zona glomerulosa of the adrenal cortex, is stimulated by angiotensin II and atrial natriuretic peptides. Because aldosterone increases renal tubular reabsorption of sodium and secretion of potassium and hydrogen by the kidney, the sodium and extracellular fluid content of the body are increased, resulting in increased blood volume and, eventually, increased blood pressure. The vasopressin system becomes effective in approximately 20 minutes. The effects of aldosterone on the circulatory system appear after several hours and are not fully effective for several days.

From review of the control mechanisms of circulation, one can see that acute disturbances in blood pressure are counteracted at the level of the resistance vessels chiefly by alterations in vessel capacity and peripheral vascular resistance. In chronic conditions, volume control hormones have the dominant effect but take longer to become fully effective. Figure 5-14 is a schematic diagram of the various control mechanisms and their interrelationships.

Functioning of Control Mechanisms

The numerous control mechanisms that regulate blood pressure do so by altering components of the following equation:

$$BP = HR \times SV \times PVR$$

Changes in heart rate can cause either an increase or a decrease in blood pressure by altering cardiac output. Elevated sympathetic tone, elicited by the baroreceptors, increases the heart rate in a hypotensive patient. In general, rates up to 150 beats per minute (bpm) are reasonably tolerated. Shortening the cardiac cycle by increasing the heart rate affects the diastolic time component but has little effect on the systolic time interval. Rates exceeding 150 bpm usually do not allow adequate diastolic filling of the ventricles in preparation for the next systole. Shortening diastole also shortens the time for cardiac perfusion, since most coronary artery blood flow occurs during diastole. A faster heart rate also increases cardiac oxygen consumption. Because the heart extracts such a high percentage of delivered oxygen, increased coronary blood flow is required to meet the increased demands. At rates over 150 bpm, oxygen demand outstrips supply. Patients with diseased coronary vessels that limit flow may reach this point at slower heart rates.

Increasing stroke volume as a mechanism of increasing cardiac output and therefore blood pressure also has mechanical and physiologic limits. Stroke volume can be augmented by enhancing contractility or preload. In resting, supine, healthy humans, stroke volume is not usually increased by augmented preload because the cardiac chambers are close to their maximum volumes. In the upright position the chamber volumes drop approximately 30%, resulting in a reserve capacity. In healthy, exercising humans, stroke volume is typically increased by altering heart rate and contractility. The cardiac reserve, or the ability of the heart to meet unusual output demands, depends not only on increases in diastolic volume but also on the positive inotropic and chronotropic effect of the sympathetic system, which effort is limited by the size of the end-diastolic volume. Stroke volume can be increased by as much as three to four times normal by these mechanisms. However, increases in stroke volume result in increased cardiac oxygen consumption, because the oxygen consumption of the heart with each beat depends on the myocardial fiber tension (Figure 5-15).

Changes in peripheral vascular resistance, as mediated by the sympathetic and hormonal control mechanisms, result in altered regional blood flow and increased systemic blood pressure. Increases in peripheral vascular resistance yield a decrease in the radius of the resistance vessels that causes decreased flow to capillary beds, since resistance and volume flow are inversely related to the fourth power of the radius. If all regional capillary beds had the same sensitivity to increased sympathetic tone, flow to all beds would be decreased at the benefit of increasing blood pressure, a paradoxic situation. A prioritization of flow occurs in which less important vascular beds are underperfused to the benefit

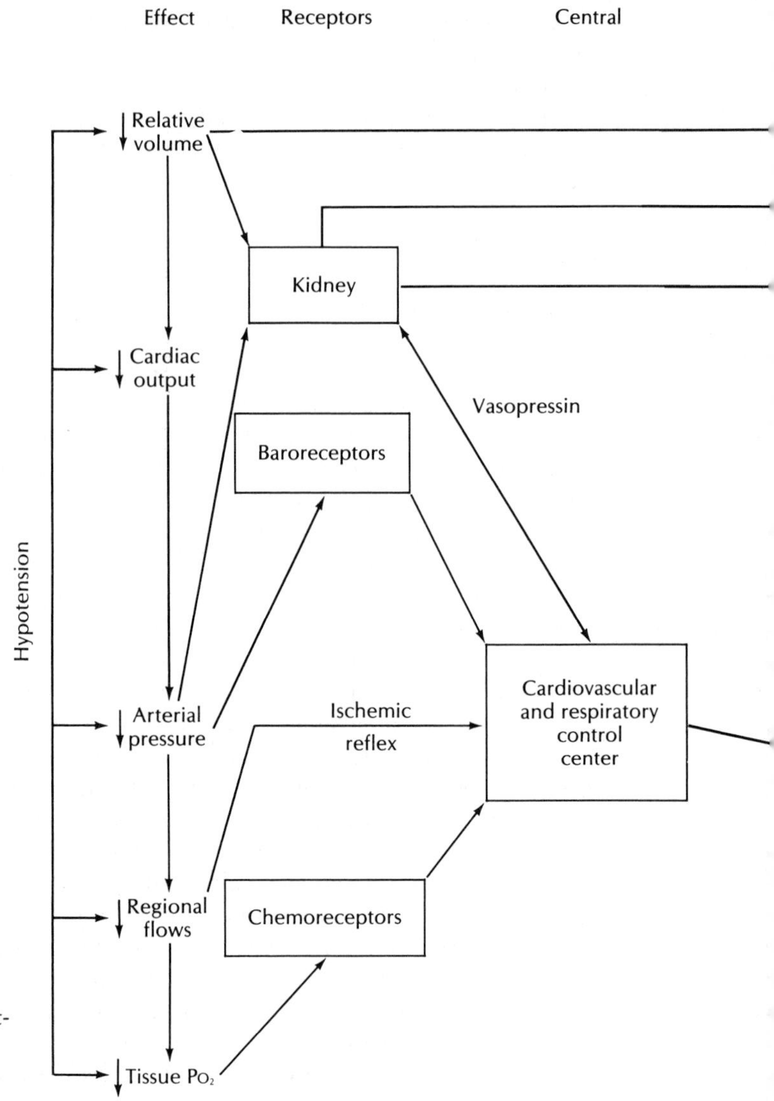

FIGURE 5-14 Composite diagram schematically representing the various control mechanisms important in restoring tissue perfusion in the patient with hypovolemic hypotension.

of perfusion of more critical areas. The order of blood flow prioritization is the brain, heart, kidneys, foregut, midgut, and hindgut, muscles, and skin.[6] The higher in the order, the less sympathetic innervation there is to the resistance vessels of that regional bed. However, maintaining flow to the brain and heart by increasing peripheral vascular resistance and decreasing flow to other regional beds is not without drawbacks. In general, increases in peripheral vascular resistance or afterload result in decreased cardiac output and increased work by the heart. Underperfusion of other beds obviously may lead to ischemic damage, especially to the kidneys.

The effects of decreased regional perfusion are related to altered nutrient delivery. Regional shifts in the distribution of cardiac output occur so that the brain and heart may be perfused at the relative expense of other systems. Hypoperfusion of vascular beds results in cellular injury, the severity of which depends on the magnitude and duration of the hypoperfusion. Prompt restoration of perfusion prevents significant cellular injury. Failure to correct perfusion leads to impaired organ function, with the possibility of multiple organ failure; these patients can have exceptionally high death rates.

SHOCK

In general, the causes of shock and hypoperfusion fall into four categories (Table 5-2): hypovolemic shock, cardiogenic shock, septic shock (failure at a cellular level in sepsis), and circulatory shock. Malperfusion and organ dysfunction are the ultimate endpoints of any shock state (Figure 5-16). Placing the patient in any one cat-

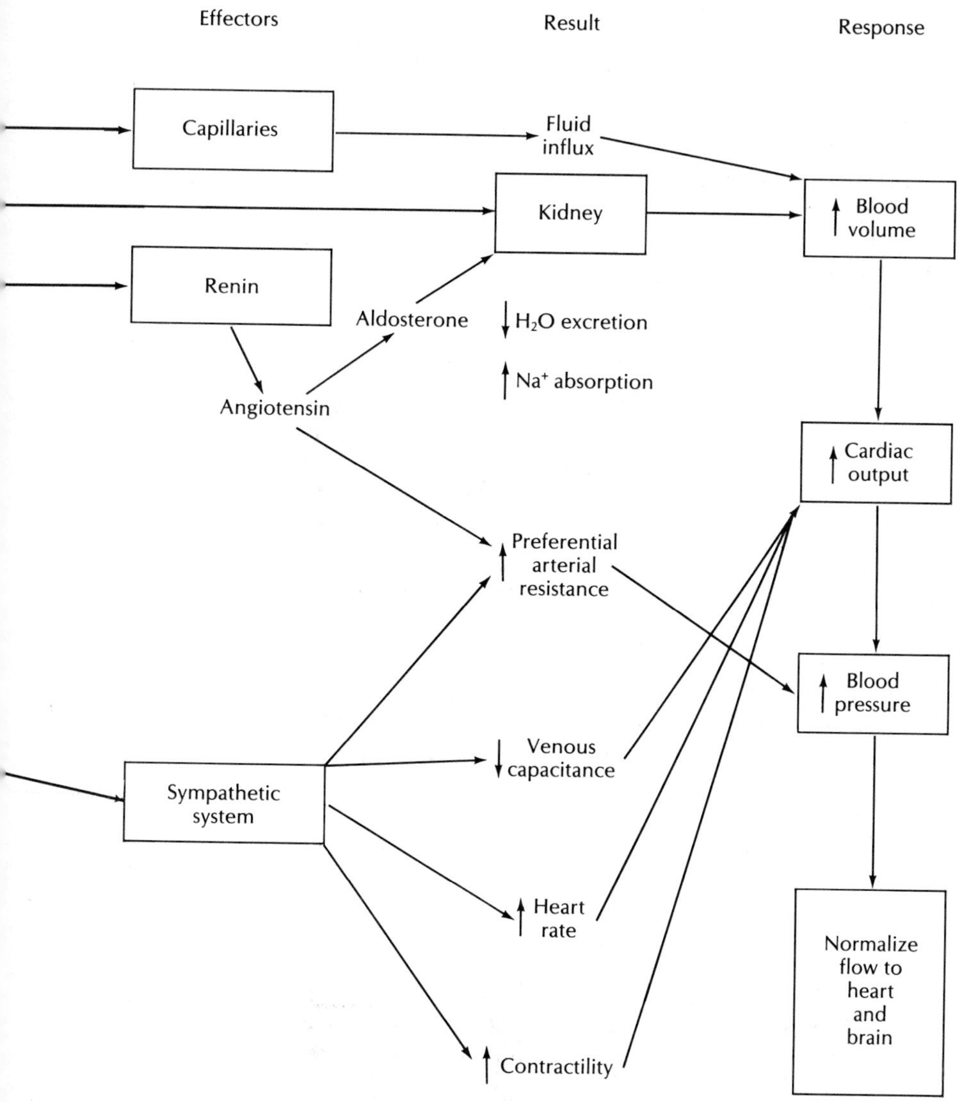

TABLE 5-2 COMPARISON OF TYPES OF SHOCK

	HYPOVOLEMIC	CARDIOGENIC	SEPTIC	CIRCULATORY
Cardiac index	↓ ↑	↓ ↓	↑ ↓	↑
Peripheral resistance	↑	↑	↓	↓ ↓
Venous capacitance	↓ ↓	↑	↓	↑
Blood volume	↓ ↓	↑	↓	→
Core temperature	→ ↓	→	↑ ↓	↓
Metabolic effects	Effect	→	Cause	→
Cellular effects	Late	→	Cause	→

Modified from Committee on Trauma, American College of Surgeons: *Early care of the injured*, ed 3, Philadelphia, 1982, WB Saunders.

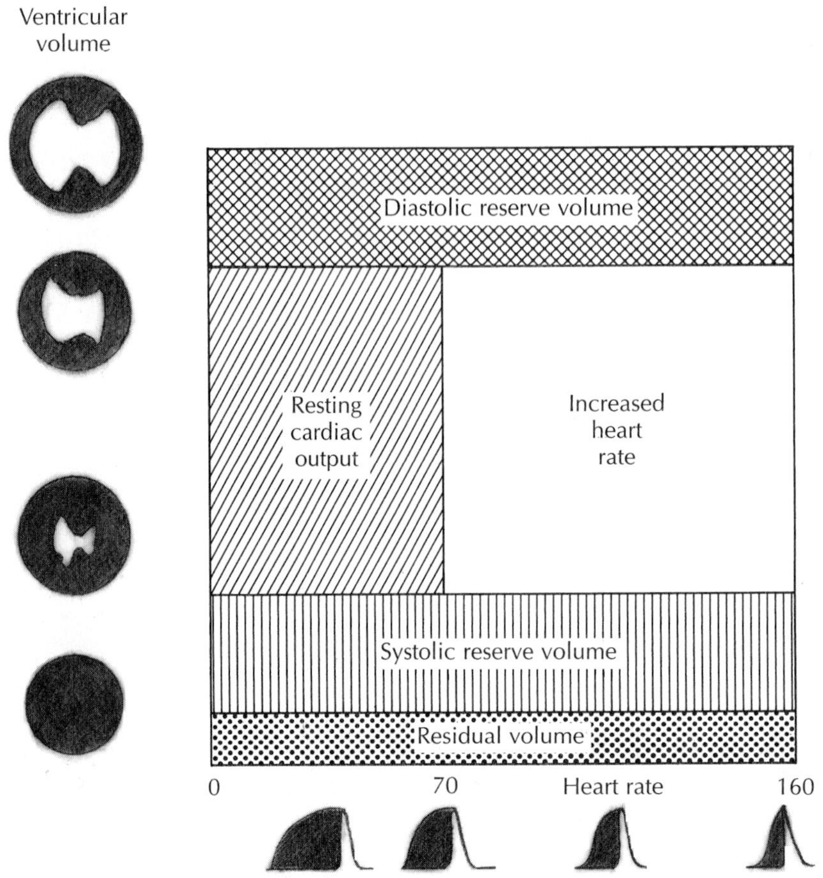

FIGURE 5-15 Ventricular volumes. Resting cardiac output (about 5 L/min) equals stroke volume (about 70 ml) × heart rate (about 72 bpm). Maximum cardiac output increase of about sixfold *(total shaded area)* can occur through elevation of heart rate and stroke volume. Stroke volume increases by encroachment on systolic and diastolic reserve volumes by changes in contractility or preload. (Redrawn from Rushmer RF: *Cardiovascular dynamics,* ed 3, Philadelphia, 1970, WB Saunders.)

egory does not exclude the possibility of other, concurrent causes. Patients in shock often are critically ill with several preexisting disorders that are superimposed upon other, acute organ dysfunctions, and they cannot tolerate a further physiologic insult. Classifying the patient's condition into one of these four categories allows the clinician to start therapy and to determine what initial monitoring and ongoing evaluation may be required.

The initial evaluation should always start with a history and an appropriate physical examination. Pertinent parts of the history are any data suggesting that the patient may be experiencing volume loss secondary to hemorrhage or third space fluid sequestration. Also, any evidence should be obtained of preexisting cardiac disease, symptoms compatible with acute myocardial events, respiratory problems, infection, recently administered drugs or anesthetics, injuries, or operations. The patient's current vital signs, orthostatic signs if appropriate, and precise fluid intake and output over the preceding hours, if available, must be noted.

During the physical examination the physician should observe the color and temperature of the skin and the color of the nail beds, evaluate the condition of the mucous membranes, and assess volume status by neck vein inspection. Assessment of the patient's neurologic status, as well as cardiac, lung, and abdominal examinations, should be performed carefully and rapidly. With this basic clinical information, the physician should begin to formulate the likely cause of the shock state and decide on appropriate initial treatment. For many patients in shock, this initial examination may be sufficient for evaluation. However, some critically ill patients may require more sophisticated evaluation.

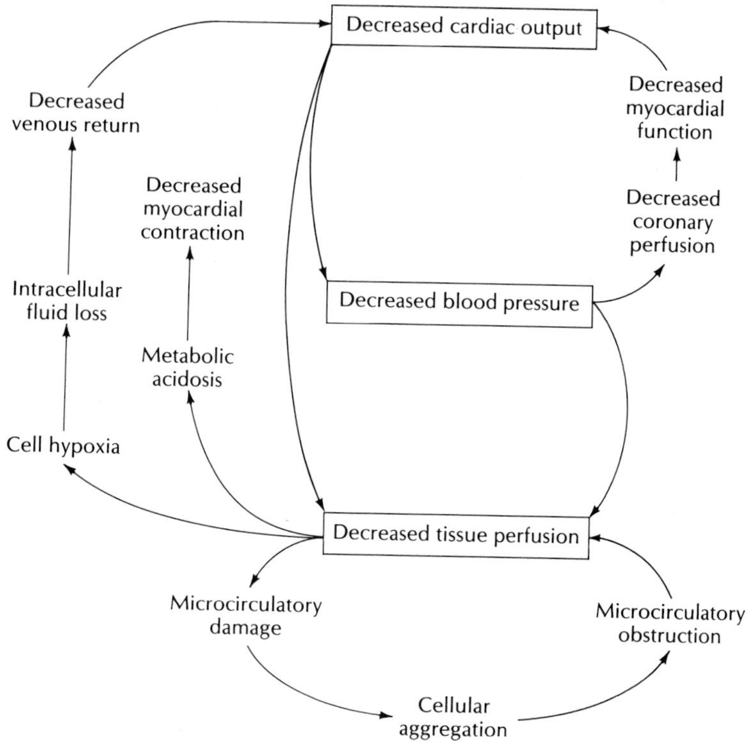

FIGURE 5-16 Vicious circles in shock. Initiation of shock can occur at any point, but the endpoint is often the same. (From Dunphy JF, Way LW: *Current diagnosis and treatment,* ed 4, Los Altos, Calif, 1979, Lange.)

HYPOVOLEMIC SHOCK

Changes in circulating volume, whether secondary to hemorrhage, excessive plasma loss (as in burns), or extracellular volume loss (i.e., third space losses that can occur in gastrointestinal obstruction), may lead to a shock state. Clinically, when volume loss is suspected of precipitating the shock state, volume restoration should be initiated immediately. The patient's signs and symptoms depend on the size of the blood volume deficit (Table 5-3). In general, uncomplicated losses up to 15% of the total blood volume result in a mild resting tachycardia of approximately 100 bpm, with normal blood pressure, pulse pressure, respiratory rate, skin color, and temperature. With losses between 15% and 30% of the blood volume, the tachycardia increases to over 100 bpm. Systolic blood pressure is normal, but the pulse pressure is decreased. The respiratory rate is slightly increased, and in the case of hemorrhage, the nail beds are pale. The patient may be anxious but otherwise have appropriate responses. With losses of 30% to 40%, or 1500 to 2000 ml in a 70 kg male, the tachycardia increases to over 120 bpm. At this point, in addition to a narrowed pulse pressure, the systolic blood pressure is also decreased. Tachypnea is evident, and the skin is cool and clammy with a pale, mottled coloration. Confusion is now associated with anxiety. Severe volume loss (greater than 40%) is associated with findings similar to those for 30% to 40% loss; in addition, the patient may be extremely lethargic. The ability of the cardiovascular compensatory mechanisms to maintain near-normal circulatory status during mild to moderate volume loss depends on optimal synchronization of these mechanisms in a healthy cardiovascular system. In older or severely ill patients, these mechanisms may fail, with smaller volume losses resulting in overt clinical shock states well before a 30% volume loss.

Consider the following patient:

PROBLEM: POSTOPERATIVE HYPOTENSION

Clinical Presentation

History (Subjective Findings)

A 72-year-old white male in generally good health 18 hours after repair of an infrarenal abdominal aortic aneurysm.

TABLE 5-3 CLINICAL SIGNS OF VOLUME LOSS

VOLUME LOSS	CLINICAL FINDINGS	
	NORMAL	ABNORMAL
15%	BP, PP, temperature, RR, mentation	P (↑)
15% to 30%	BP, temperature, RR, mentation	P (↑ ↑), PP (↓)
30% to 40%	—	P (↑ ↑ ↑), PP (↓ ↓), BP (↓), temperature (↓), RR (↑), confusion
Greater than 40%	—	Same as 30% to 40%, lethargy (↑)

BP, Blood pressure; *PP*, pulse pressure; *P*, pulse; *RR*, respiratory rate.

Physical Examination (Objective Findings)

The patient is intubated on mechanical ventilatory support. He responds to questions by opening his eyes and moves all four extremities appropriately. His blood pressure is 75/50 mm Hg, pulse is 120 bpm with a sinus tachycardia, respirations are 28/min, temperature is 38.2° C (101° F) rectally, and his urine output has been 10 ml/hr over the previous 3 hours. The physical examination with the patient supine reveals that he has cold, clammy skin and pale, mottled nail beds. His neck veins are flat; the cardiac examination reveals normal heart sounds without a gallop; the lung examination shows coarse bilateral respiratory sounds; and the abdomen is distended but has not changed appreciably since the patient was in surgery.

Assessment

By clinical criteria this patient is in shock. His blood pressure indicates a significant alteration in normal circulatory dynamics. Systolic blood pressure reflects the systemic vascular resistance (SVR), and diastolic pressure the blood volume. The pulse pressure reflects cardiac output (CO) as well as blood volume. A pulse pressure below a normal value of 40 mm Hg indicates decreased CO. Patients with pulse pressures of 20 mm Hg and a normal systolic blood pressure may have alterations in regional perfusion. A patient with a systolic pressure of 80 or 90 mm Hg but a normal pulse pressure probably has adequate blood flow. Because blood pressure reflects the product of CO and SVR, a patient with low blood pressure may have a low CO or low SVR, or both.

This patient appears to have elevated SVR, as manifested by cold, clammy skin with pale nail beds. Because blood pressure is low and peripheral vascular resistance is high, CO must be decreased. CO depends on stroke volume and heart rate. This patient's heart rate is elevated, and thus stroke volume must be low. Stroke volume reflects cardiac performance and is directly related to preload, contractility, and afterload. Because afterload is elevated secondary to elevated SVR and contractility is probably increased secondary to the effects of increased sympathetic tone, preload must be decreased. Taking all this into consideration, the patient appears to have a significant decrement in blood volume. However, one should remember that cardiac function has not been measured objectively and that cardiac dysfunction cannot be ruled out. Still, other causes of shock cannot be evaluated until the hypovolemia has been treated.

Management

Immediate Fluid Replacement

Volume loss must be corrected immediately once the diagnosis has been made. Restoration should begin with a balanced salt solution such as a lactated Ringer's solution. After further investigation to determine the cause of the hypovolemia, the physician may continue volume restoration with crystalloids, colloid solutions, or blood products. The goal should be to maintain the oxygen-carrying capacity of the blood while restoring the circulating volume.

CRYSTALLOID SOLUTIONS. Commercially available crystalloid solutions include lactated Ringer's solution and normal saline (NaCl). They are both similar to plasma in ionic composition and may be used for volume replacement. To replace pure blood loss, these solutions should be administered in a ratio of 3:1 or 4:1 of the calculated blood volume deficit, because they quickly equilibrate in the interstitial and intravascular compartments. A patient with a blood loss of 500 ml requires infusion of 2 L of a balanced salt solution to restore the circulating volume. Some researchers have proposed the use of hypertonic salt solutions for resuscitation of hypovolemic shock. The use of hypertonic saline is intended to limit the resuscitation volume required when isotonic salt solutions are used. Infusion of hypertonic solutions into the intravascular space increases intravascular volume by causing water to shift from the intercellular and interstitial compartments into the intravascular space. Large animal shock models have determined that 7.5% NaCl with 6% dextran (HTS-D) is the optimal solution for maintaining hemodynamic stability. Omission of dextran leads to a transient hemodynamic effect.[59] Several models[105] have demonstrated no hemodynamic benefit of HTS-D, compared to isotonic solutions, if the administered sodium load is the same, although the volume administered is significantly less. Isovolumic resuscitation leads to the expected findings of significant hemodynamic stability compared to isotonic solutions. The combination of head injury and hemorrhagic shock poses a significant resuscitation problem. Large volumes of isotonic solutions result in marked elevation of intracranial pressure (ICP) and a decrease in cerebral perfusion pressure (CPP). Substitution with HTS-D results in significantly lower ICP and less cerebral edema, but the effect on CPP has been inconsistent.[57,118,149] The ability to limit volume in this group of patients may prove beneficial.

Contraction of intercellular volume may be deleterious and thus limit the use of hypertonic saline solutions. Trauma patients often are dehydrated at the time of injury, and the effect of hypertonic saline in this setting has not been adequately studied (most large animal studies have been of limited duration). When hypertonic saline has been used as the sole resuscitation agent in small animal shock models, long-term follow-up has shown increased mortality compared to isotonic resuscitation.[129] Human trials of hypertonic saline have focused on small-volume boluses administered in the early phase of resuscitation, with subsequent volume administered as isotonic solutions and blood components. Although hypertonic saline has been proved safe when administered in small volumes, its superiority to isotonic solutions has not been demonstrated in a clinical trial.[65,87]

COLLOID SOLUTIONS. Colloids typically consist of albumin added to a balanced salt solution. The albumin solutions are prepared from pooled plasma proteins, from many donors, that have been pretreated at 60° C (140° F) to reduce the risk of hepatitis transmission. Colloid solutions contain no clotting factors or immunoglobulins. The rationale for colloid use is that large molecules should stay in the intravascular space, increasing the colloid osmotic pressure and reducing the amount of fluid needed for resuscitation, and thus decreasing interstitial edema.

CRYSTALLOIDS VERSUS COLLOIDS. Whether crystalloids or colloids should be used for resuscitation has been the subject of a long debate that has yet to be resolved.* Colloid enthusiasts cite the excessive volume of crystalloids needed to resuscitate hypovolemic patients. They claim that the decrease in colloid osmotic pressure and the increase in weight secondary to massive fluid volumes are detrimental to the patient. Indeed, some experimental evidence suggests a higher survival rate for animals treated with colloids rather than crystalloids in a hemorrhagic hypovolemic shock model.[29] In some hemorrhagic shock models, regional blood flow has been more effectively restored with colloid solutions than with isotonic crystalloids.[139] Hauser and associates[60] have shown a greater and more prolonged increase in plasma volume, cardiac index, blood pressure, and oxygen delivery while identifying no significant capillary leak of colloids in hypovolemic patients resuscitated with colloids.

Those favoring crystalloid administration cite the lower cost and lack of anaphylaxis or hepatitis risk, which is approximately 0.1% in commercially prepared albumin preparations. Data also show that in the acute phase of resuscitation, infused albumin rapidly equilibrates into the interstitial space.[86] Furthermore, clinical studies have shown that there is no difference in the pulmonary complications associated with large-volume infusions, whether crystalloid or colloid, in trauma patients[120,121]—data that have been corroborated in animal models.[101] Two recent meta-analyses of all human trials comparing colloids and crystalloids have concluded that there were no differences in mortality.[15,146]

These reviews, in conjunction with the large cost differential in favor of crystalloids, lead us to recommend the use of crystalloids as the initial resuscitation fluid except in a patient with extreme hypoproteinemia. Colloid use in patients with capillary leak syndrome is of no therapeutic benefit, because rapid extravasation occurs into the interstitial space. In postoperative patients without acute trauma or sepsis, colloids may be of greater benefit.

OTHER VOLUME EXPANDERS. Because of the cost and the potential for disease transmission associated with albumin preparations, other volume expanders have become available as plasma substitutes. The use of dextran, which is formulated as both a high molecular solution (70,000 molecular weight) and a low molecular solution (40,000 molecular weight), is associated with inhibition of platelet function secondary to decreased platelet adhesiveness and decreased factor VIII activity.[2,56] The risk of anaphylaxis with dextran infusion is less than 1%. Other solutions containing various forms of hydroxyethyl starch are commercially prepared in differing molecular weights. The higher molecular weight solutions act as volume expanders similar to other colloids and are at least as effective as albumin.[77] Although some investigators have reported abnormal in vitro clotting studies following infusion of hydroxyethyl starch,[137] two recent studies have shown evidence of increased bleeding when the solution is infused into postoperative surgical patients.[50,94] Elevation of serum amylase has been reported in other series.[72] Pentafraction, a higher molecular fraction of pentastarch, has been reported to be superior to hetastarch, although there are no human trials that compare these plasma substitutes.

*References 23, 93, 104, 123, 140, and 148.

BLOOD PRODUCTS. In hemorrhagic hypovolemic shock, the use of blood or blood products should be limited to patients with severe continuous hemorrhage or blood loss exceeding approximately 30% of the blood volume (1500 to 2000 ml). The red cell mass is the primary determinant of the O_2-carrying capacity of the blood, and increases in hemoglobin concentration of 2 g may increase the O_2-carrying capacity by as much as 20%. The optimal hematocrit in resuscitation of shock patients is unresolved. Increasing hematocrit concentration may result in an increase in blood viscosity at a time when flow is decreased. Although viscosity remains relatively low with hematocrit levels from 0 to 35, it increases rapidly past this point. Increasing viscosity could result in sludging in the capillaries and lead to decreased O_2 supply to the tissues despite the increased O_2-carrying capacity. The optimal hematocrit for O_2 transport in the coronary circulation is approximately 25%; it is slightly higher in the systemic circulation. In patients who can increase their cardiac output and are not hypermetabolic, hematocrit levels as low as 20% to 25% can be easily tolerated. In patients who are already hypermetabolic or who have increased cardiac demands for other reasons, a hematocrit of approximately 30% may be necessary for adequate O_2 transport. Elevating the hematocrit above this level is unnecessary and may be detrimental to the patient.

The use of type O blood is rarely indicated, except in resuscitation of a patient who has uncontrolled and severe blood loss. Type-specific blood should be available in approximately 10 minutes and saline cross-matched blood in an additional 15 to 20 minutes. Type-specific blood guarantees ABO and Rh compatibility, although minor incompatibilities may exist. Fully cross-matching blood takes up to 1 hour. Although blood transfusions should never be withheld when appropriate indications are present, transfusions can be associated with complications. Transfusion reactions and transmission of diseases such as hepatitis or acquired immune deficiency syndrome (AIDS) may be a problem, depending on the blood donor pool. The prevalence of the human immunodeficiency virus (HIV) in the current blood pools is estimated at 1 in 30,000 to 50,000 units, resulting in an incidence of HIV transmission of 1 per 156,000 transfusions; or, approximately 100 to 200 persons may develop transfusion-associated AIDS yearly. The prevalence of non A, non B hepatitis is estimated at 1% to 4%, although this should decrease significantly with the advent of wide-scale hepatitis C screening. Currently an estimated 40,000 transfusion recipients develop hepatitis annually. Recently the relationship between blood transfusion and altered immune responsiveness leading to increased risk of infection has been described,[47,143] which further complicates the decision to transfuse a patient.

Massive transfusions are associated with many potentially lethal complications. The coagulopathy identified in massively transfused hemorrhagic shock patients is complex and is secondary to a state resembling diffuse intravascular coagulation, which is related to the low-flow state and the consumption of coagulation factors. In massive transfusions (i.e., when transfusion of at least one blood volume is anticipated), administration of fresh frozen plasma or other blood components should be based on coagulation studies rather than protocol. Binding of calcium by anticoagulants in banked blood is rarely a problem, because calcium mobilization usually is adequate. However, when transfusion rates exceed 100 ml/min, calcium administration may be indicated. An appropriate dose is 0.2 g of calcium chloride (2 ml of 10% solution). The total dose given should not exceed 1 g, because hypercalcemia may result. Thermal problems may occur as a result of rapid infusion of a large amount of blood, which normally is stored at 4° C (39° F). Hypothermia can be avoided by using specially designed blood/fluid warmers, which can selectively warm more than 1 L/min of hypothermic solution.[126]

Because of the problems associated with blood transfusion, as well as the relative scarcity of blood products, many attempts have been made to generate blood substitutes. Fluorocarbon solutions, specifically Fluosol DA, are one example. These compounds carry O_2 in simple solution, with 40 ml of O_2 carried per 100 ml of solution at an oxygen pressure (PO_2) of 100 torr in vitro. In one human trial, fluorocarbons were associated with pulmonary, liver, respiratory, reticuloendothelial system, and kidney toxicity.[39] Few data currently are available by which to judge the clinical applicability of these new compounds. A 20% solution carries only three times the amount of O_2 as plasma, and O_2 exchange with these solutions is linear versus O_2 tension. To deliver 5 vol% of O_2, the arteriovenous O_2 (AVO_2) difference must be approximately 500. To obtain this AVO_2 difference, the patient must be kept on extremely high inspired O_2 levels, which involves antecedent risks. In a randomized, controlled trial of the use of Fluosol DA in severely anemic patients, dissolved O_2 content was significantly but transiently raised. The rapid elimination of the fluorocarbon solution in these patients greatly limited its usefulness.[133]

Stroma-free hemoglobin solutions are another form of blood substitute.[53] They are not associated with transmission of disease or transfusion reactions. Their oxyhemoglobin dissociation curve is the same as that for red cells. These solutions are oncotically active and act as plasma expanders. Unpolymerized Hb solutions have an extremely short half-life (less than 1 hour) and are associated with nephrotoxicity. Improved purification of hemoglobin in concert with polymerization by a variety of methods has partly corrected these problems, extending the half-life to approximately 3 hours.[41] Liposome encapsulation, as well as the recent availability of human recombinant hemoglobin, should extend the usefulness of these compounds by extending their half-life and decreasing the associated nephrotoxicity.[79]

The aggressiveness and rapidity of fluid resuscitation depend on the clinical situation. Initially a fluid bolus is administered, and the response to the bolus dictates further therapeutic and diagnostic decisions. The initial fluid bolus should be between 10 and 25 ml/kg of body weight, with the rate of administration determined by the severity of shock. The volume administered depends on the estimated volume deficit. Because crystalloid solutions must be given in a 3:1 to 4:1 ratio, the initial bolus will totally replenish the deficit in only a small percentage of cases, such as when the deficit is less than 750 ml. In patients with an estimated volume deficit greater than 20% of their total blood volume, the volume infused should be 25 ml/kg.

The same signs, symptoms, and measurements of inadequate perfusion used to diagnose the shock state are also useful parameters in following the response to therapy. Return of blood pressure, pulse pressure, and pulse rate toward normal are positive signs and indicate stabilization of the condition. Restoration of perfusion to the kidneys produces an easily quantifiable response: increased urine output. Urine output of 0.5 to 1 ml/kg/hr, if not secondary to administration of diuretics, indicates adequate perfusion and is a valid marker for restoration of regional perfusion.

One study has demonstrated that the base deficit is the most reliable indicator of the severity of shock and the adequacy of resuscitation.[30] This concept has been extended to the use of gastric tonometry, which measures intramucosal gastric pH as an index of splanchnic tissue oxygenation. Although the splanchnic bed is particularly sensitive to ischemia, the clinical utility of this measurement remains to be proven.[125]

The hemodynamic response to the initial fluid infusion normally falls into one of three categories. A few patients have a rapid improvement in blood pressure after receiving the first bolus and remain stable. They usually have sustained a volume loss of less than 20%. Further therapy should be aimed at keeping pace with ongoing losses, and simple measures of the adequacy of resuscitation, such as urine output, usually are sufficient. The second and largest group of patients has a transient response to the fluid bolus. Initially they show signs of volume restoration and improved circulation, which then deteriorate over time. Most of these patients have had an initial volume loss of 20% to 40% and additional continuous losses; they require continued administration of volume expanders and possibly surgical intervention. Another small group of patients shows minimum or no response to initial fluid boluses. The problem may be rapidly exsanguinating hemorrhage, which requires immediate surgical intervention, such as a freely ruptured aortic aneurysm. Alternatively, these patients may have a component of myocardial dysfunction or may have entered the decompensatory phase of shock, in which vascular tone is lost. The loss of vascular tone may be secondary to excessive production of nitric oxide or failure of vessels to respond to circulating vasoconstrictive substances.

The latter two groups of patients require more aggressive and sophisticated resuscitation and monitoring. Maximized volume status and cardiac function must be obtained promptly to ensure adequate O_2 delivery. Currently controversy exists over the optimum method of resuscitating these patients. The benefit of prompt restoration of normal blood pressure and volume has been demonstrated in both animal and human trials. Rapid fluid infusion using a variety of infusion devices that can administer normothermic volumes above 1.5 L/min has been demonstrated to result in a decrease in postresuscitation complications compared to conventional fluid administration practices. Presumably this is secondary to prevention of a large cellular or tissue O_2 debt. Some clinicians have recommended resuscitation to supranormal hemodynamic levels in an attempt to limit O_2 debt.[10] Such resuscitation requires placement of a Swan-Ganz catheter so that cardiac output and O_2 consumption and delivery can be monitored. Recommendations for therapy include resuscitation to a cardiac output greater than 4.5 L/min and O_2 delivery in excess of 600 ml/min/m^2,[122] or maximizing O_2 delivery until O_2 consumption plateaus.[10] Clinical support for attaining either of these goals is somewhat lacking. Observations have shown that survivors of severe shock can attain these goals through aggressive resuscitation with use of fluids and inotropes. Nonsurvivors typically are unable to be resuscitated to those levels. It may be argued that failure to reach such goals is only a marker of severe decompensation and a system that has no reserve (see the section on Cardiogenic Shock for further discussion). Large-scale clinical trials must be performed to document the efficacy of this approach.

Measurement of Volume Status

Attempts to measure volume status objectively are helpful when volume restoration is begun. A simple method of measuring volume status is determining the central venous pressure (CVP). CVP is a function of the volume of blood in the central veins, the compliance and contractility of the right side of the heart, the vasomotor activity in the veins, the intrathoracic pressure, and the intrapericardial pressure. CVP reflects the volume of blood returning to the heart and the right ventricle's ability to expel it. True CVP should reflect the volume of blood in the capacitance side of the vascular system.

Normal CVP values in a nontraumatized, nonstressed person are −2 to +4 cm H_2O. Changes in vasomotor activity as it occurs in the capacitance vessels during increased sympathetic activity may result in elevated CVP when the blood volume is low. In addition, elevated intrathoracic pressure, which occurs when positive end-expiratory ventilation is used, may falsely elevate CVP values. Inability of the right side of the heart to propel its volume load to the pulmonary circulation, as is seen in right ventricular infarctions or in cases of markedly elevated pulmonary vascular resistance, may also elevate CVP. In general, serial measurements of CVP allow assessment of the patient's volume status. Increasing CVP measurements usually reflect increasing intravascular volume.

If bolus infusion results in relatively small gains in CVP, hypovolemia is definitely a problem. However, the goal of resuscitation should not be to elevate CVP to an arbitrary predetermined level, but rather to restore organ perfusion. This may occur at a CVP of 5 cm H_2O in some cases or at 10 to 15 cm H_2O in others. These elevated levels may seem paradoxic when normal CVP readings are −2 to +4 cm H_2O. However, in a shock patient higher CVP levels may be required because of changes in the compliance of the heart and venous system, with higher filling pressures needed to effectively deliver the same blood volume to the heart. Unfortunately, CVP does not reflect the filling pressure and thus filling volumes of the left ventricle. In severely ill patients or those in whom CVP fails to respond as anticipated, placement of a Swan-Ganz catheter is necessary to ensure adequate volume restoration and optimal left ventricular performance (see the following section on Cardiogenic Shock).

Returning to the patient example, the CVP initially was 0 to 2 cm H_2O. After infusion of 1 L of lactated Ringer's solution, the CVP was 2 cm H_2O. Because the bolus of crystalloid solution resulted in a relatively small gain in CVP, the likely problem was presumed to be hypovolemia. When a second liter of lactated Ringer's solution was administered to this patient, his CVP rose to 6 cm H_2O. Also, his pulse rate decreased to 95 bpm and his blood pressure rose to 110 mm Hg systolic. During the ensuing hour his urine output was 55 ml. In this patient volume restoration apparently reversed the shock state.

The patient's hypovolemia could have been caused by many factors, and even though the hypotensive episode has been averted, his evaluation is incomplete. The physician must attempt to ascertain the reason for the hypovolemia; only after the cause of the shock state has been determined is the resuscitation complete.

HEMATOCRIT. A common mistake made in evaluating a hypovolemic patient is relying on hematocrit measurements to estimate blood loss or to diagnose shock. This is inappropriate and unreliable. Massive blood loss acutely produces only a minimal decrease in hematocrit, and changes occur only after volume resuscitation and transcapillary refilling.

Other Concerns

Although volume resuscitation is paramount in the treatment of hypovolemic shock, the entire clinical picture must not be ignored.

VENTILATION. Attention to the patient's airway and ventilatory status is of critical importance and should always precede other manipulations. Appropriate airway control and O_2 therapy, as well as mechanical ventilation if necessary, should be used to maintain adequate oxygenation and CO_2 clearance. In general, the physician should attempt to achieve an arterial O_2 level between 70 and 80 mm Hg. At this level more than 90% of the hemoglobin is saturated with O_2, helping to ensure optimal O_2 content of the blood. When the PO_2 exceeds 70 torr, hemoglobin concentration and cardiac output (CO) have a stronger influence on O_2 delivery to the tissues because of the flatness of the oxyhemoglobin dissociation curve at this level of PO_2.

ACID-BASE BALANCE. Attention to acid-base balance is also important. The metabolic acidosis that normally accompanies hypovolemic shock is best treated by restoring the circulating volume and ensuring adequate tissue perfusion, not by administering bicarbonate therapy. Lactated Ringer's solution works no better than normal saline solution in correcting acidosis in hypovolemic shock.[21] Mild metabolic acidosis is not dangerous and shifts the oxyhemoglobin dissociation curve to the right, thus helping to increase O_2 delivery to the tissues. However, severe metabolic or respiratory acidosis with a pH of 7.2 or less may be associated with cardiac dysfunction and should always be treated.

With the changes in distribution of cardiac output that accompany hypovolemic shock, the brain and heart are preferentially perfused at the expense of the skin, renal, mesenteric, and hepatic vascular beds. Restoration of renal perfusion, as manifested by adequate urine output, indicates that at least the cerebral, cardiac, and renal beds are adequately perfused. However, if urine output remains low after circulating volume and cardiac output have been restored, diuretic agents may be indicated.

RESTORATION OF PERFUSION. The use of corticosteroids in hemorrhagic shock has been advocated, because they may increase perfusion by causing capillary vasodilatation. Additional benefit has been hypothesized because of the potential for steroids to act as membrane stabilizers, thus helping to limit cell injury. Laboratory studies indicate that administering steroids late in the clinical course is not beneficial. When steroids are administered for hemorrhagic shock, pharmacologic, not physiologic, doses should be given. Because no clinical studies have shown benefit, their use cannot be advocated.

Prolonged administration of vasoconstrictive drugs in hypovolemic shock before volume restoration is contraindicated. Vasoconstrictors (which include any alpha-agonist such as norepinephrine, phenylephrine, high doses of epinephrine, and dopamine) severely constrict arterioles, increasing maldistribution of flow without altering the underlying problem of decreased blood volume. Currently animal models are being used to test the hypothesis that inhibiting nitric oxide (NO) synthesis or activity during refractory shock may result in more appropriate distribution of cardiac output because of the differential local activity of NO in various tissues.

The use of vasodilators has been recommended on the basis of animal studies in which the shock state appeared to be refractory to volume replacement.[98] The concept of blocking the vasoconstriction of the resistant vessels to possibly improve blood flow to the vascular beds is theoretically appealing but probably not pharmacologically attainable. Most drugs not only cause arteriolar dilatation but venous dilatation as well. This may lead to decreased cardiac blood return and thus a lower CO. In addition, the use of vasodilators when blood volume is inadequate may cause circulatory collapse and cardiac arrest. Vasodilators may be of value in complex cases of hypovolemic shock when cardiac dysfunction plays a major role. They also are used to increase cardiac performance after volume has been restored. Blocking peripheral vasoconstriction cannot ensure that the microcirculatory pathways being opened are appropriate or that the redistribution of CO in a compromised patient is beneficial to the coronary and cerebrovascular beds.

Summary

In traumatic and hypovolemic shock, the physician normally identifies a decrease in blood pressure, CO, CVP, blood volume, stroke volume, O_2 delivery, and O_2 consumption, in concert with an increase in heart rate, SVR, AVO_2 difference, and O_2 extraction. The vasomotor changes are secondary to sympathetic activity. In simple hypovolemic shock, when volume loss is the major factor, restoring circulating volume normally corrects the derangement in hemodynamic stability. Once the underlying cause has been reversed, the patient usually survives. However, in severe, prolonged shock secondary to hypovolemia or in a patient with preexisting cardiac disease, simple volume restoration is not always sufficient. As Wiggers demonstrated, at a certain level the shock state can no longer be reversed by simple measures. Early investigators focused on the failure of the peripheral circulation as the cause. It is now evident that loss of the circulatory control mechanism is only a manifestation of the problem, which may be secondary to sustained tissue ischemia. Treatment regimens aimed at cellular salvage following prolonged ischemia have focused on rapid restoration of cellular energy stores. Adenosine triphosphate–magnesium chloride, pyruvate, glucose/insulin, and other compounds have all been demonstrated to be of benefit in selected animal studies, but as of yet no human data are available. In addition, Pearce and colleagues have reported normal skeletal muscle energy stores during the decompensatory phase of hemorrhagic shock, further complicating the issue.

Survivors of severe hypovolemic shock often suffer from organ damage, which is compounded by the presence of various mediators of the humoral and cellular immune system. The pivotal cell resulting in end-organ damage appears to be the granulocyte.[145] Neutrophil activation, leading to adherence of the polymorphonuclear neutrophils (PMNs) to endothelium, creates a microenvironment rich in oxygen radicals and proteolytic enzymes, which damage the capillary bed. Several mechanisms can trigger neutrophil activation, including translocation of endotoxin from the gut and secretion of tumor necrosis factor (TNF) by macrophages and various other cytokines that are elaborated during stress. Treatment aimed at preventing the nonbacterial inflammatory response ranges from attempts to block activation and adherence of neutrophils to neutralization of the potent radicals and enzymes they produce. Strategies range from nonspecific therapy, such as iron chelation with deferoxamine, using oxygen radical scavengers, and administering pentoxifylline to improve membrane fluidity, to more specific approaches, such as blockading PMN priming, activation, and adherence with platelet activation factor (PAF) antagonists or monoclonal antibodies directed against TNF, interleukin-6 (IL-6), or adherence receptors. The efficacy of these approaches remains to be proven.

CARDIOGENIC SHOCK

Cardiogenic shock, or pump failure, may be either a primary cause of shock or an endpoint of progressive hypovolemic shock; it demands active intervention. More precisely, cardiogenic shock is defined as abnormal perfusion secondary to inadequate cardiac output with normal or elevated cardiac filling volumes (Table 5-4).[83] Cardiogenic shock may be secondary to noncardiac conditions that interfere with blood return to the heart, such as cardiac tamponade and tension pneumothorax. These situations require immediate diagnosis and treatment. More often cardiogenic shock is secondary to primary cardiac events such as ischemia, frank myocardial infarction, or possibly circulating myocardial depressant factors, which have been postulated in such disease processes as sepsis and burns but have eluded identification. Pump failure following myocardial infarction occurs in

TABLE 5-4 CAUSES OF CARDIOGENIC SHOCK

CARDIAC	NONCARDIAC
Ischemia	Cardiac tamponade
Infarct	Tension pneumothorax
Valvular malfunction	
Myocardial depressant factors	

approximately 10% to 15% of patients who survive long enough to reach the hospital; mortality is approximately 80%. This form of cardiogenic shock has been most extensively reviewed and studied in the literature. Clinical signs of cardiogenic shock include systemic hypoperfusion with reflex vasoconstriction and diaphoresis despite adequate volume. The mechanism inducing cardiogenic shock as a terminal event in all forms of shock is unknown. However, compromised coronary perfusion, increased cardiac metabolic requirements, changes in regional cardiac perfusion, and myocardial edema all play a role.[128]

Diagnosis

Nonmyocardial lesions that cause cardiogenic shock usually can be diagnosed by physical examination. Clinical findings of cardiac tamponade are distended neck veins associated with decreased blood pressure and occasionally mechanical and electrical alterations. Tension pneumothorax should be suspected when a shift of the trachea with absence of breath sounds on one side is associated with respiratory difficulty. If nonmyocardial causes can be excluded and the patient is not overtly hypovolemic, a direct myocardial cause is likely.

Management

The primary goal in all patients when treating cardiogenic shock is to maintain tissue oxygenation with the smallest possible increase in myocardial O_2 consumption. To achieve this, cardiac function must be manipulated to increase O_2 delivery. The goal is accomplished first by maximizing preload, then if possible by manipulating afterload, and finally by altering the cardiac contractile state with inotropic drugs. Tachyarrhythmias, which may reduce CO, must be treated. Patients in cardiogenic shock represent an extremely complex clinical problem in which several abnormalities may be affecting the cardiovascular system.

Maximizing Preload

The first step in evaluating a patient suspected of being in cardiogenic shock is to assess the patient's volume status to rule out hypovolemia and to maximize preload as a form of therapy. Does the patient's CVP accurately reflect volume status and left ventricular end-diastolic volume? CVP measurements are affected by several factors that may decrease the value of CVP as a gauge of volume status. In addition, some studies have suggested that blood volume and CVP are not always related.[84] However, elevation of CVP to 10 to 15 cm H_2O with volume infusion usually indicates restoration of the patient's volume status.

CVP readings may be elevated with right ventricular failure, increased intrathoracic pressure (as in hemopneumothorax), or positive end-expiratory pressure (PEEP) ventilation. Also, CVP adequately reflects left-sided pressure in patients with healthy hearts but not in those with cardiac dysfunction. CVP has been shown to be dissociated with left-sided pressures in myocardial ischemia,[46] sepsis,[74] respiratory failure,[144] and pulmonary embolism.[144] Because critically ill patients often show changes in the relationship of right and left ventricular hemodynamics, right-sided measurements may not indicate left-sided function. In a group of critically ill patients, Weisel and associates[150] demonstrated that CVP and pulmonary artery occlusion pressure (PAOP) are poorly correlated. However, if CVP was greater than 12 cm H_2O, PAOP was never less than 5 mm Hg. In addition, if CVP was less than 5 cm H_2O, it was unlikely that PAOP was greater than 12 mm Hg.

When attempting to maximize preload in patients with cardiogenic shock, the physician should not rely on measurements of right-sided filling pressures. More precise assessments of preload, and thus volume status, as well as a means to assess cardiac function, are needed. The Swan-Ganz flow-directed catheters, used to obtain pulmonary occlusion pressures (PAOP) as well as pulmonary artery pressures and CO, are very useful.[138] Both PAOP and pulmonary artery diastolic pressure are better estimates of left ventricular end-diastolic pressure than CVP readings.[32] In addition, reliable estimates of CO obtained by the thermodilution technique yield valuable information in the care of patients with cardiogenic shock.[132]

Although many factors may influence the ability of PAOP to satisfactorily estimate left ventricular end-diastolic volume, no better clinical tool exists at this time. The most common discrepancies are falsely elevated pressures. Falsely elevated readings during mechanical ventilation with PEEP have been thoroughly discussed in the literature.[99] Low levels of PEEP minimally change pulmonary wedge pressures, but levels above 15 torr can greatly affect PAOP.[14] With elevated levels of PEEP, patients should not be routinely disconnected from the ventilator (and thus from the PEEP) to measure pulmonary artery wedge pressure.[31] Although this may yield a clearer picture of the true volume status, it does not simulate the clinical situation under which the heart must function.

To use PAOP as an estimate preload, pressure readings must be correlated with volume. The ideal measurement in assessing preload would be left ventricular end-diastolic volume. The major factor that alters the reliability of pressure readings to reflect volume measurements is ventricular compliance. The relationship of end-diastolic pressure to end-diastolic volume is nonlinear and is affected by primary disease processes within the heart, as well as by various clinical manipulations.[20] Lewis and Gotsmann[76] have described a series of ventricular compliance curves, using the Starling relationship, similar to ventricular function curves. Figure 5-17 shows the relationship between pressure and volume readings as they relate to ventricular compliance. An increase in ventricular compliance allows more volume at lower pressures. Ventricular compliance may be elevated by chronic volume overload, cardiomyopathies, and drugs such as nitroglycerin. Decreased ventricular compliance is caused by ischemia, increases in intrathoracic pressure (as with the use of PEEP), shock states, and inotropic drugs such as dopamine.

The concept of ventricular compliance curves is important in attempting to maximize preload in cardiogenic shock. Through the recent development of fast-response thermistors, beat-to-beat cardiac output can now be measured and right ventricular end-diastolic pressure and right ventricular ejection fraction can be estimated. Although clinical experience is relatively modest, these devices should help refine the optimization of cardiac function by more precise manipulation of preload.

The Swan-Ganz catheter also allows measurement of cardiac output by the thermodilution technique, which has been correlated with the dye dilution technique.[132] Newer catheters containing a small thermistor, which emits pulses of heat, allow continuous averaged CO measurement. Although right ventricular output actually is being measured with this method, the measurement reflects left ventricular output, except in cases of right ventricular failure. CO is standardized by dividing the output reading by the body surface area to derive cardiac index. A cardiac index below 2.2 $L/min/m^2$ that is not secondary to hypovolemia is diagnostic of cardiogenic shock (Table 5-5). Because cardiac output is directly related to preload and contractility and inversely related to afterload, the physician may then attempt to maximize these variables to optimize CO.

The treatment of patients with cardiogenic shock involves restoring tissue perfusion and thus O_2 transport. Therefore the physician must be knowledgeable about the variables involved in O_2 transport to the tissues. In addition, tissue perfusion must be measured to determine the efficacy of treatment. Clinically, evidence of altered perfusion may be manifested by changes in mentation, electrocardiographic changes consistent with

TABLE 5-5 NORMAL PHYSIOLOGIC VARIABLES

	ABBREVIATION	FORMULA	UNITS	NORMAL
Volume Related				
Mean arterial pressure	MAP	—	mm Hg	90 ± 5
Central venous pressure	CVP	—	cm H_2O	5 ± 4
Pulmonary artery occlusion pressure	PAOP	—	mm Hg	10 ± 4
Flow Related				
Cardiac index	CI	CI = CO/BSA	$L/min/m^2$	3.2 ± 0.2
Stroke index	SI	SI = CI/HR	ml/m^2	46 ± 5
Left ventricular stroke work index	LVSWI	$LVSWI = \frac{(MAP - PAOP)(CI)(0.0136)}{P}$	$g/min/m^2$	30-110
Bodily Responses				
Systemic vascular resistance	SVR	$SVR = \frac{(MAP - CVP)\ 80}{CO}$	dynes mc^2/sec	800-1200
Heart rate	HR	—	—	70 ± 10
O_2 Transport Variables				
Arterial pH	pH_a	—	—	7.4 ± .02
Arterial CO_2 tension	$Paco_2$	—	mm Hg	40 ± 2
Mixed venous O_2 tension	MVo_2	—	mm Hg	38 ± 4
Arterial hemoglobin saturation	Sao_2	—	%	97 ± 1
Arteriovenous O_2 difference	AVo_2	$AVo_2 = Cao_2 - CVo_2$	ml/dl	4.6 ± 0.4

BSA, Body surface area; *HR*, heart rate; *Cao_2*, arterial O_2 content; *CVo_2*, venous O_2 content.

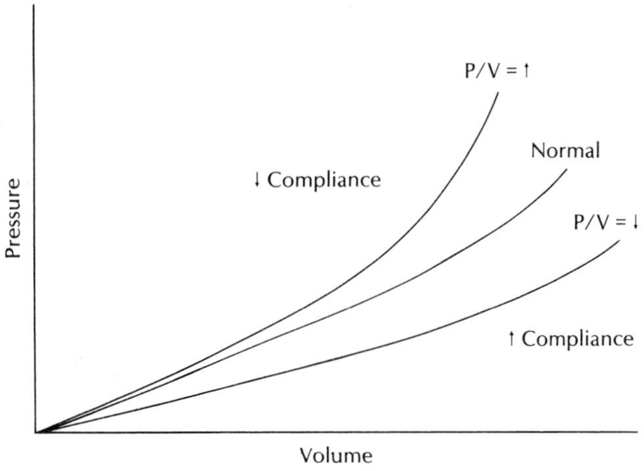

FIGURE 5-17 Relationship between end-diastolic volume and end-diastolic pressure on ventricular compliance. (Modified from Lewis BS, Gotsman MS: *Am Heart J* 99:101, 1980.) *P/V*, Pressure/volume ratio.

ischemia, or decreased urine output as an index of decreased renal perfusion. However, in critically ill patients these assessments are inadequate.

The variable that reflects the summation of tissue oxygenation for the whole body is that of mixed venous PO_2 (MVO_2). In a normal individual MVO_2 is approximately 40 mm Hg, which indicates a venous O_2 saturation (SVO_2) of approximately 75%. Abnormalities of MVO_2 are not diagnostic of a specific physiologic problem but imply a defect in the general process of O_2 delivery and consumption. Rearrangement of the Fick equation to

$$SVO_2 = SaO_2 - VO_2/(CO \times Hb \times 1.34)$$

clarifies this relationship, as SVO_2 can be estimated from MVO_2 and the oxyhemoglobin dissociation curve. A low MVO_2 may indicate increased O_2 consumption, decreased CO, decreased arterial O_2 pressure (PaO_2), or an altered oxyhemoglobin dissociation curve. Increases in MVO_2 may be secondary to decreased O_2 consumption, arteriovenous shunting, elevated PaO_2, or alterations in the oxyhemoglobin dissociation curve. Other calculated variables, such as the O_2 extraction ratio or the arteriovenous O_2 difference (AVO_2), represent similar estimates of whole body oxygen utilization. The physiologic consequences of a low MVO_2 have been previously discussed. An MVO_2 of approximately 35 mm Hg reflects a compromised system with decreased reserves; levels of 27 mm Hg or lower usually result in metabolic pathway disruption at the cellular level. An MVO_2 of 20 mm Hg is associated with an essentially irreversible shock state and ensuing death. The measurement of MVO_2 entails measuring the oxygen content of a blood sample drawn from the distal part of a Swan-Ganz catheter. Continuous monitoring of SVO_2 (and thus estimation of MVO_2) is possible, eliminating the blood sample requirement.

The major difficulty with relying on MVO_2 as an indicator of tissue perfusion is that a normal value may be the result of hyperperfusion in some tissue beds and hypoperfusion in others. More important, under conditions in which oxygen consumption is delivery dependent, increasing SVO_2 may actually be associated with a falling oxygen consumption and thus yield a false perspective of the patient's physiologic state. However, with careful interpretation, MVO_2 is the easiest and most useful indicator available for whole body perfusion.[127]

Measuring the plasma redox potential has become a popular method of assessing perfusion adequacy. The plasma lactate concentration is the most commonly used indicator, although the blood ketone/body ratio (acetoacetic acid/beta-hydroxybutyric acid) has also been used. Lactate levels below 2 mmol/L and a ketone ratio above 0.7 indicate adequate whole body perfusion. Newer potential measures of tissue oxygenation currently under study include plasma amino acid clearance, near-infrared spectroscopy, and ^{32}P nuclear magnetic resonance.

MVO_2 reflects oxygenation that may be altered not only by defects in the transport variables but also by increases in demand. Oxygen demand may be increased by agitation, shivering, seizures, increased ventilatory work, or hyperthermia. Oxygen consumption rises 10% for each degree Celsius above 38°.[24] Attempts should be made to decrease O_2 demand in these situations.

Transcutaneous PO_2 measurements are sometimes used as a measure of perfusion. If transcutaneous PO_2 is equal to PaO_2, it may be assumed that the cutaneous tissue beds are being perfused. Because the cutaneous beds are the first to become vasoconstricted (and thus underperfused) during shock, maintaining cutaneous PO_2 levels implies that perfusion to other tissue beds is adequate.

Attention directed toward O_2 transport is essential in the therapy of cardiogenic shock. Because O_2 delivery to tissues depends on arterial O_2 content as well as CO, the physician must ensure adequate oxygen-carrying capacity. Unlike in hemorrhagic hypovolemic shock, adequate red cell mass usually is available for O_2 transport in cardiogenic shock, with a hematocrit level of 30% sufficient. Maintaining the PaO_2 between 70 and 80 mm Hg ensures hemoglobin saturation above 90%. Appropriate use of ventilatory support, including intubation and mechanical ventilation, may be necessary to achieve these goals.

Optimizing CO involves manipulating three variables: preload, afterload, and contractility. The rate-pressure product, or the product of heart rate and systolic blood pressure, parallels increases in O_2 consump-

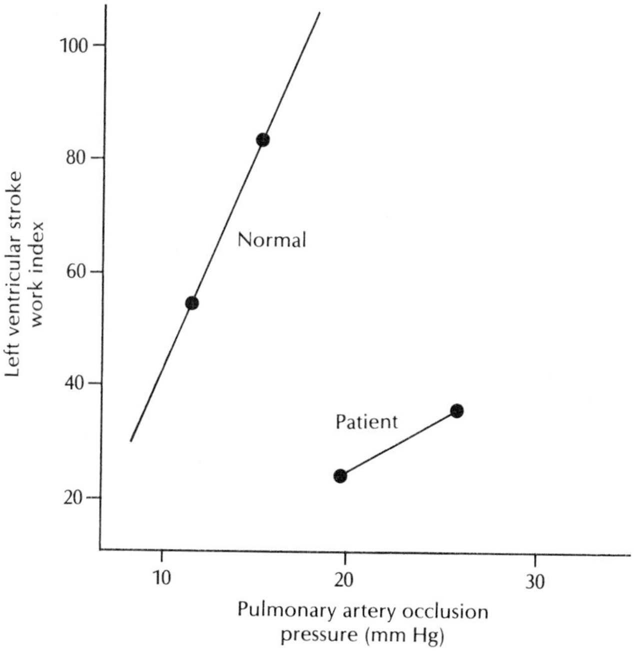

FIGURE 5-18 Relationship between left ventricular stroke work index (LVSWI) and pulmonary artery occlusion pressure (PAOP) in a normal heart. If the slope of the line is flatter than the normal curve following fluid boluses, the patient probably will not benefit from more fluid. This concept is demonstrated in the patient with cardiogenic shock. A fluid bolus increased the LVSWI from 14 to 15.5 g/min/m², whereas PAOP increased from 18 to 23 mm Hg. (See text.) (Modified from Lucas CE, Ledgerwood AM: *Surg Clin North Am* 63(2):439, 1983.)

tion by the heart; this is an easy way to determine the effect of treatment on cardiac O_2 consumption. Normal values are 8,000 to 10,000.

In the management of cardiogenic shock, optimizing preload manipulation should always precede other therapy. Increasing CO by augmenting preload results in a smaller increase in myocardial O_2 consumption and fewer deleterious side effects than pharmacologic intervention. The optimal value of PAOP when used as a measure of preload is between 15 and 18 mm Hg. However, because PAOP may not always directly correlate with filling volumes, using heart work/central filling pressure ratios may be beneficial. This method enables the physician to decide whether more volume is necessary when myocardial compliance is altered and the PAOP is between 15 and 18 mm Hg[80] (Figure 5-18). When using this method, a Swan-Ganz catheter should be placed. The method involves constructing ventricular function curves by plotting the left ventricular stroke work index (LVSWI) against the PAOP:

$$\text{LVSWI} = \frac{(\text{MAP} - \text{PAOP})(\text{CI})(0.0136)}{\text{P}} = \text{g/min/m}^2$$

in which

MAP = Mean arterial pressure
PAOP = Pulmonary artery occlusion pressure
CI = Cardiac index (mm/min)
P = Pulse rate

Normal values are 35 to 70 g/min/m².

The physician should administer small fluid boluses of 250 ml and then remeasure CO and PAOP. LVSWI is plotted against wedge pressure before and after each bolus. By comparing the slope of the line generated by the two measurements to a normal curve, one may decide whether additional volume will yield increased stroke work with minor increases in PAOP. The patient will benefit from additional volume if the slope is steep, indicating a greater increase in LVSWI than PAOP. However, if the slope is flat, indicating very little gain in stroke work but a significant increase in wedge pressure, the patient will not benefit from additional volume. Using this method, the judicious use of volume may be reflected in increased cardiac performance with minimum increases in O_2 consumption.

Reducing Afterload

If CO is still depressed after preload has been maximized, the next step should be an attempt to reduce afterload. This approach is superior to immediately altering contractility because decreasing afterload has the added effect of not increasing myocardial O_2 consumption while increasing CO. However, the physician may attempt afterload reduction if, and only if, adequate volume has first been given. Braunwald[18] has described afterload reduction as the physiologic approach to heart failure. Attempts to reduce afterload when the systolic blood pressure is below 90 to 95 mm Hg may result in a further decrease in blood pressure and tissue perfusion. Clinically, afterload usually is measured by the following equation:

$$\text{SVR} = \frac{(\text{MAP} - \text{RAP}) \times 80}{\text{CO}} = \text{dynes cm}^2\text{/sec}$$

in which

SVR = Systemic vascular resistance
MAP = Mean arterial pressure
RAP = Right atrial pressure
CO = Cardiac output

Normal values are between 800 and 1200 dynes cm²/sec but may vary considerably, depending on body size. Although this is a calculated value, it serves as a useful estimate of the impedance to ventricular ejection. Patients with a normal calculated SVR derive less benefit from afterload reduction than those with elevated values.

Most drugs used to reduce afterload also increase arteriovenous shunting. This is especially critical in the pulmonary circuit, because a further increase in arteriovenous shunting may result in marked ventilation-perfusion mismatching, causing a decrease in arterial oxygen content and, ultimately, oxygen delivery.

The drug used for afterload reduction depends on the clinical situation. Nitroprusside acts both as a systemic venodilator and as an arterial vasodilator, decreasing both preload and afterload. This dual action may be beneficial when preload is also elevated. However, prolonged use of high-dose nitroprusside (over 3 μg/kg/min) may be associated with cyanide toxicity. Evidence of confusion, hyperreflexia, unexplained metabolic acidosis, or seizures requires prompt cessation of therapy and measurement of cyanide levels. Treatment consists of chelating agents and dialysis.[28]

Pure afterload reduction, with little effect on preload, may be obtained with drugs such as phentolamine, phenoxybenzamine, and hydralazine. There is little justification for using nitrates for afterload reduction, because they primarily decrease preload by dilating systemic veins and increasing venous capacitance.[62] However, nitrates may be used in an attempt to improve coronary perfusion when myocardial ischemia is present.

Afterload reduction therapy should be titrated against the systolic blood pressure, attempting to maintain a pressure of 95 to 100 mm Hg. Once this has been accomplished, the response to therapy should be checked by remeasuring cardiac output. Diastolic blood pressure should not be reduced below 55 mm Hg, because a decrease in coronary perfusion pressure may result in ischemia.

Altering Cardiac Contractility

If an attempt to reduce afterload cannot be made after maximizing preload and the patient remains in shock, inotropic support may be needed to increase cardiac contractility. Decreased contractility may be caused by ischemia, hypoxia, edema, acidosis, hypertrophy, or circulating myocardial depressant factors. The goal of inotropic support should be maximum increases in contractility for minimum increases in myocardial O_2 consumption (Tables 5-6 and 5-7).

The most commonly used inotrope is dopamine (3,4-dihydroxyphenethylamine).[61] Its popularity reflects its variable actions, which depend on the dose infused. The inotropic effects of dopamine result from stimulation of cardiac beta-receptors. When infused at rates of 1 to 5 μg/kg/min, dopamine acts as a weak inotrope. Its principal action is peripheral vasodilatation, mainly of mesenteric and renal vessels via dopamine receptors. With dopamine infusion rates of 5 to 15 μg/kg/min, the inotropic effect increases, with increasing peripheral vasoconstriction secondary to alpha-receptor stimulation. At administration rates above 15 μg/kg/min, marked peripheral vasoconstriction occurs. Recent studies have documented a shift to the left in the dose response to dopamine in thermally injured patients, suggesting that inotropic support may be attainable at much lower infusion rates in this group of patients.

Because of the vasoconstrictive effects of high-dose dopamine, a synthetic sympathomimetic, dobutamine, has gained popularity. It acts by direct stimulation of cardiac beta-receptors, with no vasoconstrictive effect because of a lack of alpha-receptor stimulation. It may cause mild peripheral vasodilatation because of arteriolar beta-receptor stimulation. Whether dobutamine actually results in smaller increases in myocardial O_2 consumption compared to dopamine, as originally claimed, is unclear.[68,130] However, when a pure inotrope is required, dobutamine may well be the drug of choice.

In cardiogenic shock the use of isoproterenol as a beta-stimulant is probably not warranted. It is a strong beta-stimulant and a powerful chronotrope. Because of its effect on the heart rate, low-dose isoproterenol may induce tachycardia and thus increase myocardial O_2 consumption with very little increase in contractility. Isoproterenol primarily augments CO by increasing the heart rate and not the stroke volume.[73] It is mainly used in selected cases of right heart failure or to increase the heart rate in cases involving atrioventricular block.

When an inotrope and a strong vasoconstrictor is needed, use of epinephrine or norepinephrine may be

TABLE 5-6 INOTROPIC RECEPTOR ACTIVITY

CATECHOLAMINE	$BETA_1$-RECEPTOR	$BETA_2$-RECEPTOR	ALPHA-RECEPTOR	DOPAMINE RECEPTOR
Dobutamine	++	+	+	0
Dopamine	++	0	++*	++
Epinephrine	++	++	+++*	0
Isoproterenol	++	++	0	0
Norepinephrine	++	0	++	0

*Depends on dosage.

TABLE 5-7 COMMONLY USED CARDIOVASCULAR DRUGS

DRUG	ACTION	ADVERSE REACTION	DOSAGE
Inotropes			
Dobutamine*	Direct beta-inotrope	Tachycardia	2.5-10 μg/kg/min
Dopamine*	Sympathomimetic amine with action dependent on dose	Tachycardia	1-30 μg/kg/min
Epinephrine*	Chronotrope, inotrope, potent vasoconstrictor	Tachycardia, elevated SVR	1-4 μg/min
Isoproterenol	Chronotrope, inotrope, peripheral vasodilator	Marked tachycardia	0.5-5 μg/min
Vasodilators			
Diazoxide	Direct peripheral arteriolar dilator	Prolonged hypotension	1-3 mg/kg
Hydralazine	Vascular smooth muscle	Prolonged hypotension	20-40 mg IV/IM
Nitroglycerin	Vascular smooth muscle relaxation, venous first then arterial	Methemoglobinuria	0.25-4 μg/kg/min
Nitroprusside	Peripheral arterial and venous dilator	Central nervous system toxicity	0.5-8.9 μg/kg/min
Phentolamine	Adrenergic blocker	Angina, prolonged hypotension	1.5-2 μg/kg/min
Vasopressors			
Metaraminol*	Adrenergic stimulation	Tachycardia, arrhythmias	0.5-5 μg/min
Phenylephrine*	Adrenergic stimulation	Bradycardia, arrhythmias	40-60 μg/min

*Extravasation may cause tissue necrosis. Area should be infiltrated with phentolamine, 10 mg, in suspected cases.

warranted. Although both significantly increase myocardial O_2 consumption, epinephrine may be necessary in the treatment of severe cardiac dysfunction and circulatory collapse.

Another class of inotropic drugs reduces afterload by inhibiting phosphodiesterase. Amrinone, the prototype agent, is short acting and available for intravenous use. Current studies have shown marked improvement in cardiac indices when this drug was used in groups of patients with class IV chronic congestive heart failure.

Combining Therapies

Treatment of cardiogenic shock often involves manipulating preload, afterload, and contractility. Not all situations lend themselves to stepwise treatment. A common practice is simultaneous use of inotropes and afterload reduction while increasing preload. Patients with severe hypotension associated with cardiogenic shock require immediate pressor therapy to maintain perfusion to the brain and heart while volume and inotropic support is initiated.

The use of these principles is illustrated by the following case:

PROBLEM: POSTOPERATIVE HYPOTENSION

Eighteen hours after repair of an abdominal aortic aneurysm in a 72-year-old male, the following clinical situation exists.

Clinical Presentation

Physical Examination (Objective Findings)

The patient's heart rate is 100 bpm, and his systolic blood pressure is 85 mm Hg, with a mean arterial pressure of 70 mm Hg. Cardiac output is 2.8 L/min, cardiac index is 1.4 L/min/m^2, PAOP is 16 mm Hg, and CVP is 15 cm H_2O. Maximum venous oxygen consumption is 30 mm Hg, and hematocrit is 32%, with a mean arterial O_2 saturation of 94%. Arterial blood gases reflect a pH of 7.3, Po_2 of 75 mm Hg, and Pco_2 of 36 mm Hg on 40% forced inspired oxygen (FIo_2). The patient's urine output has been 10 ml over the previous 3 hours. Calculated variables are an SVR of 1571 dynes cm^2/sec, a rate-pressure product of 8500, and an LVSWI of 13.3 g/min/m^2.

Assessment

This patient does not appear to be hypovolemic. In addition, the measured variable of PAOP, which is used to estimate preload, is at the upper level of normal. However, since PAOP may not accurately reflect end-diastolic volume in a variety of circumstances, a fluid challenge with calculation of a change in stroke work index may be of benefit. The patient received a 500 ml bolus of lactated Ringer's solution over 10 minutes. After the fluid bolus, the important indices that changed were blood pressure, now 90 mm Hg systolic with a mean arterial pressure of 80 mm Hg, cardiac index, 1.5; PAOP, 20 mm Hg; and CVP, 19 cm H_2O. His SVR remained elevated at 1626 dynes cm^2/sec. The rate-pressure product increased to 9000, indicating a slight increase in myocardial O_2 consumption. The LVSWI was now 16.3 g/min/m^2. Referring to Figure 5-18, one can plot the LVSWI before and after the fluid bolus, which yields a line with a very flat slope, indicating that the patient has not benefitted from the additional fluid bolus. Management should consist of afterload reduction and inotropic support.

Management

Because of the patient's low systolic blood pressure, it was not possible to attempt afterload reduction. Therefore inotropic support was initiated with dopamine, which was titrated to a dosage of 7.5 μg/kg/min. With this therapy the patient's blood pressure increased to 105 to 110 mm Hg systolic, and his cardiac index increased to 2 L/min/m^2. His wedge pressure decreased to 18 mm Hg, and systemic vascular resistance remained elevated at 1360 dynes/cm^2/sec. A repeat MVo_2 measurement was 35 mm Hg, and the patient's urine output increased to 30 ml over the next hour. The patient apparently benefitted from inotropic support. However, his rate-pressure product increased to 11,000, indicating a further increase in myocardial O_2 consumption.

Because the patient's SVR remained elevated, afterload reduction was attempted. Nitroprusside was started and titrated to a systolic blood pressure of approximately 95 to 100 mm Hg. After stabilization, repeat measurements showed the MVo_2 had increased to 38 mm Hg, with a cardiac index of 2.8 L/min/m^2 and an SVR of 856 dynes/cm^2/sec. The patient's dopamine dosage was weaned to 5 μg/kg/min. His urine output increased to 30 to 40 ml/hr over the next several hours. The patient's systolic blood pressure was 95 mm Hg and the heart rate was approximately 100 bpm, for a rate-pressure product of 9500, indicating a decrease in myocardial O_2 consumption presumably secondary to afterload reduction.

The appropriate goals of therapy for this type of patient remain controversial. Shoemaker and colleagues[122] have reported that high-risk patients who have survived noncardiac general surgery have cardiac indices averaging 4.5 L/min/m^2, O_2 delivery (Do_2) in excess of 600 ml/min/m^2, and Vo_2 in excess of 10 ml/min/m^2. Nonsurvivors maintained relatively normal values in the immediate postoperative period. These increased levels of flow and O_2 transport, which are normal compensatory responses, have been recommended as appropriate therapeutic goals. In another report these same authors noted significant reduction in morbidity and mortality when these goals were obtained in a protocol group compared to a conventionally treated cohort.[42a]

Other clinicians have recommended that such patients should be resuscitated to the point where O_2 consumption is no longer delivery dependent. Such recommendations are based on observations in critically ill patients in whom O_2 consumption continues to increase as O_2 delivery increases (i.e., flow-dependent O_2 consumption). Under nonpathologic conditions, the critical Do_2 point is estimated to be 8 ml/kg/min, a point well below the normal Do_2 range. Stressed patients are typically hypermetabolic with Vo_2 values in the supranormal range. In some critically ill patients, the critical Do_2 point has been estimated to be in the range of 15 to 21 ml/kg/min. Clinically observed Do_2 values often fall within this range. The implication is that failure to meet this elevated demand will result in organ ischemia. Critics of this theory maintain that the methodology used to demonstrate flow-dependent O_2 consumption is flawed, and that if patients were followed with indirect calorimetry, these changes would not be observed. When Vo_2 is not directly measured but rather calculated as the product of cardiac output and arteriovenous oxygen content ($C[AV]o_2$), the expected coefficient of correlation between Vo_2 and Do_2 is 0.71. This is expected, since both Vo_2 and Do_2 have in common cardiac output and Cao_2. Therefore the significance of the coefficients comparing Vo_2 with Do_2 should be determined as greater than 0.71 rather than greater than zero. The physician should be skeptical of any calculated Vo_2 that suggests flow dependency but that is not verified by a directly measured Vo_2. Certainly patients with abnormal perfusion indices should be resuscitated to a point where perfusion is deemed adequate. The goal of therapy should be to avoid an increasing cellular O_2 debt. The value of applying these principles to patients who do not have a clinically obvious perfusion abnormality remains unproven in large clinical trials. Clearly attempts should be made to resuscitate patients to normal values; attempts to achieve supranormal levels currently remain a matter of individual prejudice.

When cardiogenic shock is diagnosed, cardiac ischemia and infarction must be suspected as a cause. A 12-lead electrocardiogram (ECG) should be examined for evidence of ischemia. If this diagnosis is made, the use of thrombolytic therapy must be considered early. Further diagnostic evaluation should be performed concurrently with therapy to determine whether definitive treatment with angioplasty or urgent bypass surgery is warranted. Mechanical assistive devices, such as the intra-aortic balloon pump, may be beneficial in augmenting coronary artery blood flow while decreasing cardiac work.

Summary

In treating a hypotensive patient, the physician must remember that fluid resuscitation is of primary importance. The concept of maximizing preload followed by judicious use of afterload reduction, sometimes with inotropic support, is also important. The physician must always remember the effects of the treatment regimen on variables such as myocardial O_2 consumption, because increased peripheral perfusion may occur at the expense of increased myocardial shock.

SEPTIC SHOCK

Septic shock, with its incidence increasing 20-fold over the past 25 years, is now the leading cause of death in intensive care units.[88,95] Because of our improved ability to support critically ill patients, many more individuals are now at risk for infection-related complications. Also, patients who are immunosuppressed because of chronic disease or drug therapy are a group at substantial risk. Any organism capable of being a pathogen can precipitate a septic shock state. Although gram-negative organisms currently are the most common cause of septic shock, shock states caused by gram-positive organisms, viruses, and fungi have recently been reported.[119,141,142]

Patients in septic shock manifest a state in which the primary defect is a cellular defect in O_2 metabolism. Although hemodynamic changes often are first recognized, Siegel and associates[124] noted that patients usually manifest metabolic derangements as a prelude to the shock state. The metabolic alterations may cause changes in cardiac and vascular function, altering perfusion and thus resulting in further derangements in cellular function. Because many patients with sepsis have altered O_2 consumption, as measured by narrow arteriovenous O_2 differences, early investigators presumed the defect to be secondary to increased regional arteriovenous shunting. However, Finley and associates[42] and Wright and colleagues[154] have shown by xenon clearance methods that very little arteriovenous shunting occurs in a septic patient, because capillary blood flow is maintained at either normal or increased levels. Mela and others[90] have demonstrated that in endotoxic shock, cellular function seems to be directly inhibited, resulting in decreased mitochondrial O_2 consumption. More recent studies have questioned the validity of this model, specifically the extremely high doses of endotoxin that were used. In addition, Ascher and coworkers have reported normal mitochodrial function during early sepsis.[7] Current theories favor a maldistribution of blood flow that may be secondary to factors such as capillary obstruction by microemboli or tissue edema and intense regional vasoconstriction. The end result is decreased O_2 consumption and a decreased O_2 extraction ratio.

The clinical hemodynamic syndrome associated with septic shock is not constant. The patients may be in either a hyperdynamic or a hypodynamic state. The syndrome recognized most often is the hyperdynamic state, in which CO measurements typically are at least twice normal (thus the term *hyperdynamic*). This patient often is hyperventilating, with a resultant respiratory alkalosis; has warm, dry extremities; and is oliguric. Physiologically, inappropirate regional vasodilatation exists, which results in a nonphysiologic distribution of CO, with accompanying systemic hypotension. In contrast, hypodynamic patients have a decreased CO, increased SVR, and cool extremities. The major determinant of the clinical findings depends on whether the peripheral vasculature is dilated or constricted. Generally, patients who are normovolemic during the onset of sepsis tend to become hyperdynamic, whereas hypovolemic patients display a hypodynamic circulation. In addition, patients in hyperdynamic shock who are left untreated, with either inadequate fluid resuscitation or failure to evaluate and treat the underlying cause, eventually succumb to their septic insult in a hypodynamic state.

Although sepsis normally produces a low systemic vascular resistance and elevated cardiac output, ample evidence suggests that myocardial function is depressed. In a group of patients in hyperdynamic sepsis, Parker and Parrillo[100] noted that in each patient, CO was elevated but ejection fractions were subnormal, a finding corroborated by Weisel and associates.[150] This was presumed to be secondary to a circulating myocardial depressant factor affecting contractility.[1,75,100] Interpretation of these and similar studies is confounded by the inability to measure contractility accurately and the difficulty in unmasking the effects of preload, afterload, heart rate, and other potential mediators of myocardial dysfunction, such as ischemia or ionic disturbances. Although such a substance has not been identified, other investigators have reported that its effect is serum transferable and reversible by hemofiltration.[51,107] In an in vitro model, DeMeules[33] has further characterized this defect and demonstrated that a serum-mediated factor causes changes in sodium fast channel conductance.

Diagnosis

Because mortality can be decreased when sepsis is diagnosed and treated before circulatory collapse,[4] the physician must be able to recognize clinical changes that may precede profound shock. Normally, glucose intolerance, tachycardia, hyperventilation, temperature changes, and neurologic signs precede circulatory collapse.[38]

One of the earliest signs of septic metabolic derangement is glucose intolerance. When a critically ill patient exhibits hyperglycemia or glycosuria without an obvious cause, sepsis should be suspected. This is an especially useful sign in patients receiving intravenous hyperalimentation. Work by Clowes and associates[25] has suggested this to be secondary to increased peripheral insulin resistance and circulating glucagon levels.

Other early signs of sepsis include hyperventilation and concomitant respiratory alkalosis. This is presumed to be secondary to an alteration in the respiratory center caused by circulating bacteria or toxins. In addition, patients often show increasing irritability and irrational behavior, which generally are unexplained by such measurements as arterial Po_2. Although hyperthermia is often present,[36] patients may be normothermic or hypothermic. The presence of hypothermia may be as important an indicator of early sepsis as sustained temperature elevation.[9] Increasing fluid requirements secondary to third space losses may be another indication of occult sepsis. In children, decreasing platelet counts have been shown to be a reliable early indicator of a preseptic state.[109]

Although all these signs and symptoms may occur early in sepsis, they also occur in other clinical states, which limits their usefulness and makes the diagnosis of early sepsis difficult. Siegel and associates[124] have systematically studied septic patients, using a series of physiologic and metabolic parameters they believe allow segregation of patients into various clinical states before obvious clinical deterioration. Treatment of a septic patient should involve a multisystem approach, because the hemodynamic consequences reflect a severe metabolic derangement.

Management

The mainstay of treatment in a septic patient should be eradication of the septic foci. Historically, MacLean and associates[85] noted that when a drainable septic site was present, there was a 48% survival rate from the septic event. The survival rate decreased to 23% if no drainable focus of infection was found. Along with debridement and drainage, the appropriate use of antibiotics is extremely important. Altemeier, Todd, and Wellfund[4] have shown that appropriate selection of antibiotics resulted in a 28% mortality from septic shock. In a similar group of patients treated with inappropriate antibiotics for the isolated pathogen, mortality was 54%. Myerowitz and coworkers[96] and McHenry and associates[89] have shown similar results, reducing mortality from 67% to 21% with appropriate use of antibiotics.

Before the pathogen is isolated, antibiotics should be chosen according to the presumed site of sepsis. If the abdomen is the suspected source, antibiotics that cover gram-negative and anaerobic bacteria should be administered. In addition, ampicillin or ampicillin/saldactin often is added for enterococcal coverage. If the genitourinary tract is the suspected septic focus, gram-negative coverage should be instituted. A Gram's stain of spun urine can provide useful information. Treatment of wound infections can also be guided by the use of Gram's stains. Wound infection associated with a high fever, shaking chills, crepitus, and a thin, watery discharge should always raise suspicion of a *Clostridium* infection. Immediate high-dose penicillin (24 million U/day) with surgical debridement is mandatory. Synergistic facial infections, such as Fournier's disease, require broad-spectrum gram-negative and anaerobic coverage and aggressive surgical therapy. Treatment for pulmonary sources usually can be guided by examination of the sputum. Outpatient-acquired infections often are gram positive, whereas inpatient infections frequently are gram negative. Gram-negative organisms, such as *Pseudomonas* species, are particularly prevalent in some critical care units. Rapidly progressive, atypical pneumonias should lead the physician to suspect Legionnaire's disease or other atypical pneumonias and to institute appropriate treatment. Immunocompromised patients are particularly susceptible to *Pneumocystis carinii* and fungal infections. In patients with neurologic changes, spinal fluid must be obtained for study.

Whether the patient is in a hyperdynamic or a hypodynamic state, treatment should follow the same principles as for other kinds of shock. The physician should first maximize intravascular volume. Fluid requirements are greater in septic shock than in other forms of shock because of increased third space losses secondary to changes in capillary permeability. For volume expansion, balanced salt solutions are probably superior to colloid solutions, because albumin may rapidly equilibrate between the interstitial and intravascular spaces. Urine output may not be a reliable indicator of renal perfusion; patients in septic shock often demonstrate a paradoxic diuresis despite hypovolemia. This is thought to be secondary to changes in intrarenal blood flow, in which blood is shunted from the juxtacortical nephrons to the juxtamedullary nephrons, resulting in decreased sodium retention and increased water clearance. Failure to maintain adequate volume despite apparently adequate urine output may result in prerenal azotemia and a renal insult acute secondary to hypovolemia.

The use of vasodilators was once a popular treatment for patients in septic shock, because the defect was presumed to be increased arteriovenous shunting secondary to intense arteriolar constriction. The vasoconstriction was thought to result from catecholamine release in response to stress and sepsis. It was believed that by releasing this arterial vasoconstriction, arteriovenous shunting would be decreased and perfusion corrected. Maldistribution of flow may potentially be corrected by judicious vasodilatation therapy, but it should not be attempted before volume correction.

Some patients require vasopressor support when shock intervenes and cardiac and cerebral perfusion are jeopardized. This form of therapy should be reserved for patients with marked hemodynamic decompensation and should be used in concert with or preceded by restoration of blood volume. Vasopressors may exacerbate the maldistribution of cardiac output, resulting in increased organ ischemia and damage. Norepinephrine appears to be the drug of choice to treat shock secondary to sepsis. Several studies have documented improved hemodynamic indices without deleterious renal effects.[34,49] Usually only those patients with normal lactate levels before therapy show improvement. Some recommend concomitant administration of renal-dose dopamine as a mechanism to maintain renal blood flow. Some evidence supports the hypothesis that nitric oxide (NO) may be the final mediator of sepsis-induced vasodilatation.[70] Administration of NO synthase inhibitors results in rapid, complete restoration of blood pressure in animals made hypotensive by TNF, IL-1, and endotoxin. Similar salutary effects have been noted in a few patients refractory to conventional pressor therapy.[103] Clinical use should be approached with caution because of the lack of adequate toxicology and pharmacology studies in animals.[97] Wide-scale NO inhibition may result in further microcirculatory derangement, rendering some organs, such as the gut, even more ischemic.

Sepsis-related mortality has remained significant despite our enhanced ability to care for critically ill patients. Failure of conservative standard treatment protocols has prompted a substantial amount of both clinical and laboratory research. The ideal agent or treatment would restore systemic arterial pressure, normalize pulmonary vascular resistance, improve cardiac function, improve organ perfusion, decrease tissue edema, inhibit neutrophil priming and activation, and ultimately stop progression of organ damage and thus improve survival. Pivotal to designing such treatments is an understanding of the basic pathophysiologic mechanisms that control the host response to infection. It is unlikely that any one therapy will be able to achieve all the above, and the successful regimen probably will be a cocktail of various agents used to block or augment various aspects of the cascading host response, which is discussed in Chapter 10. As our knowledge of this response has evolved, clinical trials of various therapies have been performed and are discussed below.

The use of steroids in septic shock is no longer controversial and should be avoided. Experimental work by Hinshaw and associates[63,64] demonstrated increased survival in septic primates who were treated with a combination of methylprednisolone sodium succinate and gentamicin after receiving a lethal dose of *Escherichia coli*. The doses of steroids used in these studies ranged from 30 to 50 mg/kg of methylprednisolone sodium succinate in bolus infusion. In a prospective, randomized study, Schumer used high-dose steroids and showed a decrease in mortality from 38% to 10% in a group of patients with sepsis.[117] Other studies have failed to show the beneficial effect of steroids in septic shock.[17,81,134,152] These prospective, randomized, blinded studies failed to duplicate Schumer's results. Steroid use was associated with improved early survival in one of the studies and occasional but short-term hemodynamic benefit, but it did not alter long-term hospital mortality in any of these more recent studies.

The use of narcotic antagonists such as naloxone is based on the work of Faden and Holiday,[40] who reported in 1978 that some hemodynamic consequences of sepsis could possibly be mediated through endorphin-like substances. They thought that by blocking these endorphins with naloxone, they might block the hemodynamic response. Experimental work has shown some improvement in hemodynamic variables in animals and humans after infusion of large doses of naloxone.[102,106,108] However, a prospective, randomized trial in early hyperdynamic septic shock was clinically efficacious in improving the hemodynamic profile of only a subgroup of those treated and did not improve survival.[111]

Recent understanding of the cascade of cytokines involved in the response to gram-negative infection presumably mediated through endotoxin,[37] along with the advent of recombinant DNA technology, has allowed the trial of several forms of antibody therapy. Two prospective trials of anti-endotoxin antibody in patients with sepsis have just been concluded.[55,155] These studies were based on Ziegler's 1984 report in which antiserum to a mutant *E. coli* strain was noted to reduce mortality in a group of septic patients.[156] Although both trials concluded that the antibody was efficacious in a subgroup of patients (a different group in each trial), design flaws and questionable data analysis techniques hinder belief in the investigators' claims of efficacy.[12,153] This, in conjunction with the cost of therapy, will limit their use until further clinical testing can be completed. Lack of clear efficacy may have been due to the brief circulating half-life of endotoxin, which may have already initiated the cytokine response, as well as by the possibile existence of other causative organisms besides gram-negative bacteria. Other targets for treating septic shock include neutralizing antibodies to C5a, TNF, and IL-1 receptors as well as platelet-activating factor antagonists, prostaglandin and leukotriene synthesis blockers,[43] and blockade of endothelial cell/leukocyte adhesion molecules.[35] Many of these agents are currently in clinical trials.[27,147]

Therapy aimed at improving cellular O_2 utilization has been less rewarding. Current interest involves maximizing oxygen delivery so that consumption is not flow dependent. As with other forms of shock, data confirming the efficacy of this approach are lacking. The administration of insulin, potassium, and glucose, as recommended by Clowes[26] and Weisul,[151] has not been proved to be beneficial.

In general, the care of a septic shock patient should involve appropriate antibiotic therapy, eradication of the septic foci, and hemodynamic support. As in the treatment of any critically ill patient, ventilatory and O_2

transport parameters should be followed and appropriate treatment instituted. Additional therapy intended to modify the host response awaits further clinical testing.

CIRCULATORY SHOCK

Previous sections discussed shock as a manifestation of loss of circulating volume in hypovolemic shock, pump failure in cardiogenic shock, and cellular dysfunction and utilization of oxygen in septic shock. However, some shock patients have an underlying defect in the circulatory or vascular system. Spinal shock secondary to loss of the resistance vessels' ability to respond to a sympathetic discharge occurs both under spinal anesthesia and in patients with spinal cord injury. The loss of sympathetic tone of the affected areas results in unopposed vasodilatation and inability to respond to appropriate stimuli with vasoconstriction. The resultant relative hypovolemia is secondary to expansion of the capacitance circuit, that is, decreased venomotor tone. Treatment for these patients, when they are hypotensive, should consist of volume loading, because they are relatively hypovolemic. Use of alpha-agonist agents is restricted to patients with deleteriously low blood pressure; these agents should be used only to ensure adequate cardiac perfusion.

Another form of circulatory failure is seen in anaphylactic shock. This is an antigen-antibody–mediated response in which released vasoactive substances cause a variety of vascular changes. Early in the disease course, vascular collapse is associated with a low SVR and a high CO. Because of increased vascular permeability, pulmonary edema may result, and a hypovolemic state ensues secondary to increased losses of plasma water. An intense bronchospasm is associated with these hemodynamic changes. Treatment of these patients should include immediate airway management and treatment with an epinephrine-type drug. This increases CO by an inotropic effect; the drug's alpha-agonist properties cause increased SVR, thus increasing blood pressure, and its beta-agonist activity results in bronchodilatation, helping to decrease bronchospasm. Additional use of other bronchodilators, such as aminophylline, is often necessary. Aside from pharmacologic treatment, resuscitation should always include volume replacement, because these patients are hypovolemic secondary to their altered vascular permeability. The time period of altered vascular permeability is short, but these patients can exhibit relatively marked hypovolemia as a result of interstitial fluid losses.

Summary

As outlined in previous sections, treatment of a patient in shock involves analysis of the hemodynamic profile to determine the immediate cause of the hypotension or decreased perfusion. Classifying the patient into one of the four major categories of shock allows the physician to begin resuscitation. Whatever the etiology of shock, however, the underlying cause cannot be adequately assessed or treated until hypovolemia has either been treated or ruled out as a cause. In critically ill patients, the physician often sees a subset of patients in whom the shock state is a manifestation of multiple abnormalities, in both blood volume and cardiac function. The preceding sections should provide a method for evaluating these patients and the means to institute appropriate therapy.

REFERENCES

1. Abel FL: Does the heart fail in endotoxin shock? *Circ Shock* 30(1):5, 1990.
2. Aberg M, Hedner U, Bergentz SE: Effect of dextran on factor VIII (antihemophilic factor and platelet function), *Ann Surg* 189:243, 1979.
3. Ahlquist RP: Adrenergic drugs. In Diel VA, editor: *Pharmacology in medicine,* vol 2, New York, 1958, McGraw-Hill.
4. Altemeier WA, Todd JC, Wellfund WI: Gram-negative septicemia: a growing threat, *Ann Surg* 166:530, 1967.
5. Archibald EW, McLean WS: Observations upon shock, with particular reference to the condition as seen in war surgery, *Ann Surg* 66:280, 1917.
6. Asch MJ, Meserol PM, Masm AD et al: Regional blood flow in the burned unanesthetized dog, *Inst Surg Res Ann Rep* 25:1, 1971.
7. Ascher EF, Garrison RN, Ratcliffe DJ et al: Endotoxin, cellular function, and nutrient blood flow, *Arch Surg* 118:441, 1983.
8. Bainbridge FA: On some cardiac reflexes, *J Physiol* 48:332, 1914.
9. Barois A, Bowdain JL: Les septicemies avec hypothermie. In Goulon M, Rapin M, editors: *Reanimation et medecine d'urgence,* Paris, 1973, Expansion.
10. Barone JE, Snyder AB: Treatment strategies in shock: use of oxygen transport measurements, *Heart Lung* 20(1):81, 1991.
11. Bauer C: On the respiratory function of hemoglobin, *Rev Physiol Biochem Pharmacol* 70:1, 1974.
12. Baumgartner JD: Monoclonal anti-endotoxin antibodies for the treatment of gram-negative bacteremia and septic shock, *Eur J Clin Microbiol Infect Dis* 9(10):711, 1990.
13. Baylis WM: On the local reactions of the arterial wall to changes of internal pressure, *J Physiol* 28:220, 1902.
14. Berryhill RE, Benumof JL: PEEP-induced discrepancy between pulmonary arterial wedge pressure and left arterial pressure: the effects of controlled vs. spontaneous ventilation and compliant vs. noncompliant lungs in the dog, *Anesthesiology* 51:303, 1979.
15. Bisonni RS, Holtgrave DR, Lawler F et al: Colloids versus crystalloids in fluid resuscitation: an analysis of randomized controlled trials, *J Fam Pract* 32(4):387, 1991.
16. Blinks JR, Koch-Weser J: Analysis of effect of changes in rate and rhythm upon myocardial contractility, *J Pharmacol Exp Ther* 134:373, 1961.
17. Bone RC, Fisher CJ Jr, Clemmer TP et al: A controlled clinical trial of high-dose methylprednisolone in the treatment of severe sepsis and septic shock, *N Engl J Med* 317(11):653, 1987.
18. Braunwald E: Vasodilator therapy: a physiologic approach to the treatment of heart failure, *N Engl J Med* 297:331, 1977.
19. Bretschneider JH, Hellige G: Pathophysiologie der Ventrikelkontraktion-Kontraktiliat, Inotropie. Suffizienzgrad, und Arbeitsokonomie des Hezzons, *Xech Dtsch Gos Kreislauffursch* 42:14, 1976.

20 Calvin JE, Driedger AA, Sibbald WJ: Does the pulmonary capillary wedge pressure predict left ventricular preload in the critically ill? *Crit Care Med* 9:437, 1981.
21 Carey LC, Lowery BD, Cloutier CT: Hemorrhagic shock, *Curr Probl Surg* 1, 1971.
22 Carr CG, Pesley TJ, Schroter RC et al: *The mechanics of circulation,* New York, 1978, Oxford University Press.
23 Carrico CJ, Canizaro PC, Shires GT: Fluid resuscitation following injury: rationale for the use of balanced salt solutions, *Crit Care Med* 4:46, 1976.
24 Clowes GH: Oxygen transport and utilization in fulminating sepsis and septic shock. In Hersay SG, Delgeurico LRM, McConn R, editors: *Septic shock in man,* Boston, 1971, Little, Brown.
25 Clowes GH, Martin H, Walji S et al: Blood insulin responses to blood glucose levels in high output septic shock, *Am J Surg* 135:577, 1978.
26 Clowes GH, O'Donnell TF, Ryan NT et al: Energy metabolism in sepsis: treatment based on different patterns in shock and high output state, *Ann Surg* 179:684, 1974.
27 Cohen J: Antibodies to tumor necrosis factor in the treatment of severe sepsis: rationale and early clinical experience, *Prog Clin Biol Res* 367:187, 1991.
28 Cohn JN, Burke LP: Nitroprusside, *Ann Intern Med* 91:752, 1979.
29 Davidson I, Gelin LE, Hedman L et al: Hemodilution and recovery from experimental intestinal shock in rats: a comparison of the efficacy of three colloids and one electrolyte solution, *Crit Care Med* 9:42, 1981.
30 Davis JW, Shackford SR, Holbrook TL: Base deficit as a sensitive indicator of compensated shock and tissue oxygen utilization, *Surg Gynecol Obstet* 173(6):473, 1991.
31 Davison R, Parker M, Harrison RA: The validity of determinations of pulmonary wedge pressure during mechanical ventilation, *Chest* 73:352, 1978.
32 DelGeurico LRM, Cohn JD: Monitoring: methods and significance, *Surg Clin North Am* 56(4):977, 1976.
33 DeMeules JE: A physiologic explanation for cardiac deterioration in septic shock, *J Surg Res* 36:553, 1984.
34 Desjars P, Pinaud M, Bugnon D et al: Norepinephrine therapy has no deleterious renal effects in human septic shock, *Crit Care Med* 17(5):426, 1989.
35 Dinarello CA: The proinflammatory cytokines interleukin-1 and tumor necrosis factor and treatment of the septic shock syndrome, *J Infect Dis* 163(6):1177, 1991.
36 Dinarello CA, Wolff SM: Pathogenesis of fever in man, *N Engl J Med* 298:607, 1978.
37 Dunn DL: Role of endotoxin and host cytokines in septic shock, *Chest* 100(suppl 3):164S, 1991.
38 Dussar J, Regnier B, Darragon T et al: Hyperkinetic shock in viral and pneumococcal pneumonias, *Int Care Med* 5:59, 1979.
39 Elliott LA, Ledgerwood AM, Lucas CE et al: Role of Fluosol-DA 20% in prehospital resuscitation, *Crit Care Med* 17(2):166, 1989.
40 Faden AI, Holiday JW: Experimental endotoxin shock: the pathophysiologic function of endorphins and treatment with opiate antagonists, *J Infect Dis* 42:229, 1980.
41 Feola M, Simoni J, Tran R et al: Nephrotoxicity of hemoglobin solutions, *Biomater Artif Cells Artif Organs* 18(2):233, 1990.
42 Finley RJ, Duff JH, Holliday RL et al: Capillary muscle blood flow in human sepsis, *Surgery* 78:87, 1975.
42a Fleming A, Bishop M, Shoemaker W et al: Prospective trial of supranormal valves as goals of resuscitation in severe trauma, *Arch Surg* 127:1175, 1992.
43 Fletcher JR, Herman CM, Ramwell PW: Improved survival in endotoxemia with aspirin and endomethacin pretreatment, *Surg Forum* 27:11, 1976.
44 Folkow B: Description of the myogenic hypothesis, *Circ Res* 1:279, 1964.
45 Folkow B, Neil E: *Circulation,* New York, 1971, Oxford University Press.
46 Forrester JS, Diamond GA, Swan HJ et al: Correlative classification of clinical and hemodynamic function after acute myocardial infarction, *Am J Cardiol* 39:137, 1977.
47 Foster RS Jr, Costanza MC, Foster JC et al: Adverse relationship between blood transfusions and survival after colectomy for colon cancer, *Cancer* 55(6):1195, 1986.
48 Frank O: Zur Dynamik des Harzmuskels, *Z Biol* 32:370, 1895.
49 Fukuoka T, Nishimura M, Imanaka H et al: Effects of norepinephrine on renal function in septic patients with normal and elevated serum lactate levels, *Crit Care Med* 17(11):1104, 1989.
50 Gold MS, Russo J, Tissot M et al: Comparison of hetastarch to albumin for perioperative bleeding in patients undergoing abdominal aortic aneurysm surgery: a prospective, randomized study, *Ann Surg* 211(4):482, 1990.
51 Gomez A, Wang R, Unruh H et al: Hemofiltration reverses left ventricular dysfunction during sepsis in dogs, *Anesthesiology* 73(4):67, 1990.
52 Green JF: Determinants of systemic blood flow. In Guyton AC, Young EB, editors: *Cardiovascular physiology III,* vol 18, Baltimore, 1979, University Park Press.
53 Greenburg AG, Schooley M, Peskin GW: Improved retention of stroma-free hemoglobin solution by chemical modification, *J Trauma* 17:501, 1977.
54 Greenfield AD: Survey of evidence for active neurogenic vasodilation in man, *Fed Proc* 25:1607, 1966.
55 Greenman RL, Schein RM, Martin MA et al: A controlled clinical trial of E5 murine monoclonal IgM antibody to endotoxin in the treatment of gram-negative sepsis. The XOMA Sepsis Study Group, *JAMA* 266(8):1097, 1991.
56 Gruber UF: Dextran and the prevention of postoperative thromboembolic complications, *Surg Clin North Am* 55:679, 1975.
57 Gunnar W, Jonasson O, Merlotti G et al: Head injury and hemorrhagic shock: studies of the blood-brain barrier and intracranial pressure after resuscitation with normal saline solution, 3% saline solution, and dextran 40, *Surgery* 103(4):398, 1988.
58 Guyton AC: *Textbook of medical physiology,* ed 6, Philadelphia, 1981, WB Saunders.
59 Halvorsen L, Gunther RA, Dubick MA et al: Dose response characteristics of hypertonic saline dextran solutions, *J Trauma* 31(6):785, 1991.
60 Hauser CJ, Shoemaker WC, Turpin I et al: Oxygen transport responses to colloids and crystalloids in criticaly ill surgical patients, *Surg Gynecol Obstet* 50:811, 1980.
61. Herbert P, Tinker J: Inotropic drugs in acute circulatory failure, *Int Care Med* 6:101, 1980.
62 Hill NS, Antman EM, Green LH et al: Intravenous nitroglycerin: a review of pharmacolgy, indications, therapeutic effects, and complications, *Chest* 79:69, 1981.
63 Hinshaw LB, Archer LT, Beller-Todd BK et al: Survival of primates in LD^{100} septic shock following steroid/antibiotic therapy, *J Surg Res* 28:151, 1980.
64 Hinshaw LB, Beller-Todd BK, Archer LT et al: Effectiveness of steroid/antibiotic treatment in primates administered LD^{100} *Escherichia coli, Ann Surg* 19:51, 1981.
65 Holcroft JW, Vassar MJ, Perry CA et al: Use of a 7.5% NaCl/6% dextran 70 solution in the resuscitation of injured patients in the emergency room, *Prog Clin Biol Res* 299:331, 1989.
66 Johnson PC: Autoregulation of blood flow, *Circ Res* 15(suppl 1):1, 1964.
67 Katz LN: The performance of the heart, *Circulation* 21:483, 1960.
68 Kersting F, Follath F, Moulds R et al: A comparison of cardio-

vascular effects of dobutamine and isoprenaline after open heart surgery, *Br Heart J* 38:622, 1976.

69 Keul J, Doll E, Steim H et al: Uber den Stoffwechsel des menschlichen Herzems. I. De Substratversorgung des gesunden menschlichen Herzens in Ruhe, während und nach körperlicher Arbeit, *Pflügers Arch Ges Physiol* 282:1, 1965.

70 Kilbourn RG, Jubran A, Gross SS et al: Reversal of endotoxin-mediated shock by NG-methyl-L-arginine, an inhibitor of nitric oxide synthesis, *Biochem Biophys Res Commun* 172(3):1132, 1990.

71 Kilmartin JV, Rossi-Bernard L: Interactions of hemoglobin with hydrogen ions, carbon dioxide, and organic phosphates, *Physiol Rev* 53:836, 1976.

72 Kohter H, Kirch W, Weihrauch JR et al: Macroamylasemia after treatment with hydroxyethyl starch, *Eur J Clin Invest* 7:205, 1977.

73 Kuhn KL, Kline HJ, Goodman P et al: Effects of isoproterenol on hemodynamic alterations, myocardial metabolism, and coronary flow in experimental acute myocardial infarction with shock, *Am Heart J* 77:772, 1969.

74 Lefcoe MS, Sibbald WJ, Holliday RL: Wedged balloon catheter angiography in the critical care unit, *Crit Care Med* 7:449, 1979.

75 Lefer AM: Properties of cardioinhibitory factors produced in shock, *Fed Proc* 37:2734, 1978.

76 Lewis BS, Gotsmann MS: Current concepts of left ventricular relaxation and compliance, *Am Heart J* 99:101, 1980.

77 Linko K, Makelainen A: Hydroxyethyl starch 120, dextran 70, and acetated Ringer's solution: hemodilution, albumin, colloid osmotic pressure, and fluid balance following replacement of blood loss in pigs, *Acta Anaesthesiol Scand* 32(3):228, 1988.

78 Lister J, McNeil JF, Marshall YC et al: Transcapillary refilling and hemorrhage in normal man: basal rates and volumes—effect of norepinephrine, *Ann Surg* 158:698, 1963.

79 Looker D, Abbott-Brown D, Cozart P et al: A human recombinant haemoglobin designed for use as a blood substitute, *Nature* 356(6366):258, 1992.

80 Lucas CE, Ledgerwood AM: The fluid problem in the critically ill, *Surg Clin North Am* 63(2):439, 1983.

81 Luce JM, Montgomery AB, Marks JD et al: Ineffectiveness of high-dose methylprednisolone in preventing parenchymal lung injury and improving mortality in patients with septic shock, *Am Rev Respir Dis* 138(1):62, 1988.

82 MacDonald DA: *Blood flow in arteries,* ed 2, London, 1974, Edward Arnold.

83 MacLean LD: Shock: causes and management of circulatory collapse. In Sabiston DC, editor: *Textbook of surgery,* ed 11, Philadelphia, 1977, WB Saunders.

84 MacLean LD, Duff JH, Scott HM et al: Treatment of shock in man based on hemodynamic diagnosis, *Surg Gynecol Obstet* 120:1, 1965.

85 MacLean LD, Mulligan WG, McLean APH et al: Patterns of septic shock in man: a detailed study of 56 patients, *Ann Surg* 166:543, 1967.

86 Marty AT: Hyperoncotic albumin therapy, *Surg Gynecol Obstet* 139:105, 1974.

87 Mattox KL, Maningas PA, Moore EE et al: Prehospital hypertonic saline/dextran infusion for post-traumatic hypotension: the USA Multicenter Trial, *Ann Surg* 213(5):482, 1991.

88 McCabe WR: Gram-negative bacteremia, *Adv Intern Med* 19:135, 1974.

89 McHenry MC, Gavin TL, Hawk WA et al: Gram-negative bacteremia: variable clinical course and useful prognostic factors, *Cleve Clin O* 42:15, 1975.

90 Mela L, Bacalzo LV Jr, Miller LD: Defective oxidative metabolism of rat liver mitochondria in hemorrhagic and endotoxic shock, *Am J Physiol* 220:571, 1971.

91 Mellander S, Louis DH: Effect of hemorrhagic shock on the reactivity of resistance and capacitance vessels and on capillary filtration transfer in cat skeletal muscle, *Circ Res* 13:105, 1963.

92 Mountcastle VB, editor: *Medical physiology,* St Louis, 1974, Mosby.

93 Moyer CA: *Fluid balance,* Chicago, 1954, Yearbook.

94 Munsch CM, MacIntyre E, Machin SJ et al: Hydroxyethyl starch: an alternative to plasma for postoperative volume expansion after cardiac surgery, *Br J Surg* 75(7):675, 1988.

95 Murray MJ, Kumar M: Sepsis and septic shock: deadly complications that are on the rise, *Postgrad Med* 90(1):199, 1991.

96 Myerowitz RL, Mederios A, O'Brien TF: Recent experience with bacillemia due to gram-negative organisms, *J Infect Dis* 124:239, 1971.

97 Nava E, Palmer RM, Moncada S: Inhibition of nitric oxide synthesis in septic shock: how much is beneficial? *Lancet* 338(8782-8783):1555, 1991.

98 Nickerson M: Sympathetic blockade in the therapy of shock, *Am J Cardiol* 12:919, 1963.

99 Pace NL: A critique of flow-directed pulmonary arterial catheterization, *Anesthesiology* 47:455, 1971.

100 Parker MM, Parrillo JE: Septic shock: hemodynamics and pathogenesis, *JAMA* 250(24):3324, 1983.

101 Pearl RG, Halperin BD, Mihm FG et al: Pulmonary effects of crystalloid and colloid resuscitation from hemorrhagic shock in the presence of oleic acid–induced pulmonary capillary injury in the dog, *Anesthesiology* 68(1):12, 1988.

102 Peters WP, Johnson MW, Friedman PA et al: Pressor effect of naloxone in septic shock, *Lancet* 1(8219):529, 1981.

103 Petros A, Bennett D, Vallance P: Effect of nitric oxide synthase inhibitors on hypotension in patients with septic shock, *Lancet* 338(8782-8783):1557, 1991.

104 Poole GV, Meredith JW, Pennell T et al: Comparison of colloids and crystalloids in resuscitation from hemorrhagic shock, *Surg Gynecol Obstet* 154:577, 1982.

105 Prough DS, Whitley JM, Taylor CL et al: Regional cerebral blood flow following resuscitation from hemorrhagic shock with hypertonic saline: influence of a subdural mass, *Anesthesiology* 75(2):319, 1991.

106 Raymond RM, Harkema JM, Stoffs WV et al: Effects of naloxone therapy on hemodynamics and metabolism following a superlethal dosage of *Escherichia coli* endotoxin in dogs, *Surg Gynecol Obstet* 152:159, 1981.

107 Reilly JM, Cunnion RE, Burch-Whitman C et al: A circulating myocardial depressant subjective is associated with cardiac dysfunction and peripheral hypoperfusion (lactic acidemia) in patients with septic shock, *Chest* 95(5):1072, 1989.

108 Reynolds DG, Gurll NJ, Vargish T et al: Blockade of opiate receptors with naloxone improves survival and cardiac performance in canine endotoxic shock, *Circ Shock* 7:39, 1980.

109 Rowe MI, Newmark BS: The early diagnosis of gram-negative septicemia in the pediatric surgical patient, *Ann Surg* 182:280, 1975.

110 Rushmore RF: *Cardiovascular dynamics,* ed 3, Philadelphia, 1970, WB Saunders.

111 Safani M, Blair J, Ross D et al: Prospective, controlled, randomized trial of naloxone infusion in early hyperdynamic septic shock, *Crit Care Med* 17(10):1004, 1989.

112 Sarnoff SJ: Symposium on regulation of performance of the heart: myocardial contractility as described by ventricular function curves: observations on Starling law of the heart, *Physiol Rev* 35:107, 1955.

113 Sarnoff SJ, Braunwald E, Welch GH et al: Hemodynamic determinants of oxygen consumption of the heart with special reference to the tension time index, *Am J Physiol* 192:148, 1958.

114 Sarnoff SJ, Mitchell JH: The control of the function of the heart.

In Hamilton WF, Down P, editors: *Circulation section: handbook of physiology*. Baltimore, 1962, Williams & Wilkins.
115 Schmid HE JR, Spencer MP: Characteristics of pressure-flow regulation by the kidney, *J Appl Physiol* 17:201, 1962.
116 Schmidt RF, Threws G, editors: *Human physiology*, New York, 1983, Springer-Verlag.
117 Schumer W: Steroids in the treatment of clinical septic shock, *Ann Surg* 184:333, 1976.
118 Shackford SR, Zhuang J, Schmoker J: Intravenous fluid tonicity: effect on intracranial pressure, cerebral blood flow, and cerebral oxygen delivery in focal brain injury, *J Neurosurg* 76(1):91, 1992.
119 Shands KN, Dan BB, Schmid GP: Toxic shock syndrome: the emerging picture, *Ann Intern Med* 94:264, 1981.
120 Shires GT, Bergentz SE, Gruber UF et al: Colloids or not for resuscitation? In Allgower M, Hardee F, editors: *State of the art surgery*, New York, 1979-1980, Springer-Verlag.
121 Shoemaker WC, Hauser CJ: Critique of crystalloid versus colloid therapy in shock and shock lung, *Crit Care Med* 7:117, 1979.
122 Shoemaker WC, Kram HB, Appel PL: Therapy of shock based on pathophysiology, monitoring, and outcome prediction, *Crit Care Med* 18(1 Pt 2):S19, 1990.
123 Shoemaker WC, Schluchter M, Hopkins JA et al: Comparison of the relative effectiveness of colloids and crystalloids in emergency resuscitation, *Am J Surg* 142:73, 1981.
124 Siegel JH, Cerra FB et al: Human response to sepsis. In Cowley RA, Trump BF, editors: *Anoxia and ischemia*, Baltimore, 1982, Williams & Wilkins.
125 Silverman HJ: Gastric tonometry: an index of splanchnic tissue oxygenation? *Crit Care Med* 19(10):1223, 1991.
126 Smith JS Jr, Snider MT: An improved technique for rapid infusion of warmed fluid using a Level 1 Fluid Warmer, *Surg Gynecol Obstet* 168(3):273, 1989.
127 Snyder JV, Carroll GC: Tissue oxygenation: a physiologic approach to a clincial problem, *Curr Probl Surg* 19(11):650, 1982.
128 Sobel BE: Cardiac and noncardiac forms of acute circulatory collapse. In Braunwald E, editor: *Heart disease: a textbook of cardiovascular medicine*, Philadelphia, 1980, WB Saunders.
129 Soliman MH, Ragab H, Waxman K: Survival after hypertonic saline resuscitation from hemorrhage, *Am Surg* 56(12):749, 1990.
130 Sonnenblick EH, Frishman WH, LeJemtel TH: Dobutamine: a new synthetic cardioactive sympathetic amine, *N Engl J Med* 300:17, 1979.
131 Sonnenblick EH, Ross J Jr, Covell JW et al: Velocity of contraction: major determinants of myocardial oxygen consumption, *J Clin Invest* 44:1099, 1965.
132 Sorenson MB, Bille-Brahe NE, Engell HC: Cardiac output measurement by thermal dilution: reproducibility and comparison with the dye-dilution technique, *Ann Surg* 183:67, 1976.
133 Spence RK, McCoy S, Costabile J et al: Fluosol DA-20 in the treatment of severe anemia: randomized, controlled study of 46 patients, *Crit Care Med* 18(11):1227, 1990.
134 Sprung CL, Panagiota VC, Marcial EH: The effects of high-dose corticosteroids in patients with septic shock, *N Engl J Med* 311:1137, 1984.
135 Stainsby WN: Local control of regional blood flow, *Annu Rev Physiol* 35:151, 1973.
136 Starling E: *The Linacre Lecture on the law of the heart*, New York, 1918, Longman.
137 Strauss RG, Stansfield C, Henriksen RA et al: Pentastarch may cause fewer effects on coagulation than hetastarch, *Transfusion* 28(3):257, 1988.
138 Swan HJ, Ganz W, Forrester J et al: Catheterization of the heart in man with the use of a flow-directed balloon-tipped catheter, *N Engl J Med* 283:447, 1970.
139 Tait AR, Larson LO: Resuscitation fluids for the treatment of hemorrhagic shock in dogs: effects on myocardial blood flow and oxygen transport, *Crit Care Med* 19(12):1561, 1991.
140 Tinker J: Shock: A pharmacological approach to the treatment of shock, *Br J Hosp Med* 261, 1979.
141 Todd J, Fishant M, Kapral F et al: Toxic shock syndrome associated with phase 1 staphylococcus, *Lancet* 2(8100):1116, 1978.
142 Torres-Martinez C, Mehta D, Butt A et al: Streptococcus-associated toxic shock, *Arch Dis Child* 67(1):126, 1992.
143 Triulzi DJ, Blumberg N, Heal JM: Association of transfusion with postoperative bacterial infection, *Crit Rev Clin Lab Sci* 28(2):95, 1990.
144 Unger KM, Shibel EM, Moser KM: Detection of left ventricular failure in patients with adult respiratory distress syndrome, *Chest* 67:8, 1975.
145 Vedder NB, Fouty BW, Winn RK et al: Role of neutrophils in generalized reperfusion injury associated with resuscitation from shock, *Surgery* 106(3):509, 1989.
146 Velanovich V: Crystalloid versus colloid fluid resuscitation: a meta-analysis of mortality, *Surgery* 105(1):65, 1989.
147 Vincent JL, Bakker J, Marecaux G et al: Administration of anti-TNF antibody improves left ventricular function in septic shock patients: results of a pilot study, *Chest* 101(3):810, 1992.
148 Virgilio RW, Rice CL, Smith DE et al: Crystalloid versus colloid resuscitation: is one better? *Surgery* 85:129, 1979.
149 Walsh JC, Zhuang J, Shackford SR: A comparison of hypertonic to isotonic fluid in the resuscitation of brain injury and hemorrhagic shock, *J Surg Res* 50(3):284, 1991.
150 Weisel RD, Vito L, Dennis RC et al: Myocardial depression during sepsis, *Am J Surg* 133:512, 1977.
151 Weisul JP, O'Donnell TF Jr, Stone MA et al: Myocardial performance in clinical septic shock: effects of isoprenaline and glucose potassium insulin, *J Surg Res* 18:357, 1975.
152 Weitzman S, Berger S: Clinical trial design in studies of corticosteroid for bacterial infections, *Ann Intern Med* 81:36, 1975.
153 Wolff SM: Monoclonal antibodies and the treatment of gram-negative bacteremia and shock, *N Engl J Med* 324(7):486, 1991.
154 Wright CJ, Duff JH, McLean APH et al: Regional capillary blood flow and oxygen uptake in severe sepsis, *Surg Gynecol Obstet* 132:637, 1971.
155 Ziegler EJ, Fisher CJ Jr, Sprung CL et al: Treatment of gram-negative bacteremia and septic shock with HA-1A human monoclonal antibody against endotoxin: a randomized, double-blind, placebo-controlled trial. The HA-1A Sepsis Study Group, *N Engl J Med* 324(7):429, 1991.
156 Ziegler EJ, McCutchan JA, Fierer J et al: Treatment of gram-negative bacteremia and shock with human antiserum to a mutant *E. coli*, *N Engl J Med* 307:1125, 1982.

CHAPTER

6

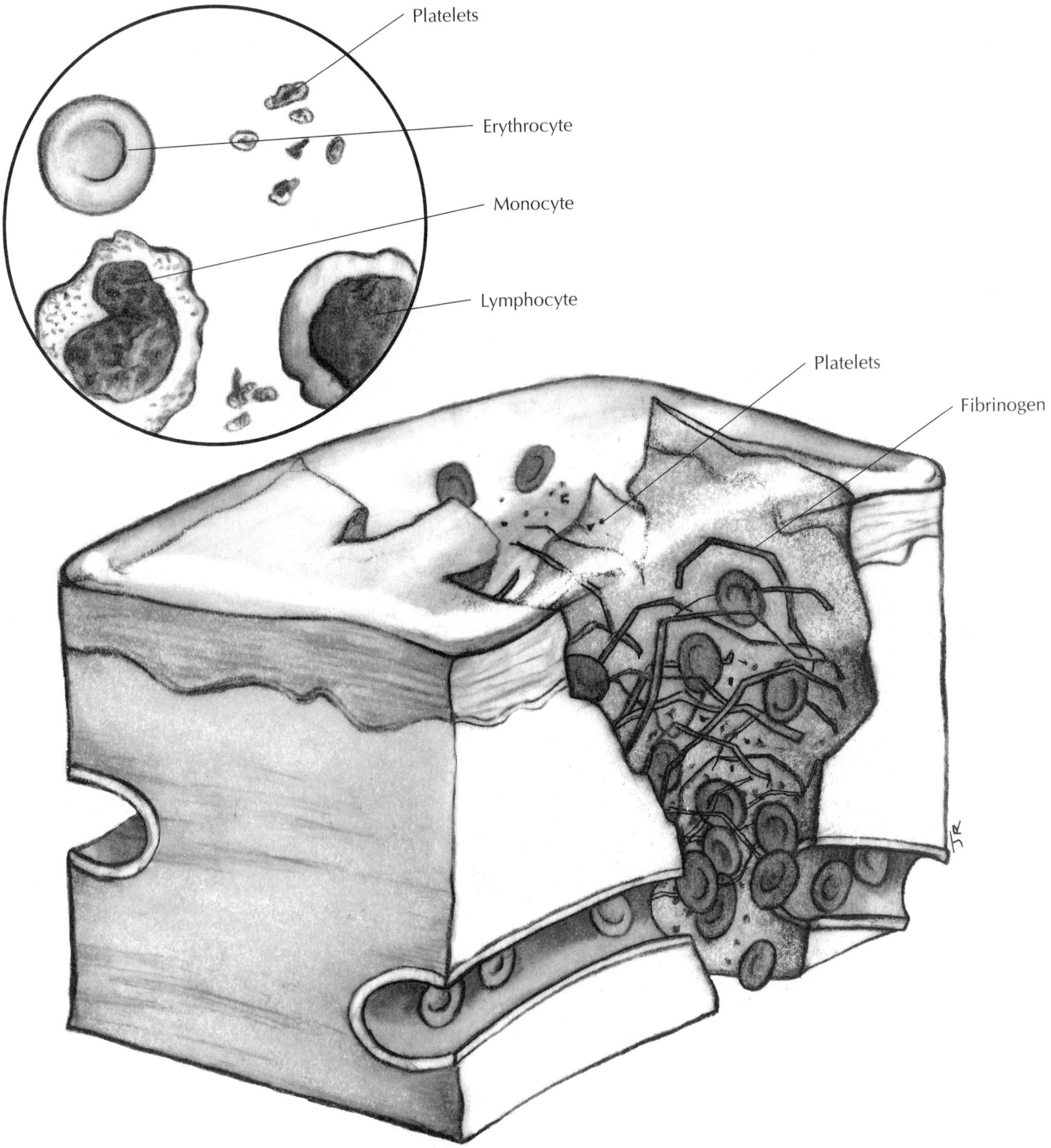

Platelets
Erythrocyte
Monocyte
Lymphocyte
Platelets
Fibrinogen
JR

BLEEDING, COAGULATION, AND BLOOD COMPONENT REPLACEMENT THERAPY

Robert Rutledge • George F. Sheldon • Samir M. Fakhry

BLEEDING AND COAGULATION

This chapter provides the surgeon with a general understanding of the basic elements of normal hemostasis. Particular consideration is given to the appropriate preoperative screening of patients for potential problems with hemostasis. Abnormalities of hemostasis, their evaluation, and treatment are also reviewed.

FUNCTIONS OF THE HEMOSTATIC SYSTEM

The hemostatic system is a complex interaction of countervailing pressures, one toward coagulation and blood clotting and the other toward anticoagulation and maintenance of blood fluidity. It is useful to consider the events of normal hemostasis in three phases. The first phase includes the immediate control mechanisms related to the vascular response and the formation of a platelet plug at the site of vessel injury. The second phase includes the long-term control mechanisms involved in the coagulation cascade. The opposing mechanisms directed toward maintaining blood fluidity and clot lysis may be considered as components of the third phase. There is considerable overlap and interaction among these three phases.

Several humoral agents act to stimulate the clotting system to stop hemorrhage. Thromboxane causes constriction of smooth muscle and is active early after vessel injury. Thromboxane is synthesized through prostaglandin metabolism, is released primarily by platelets at the site of disruption of the endothelial surface, and induces platelet aggregation. Agents such as epinephrine and norepinephrine cause vasoconstriction of larger vessels and induce platelet aggregation. Arteries are much more efficient than veins in vasoconstricting and sealing when injured. As is frequently mentioned, partial transection is more likely to lead to significant blood loss than complete transection because partial transection prevents complete vasoconstriction.

The relative composition of a thrombus is dictated largely by local blood flow conditions. In areas of sluggish blood flow where fluid shear stress is low or where eddies of the flow permit long residence of blood elements near abnormal surfaces, activation of clotting factors leads to a buildup of procoagulants and ultimately to formation of a plasma clot, the so-called red thrombus. This clot is composed of red cells trapped in fibrin strands. It predominates in peripheral veins and other areas of low flow. In regions where blood flow is brisk and the fluid shear stress is greater, as in the peripheral arteries, the so-called white thrombus is more common. The white thrombus is characteristic of arteries and other high flow areas.

Platelets

Platelets are important components of the hemostatic system. When platelets encounter exposed collagen, they aggregate and adhere to nonendothelial surfaces. Following the aggregation and adherence comes release of substances such as serotonin and thromboxane that aid in vessel contraction. In addition there is elaboration of substances that further accelerate platelet adherence, including epinephrine, adenosine diphosphate, and thromboxane. This acceleration reaction recruits other platelets, thus forming a plug in the areas of damaged blood vessels. Thrombosthenin is a contractile protein within platelets that causes platelet contraction and reinforces the clot. Furthermore, platelets release platelet factor III, a thrombogenic phospholipid that promotes coagulation, and thrombin, which contributes to local platelet aggregation and adherence.

Drug history is very important when evaluating the platelet system, particularly the identification of ingestion of aspirin-containing compounds or other nonsteroidal antiinflammatory drugs or other antiplatelet agents such as dipyridamole. Kitchen and associates[66] evaluated the effect of drug-induced platelet dysfunction on surgical bleeding. In this study, 200 patients scheduled for surgical or gynecologic procedures were evaluated with drug history and platelet aggregation studies. More bleeding than anticipated was noted in 20% of the patients who had a positive drug history (i.e., they had ingested aspirin or other nonsteroid antiinflammatory agents or had an abnormal platelet aggregation time). This is compared with a 10% incidence of abnormal bleeding in patients with a negative drug history and an 8% incidence in patients with normal platelet aggregation times. They concluded that aspirin ingestion close to the time of operation caused abnormal platelet aggregation and increased the likelihood of bleeding at the time of operation. This bleeding was significant in these patients because the total amount of blood transfused was twice as great as in patients who had negative drug history and normal platelet aggregation studies. Other studies have shown that even low doses of aspirin can cause platelet aggregation abnormality. As few as two aspirin tablets within a week before surgery were adequate to prolong the platelet aggregation study.

Alcohol has also been demonstrated to be a significant inhibitor of platelet function. Elmer and associates[33] demonstrated impairment of platelet responsiveness to collagen and adenosine diphosphate (ADP) after ingestion of 2 ml/kg bodyweight of 40% alcohol. Ingestion of this amount of alcohol did not affect coagulation or fibrinolysis.

The platelet system, which is not entirely directed toward coagulation, also has the balancing or opposing effect of maintaining blood fluidity. Prostacyclin, another product of the prostaglandin metabolic pathway, is produced by endothelium in blood vessels. Prostacyclin acts as an inhibitor of platelet aggregation and as a vasodilator.[27,29]

Coagulation Pathways

The coagulation system is made up of a system of enzymes that circulate in the inactivated precursor form and are activated by a proteolytic cascade.[42,133]

The activation requires several cofactors, of which calcium is probably the most important. The fibrin clot is formed through initiation of one of the two pathways that activate coagulation, the intrinsic and extrinsic pathways. The intrinsic pathway is a cascade that begins with factor XII (Figure 6-1). This factor is then activated to XIIA; similarly factor XI becomes XIA, factor IX becomes IXA, and factor VIII becomes VIIIA. Then with factors V and X, thrombin is activated. The extrinsic pathway begins with factor VII and then activates factors X and V once again to form thrombin from prothrombin. After thrombin has split fibrinogen to form a soluble fibrin monomer, the monomer binds to form insoluble fibrin. Factor XIII forms a firmer chemical bond and thus a stronger clot by acting on fibrin. The cascade of proteolysis that makes up the coagulation system amplifies the system's response because each enzyme tends to activate a more powerful enzyme; thus an initial small stimulus causes a large reaction.

Fibrinolytic System

The fibrinolytic system is important in opposing the tendency toward blood coagulation and maintaining the fluid characteristics of blood and the intravascular space.[103] The main product of the fibrinolytic pathway is plasmin, also called *fibrinolysin*. Plasmin, a strong proteolytic enzyme, reduces fibrin to soluble fragments. Plasmin is formed from plasminogen, another circulating precursor; a variety of plasminogen activators stimulate this formation. Tissue plasminogen activator and other activators that are found in a variety of secretions stimulate plasminogen to be lysed to form plasmin.[10] The liver is important in clearing the blood stream of activated metabolites of both fibrinolysis and coagulation. Therefore liver dysfunction from any cause may push the coagulation system in one direction or the other.

Plasmin acts not only on fibrin but also on fibrinogen and factors II, V, VIII and, as some data suggest, on factors IX and XI. This powerful serine protease effectively metabolizes a number of other proteins, including growth hormone, insulin, and adrenocorticotropic hormone (ACTH). Furthermore, it activates factor XII, and when activated through factor XII, plasmin can trigger the complement, kinin, and coagulation systems.

Kinin and Complement Systems

The coagulation system is involved in the kinin complement systems. The effect of high molecular weight kininogen is to activate factor XII.[80] Fragments of factor XIIA, generated by plasmin, stimulate the change of prekallikrein to kallikrein.[84] This change sets off the conversion of kininogen to kinin and also activates complements C1, C3, and C5. These complements may also replace factor D in the alternative complement pathway.

A variety of circulating antiproteases block the proteolytic enzymes of the complement, kininogen, and coagulation pathways. Antithrombin III is a powerful inhibitor of the coagulation system. Deficiencies in antithrombin III are associated with significant thrombotic disorders.[37,43] Other important antiproteases include alpha$_2$-macroglobulin, alpha$_1$-antitrypsin, and alpha$_2$-plasma inhibitor.[129]

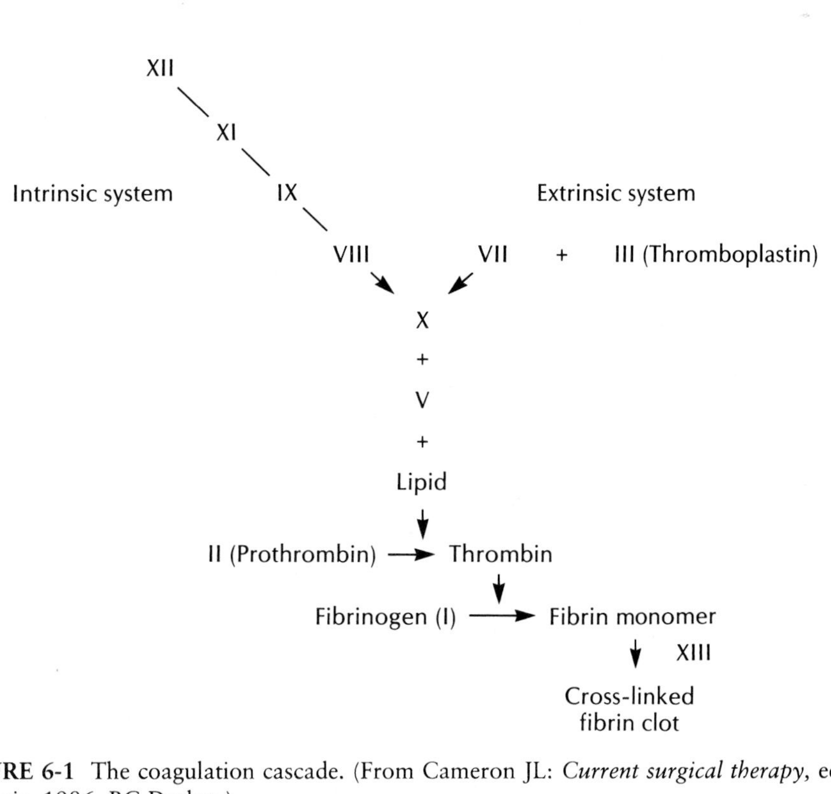

FIGURE 6-1 The coagulation cascade. (From Cameron JL: *Current surgical therapy*, ed 2, St Louis, 1986, BC Decker.)

CHANGES IN COAGULATION WITH TRAUMA

Trauma causes an increased coagulability. Platelets and damaged tissue release thromboplastic substances such as serotonin, which contributes to local vasoconstriction.[93] Acidosis and ischemia shorten the clotting time. Plasma levels of prekallikrein, Hageman factor, and antithrombin III are all reduced after trauma.* In survivors these parameters normalize in the first 5 days after injury. In fatal cases these factors remain low or decline further. Fatal cases also have elevated serum fibrin degredation products and consistently low platelet counts. The activation of the kallikrein-kinin system is part of the pathologic proteolysis that occurs in multiple trauma patients. Persistent reduction of plasma prekallikrein, Hageman factor, and antithrombin III, in addition to elevated fibrin split products and reduced platelet counts, indicate a poor prognosis.[52] Plasminogen concentrations are initially depressed in injured patients. Twenty-four hours later the plasminogen concentration rises in patients with the most severe injuries (injury severity scores ranging from 30 to 50), whereas in those patients with less severe injuries, the plasminogen concentrations return to normal.[2]

Fibrinolytic activity is increased on the day of traumatic injury, but appears to be suppressed in many patients during the next 5 days and returns to normal limits by the first week of injury.[63,101] Patients with the most severe injuries have the greatest increase in fibrinolysis initially. Twenty-four hours after injury, the fibrinolytic activity returns to normal in patients with mild to moderate injuries.† Factors II, V, VII, and X are generally within 70% to 130% of normal after trauma. Fibrinogen is markedly reduced during the first 5 days after injury and thereafter gradually normalizes.[63] After an initial period of hypercoagulability, secondary fibrinolysis develops. Patients with central nervous system (CNS) injury appear to have a propensity for coagulopathy that is absent in patients following elective CNS procedures.[64]

The use of D-dimer fibrin degradation products has been advocated as an indicator of pathologic thrombosis and hypercoagulability in injured patients.[108] When a stable clot forms, the fibrin polymers within it are crosslinked. Plasmin acts upon fibrin polymers and produces the D-dimer degradation products. D-dimer levels are more specific than fibrin degradation products because the latter result from the breakdown not only of crosslinked fibrin from stable clots, but also of fibrin monomers and uncrosslinked polymers. Elevated serum levels of D-dimer may therefore be useful as a clinical indicator of patients in whom the thrombolic process is active.

*References 14, 25, 34, 50, 54, 76, 100, and 135.
†References 25, 34, 50, 76, 100, and 135.

In patients who develop sepsis and septic shock, plasminogen activator inhibitor activity is significantly increased and may contribute to the development of depressed fibrinolysis and disseminated intravascular coagulation.[28] The use of plasma levels of this and other substances may provide useful information in the management of patients with abnormal coagulation and fibrinolysis.

CONGENITAL COAGULATION DISORDERS

Congenital coagulation disorders may appear initially as pathologic bleeding in the trauma patient. Congenital disorders of coagulation characteristically involve a single coagulation protein. The plasma concentration of coagulation proteins in general is low; therefore diagnosis depends on assay of the plasma factor level.[44]

Hemophilia

Hemophilia A is secondary to factor VIII deficiency. It is the most common congenital coagulation factor disorder and occurs in approximately 1 of 10,000 persons. Because the platelet plug is the first line of defense against bleeding and coagulation is the second, the onset of bleeding in patients with hemophilia and normal platelet function is often delayed by several hours or days after injury. Bleeding then may persist for several days or weeks because coagulation is important in maintaining the occlusion. Clinical manifestations of hemophilia vary depending on the factor VIII level. With a factor VIII level of 50% to 100% in the blood, generally no bleeding complications occur. With a level of 25% to 50%, bleeding may occur after major trauma. With a level of 5% to 25%, severe bleeding can occur after surgical procedures, and some bleeding may occur after minor trauma. In general, no spontaneous bleeding occurs at this level. At levels of 1% to 5%, severe bleeding can occur after minor injury, and there are occasional spontaneous hemorrhages such as into muscle or joints. With no measurable factor VIII level, severe hemophilia occurs with spontaneous bleeding into muscles and joints.

Diagnosis is based on family history, history of bleeding problems, an elevated partial thromboplastin time (PTT), a normal prothrombin time (PT), a normal bleeding time demonstrating normal platelet function, and low levels of factor VIII in the serum.

The treatment of the trauma patient with factor VIII deficiency should be two staged.[107,127] Initial evidence of abnormal bleeding should be treated by immediate replacement with fresh frozen plasma. This replacement will allow volume resuscitation in addition to providing factor VIII.[8] In patients who require large amounts of volume, this will provide adequate factor VIII levels. After the initial emergency, more extensive evaluations such as assaying factor levels to determine the quantity of elevated PTT, a lower factor VIII level, and other tests of platelet function may be carried out.

Von Willebrand's Disease

Von Willebrand's disease, or pseudohemophilia, is being increasingly recognized and is probably as common as true hemophilia. The bleeding manifestations of von Willebrand's disease are usually mild except after major trauma or surgery. Some patients may have had spontaneous bleeding into the skin or mucous membranes, epistaxis, or menorrhagia. The deficient von Willebrand's factor, called the factor VIII-related antigen, can cause a decrease in the activity level of factor VIII assays. Many patients with von Willebrand's disease will have a prolonged bleeding time because of platelet dysfunction.

Transfusion of fresh frozen plasma has a sustained effect on factor VIII levels in most patients with von Willebrand's disease. This effect is unlike the brief elevation in factor VIII activity seen in hemophilia.

Other Congenital Abnormalities of Coagulation

Congenital deficiency of other coagulation factors occurs, but much less commonly. The deficiency in factor XII is not associated with bleeding but is actually associated with hypercoagulability. Factor IX deficiency, or Christmas factor disease, occurs about one-sixth as frequently as factor VIII deficiency. Clinical manifestations are similar to hemophilia A. Treatment is the use of factor IX-containing concentrates. These concentrates of prothrombin complex generally contain prothrombin and factors VII, IX, and X. Many of these concentrates contain activated factors as well and if infused rapidly may lead to disseminated intravascular coagulation (DIC). The indications for use of these concentrates are severe bleeding and presence of established deficiency. In the presence of major trauma with volume loss, once again initial treatment is aggressive resuscitation with fresh frozen plasma, which will have the least potential for adverse reaction in these patients. Other deficiencies are best treated by aggressive initial resuscitation with fresh frozen plasma and then subsequent consultation with specialists in coagulation diseases.

ACQUIRED COAGULATION DEFECTS

Vitamin K Deficiency

Acquired coagulation defects are much more common than the congenital defects.[131] Probably the commonest is vitamin K deficiency. Vitamin K is essential for synthesis of prothrombin (II) and factors VII, IX, and X, the so-called vitamin K-dependent factors. The cause of vitamin K deficiency may be inadequate diet, malabsorption, lack of bile salts, obstructive jaundice, biliary fistula, oral administration of antibiotics, or parenteral alimentation.

Immediate treatment is rapid infusion of fresh frozen plasma to the volume-depleted, bleeding patient. In patients who do not have severe bleeding or who have volume overload, vitamin K may be administered parenterally. Vitamin K causes measurable correction in clotting times within 6 to 12 hours of intravenous administration. Initial treatment may be up to 5 mg given slowly intravenously. Previous preparations of vitamin K were less purified than those currently used, and anaphylaxis and death were associated with intravenous administration. The more purified forms are less likely to cause complications, but intravenous vitamin K should not be given without carefully considering this possibility and having resuscitative equipment available. Intramuscular vitamin K is appropriate when given in adequate doses; a dose of 25 mg given intramuscularly may be valuable. Repeated doses of intramuscular vitamin K will allow total body repletion, and 25 mg intramuscularly administered for 3 days should provide adequate vitamin K stores for any patient.

Oral Anticoagulants

Coumadin derivatives act by antagonizing vitamin K. Coumadin prolongs the PT, causes a slight elevation in the PTT, and reduces the levels of prothrombin (factor II) and factors VII, IX, and X. Warfarin has a half-life of 40 hours, and treatment consists of vitamin K administration or infusion of fresh frozen plasma (FFP).

A patient on therapeutic anticoagulation with Coumadin who is scheduled to undergo elective surgery can have the oral anticoagulant discontinued 3 to 4 days before the operative procedure. The patient's PT should be closely monitored and intravenous heparin started to maintain therapeutic anticoagulation. The heparin can then be discontinued 6 to 8 hours preoperatively and restarted in the postoperative period once hemostasis is secure.

Patients on oral anticoagulants who require emergent operative intervention should have their oral anticoagulant discontinued and fresh frozen plasma administered. The administration of vitamin K can provide a more prolonged reversal of the anticoagulation. The effect of vitamin K will not be seen for several hours, however, and its maximal effect will not be obtained for approximately 30 hours.

In the patient receiving therapeutic anticoagulation with Coumadin who is to undergo a major surgical procedure or other invasive procedure, the administration of fresh frozen plasma may be preferable to treatment with parenteral vitamin K. The use of fresh frozen plasma results in a more rapid and predictable response. The administration of parenteral vitamin K may result in subsequent difficulty in reestablishing adequate anticoagulation with Coumadin. The use of vitamin K without FFP will also result in a delay in the correction of the elevated PT.

Heparin

Heparin is a commonly used anticoagulant that acts to block the activation of factor X by binding with antithrombin III to the thrombin molecule and inactivating it. Heparin affects all coagulation tests, including the PT, but the PTT is most sensitive. An average dose of heparin is cleared from the blood in approximately 6 hours; but this rate is variable, depending on other factors such as liver function, body temperature, and shock. Because heparin's charge is strongly negative, it may be neutralized on a milligram for milligram basis by intravenous protamine sulfate, which carries a strongly positive charge: 100 units of heparin is equal to 1 mg of heparin. The dose of protamine given should be approximately equal to the dose of heparin given, adjusted for the half-life of heparin.

Heparin has a number of clinical uses, including prevention and treatment of venous thrombosis and pulmonary embolism and in several clinical situations with myocardial infarction. Heparin is also used to maintain the patency of vascular grafts, to prevent thrombosis in extracorporeal devices used in open heart surgery and in hemodialysis machines, to treat some cases of disseminated intravascular coagulation (DIC), and to prevent thrombosis in arterial and venous monitoring catheters.

The use of heparin for the treatment of venous thrombosis and pulmonary embolism has been examined in multiple studies. In the treatment of venous thrombosis with heparin, the rates of further thrombosis were significantly decreased as long as the patient was maintained on anticoagulation. To prevent subsequent rethrombosis, further treatment with either parenteral or oral anticoagulants is necessary. Decreased mortality after pulmonary embolism has been demonstrated using heparin followed by anticoagulation with an oral preparation.[57] Recent studies on the use of subcutaneous heparin as an alternative to continuous intravenous heparin have demonstrated equivalent efficacy, provided that adequate doses are given to achieve prolongation of the activated PTT.

A number of complications have been reported with the use of heparin. The most common is hemorrhage.[65,71,130] Thrombocytopenia following the administration of heparin is more common with bovine preparations than with porcine preparations of heparin. The rate varies between 5% and 15% of patients receiving heparin. More serious complications associated with thrombocytopenia develop in approximately 5% of patients. These complications consist of arterial and venous thrombosis and have been designated heparin-associated thrombocytopenia or "white clot syndrome" because of the development of clots rich in platelets without large numbers of entrapped red cells. This syndrome is thought to be caused by development of IgG-heparin immune complexes leading to platelet clumping. Patients who develop significant thrombocytopenia may require discontinuation of the heparin infusion. Patients who develop the more severe heparin-associated thrombocytopenia and white clot syndrome should have their heparin discontinued immediately. Even small doses of heparin such as those administered to keep arterial and venous monitoring devices open can lead to thrombocytopenia. An alternative is the use of citrate as an anticoagulant for monitoring lines, especially in critically ill intensive care unit patients. The development of low molecular weight heparins, heparin-like substances (heparinoids) and prostacycline derivatives, has provided an alternative to heparin administration.[57]

Liver Disease

Liver disease is a common cause of impaired coagulation. All types of liver disease including major hepatic trauma, cirrhosis, and biliary obstruction may cause impaired coagulation because the liver is the major site of synthesis of all the coagulation factors except factor VIII, which may be decreased with hepatic dysfunction. Hemostasis may be further impaired by thrombocytopenia and platelet dysfunction, which can occur with liver disease.

Liver disease commonly is associated with a low serum fibrinogen level, a prolonged PT, and a normal to slightly increased PTT. The thrombin time is elevated, indicating an abnormal or decreased fibrinogen. In the management of bleeding in these patients, plasma infusion is preferable to any activated concentrates because of the likelihood of inducing DIC. Heparin infusion in many patients with severe liver disease transiently increases the fibrinogen level, suggesting that chronic low-grade DIC may be a partial cause for decrease in the fibrinogen levels seen in these patients. In patients with severe liver dysfunction, whether caused by cirrhosis, shock, or hepatic trauma, extremely large volumes of fresh frozen plasma may be required to maintain adequate hemostasis, normalize clotting tests, and control bleeding (up to 2 units every 2 hours in patients with complete liver failure).

Platelet Disorders

Platelet malfunction may lead to significant bleeding in the trauma patient. One of the commonest causes of platelet malfunction in trauma is dilution secondary to massive blood loss, with infusion of platelet-poor crystalloid and blood products. The thrombocytopenia associated with massive transfusion and its treatment are discussed in the section Massive Blood Transfusion.

Normal platelet counts range from 150,000 to 400,000. A platelet count of less than 100,000 constitutes thrombocytopenia. With platelet counts greater than 40,000, bleeding may occur after injury or surgery, but spontaneous bleeding is uncommon. Spontaneous bleeding may occur with platelet counts between 10,000 and 20,000; with counts below 10,000, spontaneous bleeding is common and frequently severe. Platelet defects often lead to spontaneous bleeding into the skin, which is manifested by purpuric petechiae or confluent ecchymoses. An extensive list of causes of thrombocytopenia and platelet dysfunction should be considered, but generally the trauma patient without other problems develops thrombocytopenia on a dilutional basis alone. Some of the other causes of thrombocytopenia include production defects such as marrow failure or injury, marrow invasion by malignant processes, and defective maturation perhaps caused by vitamin B_{12} or folic acid deficiency. Sequestration of platelets may exist and occurs in splenomegaly and occasionally with hypothermia. Accelerated destruction, which can occur secondary to antibodies as in idiopathic thrombocytopenic purpura, systemic lupus erythematosus, or hemolytic anemias, may exist. Certain drugs can induce this destruction, and transfusion reactions such as posttransfusion purpura leading to production of autoantibodies that destroy platelets may develop. Nonimmunologic causes may accelerate platelet destruction, which can occur secondary to infection and sepsis or platelet interaction with prosthetic surfaces such as valves or grafts. Consumption may also occur through DIC or thrombotic thrombocytopenic purpura. Generally treatment in the acute situation is removal of the offending agent or causative factor and subsequent consultation for further evaluation of other possible causes.

Drugs with important effects on platelets include chemotherapeutic agents, thiazide diuretics, alcohol, estrogen, antibiotics such as the sulfa antibiotics, quinidine and quinine, methyldopa, and gold salts. Probably the commonest drugs that block platelet function are the prostaglandin inhibitors, particularly aspirin, indomethacin, and other nonsteroidal antiinflammatory drugs such as ibuprofen. The H_2 blockers have been associated with thrombocytopenia and impaired platelet function in some patients.

Bleeding disorders may also rarely occur secondary to vessel wall abnormalities. Infections such as sepsis, meningococcemia, typhoid fever, and subacute bacterial endocarditis may lead to abnormal platelet function and coagulation defects, as well as vascular defects and hemorrhage. Vitamin C deficiency leads to petechial hemorrhages. Steroid treatment with Cushing's syndrome leads to excessive vascular breakdown. Henoch-Schönlein purpura, senile purpura, and hereditary hemorrhagic telangiectasia may also lead to delicate blood vessels and easily damaged areas that cause increased bruising and bleeding with major or minor trauma.

HEMOSTATIC TESTING

Bleeding Time

The bleeding time is the time required for bleeding to cease from an undisturbed standard skin incision. The incision is usually made to a depth of 2 mm in the earlobe or the volar surface of the forearm. The upper limits of normal bleeding vary according to the specific technique used but usually do not exceed 5 to 10 mm.

The bleeding time represents the time for formation of the platelet plug and is thus indicative of adequate platelet function and numbers. The bleeding time is usually normal when the platelet count is greater than 75,000/mm^3. Patients with qualitative platelet defects, capillary abnormalities, or von Willebrand's disease may have prolonged bleeding times.

Platelet Counts

Platelets can be directly enumerated by counting under the microscope in a hemocytometer or by the use of an electronic particle counter. Microscopic examination of properly prepared blood smears can provide estimates of platelet counts that are satisfactory in the evaluation of most patients. The normal number of platelets per oil immersion field is 15 to 20; each platelet per field is thus roughly equivalent to 10,000/mm^3. When there is a deficiency of platelets in the smear, an actual platelet count should be performed.

Platelet Function

Among the tests used to evaluate platelet quality are aggregation tests and tests of the ability of platelets to release platelet factor III, factor IV, serotonin, or betathromboglobulin.

Activated Partial Thromboplastin Time

PTT measures the activity of the intrinsic coagulation system in the common pathway of the coagulation system. The result expressed in seconds is the time required for a fibrin clot to form after calcium and an activating agent are added to the patient's citrated platelet-poor plasma. The result is then compared with time obtained simultaneously on a normal control plasma sample or with a distribution of normal values. False-positive results can occur in polycythemia, with an inadequate volume, or when blood is contaminated with heparin from an intravenous or intraarterial line.

Prothrombin Time

PT measures the function of the extrinsic system and the common pathway. Factor VII is a vitamin K-dependent factor synthesized for the liver and has a short half-life. Thus the PT yields evidence about the current synthetic capacity of the liver, the adequacy of vitamin K absorption, and the presence of clotting factor inhibition by drugs such as warfarin. The result expressed in seconds is the time required for fibrin strands to appear after the addition of tissue thromboplastin and calcium to a patient's platelet-poor plasma. False-positive results can occur as a result of improper handling of the sample. At usual therapeutic doses, heparin has only a minimum effect on the PT. Certain levels of the coagulation system factors are needed to obtain a normal coagulation test: factor XII is unnecessary; factor XI must be present at a level of 20%; factor IX (Christmas factor) must be present at a level of 40%; factor VIII must be present at a level of 30%; extrinsic system factor VII (proconvertin) must be present at a level of 25%; factors X (Stuart factor), V (proaccelerin), and II (prothrombin) must all be present at 40% of normal value; and factor I (fibrinogen) must be present in a concentration of at least 100 mg/dl.

Thrombin Time

The clotting time of a patient's plasma after the addition of thrombin is known as the *thrombin time*. Thrombin time is a test that detects abnormalities in fibrinogen, as well as circulating anticoagulants and inhibitors of fibrin polymerization.

ROUTINE PREOPERATIVE COAGULATION SCREENING

Adequate clinical assessment including a properly obtained medical history, examination for evidence of purpura, liver disease, malabsorption, and malnutrition should be sufficiently sensitive in detecting congenital and acquired coagulopathies to obviate laboratory testing of persons with normal findings.[7,15,59,123] History should include personal or family history of known bleeding disorders; prolonged bleeding after injury, dental extraction, or other surgical procedure; and frequent or severe nosebleeds or spontaneous bleeding at other times. The history should also reveal any personal history of liver disease, malabsorption, malnutrition, and recent anticoagulation therapy, including the use of nonsteroidal antiinflammatory agents and aspirin. Physical findings should include inspection of skin and mucous membranes for petechiae, ecchymoses, and hematomas. Routine preoperative screening with either the PTT or PT in patients without clinical assessment that suggests the possibility of a bleeding disorder, liver disease, malabsorption, or malnutrition is not recommended. PTT and PT are indicated for patients whose normal coagulation may be disrupted by the planned procedure (e.g., peritoneovenous shunt, prostatectomy, or cardiopulmonary bypass). Abnormal test results warrant repetition. If the results are still abnormal, more detailed evaluation is appropriate, usually in consultation with a specialist in coagulation disease.

Cost Containment

Numerous studies suggest that physicians overuse laboratory testing. Although individual costs of the tests are low, cumulative costs are substantial. In an attempt to evaluate appropriate laboratory usage, the usefulness of preoperative laboratory screening was evaluated in 2000 patients undergoing elective surgery over a 4-month period, and randomly selected samples of patients were studied by Kaplan and associates.[62] In their study, a total of 650 PT and PTT assays were performed in a year. Approximately 77% were performed "without indications," (i.e., without any abnormalities on physical examination or history). In this evaluation, of the entire group sampled, 1.5% were abnormal. None of these abnormalities occurred in patients without a history of physical abnormalities. This result once again confirms the value of the preoperative examination and the lack of value of the PT and PTT as screening tests.

Numerous other analyses of preoperative testing have been published. Most have concluded that routine testing in the absence of a suggestive history or physical findings is not useful.

DISSEMINATED INTRAVASCULAR COAGULATION

DIC is associated with a number of the complications of severe trauma. Shock, sepsis, and extensive tissue necrosis all may be associated with extensive release of thromboplastic substances that may initiate the coagulation system, leading to DIC.* The principal site of action in DIC is fibrinogen. The enzymes that degrade fibrinogen are thrombin and plasmin. Thrombin also digests factors V and VIII and leads to platelet aggregation. The degradation products of fibrinogen acted on by plasmin are called fibrin degradation products or fibrin split products.[73] These degradation products have significant physiologic effects inhibiting the normal coagulation of blood.[81,111] They act to delay polymerization of fibrin and prolong the thrombin time. Fibrin split products may also interpose themselves between fibrin and polymers and therefore form a weak fibrin clot.[17] Platelet aggregation by adenosine diphosphate is also blocked. When a fibrin thrombus is formed, plasmin is normally thought to be absorbed into the fibrin strand. There it is free from inhibitors such as the alpha$_2$-macroglobulin and is able to digest fibrin.[17]

The normal concentration of fibrinogen reflects this balance between both synthesis and enzymatic metabolism. The hepatic synthesis of fibrinogen normally may be increased up to tenfold in response to stress.[105] The normal half-life of fibrinogen is 100 hours. Thrombin's action on fibrinogen is thought to contribute less than

*References 36, 47, 82, 88, 99, and 112.

2% to normal fibrinogen metabolism. Experimental studies have shown that rapid injection of thrombin leads to local thrombosis. Slower infusion leads to disseminated hypofibrinogenemia and usually small vessel thrombus in the kidneys and adrenals.[134] The reticuloendothelial system, particularly the liver, removes fibrin and activated coagulation factors from the circulation. Suppression of reticuloendothelial system functioning increases susceptibility to DIC. Trauma releases particulate material, which is cleared from the bloodstream after trauma. In animals, administration of intravenous gelatin, a particulate material that is removed by the reticuloendothelial system, increased susceptibility to hypotension and shock secondary to a bacterial challenge.

Diagnosis of DIC is based on clinical suspicion; diffuse bleeding from multiple sites (including venipuncture sites), skin incisions, and sites of mucosal trauma should raise concern. The thrombin time is valuable because it measures the functional fibrinogen concentration and is prolonged in DIC. The PT and PTT are generally prolonged, the platelet count is decreased, and a microangiopathic anemia is seen on blood smear. A simple screening coagulation test is to draw blood in a glass tube and determine the length of time required for clotting. Clotting in less than 10 minutes indicates an adequate fibrinogen concentration. Subsequently, lyses of the clot indicate the presence of a fibrinolysin, and concern about DIC should be heightened. Factor assays, particularly of factors V and VIII, will generally show marked decrease in these factor levels.

Treatment

Primary treatment of DIC should be directed at the underlying disease.[118] Clearly, when shock is a precipitating factor, every effort should be made to rapidly resuscitate the patient. The second line of therapy involves replacement of blood components.[118] The primary blood components effective in this situation are fresh frozen plasma and cryoprecipitate, which provide both factor VIII and fibrinogen. The dosage is empiric based on careful clinical monitoring and follow-up of the thrombin time. Platelet concentrates may be given, and vitamin K should be given to all patients because of the frequent association of vitamin K deficiency with DIC. Heparin has been shown to be effective in some animal models of DIC. Unfortunately, it is not appropriate for acutely injured patients. The dosage is arbitrary but generally ranges from 500 to 1000 units/hour.[113] Where available, a heparin assay should be used to adjust heparin levels of 0.2 to 0.3 U/ml. The antifibrinolytic agent epsilon-aminocaproic acid is not indicated. It has been associated with a variety of catastrophic complications such as thrombosis of major vessels.

MANAGEMENT OF COAGULOPATHY

Massive Blood Transfusion

If over 50% of a patient's blood volume requires replacement during a 3-hour period, sufficient alteration in the properties of the circulating blood volume occurs to develop a potential coagulation lesion. Blood in liquid preservation develops storage defects that assume greater clinical significance in massive transfusion than in low-volume elective transfusion.

The massively transfused patient undergoing a complex operation, usually as a result of traumatic injury, is a tempting candidate to receive a variety of clotting factors. The major defect in the massively transfused patient usually relates to thrombocytopenia. A platelet count above 50,000 is adequate for hemostasis in most clinical situations. If platelet counts are lower than 50,000, bleeding may well be related to this thrombocytopenia. A transfusion reaction or a consumptive coagulopathy should be considered as the potential cause of the thrombocytopenia. Factors V and VIII, the so-called labile factors, decline during liquid preservation. Frequently fresh frozen plasma is administered to the massively transfused patient, but studies by Carrico and others suggest that there is little relationship between the levels of these or other of the coagulation factors and bleeding that occurs following massive transfusion.[75,100] Their work suggests that platelets are the key components in nonmechanical bleeding after massive transfusion for injury.

Laboratory tests of clotting function take time to complete; therefore specifically targeting therapy of suspected clotting problems is often difficult. One of the best tests is a simple clotting time assay obtained by drawing blood into a glass tube, taping it to the wall or to the patient's bed, and determining how long it takes for clotting to occur. If a clot forms in less than 15 minutes, the clotting function is still adequate. If that clot lyses after 20 minutes, a circulating fibrinolysin is present, and a transfusion reaction may have occurred.

The commonest cause of intraoperative bleeding in the massive transfusion patient is inadequate surgical control of bleeding vessels. Although dilutional thrombocytopenia or altered platelet function, factors V and VII deficiency, or more likely, a combination of all these factors may have some impact on impairment of clotting time, one should assume that intraoperative bleeding is the result of a technical problem rather than a clotting defect or platelet deficiency until proved otherwise.

If more than 10 units of blood have been required and the patient has nonmechanical active bleeding, an abnormality of the coagulation system may be present. However, if no evidence of intraoperative bleeding exists, proceeding to a multiple unit resuscitation is safe. If extended transfusion is needed in excess of 25 units with anticipation of additional multiple transfusions, initiating supplemental clotting therapy by administering platelets is usually useful.

Platelet Concentrate Transfusion

Platelet transfusions can be therapeutic in thrombocytopenic patients, especially those who are bleeding because of the decrease of platelets. Some patients with abnormal platelet function also respond.

Three types of platelet concentrates are usually available. Single unit, random donor platelet concentrate is produced from a single unit of blood within 6 hours of collection. Multiple unit, single donor platelet concentrate is removed by mechanical apheresis from one donor. Each collection has as many platelets as 6 to 10 single units. This product may be obtained from donors of known human lymphocyte antigen (HLA) type to yield HLA-matched platelets or from the patient's family members.

Platelet transfusions contain sufficient amounts of other clotting factors to preclude the need for their being administered if platelets have actually been transfused. The aim of all special hemostatic therapy is to preclude bleeding regardless of what the counts are. If the patient is not bleeding, further transfusion of specific clotting factors is probably not warranted.

In addition to the observation of the hemostatic response, the importance of follow-up counts at 1, 12, and/or 24 hours should be stressed. Depending on the clinical situation, at 1 hour an increment of at least 5000 platelets/μl should be achieved for each single unit transfused. Less than the expected increment may indicate immunization. If the patient is not rapidly consuming platelets (e.g., bleeding, febrile, or in DIC state), a count at 12 and/or 24 hours will give an indication of platelet survival.

Clotting Factors

During liquid preservation, the labile factors V and VIII deteriorate during the storage of whole blood. By the end of 14 to 21 days, minimum levels of factors V and VIII are present. In addition to deteriorating during storage, factors V and VIII are often consumed in the process of coagulation because plasmin degrades them.

Although most clotting factors are potentially available for transfusion, fibrinogen is a potentially dangerous product with limited indications for use. Cryoprecipitate provides sufficient fibrinogen in an acceptably small volume for most uses and has a lower risk of transmitting hepatitis than does fibrinogen infusion. Factor V is present in normal concentrations in fresh frozen plasma. Factor VIII is also present in fresh frozen plasma but in a more concentrated form in cryoprecipitate.

BLOOD COMPONENT REPLACEMENT THERAPY

The ability to replace lost blood has made modern surgery possible; 60% of all blood products given are transfused at or near the time of surgery. Patients who are anemic or thrombocytopenic or who have coagulopathy often can be operated on successfully because they can be prepared for the procedure by transfusion of the appropriate blood component. The following section provides a general outline of the rationale for blood component therapy in a number of clinical situations.

Blood products are the most dangerous "drugs" physicians prescribe. Most clinicians are aware that a transfusion of incompatible red blood cells (RBCs) is potentially fatal, but other significant concerns exist when a patient receives a blood component. The infectious hazards associated with human blood products are well known. Despite the recent concern over the acquired immune deficiency syndrome (AIDS), non-A, non-B hepatitis remains the major infectious risk of transfusion because, on average, 1 out of 10 patients who undergo transfusion will show evidence of infection[1] (Table 6-1). The recipient risks sensitization to cellular and protein antigens present in the blood product. The antibodies that result cause problems in some patients if they require transfusion support for a prolonged period. Importantly, young girls and women of child-bearing age risk developing antibodies that may lead to hemolytic disease of the newborn if they become pregnant.

A transfusion is a "transplant" and exposes the recipient to a complex mixture of donor cells and proteins. Despite the label that says "packed red cells" or "platelet concentrate," these blood components contain viable lymphocytes capable of mounting a graft-versus-host response in the severely immunocompromised recipient.[132] Transfusion has the potential to modify the recipient's immune response, as has been amply demonstrated in the case of patients undergoing renal transplantation.[89] Thus given the spectrum of infections and immunologic

TABLE 6-1 RISK OF TRANSFUSION-TRANSMITTED INFECTION IN GENERAL BLOOD SUPPLY (I.E., COMMUNITY VOLUNTEER DONORS)

INFECTION	RISK PER UNIT
HIV	1 in 225,000
Hepatitis B	1 in 200,000
Hepatitis C	1 in 3,300
HTLV I/II	1 in 50,000
Yersinia enterocolitica, Malaria, Babesia microti, Trypanosoma cruzi	Less than 1 in 1,000,000

Data from Dodd R: The risk of transfusion-transmitted infection, *N Engl J Med* 327:419, 1992.

complications associated with transfusion, transfusion should be given only when clearly indicated.

COMPONENTS

Blood component therapy is designed to maximize their therapeutic potency and usefulness.[86] Approximately 250 ml of RBCs contain the same number of red cells as 450 ml of whole blood. The patient who is thrombocytopenic because of marrow suppression caused by chemotherapy and who needs surgery should receive platelet concentrate. The following section presents the most commonly prescribed blood components.

Methods of Component Preparation

In the 1950s, after the introduction of plastic bags and reliable centrifuges, the separation of whole blood into its constituents became routine.[85] As blood is withdrawn from the donor, it is continuously, gently mixed with a solution in which citrate prevents coagulation by binding calcium. The solutions used most commonly today are citrate phosphate dextrose (CPD) and citrate phosphate dextrose adenine (CPDA-1).* Within 6 hours of collection, the unit is gently centrifuged. This packs the RBCs and leaves about 70% of the platelets suspended in plasma. The platelet-rich plasma is expressed into a plastic satellite bag. The bag containing platelet-rich plasma is spun again at a faster speed to "pellet" the platelets. All but 50 ml of supernatant plasma is removed into a second satellite bag and rapidly frozen at less than −30° C. The platelets are resuspended in the plasma left in the first bag to yield platelet concentrate. If the frozen plasma is stored at less than −18° C, it is fresh frozen plasma (FFP). If the frozen plasma is allowed to thaw at 4° C, the precipitate that remains can be collected to yield cryoprecipitate. Proteins, such as albumin, can be isolated from the remaining supernatant "cryopocr" plasma by ethanol fractionation.[23,114]

In addition to preparation from single donations of whole blood, leukocytes, platelets, or plasma can be collected by either manual or mechanical apheresis.[85] During manual apheresis a unit of whole blood is drawn from the donor and centrifuged; plasma or platelets or both are removed, and the RBCs are returned to the donor. During mechanical apheresis the donor's blood is removed and centrifuged and portions returned in a continuous loop. The cellular component of interest is continuously removed. These systems can be used to remove large numbers of leukocytes or platelets in a relatively short period.

*Recently, solutions containing extra nutrients have been used to extend the storage life of cells. These solutions are added to the packed cells after platelets and plasma are removed. If red cells have had these solutions added, they are labeled AS-1 or AS-2, depending on the specific solution.

Guidelines for Component Therapy

The following discussion presents very general guidelines for the use of blood components (Table 6-2). The specific needs of some patients may require consultation with specialists in transfusion medicine. *Careful posttransfusion follow-up and evaluation are crucial to effective patient management.* If the expected therapeutic result is not achieved, further studies may be needed to find the optimal product for the particular patient.

Cellular Components

This section discusses the major cellular components of blood. The reader is referred to Table 6-3 for additional information of these components.

WHOLE BLOOD. Whole blood (WB) is appropriate for patients with acute blood loss who have lost over 15% of their blood volume.[19] In this situation, rapid replacement of both oxygen-carrying capacity and volume is important to prevent irreversible hemorrhagic shock. Whole blood can be stored in CPDA-1 for 35 days at 1° C to 6° C. After this time fewer than 70% of the RBCs remain in the circulation 24 hours after transfusion, the U.S. Food and Drug Administration (FDA) criterion for outdating. Because platelets degenerate at refrigerator temperatures, banked WB contains essentially no functioning platelets. The levels of activity of clotting factors V and VIII decrease appreciably over 24 hours at 1° to 6° C, but the levels of the other factors remain essentially unchanged. When both colloid and oxygen-carrying capacity are needed, giving WB instead of packed RBCs and plasma is less expensive and carries half the infectious risk of packed RBCs plus FFP, each from different donors.

PACKED RED BLOOD CELLS. Packed RBCs (PRBCs) are indicated when the patient needs oxygen-carrying capacity but does not require additional blood volume.[19] PRBCs are also indicated for the patient whose anemia cannot be corrected by iron or other therapy. The decision to transfuse and the amount to transfuse depend on the clinical situation. Many chronically anemic patients tolerate hemoglobin levels of 7 to 8 g/dl under ordinary conditions but require RBCs if they are to undergo the stress of surgery. Each unit of PRBCs usually raises the hematocrit approximately 2% to 3% in a 70 kg person.

WASHED RED BLOOD CELLS. The indications for RBCs that have been washed with normal saline are essentially the same as for the PRBCs except that removal of most plasma and leukocyte and platelet debris is also needed. Patients who may require washed RBCs include those who have febrile reactions caused by leukoagglutinins or patients with impaired renal function who cannot tol-

TABLE 6-2 USE OF BLOOD COMPONENTS

COMPONENT	MAJOR INDICATIONS	CONTRAINDICATIONS	EXPECTED RESPONSE
WB	Moderate to massive blood loss (>15% of blood volume), leading to symptoms of hypoxia and volume deficit	Condition responsive to specific component	Rise in hematocrit of 1.1%/unit transfused in 70 kg human
PRBCs	Symptomatic anemia; decreased red cell mass	Treatable anemia; coagulation deficiency	Rise in hematocrit of 2.2%/unit in 70 kg human
Washed RBCs	Febrile reactions from antibodies to leukocyte antigens; need to remove plasma	Same as PRBCs	Same as PRBCs
Deglycerolized RBCs	As for washed RBCs, also IgA sensitization; rare blood types	Same as PRBCs	Same as PRBCs
Platelet concentrate	Bleeding caused by thrombocytopenia or abnormal platelet function*	Conditions with rapid platelet destruction	Cessation of bleeding; increased platelet count; decreased bleeding time
Leukocyte concentrate	Severe neutropenia and infection unresponsive to antibiotics	Infection responsive to antibiotics	Resolution of sepsis
FFP	Deficit of labile plasma coagulation factors; thrombotic thrombocytopenic purpura	Coagulopathy responsive to specific concentrate; volume replacement	Improved hemostasis
Single-donor plasma	Deficit of stable plasma coagulation factors	As for FFP	Improved hemostasis
Cryoprecipitate	Factor VIII deficiency (hemophilia A); von Willebrand's disease; hypofibrinogenemia; factor XIII deficiency	Coagulation defect not defined	Improved hemostasis

*Pretransfusion and posttransfusion platelet counts at 1 hour, 12 hours, or 24 hours are recommended for patients receiving transfusions of platelet concentrate.

erate the potassium in the plasma of banked blood. Several options exist to treat patients with febrile reactions, such as the use of microaggregate filters, and each case should be discussed with the transfusion specialist.

DEGLYCEROLIZED RED BLOOD CELLS. Red blood cells can be stored for up to 3 years at lower than −65° C if protected by glycerol-containing media. Patients with rare blood types often must be transfused with rare units available from the frozen cell inventory. After thawing, the RBCs are washed extensively and therefore may be used in patients for whom any plasma protein is detrimental. These patients include those with IgA deficiency who have antibodies to IgA. Contrary to early reports, experience has shown that the risk for posttransfusion hepatitis from frozen blood is the same as that from other products.

PLATELET CONCENTRATE. Platelet transfusions can be therapeutic in thrombocytopenic patients, especially those who are bleeding because of the low number of platelets.[115] Some patients with abnormal platelet function also respond. Three types of platelet concentrate are usually available. Single-unit, random-donor platelet concentrate is produced from a single donation of WB within 6 hours of collection. Multiple-unit, single-donor platelet concentrate[106] is harvested from one donor by mechanical apheresis technique. Each collection has as many platelets as 6 to 10 single "random" units. This product may be obtained from donors of known human lymphocyte antigen (HLA) type to yield HLA-matched platelets[77] or may be drawn from members of the patient's family.

Basic guidelines for platelet transfusion are as follows:

1. Platelets may be given to patients with platelet counts lower than 20,000 μl.
2. Platelets may be given to patients who have microvascular bleeding or who are going to have surgery and have a platelet count lower than 60,000 μl.
3. Platelets may be given to patients who have microvascular bleeding and who have had a precipitous fall in platelet count.
4. Platelets may be given to patients with a bleeding time greater than 15 minutes who have microvascular bleeding or who are about to undergo an invasive procedure.
5. Platelets may be given to adult patients in the operating room who have had complicated procedures or have required more than 10 units of blood and have microvascular bleeding or to children whose transfused volume exceeds one blood vol-

TABLE 6-3 SUMMARY OF CELLULAR BLOOD COMPONENTS

COMPONENT	CONTENT AND VOLUME	SHELF LIFE STORAGE CONDITIONS	SPECIAL PRECAUTIONS (HEPATITIS OR AIDS RISK?)
WB	RBCs; nonfunctional, fragmented WBCs and platelets; plasma (450 ml total volume contains 200 ml of RBCs)	CPDA-1: 35 days (1° to 6° C)	Must be ABO compatible (yes)
PRBCs	RBCs; some plasma; nonfunctional, fragmented WBCs and platelets (250 to 350 ml total volume contains 200 ml of RBCs)	AS-1: 42 days CPDA-1: 35 days (1° to 6° C)	Must be ABO compatible (yes)
Washed RBCs	RBCs; minimum plasma and nonfunctional WBCs and platelets (200 ml total volume contains 170 to 190 ml of RBCs)	24 hours (1° to 6° C)	Must be ABO compatible (yes)
Deglycerolized RBCs	RBCs; no plasma, minimum WBC and platelet debris (200 ml total volume contains 170 to 190 ml of RBCs)	24 hours after deglycerolization (1° to 6° C) 3 years (<−65° C)	Must be ABO compatible (yes)
Platelet concentrate (single unit)	Platelets; some nonfunctional WBCs; few RBCs; plasma (50 to 70 ml total volume contains 5.5×10^{10} platelets; level of labile clotting factors depends on storage time)	5 days (20° to 24° C)	Should be ABO compatible; do not use microaggregate filter (yes)
Platelet concentrate (apheresis unit random donor)	As above; usually contains as many platelets as 6 to 10 single units (>30×10^{10})	Usually 24 hours; may be 5 days (20° to 24° C)	Should be ABO compatible; do not use microaggregate filter (yes)
Leukocyte concentrate	WBCs; may contain large numbers of platelets, some RBCs (600 ml total volume contains 5 to 30×10^9 granulocytes)	24 hours (20° to 24° C)	Must be ABO compatible; do not use microaggregate filter (yes)

ume. Giving platelets assumes adequate surgical hemostasis has been achieved.

6. Platelets may be given to patients who have undergone open heart surgery and whose time on cardiopulmonary bypass has exceeded 2 hours.
7. Platelets may be given to children who have undergone surgery (especially those children weighing less than 20 kg) and who are particularly prone to hemodilution because their own blood volume is small in relation to the extracorporeal circulation.
8. Platelet transfusion is probably contraindicated in patients having a diagnosis of thrombotic thrombocytopenic purpura (TTP) or posttransfusion purpura (PTP) and probably not indicated in patients with idiopathic thrombocytopenic purpura (ITP).

In addition to observation of the hemostatic response, it is important to determine follow-up platelet counts at 1 hour and then at 12 or 24 hours. Depending on the clinical situation, an increment at 1 hour of at least 5000 platelets/μl should be achieved in an average adult for each unit of random donor platelets transfused. Less than the expected increment may indicate alloimmunization and the need for platelets from a donor of HLA type similar to the patient.[51,77,116] A follow-up count at 12 or 24 hours gives an indication of platelet survival.

LEUKOCYTE CONCENTRATE. Leukocyte transfusions are indicated in profoundly granulocytopenic (less than 500/μl) patients with evidence of infection (e.g., positive blood culture, persistent temperature greater than 38.5° C) unresponsive to antibiotic therapy.[38,56,67] Once initiated, daily transfusions are given until the infection is under control or the pretransfusion granulocyte count is greater than 1000/μl. Because leukocyte concentrate is usually prepared by mechanical apheresis from donors typically premedicated with steroids to increase the number of circulating granulocytes and by a method that requires the use of hydroxyethyl starch to enhance the separation of cells, there is more risk to the donor than with a routine blood donation. Consultation with specialists in infectious disease is recommended before leukocyte concentrate is given. Decisions are made on a case-by-case basis.

TABLE 6-4 SUMMARY OF PLASMA COMPONENTS

COMPONENT	CONTENT AND VOLUME	SHELF LIFE STORAGE CONDITIONS	SPECIAL PRECAUTIONS (HEPATITIS/AIDS RISK?)
FFP	Plasma, all coagulation factors, minimum cellular debris (180-250 ml contain 0.7 to 1 Unit/ml of factor II, factor V, factor VII, factor VIII, factor IX, factor XII, factor XIII, and 500 mg of fibrinogen)	Frozen: 1 year (< −30° C) Thawed: 24 hours (1 to 6° C)	Should be ABO compatible (yes)
Cryoprecipitate (antihemophilic factor [AHF])	Fibrinogen, factor VIII, factor XIII, von Willebrand's factor, fibronectin (10-20 ml contains 80 U/ml factor VIII, 200 mg fibrinogen)	Frozen: 1 year (< −30° C) Thawed: 4 hours if pooled (20 to 24° C)	Preferably ABO compatible; keep at room temperature until infusion (yes)
Factor VIII concentrate	Factor VIII (lyophilized)	Stated on label	High hepatitis risk (no AIDS risk; reduced hepatitis risk if heat treated)
Factor IX complex	Factor II, factor VII, factor IX, factor X (lyophilized)	Stated on label	Thrombosis risk; high hepatitis risk (no AIDS risk; reduced hepatitis risk if heat treated)
Albumin	Albumin (50-250 ml contain 12.5 g albumin)	3 years (room temperature)	No hepatitis or AIDS risk
Plasma protein fraction (PPF)	Albumin and 17% globulins (250 ml contains 12.5 g protein)	3 years (room temperature)	No hepatitis or AIDS risk

Plasma Components

The reader is referred to Table 6-4 for additional information regarding the plasma components discussed in this section.

FRESH FROZEN PLASMA. The major indication for FFP is coagulopathy resulting from deficient labile clotting factors.[21] This situation may be the result of liver dysfunction, congenital absence of clotting factor, or transfusion of factor-deficient blood products. The volume and factor content of one unit of FFP are presented in Table 6-4.

CRYOPRECIPITATE. Cryoprecipitate is useful in the treatment of factor deficiency (hemophilia A), von Willebrand's disease, and hypofibrinogenemia and may aid in the treatment of uremic bleeding.[60] Each 5 to 15 ml unit contains 80 units of factor VIII and about 200 mg of fibrinogen. Fibronectin is also present. Because the proteins mentioned previously are in relatively high concentration, a smaller volume may be given than would be required if FFP were used. The infectious risk associated with this product is smaller than that of purified factor concentrates made from plasma pooled from many donors. However, heat treatment of these factor concentrates inactivates the virus associated with AIDS and significantly reduces the risk of hepatitis.[53]

PRETRANSFUSION TESTING

The most important determinant of compatibility between the donor and recipient is the ABO blood type of each. Because A and B antigens are ubiquitous in the environment, each person develops antibodies to the antigen(s) he or she lacks by about 18 months of age, even without transfusion. For example, type O persons who lack both A and B antigens develop significant levels of anti-A and anti-B and an antibody that recognizes both A and B, anti-A,B. If they receive RBCs bearing A or B antigen, potentially fatal complement-mediated intravascular hemolysis occurs. The compatibility relationships are outlined in Table 6-5. The next most important antigen in RBC transfusion is D of the Rh blood group system. Unlike anti-A and anti-B, anti-D antibody almost never develops without prior exposure to D-positive RBCs as the result of transfusion or pregnancy. Because more than 50% of D-negative patients who receive a unit of D-positive RBCs will develop the antibody, where possible, persons who lack this antigen should receive only D-negative RBCs. Therefore the first step in pretransfusion testing is to determine the recipient's ABO and D types.

Next it must be determined whether the patient has antibodies to other clinically significant RBC antigens. The test used to determine this variable is the antibody screen, or the indirect Coombs' test. The patient's serum is combined with "reagent" RBCs from two or three type O persons who possess among them the 14 clinically most significant antigens. If the patient's serum does not agglutinate or hemolyze these RBCs in the test tube under different incubation conditions, the screen is negative, and the patient is thought not to have significant antibodies. If the patient's serum reacts with one or more reagent cells, the screen is positive, and further testing

TABLE 6-5 COMPATIBILITY RELATIONSHIPS

RECIPIENT'S RBCs	RECIPIENT'S PLASMA	COMPATIBLE DONOR'S RBCs	COMPATIBLE DONOR'S PLASMA
A	Anti-B	A or O	A or AB
B	Anti-A	B or O	B or AB
AB	Neither	A, B, AB, or O	AB
O	Anti-A, anti-B, anti-A,B	O	A, B, AB, or O

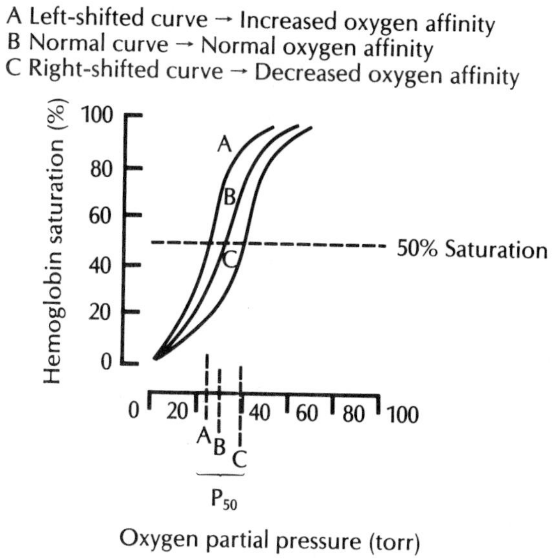

FIGURE 6-2 Oxyhemoglobin dissociation curves. Factors that shift the curve to the right include increased levels of 2,3-DPG, decreased pH, and increased P_{CO_2}. Transfusion-related (1) low 2,3-DPG levels, (2) reduced body temperature, and (3) metabolic alkalosis all result in lowering of the P_{50} value of the oxyhemoglobin dissociation curve. (From Sheldon GF: Hemotherapy in a trauma center. In Johnson W, editor: *Hemotherapy in trauma and surgery,* Arlington, Va, 1979, American Association of Blood Banks.)

is required to identify the specific antigen(s) involved. In most instances, the patient must be transfused with RBCs known to lack the antigen(s).

On average, about 3% of patients who have been transfused will have developed clinically significant antibodies to antigens other than A or B. Those most likely to have positive screens include women who have had multiple pregnancies or patients who have received many transfusions. Hence the fraction of patients with antibodies may rise to 10% to 12% in a tertiary care hospital. A detailed transfusion and obstetric history in any patient who will likely require transfusion is important. If a patient has been previously transfused or pregnant, preadmission testing may prove cost effective because antibodies can be identified early and antigen-negative units of blood can be located before admission. If the patient is not tested until the evening before surgery, a positive screen may delay the operation. To say a priori how long finding compatible blood will take in every instance is not possible.

The *crossmatch* refers to the part of compatibility testing in which the donor RBCs are combined with recipient serum or plasma in the test tube. If the antibody screen is negative and the patient has no history of a clinically significant antibody, the crossmatch may be abbreviated to confirm ABO compatibility. If the screen is positive, more extensive incubation under enhancement conditions is performed. Each blood bank may perform the crossmatch and antibody screen using a different technique within the standards set by the American Association of Blood Banks and should be consulted for details at each institution. It must be emphasized that a unit that satisfies all in vitro testing may not produce the expected therapeutic increment in vivo. Thus post-transfusion follow-up is crucial.

Not all antibodies lead to increased destruction of RBCs bearing the corresponding antigen despite the fact that they may cause a positive antibody screen and an incompatible crossmatch.[83] The most important factors in determining if an antibody is significant clinically include (1) the titer, or amount, of antibody in the patient's serum; (2) the class of immunoglobulin involved and whether it fixes complement, leading to intravascular lysis, or coats the cell, leading to extravascular phagocytosis by the reticuloendothelial system; (3) the number and mobility of antigen sites on the RBC; (4) the relative affinity of the antibody for antigen; and (5) the volume of antigen-positive blood transfused. It is beyond the scope of this chapter to discuss these mechanisms in detail, but the systems other than ABO most often involved in hemolytic transfusion reactions include Rh, Kell, Kidd, and Duffy.

PREOPERATIVE TRANSFUSION

Studies involving Jehovah's Witnesses and experiments with perfluorocarbons have made clear that anemia is an extremely well-tolerated condition. Scientists have know for a long time that a patient who is chronically anemic, such as one with hemoglobinopathy, can lead a relatively normal life despite severe anemia. We also now know that adaptation to chronic anemia, regardless of its cause, is usually associated with increased RBC glycolysis, leading to increased levels of intracellular 2,3-diphosphoglycerate (2,3-DPG) and enhanced unloading of oxygen from hemoglobin (Figures 6-2 and 6-3). Chronically uremic patients requiring kidney transplantation who are universally anemic tolerate surgery well.

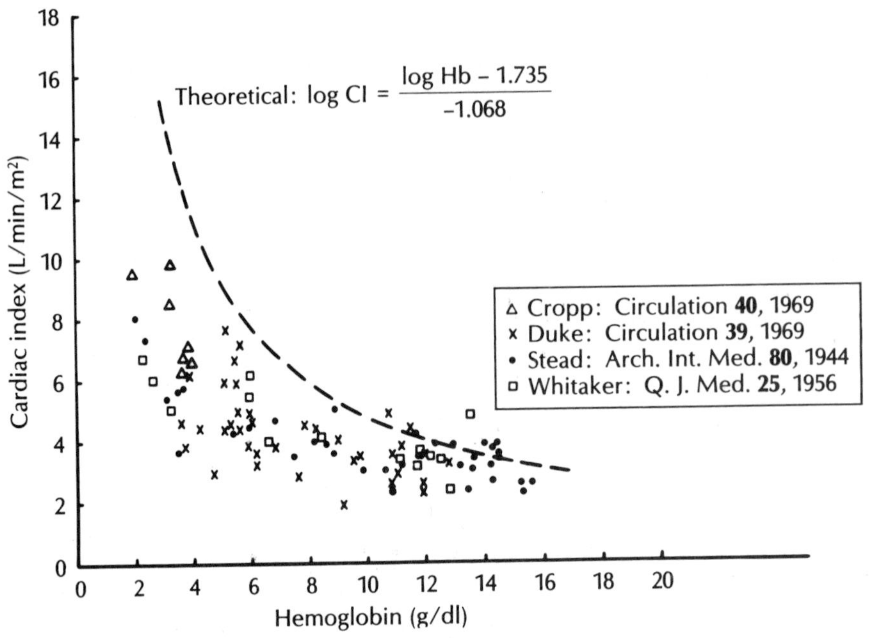

FIGURE 6-3 Cardiac output in anemia. This diagram examines the relationship of oxygen transport in chronically anemic patients using data from four published articles, which have all aspects of oxygen transport within the Fick equation available. The predicted increase in cardiac output *(dashed line)* as patients become anemic is not found in these and other studies. The measured change in cardiac output occurs at much lower hemoglobin values and does not appear to be much of a factor until the hemoglobin falls below 7.2 g/dl. Much of this adaptation is caused by an increase in 2,3-DPG and the resultant decrease in the affinity of hemoglobin for oxygen. Hence increased oxygen transport is accomplished within the function of hemoglobin without the requirement that cardiac output be increased. (Courtesy of George Watkins, M.D.)

The evaluation of an anemic patient determines the cause of the anemia. If a circulating autoantibody causes hemolysis, then specific therapy may involve splenectomy. If the anemia is caused by chronic blood loss, with the production of new RBCs lagging behind that loss, then administration of iron may be sufficient. In most cases evaluation requires a reticulocyte count, which should indicate the ability of the bone marrow to produce RBCs. If the patient is anemic and not producing RBCs, an erythropoietic signal may not be received, and transfusion may be the only way to raise the hemoglobin level before surgery (Figure 6-4).

Determining the need for transfusion begins with the clinical diagnosis, progresses to a reticulocyte count, and concludes with an evaluation of symptoms. If the patient is dyspneic and tachycardic and in need of an operation, providing transfusion preoperatively is preferred. The end point for transfusion should be the relief of symptoms in the chronically anemic patient. Although the single-unit transfusion has been justifiably condemned, if one unit is sufficient to alleviate symptoms, no additional transfusion should be given because each unit transfused adds to the risk of disease transmission.

The strategy for preoperative or intraoperative transfusion usually depends on anticipated intraoperative blood loss. Although no specific hematocrit is an indication for transfusion, an anemic patient who is anticipating a procedure that will predictably result in significant blood loss is best transfused before his operation. Transfusing the patient preoperatively allows an in vivo test of compatibility between donor blood and recipient. The surgeon thus avoids an intraoperative transfusion reaction. In addition, if the patient is transfused 24 hours or more in advance of operation, most of the stored RBCs will have regained normal physiologic function.

Friedman and associates' studies[40] have demonstrated that the use of blood products for similar disease states varies significantly in different parts of the country. Although the reasons for these differences are unclear, clinical indications for the use of blood products apparently vary according to the clinician's background. National statistics indicate that complicated peptic ulcer, fracture of the femur, traumatic injury, ischemic heart disease,

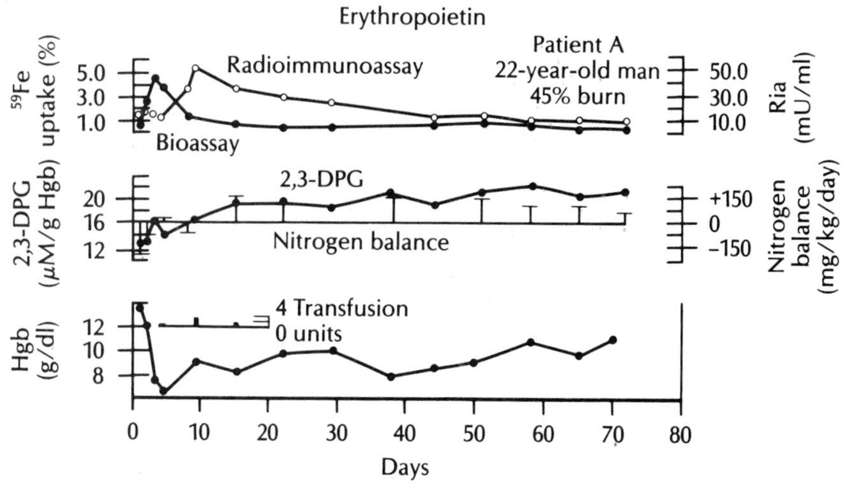

FIGURE 6-4 Erythropoietin. This study using both radioimmunoassay and mouse bioassays shows data in anemic patients who have not been massively transfused (e.g., burn patients). The data suggest that in the chronic anemia following injury, 2,3-DPG increases in the RBCs and leads to increased unloading of oxygen from hemoglobin. This phenomenon may result in the failure of a hypoxic signal to reach the kidney so that erythropoietin levels remain normal or low. Reticulocytosis does not occur. The reticulocytopenic anemic patient usually needs to be transfused unless the cause of the anemia is iron, folate, or B_{12} deficiency. (From Sheldon GF: Hemotherapy in a trauma center. In Johnson W, editor: *Hemotherapy in trauma and surgery,* Arlington, Va, 1979, American Association of Blood Banks.)

and malignant diseases account for most of the blood transfusions in the United States.

The growing use of the maximum surgical blood order schedule (MSBOS) is a rational way to minimize the use of RBC-containing products.[41] The schedule is usually based on the institution's or physician's record of transfusion for certain operative procedures. Rather than a surgeon asking for a specific amount of blood, he sends a clotted sample to the blood bank, where a "type and screen" procedure is performed to determine the patient's ABO and D types and to detect preformed antibodies to RBC antigens. If the antibody screen is negative and the probability that the patient will require blood in the operating room is less than 10%, units are not crossmatched unless the patient actually needs blood in surgery. If this is the case, an abbreviated crossmatch is performed within a few minutes and blood is released. If the probability of transfusion is greater than 10%, blood is crossmatched preoperatively. The number of units set up is a function of the usual number of units transfused during the procedure in the past. In situations in which blood is frequently used, such as open heart or vascular surgery, the minimum number of units is crossmatched, and additional units are made available if they are needed unexpectedly. Similarly, when a procedure is completed, blood is held usually for 24 to 48 hours and then automatically released for other patients. This process allows the most efficient use of blood products and avoids the time-consuming three-phase crossmatch, which need not be done in most instances.

EMERGENCY TRANSFUSION

The logistics of transfusion in the emergency situation begin with adequate vascular access with large-bore intravenous tubing. As the catheter is inserted, the blood withdrawn is sent to the blood bank so that the patient's blood type can be determined for immediate transfusion if necessary. This is *the* most important blood sample drawn from an injured patient. It must be *labeled at the side of the patient* and transported to the blood bank immediately. A fluid challenge of balanced salt solution is administered rapidly (500 ml of solution given in a 10-minute period or 2000 ml over 1 hour). If further fluid is needed to resuscitate the patient, it is administered at the same rate. As fluid therapy proceeds, blood products become available to supplement the crystalloid-containing solution. The initial blood product used can be autologous blood collected from a body cavity, especially the thorax.[16,58,136] If massive quantities of blood are immediately required, uncrossmatched type O PRBCs can be administered. In mass casualty situations, giving all casualties type O blood is theoretically safer than risking a transfusion reaction caused by ABO incompatibility, which might occur if patients of more than one ABO type are being transfused in the same area. However, in most urgent situations, type-specific blood is usually available within 5 to 10 minutes. The crossmatch is completed *after* the transfusion is given.

Because by far the most important determinants of compatibility of the donor and recipient are their respective ABO types, giving known ABO-compatible blood even without crossmatch is prudent when there is not time for a crossmatch. The safety of uncrossmatched blood has been demonstrated in both military and civilian trauma practice.[69,109] However, the patients sustaining acute trauma are predominantly young men who have not been previously transfused. In emergencies involving women who may later become pregnant and men who have a history of transfusion, the risk of using uncrossmatched blood is greater.[95]

Using crystalloid solution at a 3:1 ratio (volume to volume) with RBCs, transfusion proceeds as therapy continues. In most instances the RBC-containing blood product given is PRBC product. Because the hematocrit is usually about 80%, this product is too viscous to flow as rapidly as needed in the emergency situation. Normal saline may be added to the bag to decrease viscosity. Many centers now supply PRBCs with an additive solution that reduces the viscosity without the need for additional saline. The blood bank of each institution should be consulted to determine the local practice.

Many patients who are transfused in emergency situations receive large amounts of stored RBC-containing components.

TRANSFUSION OF THE PATIENT IN SHOCK

In World War I various theories were developed regarding vasomotor control of vascular collapse in injured patients. At that time it was unclear that vascular collapse was caused not by toxins but by loss of extravascular fluid volume in excess of the obvious shed blood. In a unique group of experiments in the 1930s, Phemister and Blalock showed that fluid loss in injured tissue often accompanied injury and was unavailable to the intravascular space for maintenance of circulation. The idea of an extra "space" in which fluid would be sequestered and therefore unavailable to the intravascular space is part of that concept.

By World War II plasma was a favored resuscitation solution. The development of other types of solutions for resuscitation, especially those containing electrolytes, grew out of experiments in children with diarrhea in whom fluid volume was critical. By the mid-1940s, advances were made in defining the metabolic and endocrine environment associated with injury. However, the concept that a limited amount of salt and water should be given to patients after operations or injury prevailed until the Korean conflict, when a series of experiments seemed to indicate that extracellular fluids shifted into the intravascular space after significant amounts of hemorrhage. Providing volume resuscitation in excess of shed blood then became an acceptable practice to maintain adequate circulation.

During World War II acute tubular necrosis (ATN) was a common consequence of hypovolemic shock. Because of the liberal use of fluid resuscitation during the Korean and Vietnam conflicts, the incidence of ATN dramatically decreased. Although the incidence of ATN secondary to hypovolemic shock has been markedly reduced, the mortality from ATN remains little different from that of predialysis days.

As ATN as a consequence of hypovolemic shock became less of a problem because of the liberalized use of fluid in resuscitation, the "shock lung" syndrome (adult respiratory distress syndrome) emerged. This syndrome resulted when fluid and blood were used aggressively in treatment. During the Vietnam conflict, various names, such as "Da Nang lung," were given to the pulmonary edema that developed in resuscitated patients. Filtering blood products through microaggregate filters was advocated because it was thought that microparticles could embolize to the lung and lead to the shock lung syndrome. Careful research has since convincingly demonstrated that, like the kidney, the lung is an end organ for shock, and the impact of the resuscitation solution on the lung has more to do with the underlying shock than with the resuscitation solution. As researchers study patients with shock more intensively, they are identifying poorly understood gastrointestinal lesions. The concept that the immune system may fail as a consequence of shock and lead to increased susceptibility to infection, general fluid sequestration, and eventually death from sepsis is the current frontier of shock research. Currently, sophisticated hemodynamic end points for treatment of hypovolemic shock have led to combined crystalloid and blood component therapy.

The therapeutic goal in the treatment of shock is timely restoration of adequate circulation and oxygen transport. Restoration of circulation allows the cell to clear products of anaerobic metabolism and restore aerobic metabolism. The American College of Surgeons Committee on Trauma has developed a classification of shock that permits useful guidelines for resuscitation. These routines rely on three units of crystalloid for every unit of RBCs administered, and therapy is monitored by hemodynamic response.[24]

Because crystalloid solutions are universally available and some delay is required to prepare blood products, crystalloid is the proper initial resuscitation fluid. Resuscitation then proceeds with the use of blood products, depending on the patient's response. For many years the use of a colloid solution such as albumin or a crystalloid solution such as lactated Ringer's solution as the preferred fluid was controversial. Both can expand the extracellular space and provide effective resuscitation. However, crystalloid solutions are favored because they are cheaper, do not need to be crossmatched with the patient, and do not transmit disease, such as hepatitis. Moreover, crystalloid solutions contain ions that move into the intracellular space or are lost in the urine of patients with acute hypovolemia. Recent evidence indicates that colloid solutions, although having the theoretic advantage of maintaining fluid longer in the intravascular space, have the immediate effect of probably causing more fluid to be maintained in interstitial tissue of the lung. Experimental data do not indicate that using colloid rather than crystalloid solutions can prevent pulmonary edema.[72,128]

Although many crystalloid solutions are available for resuscitation, pure dextrose solutions and solutions containing less-than-physiologic levels of ions are less optimal than balanced salt solutions. Lactated Ringer's solution, which contains isotonic quantities of anions, has some minor disadvantages. Although it was originally thought that the lactate in Ringer's solution might contribute to lactic acidosis commonly seen in shock, the administered lactate is now clearly known to be converted to bicarbonate if blood flow to the liver is restored. However, because lactated Ringer's solution contains calcium, if it is added to a unit of blood product when one moves from crystalloid to blood transfusion, the blood may clot in the bag. Ringer's acetate solution has the theoretic advantage of replacing the calcium with magnesium, although this divalent cation may also cause clotting of blood products. Acetate is easily metabolized to bicarbonate, and metabolic alkalosis is the net effect of acetate as well as lactate infusions.

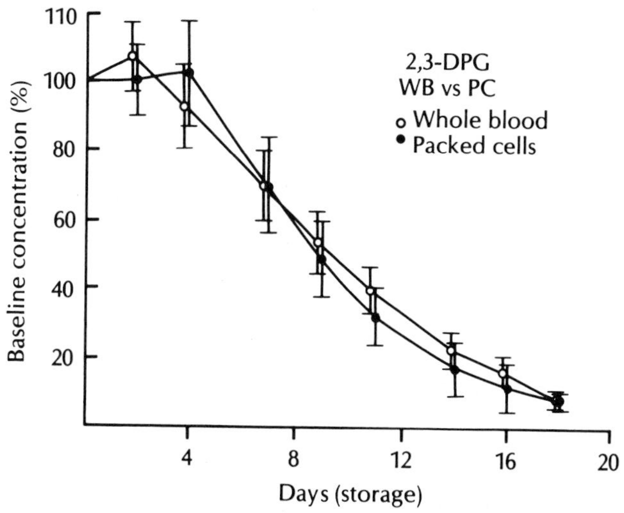

FIGURE 6-5 2,3-DPG levels diminish equally in packed cells and whole blood during liquid storage in CPD preservative. The data are expressed as a percentage of initial 2,3-DPG values. (From Sheldon GF: Hemotherapy in a trauma center. In Johnson W, editor: *Hemotherapy in trauma and surgery,* Arlington, Va, 1979, American Association of Blood Banks.)

THE MASSIVELY TRANSFUSED PATIENT

Most authors define massive transfusion as replacement of the patient's blood volume with stored RBCs in 24 hours. Few would disagree that if 50% of the patient's blood volume is replaced by stored WB or PRBCs and plasma in 3 hours, the potential exists for significant changes in the patient's metabolic status because of the infusion of large volumes of cold citrate-containing blood that has undergone changes during storage.

As blood is stored at 1° C to 6° C changes occur over time, including leakage of intracellular potassium, reduced levels of intracellular adenosine 5′-triphosphate (ATP) and 2,3-DPG in the RBCs (Figure 6-5), degeneration of functional granulocytes and platelets, and deterioration of clotting factors V and VIII. Consequently, if a large volume of stored blood is infused rapidly, significant effects may be seen in the recipient, depending on the metabolic state.

Thermal Load

A significant problem in massive transfusion is the lowering of body temperature often associated with rapid transfusion of large volumes of cold blood products. Such situations usually occur in patients who have an open thoracic or abdominal cavity, which accelerates heat loss. If the patient is able to shiver, a decrease in temperature of less than 1° C can increase oxygen consumption and cardiac output. Lowering the body temperature also increases the affinity of hemoglobin for oxygen, as does alkalosis and reduced 2,3-DPG in the transfused RBCs. Moreover, chilling impairs platelet function and increases the potential for hypocalcemia because the liver does not metabolize citrate as well. If the blood is being rapidly infused through a central line, with exit near the sinoatrial node, fatal arrhythmias can result. Patients who have a core temperature below 34° C do not clot normally, even if the levels of clotting factors and platelets are normal.

Hypothermia is best prevented by warming intravenous fluids before administration. Commercial warmers have not been uniformly effective in warming infusion products, but heat exchanges similar to those used in cardiothoracic surgery hold promise.[38] Care must be exercised to not heat RBCs to greater than 37° C because shortened survival or acute hemolysis can result.

Acid-Base Changes

Although stored RBCs and WB are intrinsically acid, usually with a pH of about 6.3 or 6.4, the early net result of successful resuscitation is posttransfusion alkalosis in the patient. The sodium citrate, which is the anticoagulant in blood products, is converted to sodium bicarbonate. The alkalosis initially increases the oxygen affinity of hemoglobin. However, because it stimulates enzymes in the Embden-Myerhof pathway of glycolysis, the net effects of alkalosis are to increase intracellular 2,3-DPG and restore RBC oxygen transport. The posttransfusion pH may range from 7.48 to 7.50 and is associated with an increased potassium excretion.

Changes Due to Citrate

Massive transfusion of citrated blood products can lead to transiently decreased levels of ionized calcium. The effects of hypocalcemia are hypotension; narrowed pulse pressure; and elevated left ventricular, end-diastolic, pulmonary artery, and central venous pressures. Commercially available electrodes now allow evaluation, but intraoperative monitoring of ionized calcium levels is still unreliable. Monitoring changes such as electrocardiographic abnormalities (e.g., prolonged QT intervals) is also unsatisfactory. However, most normothermic adults can withstand the infusion of one unit of RBCs every 5 minutes without requiring calcium supplementation. Indiscriminate calcium administration can produce transient hypercalcemia and should be strictly avoided.

Changes in Potassium

The potassium concentration in the plasma of stored WB increases by 30 to 40 mEq/L by 3½ weeks of storage. When multiple units of blood have been transfused, hyperkalemia is theoretically possible. However, unless the transfusion rate exceeds 100 to 150 ml/min, clinical problems associated with potassium are rare. Moreover, most patients requiring rapid transfusion are in shock and have an increase in aldosterone, antidiuretic hormone, and the permissive steroid hormones. Therefore most massively transfused patients are hypokalemic unless renal function ceases. However, one should remember that hyperkalemia associated with hypocalcemia may significantly alter cardiac function. Hyperkalemia, which may cause elevated peaked T waves on the electrocardiogram, may be treated by insulin and glucose.

Changes in 2,3-Diphosphoglycerate

Because 2,3-DPG is greatly reduced in RBCs after about 3 weeks of storage, large-volume transfusion of a patient with blood near the end of its storage life may result in a decrease in oxygen off-loading (Figure 6-6). This decrease is often of theoretic rather than actual concern because of the rapid correction of the cellular defect once the RBCs are transfused (Figure 6-7) and because, if cardiac function is adequate, oxygen transport is maintained. However, if the hematocrit is low and cardiac

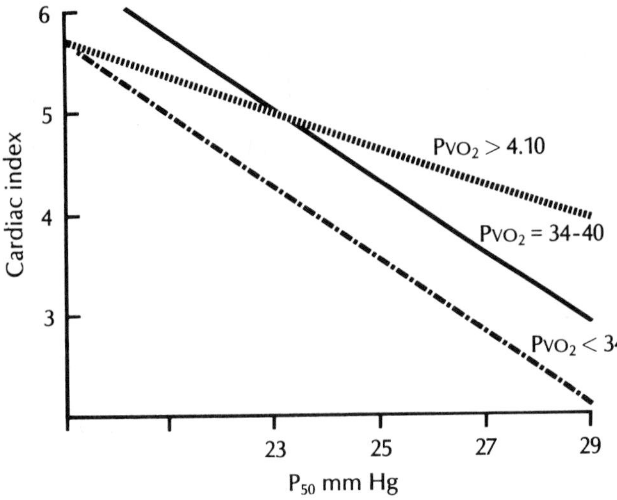

FIGURE 6-6 Posttransfusion increase in the affinity of hemoglobin for oxygen is associated with (1) low P_{50} values; (2) high cardiac index; and (3) lowered mixed oxygen tension. (From Sheldon GF: Hemotherapy in a trauma center. In Johnson W, editor: *Hemotherapy in trauma and surgery,* Arlington, Va, 1979, American Association of Blood Banks.)

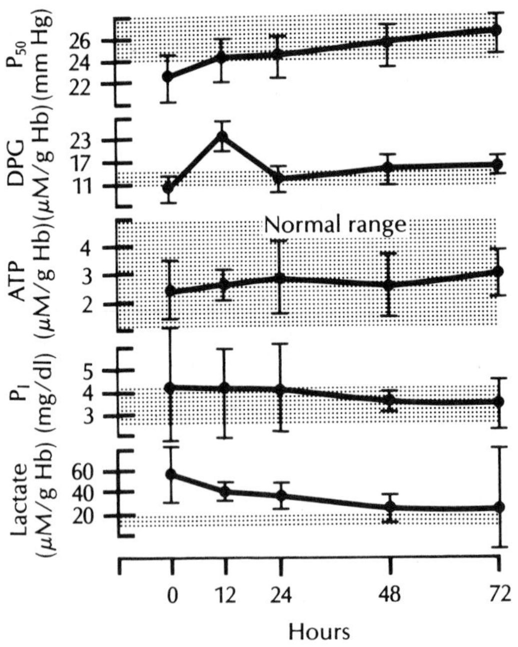

FIGURE 6-7 Metabolic data from eight massively transfused patients shows the rapid recovery of 2,3-DPG and P_{50} values in association with elevation of inorganic phosphate values. Note that lactic acidosis is cleared by 24 hours after successful resuscitation. (From Sheldon GF: Hemotherapy in a trauma center. In Johnson W, editor: *Hemotherapy in trauma and surgery,* Arlington, Va, 1979, American Association of Blood Banks.)

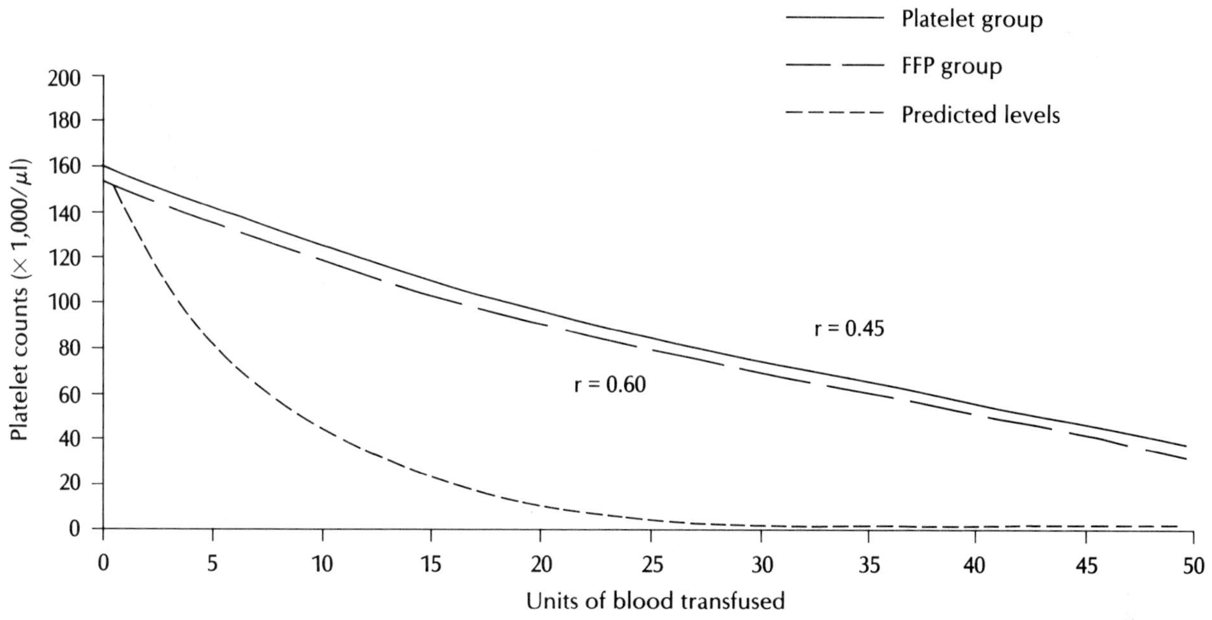

FIGURE 6-8 Exponential regression lines from platelet counts of patients treated prophylactically with either six units of platelet concentrate or two units of FFP. The dotted line is based on an exponential equation for continuous exchange transfusion with blood containing no platelets. The group that received platelets and the group that received FFP are not significantly different from each other, but both show higher platelet counts than would be expected from simple washout. (From Reed RL et al: *Ann Surg* 203:46, 1986.)

function is compromised, as is the case in elderly persons with atherosclerosis, the reduced level of 2,3-DPG may be detrimental.

Hemostasis

Dilutional thrombocytopenia may result in the massively transfused patient because the number of viable platelets is almost nil in blood stored for 24 hours at 1° C to 6° C. This is observed even though the decrease is often less than one would expect on the basis of simple dilution. The body has reserves of platelets in the spleen and can release additional platelets from the marrow (Figure 6-8).* Despite the fact that platelet counts may fall with massive transfusion, dilutional thrombocytopenia alone usually does not account for microvascular bleeding (MVB).[100] For this reason the prophylactic use of platelet concentrate in the massively transfused patient is not justified unless MVB is present. In patients who develop DIC, large doses of platelet concentrate, FFP, and cryoprecipitate may be required. One should remember that the plasma contained in platelet concentrate has good levels of all clotting factors except factor VIII, a factor often increased in trauma victims.

In summary, the major changes that one may see in the massively transfused patient are in opposition to what one might expect based on the changes that occur during the storage of RBCs. Table 6-4 outlines these changes.

*References 25, 34, 50, 76, 100, and 135.

TRANSFUSION REACTIONS

The most severe transfusion reactions result when complement-mediated RBC destruction occurs. As the RBCs are rapidly destroyed intravascularly, peptides are released from proteins of the complement system that produce hypotension, compromise renal blood flow, activate the clotting cascade, and lead to DIC. The conscious patient may become aware something is wrong almost immediately. Signs and symptoms include pain and redness along the infused vein, chest tightness and pain, a feeling of "doom," hypotension, oozing from intravenous sites, hematuria, oliguria, chills, and fever. In the unconscious patient, hypotension, hemoglobinuria, and diffuse oozing may be the only clues.

The major antigens involved in fatal hemolytic transfusion reactions are of the ABO system. Most reported fatalities have resulted when a type O person received type A RBCs because of a mishap in identification either at the time the sample was drawn, when the sample and unit were processed in the laboratory, or when the unit was administered.[20] The majority of the accidents occur in the emergency department, the intensive care unit, or the operating room, sites where more than one patient is receiving blood at the same time. Because all of these deaths are preventable, anyone associated with the drawing of blood samples, the processing of blood samples and products, and the administering of blood products must *pay meticulous attention to identification procedures, especially in the acute trauma or surgical situation.* All samples should be labeled at the patient's side to match the identification wristband; the identification of all units should be verified with the wristband before the product is given.

If a transfusion reaction is suspected, the infusion should be stopped immediately and the label on the unit checked against the recipient's wristband. To minimize the administration of the incompatible RBCs, the intravenous line should be replaced with fresh tubing from the needle or catheter to maintain intravenous access. The suspect unit, with all attached intravenous solutions and tubing and blood samples drawn from a site remote from the infusion line, should be sent to the blood bank. Urine should be tested for free hemoglobin. Technologists in the blood bank will immediately verify the identification of all samples and double-check internal records, note whether the posttransfusion plasma is pink, and perform a direct antiglobulin test. Clinically it is imperative to prevent hypotension and maintain renal blood flow by giving adequate intravenous fluids and diuretics. Mannitol can be used to maintain diuresis. Patients who die are those who develop hypotension and DIC early in the reaction.

Hemolytic reactions can also occur from hours to days after an infusion is complete, depending on the particular antibodies involved and whether the patient has been previously sensitized.[83] The development of delayed hemolysis can be particularly important in the patient whose total RBC mass has been replaced by massive transfusion. Any transfused patient who develops an unexplained fall in hematocrit, fever, or jaundice should have samples sent to the blood bank for testing. The fever seen in these patients is sometimes misinterpreted to indicate abscess or postoperative infection.

The most common types of transfusion reactions are nonhemolytic and are caused by antibodies against white cells or plasma proteins. The former usually cause chills and fever, whereas the latter lead to allergic symptoms such as urticaria or anaphylaxis. Febrile reactions can be prevented by transfusing leukocyte-poor RBCs or by premedicating the patient with acetaminophen before giving non–RBC-containing components such as platelet concentrate. Allergic reactions are usually prevented by premedication with diphenhydramine.

AUTOLOGOUS BLOOD

This section describes the use of autologous blood for the patient undergoing elective surgery.[48,87] The advantages of autologous blood are many.[45] It exposes the patient to no additional risk for hepatitis or AIDS, prevents alloimmunization, and is completely compatible. Because the only concern is the safety of donation for the donor, any patient who can undergo elective surgery should be able to undergo the phlebotomy necessary to predonate. Age is no limitation; children and elderly persons can be evaluated. The minimum hematocrit is less than that required for homologous donation. Many patients can have blood withdrawn every 3 to 4 days until 3 days before surgery. Autologous donors must receive iron supplementation and should maintain good nutrition. Patients ordinarily thought to be at high risk, such as those with cardiac disease, have successfully predonated.[74] When the surgeon and staff of the blood bank work together, autologous predonation is very well received by patients and can significantly reduce the risks of blood transfusion. On rare occasions, autologous blood may be the only compatible blood for the patient.

REFERENCES

1 Aach RD, Szmuness W, Mosley JW et al: Serum alanine aminotransferase of donors in relation to the risk of non-A, non-B hepatitis in recipients, *N Engl J Med* 304:989, 1981.

2 Aasen A, Kierulf P, Vaage J et al: Determination of components of the plasma proteolytic enzyme systems gives information of prognostic value in patients with multiple trauma, *Adv Exp Med Biol* 156:1037, 1983.

3 Alter H, Tabor E, Meryman H et al: Transmission of hepatitis B virus infection by infusion of frozen deglycerolised red blood cells, *N Engl J Med* 238:637, 1978.

4 American Association of Blood Banks: *Standards for blood banks and transfusion services,* ed 10, Washington, DC, 1981, The Association.

5 American Association of Blood Banks: *Technical manual,* Washington, DC, 1981, The Association.

6 American Association of Blood Banks: *Plasma products: use and management,* Anaheim, Calif, 1982, The Association.

7 Ampel LL, Marshall S, Caprini JA: Etiology, diagnosis, and treatment of recovery room bleeding hemorrhage, *Heart Lung* 14(6):556, 1985.

8 Andes W, Wulff K, Smith W: Head trauma in hemophilia: a prospective study, *Arch Intern Med* 144:1981, 1984.

9 Arnow P, Weiss L, Weil D et al: *Escherichia coli* sepsis from contaminated platelet transfusion, *Arch Intern Med* 146:321, 1986.

10 Bachman F, Kruithof I: Tissue plasminogen activator: chemical and physiology aspects, *Semin Thromb Hemost* 10:6, 1984.

11 Barker L: Posttransfusion hepatitis: epidemiology, experimental studies and U.S. perspectives, *Bibl Haematologica* 46:3, 1980.

12 Barton J: Nonhemolytic, noninfectious transfusion reactions, *Semin Hematol* 18:95, 1981.

13 Bennett B, Towler H: Haemostatic response to trauma, *Br Med Bull* 41:274, 1985.

14 Berry TK, Flynn TC, Miller PW, Fischer RP: Diagnostic peritoneal lavage in blunt trauma patients with coagulopathy, *Ann Emerg Med* 13(10):879, 1984.

15 Blanchard SA, Sirridge M: Deep venous thrombosis in surgical patients: possible laboratory predictors, *South Med J* 78(10): 1161, 1985.

16 Bull BS, Bull MH: Enhancing the safety of intraoperative RBC salvage, *J Trauma* 29(3):320, 1989.

17 Buller H, Ten-Cate J: Antithrombin III infusion in patients undergoing peritoneovenous shunt operation: failure in the preven-

tion of disseminated intravascular coagulation, *Semin Thromb Hemost* 49:128, 1983.

18 Caggiano V: Red blood cell transfusions. In Silver H, editor: *Blood, blood components and derivatives in transfusion therapy,* Washington, DC, 1980, American Association of Blood Banks.

19 Caggiano V: Red blood cell transfusions. In Silver H, editor: *Blood, blood components and derivatives in transfusion therapy,* Washington, DC 1980, American Association of Blood Banks.

20 Camp FR, Monsghan WP: Fatal blood transfusion reactions, *Am J Forensic Med Pathol* 2:143, 1981.

21 Cederbaum AI: The appropriate use of plasma and plasma components in clinical medicine. In Silver H, editor: *Blood, blood components and derivatives in transfusion therapy,* Washington, DC, 1980, American Association of Blood Banks.

22 Chaimoff C, Creter D, Djaldetti M: The effect of pH on platelet and coagulation factor activities, *Am J Surg* 136(2):257, 1978.

23 Cohn E, Strong LE, Hughes WL: Preparation and properties of serum and plasma proteins. IV. A system for the separation into fractions of the protein and lipoprotein components of biological tissues and fluids, *J Am Chem Soc* 68:459, 1946.

24 Committee on Trauma, American College of Surgeons: *Resources for the optimal care of the injured patient,* ed 3, Philadelphia, 1982, WB Saunders.

25 Counts RB, Haisch C, Simon TL et al: Hemostasis in massively transfused trauma patients, *Ann Surg* 190(1):91, 1979.

26 Davis JM, Demling RH, Lewis FR et al: The Surgical Infection Society's Policy on Human Immunodeficiency Virus and Hepatitis B and C Infection: the ad hoc committee on acquired immunodeficiency syndrome and hepatitis, *Arch Surg* 127:218, 1992.

27 DeRie M, Van der Plas van Dalen CM, Engelfriet C et al: The serology of febrile transfusion reactions, *Vox Sang* 49:126, 1985.

28 Dofferhoff AS, Bomv JJ et al: Patterns of cytokines, plasma endotoxin, plasminogen activator inhibitor and acute phase proteins during the treatment of severe sepsis in humans, *Crit Care Med* 20:185, 1992.

29 Dutta R, Ray T, Sinha A: Prostacyclin stimulation of the activation of blood coagulation factor X by platelets, *Science* 231:385, 1986.

30 Effeney D, Blaisdell F, McIntyre K et al: The relationship between sepsis and disseminated intravascular coagulation, *J Trauma* 18:689, 1978.

31 Eika C, Havig O, Godal HC: The value of preoperative haemostatic screening, *Scand J Haematol* 21(4):3459, 1978.

32 Eisenberg JM, Clarke JR, Sussman SA: Prothrombin and partial thromboplastin times as preoperative screening tests, *Arch Surg* 117(1):48, 1982.

33 Elmer O, Goransson G, Zoucas E: Impairment of primary hemostasis and platelet function after alcohol ingestion in man, *Haemostasis* 14(2):223, 1984.

34 Ferrara A, MacArthur JD, Wright HK et al: Hypothermia and acidosis worsen coagulopathy in the patient requiring massive transfusion, *Am J Surg* 160:515, 1990.

35 Fish K, Sarnquist F, Van Steennis C et al: A prospective, randomized study of the effects of prostacyclin on platelets and blood loss during coronary bypass operations, *J Thorac Cardiovasc Surg* 91(3):436, 1986.

36 Fisher D, Yawn D, Crawford E: Preoperative disseminated intravascular coagulation associated with aortic aneurysms, *Arch Surg* 118:1252, 1983.

37 Freed D, Buisseret P, Lloyd M et al: Angioedema responding to antiprotease treatment but without abnormalities of the complement system, *Clin Allergy* 10(1):21, 1980.

38 Freireich EJ: Granulocyte transfusion: an overview. In Mielke CH Jr, editor: *Apheresis: development, applications, and collection procedures,* New York, 1981, Alan R Liss.

39 Fried SJ, Bhagwan S, Zeeb P: Normothermic rapid volume replacement for hypovolemic shock: an in vivo and in vitro study utilizing a new technique, *J Trauma* 26:183, 1986.

40 Friedman BA, Burns TL, Schork MA: A study of blood utilization by diagnosis, month of transfusion, and geographic region of the United States, *Transfusion* 19:511, 1979.

41 Friedman BA, Oberman HA, Chadwick R, Kingdon I: The maximum surgical blood order schedule and surgical blood use in the United States, *Transfusion* 16:380, 1976.

42 Furie B, Furie BC: Molecular and cellular biology of blood coagulation, *N Engl J Med* 326:800, 1992.

43 Gallimore M: Serum inhibitors in fibrinolysis, *Br J Haematol* 31:217, 1975.

44 Giles A: Disseminated intravascular coagulation. In Rakel R, editor: *Conn's current therapy,* Philadelphia, 1985, WB Saunders.

45 Giordano GF, Giordano DM, Wallace BA et al: An analysis of 9,918 consecutive perioperative autotransfusions, *Surg Gynecol Obstet* 176(2):103, 1993.

46 Gleysteen JJ, Klamer TW: Peritoneovenous shunts: predictive factors of early treatment failure, *Am J Gastroenterol* 79(8):654, 1984.

47 Goldenberg S, Fenster H, Perler Z et al: Disseminated intravascular coagulation in carcinoma of prostate: role of estrogen therapy, *Urology* 22:130, 1983.

48 Goodnough LT, Rudnick S, Price TH et al: Increased preoperative collection of autologous blood with recombinant human erythropoietin therapy, *N Engl J Med* 321(17):1163, 1989.

49 Gruber UF, Rem J, Meisner C, Gratzl O: Prevention of thromboembolic complications with miniheparin-dihydroergotamine in patients undergoing lumbar disc operations, *Eur Arch Psychiatry Neurol Sci* 234(3):157, 1984.

50 Harrigan C, Lucas CE, Ledgerwood AM et al: Serial changes in primary hemostasis after massive transfusion, *Surgery* 98(4):836, 1985.

51 Hecht T, Wolf JL, Niraz L et al: Platelet transfusion therapy in an alloimmunized patient. The value of crossmatch procedures for donor selection, *JAMA* 248:2301, 1982.

52 Hedner U, Martinsson G, Bergqvist D: Influence of operative trauma on factor XII and inhibitor of plasminogen activator, *Haemostasis* 13:219, 1983.

53 Heldebrant CM, Gomperts ED, Kasper CK et al: Evaluation of two viral inactivation methods for the preparation of safer factor VIII and factor IX concentrates, *Transfusion* 25:510, 1985.

54 Hewson J: Homeostatic alterations with major trauma: massive transfusion, *Can Anaesth Soc J* 32:239, 1985.

55 Heymann SJ, Brewer TF, Fineberg HV et al: How safe is safe enough? New infections and the US blood supply, *Ann Intern Med* 117(7):612, 1992.

56 Higby DJ: Granulocyte transfusions. In Silver H, editor: *Blood, blood components and derivatives in transfusion therapy,* Washington, DC, 1980, American Association of Blood Banks.

57 Hirsh J: Drug therapy: heparin, *N Engl J Med* 324:1565, 1991.

58 Horst HM, Dlugos S, Fath JJ et al: Coagulopathy and intraoperative blood salvage (IBS), *J Trauma* 32(5):646, 1992.

59 Hughes CF, Grant AF, Leckie BD, Baird DK: Cardioplegic solution: a contamination crisis, *J Thorac Cardiovasc Surg* 91(2):296, 1986.

60 Janson PA, Jubelirer SJ, Weinstein MJ, Deykin D: Treatment of the bleeding tendency in uremia with cryoprecipitate, *N Engl J Med* 303:1319, 1980.

61 Kambayashi J, Ohshiro T, Mori T, Kosaki G: Hemostatic defects in experimental obstructive jaundice, *Jpn J Surg* 15(1):75, 1985.

62 Kaplan EB, Sheiner LB, Boeckmann AJ et al: The usefulness of preoperative laboratory screening, *JAMA* 253(24):3576, 1985.

63 Kapsch D, Metzler M, Harrington M et al: Fibrinolytic response to trauma, *Surgery* 95:473, 1984.

64 Kearney TJ, Bentt L, Grode M et al: Coagulopathy and catecholamines in severe head injury, *J Trauma* 32:608, 1992.

65 King DJ, Kelton JG: Heparin associated thrombocytopenia, *Ann Intern Med* 100:535, 1984.

66 Kitchen L, Erichson RB, Sideropoulos H: Effect of drug-induced platelet dysfunction on surgical bleeding, *Am J Surg* 143(2):215, 1982.

67 Klock JC: Granulocyte transfusion physiology. In Mielke CH Jr, editor: *Apheresis: development, applications and collection procedures,* New York, 1981, Alan R Liss.

68 Kobayashi H, Honda Y: Intraocular hemorrhage in a patient with hemophilia, *Metab Ophthalmol* 8:27, 1984.

69 Lefebre J, McLellan BA, Coovadia AS: Seven years experience unmatched packed red regional trauma unit, *Ann Emerg Med* 16(12):1344, 1987.

70 Lefemine AA, Lewis M: Activated clotting time for control of anticoagulation during surgery, *Am J Surg* 51(5):274, 1985.

71 Levine M, Hirsch J: Hemorrhagic complications of anticoagulant therapy, *Semin Thromb Hemost* 12:39, 1986.

72 Lewis FR, Elings VB, Sturm JA: Bedside measurement of lung water, *J Surg Res* 27:250, 1979.

73 Mammen E, Miyakawa T, Phillips T et al: Human antithrombin concentrates and experimental disseminated intravascular coagulation, *Semin Thromb Hemost* 11:373, 1985.

74 Mann M, Sacks HJ, Goldfinger D: Safety of autologous blood donation prior to elective surgery for a variety of potentially "high-risk" patients, *Transfusion* 23:229, 1983.

75 Martin DJ, Lucas CE, Ledgerwood AM et al: Fresh frozen plasma supplement to massive red blood cell transfusion, *Ann Surg* 202(4):505, 1985.

76 Martin DJ, Lucas CE, Ledgerwood AM et al: Fresh frozen plasma supplement to massive red blood cell transfusion, *Ann Surg* 202(4):505, 1985.

77 McCredie KB: Indications for HLA typing in granulocyte and platelet concentrate transfusions. In Mielke CH Jr, editor: *Apheresis: development, applications, and collection procedures,* New York, 1981, Alan R Liss.

78 McKenna P, Scheinman H: Transient coagulation abnormalities after incompatible blood transfusion, *Crit Care Med* 3(1):8, 1975.

79 McLeod B, Sassetti R, Weens J et al: Haemolytic transfusion reaction due to ABO incompatible plasma in a platelet concentrate, *Scand J Haematol* 28:193, 1982.

80 Meier H, Pierce J, Colman R et al: Activation and function of human Hageman factor, *J Clin Invest* 60:18, 1977.

81 Menitove J, McElligott M, Aster R: Febrile transfusion reaction: what blood component should be given next? *Vox Sang* 42:318, 1982.

82 Miner M, Kaufman H, Graham S et al: Disseminated intravascular coagulation fibrinolytic syndrome following head injury in children: frequency and prognostic implications, *J Pediatr* 100:687, 1982.

83 Mollison PL: *Blood transfusion in clinical medicine,* ed 7, Oxford, 1983, Blackwell Scientific Publications, Ltd.

84 Movat H: Kinins and the kinin system as inflammatory mediators, *Handbook of Inflammation* 1:47, 1979.

85 Murphy C, Tishkoff GH: Preparation of components and their characteristics: plasmapheresis and cytapheresis. In Petz ID, Swisher SN, editors: *Clinical practice of blood transfusion,* New York, 1981, Churchill Livingstone.

86 Myhre BA, Harris GE: Blood components for hemotherapy, *Clin Lab Med* 2(1), 1982.

87 The National Blood Resource Education Program Expert Panel: The use of autologous blood, *JAMA* 263(3):414, 1990.

88 Ohsato K, Takaki A, Takeda S et al: A clinical study on surgical patients with disseminated intravascular coagulations: with special reference to the occurrence of major organ failures, *Nippon Geka Gakkai Zasshi* 84:860, 1983.

89 Opelz G, Sengar DPS, Mickey MR, Terasaki PI: Effect of blood transfusion on subsequent kidney transplants, *Transplantation* 5:253, 1973.

90 O'Reilly R, Lombard C, Azzi R: Delayed hemolytic transfusion reaction associated with Rh antibody anti-f, first reported case, *Vox Sang* 49:336, 1985.

91 Ottensen S, Stormorken H, Hatteland K: The value of activated coagulation time in monitoring heparin therapy during extracorporeal circulation, *Scand J Thorac Cardiovasc Surg* 18(2):123, 1984.

92 Patten E, Reddi C, Riglin H et al: Delayed hemolytic transfusion reaction caused by a primary immune response, *Transfusion* 22:248, 1982.

93 Pedersen P, Biber B, Martinelli S et al: Hemodynamic and hematologic changes in a standardized trauma-sepsis model in rats, *Circ Shock* 14:13, 1984.

94 Perinovic D, Muminagic S, Boskovic S et al: Orthopedic and trauma surgery in hemophilia with a case report, *Med Arch* 36:41, 1982.

95 Pineda A, Brzica S, Taswell H: Hemolytic transfusion reaction: recent experience in a large blood bank, *Mayo Clin Proc* 53:378, 1978.

96 Pineda A, Taswell H, Brzica S: Transfusion reaction: an immunologic hazard of blood transfusion, *Transfusion* 18:1, 1978.

97 Preiss DU, Schmidt-Bleibtreu H, Berguson P, Metz G: Blood transfusion requirements in coronary artery surgery with and without the activated clotting time (ACT) technique, *Klin Wochenschr* 63(6):252, 1985.

98 Rao S, Bhagavath S, Chen C et al: Mesenchymal hamartoma of the liver in an older child: association with disseminated intravascular coagulation, *Med Pediatr Oncol* 12:112, 1984.

99 Raphael B, Lackner H, Engler G: Disseminated intravascular coagulation during surgery for scoliosis, *Clin Orthop* 162:41, 1982.

100 Reed RL, Giavarella D, Heimbach DM et al: Prophylactic platelet administration during massive transfusion: a prospective, randomized, double-blind clinical study, *Ann Surg* 203:40, 1986.

101 Risberg B, Medegard A, Heideman M et al: Early activation of humoral proteolytic systems in patients with multiple trauma, *Crit Care Med* 14:917, 1986.

102 Roseman B: Disseminated intravascular coagulation: a review, *Oral Surg* 59:551, 1985.

103 Rosenberg R, Rosenberg J: Natural anticoagulant mechanisms, *J Clin Invest* 74:1, 1984.

104 Rush B, Lee N: Clinical presentation of nonhaemolytic transfusion reactions, *Anaesth Intensive Care* 8:125, 1980.

105 Salem H, Koutts J, Handley C et al: The aggregation of human platelets by ascitic fluid: a possible mechanism for disseminated intravascular coagulation complicating LeVeen shunts, *Am J Hematol* 11:153, 1981.

106 Schiffer CA, Slichter SJ: Platelet transfusions from single donors, *N Engl J Med* 307:245, 1982.

107 Schiller W, Hartmann G, Remde W: Causes of death in hemophilia patients in East Germany, *Folia Haemotol* 112:845, 1985.

108 Schmidt U, Enderson BL, Chen JP, Maull KI: D-Dimer levels correlate with pathologic thrombosis in trauma patients, *J Trauma* 33:312, 1992.

109 Schwab CW, Shayne JP, Turner J: Immediate trauma resuscitation with type O uncrossmatched blood: a two-year prospective experience, *J Trauma* 26(10):897, 1986.

110 Sheldon GF: Hemotherapy in a trauma center. In Johnson W, editor: *Hemotherapy in trauma and surgery,* Committee on Technical Workshops, Arlington, Va, 1979, American Association of Blood Banks.

111 Shikimori M, Oka T: Disseminated intravascular coagulation syndrome, *Int J Oral Surg* 14:451, 1985.
112 Shinagawa S, Kagiya A, Kikuchi M et al: Gynecological malignancies and disseminated intravascular coagulation, *Nippon Sanka Fujinka Gakkai Zasshi* 36:108, 1984.
113 Siegal T, Seligsohn U, Aghai E et al: Clinical and laboratory aspects of disseminated intravascular coagulation (DIC): a study of 118 cases, *Thromb Haemost* 39(1):122, 1978.
114 Silver H: Normal serum albumin and plasma protein fraction. In Silver H, editor: *Blood, blood components and derivatives in transfusion therapy,* Washington, DC, 1980, American Association of Blood Banks.
115 Silvergleid AJ: Clinical platelet transfusions. In Silver H, editor: *Blood, blood components and derivatives in transfusion therapy,* Washington, DC, 1980, American Association of Blood Banks.
116 Slichter SJ: Controversies in platelet transfusion therapy, *Annu Rev Med* 31:509, 1980.
117 Soper D: Delayed hemolytic transfusion reaction: a cause of late postoperative fever, *Am J Obstet Gynecol* 153:227, 1985.
118 Spero J, Lewis J, Hasiba U: Disseminated intravascular coagulation: findings in 346 patients, *Thromb Haemost* 43:28, 1980.
119 Starling EH: On the absorption of fluids from the connective tissue spaces, *J Physiol* (Lond) 19:312, 1896.
120 Suchman AL, Griner PF: Diagnostic uses of the activated partial thromboplastin time and prothrombin time, *Ann Intern Med* 104(6):810, 1986.
121 Taddie S, Barrasso C, Ness P: A delayed transfusion reaction caused by anti-K6, *Transfusion* 22:68, 1982.
122 Takaki A, Kato H, Takeda S et al: The role of disseminated intravascular coagulation in shock induced by transfusion of human blood in dogs, *Transfusion* 19:404, 1979.
123 Talbot RW, Heppell J, Dozois RR, Beart RW Jr: Vascular complications of inflammatory bowel disease, *Mayo Clin Proc* 61(2):140, 1986.
124 Towne JB, Bandyk DF, Hussey CV, Tollack VT: Abnormal plasminogen: a genetically determined cause of hypercoagulability, *J Vasc Surg* 1(6):896, 1984.
125 Turinetto B, Cahsai G, Dozza F et al: Early thrombosis of an aortic St. Jude valve in spite of effective anticoagulant treatment, *J Cardiovasc Surg* 25(2):182, 1984.
126 Urban AE, Popov-Cenic S, Noe G, Kulzer R: Aprotinin in open-heart surgery of infants and children using the heart-lung machine, *Clin Ther* 6(4):425, 1984.
127 Verstraete M: Clinical application of inhibitors of fibrinolysis, *Drugs* 29:236, 1985.
128 Von Fliedner V, Higby DJ, Kim U: Graft-versus-host reaction following blood product transfusion, *Am J Med* 72:951, 1982.
129 Walker I, Davidson J, Young P et al: Effect of anabolic steroids on plasma antithrombin III, $alpha_2$ macroglobulin and $alpha_1$ antitrypsin levels, *Thromb Diath Haemorrh* 34:106, 1975.
130 Warkentin TE, Kelton JG: Heparin induced thrombocytopenia, *Annu Rev Med* 40:31, 1989.
131 Weiss HJ: Bleeding disorders due to abnormal platelet function, *Med Clin North Am* 37(2):517, 1973.
132 Widman FK, editor: *Technical manual of the American Association of Blood Banks,* ed 9, Arlington, Va, 1985, American Association of Blood Banks.
133 Williams W et al, editors. Hematology. In *Hemostasis,* New York, 1982, McGraw-Hill.
134 Winkler M, Trunkey D: Dopamine gangrene: association with disseminated intravascular coagulation, *Am J Surg* 142:588, 1981.
135 Wudel JH, Morris JA, Yates K et al: Massive transfusion: Outcome in blunt trauma patients, *J Trauma* 31(1):1, 1991.
136 Zulim RA, Rocco M, Goodnight JE et al: Intraoperative autotransfusion in hepatic resection for malignancy: is it safe? *Arch Surg* 128:206, 1993.

CHAPTER

7

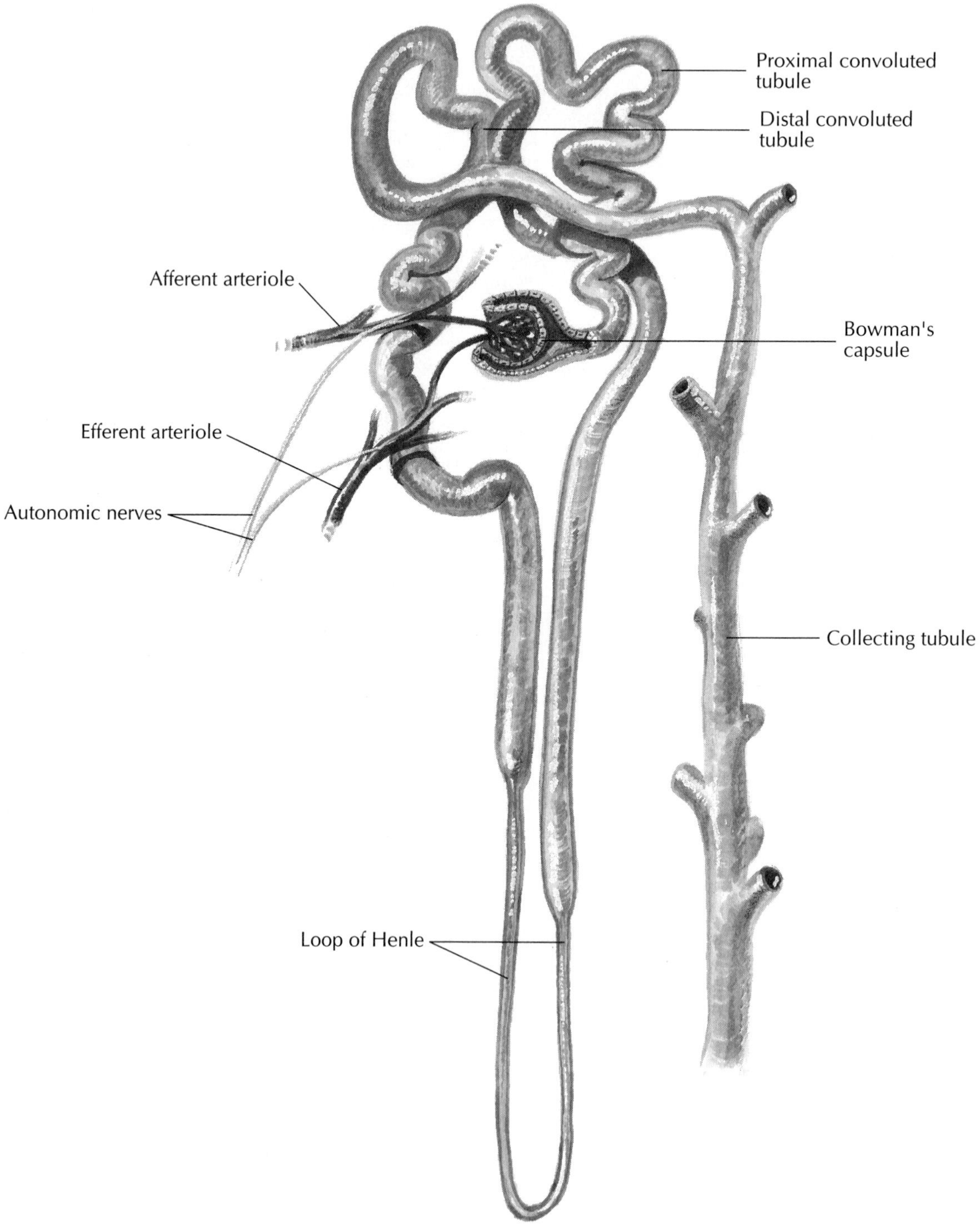

Proximal convoluted tubule
Distal convoluted tubule
Afferent arteriole
Bowman's capsule
Efferent arteriole
Autonomic nerves
Collecting tubule
Loop of Henle

RENAL FUNCTION AND ACUTE RENAL FAILURE

Geoffrey Silver • Richard L. Gamelli

RENAL DEVELOPMENT AND ANATOMY

The kidney is a complex organ that performs an abundance of endocrine, metabolic, and regulatory functions. It is the site of erythropoietin production, it participates in the metabolism of vitamin D, it produces glucose during periods of starvation, and it continuously performs homeostatic tasks in a dynamic environment of neural, hormonal, hemodynamic, and metabolic signals. During the adverse conditions imposed by injury, sepsis, and organ failure, the kidney responds predictably and effectively to maintain homeostasis. If metabolic or hemodynamic limits are exceeded or the renal parenchyma is damaged, the renal homeostatic response is impaired or lost, and acute renal failure ensues.

Acute renal failure in critical illness, both with and without other organ failure, is relatively common and has an associated mortality of 50% or higher.[25] Mortality and morbidity are directly related to the severity of the underlying disease, the presence of infection, and the number of other organ systems involved.[29,77] In patients who develop acute renal failure, preventing associated complications and starting therapy quickly are critical to improving the outcome.

Embryology

The kidney develops in three sequential, overlapping stages: the pronephros, the mesonephros, and the metanephros (Figure 7-1).[76] As each stage develops, it affects the development of the subsequent stage. The first of these stages, the pronephros, is transient and regresses early in embryonic life. The second stage, the mesonephros, results in the mesonephric duct, which in turn gives rise to the metanephric diverticulum. The metanephric diverticulum, or ureteric bud, develops into the collecting system.[60,100] The ureter arises from the cranial end of the metanephric diverticulum, which by repeated splitting gives rise to the renal pelvis, calices, and collecting tubules. Each collecting tubule is surrounded by the metanephric mesoderm, which forms the tubular nephron. The distal end of the primitive nephron forms an open connection with the collecting tubules. The proximal end of the nephron forms Bowman's capsule. The various segmental divisions of the nephron are formed by further elongation and differentiation.

The vascular supply develops in concert with the collecting system and nephron. The glomerular capillaries develop in situ directly from mesoderm with Bowman's capsule.[59,64,88] These capillaries multiply by luminal

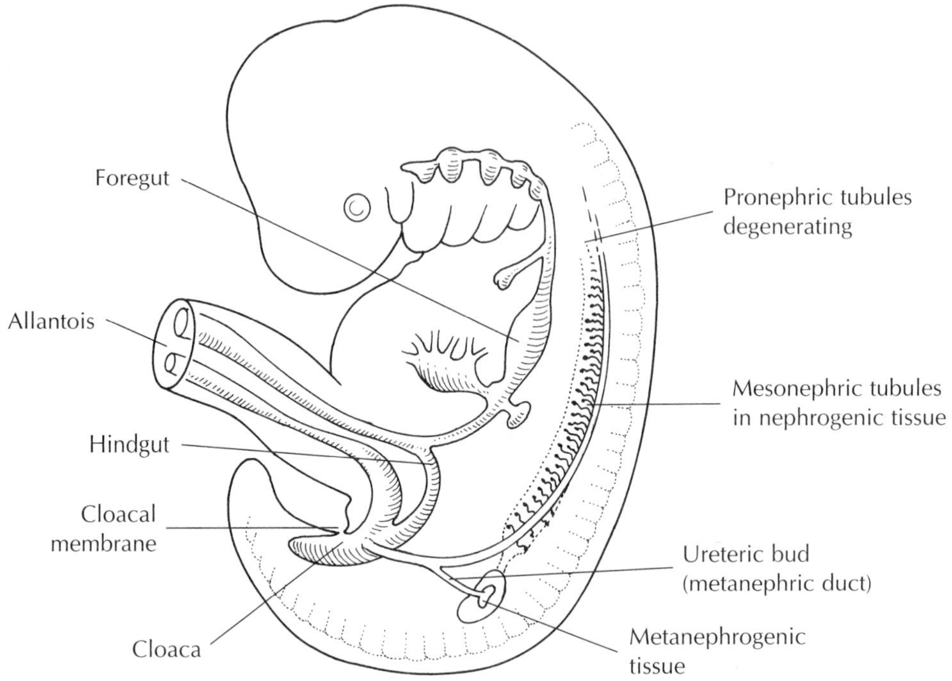

FIGURE 7-1 Developing embryo, showing the anatomic correlates of the three overlapping stages of renal development. (From Netter F: *The CIBA Collection of Medical Illustrations,* vol 6, New Jersey, 1973, CIBA.)

subdivision, forming the glomerular capillary bed.[4] Branches of the afferent arteriole connect with the previously formed capillaries of the glomerulus, establishing continuity of the renal circulation with the systemic circulation. An efferent vessel leaves the glomerulus to subdivide again to form the meshwork of capillaries surrounding the nephron. This process of glomerular formation continues at least to the thirty-fifth week of gestation.

The primitive kidney originates in the fetal pelvis, receiving its blood from the regional arterial supply. As the ureteric bud lengthens, the kidney migrates cranially. By the third month the kidney is at the level of the second lumbar vertebra, and a distinct renal artery has emerged, derived from caudal branches of the embryonic lateral splanchnic arteries.

Anatomy

The final result of embryonic differentiation is the complex architecture of the functioning human kidney. The structural arrangement of the vascular and tubular elements has a profound effect on the integrity of renal homeostatic functions. The renal arteries arise directly from the abdominal aorta at the second lumbar vertebra. The origin is approximately 1 cm below the origin of the superior mesenteric artery. The right renal artery is longer and passes behind the inferior vena cava and right renal vein, posterior to the head of the pancreas and the second part of the duodenum. The left renal artery passes behind the renal vein posterior to the body of the pancreas and splenic vein. Before entering the renal parenchyma, the renal arteries give off an inferior suprarenal artery. Branches of this artery supply the inferior portion of the suprarenal gland, as well as the perinephric tissue, the renal capsule, the renal pelvis, and the proximal ureter. At the level of the renal hilum, each artery divides into an anterior and posterior division supplying separate vascular segments of the kidney. There are five segments: the apical, the upper anterior, the middle anterior, the lower, and the posterior. The anterior division of the renal artery gives rise to the upper, middle, and lower segmental arteries. The posterior division supplies the posterior segment. The apical segment is supplied by either the anterior or posterior division. Arising from these primary branches are the lobar, interlobar, arcuate, and interlobular arteries. The lobar arteries are distributed one to each pyramid (the pyramids contain part of the secreting tubules and the collecting tubules). Just before entering the parenchyma, the lobar arteries divide into two or three interlobar arteries that run toward the cortex along the renal pyramids. At the junction between the cortex and the medulla, the interlobar arteries divide at right angles into several arcuate arteries, which course between the cortex and the medulla. These branch and

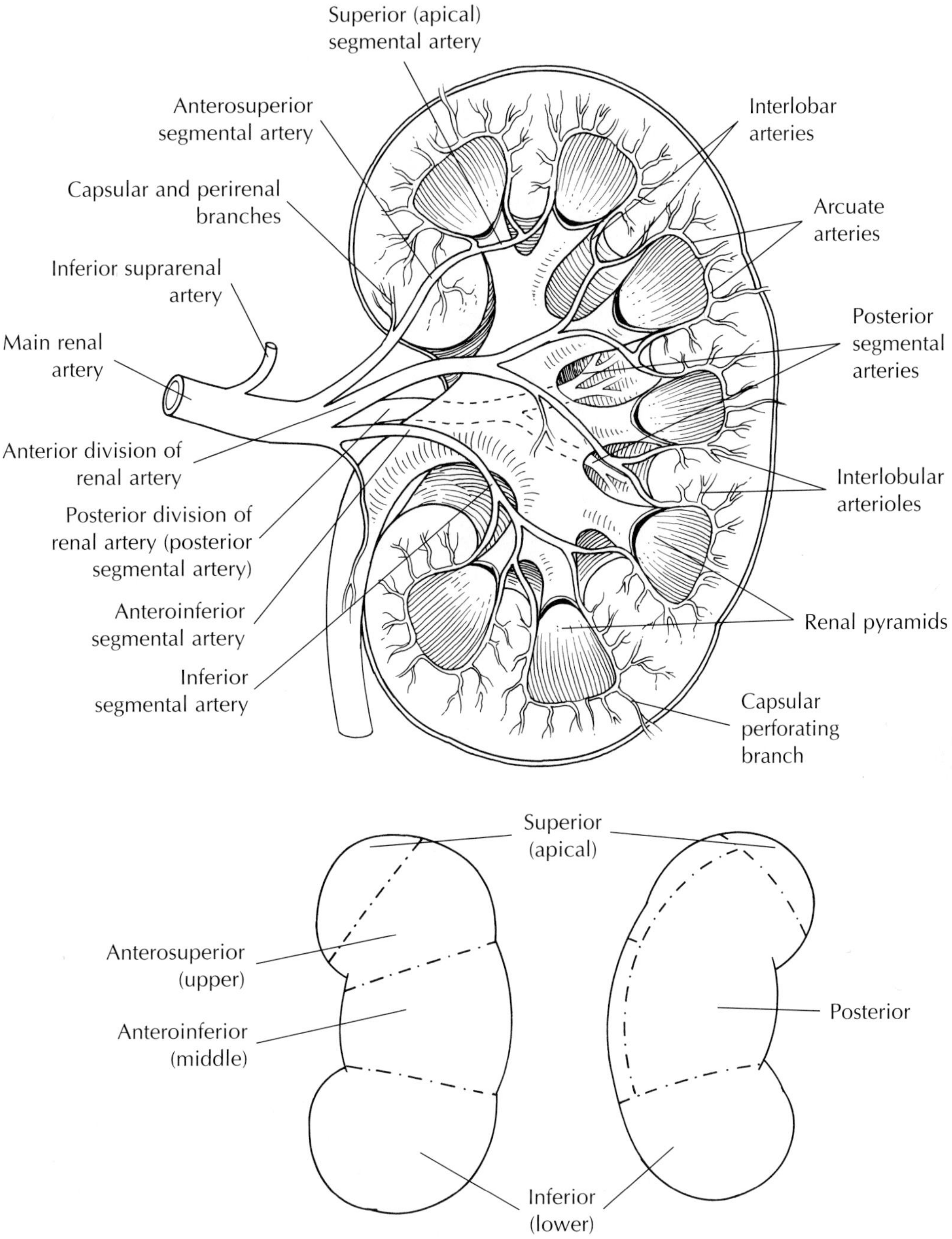

FIGURE 7-2 Arterial supply to the kidney. The segmental anatomy is depicted in the lower half of the figure. (From Netter F: *The CIBA Collection of Medical Illustrations,* vol 6, New Jersey, 1973, CIBA.)

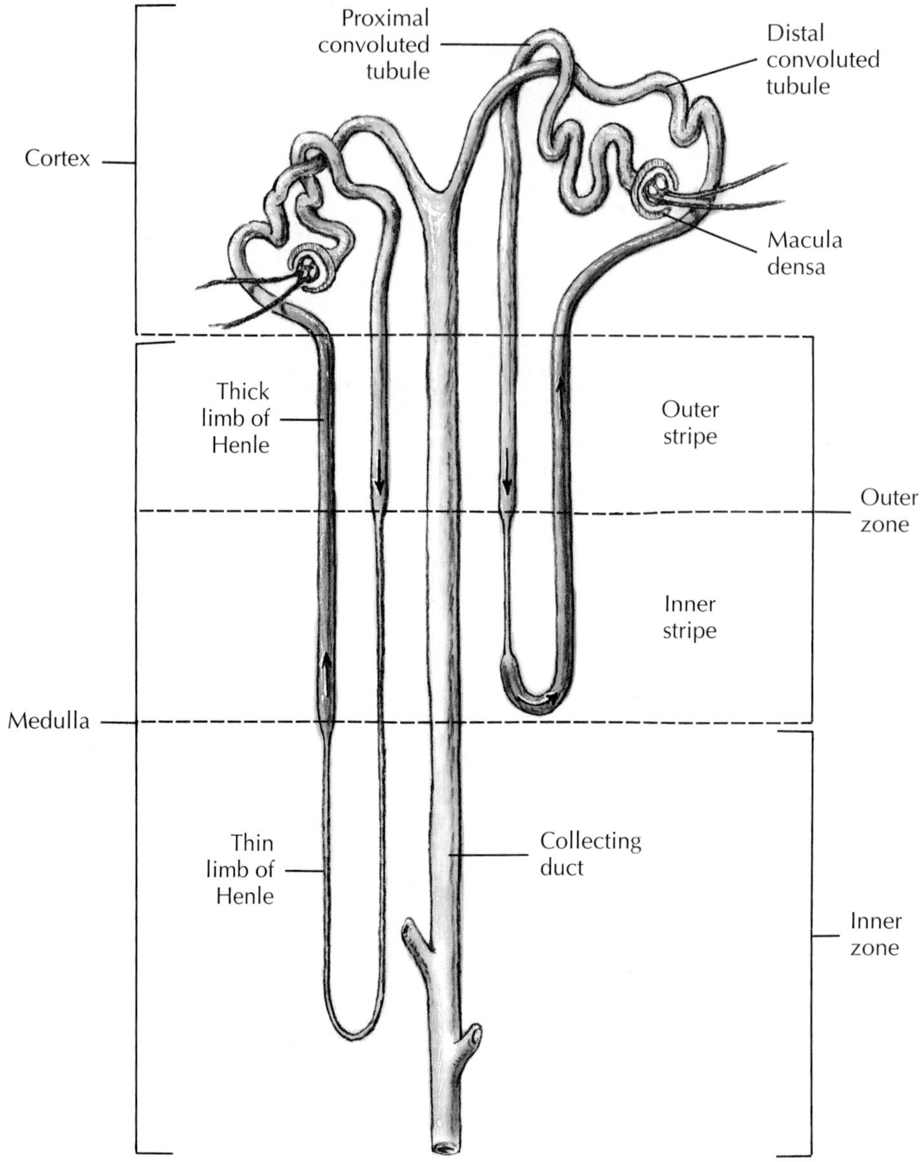

FIGURE 7-3 The nephron, the functional unit of the kidney. (From Gamelli RL, Silver GM: Acute renal failure. In Deitch E, editor: *Multiple organ failure,* New York, 1990, Thieme.)

form the nonanastomosing interlobular arteries, which give rise to the afferent arterioles (Figure 7-2). The glomerulus, which is a system of branching capillaries, lies between the afferent and efferent arterioles.

The nephron is considered the functional unit of the kidney. It comprises the glomerular capillaries connected to a continuum of specialized tubular segments spatially oriented to each other, to vascular elements, and to other nephrons. The afferent arterioles, the glomerular capillaries, and the efferent arterioles are in intimate contact with the nephron. The peritubular capillaries of the renal cortex are derived from the efferent arterioles. The efferent arterioles within the inner one third of the cortex are the origin of the descending and ascending vasa recta. The vasa recta are arranged in dense, parallel, hairpin-shaped loops that are close to the nephron and that descend deep into the medulla. This anatomic arrangement helps to preserve medullary hypertonicity through the countercurrent exchange mechanism.[35,90]

The segmental divisions of the nephron (Figure 7-3), often the source of controversy, are based on both structure and function. The divisions are (1) the glomerulus; (2) the proximal tubule; (3) the loop of Henle; and (4) the distal nephron. Each of these segments can be further subdivided according to structure and function.

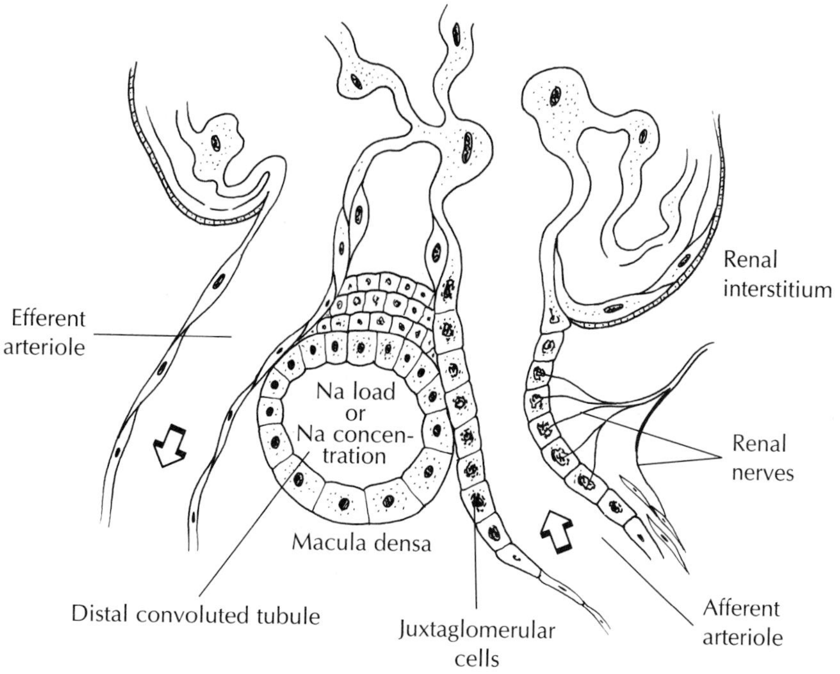

FIGURE 7-4 Diagrammatic representation of an electron micrograph of the human renal glomerulus. Note the proximity of the distal convoluted tubule to the afferent and efferent arterioles. This anatomic arrangement allows for feedback regulation of the glomerular filtration rate. (From Davis JD: *Circ Res* 28:301, 1971.)

RENAL FUNCTION

Glomerulus

The glomerulus is surrounded by Bowman's space, which is the beginning of the proximal tubule (Figure 7-4). The glomerulus is a set of specialized capillaries situated between the tonically active afferent and efferent arterioles. These arterioles are regulated by several factors, including neural and hormonal influences, that assist in maintaining hydrostatic pressure to drive glomerular filtration. The glomerular hydrostatic pressure is maintained between 30% and 50% of systemic mean arterial pressure.[34] This relationship generally obtains until mean arterial pressure approaches 80 mm Hg, at which point glomerular filtration and urine output drop precipitously.[74]

Starling elucidated the basics of glomerular filtration in the nineteenth century. He stated that filtration was the net result of opposing hydrostatic and oncotic forces. Forces that favor filtration are the glomerular capillary hydrostatic pressure and the oncotic pressure of Bowman's space. Forces that oppose filtration are the hydrostatic pressure within Bowman's space and the oncotic pressure of the glomerular capillary. For any single nephron, this relationship can be expressed quantitatively by the following equation:

$$\text{SNGFR} = K_f[(\text{Pgc} - \text{Pb}) - (\text{pgc} - \text{pb})]$$

in which SNGFR = single nephron glomerular filtration rate

K_f = Filtration coefficient
Pgc = Glomerular capillary hydrostatic pressure
Pb = Hydrostatic pressure of Bowman's space
pgc = Oncotic pressure of glomerular capillary
pb = Oncotic pressure of Bowman's space

The filtration coefficient (K_f) depends on the permeability of the membrane and the total glomerular surface area available for filtration.[12] The glomerular capillary membrane acts as a filter, allowing molecules to pass into Bowman's space on the basis of size and charge.[81] The glomerular membrane normally is permeable to neutral solutes up to a molecular weight of 50,000 daltons. Because it is negatively charged, the glomerular membrane is less permeable to polyanions (e.g., albumin).[15,56]

Proximal Tubule

The proximal tubule can be subdivided into the proximal convoluted tubule and the proximal straight tubule (Figure 7-5). Approximately 180 L of filtrate enters the sum of proximal tubules in a normal individual each day. Approximately two thirds of this filtrate is reclaimed by the proximal tubule isotonically. Sodium is actively transported from the tubular lumen by a sodium- and potassium-activated adenosine triphosphatase (ATPase).[67,79] This is followed by passive reabsorption of water and other solutes driven to maintain

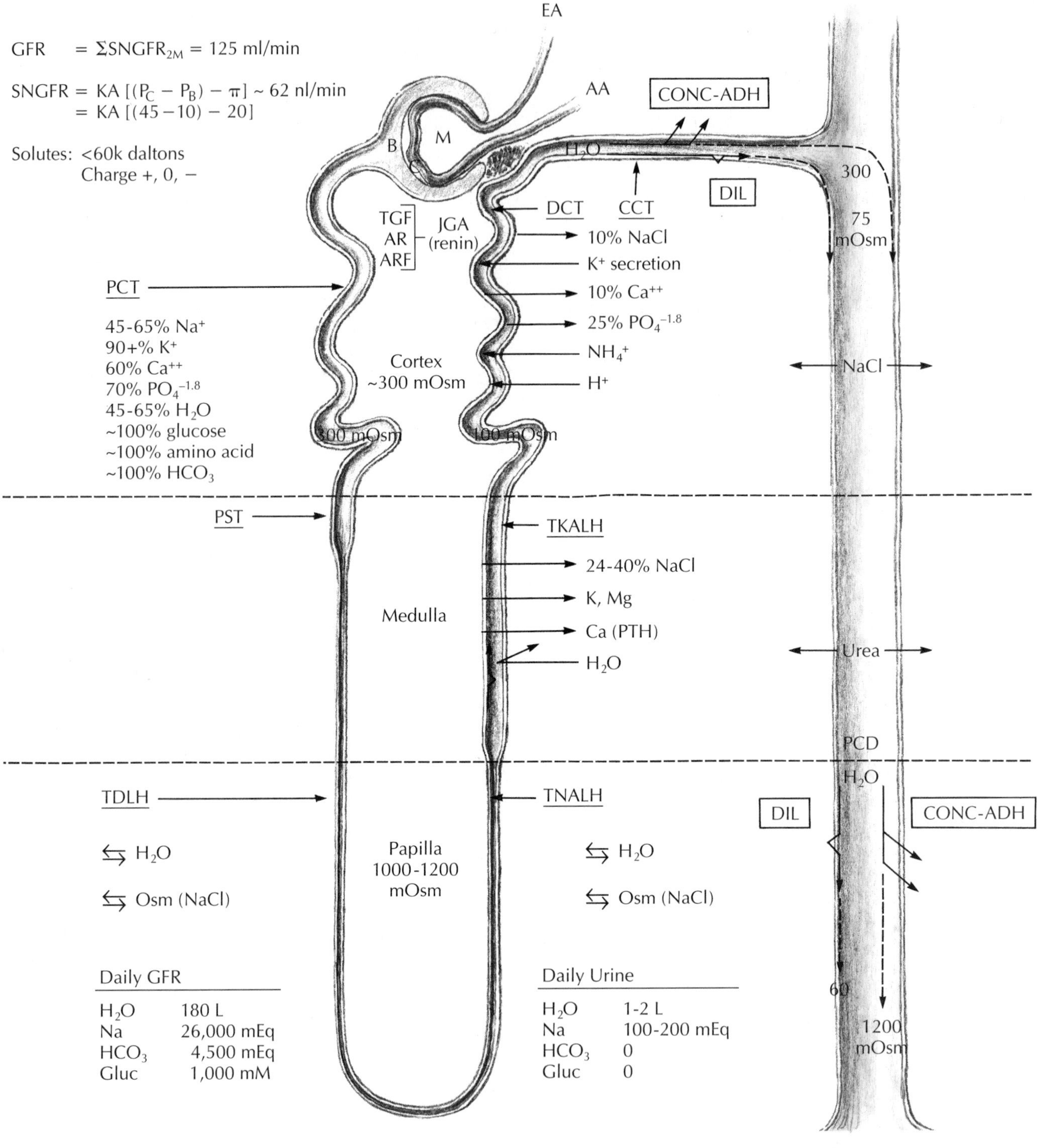

FIGURE 7-5 Glomerulus, nephron, and collecting ducts. The functional regions and sites of action of various hormones are depicted. *EA,* Efferent arteriole; *AA,* afferent arteriole; *B,* Bowman's space; *PCT,* proximal convoluted tubule; *PST,* proximal straight tubule; *TDLH,* thin descending limb of Henle; *TNALH,* thin ascending limb of Henle; *TKALH,* thick ascending limb of Henle; *DCT,* distal convoluted tubule; *CCT,* cortical collecting tubule; *JGA,* juxtaglomerular apparatus.

osmotic and electrostatic equilibrium as the plasma flows toward the loop of Henle.

Fifty to seventy percent of the total filtered calcium is reabsorbed in the proximal tubule under the control of parathyroid hormone (PTH).[62] The remaining filtered calcium is reabsorbed in the ascending limb of Henle and the collecting duct, with less than 3% excreted.

The principal function of PTH is to regulate calcium (Ca^{++}) in the extracellular fluid compartment. Through a cyclic adenosine monophosphate (cAMP) mechanism, PTH increases CA^{++} reabsorption and decreases sodium-dependent phosphate, bicarbonate, and fluid reabsorption in the proximal tubule, the thick ascending limb of Henle, and the collecting duct.[23,72] This decreased absorption of solute can be compensated for by increased reabsorption more distally.

Loop of Henle

There are three types of Henle's loops: cortical, short, and long. The cortical loops originate from superficial glomeruli and do not enter the medulla. The other two types of loops arise from juxtamedullary glomeruli and can be further characterized by the extent to which they penetrate the medulla. The loop of Henle can be divided into descending and ascending limbs. The ascending limb has both a thin and a thick portion. The descending limb receives the isotonic filtrate from the proximal tubule. In the descending limb the functional characteristics of the tubular cells change. Sodium is no longer transported actively, and the cells are more permeable to water and less permeable to solute. The net result is the passive movement of water out of the lumen into the medullary interstitium, which is rendered hypertonic by the proximal tubules of surrounding nephrons and the thick ascending limb. The luminal filtrate is therefore concentrated. As the descending limb changes to the ascending limb, the permeability of solutes increases and permeability to water decreases abruptly.[47] This causes solutes to diffuse out of the lumen, thereby decreasing the tonicity of the filtrate. As the thick segment is reached, the active transport of sodium resumes, whereas the tubule remains impermeable to water. This has two consequences: the luminal filtrate is further diluted, and medullary hypertonicity is maintained.[41] Calcium is reabsorbed in the thick segment as well.

The structural and functional aspects of Henle's loop allow for the production of high intramedullary tonicity by countercurrent multiplication. The necessary components of this system are (1) the production of osmotic pressure differences between the ascending and descending limbs of the loop; (2) differential permeability, allowing solute diffusion from the ascending limb to the descending limb; and (3) sufficient length, along which small concentration changes can be multiplied and maintained. The loop of Henle has all of these characteristics inherent in its structure. The thick ascending limb transports sodium actively and can maintain a gradient of 200 mOsm. The descending limb is freely permeable to water and slightly permeable to solute. Together these two features allow production of a concentration gradient that causes successive increases in descending solute concentration by both equilibration and net solute flow from the thick ascending limb to the thin descending limb. As successively higher concentrations reach the site of transport in the thick ascending limb, the same 200 mOsm concentration gradient is maintained, thereby establishing higher medullary tonicity. The mechanism is very effective, permitting maximum concentrations near the hairpin portion of Henle's loop to reach 1400 mOsm. This high tonicity is supported by a second countercurrent multiplication system provided by the anatomic arrangement of the vasa recta. The ascending and descending vasa recta run parallel and close to each other and the loop of Henle. The capillary membranes of the vasa recta are freely permeable to solute, allowing passive flow of solute from the highly concentrated plasma of the ascending vasa recta to the lower concentration of the descending vasa recta.[35] This arrangement supports and maintains the concentration gradient from the cortex to the deep medulla created by the loop of Henle.

Juxtaglomerular Apparatus

The juxtaglomerular apparatus consists of the macula densa; the extraglomerular mesangial cells, which fill the angle between the afferent and efferent arterioles; the afferent arteriole; and the efferent arteriole (see Figure 7-3).[18] The macula densa is a group of densely packed cells, found at the site of contact between the ascending limb and the afferent and efferent arterioles, that are different from the usual epithelial cells of the thick ascending limb. The end portion of the thick ascending limb returns to the cortex, where it comes close to its own glomerulus. The thick ascending limb passes through the angle formed by the afferent and efferent arterioles and makes intimate contact with each, as well as with the capillaries of the glomerular tuft. This site is the location of the juxtaglomerular apparatus. The macula densa is believed to function as a tubular sensor, which can respond to changes in the luminal flow rates of the thick ascending limb by influencing the glomerular filtration rate (GFR).[37]

Distal Convoluted Tubule

The filtrate reaching the distal convoluted tubule is hypotonic by virtue of the active transport along the length of the thick ascending limb of Henle's loop. This filtrate represents 20% of the original protein-free filtrate. At the level of the distal convoluted tubule, additional sodium is reabsorbed actively, the rate being regulated by the influence of aldosterone. Potassium is also secreted in the distal convoluted tubule and is linked with both the rate of sodium reabsorption and hydrogen ion secretion.

Collecting Duct

Nearly 30 L of hypotonic filtrate reaches the collecting ducts each day. Under the influence of antidiuretic hormone (ADH), the cells of the distal convoluted tubule and the collecting duct become more permeable, allowing passive water reabsorption and concentration of urine. This passive reabsorption of water is driven by the high tonicity of the medullary interstitium created by countercurrent multiplication. The deeper the collecting tubule penetrates the medulla, the higher the medullary tonicity, allowing maintenance of a concentration gradient between the increasing tonicity of the luminal contents of the collecting duct. In water-depleted states, urine osmolarity can reach 1400 mOsm by this process. This number represents the physiologic maximum concentrating ability of the human kidney. With an obligate solute turnover of approximately 700 mOsm/day, an obligate urine volume of approximately 400 ml/day is required to maintain homeostasis. Less urine production per day results in accumulation of solutes.

Renal Regulation of Acid-Base Balance

Both renal and respiratory mechanisms are responsible for maintaining blood pH. The respiratory response occurs through changes in the ventilatory rate, which cause rapid adjustments in the partial pressure of carbon dioxide PCO_2. The renal response occurs through the excretion of titratable acid and through the variable filtration of bicarbonate. The filtered load of bicarbonate is approximately 4500 mEq/day. The bulk of bicarbonate is reabsorbed in the proximal tubule. In this process sodium is actively reabsorbed in exchange for hydrogen ions, which are buffered in the tubule lumen by available bicarbonate. The H_2O and CO_2 formed are reabsorbed into the cell, where the formation of bicarbonate is catalyzed by carbonic anhydrase. Factors causing increased bicarbonate reabsorption are extracellular fluid (ECF) volume depletion, increased PCO_2, and hypokalemia. The distal nephron also helps regulate acid-base balance by reabsorbing bicarbonate, forming titratable acidity, and producing ammonium ion.

As nonvolatile acids are formed from metabolic processes, bicarbonate is consumed by buffering the acid in the ECF. The sodium salt of the acid anions is filtered at the glomerulus. In the distal nephron, hydrogen ions are secreted into the tubular lumen and a bicarbonate ion is formed for each acid anion filtered. Sodium is reabsorbed from the tubular lumen, and bicarbonate is secreted by the tubular cell into the bloodstream. Secreted protons form ammonium ions in combination with ammonia (NH_3) and in turn combine with acid anions to be excreted. Approximately 50 to 70 mEq of acid is processed in this fashion each day.

Diuretics

Diuretics are drugs that increase the rate of urine formation. In addition, diuretics have a wide variety of both renal and systemic effects. Diuretics may be classified according to their site of their proposed action.

The osmotic diuretics (e.g., mannitol) exert their primary effects throughout the nephron. They are freely filtered at the glomerulus and are poorly reabsorbed by the renal tubule. In addition, they are pharmacologically inert and can therefore be administered in quantities sufficient to increase the osmolality of the plasma and the osmotic load of the filtrate reaching the nephron.[96] The increased osmotic load causes an increase in urine volume, thereby increasing the rate of excretion of sodium, potassium, and chloride. The filtrate volume is subject to modification by the action of ADH on the collecting tubule.

Carbonic anhydrase inhibitors (e.g., acetazolamide) have several sites of action, including the kidney, intraocular structures, gastrointestinal tract, and central nervous system. In the kidney, inhibition of carbonic anhydrase reduces reabsorption of bicarbonate ion in the proximal tubule. Micropuncture studies of isolated nephrons also show decreased reabsorption of sodium and chloride. The overall mechanism is poorly understood, but clearly the net effect is increased solute load in the tubule lumen. The effects of this decreased reabsorption are partly compensated for by an increase in solute reabsorption by the distal nephron, which limits the efficiency of the diuretic effect.

The thick ascending limb of Henle is the site of action of the "loop diuretics." This class of diuretics includes furosemide, ethacrynic acid, and bumetanide. At the usual therapeutic doses, these diuretics do not have appreciable systemic effects. Higher doses have been known to cause hearing loss. Their potency is the product of at least two different effects: they block active transport of chloride and inhibit tubuloglomerular feedback.[102] In so doing they increase the solute load reaching the distal tubules without decreasing the GFR. This dual effect greatly increases their diuretic efficiency. Administration of furosemide or ethacrynic acid does not alter renal oxygen consumption despite reducing sodium reabsorption by approximately one third.[33]

The distal tubule is the site of action of the thiazide diuretics, chlorthalidone and metolazone. These diuretics decrease sodium reabsorption in the cortical portion of the ascending limb and distal convoluted tubule. The overall effects of the thiazides are similar to those of the loop diuretics except with respect to calcium. The loop diuretics are calciuric, whereas the thiazides are hypocalciuric and cause elevated serum calcium levels with prolonged use.

The distal tubule is the site of action of the potassium-sparing diuretics, which are divided into two groups. The triamterine group causes the formation of a positive potential difference in the distal tubule, which inhibits secretion of potassium ion. These diuretics also decrease sodium permeability, inhibiting reabsorption. The spironolactone group acts by competitive inhibition of aldosterone activity at the receptor level[26]; this inhibits sodium reabsorption and in turn potassium secretion.

Hormonal Regulation of Renal Function

To maintain homeostasis, the kidney must respond appropriately to the myriad perturbations of the organism's internal milieu. With injury and sepsis, these changes may be quite drastic, causing a complex series of responses aimed at restoring homeostasis. This task is accomplished through both systemic and local responses mediated by neural and hormonal signals. It is beyond the scope of this chapter to review all of the hormonal interactions involved in renal homeostasis. Those of particular relevance to the homeostatic perturbations found with impaired renal perfusion are reviewed in this section.

Renin-Angiotensin-Aldosterone System

Renin is a 40 kilodalton glycoprotein stored by the juxtaglomerular cells of the afferent arteriole. It is secreted by the juxtaglomerular cells in response to decreased tubular sodium chloride (NaCl) concentration during hypovolemia or other low perfusion states. A diminished effective perfusion volume decreases NaCl flux through the distal tubule, which is sensed by the macula densa, causing the release of renin from the juxtaglomerular cells. Systemically, renin frees angiotensin I from alpha$_2$-globulin. Angiotensin I, a decapeptide, is then cleaved by a converting enzyme to angiotensin II. Angiotensin II is a potent arteriolar vasoconstrictor. In low concentrations it causes constriction of the efferent arteriole. Higher concentrations cause a more global response, resulting in increased systemic resistance and increased arterial pressures at the expense of GFR. Recent evidence suggests that both renin and angiotensin I are present in juxtaglomerular cells. These hormones may then act as paracrine substances, being released and then acting on the renal vasculature locally.[45]

Angiotensin II and its metabolite, angiotensin III, stimulate the adrenal gland to secrete aldosterone.[22] Aldosterone acts at the cortical and medullary collecting tubules, helping to maintain extracellular fluid balance by increasing sodium reabsorption.

Antidiuretic Hormone

In hypovolemia, the kidney also responds to conserve free water; this is accomplished through the release of antidiuretic hormone (ADH). The release of ADH is controlled by both the plasma osmolality and the ECF volume. The primary stimulus is osmolality. The release of ADH occurs above a plasma threshold value of approximately 280 mOsm/kg.[83] Alternatively, a significant decrease in ECF is necessary to stimulate ADH secretion.[48,82] ADH acts through a receptor-dependent CAMP mechanism, which causes a cell permeability change that facilitates the transcellular movement of water.

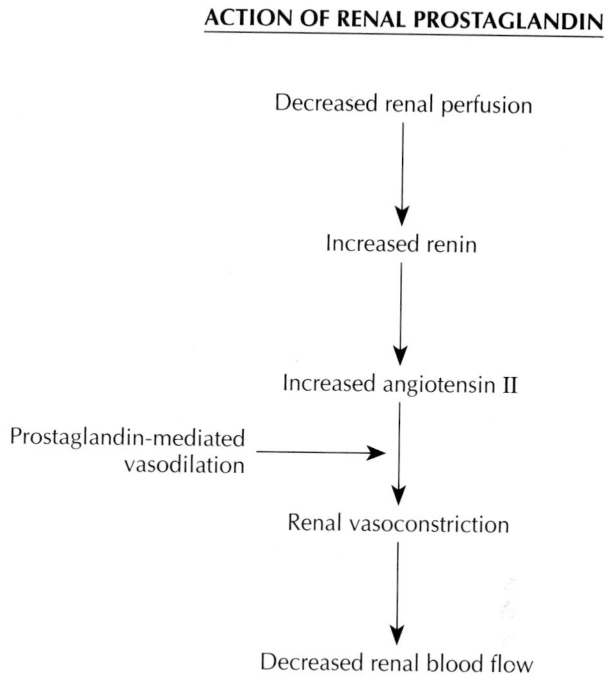

FIGURE 7-6 Modulating effect of prostaglandins on the vasoconstricting activity of angiotensin II. The effect is locally mediated at or near the site of action of angiotensin II.

Prostaglandins

Prostaglandins are products of arachidonic acid metabolism. They are produced throughout the body and initiate a wide range of locally mediated effects. The kidney is a major site of prostaglandin synthesis and action. In the renal cortex, prostaglandins are produced by cells of both the glomerulus and the arterioles.[73] Prostaglandins locally affect renin release, renal blood flow, and GFR. They also modulate the function of other hormones and influence salt and water permeability. In compromised renal perfusion, locally released prostaglandins act to prevent the vasoconstriction caused by angiotensin II and norepinephrine, thereby attenuating a fall in GFR (Figure 7-6).[30]

Atrial Natriuretic Factor

Atrial natriuretic factor (ANF) is a family of low-molecular-weight peptides that affect water balance by regulating sodium excretion.[28] The stimuli for release of ANF are atrial distention or sodium concentration, or both. ANF is a fast-acting hormone that has numerous effects on both the systemic and renal vasculature. The site and mechanism of action currently are poorly understood.

Endothelin

Endothelin, a 21-amino acid peptide, is a potent vasoconstrictor produced by vascular endothelial cells.[103] Administration of this peptide has been shown to cause intense intrarenal vasoconstriction.[52] It is thought that endothelin is released when endothelial damage occurs, and that it may play a role in the pathogenesis of acute renal failure.[97] Tomita and associates measured plasma endothelin levels in seven patients with acute renal failure and found significant elevations.[91] Further investigation is needed to define the role of this hormone in acute renal failure.

Renal Responses to Decreased Perfusion

Renal responses to injury and sepsis are primarily the result of changes in renal perfusion. The integration of systemic and renal responses to decreased perfusion is an adaptive spectrum of survival events initiated through changes in renal vascular resistance, blood flow distribution, glomerular filtration, solute reabsorption, and water excretion. This response is a graded continuum in which progressively severe perfusion deficits are counteracted by increased renal and systemic responses. In the euvolemic state, an equilibrium is established by a balance of vasoconstrictors, vasodilators, prostaglandins, and neural tone.[7,55,61] In mild states of hypovolemia (less than 15% hemorrhage), the kidney responds by attempting to restore effective plasma volume while preserving renal function. The initial response is a reflex decrease in afferent arteriolar tone, maintaining flow to the glomerulus. This is a remarkably effective process of autoregulation that maintains GFR over a significant range of perfusion pressures.[104] Eventually, progressive perfusion deficits cause progressive increases in renal vascular resistance to maintain systemic perfusion. As 20% to 30% of cardiac output is directed to renal perfusion, substantial gains to systemic perfusion become available. During this process intrinsic renal blood flow is shunted from the outer cortex to the juxtamedullary region and medulla in an effort to maintain the GFR.[36,51] As renal vascular resistance increases, deficits in renal function occur, manifested by oliguria caused by diminished glomerular filtration.[43] This begins to occur at moderate volume deficits (15% to 30% hemorrhage).[68] As mean arterial pressure falls below 80 mm Hg, renal blood flow and GFR fall precipitously. In severe hemorrhage (over 40%), renal blood flow virtually ceases and cell damage results if the condition is not quickly reversed.

The above responses are mediated by the interaction of the sympathetic nervous system, locally and systemically released hormones, and locally released prostaglandins.[42] Reductions in perfusion pressure at the glomerulus cause reductions in filtration. This results in decreased sodium delivery to the thick ascending limb of Henle. The change in sodium delivery is monitored at the macula densa, which in turn stimulates the release of renin from the granular epithelial cells of the juxtaglomerular apparatus. As described above, renal renin production causes the conversion of angiotensin I to angiotensin II, which in turn triggers the release of aldosterone, augmenting sodium reabsorption. Angiotensin II also works to increase arteriolar tone, both systemically and at the efferent arteriole.[46] Angiotensin II preferentially increases efferent arteriolar tone, thereby increasing renal vascular resistance while maintaining GFR.[30,55,104]

A fall in perfusion pressure also stimulates increased systemic release of antidiuretic hormone (ADH) by the posterior pituitary. Vasopressin causes both systemic and renal vasoconstriction. The renal effects of vasopressin appear to be modified by local release of vasodilator prostaglandins, which inhibit vasoconstriction of the arterioles in the juxtamedullary region.[24] The overall result of this complex interaction is the finely controlled, progressive response of the renal vasculature to decreasing perfusion. This is a dynamic response that allows the progressive increase of renal vascular resistance and the preservation of glomerular filtration.

As described above, both ADH and aldosterone are released during depletion of extracellular fluid volume. Aldosterone release is triggered by rising levels of angiotensin II and falling levels of atrial natriuretic factor.[6,70] Aldosterone and ADH function together to restore extracellular fluid volume by increasing sodium and free water reabsorption respectively.

ACUTE RENAL FAILURE

Acute renal failure (ARF) can be defined as a syndrome characterized by an abrupt reduction in renal function that results in the accumulation of nitrogenous wastes.[3,4,99] The origins of the syndrome are diverse and often involve a number of factors. There are two forms of ARF, oliguric and nonoliguric. The oliguric form is associated with 24-hour urine volumes of less than the obligate minimum output of approximately 400 ml. The nonoliguric form may have urine outputs as high as 2 L/day.[5] The combined incidence is reported to be as high as 4.9% of all hospital admissions.[44] The associated mortality from acute renal failure after severe trauma, prolonged surgery, burns, and sepsis is greater than 50%. The most common cause of death in acute renal failure is infection.

Etiology

There are several methods of classifying acute renal failure. The origin can be classified into three anatomic types: prerenal, renal, and postrenal. The major causes of the three types are shown in the boxes on p. 204. Prerenal causes are attributed primarily to decreases in effective plasma volume, impaired cardiac output, or renal vascular obstruction. Renal causes are due to parenchymal lesions of the glomerulus or tubules caused by numerous factors, including nephrotoxins and prolonged prerenal or postrenal states. Thus it is important to identify prerenal causes early, because improving intravascular volume prevents acute renal failure. Postrenal causes stem from obstruction of the urinary tract.

Classification

Prerenal Acute Renal Failure

Prerenal acute renal failure is common in trauma and burn patients. In trauma patients, early acute renal failure is attributed to decreased effective volume status caused by hemorrhage, fluid sequestration, and nasogastric or biliary drainage. In burn patients, dermal losses of salt and water, as well as fluid sequestration, can contribute to volume depletion and prerenal failure.[13]

Nephrotoxic Acute Renal Failure

The aminoglycosides are the chief cause of nephrotoxic acute renal failure, accounting for 16% of all such cases.[49] Early aminoglycoside toxicity is evidenced by reduced urinary concentrating ability and electrolyte abnormalities. This is sometimes broadcast by a rising serum trough level in patients on a constant dose.[27] More pronounced nephrotoxicity is associated with increasing proteinuria and azotemia. Toxicity usually is gradual in onset and, if identified early, is self-limiting. Mild toxicity manifests as nonoliguric acute renal failure. More severe toxicity causes oliguria and may require dialysis.

Amphotericin B, cisplatin, cyclosporine, nonsteroidal anti-inflammatory drugs, and heme pigments all can cause acute renal failure. Amphotericin B manifests a predictable, cumulative nephrotoxicity that causes necrosis of cells in the proximal and distal tubules.[21] Cisplatin also causes cumulative, dose-dependent renal toxicity.[11] Acetaminophen causes renal tubular necrosis by means of an active metabolite that binds to macromolecules of the tubule cells. Cyclosporine causes dose-dependent renal toxicity.[10]

Radiocontrast agents are responsible for approximately 10% of cases of acute renal failure.[59] The current contrast agents responsible for acute renal failure are iodinated derivatives of benzoic acid, which are excreted unchanged by the kidneys. The incidence of acute renal failure arising from use of contrast agents depends on the presence or absence of various risk factors. Patients with several risk factors are at the highest risk.[39,40] Diabetes and preexisting chronic renal insufficiency are the two best-documented risk factors. Other possible risk factors are decreased plasma volume, concurrent use of other nephrotoxic drugs, hypertension, peripheral vascular disease, and age.

Nonsteroidal anti-inflammatory drugs have been implicated as causative agents in acute renal failure.[95] Inhibition of prostaglandin synthesis causes increased renal vasoconstriction. In addition, the vasoconstrictor action of angiotensin II is significantly increased in the presence of cyclooxygenase inhibitors.[1] It follows that using nonsteroidal anti-inflammatory drugs in patients with elevated angiotensin II levels (i.e., those with decreased effective plasma volume) and congestive heart failure poses a significant risk of impairing renal function.

Myoglobin, an oxygen-carrying protein with a molecular weight of 17,000, is released from necrotic muscle. It is filtered at the glomerulus and forms hematin when the urine pH falls below 5.6.[14] Hematin is toxic to the kidneys and is thought to be responsible for tubular damage. Myoglobin also precipitates in the tubules, causing obstruction. Hypotension and hemoconcentration often follow sequestration of fluid at the site of tissue injury, particularly in burn or crush injuries, exacerbating the effects of myoglobin. The clinical course shows a rapid rise in serum creatinine, sometimes as high as 2 mg/dl/day. Acute renal failure resulting from myoglobinuria often is associated with hyperphosphatemia caused by the release of phosphates from necrotic muscle. Mannitol has been shown to prevent acute renal failure in rat models of pigmenturia if given before or shortly after the onset of pigmenturia.[101] Mannitol is thought to act by inducing an osmotic diuresis, preventing intratubular obstruction by precipitated pigments. Hypovolemia and hypotension should be avoided by adequate resuscitation. Alkalinization of the urine may prevent formation of hematin and thus acute renal failure.

Postrenal Acute Renal Failure

Frequent causes of postrenal acute renal failure are shown in the box on p. 204. It is important to note that this form of ARF often is caused by an anatomic obstruction that may be discovered by careful physical examination and relieved by timely intervention.

Pathophysiology

The renal manifestations associated with parenchymal disease are the result of four broad categories of pathophysiology: renal ischemia, chemical injury, blood vessel disease, and glomerular disease. The lesions caused by

COMMON CAUSES OF PRERENAL ACUTE RENAL FAILURE

Trauma
Hemorrhage
Peritonitis
Burns
Crush injury
Sepsis

Gastrointestinal Losses
Vomiting
Diarrhea
Fistulae
Nasogastric suction

Dehydration

Cardiac insults
Myocardial infarction
Tamponade
Cardiac failure

COMMON CAUSES OF NEPHROTOXIC ACUTE RENAL FAILURE

Antibiotics
Aminoglycosides
Penicillins
Amphotericin B

Myoglobin (hematin)
Contrast media
Uric acid
Nonsteroidal anti-inflammatory drugs

Organic Solvents
Carbon tetrachloride
Ethylene glycol

Heavy Metals
Mercury
Arsenic
Lead

COMMON CAUSES OF POSTRENAL OBSTRUCTIVE UROPATHY

Ureter
Calculus
Blood clot
Stricture
Neoplasm (intraperitoneal or retroperitoneal)
Abdominal aortic aneurysm

Bladder
Blood clot
Calculus
Carcinoma

Urethra
Urethral stricture
Prostate (hypertrophy or carcinoma)
Traumatic injury

ischemic and chemical injury are commonly referred to as acute tubular necrosis, although the pathologic process may not be limited to this site or may not be identifiable. Post ischemic injury is the most common form of acute renal failure found in surgical patients. This can be caused by several factors, generally including those responsible for prerenal azotemia.

The difference between prerenal azotemia and renal failure caused by ischemia is one of severity, and the distinction between the two is not always clear. Prerenal azotemia generally can be reversed by correcting the underlying pathologic condition. When the cause is allowed to persist, the resulting pathologic damage is more severe and may progress to cell injury and necrosis. The renal medulla is susceptible to ischemic damage because of the high metabolic rate and subsequent high oxygen consumption of the resident cells.[16] Also, medullary blood flow remains reduced after resuscitation, further aggravating the acute injury.[32] When blood flow is no longer adequate to maintain metabolic demands, ischemic damage follows.

It is important to distinguish between ischemic and hypoxic causes, because there may be mechanistic differences. In the clinical picture, elements of both reduced oxygen tension and reduced blood flow are likely to exist simultaneously. In experimental models, early injury has been located at the proximal convoluted tubules. Venkatachalam and colleagues demonstrated loss of the brush border from this site upon reperfusion of rat kidneys after mild ischemia.[92,93] In an isolated perfusion model of rat kidneys, several investigators have demonstrated selective damage to the thick ascending limb of Henle.[2,17] This cellular injury is mediated by several factors, including depletion of adenosine triphosphate (ATP) precursors, acidosis, increased free Ca^{++}, oxygen free radicals, and phospholipase.[93] Together these mediators cause cell permeability changes, which in turn cause swelling upon reperfusion secondary to the influx of calcium.[19,20]

Tubule cell damage leads to cell sloughing, causing loss of tubular integrity and tubule obstruction. These events are thought to be responsible for the build-up of nitrogenous wastes. Morphologically, the lesion is characterized by tubule cell necrosis and cast formation.[75] The loss of tubular integrity causes back leakage of filtered solute. Tubular obstruction may contribute to the observed decreases in glomerular filtration by causing an increased hydrostatic pressure in Bowman's space. Both of the proposed mechanisms effectively inhibit the clearance of nitrogenous wastes and other solutes, and the result is seen clinically as a decrease in GFR.

The pathologic lesions of nephrotoxic acute tubular necrosis are similar to those found in ischemic acute tubular necrosis (ATN). There is proximal tubule cell necrosis and obstruction of the lumen by casts. However, the distribution of the lesions is different from that in ischemic injury, and the mechanism of induction varies

TABLE 7-1 LABORATORY ASSESSMENT OF ACUTE RENAL FAILURE

	PRERENAL	RENAL	POSTRENAL
Urinalysis			
Protein	—	2—4+	—
White blood cells (WBCs)	—	2—4+	1+
Red blood cells (RBCs)	—	2—4+	±
Casts	Few hyaline	Pigmented, epithelial, WBC	—
Chemistry			
Urinary osmolality (U_{Osm})	>500 mOsm/L	= Plasma	Variable
U_{Osm}/Plasma osmolality (P_{Osm})	<1.5	>1.5	Variable
Urinary sodium (U_{Na})	20 mOsm/L	50 mOsm/L	Variable
Fractional excretion of sodium (FE_{Na})	<1%	>3%	Variable

from agent to agent. In ischemic ATN the lesions are primarily medullary and juxtamedullary, whereas in nephrotoxic ATN the lesions are evenly distributed throughout the nephron population.[57]

Differential Diagnosis of Acute Renal Failure

A systematic approach is necessary to facilitate accurate and timely diagnosis of acute renal failure. In most cases prompt diagnosis and institution of the appropriate therapy will reverse or lessen the degree of insult. Acute renal failure can evolve from diminished renal blood flow, parenchymal damage, or obstruction of urine outflow. The first step in assessing the cause of ARF is to anatomically localize the disease as prerenal, renal, or postrenal. Prerenal, renal, and postrenal causes of acute renal failure all cause azotemia differently. These variations can be measured, which allows the physician to distinguish among the three anatomic locations.

History and Physical Examination

A thorough history, physical examination, and chart review are essential in determining the cause of acute renal failure. The clinician must determine the presence of preexisting renal disease, risk factors, exposure to nephrotoxins, infection, cardiac failure, and hemodynamic instability. The physical examination may yield information relevant to volume status, cardiac dysfunction, or the presence of sepsis. A pelvic or rectal examination, or both, may reveal a large obstructing mass or an enlarged prostate as a potential cause of postrenal obstruction.

Urinalysis

Chemical and microscopic analysis of the urine yields diagnostic information in most patients with new-onset renal dysfunction (Table 7-1).[59] In prerenal azotemia the urine is concentrated (urine osmolarity is above 350 mOsm). The microscopic examination is unremarkable, containing few findings except for hyaline casts.

Patients with intrinsic renal failure have more than 2 or 3 red cells/high-power field. Brown pigmented casts and renal tubular epithelial cells are observed in most cases. Both hemolysis and rhabdomyolysis produce a positive result on tests for occult blood, but the urine contains no red cells. Patients with hemoglobinuria have pink-colored plasma. The presence of urate crystals is diagnostic of uric acid nephropathy.

In obstructive uropathy the urine is not concentrated and usually is unremarkable. Sediment is normal as well. Sterile catheterization of the bladder should be performed early, because this will resolve a bladder obstruction. Dilatation of the collecting system can also be detected by ultrasonography, which is easily performed and poses no further risk to the patient.

Urine Flow Rate

Oliguria is defined as a total urine output of less than 400 ml/day. *Anuria* is defined as an output of less than 50 ml/day, or by the absence of urine upon catheterization. Sustained anuria suggests obstructive uropathy, mechanical obstruction of the renal arteries, or renal cortical necrosis.

Progressive azotemia can occur without oliguria. This syndrome, aptly called nonoliguric renal failure, is relatively common. Anderson and colleagues showed that more than 59% of the ARF patients in their study population had progressive azotemia without oliguria.[5] This occurs quite frequently after traumatic injuries and burns.[9,94] In patients with severe burns, the incidence may approach 40%.[78] Patients with nonoliguric acute renal failure may have a significantly better prognosis in terms of morbidity and mortality, and less morbidity from infection and gastrointestinal bleeding.[5]

Urine Chemistry

Spot urine sodium samples aid in the diagnosis of renal failure. In prerenal states the kidney avidly retains sodium in an attempt to correct the volume deficit.

Therefore urine concentration is less than 10 mEq/L. A more accurate expression is the fractional excretion of sodium (FE_{Na}), which can be expressed by the following equation:

$$FE_{Na} = \frac{U_{Na}}{P_{Na}} \div \frac{U_{Cr}}{P_{Cr}} \times 100\%$$

in which

U_{Na} = Urinary sodium
P_{Na} = Plasma sodium
U_{Cr} = Urinary creatinine
P_{Cr} = Plasma creatinine

FE_{Na} is defined as the urine-to-plasma sodium ratio divided by the urine-to-plasma creatinine ratio multiplied by 100%. FE_{Na} is a useful measurement in the oliguric patient. In prerenal states FE_{Na} is less than 1% (see Table 7-1). In renal parenchymal injury the concentrating ability of the kidney is lost, and FE_{Na} is greater than 3%. This analysis is about 90% sensitive and specific in differentiating between prerenal azotemia and ATN.[71]

Blood Chemistry

Decreased GFR causes accumulation of nitrogenous wastes. Blood urea nitrogen (BUN) and serum creatinine (Cr) concentrations rise. The rate of the increase depends on the patient's catabolic rate. An elevated BUN commonly is seen in patients with trauma, infection, rhabdomyolysis, or gastrointestinal hemorrhage. In patients with severe muscle necrosis, as in crush injuries, electrical injuries, extensive burns, or burns with deep extension, an inordinate rise in serum creatinine is observed as well. This is because creatine is released from injured muscle and converted to creatinine spontaneously in the bloodstream. Hyperkalemia is one of the severest complications of acute renal failure, and it occurs most frequently in patients with both oliguria and tissue injury.[54] Diabetics and patients with myonecrosis run the greatest risk of developing hyperkalemia.

Management of Acute Renal Failure

Clinical Course

The clinical course of acute renal failure can be subdivided into three phases: the initiation phase, the maintenance phase, and the recovery phase. The initiation phase corresponds to the period during which renal function begins to deteriorate, before the onset of irreversible renal damage. It is in this period that preventive or therapeutic measures have significant impact. This phase often is heralded by falling urine output. If recognized, immediate therapeutic measures may result in reversal and avoidance of more serious injury. Unfortunately, this period often goes unrecognized, because nonoliguric forms of acute renal failure often precede oliguric renal failure, and because this phase often is of short duration.

The maintenance phase begins at the point where the renal insult is no longer readily reversible and parenchymal damage has occurred. The duration of this phase varies, depending on the severity of the insult. The oliguric forms may vary from a few days in duration to several months, whereas the nonoliguric form typically lasts for 5 to 7 days.

The onset of the recovery phase is marked by stabilization of BUN and creatinine levels and improvement in GFR. In oliguric patients the onset of this phase is associated with improved urine output. In nonoliguric patients this phase is associated with stabilization of BUN and creatinine levels.

Complications

Renal excretion of nitrogenous wastes, water, electrolytes, and acids is impaired during acute renal failure. The magnitude of impairment depends on whether the patient is oliguric or nonoliguric. The patient's catabolic state is important, because patients with high catabolic states produce more nitrogenous wastes. For this reason patients with severe trauma, burns, or sepsis are difficult to manage if they are oliguric and require dialysis.

The rate of progression of azotemia is directly proportional to the degree of renal failure and the catabolic rate. In noncatabolic patients, the rate of rise of BUN is 10 to 20 mg/dl/day. In patients who are severely catabolic, the BUN may rise extremely rapidly. Patients with major thermal burns catabolize more than 100 g of protein a day, corresponding to a rise of more than 40 mg/dl/day in BUN and 2 mg/dl/day in creatinine.

One common complication of acute renal failure is fluid overload.[63,69] Fluid resuscitation during hypovolemic shock is aimed at restoring cardiac output and maintaining renal blood flow. During this process substantial third space accumulation of fluid occurs, particularly in patients with substantial tissue injury. At the point in the patient's clinical course where sequestered fluid is mobilized, symptoms of volume overload may result from the loss of volume regulatory function by the impaired kidney. During these fluid shifts the risk of pulmonary edema is high and warrants the use of invasive monitoring, hemofiltration, or dialysis to avoid volume overload.

Hyponatremia in acute renal failure is primarily due to free water intake in excess of excretion, not sodium depletion. In addition, hyponatremia may arise from water production as a byproduct of metabolism or the release of water from injured cells. Water intake should be restricted when ARF is recognized.

Hyperkalemia is a common cause of death in acute renal failure; it occurs in 50% of ARF patients. Hyperkalemia is caused by impaired excretion, cellular release, metabolic acidosis, and exogenous administration. Intracellular potassium is in high concentration. Muscle cells contain 155 mEq/L of potassium. During cell damage and necrosis, as occurs in a crush injury, large amounts of potassium are liberated into the blood. Acidemia aggravates this complication by causing further shifts of potassium out of the cell in exchange for hydrogen. Hyperkalemia usually remains asymptomatic until the serum concentration reaches 6 mEq/L. Serum concentrations in this range are associated with electrocardiographic abnormalities. The ECG shows characteristic changes, beginning with tented or peaked T waves and progressing to prolonged P-R interval, A-V block, and ventricular fibrillation.

In catabolic patients with acute renal failure, fixed acid production is increased. Sulfuric and phosphoric acid are derived from catabolism at a rate of 50 to 100 mEq/day.[80] The plasma bicarbonate levels are inversely proportional to the catabolic rate. This relationship can be modified by administration of alkali or through gastric acid loss.

Acute renal failure is associated with blood abnormalities on several levels. Anemia, hemorrhage, hemolysis, and iatrogenic losses occur. Thrombocytopenia and qualitative platelet function defects also result. The primary cause of the anemia is a decrease in erythropoietin; however, with severe azotemia, hemolysis contributes as well. The development of anemia exacerbates cardiac, respiratory, and wound healing problems.

Acute gastrointestinal hemorrhage is the second leading cause of death in acute renal failure.[89] The bleeding is caused by stress ulceration and gastritis, both of which are increased in acute renal failure. During acute renal failure, the clearance of gastrointestinal hormones is reduced.[38,86] In particular, elevated gastrin levels were noted in 50% of patients in one study.[98] This, in addition to platelet dysfunction and the use of anticoagulation during dialysis, probably is responsible for the increased risk of hemorrhage in ARF.

Infectious complications of acute renal failure occur in more than 50% of patients in association with trauma or surgery.[66] The incidence of infection was 89% in Vietnam casualties who had acute renal failure. In this study infection accounted for 72% of the deaths. There are several common manifestations of infection. The three most serious are septicemia, pneumonia, and peritonitis. Together these infectious complications account for most of the mortality attributed to infection.[84] Other causes of infection are wound infection and urinary tract infection. Urinary tract infections are very common and may contribute indirectly to the high mortality rate by causing septicemia.

Therapy

The goal of the therapeutic plan should be to restore renal blood flow, increase tubular urine flow, and stop ongoing injury. Reversible causes of renal damage should be excluded. All prerenal factors must be corrected and attempts made to establish a urine output. The physician must optimize the clinical parameters to prevent complications. The intake of nitrogen, water, and electrolytes should be adjusted to prevent imbalances. Enough calories must be provided to prevent muscle wasting. Drug therapy must be adjusted to account for changes in metabolism and clearance. The patient's hemodynamic status, body weight, and biochemical parameters must be evaluated frequently, and abnormalities must be corrected early to prevent complications. Regardless of the effectiveness of the therapeutic plan, certain patients will require dialysis for variable periods of time, depending on the severity of the insult.

Preventing acute renal failure is an important aspect of treatment. Early intervention in the ischemic process may prevent or decrease the renal injury. Establishing hemodynamic stability is of primary importance at the outset. Hemodynamic monitoring is necessary and may be facilitated by the use of a Swan-Ganz catheter for measuring cardiac index and wedge pressures as a guide to adequate restoration of effective volume status.

After resuscitation is complete and prerenal causes have been excluded or treated, potential nephrotoxins discontinued, and obstructive uropathy ruled out, diuretics may be used in an attempt to establish urine output. It has been proposed that administering furosemide and/or mannitol in oliguric acute renal failure may cause a shift to a more benign nonoliguric form, a condition that is easier to manage and that carries a lower mortality.[8] The use of furosemide and/or mannitol in this setting has met with inconsistent success. Studies of diuretic use in patients with established renal failure and in patients requiring dialysis do not show convincing evidence of improvement in decreasing the need for dialysis or in mortality.

Dopamine is thought to cause selective renal vasodilatation and increased renal blood flow through stimulation of dopaminergic receptors.[85] Low-dose dopamine (2 to 5 μg/kg/min) increases cortical perfusion, GFR, and urine output. However, it is not clear whether this effect is secondary to stimulation of dopaminergic receptors or to the drug's inotropic effects. Use of low-dose dopamine in ARF therefore must be done with caution. Care must be taken to ensure that the patient is appropriately resuscitated and monitored. If the desired effect from the application of low-dose dopamine is not achieved, then it should be discontinued. Evidence supporting the use of dopamine for prophylaxis of ARF is sparse and remains controversial.

Prevention of Complications

Since the advent of dialysis, death from uremia and electrolyte abnormalities has decreased. Still, complications of ARF are common, particularly in hypercatabolic patients and those with extensive tissue insults, as seen in crush injury and burns. Hyperkalemia must be prevented through potassium restriction, frequent measurement of serum potassium, ECG monitoring, and the use of hemofiltration or dialysis as often as necessary. Even with these measures hyperkalemia may occur acutely and necessitates immediate treatment. Acute treatment of hyperkalemia is designed to remove excess potassium from the body, restore the transcellular gradient, and reverse membrane abnormalities.[58] If life-threatening conduction disturbances occur, 10 ml of intravenous 10% calcium gluconate should be administered. This is effective in restoring membrane potential and temporarily reversing conduction abnormalities. Continued treatment is necessary. Administering 50% dextrose and insulin causes a shift of potassium toward the intracellular compartment. However, neither method changes total body potassium, necessitating the use of dialysis, hemofiltration, or cation exchange resins. Sodium polystyrene sulfonate (Kayexalate) (30 to 50 g in 100 ml of 35% sorbitol) may be given as an enema at 6-hour intervals. Preventing hyperkalemia is the most successful treatment, and early use of dialysis is advisable.

Surgical complications must be treated immediately. It is inadvisable to wait for ARF to subside before draining abscesses or removing necrotic tissue, because these exacerbate the course of ARF and cause further complications.

Preventing infection can become a difficult problem. With severe trauma and burns, immunosuppression is always present. This is further complicated by the addition of renal failure and varying degrees of malnutrition. In addition, the onset of infection often is difficult to diagnose because of the antipyretic effects of uremia and a blunted white cell response.[50] Prevention therefore becomes paramount. Once the patient's condition has been stabilized, indwelling catheters should be removed. Those that must remain require constant inspection. Antibiotic treatment should be selective by clinical criteria or positive sputum, blood, or urine cultures. If an aminoglycoside antibiotic is required, the dosage must be carefully managed through predialysis and postdialysis determinations to prevent further nephrotoxicity. In the future it may be possible to use recombinant human hematopoietic factors as an adjunct to antibiotic therapy and thereby reduce the incidence of superimposed nephrotoxicity.[87]

Hemodialysis is the treatment of choice for a hypercatabolic patient with acute renal failure. The use of hemodialysis for ARF in battle casualties in the Korean War diminished mortality from 95% to approximately 65%.[53] Although hemodialysis requires a vascular access procedure and periodic anticoagulation, the benefits are clearly worthwhile. Dialysis should be instituted early to prevent uremic complications.

Continuous peritoneal dialysis may be used as an alternative to hemodialysis. The theoretical advantages are less associated hypotension, no need for anticoagulation, and technical feasibility. However, there is a risk of peritonitis, and the procedure is contraindicated in patients with recent laparotomies.

Nutritional Supplementation

Nutritional therapy in a patient with acute renal failure and multiple organ failure represents a difficult clinical challenge. Adequate nutritional support is especially important in such patients because of their high catabolic rate and increased susceptibility to infection. In patients with acute renal failure, plasma total protein, albumin, and free amino acid levels are depressed. If patients with trauma, thermal injury, or multiple organ failure suffer ARF, the metabolic derangements are compounded. Feinstein and associates demonstrated severe protein losses (up to approximately 12 g/day) in patients with acute renal failure secondary to sepsis, hypotension, or rhabdomyolysis.[31] These patients are in chronic negative nitrogen balance, the results of which are fragile host defenses and poor wound healing.

Adequate calories must be supplied to match the metabolic rate. If caloric supplementation is inadequate, the protein catabolism is exacerbated. The caloric requirement should be based on the predicted energy needs. Estimating the resting metabolic expenditure (RME), as recommended by Long, is helpful for predicting caloric requirements in injured patients.[65] Also, bedside indirect calorimetry techniques can more precisely predict an individual patient's needs. Combinations of glucose and lipid may be used to supply the caloric requirements. Giving carbohydrates in large amounts results in excess CO_2 production. Current guidelines suggest that for a 70 kg individual, carbohydrate calories should be limited to 1700 to 2500 kcal/day, using the lower limit for patients with greater degrees of stress.

Amino acids must be supplied to ensure positive nitrogen balance. A catabolic patient may require 1 to 1.5 g protein/kg/day. Whenever possible enteral feeding should be used. If this is not possible, parenteral infusion should be used, and the solution should contain both essential and nonessential amino acids. Although the capability to synthesize the nonessential amino acids may be present, this may be impaired in a patient with high metabolic demands. Whenever possible nitrogen losses should be estimated in order to estimate nitrogen requirements and avoid unnecessary elevation in urea nitrogen. Dialysis should be used as often as necessary to prevent uremic complications, volume overload, and electrolyte abnormalities.

Metabolic derangements are common in a patient with acute renal failure who is receiving total parenteral nutrition (TPN). Electrolyte abnormalities, hyperglycemia, hypophosphatemia, and hypomagnesemia most often occur at the beginning of TPN therapy. Hyperglycemia can be managed by adding insulin to the TPN solution or by an insulin drip. Enough insulin should be infused to keep the serum glucose level below 200 mg/dl. Septic patients require substantial amounts of insulin and may be most appropriately managed with an insulin drip. The infusion of glucose and insulin causes shifts of potassium, phosphate, and magnesium intracellularly. This often occurs to a significant degree and may necessitate supplementation between dialysis treatments to prevent complications. In an unstable patient the serum values of these electrolytes must be measured frequently.

Hypophosphatemia in a patient with ARF can be seen during the initiation of total parenteral nutrition and on occasion after soft tissue injury, as with extensive burns. Severe hypophosphatemia (levels below 1.5 mg/dl) may be associated with tissue hypoxia, rhabdomyolysis, myocardial depression, peripheral neuropathy, or respiratory muscle failure. Therapy should be directed toward maintaining serum phosphorus levels between 3 and 4 mg/dl. Phosphorus can be given both orally and intravenously. In severe hypophosphatemia, intravenous phosphate can be given as sodium or potassium phosphate. In children up to 12 to 15 years of age, 1 to 1.5 mM phosphate/kg in a 24-hour period may be required. In cases of severe hypophosphatemia, this can be increased up to 2.5 mM phosphate/kg in a 24-hour period. In adults, phosphate needs can approach 1 mM/kg in a 24-hour period. If potassium phosphate is given, for every 3 mM of phosphate given, 4.4 mEq of potassium is be administered; with sodium phosphate, 4 mEq of sodium is administered for each 3 mM of phosphate. The effect of additional sodium, and particularly potassium, must be carefully assessed in the individual patient. Levels should be measured frequently, and care should be taken to avoid hyperphosphatemia.

Prognosis

The overall mortality rate for acute renal failure ranges from 40% to 60%. The nonoliguric form is associated with a lower rate (26%) than the oliguric form (50%).[58] Factors associated with increased mortality are the underlying disease, associated multiple organ dysfunction, and the development of complications. Age, sex, and the length of time dialysis is required are less consistently related to mortality. The basic underlying disease is the most important factor in survival. Patients without severe underlying illness or ARF secondary to nephrotoxins may have a very low mortality rate, whereas ARF secondary to trauma and major surgery are associated with a mortality rate of 62%.[32] The involvement of other organ systems and the development of complications significantly dim the prognosis.

REFERENCES

1 Aiken JW, Vane JR: Intrarenal prostaglandin release attenuates the renal vasoconstrictor activity of angiotensin, *J Pharmacol Exp Ther* 184:678, 1973.

2 Alcorn D, Emslie KR, Ross BD et al: Selective distal nephron damage during isolated perfused kidney, *Kidney Int* 19:638, 1980.

3 Anderson RJ, Schrier RW: Acute tubular necrosis. In Schrier RW, Gottschalk CW, editors: *Diseases of the kidney,* ed 4, Boston, 1988, Little, Brown.

4 Anderson RJ, Schrier RW: Clinical spectrum of oliguric and nonoliguric acute renal failure. In Brenner BM, Stein JH, editors: *Acute renal failure (contemporary issues in nephrology),* vol 6, New York, 1980, Churchill Livingstone.

5 Anderson RJ, Linas SL, Berns AS et al: Nonoliguric acute renal failure, *N Engl J Med* 296(20):1134, 1977.

6 Atarashi K, Mulrow PJ, Franco-Saenz R: Effect of atrial peptides on aldosterone production, *J Clin Invest* 76:1807, 1985.

7 Badr KF, Ichikawa I: Prerenal failure: a deleterious shift from renal compensation to decompensation, *N Engl J Med* 319(10):623, 1988.

8 Barry KG, Malloy JP: Oliguric renal failure: evaluation and therapy by the intravenous infusion of mannitol, *JAMA* 179:510, 1962.

9 Baxter CR, Zelditz WD, Shires GT: High output acute renal failure complicating traumatic injury, *J Trauma* 4:567, 1964.

10 Bennet WM, Pulliam JP: Cyclosporine nephrotoxicity, *Ann Intern Med* 99:851, 1983.

11 Blachley JD, Hill JB: Renal and electrolyte disturbances associated with cisplatin, *Ann Intern Med* 95:628, 1981.

12 Blantz RC: Dynamics of glomerular ultrafiltration in the rat, *Fed Proc* 36(12):2602, 1977.

13 Boswick JA, Thompson JD, Kershner CJ: Critical care of the burned patient, *Anesthesiology* 47:164, 1977.

14 Braun SR, Weiss FR, Keller AI et al: Evaluation of the renal toxicity of heme proteins and their derivatives: a role in the genesis of acute tubular necrosis, *J Exp Med* 131:443, 1970.

15 Brenner BM, Baylis C, Deen WM: Transport of molecules across renal glomerular capillaries, *Physiol Rev* 56:502, 1976.

16 Brezis M, Rosen S, Silva P, Epstein FH: Renal ischemia: a new perspective, *Kidney Int* 26:375, 1984.

17 Brezis M, Rosen S, Silva P et al: Selective vulnerability of the thick ascending limb to anoxia in the isolated perfused rat kidney, *J Clin Invest* 73:182, 1984.

18 Bulger RE, Hebert SC: Structural-functional relationships in the kidney. In Schrier RW, Gottschalk CW, editors: *Diseases of the kidney,* ed 4, Boston, 1988, Little, Brown.

19 Burke TJ, Arnold PE, Gordon JA et al: Protective effect of intrarenal calcium blockers before or after renal ischemia: functional, morphological, and mitochondrial studies, *J Clin Invest* 74:1830, 1984.

20 Burke TJ, Cronin RE, Duchin KL et al: Ischemia and tubule obstruction during acute renal failure in dogs: mannitol protection, *Am J Physiol* 238:F305, 1980.

21 Butler WT, Hill GJ, Szwed CF, Knight V: Amphotericin B renal toxicity in the dog, *J Pharmacol Exp Ther* 143:47, 1964.

22 Campbell WB, Schmitz JM, Itskovitch R: (Des-Asp)-angiotensin I: a study of its pressor and steroidogenic activity in conscious rats, *Endocrinology* 100(1):46, 1977.

23 Chabardes D, Gagnan-Burnette M, Imbert-Teboul M et al: Adenylate cyclase responsiveness to hormones in various portions of the human nephron, *J Clin Invest* 65(2):439, 1980.

24 Chapnick BM, Panstian PW, Klanier E: Influence of prostaglandin synthesis on renal vascular responses to vasopressor and vasodilator agents in the cat, *J Pharmacol Exp Ther* 196:44, 1976.

25 Cioffi GW, Ashikaga T, Gamelli RL: Probability of surviving postoperative acute renal failure: development of a prognostic index, *Ann Surg* 200(2):205, 1984.

26 Corvol P, Claire M, Oblin ME et al: Mechanism of the antimineralocorticoid effects of spironolactones, *Kidney Int* 20:1, 1981.

27 Dahlgren JG, Anderson ET, Hewitt WL: Gentamicin blood levels: a guide to nephrotoxicity, *Antimicrob Agents Chemother* 8:58, 1975.

28 De Bold AJ, Borenstein HB, Veress AT et al: A rapid and potent natriuretic response to intravenous injection of atrial myocardial extract in cats, *Life Sci* 28(1):89, 1981.

29 DeCamp MM, Demling RH: Post-traumatic multisystem organ failure, *JAMA* 260(4):530, 1988.

30 Dibona GF: Prostaglandins and nonsteroidal anti-inflammatory drugs: effects on renal hemodynamics, *Am J Med* 80(suppl 1a):12, 1986.

31 Feinstein EI, Blumenkrantz MJ, Healy H et al: Clinical and metabolic responses to parenteral nutrition in acute renal failure: a controlled double-blind study, *Medicine* 60:124, 1981.

32 Finn WF, Chevalier RL: Recovery from acute renal failure, *Kidney Int* 16:113, 1979.

33 Fleming JS, Rennie DW: Effects of osmotic diuresis on sodium reabsorption and oxygen consumption in the kidney, *Am J Physiol* 210(4):751, 1966.

34 Fried AF, Stein JH: Glomerular dynamics, *Arch Intern Med* 143:787, 1983.

35 Gottschalk CW, Lassiter WE, Mylle M: Studies of the composition of vasa recta plasma in the hamster kidney, *Excerpta Med* (International Congress Services) 47:375, 1962.

36 Gransjo G, Wogast M: The pressure/flow relationship in renal, cortical, and medullary circulation, *Acta Physiol Scand* 85:228, 1972.

37 Guyton AC, Langston JB, Navar G: Theory for renal autoregulation by feedback at the juxtaglomerular apparatus, *Circ Res* 15(suppl 1):187, 1964.

38 Hansky J: Effect of renal failure on gastrointestinal hormones, *World J Surg* 3(4):463, 1979.

39 Harkonen S, Kjellstrand CM: Exacerbation of diabetic renal failure following intravenous pyelography, *Am J Med* 63:939, 1977.

40 Harkonen S, Kjellstrand CM: Contrast nephropathy, *Am J Nephrol* 1:69, 1981.

41 Hebert SC, Andreoli TE: Control of NaCl transport in the thick ascending limb, *Am J Physiol* 246:F745, 1984.

42 Henrich WL, Berl T, McDonald KM et al: Angiotensin II, renal nerves, and prostaglandins in renal hemodynamics during hemorrhage, *Am J Physiol* 235:F46, 1978.

43 Hishaw LB, Page BB, Brake CM et al: Mechanism of intrarenal hemodynamic changes following acute arterial occlusion, *Am J Physiol* 205:1033, 1963.

44 Hou SH, Bushinsky DA, Wish JB et al: Hospital-acquired renal insufficiency: a prospective study, *Am J Med* 74:243, 1983.

45 Hunt MK, Ramos SP, Geary KM et al: Colocalization and release of angiotensin and renin in renal cortical cells, *Am J Physiol* 263(3):F363, 1992.

46 Ichikawa I, Brenner BM: Importance of efferent arteriolar vascular tone in regulation of proximal tubule fluid reabsorption and glomerulotubular balance in the rat, *J Clin Invest* 65:1192, 1980.

47 Jamison RL: Micropuncture studies of segments of thin loop of Henle in the rat, *Am J Physiol* 215(1):236, 1968.

48 Johnson JA, Zahr JE, Moore WW: Effects of separate and concurrent osmotic and volume stimuli on plasma ADH in sheep, *Am J Physiol* 218:1273, 1970.

49 Kahlmeter G, Dahlager J: Aminoglycoside toxicity: a review of clinical studies published between 1975 and 1982, *J Antimicrob Chemother* 13:9, 1984.

50 Kaplow LS, Goffinet JA: Profound neutropenia during the early phase of hemodialysis, *JAMA* 203(3):1133, 1968.

51 Kelleher SP, Robinette JB, Conger JD: Sympathetic nervous system in the loss of autoregulation in acute renal failure, *Am J Physiol* 246:F379, 1984.

52 King A, Brenner BM, Anderson S: Endothelin: a potent renal and systemic vasoconstrictor peptide, *Am J Physiol* 256:F1051, 1989.

53 Kjellstrand CM, Berkseth RO: Treatment of acute renal failure. In Schrier RW, Gottschalk CW, editors: *Diseases of the kidney,* ed 4, Boston, 1988, Little, Brown.

54 Knochel JP: Biochemical, electrolyte, and acid-base disturbances in acute renal failure. In Brenner BM, Lazarus JM, editors: *Acute renal failure,* ed 2, New York, 1988, Churchill Livingstone.

55 Kon V, Yared A, Ichikawa I: Role of renal sympathetic nerves in mediating hypoperfusion of renal cortical microcirculation in experimental congestive heart failure and acute extracellular fluid volume depletion, *J Clin Invest* 76:1913, 1986.

56 Koushanpour E, Kriz W: *Renal physiology: principles, structure, and function,* ed 2, New York, 1986, Springer-Verlag.

57 Kreisberg JI, Venkatachalam MA: Morphologic factors in acute renal failure. In Brenner BM, Lazarus JM, editors: *Acute renal failure,* ed 2, New York, 1988, Churchill Livingstone.

58 Kunis CL, Lowenstein J: The emergency treatment of hyperkalemia, *Med Clin North Am* 65(1):165, 1981.

59 Kurtz SM, McManus JF: A reconsideration of the development, structure, and disease of the human renal glomerulus, *Am Heart J* 58(3):357, 1959.

60 Langman J: *Medical embryology,* ed 4, Baltimore, 1981, Williams & Wilkins.

61 Laragh JH: Atrial natriuretic hormone, the renin-angiotensin axis, and blood pressure–electrolyte homeostasis, *N Engl J Med* 313(21):1330, 1985.

62 Lassiter WE, Gottschalk CW, Mylle M: Micropuncture study of renal tubular reabsorption of calcium in normal rodents, *Am J Physiol* 204:771, 1963.

63 Ledgerwood AM, Lucas CE: Postresuscitation hypertension: etiology, morbidity, and treatment, *Arch Surg* 108:531, 1974.

64 Lewis OJ: The development of the blood vessels of the metanephros, *J Anat* 92:84, 1958.

65 Long C: Metabolic response to injury and illness: estimation of energy and protein needs from indirect calorimetry and nitrogen balance, *J Parenter Enteral Nutr* 185:417, 1977.

66 Lordon RE, Burton JR: Post-traumatic renal failure in military personnel in Southeast Asia, *Am J Med* 53:137, 1972.

67 Lorenzen M, Lee CO, Windhager EE: Cytosolic Ca^{++} and Na^{+} activities in proximal tubules of *Necturus* kidney, *Am J Physiol* 247:F93, 1984.

68 Lucas CE: Renal considerations in the injured patient, *Surg Clin North Am* 62(1):133, 1982.

69 Lucas CE, Ledgerwood AM, Shier MR et al: The renal factor in the post-traumatic "fluid overload" syndrome, *J Trauma* 17(9):667, 1977.

70 Maack T, Marion DN, Camargo MJF et al: Effects of auriculin on blood pressure, renal function, and the renin-aldosterone system in dogs, *Am J Med* 77:1069, 1984.

71 Miller TR, Anderson RJ, Berns AS: Urinary diagnostic indices in acute renal failure: a prospective study, *Ann Intern Med* 89(1):47, 1978.

72 Morel F: Regulation of kidney function by hormones: a new approach, *Recent Prog Horm Res* 39:271, 1983.

73 Morrison AR: Biochemistry and pharmacology of renal arachidonic acid metabolism, *Am J Med* 80(suppl 1a):3, 1986.

74 Navar LG, Marsh DJ, Blantz RC et al: Intrinsic control of renal hemodynamics, *Fed Proc* 41(14):3022, 1982.

75 Oliver J, MacDowell M, Tracy A: The pathogenesis of acute

renal failure associated with traumatic and toxic injury: renal ischemia, nephrotoxic damage, and the ischemuric episode, *J Clin Invest* 30:1307, 1951.

76 Osathanondh V, Potter EL: Development of the human kidney as shown by microdissection. Parts I, II, and III, *Arch Pathol* 76:271, 1963.

77 Pine RW, Wertz MJ, Lennard ES et al: Determinants of organ malfunction or death in patients with intra-abdominal sepsis, *Arch Surg* 118(2):242, 1983.

78 Planas M, Wachtel T, Frank H et al: Characterization of acute renal failure in the burned patient, *Arch Intern Med* 142:2087, 1982.

79 Reeves BW, Andreoli TE: Tubular sodium transport. In Schrier RW, Gottschalk CW, editors: *Diseases of the kidney,* ed 4, Boston, 1988, Little, Brown.

80 Relman, AS: Renal acidosis and renal excretion of fixed acids in health and disease, *Adv Intern Med* 12:295, 1964.

81 Rennke HG, Venkatachalam MA: Glomerular permeability: in vivo tracer studies with polyionic and polycationic ferritins, *Kidney Int* 11:44, 1977.

82 Robertson GL: The regulation of vasopressin function in health and disease, *Recent Prog Horm Res* 33:333, 1970.

83 Robertson GL, Athar S: The interaction of blood osmolality and blood volume in regulating plasma vasopressin in man, *J Clin Endocrinol Metab* 42(4):613, 1976.

84 Routh GS, Briggs JD, Mone JG et al: Survival from acute renal failure with and without multiple organ dysfunction, *Postgrad Med J* 56:244, 1980.

85 Schwartz LB, Gewertz BL: The renal response to low-dose dopamine, *J Surg Res* 45:574, 1988.

86 Shapira N, Skillman JJ, Steinman TI et al: Gastric mucosal permeability and gastric acid secretion before and after hemodialysis in patients with chronic renal failure, *Surgery* 83:528, 1978.

87 Silver GM, Gamelli RL, O'Reilly M: The beneficial effect of granulocyte colony stimulating factor (G-CSF) in combination with gentamicin on survival following *Pseudomonas* burn wound infection, *Surgery* 106(2):452, 1989.

88 Speller AM, Moffat DB: Tubulovascular relationships in the developing kidney, *J Anat* 123:487, 1977.

89 Steinman TI, Lazarus JM: Organ system involvement in acute renal failure. In Brenner BM, Lazarus JM, editors: *Acute renal failure,* ed 2, New York, 1988, Churchill Livingstone.

90 Thurau K, Levine A: The renal circulation. In Rouiller C, Muller AF, editors: *The kidney: morphology, biochemistry, physiology,* New York, 1971, Academic Press.

91 Tomita K, Ujiie K, Nakanishi T et al: Plasma endothelin levels in patients with acute renal failure (letter), *N Engl J Med* 321(16):1127, 1989.

92 Venkatachalam MA, Bernard DB, Levinsky NG: Ischemic damage and repair in the rat proximal tubule: differences among the S1, S2, S3 segments, *Kidney Int* 14:31, 1978.

93 Venkatachalam MA: Mechanism of proximal tubule brush border loss and regeneration following mild ischemia, *Lab Invest* 45(4):355, 1981.

94 Vertel RM, Knochel JP: Nonoliguric acute renal failure, *JAMA* 200:598-602, 1967.

95 Walshe JJ, Venuto RC: Acute oliguric renal failure induced by indomethacin: possible mechanism, *Ann Intern Med* 91(1):47, 1979.

96 Warren SE, Blantz RC: Mannitol, *Arch Intern Med* 141(4):493, 1981.

97 Weitzberg E, Lundberg JM, Rudehill A: Elevated plasma levels of endothelin in patients with sepsis syndrome, *Circ Shock* 33:222, 1991.

98 Wesdorp RI, Falcao H, Banks PB et al: Gastrin and gastric acid secretion in renal failure, *Am J Surg* 141:334, 1981.

99 Wilkes BM, Mailloux LU: Acute renal failure: pathogenesis and prevention, *Am J Med* 80:1129, 1986.

100 Williams PL, Warwick R: *Gray's anatomy,* ed 36, Philadelphia, 1980, WB Saunders.

101 Wilson DR, Thiel G, Arce ML et al: Glycerol-induced hemoglobinuric acute renal failure in the rat. III: Micropuncture study of the effects of mannitol on individual nephron function, *Nephron* 4:337, 1967.

102 Wright FS, Schnermann J: Interference with feedback control of glomerular filtration rate by furosemide, triflocin, and cyanide, *J Clin Invest* 53:1695, 1974.

103 Yanagissawa M, Kurihara S, Kimura Y et al: A novel, potent vasoconstrictor peptide produced by vascular endothelial cells, *Nature* 332:411, 1988.

104 Yared A, Kon V, Ichikawa I: Mechanism of preservation of glomerular perfusion and filtration during acute extracellular fluid volume depletion, *J Clin Invest* 75:1477, 1985.

CHAPTER

8

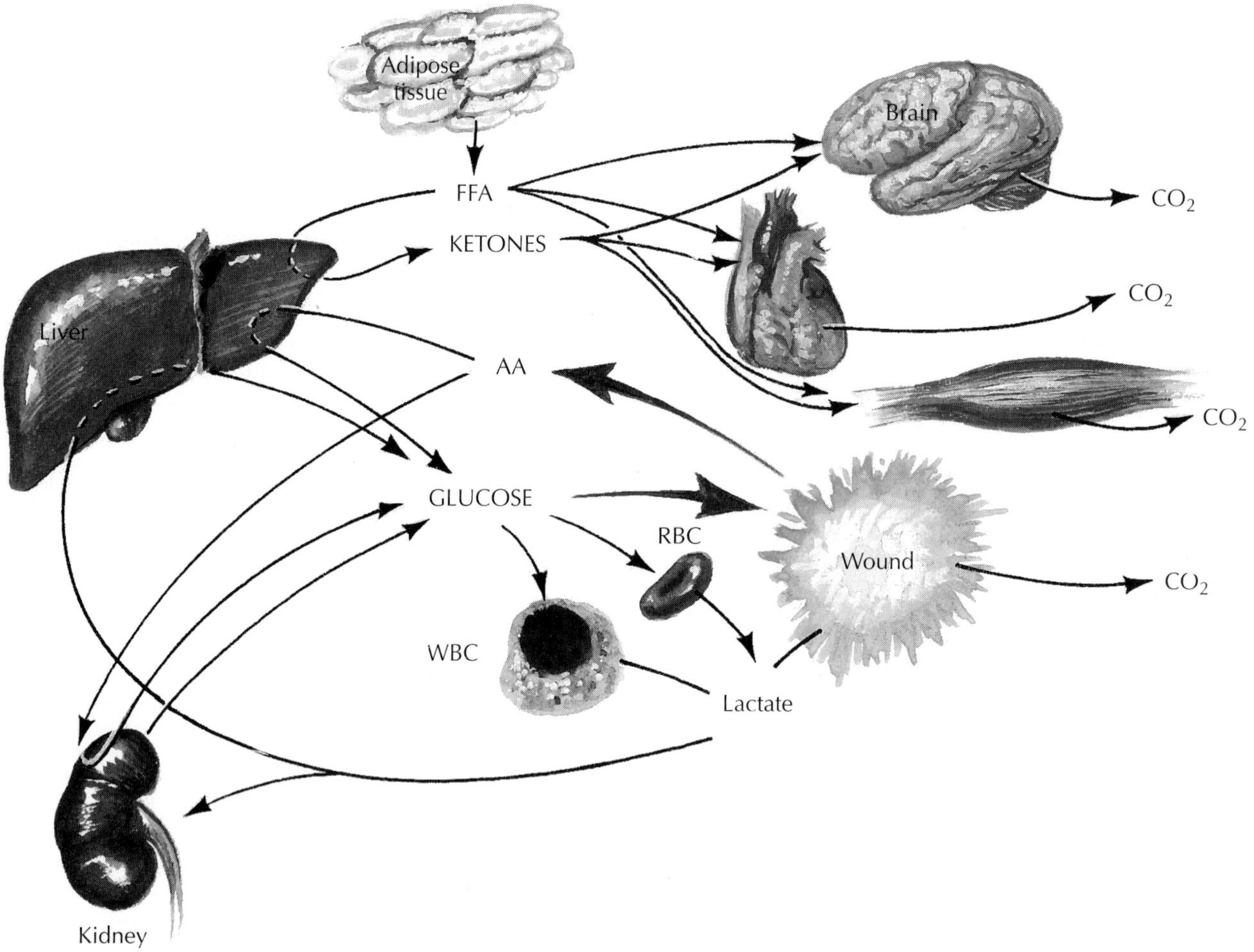

Adipose tissue
Brain
FFA
KETONES
Liver
AA
GLUCOSE
RBC
Wound
WBC
Lactate
Kidney
CO_2
CO_2
CO_2
CO_2

THE BIOLOGIC RESPONSE TO INJURY

Donald S. Gann • Andrew H. Foster

RELATED MATERIAL APPEARS IN CHAPTERS 3, 5, AND 9

FOR A SUMMARY OF THIS CHAPTER, TURN TO PAGE 278

The human response to injury is enacted through communication networks and dynamic biologic systems. Bernard believed that the "stability of the milieu interior" was the primary condition for existence,[54] but the idea of an active chemical messenger in the blood was not introduced until Brown-Sequard.[93] Cannon later introduced the term *homeostasis,* which he defined as "the coordinated physiological process which maintains most of the steady states in the organism."[105] Currently, the panoramic horizon of measurable homeostastic responses is vast. Homeostasis encompasses innumerable processes that maintain regulation on and between levels reaching from mitochondrial proton transfer to thermogenesis by shivering of large skeletal muscles. We now know that input is constantly modulated, that *change,* not *stasis,* is the process essential for maintaining steady-state conditions. For this reason, Yates' concept of *homeodynamic stability*[690,691] is a more accurate description. For the safe surgeon (who is consequently a human physiologist), understanding of the dynamic temporal relationship of the body's biologic response to injury is essential. Injury, operation, illness, aging—each circumstance engages multiple interacting systems with individual trajectories in time that must be directed by the surgeon to achieve healing and functional recovery of the surgical patient.

The magnitude and nature of the injury, as well as other variables, determine the responses of these dynamic systems. Of the physiologic "subsystems" involved in the injury response, those of the neuroendocrine reflexes have been relatively well characterized, and they demonstrate how multiple levels interact in the stimulus response.

The least complex response to injury is that of the simple neuronal reflex arc that passes to the spinal cord level, producing withdrawal with very rapid response times. However, the responses considered in this chapter involve multiple interactions and more complex central regulation and control. Specialized peripheral and central receptors transduce the stimulus into a discrete set of afferent neural inputs that are transmitted to the central nervous system via specific neural pathways. In the higher level neural centers, the inputs are integrated and modulated with other signals, creating a discrete set of efferent neural outputs that produce numerous, widespread effector signals by means of hormone secretion and potentiation effects, with longer response times and duration of action (e.g., nuclear transcription for de novo protein synthesis, immunologic activation, and cellular proliferation). The stimuli also affect the highest order cortical neuronal activity, causing conscious and unconscious thoughts that result in complex behavioral responses, such as avoidance, formulation of a plan of attack or, with great injury, even thoughts of the afterlife.

On a cellular level, the stimuli caused by injury provoke rapid secretion of many substances, such as endothelial cell nitric oxide, which maintains vascular tone and allows continued delivery of oxygen. The immediate need for energy may deplete constituitive energy depots and shunt to nonoxidative metabolism. Other responses by different types of cells include cytokine secretion, acute-phase protein release, abrupt changes in coagulation proteins, ion shifts, and rapid transcription and protein synthesis. In the absence of significant injury, sepsis, or starvation, the physiologic alterations are minor and the adjustments required to maintain homeostasis are easily and successfully made. In the presence of significant injury, sepsis, or starvation, the stimuli are multiple and intensified and the responses are directed to preserve oxygen delivery, mobilize energy substrates, and minimize pain. When subsequent compensation becomes inadequate or poorly modulated, the inexorable progression of profound shock or syndrome of multiple organ dysfunction may result and death may supervene.

SYSTEMIC NEUROENDOCRINE REFLEXES

Neuroendocrine reflexes require intact signal receptors, signal transduction, rapid changes in transmembrane potential, and integration and modulation; and these must be followed by afferent neural transmission to target endocrine organs. This fact is demonstrated by the absence of adrenocortical stimulation from laparotomy or a burn when the stimulated areas are denervated[191,333]

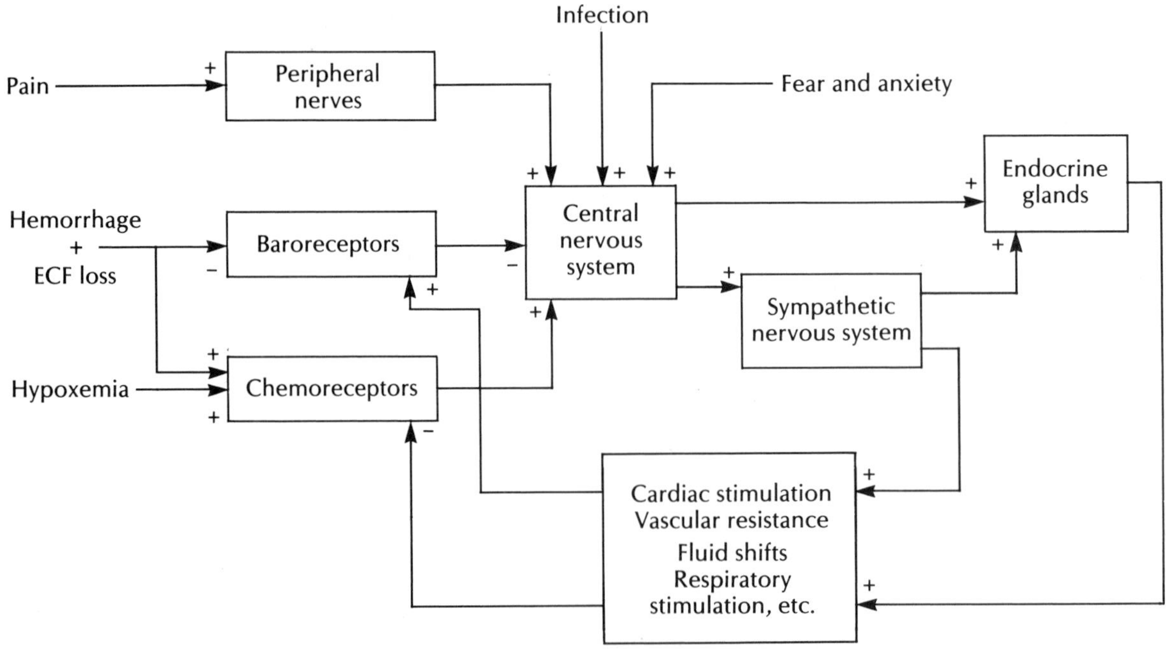

FIGURE 8-1 Overview of the neuroendocrine reflexes induced by shock and trauma. A reduction in effective circulating volume is of central importance because this stimulus is present in most cases of severe injury.

or when they are below the level of cord transection in paraplegic patients.[331] Most surgeons make use of this simple principle by using local anesthetics to modulate the stress response during minor surgery. The effects of general anesthetics are more complex, because these agents have shown an inherent ability to modulate neuroendocrine reflexes in both experimental cases[415,697] and clinical circumstances.[660]

Stimuli for Neuroendocrine Reflexes

The major stimuli for neuroendocrine reflexes are changes in (1) effective circulating fluid volume; (2) concentration of hydrogen ion in the blood; partial pressure of oxygen (PaO_2) or carbon dioxide ($PaCO_2$); (3) emotional state; (4) substrate availability; (5) ambient or core temperature; and (6) the presence of pain or (7) infection (Figure 8-1).

The effective circulating volume may be diminished by any type of injury.[79] The condition may arise from direct loss of blood (hemorrhage), loss or sequestration of plasma (dehydration, third spacing, or burn injury), or inability of the blood to circulate (cardiac tamponade or pulmonary embolism). Loss of effective circulating volume is sensed by high-pressure baroreceptors in the aorta, carotid arteries, and kidneys, and by low-pressure stretch receptors in the atria[33,263,373] (Figure 8-2).

Arterial baroreceptors sense the magnitude and rate of change in arterial pressure.[373] Stretch receptors sense the atrial volume and its rate of change.[380] Afferent signals from high-pressure baroreceptors in the carotid arteries and aorta and from low-pressure stretch receptors in the atria exert tonic inhibition of hormonal release and activities of the central nervous system (CNS) and the autonomic nervous system (ANS). When the effective circulating volume decreases, baroreceptor and stretch receptor activity decreases, reducing tonic inhibition.[263]

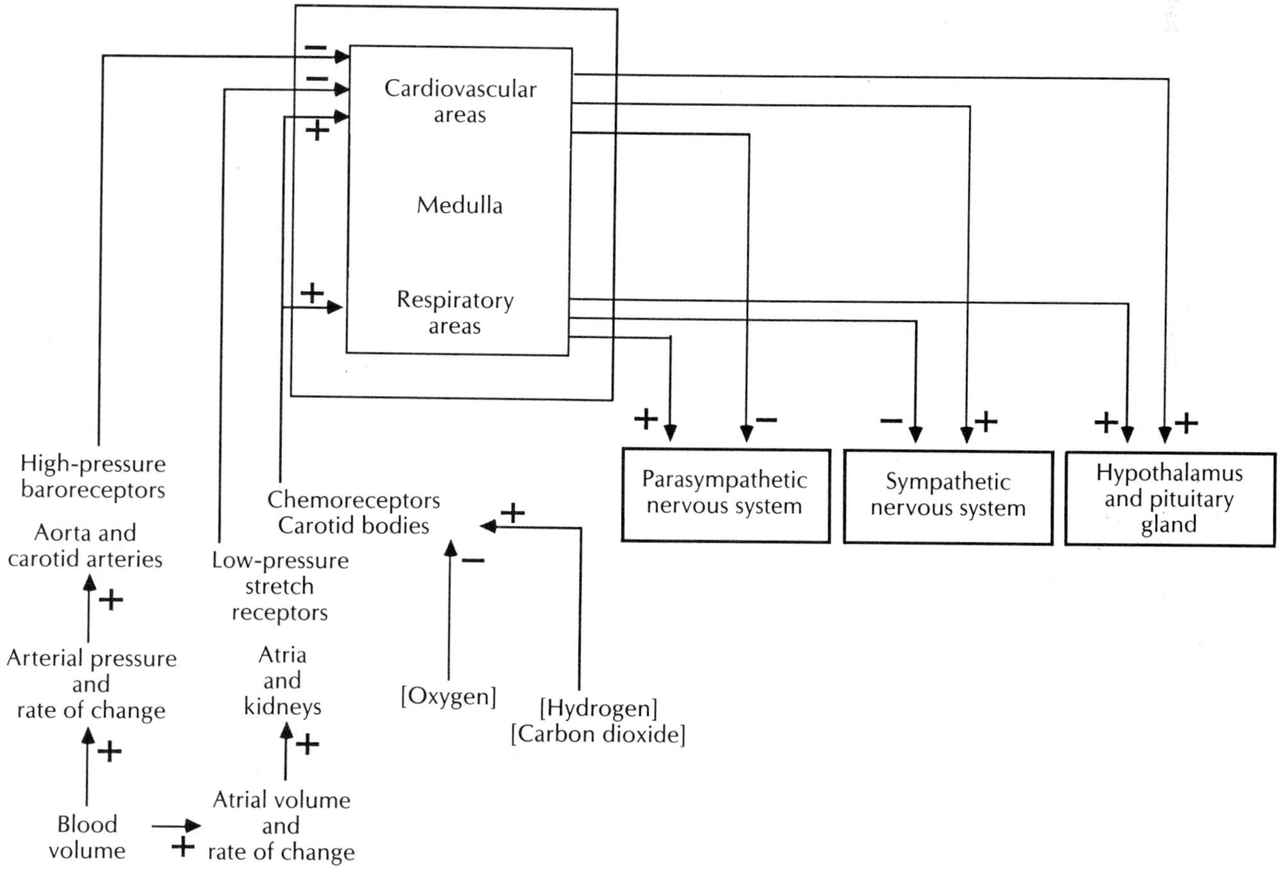

FIGURE 8-2 Baroreceptor and chemoreceptor reflexes elicited by injury. An increase in the stimulus leads to an increase (+) or decrease (−) in the activity of the receptor of the projected medullary areas and in target-site activities *(heavy boxes)*. For example, an increase in effective circulating volume increases the activity of baroreceptors, which inhibits the cardiovascular areas of the medulla. As a result of this inhibition, the activity of the sympathetic nervous system decreases, hypothalamic secretion declines, and the activity of the parasympathetic nervous system increases.

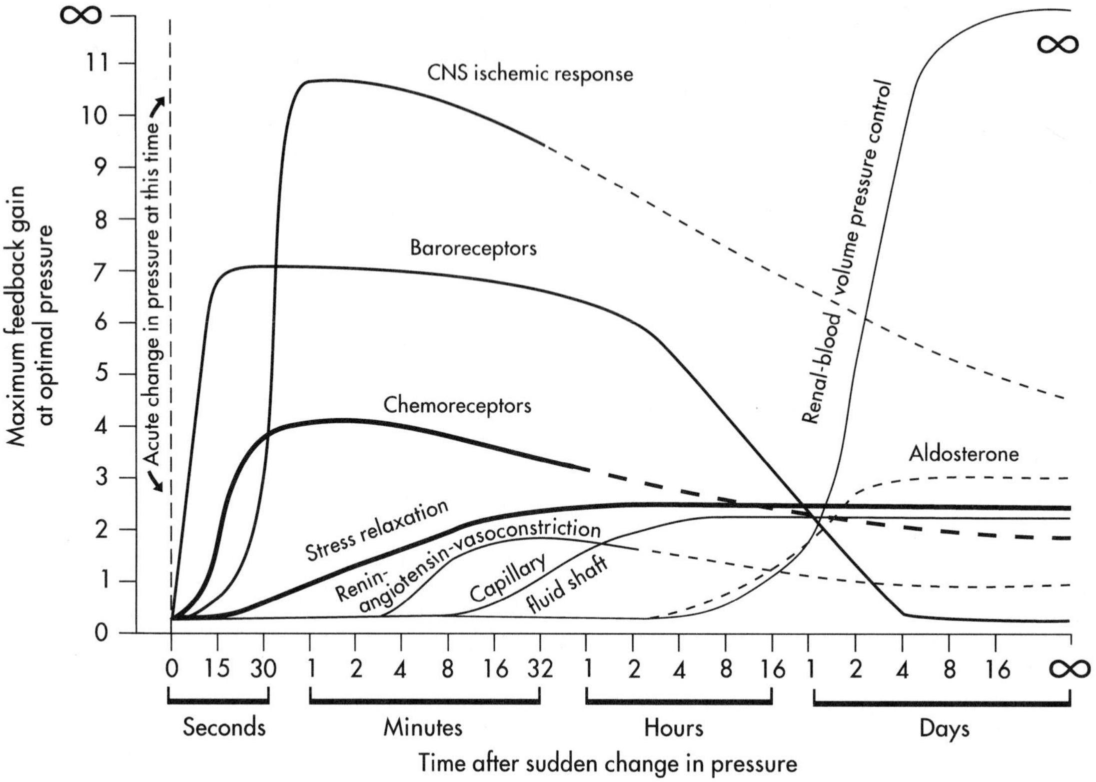

FIGURE 8-3 Approximate potency of mechanisms for controlling arterial blood pressure at different time intervals after blood pressure perturbation. (From Guyton AC: *Arterial pressure and hypertension*, Philadelphia, 1980, WB Saunders.)

The vagus carries afferent nerves from the baroreceptors to the tractus solitarius of the medulla, then through the reticular formation to the brainstem and hypothalamus, where further modulation and integration occur. Further neuroendocrine stimulation ensues, including secretion of angiotensin via renin[517]; secretion of aldosterone via angiotensin II and adrenocorticotropic hormone (ACTH)[553]; secretion of cortisol via ACTH[263]; secretion of glucagon via epinephrine[268]; and reduced secretion of insulin via epinephrine effect.[532]

Decreases in effective circulating volume sensed by stretch receptors in the kidneys' juxtaglomerular complexes also lead to secretion of renin, and therefore to formation of angiotensin and secretion of aldosterone.[236] The decrease in baroreceptor and stretch receptor discharge also stimulates the heart rate, cardiac contractility, and vasoconstriction by means of increases in sympathetic nervous system (SNS) output and decreases in parasympathetic nervous system (PNS) output.[287] The relative sensitivity of these interactions to changes in blood pressure is shown in Figure 8-3. The maximum sensitivity for baroreceptor responses occurs at approximately 80 mm Hg.[286]

Changes in PaO_2, $PaCO_2$, and hydrogen ion concentration initiate cardiovascular, pulmonary, and neuroendocrine responses by activating peripheral chemoreceptors. The peripheral chemoreceptors are 1 to 2 mm in size and are composed of dopamine-containing, richly vascularized tissue (glomus cells), which are found primarily in the carotid bodies at the bifurcation of the common carotid arteries and in the aortic bodies located above and below the aortic arch. The primary receptors are those of the carotid bodies.[144] Carotid glomus cells are activated by a decrease in oxygen and, to a lesser extent, by an increase in $PaCO_2$ and by an increase in hydrogen ions.[663] As a result of the extremely high blood flow through the chemoreceptors, the oxygen content of arterial blood, glomus cells, and venous blood is nearly equal. As a consequence of the low arteriovenous difference, decreases in both arterial blood flow and arterial oxygen tension result in increased extraction of oxygen by the chemoreceptor tissue, cause decreased venous oxygen content, and elicit receptor activation.

Chemoreceptors respond most rapidly when PaO_2 falls below 50 torr.[663] Activation of the chemoreceptors stimulates the hypothalamus and the vascular component of the sympathetic nervous system that increases heart rate and cardiac contractility. It also stimulates the respiratory center by means of central receptors, leading to an increase in respiratory rate. Interactions occur, so that increases in chemoreceptor activity that are caused by reduced oxygen tension are further potentiated by hypercarbia and acidosis. Hypovolemia is usually accompanied by hyperventilation due to chemoreceptor activation.

A complex interplay of vagally mediated and sympathetic afferent reflexes occurs when chemoreceptors are activated by endogenous substances such as prostaglandin and kinins.[144] Oxygen-sensitive potassium channel receptors sensitive to hypoxia have been recently found in the respiratory tree.[694] The most important central chemoreceptors are those situated just below the ventral medulla and are surrounded by cerebrospinal fluid (CSF). These receptors are sensitive to $Pa{CO_2}$ and by diffusion to resultant changes in the hydrogen ion concentration.

Pain and emotional arousal are characteristic of most injuries and cause neuroendocrine activation. Pain results in stimulation of the thalamus and hypothalamus through projections of peripheral nociceptive fibers.[260] Emotional arousal is produced by the perception or threat of injury and through the limbic areas of the brain evokes anger, fear, or anxiety.[105] Emotion stimulates neuroendocrine reflexes through projections from the limbic system to hypothalamic and lower brainstem nuclei. As a result, both pain and emotional arousal cause secretion of catecholamines, ACTH, cortisol, aldosterone, arginine vasopressin (AVP), endogenous opiates, and increased autonomic nervous system activity.

A change in the plasma glucose concentration is the primary substrate alteration that causes neuroendocrine activation; however, amino acid changes also cause hormone secretion.[243] Receptors in the ventromedial nucleus of the hypothalamus and in the pancreas sense the change in glucose concentration.[267] A decrease in the plasma glucose concentration stimulates the release of catecholamines, growth hormone, cortisol, ACTH, beta-endorphin, and vasopressin through central pathways (hypothalamus and ANS) and stimulates the release of glucagon through autonomic and pancreatic activation.[243,267] Insulin secretion is inhibited through pathways mediated by the autonomic nervous system[446] and by pancreatic cells.[449,532]

The effects of amino acids on hormone secretion are partly mediated by cell-surface receptors and are structure specific; for example, arginine is a potent stimulus to the secretion of insulin and glucagon; leucine also stimulates secretion of insulin but does not stimulate secretion of glucagon.[531] Local concentrations of amino acids are also known to enhance the activity of growth factors in wounds.[660] Amino acids are parent compounds for a number of hormones and neurotransmitters, including thyroxine (T_4), peptide hormones, catecholamines, histamine, and serotonin.

Changes in the core body temperature, which are sensed in the preoptic area of the hypothalamus,[56,310] alter the secretion of hormones, including ACTH, cortisol, AVP, growth hormone, catecholamines, aldosterone, and T_4.[192,332,681] Core temperature may be altered by changes in ambient temperature, loss of thermal insulation (burn injury), inadequate hepatic blood flow (hypovolemia), inadequate substrate (starvation), or inadequate vasomotor control (sepsis).

Infection may stimulate the neuroendocrine system directly, through the action of endotoxin,[190] or indirectly, through secondary changes in blood volume, oxygen concentration, substrate concentrations, and pain. The ubiquitous interactions of the cytokine proteins with the neuroendocrine system have been reviewed recently.[80,410,680]

Integration and Modulation

As a result of the integration of sensory inputs into the CNS and the modulation of efferent signals from the CNS, the neuroendocrine response to a given stimulus is graded and varies, depending on several factors. The particular response depends on the magnitude and duration of the stimulus; the presence and timing of simultaneous and sequential stimuli; circadian effects; and overall physiologic conditions, including concomitant disease, age, nutrition, immunologic competence, and the effects of long-term or acute drug therapy.

The dependence of the response on the intensity and duration of the stimulus, and the importance of CNS integration, have been well described for cardiopulmonary reflexes and adrenomedullary secretion of catecholamines. In contrast to the potent activation of the sympathetic nervous system by small, nonhypotensive hemorrhages,[487,520] adrenomedullary secretion of catecholamines occurs only when hypotension develops. This suggests that inactivation of cardiac stretch receptors alone is not enough to activate catecholamine release, because nonhypotensive hemorrhages have little if any effect on arterial baroreceptors. Similarly, activation of chemoreceptors alone,[1] or inactivation of baroreceptors alone,[214] has a potent effect on SNS activity but a minor effect on catecholamine secretion. Catecholamine secretion occurs during hypotensive hemorrhages that activate both high- and low-pressure baroreceptors.

Besides intensity and duration, the rate of stimulation is important to the modulation of efferent signals. For example, in experimental hemorrhage, the plasma epinephrine concentration is significantly higher after rapid blood loss than with slow hemorrhage to an equal remaining blood volume.[50]

Stimulus transduction is influenced by concomitant neuroendocrine input. For example, the set point and gain of central hypothalamic osmoreceptors are changed by baroreceptor input and by baroreceptor-mediated secretion of AVP.[69,585] Similarly, the set point and gain of

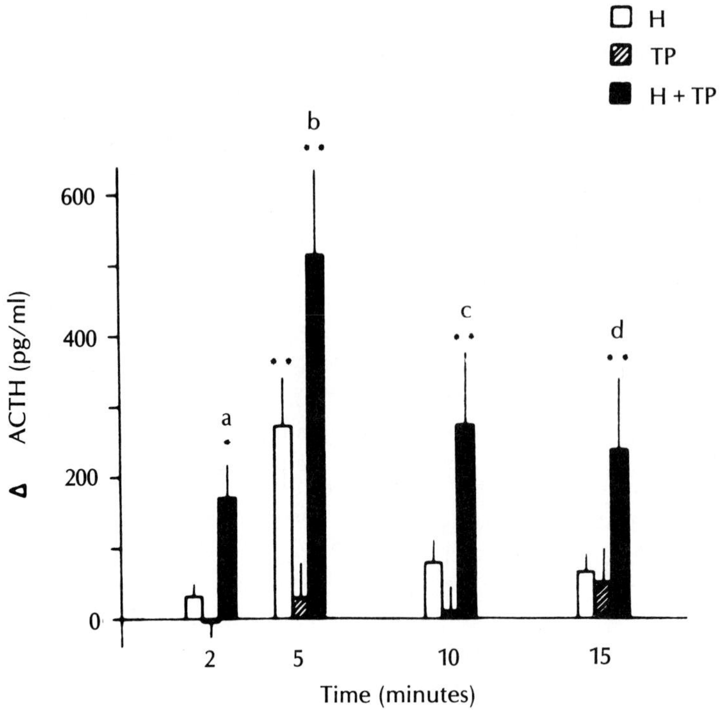

FIGURE 8-4 Potentiation of the adrenocorticoptropic hormone (ACTH) response to hemorrhage by simultaneous nerve stimulation. Cats subjected to a 10 ml/kg hemorrhage demonstrated a transient increase in plasma ACTH concentration 5 minutes after hemorrhage. The concentration did not change with tooth pulp stimulation. In contrast, combining a hemorrhage of the same magnitude with tooth pulp stimulation produced a statistically significant increase in the intensity and duration of plasma ACTH. *H,* Hemorrhage; *TP,* tooth pulp; (*), $P < 0.05$ versus baseline; (**), $P < 0.01$ versus baseline. (From Guyton AC: *Arterial pressure and hypertension,* Philadelphia, 1980, WB Saunders.)

baroreceptors may be changed when viscerosomatic and somatosensory afferents converge with baroreceptor inputs in the cardiovascular areas of the medulla,[373,538,576] and baroreceptor responsiveness may be increased by catecholamines, AVP, and angiotensin.[148,280,327] The sensitivity of some receptors, such as those of the adrenal cortex, may also change with the time of day.[200] Thus a particular stimulus may produce different effects under different circumstances.

In clinical circumstances, the stimuli accompanying injury, sepsis, and starvation rarely occur alone. The neuroendocrine response to injury is the sum of all stimuli, which often is different from the response to any single stimulus[49,503] (Figure 8-4).

Multiple stimuli or injuries may occur sequentially. Under most circumstances, the response to the second set of stimuli is unchanged; however, it may be amplified by the process of potentiation. The mechanism by which potentiation occurs is not well understood, but for the hypothalamic-pituitary axis, it appears to require 60 to 90 minutes to offset cortisol feedback inhibition, and it persists for approximately 24 hours.[259] Physiologic potentiation for cortisol and catecholamines has been demonstrated in response to sequential hemorrhages and sequential operations (Figure 8-5).[408,409] Some researchers have demonstrated potentiation of the adrenocortical response to hypoxia and the timing of surgery[541] and the effect of temperature on the secretion of ACTH, corticosteroids, and vasopressin.[681] The initial neuroendocrine responses to trauma, shock, and sepsis consequently modify the changes induced by subsequent surgery.

Efferent Output

The efferent limb of the reflex neuroendocrine response to injury comprises many nested layers, which can be broadly subdivided into the hormonal response, the mediator response, and the intracellular response. These divisions are arbitrary, but useful for giving a general structure to the biologic response to injury, making it easier to understand. The neural reflex response that originates predominantly in the brainstem centers also

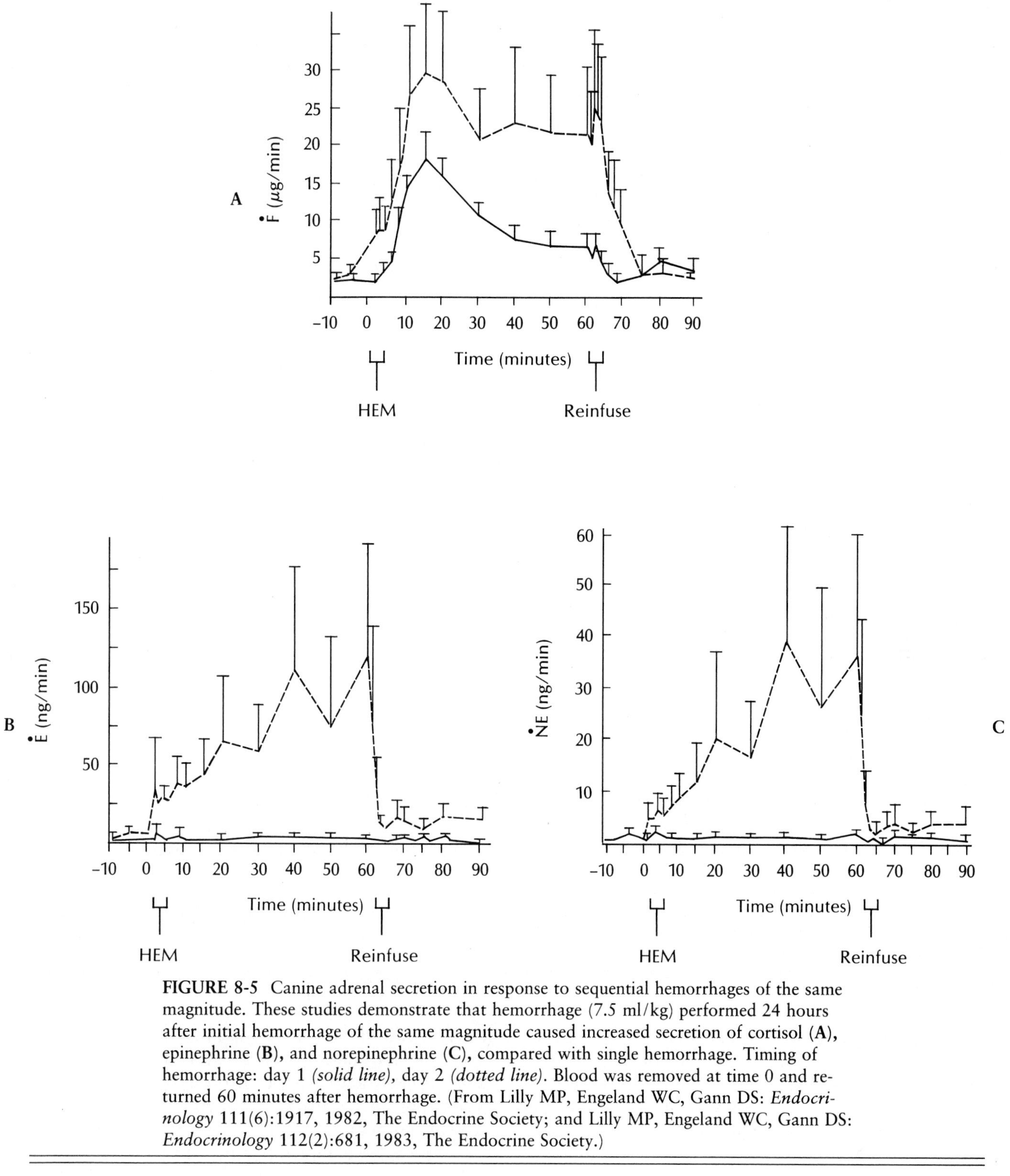

FIGURE 8-5 Canine adrenal secretion in response to sequential hemorrhages of the same magnitude. These studies demonstrate that hemorrhage (7.5 ml/kg) performed 24 hours after initial hemorrhage of the same magnitude caused increased secretion of cortisol (**A**), epinephrine (**B**), and norepinephrine (**C**), compared with single hemorrhage. Timing of hemorrhage: day 1 *(solid line)*, day 2 *(dotted line)*. Blood was removed at time 0 and returned 60 minutes after hemorrhage. (From Lilly MP, Engeland WC, Gann DS: *Endocrinology* 111(6):1917, 1982, The Endocrine Society; and Lilly MP, Engeland WC, Gann DS: *Endocrinology* 112(2):681, 1983, The Endocrine Society.)

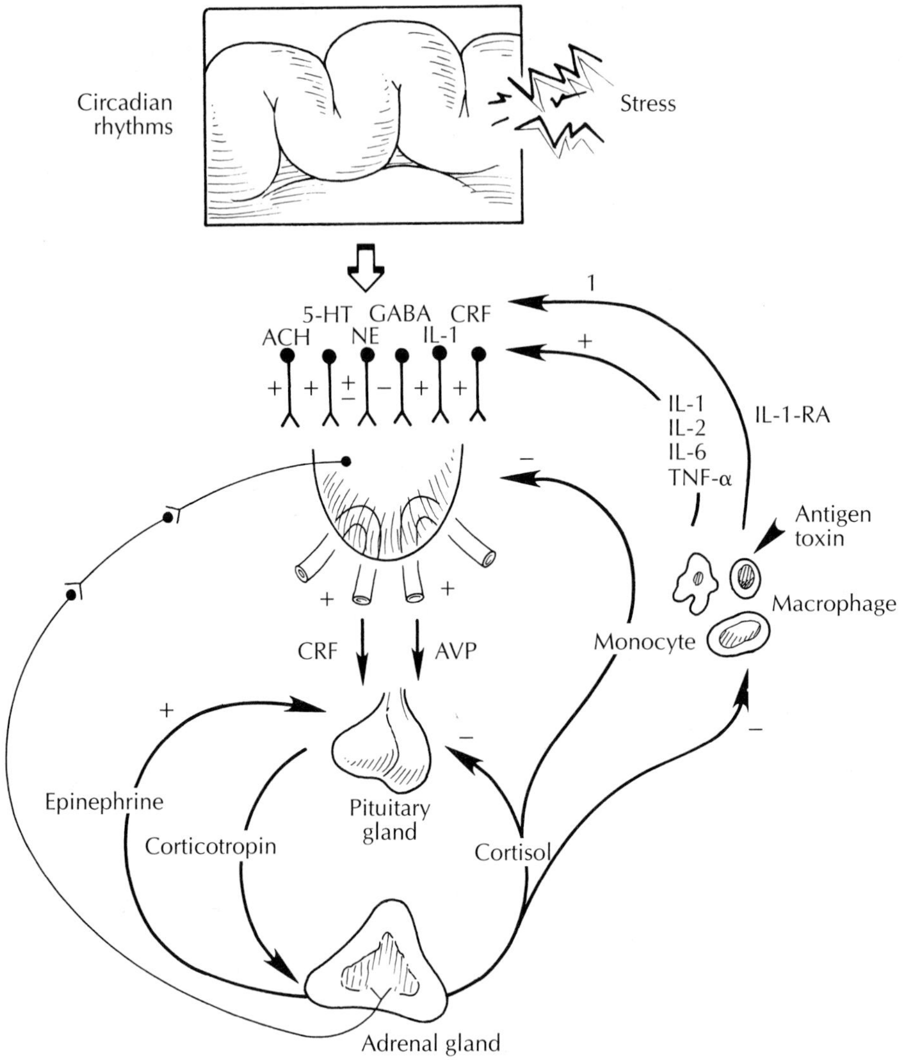

FIGURE 8-6 Interactions between hypothalamic, pituitary, and immunocompetent cells are bidirectional. Neural elements are modulated by external factors (e.g., circadian rhythm, emotional stress, injury) and by activated immunocompetent cells en passant that secrete cytokines and other factors. Cytokines induce the hypothalamic release of corticotropin-releasing factor (CRF) and arginine vasopressin (AVP), stimulating secretion of corticotropin. Circulating adrenal epinephrine acts synergistically with CRF and AVP. Cortisol inhibits activation of lymphocytes and other white blood cells and modulates further secretion of cytokines and other mediators. *ACH,* Acetylcholine; *5-HT,* serotonin; *NE,* norepinephrine; *GABA,* gamma-aminobutyric acid; *IL,* interleukin; *IL-1-RA,* interluekin-1-receptor antagonist; *TNF-α,* tumor necrosis factor alpha. (From Reichlin S: *N Engl J Med* 329:1249, 1992.)

activates central hypothalamic regions and distal innervated endocrine organs. Similarly, the mediator response, which includes secretion of cytokines such as interleukins (ILs) and tumor necrosis factors (TNFs), has systemic physiologic consequences in certain circumstances and may produce systemic effects in addition to localized or paracrine changes. The bidirectional interactions of neuroendocrine hormones and mediator substances are complex and have yet to be fully explained (Figure 8-6).[552]

The neuroendocrine response may be further subdivided into substances controlled by the hypothalamic-pituitary axis and those controlled by the autonomic regions of the brainstem. Secretion of cortisol, T_4, growth hormone, and AVP primarily is controlled by the hypothalamic-pituitary axis; secretion of insulin, glucagon, and catecholamines primarily is controlled by the autonomic regions of the brainstem. The mediator response involves cytokines, growth factors, eicosanoids, complement proteins, and endothelial cell prod-

TABLE 8-1 NEUROENDOCRINE AND MEDIATOR RESPONSE TO INJURY

HORMONES	MEDIATORS
INCREASED RELEASE	
Epinephrine	Interleukin-1 (IL-1)
Norepinephrine	Interleukin-2 (IL-2)
Dopamine	Interleukin-6 (IL-6)
Glucagon	Interleukin-8 (IL-8)*
Renin	Tumor necrosis factor–alpha (TNF-alpha)
Angiotensin II	Prostaglandin E_2 (PGE_2)
Arginine vasopressin (AVP)	Leukotriene B_4 (LTB_4)
Adrenocorticotropic hormone (ACTH)	Kinins
Cortisol	
Aldosterone	Histamine
Beta-endorphin	Serotonin
	Platelet-activating factor (PAF)
Enkephalins	Complement
Growth hormone	Endothelins
Prolactin	Nitric oxide (NO)
DECREASED RELEASE	
Insulin	IL-8*
Somatomedins†	Interferon-gamma (IFN-gamma)‡
Insulin-like growth factor (IGF)†	
Thyroxine (T_4)	
Triiodothyronine (T_3)	
Luteinizing hormone (LH)	
Testosterone	
Estrogen	
Follicle-stimulating hormone (FSH)	

*IL-8 changes are not clearly known.
†Reduced secretion of somatomedin and IGF appears to correlate with a reduction in insulin.
‡PGE_2 inhibits secretion of IFN.

ucts. Injury causes the release of all hypothalamic-pituitary hormones and all hormones mediated by the autonomic nervous system, except for thyroid hormones, gonadotropins, and insulin (Table 8-1). Injury (particularly sepsis or endotoxemia) also causes the release of most mediators. Many arms of the afferent limbs have not yet been identified and characterized.

Hormones secreted by endocrine organs, mediator substances released by cells, and neurotransmitters released at nerve terminals fall into one of three chemical classes: proteins; fatty acid derivatives of cholesterol or arachidonic acid; and amino acid derivatives (see the box at upper right). These substances act on receptors on the cell membrane's surface or in the cell cytoplasm. The density and affinity of receptors can be modulated

CHEMICAL CLASSES OF SOME HORMONES AND MEDIATORS

Proteins (Polypeptides, Small Peptides, Glycoproteins)

Insulin	Thyroid-stimulating hormone (TSH)
Glucagon	FSH
AVP	LH
Renin	Thyrotropin-releasing hormone (TRH)
Angiotensin	Luteinizing hormone–releasing hormone (LHRH)
Growth hormone	Endothelins
Somatomedin	Interleukins
Atrial natriuretic peptides (ANP)	TNF

Fatty Acid Derivatives (Lipid Soluble)

Cholesterol	Arachidonic acid
Cortisol	Eicosanoids
Testosterone	Leukotrienes
Aldosterone	
Platelet-activating factor (PAF)	

Amino Acid Derivatives

Epinephrine	T_3
Norepinephrine	Serotonin
Dopamine	Histamine

by factors such as conformational change at different sites on either side of the cell membrane[352]; by the effects of circulating receptor antagonists; and by postbinding changes within the target cell.[136]

Signal Transduction

The mechanisms by which hormones, mediators, and neurotransmitters (ligands) effect intracellular change depend on the lipid and water solubility of both the signaler and the cell membrane. Generally, the signaling ligand changes ion membrane permeability or genomic transcription, or both. Ligands that nearly directly alter transcription tend to be lipid soluble and are permeable to the lipid bilayer of cell membranes. Other ligands change ion transport by attaching to membrane receptors, either directly, at the channel, or indirectly, by coupling to guanine nucleotide–binding proteins (G proteins), intracellular calcium, or other modulators of the cell signal. These hormones act through secondary changes in the intracellular cyclic adenosine 3′,5′-monophosphate (cAMP) through influx or mobilization (or both) of calcium or through hormone-receptor protein kinase activity.[352,622] Polypeptides such as interferon-gamma (IFN-gamma)[130] and some interleukins[601] bind to unique cell-surface receptors, which signal activation of specific cytosolic factors that effect genomic transcription.

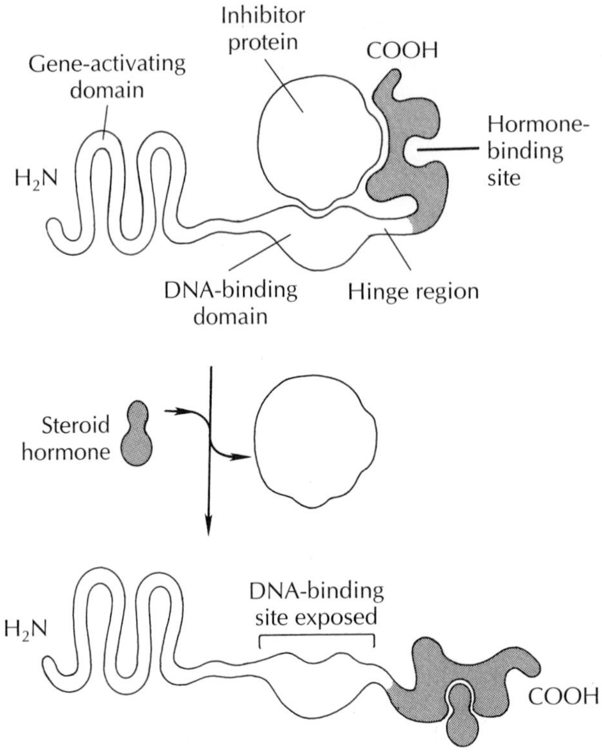

FIGURE 8-7 Model of a steroid-hormone receptor protein based on cortisol. The receptors for estrogen, testosterone, progesterone, aldosterone, thyroid hormone, retinoic acid, and vitamin D have a similar structure and together form the steroid receptor superfamily. In the inactive state, the receptor is bound to an inhibitor protein that blocks the DNA-binding domain of the receptor (believed to be the 90,000 dalton heat-shock protein hsp90 in the case of cortisol). The binding of hormone to the receptor causes the inhibitor protein to dissociate and activate the receptor. (From Alberts B, Bray J, Lewis J et al: *Molecular biology of the cell,* ed 2, New York, 1989, Garland.)

The precise signaling mechanisms for some substances are still unknown, but the search is intriguing. For example, recent studies of tumor necrosis factor–alpha (TNF-alpha)[180] and IL-1[428] have suggested mechanisms such as activation of membrane-bound sphingomyelinase to generate ceramide as a second messenger. An additional mechanism for TNF-alpha action may involve intrinsic ion channel–forming activity of the TNF-alpha molecule.[350]

Mechanisms of Hormone Action

Nuclear Hormone Signal Transduction

The primary actions of steroids, thyroid hormones, retinoic acid, and vitamin D are mediated by receptor proteins that bind to specific genes after free diffusion through the lipid bilayer of the cell membrane.[136] After rapid diffusion, steroid hormones bind to cytosolic receptors,[491,500,617] and the steroid hormone–receptor complex, known as the steroid receptor superfamily,[205] (Figure 8-7) migrates to the cell nucleus, where genomic action modulates the transcription of messenger RNA (mRNA) for protein synthesis[136,249] (Figure 8-8). Nuclear mechanisms also account for most actions of triiodothyronine (T_3),[162] which explains the 1- to 2-hour interval before the primary actions of membrane-soluble hormones can be detected. More quickly detectable actions of steroids[477] and T_3[587] may also be mediated through the cell membrane. Thyroid hormones do not appear to bind to cytosolic receptors after diffusing through the cell membrane. Unbound thyroid hormone passes to the nucleus, where it binds to nonhistone proteins of the nuclear chromatin, activating gene expression.[162]

Recent identification of a specific protein transcription factor coupled to tyrosine kinase and activated by INF-gamma[581,601] suggests that additional factors act via direct nuclear signal pathways and may account for some of the observed nonpromiscuous actions of mediators.

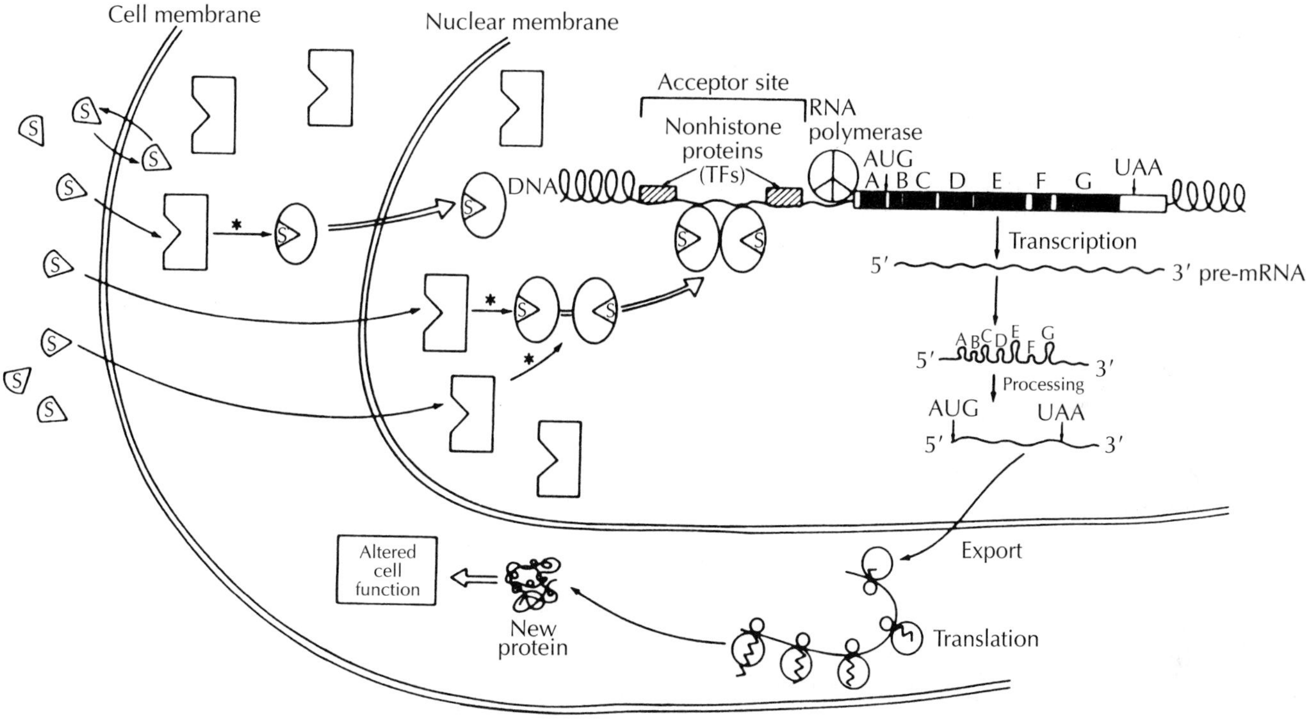

FIGURE 8-8 Molecular pathway for the action of steroid hormones. Diffusion of steroid through the cell membrane lipid bilayer to bind to cytosolic or nuclear receptor proteins causes displacement of heat-shock protein and activation of the receptor to allow nonhistone protein binding and DNA transcription by RNA polymerase. After RNA processing and export to the cytosol, new proteins are produced that alter cell function. (From Wilson JD, Foster DW, editors: *Williams textbook of endocrinology,* ed 8, Philadelphia, 1992, WB Saunders.)

Membrane-Active Hormone Signal Transduction

Water-soluble protein and amino acid–derivative hormones bind to receptors on the surface of the cell membrane. There are three major classes of cell membrane receptors for these hormones and neurotransmitters: (1) those with intrinsic tyrosine kinase activity; (2) those coupled through G proteins to adenylate cyclase or phosphatidylinositol turnover; and (3) those associated with ligand-gated ion channels (Figure 8-9). After receptor-ligand interaction, the hormone-receptor complex may directly phosphorylate the tyrosine residue of the protein (tyrosine-specific protein kinase), as in the case of insulin and growth factors. Other hormones (e.g., peptides, neurotransmitters and prostaglandins) activate protein kinases through G protein–regulated pathways[273,274] that involve intermediate formation of cAMP by the membrane adenylate cyclase complex or by intracellular release of calcium (Figure 8-10). Ion channels that control the flux of potassium, sodium, chloride, and calcium at the membrane may be charge or ligand regulated. The ligand-gated channels include the nicotinic cholinergic receptors (Figure 8-11) and, as in the beta-adrenergic calcium channel and the cholinergic muscarinic potassium channels in the heart, also may involve G proteins as signal transducers.[76] These second messengers modulate the activity of regulatory proteins and enzymes to cause cellular effects that usually are more quickly detected than those directed by lipid-soluble, nuclear-acting ligands.

G proteins modulate the activity of cell surface hormone receptors with membrane-bound enzymes such as adenylate cyclase, phospholipases A_2 and C, and ligand-gated potassium and calcium channels.[75,134,620] G proteins have a stimulatory (G_S) or an inhibitory (G_i) effect[476] (Figure 8-12). In the absence of ligand binding, the G protein (heterotrimer–alpha-beta-gamma) binds guanosine diphosphate (GDP) via the alpha-subunit. Formation of the ligand-receptor complex in the presence of magnesium results in receptor and G-protein interaction and replacement of GDP with guanosine triphosphate (GTP). The GTP-bound, activated alpha-subunit then dissociates from the beta-gamma–dimer subunit to modulate the activities of the membrane-bound enzyme or ion channel. The inherent guanosine tri-

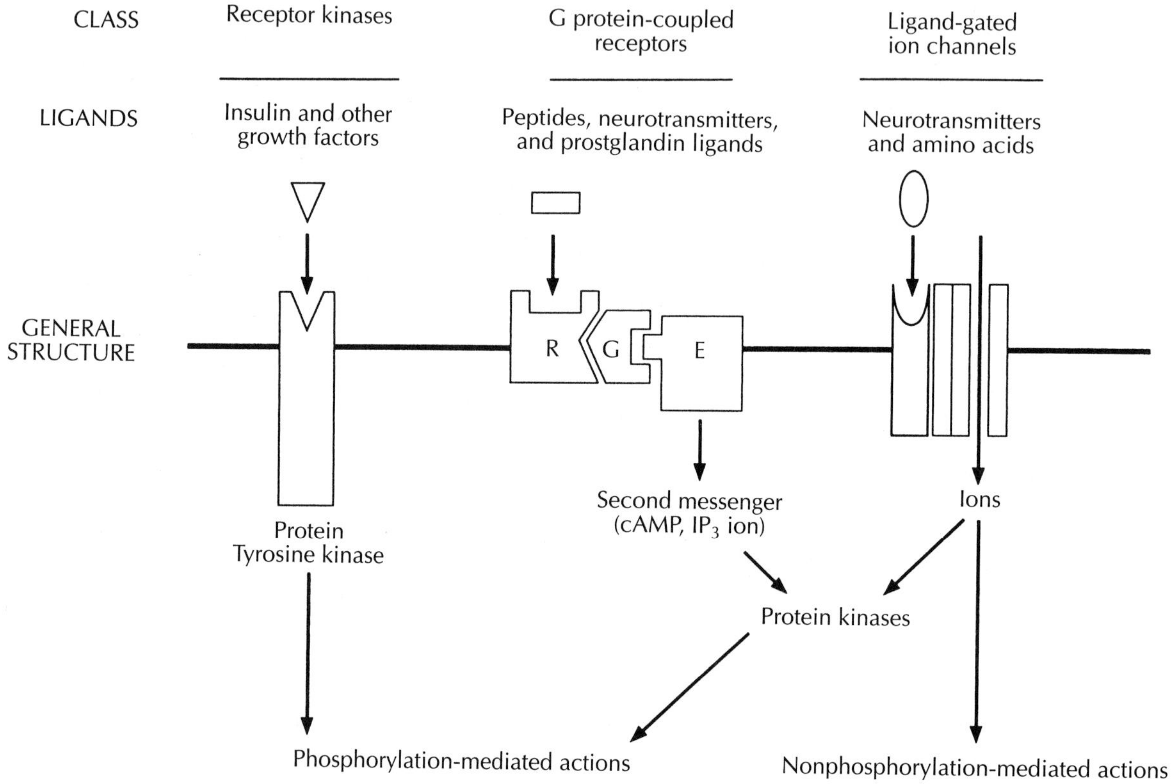

FIGURE 8-9 Membrane receptors for hormones and neurotransmitters may be classified into three major categories. Those in the first category (insulin and other growth factors) bind to cell-surface receptors that stimulate the phosphorylation of proteins on tyrosine residues (protein tyrosine kinases). Those in the second category (peptides, neurotransmitters, and prostaglandin ligands) bind to receptors *(R)* that are coupled to effector *(E)* enzymes and produce second messengers that activate distinct proteins (generally serine/threonine kinases). The third major category comprises ligand-gated ion channels, which also may be coupled to G proteins. (From Wilson JD, Foster DW, editors: *Williams textbook of endocrinology,* ed 8, Philadelphia, 1992, WB Saunders.)

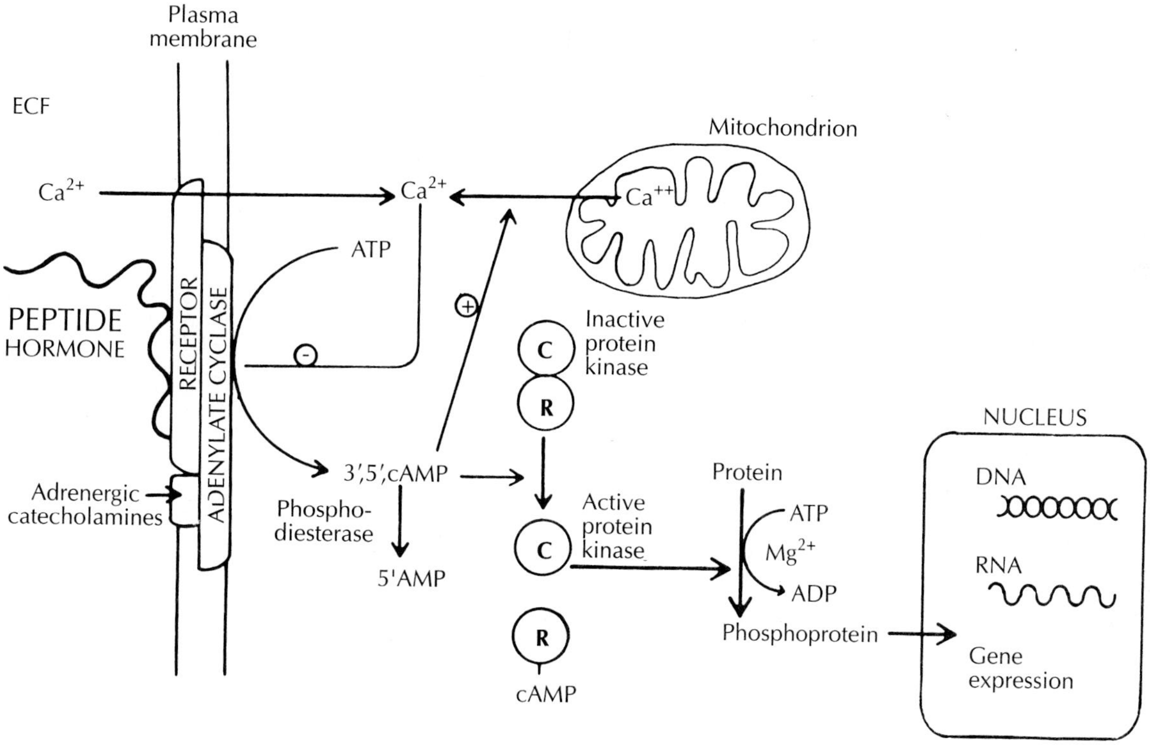

FIGURE 8-10 Proposed cellular mechanism for peptide hormone activation of gene expression in an endocrine cell. Binding of the peptide to the plasma membrane receptor activates adenylate cyclase, which leads to formation of 3′,5′-cAMP, activation of protein kinases, and phosphorylation of specific proteins. The final active phosphoprotein interacts with regulatory sites on the gene to allow transcription and expression. *C* and *R* refer to catalytic and regulatory (cAMP-receptor) subunits of protein kinase, respectively. Calcium is released from mitochondrial stores and by extracellular influx to modulate the formation of cAMP. (From Wilson JD, Foster DW, editors: *Williams textbook of endocrinology,* ed 8, Philadelphia, 1992, WB Saunders.)

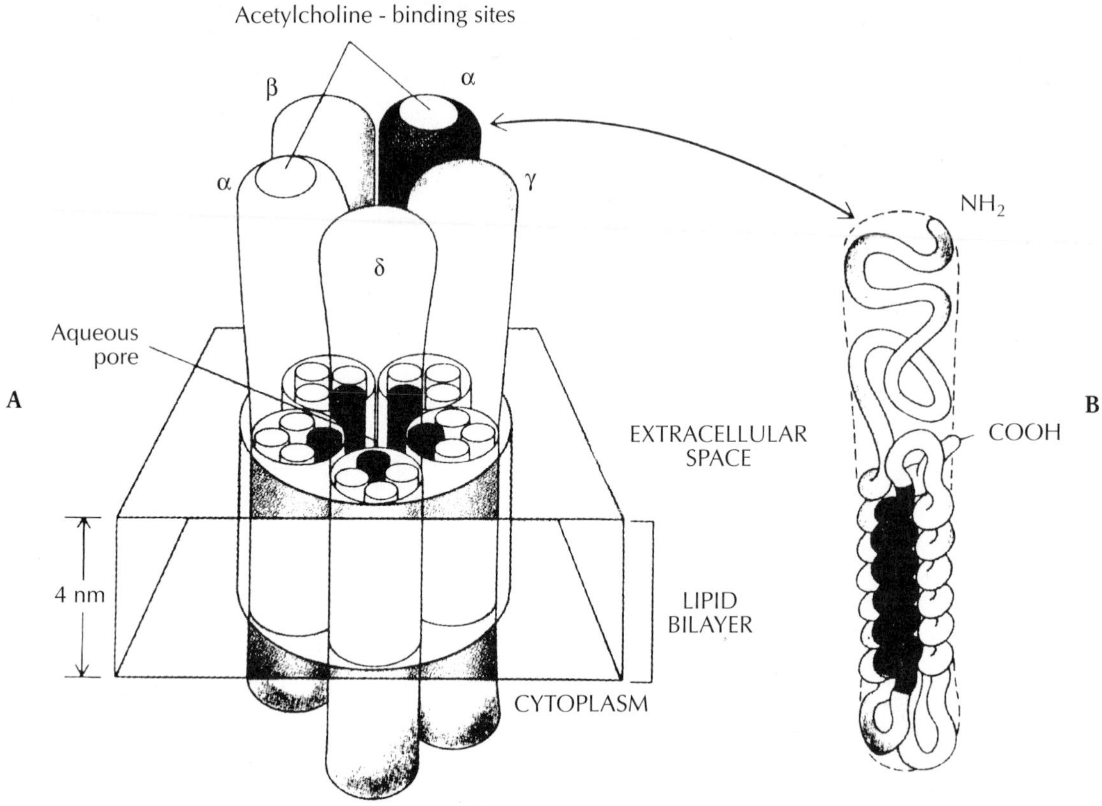

FIGURE 8-11 Composition of the nicotinic acetylcholine receptor. **A,** The receptor is made up of five subunits grouped in a pentagonal array to form the aqueous pore. The two alpha subunits interact with the ligand. **B,** Each subunit contains alpha-helical regions that span the plasma membrane with the four hydrophobic domains. There is also a long NH_2-terminal extracellular region. One transmembrane region in each subunit lines the aqueous pore. (From Wilson JB, Foster DW, editors: *Williams textbook of endocrinology*, ed 8, Philadelphia, 1992, WB Saunders.)

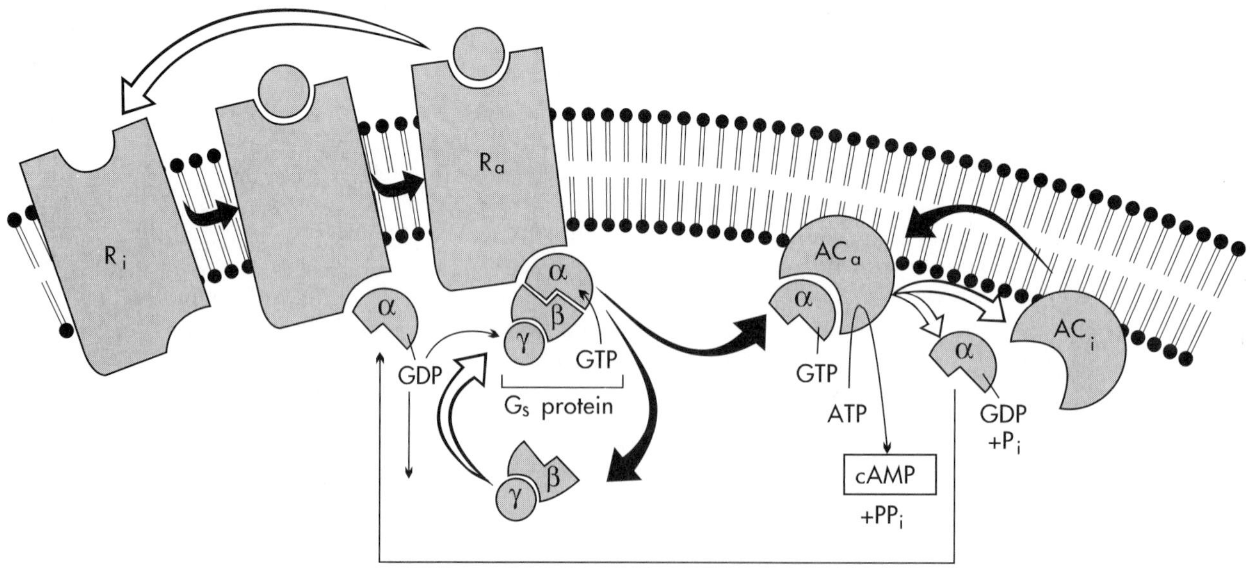

FIGURE 8-12 Activation of adenylate cyclase and cyclic adenosine monophosphate (cAMP)-dependent protein kinase. Receptors that generate this response include those for epinephrine, adrenocorticotropin, and thyrotropin. See text for discussion. R_i, inactive receptor; R_a, active receptor; AC_i, inactive adenylate cyclase; AC_a, active adenylate cyclase. (From Widnell CC, Pfenninger KH: *Essential cell biology*, Baltimore, 1990, Williams & Wilkins.)

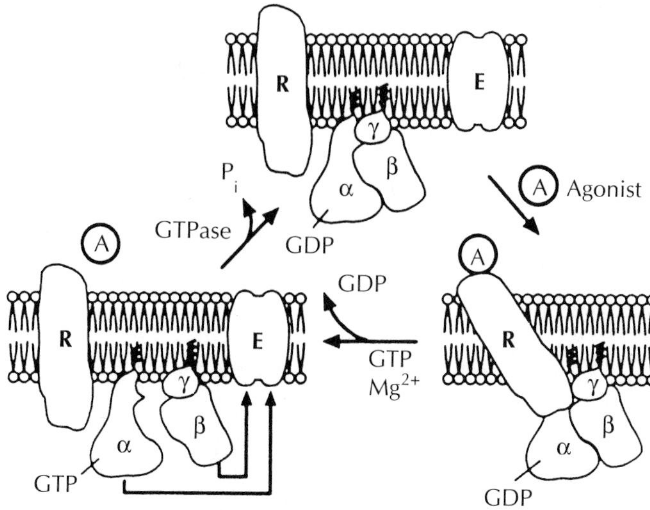

FIGURE 8-13 Both subunits of the guanosine diphosphate (GDP)–bound G-protein heterotrimer interact with the receptor. The agonist-bound receptor catalyzes the exchange of guanosine triphosphate (GTP) for GDP on the G–alpha-subunit. GTP-liganded G-alpha presumably dissociates from G–beta-gamma. (From Clapham DE, Neer EJ: *Nature* 365:404, 1993.)

phosphatase (GTPase) activity of the alpha-subunit hydrolyzes GTP to GDP, to terminate hormone signaling. Receptors for beta-adrenergic catecholamines, ACTH, thyroid-stimulating hormone (TSH), and glucagon are coupled to stimulatory G proteins and affect adenylate cyclase and calcium channels. Receptors for alpha-adrenergic catecholamines, somatostatin, and perhaps insulin, as well as muscarinic receptors, are coupled to inhibitory G proteins that reduce either the activity of adenylate cyclase or the likelihood that potassium or calcium channels will open.[352]

The complexity of G-protein regulation is underscored by recent discoveries, which have established active effector roles for the beta-gamma–dimer subunit as well as for the alpha-subunit.[134] Regulation by the G protein beta-gamma–dimer subunit has been described for adenylate cyclase (synergistic and antagonistic),[624] muscarinic receptor kinase,[294] phospholipase A_2,[346] and potassium channels.[412] It now appears that both subunits are involved in GDP-bound G-protein interactions with the hormone receptor (Figure 8-13). Oncogene transcripts (*ras* proteins, so called because they were first isolated from viruses that caused rat sarcoma) and the effects of growth factors on cell proliferation are believed to involve G protein–coupled signal transduction and protein–tyrosine kinase action.[433]

Changes in intracellular calcium, which are crucial to many cellular functions, are achieved through G protein–coupled membrane receptors (Figure 8-14) via the inositol triphosphate (IP_3) receptor pathways and voltage-activated mechanisms (Figure 8-15).[58,61] The bifurcating messenger inositol lipid system produces IP_3, which mobilizes calcium from internal stores and produces diacylglycerol (DAG), which activates protein kinase C (PKC).[483] As an intracellular messenger, IP_3 may have a greater range of action than intracellular calcium ion.[8] Recent evidence of control of intracellular calcium stores may implicate cyclic adenosine diphosphate ribose (cADPR) as a second messenger[253,395] and may betoken the existence of additional second messengers.[510,545] These transduction mechanisms for intracellular calcium metabolism may help synthesize the effects of diverse factors, such as nitric oxide (NO)[59] (Figure 8-16), endothelin[426] (Figure 8-17), and mechanisms for insulin release.[623] Intracellular calcium is finely regulated by transport mechanisms across plasma membrane, endoplasmic or sarcoplasmic reticulum, mitochondria, and a specialized calcium-sequestering compartment.[107]

The continuous, rapid removal of the second messengers, cAMP, and calcium from the cytosol allows rapid cellular response to extracellular signals. These substances interact within the cell to further modulate signal transduction. Besides cAMP and calcium, cyclic guanosine monophosphate (cGMP) and cADPR also may act as second messengers. Intracellular changes in cAMP cause activation of protein kinase A (PKA) and mediate the actions of several hormones, including ACTH, TSH, catecholamines, parathormone, AVP, insulin, and glucagon. The ubiquitous intracellular effects of calcium include neuronal, endocrine, and exocrine

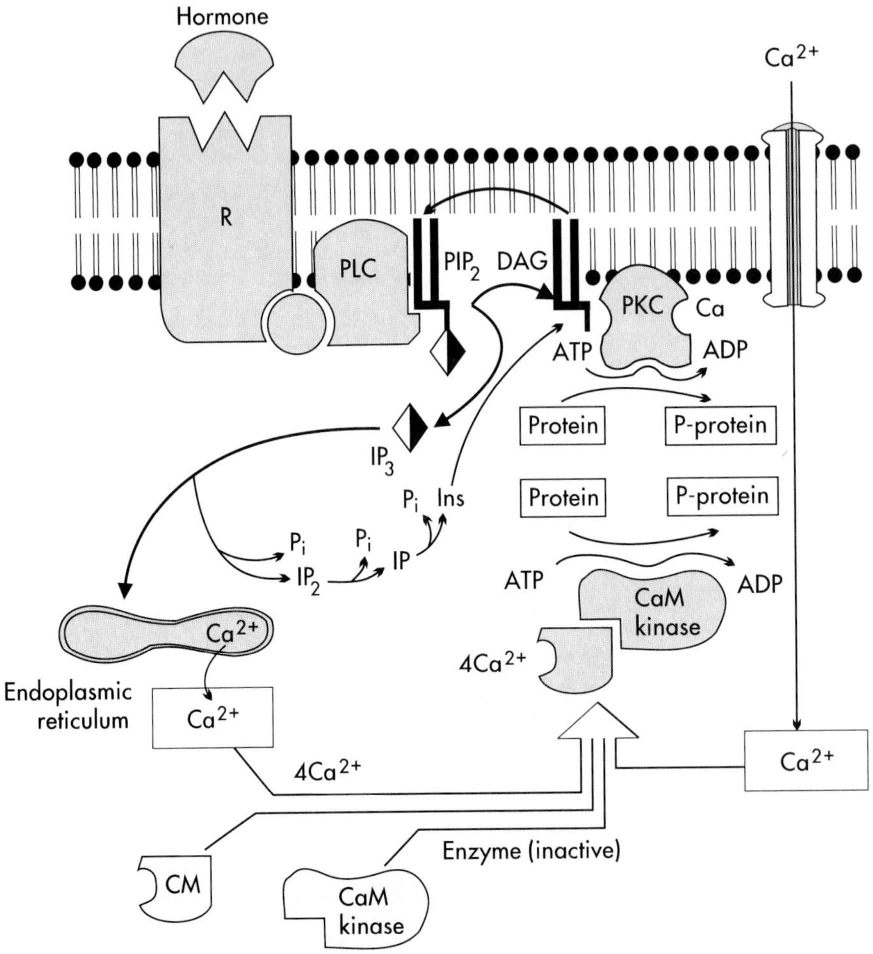

FIGURE 8-14 Calcium-mediated signal transduction. Arginine vasopressin, angiotensin, and alpha$_1$-adrenergic receptors function by this mechanism. *CaM kinase*, Calcium/calmodulin-dependent kinase; *CM*, calmodulin; *IP, IP_2, IP_3*, inositol monophosphate, diphosphate, and triphosphate, respectively; *DAG*, diacylglycerol; *PIP*, phosphatidylinositol; *PKC*, protein kinase C; *PLC*, phospholipase C. (From Widnell CC, Pfenninger KH: *Essential cell biology*, Baltimore, 1990, Williams & Wilkins.)

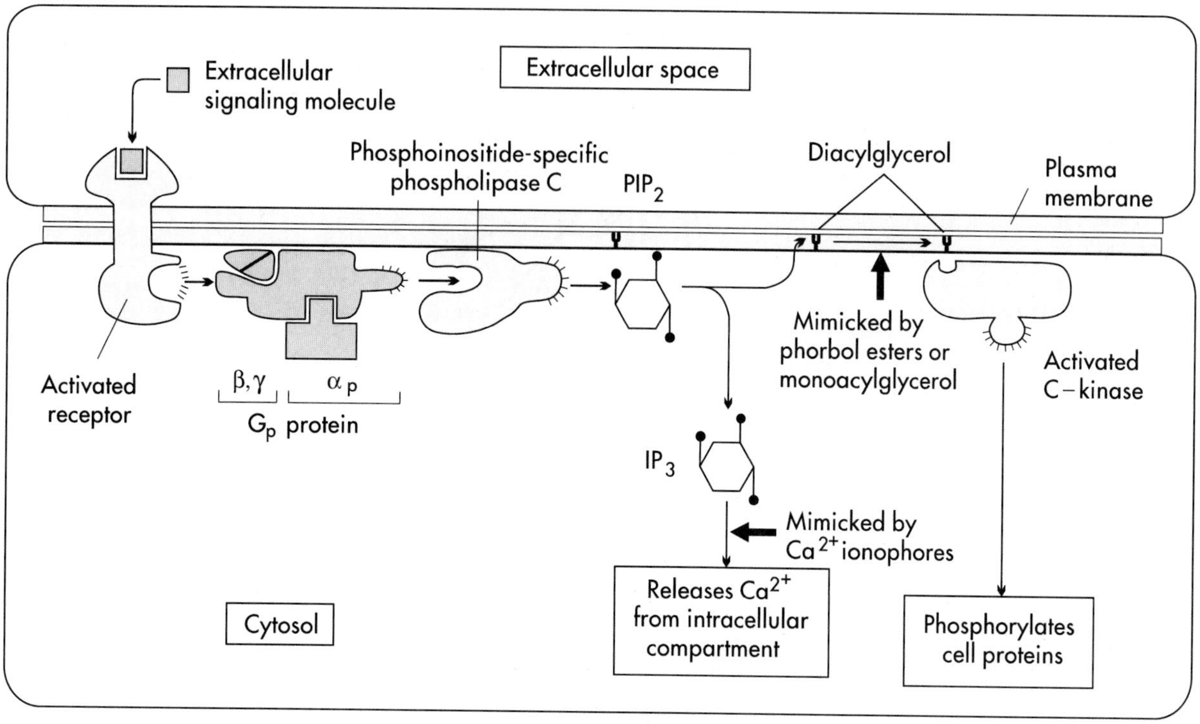

FIGURE 8-15 The two branches of the inositol phospholipid pathway. The activated receptor binds to a specific G protein (G_p), causing the alpha-subunit to dissociate and activate phospholipase C to generate inositol triphosphate (IP_3) and diacylglycerol from phosphatidylinositol biphosphate (PIP_2). Diacylglycerol and calcium activate protein kinase (PKC). IP_3 causes release of intracellular calcium. (From Alberts B, Bray D, Lewis J et al: *Molecular biology of the cell,* ed 2, New York, 1989, Garland.)

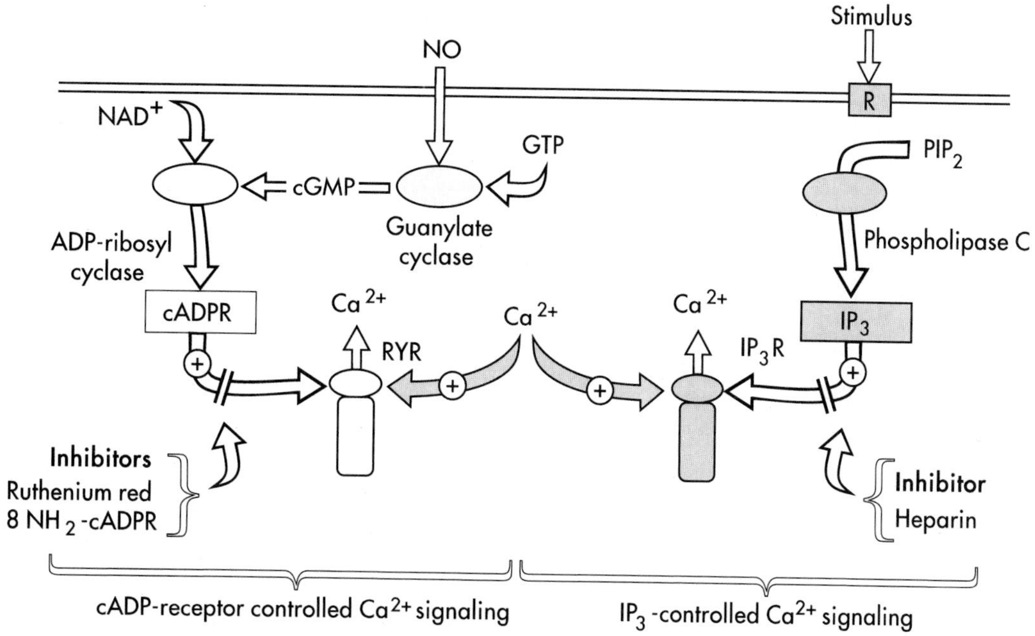

FIGURE 8-16 Calcium-mobilizing second messengers. Two separate signaling pathways activate the ryanodine receptor (RYR) and the inositol triphosphate receptor (IP_3R). *cADPR,* Cyclic adenosine diphosphate (ADP) ribose; *NO,* nitric oxide; *PIP_2,* phosphatidylinositol biphosphate. (From Berridge MJ: *Nature* 365:388, 1993.)

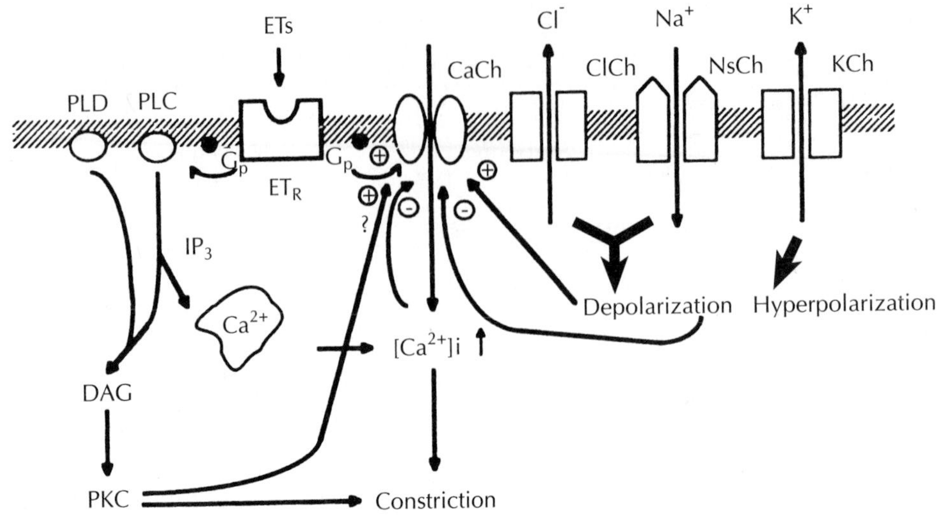

FIGURE 8-17 Intracellular signaling mechanism for endothelins (ETs). ETs cause release of intracellular calcium by activating phospholipases C and D and by the actions of inositol triphosphate and diacylglycerol. ETs also cause the influx of extracellular calcium directly (by stimulating calcium channels) and indirectly (by activating protein kinase C, opening nonselective cation channels and chloride channels, and depolarizing the cell membrane). ETs oppose calcium release by opening potassium channels (hyperpolarization), which inhibits calcium channels. Increased intracellular calcium mediates vasoconstriction. *ET_R*, Endothelin receptors; *G_p*, G protein; *PLC*, phospholipase C; *PLD*, phospholipase D; *IP_3*, inositol triphosphate; *DAG*, diacylglycerol; *PKC*, protein kinase C; *$Ca^{2+}i$*, concentration of intracellular free calcium; *CaCh*, calcium channel; *ClCh*, chloride channel; *NsCh*, nonselective cation channel; *KCh*, potassium channel. (From Masaki T: *Endocr Rev* 14:295, 1993.)

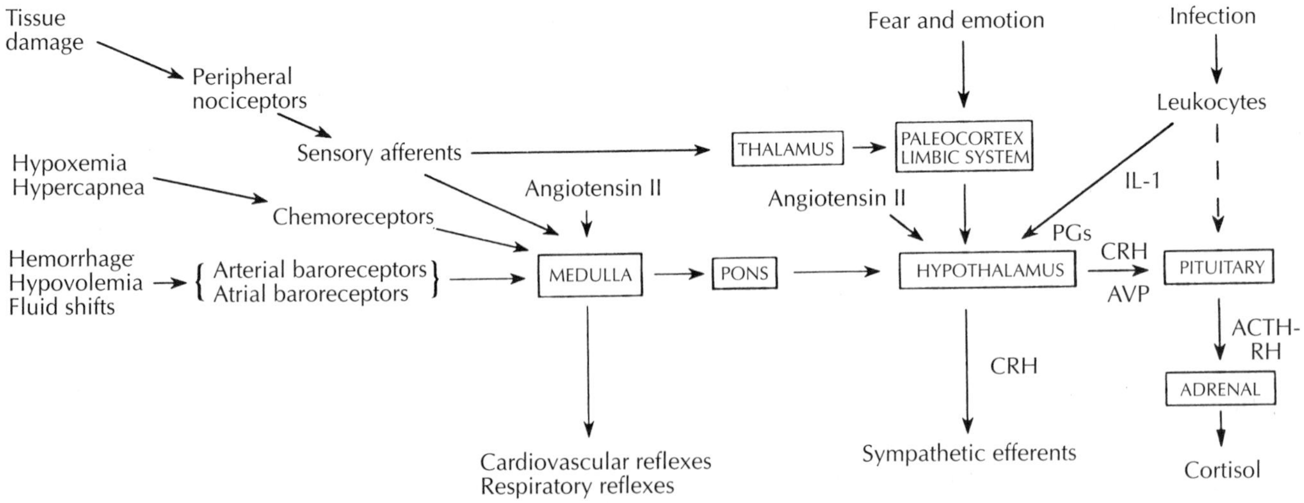

FIGURE 8-18 Hypothalamic-pituitary-adrenal system, showing afferent inputs, neural pathways, and endocrine and mediator interactions. *PGs*, Prostaglandins; *IL-1*, interleukin-1; *CRH*, corticotropin-releasing hormone; *AVP*, arginine vasopressin; *ACTH-RH*, adrenocorticotropin hormone–releasing hormone. (From Lilly MP, Gann DS: *Arch Surg* 127:1463, 1992.)

cell exocytosis; cell motility; excitation-contraction coupling; neuronal transport; smooth muscle contraction; platelet aggregation; and a host of biochemical effects such as regulatory binding to calmodulin and subsequent activation of calcium kinases. Intracellular changes in cGMP are caused by endothelial NO and atrial natriuretic peptides (ANP). The potential interactions of cADPR with calcium release and perhaps NO metabolism (see Figure 8-16) highlight the complexity and speed of subcellular and molecular research advances in signal transduction and neuroendocrine modulation.

NEUROENDOCRINE RESPONSE TO INJURY

Hormones Controlled by the Hypothalamic-Pituitary Axis[501]

Corticotropin-Releasing Factor; Adrenocorticotropic Hormone; Cortisol

The synthesis and release of cortisol from the adrenal zona fasciculata is controlled primarily by adrenocorticotropic hormone (ACTH), which in turn is controlled by pituitary secretion of corticotropin-releasing factor (CRF), also called corticotropin-releasing hormone (CRH).[551] When an injury occurs, the effector hormone, cortisol, is secreted to establish the metabolic availability of glucose from the liver, skeletal muscle, and adipose tissue. Cortisol has permissive effects that, combined with the action of other hormones,[193,218] are essential to restitution of blood volume.[526] Cortisol also has immunologic effects that have not yet been completely described.[410,552] The hypothalamic-pituitary-adrenal system comprises numerous afferent pathways, neural inputs, and neuroendocrine and neuroimmune interactions (Figure 8-18).

CRF, a 41-amino acid polypeptide, is synthesized primarily in hypothalamic cells of the paraventricular nucleus, which are found near cells that secrete arginine vasopressin (AVP), formerly called antidiuretic hormone. Release of CRF into the hypophyseal–portal venous system is induced by neurogenic hypothalamic input and potentiated by AVP.[19]

ACTH is synthesized, stored, and released by chromophobe cells of the anterior pituitary gland as a fragment of a larger molecule, proopiomelanocortin (POMC). POMC contains gamma- and beta-lipotropin, alpha–melanocyte-stimulating hormone (alpha-MSH), and beta-endorphin (Figure 8-19). ACTH binds to all surface receptors, and signals for cortisol release through intracellular changes in cAMP. Pituitary release of ACTH is stimulated by CRF and modulated by AVP[421] and possibly by oxytocin.[178] Mediator cytokines such as IL-1[174,186] and IL-2[92] also stimulate pituitary release of ACTH.[53,62] In addition, a protein released by the pituitary, called macrophage inhibitory factor (MIF), has been identified. MIF has potentiated lethal endotoxemia in experimental models, providing additional evidence of central neuroimmunomodulation through the hypothalamic-pituitary axis.[55]

Release of ACTH is inhibited by cortisol and by ACTH itself, by means of long and short feedback loops, respectively.[551] ACTH stimulates lipolysis in fat cells and amino acid and glucose uptake in skeletal muscle cells.[244]

Cortisol has widespread effects on the metabolism of carbohydrates, amino acids, and fatty acids. In the liver, cortisol inhibits the pentose phosphate shunt, the action of insulin, and regulatory glycolytic enzymes (glucokinase, phosphofructokinase, and pyruvate kinase). Cortisol stimulates glycogen synthetase activity, amino acid uptake, amino acid transaminase activity, and the activity and de novo synthesis of several regulatory gluconeogenetic enzymes, including pyruvate carboxylase, phosphoenolpyruvate carboxykinase (PEPCK), and glucose-6-phosphatase.* In conjunction with the release of epinephrine and ACTH, pyruvate dehydrogenase activity is reduced, which increases the availability of pyruvate for gluconeogenesis. Cortisol also potentiates the effects of glucagon and epinephrine on the liver.[218]

Despite these major effects on hepatic carbohydrate metabolism, adrenalectomized animals do not show marked changes in carbohydrate metabolism if food is constantly available.[203] However, with injury or starvation, adrenalectomized animals do show marked changes in hepatic carbohydrate metabolism, resulting in rapid hypoglycemia and reduced release of nonglucose solute from the liver.[135] However, the absence of cortisol-mediated induction of de novo synthesis of hepatic enzymes is not enough to explain the reduction in serum glucose because enzyme synthesis requires several hours.[307] Furthermore, perfusion of the livers of adrenalectomized animals in the absence of any gluconeogenetic hormones (e.g., epinephrine or glucagon) reveals no difference in the gluconeogenetic conversion of lactate or alanine to glucose compared with control animals.[125] However, total glucose release is impaired, and glycogen stores are virtually absent.[11] Also, in the presence of glucagon or epinephrine, the perfused livers of adrenalectomized animals show a marked impairment of gluconeogenesis.[125] Thus stress-induced hypoglycemia in adrenalectomized animals appears to be at least partly the result of the inability to store glycogen and the absence of the permissive action of corticosteroids on glucagon- and epinephrine-mediated gluconeogenesis.

In skeletal muscle tissue, cortisol has no direct effect on glucose uptake or gluconeogenesis, but it does inhibit insulin-mediated glucose uptake.[101,193] Cortisol reduces the uptake and increases the release of amino acids by skeletal muscle.[101] The release of amino acids from skeletal muscle that is mediated by cytokines such as TNF, IL-1, IFN, and prostaglandin E (PGE) appears to be mediated by cortisol to varying degrees.[223] In the absence

*References 307, 309, 349, 382, and 692.

of cortisol, amino acid release decreases. Consequently, cortisol maintains euglycemia during stress by releasing gluconeogenetic substrates from skeletal muscle and by increasing the activity of gluconeogenetic pathways in the liver.

In adipose tissue, cortisol reduces glucose uptake and potentiates the lipolytic actions of ACTH, epinephrine, glucagon, and growth hormone.[208,210,211] The concentrations of free fatty acids and glycerol increase.

Cortisol impairs the functions of lymphocytes, monocytes, and polymorphonuclear cells (PMNs) when administered in supraphysiologic amounts.[466,513] Administering corticosteroids increases the circulating concentrations of lymphocytes and neutrophils and decreases the circulating concentrations of monocytes and eosinophils. Corticosteroids markedly reduce accumulation of PMNs, monocytes, macrophages, and lymphocytes at inflammatory sites. At physiologic concentrations, cortisol reduces lymphocyte glucose uptake and the release of amino acids; decreases prostaglandin and leukotriene synthesis by inhibiting phospholipase A; and suppresses leukocyte production of IL-1, IL-2, IFN-gamma, beta-endorphin, kinins, and proteases associated with inflammation.[552,661] A new appreciation of the

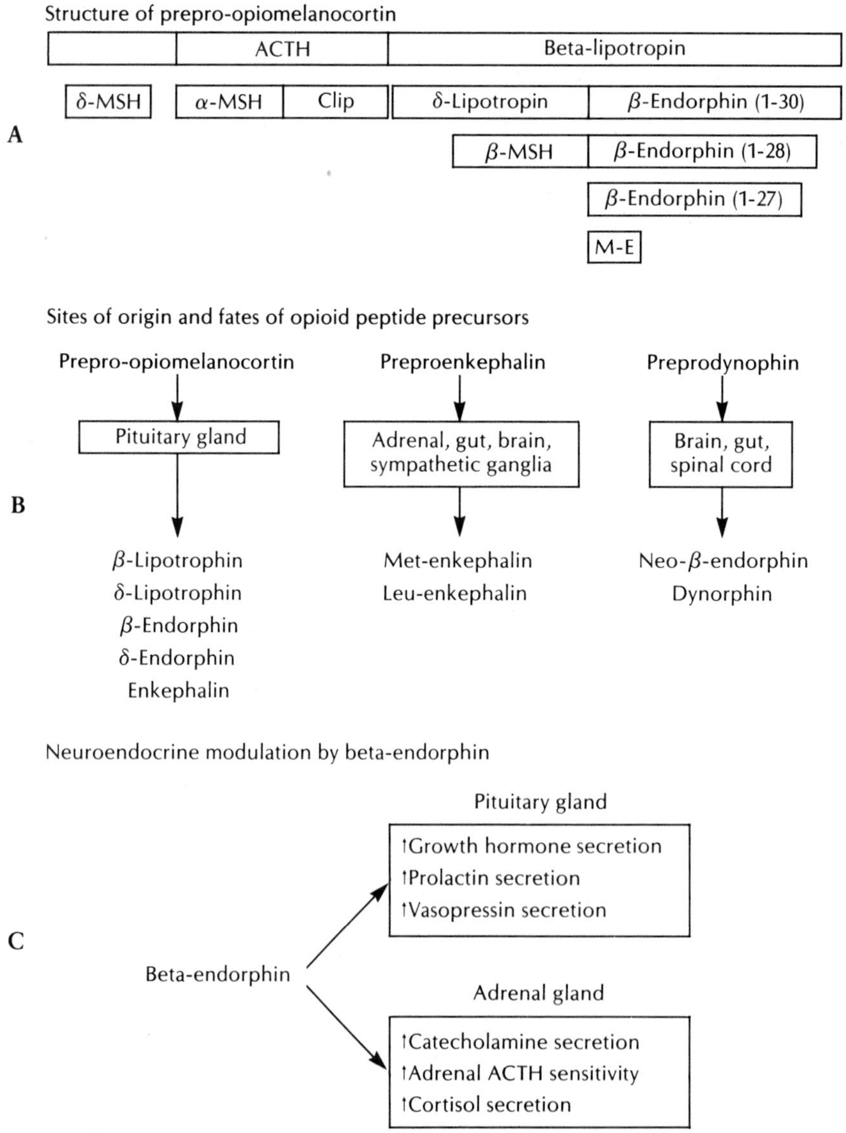

FIGURE 8-19 Endogenous opiates. **A,** Structure of prepro-opiomelanocortin and its relationship to ACTH and endorphins. **B,** Sites of origin and fates of opioid peptide precursors. **C,** Neuroendocrine modulation in the pituitary and adrenal glands by beta-endorphin.

role of cytokines in the pathogenesis of multiple organ dysfunction syndrome[166] is reflected by recent use of the term *systemic inflammatory response syndrome*[83] in describing treatments directed toward modulating pituitary-mediator interactions.[175]

Injury stimulates secretion of CRF, ACTH, and cortisol. Cortisol typically remains elevated for up to 4 weeks after thermal injury, for less than 1 week after soft tissue trauma, and for days after hemorrhage. The increase is accompanied by loss of circadian rhythm. In pure hypovolemia, plasma cortisol normalizes when blood volume is restored. Infection prolongs the cortisol response to injury. Persistent elevation of serum cortisol is associated with a reduced chance of survival.

Growth Hormone

Growth hormone (GH) is synthesized and released by acidophilic cells of the anterior pituitary gland. GH release is stimulated primarily by hypothalamic growth hormone–releasing hormone (GHRH) and is inhibited by somatostatin and cortisol. GH release is also stimulated by ACTH, AVP, T_4, alpha-MSH, testosterone, estrogens, alpha-adrenergic stimulation, and increasing amino acid concentrations. It is also inhibited by beta-adrenergic stimulation, hyperglycemia, and increasing plasma fatty acid concentrations. Besides the direct effects of GH, secondary release of insulin-like growth factors (IGF-1), also mediates the effects of GH. These peptides, formerly called somatomedins, are released primarily in the liver and have important metabolic effects on hepatic and skeletal muscle cells.[312]

GH increases amino acid uptake and protein synthesis in hepatocyte and skeletal muscle cells and inhibits hepatocyte ureagenesis[662] and glucose transport, partly by inhibiting the action of insulin and reducing the activity of glucokinase.[243] In adipose tissue, growth hormone stimulates lipolysis and potentiates the actions of catecholamines; in the liver, it promotes ketogenesis. IGF-1 mediates much, but not all, of the hepatic suppression of proteolysis, increased amino acid uptake, and cellular proliferation in liver and skeletal muscle[247]; also, with other growth factors, it has a profound effect on wound healing.[437] Interestingly, recent work suggests that growth factors, such as GH, and peptide mediators, such as IL-6, have a structural similarity in cell receptors, together constituting a hematopoietic receptor superfamily.[45]

Secretion of GH increases after hemorrhage, injury, and anesthesia.[481,687] Paradoxically, IGF-1 levels decrease after injury, correlating with injury-induced reduction in insulin secretion and observed negative nitrogen balance.[306] GH infusion raises IGF-1 levels and can cause up-regulation of IGF-1 receptors. Recent clinical studies using recombinant GH and IGF-1 infusions indicated that complex interactions occurred among hepatocyte membrane transport mechanisms,[504] skeletal-muscle protein catabolism, and levels of GH, IGF-1, and insulin in patients who underwent surgery and had sepsis[651] or cancer.[678]

Thyrotropin-Releasing Hormone; Thyroid-Stimulating Hormone; Triiodothyronine; Thyroxine

Hypothalamic thyrotropin-releasing hormone (TRH) stimulates the release of thyroid-stimulating hormone (TSH), which is released by basophilic cells in the anterior pituitary gland. TSH stimulates the release of thyroxine (T_4) from the thyroid. T_4 is converted to the most biologically potent form, triiodothyronine (T_3), in peripheral tissues. Hypothalamic release of TRH and pituitary release of TSH are inhibited by T_3 and T_4.[393,578] Pituitary release of TSH is stimulated by estrogens and inhibited by T_3, cortisol, GH, and somatostatin, and by fasting.[162,502,649]

T_3 and T_4 have acute cellular effects that may be mediated by extranuclear receptors,[587] but genomic signal transduction mechanisms predominate (i.e., T_3 binds to nonhistone proteins of the nuclear chromatin, activating gene expression).[162] Thyroid hormones increase oxygen consumption, heat production,[189] and SNS activity.[617] Excessive thyroid hormone, such as occurs in thyroxicosis, stimulates glycolysis, gluconeogenesis, glycogenolysis, proteolysis, lipolysis, and ketogenesis.[162]

Even though the plasma concentrations of free and total T_3 often are lower after injury or surgery, TSH secretion does not increase, because T_4 is quickly converted to T_3 in the thyrotropic cells of the anterior pituitary gland,[338] and T_4 and T_3 become equipotent inhibitors of TSH secretion after injury.[127] The reduced serum concentration of TSH seen in burn patients paradoxically is associated with low serum concentrations of both free T_4 and free T_3.[594] This situation is similar to euthyroid sick syndrome, seen in critically ill, nonsurgical patients, and may be the result either of impaired hypothalamic or pituitary secretion or of changes in peripheral hormone binding.

With injury, burns, and major surgery, peripheral conversion of T_4 to T_3 is impaired, resulting in reduced circulating concentrations of both free and total T_3.[29,544] This is partly the result of cortisol-mediated blockage of the conversion of T_4 to T_3[544] and of increased conversion of T_4 to the biologically inactive molecule, reverse T_3 (rT_3).[119] An increase in rT_3 is also characteristic of injury. Plasma total T_4 may be reduced after injury, but free T_4 concentrations usually are normal. In fact, depressed concentrations of free T_4 are associated with a poor outcome in injured, burned, and critically ill patients.

Gonadotropins: Follicle-Stimulating Hormone and Luteinizing Hormone

Follicle-stimulating hormone (FSH) and luteinizing hormone (LH) are glycoproteins composed of similar alpha-chains and dissimilar beta-chains that are synthesized and secreted by basophilic cells of the adenohypophysis. Release of these hormones is governed by the stimulatory influence of luteinizing hormone–releasing hormone (LHRH) and estrogens, and the inhibitory influence of estrogens, progestins, prolactin, and androgens.[234] Secretion of FSH and LH is suppressed after surgery, emotional stress, and burns.* Decreased serum testosterone also has been reported after injury.[21,114] Changes in the secretion of gonadotropin may account for the menstrual dysfunction that is common after injury. Administering testosterone or conjugated estrogens shortly before inducing shock has been shown to improve survival,[486] but the significance of this finding is not fully understood. There is evidence of interaction between the gonadal and immunologic systems, including cytokine-induced release of gonadotropin-releasing hormone (GnRH) and gonadotropin-mediated changes in immune competence.[284,512]

Prolactin

Prolactin is synthesized and secreted by acidophilic cells of the anterior pituitary gland in response to various emotional and physical stressors. The release of prolactin, like that of GH, is controlled by stimulatory and inhibitory influences. Secretion is stimulated by CRF, TRH, GHRH, and vasoactive intestinal peptide and inhibited by GnRH and gonadotropin-associated peptide. A specific prolactin-stimulating hormone appears to operate through a serotonergic mechanism. Inhibition is mediated by a dopaminergic pathway.[270] With injury, the serum concentration of prolactin increases,[127] correlating to the extent of injury.[485] This increase seems to stem from direct stimulation rather than suppression of tonic inhibition.

Although prolactin appears to act primarily on the breast to induce lactation and mammary development, prolactin receptors also have been identified in the kidneys and liver.[244] The presence of these receptors may explain the changes prolactin causes in the metabolism of fluids, electrolytes, carbohydrates, and nitrogen. Prolactin stimulates the retention of salt, water, and potassium.[244,328] Administering prolactin or inducing hyperprolactinemia produces metabolic effects similar to those caused by GH (i.e., increased nitrogen retention and lipid mobilization and carbohydrate intolerance).[244] Recently, prolactin has been reported to have a stimulatory effect on lymphocyte function.[121]

Opioid Peptides

Endogenous opioids are secreted by many cells, including those in the central nervous system, hypothalamus, intermediate lobe of the pituitary gland, spinal cord, sympathetic autonomic neurons, intestinal wall, and adrenal medulla.[551] These opioids derive from three precursor molecules: prepro-opiomelanocortin, preproenkephalin A, and preprodynorphin (see Figure 8-19).[326,635] Prepro-opiomelanocortin is found primarily in the anterior pituitary gland and also is present in other cell types.[163] Prepro-opiomelanocortin contains the amino acid sequences for ACTH and gamma–melanocyte-stimulating hormone (gamma-MSH), as well for the opioids, beta-lipotropin, and beta- and gamma-endorphin (see Figure 8-19).[635] Consequently, ACTH and beta-endorphin are cosecreted by the pituitary gland in response to a variety of stressors.[285,410] Elevated plasma concentrations of beta-endorphin have been documented after surgery, sepsis, trauma, and hemorrhagic and septic shock.[149,184,404,563]

Preproenkephalin A is found in the adrenal gland, brain, gut, and sympathetic ganglia[635] (see Figure 8-19, *B*). It is a polyenkephalin from which the pentapeptides methionine enkephalin (met-enkephalin) and leucine enkephalin (leu-enkephalin) derive in a 4:1 ratio.[124,484] The concentrations of both these hormones have been noted to increase after acute hypotension or hemorrhage.[213,391] Preprodynorphin is found primarily in the brain, spinal cord, and gut.[635] Cleavage of preprodynorphin yields neo-beta-endorphin and dynorphin. The physiologic significance of these compounds has not yet been determined.

Receptor subtypes mu, delta, and kappa have been identified for opioids.[515] Morphine and fentanyl bind primarily to mu-receptors; met-enkephalin and leu-enkephalin bind to delta-receptors; and dynorphin binds to kappa-receptors. Receptor binding for opiates sometimes overlaps, as with beta-endorphin, which acts at both mu- and delta-receptors.[515]

Endogenous opiates affect sensory perception, cardiovascular function, intermediary metabolism, neuroendocrine modulation, and immunologic function.[149,410,524] Analgesic activity is found at both mu- and delta-receptors but not at kappa-receptors.[515]

Interest in opioid peptides stems from the finding that blocking mu-receptors with naloxone improves hemodynamics and survival following hemorrhagic,[57] septic,[300] and spinal shock.[156,324,325] Endorphins, enkephalins, and morphine (via mu- and delta-receptors) have significant cardiovascular activity: beta-endorphin causes hypotension mediated through serotonergic pathways[399]; enkephalins cause hypertension and tachycardia that appear to be mediated through sympathetic reflexes[580]; and morphine causes hypotension but is not as potent as beta-endorphin.[187]

Like morphine, centrally administered beta-endorphin causes hyperglycemia.[643] Beta-endorphin stimulates pancreatic release of insulin and glucagon[215,339] and appears to modulate glucose kinetics by central mechanisms.[243] Nonspecific blockade of opioid receptors with naloxone increases glucose uptake in skeletal muscle,[10]

*References 88, 114,127,621, and 684.

decreases gluconeogenesis in the liver, and blunts the hyperglycemic response to injury.[14,49] The fact that physiologic concentrations of beta-endorphin apparently do not affect hepatic neogenesis and glucose uptake by skeletal muscle[13] suggests the presence of complex interactions among central, peripheral, and intermediary metabolic mechanisms.

Endogenous opiates modulate neuroendocrine activity (see Figures 8-18 and 8-19, *C*).[80,410] Beta-endorphin potentiates the release of GH, AVP, and prolactin and inhibits the release of ACTH.[524] Blocking receptors with naloxone suppresses hypoglycemia-induced increases in GH and prolactin and potentiates the release of ACTH. Endogenous opioids increase the release of adrenal catecholamines and the secretion of adrenocortical cortisol.[420,643] Administering morphine or its analogs stimulates release of GH[459] and AVP[283] and inhibits release of gonadotropins and TSH.[551]

The immunologic effects of opioids are not yet fully understood. In vivo suppression of lymphocyte cytotoxicity may be due to centrally mediated effects, because the effects of opioids on peripheral leukocytes enhance many immunologic functions.[625] Opioid peptides are believed to influence the suppression of cytotoxicity that can accompany trauma[591] and septic shock.[300] Elevated plasma levels of circulating opioids may influence leukocyte function after trauma[404] and thermal injury.[165] On the cellular level, the intriguing possibility has been postulated that a vitronectin-endorphin–complex feedback loop induces the release of cytokines.[625] Beta-endorphin binds through nonopioid sites to vitronectin (S protein) in a highly specific manner after vitronectin, a coagulation and complement system protein secreted by monocytes, is activated by glycosaminoglycans or terminal complement factor complexes.[316,317] Because the N-terminus of endorphin exerts chemotactic effects,[641] and because vitronectin enhances monocyte phagocytosis,[511] this complex may activate leukocytes to secrete cytokines, which in turn might stimulate additional release of pituitary or leukocyte beta-endorphins.[625] The complex actions of these ubquitous peptides are clinically relevant to the effect of immunologic depression and penetrating injury in addicted individuals using exogenously administered opioids.

Arginine Vasopressin

Certain hormones, such as arginine vasopressin (AVP) and oxytocin, are synthesized by hypothalamic cells before being stored in cells of the posterior pituitary gland or neurohypophysis. AVP (formerly called antidiuretic hormone, or ADH) is synthesized by cells of the supraoptic and paraventricular nuclei before being transported to the posterior pituitary gland (see Figure 8-6).[548,551]

The primary stimulus to secretion of AVP is an increase in plasma osmolality.[373,380,551] Changes in plasma osmolality are sensed by sodium-sensitive osmoreceptors in the hypothalamus near the third ventricles and by extracerebral osmoreceptors in the liver or portal circulation.[288,373,577] Hyperglycemia stimulates secretion of AVP but does so through a nonosmotic pathway.[44]

Changes in effective circulating volume also stimulate AVP release through baroreceptor, atrial stretch receptor, and chemoreceptor reflexes.[15,380] A reduction in the effective circulating volume of as little as 10% (equivalent to a change from the supine to the upright position) can produce twofold to threefold increases in AVP.[15]

AVP also interacts with many hormones.[606,611] AVP's control over pituitary secretion of ACTH currently is receiving considerable attention.[19] Angiotensin II potentiates the release of AVP through central action (see Figure 8-18).[465,606] Cortisol, catecholamines, opioid peptides, insulin, and histamine affect AVP secretion through changes in blood volume, plasma osmolality, and blood glucose concentration.[323,551] Numerous other factors enhance release of AVP, including beta-adrenergic agents, prostaglandin E_2 (PGE_2), hypoxia, hypercapnia, histamine, morphine, anesthetic agents, pain, emotional arousal, and exercise.[362,380,548]

The actions of AVP affect osmoregulation, vasoregulation, and glucose metabolism. AVP's solute-free water resorption action on renal distal tubules and collecting ducts is mediated by signal transduction via cell-surface receptors through G-protein activation of adenylate cyclase[613] and protein kinase, which causes microtubule-dependent insertion of membrane patches containing water channels or ion-specific transport channels into apical cell membranes.[90,638] AVP causes peripheral vasoconstriction, especially in the splanchnic bed.[148] Physiologic concentrations of AVP stimulate hepatic glycogenolysis through a calcium-dependent, cAMP-independent mechanism[374]; enhance hepatic gluconeogenesis[382]; and inhibit hepatic ketogenesis.[670]

Secretion of AVP increases after major surgery, trauma, hemorrhage, sepsis, and burns.[137,142,589] Early release of AVP is mediated by reflexes related to changes in blood volume. In the absence of changes in osmolality or blood volume, prolonged elevation of AVP (5 to 7 days) after major surgery is believed to stem from emotional arousal, narcotics, and incisional pain. The increased secretion of AVP seen after thermal injury is related to significant reduction in blood volume in these patients.[133] The increased secretion of AVP seen with hemorrhage is important in blood pressure control and has been implicated in the pathophysiology of splanchnic vasoconstriction, which predisposes the patient to intestinal ischemia and bacterial translocation in the gut. The metabolic actions of AVP contribute to the hyperglycemia that follows injury; on a molar basis, AVP is more active than glucagon in this regard.[309,382] The osmotic effects of hyperglycemia help restore effective circulating blood volume through Starling forces.

Hormones Controlled by the Autonomic Nervous System

Catecholamines

The division between the nervous system and the endocrine system is arbitrary, because many hormones and neurotransmitters (e.g., catecholamines) have interchangeable and overlapping functions.[153,389] Epinephrine, which is produced almost exclusively by the adrenal medulla, functions primarily as a hormone. Norepinephrine and dopamine, which are released primarily at nerve terminals, function as neurotransmitters and make their way into the plasma by spillover from the synaptic cleft.[204,410]

The adrenal medulla may be viewed as a collection of postganglionic sympathetic neurons without axons that release their neurotransmitters into the general circulation.[153] These neurotransmitters (primarily epinephrine) are stored in chromaffin granules, where they are tightly bound to adenosine triphosphate (ATP). When adrenal chromaffin cells are stimulated, the chromaffin granules are released into the extracellular fluid through the fusion with the plasma membrane.[154] As a result, the adrenal medulla releases catecholamines in a quantum fashion as granule packets are released. The signal for fusion and rupture of the chromaffin granules appears to be mediated through an increase in the concentration of intracellular calcium.[154] Besides catecholamines, chromaffin granules release dopamine, beta-hydroxylase, ascorbic acid, met-enkephalin, leu-enkephalin, ATP, and chromogranins.[669]

Although numerous stimuli cause secretion of catecholamines (e.g., hypoxia, hypovolemia, hypoglycemia, pain, and fever), the exact mechanisms of adrenomedullary control of catecholamine secretion are still poorly understood.[261] As noted previously, small, nonhypotensive hemorrhages, which are potent stimuli for activation of the sympathetic nervous system, do not increase adrenomedullary secretion of catecholamines.[696] The latter occurs only when some degree of hypotension develops.[201] Increased chemoreceptor drive and decreased high-pressure baroreceptor drive may have minimal effects on adrenomedullary secretion of catecholamines when the reflexes alone are examined.[1,214] Conversely, SNS-mediated adrenomedullary secretion of catecholamines can occur in the absence of increased cardiac or renal SNS activity.[256] The activation of the sympathetic nervous system can be graded and may be distinct from adrenomedullary activation.

The hormonal actions of epinephrine and norepinephrine may be broadly classified as metabolic, hemodynamic, or modulatory. In the liver, epinephrine stimulates glycogenolysis (alpha$_1$-mediated stimulation of glycogen phosphorylase *a* and inhibition of glycogen synthesis)[209]; gluconeogenesis (inhibition of phosphofructokinase and hexokinase by the products of lipolysis and glycogenolysis)[480,693]; lipolysis (beta$_1$ activation of triacylglycerol lipase); and ketogenesis (beta$_1$—see the section on glucagon).[480] Among these hepatic actions, epinephrine appears to be most potent in stimulating glycogenolysis.[218]

In adipose tissue, epinephrine increases lipolysis (beta$_1$ activation of triacylglycerol lipase).[210] In skeletal muscle, it increases glycogenolysis (alpha$_1$-mediated stimulation of glycogen phosphorylase *a* and inhibition of glycogen synthetase) and inhibits insulin-stimulated glucose uptake (beta$_2$ and alpha$_1$).[123] As a result of these actions, epinephrine appears to mediate insulin resistance (stress-induced hyperglycemia) by increasing hepatic production of glucose and decreasing peripheral glucose uptake.

The hormonal effects of catecholamines include a beta-receptor–mediated increase in renin[348]; release of parathyroid hormone (PTH)[386]; alpha-receptor–mediated inhibition of insulin and glucagon secretion[532]; and beta-receptor–mediated stimulation of insulin and glucagon.[636] These hormonal effects depend on the receptor density or sensitivity of the effector cells. For example, pancreatic alpha- and beta-islet cells, which secrete glucagon and insulin, respectively, contain both alpha- and beta-adrenergic receptors. Because the density of the alpha-adrenergic receptors of the beta-islet cells is greater than that of the alpha-islet cells, catecholamine and SNS stimulation of the pancreas increases the secretion of glucagon and decreases the secretion of insulin.

The hemodynamic effects of catecholamines, which are dose dependent, include alpha$_1$-mediated venous and arterial vasoconstriction; beta$_2$-mediated arterial vasodilatation; and beta$_1$-mediated increases in the myocardial rate, contractility, and conductivity.[154] In low doses, epinephrine acts primarily at beta$_1$- and beta$_2$-receptors, whereas at high doses it acts primarily at alpha$_1$-receptors. In normal physiologic circumstances, norepinephrine is most important in the beta$_1$ and alpha$_2$ actions of catecholamines, whereas epinephrine is responsible for beta$_2$ effects.[210]

The hemodynamic effects of dopamine are mediated through both dopaminergic and adrenergic receptors. In low circulating concentrations or low doses, dopamine causes renal vasodilatation through dopaminergic receptor action. At higher concentrations, dopamine acts at beta-receptors and eventually at alpha-receptors.[279]

Renin and Angiotensin

Renin exists in an inactive form, prorenin, in the myoepithelial cells of the renal afferent arterioles.[337] Proteolytic cleavage of the zymogen and release of renin are controlled by three intrarenal receptors and influenced by several hormones and ions.[236] The macula densa receptor senses the concentration of chloride in tubular fluid as it passes through the distal nephron. When the chloride concentration of the tubular fluid decreases, release of renin increases. The neurogenic receptor of the juxtaglomerular apparatus is the second renal receptor involved in the release of renin. This receptor responds to beta-adrenergic stimulation by increasing the release of renin. The third renal receptor is the juxtaglomerular cell itself, which acts as a stretch receptor. Increases in stretch and therefore in blood pressure reduce the secretion of renin, whereas decreases in stretch increase the secretion of renin. Hormones and ions that alter the secretion of renin include ACTH, vasopressin, prostaglandins, glucagon, potassium, magnesium, and calcium.[33]

When renin is released into the circulation, it converts renin substrate into angiotensin I. Secretion of renin substrate, which is produced by the liver, is increased by ACTH, corticosteroids, and angiotensin II.[517] Angiotensin I acts primarily as the precursor for formation of angiotensin II, a process that is mediated in the pulmonary circulation by angiotensin-converting enzyme, a carboxypeptidase. It also potentiates the release of catecholamines by the adrenal medulla and is a selective renal vasoconstrictor, which redistributes blood flow to the renal cortex by decreasing blood flow to the medullary areas of the kidney[32] (Figure 8-20).

The actions of angiotensin II can be broadly classified according to the effect on hemodynamics, fluid-electrolyte balance, hormone regulation, metabolism, and paracrine effects. Angiotensin II is a potent vasoconstrictor[31] that is vital to maintaining normal blood pressure and also plays a major role in the pathogenesis of hypertension. Additional hemodynamic effects are tachycardia and increased contractility and vascular permeability.[517] The profound effects of angiotensin II on fluid and electrolyte homeostasis are mediated by potent stimulation of the synthesis and secretion of aldosterone, increased secretion of vasopressin,[517] and regulation of thirst.[604] Angiotensin II increases the release of CRH and, by increasing the release of ACTH,[303] potentiates the effects of ACTH on the adrenal cortex.[554] Angiotensin II also potentiates the release of epinephrine by the adrenal medulla[303] and increases sympathetic neurotransmission.[517] The metabolic actions of angiotensin II include stimulating glycogenolysis and gluconeogenesis in the liver through a cAMP-independent, calcium-dependent mechanism.[382] In addition, recent studies have demonstrated that the renin–angiotensin II system has a blood flow–dependent effect on insulin action and whole-body glucose utilization.[95] The fact that insulin and IGF-1 are secretagogues for angiotensin II provides evidence that the renin system has other metabolic effects as well.[20] Evidence that the renin system is involved in immunologic interactions arises from the fact that both TNF and IL-1 act as secretagogues for renin release. Interestingly, recent research has shown that another

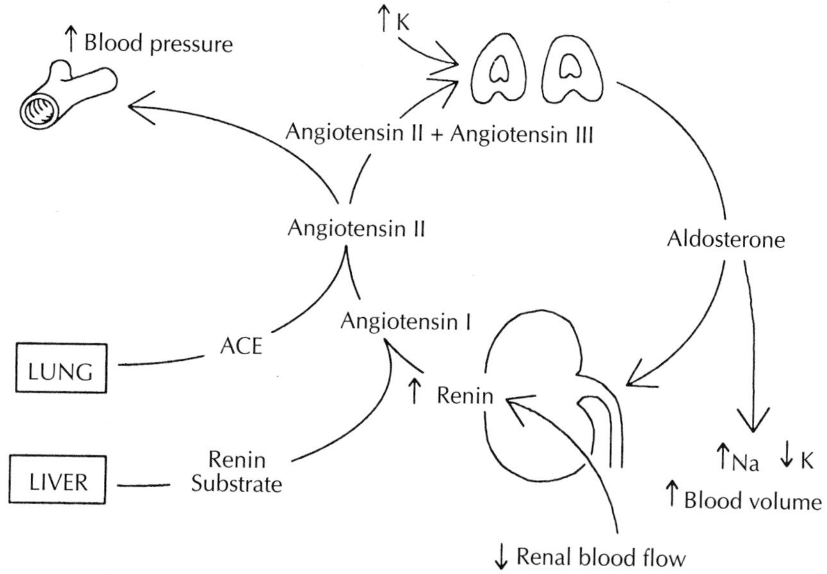

FIGURE 8-20 Normal renin-angiotensin-aldosterone regulatory system. Renin, secreted by the kidneys, cleaves angiotensin I from renin substrate (angiotensinogen), an alpha$_2$-globulin produced by the liver. Angiotension I is converted into biologically active angiotensin II by angiotensin-converting enzyme (ACE), primarily in the lungs. Angiotensin II increases peripheral vascular resistance and, with angiotensin III, stimulates secretion of aldosterone, which causes sodium retention, potassium loss, and increased plasma volume. (From Wilson JD, Foster DW, editors: *Williams textbook of endocrinology,* ed 8, Philadelphia, 1992, WB Saunders.)

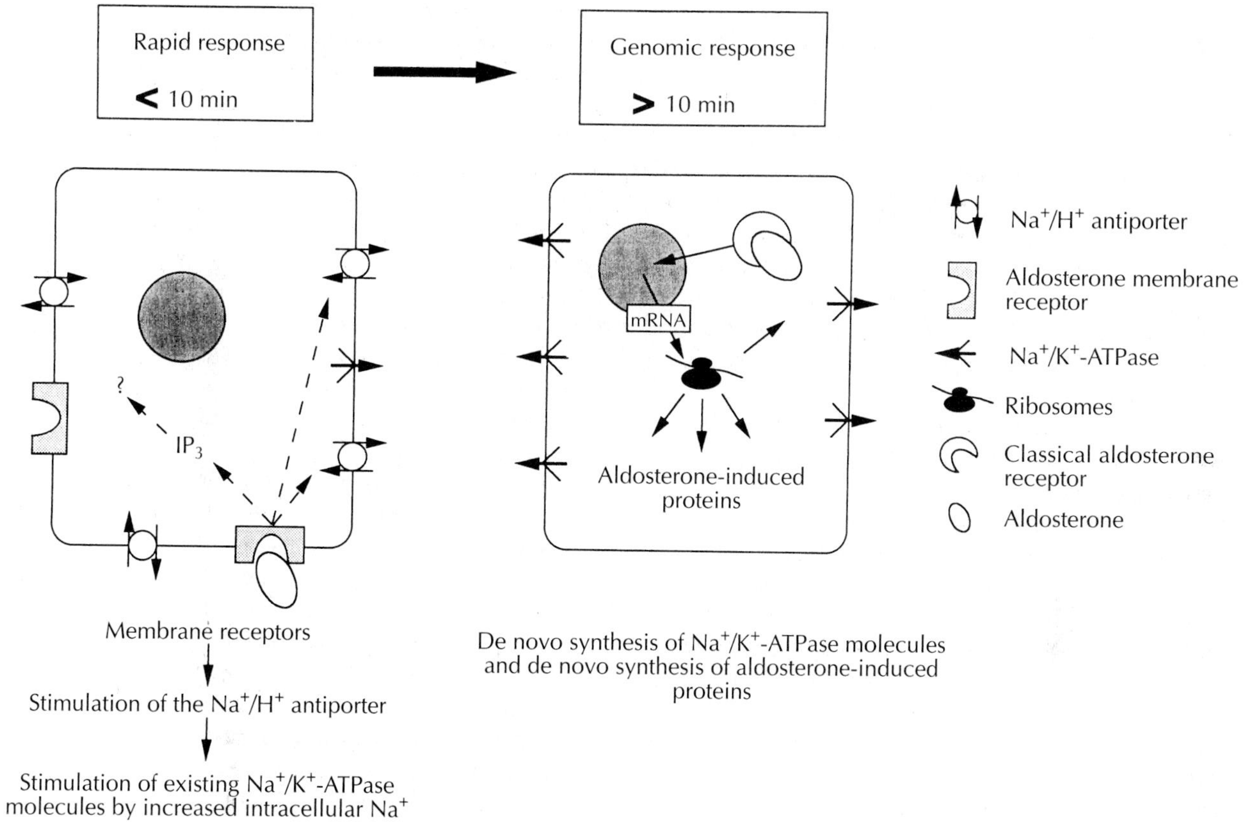

FIGURE 8-21 Initial steps of mineralocorticoid action (activation of Na^+/H^+ exchanger) and subsequent effects on Na^+/K^+ fluxes and Na^+/K^+-ATPase. *IP_3*, Inositol triphosphate. (From Wehling M, Eisen C, Christ M: *News Physio Sci* 8:241, 1993.)

Somatostatin is a potent inhibitor of insulin secretion through direct action on the beta-islet cells.[550] In contrast, beta-endorphin,[215] glucagon,[637] gastrointestinal hormones (see the section on Glucagon), cortisol,[193] estrogen, progesterone, and parathyroid hormone all produce hyperinsulinism.[193,215,217,531] Whereas glucagon, beta-endorphin, and the gastrointestinal hormones increase insulin secretion through direct action on pancreatic beta-cells, the latter hormones appear to increase the secretion of insulin by interfering with the peripheral action of insulin.[217] In addition, cortisol appears to play an important role in the development of insulin resistance, but the physiologic significance of estrogen and progesterone in this regard is unknown. Recent work also suggests that the release of insulin may be mediated by nitric oxide and may account for the secretagogue properties of arginine.

By promoting the storage of carbohydrate, protein, and lipid, insulin serves as the body's primary anabolic hormone. Insulin acts primarily on the liver, skeletal muscle, and adipose tissue, but it affects most tissues, with the notable exceptions of hematopoietic, CNS, and wounded tissues. Insulin promotes the entry of glucose into cells by stimulating membrane transport of glucose. The increased intracellular concentrations of glucose are used in glycogenesis (stimulation of glycogen synthetase and inhibition of glycogen phosphorylase)[480] and in glycolysis (stimulation of glucokinase, phosphofructokinase, and pyruvate kinase).[480] By stimulating both these processes concurrently, the energy needed for glycogen synthesis is made available by glycolysis. Insulin also inhibits gluconeogenesis in the liver by inhibiting phosphoenolpyruvate carboxylase and by stimulating phosphofructokinase and pyruvate kinase.[206,382]

The major action of insulin in protein metabolism is promoting protein synthesis. This synthesis is accomplished by increasing the transport of amino acids into the liver and other peripheral tissues and by inhibiting gluconeogenesis and amino acid oxidation.[217] Insulin's action on lipid metabolism is directed toward stimulating lipid synthesis and inhibiting lipid degradation. By stimulating lipoprotein lipase, insulin makes triglycerides more available for uptake from the plasma by adipose tissue and the liver. Glycerol synthesis from glucose and the pentose phosphate shunt also are stimulated by insulin, thereby providing the elements needed for synthesis of lipids.

Glucagon

Synthesis and secretion of glucagon by the alpha-islet cells of the pancreas are controlled by three major mechanisms: the concentrations of circulating substrates (glucose, amino acids, and fatty acids); the efferent activity of the autonomic and central nervous systems; and the action of circulating and local hormones. Under normal conditions, the primary stimuli are the plasma concentrations of glucose and amino acids and exercise.[382] Glucose alters glucagon secretion in an inverse manner; hyperglycemia inhibits secretion of glucagon, and hypoglycemia stimulates it. These phenomena appear to result primarily from direct action of glucose on the alpha-cell, either through a glucoreceptor on the cell's surface or through intracellular metabolism of glucose.[637]

The potency of different amino acids in stimulating the secretion of glucagon varies and is not related to their ability to stimulate the secretion of insulin. In general, the gluconeogenic amino acids have a greater stimulatory effect than the nongluconeogenic amino acids.[531] As noted previously, it is not completely known how amino acids stimulate the synthesis and secretion of glucagon, but some evidence supports mediation by cell-surface receptors and by intracellular metabolism.

The ability of amino acids to stimulate secretion of glucagon is critical for maintaining euglycemia when a protein meal is ingested. If amino acids were unable to stimulate glucagon secretion, their unopposed stimulation of insulin secretion after a protein meal would result in hypoglycemia through decreased production of hepatic glucose, increased protein synthesis, and increased glucose uptake in skeletal muscle. However, in the presence of glucagon, the liver increases its production of glucose, thereby allowing the action of insulin to be opposed and glucose homeostasis to be maintained.[219]

The potency of glucose and amino acids in changing the secretion of glucagon and insulin depends on the route of administration. Ingesting a protein meal produces a greater increase in glucagon and insulin secretion than intravenous administration of similar concentrations of amino acids.[438] Ingesting glucose produces greater changes in insulin and glucagon secretion than intravenous administration of a similar glucose load.[547] These phenomena may be mediated through presentation of a greater concentration of substrate to the pancreas when the substrates enter through the GI tract; through potentiation by gastrointestinal hormones of substrate-induced pancreatic secretion; or through the effects of neural inputs to the pancreas activated by eating.[531] For example, cholecystokinin, gastrin, vasoactive intestinal peptide, substance P, neurotensin, and gastric inhibitory peptide (GIP) all increase secretion of glucagon and insulin when administered pharmacologically.[531,550,637] Although the physiologic role of these hormones in the modulation of pancreatic hormonal secretion is uncertain, gastrin in physiologic concentrations appears to potentiate amino acid–stimulated release of glucagon and insulin, and GIP appears to potentiate glucose-mediated inhibition of glucagon secretion and stimulation of insulin secretion.[637]

Other hormones that increase the secretion of glucagon are beta-endorphin, insulin, and cortisol.[215,637] Somatostatin is the major hormone that inhibits glucagon secretion.[550]

The ANS mechanisms that control the release of glucagon are opposite to those for insulin; that is, activation of alpha-adrenergic receptors stimulates glucagon secretion, whereas activation of beta-adrenergic receptors or the parasympathetic efferents to the pancreas inhibits glucagon release.[531] However, unlike the beta-islet cell, the alpha-islet cell has a much greater density of alpha-adrenergic receptors than of beta-adrenergic receptors. As a result, increased circulating concentrations of epinephrine or norepinephrine or SNS stimulation of the pancreas increase rather than decrease the secretion of glucagon.

The physiologic actions of glucagon are limited primarily to the liver and are mediated through an increase in cAMP.[382,480] These physiologic actions include activation of glycogen phosphorylase *a* and inhibition of glycogen synthetase; this promotes glycogenolysis and activation of phosphoenolpyruvate carboxykinase, as well as amino acid transanimation, thereby promoting gluconeogenesis.[382,480] Although it does not increase transport of amino acids into the liver per se, it does direct amino acids toward gluconeogenesis.[122] The net result is an increase in hepatic production of glucose that, under basal conditions, accounts for 75% of the glucose produced by the liver.[637] Although in the absence of cortisol the peak action of glucagon is very brief, in the presence of cortisol the action of glucagon lasts longer and the initial increase in hepatic glucose is greater.[191] Nevertheless, the effects of glucagon do not last long.[233] After 30 to 60 minutes, the activity assigned to glucagon decreases even if the plasma glucagon concentration remains elevated. However, if the concentration of glucagon increases further, the activity of glucagon does increase. Therefore it appears that an increase in the concentration of glucagon, rather than the absolute amount of glucagon present, determines the hormone's activity.[233] This burst effect also appears to be true of other cAMP-mediated hormones.

Glucagon stimulates lipolysis in the liver and in adipose tisue.[233] It also inhibits acetyl-CoA carboxylase, the enzyme that converts acetyl-coenzyme A (acetyl-CoA) to malonyl-CoA.[531] In turn, the reduction in malonyl-CoA produces inhibition of triglyceride synthesis and activation of carnitine acyltransferase. The latter effect increases the transfer of fatty acids into the mitochondria, thereby increasing acetyl-CoA oxidation and ketogenesis. As a result, glucagon is very important during starvation and injury because of its ability to increase hepatic production of glucose and ketogenesis.

Somatostatin

Somatostatin, a tetradecapeptide, is a potent inhibitor of the secretion of both insulin and glucagon.[550,636] Somatostatin is found in pancreatic D cells and in the hypothalamus, limbic system, brainstem, spinal cord, other neural tissue, salivary glands, and parafollicular thyroid cells, as well as in kidney and gastrointestinal tissue.[550] Although somatostatin originally was named for its ability to inhibit secretion of growth hormone, it now is known to inhibit secretion of TSH, renin, calcitonin, gastrin, secretin, cholecystokinin, insulin, and glucagon.[550] In addition, somatostatinergic nerve fibers are involved in the projection of impulses from peripheral sensory organs to the neuroaxis.[550]

The precise role somatostatin plays in the physiologic regulation of insulin and glucagon secretion is not known. The alpha-, beta-, and delta-cells all have somatostatin receptors that, when activated, inhibit secretion of glucagon, insulin, and somatostatin, respectively. Somatostatin's mechanism of action is thought to be mediated primarily by local diffusion of somatostatin from delta-cells to alpha- and beta-cells (the so-called paracrine function).[550,636] However, recent evidence suggests that somatostatin that reaches the pancreas through the bloodstream may be more important in the modulation of pancreatic secretion than that produced locally. The effects of somatostatin on alpha-cells are transient, but the effects on beta-cells are persistent.[636] This difference may account for the relative hyperglycemia that occurs in patients with somatostatinomas or after long-term administration of somatostatin.[636]

Parathyroid Hormone

Parathyroid hormone (PTH), which is synthesized in the parathyroid glands, is not stored in large quantities.[291] As a result, large increases in secretion of PTH must be accompanied by an increase in its synthesis. The major regulator of PTH synthesis and secretion is the serum concentration of ionized calcium[146]; secretion of PTH varies inversely with the ionized calcium concentration.[290] Within the normal range of serum calcium, small changes in the serum calcium concentration produce small, inverse changes in the secretion of PTH. In contrast, outside the normal range of calcium, small changes in the serum calcium concentration are accompanied by large, inverse changes in the secretion of PTH. Although the exact mechanism by which changes in the serum calcium concentration affect secretion of PTH is not known, the process is at least partly mediated through changes in the intracellular concentration of cAMP. The process is also influenced by the serum magnesium concentration.[290] Both hypomagnesemia and hypermagnesemia are associated with an impairment of PTH secretion. However, within the normal range, the magnesium concentration does not affect secretion of PTH in response to calcium. In contrast, changes in the concentration of inorganic phosphorus do not directly affect the response of the parathyroid glands to changes in the serum calcium concentration.[290]

Although there is no direct evidence that the innervation of the parathyroid glands is important in their secretory response, beta-adrenergic receptors have been identified on parathyroid cells, and epinephrine and isoproterenol have been shown to increase the release of PTH.[222,386] Unlike with glucagon and calcitonin, which appear to stimulate PTH secretion through a decrease in extracellular calcium, increases in PTH secretion brought about by epinephrine appear to occur independently of changes in the extracellular calcium and may be mediated through an increase in the intracellular concentration of cAMP.[290,386] The physiologic importance of catecholamine-mediated secretion of PTH is not known.

The primary target organs for PTH are the kidneys and bone.[290,558] In the kidneys, PTH mediates three processes. First, it increases the distal tubular (but not the proximal tubular) resorption of calcium. Because only 10% of the normally filtered load of calcium reaches the distal tubule, regulation of distal tubular resorption of calcium serves to fine-tune calcium balance. The cellular mechanism for the increase in calcium resorption is unknown. Second, PTH decreases the proximal resorption of phosphorus through a cAMP-dependent mechanism, thereby producing phosphaturia. Third, PTH stimulates the conversion of 1-hydroxyvitamin D to 1,25-dihydroxyvitamin D (calcitriol) in the kidney, which in turn stimulates intestinal absorption of calcium and phosphorus. In bone, PTH stimulates calcium mobilization, bone resorption, and bone remodeling through a series of complex actions.

MEDIATOR RESPONSE

The sophisticated cellular and molecular techniques that have emerged over the past decade have led to identification and preliminary understanding of the substances, known as factors, released by activated cells. On a very basic level, these factors act as messengers in cellular communication (cytokines), at times spilling over into the circulation to function as hormones in response to hemorrhage, sepsis, inflammation, and other types of injury. Among these mediators are the cytokines, eicosanoids, and endothelial cell factors.

Mediator substances act locally as paracrine substances (e.g., lymphokines acting on lymphocytes) and may also act on distant cells or organs, causing them to function as hormones. Some factors stored within cells are released from preformed intracellular packets through the process of exocytosis; others exert their effects during the complex process of phagocytosis. Mediators may be released as a consequence of cell death and may exert their effects by diffusion. Other mediators are not carried within cells, but rather circulate as inactive forms in plasma. They exert their actions instantly when triggered by local activation processes (e.g., the complement, coagulation, kinin and angiotensin systems), contributing to the development of pathologic conditions such as adult respiratory distress syndrome (ARDS), acute renal failure, and multiple organ dysfunction syndrome.

IL-1 acts as an immunologic adjuvant, because it causes T-cell proliferation by enhancing production of IL-2[609] and expression of IL-2 receptors, and by stimulating production of IL-6 and IL-8. IL-1 also[407] induces fever by stimulating local release of prostaglandins in the anterior hypothalamus[658]; induces anorexia by acting directly on the satiety center[498]; lessens the perception of pain by stimulating the release of beta-endorphins[207]; and up-regulates central opiate-like receptors.[668] In addition, IL-1 increases the basal metabolic rate and oxygen consumption.[173]

IL-1 also causes metabolic responses. It acts with IL-6, TNF, IFN, and cortisol to promote rapid synthesis of hepatic acute-phase proteins.[40,543] Energy and substrate demands for increased hepatic synthesis also may be partly modulated by actions of IL-1. The precise action of IL-1 on skeletal muscle metabolism has not yet been delineated, but it has been clearly established that a breakdown fragment of IL-1 promotes skeletal muscle proteolysis,[138,140,172] an effect that may require PGE_2.[37,278,450] An infusion of IL-1-alpha in humans promotes skeletal muscle proteolysis,[229] but induction of endogenous IL-1 by injection of etiocholanolone does not change protein metabolism.[659] Although the physiology of cytokine infusion may be different from that of locally stimulated cytokine release, it does appear that IL-1, IL-6, TNF, IFN, and cortisol play important roles in modulating protein metabolism to meet the demands of injury, by inducing hepatic acute-phase protein synthesis and promoting breakdown of skeletal muscle to amino acids.

It should be noted that the increase in hepatic protein synthesis caused by IL-1 is not global. For example, the synthesis of albumin decreases during the acute-phase response, and overall hepatic protein synthesis decreases early after injury.[173] The amino acids released after injury appear to be used for hepatic energy as well as protein synthesis, because much of the amino acid released is oxidized.

The metabolic effects of IL-1 also may be partly related to central actions, such as those on the hypothalamic-pituitary axis that cause stimulation of CRH[92,575] and ACTH[417,680] (see Figure 8-18). Blood levels of growth hormone, alpha-MSH, and prolactin are not markedly affected by IL-1, and catecholamines increase only marginally.[52]

IL-1 also may act on pancreatic islet cells to stimulate the secretion of insulin and glucagon.[266] IL-1 and TNF have been described as having cytotoxic effects on insulin-producing beta-cells[174]; however, because central noradrenergic pathways are stimulated by IL-1,[186] it may be that central mechanisms mediate the carbohydrate effects of IL-1. The effect of IL-1 on glucose metabolism, which is a mild hypoglycemic response, is related to a central change in the glucose set point because IL-1 action appears to take place independent of pancreatic endocrine cell function, peripheral insulin sensitivity, and the serum glucose concentration.[63]

Cytokines[91,231,623]

Cytokines compose vast sets of small polypeptides and glycoproteins (less than 30 kDa monomers) with specific, high-affinity cell-surface receptors (K_d 10^{-9}-10^{-12} M). Cytokines are chiefly involved in cell-to-cell communication.

Redundancy crept into the naming of these substances because many independent research groups focused on different biologic actions of what later proved to be identical compounds. The extraordinary number of experimental studies and the vast complexity of cytokine biology prevent an exhaustive understanding of the clinical ramifications of these substances. The limited summary that follows is intended to introduce cytokines and other mediators so that as their roles in the response to injury become more fully defined, the reader may understand their basic biologic properties.

Interleukins

Some interleukins (e.g., IL-2) are lymphokines in that their effects are limited to the immunologic system. Other interleukins (e.g., IL-1, IL-3, IL-6, and IL-8) have more pleotrophic effects and are more properly called cytokines.

INTERLEUKIN-1. Interleukin-1 (IL-1) was first described in 1970 as an activity that augmented human mixed lymphocyte responses, and later as the activities of lymphocyte-activating factor (LAF) and endogenous pyrogen.[30] IL-1 activity is mediated by two peptide molecules,[424] IL-1-alpha and IL-1-beta, which are secreted by activated mononuclear phagocytes and epithelial and endothelial cells. IL-1-beta is produced in tenfold greater amounts and is more biologically active than IL-1-alpha.[30] The two forms of IL-1 have different mechanisms of action and bioactive states and are translated in precursor form. Bioactive precursor IL-1-alpha is degraded rapidly to a smaller form that is principally membrane bound[384]; it induces killer cell cytotoxicity and other T-cell functions through cell contact.[64,495] The precursor form of IL-1-beta is not bioactive. Most of it is degraded to the active, smaller species by tissue proteases when cell death and lysis occur.[429] Non-bound IL-1 species have a circulating half-life of approximately 6 minutes. The precise transduction mechanism or mechanisms have not been fully elucidated. Besides a prostaglandin-related pathway, another mechanism has been described that acts through a calcium-mediated process involving cAMP, whereby IL-1 binds to the membrane receptor is internalized and binds to the genome in the nucleus.[72] Both IL-1 species bind to either of two cell-surface IL-1 receptors that have been described, with varied tissue distribution.[176] A third IL-1 species, called IL-1 receptor antagonist (IL-1ra), has no agonist activity but appears to act as an IL-1–specific inhibitor by blocking the binding of IL-1 to cell-surface receptors.[116,220] IL-1ra is produced by human monocytes.[23,586]

The stimuli for the release of IL-1 have been thought to include nearly all inflammatory, infectious, and immunologic processes. The fact that IL-1-alpha has not been detected in human circulation is consistent with the membrane-binding properties of this compound and its paracrine effects. Circulating IL-1-beta has been found sporadically with sepsis[275,652] and in certain chronic diseases.[430,536] IL-1 forms were not found in the circulation of volunteers after intravenous administration of endotoxin, whereas other cytokines (e.g., tumor necrosis factor,[447] interferon, and IL-6) were readily detected.[230]

INTERLEUKIN-2. Interleukin-2 (IL-2), originally isolated as a T-cell growth factor (TGF), is a true lymphokine. It is produced by $CD4^+$ and $CD8^+$ T cells and acts principally as an immunostimulant. Antigen stimulation of lymphocytes triggers increased transcription of the genes for both IL-2 and IL-2 receptors. Recombinant human IL-2 is a nonglycosylated protein molecule with a serum half-life of 6 to 10 minutes when administered intravenously. Investigations are underway into the use of IL-2 to generate lymphokine-activated killer (LAK) cells for the treatment of malignant disease. The body's production of IL-2 is impaired after trauma[559] and thermal injury.[682] Excessive or persistent T-cell stimulation leads to shedding of IL-2 receptors, which raises the possibility of using these receptors as markers for rejection and sepsis.

INTERLEUKIN-4. Interleukin-4 (IL-4), which is produced by $CD4^+$ T cells, activates IgE production for B cells and T-cell adhesion by endothelial cells. IL-4 modulates the production of several cytokines in cell-specific fashion. For example, IL-4 induces or increases secretion of IL-6 and TNF by B lymphocytes, yet decreases TNF secretion by natural killer (NK) cells and macrophages, and decreases secretion of IL-6 by macrophages and fibroblasts. The proliferation and induction effects of IL-4 are also cell-type specific. The major biologic actions of IL-4 are antitumor and anti-inflammatory.

INTERLEUKIN-6. Interleukin-6 (IL-6) is a family of glycoproteins also known as hepatocyte stimulatory factor, interferon-beta$_2$ (IFN-beta$_2$), and B-cell stimulatory factor-2. IL-6 is quickly released by a variety of cell types, including monocytes, fibroblasts, and endothelial cells, in response to bacterial products, viruses, and the cytokines IL-1 and TNF. The primary biologic roles of IL-6 compounds appear to be enhancing immune function and acting with IL-1 to promote synthesis of hepatic acute-phase proteins. Hepatocyte protein synthesis after injury may be mediated by the cytokine-induced release of nitric oxide from Kuppfer's cells.[155] In the modulating presence of cortisol and perhaps IL-1, TNF, and IFN, acute-phase proteins are induced (e.g., ceruloplasmin, fibrinogen, haptoglobin, C-reactive protein, complement factors, alpha$_1$-antitrypsin, and alpha$_2$-macroglobin), and the synthesis of albumin is suppressed. The liver is stimulated to accumulate amino acids, zinc, and iron from plasma pools. Copper is released and combines with ceruloplasmin to clear oxygen free radicals and to donate copper to necessary enzyme systems, such as lysyl oxidase, which is essential for collagen cross-linkage.

The acute-phase proteins alpha$_1$-antitrypsin and alpha$_2$-macroglobulin are protease inhibitors. C-reactive protein plays a role in bacterial opsonization, complement activation, and phagocytosis. IL-6 also may have central hormonal modulating effects (e.g., causing prostaglandin-mediated stimulation of CRF).[469] Unlike many other cytokines, IL-6 is more readily detected in the systemic circulation, and is present within 60 minutes of intravenous administration of endotoxin. IL-6 is stimulated after elective surgery,[593] thermal injury,[482] and transplant rejection.[644]

INTERLEUKIN-8. The interleukin-8 (IL-8) proteins have biologic effects similar to those of substances such as anaphylatoxin C5a, leukotriene B_4 (LTB_4), and platelet-activating factor (PAF). Like IL-6, IL-8 is produced by a variety of cell types, including activated monocytes, fibroblasts, and endothelial cells. IL-1 and TNF induce IL-8 by fibroblasts and endothelial cells. The functions of IL-8 may include chemotaxis; inducing neutrophil degranulation; stimulating respiratory burst; releasing LTB_4; recruiting neutrophils during lung injury; and angiogenesis.[161]

Tumor Necrosis Factor[627]

Tumor necrosis factor–alpha (TNF or TNF-alpha), also called cachectin, is a cytokine that was isolated for its ability to produce hemorrhagic necrosis of methylcholanthrene-transformed sarcoma in mice.[4,67,115] Human pro-TNF undergoes proteolysis to exist in dimer, trimer, or pentamer forms in solution.[4,65,66] Intermediate species are stable, bioactive, and cell associated[364,384] and have a circulating half-life of 14 to 18 minutes in humans.[81] Many cell types produce TNF within minutes of stimulation, including monocytes, lymphocytes, NK cells, mast cells, astrocytes and glial cells, pulmonary and peritoneal macrophages, Kupffer's cells, smooth muscle cells, and endothelial cells. The release of TNF is stimulated by endotoxin, viruses, IL-1, IL-2, IFN, complement activation products, and indomethacin.[3,608] TNF is suppressed by IL-4, IL-6, PGE_2, TGF-beta, PAF receptor antagonists, and cyclosporin A. TNF binds to either of two specific cell receptors, and although the precise mechanism of signal transduction is unknown, TNF may act by means of ion channel formation by the TNF molecule.[350]

TNF is believed to act synergistically with IL-1 to induce hypotension, tissue injury,[496] and death in animals subjected to experimental sepsis. The hypotension induced by TNF may be partly mediated by the production of nitric oxide.[366,367] TNF induces release of PGE_2, aggregation of neutrophils, synthesis of thromboxane, and cytotoxicity for insulin-producing beta-cells.[174] TNF and IL-1 induce eicosanoids[397] and PAF.[177] TNF also acts to suppress the activity of lipoprotein lipase in adipose cells and to cause a fall in transmembrane potential in skeletal muscle.[630] TNF is not believed to have direct effects on proteolysis; rather, its actions are mediated by corticosteroids.[440,450]

Experimental work suggests that TNF mediates the early hypotension of sepsis and IL-1, or factors induced by IL-1 may participate in later phases of sepsis-induced hemodynamic collapse.[654] Endogenous protein inhibitors of TNF have been found in the serum of patients with sarcoidosis and tuberculosis,[228] in the urine,[202,518] and with pleural effusions.[39]

Because many of the deleterious effects of TNF (cachexia, tissue injury, irreversible shock) are correlated with serum levels of TNF, use of monoclonal antibodies as treatment is most compelling. A large body of experimental work provides a rationale for anti-TNF therapy as a means to ameliorate shock through primary blockade of TNF,[628] secondary reduction of TNF-induced cytokines (e.g., IL-1 and IL-6),[30] and minimization of TNF-induced changes in effective blood volume.[521]

Interferon

Interferon-gamma (IFN or IFN-gamma) is a glycoprotein released by activated T lymphocytes and IL-2.[648] IFN-gamma activates macrophages to release IL-1 and TNF[145]; increases monocyte IL-2 receptors; induces the enzymes required for leukocyte respiratory burst; increases expression of the major histocompatibility complex; and, most importantly, inhibits replication of viruses. IFN acts synergistically with IL-6 and cortisol to modulate the synthesis of acute-phase proteins. Elevated levels of IFN have been observed in patients with pelvic inflammatory disease. The release of cortisol has been observed after infusion of IFN in cancer patients, but the mechanism is not well-understood. Secretion of IFN is reduced early after injury; this suppression may be mediated by the inhibitory effects of PGE_2.

Eicosanoids[468]

Eicosanoids, or phospholipid mediators, are 20-carbon cyclic fatty acids derived primarily from arachidonic acid and synthesized by most cell types. The arachidonic acid used to synthesize eicosanoids is derived from phosphatidylcholine, phosphatidylinositol, and cell membrane phospholipids, through the action of phospholipase A.[396] Subsequent metabolism yields four major groups: prostaglandins (PGE, PGF), prostacyclins (PGI_2), thromboxanes (TXA_2, TXB_2), and leukotrienes (Figure 8-22). Endothelium converts arachidonic acid primarily to PGI_2, and platelets convert arachidonic acid primarily to TXA_2,[522] largely because of enzyme-cell specificity.

Prostaglandins are not stored; rather, they require de novo synthesis. Numerous stimuli can trigger the synthesis and release of prostaglandins, although many of these stimuli have not yet been pinpointed. Some of the better known stimuli are hypoxia, ischemia, and tissue injury; pyrogen, endotoxin, collagen, and thrombin; neural stimulation; and hormonal stimulation (serotonin, acetylcholine, histamine, norepinephrine, vasopressin, angiotensin II, and bradykinin).[246,396] These stimuli are relatively nonspecific because they cause the release of several prostaglandins that are cell specific rather than stimulus specific. Because of the varied nature of the stimuli, it is no surprise that plasma concentrations of prostaglandins increase during hemorrhagic, septic, and endotoxic shock.

Eicosanoids have a very short half-life and duration of action. Metabolism occurs primarily at the site of release and secondarily in the lung,[396] resulting in production of inactive fragments. The synthesis of prostaglandins has been linked to phosphatidylinositol breakdown in calcium-dependent hormonal regulation ($alpha_1$ type of second-messenger action).[209] The increase in prostaglandins may stimulate the degradation of phosphatidylinositol, thereby augmenting the hormonal response.

The biologic actions of prostaglandins also are closely linked to changes in the intracellular concentration of cAMP. In general, when a prostaglandin leads to an increase in the concentration of cAMP in a target cell, the target cell action is stimulated; conversely, when a

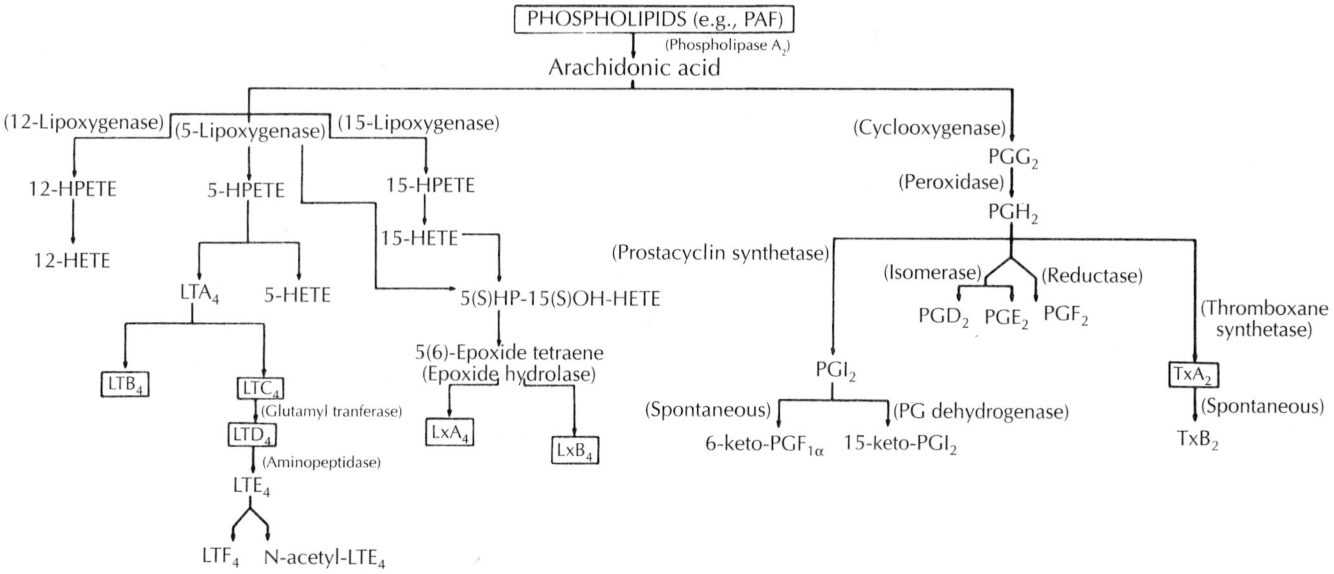

FIGURE 8-22 Biosynthetic pathway of lipid mediators. *HPETE*, Hydroxy-eicosatetraenoic acid; *LT*, leukotriene; *PG*, prostaglandin; *Tx*, thromboxane; *Lx*, lipoxin. (From Lefer AM et al: *Circ Shock* 27:3, 1989.)

prostaglandin leads to a decrease in cAMP, the target cell action is inhibited. However, a specific prostaglandin does not always lead to a specific change in the intracellular concentration of cAMP. Thus the same prostaglandin that inhibits the formation of cAMP in one tissue may stimulate it in another.

The biologic actions of prostaglandins are the most varied of any naturally occurring compound. Generally, for every action produced by one prostaglandin, an antagonistic action is produced by another prostaglandin. TXA_2 is the most potent endogenous vasoconstrictor known, whereas PGI_2 and PGE_2 are potent vasodilators.[475,573] These effects occur in both small and large vessels and in virtually all circulatory beds. Prostacyclin is also a potent inhibitor of platelet aggregation, whereas TXA_2 is a potent stimulator.[281,475]

The antagonistic actions of prostaglandins produced by vascular endothelium and platelets suggest that an imbalance in the production of these substances may be involved in the pathogenesis of abnormal conditions that arise after injury. For example, an increase in the release of TXA_2 or a decrease in the production of PGI_2 would favor platelet aggregation and vasoconstriction, features characteristic of adult respiratory distress syndrome (ARDS). In fact, an increase in the ratio of TXB_2 (the major metabolite of TXA_2) to 6-keto-F_1-alpha (the major metabolite of PGI_2) is greater in the plasma of patients with sepsis and ARDS than in patients with sepsis alone.[607] In contrast, sepsis alone is associated with parallel increases in both TXB_2 and PGI_2 that correlate with the fall in blood pressure during septic shock.[111]

The E family of prostaglandins (PGE_1 and PGE_2) causes bronchodilatation, whereas PGF_2-alpha causes bronchoconstriction.[516] In contrast, PGE_2 and PGF_2-alpha increase pulmonary vascular resistance and capillary permeability but decrease systemic vascular resistance.[475,573] These substances have been implicated in the redistribution of renal blood flow from the outer cortical areas to the inner cortical and outer medullary areas during periods of reduced renal blood flow, and in the pathogenesis of septic shock[226,227] and ARDS.[84,494,509]

Leukotrienes are important mediators of the inflammatory response that may play an important role in the development of cell and tissue injury during shock and ischemia.[397] Leukotrienes are produced by a variety of cell types, including pulmonary parenchymal cells, macrophages, mast cells, leukocytes, smooth muscle cells, and connective tissue cells.[276,298] Leukotrienes increase vascular permeability, stimulate leukocyte adherence,[159] and cause bronchoconstriction and vasoconstriction.[330,523] Leukotriene-induced vasoconstriction occurs in a variety of vascular beds, including those of the skin, intestine, and heart,[523] and it may impair cardiac contractility.

Plasma concentrations of leukotrienes increase moderately during shock.[397] Experimental infusion of lipoxygenase, the enzyme required for leukotriene formation, produces an increase in pulmonary vascular permeability and pulmonary edema, suggesting that leukotrienes are involved in the pathogenesis of ARDS.[631]

Serotonin

Serotonin (5-hydroxytryptamine) is a neurotransmitter that acts primarily on smooth muscle and nerve endings.[443] It is formed from tryptophan by tryptophan hydroxylase, a rate-limiting enzyme. Of the total serotonin stored in the body, 90% normally is found in enterochromaffin cells of the gut. The remaining 10% is found in platelets and the brain.

The actions of serotonin include bronchoconstriction, venoconstriction, arterial vasodilatation, platelet aggregation, and positive myocardial inotropy and chronotropy.[164] Serotonin is released in response to tissue injury and is an important mediator of the inflammatory response. Elevated plasma concentrations have been noted during septic shock, and this may stem from direct action of endotoxin.[196]

Histamine

Histamine is synthesized from histidine by histidine decarboxylase. In tissue, histamine is chiefly stored in mast cells; in blood, it is mainly stored in basophils.[443] Histamine is also stored in the gastric mucosa, neurons, and epidermis.[443] The stimuli that elicit the release of histamine from these tissues are not known with certainty, but a decrease in the intracellular concentration of cAMP and an increase in intracellular calcium are associated with the release of histamine from basophils and mast cells. Elevated concentrations have been seen after hemorrhagic and septic shock and thermal injury.[425,542]

Histamine acts on cell-surface receptors, which can be categorized as H_1 and H_2. H_1 receptors mediate an increase in the uptake of L-histidine (precursor of histamine) into cells, and actions such as bronchoconstriction, increased myocardial contractility, and intestinal contractions.[443] H_2 receptors inhibit the release of histamine and mediate changes in gastric secretion, cardiac rate, and immunologic function.[443] Both H_1 and H_2 receptors appear to mediate small-vessel vasodilatation and increased vascular permeability. Stimulation of H_1 receptors is associated with an increase in cyclic 3′,5′-guanosine monophosphate (cGMP), whereas stimulation of H_2 receptors is associated with an increase in cAMP. However, it is not known whether these cyclic nucleotides act as second messengers in a histamine-mediated response.

Somatomedins and Insulin-like Growth Factors

Somatomedins are a family of polypeptides that stimulate proteoglycan synthesis in cartilage and DNA synthesis and cell replication in a variety of cell types.[695] Somatomedins were so named because of their ability to mediate some of the actions of growth hormone, such as sulfation of cartilage and other aspects of cell growth. Somatomedins also demonstrate insulin-like actions, including increased glucose uptake and protein synthesis in skeletal muscle[452,529]; increased glucose uptake and oxidation, and lipid synthesis in adipose tissue[695]; increased protein synthesis and glycogenesis in the liver[43,667]; and decreased glucagon-stimulated hepatic gluconeogenesis.[234]

Concurrent with the discovery of somatomedins, researchers discovered that human plasma has large amounts of insulin-like activity that does not reside in insulin itself, because human plasma treated with insulin antibodies still demonstrates insulin-like actions.[695] This nonsuppressible, insulin-like activity (NSILA) contains all the known metabolic actions of insulin and can be divided into two chemically and biologically related polypeptides, NSILA-I and NSILA-II. In addition to their insulin-like effects, these two proteins have marked effects on cell growth. As a result, they are now called insulin-like growth factor I (IGF-I) and insulin-like growth factor II (IGF-II). Currently, it appears that somatomedin C, somatomedin A, and IGF-I, all of which require growth hormone for their effects on cartilage sulfation, are the same molecule,[197] and that somatomedin B is the same molecule as epidermal growth factor. However, a relationship between IGF-II and the other somatomedins has not been established.

Large amounts of the insulin-like growth factors are found in human plasma, primarily in an inactive, bound form. These molecules have been isolated from the liver, muscle, fibroblasts, and kidneys and have been shown to have a molecular weight of less than 10,000.[522] The exact physiologic role of the somatomedins and insulin-like growth factors has not yet been fully clarified.

After injury, the plasma concentrations of somatomedins and IGF are decreased.[237] This may largely be due to the starvation that accompanies injury because the plasma concentration of these substances is also depressed during fasting.[445] Nonetheless, the concentration of insulin-like growth factors increases during the late stages of endotoxicosis[221]; this may explain the paradoxic increase in peripheral use of glucose and the depression in hepatic gluconeogenesis noted during late endotoxicosis in association with a reduced plasma concentration of insulin.[221]

Atrial Natriuretic Peptides

Atrial natriuretic peptides (ANP) are released by the central nervous system and by neurosecretory granules in left atrial myocytes in response to changes in atrial wall tension.[551] Centrally, ANP reduces the secretion of AVP from the posterior pituitary[530] and also inhibits peripheral action of AVP.[171] AVP stimulates the secretion of ANP.[423] These peptides are potent inhibitors of aldosterone secretion, and they block resorption of sodium in the perirenal tubules, but their role in the normal control of fluid and electrolyte balance remains controversial.[277] ANP is unaffected by coronary artery bypass surgery[151] but does change after atrial reconstructions.[618] Fluid resuscitation does not appear to change plasma

ENDOTHELIAL CELL–DERIVED FACTORS AND RESPONSES

Anticoagulation	Prostacyclin (PGI_2)
	Tissue plasminogen activator
	Glycosaminoglycans
	Thrombomodulin
	Proteins S and C
	Nitric oxide (EDRF)
Procoagulation	Thromboxane (TXA_2)
	Tissue factor
	Plasminogen activator inhibitor-1
	Factor V
	Platelet-activating factor
	Factors V and XII activators
	Von Willebrand factor
	Fibronectin
	Factor IXa binding protein
Leukocyte interactions	IL-1-beta
	IL-6
	IL-8
	TNF-alpha
	ICAM-1 and ICAM-2
	ELAM-1
	PECAM-1
	VCAM-1
	P and E selectin
	Class I and class II MHC antigens
	Colony-stimulating factors
	Reactive oxygen intermediates
	oxLDL
Growth factors	TGF-beta
	PDGF
	IGF-1
Vasorelaxation	PGE_2
	Nitric oxide
	Atrial naturietic peptides
	Other EDRFs
Vasoconstriction	Endothelins
	Angiotensin II

EDRF, Endothelium-derived relaxation factor; *IL,* interleukin; *ICAM,* intercellular adhesion molecule; *ELAM,* endothelial leukocyte adhesion molecule; *PECAM,* platelet cell adhesion molecule; *VCAM,* vascular cell adhesion molecule; *MHC,* major histocompatibility complex; *oxLDL,* oxidized low-density lipoprotein; *TGF,* transforming growth factor; *PDGF,* platelet-derived growth factor; *IGF,* insulin-like growth factor.

(Modified from Palombo JD, Blackburn GL, Forse RA: *Surg Gynecol Obstet* 173:505, 1991; Gerritsen ME, Bloor CM: *FASEB J* 7:523, 1993; Ross R: *Nature* 362:801, 1993.)

ANP levels after experimental hemorrhage.[252] The role of ANP in postinjury responses is not yet clear.

Other stimuli that cause the release of atrial ANP are acute volume loading, congestive heart failure, atrial arrhythmias, and acute and chronic renal failure. Secretion of ANP also is stimulated by angiotensin, AVP, alpha- and beta-agonists, and endothelin controlled by the autonomic nervous system.

Metabolic effects of ANP are suggested by the finding that these peptides modulate the response of ACTH, AVP, and angiotensin II to acute hypoglycemia.[677] The precise physiologic role of ANP in fluid balance and metabolic response to injury is not yet fully understood.

Endothelial Cell Mediators[507,527]

The paracrine actions of endothelial cell products span the entire spectrum of neuroendocrine, vasoactive, coagulative, cell proliferative, and immunologic functions (see the box at left).[269,507,562,567] In some abnormal conditions, plasma or urinary levels of some endothelial factors increase, suggesting that these substances also may have systemic or pathophysiologic effects. The endothelium could be considered an endocrine organ in its own right, because it responds to external stimuli by producing paracrine hormones and growth factors that act on neighboring smooth muscle cells, monocytes, macrophages, fibroblasts, and organ-specific cells.[18] Endothelial cell products also may modulate cardiovascular functions by acting on central cardiovascular, baroreceptor, and neuroeffector systems (Figure 8-23).[564] However, the primary actions of endothelial-derived substances are believed to be local vasomotor regulation and modulation of coagulation.

Recent studies also suggest that endothelial cells act on immune function through elaboration of substances such as intercellular adhesion molecules, endothelial leukocyte adhesion molecules, and other molecules that promote platelet and lymphocyte binding, with secretion of many of these factors as cytokines such as IL-1, TNF, and IFN. The vascular system may thereby be considered an immunologic organ as well (Figure 8-24). The box at left lists the many substances expressed by endothelial cells that interact with coagulation, leukocyte function, and smooth muscle function.[269,507,562] Cytokines such as IL-1 and TNF-alpha activate endothelial cells to lose anticoagulant properties and to activate the extrinsic clotting pathway.[528] Cell-surface receptors such as E-selectin, P-selectin, and intracellular adhesion molecule-1 promote adherence of leukocytes.[188,301] Reactive oxygen intermediates also are induced by cytokines in endothelial cells.[241] Oxidized low-density lipoprotein causes monocyte chemotaxis and endothelial transmigration.[118,539]

Nitric Oxide

It is well established that endothelial cells are required for the mascurinic receptor, vasodilatory action of acetylcholine, through the release of a substance previously *called endothelium-derived relaxing factor (EDRF) but now known as nitric oxide (NO).*[334,506] Like the nitrovasodilatory drugs in clinical use, NO acts through stimulation of soluble guanylate cyclase, formation of cGMP, activation of cGMP-dependent protein kinases, and dephosphorylation of myosin light chains to pro-

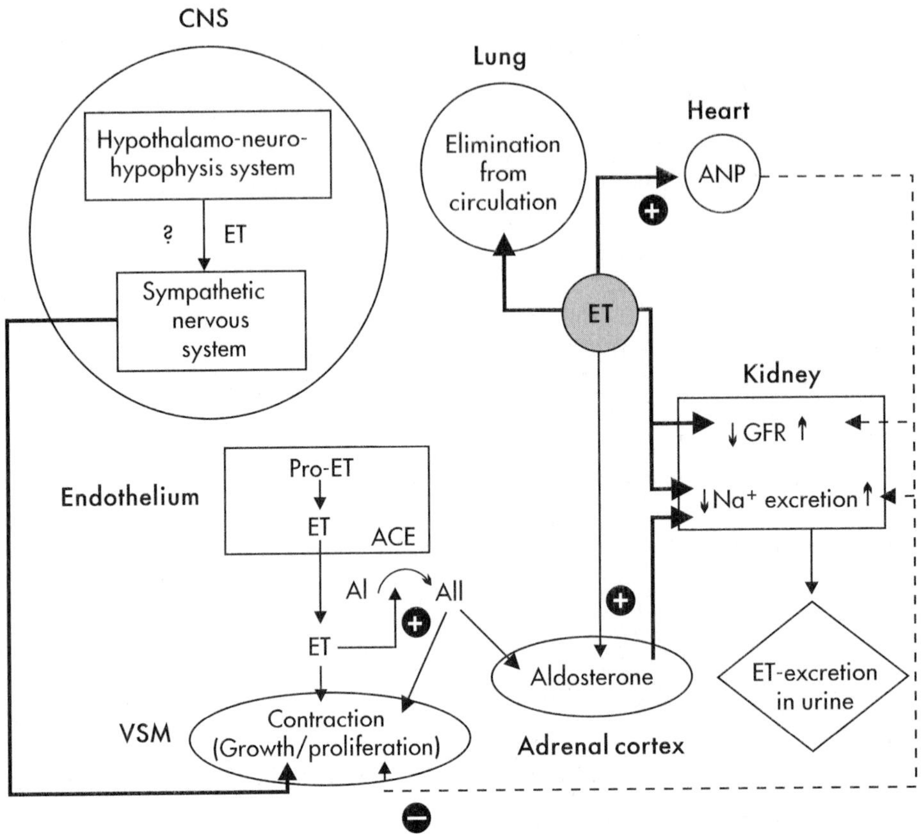

FIGURE 8-23 Hypothetical cardiovascular actions of endothelin (ET). ET may indirectly modulate cardiovascular and renal function. Circulating ET *(shaded circle)* is removed by the lungs and excreted by the kidneys. *VSM,* Vascular smooth muscle; *Pro-ET,* precursors of ET; *ACE,* angiotensin-converting enzyme; *AI,* angiotensin I; *AII,* angiotensin II; *ANP,* atrial natriuretic peptide; *GFR,* glomerular filtration rate. (From Rubanyi GM et al: *FASEB J* 5:2717, 1991.)

duce muscle relaxation. NO is formed through nitric oxide synthase (NOS) by conversion of L-arginine to citrulline and is released by many cell types besides endothelium, such as neutrophils, macrophages, cerebellar neurons, renal cells, and Kupffer's cells.[451]

There is evidence that blood vessels are dilated continuously by endothelial-generated EDRF-NO; this substance acts as a true paracrine compound, with immediate inactivation by hemoglobin in the bloodstream (half-life is 6 seconds) and synergistic vasodilatory actions by prostacyclin through adenylate cyclase (see Figure 8-24). The vasodilatory actions of these compounds appear to be countered by the potent endothelial cell products called endothelins (ETs), which are described below.

The physiologically relevant effects of NO in humans are active areas of investigation at this time.[640] Although all sources of nitric oxide have not yet been clearly identified, NO synthase in human hepatocytes recently was cloned and expressed.[265] The three forms of NOS are the products of distinct genes. Constitutive NOS enzymes (cNOS; two human forms—neuronal and endothelial) are always present and activate quickly to produce small amounts of NO. Inducible NOS enzymes (iNOS; hepatocyte type) can be produced experimentally after stimulation with lipopolysaccharide, IL-1, IL-2, TNF, and IFN. iNOS is important, because it can generate NO in 1000-fold greater quantities than the cNOS isoform, and it may be implicated in some of the exaggerated hemodynamic and metabolic responses to injury and infection. Consequently, modulating iNOS may be a logical therapeutic target with severe shock and sepsis. Significant positive correlations between an elevated NO level, the presence of endotoxin, and a clinical state of low vascular resistance have been observed in patients after trauma and during sepsis.[492]

Besides vascular endothelium, other cell types produce nitric oxide and may be affected by it, including

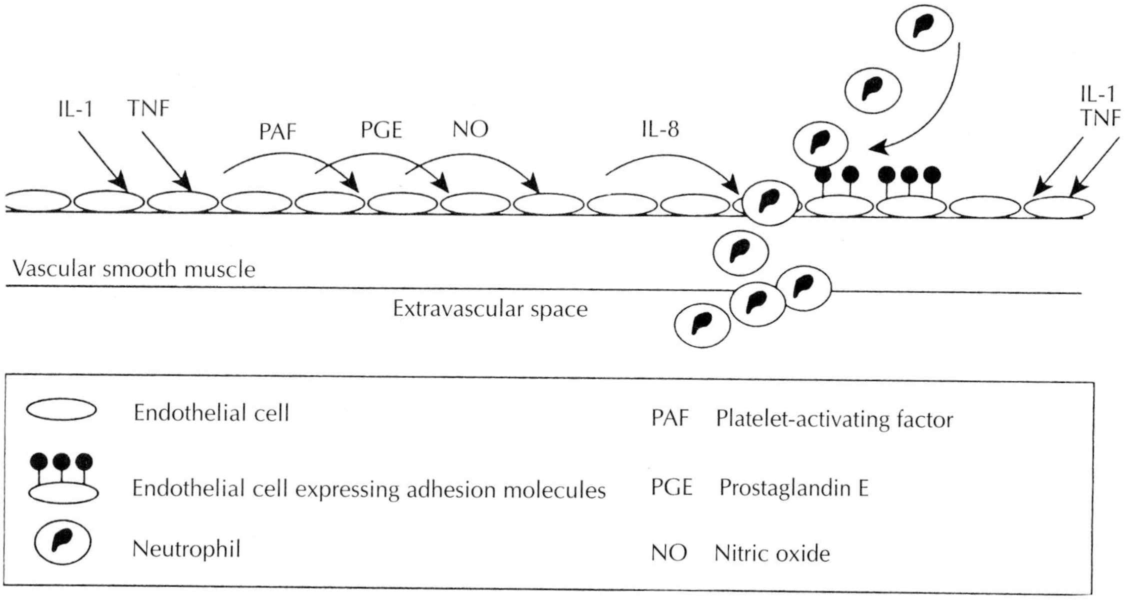

FIGURE 8-24 Effect of interleukin-1 (IL-1) and tumor necrosis factor (TNF) on the endothelium. IL-1 and TNF stimulate synthesis of platelet-activating factor (PAF), prostaglandin E (PGE), and nitric oxide (NO), resulting in vasodilatation and hypotension. Hypotension may result in inadequate organ perfusion, acidosis, and organ failure. IL-1 and TNF stimulate the synthesis of endothelial adhesion molecules, which facilitate adherence of circulating neutrophils. IL-1 and TNF also induce production of interleukin-8 (IL-8) from the endothelium. IL-8 attracts neutrophils adhering to the endothelial surface to emigrate into the extravascular space and release enzymes and oxygen-reactive radicals, causing cytotoxicity. (From Dinarello CA, Gelfand JA, Wolff SM: *JAMA* 269,1830, 1993.)

hepatocytes,[155] Kupffer's cells,[70] macrophages,[314] neutrophils,[582] and cerebellar neurons[376]; this suggests a wide spectrum of possible physiologic effects. As previously described, NO mediates protein synthesis in hepatocytes[155] and electron transport in hepatocyte mitochondria. NO also exerts immunomodulatory effects that may be important in graft-versus-host disease.[322,392]

Endothelins

In response to injury, vascular endothelial cells produce peptides called endothelins (ETs),[688] which are extremely potent vasoconstrictors.[571] Endothelins originate from a large prepropeptide, from which a 38-amino acid peptide (called big ET) is generated by proteolytic cleavage and in turn is transformed into more active forms. Isopeptide ET forms have been found with different activities, tissue distribution, and receptors.

ET-1 is the most biologically active form of ET and the most potent vasoconstrictor known; it is approximately 10 times more potent than angiotensin II. The putative mechanism of ET action is complex[426,473] (see Figure 8-17). ETs also have been shown to enhance phosphorylation of protein tyrosine in a manner similar to other growth factors, which may explain the cell proliferative effects of ETs.

Increased serum endothelin correlates with the severity of injury in patients after major trauma[378] and major surgery,[319,340] and in those in cardiogenic shock or who have sepsis.[120] It is believed that the primary actions of ETs are paracrine,[35] because the picogram concentrations of circulating ETs are too low to cause systemic effects.[645] Recent development of an oral antagonist to specific ET receptors suggests that blockade may have therapeutic benefits in renal ischemia-reperfusion vasoconstriction, and in cerebral spasm of subarachnoid hemorrhage in animals.[141]

Factors that affect the release of endothelin include thrombin, catecholamines, and anoxia. ETs may be involved in counteracting basal levels of EDRF-NO and prostacyclins at the smooth muscle level of blood vessels to maintain physiologic tone. Endothelial cells also are stimulated by mediators such as IL-1, TNF, and endotoxin (see Figure 8-24). Endothelin, nitric oxide,[366,572] and substances such as endothelial leukocyte adhesion molecule-1[68] and oxygen free radicals[87] are produced and released by endothelium in the presence of cytokines such as IL-1, TNF, and endotoxins. Endothelin may also modulate the recently described mitogenic effects of angiotensin II.

Prostaglandins

As discussed in the section on eicosanoids, endothelial cells synthesize predominantly prostacyclin and PGE_2, and only small amounts of TXA_2. These products act to promote vasodilatation and reduce platelet aggregation. The primary prostaglandin products of platelets, TXA_2 and 12-hydroxy-eicosatetraenoic acid (12-HETE), have opposite effects.

Platelet-Activating Factor

Stimulation of endothelial cells by TNF, IL-1, AVP, and angiotensin II causes the formation and release of platelet-activating factor (PAF), a phospholipid constituent of cell membranes (see Figure 8-24).[104,535] PAF (acetyl glyceryl ether phosphoryl choline [AGEPC]) binds to surface-membrane receptors on platelets and other cell types to induce platelet aggregation and adhesion of platelets to endothelial cells, and to stimulate the release of vasoconstrictors.[657] These actions may be mediated by phospholipase A_2 and share features common to the production of eicosanoids.[131] PAF also mediates cytoskeletal changes in endothelial cells, increasing barrier permeability to albumin.[97] Among other potential actions, PAF is thought to be a possible mediator of the hemodynamic and metabolic effects of endotoxin.[225] Experimental infusion of PAF changes glucose kinetics, suggesting that PAF promotes the release of glucagon and catecholamines.[390]

Plasminogen Activators

Endothelial cells also synthesize tissue plasminogen activator (t-PA), which catalyzes the formation of plasmin, a protease that activates platelets. Activated platelets can release plasminogen activator inhibitor type 1 (PAI-1), which neutralizes endothelium-associated plasminogen activator. Endothelial cells also can secrete PAI-1 in response to other platelet products. The changes in PAI-1 caused by elective surgery and trauma may contribute to a fibrinolytic shutdown in these cases and may play as yet undefined additional roles in the biologic response to injury.

Endothelial Cell Function in Disease

It is important to realize that the endothelium of atherosclerotic vessels responds pathologically to platelet interactions and vasoactive substances.[562,656] Platelet aggregation, with resultant release of TXA_2, serotonin, and ADP, induces the formation of EDRF, which is attenuated in diseased vessels.[239] Leukocyte-derived oxygen free radicals, present in the media of atherosclerotic vessels, also inactivate EDRF and nitric oxide. The response to nitric oxide also is reduced with clinical diabetes[570] and hypercholesterolemia.[385]

Plasma Protein Cascades

The plasma cascades involve protein and polypeptide factors that circulate in inactive forms. Activation of these cascades (e.g., the kallikrein-kinin system and the complement and coagulation cascades) can occur when inactive proteins are activated, proenzymes are cleaved, or the release of circulating inhibitors is reduced. These substances also interact with and modulate the release of other mediators.

Kallikrein-Kinins

The kinins are formed by the serine protease kallikrein in plasma and tissues to produce bradykinin and kallidin, respectively.[354] In plasma, kallikrein acts on a 100,000 kDa kininogen (also called Fitzgerald factor) to form the nonapeptide bradykinin. In glandular tissue, kallikrein acts on a 50,000 kDa kininogen to produce the decapeptide kallidin (lysyl-bradykinin).[354,579] Plasma kallikrein circulates in the inactive form (called prekallikrein or Fletcher factor), which is activated by Hageman factor of the coagulation cascade. When Hageman factor is activated by exposure to a negatively charged surface, prekallikrein is converted to kallikrein, which generates bradykinin through proteolysis and acts as a coagulation factor.[354] Kallikrein is inactivated by plasma inhibitors (i.e., alpha$_2$-macroglobulin, C1-anaphylatoxin inactivator, alpha$_1$-antitrypsin, and antithrombin III). Plasma kinins are inactivated by kinase I and kinase II.[549] Kinase I is a carboxypeptidase identical to the anaphylatoxin inactivator that degrades C3a, C4a, and C5a anaphylatoxins.[82] Kinase II is a dipeptidase identical to angiotensin-converting enzyme.[32]

In inflammatory conditions, the kinins are potent vasodilators that increase capillary permeability, produce edema, evoke pain, increase bronchial resistance, and enhance the clearance of glucose.[549] Kinins also cause renal vasodilatation,[402] reduce renal blood flow,[405] increase the formation of renin,[224] and increase sodium and water retention when administered in pharmacologic doses.[246,615]

Increased plasma concentrations of kallikrein and bradykinin are seen in hemorrhagic shock,[60] endotoxemia, sepsis, and tissue injury.[289] With sepsis, plasma prekallikrein decreases and kallikrein activity increases. A gradual increase in prekallikrein was observed in survivors of sepsis, whereas prekallikrein levels remained low in those who died. In ARDS, the resultant endothelial damage may inhibit the formation or action of kinase II, causing bradykinin to accumulate and reducing angiotensin II.[169] These changes may be important in the systemic as well as local manifestations of acute respiratory distress syndrome.

Coagulation Cascade

Activation of the coagulation pathways by Hageman factor causes activation of prekallikrein through formation of a complex with plasma kininogen, as described previously. This activation generates active kallikrein, which is a chemoattractant, as well as bradykinin. Kallikrein also cleaves plasma plasminogen to produce plasmin and cause fibrinolysis. Decreased levels of Hageman factor, antithrombin III, and plasminogen activator inhibitor have been found after surgery. The occurrence of disseminated intravascular coagulation (DIC) after severe trauma, infection, or sepsis, and of fibrinolysis after open heart surgery highlight the central role of this cascade in maintaining homeostasis and producing the biologic response to injury. Understanding the precise role of the coagulation cascade in these clinical circumstances is complicated by the frequent need for transfusion of blood, platelets, and blood products, and by administration of confounding exogenous substances such as aspirin, heparin, and protamine.

Complement Cascade

Complement systems consist of more than 20 distinct plasma proteins that interact in sequence to cause cell lysis. Activation of this cascade leads to production of biologically active fragments through enzymatic cleavage, amplification, immunoglobulin interaction, and formation of membrane attack complexes (Figure 8-25), as well as by interaction with the coagulation cascade, endothelial cells, and inflammatory cells. Two systems, known as the classical and alternative pathways, have been described for complement activation. The classical pathway usually is initiated by active C1 in association with antigen interactions; the alternative pathway is not antibody dependent, is activated by endotoxin and gram-positive bacterial cell-wall components, and appears to be most important in sepsis and injury. C3 is the central component for activation of both pathways.

Lysis of target cells occurs when the C5b-9 attack complex is generated by cleavage of C3 (Figure 8-25). Many of the active complement proteins cause neutrophil, macrophage, and monocyte chemoattraction, degranulation, activation, and adherence. Activated complement fragments can cause lysis of microbes and of host cells by release of oxygen free radicals and lysosomal enzymes. Increased concentrations of active complement have been associated with increased mortality in patients with sepsis.[292] Studies using monoclonal antibodies directed at leukocyte-complement receptors may reveal a way to mitigate the vascular and tissue damage that often follows severe injury and infection.[168,254]

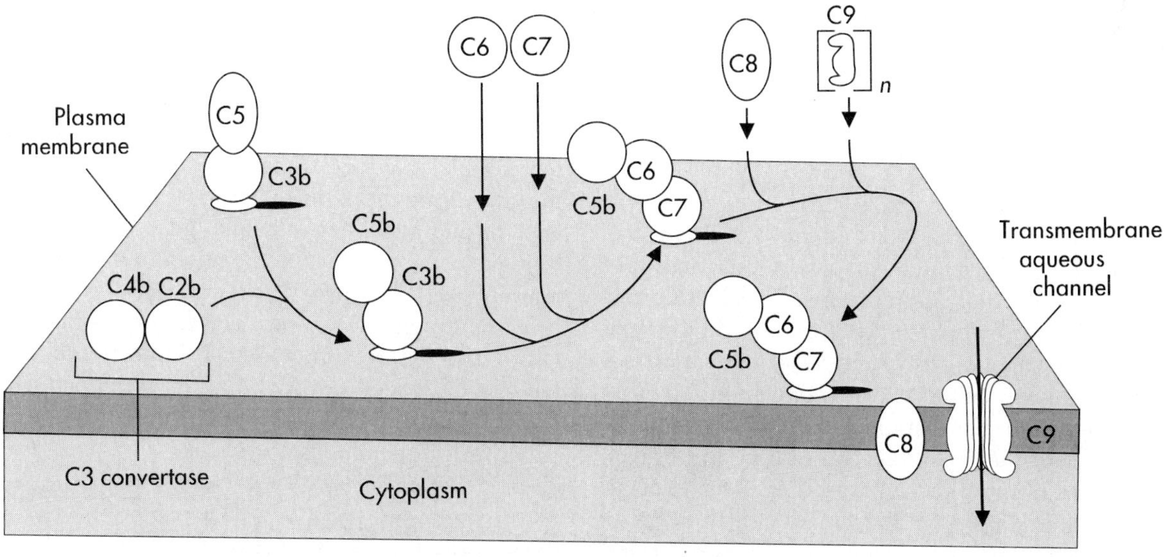

FIGURE 8-25 Late complement components assemble to form a membrane attack complex by binding of C9 to C5678, which inserts C9 into the lipid bilayer of the target cell, next to C8. A chain reaction ensues in which the altered C9 binds a second molecule of C9, which then inserts into the bilayer, where another molecule of C9 is bound, and so on. A chain of C9 molecules thereby forms a large transmembrane channel. The final $C56789(9)_n$ complex can contain as many as 18 C9 molecules, yielding a molecular weight of almost 2 million. The C5678 complexes also produce smaller transmembrane pores. (From Alberts B, Bray D, Lewis J et al: *Molecular biology of the cell,* ed 2, New York, 1989, Garland.)

Single-Cell Products (Intracellular Factors)

Heat-Shock Proteins[411]

Originally named because of their expression after heat stimulation, intracellular heat-shock proteins (HSPs) are highly conserved groups of proteins that are induced after a variety of experimental stress, such as hypoxia, ether anesthesia, trauma, and hemorrhage.[458,633,634] HSPs are also part of nonstressed cellular responses; for example, they act in the inhibition of steroid-inhibitor protein for cortisol and estrogen (see Figure 8-7). It is believed that HSPs interact with a variety of intracellular proteins, serving as molecular chaperones to assist in assembly, disassembly, stability, and intracellular transport.[112,132]

The role of HSPs in the human cellular response to stress has not yet been fully defined. In experimental models, expression of the HSP gene increases parallel with activation of the hypothalamic-pituitary axis. Some HSP expression may be specific to adrenocortical cells and vascular endothelium and may be ACTH sensitive and age dependent.[78] Preliminary experimental work suggests that synthesis of HSPs during shock may modulate the synthesis of hepatic acute-phase proteins.[583] Given the ubiquity of these molecular chaperones, the full role of HSPs in the injury response will be difficult to fully characterize. Recent investigations of preconditioning (e.g., induction of endogenous tolerance to ischemia-reperfusion injury in the myocardium) may implicate the accumulation of stress-induced HSPs,[546] in addition to intracellular accumulation of metabolites (e.g., adenosine) or induction of enzymes (e.g., protein kinase C), as a mechanism for this intriguing phenomenon.[442]

Reactive Oxygen Metabolites[295]

Endogenous formation of short-lived, highly reactive molecular oxygen species with unpaired outer-orbit electrons (oxygen free radicals [OFR]) can occur as a byproduct of oxidative metabolism, arachidonic acid metabolism, and iron-catalyzed reactions, as well as during the respiratory burst of phagocytic cells. Normally generated oxygen metabolites are necessary for electron transport in mitochondria, enzyme activation, and enzyme function. Oxygen metabolites are also produced as byproducts of the cyclo-oxygenase reaction in prostaglandin synthesis; the lipoxygenase step in leukotriene synthesis; the oxidation of catecholamines, thiols, and flavins in plasma; and the conversion of hypoxanthine to xanthine by endothelial xanthine oxidase.[238,432]

Nitric oxide is an oxidized metabolite of oxygen that is generated by nitric oxide synthase enzymes, which are analogous to cytochrome P450. In the presence of molecular oxygen, NO is unstable, having a half-life of 4 to 50 seconds (see the section on Nitric Oxide for a more complete discussion). The most abundant OFRs are those based on molecular oxygen: the superoxide radical O_2^- is produced in the respiratory burst of neutrophils. The hydroxyl radical is highly unstable and extremely toxic. Host cells are damaged primarily by OFR peroxidation of cell-membrane unsaturated fatty acids.[238] OFR interaction with the plasma membrane results in increased membrane permeability and inability to maintain normal transmembrane ion gradients. The cell injury and death induced by irradiation and some antibiotics and antineoplastic drugs is mediated through generation of OFRs.[432]

OFR species that contribute to radical-mediated damage (e.g., O_2^-, the hydroxyl radical, and endogenous hydrogen peroxide) are produced after ischemia and shock by activated granulocytes and by oxidases found in endothelium (e.g., xanthine oxidase). Comprehension of this ischemia-reperfusion injury response is critical to successful results after resuscitation from shock; revascularization of the heart, limb, or gut; and in organ preservation and transplantation.

Various mechanisms are necessary and available to protect against OFRs. Endogenous antioxidants include enzymatic compounds such as cytochrome oxidase, superoxide dismutase (SOD), catalase, and glutathione peroxidase. Nonenzymatic compounds include lipid phase alpha-tocopherol (vitamin E) and beta-carotene (vitamin A precursor), aqueous phase ascorbic acid (vitamin C), albumin, bilirubin, ceruloplasmin, and transferrin. In the intracellular space, SOD is present in high concentrations to react with the superoxide radical during the formation of hydrogen peroxide and oxygen. Catalase and glutathione peroxidase decompose hydrogen peroxide to water. In the extracellular space, SOD-like activity is very low and has an affinity for endothelium.[356] The fact that endothelium-derived relaxing factor is inactivated by superoxide anions[564] may be important to the mechanisms of local regulation of blood flow during and after ischemia and shock.[644] Administering exogenous substances known to inhibit OFR formation (e.g., allopurinol, which inhibits xanthine oxidase; mannitol, which acts as a hydroxyl radical scavenger; and deferoxamine, which binds free Fe^{+++} ion) has had beneficial effects in organ preservation and in some cases has reduced bacterial translocation during experimental hemmorhagic shock.[167]

INJURY-INDUCED CHANGES IN SUBSTRATE AND ENERGY

Intermediary Metabolism: Basic Concepts

The body's minimal metabolic requirements include energy for daily activities and obligate metabolic processes; glucose for glucose-dependent tissues; essential amino acids for obligate protein synthesis; and essential fatty acids for membrane lipid synthesis (Figure 8-26). In re-

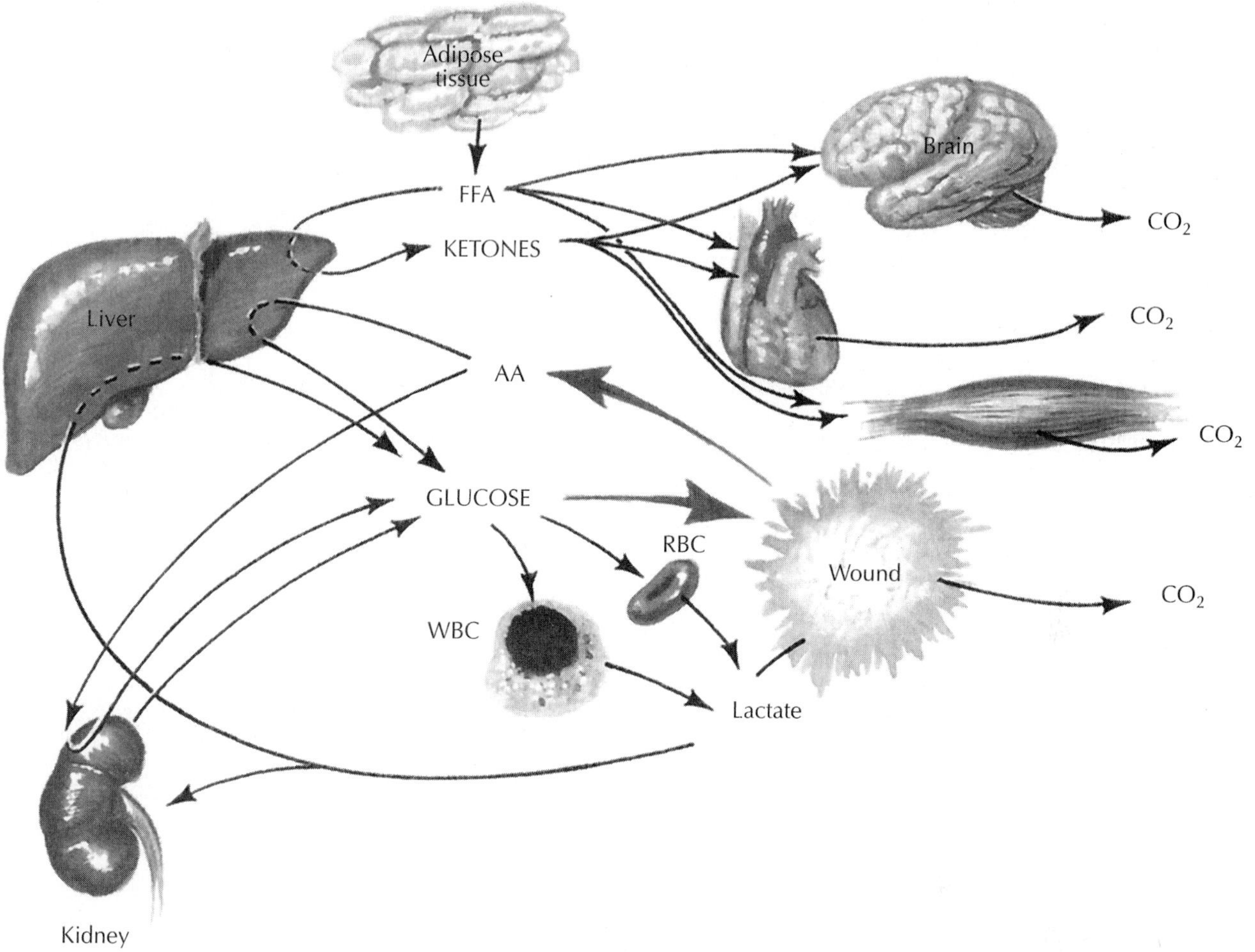

FIGURE 8-26 Metabolic requirements.

sponse to injury (and to concomitant starvation if substrates are unavailable), signals interact to direct both anabolic and catabolic metabolic pathways. Needed energy must be produced, and particular substrates must be provided for coagulation, fluid shifts, inflammation, immunologic response, and de novo synthesis of protein for cellular repair and regeneration. The balance between energy-yielding catabolic processes and energy-requiring anabolic metabolism is guided by intracellular high-energy phosphate economy.

Intermediary metabolism is regulated through the effects of substrates and through paracrine, endocrine, and autonomic signals that change membrane transport properties and regulate intracellular enzyme activity. For example, insulin increases membrane transport properties for glucose,[480] whereas epinephrine inhibits insulin-stimulated glucose transport.[127] The activity or synthesis of the key rate-limiting regulatory enzymes is modulated by glucagon. Glucagon increases the activity of phosphoenolpyruvate carboxykinase (PEPCK) in the liver, which increases the rate of gluconeogenesis. Insulin decreases the activity of PEPCK, which decreases gluconeogenesis[206] (Figure 8-27).

Most hormones and factors act through more than one of these mechanisms. For example, insulin stimulates glucose uptake, phosphofructokinase (PFK) activity, and glycogen synthetase activity.[480] Thus insulin simultaneously promotes glucose transport and energy production through glycolysis, and increases the activity of enzymes for glycogen synthesis (Figure 8-27). Most neuroendocrine effectors stimulate one intracellular metabolic pathway while inhibiting the opposing pathway through direct enzymatic action and reaction metabolites. Glucagon directly inhibits acetyl-CoA carboxylase, the enzyme that converts acetyl-CoA to malonyl-CoA. The reduction in malonyl-CoA inhibits the synthesis of triglycerides and activates carnitine acetyltransferase I, which promotes transfer of fatty acids into the mitochondria and increases the oxidation of fatty acids (Figure 8-28).

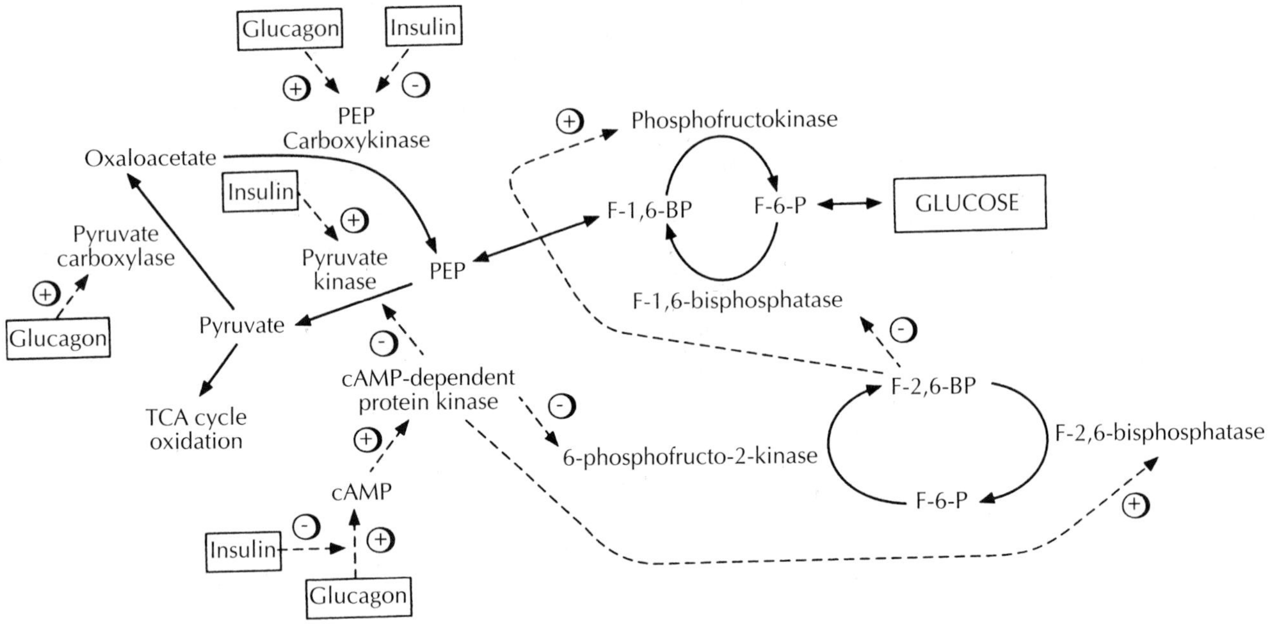

FIGURE 8-27 Regulation of gluconeogenesis by insulin and glucagon. Plus sign (+) indicates a positive regulatory effect; minus sign (−) indicates an inhibitory effect. *F-6-P,* Fructose-6-phosphate; *F-1,6-BP,* fructose-1,6-biphosphate; *PEP,* phosphoenolpyruvate; *TCA,* tricarboxylic acid. (From Wilson JD, Foster DW, editors: *Williams textbook of endocrinology,* ed 8, Philadelphia, 1992, WB Saunders.)

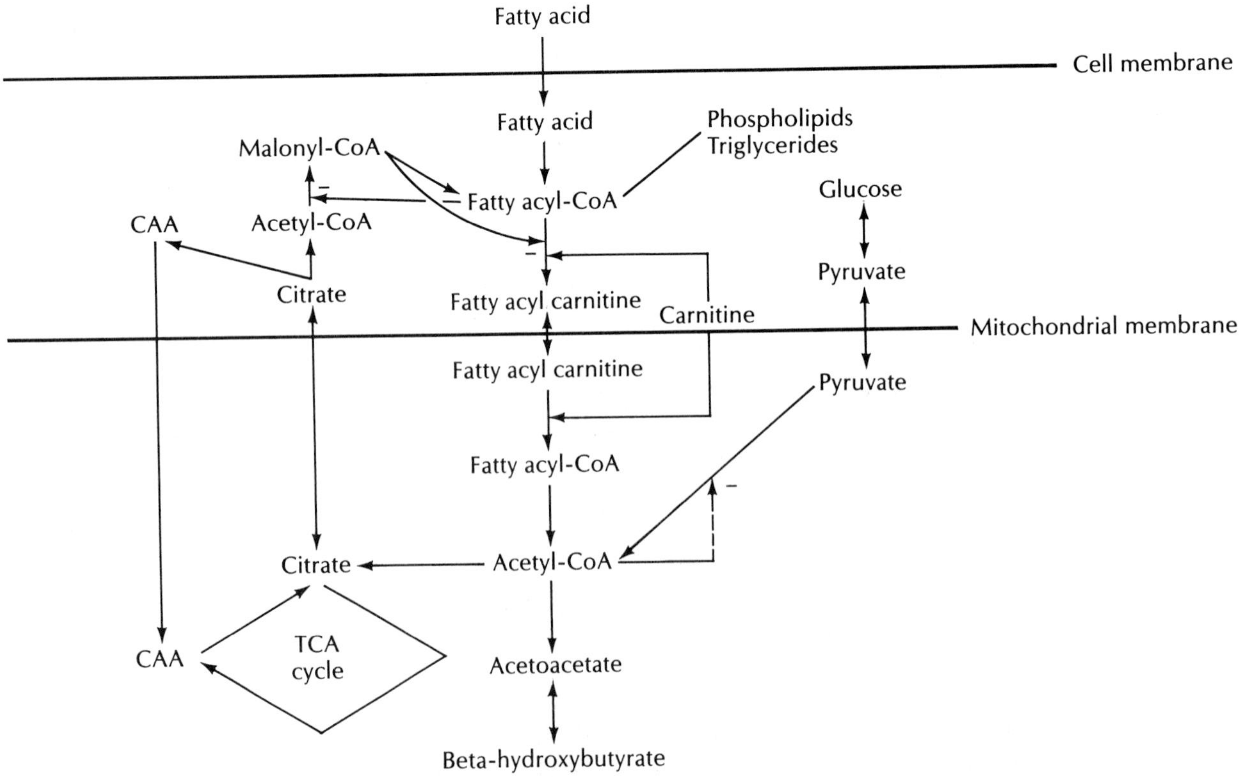

FIGURE 8-28 Metabolic pathways for fatty-acid oxidation and synthesis in the liver.

Energy Balance

The energy present in all biologic molecules is released by cytoplasmic degradation into small carbon fragments. For carbohydrates, this occurs through glycolysis; for proteins, through protein breakdown, amino acid transamination, and amino acid oxidation; and for lipids, through beta-oxidation. The remaining energy is then released by intramitochondrial oxidation of the small carbon fragments in the tricarboxylic acid cycle (Krebs, or TCA, cycle) (Figure 8-29).

Carbohydrates, proteins, and lipids enter through the common pathway of the TCA cycle by means of acetyl-CoA. Each acetyl-CoA molecule is completely oxidized in the TCA cycle to yield 12 high-energy phosphate bonds. As noted in Figure 8-28, amino acids also can enter the TCA cycle by means of succinylcoenzyme A (succinyl-CoA) and alpha-ketoglutarate.

The phosphate bonds of adenosine triphosphate (ATP) serve as the carrier of chemical energy in all living cells, whereas the phosphate bonds of creatine phos-

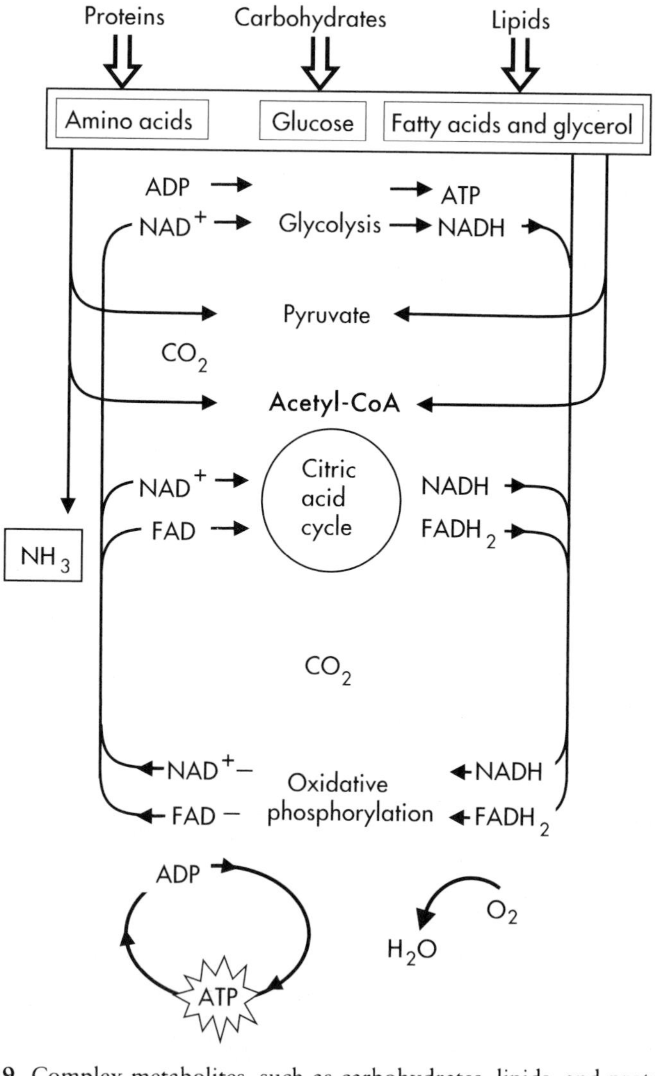

FIGURE 8-29 Complex metabolites, such as carbohydrates, lipids, and proteins, first are degraded to their monomeric units (chiefly glucose, fatty acids, glycerol, and amino acids) and then to the common intermediate, acetyl coenzyme A (acetyl-CoA). The acetyl group is then oxidized to carbon dioxide by means of the citric acid cycle, with concomitant reduction of oxidized sodium dialysate (NAD^+) and flavin adenine dinucleotide (FAD). Reoxidation of these latter coenzymes via the electron-transport chain and oxidative phosphorylation yields water and adenosine triphosphate (ATP). (From Voet D, Voet, JG: *Biochemistry*, New York, 1990, Wiley.)

phate serve as an energy reservoir.[398] Intracellular concentrations of ATP are tightly regulated and quickly depleted. When intracellular ATP is elevated, high-energy bonds are transferred to phosphagens; when ATP is low, phosphagens transfer the high-energy bonds to adenosine 5′-diphosphate (ADP). Consequently, intracellular adenine nucleotide concentrations provide the cell with a sensitive control mechanism for regulating energy-requiring and energy-yielding reactions.[26]

Regulatory Sites for Intermediary Metabolism

CARBOHYDRATE METABOLISM. Carbohydrates serve as the body's energy source when energy is quickly needed, providing 4 kcal/g of oxidized carbohydrate. In addition, some tissues are glucose dependent (e.g., the brain, erythrocytes, leukocytes, and wounds). Glucose is derived from food, pyruvate and lactate, gluconeogenic amino acids, and the glycerol moiety of lipids, as well as from the storage form, glycogen.

Most of the body's glycogen is stored in the liver, skeletal muscle, and cardiac muscle. Hepatic glycogen is used primarily to provide glucose to glucose-dependent tissue. Muscle glycogen is not available for free release to other tissues, because glucose-6-phosphatase is not present in muscle.[480] Insulin and the action of steroids activate glycogen synthetase, through a poorly understood process. Epinephrine inhibits the enzyme through cAMP-dependent stimulation of a protein kinase. The breakdown of glycogen is initiated by the enzyme glycogen phosphorylase (phosphophosphorylase), which yields glucose-1-phosphate and a glycogen molecule that has one fewer glucose molecule.[302] Phosphoglucomutase converts glucose-1-phosphate to glucose-6-phosphate, which enters glycolysis. Glycogen phosphorylase is stimulated by AVP and angiotensin II through calcium, and by glucagon and epinephrine through a cAMP-dependent mechanism.[313]

As noted in Figure 8-30, glycolysis involves three nonreversible reactions: conversion of glucose to glucose-6-phosphate (by hexokinase); conversion of fructose-6-phosphate to fructose-1,6-diphosphate (by PFK); and conversion of phosphoenolpyruvate to pyruvate (by pyruvate kinase). These irreversible reactions are ideally suited to control the rate of glycolysis.[480] The activities of the corresponding enzymes are modified by hormones and substrates, including insulin, adenosine monophosphate (AMP), ADP, pyrophosphate, fructose-1,6-biphosphate, fructose-2,6-biphosphate, glucose-1,6-biphosphate, ammonium ion, phosphorus (increases PFK activity), ATP, citrate, 2,3-phosphoglycerate, and alpha-glycerophosphate (decreases PFK activity).[47,480] Hexokinase activity appears to be inhibited by glucose-6-phosphate[480] and, to a lesser extent, by ATP and AMP. Although pyruvate kinase activity in human muscle appears to have few regulatory properties, pyruvate kinase in the liver and adipose tissue is inhibited by ATP and citrate.[47]

Regulation of PFK is linked to hexokinase. For example, inhibition of phosphofructokinase leads to accumulation of glucose-6-phosphate, which inhibits hexokinase.[480] Inhibition of hexokinase causes intracellular accumulation of glucose and inhibits glucose transport. Consequently, inhibition of either PFK or hexokinase decreases glucose uptake.

In the absence of inhibition, glucose catabolism rapidly proceeds to pyruvate. Under aerobic conditions, most tissues oxidatively decarboxylate pyruvate, by means of pyruvate dehydrogenase, to acetyl-CoA and then oxidize the acetyl-CoA in the TCA cycle. However, because this reaction requires oxygen, under anaerobic conditions, the pyruvate formed must be converted to lactate. As a result, elevated tissue and plasma concentrations of lactate, generated by anaerobic glycolysis, are characteristic of ischemia and anoxia. Furthermore, some tissues (e.g., erythrocytes and leukocytes) can only convert pyruvate to lactate, even if abundant oxygen is present. Although these cells derive their energy entirely from glycolysis, it is aerobic rather than anaerobic.

Because of their metabolic needs, glucose-dependent tissues must have glucose available at all times. Glucose is derived from hepatic glycogen, from exogenously ingested glucose, and from the synthesis of glucose. Gluconeogenesis can proceed from lactate, pyruvate, glycerol, and amino acids. However, comparison of Figure 8-30 with Figure 8-31 should not suggest that gluconeogenesis can occur by reversing glycolysis; gluconeogenesis and glycolysis have the same intermediates.

Glycolysis requires three unidirectional steps, which are bypassed primarily in the liver and secondarily in the kidneys, due to the presence of four regulated enzymes (Figure 8-31).[368,382] The first of these enzymes is pyruvate carboxylase; in the presence of ATP, carbon dioxide (CO_2), and biotin, it converts pyruvate to oxaloacetate in the mitochondria. Oxaloacetate is then converted to phosphoenolpyruvate by the cytoplasmic enzyme PEPCK. Oxaloacetate must cross the mitochondrial membranes into the cytoplasm, because oxaloacetate is formed in the mitochondria, and PEPCK is formed in the cytoplasm. Because oxaloacetate cannot permeate the mitochondrial membrane, it must be shuttled across as aspartate or malate before reconversion to oxaloacetate in the cytoplasm.[126]

Once phosphoenolpyruvate is formed, glycolysis can proceed quickly in the reverse direction to fructose-1, 6-biphosphate, at which point the enzyme fructose-1,6-biphosphatase forms fructose-6-phosphate. This enzyme, which is present primarily in the liver, kidneys and, to a lesser extent, in skeletal muscle, is not present in adipose tissue or cardiac and smooth muscle. Fructose-6-phosphate then proceeds to glucose-6-phosphate.

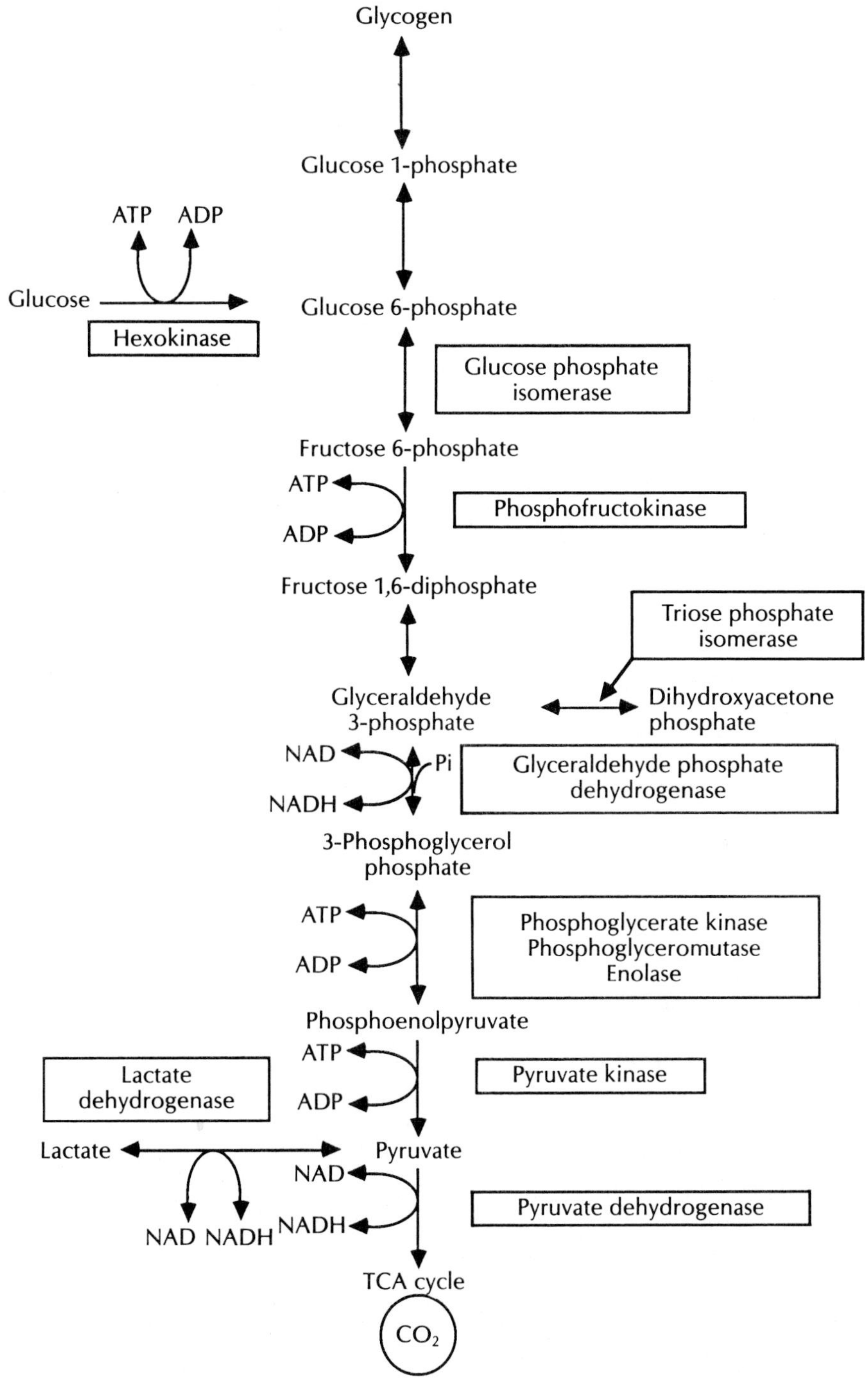

FIGURE 8-30 Glycolysis.

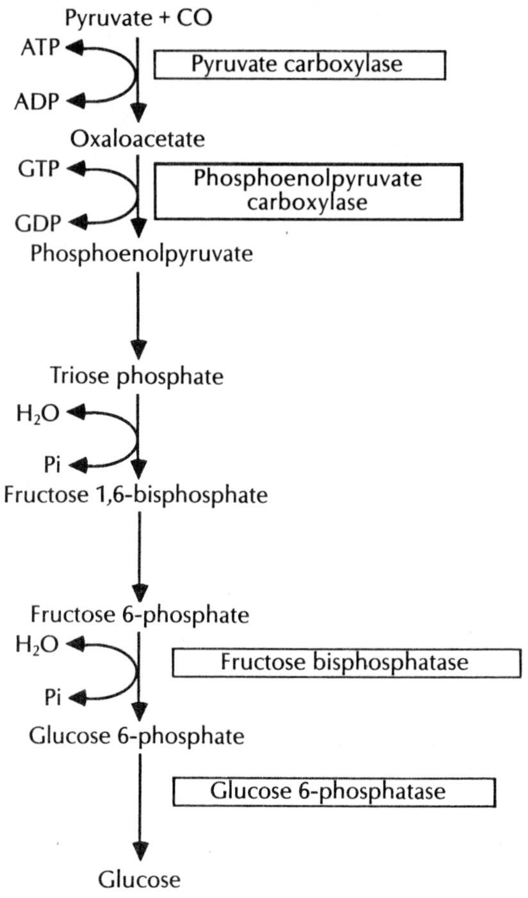

FIGURE 8-31 Gluconeogenesis in the liver and kidneys.

Conversion of the latter intermediate to glucose requires the presence of the fourth gluconeogenic enzyme, glucose-6-phosphatase. This enzyme is present in liver and kidney tissue but not in skeletal muscle. Consequently, free glucose can be released from the liver and kidneys but not from other tissues.

Constant production of lactate and pyruvate in aerobic glycolytic tissues ensures a constant supply of lactate and pyruvate to the liver for gluconeogenesis. The newly formed glucose is available for metabolism by glucose-dependent tissues through reconversion to lactate in the Cori or glucose-lactate cycle (Figure 8-32). Although no additional glucose carbon is provided by the Cori cycle (the glucose formed is derived from lactate that previously existed as glucose), it is important to glucose homeostasis. Under anaerobic conditions, this process assumes even greater importance, because glucose is converted to lactate by ischemic and anoxic tissues, which under aerobic conditions convert glucose to CO_2.

Protein Metabolism

Proteins are essential components of all living cells. They are necessary for growth; metabolism (enzymes); regulation (protein kinases, receptors, and transport systems); replication (spindles, cell membranes); protection (immunoglobins, lymphokines, and membranes); repair (collagen); communication (hormones, neurotransmitters); and motion of individual cells (contractile elements), as well as for coordinated functioning of the entire organism. Consequently, it is striking that, excluding connective tissue and bone, cellular protein accounts for only 11% of the total body weight of a 70 kg man, 87% of which occurs in the form of skeletal muscle.[455,639] Although protein has no true storage form, energy and glucose can be derived from the metabolism of amino acids. Protein catabolism is accompanied by the loss of body function when the amino acids are drafted from skeletal muscle stores or derived from the diet.

In general, the catabolism of all amino acids involves removal of the alpha-amino group from the carbon skeleton of the amino acid to form ammonia and an alpha-keto acid, followed by conversion of ammonia to urea and of alpha-keto acids to intermediates or precursors of the TCA cycle.[383] Although deamination and transformation of all alpha-amino acids to alpha-keto acid

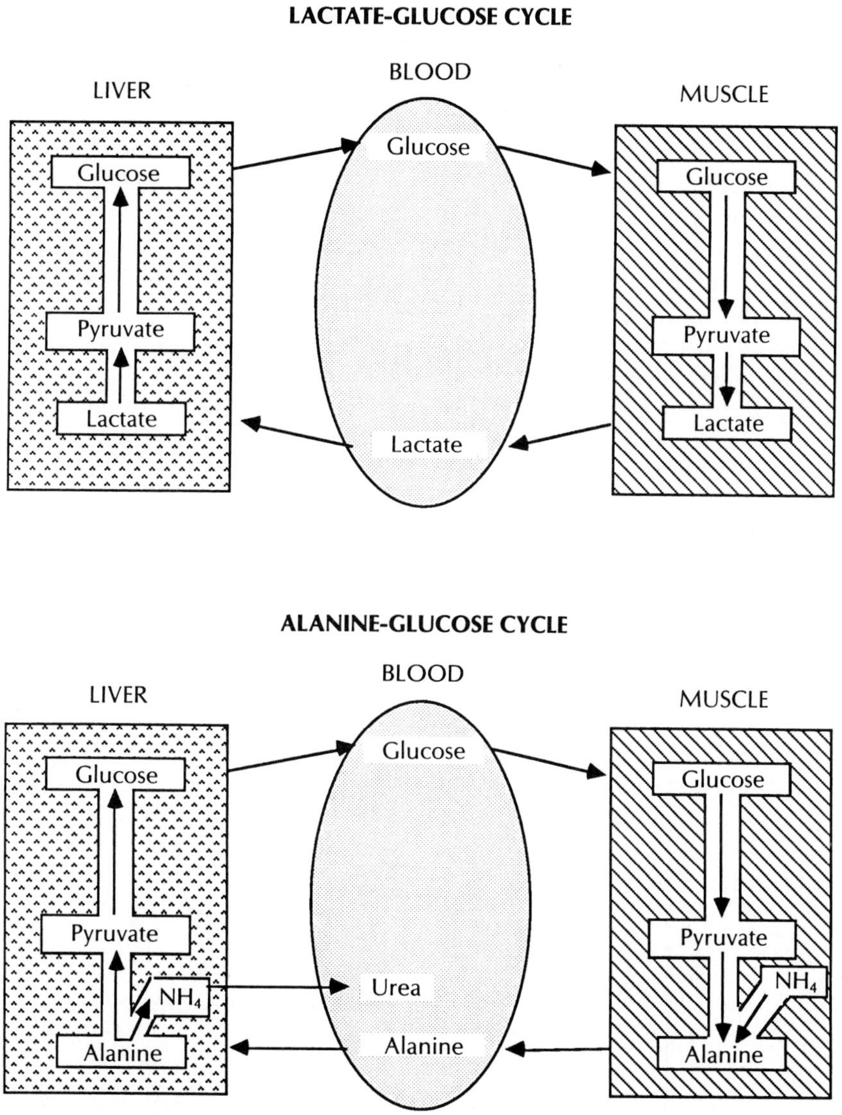

FIGURE 8-32 Glucose-lactate and glucose-alanine cycles.

secretagogue for renin release is mitogen action for angiotensin II for human mesangial cells, an action that is partly mediated by endothelin.[35]

Aldosterone

Aldosterone is synthesized and secreted by cells of the adrenal zona glomerulosa in response to at least three stimuli: angiotensin II, ACTH, and an increase in the potassium ion concentration.

Angiotensin II is a potent stimulator of aldosterone secretion, which acts through calcium-dependent, cAMP-independent enhancement[212,248] of the conversion of cholesterol to pregnenolone and of corticosterone to 18-hydroxycorticosterone and aldosterone.[355] Of these steps, early conversion of cholesterol to pregnenolone appears to be the most important to the stimulation of aldosterone secretion by angiotensin II.[5]

ACTH stimulates the secretion of aldosterone through a calcium-dependent, cAMP-dependent pathway.[212,248,355] Like angiotensin, ACTH stimulates early conversion of cholesterol to pregnenolone,[5] but it does not appear to stimulate the later steps of aldosterone biosynthesis in humans.[5]

A rise in serum potassium also produces stimulation of aldosterone secretion.[669] This occurs through a calcium-dependent, cAMP-independent increase in the conversion of cholesterol to pregnenolone.[212,248]

There is evidence that humans have an aldosterone-stimulating hormone (ASH) that is produced by the pituitary gland.[588] This glycoprotein (which has been isolated in the urine of normal individuals but not in that of patients who have undergone hypophysectomy) stimulates the secretion of aldosterone in vitro.[86] ASH also has caused hypertension and hyperaldosteronism in experimental models. Immunofluorescent studies have located it in the anterior pituitary gland,[588] but the exact structure has not yet been determined.

On a molar basis, ACTH is the most potent stimulator of aldosterone production.[669] As a result, stress-induced increases in aldosterone probably are mediated through ACTH. However, ACTH's stimulatory effect on aldosterone production is short lived, a phenomenon that has been attributed either to down-regulation of ACTH on zona glomerulosa cells or to inhibition of angiotensin II synthesis by an increase in the effective circulating volume.[42,669] This short-lived potency suggests that ACTH plays a minor role in the overall control of aldosterone secretion in chronic states.[669] In chronic conditions, angiotensin II most likely is the primary stimulus for aldosterone secretion. This premise is supported by the finding that sodium restriction in ACTH-deficient individuals evokes an appropriate increase in the release of aldosterone.[42,361]

The existence of an inhibitory dopaminergic pathway that blocks the later stages of aldosterone synthesis has been suggested.[669] This may explain the fact that metaclopropramide, a dopamine antagonist, causes increased secretion of aldosterone, whereas bromocriptine, a dopamine agonist, inhibits the secretion of aldosterone stimulated by ACTH or angiotensin II but does not change the basal secretory rate of aldosterone.[439] This pathway may be important in mediating changes in aldosterone secretion that occur in response to changes in the plasma sodium concentration or the effective circulating volume.[7,110]

The primary actions of aldosterone are increasing reabsorption of sodium and chloride in the early distal convoluted tubule of the kidney epithelia and the gastrointestinal (GI) tract. Aldosterone also promotes sodium reabsorption and potassium secretion in the late distal convoluted tubules and the early collecting ducts.[42,501] On a cellular level, aldosterone acts at surface receptors (rapid response) and by forming activated, nuclear-bound complexes similar to those of other steroids (genomic response). The proteins induced by aldosterone stimulate an increase in the number of membrane sodium-specific channels and in the activities of mitochondrial enzymes that generate ATP[136] (Figure 8-21).

Insulin

Synthesis and secretion of insulin by the beta-islet cells of the pancreas are controlled by at least three mechanisms: the concentration of circulating substrate (glucose, amino acids, and free fatty acids); the activity of the autonomic nervous system; and the direct and indirect effects of several hormones. An increase in the plasma concentration of glucose stimulates the secretion of insulin through central glucoreceptors and direct pancreatic beta-cell activation. A decrease in the glucose concentration inhibits the secretion of insulin through similar pathways.[636] Insulin secretion is also stimulated by an increase in the plasma concentration of amino acids and possibly by an increase in the concentration of free fatty acids and ketone bodies. Under normal physiologic conditions, the plasma concentration of glucose is the most important controller of insulin secretion. However, during injury and stress, the effect of glucose is blunted by neural and humoral mechanisms (the so-called insulin resistance).[9]

As noted previously, beta-islet cells have a greater density of alpha-adrenergic receptors (which inhibit insulin secretion) than of beta-adrenergic receptors (which stimulate insulin secretion). As a result, stimulation of the sympathetic innervation of the pancreas or an increase in the circulating concentration of epinephrine or norepinephrine produces an inhibition of the secretion of insulin. In contrast, infusion of isoproterenol, a pure beta-agonist, produces an increase in insulin secretion. Parasympathetic stimulation of the pancreas increases insulin secretion.[532]

derivatives can occur in most tissues, complete oxidation of alpha-amino acids to urea and CO_2 occurs primarily in the liver and, to a lesser extent, in the kidneys (Figure 8-33).

The alpha-amino group of amino acids can be removed through one of three processes. The most common mechanism involves transamination between a pair of alpha-amino acids and a pair of alpha-keto acids, with at least 12 of the alpha-amino acids undergoing transamination.[383] These reactions, which require the presence of pyridoxal phosphate and an amino acid–specific transaminase, are freely reversible and consequently function in both amino acid synthesis and catabolism. Through the collective action of all the transaminases, the alpha-amino groups are collected in the peripheral tissues in the form of glutamate or alanine and transported to the liver.

In the liver, alpha-ketoglutarate accepts the alpha-amino group from all amino acids that are transaminated, including alanine. The movement of transaminated amino acids from peripheral tissues is the basis of the glucose-alanine cycle, which is analogous to the glucose-lactate cycle[216,422] (see Figure 8-32). According to this theory, alpha-amino acids are transaminated with pyruvate in peripheral tissues to form alanine and an alpha-keto acid. The alanine is then transported to the liver, where it is transaminated with alpha-ketoglutarate to form pyruvate and glutamate. The pyruvate can then serve as a substrate for gluconeogenesis to form new glucose, which is available for reuptake by peripheral tissues and reconversion to pyruvate.[216]

As is apparent, transamination does not eliminate the alpha-amino group; it only transfers it to another carbon skeleton to form a new alpha-amino acid. The process of oxidative deamination is an important mechanism for eliminating the alpha-amino group in general and for regenerating alpha-ketoglutarate in particular. In this process, the alpha-amino group of the amino acid is oxidatively removed by an amino acid–specific oxidase, resulting in the formation of an alpha-keto acid and free ammonia. Although amino acid oxidases are found in both the liver and kidneys for a variety of amino acids, the only one of physiologic importance in humans is glutamate oxidase, which generates alpha-ketoglutarate from glutamate.[383]

A few amino acids use nonoxidative deamination to eliminate the alpha-amino group. Serine and threonine undergo nonoxidative deamination by dehydration, and histidine undergoes direct deamination.

The free ammonia generated during deamination must be eliminated, because it is poorly tolerated by cells, even in small concentrations. The primary mechanism

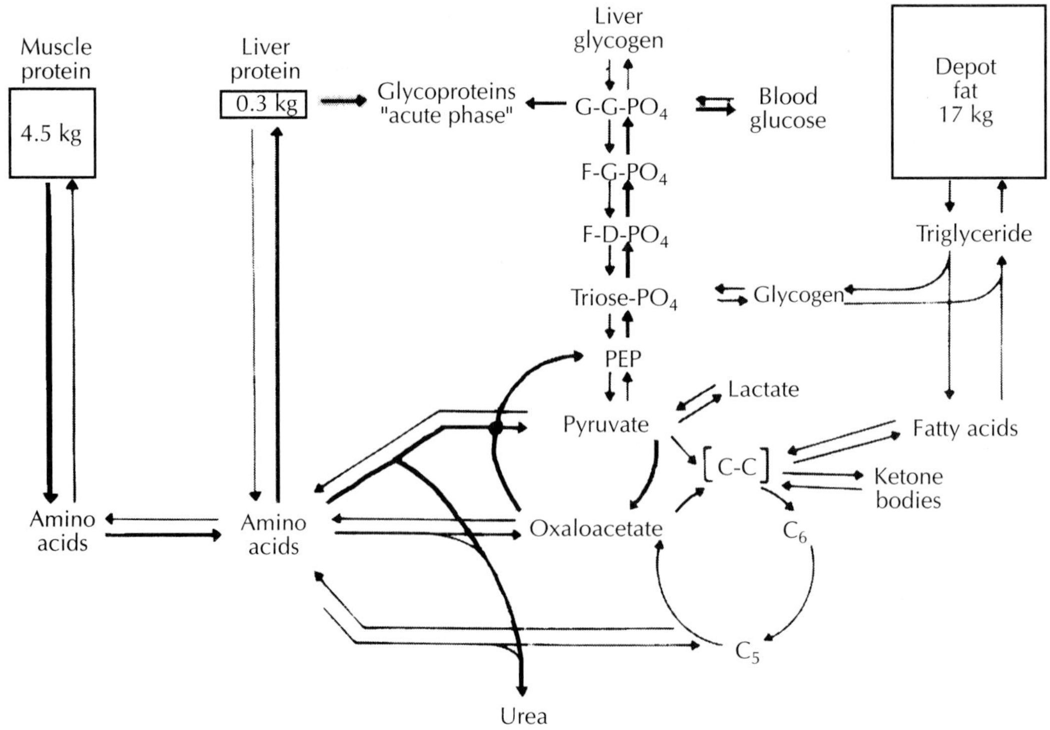

FIGURE 8-33 A major feature of catabolism is the breakdown of muscle protein to provide amino acids, which can be deaminated for gluconeogenesis or taken up directly by viscera (e.g., the liver) for synthesis of new protein.

in brain and muscle cells involves adding ammonia to glutamate, which forms glutamine. The free ammonia may also be eliminated by adding it to alpha-ketoglutarate in a freely reversible reaction that is catalyzed by glutamate synthetase. The resulting glutamate can be used in the synthesis of proteins, citrulline, and arginine, or as an alpha-amino donor in transamination reactions.

Although these two ammonia-clearing reactions can account for a substantial amount of ammonia, most ammonia formed is cleared by the liver in the urea (Krebs-Henseleit) cycle (Figures 8-34 and 8-35) or by the kidneys through excretion of free ammonia. Two thirds of the ammonia excreted by the kidneys is derived from the amide nitrogen of glutamine in renal arterial blood, and one third is derived from the alpha-amino nitrogen of renal arterial amino acids.[665]

The carbon skeletons remaining after amino acid deamination or transamination are converted either to intermediates of the TCA cycle or to precursors of acetyl-CoA, such as pyruvate and oxaloacetate. As a result, all the carbon skeletons of alpha-amino acids can be oxidized in the TCA cycle to provide energy or can be converted either to glucose through gluconeogenesis or to fat through lipogenesis. The carbon skeletons of seven of the 22 most common amino acids found in proteins (alanine, serine, glycine, cysteine, cystine, threonine, and hydroxyproline) are converted to pyruvate. Depending on the oxidation-reduction state of the cell, these carbon skeletons can then be used in gluconeogenesis or lipogenesis, or for energy. The carbon skeletons of five amino acids (leucine, lysine, phenylalanine, tyrosine, and tryptophan) form acetoacetate. As a result, these amino acids can be used either for energy (TCA cycle) or for lipogenesis. However, they cannot be used for gluconeogenesis because by the time the acetyl-CoA gets to malate, the molecule of acetyl-CoA that entered the TCA cycle has been completely oxidized. In contrast, amino acids whose carbon skeletons can enter the TCA cycle after the acetyl-CoA step can be used for gluconeogenesis but not for lipogenesis. Even though phenylalanine, tyrosine, tryptophan, and lysine are cleaved into acetoacetate, they also produce molecules that can enter the TCA cycle at non-acetyl-CoA steps (fumarate and pyruvate). As a result, they can donate carbon atoms for both gluconeogenesis and lipogenesis. Other amino acids that can be used for either energy or gluconeogenesis are isoleucine, methionine, and valine (which are cleaved into succinyl-CoA); aspartate and arginine (which are cleaved into oxaloacetate), and glutamate, glutamine, proline, histidine, and arginine (which are cleaved into alpha-ketoglutarate).

Lipid Metabolism

Lipids, which are stored in adipose tissue as triglycerides, constitute the largest energy source in the body, providing 9.4 kcal/g of lipid oxidized. These molecules are used by all tissues that are not glucose dependent for energy, including cardiac and skeletal muscle, adipose tissue, and the liver, pancreas, and lungs. Triglycerides are composed of three fatty acid chains linked together by a glycerol molecule. During lipolysis, the fatty acids are sequentially cleaved off the glycerol moiety by lipases. The remaining glycerate is then used in the synthesis of new glucose or converted to pyruvate for oxidation in the TCA cycle.

The catabolism of fatty acids can be divided into two stages: beta-oxidation in the outer mitochondrial membrane to produce multiple molecules of acetyl-CoA, followed by processing of the acetyl-CoA in the mitochondria to produce either ketone bodies (through ketogenesis) or CO_2 and energy (through the TCA cycle)[400,427] (see Figure 8-28). Only the first step in this process,

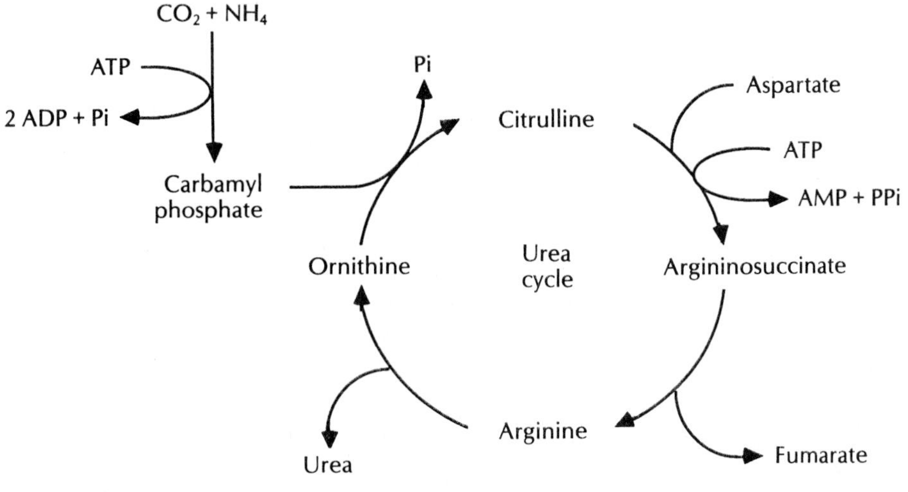

FIGURE 8-34 Urea cycle.

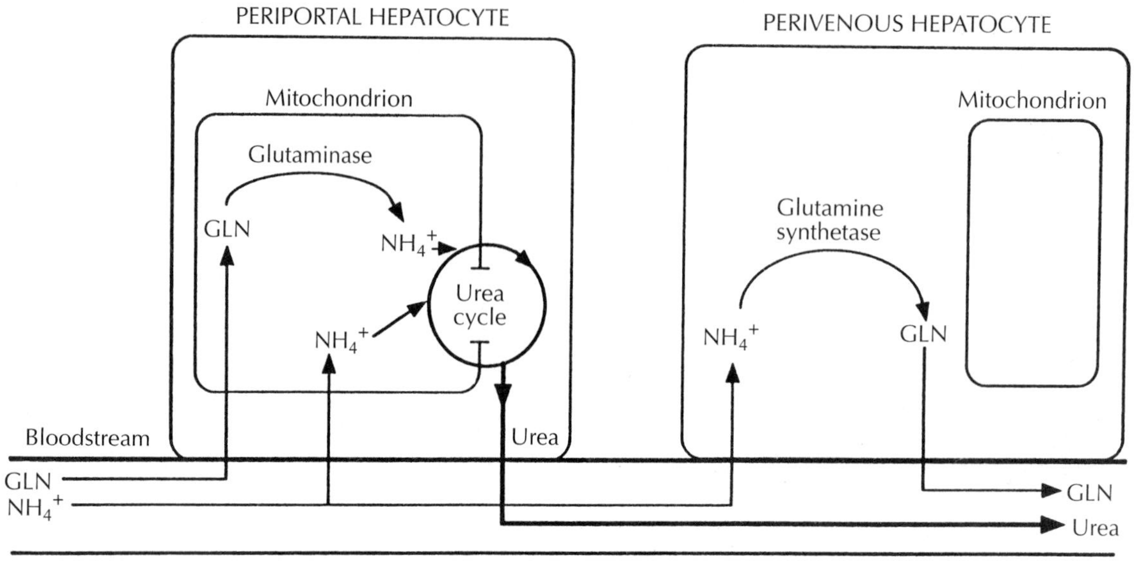

FIGURE 8-35 Hepatocyte heterogeneity in the liver. Periportal hepatocytes contain glutaminase and urea cycle enzymes; the perivenous cells express glutamine synthetase. Glutaminase, which is activated by ammonia in the periportal cells, can control the urea cycle. Glutamine synthetase acts as a downstream scavenger by converting ammonia to glutamine and preventing ammonia intoxication (From Souba WW: *Annu Rev Nutr* 11:285, 1991.)

catalyzed by thiokinase, requires energy; thus it serves as a major regulator of the rate of lipolysis. In beta-oxidation, thiokinase adds coenzyme A (CoA) to a fatty acid, forming a fatty acyl-CoA, which then undergoes a sequence of reversible reactions until the final two carbons, along with the CoA group, are cleaved off; this produces an acetyl-CoA group, five high-energy phosphate bonds, and a new fatty acyl-CoA that is two carbons shorter than the parent fatty acid. With even-numbered fatty acids, this process continues until the entire fatty acid has been sequentially cleaved. With odd-numbered fatty acids, the process continues until a three-carbon fragment (propionyl-CoA) remains. Propionyl-CoA is converted to succinyl-CoA and used in the TCA cycle.

As a result of their ultimate breakdown to acetyl-CoA, lipids cannot be converted to glucose and are used only as a source of energy and ketone bodies, or to form new lipids. Ketone bodies, which are formed exclusively in the liver, can be used by a variety of tissues, including the brain, as a source of energy through conversion to acetyl-CoA. Formation of ketone bodies in the liver is catalyzed by the enzyme thiolase in a readily reversible reaction that combines two molecules of acetyl-CoA to form a molecule of acetoacetyl-CoA.[99] Acetoacetyl-CoA is then converted to 3-hydroxy-3-methylglutaryl-CoA, the precursor for cholesterol synthesis and formation of the three ketone bodies (acetoacetate, beta-hydroxybutyrate, and acetone) in the Lynen cycle. The enzyme that catalyzes this reaction, 3-hydroxy-3-methylglutaryl-CoA synthetase, appears to be the regulatory enzyme in the synthesis of ketone bodies and cholesterol, but little is known about the factors that inhibit or stimulate it. Under conditions in which the liver's glycogen content is high, beta-hydroxybutyrate predominates, whereas under conditions in which the liver's glycogen content is low, acetoacetate predominates. As a result, the ratio of beta-hydroxybutyrate to acetoacetate in the liver (normally 3:1) can be used as a reflection of hepatic glycogen stores and the oxidation-reduction state of mitochondria in the liver.

In addition to the TCA and Lynen cycles, acetyl-CoA formed from lipolysis or other sources can be used in the synthesis of new fatty acids and, ultimately, triglycerides. Lipogenesis is a cytoplasmic process that requires malonyl-CoA, which is formed from acetyl-CoA by acetyl-CoA carboxylase. This enzyme is the rate-limiting enzyme in lipogenesis. When the intracellular concentrations of free fatty acids are low, acetyl-CoA carboxylase is stimulated, leading to increased formation of malonyl-CoA.[379] In turn, the increase in the concentration of malonyl-CoA inhibits carnitine acetyltransferase (the enzyme necessary for the transport of acetyl-CoA into the mitochondria), resulting in an increase in the cytoplasmic concentration of acetyl-CoA, which can be used for the synthesis of more malonyl-CoA.[436] In con-

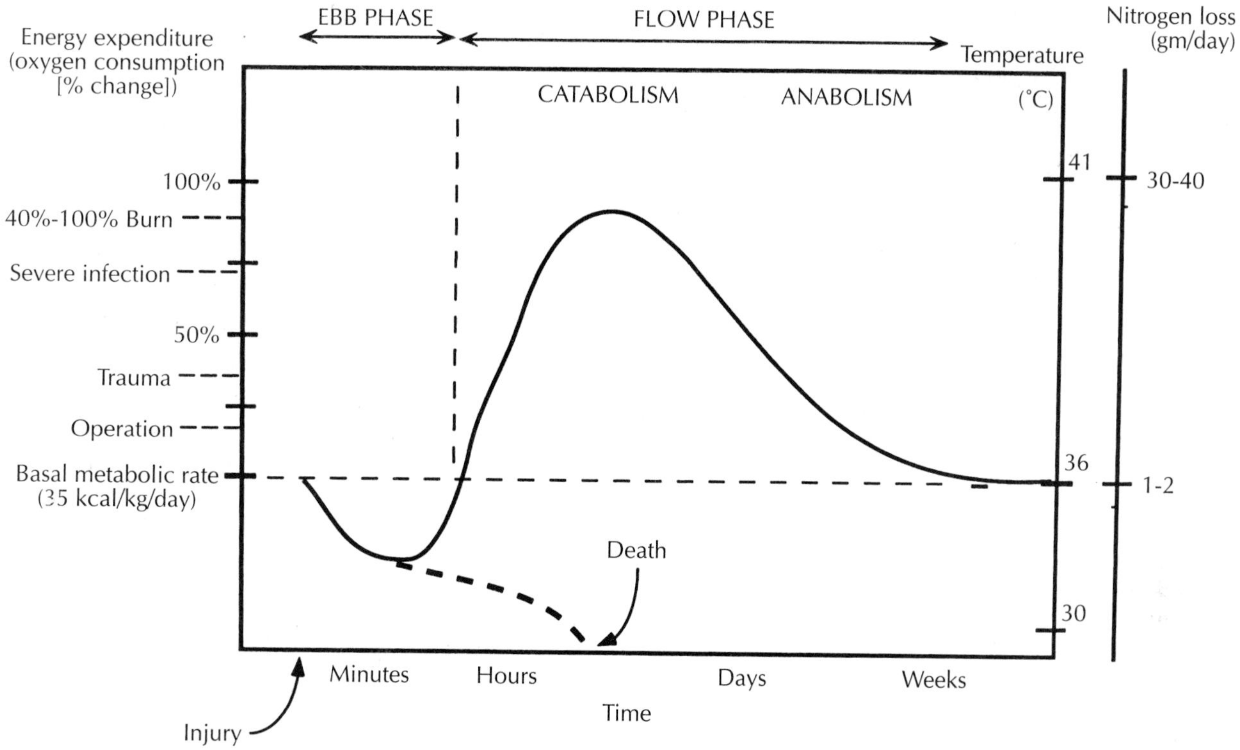

FIGURE 8-36 Ebb and flow phases of the metabolic response to injury. Corresponding changes in energy expenditure (oxygen consumption), body temperature, and nitrogen loss are elicited by major injury (near 100% full-thickness burn). Inadequate biologic compensation results in death.

trast, when the intracellular concentrations of free fatty acids are high, acetyl-CoA carboxylase is inhibited, leading to a decrease in the formation of malonyl-CoA; this stimulates carnitine acetyltransferase, increasing the transport of acetyl-CoA into the mitochondria for oxidation and ketogenesis, and inhibiting lipogenesis.[435]

Another feature of the inhibition of acetyl-CoA carboxylase is the accumulation of cytoplasmic citrate, which as noted previously, can inhibit glycolysis by inhibiting phosphofructokinase (the Randle effect).[480]

Metabolism in Injured Patients

The posttraumatic state is characterized by immobilization, starvation, and repair. Although starvation and immobilization are associated with a reduction in energy requirements, reparative processes are associated with an increase in energy needs. As a result, overall energy requirements increase for traumatized, septic, and burned individuals. Also, an increased amount of glucose is needed after injury because of an increase in the number and metabolism of inflammatory cells and fibroblasts and because of the increased glucose uptake of wounded tissue. To meet the demand for glucose, protein catabolism also must increase after injury. As a result, the metabolic response to injury is characterized by generalized catabolism, negative nitrogen balance, increased heart production and, paradoxically, hyperglycemia.

In his classic studies of the metabolic response to long-bone fractures, Cuthbertson[157] divided this metabolic response into two parts, the ebb and the flow phases (Figure 8-36). Subsequently, Moore[453] divided the flow phase into catabolic and anabolic stages.

The ebb phase encompasses the first several hours after injury and is characterized by hyperglycemia, and restoration of circulating volume and tissue perfusion. Once tissue perfusion has been restored, reparative processes can take place, and the flow phase begins.

The flow phase is characterized by generalized catabolism, negative nitrogen balance, hyperglycemia, and heat production. This phase may last from days to weeks, depending on the severity of injury, the patient's previous health, and medical intervention. Once volume deficits have been corrected, infection has been controlled, pain has been eliminated, and complete oxygenation has been restored, the anabolic phase begins.

The anabolic phase is associated with a slow but progressive reaccumulation of protein followed by the reaccumulation of body fat. This phase usually lasts considerably longer than the catabolic phase because the rate of protein catabolism may exceed 15 g/day, but the rate of protein synthesis cannot exceed 3 to 5 g/day.[467]

Energy Metabolism

Loss of body weight is a characteristic feature of injury and sepsis that derives from an increase in energy expenditure in the face of reduced or absent food intake. The increase in energy needed varies directly with the severity of injury.

Using indirect calorimetry, Kinney and Roe[369,372] have determined that in healthy individuals who undergo uncomplicated elective surgery, the resting energy expenditure (REE) increases by no more than 10%, and that patients with multiple skeletal injuries have a 10% to 25% increase. However, a febrile complication increases these requirements significantly.[187,372] Kinney and Roe[372] have estimated that REE increases 7% for each degree Fahrenheit of fever. More serious infections (e.g., peritonitis, intra-abdominal abscesses) are associated with an increase in REE (20% to 50%) that is even greater than one would predict on the basis of temperature elevation alone, and this condition persists as long as the inflammation remains. In this regard, the most severe complication is sepsis, and the most severe injury is a burn (Figure 8-37). In fact, the only surgical disorder in which the REE can exceed 50% is a major third-degree burn, and increases above 100% have been noted in these cases.[372,675] In general, the increase in REE after burns, as in other injuries, is proportional to the size and degree of the burn.

The increase in REE also depends on the person's size. The largest increases are seen in heavily muscled, well-nourished young men and the smallest in poorly nourished, elderly women. This difference reflects the larger body cell mass in the former group because REE is linearly related to body cell mass.[370]

Changes in environmental temperature also alter the REE. Cuthbertson and Tilstone[158] noted a decrease in the energy requirement of patients with long-bone fractures who were treated at 30° C (86° F) rather than 20° C (68° V).

The energy the body needs can be derived from carbohydrates, protein, or fat (Figure 8-38). However, the available stores of carbohydrate are small and without adequate nutritional intake are insufficient to supply the glucose required for glucose-dependent tissues. Similarly, protein has no storage form, and any degradation of protein for energy requires the loss or reduction of some body function. Consequently, the primary source

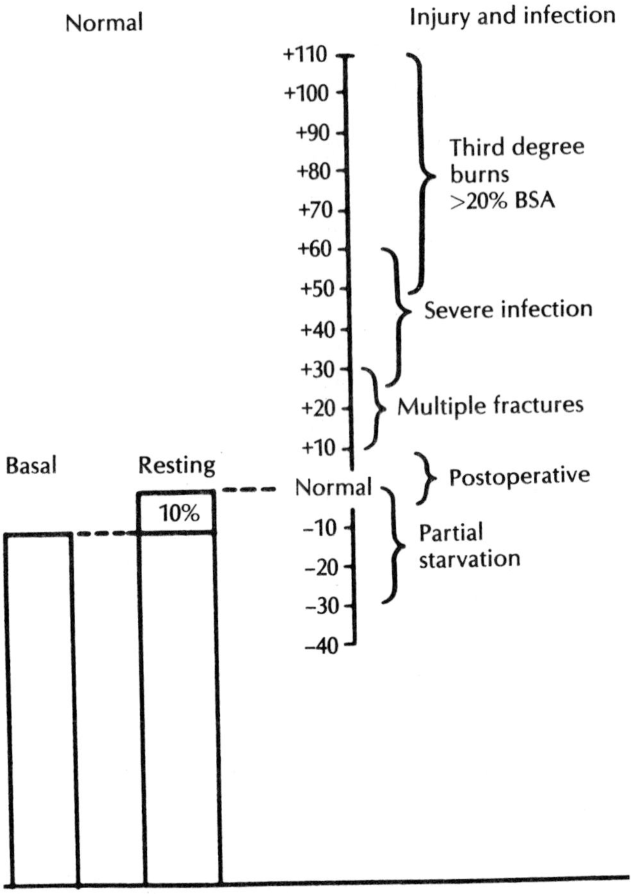

FIGURE 8-37 Changes in the resting energy expenditure of adult patients with major injuries and sepsis. (From Kinney JM, Roe CF: *Ann Surg* 156:610, 1962.)

for energy during injury is fat, which is reflected in the low respiratory quotients noted after injury and sepsis. Wilmore and associates[673] found respiratory quotients of 0.7 to 0.76 after severe burns. In addition, septic injury appears to involve a greater dependence on lipids for energy than does nonseptic injury.[27,470]

With regard to energy metabolism for specific tissues and injuries, a significant reduction in energy charge and ATP content has been noted during severe hemorrhagic shock, hypoxemia, and total ischemia in the liver, kidneys, skeletal muscle, and cardiac muscle.[128,308,321,514] These reductions, which are related to the severity of the hemorrhage or hypoxic insult, usually occur in the liver and kidneys before those in cardiac and skeletal muscle.

The different responses of these tissue types may be partly the result of the differences in blood flow and in the metabolic activity of the specific tissue examined. For example, for a given degree of hemorrhage, hepatic blood flow is reduced more than myocardial blood flow.[574,600] Furthermore, although the reduction in blood flow to skeletal muscle may be greater than that to the

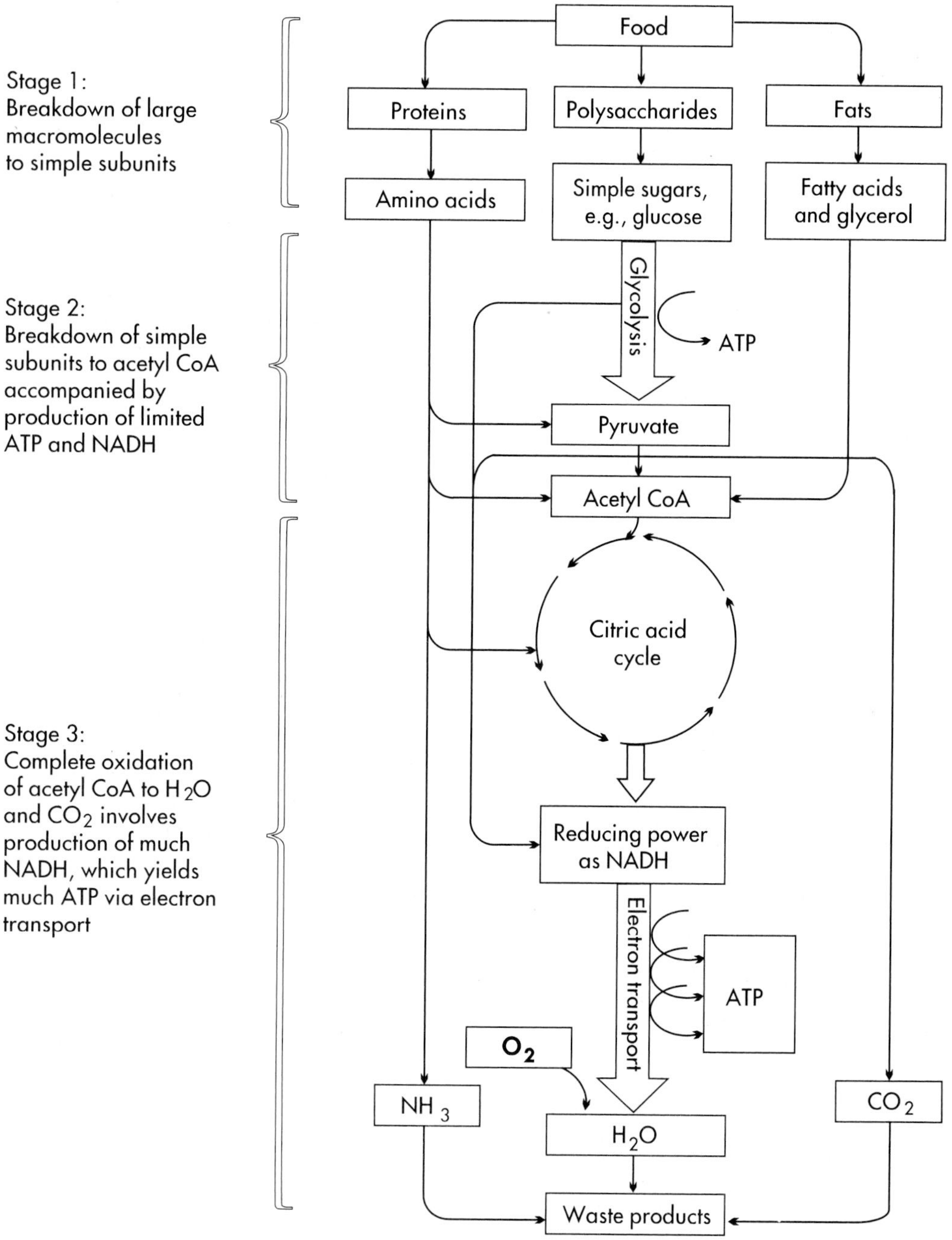

FIGURE 8-38 Stages of catabolism. Food is ultimately degraded to waste products. Cellular energy (ATP) is derived by oxidation of acetyl CoA and electron transport. (From Alberts B, Bray D, Raff LJ et al: *Molecular biology of the cell,* ed 2, New York, 1989, Garland.)

liver during hemorrhage, skeletal muscle has considerably less metabolic activity than does the liver. As a result, the energy charge of the liver is affected early in hemorrhage, whereas skeletal and cardiac muscles are more resistant. Nonetheless, a reduction in the energy charge and ATP and creatine phosphate content of all tissues eventually occurs if compensation for the hemorrhage is insufficient.

Characteristically, wounded tissue also shows a reduction in energy charge, ATP, and creatine phosphate during early healing.[336,674] Traditionally, this phenomenon has been attributed to a decrease in the production of high-energy phosphate compounds resulting from anaerobic metabolism of wounded tissue.[336,674] However, oxygen consumption and the oxidation of glucose and other substrates are not reduced in wounded tissue.[102,674] Furthermore, as is discussed subsequently in greater detail, the metabolism of wounded tissue appears to be aerobic rather than anaerobic.[102] These findings imply that wounded tissue has the same capacity for producing high-energy phosphates as normal tissue.

In addition to the decrease in production of high-energy phosphates, the reduction in the energy charge of wounded tissue could be the result of an increase in the degradation of high-energy phosphates or an artifact that results from the compartmentalization of high-energy phosphates in wounded tissue. Wounded tissue is composed of normal and injured resident tissue and an intense inflammatory infiltrate, which is composed primarily of polymorphonuclear leukocytes (PMNs) immediately after wounding, and of macrophages 5 days after wounding. These inflammatory cells, which contain few high-energy compounds, account for as much as 50% of the deoxyribonucleic acid (DNA) (and therefore 50% of the cells) present in wounded tissue.[460] This infiltrate may dilute the high-energy phosphate content of wounded tissue, even though high-energy phosphate content is normal or actually has increased. In fact, Morris and associates[460] recently demonstrated this to be the case. They also have demonstrated the presence of a macrophage-mediated factor that increases the high-energy phosphate content of wounded skeletal muscle.[463] Thus the high-energy content of resident injured tissue does not appear to be reduced after wounding and may actually be greater.

A reduction in the high-energy phosphate content of tissue has also been demonstrated for sepsis, and this is attributed to reduced production of high-energy phosphate stemming from the anaerobic metabolism that accompanies a reduction in blood flow.[12,335,406,597] Accordingly, a reduction in high-energy charge is noted only with marked reductions in blood flow. Similarly, the high-energy phosphate content of septic tissue is usually reduced.[129] This reduction also has been attributed to a decrease in the production of high-energy phosphates that occurs secondary to anaerobic metabolism. In light of the findings in nonseptic wounded tissue, one might speculate that this reduction is also dilutional, because septic tissue has an increased amount of inflammatory cell infiltrate. However, no evidence has yet been presented to support this theory.

Carbohydrate Metabolism

Unlike fasting and starvation, which are associated with hypoglycemia, the conditions of injury, sepsis, and stress are characterized by hyperglycemia. An increase in the concentration of blood glucose occurs during both the ebb and flow phases of injury and is proportional to the severity of the injury.[109,441] In addition, plasma concentrations increase for lactate, pyruvate, organic phosphates, total amino acids, glycerol, and free fatty acids. These changes in the concentrations of lactate, pyruvate, and alanine also correlate with the severity of injury.[499] The rise in the concentrations of glucose and other solutes contributes to an elevated plasma osmolality after hemorrhage and injury that is thought to be critical in the complete restitution of blood volume and plasma proteins.[181,255,257,363] In addition, the increase in blood glucose is thought to be critical in maintaining normal function in glucose-dependent tissues.

The changes in carbohydrate metabolism that occur during injury, stress, and sepsis arise primarily as the result of the actions and interactions of catecholamines, cortisol, glucagon, insulin, growth hormone, vasopressin, angiotensin II, and somatostatin.* It is well documented that the elevation in blood glucose concentration results from increased hepatic production and impaired peripheral uptake of glucose, which are at least partly under endocrine control. However, despite hyperglycemia, increased gluconeogenesis, and hepatic and peripheral insulin resistance during both the ebb and flow phases, the endocrine mechanisms involved in these carbohydrate "abnormalities" are different. During the ebb phase, plasma insulin is clearly depressed in relation to the degree of hyperglycemia.[315,464,676] This results from a reduction in B-cell sensitivity to glucose that is secondary to production of catecholamines, somatostatin, reduced pancreatic blood flow, and increased activity of the sympathetic nervous system.† An intact adrenal gland is also necessary for this response because the blunting of insulin secretion can be eliminated by adrenalectomy.[315] During the flow phase, B-cell sensitivity returns to normal, and insulin concentrations rise to more appropriate values. Nevertheless, hyperglycemia persists.[351,676]

Both the ebb and the flow phases show delayed assimilation of a glucose load, glucosuria, and resistance to exogenously administered insulin.[6,77,108] Despite this "diabetes of injury," glucose uptake and use by periph-

*References 108, 109, 193, 209, 555, and 556.
†References 77, 183, 297, 315, 505, and 532.

eral tissues in both the ebb and the flow phases have been demonstrated consistently to be greater in the ebb and flow phases of injury than under normal circumstances.* The resistance to insulin is manifested in decreased clearance of glucose. Consequently, the high plasma glucose concentration and the attendant increase in the plasma-to-tissue glucose concentration gradient appear to overcome the peripheral tissues' resistance to the entry of glucose, allowing for normal or increased glucose uptake in peripheral tissues.

Hepatic carbohydrate metabolism is also affected by insulin resistance. During the ebb phase, elevated concentrations of catecholamines, cortisol, and glucagon, and a decrease in the concentration of insulin result in rapid glycogenolysis and an outpouring of glucose from the liver. These hormonal alterations also stimulate gluconeogenesis from alanine and lactate. Growth hormone becomes involved in hepatic insulin resistance by inhibiting glucose uptake through inhibition of glucokinase. During the flow phase, gluconeogenesis persists despite near-normal concentrations of insulin.[351,676] This appears to result from insulin resistance and produces a continued flow of glucose from the liver. Therefore the hyperglycemia that occurs after injury results from a combination of increased hepatic production and release of glucose and peripheral resistance to the entry of glucose. Because production supersedes use, hyperglycemia persists. However, if the rate of gluconeogenesis decreases through a reduction in either gluconeogenic precursors or gluconeogenic enzymatic function, hepatic glucose production declines and hypoglycemia ensues, as is seen in terminal injuries and with prolonged sepsis.

Although the mechanisms in this process are not fully understood, Moore, Goodrum, and Berry[456] have suggested that the reduction in gluconeogenesis during sepsis is produced by a Kupffer cell-mediated monokine that inhibits the ability of cortisol to stimulate PEPCK. However, this is not sufficient to explain the defect because the in vitro activity of PEPCK is reduced during sepsis even though in vivo hepatic glucose production is increased, which presumably is the result of the ability of high substrate concentrations to drive gluconeogenesis in vivo, even though the in vitro activity of the enzyme is reduced. Thus it appears that a reduction in substrate is more important than a reduction in the activity of the enzyme because the high substrate concentrations can override the enzymatic inhibition produced by the monokine or other agent.[382]

Traditionally, the insulin resistance that develops after injury has been thought to arise from a reduction in the release of insulin from the pancreas and from an inhibition of insulin action on peripheral tissue that is mediated by the sympathetic nervous system, catecholamines, and cortisol.* In fact, in vitro[123] and in vivo[193,218,505] studies have consistently demonstrated the ability of these agents to blunt the release and action of insulin. However, other unidentified factors have been thought to be involved in this response. Recently, Pekala and associates[519] have demonstrated a reduction in insulin action on adipose tissue by a macrophage-mediated monokine.

After injury and during sepsis, glucose must be provided not only to red cells, white cells, renal medulla, and neural tissues but also to wounded tissues.[108,315,632] In fact, glucose uptake and lactate production in wounded tissue are increased by as much as 100% and are proportional to the circulating concentration of glucose present.[9,488] For example, in the absence of insulin, rat skeletal muscle demonstrates maximum glucose uptake at a circulating glucose concentration of 5 mM; wounded skeletal muscle does not reach maximum glucose uptake until the circulating glucose concentration exceeds 20 mM.[9]

The increase in glucose uptake in wounded tissue is associated with an increase in the activity of phosphofructokinase,[461] a major rate-limiting enzyme in glycolysis. The increase in the activity of phosphofructokinase is associated with an increase in the positive effectors of its activity (AMP, ADP, pyrophosphate, fructose-1,6-biphosphate, fructose-2,6-biphosphate, glucose-1,6-biphosphate, ammonium ion, and phosphorus) and a decrease in the negative effectors (ATP, citrate, 2,3-phosphoglycerate, and alpha-glycerolphosphate).

Despite the increase in glucose uptake and phosphofructokinase activity, wounded and burned tissues demonstrate a lack of insulin sensitivity and do not increase their glucose uptake or glycogenesis in response to insulin.[478,479,674] However, the accelerated glucose uptake in wounded and burned tissues does correlate with the degree of inflammatory cellular infiltrate.[632,674] Our laboratories have recently demonstrated that at least 80% of the glucose uptake of wounded tissue and most of the increase above the resting rate of nonwounded muscle can be explained by glucose uptake in the inflammatory cells. Furthermore, the inflammatory infiltrate may actually mediate an increase in glucose uptake of the wounded noninflammatory tissue itself because the uptake of glucose by muscle in the presence of macrophages is greater than that of muscle not exposed to macrophages.[462]

Traditionally, the increase in glucose uptake and lactate production by wounded, burned, and septic tissue has been attributed to anaerobic glycolysis that results from local tissue hypoxia and a reduction in local tissue perfusion.[336,674] For this to be true, at least three findings should be consistently demonstrated: oxygen consump-

*References 182, 414, 566, 639, and 676.

*References 123, 193, 218, 464, 505, and 555.

tion of wounded tissue should be less than that of nonwounded tissue; glucose oxidation should be less in wounded tissue; and an increase in the supply of oxygen to wounded tissue should result in an increase in oxygen consumption and glucose oxidation and a decrease in lactate production.

In fact, none of these findings has been consistently demonstrated in wounded and burned tissue. Wilmore and associates[674] and Turinsky[632] studied burned tissue, and Caldwell and associates[102] studied wounded muscle tissue; these researchers found no difference between injured and healthy tissue in the consumption of oxygen or the oxidation of glucose, despite an increase in glucose use by the injured tissue. Turinsky[632] found an increase in lactate production when the oxygen content of burned tissue was reduced, which implies that at least some of the glucose metabolism of wounded tissue is aerobic. However, Wilmore and associates[674] were not able to reduce the lactate production of burned tissue when the oxygen supply to wounded tissue was increased.

Together these data strongly suggest that glucose metabolism in wounded and burned tissue is aerobic and *not* anaerobic, as was traditionally thought. In aerobic glycolysis, glucose proceeds to lactate in the presence of adequate concentrations of oxygen and normal substrate oxidation. Thus oxygen consumption and CO_2 production are normal, but lactate production is increased.

The presence of aerobic glycolysis has been demonstrated in the lambda-carrageenan–wounded hindlimb model used in our laboratory.[102] The oxygen consumption of wounded hindlimbs was no different from that of nonwounded hindlimbs. Furthermore, the ability of the wounded tissue to oxidize glucose, pyruvate, leucine, and palmitate was the same. Thus in the face of normal oxygen consumption and an equal potential to oxidize various substrates, the glycolysis of wounded tissue is aerobic rather than anaerobic, and from the available data it can also be inferred that this is true for burned tissue.

Although the exact mechanisms for aerobic glycolysis are not known, they may be related to an inability of the reduced nicotinamide adenine dinucleotide (NADH) shuttle to transfer reducing equivalents from the cytoplasm to the mitochondria.[321,474] Aerobic glycolysis is characteristic of the cellular inflammatory infiltrate that accompanies wounds and burns.[561,619]

Under normal conditions, resting PMNs, monocytes, and macrophages, when stimulated by a variety of agents, increase their conversion of glucose to lactate aerobically. Teleologically, one can speculate that this gives the white cell the ability to save oxygen for its important phagocytic functions by providing energy through a nonoxidative pathway. Furthermore, because the lactate released by white cells can be reconverted to glucose in the liver and used locally by a variety of tissues,[12] the white cells can provide their energy without depleting the potential glucose available. Although this is less fuel efficient than the oxidative pathway, it does tend to ensure that white cells do not become energy rich, oxygen poor, and unable to carry out their phagocytic functions.

Concerning wounded tissue, current data favor the viewpoint that the increase in glucose uptake and lactate release, as manifested in aerobic glycolysis, is the result of aerobic metabolism in the inflammatory infiltrate because most of the increase in glucose uptake in wounded tissue is attributable to the white cells present in the wound. However, there may also be augmentation of glucose uptake in the wounded, noninflammatory tissue that is mediated by the infiltrate, but it is not known if this is oxidative, nonoxidative aerobic, or nonoxidative anaerobic metabolism.

Metabolic derangements suggestive of aerobic glycolysis have also been seen in septic and endotoxic tissue.[560] Classically, sepsis and endotoxicosis are associated with an increase in peripheral glucose use and lactate production, and no change in glucose oxidation or oxygen consumption. For example, Romanosky and associates[560] found that, 1 hour after in vivo administration of a small dose of endotoxin, increases in glucose uptake and lactate production occurred in the gracilis muscle of a dog that were not associated with any change in oxygen consumption. They concluded that endotoxin had mediated a direct increase in glucose uptake in skeletal muscle that was secondary to anaerobic glycolysis. Because there was no detectable difference in blood flow, it appeared that this was the result of a defect in the ability of this muscle to use oxygen. In fact, the increase in glucose uptake and lactate production during sepsis and endotoxicosis typically has been ascribed to inadequate tissue perfusion and hypoxia or to a defect in the cells' ability to use oxygen.[603]

It is apparent that these findings can be equally explained by aerobic rather than by anaerobic glycolysis. Our laboratory has attempted to demonstrate this by using an isolated perfused hindlimb model.[12] Unexpectedly, low-dose endotoxin did not alter glucose uptake in skeletal muscle. This finding suggests that endotoxin does not directly change glucose uptake in skeletal muscle. The difference in our findings compared to those of Romanosky and associates[560] may be the result of the absence of leukocytes from the perfusate of the hindlimb preparation. As noted previously, leukocytes are one of the few tissues in the body that normally convert glucose to lactate aerobically rather than anaerobically. Furthermore, endotoxin's ability to stimulate aerobic glycolysis in PMNs and macrophages is well documented.[143]

Protein Metabolism

As one might expect, negative nitrogen balance and net proteolysis are characteristic of the shock, posttraumatic, and septic states.[2,157,453,603] However, only 20% of the protein broken down is used for calories.[185] The remainder is used by the liver and kidneys to produce glucose, which is reflected in the accelerated ureagenesis that is noted after injury.[454] As noted previously, this results primarily from an increase in the circulating concentrations of cortisol, glucagon, and catecholamines and the decreased effectiveness of insulin.

The rise in urinary nitrogen concentration is associated with increased excretion of urea, sulfur, phosphorus, potassium, magnesium, and creatinine, suggesting the breakdown of intracellular materials.[157,235] Isotope dilution studies suggest that this loss of protein results from a decrease in cell mass rather than cell number.[157,453] The nitrogen/sulfur and nitrogen/potassium ratios suggest that this loss is mainly from muscle.[157] The marked increase in the urinary excretion of 3-methylhistidine during trauma, sepsis, and burns also suggests the importance of skeletal muscle in this response.[71,413,671] Analysis of the protein content and the incorporation of radiolabeled amino acids in visceral tissues and skeletal muscle confirms that skeletal muscle is depleted while visceral tissues (liver, kidneys) are spared, which is the opposite of nonstressed starvation in which visceral proteins appear to be used more than muscle proteins, a phenomenon called *visceral translocation of protein*.[368,568]

The net catabolism of protein can result from increased catabolism, decreased synthesis, or a combination of these factors. Available data on total body protein turnover suggest that after injury, the net changes in catabolism and synthesis depend on the severity of the injury.[73] Elective surgery and minor injury appear to result in a decreased rate of synthesis with a normal rate of protein catabolism.[150,490] Severe trauma, burns, and sepsis appear to be associated with increases in both synthesis and catabolism, but a greater increase in the latter results in net catabolism.[73,365,413,616] Accelerated proteolysis and a high rate of gluconeogenesis persist after major injury and during sepsis, apparently as a result of inhibition of ketoadaptation.[139,489] Unlike in starvation, ketogenesis is not prominent, and it does not fuel the brain in significant amounts after major injuries and sepsis. As a result, a high requirement for glucose and therefore for gluconeogenesis persists.

The mechanism for this inhibition of ketoadaptation is not yet understood. Based on studies of in vitro muscle incubations, Barakos and associates[38] have proposed that interleukin-1 may be responsible for the accelerated proteolysis that accompanies fever and sepsis and that the action of interleukin-1 is mediated by PGE_2. Clowes and associates[138] have presented evidence suggesting the involvement of a circulating peptide containing 33 amino acids. However, in vivo infusions of interleukin-1 and PGE_2 in dogs have failed to demonstrate any change in skeletal muscle protein metabolism,[672] and in vitro blockade of prostaglandins in burned rat muscle has failed to produce any change in muscle proteolysis.[493]

The net catabolism of protein that occurs after any injury depends on the severity of the injury. Young healthy men lose more protein in response to an injury than do women or elderly individuals.[371] In addition, the urinary excretion of nitrogen is less after a second operation if it closely follows the first, which presumably is the result of a reduction in available protein stores.[94,329] Finally, negative nitrogen balance can be reduced or virtually eliminated by high-calorie nitrogen supplementation.[318,537,599,616] Together these facts suggest that the loss of protein that occurs after injury is not entirely obligatory to the injury but is also a manifestation of acute starvation.[592,618]

The changes in plasma amino acids during the ebb and flow phases of shock are not well defined yet. During the ebb phase, Engel[198] and McCoy and associates[434] noted increases in the plasma concentrations of most amino acids; Levenson, Howard, and Rosen,[401] as well as Rose,[561] noted increases only in the plasma concentrations of alanine, cystine, taurine, and the aromatic amino acids; and Elwyn and associates[195] noted little change in total amino acid concentrations until the late phases of shock or the flow phase, when the concentrations of most amino acids increased.

Elwyn and associates[195] concluded that most of the changes noted resulted primarily from a decrease in hepatic uptake, and not from an increase in peripheral and hepatic proteolysis or an increase in the release of amino acids from these tissues, as was previously thought. The decrease in hepatic uptake of most amino acids may be related to marked reduction of hepatic blood flow during severe hemorrhage.[198,375]

Despite the decrease in hepatic uptake, ureagenesis does increase, which probably reflects the catabolism of hepatic protein rather than the catabolism of peripheral amino acids that have been transferred to the liver.[195] However, peripheral catabolism of protein and transport of amino acids to the liver during hemorrhage do occur, as is reflected in the increased release and hepatic uptake of phenylalanine and glutamine. The interorgan flux of specific amino acids during the ebb and the flow phases occurs in opposite directions. For example, during the flow phase, seven amino acids (valine, leucine, isoleucine, methionine, glutamate, aspartate, and taurine) move primarily from the liver to the periphery, whereas eight amino acids (phenylalanine, tyrosine, lysine, histidine, threonine, serine, alanine, and glutamine) move primarily from the periphery to the liver.[195]

Together these data suggest that the negative correlation between survival and the plasma concentration of amino acids (noted in animals[199] and humans[388,401] in hemorrhagic shock) and the variations noted in the plasma concentrations of specific and total amino acids during shock are related to the severity of hemorrhage and the time after hemorrhage that the plasma concentrations were determined.

Because the ebb phase of sepsis, trauma, and thermal injury is a hypovolemic period that results from the loss of plasma or blood from the intravascular space, the changes in plasma amino acids for the most part should be similar to those seen during the ebb phase of hemorrhagic shock. During the flow phase of sepsis, burns, and nonthermal injury, changes in plasma amino acids also appear to be related to how long after injury the plasma concentrations of amino acids are determined and the degree of starvation present.* For example, negative nitrogen balance, weight loss, and the plasma amino acid concentrations of wounded animals are in the same direction and of the same magnitude as those that occur in nonwounded animals pair-fed to the reduced intake of nonwounded animals.[6] Although this suggests that the changes in proteolysis and amino acid metabolism are solely the result of starvation, it is noteworthy that in the same study, the intracellular skeletal muscle concentrations of specific amino acids differed greatly between groups.

The importance of when a specific amino acid concentration is measured after injury in determining the response of that amino acid is best exemplified by alanine. Early in the flow phase, the concentration of alanine in plasma is increased, but as the injury persists, serum alanine concentration decreases, presumably as a result of its lack of availability in peripheral tissues and its continued hepatic uptake. This pattern for alanine is noted in most forms of injury.

Two basic schools of thought exist on the effect the type and severity of injury has on changes in amino acid metabolism. On the one hand, evidence has been presented to support the hypothesis that changes in amino acid metabolism do not depend on the type or severity of injury. For example, in many studies the direction of changes in the plasma concentrations of specific amino acids is similar after major thermal injury,[250] elective surgery,[650] trauma,[6] and sepsis, but the magnitude of changes is often greater in sepsis. Similarly, changes in the intracellular concentrations in muscle and the muscle/plasma ratios of specific amino acids appear to be greater in septic states than in nonseptic states.

Despite the evidence favoring this viewpoint, some studies have noted marked differences in plasma and muscle amino acid patterns during sepsis and other injuries that appear to be related to the severity of the injury or infection and to the offending microorganism.[139,240,655,683] This evidence has been used to support the hypothesis that these factors do matter in the overall response of amino acids. As a result, considerable controversy exists over the specific effects injury and sepsis have on amino acid metabolism and what can be done to ameliorate the injury from the standpoint of nitrogen metabolism. Glutamine, for example, has been shown to be vital to proper cellular function during stress, particularly for intestinal cells. It has now been shown that differential utilization of amino acids (Figure 8-39) and cellular amino acid metabolism (Figure 8-40) are changes by the nature and magnitude of injury (Figure 8-41).

The difference in the two schools of thought are best exemplified in the controversy surrounding the metabolism of branched-chain amino acids. It has been hypothesized by O'Donnell and associates[489] and Ryan and associates[569] that because the rate of oxidation of branched-chain amino acids appears to determine the overall rate of protein synthesis,[96,493] a peripheral energy deficit exists during sepsis that stimulates branched-chain amino acid oxidation to overcome this deficit. An increase in the rate of branched-chain amino acid oxidation during sepsis or severe injury would limit not only the availability of branched-chain amino acids but also the availability of other amino acids necessary for protein synthesis. Increased oxidation of branched-chain amino acids also would result in an increase in the intracellular concentrations of amino acids that are not metabolized in muscle and eventually produce an increase in the release of these amino acids.[489,569] Finally, the increase in the amino groups made available from the oxidation of branched-chain amino acids, coupled with an impairment in glycolysis, should lead to an increase in the formation and release of alanine because these amino groups are transaminated with pyruvate.[489,493,569]

In support of this hypothesis, Ryan and associates[569] have noted an increased rate of leucine oxidation in muscle during hemorrhagic shock and sepsis in experimental animals, and other studies have noted an increase in the release of alanine from muscle tissue during injury or sepsis.[6,25,493]

On the basis of this hypothesis, one would predict that the intracellular concentrations of branched-chain amino acids should be low. However, many studies have noted an increase in the intracellular muscle concentrations and the muscle/plasma ratios of branched-chain amino acids in traumatized, thermally injured, and septic individuals and animals.[6,25,26,650] Furthermore, as noted previously, the peripheral energy deficit may be the result of an inflammatory cell infiltrate and may not represent an actual deficit of energy in skeletal muscle. Finally, at least in wounded tissue[28,211] and normal skeletal muscle,[264] the release of alanine does not appear to be related to the rate of glycolysis.

*References 6, 157, 160, 240, 454, and 683.

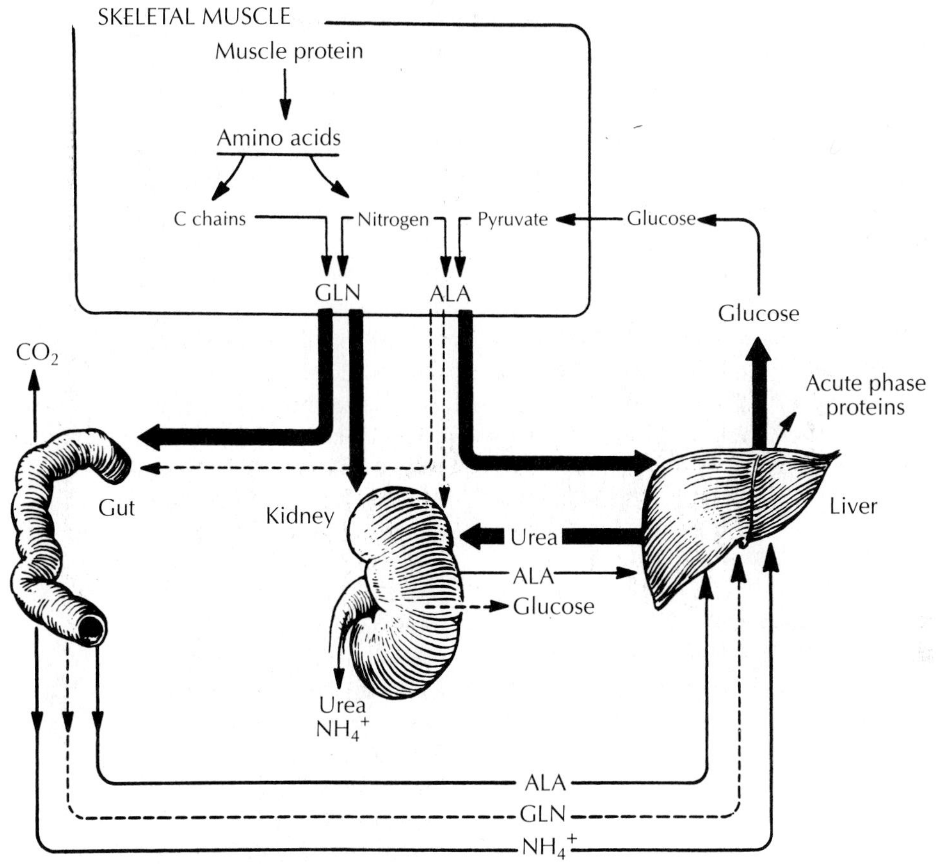

FIGURE 8-39 In catabolic states, the net increase in skeletal muscle proteolysis results in efflux of alanine (ALA) and glutamine (GLN). Consumption of these amino acids by visceral organs yields urea and ammonia and causes loss of nitrogen. (From Souba WW, Smith RJ, Wilmore DW: *JPEN* 9:612, 1985.)

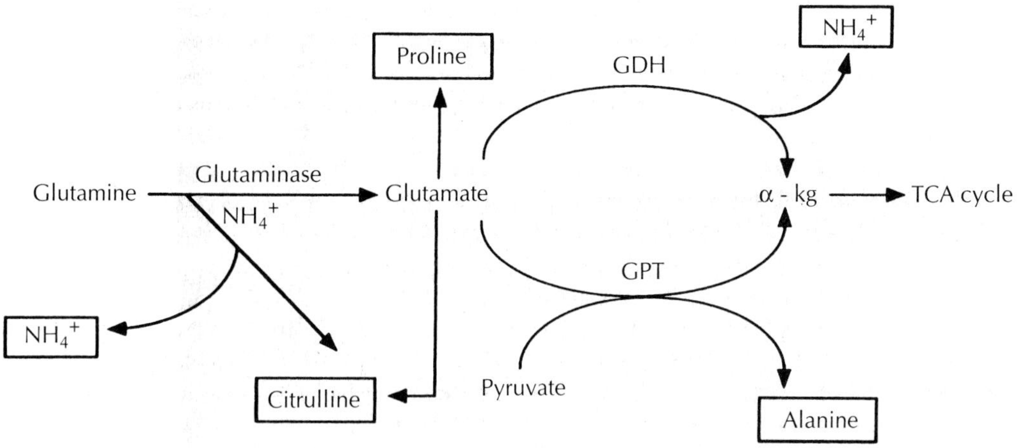

FIGURE 8-40 Pathways of glutamine metabolism in the enterocyte of the small intestine. Glutamine metabolism is not affected by whether the cell is entered from the lumen or the bloodstream. Two thirds of glutamine carbons are oxidized to carbon dioxide by the tricarboxylic acid (TCA) cycle. Glutamine-derived nitrogen is released into the portal circulation as ammonia, citrulline, alanine, and proline. Ammonia and alanine are extracted in large part by the liver. Citrulline is used by the kidneys for biosynthesis of arginine. (From Souba WW: *Annu Rev Nutr* 11:285, 1991.)

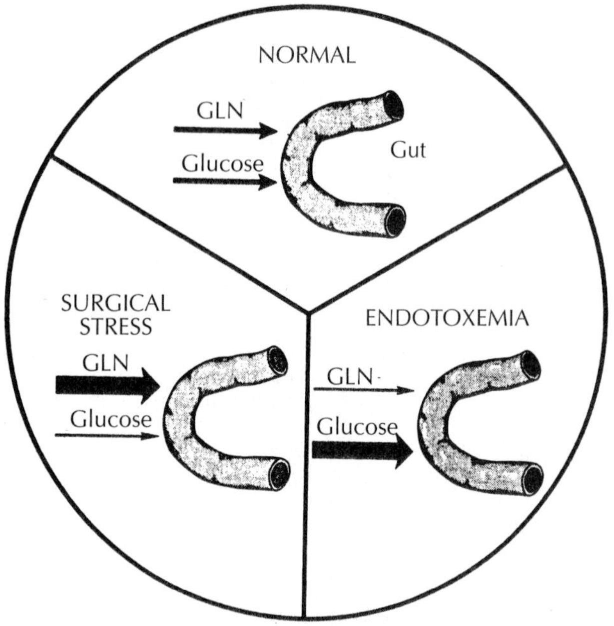

FIGURE 8-41 Relative rates of glutamine (GLN) and glucose consumption by the gut in normal conditions, after surgery, and in endotoxemia. (From Souba WW: *Annu Rev Nutr* 11:285, 1991.)

The intracellular muscle concentrations and the muscle/plasma ratios of glutamine are greatly reduced in most studies of sepsis, wounds, and thermal injury.* In general, the release of glutamine is greater than can be predicted from its relative abundance in muscle tissue protein,[6,565] and evidence has been presented for its synthesis in muscle.[565] However, the release of glutamine from wounded and nonwounded muscle is no different,[6] and if the release of glutamine is expressed as a ratio to the phenylalanine released, the release rate is lower in wounded than in nonwounded tissue.[6] Because phenylalanine is not catabolized or synthesized in muscle,[457] a lower glutamine/phenylalanine ratio suggests that either the synthesis of glutamine in wounded tissue is reduced, or local catabolism in wounded muscle is increased. Glutamine is a major energy source for lymphocytes[22] and fibroblasts.[179] Thus accelerated use of glutamine by the cellular infiltrate in wounded or septic tissue could explain the decreased concentrations noted at the site of injury.[6]

The importance of leukocyte and lymphocyte interactions with parenchymal cells in protein metabolism has been demonstrated by Keller and associates[359,360] and West and associates.[664] In their studies, isolated hepatocytes were cultured in the presence of nonparenchymal hepatic cells (Kupffer's cells), peritoneal macrophages, or conditioned media in which nonparenchymal cells had been previously cultured; the hepatocytes demonstrated a marked reduction in protein synthesis, as evidence by a reduced rate of incorporation of radiolabeled leucine. This response was even greater when the hepatocyte nonparenchymal cell mixture was coincubated with endotoxin. Corroborating our findings about the absence of a direct effect of endotoxin on glucose metabolism in skeletal muscle,[12] incubation of hepatocytes alone with endotoxin had no effect on protein synthesis. These data suggest the existence of a macrophage-Kupffer cell–mediated factor that affects protein metabolism in hepatocytes.

Despite phagocytic cells' ability to reduce protein synthesis in the liver; a negative nitrogen balance; a negative energy balance; and reduced tissue and plasma concentrations of zinc, thiamine, riboflavin, vitamin C, and vitamin A, most wounds do heal.* Moore[453] has called this ability of wound healing to proceed in the presence and absence of abundant substrate supply the *biologic priority of wound healing*. However, this term should not be taken to mean that wound healing is normal in a severely injured patient. As Levenson, Seifter, and Van Winkle have noted, "Whereas the healing of a wound after injury appears satisfactory, it may be neither normal nor optimal."[402] In examining the healing of laparotomy wounds in normal and burned (35%) rodents, Levenson and associates[400] noted a distinct delay in the wound healing of burned animals. Similarly, the skin incisions in rodents with a fractured femur did not heal as well as those in rodents with a skin incision alone.

The biologic priority of wound healing also does not mean that wound healing cannot be improved in severely injured patients. Large, open wounds, such as burns, are associated with inhibition of nitrogen anabolism of the host and may result in protein malnutriton and death if the substrate demands of the wounds are not met exogenously. It is not clear whether administering protein improves wound healing per se. However, it has been shown to reduce negative nitrogen balance. Some investigators[305,377,672] have also noted an improvement in wound healing with protein supplementation, but others[672] have been unable to document any change.

Changes in the ambient temperature of experimental animals have been shown to result in accelerated wound healing and diminished excretion of urinary nitrogen after thermal injury, skin wounding, or leg fracture,[100,103,152] but similar findings in humans have not been confirmed.[675]

In summary, generalized catabolism, hyperglycemia, persistent gluconeogenesis, protein wasting, negative nitrogen balance, heat production, and loss of body mass, all paralleling the severity of the injury, are characteristic after trauma and during sepsis. Most of the energy necessary for biologic processes to proceed is derived from

*References 6, 25, 26, 139, 240, 250, 650, and 683.

*References 311, 400, 402, 418, 419, 453, 642, and 672.

fat. Net catabolism of 300 to 500 g of lean body cell mass per day apparently is required as a source of amino acids for gluconeogenesis. If the injury (particularly sepsis) persists, unknown mechanisms cause inhibition of the usual adaptive mechanisms in starvation, resulting in persistence of a highly catabolic state. This high catabolic state in turn leads to protein wasting and malnutrition and ultimately to multiple organ failure and death[621] if the stimuli are not eliminated.

Lipid Metabolism

Increased lipolysis generally is seen during both the ebb and flow phases of the metabolic response to injury. During the ebb phase, elevated concentrations of cortisol, catecholamines, glucagon, growth hormone, and ACTH; increased SNS activity, and depressed concentrations of insulin favor lipolysis. Cortisol appears to be necessary for the remainder of these hormonal agents to be effective.[211,590]

Elevated concentrations of glycerol and free fatty acids are well documented during the ebb phase.* However, Kovach and associates[381] and Spitzer and associates[612] have noted that plasma concentrations of free fatty acids may not increase during severe hemorrhage or during severe endotoxic shock, possibly because of intense vasoconstriction that allows minimum blood flow in adipose tissue and/or because of an increase in the reesterification rate of free fatty acids in the presence of high concentrations of lactate.[245] The latter hypothesis is supported by the rise in the plasma concentrations of glycerol and lactate seen in both studies despite the absence of a change in the concentration of free fatty acids.

Other factors that may affect the mobilization of lipids from storage depots in response to injury include a decrease in pH,[320] hyperglycemia,[602] and some types of anesthetic.[679] For example, Wolfe, Shaw, and Durkot[679] have pointed out that lipolysis is directly inhibited by the anesthetic pentobarbital, and that hemorrhage in the presence of pentobarbital usually results in a fall in the plasma concentrations of free fatty acids and ketone bodies. In contrast, hemorrhage experiments using other types of anesthetics or in awake animals produce a rise in free fatty acids and ketone bodies.

The exact mechanism by which pentobarbital reduces lipolysis is not known, but it may be related to the drug's ability to reduce the SNS response to stress. In fact, the sympathetic nervous system is of paramount importance in the lipolytic response to stress, because SNS blockade causes a marked reduction in lipolysis.[297,679] However, stimulating the sympathetic nervous system is a double-edged sword, because a large increase in SNS activity inhibits blood flow, thus reducing the release of fatty acids from adipose tissue. The consequent increase in the intracellular concentration of fatty acids in adipose tissue inhibits further lipolysis and actually may injure the cell.[245,320]

During the flow phase, net lipolysis persists despite an increase in the concentration of insulin. Lipolysis is reflected in increased concentrations of plasma free fatty acids or in increased clearance of fatty acids, both of which have been noted during the flow phase of trauma, burns, and sepsis.[74,431,499,610] As long as sufficient oxygen is available, most tissues in the body, including cardiac and skeletal muscle, can oxidize the fatty acids released to produce energy. In fact, normal or elevated rates of fatty acid oxidation have been noted during sepsis, endotoxemia, wounding, and thermal injury.

Therefore, if the rate of clearance of fatty acids is equal to the rate of appearance, the plasma concentration does not increase; if the rate of clearance is greater than the rate of appearance, the concentration decreases.[679] For example, although there does appear to be an increase in the rate of appearance and oxidation of free fatty acids during sepsis and endotoxemia, a rise in the plasma free fatty acid concentration is not always noted. An analogous situation is true for the hypertriglyceridemia that is characteristic of sepsis and endotoxemia. This condition may be the result either of increased release of triglycerides beyond the tissues' ability to clear them[679] or of a normal rate of release with a decrease in the tissues' ability to break down the molecules.[34,357] There is evidence to support both points of view, which highlights the controversy over metabolism of lipids during injury.

In both the ebb and flow phases, the high concentrations of intracellular fatty acids and the elevated concentration of glucagon inhibit acetyl-CoA carboxylase, thereby decreasing malonyl-CoA concentrations and the synthesis of fatty acids. In hepatocytes this also stimulates carnitine acyltransferase, increasing the transport of acetyl-CoA into the mitochondria for oxidation and ketogenesis. However, the activity of ketogenesis after shock, injury, and sepsis varies and correlates with the severity of injury.[34,357,499,610]

After major injury, severe shock, and sepsis, ketogenesis is low or absent, whereas after minor injury or mild infection, it is increased but to a lesser extent than that seen during nonstressed starvation.[431,679] This appears to be at least partly the result of inhibition of ketogenesis during severe injury and sepsis by elevated concentrations of malonyl-CoA.[647] In contrast, minor inflammation or injury is not associated with an increase in malonyl-CoA. Injuries in which ketogenesis is low also appear to be associated with a small or no increase in the plasma concentration of free fatty acids. Thus the absence of ketogenesis in these situations may stem from the absence of an increase in intracellular concentrations of free fatty acids and therefore of malonyl-CoA.

During starvation, inhibition of acetyl-CoA carbox-

*References 147, 297, 490, and 605.

ylase also results in accumulation of cytoplasmic citrate, which in turn inhibits glycolysis through inhibition of phosphofructokinase (the Randle effect).[480] Controversy has existed as to whether this fatty acid–induced inhibition of glycolysis through citrate occurs in vivo or whether it is only an in vitro phenomenon. Wolfe, Shaw, and Durkot[679] recently provided evidence in conscious, burned dogs that the Randle effect does occur in vivo and that it may be a major mechanism for reducing glycolysis that occurs in nonseptic injury during the flow phase. An increase in the cytoplasmic concentration of citrate is seen during mild inflammation and injury. However, after shock and major injury, citrate does not appear to accumulate,[461] which may be an important factor in the persistence of glycolysis after injury.

FLUID AND ELECTROLYTE METABOLISM AFTER INJURY

Almost all acute injuries are associated with changes in fluid and electrolyte metabolism, acid-base status, and renal function. These changes are primarily the result of reductions in the effective circulating volume. A reduction in effective circulating volume after injury may be caused by loss of blood (hemorrhage), loss of vascular tone (sepsis), pump failure (cardiac tamponade), inadequate oral intake (coma), excessive unreplaced extrarenal losses (diarrhea, vomiting, and drainage of fistulae), or sequestration of fluids (third-space losses).

The third space results from injury, ischemia, or inflammation and represents sequestered extracellular fluid. Because the fluid and electrolytes in the third space are derived from the functional extracellular fluid, an increase in the size of the third space reduces the functional extracellular fluid volume. In addition, the fluid that accumulates in the third space is equivalent in electrolyte composition to the extracellular fluid. Thus, for each liter of fluid sequestered in a third space, approximately 150 mEq of sodium, 112 mEq of chloride, and 4.6 mEq of potassium is lost from the functional extracellular fluid.

The volume of the third space is directly proportional to the severity of injury.[598] Thus minor surgical procedures, such as an appendectomy, are associated with considerably less fluid sequestration than are major procedures, such as extensive retroperitoneal dissection. Similarly, minor traumatic injuries, such as an isolated, simple limb fracture, are associated with less fluid sequestration than are major injuries, such as burns. The most extensive third-space accumulations are those that follow burns and sepsis.

Blalock[79] was the first to demonstrate that traumatic injury to an extremity resulted in mobilization of fluid and electrolytes to the area of injury, reducing the functional extracellular fluid volume. With nonthermal traumatic injury, the third space forms immediately and reaches its maximum after 5 to 6 hours. It resolves more slowly, possibly taking longer than 10 days.[558]

Hypovolemic shock is also associated with a reduction in the exchangeable extracellular fluid volume that exceeds the amount lost from the body through hemorrhage or dehydration. Studies by Shires, Carrico, and Cannizaro[595] have demonstrated that when shed blood alone is replaced after hemorrhage, the red cell mass and blood volume return to normal, but a deficit persists in the functional extracellular fluid volume. In contrast, when shed blood and additional lactated Ringer's solution are administered, the red cell mass, blood volume, and extracellular fluid volume return to normal.

Third-space formation appears to occur in the intracellular space, because hemorrhages that exceed 30% of the total blood volume are associated with a contraction of the intracellular space and an increase in intracellular volume.

Major burns affect the capillary integrity of the burned tissue, resulting in exudation of plasma and evaporative water loss.[24,170] Also, fluid flux across capillaries in unburned tissue increases.[24,170] edema appears to form in burned tissue as the result of an increase in capillary permeability, whereas it seemingly develops in unburned tissue as a result of hypoproteinemia rather than a direct increase in capillary permeability.[170,299] Edema forms primarily in the first 24 hours, and the greatest losses occur during the first 8 hours.[41]

In sepsis a generalized capillary leakage develops that results in edema and a decrease in the effective circulating volume.[194,626] As the sepsis persists, the associated protein malnutrition produces hypoproteinemia, which in turn may increase the formation of edema.

Thus any traumatic injury produces rapid changes in the functional extracellular fluid volume, the plasma volume, and the osmolality and electrolyte composition, all of which trigger renal compensatory mechanisms aimed at improving salt and water balance. The degree of impairment of these parameters depends partly on the severity of the injury; the quality and quantity of fluid given; the patient's age, preexisting illnesses, and concurrent medications; and the anesthetic used.

Renal Conservation of Salt and Water

Because the formation of tubular fluid at the glomerulus depends on the forces described in Starling's hypothesis of capillary equilibrium, it is apparent that the quantity of filtrate formed depends on the renal perfusion pressure at the glomerulus. Thus a reduction in the renal perfusion pressure should result in a reduction in the amount of glomerular ultrafiltrate that is formed. However, even when renal perfusion pressure is reduced to 90 mm Hg, renal blood flow and glomerular filtration remain unchanged[471] (Figure 8-42).

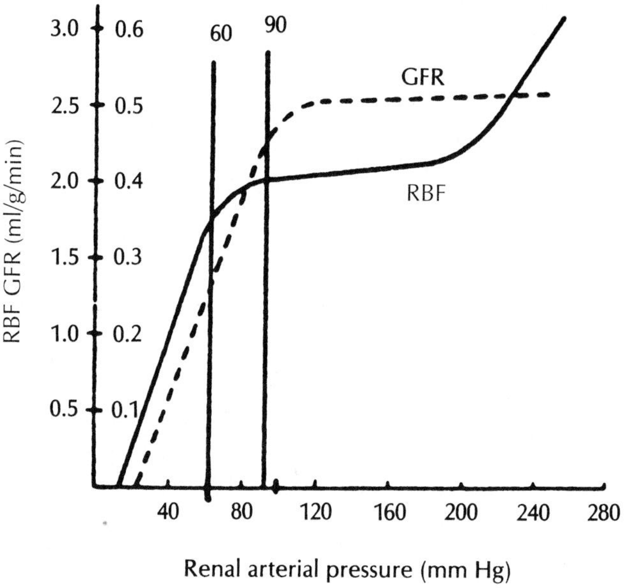

FIGURE 8-42 Autoregulation of renal blood flow. Despite a reduction in renal arterial pressure of 90 mm Hg, renal blood flow (RBF) and the glomerular filtration rate (GFR) are maintained. (From Powers RS: In Sabiston DC, editor: *Davis-Christopher textbook of surgery*, Philadelphia, 1981, WB Saunders.)

The process by which renal blood flow and the glomerular filtration rate (GFR) remain unchanged is called intrinsic autoregulation. Although the exact mechanisms are not known, the process is thought to involve tubuloglomerular feedback; that is, individual nephrons sense their tubular fluid flow and change the rate of glomerular filtration by changing the glomerular capillary pressure, primarily at the efferent arteriole.[472] Decreases in tubular fluid flow lead to an increase in efferent arteriolar resistance. This increases the fraction of peritubular blood filtered at the glomerulus, allowing the total GFR to be maintained.[685]

Tubuloglomerular feedback also is thought to involve the sensing of tubular chloride or sodium at the macula densa,[472] and the sympathetic nervous system and renin-angiotensin system are thought to play an important role in this process.[32,584]

The increase in the filtration fraction produces an increase in the oncotic pressure of the peritubular capillary blood perfusing the proximal tubule because of the impermeability of the glomerular basement membranes to protein. In turn, the increase in peritubular oncotic pressure produces an increase in the net transfer of water, sodium, chloride, and bicarbonate from the proximal tubular filtrate to the peritubular blood. In addition, SNS activity may directly increase the proximal tubular transport of sodium[271,272] and suppress the release of cerebral natriuretic hormone[358] and atrial natriuretic factor.[106]

The net result of these changes is a decrease in the delivery of sodium, chloride, and filtered fluid to Henle's loop. Because maintaining the normal medullary osmotic gradient requires adequate delivery of sodium and chloride to the long loops of Henle, a fall in medullary hyperosmolarity frequently follows injury, from which a defect in urinary-concentrating ability may develop.[606,686] This defect results in the need to excrete a larger amount of urine to eliminate the same amount of solute. This paradoxic increase in free water clearance has been called polyuric renal failure,[448] and it may be involved in the genesis of acute renal failure, particularly of the nonoliguric type.[17] Recently, in a rodent model, Anderson and associates[16] demonstrated ischemia-induced, nonoliguric renal failure in which a defect in the inner medullary interstitial solute was indeed responsible for the impairment in urinary-concentrating ability.

Concomitant with the compensatory mechanisms for enhancing sodium resorption, blood flow is redistributed from the superficial cortical nephrons to the juxtamedullary glomeruli,[614] which increases sodium resorption by shifting blood flow to the juxtamedullary nephrons that have long loops of Henle. Various hormonal mediators have been implicated in this redistribution, including catecholamines,[584] angiotensin I,[341] angiotensin II,[296] PGE_2,[342] and vasopressin.[347] Current evidence supports the idea that the redistribution is the result of PGE_2-mediated medullary vasodilatation combined with angiotensin I–mediated cortical vasoconstriction.[32]

Because sodium resorption in the ascending limb of Henle's loop follows chloride passively, sodium delivery to the distal tubules increases when chloride delivery to the loop is inadequate. This produces potassium wasting and metabolic alkalosis, and it is augmented by the secretion of aldosterone that accompanies hypovolemia and injury. Conversely, if sodium delivery to the distal tubules is inadequate, potassium is not excreted, even in the presence of aldosterone, and hyperkalemia and metabolic acidosis may ensue.

In hypotension and injury, secretion of vasopressin is stimulated by osmotic and nonosmotic (baroreceptor) pathways.[585] This increase normally lasts 3 to 5 days after injury and usually results in water retention. However, when the countercurrent mechanism is disrupted by a fall in medullary osmolality, the action of vasopressin is impaired, resulting in loss of free water. Consequently, a normal or increased urine output in a hypotensive or injured patient does not necessarily reflect an adequate blood volume. Similarly, reduced urine output does not reflect inadequate blood volume or inappropriate secretion of vasopressin because numerous nonosmotic stimuli (e.g., pain) may be present that lead to increased secretion of vasopressin, despite a normal

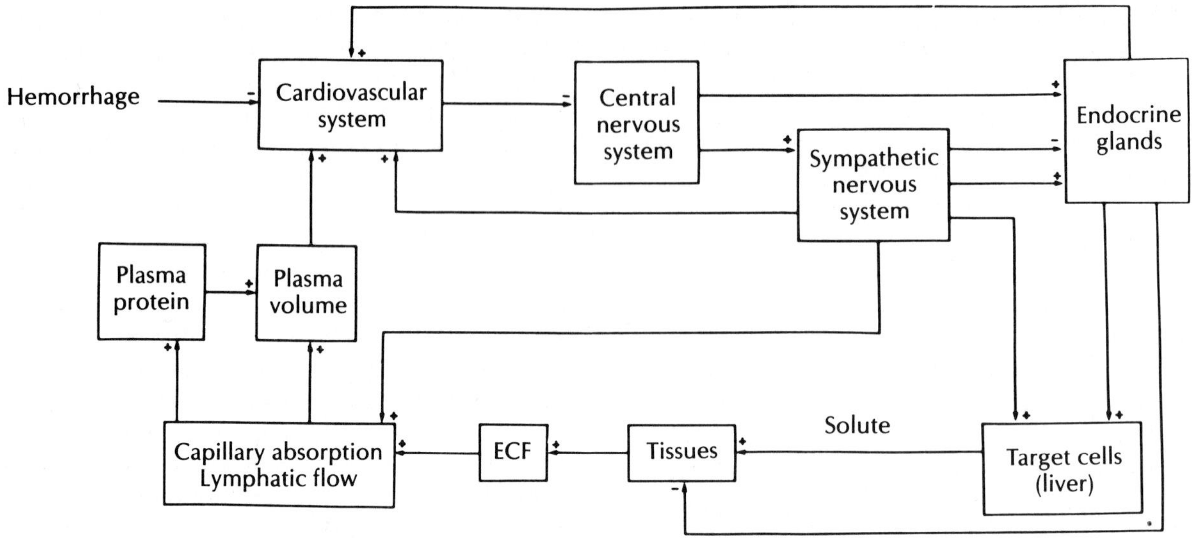

FIGURE 8-43 Restitution of blood volume. (From Gann DS, Amaral JF: The pathophysiology of trauma and shock. In Zuidema GD, Rutherford WF, Ballinger WF, editors: *The management of trauma,* Philadelphia, 1985, WB Saunders.)

plasma osmolality and blood volume.

The return of vasopressin secretion to normal is signaled by the brisk diuresis of free water seen in most surgical patients on the third to fifth postoperative day. This diuresis is the *fluid mobilization* phase of injury.

Finally, all the mechanisms involved in renal conservation of salt and water are directed at preventing further losses of circulating volume through renal excretion. However, even in the complete absence of renal excretion, no increase in the functional extracellular fluid volume can occur. For effective circulating volume, cardiac output, and vascular resistance to return to normal during hypovolemia, the blood volume must be restored.

Restitution of Blood Volume

Blood volume can be restored by administering exogenous fluids. If these fluids are given intravenously, the increase in blood volume is direct. If the fluids are given orally, blood volume increases through intestinal absorption, a process that is partly mediated by glucagon. If exogenous fluids are not given, the blood volume must be restored from fluids in the interstitial fluid and the cells. This process may be thought of as occurring in two overlapping phases: the first involves the movement of essentially protein-free fluid from the interstitium to the plasma, and the second involves the restitution of plasma protein, which brings about the complete restitution of blood volume[255] (Figure 8-43).

The first phase involves a net movement of protein-free fluid from the interstitium to the vascular space, which is mediated by a fall in capillary pressure.[293] The decrease in capillary pressure is initiated by hypotension and augmented by reflex sympathetic vasoconstriction.[255] According to the current concept of Starling's hypothesis of capillary equilibrium,[508] the direction of fluid movement between the vascular space and the interstitial space is determined by three factors: the capillary (P_c) and interstitial (P_i) hydrostatic pressure; the capillary (π_c) and interstitial (π_i) colloid oncotic pressure; and the permeability (k) and area (A) of the capillary membranes. The forces causing the net movement of fluid out of the capillary beds are P_c and P_i, and the forces causing fluid movement into the capillary beds are P_i and P_c. Net flux (F) is described by the equation:

$$F = kA[(P_c - P_i) - (\pi_c - \pi_i)] = kA[(P_c + \pi_i) - (\pi_c + P_i)]$$

As capillary hydrostatic pressure decreases during hypovolemic shock, the steady-state flux of fluid changes, resulting in net movement of the fluid into the capillary bed. This results in restoration of 20% to 50% of the blood volume lost.[98] Because this fluid is protein free, plasma colloid oncotic pressure decreases. Interstitial hydrostatic pressure also decreases as fluid leaves a compartment with finite compliance. This results in establishment of a new steady state in which further restitution of blood volume is impossible.

Complete restitution of blood volume depends on the second phase, which is associated with restitution of plasma protein and a shift of fluid from cells via the interstitial space to the capillary bed.[255,257] This movement of water appears to be mediated by a hormonally induced increase in extracellular osmolality.[181,255,257] The protein involved in this process is primarily in the form of albumin. Because the synthesis of albumin takes at least 48 hours, the increase in plasma albumin must derive from the interstitium itself.[525]

Two mechanisms move protein from the interstitium to the capillary space—the lymphatics and the fenestrae of the capillary membrane.[117,525] For either to be effective, interstitial pressure must increase.[525] Because the compliance of the interstitium is fixed, an increase in volume leads to an increase in interstitial pressure. Because plasma water is reduced in hypotension, an increase in interstitial volume must come from cells. Fluid moves out of cells only down an osmotic gradient, which implies that an osmotic gradient exists between the intracellular and extracellular spaces in hypotension and hypovolemia.

Bergentz and Brief[51] and Brooks and associates[89] were the first to observe that hemorrhage in experimental animals was associated with a rise in plasma osmolality, a finding later confirmed in humans by Boyd and Mansberger.[85] These investigators believed that the increase in plasma osmolality reflected a change in metabolism resulting from inadequate tissue perfusion; however, Jarhult and associates[343] suggested that the hyperosmolar response to hemorrhage and hypovolemia is an important compensatory mechanism for increasing plasma volume. The increase in serum osmolality occurs promptly after hemorrhage and correlates with the rate and degree of hemorrhage and the severity of injury.[258,262,363]

The osmotic gradient is produced transiently by a complex set of mechanisms that clearly depend on the neuroendocrine response. An increase in cortisol is necessary but not sufficient to produce the increase in osmolality.[262] The process also requires an adrenal factor (? catecholamines), a pituitary factor (probably vasopressin), and glucagon.[256] The viscera (primarily the liver) is the source of solute production.[257] These solutes, including glucose, phosphate, lactate, and pyruvate, are then delivered to the peripheral tissues (primarily muscle), where they increase interstitial osmolality. Because the constituent molecules are relatively unable to permeate to cell membranes, an osmotic gradient is established, and fluid moves from cells to the interstitium. In turn, the increase in interstitial osmolality leads to the movement of water out of the cells and into the interstitium. The increase in interstitial volume results in an increase in interstitial pressure, which opens the capillary fenestrae, allowing protein to move through the capillary membrane and the lymphatics.

The rise in osmolality also appears to contribute to the phase of transcapillary refill.[257] The solute is delivered to the peripheral tissues, where it mediates the movement of water from cells to the interstitium, as is the case in the plasma protein restitution phase. Thus by increasing the interstitial pressure, the hyperosmolality also augments the transcapillary refill phase.

Nutritional status plays an important role in the hyperosmolality seen after hemorrhage. Fasted animals show a lower degree of hyperglycemia and a slower rise in plasma osmolality than fed animals.[242,656] This difference is associated with less blood volume restitution in animals that are fasted than in those that are fed.[242] However, this difference was eliminated by administering hyperosmolar glucose or xylose to the fasted animals.[444,540] Because xylose cannot be metabolized, these results suggest that glucose acts primarily as an osmotic agent rather than as an energy source.

On the basis of these data, one would predict that the higher the serum glucose concentration, the more favorable the response, a prediction in contrast to the association of a high glucose concentration with high mortality, as in the study of combat injuries done by Carey, Lowery, and Cloutier.[109]

It is important to note that the changes described result from an increase in the production of solute by the liver and its subsequent delivery to the interstitium bathing the skeletal muscle. Given the same increase in solute production, changes in plasma solute concentrations are smaller if muscle perfusion is adequate than if it is decreased by intense vasoconstriction. Thus a very high increase in the serum glucose concentration may be the result of inadequate tissue perfusion rather than an accelerated rate of glucose production. In these cases, restitution would be significantly impaired and an increase in mortality would be expected. In fact, although the second phase of restitution is present during all hemorrhages, the restitution in large hemorrhages (more than 25% of the total blood volume) is no greater than that seen in small hemorrhages of 10% of total blood volume.[258] Furthermore, this finding correlates with the appearance of a decrease in transmembrane potential, cell swelling, and eventually cell death.[596]

CONSEQUENCES OF THE METABOLIC RESPONSE TO INJURY

This chapter has integrated the neuroendocrine response that results from the stimuli elicited by injury and starvation with the changes that response produces in intermediary and fluid and electrolyte metabolism. As such, the metabolic changes that accompany injury are the consequence of the neuroendocrine response rather than the injury itself. Furthermore, it is apparent that the inflammatory response also may significantly modify or augment the metabolic response.

In general, the combined result of the neuroendocrine and inflammatory responses to injury is a change in the enzymatic activity and substrate supply throughout the body, triggering hyperglycemia, increased production of lactate, production of glucose, mobilization and oxidation of fatty acids, degradation of protein, and conservation of fluids and electrolytes. These changes in intermediary and fluid and electrolyte metabolism are critical for generating other important events during injury and sepsis (e.g., restitution of blood volume, conservation of salt and water, and delivery of glucose to injured tissue), which appear to be necessary to survival. However, other results of the metabolic and neuroendocrine responses appear to be detrimental, including inhibition of the inflammatory response, development of a urinary-concentrating defect, and production of negative nitrogen balance during wound healing. It remains for future study to determine whether interrupting the neuroendocrine-metabolic response to injury by substituting its identified beneficial effects may prove therapeutically useful for critically ill patients.

SUMMARY

Systemic Neuroendocrine Reflexes

The biologic response to injury is transmitted through neuroendocrine changes, the release of mediator substances, and alterations in cellular and intermediary metabolism that are tailored to the magnitude and nature of the injury. The primary stimuli for this response include changes in effective circulating volume; changes in the concentration of oxygen, carbon dioxide, or hydrogen ions; the presence of pain; changes in substrate availability; changes in temperature; and ongoing infection.

These stimuli are transduced by specialized receptors that form efferent signals, which are further modulated and integrated by the peripheral and central nervous systems. Afferent output then is enacted through multiple coordinated systems, including the hypothalamic-pituitary-adrenal axis, autonomic nervous system, and neuroimmunologic axes, which control the release of mediators, the activation of coagulation proteins, and the secretion of endothelial cells.

The actions of endocrine hormones, mediator substances, paracrine growth factors, and endothelial cell products occur through signal transduction mechanisms that either act directly on genomic transcription (e.g., lipid-permeable hormones such as steroids and thyroid hormones); or by binding to cell-surface receptors (e.g., as with catecholamines, insulin, and interleukins); or through a combination of both mechanisms (e.g., interferon). Binding of ligands to cell-surface receptors causes intracellular action through mechanisms that include direct enzyme action (e.g., phosphorylation), guanine nucleotide-binding proteins (G proteins), and/or ligand-gated ion channels. Intracellular second messengers include cAMP, cGMP, and free calcium ions.

Neuroendocrine Response

Endocrine hormones may be broadly classified as those under hypothalamic-pituitary control and those directed by the autonomic nervous system. Hormones of the hypothalamic-pituitary axis include corticotropin-releasing factor (CRF), adrenocorticotropin hormone (ACTH) and cortisol, growth hormone, thyroid hormones, gonadotropins, prolactin, opioid peptides, and arginine vasopressin (AVP). Hormones under ANS control include catecholamines, renin and angiotensin, aldosterone, insulin, glucagon, somatostatin and, to some extent, parathyroid hormone. In general, injury causes increased release of all hypothalamic-pituitary axis hormones except for thyroid hormones and the gonadotropins. Hormones primarily controlled by the autonomic nervous system are also increased early after injury, except for insulin and the insulin-like growth factors.

Mediator, Endothelial, and Intracellular Response

Mediator substances that are found in the circulation in only small amounts have profound effects at the site of origin (paracine effects). Mediators include the cytokines, eicosanoids (also called phospholipid mediators), kallikrein-kinins, serotonin, histamine, growth factors, and plasma proteins of the coagulation and complement systems. Cytokines are small peptide intercellular messengers that include the interleukins, tumor necrosis factors, and interferons. Cytokines play critical roles in the processes of immunologic defense, inflammation, acute-phase protein release, and activation of endothelial cells. Multiple organ dysfunction syndrome, which can be observed after severe injury, may be related to sustained release of certain mediators.

Just as the lymphocyte is the key to immunologic processes, the endothelial cell is pivotal to the biologic response to injury. The presence of endothelium in all organs constitutes a collective cellular mass of equal physiologic importance to that of more traditionally recognized endocrine organs. Endothelial cell responses to injury include interactions with blood-borne white cells and coagulation and complement factors; endothelial secretion of cytokines and other mediators; and modulation of smooth muscle contraction and permeability by eicosanoids, platelet-activating factor, and endothelin, and by the release of nitric oxide. Certain genetic and environmental factors predispose a person to disease states (e.g., atherosclerosis) that may critically affect the physiologic response to injury by the heart, lungs, and kidneys; proper functioning of these tissues is vital during periods of extreme physiologic compensation. Intracellular products of metabolism (e.g., oxygen free-radicals that are released after postischemic reperfusion) and induction of heat-shock proteins after periods of stress are evolving therapeutic targets for reducing injury-induced cellular damage.

Substrate and Energy Changes

Changes in intermediary metabolism and the whole-body energetic response to injury has been considered to occur in two phases. The early, or ebb, phase corresponds to the first hours after injury and is characterized by hyperglycemia and restoration of circulating volume and tissue perfusion. After tissue perfusion has been restored, the reparative process occurs characterized by protein catabolism, negative nitrogen balance, hyperglycemia, and heat production and is called the late, or flow, phase and requires days to weeks to complete.

The local and total energy requirement for the biologic response to injury varies with the magnitude, duration, and nature of the stimuli. In general, patients who have had elective surgery show a 10% increase in overall resting energy expenditure; patients with multiple skeletal injuries show increases up to 25% and incur additional energy demands from concomitant fever, inflammation, or sepsis. Thermal injuries affecting a large surface area cause the greatest increase in metabolic rate, to as much as 50% to 100% above basal energy expenditure.

Limited carbohydrate stores and interactions between catecholamines, cortisol, and glucagon result in a significant draft on skeletal muscle protein and negative nitrogen balance. However, only 20% of the protein is used directly for energy requirements. The remainder is used by the liver and kidneys to produce glucose, reflected by the accelerated production of urea observed after injury. Obligate glucose utilization by brain and blood cells requires that glucose be available beyond the period when limited hepatic glycogen stores are depleted.

During the ebb phase, increases in hormone secretion and SNS activity favor lipolysis. Increased concentrations of glycerol and free fatty acids persist even during the flow phase, when net lipolysis continues despite increased secretion of insulin. During the flow phase, end-organ insulin resistance and secretion of catecholamines promote metabolic pathways that counter protein synthesis. Substrate cycling (alanine, ketones, and glucose) occurs between skeletal muscle, liver, intestine, and wounded tissue. Amino acids are shunted to the liver for glucose formation and acute-phase protein synthesis. Glutamine is metabolized preferentially during catabolic states to serve as a major source of energy for the gastrointestinal tract, lymphocytes, and fibroblasts after injury. During catabolic states, glutamine may act as an essential amino acid, because depletion of this substrate has pronounced negative effects on enterocytes and the integrity of the intestinal mucosa. Failure to supply additional glutamine during severe stress has been implicated in the pathogenesis of bacterial translocation and the development of multiple organ dysfunction syndrome.

Fluid and Electrolyte Shifts

Changes in restitution of blood volume and in fluid and electrolyte metabolism are of primary physiologic importance because almost all severe injuries involve a change in effective blood volume. Effective circulating volume may be reduced through blood loss, loss of vascular tone and capillary leakage, cardiac failure, excessive unreplaced extrarenal fluid loss, gastrointestinal disturbances, or drainage of fistulae. The overall response to the loss of effective circulating volume is a coordinated physiologic effort to prevent unnecessary further loss; this is accomplished through activation of coagulation proteins, renal conservation of salt and water, movement of protein-free fluid from the interstitium to the vascular space, and (ultimately to restore blood volume) movement of protein from the interstitium.

The biologic response to reductions in blood volume is mediated through reflex responses of the cardiovascular system, central nervous system, and autonomic nervous system; secretion of endocrine gland substances; and release of endothelial cell factors. Baroreceptor and chemoreceptor system reflexes initiate endocrine responses, which include secretion of renin-angiotensin, arginine, vasopressin, cortisol, and catecholamines; release by endothelial cells of prostaglandins and endothelins; and reduced formation of nitric oxide.

The increase in serum osmolality that occurs promptly after hemorrhage is mediated by cortisol, catecholamines, arginine vasopressin, and glucagon and is derived primarily from hepatic substrates, including glucose, phosphate, lactate, and pyruvate. The response is further modulated by nutritional status. The movement of fluid out of the cells via the interstitial space to the capillary bed is mediated by increases in extracellular solute and is critical for restitution of blood volume. This mechanism may be offset by decreases in transmembrane potential and the accompanying cell swelling. These cellular derangements may be caused by rapid activation of circulating proteins that have yet to be fully characterized and may be critical to the understanding and medical amelioration of some aspects of the biologic response to injury.

REFERENCES

1 Achtel RA, Downing S: Ventricular responses to hypoxemia following chemoreceptor denervation and adrenalectomy, *Am Heart J* 84:377, 1982.

2 Abbott NE, Anderson K: The effect of starvation, infection, and injury on the metabolic processes and body composition, *Acad Sci* 110:941, 1963.

3 Aggarwal BB: Comparative analysis of the structure and function of TNF. In Aggarwal BB, editor: *Tumor necrosis factor,* New York, 1992, BC Dekker.

4 Aggarwal BB, Kohr WJ, Haas PE et al: Human tumor necrosis factor: production, purification, and characterization, *J Biol Chem* 23:45, 1985.
5 Aguilera G, Catt KJ: Loci of action of regulators of aldosterone biosynthesis in isolated glomerulosa cells, *Endocrinology* 104:1046, 1980.
6 Albina JE, Shearer JD, Mastrofancesco B et al: Amino acid metabolism following lambda-carrageenan injury to rat skeletal muscle, *Am J Physiol* 250:E24, 1985.
7 Alexander RW, Gill JRJ, Yambe H: Effects of dietary sodium and of acute saline infusion on the interrelationship between dopamine excretion and adrenergic activity in man, *J Clin Invest* 54:194, 1974.
8 Allbritton NL, Meyer T, Stryer L: Range of messenger action of calcium ion and inositol 1,4,5-triphosphate, *Science* 258:1812, 1992.
9 Allison SP, Hinton P, Chamberlain MJ: Intravenous glucose tolerance, insulin, and free fatty acid levels in burn patients, *Lancet* 2:1118, 1968.
10 Amaral JF, Caldwell MD, Gann DS: Effect of naloxone on glucose metabolism in skeletal muscle, *Surg Forum* 35:52, 1984.
11 Amaral JF, Shearer JD, Caldwell MD: Hepatic metabolism following injury and adrenalectomy, Providence, RI, 1987 (unpublished observation).
12 Amaral JF, Shearer JD, Caldwell MD: High-dose endotoxin decrease–glucose uptake in skeletal muscle, *Arch Surg* 1987.
13 Amaral JF, Shearer JD, Gann DS et al: Do physiological concentrations of beta endorphin alter glucose metabolism in the periphery? *Metabolism* (in press).
14 Amir S, Berstein M: Endogenous opiates interact in stress-induced hyperglycemia in mice. In *Physiology and behavior,* Elmsford, NY, 1982, Pergamon.
15 Anderson B: Regulation of body fluids, *Annu Rev Physiol* 39:185, 1977.
16 Anderson RJ, Gordon JA, Kim J: Renal concentration defect following nonoliguric acute renal failure in the rat, *Kidney Int* 21:583, 1982.
17 Anderson RJ, Kinas SL, Berns AS et al: Nonoliguric renal failure, *N Engl J Med* 296:1134, 1977.
18 Anggard EE: The endothelium: the body's largest endocrine gland? *J Endocrinol* 127:371, 1990.
19 Antoni FA: Vasopressinergic control of pituitary adrenocorticotropin secretion comes of age, *Front Neuroendocrinol* 14:76, 1993.
20 Antonipillai I, Horton R: Paracrine regulation of the renin-angiotensin system, *J Steroid Bioch Mol Biol* 45:27, 1993.
21 Aono T, Kurachi K, Miyata M et al: Influence of surgical stress under general anesthesia on serum gonadotropin levels, *J Clin Endocrinol Metab* 42:144, 1976.
22 Ardawi MSM, Newsholme EA: Glutamine metabolism in lymphoid tissue. In Haussinger D, Sies H, editors: *Glutamine metabolism in mammalian tissues,* New York, 1984, Springer-Verlag.
23 Arend WP, Joslin FG, Massoni RJ: Effects of immune complexes on production by human monocytes of interleukin-1 or interleukin-1 inhibitor, *J Immunol* 134:3868, 1986.
24 Arturson G: Microvascular permeability to macromolecules in thermal injury, *Acta Physiol Scand* 463:111, 1979.
25 Askanazi J, Carpentier YA, Michensen CB et al: Muscle and plasma amino acids following injury: influence of intercurrent infection, *Ann Surg* 182:78, 1980.
26 Askanazi J, Elwyn DH, Kinney JM et al: Muscle and plasma amino acids after injury: the role of inactivity, *Ann Surg* 188:797, 1978.
27 Askanazi J, Elwyn DH, Silverberg PA et al: Respiratory distress secondary to a high carbohydrate load, *Surgery* 86:596, 1980.
28 Aulick LH, Wilmore DH: Increased peripheral amino acid release following burn injury, *Surgery* 85:560, 1979.
29 Aun F, Young RN et al: The effect of major trauma on the pathways of thyroid hormone metabolism, *J Trauma* 23:1048, 1983.
30 Auron PE, Webb AC, Rosenwasser LJ et al: Nucleotide sequence of human monocyte interleukin-1 precursor cDNA, *Pro Natl Acad Sci USA* 81:7907, 1984.
31 Averill DB, Scher AM, Feigl ED: Angiotensin causes vasoconstriction during hemorrhage in baroreceptor-denervated dogs, *Am J Physiol* 245:H667, 1983.
32 Baer PG, McGiff JC: Hormonal systems and renal hemodynamics, *Annu Rev Physiol* 42:589, 1980.
33 Baertschi AJ, Ward DG, Gann DS: Role of atrial receptors in the control of ACTH, *Am J Physiol* 231:692, 1976.
34 Bagby GJ, Coril CB, Martinez RR: Triglyceride and free fatty acid turnover in *E. coli* endotoxin–treated rats, *Circ Shock* 16:76, 1980.
35 Bakris GL, Re RN: Endothelin modulates the angiotensin II–induced mitogenesis of human mesangial cells, *Am J Physiol* 264:F937, 1993.
36 Banchereau J: Interleukin-4. In Thomson AW, editor: *The cytokine handbook,* London, 1991, Academic Press.
37 Baracos V, Rodemann HP, Dinarello CA et al: Stimulation of muscle protein degradation and prostaglandin E_2 release by leukocyte pyrogen (interleukin-1), *N Engl J Med* 253:5532, 1983.
38 Baracos V, Rodemann HP, Dinarello CA et al: Stimulation of muscle protein degradation and prostaglandin E_2 release by leukocyte pyrogen (interleukin-1), *N Engl J Med* 308:553, 1983.
39 Baughman RP, Lower EE: An inhibitor of tumor necrosis factor found in pleural effusions, *J Lab Clin Med* 118:326, 1991.
40 Baumann H, Isseroff H, Latimer JJ et al: Phorbol ester–modulated interleukin-6 and interleukin-1–regulated expression of acute-phase plasma proteins in hempatoma cells, *J Biol Chem* 263:17369, 1988.
41 Baxter CR, Shires T: Physiological response to crystalloid resuscitation of severe burns, *Ann NY Acad Sci* 150:874, 1968.
42 Baxter JD, Tyrell JB, Felig P et al: The adrenal cortex. In Felig P, Baxter JD, Brodus AE, Frohman LA, editors: *Endocrinology and metabolism,* New York, 1981, McGraw-Hill.
43 Baxter RC, Turtle JR: Stimulation of protein synthesis in isolated hepatocytes by somatomedin, *Metabolism* 27:503, 1978.
44 Baylis PH, Zepre RL, Robertson GL: Arginine vasopressin response to insulin-induced hypoglycemia in man, *J Clin Endocrinol Metab* 53:935, 1981.
45 Bazan JF: Haemopoietic receptors and helical cytokines, *Immunol Today* 11:350, 1990.
46 Beisel WR, Pekarek RS, Wannemacher RW: Homeostatic mechanisms affecting plasma zinc levels in acute stress. In Prasad AS, editor: *Trace elements in human health and disease,* New York, 1976, Academic Press.
47 Belfiore F: *Enzyme regulation and metabolic disease,* New York, 1980, Karger.
48 Bereiter DA, Plotsky PM, Gann DS: Tooth pulp stimulation potentiates the ACTH response to hemorrhage in cats, *Endocrinology* 111:1127, 1982.
49 Bereiter DA, Plotsky PM, Gann DS: Selective opiate modulation of the physiological responses to hemorrhage in the cat, *Endocrinology* 113:1439, 1983.
50 Bereiter DA, Zaid AM, Gann DS: Effect of rate of hemorrhage on sympathoadrenal catecholamine release in cats, *Am J Physiol* 250:E69, 1986.
51 Bergentz SE, Brief DD: The effect of pH and osmolality on the production of canine hemorrhagic shock, 58:412, 1965.
52 Berkenbosch F, De Goeij EC, Del Rey A et al: Neuroendocrine,

sympathetic, and metabolic responses induced by interleukin-1, *Neuroendocrinology* 50:570, 1989.
53 Berman A, Singh A, Kral T et al: The immune-hypothalamic-pituitary-adrenal axis, *Endocrinol Rev* 10:92, 1989.
54 Bernard C: *Introduction to the experimental study of medicine,* New York, 1927, Macmillan.
55 Bernhagen J, Calandra T, Mitchell RA et al: MIF is a pituitary-derived cytokine that potentiates lethal endotoxemia, *Nature* 365:756, 1993.
56 Bernheim HA, Block LH, Atkins E: Fever: pathogenesis, pathophysiology, and purpose, *Ann Intern Med* 91:261, 1979.
57 Bernton EW, Long J, Holaday JW: Opioids and neuropeptides: mechanisms in circulatory shock, *Fed Proc* 44:290, 1985.
58 Berridge MJ: Inositol triphosphate and calcium signaling, *Nature* 361:315, 1993.
59 Berridge MJ: A tale of two messengers, *Nature* 365:388, 1993.
60 Berry HE, Collier JG, Vane JR: The generation of kinins in the blood of dogs during hypotension due to hemorrhage, *Clin Sci* 39:349, 1970.
61 Bers DM: *Excitation-contraction coupling and cardiac contractile force,* Dordrecht, Germany, 1991, Kluwer Academic Publishers.
62 Besedovsky HO, Del Rey A: Immunoregulatory feedback between interleukin-1 and glucocorticoid hormones, *Science* 233:652, 1986.
63 Besedovsky HO, Del Rey A: Metabolic and endocrine actions of interleukin-1: effects on insulin-resistant animals, *Ann NY Acad Sci* 594:214, 1990.
64 Beuschler HU, Fallon R, Colten HR: Macrophage membrane interleukin-1 regulates the expression of acute-phase proteins in human hepatoma Hep 3B cells, *J Immunol* 139:1896, 1987.
65 Beutler B, Cerami A: Cachectin and tumor necrosis factor as two sides of the same biologic coin, *Nature* 1986:584, 1986.
66 Beutler B, Cerami A: Cachectin: more than a tumor necrosis factor, *N Engl J Med* 316:379, 1987.
67 Beutler B, Mahoney J, Le Tang N et al: Purification of cachectin, a lipoprotein lipase–suppressing hormone secreted by endotoxin-induced RAW 264.7 cells, *J Exp Med* 161:379, 1985.
68 Beveilacqua MP et al: Endothelial leukocyte adhesion molecule-1: an inducible receptor for neutrophils related to complement regulatory proteins and lectins, *Science* 243:1160, 1989.
69 Bie P: Osmoreceptors, vasopressin, and control of renal water excretion, *Physiol Rev* 60:961, 1980.
70 Billiar TR, Curran RD, Stuehr DJ et al: An L-arginine–dependent mechanism mediates Kupffer cell inhibition of hepatocyte protein synthesis in vitro, *J Exp Med* 170:1769, 1989.
71 Bilmazer C et al: Quantitative contribution by skeletal muscle to elevated ratio of whole-body protein breakdown in burned children as measured by 3-MEH output, *Metabolism* 27:671, 1978.
72 Bird TA, Saklatvala J: Studies on the fate of receptor-bound ^{125}I-interleukin-1-beta in porcine synovial fibroblasts, *J Immunol* 139:92, 1987.
73 Birkhain RH et al: Effects of major skeletal trauma on whole-body protein turnover in man measured by (14-C) leucine, *Surgery* 888:294, 1980.
74 Birkhain RH, Long CL, Fitkin DL et al: A comparison of the effects of skeletal trauma and surgery on the ketosis of starvation in man, *J Trauma* 1:513, 1981.
75 Birnbaumer L: Transduction of receptor signal into modulation of effector activity by G proteins, *FASEB J* 4:3179, 1990.
76 Birnbaumer L, Codina J, Yatani Y: Molecular basis of regulation of ionic channels by G protein–coupled receptors, *Recent Prog Horm Res* 45:121, 1989.
77 Black PR, Brooks DC, Bessey PQ et al: Mechanisms of insulin resistance following injury, *Ann Surg* 196:420, 1982.
78 Blake MJ, Udelsman R, G.J. F et al: Stress-induced heat-shock protein 70 expression in the adrenal cortex: an adrenocorticotropic hormone-sensitive, age-dependent response, *Proc Natl Acad Sci USA* 88:9873, 1991.
79 Blalock A: Experimental shock: the cause of low blood pressure caused by muscle injury, *Arch Surg* 20:959, 1930.
80 Blalock JE: A molecular basis for bidirectional communication between the immune and neuroendocrine systems, *Physiol Rev* 69:1, 1989.
81 Blick M, Sherwin SA, Rosenblum M et al: Phase 1 study of recombinant tumor necrosis factor in cancer patients, *Cancer Res* 47:286, 1987.
82 Bokisch V, Muller-Eberhard HJ: Anaphylatoxin inactivator of human plasma: its isolation and characterization, *J Clin Invest* 49:2427, 1970.
83 Bone RC: Toward an epidemiology and natural history of SIRS (systemic inflammatory response syndrome), *JAMA* 268:3452, 1992.
84 Bowers RE, Ellis EF, Brigham KL et al: Effects of prostaglandin cyclic endoperoxides on the lung circulation of unanesthetized sheep, *J Clin Invest* 633:131, 1979.
85 Boyd DR, Mansberger AR: Serum water and osmolar changes in hemorrhagic shock, *Am Surg* 34:744, 1968.
86 Bravo EL, Saito F, Zaella T et al: In vitro steroidogenic properties of a new hypertension-producing compound from normal human urine, *J Clin Endocrinal Metab* 51:176, 1980.
87 Brigham KL, Meyrick B, Berry LC Jr et al: Antioxidants protect cultured bovine lung endothelial cells from injury from endotoxin, *J Appl Physiol* 63:840, 1987.
88 Brizio-Molteni L, Molteni A, Warpeha RL et al: Prolactin, corticotropin, and gonadotropin concentrations following thermal injury in adults, *J Trauma* 24:1, 1984.
89 Brooks DK, Williams WG, Manley RW et al: Osmolar and electrolyte changes in hemorrhagic shock, *Lancet* 1:521, 1963.
90 Brown D: Membrane recycling and epithelial cell function, *Am J Physiol* 256:F1, 1989.
91 Brown JM, Grosso MA, Harkin AH: Cytokines, sepsis, and the surgeon, *Surg Gynecol Obstet* 169:568, 1989.
92 Brown SL, Smith LR, Blalock JE: Interleukin-1 and interleukin-2 enhance pro-opiomelanocortin gene expression in pituitary cells, *J Immunol* 139:3181, 1987.
93 Brown-Sequard E: Des effets produits chez l'homme par des injections sous-cutanees d'un liquide retire des testicules frais de cobaye et de chien, *Compt Societ Biol (Paris)* 41:415, 1889.
94 Browne JSL, Schneker L: Conference on metabolic aspects of convalescence, including bone and wound healing: transactions of the third meeting, New York, 1943, Josiah Macy Jr.
95 Buchanan TA, Thawani H, Dades W et al: Angiotensin II increases glucose utilization during acute hyperinsulinemia via a hemodynamic mechanism, *J Clin Invest* 92:720, 1993.
96 Buse MG, Reid SS: Leucine: a possible regulator of protein turnover in muscle, *J Clin Invest* 56:1250, 1975.
97 Bussolino E, Camussi G, Aglietta M et al: Human endothelial cells are targets for cytoskeleton structures, *J Immunol* 139:2493, 1987.
98 Byrnes GJ, Pirkle JC Jr, Gann DS: Cardiovascular stabilization after hemorrhage depends upon restitution of blood volume, *J Trauma* 18:623, 1978.
99 Cahill GF: Ketosis, *JPEN* 1981.
100 Caldwell FT Jr: Metabolic responses to thermal trauma. II. Nutritional studies with rats at two environmental temperatures, *Ann Surg* 155:119, 1962.
101 Caldwell MD, Lacy WW, Exton JH: Effects of adrenalectomy on the amino acid and glucose metabolism of perfused rat hindlimbs, *J Biol Chem* 253:6837, 1978.
102 Caldwell MD, Shearer J, Morris A et al: Evidence for aerobic

glycolysis in lambda-carrageenan–wounded skeletal muscle, *J Surg Res* 37:63, 1984.
103 Calloway DH, Grossman MI, Bowman J et al: Effect of previous level of protein feeding on wound healing and on metabolic response to injury, *Surgery* 37:935, 1955.
104 Camussie G, Aglietta M, Malavasi F et al: The release of platelet activating factor from human endothelial cells in culture, *J Immunol* 131:2397, 1983.
105 Cannon WB: *The wisdom of the body,* New York, 1939, Norton.
106 Cantin M, Genest J: The heart and atrial natriuretic factor, *Endocr Rev* 6:1, 1985.
107 Carafoli E: Intracellular calcium homeostasis, *Annu Rev Biochem* 56:395, 1987.
108 Carey LC, Cloutier CT, Lowery BD: Growth hormone and adrenal cortisol response to shock and trauma in the human, *Ann Surg* 174:451, 1971.
109 Carey LC, Lowery BD, Cloutier CT: Blood sugar and insulin response in human shock, *Ann Surg* 172:342, 1970.
110 Carey RM, VanLoon GR, Baines AD et al: Decreased plasma and urinary dopamine during dietary sodium depletion in man, *J Clin Endocrinol Metab* 52:903, 1981.
111 Caromona OA, Tsao RC, Trunkey DD et al: The role of prostacyclin and thromboxane in sepsis and septic shock, *Arch Surg* 119:189, 1984.
112 Carper SW, Duffy JJ, Gerner EW: Heat shock–related proteins in thermotolerance and other cellular processes, *Cancer Res* 47:5429, 1987.
113 Carretero OA, Scicli AG: The renal kallikrein-kinin system. In Dunn MJ, editor: *Renal endocrinology,* Baltimore, 1983, Williams and Wilkins.
114 Carstensen H et al: Testosterone, luteinizing hormone, and growth hormone in blood following surgical trauma, *Acta Chir Scand* 138:1, 1972.
115 Carswell EA: An endotoxin-induced serum factor that causes necrosis of tumors, *Proc Natl Acad Sci USA* 72:3666, 1975.
116 Carter DB, Deibel MR, Dunn CJ et al: Purification, cloning, expression, and biological characterization of an interleukin-1 receptor antagonist protein, *Nature* 344:633, 1990.
117 Casley-Smith JR: The functioning and interrelationships of blood capillaries and lymphatics, *Experientia* 32:1, 1976.
118 Cathcart MK, Morel DW, Chisolm GM: *J Leuk Biol* 38:341, 1985.
119 Cavalieri RR, Rappoport B: Impaired peripheral conversion of thyroxine to triiodothyronine, *Annu Rev Med* 28:57, 1977.
120 Cernacek P, Stewart DJ: Immunoreactive endothelin in human plasma: marked elevation in patients in cardiogenic shock, *Biochem Biophys Res Commun* 161:562, 1989.
121 Cerra FB: Nutrient modulation of inflammatory and immune function, *Am J Surg* 161:230, 1991.
122 Chaisson JL, Liljenquist JE, Sinclair-Smith BC et al: Gluconeogenesis from alanine in normal postabsorptive man: intrahepatic stimulatory effect of glucagon, *Diabetes* 24:574, 1975.
123 Chaisson JL, Shikama H, Chu DTW et al: Inhibitory effect of epinephrine on insulin-stimulated glucose uptake by rat skeletal muscle, *J Clin Invest* 68:706, 1981.
124 Chaminade M, Fortz AS, Rossier J: Co-release of enkephalins and precursors with catecholamines from the perfused cat adrenal gland in situ, *J Physiol* 353:157, 1984.
125 Chan TM: The permissive effects of gluococorticoids on hepatic gluconeogenesis, *J Biol Chem* 259:7426, 1984.
126 Chappell JB: Systems used for the transport of substances into mitochondria, *Br Med Bull* 24:150, 1968.
127 Charters AC, O'Dell MWD, Thompson JC: Anterior pituitary function during surgical stress and convalescence, *J Clin Endocrinol Metab* 29:63, 1969.
128 Chaudry IH, Sayeed MM, Baue AE: Depletion and restoration of tissue ATP in hemorrhagic shock, *Arch Surg* 108:208, 1974.
129 Chaudry IH, Wichterman KA, Baue AE: Effect of sepsis on tissue adenine nucleotid levels, *Surgery* 85:205, 1979.
130 Chiba T, Nagata Y, Machide M et al: Tyrosine kinase activation through the extracellular domains of cytokine receptors, *Nature* 362:646, 1993.
131 Chilton FH, O'Flaherty JT, Ellis JM et al: Metabolic rate of platelet activating factor in neutrophils, *J Biol Chem* 258:7268, 1983.
132 Chirico WJ, Waters MG, Blobel G: 70k heat shock–related proteins stimulate protein translocation into microsomes, *Nature* 322:85, 1991.
133 Cioffi WGJ, Vaughan GM, Heironimus JD et al: Dissociation of blood volume and flow in regulation of salt and water balance in burn patients, *Ann Surg* 214:213, 1991.
134 Clapham DE, Neer EJ: New roles for G protein beta-gamma-dimers in transmembrane signaling, *Nature* 365:403, 1993.
135 Clark EJ, Rossiter R: Carbohydrate metabolism after burning, *Q J Exp Physiol* 32:279, 1944.
136 Clark JH, Schrader WT, O'Malley BW: Mechanisms of action of steroid hormones. In Wilson JD, Foster DW, editors: *Williams textbook of endocrinology,* ed 8, Philadelphia, 1992, WB Saunders.
137 Claybaugh JR, Share L: Vasopressin, renin, and cardiovascular responses to continuous slow hemorrhage, *Am J Physiol* 224:519, 1973.
138 Clowes G, George BC, Villee CA et al: Muscle proteolysis induced by a circulation peptide in patients with sepsis or trauma, *N Engl J Med* 308:545, 1983.
139 Clowes G, Randall H, Cha C: Amino acid and energy metabolism in septic and traumatized patients, *JPEN* 4:195, 1980.
140 Clowes GHA Jr, Hirsch E, George B et al: Survival from sepsis: the significance of altered protein metabolism regulated by proteolysis-inducing factor, the circulating cleavage product of interleukin-1, *Ann Surg* 202:446, 1985.
141 Clozel M, Breu V, Burri K et al: Pathophysiological role of endothelin revealed by the first orally active endothelin-receptor antagonist, *Nature* 365:759, 1993.
142 Cochrane JPS, Forsling ML, Gow NM et al: Arginine vasopressin release following surgical operations, *Br J Surg* 68:209, 1981.
143 Cohn ZA, Morse SI: Functional and metabolic properties of polymorphonuclear leukocytes, *J Exp Med* 111:689, 1960.
144 Coleridge JCG, Coleridge HM: Chemoreflex regulation of the heart. In Berne RM, editor: *Handbook of physiology,* Baltimore, 1979, Williams & Wilkins.
145 Collort MA, Belin D, Vassalli JD et al: Gamma-interferon enhances macrophage transcription of the tumor necrosis factor/cachectin, interleukin-1, and urokinase genes, which are controlled by short-lived repressors, *J Exper Med* 164:2113, 1986.
146 Coop DH: Parathyroids, calcitonin, and control of plasma calcium, *Recent Prog Horm Res* 20:59, 1964.
147 Coran AG, Cryer PE, Horwitz DL et al: Fat and carbohydrate metabolism during hemorrhagic shock in the unanesthetized baboon, *Surg Forum* 9:10, 1971.
148 Cowley AW, Quitlen EW, Skelton MM: Role of vasopressin in cardiovascular regulation, *Fed Proc* 42:3170, 1983.
149 Cox BM, Baizman ER: Physiological functions of the endorphins. In Malick JB, Bell RMS, editors: *Endorphins: chemistry, physiology, pharmacology, and clinical relevance,* New York, 1982, Dekker.
150 Crane CW et al: Protein turnover in patients before and after elective orthopedic operations, *Br J Surg* 64:129, 1977.
151 Cross JS, Gruber DP, Gann DS et al: Hypertonic saline attenuates the hormonal response to injury, *Ann Surg* 209:684, 1989.
152 Crowley CV, Seifter E, Kriss P et al: Effects of environmental temperature and femoral fracture on wound healing in rats, *J Trauma* 17:436, 1977.

153 Cryer PE: Physiology and pathophysiology of the human sympathoadrenal neuroendocrine system, *N Engl J Med* 303:436, 1980.
154 Cryer PE: Disease of the adrenal medullae and sympathetic nervous system. In Felig P, Baxter JD, Broadus AE, Frohman LA, editors: *Endocrinology and metabolism,* New York, 1981, McGraw-Hill.
155 Curran RD, Billiar TR, Stuehr DJ et al: Multiple cytokines are required to induce hepatocyte nitric oxide production and inhibit total protein synthesis, *Ann Surg* 212:462, 1989.
156 Curtis T, Lefer A: Protective actions of naloxone in hemorrhagic shock, *Am J Physiol* 239:H416, 1980.
157 Cuthbertson DP: Observations on the disturbances of metabolism by injury to the limbs, *Q J Med* 1:233, 1932.
158 Cuthbertson DP, Tilstone WJ: Effects of environmental temperature on the closure of full-thickness skin wounds in the rat, *Q J Exp Physiol* 52:249, 1967.
159 Dahlen S, Bjork J, Hedquist P et al: Leukotrienes promote capillary leakage and leukocyte adhesions in postcapillary venules: in vivo effects with relevance to acute inflammatory response, *Proc Natl Acad Sci USA* 70:3887, 1981.
160 Dale G et al: The effect of surgical operation on venous plasma free amino acids, *Surgery* 81:295, 1977.
161 Damme JV: Interleukin-8 and related molecules. In Thomson A, editor: *The cytokine handbook,* London, 1991, Academic Press.
162 Davis PJ: Cellular actions of thyroid hormone. In Utiger RD, editor: *Werner and Ingbar's the thyroid,* Philadelphia, 1991, JB Lippincott.
163 DeBold CR, Menefee JK, Nicholson WE et al: Pro-opiomelanocorticotropin gene is expressed by many normal human tissues and in tumors not associated with ectopic adrenocorticotropin syndrome, *Mol Endocrinol* 2:862, 1989.
164 DeClerck FF, Herman AG: 5-Hydroxytryptamine and platelet aggregation, *Fed Proc* 42:228, 1983.
165 Deitch EA, Xo D, Bridgs R: Opioids modulate neutrophil lymphocyte function: thermal injury alters plasma beta-endorphin levels, *Surgery* 104:41, 1988.
166 Deitch EA: Multiple organ failure: pathophysiology and potential future therapy, *Ann Surg* 216:117, 1992.
167 Deitch EA, Bridges W, Baker J et al: Hemorrhagic shock–induced bacterial translocation is reduced by xanthine oxidase inhibition or inactivation, *Surgery* 104:191, 1988.
168 Deitch EA, Mancini MC: Complement receptors in shock and transplantation, *Arch Surg* 128:1222, 1993.
169 Demling RH: Respiratory failure after trauma and sepsis, *Surg Clin North Am* 56:1373, 1980.
170 Demling RH, Kramer G, Harms B: Role of thermal injury–induced hypoproteinemia on fluid flux and protein permeability in burned and unburned tissue, *Surgery* 95:136, 1984.
171 Dillingham MA, Anderson RJ: Inhibition of vasopressin action by atrial natriuretic factor, *Science* 231:1572, 1986.
172 Dinarello C, Clowes GHA Jr, Gordon AH et al: Cleavage of human interleukin-1: isolation of a peptide fragment from plasma of febrile humans and activated monocytes, *J Immunol* 133:1332, 1984.
173 Dinarello CA: Interleukin-1 and the pathogenesis of the acute-phase response, *N Engl J Med* 311:1413, 1984.
174 Dinarello CA: Interleukin-1 and its biologically related cytokines, *Adv Immunol* 44:153, 1989.
175 Dinarello CA, Gelfand JA, Wolff SM: Anticytokine strategies in the treatment of systemic inflammatory response syndrome, *JAMA* 269:1829, 1993.
176 Dinarello CA, Savage N: Interleukin-1 and its receptor, *CRC Crit Rev Immunol* 9:1, 1989.
177 Doebber TW, Wu MS, Robbins JC et al: Platelet-activating factor involvement in endotoxin-induced hypotension in rats: studies with PAF-receptor antagonist kadsurenone, *Biochem, Biophys Res Commun* 127:799, 1985.
178 Dohanics J, Linton EA, Lowry PJ et al: Osmotic stimulation affects neurohypophysial corticotropin-releasing factor 41 content: effect of dexamethasone, *Peptides* 11:51, 1990.
179 Donnely M, Sheffer E: Energy metabolism in respiration-deficient and wild type Chinese hamster fibroblast in culture, *J Cell Physiol* 89:39, 1976.
180 Dressler KA, Mathias S, Kolesnick RN: Tumor necrosis factor-alpha activates the sphingomyelin signal transduction pathway in a cell-free system, *Science* 255:1715, 1992.
181 Drucker WR, Chadwick CDJ, Gann DS: Transcapillary refill in hemorrhage and shock, *Arch Surg* 116:1344, 1981.
182 Drucker WR, Dekieweit JC: Glucose uptake by diaphragms from rats subjected to hemorrhagic shock, *Am J Physiol* :317, 1964.
183 Drucker WR, Gallie BL, Lau TS et al: *Neurohumoral and metabolic response to injury,* New York, 1978, Plenum.
184 Dubois M, Pickar D, Cohen MR et al: Surgical stress in humans is accompanied by an increase in plasma beta-endorphin immunoreactivity, *Life Sci* 29:1249, 1981.
185 Duke JH, Jorgensen BS, Broell JR et al: Contribution of protein to caloric expenditure following injury, *Surgery* 68:168, 1970.
186 Dunn A: Systemic interkeukin-1 administration stimulates hypothalamic norepinephrine metabolism paralleling the increased plasma corticosterone, *Life Sci* 1988:429, 1988.
187 Eckenhoff JE, Oech SR: The effects of narcotics and antagonists upon respiration and circulation in man, *Clin Pharmacol Ther* 1:483, 1960.
188 Edelman GM: *Topobiology: an introduction to molecular embryology,* New York, 1988, Harper Collins.
189 Edelman IS, Ismail-Beigi F: Thyroid thermogenesis and active sodium transport, *Recent Prog Horm Res* 30:235, 1974.
190 Egdahl RH: The differential response of the adrenal cortex and medulla to bacterial endotoxin, *J Clin Invest* 38:1120, 1959.
191 Egdahl RH: Pituitary-adrenal response following trauma to the isolated leg, *Surgery* 46:9, 1959.
192 Egdahl RH, Nelson DH, Hume DM: Adrenal cortical function in hypothermia, *Surg Gynecol Obstet* 101:15, 1955.
193 Eigler N, Sacca L, Sherwin RS: Synergistic interactions of physiologic increments of glucagon, epinephrine, and cortisol in the dog, *J Clin Invest* 63:114, 1979.
194 Elder JM, Miles AA: The action of the lethal toxins of gas gangrene clostridia on capillary permeability, *J Pathol* 74:133, 1957.
195 Elwyn DH, Parikh HC, Stahr LJ et al: Interorgan transport of amino acids in hemorrhagic shock, *Am J Physiol* 231:377, 1976.
196 Emerson TW: Participation of endogenous vasoactive agents in the pathogenesis of endotoxic shock, *Adv Exp Med Biol* 23:25, 1974.
197 Enberg G, Carlquist M, Jornvall H et al: The characterization of somatomedin A, isolated by microcomputer-controlled chromatography, reveals an apparent identity to insulin-like growth factor I, *Eur J Biochem* 143:117, 1984.
198 Engel FL: The significance of the metabolic changes during shock, *Ann NY Acad Sci* 55:383, 1956.
199 Engel FL, Winton MG, Long CHH: Biochemical studies on shock. I. The metabolism of amino acids and carbohydrates during hemorrhagic shock in the rat, *J Exp Med* 77:397, 1942.
200 Engeland WC, Byrnes GJ, Gann DS: The pituitary adrenocortical response to hemorrhage depends on the time of day, *Endocrinology* 110:1856, 1982.
201 Engeland WC, Demsher DP, Byrnes GJ et al: The adrenal medullary response to graded hemorrhage in awake dogs, *Endocrinology* 109:1539, 1981.
202 Engelmann H, Aderka D, Rubinstein M et al: A tumor necrosis

factor–binding protein purified to homogeneity from human urine protects cells from tumor necrosis factor toxicity, *J Biol Chem* 264:11974, 1989.
203 Engels FL, Fredericks J: Contribution to understanding of the mechanism of permissive action of corticoids, *Proc Soc Exp Biol Med* 95:593, 1957.
204 Esler M, Jennings G, Lamberg G et al: Overflow of catecholamine neurotransmitters to the circulation: source, rate, and functions, *Physiol Rev* 70:963, 1992.
205 Evans RM: The steroid and thyroid hormone receptor superfamily, *Science* 240:889, 1988.
206 Exton JH: Gluconeogenesis, *Metabolism* 21:945, 1972.
207 Fagarasan MO, Eskay R, Axelrod J: Interleukin-1 potentiates the secretion of beta-endorphin induced by secretagogues in a mouse pituitary cell line (AtT-20), *Proc Natl Acad Sci USA* 86:2070, 1989.
208 Fain JN: Inhibition of glucose transport in fat cells and activation of lipolysis by glucocorticoids. In Baxter JD, Rousseau GG, editors: *Glucocorticoid hormone action,* New York, 1979, Springer-Verlag.
209 Fain JN: Involvement of phosphatidylinositol breakdown in elevation of cytosol CA^{++} by hormones and relationship to prostaglandin formation. In Kohn LD, editor: *Hormone receptors,* New York, 1982, Wiley & Sons.
210 Fain JN, Garcia-Sainz JA: Adrenergic regulation of adipocyte metabolism, *J Lipid Res* 24:945, 1983.
211 Fain JN, Kovacev VP, Scow RO: Effect of growth hormone and dexamethasone on lipolysis and metabolism in isolated fat cells of the rat, *J Biol Chem* 240:3522, 1965.
212 Fakunding JL, Chow R, Catt KJ: The role of calcium in the stimulation of aldosterone production by ACTH, angiotensin II, and potassium in isolated glomerulosa cells, *Endocrinology* 105:327, 1979.
213 Farrell LD, Harrison TS, Demers LM: Immunoreactive met-enkephalin in the canine adrenal: response to acute hypovolemia, *Proc Soc Exp Biol Med* 173:515, 1983.
214 Fater DC, Sundet WD, Schultz HD et al: Arterial baroreceptors have minimal physiological effects on adrenal medullary secretion, *Am J Physiol* 224:H194, 1983.
215 Feldman M, Kiser RS, Unger RH et al: Beta-endorphin and the endocrine pancreas, *N Engl J Med* 308:350, 1983.
216 Felig P: The glucose-alanine cycle, *Metabolism* 22:179, 1973.
217 Felig P: The endocrine pancreas: diabetes mellitus. In Felig P, Baxter JD, Broadus AE, Frohman LA, editors: *Endocrinology and metabolism,* New York, 1981, McGraw-Hill.
218 Felig P, Sherwin RS, Soman V et al: Hormonal interactions in the regulation of blood glucose, *Recent Prog Horm Res* 35:501, 1979.
219 Felig P, Wahren J, Hendler R: Influence of physiologic hyperglucagonemia on basal and insulin-inhibited splanchnic glucose output in normal man, *J Clin Invest* 58:761, 1976.
220 Fernandez-Botran R: Soluble cytokine receptors: their role in immunoregulation, *FASEB J* 5:2567, 1991.
221 Filkins JP: Glucoregulation of the RES. In Reichard SM, Filkins JM, editor: *The reticuloendothelial system: a comprehensive treatise,* New York, 1984, Plenum.
222 Fisher JA, Blum JW et al: Acute parathyroid hormone response to epinephrine in vivo, *J Clin Invest* 52:2434, 1973.
223 Fisher JE, Hasselgren PO: Cytokines and glucocorticoids in the regulation of the heptatico-skeletal muscle axis in sepsis, *Am J Surg* 162:266, 1991.
224 Flamenbaum W, Gasgon J, Ramwell P: Bradykinin-induced renal hemodynamic alterations: renin and prostaglandin relationships, *Am J Physiol* 237:F433, 1979.
225 Fletcher JR, DiSimone AG, Earnest MA: Platelet-activating factor receptor antagonist improves survival and attenuates eicosanoid release in severe endotoxemia, *Ann Surg* 211:312, 1990.
226 Fletcher JR, Ramwell PW, Herman CW: Prostaglandins and the hemodynamic course of endotoxin shock, *J Surg Res* 20:589, 1976.
227 Fletcher JR, Short BL, Walker RI et al: Prostaglandins as mediators of the hemodynamic abnormalities in endotoxemia and sepsis. In McConn R, editor: *Role of chemical mediators in the pathophysiology of acute illness and injury,* New York, 1982, Raven.
228 Foley NM, McNicol MW, Rook GAW et al: Effect of serum from patients with sarcoidosis and tuberculosis on TNF-induced killing of murine cells, *Am Rev Respir Dis* 139:A58, 1989.
229 Fong Y, Moldawer LL, Marano M et al: Cachectin/TNF or IL-1-alpha induces cachexia with redistribution of body protein, *Am J Physiol* 256:R659, 1989.
230 Fong Y, Moldawer LL, Marano MA et al: Endotoxemia elicits increased circulating 20-IFN/IL-6 in man, *J Immunol* 142:2321, 1989.
231 Fong Y, Moldawer LL, Shires GT et al: The biological characteristics of cytokines and their implication in surgical injury, *Surg Gynecol Obstet* 170:363, 1990.
232 Fong Y, Tracey KJ, Moldawer LL et al: Antibodies to cachectin/TNF reduce interleukin-1 and interleukin-6 appearance during lethal bacteremia, *J Exp Med* 170:167, 1989.
233 Fradkin J, Shamoon H, Felig P et al: Evidence of an important role for changes in, rather than absolute concentration of, glucagon in the regulation of glucose production in humans, *J Clin Endocrinol Metab* 50:698, 1980.
234 Franchimont P: The regulation of follicle-stimulating hormone and luteinizing hormone secretion in humans. In Martini L, Ganong WF, editors: *Frontiers in neuroendocrinology,* New York, 1971, Oxford University Press.
235 Frawley JP, Artz CP, Howard JM: Muscle metabolism and catabolism in combat casualities, *Arch Surg* 71:612, 1955.
236 Fray JCS, Luch DJ, Valentine A: Cellular mechanisms of renin secretion, *Fed Proc* 42:3250, 1983.
237 Frayn KN, Prete DA, Maycock PF et al: Plasma somatomedin activity after injury in man and its relationship to other hormonal and metabolic changes, *Clin Endocrinol* 20:179, 1984.
238 Freeman BA, Crapo JD: Free radicals and tissue injury. In Rubill E, Damjaniv I, editors: *Advances in the biology of disease,* Baltimore, 1984, Williams & Wilkins.
239 Freiman PC, Mitchell GG, Heistad DD et al: Atherosclerosis impairs endothelium-dependent vascular relaxation to acetylcholine and thrombin in primates, *Circ Res* 58:783, 1986.
240 Freund HR, Ryan JA, Fischer JE: Amino acid derangements in patients with sepsis: treatment with branched-chain amino acid–rich infusions, *Ann Surg* 188:423, 1978.
241 Friedl HP, Till GO, Ryan US et al: Mediator-induced activation of xanthine oxidase in endothelial cells, *FASEB J* 3:2512, 1989.
242 Friedman SG, Pearce FJ, Drucker WR: The role of blood glucose in the defense of plasma volume during hemorrhage, *J Trauma* 22:86, 1982.
243 Frohman JC: CNS peptides and glucoregulation, *Annu Rev Physiol* 45:95, 1983.
244 Frohman L: Diseases of the anterior pituitary. In Felig P, Barter JD, Broadus AE, Frohman LA, editors: *Endocrinology and metabolism,* New York, 1981, McGraw-Hill.
245 Froholm BB: The effect of lactate in canine subcutaneous adipose tissue in situ, *Acta Physiol Scand* 81:110, 1971.
246 Frolich JC, Margolius HS: Prostaglandins, the kallikrein-kinin system: Bartter's syndrome and the carcinoid syndrome. In Felig P, Barter JD, Broadus AE, Frohman LA, editors: *Endocrinology and metabolism,* New York, 1981, McGraw-Hill.

247 Fryburg DA, Gelfand RA, Barrett EJ: Growth hormone acutely stimulates forearm muscle protein synthesis in normal humans, *Am J Physiol* 260:E499, 1991.
248 Fujita K, Aguilera G, Catt KJ: The role of cAMP in the aldosterone production by isolated zona glomerulosa cells, *J Biol Chem* 254:8567, 1979.
249 Funder JW: Mineralocorticoids, glucocorticoids, receptors, and response elements, *Science* 259:1132, 1993.
250 Furst P, Bergstrom S, Chao L: Influence of amino acid sulphur on nitrogen and amino acid metabolism in severe trauma, *Acta Chir Scand (Suppl)* 494:136, 1979.
251 Gabow PA, Peterson LN: Disorders of potassium metabolism. In Schrier RW, editor: *Renal and electrolyte disorders,* Boston, 1980, Little, Brown.
252 Gala GJ, Lilly MP, Thomas SE et al: Interaction of sodium and volume in fluid resuscitation after hemorrhage, *J Trauma* 31:545, 1989.
253 Galione A: Cyclic-ADP ribose: a new way to control calcium, *Science* 259:325, 1993.
254 Gallinaro R, Cheadle WG, Applegate K et al: The role of the complement system in trauma and infection, *Surg Gynecol Obstet* 174:435, 1992.
255 Gann DS: Endocrine control of plasma protein and volume, *Surg Clin North Am* 56:1135, 1976.
256 Gann DS, Amaral JF: The pathophysiological response to injury. In Zuidema G, Rutherford R, Ballinger WF, editors: *The management of trauma,* Philadelphia, 1985, WB Saunders.
257 Gann DS, Carlson DE, Byrnes GJ et al: Role of solute in the early restitution of blood volume after hemorrhage, *Surgery* 94:439, 1983.
258 Gann DS, Carlson DE, Byrnes GJ: Impaired restitution of blood volume after large hemorrhage, *J Trauma* 21:598, 1981.
259 Gann DS, Cryer GL, Pirkle JC Jr: Physiological inhibition and facilitation in adrenocortical response to hemorrhage, *Am J Physiol* 232:R5, 1977.
260 Gann DS, Dallman MF, Engeland WC: Reflex control and modulation of ACTH and corticosteroids. In McCann SM, editor: *Endocrine physiology III: international review of physiology,* Baltimore, 1981, University Park Press.
261 Gann DS, Lilly MP: The neuroendocrine response to multiple trauma, *World J Surg* 7:101, 1983.
262 Gann DS, Pirkle JC: Role of cortisol in the restitution of blood volume after hemorrhage, *Am J Surg* 130:565, 1975.
263 Gann DS, Ward DG, Baertschi AJ et al: Neural control of ACTH release in response to hemorrhage, *Ann NY Acad Sci* 297:477, 1977.
264 Garber AJ, Karl IE, Kipnis DM: Alanine and glutamine synthesis and release from skeletal muscle. I. Glycolysis and amino acid release, *J Biol Chem* 251:826, 1976.
265 Gellar DA, Lowenstein CJ, Shapiro RA et al: Molecular cloning and expression of inducible nitric oxide synthase from human hepatocytes, *Proc Natl Acad Sci USA* 90:3491, 1993.
266 George DT, Abeles FB, Mapes CA et al: Effect of leukocyte endogenous mediators on endocrine pancrease secretary response, *Am J Physiol* 233:E240, 1977.
267 Gerich JE, Charles MA et al: Regulation of pancreatic insulin and glucagon secretion, *Annu Rev Physiol* 38:353, 1976.
268 Gerich JE, Karam JH, Forsham PH: Stimulation of glucagon secretion by epinephrine in man, *J Clin Endocrinol Metab* 253:157, 1975.
269 Gerritsen ME, Bloor CM: Endothelial cell gene expression in response to injury, *FASEB J* 7:523, 1993.
270 Gibbs DM: Measurement of hypothalamic releasing factors in hypophyseal-portal blood, *Regul Pept* (in press).
271 Gill JR Jr, Casper AGT: Role of sympathetic nervous system in the renal response to hemorrhage, *J Clin Invest* 48:915, 1969.
272 Gill JR Jr, Casper AGT: Effect of renal alpha-adrenergic stimulation on proximal sodium resorption, *Am J Physiol* 223:1201, 1972.
273 Gilman AG: G proteins and dual control of adenylate cyclase, *Cell* 36:577, 1984.
274 Gilman AG: G proteins: transducers of receptor-generated signals, *Annu Rev Biopchem* 56:615, 1987.
275 Girardin E, Grau JM, Dayer JM et al: Tumor necrosis factor and interleukin-1 in the serum of children with severe infectious purpura, *N Engl J Med* 319:397, 1988.
276 Goetel EJ: Leukocyte recognition and metabolism of leukotrienes, *Fed Proc* 42:3128, 1983.
277 Goetz KL, Wang BC, Greer PG et al: Atrial stretch increases sodium excretion independently of release of atrial peptides, *Am J Physiol* 250:R946, 1986.
278 Goldberg AL, Kettlehut IC, Furuno K et al: Activation of protein breakdown and prostaglandin E_2 production in rat skeletal muscle in liver is signaled by a macrophage product distinct from interleukin-1 and other known cytokines, *J Clin Invest* 81:378, 1988.
279 Goldberg LI: Dopamine: clinical uses of an endogenous catecholamine, *N Engl J Med* 291:707, 1974.
280 Goldman WF, Saum WR: A direct excitatory action of catecholamines on rat aortic baroreceptors in vitro, *Circ Res* 55:18, 1984.
281 Gorman RR: Mechanism of action of prostacyclin and thromboxane A_2. In Wu K, Rossi EC, editors: *Prostaglandins in clinical medicine: cardiovascular and thrombotic disorders,* New York, 1982, Mosby.
282 Grbic JT, Mannick JA, Gough DB et al: The role of prostaglandin E_2 in immune suppression following injury, *Ann Surg* 214:253, 1991.
283 Grossman A: Brain opiates and neuroendocrine function, *Clin Endocrinol Metab* 12:725, 1983.
284 Grossman CJ: Regulation of the immune system by sex steroids, *Endocr Rev* 5:435, 1984.
285 Guillmen R, Vargo T, Rossier J et al: Beta-endorphin and adrenocorticotropin are secreted concomitantly by the pituitary gland, *Science* 197:1367, 1977.
286 Guyton AC: *Arterial pressure and hypertension,* Philadelphia, 1980, WB Saunders.
287 Guyton AC: Arterial pressure regulation. I. Rapid pressure control by nervous reflexes and other mechanisms. In Guyton AC, editor: *Textbook of medical physiology,* Philadelphia, 1986, WB Saunders.
288 Haberich FJ: Osmoreception in the portal circulation, *Fed Proc* 27:1137, 1968.
289 Haberland GL: The role of kininogenases, kinin formation, and kininogenase inhibition in post-traumatic shock and related conditions, *Klin Wochenschr* 56:325, 1978.
290 Habner JF, Potts JT: Chemistry, biosynthesis, secretion, and metabolism of parathyroid hormone. In Aurbach GD, editor: *Handbook of physiology,* Washington DC, 1976, American Physiological Society.
291 Habner JF, Potts JT: Biosynthesis of parathyroid hormone, *N Engl J Med* 299:580, 1978.
292 Hack CE, Nuijens JH, Felt-Bersma RJ et al: Elevated plasma levels of the anaphylatoxins C3a and C4a are associated with fatal outcome in sepsis, *Am J Med* 86:20, 1989.
293 Haddy FJ, Scott JB, Molnar JJ: Mechanisms of volume replacement and vascular constriction following hemorrhage, *Am J Physiol* 208:169, 1965.
294 Haga K, Haga T: *J Biol Chem* 267:2222, 1992.
295 Haglund U, Gerdin B: Oxygen free radicals and circulatory shock, *Circ Shock* 34:405, 1991.

296 Hall JE, Guvton AC, Cowley AW Jr: Control of glomerular filtration rate by renin-angiotensin system, *Am J Physiol* 232:F215, 1979.
297 Halmaagyi DFJ, Irving MH, Varga D: Effect of adrenergic blockade on the metabolic response to hemorrhagic shock, *J Appl Physiol* 25:384, 1968.
298 Hammarstrom S: Leukotrienes, Annu Rev Biochem 52:355, 1983.
299 Hams B, Bodai B, Kramer G et al: Microvascular fluid and protein flux in pulmonary and systemic circulations after thermal injury, *Microvasc Res* 23:77, 1982.
300 Harbour DV, Galin FS, Hughes TK et al: Role of leukocyte-derived pro-opiomelanocortin peptides in endotoxic shock, *Circ Shock* 35:181, 1991.
301 Harlan JM, Liu DM: Adhesion: its role in inflammatory disease. In *Breakthroughs in molecular biology,* New York, 1991, Freeman.
302 Harper HA, Rodwell VW, Mayes PA: *Review of physiological chemistry,* ed 16, Los Altos, Calif, 1977, Lange.
303 Harrison RS, Birbari A, Seaton JF: Reinforcement of reflex epinephrine release by angiotensin II, *Am J Physiol* 224:31, 1973.
304 Hartl WH, Herndon DN, Wolfe RR: Kinin/prostaglandin system: its therapeutic value in surgical stress, *Crit Care Med* 18:1167, 1990.
305 Harvey SC, Howes EZ: Effect of high-protein diet on the velocity of growth of fibroblasts in the healing wound, *Ann Surg* 91:641, 1930.
306 Hawker FH, Stewart PM, Baxter RC et al: Relationship of somatomedin C/insulin-like growth factor I levels to conventional nutritional indices in critically ill patients, *Crit Care Med* 15:732, 1987.
307 Haynes RC, Larner J: Andrenocorticotropic hormone: adrenocortical steroids and their synthetic analogs. In Goodman LS, Gilman A, editors: *The pharmacological basis of therapeutics,* New York, 1975, Macmillan.
308 Hems DA, Brosnan JT: Effects of ischemia on content of metabolites in rat liver and kidney in vivo, *Biochem J* 120:105, 1970.
309 Hems DA, Whitton PD: Control of hepatic glycogenolysis, *Physiol Rev* 60:1, 1980.
310 Hensel H: Neural processes in thermoregulation, *Physiol Rev* 53:948, 1973.
311 Henzel JG, DeNeese MS, Lichti EL: Zinc concentration within healing wounds, *Arch Surg* 100:349, 1970.
312 Herndon DN, Nguyen TT, Gilpin DA: Growth factors, *Arch Surg* 128:1227, 1993.
313 Hers HG: The control of glycogen metabolism in the liver, *Annu Rev Biochem* 45:167, 1976.
314 Hibbs JB Jr, Taintor R: Nitric oxide: a cytotoxin-activated macrophage effector molecule, *Biochem Biophys Res Commun* 156:87, 1988.
315 Hiebert JM, Celik Z, Soeldner JS et al: Insulin response to hemorrhagic shock in the intact of an adrenalextomized primate, *Am J Surg* 125:501, 1973.
316 Hildebrand A: *Biochem Biophys Res Commun* 159:799, 1989.
317 Hildebrand A, Preissner KT, Muller-Barghaus G et al: *J Biol Chem* 264:15429, 1989.
318 Hinton P, Allison SP, Littlejohn S et al: Insulin and glucose to reduce catabolic response to injury in burned patients, *Lancet* 1:767, 1971.
319 Hirata Y, Itoh K, Ando K et al: Plasma endothelin level during surgery, *N Engl J Med* 321:1686, 1989.
320 Hjemdahl L: Studies on the antilipolytic effect of acidosis, *Acta Physiol Scand (Suppl)* 434:1, 1976.
321 Hochachka PW: *Living without oxygen,* Cambridge, 1980, Harvard University Press.
322 Hoffman RA, Langrehr JM, Wren SM et al: Characterization of the immunosuppressive effects of nitric oxide in graft vs host disease, *J Immunol* 151:1508, 1993.
323 Holaday JW, Black LE, Long JB: Neuropeptides in shock and trauma. In Gellhoed GW, Chernow B, editor: *Endocrine aspects of acute illness,* New York, 1985, Churchill Livingstone.
324 Holaday JW, Faden AI: Naloxone acts at central opiate receptors to reverse hypotension, hypothermia, and hypoventilation in spinal shock, *Brain Res* 189:295, 1980.
325 Holaday JW, Faden AI: Naloxone reversal of endotoxin hypotension suggests role of endorphines in shock, *Nature* 275:450, 1980.
326 Hollt V: Multiple endogenous opioid peptides, *Trends Neurosci* 6:24, 1983.
327 Holmes AE, Ledsome JR: Effect of norepinephrine and vasopressin on carotid sinus baroreceptor activity in the anesthetized rabbit, *Experientia* 40:825, 1984.
328 Horrobin DF: Prolactin as a regulator of fluid and electrolyte metabolism in mammals, *Fed Proc* 39:2567, 1980.
329 Howard JE, Bingham RS Jr, Mason RE: Studies on convalescence: in nitrogen and mineral balances during starvation and graduated feeding in healthy young males on bed rest, *Trans Assoc Ann Physicians* 59:242, 1946.
330 Hozroyde MC, Altounyan REC, Cole M et al: Bronchoconstriction produced in man by leukotrienes C and D, *Lancet* 2:17, 1981.
331 Hume DM, Bell CL, Bartter F: Direct measurement of adrenal secretion during operative trauma and convalescence, *Surgery* 52:174, 1962.
332 Hume DM, Egdahl RH: Effect of hypothermia and of cold exposure on adrenal cortical and medullary secretion, *Ann NY Acad Sci* 80:435, 1959.
333 Hume DM, Egdahl RH: The importance of the brain in the neuroendocrine response to injury, *Ann Surg* 150:697, 1959.
334 Ignarr LJ, Buga GM, Wood KS et al: Enothelium-derived relaxing factor produced and released from artery and vein is nitric oxide, *Proc Natl Acad Sci USA* 84:9265, 1987.
335 Illner HP, Shires T: Membrane defect and energy status of rabbit skeletal muscle cells in sepsis and septic shock, *Arch Surg* 116:1302, 1981.
336 Im MJC, Hoopes JE: Energy metabolism in healing skin wounds, *J Surg Res* 10:459, 1970.
337 Inagami R, Chang JJ, Dykes CW et al: Renin: structural features of active enzyme and inactive precursor, *Fed Proc* 42:2729, 1983.
338 Ingenbleck Y: Thyroid function in nonthyroid illness. In De-Visscher M, editor: *The thyroid gland,* New York, 1980, Raven.
339 Ippe E, Dobbs R, Unger RH: Morphine and beta-endorphin influence the secretion of the endocrine pancreas, *Nature* 276:190, 1978.
340 Itoh K, Goseki N, Endo M et al: Intraoperative hemorrhage affects endothelin-1 concentrations, *Am J Gastroenterol* 86:118, 1991.
341 Itskovitz HD, McGiff JC: Hormonal regulation of renal circulation, *Circ Res* 34-35(suppl 1):165, 1974.
342 Itskovitz HD, Terragno NA, McGiff JC: Effect of renal prostaglandin on distribution of blood flow in isolated canine kidney, *Circ Res* 34:770, 1974.
343 Jarhult J, Lundvall J, Mellander S et al: Osmolar control of plasma volume during hemorrhagic hypotension, *Acta Physiol Scan* 85:F111, 1972.
344 Jauch KW, Gunther B, Hartl WH et al: Improvement of impaired postoperative insulin action by bradykinin, *Biol Chem Hoppe Seyler* 367:27, 1986.
345 Jauch KW, Hartl WH, Feorgieff M et al: Low-dose bradykinin infusion reduces endogenous glucose production in surgical patients, *Metabolism* 37:185, 1988.

346 Jelsema CL, Axelrod J: *Proc Natl Acad Sci USA* 84:3623, 1987.
347 Johnson MD, Park CS, Malrin RL: Antidiuretic hormone and the distribution of renal cortical blood flow, *Am J Physiol* 232:F111, 1977.
348 Johnson MD, Shier DN, Barger AC: Circulating catecholamines and control of plasma renin activity in conscious dogs, *Am J Physiol* 236:H463, 1979.
349 Jones HT: Control of adrenocortical hormone secretion. In James VHT, editor: *The adrenal gland,* New York, 1979, Raven.
350 Kagan BL, Baldwin RL, Munoz D et al: Formation of ion-permeable channels by tumor necrosis factor—alpha, *Science* 255:1427, 1992.
351 Kahn CR: Insulin resistance, insulin insensitivity, and insulin unresponsiveness: a necessary definition, *Metabolism* 27:1893, 1973.
352 Kahn CR, Smith RJ, Chin WW: Mechanism of action of hormones that act at the cell surface. In Wilson JD, Foster DW, editors: *Williams textbook of endocrinology,* ed 8, Philadelphia, 1992, WB Saunders.
353 Kampschmidt RF: Leukocytic endogenous mediator, *J Reticuloendothel Soc* 23:287, 1978.
354 Kaplan AP: Hageman factor–dependent pathways: mechanisms of initiation and bradykinin formation, *Fed Proc* 42:3123, 1983.
355 Kaplan NM: The biosynthesis of adrenal steroids: effects of angiotensin II, adrenocorticotropin, and potassium, *J Clin Invest* 44:2029, 1965.
356 Karlsson K, Marklund SL: Extracellular superoxide dismutase in the vascular system of mammals, *Biochem J* 255:223, 1988.
357 Kaufman RL, Matson CE, Beisel WR: Hypertriglyceridemia produced by endotoxin: role of impaired triglyceride disposal mechanisms, *J Infect Dis* 133:548, 1976.
358 Keeler R: Natriuresis after unilateral stimulation of carotid receptors in unanesthetized rats, *Am J Physiol* 226:507, 1974.
359 Keller GA, West MA, Cerra FB et al: Hepatocellular modulation by macrophage/Kupffer cells in vitro. II. Effect of dexmethasone, *Surg Forum* 201:47, 1985.
360 Keller GA, West MA, Cerra FB et al: Multiple system organ failure: modulation of hepatocyte protein synthesis by endotoxin-activiated Kupffer cells, *Ann Surg* 201:87, 1985.
361 Kem DL, Gomez-Sanchez C, Kramer WJ: Plasma aldosterone and renin activity response to ACTH infusion in dexamethasone-suppressed normal and sodium-depleted man, *J Clin Endocrinol Metab* 40:116, 1975.
362 Kendler KS, Weitzman RE, Fisher DA: The effect of pain on plasma arginine vasopressin concentration in man, *Clin Endocrinol* 8:89, 1978.
363 Kenney PR, Allen-Rowlands CF, Gann DS: Glucose and osmolality as predictors of injury severity, *J Trauma* 23:712, 1983.
364 Keogh C, Fong Y, Marrano MA et al: Identification of a novel tumor necrosis factor/cachectin from the livers of burned and infected rats, *Arch Surg* 125:769, 1990.
365 Kien CL, et al: Increased rates of whole body protein synthesis and breakdown in children recovering from burns, *Ann Surg* 187:383, 1978.
366 Kilbourn R, Belloni P: Endothelial cell production of nitrogen oxides in response to interferon-gamma in combination with tumor necrosis factor, interleukin-1, or endotoxin, *J Natl Cancer Inst* 82:772, 1990.
367 Kilbourn RG, Gross SS, Jubran A et al: N-methyl-L-arginine inhibits tumor necrosis factor–induced hypotension: implications for the involvement of nitric oxide, *Proc Natl Acad Sci USA* 87:3629, 1990.
368 Kinney JM: Energy requirements in injury and sepsis, *Acta Anaesthesiol Scand* 55:15, 1974.
369 Kinney JM: Energy metabolism. In Fisher JE, editor: *Surgical nutrition,* Boston, 1983, Little, Brown.
370 Kinney JM, Lister J, Moore FD: Relationship of energy expenditure to total exchangeable potassium, *Ann NY Acad Sci* 110:722, 1963.
371 Kinney JM, Long CL, Gump FE et al: Tissue composition of weight loss in surgical patients. I. Elective operations, *Ann Surg* 168:459, 1968.
372 Kinney JM, Roe CF: Caloric equivalents of fever: patterns of postoperative response, *Ann Surg* 156:610, 1962.
373 Kircheim HR: Systemic arterial baroreceptor reflexes, *Physiol Rev* 56:100, 1976.
374 Kirk CJ, Rodrigues LM, Hems DA: The influence of vasopressin and related peptides on glycogen phosphorylase activity and phosphotidylinositol metabolism in hepatocytes, *Biochem J* 1978:493, 1979.
375 Kline DL: The effect of hemorrhage on the plasma amino acid nitrogen of the dog, *Am J Physiol* 146:654, 1946.
376 Knowles RG, Palacios M, Palmer RMJ et al: Formation of nitric oxide from L-arginine in the central nervous system: a transduction mechanism for stimulation of soluble guanylate cyclase, *Proc Natl Acad Sci USA* 86:5159, 1989.
377 Kobak MW, Bendittk EP, Wissler RW et al: The relation of protein deficiency to experimental wound healing, *Surg Gynecol Obstet* 85:751, 1947.
378 Koller J, Mair P, Wieser C et al: Endothelin and big endothelin concentrations in injured patients, *N Engl J Med* 325:325, 1991.
379 Korchak HM, Masoro EJ: Changes in the level of the fatty acid–synthesizing enzymes during starvation, *Biochem Biophys Acta* 58:354, 1962.
380 Korner PI: Integrative neural cardiovascular control, *Physiol Rev* 51:312, 1971.
381 Kovach AGB, Russell S, Sandor P et al: Blood flow, oxygen consumption, and free fatty acid release in subcutaneous adipose tissue during hemorrhagic shock in control and phenoxygenzamine-treated dogs, *Circ Res* 26:733, 1970.
382 Kraus-Friedmann H: Hormonal regulation of hepatic gluconeogenesis, *Physiol Rev* 64:170, 1984.
383 Krebs HA: The metabolic rate of amino acids. In Munro HN, Allison JB, editors: *Mammalian protein metabolism,* New York, 1964, Academic Press.
384 Kriegler M, Perez C, DeFay K et al: A novel form of TNF/cachectin is a cell surface cytotoxic transmembrane protein: ramifications for the complex physiology of TNF, *Cell* 53:45, 1988.
385 Kugiyama K, Kerns SA, Morrisett JD et al: Impairment of endothelium-dependent arterial relaxation by lysolecithin in modified low-density lipoproteins, *Nature* 344:160, 1990.
386 Kukreja SC, Hargis GK, Bowser EN et al: Role of adrenergic stimuli in parathyroid secretion in man, *J Clin Endocrinol Metab* 40:478, 1978.
387 Kurt-Jones EA, Beller DI, Mizel SB set al: Identification of a membrane-associated interleukin-1 in macrophages, *Proc Natl Acad Sci USA* 82:1204, 1985.
388 LaBrosse EH, Beech JA, McLaughlin JS et al: Plasma amino acids in normal humans and patients with shock, *Surg Gynecol Obstet* 125:516, 1967.
389 Landsberg L, Young JB: Catecholamines and the adrenal medulla. In Wilson JD, Foster DW, editors: *Willams textbook of endocrinology,* ed 8, Philadelphia, 1992, WB Saunders.
390 Lang CH, Dobrescu C, Hargrove DM et al: Platelet activating factor–induced increases in glucose kinetics, *Am J Physiol* 254:E193, 1988.
391 Lang RE, Bruckner UB, Hermann K et al: Effect of hemorrhagic shock on the concomitant release of endorphin and enkephalin-like peptides from the pituitary and adrenal gland in the dog. In Costa E, Trabucchi R, editors: *Regulatory peptides: from molecular biology to function,* New York, 1982, Raven.
392 Langehr JM, Hoffman RA, Lancaster JRJ et al: Nitric oxide: a

new endogenous immunomodulator, *Transplantation* 55:1205, 1993.

393 Larsen PR: Thyroid-pituitary interaction, *N Engl J Med* 23:32, 1982.

394 Le J, Frederickson G, Reis LFL et al: Interleukin-2–dependent and interleukin-2–independent pathways of regulation of thymocyte function by interleukin, *Proc Natl Acad Sci USA* 85:8643, 1988.

395 Lee H, Walseth GT, Bratt GT et al: *J Biol Chem* 264:1608, 1989.

396 Lee JB: The prostaglandins. In Williams RH, editor: *Textbook of endocrinology,* Philadelphia, 1981, WB Saunders.

397 Lefer AM: Eicosanoids as mediators of ischemia and shock, *Fed Proc* 44:275, 1985.

398 Lehninger AL: *Bioenergetics,* ed 2, Menlo Park, Calif, 1972, Benjamin-Cummings.

399 LeMaire R, Tseng R, LeMaire S: Systemic administration of beta-endorphin: potent hypotensive effect involving a serotonergic pathway, *Proc Natl Acad Sci USA* 75:6240, 1978.

400 Levenson SM, Green RW, Taylor FH et al: Ascorbic acid, riboflavin, thiamine, and nicotinic acid in relation to severe injury, hemorrhage, and infection in humans, *Ann Surg* 124:840, 1946.

401 Levenson SM, Howard J, Rosen J: Studies of the plasma amino acids and amino conjugates in patients with several battle wounds, *Surg Gynecol Obstet* 101:35, 1955.

402 Levenson SM, Seifter E, Van Winkle W: Nutrition. In Hunt TK, Dunphy JE, editors: *Fundamentals of wound management,* New York, 1954, Appleton-Century-Crofts.

403 Levinsky NG: The renal kallikrein-kinin system, *Circ Res* 44:441, 1978.

404 Levy EM, McIntosh T, Block PH: Elevation of circulatory beta-endorphin levels with concomitant depression of immune parameters after traumatic injury, *J Trauma* 26:246, 1986.

405 Levy SB, Lilley JJ, Frigon RP et al: Urinary kallikrein and plasma renin activity as determinants of renal blood flow, *J Clin Invest* 60:129, 1977.

406 Liaw KY, Askanazi J, Michelson CB et al: Effect of injury and sepsis on high-energy phosphates in muscle and red cells, *J Trauma* 20:755, 1980.

407 Linares OA, Jacquez JA, Zech LA et al: Norepinephrine metabolism in humans: kinetic analysis and model, *J Clin Invest* 80:1332, 1987.

408 Lilly MP, Engeland WC, Gann DS: Adrenal response to repeated hemorrhage: implications for studies of trauma, *J Trauma* 22:809, 1982.

409 Lilly MP, Gann DS: The effect of repeated operation on the response of the adrenal cortex to infused ACTH, *Surg Forum* 33:10, 1982.

410 Lilly MP, Gann DS: The hypothalamic-pituitary-adrenal-immune axis, *Arch Surg* 127:1463, 1992.

411 Lindqust S, Craig EA: The heat-shock proteins, *Annu Rev Genet* 22:631, 1988.

412 Logothetis DEK, Galper J, Neer EJ et al: *Nature* 325:321, 1987.

413 Long CL, Schiller WR, Blakemore WS et al: Muscle protein catabolism in the septic patient as measured by 3-methylhistidine exertion, *Am J Clin Nutr* 30:1349, 1977.

414 Long CL, Spencer JL, Kinney JM et al: Carbohydrate metabolism in men: effect of elective operations and major injury, *J Appl Physiol* 31:110, 1971.

415 Longnecker DE, McCoy S, Drucker WR: Anesthetic influence on response to hemorrhage in rats, *Circ Shock* 6:55, 1979.

416 Lotz M, Jurik F, Kabouridis P et al: B-cell stimulating factor 2/interleukin-6 is a costimulant for human thymocytes and T lymphocytes, *J Exp Med* 167:1253, 1988.

417 Lumpin MD: The regulation of ACTH secretion by IL-1, *Science* 238:452, 1987.

418 Lund CC, Crandon JH: Ascorbic acid and human wound healing, *Ann Surg* 114:776, 1941.

419 Lund CL, Levenson SM, Green RW et al: Ascorbic acid, thiamine, riboflavin, and nicotinic acid in relation to acute burns in man, *Arch Surg* 55:557, 1947.

420 Lymangrover JR, Dokas LA, Kong A et al: Naloxone has a direct effect on the adrenal cortex, *Endocrinology* 109:1132, 1981.

421 Makara GB: The relative importance of hypothalamic releasing neurons containing corticotrophin-releasing factor or arginine vasopressin in regulation of ACTH secretion, *Ciba Found Symp* 168:43, 1992.

422 Mallette LE, Exton JH, Park CR: Control of gluconeogenesis from amino acids in the perfused rat liver, *J Biol Chem* 244:5713, 1969.

423 Manning PT, Schwartz D, Katsube NC et al: Vasopressin-stimulated release of atriopeptin: endocrine antagonists in fluid homeostasis, *Science* 229:395, 1985.

424 March CJ, Mosley B, Larsen A et al: Cloning, sequence, and expression of two distinct human interleukin-1 complementary DNAs, *Nature* 315:641, 1985.

425 Markley K, Horakova Z, Smallman ET et al: The role of histamine in burn, tourniquet, and endotoxic shock in mice, *Eur J Pharmacol* 33:255, 1975.

426 Masaki T: Endothelins: homeostatic and compensatory actions in the circulatory and endocrine systems, *Endocr Rev* 14(3):253, 1993.

427 Masoro EJ: Lipids and lipid metabolism, *Annu Rev Physiol* 39:301, 1977.

428 Mathias S, Younes A, Kan C et al: Activation of the sphingomyelin signaling pathway in intact EL4 cells and in cell-free systems by IL-1b, *Science* 259:519, 1993.

429 Matsuchima K, Taguchi M, Kovacs EJ et al: Intracellular localization of human monocyte–associated interleukin-1 activity and release of biologically active IL-1 from monocytes by trypsin and plasmin, *J Immunol* 135:2883, 1986.

430 Maury CPJ, Salo E, Pelkonen P: Circulating interleukin-1 beta in patients with Kawasaki disease, *N Engl J Med* 319:1670, 1988.

431 May ET: The effect of surgical stress on plasma free fatty acids, *Surg Res* 10:315, 1970.

432 McCord JW: Oxygen-derived free radicals in postischemic tissue injury, *N Engl J Med* 312:159, 1985.

433 McCormick F: How receptors turn ras on, *Nature* 363:15, 1993.

434 McCoy S, Case SA, Swerchick RA et al: Determinants of blood amino acid concentration after hemorrhage, *Ann Surg* 43:787, 1977.

435 McGarry JD, Foster DW: The metabolism of (minus) octanoylcarnitine in perfused livers from fed and fasted rats: evidence for a possible regulatory role of carnitine acyltransferase in the control of ketogenesis, *J Biol Chem* 249:7984, 1975.

436 McGarry JD, Foster DW: Hormonal control of ketogenesis: biochemical consideration, *Arch Intern Med* 137:495, 1977.

437 McGrath MH: Peptide growth factors and wound healing, *Clin Plast Surg* 17:421, 1990.

438 McIntyre J et al: Intestinal factors in the control of insulin secretion, *J Clin Endocrinol* 25:1317, 1965.

439 McKenna TJ, Island DP, Nicholson WE et al: Dopamine inhibits angiotensin-stimulated aldosterone biosynthesis in bovine adrenal cells, *J Clin Endocrinol Metab* 40:125, 1975.

440 Mealy K, Van Lanschot JJB, Robinson BG et al: Are the catabolic effects of tumor necrosis factor mediated by glucocorticoids? *Arch Surg* 125:42, 1990.

441 Meguid MM, Brennan MF, Aoki II et al: Hormone-substrate interrelationships following trauma, *Arch Shock Res* 109:776, 1974.

442 Meldrum DR, Mitchell MB, Banerjee A et al: Cardiac preconditioning, *Arch Surg* 128:1208, 1993.

443 Melon KL: The endocrinologic function of selected autocoids: catecholamines, acetylcholine, serotonin, and histamine. In Wil-

liams RH, editor: *Textbook of endocrinology,* Philadelphia, 1981, WB Saunders.

444 Menguary R, Master YF: Influence of hyperglycemia on survival after hemorrhagic shock, *Adv Shock Res* 1:43, 1979.

445 Merimer TJ, Zapf MJ, Froesch ER: Insulin-like growth factors in the fed and fasted states, *J Clin Endocrinol Metab* 55:999, 1982.

446 Metz SA, Halter JB, Robertson RP: Induction of defective insulin secretion and impaired glucose tolerance uptake by clonidine: selective stimulation of metabolic alpha-adrenergic pathways, *Diabetes* 27:554, 1978.

447 Michie HR, Manogue KR, Spriggs DR et al: Detection of circulating tumor necrosis factor after endotoxin administration, *N Engl J Med* 318:1481, 1988.

448 Miller PD, Krebs RA, Neal BJ et al: Polyuric prerenal failure, *Arch Intern Med* 140:907, 1979.

449 Miller RE: Pancreatic neuroendocrinology: peripheral neural mechanisms in the regulation of the islets of Langerhans, *Endocrinol Rev* 4:417, 1981.

450 Moldawer L, Svaninger G, Gelin J et al: Interleukin-1 and tumor necrosis factor do not regulate protein balance in skeletal muscle, *Am J Physiol* 253:C766, 1987.

451 Moncada S, Palmer RN, Higgs EA: Biosynthesis of nitric oxide from L-arginine: a pathway for the regulation of cell function and communication, *Biochem Pharmacol* 38:1709, 1989.

452 Monier S, LeCam A, LeMarchand-Brustel W: Insulin and insulin-like growth factor I: effects on protein synthesis in isolated muscles from lean and gold thiogluce–obese mice, *Diabetes* 32:392, 1982.

453 Moore FD: Bodily changes during surgical convalescence, *Ann Surg* 137:289, 1953.

454 Moore FD, Brennan MF: Surgical injury: body composition, protein metabolism, and neuroendocrinology. In Ballinger WF, Collins JA, Drucker WR et al, editors: *Manual of surgical nutrition,* Philadelphia, 1975, WB Saunders.

455 Moore FM: *Metabolic care of the surgical patient,* Philadelphia, 1959, WB Saunders.

456 Moore RN, Goodrum KJ, Berry LJ: Mediation of an endotoxic effect by macrophages, *J Reticuloendothel Soc* 17:187, 1976.

457 Morgan HE, Earl DCN, Broadus A et al: Regulation of protein synthesis in heart muscle, *J Biol Chem* 251:2151, 1971.

458 Morimoto RI, Tissieres A, Georgeopoulous C: The stress response, function of the proteins, and perspectives. In Morimoto RI, Tissieres A, Georgeopoulous C, editors: *Stress proteins in biology and medicine,* Cold Spring Harbor, NY, 1990, Cold Spring Harbor Press.

459 Morley JE: Neuroendocrine effects of endogenous opioid peptides in human subjects: a review, *Psychoneuroendocrinology* 8:361, 1983.

460 Morris AS, Henry W, Shearer JD et al: Macrophage interaction with skeletal muscle: a potential role of macrophages in determining the energy state of healing wounds, *J Trauma* 25:751, 1985.

461 Morris AS, Shearer JD, Albina JE et al: Increased PKF activity in wounded tissue, *Am J Physiol* in press 1986.

462 Morris AS, Shearer JD, Caldwell MD: The role of the cellular infiltrate on glucose metabolism in wounded tissue, *Surg Forum* 1985.

463 Morris AS, Shearer JD, Henry W et al: A macrophage-mediated factor that increases the right energy phosphate content of skeletal muscle, *J Surg Res* 38:373, 1985.

464 Moss GS, Cerchio GM, Siegel DC et al: Serum insulin response in hemorrhagic shock in baboons, *Surgery* 68:34, 1970.

465 Mouw D, Bonjour J, Malvin RL et al: Central action of angiotensin in stimulating ADH release, *Am J Physiol* 220:239, 1971.

466 Munck A, Guyre PM, Holbrook NJ: Physiological functions of glucocorticoids in stress and their relation to pharmacological actions, *Endocr Rev* 5:25, 1984.

467 Munro HN, Crim MC: The proteins and amino acids. In Goodhart RS, Shils ME, editors: *Modern nutrition in health and disease,* Philadelphia, 1980, Lea & Febiger.

468 Myers A, Uotila P, Foegh ML et al: The eicosanoids: prostaglandins, thromboxane, and leukotrienes. In DeGroot, editor: *Endocrinology,* Philadelphia, 1989, WB Saunders.

469 Naitoh Y, Fukata J, Tominaga T et al: Interleukin-6 stimulates the secretion of adrenocorticotropic hormone in conscious, freely moving rats, *Biochem Biophys Res Comm* 155:1459, 1988.

470 Nanni G, Siegel JH, Coleman B et al: Increased lipid fuel dependence in the critically ill septic patient, *J Trauma* 24:14, 1983.

471 Navar LG: Renal autoregulation: perspectives from whole kidney and single nephron studies, *Am J Physiol* 234:F357, 1978.

472 Navar LG, Ploth DW, Bell PD: Distal tubular feedback control of renal hemodynamics and autoregulation, *Ann Rev Physiol* 42:557, 1980.

473 Naylor W: *Europ Pharmacol Sci* 11:96, 1990.

474 Needham AE: Regeneration in wound healing. In Alberchrombie M, editor: *Methuen's monographs on biological subjects,* New York, 1952, Wiley & Sons.

475 Needleman P: Blood cells, platelets, and prostaglandins. In Wu KK, Rosi EC, editors: *Prostaglandins in clinical medicine: cardiovascular and thrombotic disorders,* New York, 1982, Mosby.

476 Neer EJ, Clapham DE: Roles of G-protein subunits in transmembrane signaling, *Nature* 33:129, 1988.

477 Nelson DH: Corticosteroid-induced changes in phospholipid membranes as mediators of their action, *Endocr Rev* 1:180, 1980.

478 Nelson KM, Turinsky J: Local effect of burn on skeletal muscle insulin responsiveness, *J Surg Res* 31:288, 1981.

479 Nelson KM, Turinsky J: Analysis of postburn insulin unresponsiveness in skeletal muscle, *J Surg Res* 31:404, 1981.

480 Newsholme EA, Start C: *Regulation in metabolism,* New York, 1973, Wiley & Sons.

481 Newsome HH, Rose JC: The response of adrenocorticotrophic hormone and growth hormone to surgical stress, *J Clin Endocrinol Metab* 33:481, 1971.

482 Nijsten MWN, DeGroot ER, TenDuis HJ et al: Serum levels of interleukin-6 and acute-phase response, *Lancet* 2:921, 1987.

483 Nishizuka Y: *Nature* 334:661, 1988.

484 Noda M, Furntani Z, Takahashi H et al: Cloning and sequence analysis of cDNA for bovine adrenal preproenkephalin, *Nature* 295:202, 1982.

485 Noel GL, Suh HK, Stone JG et al: Human prolactin and growth hormone release during surgery and other conditions of stress, *J Clin Endocrinol Metab* 35:840, 1972.

486 Novelli GP, Marsili M, Pieraccioli E: Antishock action of steroids other than cortisone, *Eur Surg Res* 5:169, 1973.

487 O'Berg B, White S: Circulatory effects of interruption and stimulation of cardiac vagal afferents, *Acta Physiol Scand* 80:383, 1970.

488 O'Connor J, Scott R, Mellick P et al: Perfused rat hindlimb wound model, lambda-carrageenan induced, *J Biol Chem* 249:R570, 1982.

489 O'Donnell TF, Clowes GHA, Blackburn GL et al: Proteolysis associated with a deficit of peripheral energy fuel substrates in septic man, *Surgery* 80:192, 1976.

490 O'Keefe SJD, Sender PM, James WPT: Catabolic loss of body nitrogen in response to surgery, *Lancet* 2:1035, 1974.

491 O'Malley BW, Schrader WT: The receptors of steroid hormones, *Sci Am* 234:32, 1976.

492 Ochoa JB, Udekwu AO, Billiar TR et al: Nitrogen oxide levels in patients after trauma and during sepsis, *Ann Surg* 214:621, 1991.

493 Odessey R, Khairallah EA, Goldberg AL: Origin and probable

significance of alanine production by skeletal muscle, *J Biol Chem* 249:7623, 1974.
494 Ogletree ML, Brigham KL: Arachidonate raises vascular resistance but not permeability in lungs of awake sheep, *J Appl Physiol* 48:581, 1980.
495 Okubo A, Sone S, Tanaka M et al: Membrane-associated interleukin-1-alpha as a mediator of tumor cell killing by human blood monocytes fixed with paraformaldehyde, *Cancer Res* 49:265, 1989.
496 Okusawa S, Gelfand JA, Ikejima T et al: Interleukin-1 induces a shocklike state in rabbits: synergism with tumor necrosis factor and the effect of cyclo-oxygenase inhibition, *J Clin Invest* 81:1162, 1988.
497 Okusawa S, Yancey KB, van der Meer JWM et al: C5a stimulates secretion of tumor necrosis factor from human mononuclear cells in vitro, *J Exp Med* 168:43, 1988.
498 Oomura Y: Chemical and neuronal control of feeding motivation, *Physiol Behav* 44:555, 1988.
499 Oppenheim W, Williamson D, Smith R: Early biochemical changes and severity of injury in man, *J Trauma* 20:135, 1980.
500 Oppenheimer JH: Thyroid hormone action at the cellular level, *Science* 203:971, 1979.
501 Orth DN, Kovacs WJ, DeBold CR: The adrenal cortex. In Wilson, JD, Foster DW, editors: *Williams textbook of endocrinology,* ed 8, Philadelphia, 1992, WB Saunders.
502 Otsuki M, Dakoda M, Baba S: Influence of glucocorticoids on TRF-induced TSH response in man, *J Clin Endocrinol Metab* 36:945, 1973.
503 Overman RR, Wang SG: The contributory role of the afferent nervous factor in experimental shock: sublethal hemorrhage and sciatic nerve stimulation, *Am J Physiol* 148:289, 1947.
504 Pacitti AJ, Yoshifumi I, Plumley DA et al: Growth hormone regulates amino acid transport in human and rat liver, *Ann Surg* 216:353, 1992.
505 Palmer BQ, Brooks DC, Black PR et al: Epinephrine acutely mediates skeletal muscle insulin resistance, *Surgery* 94:172, 1983.
506 Palmer RMJ, Ferrife AG, Moncada S: Nitric oxide release accounts for the biological activity of endothelium-derived relaxing factor, *Nature* 327:524, 1987.
507 Palombo JD, Blackburn GL, Forse RA: Endothelial cell factors and response to injury, *Surg Gynecol Obstet* 173:505, 1991.
508 Pappenheimer JR, Soto-Rivera A: Effective osmotic pressure of the plasma proteins and other quantities associated with capillary circulation in the hindlimbs of cats and dogs, *Am J Physiol* 152:471, 1948.
509 Paratt JR, Coker SJ, Hughes B et al: The possible role of prostaglandins and thromboxanes in the pulmonary consequences of experimental endotoxin shock and clinical sepsis. In McCann R, editor: *Role of chemical mediators in the pathophysiology of acute illness and injury,* New York, 1982, Raven.
510 Parekh AB, Terlau H, Stuhmer W: Depletion of $InsP_3$ stores activates a calcium and potassium current by means of a phosphatase and a diffusible messenger, *Nature* 364:814, 1993.
511 Parker CJ, Frame MR, Elstad MR: *Blood* 71:86, 1988.
512 Parker RC, Baxter CR: Divergence in adrenal steroid secretory pattern after thermal injury in adult patients, *J Trauma* 25:508, 1985.
513 Parrillo JE, Fauci AS: Mechanisms of glucocorticoid action on immune processes, *Annu Rev Pharmacol Toxicol* 19:179, 1979.
514 Pass LJ, Schloerg PR, Chow FT et al: Liver adenosine triphosphate (ATP) in hypoxia and hemorrhagic shock, *J Trauma* 22:730, 1982.
515 Paterson SJ, Robson LE, Kosterlitz HW: Classification of opioid receptors, *Br Med J* 39:31, 1983.
516 Patterson R, Harris KE: Role of prostaglandins in asthma. In Wu KK, Rossi EC, editors: *Prostaglandins in clinical medicine: cardiovascular and thrombotic disorders,* New York, 1982, Mosby.
517 Peach MJ: Renin-angiotensin system: biochemistry and mechanism of action, *Physiol Rev* 57:313, 1977.
518 Peetre C, Thysell H, Grubb A et al: A tumor necrosis factor–binding protein is present in human biological fluids, *Euro J Haematol* 41:414, 1988.
519 Pekala P, Kawakami M, Vire W et al: Studies of insulin resistance in adipocytes induced by a microphage mediator, *J Exp Med* 157:1360, 1983.
520 Pelletier LL, Edis AJ, Shepard JT: Circulatory reflex from vagal afferents in response to hemorrhage in the dog, *Circ Res* 29:626, 1971.
521 Pellicane JV, DeMaria E, S.K. W et al: Tumor necrosis factor antibody (MOABTNF) improves survival following hemorrhagic shock in awake rats, 1992, The Shock Society.
522 Perdue JF: Chemistry structure and function of insulin-like growth factors and their receptors: a review, *Can J Biochem Cell Biol* :1237, 1984.
523 Pfeffer MA, Pfeffer JM, Lewis RA et al: Systemic hemodynamic effects of leukotrienes C4 and D4 in the rat, *Am J Physiol* 244:H628, 1983.
524 Pfeiffer A, Herz A: Endocrine action of opioids, *Horm Metab Res* 16:386, 1984.
525 Pirkle JC Jr, Gann DS: Expansion of interstitial fluid is required for full restoration of blood volume, *J Trauma* 16:937, 1977.
526 Pirkle JC Jr, Gann DS: Restitution of blood volume after hemorrhage: role of the adrenal cortex, *Am J Physiol* 230:1683, 1976.
527 Pober JS, Cotran RS: Cytokines and endothelial cell biology, *Physiol Rev* 70:505, 1990.
528 Pober JS, Cotran RS: Cytokines and endothelial cell biology, *Physiol Rev* 70:427, 1990.
529 Poggi C, Marchand-Bruster Y, Zapf J et al: Effects of binding of IGF-1 in the isolated soleus muscle of lean and obese mice: comparison with insulin, *Endocrinology* 105:723, 1979.
530 Poole CJM, Carter DA, Vallejo M et al: Atrial natriuretic factor inhibits the stimulated in vivo and in vitro release of vasopressin and oxytocin in the rat, *J Endocrinol* 112:97, 1987.
531 Porte DJ, Halter JB: The endocrine pancreas and diabetes mellitus. In Williams RH, editor: *Textbook of endocrinology,* Philadelphia, 1981, WB Saunders.
532 Porte DJ, Smith PH, Ensinck JW: Neurohumoral regulation of the pancreatic islet A and B cells, *Metabolism* 25:1453, 1976.
533 Powanda MC, Bersil WR: Hypothesis: leukocytic endogenous mediator/endogenous pyrogen/lymphocyte-activating factor modulates the development of nonspecific and specific immunity and affects nutritional status, *Am J Clin Nutr* 35:762, 1982.
534 Powanda MC, Moyer ED: Plasma proteins and wound healing, *Surg Gynecol Obstet* 153:749, 1982.
535 Prescott SM, Zimmerman FA, McIntyre TM: Platelet activating factor, *J Biol Chem* 265:17381, 1990.
536 Prieur AM, Jaufmann MT, Griscelli C et al: Specific interleukin-1 inhibitor in serum and urine of children with systemic juvenile chronic arthritis, *Lancet* 2:1240, 1987.
537 Pruitt BA: Postburn hypermetabolism and nutrition in burn patients. In Ballinger WF, Collins JA, Drucker WR et al: *Manual of surgical nutrition,* Philadelphia, 1975, WB Saunders.
538 Quest JA, Gebber GL: Modulation of barorecepor reflexes by somatic afferent nerve stimulation, *Am J Physiol* 222:1251, 1972.
539 Quinn MT, Artjasaratjy S, Steomberg D: *Proc Natl Acad Sci USA* 85:2805, 1988.
540 Quiros G, Ware J: Modification of cardiovascular responses to hemorrhage by induced hyperosmolality in the rat, *Acta Physiol Scand* 117:391, 1983.

541 Raff H, Sinsako J, Sallman MF: Surgery potentiates adrenocortical responses to hypoxia in dogs, *Proc Soc Exp Biol Med* 172:400, 1983.

542 Rai V, Paandey SK, Singh RH et al: Systemic histamine and histaminase changes during hemorrhagic shock, *Indian J Exp Biol* 14:187, 1976.

543 Ramadori G, Sipe JD, Dinarello CA et al: Pretranslational modulation of acute-phase hepatic protein synthesis by murine recombinant interleukin-1 (IL-1) and purified human IL-1, *J Exp Med* 162:930, 1985.

544 Ramsden DB, Askew RD, Bradwell RA et al: Glucocorticoids and peripheral monodeiodination of thyroxine after stress. Proceedings of the Sixth International Congress of Endocrinology, No. 363, 1980.

545 Randriamampita C, Tsien RY: Emptying of intracellular calcium stores releases a novel small messenger that stimulates calcium influx, *Nature* 364:809, 1993.

546 Rappaport L, Contard F, Dubus I et al: Stress-induced protooncogenes in the myocardium. In Proschek L, Jasmin G, editors: *Systemic effects of stress,* Basel, 1991, Karger.

547 Raptis S, Dollinger HC, Schroder KE et al: Differences in insulin, growth hormones, and pancreatic enzyme secretion after intravenous and intraduodenal administration of mixed amino acids in man, *N Engl J Med* 288:1199, 1973.

548 Reeves WB, Andreoli TE: The posterior pituitary and water metabolism. In Wilson JD, Foster DW, editors: *Williams textbook of endocrinology,* ed 8, Philadelphia, 1992, WB Saunders.

549 Regoli D, Barabe J: Pharmacology of bradykinin and related kinins, *Pharmacol Rev* 32:1, 1980.

550 Reichlin S: Somatostatin, *N Engl J Med* 309:1495, 1983.

551 Reichlin S: Neuroendocrinology. In Wilson JD, Foster DW, editors: *Williams textbook of endocrinology,* ed 8, Philadelphia, 1992, WB Saunders.

552 Reichlin S: Neuroendocrine-immune interactions, *N Engl J Med* 329(17):1246, 1993.

553 Reid IA, Ganong WF: Control of aldosterone secretion. In Genest J, Kolw E, Kuchel O, editors: *Hypertension,* New York, 1977, McGraw-Hill.

554 Riviere C, Vale W: Effect of angiotensin II on ACTH release in vivo: role of corticotropin-releasing factor, *Regul Pep* 7:253, 1983.

555 Rizza RA, Cryer PE, Haywood MW et al: Adrenergic mechanisms for the effect of epinephrine on glucose production and clearance in man, *J Clin Invest* 65:682, 1950.

556 Rizza RA, Madarino LJ, Gerich JE: Cortisol-induced insulin resistance in man: impaired suppression of glucose production and stimulation of glucose utilization due to a postreceptor defect of insulin action, *J Clin Endocrinol Metab* 54:131, 1982.

557 Roberts LJ, Oates JA: Disorders of vasodilator hormones: the carcinoid syndrome and mastocytosis. In Wilson JD, Foster DW, editors: *Williams textbook of endocrinology,* ed 8, Philadelphia, 1992, WB Saunders.

558 Rocchio MA, Randall HT: Wound kinetics: water and electrolyte changes from zero to 60 days in clean wounds, *Am J Surg* 121:4600, 1972.

559 Rodrick ML, Wood JJ, O'Mahoney JB et al: Mechanisms of immunosuppression associated with severe nonthermal traumatic injuries in man: production of interleukin-1 and -2, *J Clin Immunol* 6:310, 1986.

560 Romanosky AJ, Bagby GJ, Bockman EL et al: Increased muscle glucose uptake and lactate release after endotoxin administration, *Am J Physiol* 239:E311, 1980.

561 Ross R: The fibroblast and wound repair, *Biol Rev* 43:51, 1968.

562 Ross R: The pathogenesis of atherosclerosis: a perspective for the 1990s, *Nature* 362:801, 1993.

563 Rossier J, French ED, Rivier C et al: Heat shock–induced stress increases beta-endorphin levels in blood but not brain, *Nature* 270:618, 1977.

564 Rubanyi GM, Vanhoutte PM: Superoxide anions and hyperoxia inactivate endothelium-derived relaxing factor, *Am J Physiol* 250:H822, 1986.

565 Rudermna NB, Berger M: The formation of glutamine and alanine in skeletal muscle, *J Biol Chem* 249:5500, 1974.

566 Russell JA, Long CH, Engel FL: Biochemical studies of shock: the role of peripheral tissues on the metabolism of protein and carbohydrate during hemorrhagic shock in the rat, *J Exp Med* 79:1, 1944.

567 Ryan JS: *Endothelial cells,* Boca Raton, La, 1988, CRC Press.

568 Ryan NT: Biochemical studies of shock: the role of peripheral tissues in the metabolism of protein and carbohydrate during hemorrhagic shock in the rat, *J Exp Med* 79:1, 1976.

569 Ryan NT, George BC, Egadahl DM et al: Chronic tissue insulin resistance following hemorrhagic shock, *Ann Surg* 80:402, 1974.

570 Saenz de Tejeda I, Foldstein I, Azadzoi K et al: Impaired neurogenic and endothelium-dependent relaxation of penile smooth muscle from diabetic men with impotence, *N Engl J Med* 320:1025, 1989.

571 Saide K, Mitsui Y, Ishida N: A novel peptide, vasoactive intestinal contractor of a new (endothelin) peptide family, *J Biol Chem* 264:14613, 1989.

572 Salvemini D, Korbut R, Anggard E et al: Immediate release of a nitric oxide–like factor from bovine aortic endothelial cells by *Escherichia coli* lipopolysaccharide, *Pro Natl Acad Sci USA* 87:2593, 1990.

573 Samuelsson B: Prostaglandins and thromboxanes, *Recent Prog Horm Res* 34:239, 1978.

574 Sapirstein LA, Sapirstein EA, Bredemyer A: Effect of hemorrhage on cardiac output and its distribution in the rat, *Circ Res* 8:135, 1960.

575 Sapolsky R, Rivier C, Yamamoto F et al: Interleukin-1 stimulates the secretion of hypothalamic corticotropin-releasing factor, *Science* 238:522, 1987.

576 Sato A, Schmidt RF: Somatosympathetic reflexes: afferent fibers, central pathways, discharge characteristics, *Physiol Rev* 53:916, 1973.

577 Sawchenko PE, Friedman MI: Sensory functions of the liver: a review, *Am J Physiol* 236:R5, 1979.

578 Scanlon MF, Lewis M, Weightman DR et al: The neuroregulation of human thyrotropin secretion. In Martini L, Ganong WF, editors: *Frontiers in neuroendocrinology,* New York, 1980, Raven.

579 Schachter M: Kallikreins (kininogenases): a group of serine proteases with bioregulatory actions, *Pharmacol Rev* 31:1, 1980.

580 Schaz K, Stock G, Simon W et al: Enkephalin effects on blood pressure, heart rate, and baroreceptor reflex, *Hypertension* 2:395, 1979.

581 Schindler, Darnell: *Science* 257:809, 1992.

582 Schmidt HHHW, Seifert R, Bohme E: Formulation and release of nitric oxide from human neutrophils and HL-60 cells induced by a chemotactic peptide, platelet activating factor, and leukotriene B_4, *FEBS Lett* 244:357, 1989.

583 Schoeniger LO, Reilly PM, Bulkley GB et al: Heat-shock gene expression excludes acute-phase gene expression following resuscitation from hemorrhagic shock, *Surgery* 112:355, 1992.

584 Schrier RW: Effects of adrenergic nervous system and catecholamines on systemic and renal hemodynamics, sodium and water excretion, and renin secretion, *Kidney Int* 6:291, 1974.

585 Schrier RW, Berl WT, Anderson RJ: Osmotic and nonosmotic control of vasopressin release, *Am J Physiol* 236:F321, 1979.

586 Seckinger P, Williamson K, Balavoine JF et al: A urine inhibitor of interleukin-1 activity affects both interleukin-alpha and -beta

but not tumor necrosis factor–alpha, *J Immunol* 139:1541, 1987.

587 Segal J: A rapid, extranuclear effect of 3'5,3'-triiodothyronine on sugar uptake by several tissues in the rat in vivo, *Endocrinology* 124:2755, 1989.

588 Sen S, Bravo EL, Bumpus FM: Isolation of hypertension-producing compound from normal human urine, *Circ Res* 1:5, 1977.

589 Share L: Control of plasma ADH titer in hemorrhage: role of atrial and arterial receptors, *Am J Physiol* 215:1384, 1968.

590 Sharfrir E, Steinberg D: The essential role of the adrenal cortex in the response of plasma free fatty acids, cholesterol, and phospholipids to epinephrine injection, *J Clin Invest* 39:310, 1960.

591 Shavit Y, Lewis J, Terman G et al: Opioid peptides mediate the suppressive effect of stress on natural killer cell cytotoxity, *Science* 223:188, 1984.

592 Shearer JD, Morris AJ, Alvina JE et al: Effect of starvation on the local and systemic metabolic effects of the lambda-carrageenan wound, *Am J Surg* 147:456, 1984.

593 Shenkin A, Fraser WB, Series J et al: The serum interleukin-6 response to elective surgery, *Lymphokine Res* 8:123, 1989.

594 Shirani KZ, Vaughan GM, Pruitt BA et al: Reduced serum T_4 and T_3 and their altered transport binding after burn injury in rats, *J Trauma* 25:953, 1985.

595 Shires GT, Carrico J, Cannizaro P: Response of the extracellular fluid. In Shires GT, editor: *Shock: modern problems in clinic surgery,* Philadelphia, 1973, WB Saunders.

596 Shires GT, Cunningham JN, Baker CRF et al: Alterations in cellular membrane function during hemorrhagic shock in primates, *Ann Surg* 176:288, 1972.

597 Shires GTI, Peitzman AB, Illner H et al: Change in red blood cells' transmembrane potential in hemorrhagic shock, *Surg Forum* 32:5, 1981.

598 Shires T, Williams J, Brown L: Acute changes in extracellular fluids associated with major surgical procedures, *Ann Surg* 154:803, 1961.

599 Shizgal HM, Milne CA, Sapiner HA: The effect of nitrogen-sparing, intravenously administered fluids on postoperative body composition, *Surgery* 86:60, 1979.

600 Shoemaker WC, Stahr LJ, Kuir SI et al: Sequential circulatory and metabolic changes in the liver and whole body during hemorrhagic shock, *Adv Exp Med Biol* 33:293, 1973.

601 Shuai K, Schindler C, Prezioso VR et al: Activation of transcription by IFN-gamma: tyrosine phosphorylation of a 91-kDa DNA-binding protein, *Science* 258:1808, 1992.

602 Shulman GI, Williams PE, Liljanguest JE et al: Effect of hyperglycemia independent of changes in insulin or glucagon on lipolysis in the conscious dog, *Metabolism* 29:317, 1980.

603 Siegel JH, Cerra FB, Coleman B et al: Physiological and metabolic correlations in human sepsis, *Surgery* 86:163, 1979.

604 Simpson JB, Routtenberg A: Subfornical organ: site of drinking elicitation by angiotensin II, *Science* 181:1172, 1973.

605 Skillman JJ, Hedlye-White J, Pallotta JA: Hormonal, fuel, and respiratory relationships after acute blood loss in man, *Surg Forum* 21:23, 1970.

606 Sklar AH, Schrier RW: Central nervous system mediators of vasopressin release, *Physiol Rev* 63:1243, 1983.

607 Slotman GJ, Burchard KW, Gann DS: Thromboxane and prostacyclin in clinical acute respiratory failure, *J Surg Res* (in press).

608 Smedegard G, Lachman LB, Hugli TE: Endotoxin-induced shock in the rat: a role for C5a, *Am J Pathol* 135:489, 1989.

609 Smith KA, Lachman LB, Openheim JJ et al: The functional relationship of the interleukins, *J Exp Med* 151:1551, 1980.

610 Smith R, Fuller DJ, Wedge J et al: Initial effect of injury on ketone bodies and other blood metabolities, *Lancet* 1:1, 1975.

611 Spiegel AM, Downs RW Jr: Guanine nucleotides: key regulators of hormone receptor–adenylate cyclase interaction, *Endocrinol Rev* 2:275, 1981.

612 Spitzer JA, Kovach AGB, Rosues T et al: Influence of endotoxin on adipose tissue metabolism, *Adv Exp Med Biol* 33:337, 1974.

613 Star RA, Nonoguchi H, Balaban R et al: Calcium and cyclic adenosine monophosphate as second messengers for vasopressin in the rat inner medullary collecting tubule, *J Clin Invest* 81:1879, 1988.

614 Stein JH, Boonjarten S, Maux RC et al: Mechanism of the redistribution of renal cortical blood flow during hemorrhagic hypotension in the dog, *J Clin Invest* 52:39, 1973.

615 Stein JH, Congblay RC, Karsh DL et al: The effect of bradykinin on proximal tubular reabsorption in the dog: evidence for functional nephron heterogeneity, *J Clin Invest* 51:1709, 1972.

616 Stein TP, Leskin MJ, Wallace HW et al: Changes in protein synthesis after trauma: importance of nutrition, *Am J Physiol* 233:E348, 1976.

617 Sterling K: Thyroid hormone action at the cell level, *N Engl J Med* 300:117, 1979.

618 Stewart JM, Gewitz MH, Clark BJ et al: The role of vasopressin and atrial natriuretic factor in postoperative fluid retention after the Fontan procedure, *J Thorac Cardiovasc Surg* 102:821, 1991.

619 Stjernholm RL: Carbohydrate metabolism. In Sbarra AJ, Strauss RR, editors: *The reticuloendothelial system: a comprehensive treatise,* New York, 1980, Plenum.

620 Stryer L, Bourke HR: G proteins: a family of signal transducers, *Annu Rev Cell Biol* 2:391, 1986.

621 Studley HO: Percentage of weight loss: a basic indicator of surgical risk, *JAMA* 106:458, 1936.

622 Sutherland EW: Studies on the mechanism of hormone action, *Science* 177:401, 1972.

623 Takasawa S, Nata K, Yonekura H et al: Cyclic-ADP ribose in insulin secretion from pancreatic β cells, *Science* 259:370, 1993.

624 Tang WJ, Gilman AG: *Science* 254:1500, 1991.

625 Teschemacher H, Koch G, Scheffler H et al, editors: Opioid peptides: immunological significance? *NY Acad Sci* 594:66, 1990.

626 Tom WW, Villalba M, Szlabick RE et al: Fluorophotometric evaluation of capillary permeability in gram-negative shock, *Arch Surg* 118:636, 1983.

627 Tracey KJ: Tumor necrosis factor (cachectin) in the biology of septic shock syndrome, *Circ Shock* 35:123, 1991.

628 Tracey KJ, Fong Y, Hesse DG et al: Anti-cachectin/TNF monoclonal antibodies prevent septic shock during lethal bacteremia, *Nature* 330:662, 1987.

629 Tracey KJ, Lowery SF: The role of cytokine mediators in septic shock, *Adv Surg* 23:21, 1990.

630 Tracey KJ, Lowry SF, Beutler B et al: Cachectin/tumor necrosis factor mediates changes in skeletal muscle plasma membrane potential, *J Exp Med* 164:1368, 1986.

631 Tranbaugh RF, Lewis FR: Mechanisms and etiologic factors of pulmonary edema, *Surg Gynecol Obstet* 158:193, 1958.

632 Turninsky J: Glucose metabolism in the region recovering from burn injury, *Endocrinology* 113:1370, 1983.

633 Udelsman R, Blake MJ, Holbrook NJ: Molecular response to surgical stress: specific and simultaneous heat-shock protein induction in the adrenal cortex, aorta, and vena cava, *Surgery* 110:1125, 1991.

634 Udelsman R, Blake MJ, Stagg CA et al: Vascular heat-shock protein expression in response to stress, *J Clin Invest* 91:465, 1993.

635 Udenfriend S, Kilpatrick DG: Biochemistry of the enkephalins and enkephalin-containing peptides, *Arch Biochem Biophys* 221:309, 1983.

636 Unger RH, Dobbs RE: Insulin, glucagon, and somatostatin secretion in the regulation of metabolism, *Annu Rev Physiol* 40:307, 1978.

637 Unger RH, Orchi L: Glucagon and the A cell: physiology and pathophysiology, *N Engl J Med* 304:1518, 1981.
638 Valenti G, Hugon JS, Bourguet J: To what extent is microtubular network involved in antidiuretic response? *Am J Physiol* 255:F1098, 1988.
639 Valgeirsdottir K, Munroe HM: Protein and amino acid metabolism. In Fischer JE, editor: *Surgical nutrition,* Boston, 1983, Little, Brown.
640 Vallance P, Collier J, Moncada S: Effects of endothelium-derived nitric oxide on peripheral arteriolar tone in man, *Lancet* 2:997, 1989.
641 Van Epps DE, Saland L: *J Immunol* 132:3046, 1984.
642 Van Lancker JL: Vitamin deficiency. In Van Lancker JL, editor: *Molecular and cellular mechanisms in disease,* New York, 1976, Springer-Verlag.
643 Van Loon GR, Appel NA: Beta-endorphin–induced increases in plasma dopamine, norepinephrine, and epinephrine, *Res Commun Chem Pathol Pharmacol* 27:607, 1980.
644 Van Oers MJH, Van der Heyden APAM, Aarden LA: Interleukin-6 in serum and urine of renal transplant patients, *Clin Exp Immunol* 71:314, 1988.
645 Vane JR, Anggard EE, Botting RM: *N Engl J Med* 1990.
646 Vanhoutte PM: Endothelial cell control of vascular function, *Hypotension* 13:658, 1989.
647 Vary TC, Siegle JH, Nakatani T et al: Potential regulatory mechanism for depression of ketogenesis in sepsis, *Circ Shock* 16:78, 1985.
648 Vilcek J, Gray PW, E. R, et al: Interferon-gamma: a lymphokine for all seasons, *Lymphokine Res* 11:1, 1985.
649 Vinik AI, Kalk JW, McLaren H et al: Fasting blunts the TSH response to synthetic TRH, *J Clin Endocrinol Metab* 40:509, 1975.
650 Vinnars E, Bergstrom J, Furst P: Influence of postoperative state in the intracellular free amino acids in human muscle tissue, *Ann Surg* 182:665, 1975.
651 Voerman HJ, S.R.J.M. vS, Groeneveld ABJ et al: Effects of recombinant human growth hormone in patients with severe sepsis, *Ann Surg* 216:648, 1992.
652 Waage A, Brandtzaeg P, Halstensen A et al: The complex pattern of cytokines in serum from patients with meningococcal septic shock, *J Exp Med* 169:333, 1989.
653 Wagner F: *J Biol Chem* 267:16066, 1991.
654 Wakabayashi G, Gelfand JA, Burke JF et al: Specific receptor antagonist for interleukin-1 prevents *Escherichia coli*–induced shock in rabbits, *FASEB J* 5:338, 1991.
655 Wannemacher RW, Powanda MC, Dinterman RE: Amino acid flux and protein synthesis after exposure of rats to either *Diplococcus pneumoniae* or *Salmonella typhimurium, Immun* 10:60, 1974.
656 Ware J, Ljanquist O, Norberg KA et al: Osmolar changes in hemorrhage: the effect of an altered nutritional status, *Acta Chir Scand* 35:44, 1982.
657 Ware JA, Heistad DD: Platelet-endothelium interactions, *N Engl J Med* 328:628, 1993.
658 Water JS, Meyers P, Kruger JM: Microinjection of interleukin-1 into brain: separation of sleep and fever responses, *Physiol Behav* 45:169, 1989.
659 Watters JM, Bessey PQ, Dinarello CA et al: The induction of interleukin-1 in humans and its metabolic effects, *Surgery* 98:298, 1985.
660 Weissman C, Holinger I: Modifying systemic responses with anesthetic techniques, *Anesthesiol Clin North Am* 6:221, 1988.
661 Weissman G, Thomas L: The effects of corticosteroids upon connective tissue and lysosomes, *Recent Prog Horm Res* 20:215, 1964.
662 Welbourne T, Joshi S, McVie R: Growth hormone effects on hepatic glutamate handling in vivo, *Am J Physiol* 257:E959, 1989.
663 West JB: Control of ventilation. In West JB, editor: *Physiological basis of medical practice,* Baltimore, 1985, Williams and Wilkins.
664 West MA, Keller GA, Cerra FB et al: Mechanism of hepatic insufficiency in septic multiple system organ failure, *Surg Forum* 35:44, 1984.
665 White A, Handler P, Smith EL: *Principles of biochemistry,* New York, 1973, McGraw-Hill.
666 Wicklmayr M, Dietze G, Gunther B et al: Improvement of glucose assimilation and protein degradation by bradykinin in maturity-onset diabetes and in surgical patients, *Adv Exp Med Biol* 12:569, 1979.
667 Widner U, Schmid C, Zepf J et al: Effects of insulin-like growth factors on chick embryo hepatocytes, *Acta Endocrinol (Copenh)* 108:237, 1985.
668 Wiedermann CJ: Interleukin-1 interaction with neuroregulatory systems: selective enhancement by recombinant human and mouse interleukin-1 of in vitro opioid peptide receptor binding in rat brain, *J Neurosci Res* 22:172, 1989.
669 Williams GH: Aldosterone. In Dunn MJ, editor: *Renal endocrinology,* Baltimore, 1983, Williams & Williams.
670 Williamson DH: Regulation of ketone body metabolism and the effects of injury, *Acta Chir Scand (Suppl)* 507:22, 1982.
671 Williamson OH et al: Muscle-protein catabolism after injury in man, as measured by urinary excretion of 3-methylhistidine, *Clin Sci Mol Med* 52:527, 1977.
672 Wilmore DM: Interleukin-1 does not increase proteolysis in skeletal muscle. In 1985.
673 Wilmore DM, Goodwin CW, Aulick LH et al: Effect of injury and infection on visceral metabolism and circulation, *Ann Surg* 192:491, 1980.
674 Wilmore DW, Aulick LH, Mason AD et al: Influence of the burn wound on local and systemic responses to injury, *Ann Surg* 186:444, 1977.
675 Wilmore DW, Long JM, Mason AD et al: Catecholamines: mediators of the hypermetabolic response to thermal burn patients, *Ann Surg* 180:653, 1974.
676 Wilmore DW, Mason AD, Pruitt BA: Insulin response to glucose in hypermetabolic burn patients, *Ann Surg* 183:314, 1976.
677 Wittert GA, Espiner EA, Richards AM et al: Atrial natriuretic peptide reduces the vasopressin and angiotensin II but not the ACTH response to acute hypoglycemia in normal men, *Clin Endocrinol* 38:183, 1993.
678 Wolf RF, Pearlstone DB, Newman E et al: Growth hormone and insulin reverse net whole body and skeletal muscle protein catabolism in cancer patients, *Ann Surg* 216:280, 1992.
679 Wolfe RR, Shaw HF, Durkot MJ: Energy metabolism in trauma and sepsis: the role of fat. In Schumer W, Spitzer JJ, Marshall BE, editors: *Molecular and cellular aspects of shock and trauma,* New York, 1983, Liss.
680 Woloski BM, Smith EM, Meyer WJ et al: Corticotropin-releasing activity of monokines, *Science* 230:1035, 1985.
681 Wood CE, Shinsako J, Keil LC et al: Hormonal and hemodynamic responses to 15 ml/kg hemorrhage in conscious dogs: responses correlate to body temperature, *Pro Soc Exp Biol Med* 167:15, 1981.
682 Wood JJ, Rodrick ML, O'Mahoney JB et al: Inadequate interleukin-2 production: a fundamental immunologic deficiency in patients with major burns, *Ann Surg* 200:311, 1984.
683 Woolfe LIU: Arterial plasma amino acids in patients with serious postoperative infections and in patients with major fractures, *Surgery* 79:283, 1976.
684 Woolfe PD, Hammill RW, McDonald JV et al: Transient hypogonadotropic hypogonadism caused by critical surgical illness, *J Clin Endocrinol Metab* 66:444, 1985.

685 Wright FS, Briggs JP: Feedback control of glomerular blood flow, pressure, and filtration rate, *Physiol Rev* 59:958, 1979.
686 Wright HK, Gann DS: A defect in urinary concentrating ability during postoperative antidiuresis, *Surg Gynecol Obstet* 121:47, 1965.
687 Wright PD, Johnston IDA: The effect of surgical operation on growth hormone levels in surgery, *Surgery* 77:479, 1975.
688 Yanagisawa M, Kurihara H, Kimura S et al: A novel potent vasoconstrictor peptide produced by vascular endothelial cells, *Nature* 332:411, 1988.
689 Yang RD, Modlawer LL, Sakamoto A et al: Leukocyte endogenous mediator alters protein dynamic in rats, *Metabolism* 32:654, 1983.
690 Yates FE: Order and complexity in dynamical systems: homeodynamics as a generalized mechanism for biology. In Mikulecky DC, Witten M, editors: *Dynamics and thermodynamics of complex systems,* New York, 1993, Pergamon.
691 Yates FE: Self-organizing systems. In Boyd CAR, Noble D, editors: *The logic of life,* Oxford, 1993, Oxford University Press.
692 Yates FE, Marsh DJ, Maran JW: The adrenal cortex. In Mountcastle VB, editor: *Medical physiology,* ed 14, St Louis, 1980, Mosby.
693 Young JB, Landsberg L: Catecholamines and intermediary metabolism, *Clin Endocrinol Metab* 6:599, 1977.
694 Youngston C, Nurse C, Yeger H et al: Oxygen sensing in airway chemoreceptors, *Nature* 365:153, 1993.
695 Zapf J, Schoenle E, Froesch ER: Insulin-like growth factors I and II: some biological actions and receptor-binding characteristics of two purified constituents of nonsuppressible insulin-like activity of human sera, *Eur J Biochem* 87:285, 1978.
696 Zileli MS, Gedik P, Adalar N et al: Adrenal medullary response to removal of various amounts of blood, *Endocrinology* 95:1477, 1974.
697 Zimpfer M, Manders WT, Barger AC et al: Pentobarbital alters compensatory neural and humoral mechanisms in response to hemorrhage, *Am J Physiol* 243:H713, 1982.

KEY REFERENCES

1 Anggard EE: The endothelium—the body's largest endocrine gland? *J Endocrinol* 127:371, 1990.
2 Berridge MJ: Inositol triphosphate and calcium signalling, *Nature* 361:315, 1993.
3 Besedovsky HO, Del Rey A: Immune-neuroendocrine circuits: integrative role of cytokines, *Front Neuroendocrinol* 13:61, 1992.
4 Blalock A: Acute circulatory failure as exemplified by shock and hemorrhage, *Surg Gynecol Obstet* 58:551, 1934.
5 Blalock JE: A molecular basis for bidirectional communication between the immune and neuroendocrine systems, *Physiol Rev* 69:1, 1989.
6 Brown JM, Grosso MA, Harken AH: Cytokines, sepsis and the surgeon, *Surg Gynecol Obstet* 169:568, 1989.
7 Cunningham JNJ, Carter NW, Rector FCJ: Resting transmembrane potential difference of skeletal muscle in normal subjects and severely ill patients, *J Clin Invest* 50:49, 1971.
8 Deitch EA, Bridges W, Baker J et al: Hemorrhagic shock–induced bacterial translocation is reduced by xanthine oxidase inhibition or inactivation, *Surgery* 104:191, 1988.
9 Fletcher JR: Eicosanoids: critical agents in the physiological process and cellular injury, *Arch Surg* 128(11):1192, 1993.
10 Gann DS, Ward DG, Carlson DE. Neural control of ACTH: a homeostatic reflex, *Recent Progr Hormone Res* 35:357, 1978.
11 Geller DA, Billiar TR: Should surgeons clone genes? The strategy behind the cloning of the human inducible nitric oxide synthase gene, *Arch Surg* 128:1212, 1993.
12 Gerritsen ME, Bloor CM: Endothelial cell gene expression in response to injury, *FASEB J* 7:523, 1993.
13 Gilman AG: G proteins: transducers of receptor-generated signals, *Annu Rev Biochem* 56:615, 1987.
14 Hume DM, Egdahl RH: The importance of the brain in the neuroendocrine response to injury, *Ann Surg* 150:697, 1959.
15 Lilly MP, Gann DS: The hypothalamic-pituitary-adrenal-immune axis, *Arch Surg* 127:1463, 1992.
16 Masaki T: Endothelins: homeostatic and compensatory actions in the circulatory and endocrine systems, *Endocr Rev* 14(3):253, 1993.
17 Moncada S, Palmer RN, Higgs EA: Biosynthesis of nitric oxide from L-arginine: a pathway for the regulation of cell function and communication, *Biochemistry Pharmacology* 38:1709, 1989.
18 Pober JS, Cotran RS: Cytokines and endothelial cell biology, *Physiol Rev* 70:505, 1990.
19 Reilly PM, Schiller HJ, Bulkley GB: Reactive oxygen metabolites in shock. In Wilmore DW, Brennan MF, Harken AH et al, editors: *Care of the Surgical Patient.* New York, 1992, Scientific American.
20 Shires GT, Cunningham JN, Baker CRF et al: Alterations in cellular membrane function during hemorrhagic shock in primates, *Ann Surg* 176:288, 1972.
21 Souba WW: Glutamine: a key substrate for the splanchnic bed, *Annu Rev Nutr* 11:285, 1991.
22 Tracey KJ, Lowry SF: The role of cytokine mediators in septic shock, *Adv Surg* 23:21, 1990.

CHAPTER

9

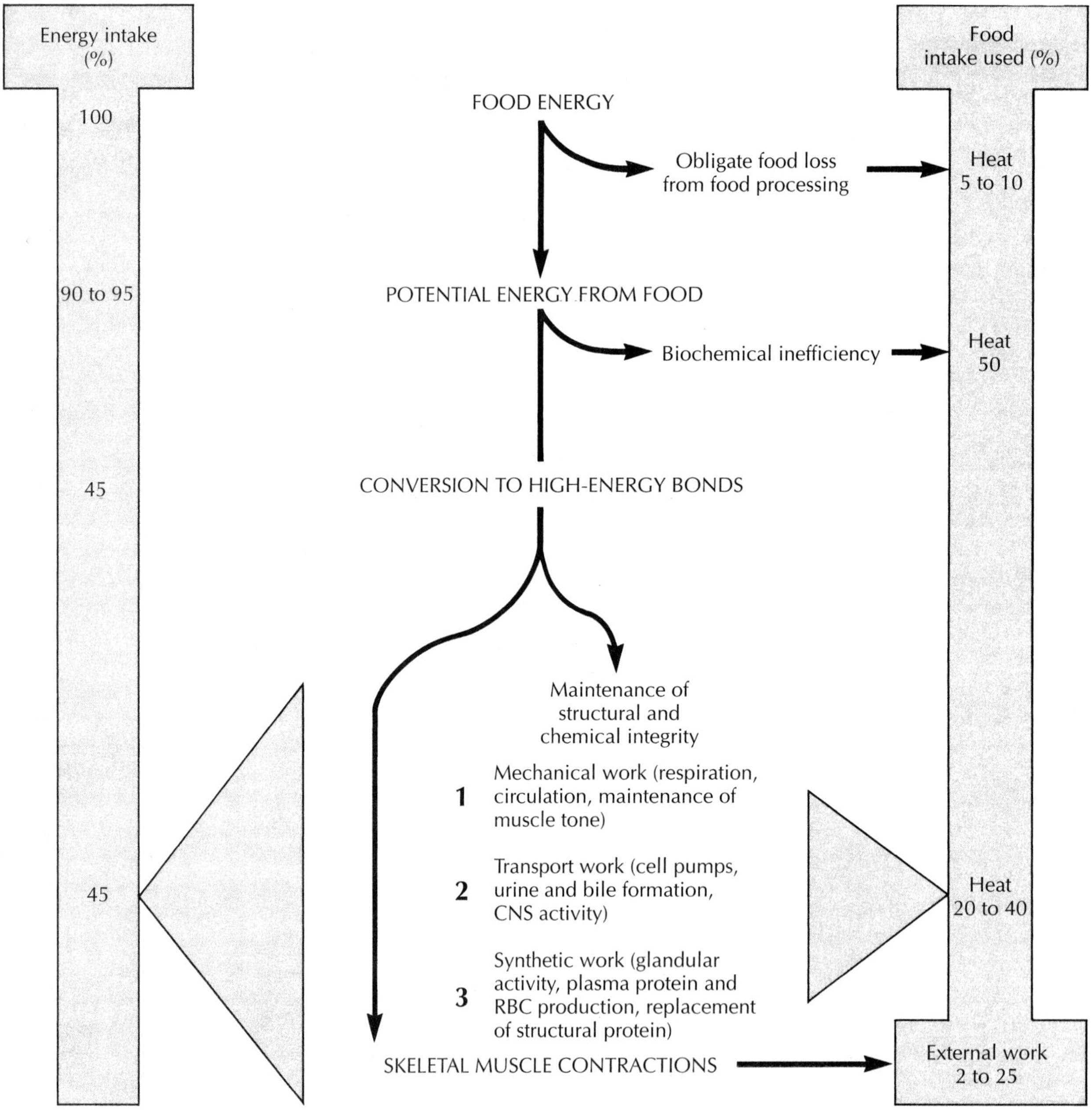
Energy intake (%)
100
90 to 95
45
45
FOOD ENERGY
Obligate food loss from food processing
POTENTIAL ENERGY FROM FOOD
Biochemical inefficiency
CONVERSION TO HIGH-ENERGY BONDS
Maintenance of structural and chemical integrity
1 Mechanical work (respiration, circulation, maintenance of muscle tone)
2 Transport work (cell pumps, urine and bile formation, CNS activity)
3 Synthetic work (glandular activity, plasma protein and RBC production, replacement of structural protein)
SKELETAL MUSCLE CONTRACTIONS
Food intake used (%)
Heat 5 to 10
Heat 50
Heat 20 to 40
External work 2 to 25

NUTRITIONAL SUPPORT

Thomas P. Paxton • Richard L. Gamelli • Mark J. Koruda

MALNUTRITION

Malnutrition, in the form of inadequate caloric intake or lack of protein of "high biologic value," continues even today as a major cause of morbidity and mortality worldwide. Although deficient nutrient intake, leading to protein-calorie malnutrition (PCM), is a greater problem in developing countries, it is also of critical importance in industrialized nations. Random population surveys in both the United States and Canada have demonstrated a high occurrence of PCM, especially in impoverished segments of society.[98]

The relationship between nutrition and health has long been recognized and is well documented. However, Scrimshaw and associates [139,298,299] were the first to consider a synergistic action between nutritional deficiencies and impairment of host immune responsiveness. The concept has evolved of a dynamic equilibrium among nutrition, immunocompetence, and infection. Nowhere could this equilibrium be of greater importance than in surgical patients, in whom hypercatabolism, sepsis, malignancy, organ failure, and/or the demands of a healing wound, combined with a depressed immunoresponsive state, lead to increased morbidity and mortality.

Rhoads and Alexander[268] suggested that surgical patients may be particularly prone to the ravages of protein or calorie malnutrition as a result of preoperative impairments, postoperative dysfunction or complications, and postsurgical stress. Also, surgical procedures and anesthesia may further compromise the patient's immune response. The surgical patient can be particularly prone to disruption of the steady state that exists among nutrition, immunocompetence, and infection. Impaired nutritional status, as a consequence of concurrent illness, trauma, surgery, anesthesia, or other therapeutic interventions, can develop quickly, even in a previously well-nourished surgical patient. For example, Mullen and associates[238] found that patients who had depressed levels of serum albumin or serum transferrin, or delayed hypersensitivity before surgery had a twofold to fivefold increase in the incidence of complications. These researchers developed a multiparameter model to identify patients at increased risk of developing complications based on nutritional indices. They found that patients who had poor nutritional status had a 46% incidence of all complications, a 26% incidence of major septic events, and an overall mortality of 33%.[62] Harvey and associates[150] found a similar ability to identify patients at risk for developing septic complications and death.

The changes in humoral and cell-mediated immunity that accompany PCM may stem from a reduction in the numbers of circulating macrophages, T cells, and B cells. Chemotactic, phagocytic, antigen-presenting, and antibody-producing capabilities may also be detrimentally affected.[332] Malnutrition may alter gut mucosal function and host immunity by reducing gut mucosal mass and increasing mucosal permeability.[97,287]

In examining the effects of PCM on the humoral component of host defense, Cannon and associates[64,65] established the concept of a dynamic balance among antibody synthesis, body protein stores, and nutritional intake of protein of "biologic value." They demonstrated a decrease in antibody production and an increase in susceptibility to infection, as well as altered states of natural resistance and impaired resistance to infection, as results of PCM. They documented that when the host was nutritionally repleted, the defect in antibody elaboration could be corrected, and survival improved following infectious challenge.* A decrease in tonsillar and splenic weights, along with a decline in delayed-type hypersensitivity, have also been demonstrated with PCM.[218] Again, evidence exists that this depression of the humoral immune response may also be reversible with provision of a balanced nutritional formula.[88,199]

Cell-mediated immunity may also be severely affected by PCM. Thymus weights are reduced.[90] Lymph node germinal centers and paracortical areas show diminished cellularity.[313] In children, the percentage of circulating T cells is reduced, correlating with an increase in nosocomial infections. Also in pediatric patients, varying degrees of protein and protein-calorie malnutrition have reduced complement factor levels, possibly by increasing their peripheral consumption or decreasing their production.[222,312] Additionally, neutrophils from patients with PCM have deranged chemotaxis and may have altered phagocytosis.[14,99,305,348] Intrabactericidal killing by neutrophils may be depressed, as evidenced by a change in the hexose monophosphate shunt, a critical element for bactericidal activity.[304,305] The function of mononuclear phagocytic cells has been shown to be depressed with PCM.[253] In addition to qualitative defects, the generation of bone marrow precursor elements of the phagocytic cells was found to be defective after chemotherapeutic treatments in animals fed a protein-free diet.[127]

It would seem therefore that a variety of changes in host defense accompany defective nutrient intake. Whether these deficits are solely a result of protein or calorie deficiency or of a selective nutrient deficiency (such as a vitamin or trace mineral) remains to be determined. Furthermore, it is unclear whether the various defects described in clinical studies are strictly related to nutritional inadequacies, or whether they are a consequence of disease plus malnutrition. In any case, it does appear that when nutritional deficiencies exist in concert with disease, the outcome is likely to be an increased incidence of complications and possibly death.

*References 35, 64, 65, 198, 324, 361, and 362.

EVALUATION OF NUTRITIONAL STATUS

Because PCM (or one of its variants) appears to lead to an increased incidence of complications in hospitalized patients, patients suffering from PCM should be identified so that nutritional support may be used therapeutically. If this is done, the reversal of malnutrition can be documented and, ideally, a decrease in the complications and improved patient response. The need for nutritional support in a surgical patient is a balance of (1) nutritional status; (2) metabolic rate; and (3) length of time the patient will be unable to eat:

$$\text{Need for nutritional support} = \frac{(\text{Metabolic rate}) \times (\text{Duration of} \downarrow \text{intake})}{\text{Nutritional status}}$$

Nutritional Anatomy

To be able to assess a patient's nutritional status, the clinician must have a general understanding of nutritional reserves. In a "normal" 70 kg healthy subject, approximately 60% of the total body weight is made up of bone, minerals, and water. Although critical to the maintenance of homeostasis, these elements contribute nothing to energy or protein reserves. The energy and protein reserves are found in the fat, protein, and carbohydrate stores of the body, which make up the remaining 40% of total body weight. The fat stores (25% of body weight), the major calorie stores, contain 150,000 kcal of energy reserves. Carbohydrates on the average constitute 50% of a "normal" diet, but they account for only 1% of body weight. They are found primarily in the liver, muscle glycogen, and circulating blood glucose and contribute only 1400 kcal to the energy reserves. Protein (15% of body weight) is a significant source of calorie reserve, in the range of 42,000 kcal. It must also be considered the structural element of the body. Proteins are available for potential caloric supply, but they can be used only to a limited degree before complications begin to develop (Table 9-1).

Nutritional History

A variety of techniques are used in assessing a patient's nutritional status, ranging from the history and physical examination to laboratory testing. Through the nutritional history, the clinician attempts to identify patients who are likely to have a nutritional deficit. The history

TABLE 9-1 NUTRITIONAL RESERVES

TISSUE	BODY WEIGHT (%)	WEIGHT (70 kg SUBJECT)	KCAL (70 kg SUBJECT)
Fat	25%	17.5 kg	150,000
Protein	15%	10.5 kg	42,000
Glycogen	1%	250 g (musle)	1,000
		100 g (liver)	400
Bone			
Minerals	5%	3.5 kg	—
Water	54%	38.5 kg	—

TABLE 9-2 EVALUATION OF WEIGHT CHANGE*

TIME	SIGNIFICANT WEIGHT LOSS	SEVERE WEIGHT LOSS
1 week	1% to 2%	>2%
1 month	5%	>5%
3 months	7.5%	>7.5%
6 months	10%	>10%

*Values charted are for percent weight change:

$$\text{Percent weight change} = \frac{(\text{Usual weight} - \text{Actual weight}) \times 100}{\text{Usual weight}}$$

specifically focuses on inadequacies of intake as a result of diet, impaired absorption, decreased appetite, and increased requirements associated with illness. Particularly important in a surgical patient are changes in absorption of vitamin B_{12}, iron, and folate that can occur after surgical procedures, resulting in either short-gut syndrome or selective resection, such as follows gastrectomies or distal ileal resection. Broad-spectrum antibiotics or warfarin-like anticoagulants may result in defective coagulation secondary to reduced levels of vitamin K–dependent coagulation factors, and chronic ingestion of ethanol produces thymidine deficits as a consequence of decreased absorption, storage, and use resulting from liver disease. Patients may lose considerable amounts of protein with repeated ascitic or pleural taps or with chronic peritoneal dialysis. Selective nutrient loss should be suspected in patients with uncontrolled diarrhea and in patients with draining small bowel fistulae who, in addition to increased water and electrolyte loss, may have selective deficiencies (particularly zinc). Deficits of calories or proteins may have evolved in patients with a history of continuous illness or injury if intake has not been balanced against needs, and selective deficiencies of vitamins or minerals may be present as well.

A fairly simple but critical element of the history is how the patient's weight has varied over the recent past. The patient's usual weight and highest weight as an adult should be recorded and compared with the current weight. Any patient who has had a weight loss greater than 10%, particularly if this has occurred within the last 6 months, should be considered as potentially suffering from PCM or one of its variants. Blackburn and associates[44] have suggested the guidelines listed in Table 9-2 as reasonable indicators of the severity of weight change.

Physical Examination

Determining the patient's current weight and height should be a standard part of any admission physical examination. These values can be correlated with standard weight-for-height tables (Table 9-3).[348] In general, patients who are either 20% above or below the standard weight for height should be considered as having abnormalities of protein or calorie balance. Obesity is not necessarily associated with good nutritional status. A patient who has recently been ill or on a diet may have selective nutrient deficiencies despite a surfeit of calories. The physical examination should include attention to the presence or absence of jaundice, cheilosis, glossitis, loss of subcutaneous fat, muscle wasting, or edema. The patient also should be examined for signs of poor wound healing, cutaneous lesions, loss of muscle strength, or hair loss. Although the surgeon cannot always predict the specific nutrient deficiency through such examination, the question can be raised whether the patient's nutritional status should be evaluated further.

Certainly finding abnormalities on the initial dietary history and physical examination establishes the need to proceed with a more detailed analysis of the patient's nutritional status.

Calorie Reserve

Fat Stores

Compartmental analysis of the individual components of a patient's nutritional status is performed by examining the major nutrient reserves of the body: fat and protein stores. The calories stored in the body's fat reserves can be estimated by using the anthropometric technique of measuring skinfold thickness. The rationale is that approximately 50% of adipose tissue is found in the subcutaneous areas of the body. A variety of skinfolds can be measured. The triceps skinfold is most commonly chosen, but subscapular, abdominal, hip, and thigh skinfolds also can be used. Serial measurements can be used to assess gains or losses within the fat compartment over time. In general, however, changes in this compartment are relatively slow, and in hospitalized patients are not measured more often than weekly. Some clinicians advocate measuring them no more than once or twice a month.

The triceps skinfold is measured with calipers that have a precisely calibrated spring tension. The skinfold

TABLE 9-3 WEIGHT-HEIGHT REFERENCE CHART (ADULTS)

HEIGHT		WOMEN FRAME*			HEIGHT		MEN FRAME*		
Ft	In	SMALL	MEDIUM	LARGE	Ft	In	SMALL	MEDIUM	LARGE
4	10	102-111	109-121	118-131	5	2	128-134	131-141	138-150
4	11	103-113	111-123	120-134	5	3	130-136	133-143	140-153
5	0	104-115	113-126	122-137	5	4	132-138	135-145	142-156
5	1	106-118	115-129	125-140	5	5	134-140	137-148	144-160
5	2	108-121	118-132	128-143	5	6	136-142	139-151	146-164
5	3	111-124	121-135	131-147	5	7	138-145	142-154	149-168
5	4	114-127	124-138	134-151	5	8	140-148	145-157	152-172
5	5	117-130	127-141	137-155	5	9	142-151	148-160	155-176
5	6	120-133	130-144	140-159	5	10	144-154	151-163	158-180
5	7	123-136	133-147	143-163	5	11	146-157	154-166	161-184
5	8	126-139	136-150	146-167	6	0	149-160	157-170	164-188
5	9	129-142	139-153	149-170	6	1	152-164	160-174	168-192
5	10	132-145	142-156	152-173	6	2	155-168	164-178	172-197
5	11	135-148	145-159	155-176	6	3	158-172	167-182	176-202
6	0	138-151	148-162	158-179	6	4	162-176	171-187	181-207

Based on a weight-height mortality study conducted by the Society of Actuaries and the Association of Life Insurance Medical Directors of America, Metropolitan Life Insurance Company, revised 1983.
*Weights at ages 25 to 59 based on lowest mortality. Height includes 1-inch heel. Weight for women includes 3 lb. for indoor clothing. Weight for men includes 5 lb. for indoor clothing.

is determined by applying the calipers at the midpoint of the nondominant arm after the skinfold is grasped on the posterior aspect of the arm. The value is recorded three times, each time 3 seconds after the calipers are applied, and the average of the three values also is recorded. This average is compared with a series of standards for men and women (a 100% standard thickness of 12.5 mm in men and 16.5 mm in women is used). Patients over 60% of standard are considered to have little or no deficit of fat calorie stores. This technique is the only practical and widely applicable means of assessing fat stores in hospitalized patients, since methods such as underwater weighing and water displacement cannot routinely be used with sick patients.

Protein Stores

The protein stores, the other source of calories available to the body, conceptually are subdivided in two categories, that within skeletal muscle (somatic protein stores) and that within the viscera (visceral protein stores). Generally, these protein compartments are not directly measured. Rather, as with fat stores, the compartment size is assessed through indirect techniques.

SKELETAL MUSCLE (SOMATIC) PROTEIN STORES. The protein in the skeletal muscle mass can be assessed through anthropometric techniques in which the arm muscle circumference is used as an index of bodywide protein stores. The circumference of the nondominant arm at its midpoint is measured with a soft tape, and the midarm muscle circumference (MAMC) is determined by subtracting the contribution of subcutaneous fat to arm circumference:

$$\text{MAMC} = \text{Arm circumference (cm)} - (3.14 \times \text{triceps skinfold [cm]})$$

The derived numbers are then compared with standards for men and women. MAMC at 100% of standard is 25.5 cm for men and 23 cm for women. A value below 60% of standard is considered abnormal.

The mass of muscle protein also can be assessed by determining the amount of creatinine excreted in the urine. Creatinine is generated as a by-product of muscle metabolism, and a person's height can be correlated to an ideal creatinine excretion. Creatinine excretion correlates well with measurements of lean body mass, and creatinine excretion increases proportionally with increases in muscle mass. Creatinine-height indices below 60% of predicted are thought to show significant deficits of somatic protein stores (Table 9-4).[44] A product of actin and myosin metabolism, 3-methyl-histidine, is excreted without being recycled and is supported by some as a measure of protein status. However, it is not widely used on a clinical basis, because it tends to increase during refeeding of starved patients, and laboratory determinations of 3-methyl-histidine are complex.

VISCERAL PROTEIN STORES. The status of the proteins in the viscera is determined by using a series of markers that have been identified as assessors of the visceral pro-

TABLE 9-4 IDEAL URINARY CREATININE VALUES*

MEN		WOMEN	
HEIGHT (cm)	IDEAL CREATININE (mg)	HEIGHT (cm)	IDEAL CREATININE (mg)
157.5	1288	147.3	830
160.0	1325	149.9	851
162.6	1359	152.4	875
165.1	1386	154.9	900
167.6	1426	157.5	925
170.2	1467	160.0	949
172.7	1513	162.6	977
175.3	1555	165.1	1006
177.8	1596	167.6	1044
180.3	1642	170.2	1076
182.9	1691	172.7	1109
185.4	1739	175.3	1141
188.0	1785	177.8	1174
190.5	1831	180.3	1206
193.0	1891	182.9	1240

*Creatinine coefficient: (men) = 23 mg/kg ideal body weight; (women) = 18 mg/kg ideal body weight.

From Blackburn GL et al: *JPEN* 1:11, American Society of Parenteral and Enteral Nutrition, 1977.

tein–containing compartment. The integrity of the visceral protein stores can be estimated by determining serum albumin and transferrin concentrations, retinol-binding protein and thyroxine-binding prealbumin levels, absolute lymphocyte count, and the status of immune responsiveness, assessed by delayed cutaneous hypersensitivity testing. PCM causes a decrease in virtually all of the plasma proteins; the degree to which the various protein levels change is related to their half-lives. However, changes occur that do not reflect altered nutritional status, such as acute loss, hemodilution, or elevation as an acute-phase reactant.

Serum albumin is most commonly used as an assessor of the visceral protein stores. The liver produces albumin, which is distributed within the intravascular and extravascular spaces. The albumin pool is approximately 4 to 5 g/kg in an adult, one third of which is found in the intravascular space. Albumin is broken down and turned over at the rate of approximately 15 g/day. Because the half-life of plasma albumin is 20 days, changes in nutritional status that occur over a short period are unlikely to reflect a change in the albumin level or even a clearly abnormal level. The albumin level's greatest value is in assessing more chronic nutritional deficiencies; this is the single most important laboratory test in the diagnosis of PCM, with a level below 3 g/dl considered abnormal.

Another component commonly used as an identifier of the visceral protein compartment is transferrin. Transferrin is a beta$_{1c}$-globulin protein with a molecular weight of approximately 90,000 daltons. It is partly synthesized by the liver and is a major transport protein for plasma iron. The body's pool of transferrin is approximately 5 g, and the protein has a serum half-life of 8 to 10 days. Because of it's shorter half-life, compared to albumin, transferrin is measured as an earlier index of changes in the visceral protein compartment. If not directly measured, transferrin, as a derived value, can be determined based on the total iron-binding capacity (TIBC)[44]:

$$\text{Transferrin} = (0.8 \times \text{TIBC}) - 43$$

However, studies[224] have suggested that a universal conversion factor for all patients is not feasible; either the formula may need to be modified, or transferrins should be measured directly. Serum transferrin levels below 200 mg/dl have been postulated as indicators of mild visceral protein malnutrition, levels below 150 mg/dl as moderate depletion, and levels below 100 mg/dl as severe depletion. As with serum albumin, the serum transferrin level is a balance between synthesis and degradation. With acute illness, there may be an increased rate of breakdown that may not reflect the true size of the visceral protein–containing compartment. Transferrin levels are increased with iron deficiency. This change must be kept in mind, because iron deficiency is one of the more common selective nutrient defects. Transferrin's shorter half-life makes it more effective as an assessor of acute change; in patients receiving supplemental albumin therapy, transferrin can be followed as an index of visceral protein status.

Two other circulating proteins that are synthesized by the liver and secreted into the circulation are the retinol-binding protein (RBP) and thyroxine-binding prealbumin (TBPA). Shetty and associates[308] demonstrated that changes in both TBPA and RBP were quite rapid and sensitive and could be used to detect subclinical malnutrition and monitor the effectiveness of dietary treatment. RBP, which has a half-life of 12 hours, responds to either protein or energy restriction, whereas TBPA, with a half-life of 2 days, responds to combined energy and protein restriction. However, both of these proteins promptly fall with acute metabolic stress with increased demands for protein synthesis, and RBP is filtered and metabolized by the kidney.[308] The acute changes that occur, although they may represent a selective depletion of these visceral proteins, might not allow accurate assessment of the size of the visceral protein compartments.

The number of circulating lymphocytes has been used by many as an assessment of the visceral protein–containing compartment, the rationale being that most of the circulating lymphocytes are T cells, and the thymus is sensitive to PCM. A level below 1800 total circulating lymphocytes/mm^3 is thought to indicate a degree of visceral protein malnutrition. However, many factors interfere with interpretation of this value (e.g., infection, immunosuppressive drugs), which makes this marker fairly imprecise, nonspecific, and a poor predictor of outcome.

Measuring delayed cutaneous hypersensitivity (DCH) is the most practical in vivo test for assessing immunocompetence, and it has a correlation with the integrity of the visceral protein–containing compartment. Generally, a standard three-battery intradermal injection of 0.1 ml of *Candida,* purified protein derivative of *Mycobacterium tuberculosis* (PPD), and mumps antigen is used as the recall panel. The DCH reaction results from the sequential processing of the antigen by macrophages, recognition of the antigen by T cells previously sensitized, and generation of an immune response, resulting in local erythema and induration of the skin at the site of inoculation. Failure to respond to any of the antigens with at least a 5 mm zone of induration after 24 to 72 hours is thought to indicate a state of anergy. Failure to respond may well be related to PCM but also may occur secondary to an underlying illness (such as lymphoma), the use of immunosuppressive drugs, or improper application of the antigenic challenge. In general, as the serum albumin level decreases, the likelihood of failure to respond increases; patients with an albumin level below 2.2 g/dl usually fail to demonstrate any DCH response.

Nutritional Assessment in Perspective

Using the previously described techniques, the surgeon can obtain a caricature of the patient's protein-calorie status. Using anthropometric techniques, individual serum protein determinations, assessments of immunocompetence, and weight, the patient's nutritional status can be assessed—at a single point in time. Changes in weight over time, changes in serum proteins, and serial tests of immunocompetence can be used to predict a change in the patient's nutritional status as a consequence of disease, illness, or therapeutic intervention.

It is not necessary to perform all of these tests on every patient admitted. As always, there is no substitute for sound clinical judgment. The minimum assessment for all patients should include a history and physical examination, as outlined above, and measurement of the serum albumin and lymphocyte levels. A serum albumin level below 3 g/dl or a total lymphocyte count below 1200 mm^3 indicates a need for more extensive nutritional evaluation, particularly if this might affect the patient's treatment.

The potential effect of nutritional status on outcome can be predicted with the prognostic nutritional index (PNI):

$$\text{PNI (\%)} = 158 - 16.6\ (\text{ALB}) - 0.78\ (\text{TSF}) - 0.2\ (\text{TFN}) - 5.8\ (\text{DCH})$$

where:

ALB = Serum albumin (g/dl)
TSF = Triceps skinfold (mm)
TFN = Serum transferrin (mg/dl)
DCH = Delayed cutaneous hypersensitivity responsiveness to mumps, PPD, and *Candida* injections (rated as 0, nonreactive; 1, <5 mm induration; 2, ≥5 mm of induration)

Using this approach, Mullen and associates[238] found a low risk of complications and death in patients undergoing gastrointestinal surgery with a PNI below 40%. In patients with an intermediate risk (PNI 40% to 49%), they found a 30% incidence of complications, two thirds of which were septic, and a mortality rate of 4.3% Their "high-risk" patients (PNI 50% or above) showed a 46% incidence of all complications, a 26% incidence of major septic conditions, and a mortality rate of 33%.[62]

Nutrient status and the development of complications in patients may or may not be causally related. However, this much appears to be clear: In patients who are ill or are to undergo stressful treatments (e.g., surgery, chemotherapy) and who also are malnourished, the incidence of inferior outcome is significantly increased. The surgeon must keep in mind two facts: (1) with progressive erosion of lean body mass, the body's organ systems progressively lose their ability to perform, and (2) a patient losing protein from the arm is also losing protein from other muscle compartments, such as the diaphragm, intercostal muscles, myocardium, and gastrointestinal tract. As serum proteins decrease, the proteins available for the body's biosynthetic functions also decline. Loss of lean body mass approaching 30% has a high association with the development of complications, particularly sepsis and death. When a series of complications develops in a patient, the surgeon must distinguish disease-specific complications from those arising from nutritional failure. Once able to identify which patients are at increased risk of developing complications that might be avoidable through nutritional support, the clinician can plan a rational, integrated approach to patient care, incorporating restoration of nutritional status with treatment of the primary disease.

Metabolic Needs and Fuel Flow

Determining a patient's needs and detecting nutrient deficits are fundamental to nutritional support. The clinician must at least have a concept of what it takes to keep the patient in balance before he can determine the degree of support necessary. In health or sickness, the body has an obligate requirement for energy. In health this is referred to as the *basal energy expenditure* (BEE), the energy required to maintain basic metabolic functions in a resting, unstressed state. BEE is the amount of energy a person would consume (in a temperate environment) doing no physical activity and having limited sensory input. Obviously, a sick, hospitalized patient rarely can be considered at a level of BEE even when at rest. In general, the degree of lowest energy expenditure is the *resting metabolic energy expenditure* (RME). RME takes into account the BEE and any increases that have occurred as a consequence of illness, injury, or therapy. A reasonable approach to begin with is to consider energy and fuel flow in simple starvation without stress.

Cahill and associates[63] have examined this area in great detail and have clearly elucidated the changes that occur in starvation. With simple starvation, there is no longer an exogenous source of nutrients. The body has an ongoing need, particularly for glucose, to supply the brain, which has a high glucose requirement. Early in starvation this need is satisfied by means of the gluconeogenic function of the liver, which processes the gluconeogenic substrates in the form of amino acids from the periphery, primarily muscle. A small contribution comes from the breakdown of stored adipose tissue, a process that liberates fatty acids and glycerol (the glycerol is an additional source of gluconeogenic precursors). Ketones are excreted in relatively high amounts in the urine from the breakdown of fatty acids, with a relatively modest use of ketones as an energy source. However, after the first week of uncomplicated starvation, the body's need for glucose progressively decreases to approximately one third of early starvation needs; a relative stability in the size of the glucose pool ensues, with no further net loss of carbohydrates from the body and a shift away from gluconeosynthesis. At this time the relative contribution of amino acids to the body's energy needs is greatly reduced, and a far greater dependency on adipose tissues emerges. Fatty acids and glycerol are released in much greater quantities; the brain's need for glucose decreases, because it is using ketones for fuel; and the body as a whole more effectively uses ketones as an energy source, with a decreased relative loss of ketones in the urine. Nitrogen loss in the urine may be taken as a reflection of the breakdown and lysis of lean body mass for gluconeosynthesis. Early on, nitrogen loss may range from 16 to 20 g/day; with the adaptations to starvation, by the second week nitrogen loss may approach 4 to 6 g/day.[63,115]

The major adaptation that occurs with starvation is the body's shift away from a high need for glucose toward conserving protein and increased use of adipose tissue as a primary energy source. Although the triglycerides released from the breakdown of adipose tissues are hydrolyzed to glycerol and fatty acids (the glycerol is converted primarily to glucose in the liver), this accounts for only a small fraction of the total energy supplied by adipose tissue. The free fatty acids become the body's major fuel source during starvation. The ketone bodies, which are metabolites of the free fatty acids, become a substitute source of energy for the brain during starvation.[247] The brain, which normally derives 100% of its energy from glucose, will substitute ketones to the extent of 70% of its energy requirements with the adaptation to starvation.[248] Similarly, the liver shifts to free fatty acids for its energy requirements, as does skeletal muscle. This shift in the body's fuel use from that supplied by carbohydrates, protein, and fat to predominant use of fat results in a change in the respiratory quotient from 0.84 (mixed substrate oxidation) to 0.7 (primarily fat oxidation) (Table 9-5).

TABLE 9-5 APPROXIMATE BODY FUEL RESERVES, DAILY FUEL CONSUMPTION, AND COMPARTMENTALIZATION OF FUEL CONSUMPTION*

	OVERNIGHT FAST (KCAL)	8-DAY FAST (KCAL)	40-DAY FAST (KCAL)
Body stores at end of period			
Fat	100,000	88,000	42,000
Carbohydrate	680	380	380
Protein	25,000	23,000	18,500
TOTAL	125,680	111,380	60,880
Daily loss (last day of period)			
Fat	1200	1400	1350
Carbohydrate	200	0	0
Protein	300	200	75
TOTAL	1700	1600	1425
Fuel consumption			
Brain: gluose	400	100-150	50-75
ketone	50	300-350	375-400
Carcass	1250	1100	975
TOTAL	1700	1600	1425

*In healthy individuals, basal energy expenditure.

Concomitant with the changes in substrate use are changes in the hormonal milieu, with insulin playing a critical role in the adaptation to fasting. As the insulin level falls, more free fatty acids are released, and release of amino acids from muscle is facilitated. Early in the fasting period catecholamine excretion increases, possibly because of the initial fall in serum glucose.[228] Subsequently, catecholamine levels fall later in starvation and remain low throughout the remainder of the fast.[51] The decline in serum glucose is accompanied by increases in serum glucagon and a reversal in the insulin/glucagon molar ratio, favoring hepatic gluconeogenesis. Although production of other hormones is altered (e.g., adrenocorticotropic hormone, thyroid-stimulating hormone, and growth hormone) they probably play a relatively minor role overall in the adaptation to starvation.

During injury or illness the body's need for energy increases markedly, with catabolism of the body's nutrient stores. The metabolic adaptation that occurs with uncomplicated starvation cannot occur when starvation is complicated by illness. With injury or illness, the body increases production of catecholamines, glucocorticoids, glycogen, growth hormone, insulin, adrenocorticotropic hormone (ACTH), renin, and aldosterone. As a consequence of the hormonal response to injury or illness, the body's ability to use adipose tissue as its primary fuel substrate is dramatically reduced. The brain continues to use glucose as a major source of energy during stress. White cells also have a high obligate need for glucose, as does the renal medulla. With injury a wound is present, which has a very selective nutrient requirement. The wound primarily employs anaerobic metabolism and uses glucose as a selective substrate. However, anaerobic metabolism is not an efficient use of glucose and leads to the production of lactate, which must then be recycled via the Cori cycle in the liver (an energy-dependent process). Catecholamines, glucocorticoids, and glycogen facilitate the liver's ability to use proteins released from the periphery as gluconeogenic substrates. In addition to increased proteolysis of the skeletal muscle mass to supply the substrates for gluconeogenesis, the body has greater need of amino acid precursors for new protein synthesis, which leads to further lysis of protein stores. Although lipolysis increases after injury, so does the serum glucose level. When starvation is complicated by stress, fat still serves as an energy source for cardiac and skeletal muscle, but unlike in simple starvation, the body is unable to shift away from its need for continuous gluconeogenesis. The extent to which these various processes occur with injury or illness is largely related to the magnitude of the insult.

ESTIMATING ENERGY REQUIREMENTS FOR CRITICALLY ILL PATIENTS

The degree to which trauma, sepsis, or infection increases the body's energy needs is related to the severity of the pathologic condition. Willmore[357] has suggested a near dose-response relationship between the size of the insult and the increased expenditure. In general, energy expenditure increases only slightly with uncomplicated surgery; with infection or a single long-bone fracture, energy expenditure may increase 20% to 30%; with severe multiple trauma or infection, the increase may be as high as 50% to 60%. In burn patients, energy expenditure increases progressively as burn size increases, reaching a near doubling of energy needs with burns of 50% of the total body surface area (BSA). However, there is a limit to which energy expenditure can be increased, a figure considered to be two to two and one half times the BEE (Figure 9-1).[357]

The underlying disease also may affect energy expenditure. It has long been a point of argument whether malnutrition in cancer patients is a consequence of lack of nutrient intake secondary to the tumor or antitumor

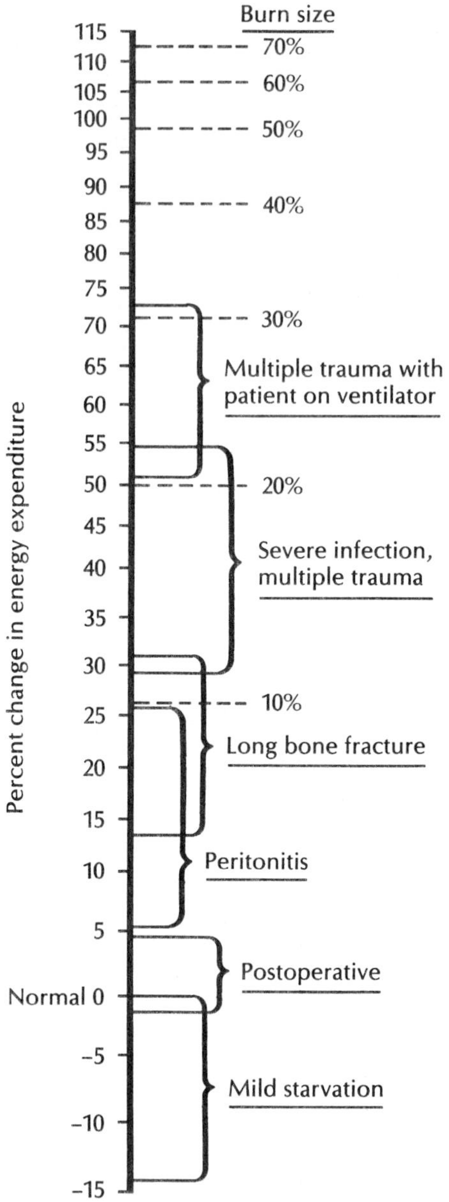

FIGURE 9-1 Percentage increase in energy expenditure with illness or injury. (Redrawn from Wilmore DW: *The metabolic management of the critically ill,* New York, 1977, Plenum.)

therapy, or of changes in nutrient use. Tumors potentially could work as selective nutritional sinks for key critical elements, or they could affect overall energy expenditure. Warnold and colleagues[347] have reported that although cancer patients have a somewhat decreased nutrient intake, they have a significant increase in RME when compared with noncancer controls. Obviously, in any patient all factors must be considered for the sum of their effect on the energy needs that must be met to maintain or restore nutritional balance.

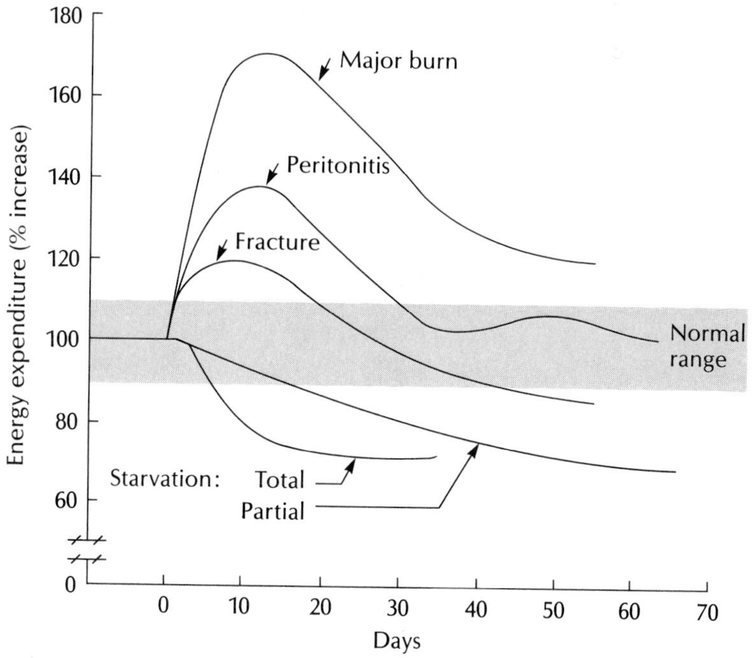

FIGURE 9-2 The duration of need and extent of increased energy expenditure with injury or illness. (Redrawn from Long C: *JPEN* 3:452, American Society of Parenteral and Enteral Nutrition, 1979.)

Besides injury or illness, other events have a bearing on the patient's energy expenditure. An increase in body temperature above 37° C (98° F) is associated with a 10% increase in the metabolic rate for each degree the temperature rises in a 24-hour period. The patient's activity also affects energy expenditure. A 70 kg man expends 1.2 kcal/min when sitting and 4.8 kcal/min when walking. With intense exertion, the same man may expend up to 24.2 kcal/min. The patient's environment can also have an effect on resting energy expenditure. When burn patients are placed in a thermal environment that more closely approaches their newly "reset" thermal regulatory mechanisms, their energy requirement is decreased compared to what it would be in a colder environment.[357]

Another factor that must be considered, along with increased energy expenditure and rate of autocatabolism, is the duration of the extraordinary needs. In general, the duration of the needs is directly related to the presence of the insult or injury. A burn patient may have increased needs for months, with these needs decreasing as the wound is closed. Patients with severe intra-abdominal sepsis may have increased needs for up to a month (Figure 9-2).[204] These increased needs and the time-course response must be compared and contrasted with the dynamics of continuous starvation, in which energy expenditure progressively decreases.

The energy and substrate needs of an ill or injured patient can be determined directly or estimated. Energy expenditure can be measured directly by using calorimetric techniques. Heat loss is determined by placing the patient in a metabolic chamber and performing direct calorimetry. However, this technique generally is not used with ill patients. Energy expenditure more commonly is determined by indirect calorimetry.

The fundamental hypothesis for the validity of indirect calorimetry is that during the period of observation and measurement, the patient is in a steady state, and the oxygen consumed and the carbon dioxide produced are related to the release of energy from the body. A good approximation is that 4.83 kcal is generated per liter of oxygen consumed during the processing of foodstuffs. Although not all foodstuffs require the same amount of energy, the estimate is probably accurate within 10%. Assessment of energy expenditure by indirect calorimetry relates the volume of oxygen consumed ($\dot{V}O_2$) and the volume of carbon dioxide produced ($\dot{V}CO_2$). Estimates of energy consumption can be further refined if the volumes of gas exchanges are correlated with the urinary nitrogen. The formula derived by Weir[349] can then be used to estimate energy expenditure:

$$\text{Energy expenditure} = 3.94\,(\dot{V}O_2) + \dot{V}CO_2 - 2.7\,(\text{Urinary nitrogen})$$

Alternatively, indirect methods may be used to estimate the patient's energy expenditure. The starting point for this is the Harris-Benedict equation, which uses weight (W), height (H), and age (A) to predict the BEE:

$$\text{BEE (men)} = 66 + (13.7 \times W) + (5 \times H) - (6.8 \times A)$$
$$\text{BEE (women)} = 655 + (9.6 \times W) + (1.7 \times H) - (4.7 \times A)$$

These equations were derived from human studies using direct calorimetry.[151] Using the result of this equation, the clinician can estimate or assign a percentage increase based on the patient's degree of activity or injury. Long[204] has suggested that patients be considered to have an RME that is a modification of the Harris-Benedict equation, in which the BEE is multiplied by an activity factor and an injury factor. A 20% to 30% increase is assigned for in-hospital activity, and up to a doubling of energy expenditure for severe injury:

$$\text{RME (men)} = [66 + (13.7 \times W) + (5 \times H) - (6.8 \times A)] \times \text{Activity factor} \times \text{Injury factor}$$

$$\text{RME (women)} = [665 + (9.6 \times W) + (1.8 \times H) - (4.7 \times A)] \times \text{Activity factor} \times \text{Injury factor}$$

The surgeon can estimate the degree of increase as a consequence of the injury or illness by examining the nitrogen excretion in a 24-hour urine collection (Figure 9-3). Nitrogen can be measured directly, using the Kjeldahl nitrogen method, or estimated by measuring the urine urea nitrogen (UUN) and adding a correction factor of 3 g to make up for the non–urea-containing nitrogen in the urine.

$$\text{Nitrogen balance} = (\text{Protein intake [g]} \div 6.25^{*}) - (\text{UUN} + 3)$$
$$^{*}\text{Nitrogen (g)} = \frac{\text{Protein (g)}}{6.25}$$

Patients who lose 8 g of nitrogen or less in a 24-hour period can be considered to have little stress; those who lose 15 g or more are under severe stress. The magnitude of stress can imply the degree to which the patient's energy expenditure is increased over resting BEE and allows selection of an appropriate injury factor in the Long modification of the Harris-Benedict equation. One difficulty with using the 24-hour nitrogen excretion assay is that it reflects total protein catabolism, arising from both dietary and endogenous sources of protein. This is not a concern if the patient is being given no protein and is receiving at least 100 g of carbohydrates per day when the nitrogen excretions are determined. Bistrian[41] has proposed the use of a catabolic index that divides total urea excretion into that resulting from dietary protein intake and obligatory urea excretion and that resulting from an increase in endogenous protein catabolism. The catabolic index (CI) can be calculated thus:

$$\text{CI} = \text{24-hour UUN} - (0.5\ \text{Dietary protein intake} + 3\ \text{g})$$

A result below zero indicates no significant stress; 0 to 5, moderate stress; and over 5, severe stress.[41]

Expected increases in energy expenditure can be summarized as follows: major elective surgery, 10% to 25%; fractures, 15% to 35%; sepsis, 50% to 60%; major burns, 100%. It must be remembered that there are major metabolic differences between fasting and postinjury states. A post-traumatic hypermetabolic patient has elevated glucose requirements and serum levels compared with the nonstressed person. Ketosis is not a metabolic feature of stress, as it is of starvation. Protein catabolism accelerates with injury or illness, compared with uncomplicated starvation, and the resting energy expenditure (REE) increases rather than decreases.

A patient's needs can be further specified as those that are strictly for maintenance (which covers resting metabolic activity and some limited physical activity). In a 24-hour period, adult patients require 30 kcal/kg and 0.7 g of protein per kilogram of lean body mass (LBM). With mild trauma or in a malnourished patient who is being repleted, energy requirements increase to 35 to 40 kcal/kg/24 hours, with protein requirements ranging up to 1.75 g/kg LMB/24 hours. In severely injured patients, energy requirements are in the range of 45 to 50 kcal/kg/24 hours, and protein requirements may be as high as 2 to 2.5 g/kg LBM/24 hours. It should be emphasized that there is a limit to the rate at which the body can use nutrients. More and more, complications of overfeeding are coming to light, and these can lead to disastrous complications from inappropriate and excessive nutritional support.

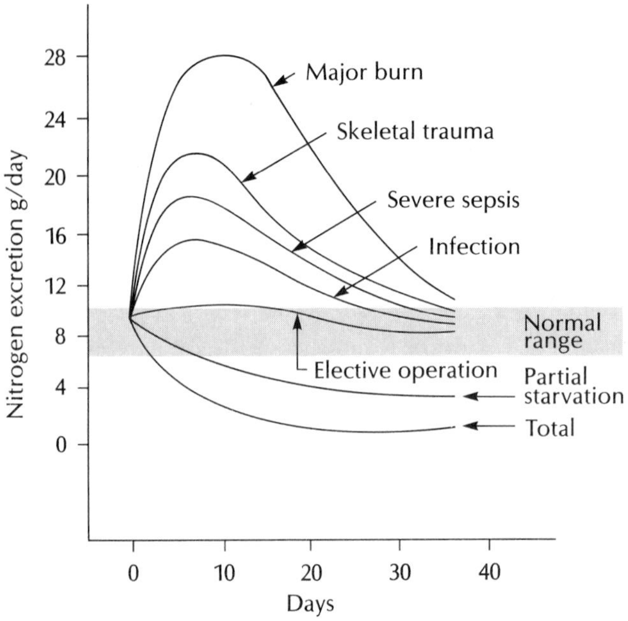

FIGURE 9-3 The effects of injury, illness, or starvation on nitrogen excretion. (From Long C: *JPEN* 3:452, American Society of Parenteral and Enteral Nutrition, 1979.)

PARENTERAL ALIMENTATION

Use of Parenteral Alimentation

Use of the intravenous route to deliver nutrients into the body can be traced to the seventeenth century. Soon after William Harvey discovered the circulation of blood in 1616, some began injecting a variety of substances intravenously into animals. Infusions of ale, urine, and opium were administered to dogs by Francesco Felli (1654) and Sir Christopher Wren (1656). Latta delivered salt solutions intravenously to patients stricken with cholera in 1831.[356] Others, in the nineteenth century, demonstrated that sugar solutions and even fresh cow's milk could be given intravenously.[334] With the concomitant developments in microbiology and advances in both chemistry and biochemistry, the importance of a more balanced solution increasingly became evident; however, crude protein preparations were associated with strong allergic reactions. It was the work of Henriques and Anderson, leading to the use of hydrolyzed casein, that provided a nonallergic source of protein, amino acids, and simple peptides.[158] Advances have continued in the use of protein substrates, including the use of refined mixtures of synthetic crystalline amino acid solutions to more precisely optimize the ratio of the various amino acid components.[254] With these developments the need arose to control the large volumes administered; a recurrent problem with more concentrated solutions in attempting to avoid the fluid overload was venous thrombosis, because these preparations were delivered primarily via the peripheral veins. Dudrick advanced intravenous alimentation by capitalizing on the work of the French surgeon Aubiniac, who had used a technique of percutaneous puncture to gain access to the subclavian vein. In 1966, working at the University of Pennsylvania, Dudrick demonstrated that energy and protein balance could be achieved by delivering concentrated solutions of glucose and amino acids via subclavian vein access. Using this technique, Dudrick was able to deliver highly concentrated solutions with a calorie/nitrogen ratio of 150 to 250:1 and totally support normal growth and development of young beagle puppies.[104] Shortly thereafter, he also reported total intravenous nutritional support in a child with essentially no functioning gastrointestinal tract.[105] Since these initial reports, there has been an explosion in the use and application of intravenous nutritional support; these uses now include treatment of patients with a variety of specific diseases, nutritional repletion of patients before surgery or therapy, and long-term nutritional support when the gastrointestinal tract is nonfunctional.

Although the development and application of intravenous nutritional support unquestionably represent significant advances, the question of what the optimum route is should always be asked, once it has been decided that the patient needs nutritional support. Selection of the route should be guided by the patient's needs and the status of the gastrointestinal tract. From the perspectives of cost, risk to the patient, efficacy of nutritional retention, and development of complications, the gastrointestinal tract is without doubt the preferred route. However, if the gastrointestinal tract is nonfunctional or the patient requires gastrointestinal rest, the intravenous route is the only alternative. The direct cost of the parenteral solutions alone easily may reach $500 a day (plus the indirect costs), but the alternatives—inadequate nutritional support and the development of complications leading to failure of the primary therapy and possibly death—make intravenous nutritional support the only reasonable alternative.

■ Parenteral Alimentation section contributed by Thomas P. Paxton and Richard L. Gamelli.

TABLE 9-6 RECOMMENDED DAILY ALLOWANCES OF WATER, ENERGY, AMINO ACIDS, AND MINERALS FOR PATIENTS ON COMPLETE INTRAVENOUS NUTRITION

	ALLOWANCE/KG BODY WEIGHT FOR ADULTS		
	BASAL AMOUNTS	MODERATE AMOUNTS	HIGH DOSE
Water	30 ml	50 ml	100-150 ml
Energy	30 kcal	35-40 kcal	50-60 kal
Amino acids	0.6 g	1.4-2 g	2.8-3.5g
Nitrogen	90 mg	0.2-0.3 g	0.4-0.5 g
Sodium	1-1.4 mEq	2.3 mEq	3-4 mEq
Potassium	0.7-0.9 mEq	2 mEq	3-4 mEq
Calcium	4.40 mg	6 mg	8 mg
Magnesium	0.96 mg	3.6-4.8 mg	7.2-9.6 mg
Chlorine	45.5-66.5 mg	70-105 mg	106-140 mg
Phosphorus	4.6 mg	12.4 mg	18.6-31 mg

Essential Nutrients

Water

It has been estimated that up to 45 individual nutrients are necessary for continuing health.[300] Water, macrominerals, amino acids, fats, a source of calories, vitamins, and trace metals are necessary parts of a balanced, intravenous nutritional diet (Table 9-6).

Water is second only to oxygen as the nutrient of which the body can least tolerate being deprived. Fluid is lost from the body each day in the form of measurable and insensible losses. The measurable losses comprise urinary output and losses from the gastrointestinal tract. There is a limit to which the kidney can concentrate the end products of metabolism for excretion, and water is necessary to carry the solute load from the body. Insensible losses occur primarily through the respiratory tract, with some small additional losses through the skin. Individual fluid requirements can be calculated with a variety of formulas. A standard approach is to give 100 ml/kg for the first 10 kg of body weight, 50 ml/kg for the next 10 kg, and 20 ml/kg for each additional kilogram. Calculation of fluid requirements may need to be modified based on the clinical situation, such as those involving extraordinary losses from the gastrointestinal tract or those in which the patient cannot tolerate "normal fluid loads" (such as cardiac, hepatic, or renal failure). In general, hypermetabolic states associated with increase in caloric need are similarly associated with an increase in fluid needs. A normal water/calorie ratio is about 1:1, although the ultimate fluid requirement must be balanced against the patient's needs or ability to tolerate a fluid load.

Macrominerals

Macrominerals, particularly sodium, potassium, and chloride, are next in order as elements of which the body cannot long be deprived. The maintenance requirements for sodium are in the range of 1 to 1.5 mEq/kg; those for potassium, 0.7 to 1 mEq/kg; and those for chloride, 1.5 to 2 mEq/kg. Alternatively, the need for macrominerals can be determined on the basis of the patient's calorie and nitrogen requirement, assuming that if the patient is to become anabolic, there is a proportional need for these macrominerals. Using this approach, for each gram of nitrogen infused, 6 mEq each of sodium and chloride, 4 mEq of potassium and, initially, as much as 4 mmoles of phosphorus would be provided. The individual needs for macrominerals must be balanced against the patient's metabolic status, as well as greater than normal losses.

Also, when patients are rapidly becoming anabolic, phosphorus and potassium may be required in larger amounts than originally calculated. Administration of large glucose loads, with the stimulation of endogenous insulin (or with exogenous insulin), is a potent stimulus for the movement of potassium and phosphorus intracellularly. Therefore both of these elements should be titrated to the patient's daily needs based on laboratory results.

The chloride load should be maintained in a ratio of 1:1 with sodium as a starting point; however, chloride may need to be increased, particularly with large gastric losses. This can be done by adding the sodium or potassium salt of chloride or, alternatively, as 0.1 N-hydrochloric acid.

Calcium requirements during parenteral alimentation are in the range of 0.2 to 0.3 mEq/kg/day. Because calcium is not a major intracellular ion, daily needs are not particularly affected by the patient's anabolic or catabolic state.

Intravenous magnesium requirements in most patients range from 0.35 to 0.45 mEq/kg/day. However, because magnesium losses can be excessive, especially with large gastrointestinal losses, the actual daily requirements should be based on serum values.

TABLE 9-7 CARBOHYDRATE CALORIES AND OSMOLARITY

CONCENTRATION	CALORIES/L OF DEXTROSE	OSMOLARITY (mOsm/kg H_2O)
5%	170	278
10%	340	523
20%	680	1250
25%	850	1900
50%	1700	3800

Carbohydrates

Glucose continues to be the most widely used source of carbohydrates and a primary source of energy in parenteral alimentation. The six-carbon skeleton of glucose can undergo oxidation within the Embden-Meyerhof pathway to pyruvate or lactate and then subsequently enter the citric acid cycle, which is the final common pathway for the oxidation of not only carbohydrates but also fats and proteins, leading to the formation of carbon dioxide and water. As an alternative to the glycolytic pathway of the Embden-Meyerhof scheme, glucose can be oxidized by the hexose monophosphate shunt that occurs primarily in the liver, lactating mammary gland, and adipose tissues. Although other carbohydrate sources (e.g., fructose, xylitol, and sorbitol) have been successfully used in clinical studies, it appears that these ultimately are converted to glucose, an energy-requiring process, and each may be associated with specific contraindications, such as increased production of lactate from fructose and hepatotoxicity secondary to xylitol. Also, blood and urinary glucose levels are quite easily determined, which is not the case for the other carbohydrate sources.

Glucose is available in highly concentrated solutions and is an extremely cost-effective form of calories. A 5% concentration of glucose, which is isotonic, provides only 170 kcal/L; however, a 25% solution, which has an osmolarity of 1900, supplies 850 kcal/L (Table 9-7). The conversion factor for glucose to energy, supplied as monohydrate glucose, is 3.4 kcal/g. The higher concentrations of glucose, which have the advantage of an increased calorie/volume density, also have an attendant increase in osmolarity; this means that they must be delivered in a rapid high-flow environment, which is achieved by using the central venous route. Adjusting the total daily glucose load (not the percentage concentration of the glucose infusion) is critical to preventing complications secondary to carbohydrate excess.

In examining glucose metabolism in humans and the response of intravenous glucose infusion, Wolfe and associates[363] demonstrated that although glucose infusions can suppress endogenous glucose production, the effectiveness of this suppression and the extent to which the body can directly oxidize the glucose load are limited. Follow-up studies by these investigators and others have produced the practical recommendation that to prevent complications, the total carbohydrate load in adults should not exceed 100 g/10 kg LBM in a 24-hour period. In patients who are glucose intolerant, this limit may be further reduced to prevent the complications of hyperglycemia and glycosuria.

Protein

Although supplying 100 g of carbohydrates daily can dramatically decrease protein loss from the body, it cannot achieve nitrogen balance or make the patient anabolic. The body has an obligate need for a series of amino acids that cannot be endogenously synthesized. Rose and associates[275,276] defined the essential amino acids as phenylalanine, methionine, lysine, threonine, tryptophan, valine, leucine, and isoleucine. Furthermore, the amino acids arginine and histidine may not be synthesized in sufficient quantities in infants or patients with renal failure.[38] The L-isomer of amino acids, both essential and nonessential, is the isomer that the body can successfully use and is the composition of commercial crystalline amino acid solutions.

Intravenously supplied protein can serve as an energy source and as a source of amino acids for protein synthesis. Thus the amount of protein that must be infused daily must be related to the patient's total calorie requirement and to other sources of protein being supplied. Patients can be placed into zero nitrogen balance with high protein loads in which the administered protein serves as a source of amino acids and three carbon fragments for energy needs. However, if calories in the form of carbohydrates are supplied and the patient is not hypermetabolic, as little as 0.5 g/kg body weight of crystalline amino acids may achieve nitrogen equilibrium.[18] In general, protein requirements can be related to the total calorie requirements with continuous intravenous feedings in a ratio of 100 to 250 : 1.[235,284,365] However, with renal or liver failure, much larger calorie/nitrogen ratios will produce the best net protein use.[159]

Achieving nitrogen retention is not the only desirable goal with delivery of protein substrates. Although the patient may be in a more "positive" nitrogen balance when the blood urea nitrogen (BUN) level increases gradually, this change does not equal improved health. If the patient receives inadequate amounts of energy to fuel the body's biosynthetic needs, catabolism proceeds unchanged and the body uses the administered protein as an energy source and continues the autocatabolism of its own protein stores. The mixture of fuels supplied can influence the site of the administered protein's incorporation. Using a carbohydrate-only energy source leads to a more prominent incorporation of administered protein into muscle protein under the influence of insulin, whereas using a mixed fuel source, such as fat and carbohydrates, leads to distribution in both the periphery and viscera, particularly the liver.[112] Similarly, the distribution of the individual amino acids can affect the use of proteins. Obviously, if the amount of essential amino acids is insufficient, regardless of the total protein load, nitrogen cannot be sufficiently used. In certain disease states, such as trauma, sepsis, and liver failure, administering specially formulated amino acid mixtures that are particularly high in the branched-chain amino acids, valine, leucine, and isoleucine may have unique properties for retention and use of supplied protein (Table 9-8).

TABLE 9-8 GUIDELINES FOR PROTEIN ADMINISTRATION

CONDITION	PROTEIN (g/kg/day)*
Renal failure, not on dialysis	0.8
Renal failure, on dialysis	1
Renal failure, on peritoneal dialysis	1.2
Malnourished, not metabolically stressed	1-1.2
Postoperative, no organ failure	1.2-1.5
Severely catabolic, no renal or organ failure	1.5-2

*Based on current dry weight unless patient is >140% of desirable weight, in which case the mean of actual and desirable weights is used.

Adapted from Heizer WD, Holcombe B: Approach to the patient requiring nutritional supplementation. In Yamada T, editor: *Textbook of gastroenterology*, Philadelphia, 1991, JB Lippincott.

Fats

Linoleic acid and its biologic derivative, arachidonic acid, are the essential fatty acids that contribute to the body's function both structurally and physiologically. They make up cell membranes and subcellular units and are important in the biosynthesis of prostaglandins.[112,156] Although they can be supplied orally in the form of unsaturated fats (e.g., safflower or corn oil), they must be supplied intravenously as fat emulsions when the gastrointestinal tract is not available. Essential fatty acid deficiencies can be prevented if 4% of the total calories administered per week are given as fats.

Using fats for more than supplying an essential nutrient or as a major calorie source is not universally accepted. As an energy source, fat may be advantageous for at least two reasons: (1) fat is a normal part of the average diet, and may have as yet undiscovered beneficial effects in the diet; and (2) intravenous calories as fats, which can be delivered at up to 2 calories/ml, are not significantly hypertonic and, as noted above, may have a positive effect on the distribution and use of supplied proteins. The argument against the use of fats centers on whether fats can be used effectively as an energy source, particularly in hypercatabolic states. Jeejeebhoy and associates[173] and Bivins[42] have suggested that fats can be a suitable source of nonprotein calories and spare nitrogen, but others, such as Long,[206,320] have not found fats to be as beneficial as glucose in supplying calories during stress. Also, in most institutions fats are a more costly source of calories, which may exceed by a factor of 10 the cost of glucose calories.

Fats must be supplied to prevent the development of essential fatty acid deficiency. If fat-free intravenous nutritional support is given to patients who are receiving no alternate source of essential fatty acids, chemical evidence of deficiency may be present as early as 1 week after therapy is begun.[138,352] Clinically obvious manifestations of essential fatty acid deficiency may appear by 3 to 4 weeks. These manifestations include dry, scaly dermatitis, hair loss, delayed wound healing, changes in red cell membrane characteristics, and potential deficits in prostaglandin synthesis. Administering 500 ml of a 10% intravenous fat emulsion twice weekly, or 25 to 50 ml/day of any unsaturated fat via the gastrointestinal tract, will prevent deficiency.

If fats are used as a primary energy source, such as in the "lipid systems," in which up to 50% of the total calories may be supplied as fats, fat overload syndrome must be prevented. The general recommendation is that no more than 2 g/kg LMB be given as fat in adults and possibly as much as 4 g/kg in children. Use of the 20% formulations in neonates has raised some concern because of the particle size of the fat emulsion. It may be more difficult for neonates to clear lipid from the circulation, and thus it becomes sequestered in the lung, liver, and spleen.

Vitamins

Minute amounts of vitamins are essential to maintain normal nutritional health, but because the body cannot synthesize them, they must be provided from an exogenous source. The most recent statement as to which vitamins are essential for humans included the four fat-soluble vitamins—A (retinol), D (ergocalciferol), E (alpha-tocopherol), and K (phytylmenaquinone)—and the nine water-soluble vitamins—ascorbic acid (vitamin C), thiamine (B_1), riboflavin (B_2), niacin, pyridoxine (B_6), pantothenic acid, folic acid, cyanocobalamin (B_{12}), and biotin. The need for various vitamins in states of altered metabolism is poorly understood. Most workers in the field tend to give relatively large quantities of the nontoxic B and C vitamins with disease and injury and only limited quantities of the fat-soluble vitamins, which may be associated with complications if given in excess. The essential vitamins may safely be added to the daily parenteral nutrition mixture. This has been our standard practice, and it has not been associated with the development of complications.

The amounts of the individual vitamins present in the various commercial solutions are based on the Recommended Dietary Allowance (RDA) of the National Academy of Sciences–National Research Council (NAS-NRC).[168] However, use of the vitamin and the rate of excretion may differ with the route of administration, and the RDA for some vitamins is based on inefficiencies of absorption (e.g., vitamin A). Also, the RDA may need to be exceeded to meet the patient's clinical requirements. The recommended formulations for dosages of the daily maintenance vitamins for patients receiving parenteral nutrition are shown in Table 9-9. If the patient has specific vitamin deficiencies, supplemental single vitamins may need to be administered.

Trace Minerals

Trace minerals, another class of nutrients, must be provided when the patient is fed intravenously, particularly with long-term intravenous nutritional support. Table 9-10 lists the trace minerals currently recognized as essential in mammals. The patient's underlying disease states may deplete the body's stores of trace minerals. In addition to the individual component deficits, the ratio of trace minerals, such as zinc to copper, may also be important.

Deficits of zinc, a component of more than 120 enzyme systems, are associated with poor wound healing, dermatitis, alopecia, and disturbances in taste.[341] Studies in animals by Fernandes and associates[116] have shown that zinc deficiency leads to loss of immune competence and defective T-cell function. Because significant quantities of zinc are present in intestinal secretions (12.2 mg/L of small bowel fluid and 17.1 mg/kg of stool or ileostomy output),[146] patients with high-output intestinal fistulae are at increased risk for the development of zinc deficiency.

Although in a healthy person the body stores of iron are large enough to replace one third of the iron contained in the red cells of a nonanemic person, with repetitive blood loss, iron deficiency may develop. In addition to the clinical manifestation of anemia, the patient may have glossitis, a burning sensation of the tongue, headaches, and paresthesia. Worldwide, iron deficiency is one of the commonest nutrient abnormalities. Measuring the serum ferritin level provides a sensitive and early index of iron depletion. Changes in red cell mass may indicate iron depletion; however, a patient receiving parenteral nutrition may have reduced hemoglobin and red cell volume for other notable reasons. Although an obligate loss of iron from the body occurs each day (via skin, gastrointestinal tract, and genitourinary tract),[142] no mechanism exists to excrete excessive amounts of

TABLE 9-9 RECOMMENDED DAILY ALLOWANCES OF VITAMINS FOR PATIENTS ON COMPLETE INTRAVENOUS NUTRITION

VITAMIN	CHILDREN UNDER AGE 11	ADULTS	FUNCTION	SIGNS OF DEFICIENCY
Fat Soluble				
A	2300 IU	3300 IV	Normal vision; mucopolysaccharide snythesis; protease release; entry of macrophages and leukocytes into an acute wound; immune stimulation and mucosal integrity	Dermatitis; night blindness; keratomalacia; xerophthalmia
D	400 IU	200 IV	Calcium and phosphorus homeostasis	Rickets; osteomalacia
E	7 IU	10 IV	Antioxidant	Hemolysis
K	0.2 mg	2μg	Clotting factors II, VII, IX, and X	Bleeding
Water Soluble				
Niacin	17 mg	40 mg	Component of the coenzymes NAD and NADP, which play a role in oxidation-reduction reactions and in the oxidative catabolism of carbohydrates, proteins, and lipids; biosynthesis of fatty acids	Pellagra; dermatitis; dementia; glossitis; diarrhea; loss of memory; headaches
Folate	140 μg	400 μg	Transfer of single carbon units; deoxyribonucleic acid (DNA) synthesis	Megaloblastic anemia; diarrhea; glossitis
B_{12}	1 μg	5 μg	Maintains normal folate metabolism; coenzyme in reactions involving isomerizations and reductions; participates in metabolism of fat, carbohydrate, protein, and myelin synthesis	Pernicious anemia; glossitis; spinal cord degeneration; peripheral neuropathy
Thiamine	1.2 mg	3 mg	Carbohydrate metabolism coenzyme in oxidative decarboxylation failure; Wernicke-Korsakoff syndrome	Paresthesia; nystagmus; impaired memory; congestive heart syndrome
Riboflavin (B_2)	1.4 mg	3.6 mg	Electron transport as flavin nucleotides	Mucositis; dermatitis; cheilosis; vascularization of cornea; photophobia; lacrimation and decreased vision; impaired wound healing
Pyridoxine (B_6)	1 mg	4 mg	Coenzyme in transformations of amino acids	Dermatitis; neuritis; convulsions
Pantothenic acid	5 mg	15 mg	Precursor of coenzyme A (Krebs cycle)	Fatigue; malaise; headache; insomnia; vomiting; abdominal cramps
Biotin	20 μg	60 μg	Coenzyme for carboxylation reactions	As with other B vitamins (normally synthesized and absorbed from gut)

this metal, and the potential exists for progressive iron accumulation and organ damage[136] if iron is inappropriately administered.

Copper is a critical trace mineral in patients who receive long-term parenteral alimentation. Neutropenia and a microcytic, hypochromic anemia have occurred in patients who received copper-free solutions.[317] Copper plays an important role in iron absorption and transport because it is a component of ceruloplasmin. The anemia of copper deficiency is secondary to deranged iron transport and can occur despite abundant iron stores.

Chromium deficiencies are associated with the development of an insulin-insensitive diabetic state in association with a peripheral neuropathy.[174] As with zinc and copper, significant chromium losses may occur with increased intestinal losses.

Deficits in selenium have been related to a clinical syndrome of congestive cardiomyopathy. Selenium is a component of mammalian glutathione peroxidase, an enzyme that destroys peroxidases.[279] Other nonspecific complaints such as myalgia, muscle tenderness, and changes in pancreatic function have been ascribed to deficiencies of selenium.[215]

TABLE 9-10 DAILY REQUIREMENTS OF TRACE MINERALS CURRENTLY RECOGNIZED AS HAVING DEFICIENCY STATES

MINERAL	FUNCTION	SYMPTOMS OF DEFICIENCY	CHILDREN
Zinc	Essential for the function of many enzymes and a component of lipid, protein, carbohydrate, and nucleic acid metabolism; cell replication and connective tissue synthesis	Dermatitis; impaired wound healing; depressed cell-mediated immunity; taste acuity and dark adaptation; sexual retardation; alopecia; depressed visceral protein status	100 μg/kg
Copper	Metalloenzyme biochemical processes; component of ceruloplasmin; connective tissue metabolism; cell replication; connective tissue synthesis	Anemia; leukopenia; neutropenia; depigmentation of skin	20 μg/kg
Chromium	Glucose tolerance; possible role in maintenance of normal serum lipid levels	Elevated serum lipid levels; insulin-resistant glucose intolerance	.14-0.2 mg/kg
Selenium*	Component of glutathione peroxidase (antioxidant)	Cardiomyopathy; myalgia; muscle tenderness; pancreatic degeneration	3 μ/kg
Molybdenum	Component of enzyme systems involved in oxidation-reduction	Headache; night blindness; irritability; lethargy; coma	—
Manganese	Oxidation phosphorylation; fatty acid metabolism; protein and mucopolysaccharide synthesis	Growth retardation; bony abnormalities; central nervous system dysfunction	2-10 μg/kg
Iron	Constituent of hemoglobin, myoglobin, and cytochrome enzymes	Microcytic hypochromic anemia; decreased serum iron; fatigue; faulty digestion	112 μg/kg
Iodine	Thyroid hormone formation	Symptoms of hypothyroidism goiter	5.08 μg/kg

*Selenium approximately 50% excreted via gastrointestinal tract, with reduced fecal loss 25 to 30 μg/day may be appropriate to maintain individual safe levels to avoid toxicity.

†Current data suggest potential for increased losses of both selenium and manganese via the gastrointestinal tract.

The trace mineral molybdenum is a component of enzyme systems involved in oxidation-reduction reactions involving organic sulfur and degradation of nucleic acids. Molybdenum deficiencies have been thought to cause a syndrome of nonspecific complaints of headache, night blindness, irritability, lethargy, and coma.[5]

Manganese is a component of a variety of metal enzymes that activate a large number of enzyme systems, particularly those involved with polysaccharide synthesis. Manganese has been established as an essential trace nutrient based primarily on animal experimentation. Manganese acts as a cofactor for pyruvate carboxylases and mitochondrial superoxide dismutase.[301,350] Most of the described syndromes in animals have consisted of impaired reproduction, skeletal abnormalities, and ataxia,[200] and in certain species, defects in carbohydrate and lipid metabolism.[17,33,111] There has been a single case report of a human deficiency of manganese.[101]

The only known function of iodine in the body is in thyroid hormone production. Approximately 25% of the total body iodine is contained within the thyroid gland. Symptoms of iodine deficiency are those primarily associated with abnormalities of thyroid function. Deficiencies to date in humans have not been described for vanadium, nickel, arsenic, silicon, or fluoride; currently, the possible importance of these elements in human health and nutrition is based primarily on experimental studies in animals.

Route of Intravenous Alimentation

After the surgeon decides that a patient requires intravenous nutritional support, he should ask himself the following questions: (1) Is the patient to be totally supported by the intravenous route? (2) How long will the intravenous therapy be needed? (3) What are the patient's needs (i.e., is the patient hypercatabolic)? and (4) What are the available sites of vascular access?

If the patient can maintain some element of gastrointestinal function, supplemental nutritional support can be given by the intravenous route. The surgeon calculates the patient's total requirements, determines what percentage is being met by the enteral route, and designs a formulation that, in all likelihood, will not be hypertonic and can be given peripherally. This approach can supply an additional 800 to 1200 calories and up to 15 g of nitrogen per day parenterally. However, caution must be exercised with this approach, because frequently patients do not meet the enteral goal on a consistent daily basis, and the hypocaloric supplement intravenous nutrition becomes the primary nutritional support. Elec-

ADULTS		
STABLE	ACUTE CATABOLIC STATE	STABLE WITH INTESTINAL LOSS
2.5-4 mg	Additional 2 mg	Add 12.2 mg/L small bowel fluid lost; 17.1 mg/L of stool or ileostomy output
0.5-1.5 mg	—	—
10-15 μg	—	20μg
40-60 μg	Decreased with renal failure	†
20-120 μg		
0.15-0.8 mg		†
14μg/kg	56 μg/kg	56 μg/kg
1.9 μg/kg		

trolyte imbalances often are corrected by adding higher than maintenance amounts of potassium and sodium, which makes the mixture hypertonic and irritating to the peripheral veins. The peripheral route may be of use in patients who might be able to support their nutritional needs effectively within 5 to 7 days. In this situation, 2.5 L/day of a mixed carbohydate and fat source can be provided with appropriate additional nutrients to achieve 1600 kcal/day and up to 100 g of crystalline amino acids.

It is true that the intravenous fat emulsions are isotonic, and if delivered in conjunction with the glucose-protein solution through a Y connector can decrease the tonicity of the carbohydrate–amino acid–electrolyte mixtures; however, in time most patients experience significant venous irritation and require rotation of the IV site or eventual placement of a central venous catheter. Currently, in the United States, mixing the carbohydrate, amino acid, and electrolyte solutions with the fat emulsions directly in a single container is not recommended because of the possibility of destabilizing the lipid emulsion. However, work from Sweden has suggested that it may be possible to have a single-solution system for delivering total intravenous nutritional support.[170]

A relative indication for the peripheral route is lack of expertise in gaining access to the central venous pool or lack of experience in caring for a central venous alimentation catheter. However, in such situations the patient would be better cared for by individuals experienced in maintaining optimum nutritional support.

Central parenteral nutritional support with hypertonic solutions is indicated when therapy is expected to exceed 7 days, when energy requirements exceed basal levels, when the need exists to make the patient anabolic by the intravenous route and, as a relative indication, when peripheral veins are poor.

Following are patient examples of the use of intravenous nutritional support.

Complications of Parenteral Alimentation

Mechanical Complications

Most mechanical complications of parenteral alimentation are related to catheterization of the subclavian vein (see the box on p. 314). The overall complication rate for catheter insertions from various reports has been given as 4.2% to 15.2%, with the incidence of major complications ranging from 2.4% to 3.7%.[59] The more common technical complications that occur with central venous catheterization are discussed below.

PNEUMOTHORAX. Pneumothoraces, which occur at the time of subclavian vein catheterization, generally are small and do not progress. However, progressive enlargement of a pneumothorax does occur in some cases. If the parietal pleura is penetrated when the needle is inserted for vein puncture, the patient may complain of sharp chest pain and even cough as a result of pleural irritation. The procedure should be stopped immediately to avoid puncturing the lung. The chosen landmarks must be reassessed carefully before any additional attempts at subclavian vein puncture.

Catheterization should be abandoned if the patient notes progressive pain or dyspnea, in which case the patient should be evaluated for a pneumothorax. A common problem is a small pneumothorax in a patient who is to undergo general endotracheal anesthesia with positive pressure ventilation. Because of the potential for rapid expansion of the pneumothorax, a "prophylactic" chest tube should be inserted.

AIR EMBOLUS. An air embolus may occur when the syringe is removed from the needle at vein puncture, when the intravenous tubing is changed, if the tubing is inadvertently disconnected from the catheter, or if a tract through the subcutaneous tissue persists after the catheter is removed. Most subclavian vein punctures are carried out with relatively large-bore needles, and as Flanagan and colleagues[118] have demonstrated, up to 100 ml of air per second can pass through a 14-gauge needle. Although the catheters inserted are somewhat smaller and longer than the insertion needle, a significant amount of air can still enter the central veins through an "open" catheter, particularly if the patient is carrying out maximum inspirations. Small amounts of aspirated air usually are asymptomatic; however, larger amounts

COMPLICATIONS OF CENTRAL VENOUS CATHETERIZATION

Pneumothorax	Arterial puncture
Air embolism	Hemothorax
Improper catheter location	Hydrothorax
Venous thrombosis	Catheter embolus
Failure to cannulate	Brachial plexus injury
Bent or occluded catheter	Skin bleeding/local hematoma
Thoracic duct injury	Subcutaneous emphysema
Hemomediastinum	

may cause the patient to become dyspneic, which can progress to cyanosis and altered mental status. The patient may become tachycardic and develop a marked rise in central venous pressure associated with a drop in systemic blood pressure as the heart becomes filled with air on the right side, which blocks blood flow. On physical examination the patient may have a loud crunching murmur over the precordium.

Emergency treatment consists of placing the patient in a left lateral decubitus position with the head down. If the catheter is still in place, a large syringe can be used to attempt aspiration of the air. Additional techniques include emergency thoracotomy with needle aspiration of the right ventricle followed by direct cardiac massage.[106]

CATHETER EMBOLUS. Relatively minimal efforts at catheter withdrawal through an insertion needle can lead to shearing off, with subsequent embolization of the central venous catheter. Because catheter embolization can serve as a nidus for infection, thrombosis, and induction of cardiac arrhythmias, it usually requires removal. The safest policy is never to withdraw the catheter without withdrawing the needle and catheter as a unit. Inserting or changing a catheter over a guide wire without an insertion needle poses little risk of catheter embolization and is the preferred technique for manipulating subclavian catheters.

ARTERIAL PUNCTURE. Arterial puncture of the subclavian artery during infraclavicular catheterization, or of the carotid artery with internal jugular approaches to central veins, results in few complications if the needle is removed immediately and direct pressure is applied. The patient should be observed frequently for ongoing bleeding; if necessary, chest radiographs should be obtained to evaluate any mediastinal bleeding. The potential for disastrous complications from arterial puncture is increased in a patient with disordered coagulation. Similarly, a significant hemothorax can occur if the lung has been inadvertently lacerated. Occasionally patients have significant bleeding from small skin arterials that require direct pressure for a prolonged period or suture of the skin insertion site.

IMPROPER LOCATION OF THE CATHETER. The proper location of the subclavian catheter for parenteral feedings is in the superior vena cava. Catheters often find their way into the internal jugular vein or the opposite subclavian vein, or they are inserted too deeply into the right atrium or ventricle. None of these sites should be considered adequate for long-term intravenous feeding, because they increase the incidence of complications, including phlebitis, thrombosis, arrhythmias, and perforation of the cardiac chamber. A chest radiograph obtained immediately after placement of any catheter should be examined closely, not only for complications secondary to the puncture of the subclavian vein but also for the catheter's position; when the catheter is in one of the previously mentioned locations, it is fairly easy to determine the problem and either manipulate or reinsert the catheter. However, the clinician must be ever observant for the possibility of a seemingly "good catheter position" that in fact is extravascular. The chest radiograph may show a relatively normal course, with a catheter curving along the inner aspect of the thoracic mediastinal pleura or one that is within the mediastinum. Infusion of hypertonic solutions in this situation quickly leads to a compromising hydrothorax or hydromediastinum as the hypertonic fluid results in further fluid accumulation. Catheters that have been in place may infrequently penetrate the superior vena cava. The intravascular location of a catheter can be checked by looking for blood flashback when the fluid administration set is lowered below the level of the right atrium or when blood can be aspirated from the catheter with a syringe.

VENOUS THROMBOSIS. Thrombosis of the subclavian vein or even the superior vena cava after subclavian vein catheterization has been thought to be relatively infrequent. However, an increased incidence of subclavian thrombosis and total venous occlusion of the subclavian vein has been recognized.[81] Any patient with a subclavian venous catheter who develops unilateral edema of the arm, neck, or face should be suspected of having subclavian vein thrombosis. Superior vena caval thrombosis may manifest with bilateral facial, arm, and neck edema. Such patients should have the catheter removed immediately and should be given heparin therapy. Septic thrombophlebitis of the subclavian vein or superior vena cava is a difficult problem. A variety of approaches have been recommended, including long-term intravenous antibiotics, anticoagulants, and venous thrombectomy.

ADDITIONAL MECHANICAL COMPLICATIONS. Additional mechanical complications of central venous catheterization include failure to cannulate the subclavian vein on either the right or left side by percutaneous technique, which occurs in approximately 1% of cases. The catheter may bend or become occluded as it exits through the subcutaneous tunnel or dives deep to the clavicle, which is a more common complication in obese or muscular patients. Injury to the thoracic duct with left-sided supraclavicular approaches to the subclavian vein has been recognized and makes this approach more hazardous.

Metabolic Complications

Metabolic complications of intravenous nutritional support mainly are related to inadequate replacement of essential nutrients or infusion of nutrients in excess of the body's ability to use them. There is no accurate data on the frequency of such occurrences, but clearly failure to recognize the broad range of essential nutrients or to tailor nutritional support to the individual patient can lead to an increased incidence of problems.

CARBOHYDRATES

Glucose intolerance. Complications related to infusion of a carbohydrate load are glucose intolerance and the metabolic fate of glucose. Although a normal adult's tolerance for glucose can be increased from 400 to 500 g to as much as 1500 g/day without evidence of glucose intolerance, this may not be true for critically ill patients. In patients receiving hypertonic dextrose infusions, it is common to see an initial mild glucose intolerance that usually is corrected by augmented release of endogenous insulin. Insulin secretion can increase four to six times over basal rates and establish a new steady state that is proportional to the infused glucose load, which results in a return to more normal levels of serum glucose. Subsequently, serum insulin will fall, possibly because peripheral tissues adapt for glucose uptake.

Patients who are severely stressed, significantly malnourished, very young or very old, or insulin-dependent diabetics may not adapt to the increased glucose load. In addition to becoming significantly hyperglycemic, these patients will exceed their renal threshold for glucose resorption and have persistent glycosuria. High concentrations of glucose in the urine will serve as an osmotic diuretic and cause an inappropriate loss of free water from the body. If this situation is not corrected, the patient will develop a hyperosmolar, nonketotic acidosis, with serum glucose levels of 700 to 800 mg/dl or higher, dehydration, excessive urinary output, and massive glycosuria. The patient initially may complain of headache, which is followed by convulsions associated with confusion and stupor, rapidly progressing to coma. Failure to recognize this syndrome and correct it frequently is fatal. The condition can be reversed by reexpanding the patient's volume, normalizing serum glucose over an 18- to 24-hour period, and reversing the systemic acidosis by administering bicarbonate. The serum glucose level should not be reversed rapidly, because blood and CNS glucose levels equilibrate slowly. Cerebral edema may result, with a precipitous drop in the serum glucose level. Concomitant with administration of insulin, serum potassium must be measured and potassium appropriately replaced to prevent hypokalemia.

New onset of glycosuria measuring above 2+ on urine dipstick testing should be followed by a blood glucose determination. If a normally euglycemic patient is found to be hyperglycemic, particularly if the serum glucose exceeds 200 mg/dl, evaluation and therapy should be started. One of the commonest causes of new-onset glucose intolerance in a previously stable patient is a sudden increase in the infusion rate. This may occur as a consequence of inappropriate adjustment of the infusion apparatus or of an increased rate of infusion. If a patient's infusion rate is behind, no attempt should be made to "catch up" the infusion rate. In patients who have been receiving insulin, failure to administer the insulin will lead to glucose intolerance and must be corrected. Many medications (e.g., glucocorticoids, diuretics, phenothiazines, phenytoins) affect glucose tolerance.* If no precipitating events can be found, the patient should be carefully evaluated for an incipient septic episode, even if no other signs of developing sepsis are present. Recent onset of glucose intolerance may precede the more routine clinical findings of a septic episode by up to 12 hours. Finally, if none of the above appear to be germane, the hyperglycemia may be a consequence of nutrient interaction. A potassium deficiency can result in glucose intolerance and glycosuria.[128,134,137,263] Occasionally patients who have been receiving insulin will manifest insulin resistance, a consequence of antibody formation to insulin; this can be rectified by switching to human recombinant insulin. Insulin resistance may occur secondary to a chromium deficiency, particularly in chronically alimented patients or in those with extraordinary gastrointestinal losses.

Carbohydrates in excess of energy use. Another aspect of glucose tolerance is the influence of the carbohydrate load on fuel use. Delivery of carbohydrates in excess of energy expenditure in normal and depleted patients is associated with a rise in the nonprotein respiratory quotient (RQ) to 1 or higher. Patients who have underlying respiratory compromise and are receiv-

*References 81, 177, 255, 281, 306, 335, and 337.

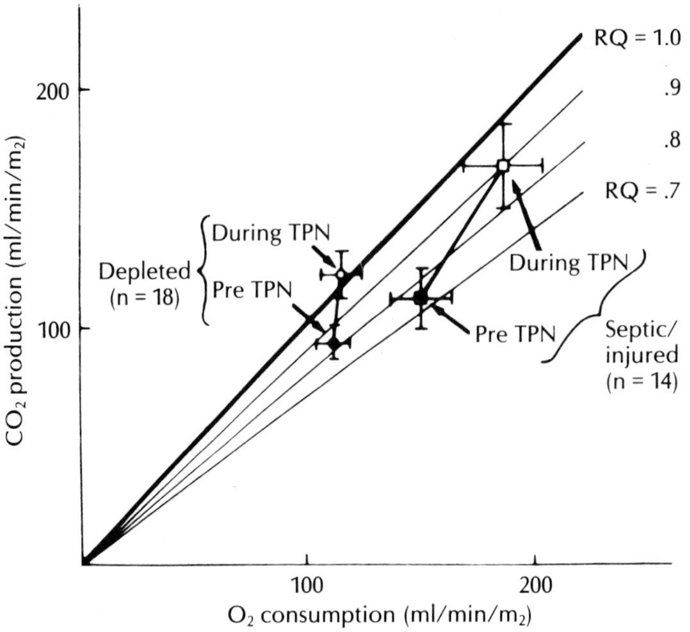

FIGURE 9-4 Changes in gas exchange that occur secondary to total parental nutrition (TPN). Clearly, two different responses are seen: depleted patients show a respiratory quotient (RQ) greater than 1 with a small increase in the volume of oxygen consumed (Vo_2), whereas hypermetabolic patients have an RQ less than 1 with a marked increase in Vo_2. Both groups showed a large increase in the production of carbon dioxide. (From Askanazi J et al: *Ann Surg* 191(1):42, 1980.)

ing high rates of glucose infusion (more than 100 g/10kg LMB/24 hours) could develop progressive problems with carbon dioxide (CO_2) retention. A rise in the RQ above 1 indicates net fat synthesis with no net fat oxidation. In a septic and depleted patient receiving carbohydrate infusions, glucose intake in excess of energy expenditure has been associated with an increase in the nonprotein RQ (which remained below 1), increased urinary catecholamine excretion, and further increase in energy expenditure.[23] In both depleted and stressed patients, the surgeon must consider this aspect of carbohydrate tolerance and avoid providing calories in excess of twice the estimated or calculated energy expenditure (Figure 9-4).

Hypoglycemia. Hypoglycemia may occur in patients receiving intravenous nutritional support if the infusion is suddenly interrupted. Hypoglycemia obviously would be more of a concern in patients who had been receiving subcutaneous insulin—which points out the advantage of administering insulin with the alimentation fluid so that a matched infusion of glucose and insulin is given. Nevertheless, even with a combined infusion, associated high production of endogenous insulin can lead to a precipitous fall in serum glucose if the infusion is stopped. Theoretically, the half-life of circulating insulin is relatively short. However, there have been several reports of hypoglycemia developing when glucose infusions were tapered rapidly; this may occur through a mechanism other than insulin-mediated glucose uptake. Medication errors, with inappropriate insulin dosages, must also be considered. When intravenous hypertonic glucose infusions are being tapered, hypoglycemia with termination of infusions can be avoided by tapering the infusion over several days, decreasing the infusion load by 600 to 1000 kcal/day as the patient progressively returns to enteral intake. When the patient is taking 1000 to 1500 kcal/day by mouth, the infusion can be further tapered by administering 5% to 10% glucose for an additional 10 to 12 hours after the hypertonic dextrose infusion is terminated. This tapering allows further adaptation and results in a low incidence of problems.

POTASSIUM. The body's need for potassium increases with the administration of glucose, which stimulates increased release of endogenous insulin. Problems with potassium can be further compounded by excessive renal or gastrointestinal losses. Signs of potassium deficiency can develop rapidly and are related to failure of normal contractility of skeletal, cardiac, and smooth muscle. Patients show progressive muscle weakness, decreased to no deep tendon reflexes, and paralytic ileus. Hypokalemic patients have a markedly increased cardiac sensitivity to digitalis compounds and a greater likelihood of arrhythmias. Electrocardiographic signs of low voltage, flattening of the T waves, and depression of ST segments are characteristic findings with hypokalemia. Patients receiving parenteral alimentation may require larger amounts than anticipated of supplemental potassium to restore depleted body stores and to meet the requirements for new tissue synthesis.

PHOSPHORUS. Similar to potassium, phosphorus is stimulated to move intracellularly in the presence of glucose and insulin. Also, new tissue synthesis increases the body's requirements for phosphorus. Patients receiving phosphate-free hyperalimentation fluid quickly can become hypophosphatemic and show laboratory and clinical evidence of hypophosphatemia within the first day of therapy. Clinical symptoms usually are present with phosphorus levels below 1 mg/dl. Patients demonstrate progressive weakness, tremors, and decreased deep tendon reflexes, and complain of pain, particularly over the long bones. If undetected and allowed to progress, hypophosphatemia can lead to altered mental status, generalized seizures, and respiratory failure.[240] Hypophosphatemia is associated with depressed myocardial performance[243]; altered erythrocyte function, leading to hemolysis; abnormalities of glucose metabolism; and impaired leukocyte function.[179] Shifts in the body's distribution of phosphate may further depress serum phosphate. Alkalosis stimulates glycolysis, leading to increased intracellular phosphorylation of carbohydrate compounds, which additionally depresses serum phosphorus concentrations.[281] The use of antacids containing aluminum, which bind phosphate, can increase intestinal loss of phosphate. Large amounts of phosphate can be lost in the urine with hyperparathyroidism, hypomagnesemia, and severe hypokalemia. Preventing hypophosphatemia is preferable to treating it. Phosphate, as well as calcium and magnesium, should be administered routinely to all patients receiving intravenous nutritional support. Serum phosphate levels should be monitored frequently during the induction and stabilization periods of intravenous nutrition, particularly in patients with altered renal function. Patients receiving intravenous nutritional support should be given a minimum of 7 to 9 mmole of phosphate per 1000 carbohydrate kilocalories or, alternatively, 4 mmole/g infused nitrogen. Each patient's phosphate requirements are a balance of basal needs, total body depletion, degree of stress, and losses. Often a patient's phosphate requirement is larger than anticipated during the initiation and stabilization phases; this can be decreased after the first 3 to 5 days and replacement based on serum levels. Hypophosphatemia can be treated with sodium or potassium phosphate given parenterally or enterally. The serum phosphate level will recover within 12 to 24 hours of slowing of the glucose infusion. Hypophosphatemic patients should be evaluated for secondary factors such as respiratory alkalosis, which has a more profound effect on phosphate shifts than does metabolic alkalosis. Respiratory alkalosis may be an early manifestation of incipient sepsis, and hypophosphatemia may be a premonitory sign of an occult septic event.

MAGNESIUM. The symptoms of hypomagnesemia, which occurs when the serum concentration falls below 1 mEq/L, are primarily neuromuscular. Magnesium also has a significant effect on the metabolism of potassium, calcium, and phosphorus. Combination deficiencies can act synergistically, giving rise to complications. Hypomagnesemia accentuates digitalis toxicity, which can be compounded by hypokalemia.[34] The combination of hypophosphatemia and hypomagnesemia can lead to progressive myoneural irritability and seizures. Patients particularly at risk for development of hypomagnesemia are those with malabsorption syndromes, extensive small-bowel resections, intestinal fistulae, prolonged nasogastric suction, and alcoholic cirrhosis. An alcoholic patient who is hyponatremic should be evaluated for concomitant hypomagnesemia. As with phosphorus, the need for magnesium replacement may be greatest early in the initiation and stabilization phases of parenteral alimentation, with requirements as high as 0.4 mEq/kg/day and additional replacements needed for excessive urinary and gastrointestinal losses. In unstable patients receiving parenteral alimentation, serum magnesium levels should be checked two or three times a week to determine proper replacement.

Hepatic Complications

Hepatic dysfunction in patients receiving intravenous hyperalimentation is a commonly seen but poorly understood event. In patients receiving parenteral alimentation, serum glutamic-oxaloacetic transaminase (SGOT), serum glutamic-pyruvic transaminase (SGPT), and alkaline phosphatase frequently are elevated; less frequently hyperbilirubinemia may also occur. Abnormal results on liver function tests are not restricted to patients with underlying liver dysfunction. As many as one third of normal patients have been found to have elevated values on liver function tests when receiving parenteral alimentation.[207] The abnormal values usually stabilize during the course of parenteral alimentation and resolve within 2 weeks of discontinuation of therapy.

Sheldon and colleagues[307] did a study on a series of 26 patients receiving intravenous hyperalimentation who underwent liver biopsies when abnormal values appeared on liver function tests. The researchers found evidence of intrahepatic cholestasis, bile duct proliferation, and bile plugs in the liver. In a series of studies by Maini and associates,[214] patients receiving 4000 to

6000 kcal of a 30% dextrose–amino acid solution experienced fatty metamorphosis after 6 weeks or longer of intravenous feedings. The hypothetical causes of these changes are increased liver synthesis of lipid, increased release of free fatty acids from peripheral adipose tissue, decreased oxidation of fatty acids in the liver, and impairment of lipid transport from the liver.[209] These changes also could be related to a deficiency of essential fatty acids in patients who are not receiving appropriate fat replacement. In patients receiving large lipid infusions, a progressive cholestasis has been reported, which responded to a decrease in the infusion load from 3 g/kg/day to 1 g/kg/day.[10] Besides excess glucose and lipid infusions, amino acid solutions have been implicated as causing liver dysfunction. Grant[141] has suggested that an oxidant (sodium bisulfate) in commercial amino acid solutions may result in breakdown products of tryptophan, which produce a toxic hepatitis.[11] The changes in liver function values, particularly elevated transaminase levels indicative of hepatitis, may precede fatty infiltration of the liver.

If liver function values rise and the patient is receiving large lipid loads, the infusion should be lowered to 2 g/kg/day or less. In patients receiving standard 25% dextrose and 4.25% amino acid solutions, consideration should be given to lowering the dextrose concentration to 15% while maintaining the same infusion rate of amino acids. Liver function values generally return to normal within 10 to 14 days of lowering the nutrient infusion rate.

Additional metabolic complications of parenteral alimentation may result from inappropriate replacement of essential fatty acids, vitamins, and trace minerals, with deficiency syndromes occurring as described previously in the section on essential nutrients. Similarly, fluid and acid-base disturbances may occur, as in any patient receiving intravenous fluid and electrolyte support. In many institutions large loads of acetate are given to balance the parenteral solutions; although this is not a particular problem in most patients, it can lead to a progressive metabolic alkalosis in some, which can be further compounded by inappropriate chloride replacement.

Infectious Complications

Infectious complications of intravenous nutritional support are primarily caused by central venous catheter sepsis. Patients receiving intravenous nutritional support frequently are malnourished, receiving broad-spectrum antibiotics, have remote sites of infection or immunosuppressive treatments, and are predisposed to the development of infectious complications. The incidence of septic complications related to parenteral nutrition has been reported to range from 2% to 33%.[11,251,297] Currently the most common pathogens are the gram-positive and gram-negative bacteria, whereas historically *Candida* species was more common. Recent reports have cited the increasing frequency of infections caused by *Staphylococcus aureus, Staphylococcus epidermidis,* and the Enterobacteriaceae.[288]

Sepsis in patients receiving intravenous nutritional support may be caused by the nutrient delivery system or a concomitant infectious process. Although the infusion of contaminated intravenous nutritional solution is potentially a mechanism of infection, it is an extremely rare occurrence when strict aseptic technique is used in preparing and handling of the nutritional fluids. If the parenteral alimentation is the source of sepsis, the central venous catheter is the most likely cause. The catheter may become colonized with bacteria as a consequence of transcatheter migration of bacteria down the side wall of the catheter from the skin-catheter junction.[259,260] The catheters may also become seeded because of a concomitant infectious process that has caused a bacteremia. In any event, once the catheters have become colonized, they can serve as a source of repeated blood-borne contamination that will not resolve until the catheter is removed. The more common of these two mechanisms is introduction of bacteria at the skin-catheter junction. Septic complications during parenteral nutrition are clearly inversely related to the extent that aseptic technique is followed during insertion and care of the catheter. A significant reduction in septic complications has been reported when rigorous nursing care of the catheter insertion sites is introduced.[181] It is a routine practice in most institutions delivering parenteral nutritional support to have a member of the nursing service assume primary responsibility for the care of the catheter insertion site, following protocols incorporating infection control. This approach has resulted in infection rates of 3% or less.[252,286,289] Obviously the intensive nursing care cannot compensate for breaks in aseptic technique during the initial catheter insertion. The insertion of the hyperalimentation catheter must be approached as the placement of a chronic indwelling intravascular device. Strict aseptic technique must be followed at the time of insertion, and the catheter should not be used for any purpose other than hyperalimentation. A relatively new development in catheter design incorporates a barrier or antimicrobial cuff between the subcutaneous tissue and skin, hopefully to lessen bacterial colonization of the fibrin sheath that develops around indwelling catheters.

Bacteremic seeding of the catheters by organisms from other infectious sites probably occurs in only 5% to 7% of patients.[141] Attempts to reduce the incidence of catheter-related infectious complications by subcutaneous tunneling of the catheter probably do not result in reductions above what can be achieved with aseptic nursing care, but the technique may reduce the sepsis rate when nursing care is suboptimal.[200]

When evaluating fever in any patient receiving parenteral nutrition, the clinician must consider all potential causes of infection. The patient should be evaluated for pulmonary sources of the fever, wound infection, urinary tract infection, thrombophlebitis, or catheter-related sepsis. In the past, allergic-type reactions secondary to the protein source, casein hydrolysate, had been reported; however, with the widespread use of crystalloid amino acids, this is an unlikely cause of fever. If the surgeon evaluating a febrile patient can find no sites of infection and the catheter insertion site is healthy, the patient must be evaluated for occult catheter or infusion-related sepsis. This is particularly important if the patient's temperature is above 38.5° C (101° F), and he has shaking fevers and chills, glucose intolerance, and leukocytosis with an increase in polymorphonuclear leukocytes.

If the patient is clearly septic or has failed to respond to the initial changing of the fluid and administration setup, the catheter should be removed, the tip cultured, and cultures of the patient's blood obtained. A septic episode in which no other site of infection is present and that resolves on removal of the catheter, with cultures of the catheter and peripheral blood yielding the same organism, establishes the diagnosis of central venous catheter sepsis.

After the catheter is removed and the infusion is discontinued, a peripheral intravenous line is inserted and the patient is given a 10% glucose and electrolyte solution at a rate sufficient to maintain fluid and electrolyte balance. After 24 to 48 hours, the infusion should be discontinued and the catheter removed if the patient's septic episode has resolved. If intravenous nutritional support is still needed, it should be provided through a clean insertion site, a new catheter should be inserted, and the infusion should be resumed at the previous concentration and rate. Usually it is not necessary to reaccommodate patients who were receiving their goal infusion rate and concentration of nutrients before the septic episode.

Another technique may serve as an alternative to discontinuing the infusion and removing the catheter. Bozzetti and associates[54] have conducted a prospective controlled trial on preventing and treating central venous catheter sepsis by using the technique of guide wire catheter exchange. Their approach is particularly attractive in a critically ill patient receiving parenteral alimentation who may well be febrile from sources other than the catheter, and it offers a simple approach to evaluating potential catheter sepsis. The exchange of catheters over a guide wire avoids the risk of new catheter insertion, preserves venous access in patients with limited sites, and maintains delivery of nutritional support.

In the infrequent cases in which the catheter and blood tests are positive for *Candida* species, patients must be evaluated for the complications of candidemia, and it must be documented that *Candida* organisms have been cleared from the bloodstream before parenteral nutrition is reinstituted. Often in patients with uncomplicated candidemia, the septic episode will resolve spontaneously with removal of the catheter, and no specific therapy will be required.[54]

The use of semiquantitative culture techniques allows the distinction to be made between catheter infection and catheter contamination. Finding more than 15 colonies on the semiquantitative culture from the catheter tip establishes the diagnosis of an infected catheter. If positive blood cultures are obtained for the same organism and no remote site is found, the catheter is the likely site of the septic episode. Local inflammation at the insertion site is associated with high-density colonization on semiquantitative culture, and its presence should heighten suspicion of a catheter-related septicemia.[215]

Special Clinical Considerations

Acute Renal Failure

The management of acute renal failure from a nutritional standpoint involves an initial nutritional assessment that takes into consideration the degree of catabolism and initial blood urea nitrogen levels. The desired therapeutic endpoint is to provide enough calories and protein to promote a positive nitrogen balance while not compounding the uremic state by increasing blood urea nitrogen (BUN). The goal is to provide enough calories in the form of carbohydrate or lipids to reduce endogenous protein breakdown and promote protein synthesis by providing protein in the form of essential amino acids (EEAs) or a balanced mixture of essential and nonessential amino acids (EEA-NEAAs). Which form of protein administration is more effective in decreasing azotemia and promoting protein synthesis is still a matter of controversy. Other factors, such as daily urine output, gastrointestinal function, other previous or active disease states, and the need for dialysis, are also important considerations when designing parenteral nutritional support for a patient with acute renal failure.

The production of urea stems from the intake of dietary amino acids or protein and the breakdown of endogenous protein stores. The well-recognized work of Giordano[132] and of Giovanetti and Maggiore[133] supports the use of "high biologic value" protein, consisting mainly of essential amino acids, in the clinical treatment of acute renal failure. Using a solution of essential amino acids and hypertonic dextrose, Wilmore and Dudrick[358] demonstrated an increase in serum albumin and restoration of positive nitrogen balance with a concomitant decrease in serum urea nitrogen, potassium, and phosphorus. In 1975 Abel and colleagues[2,3] confirmed the beneficial role of EAA-dextrose solutions in a prospective, double-blind, clinically controlled trial by demonstrating an increase in survival and a shorter period of renal failure compared with patients receiving isocaloric dextrose solutions alone. They also demonstrated significant decreases in serum urea nitrogen, potassium, magnesium, and phosphorus without the aid of dialysis when EAA-dextrose formulas were used. However, the finding of increased survival was not supported in work by Sofio and Nicora.[316]

Several clinical studies in recent years have compared the EAA-dextrose formulas with the balanced EAA-NEAA-dextrose solutions and found no demonstrable difference in their ability to lower blood urea nitrogen or achieve nitrogen balance. In comparing EAA-dextrose and EAA-NEAA-dextrose solutions, Mirtallo and associates[227] reported no significant differences in net protein usage or nitrogen balance. In the rate of decrease in BUN and urea appearance was not significantly different, and a positive nitrogen balance was achieved in both groups.[227] The parenteral solution currently recommended for nonoliguric patients who do not require dialysis is an EAA-dextrose solution, because some investigators still believe these solutions are more effective in lowering BUN. However, in oliguric patients who require dialysis, a greater negative nitrogen balance has been observed, as well as an increased loss of protein across the dialysis membrane. This increased loss of protein, in the form of EAAs and NEAAs, is best addressed with a balanced amino acid solution.[47,124,355]

A patient with acute renal failure who is receiving parenteral nutritional support must be closely monitored. Changes in body weight and accurate assessment of fluid balance should be recorded daily. Daily measurement of serum electrolytes, including sodium, potassium, phosphorus, magnesium, BUN, and creatinine, is an absolute requirement. Supplemental potassium, phosphorus, and magnesium usually are not required when initiating parenteral nutritional support, but after several days of parenteral support, it frequently becomes necessary to include these electrolytes in the nutritional regimen.[114] As with any course of parenteral nutritional support, serum glucose levels must be monitored every 6 hours until the blood glucose stabilizes. Insulin can be administered by sliding scale for serum glucose levels above 200 mg/dl, or it can be included as part of the parenteral solution at two thirds of the total daily dosage required during the previous 24 hours. After appropriate control of serum glucose has been attained, blood glucose determination twice daily should suffice.

Blood urea nitrogen levels do not directly reflect endogenous protein breakdown or consumption of exogenously administered amino acids. A rising BUN, despite administration of an appropriate renal formula, suggests deteriorating renal function, a possible increase in protein catabolism, or excessive provision of exogenous amino acids, particularly in dialysis patients.[202] Urea production can be regulated in a critically ill patient by restricting exogenously administered amino acids and providing adequate caloric intake primarily in the form of carbohydrates. Glucose is available in highly concentrated solutions (50% to 70%) which are ideal sources of fluid replacement in patients with rigid fluid restrictions. More importantly, in a catabolic patient, using glucose as the primary source of calories has a much greater protein-sparing effect than fat and reduces urea production.[206] However, as with concentrated glucose, lipid emulsion provides an excellent source of concentrated calories in patients with fluid restriction and can be given to meet 30% to 40% of total caloric requirements. The surgeon should keep in mind that lipid emulsions do contain phosphate (15 mmole/L) and may be contraindicated in renal patients with hyperphosphatemia.[102,270]

Vitamin mixtures can be administered daily, and patients requiring dialysis may need additional supplementation of water-soluble vitamins. To correct the metabolic acidosis commonly seen in uremic patients, sodium or potassium acetate may also need to be added to the parenteral formula. Furthermore, in anuric patients, trace elements should be withheld initially until serum levels have been checked and, if needed, should be given on days the patient does not undergo hemodialysis. Using BUN levels, individual energy requirements, and fluid balance, an appropriate parenteral formula can be provided.

Acute Hepatic Failure

The nutritional management of patients with hepatic failure continues to be challenging as well as controversial. These patients tend to be critically ill and are often malnourished, immunosuppressed, and commonly have life-threatening illnesses, such as bleeding esophageal varices, sepsis, or multiple system organ failure. Parenteral nutritional support of patients with liver disease often is vital to facilitating recovery of hepatic function. However, these patients frequently are intolerant of the protein administration in standard (4.25%/L) parenteral amino acid solutions.

In general, hepatic failure can be classified as acute, chronic, or acute-on-chronic. Acute hepatic failure is the result of rapid hepatocellular necrosis, most commonly following fulminant viral hepatitis. Other causes, although much less common, are toxicities from drugs such as isoniazid, rifampin, halothane, acetaminophen, and tetracycline. Patients with acute hepatic failure frequently have rapid onset of encephalopathy or coma, and the prognosis is poor. The role of parenteral nutritional support in these patients has been very limited, due to their severe hyperaminoacidemia and widespread hepatocellular destruction, and thus it will not be discussed further.[166] Chronic hepatic failure is a progressive deterioration in hepatic function and in the United States is most commonly the result of prolonged ethanol abuse, although there are less common causes.[242] The most common role for parenteral nutritional support in hepatic disease lies with "acute-on-chronic" episodes of hepatic insufficiency brought about by dehydration, sepsis, surgery, or gastrointestinal bleeding and frequently complicated by hepatic encephalopathy.[166]

Encephalopathy is graded on a scale of 0 to 4[328]: grade 0—no encephalopathy; grade 1—intermittent confusion; grade 2—impending stupor; grade 3—stupor; grade 4—coma (unresponsive to painful stimuli). Various theories exist as to the primary cause of hepatic encephalopathy. Discussions in the literature tend to favor increased levels of ammonia or a change in the systemic amino acid profile as the principal cause of the encephalopathic state.[292,368] Ammonia, which is produced by enteric flora as a by-product of nitrogen metabolism, accumulates in the serum as hepatic metabolic function declines and may have a toxic effect on the central nervous system. The precise mechanism by which hyperammonemia exerts its toxic effects is still undefined. However, not all encephalopathic patients have an elevated serum ammonia, and the degree of encephalopathy has never correlated well with either venous or arterial ammonia levels.*

The second major theory stems from a change in the ratio of branched-chain amino acids to aromatic amino acids. In the hypercatabolic state complicated by hepatic insufficiency, a persistent hyperinsulinemia, caused by decreased hepatic clearance of insulin and accompanied by increased levels of glucagon, epinephrine, and adrenocortical steroids, worsens the degree of protein catabolism, because the liver is unable to produce sufficient glucose or ketone bodies to meet the patient's energy requirements. The plasma concentration of the branched-chain amino acids (BCAAs) valine, leucine, and isoleucine declines as they are consumed by fat and muscle for local energy needs. Because the catabolism of the aromatic amino acids (AAAs) depends on adequate liver function, the plasma concentration of AAAs such as phenylalanine, methionine, tyrosine, and tryptophan rises.[109,277,315] Therefore, the usual ratio of BCAA to AAA (3.5 : 1) may decrease to 1 : 1. Because of the decrease in the BCAA/AAA ratio, larger amounts of AAAs are transported across the blood-brain barrier and accumulate in the brain. Increased levels of phenylalanine and tyrosine in the brain may be responsible for reduced levels of normal neurotransmitters, specifically norepinephrine and dopamine, and increased production of "false" or inhibitory neurotransmitters such as octopamine and serotonin.[122,226] Accumulation of these false and inhibitory neurotransmitters may lead to the neurologic impairments typical of hepatic encephalopathy.

*References 53, 166, 292, 344, and 368.

Encephalopathic patients incapable of airway protection or having factors precluding enteral feeding are good candidates for parenteral nutritional support. Before parenteral support is begun, however, routine determination of BUN, glucose, electrolytes, creatinine, calcium, magnesium, and phosphorus; a complete blood count; and a standard coagulation profile are mandatory. A liver profile is also required, comprising total protein, albumin, globulin, bilirubin, SGOT, and alkaline phosphatase. Obtaining a venous ammonia level and plasma amino acid profile is highly recommended. Total urinary nitrogen can be determined using the Kjeldahl method, and nitrogen balance calculated.

An adequate calorie and protein intake is necessary for recovery of hepatic function and also lessens the catabolism of lean body mass. Despite the fact that most of these patients have some degree of protein intolerance, a trial of a standard parenteral formula containing 25% dextrose and 4.25% amino acids per liter is recommended. If the patient requires fluid restriction, 70% dextrose can be substituted. Lipid emulsions can be used for glucose-intolerant patients. Sodium restriction may be necessary in cirrhotic patients with ascites. With cholestasis or biliary obstruction, serum copper and manganese levels must be monitored carefully. If a patient cannot tolerate a normal protein intake, it may be necessary to restrict protein to 50 g/day or less, using a 2.25% amino acid solution, until hepatic recovery allows an increased protein intake.[344]

If one accepts the plasma amino acid/false neurotransmitter theory as a viable explanation for hepatic encephalopathy, it follows that providing protein in the form of BCAA-enriched solutions may ameliorate the encephalopathic state. Several theoretical advantages support the use of such solutions in patients with hepatic insufficiency: (1) BCAAs could supply a greater portion of energy needs, because muscle, heart, liver, and brain use BCAAs directly for energy production; (2) BCAAs decrease muscle proteolysis and increase muscle protein synthesis; (3) BCAAs increase hepatic protein synthesis and normalize plasma amino acid profiles by using the AAAs for protein synthesis; (4) increased plasma levels of BCAAs provide greater competition for AAAs and prevent their transport across the blood-brain barrier; and (5) BCAAs increase ammonia metabolism in muscle by donating an amino group for glutamine synthesis.[80,130,166]

Despite these theoretical advantages, few randomized, prospective studies have examined the use of BCAAs in patients with hepatic encephalopathy. Rossi-Fanelli and associates[278] randomized 40 patients with acute or acute-on-chronic hepatic encephalopathy (grades 3 and 4) to receive either hypertonic 20% dextrose and lactulose or 57 g of BCAAs in an isocaloric amount of hypertonic dextrose. Although the two groups showed no difference in survival, an increased level of consciousness was evident in 70% of the patients treated with BCAAs versus 49% in the lactulose group. Fiaccadori and others,[117,239] also using a BCAA-enriched formula and hypertonic dextrose, significantly improved arousal and decreased mortality in encephalopathic patients compared to the lactulose-treated group. Perhaps one of the best known studies to date was that performed by Cerra and colleagues.[77] In a multicenter, randomized, prospective, double-blind trial, 75 patients with at least grade 2 encephalopathy were divided between two treatment groups. The control group received 25% glucose by a central venous catheter plus 4 g/day of neomycin via the gastrointestinal tract. The experimental group received a neomycin placebo, isocaloric dextrose, and a modified amino acid solution enriched with 36% BCAAs and deficient in AAAs. The overall results noted a significant improvement in arousal time, nitrogen balance, and survival in the BCAA-treated group compared to controls. Although these results are impressive, other studies have not been able to confirm significant improvement in arousal or survival.[135,328]

Sepsis

The normal metabolic response to surgery, trauma, or sepsis peaks on day 3 and subsides by day 7 to day 10.[75] However, in some patients the hypermetabolic response does not abate; this results in a persistent hypermetabolic state frequently accompanied by multiple system organ failure (MOF).[72,211,323] Two clinical courses are definable from this point. In one, lung injury predominates, with organ failure being a preterminal event. In the second, lung, liver, and renal dysfunction are evident early in the clinical course; a stable phase of 7 to 10 days ensues, followed by progressive deterioration of liver and renal function in patients who ultimately die.[80] Cerra and others[31,72,74,211,323] have repeatedly described identifiable risk factors for the transition to hypermetabolism and organ failure. The hypermetabolic state usually is a consequence of severe perfusion insults (e.g., ruptured abdominal aortic aneurysm), septic shock, episodes of severe inflammation (e.g., pancreatitis), and the presence of dead or injured tissue. Organ failure can result from persistent perfusion deficits, persistent sources of infection and inflammation, traumatized or necrotic tissue, and the combination of sepsis and persistent hypoperfusion.

The metabolic consequences of a persistent hypermetabolic state that follows sepsis or trauma differ markedly from those of starvation. An increase in the respiratory quotient (0.85) demonstrates a greater dependence on a mixed carbon source of fatty acids, amino acids, and glucose for energy production instead of ketones. Systemic differences include increased cardiac output, increased oxygen consumption (V_{O_2}), and decreased systemic vascular resistance. Resting energy expenditure is 1.5 to 2.5 times that of basal.[70,310]

Although the process is not fully understood, a combination of local and systemic mediators is responsible for the complex metabolic response to injury, sepsis, or septic shock. In response to the shock phase of injury, changes in the microcirculatory environment result in tissue hypoxia-anoxia, acidosis, and accumulation of organic acids. These environmental changes, combined with direct tissue injury, activate cellular elements of the host immune system, potentially causing further parenchymal injury.[69] After resuscitation, the products of activated platelets, primed endothelial cells, and adherent macrophages result in oxidant-induced injury by endothelial cells and surrounding parenchymal tissue. Subsequent to this local inflammatory reaction, a host of mediator substances such as interleukins, cytokines, tumor necrosis factor (TNF), and prostaglandin E_2 (PGE_2) are released from activated macrophages and hepatic Kupffer cells.[69] Cellular products such as these, when released into the systemic circulation, cause distant inflammatory reactions and endothelial cell injury, as is seen in adult respiratory distress syndrome (ARDS). Interleukin-1 (IL-1), an endogenous pyrogen, causes fever by resetting the hypothalamic temperature-regulating center; directly activates increased endocrine production of catecholamines, glucagon, and corticosteroids; activates B cells; and increases protein breakdown.[234] Hepatic acute-phase protein synthesis is almost completely dependent on interleukin-6.[186] The effects of TNF include increased vascular permeability, lactic acidosis, fever, and altered perfusion.[234] PGE_2 may be partly responsible for postinjury and sepsis-induced immunosuppression, a decrease in arginine availability, and a reduction in proliferative factors such as purines and pyrimidines.[28,113,195]

Carbohydrate Metabolism

Hyperglycemia is a clinical finding commonly associated with infection or a septic state. The breakdown of hepatic glycogen stores and an accelerated rate of hepatic gluconeogenesis cause peripheral blood sugar levels to rise. Glucagon, cortisol, catecholamine, and growth hormone are all increased, resulting in increased hepatic adenylate cyclase activity and heightened hepatic production and release of glucose.[32] Septic patients have an obligate need for accelerated glucose production to fuel the metabolic processes of multiple tissue compartments such as the central nervous system, host defense system, and healing wounds. Accelerated use and breakdown of carbohydrate and protein stores increase available gluconeogenic precursors such as alanine, glycerol, pyruvate, and lactate. Gump and associates[147] found that alanine uptake predominated over other amino acids and was associated with increased hepatic production of glucose and urea. Long and others,[205] using ^{14}C-L-alanine, demonstrated a marked increase in glucose production in septic patients that was not changed by administration of exogenous glucose. The hyperglycemic state is unique in that higher than normal insulin levels are typical, and the elevated blood sugar levels are not suppressable by administration of exogenous glucose.[85,205] In fact, glucose given in excess of 5 g/kg/day has been associated with hyperosmolar complications, net fat synthesis, and fatty liver syndrome.[80] Several possible explanations for this insulin-resistant state have been offered. Clowes and associates[85] suspected a circulating substance of moderate molecular size as the cause of insulin resistance, whereas Black and others[43] have postulated a postreceptor defect as the cause. Popular opinion holds with a decrease in the number of membrane receptors or loss of affinity as the most probable cause. Further research is needed.

Lipid Metabolism

Many changes occur in lipid metabolism in the hyperdynamic setting of sepsis. Unlike with starvation, ketone bodies are not a preferred fuel source, because lipoprotein lipase activity tends to favor use of fatty acids and triglycerides as a primary energy substrate, especially by cardiac and skeletal muscle. A marked increase in mobilization of fatty acids from adipose tissue, concomitant with increased hepatic production of fatty acids and triglycerides, provides a major source of substrate material for the hypermetabolic demands of sepsis.[293,322] Plasma levels of free fatty acids decline in response to (1) a reduction in transport protein (ie., albumin) concentrations; (2) increased uptake and use of free fatty acid by the liver; and (3) a possible reduction in the mobilization of triglyceride stores.[32] Peripheral triglyceride clearance is decreased, requiring frequent routine monitoring of serum triglyceride levels.[70] This decrease in clearance is important, because overadministration of omega-6 fatty acids can cause hypoxia and impair cell-mediated immunity. Lipid-laden macrophages have impaired phagocytic capabilities and can produce excessive amounts of immunosuppressive prostaglandins.[70,76]

Bagby and Spitzer[25] have noted that as sepsis continues, the availability of lipid substrates to peripheral tissues may decline. Mobilization of fatty acids from adipose tissue stores decreases because microcirculation is impaired with sepsis or septic shock. Subsequently, with the change in substrate availability, tissues may preferentially use other fuel substrates, such as lactate. Also, cytokines produced by activated macrophages (e.g., TNF, IL-1) may reduce tissue lipoprotein lipase activity and subsequent use of free fatty acids and triglycerides for energy production.

Protein Metabolism

In the septic state, the protein of the lean body mass, which resides primarily in skeletal muscle, is rapidly mobilized to provide nitrogen and carbohydrate substrates to areas of active synthetic function. These areas include the skeletal muscle itself, which oxidizes amino acids for fuel, and the liver, which oxidizes amino acids during gluconeogenesis and produces acute phase reactants, mononuclear cells that utilize released amino acids in protein synthesis and in wound healing. Despite these areas of active protein synthesis, total body catabolism prevails; the autocannibalization of the skeletal muscle compartment reaches critical levels in 10 to 14 days. A net negative nitrogen balance ensues, with rapid development of malnutrition and possibly starvation if nutritional support is not provided.[70] Exogenous administration of amino acids at 1.5 to 2 g/kg does not effectively reduce the rate of catabolism, but it can balance the rate of total body protein catabolism with that of protein synthesis, thus achieving nitrogen equilibrium.[70]

Protein stores are catabolized in proportion to the severity of injury or sepsis. Protein, primarily in the form of skeletal muscle, can be catabolized at a rate of 75 to 150 g/day, resulting in a loss of up to 300 to 600 g of lean body mass per day. This mobilization of protein stores results in a relative deficiency of essential amino acids, particularly the branched-chain amino acids valine, leucine, and isoleucine. The BCAAs are preferentially used by skeletal muscle as an energy source and substrate for gluconeogenesis.[123] Teasley and Buss[331] concluded that parenteral solutions enriched with BCAAs improve immune function parameters, increase visceral protein synthesis, increase nitrogen retention, and help normalize plasma amino acid profiles. Despite these conclusions, research concerning BCAA formulas has failed to demonstrate a significant reduction in morbidity and mortality associated with the hypermetabolic state. Exogenous administration of BCAAs does not decrease the catabolic rate, nor does it totally prevent skeletal muscle breakdown. Exogenous BCAAs may stimulate muscle protein synthesis and decrease systemic proteolysis, thereby improving the patient's ability to achieve and maintain nitrogen equilibrium.[61,125,244] Current research continues to explore the therapeutic potential of this highly efficient protein source.

Metabolic Support

Moore and Cerra[234] have offered recommendations for starting nutritional support in a septic patient. Lipid emulsions should be provided at 1 g/kg/day. Carbohydrate should be administered as glucose and should not exceed 5 g/kg/day. Amino acid formulations should provide 2 g/kg/day, and vitamins and trace metals can be administered daily as clinically indicated.

Weekly monitoring of nitrogen balance is strongly

recommended. In a stressed patient, nitrogen balance should be measured as total urine nitrogen rather than urine urea nitrogen, because non-urea nitrogen commonly is substantial, and a readily available correction factor is not known. BUN, albumin, and serum transferrin should be monitored every 5 to 7 days. Serum electrolytes, liver function, and trace elements must be checked daily in the initial phases of parenteral nutritional support.[234]

An appropriate parenteral nutritional formula helps to support and build lean body mass and organ function. Also, preventing specific nutrient deficiencies may favorably modulate the host defense system, prevent substrate-limited metabolism, and promote reparative processes.[234]

Future Directions

It is becoming increasingly evident that three factors are responsible for reducing morbidity and mortality associated with hypermetabolism–multiple organ failure (HMOF) syndrome: improved control of the initiating event; better resuscitation techniques, with restoration of cardiac output and oxygen transport; and early nutritional support.[80] However, these treatment modalities have not changed the HMOF disease process itself in a way that significantly improves outcome. New areas of research are focusing on ways to directly influence the production of inflammatory cytokines and mediators of the host immune response. It may be possible to use nutrient pharmacology to alter mononuclear cell-cell communication, modulate the production of inflammatory mediators, or prevent gut mucosal atrophy and translocation of enteric flora, thereby directly affecting the HMOF disease process. Specialty nutrients such as arginine, ribonucleic acid (RNA), and n-3 polyunsaturated fatty acids (PUFA) have been shown to play an integral part in second-messenger generation, eicosanoid production and release, and the lymphoproliferative response to antigenic stimuli.[73] In addition, glutamine reportedly prevents the gut mucosal atrophy seen in critically ill patients and may reduce translocation of enteric bacteria.[269,346]

Arginine

Arginine is defined as a nitrogen-dense amino acid that is semi-essential in nature, being necessary for growth but not the viability of cells in vitro. Also, in vitro cytokine production and release can occur in the absence of arginine. Arginine is needed for growth because it is an essential component of polyamine and nucleic acid synthesis, both obligatory for mitotic reproduction.[249] In addition, arginine has been shown to stimulate the release of growth hormone, insulin, prolactin, and glucagon.[27] Arginine has also been identified as a major source of nitrous acid and nitric acid, both in vitro and in vivo.[327] It is well known that nitrous acid and nitric acid are important mediators of vascular dilation, hepatic protein synthesis, and electron transport in hepatocyte mitochondria.[73,327] Barbul[27] reported several in vivo immune effects with administration of arginine, including increased survival of septic animals; increased survival of tumor-bearing animals; an increase in the number of T cells and improvement in delayed-type hypersensitivity responses in athymic nude mice; increased allograft rejection in rodents; and an increase in the number of thymic and peripheral blood lymphocytes in in vitro assays of mitogen-induced blastogenesis. Madden and associates[210] reported an increased survival rate in rats when arginine was supplemented orally before sepsis, or intravenously after cecal ligation and puncture. In humans, mitogen-induced blastogenesis, with an increase in the number of thymic and peripheral blood lymphocytes, has been demonstrated both in vitro and in surgical and surgical intensive care patients.[267]

Ribonucleic Acid (RNA)

Purines and pyrimidines, being precursory elements of RNA and deoxyribonucleic acid (DNA), are necessary for mitotic cell division and protein synthesis. Evidence exists that under periods of stress, supplementation of these nucleotides may prove beneficial in restoring host immune response to mitogenic stimulation.[258] In discussing the effects of dietary nucleotides on immune response to bacterial infections, Kulkarni and associates[195] reported that restricting nucleotides suppressed cellular immune response and prolonged survival of rodent allografts. A possible explanation lies in the inability of T cells to undergo blastogenesis and respond to antigenic stimuli. In murine experiments, administration of uracil restored delayed-type hypersensitivity responses to foreign antigens, stimulated T-cell proliferative responses under antigenic stimulation, and reduced abscess formation caused by gram-positive organisms. Also, administration of dietary nucleotides may augment macrophage activation of T helper/inducer cells. Cerra[73] suggested that these observations support the position of an additional dietary requirement for purines and pyrimidines, or at least uracil, during times of metabolic stress. Ineffective salvage pathways, decreased nucleotide synthesis, and/or greater than normal requirements in the hypermetabolic state were offered as possible explanations for these phenomena.

n-3 Polyunsaturated Fatty Acids (n-3 PUFA)

The polyunsaturated fatty acids are a major component of cell membranes. The composition of cell membranes can be changed by exogenous administration of lipid emulsions. By altering the phospholipid composition of the membrane, one can change membrane fluidity and signal transduction, as well as the type of prostanoid/leukotriene released in response to various stimuli.[69,76] Human cell membranes are primarily made up of n-6 PUFA, as are currently available lipid emulsions. The n-6 PUFA are precursor elements of the macrophage-derived dienoic series of prostaglandins (PGE_2) and cytokines such as interleukin-1 and interleukin-6, as well as tumor necrosis factor.[184] Given in excess, n-6 PUFA are associated with fatty liver syndrome, periportal inflammation, cholestatic jaundice, decreased pulmonary diffusion capacity, reduced cell-mediated immunity, decreased phagocytic and bactericidal capabilities, and a decreased lymphoproliferative response to antigenic stimuli.[184] The amount of PGE_2, IL-1, and TNF released by the macrophage is directly related to the n-6/n-3 ratio, total n-3 and n-6 PUFA content, and the relative PUFA membrane composition. As the n-6 content increases, and the n-6/n-3 ratio exceeds 1, more inflammatory cytokines are released from the cell membranes.[76,86] The potential benefit of the n-3 PUFA may lie in their ability to preferentially replace n-6 PUFA and decrease the n-6/n-3 ratio, thereby altering the physiologic makeup and response of the cell membrane to antigenic stimuli.[40] Increasing the n-3 PUFA content and decreasing the n-6/n-3 ratio promotes the formation of trienoic prostaglandins and leukotrienes, reduces thrombogenesis, and blunts the inflammatory response by decreasing production of IL-1, PGE_2, and TNF.[76,79,338]

Glutamine

In many critically ill patients, following cardiovascular instability and hypotension, the protective barrier function of the intestinal wall is lost due to mucosal sloughing, decreased production of mucus, intermittent areas of superficial necrosis, increased permeability of epithelial cell tight junctions, and mucosal edema.[50,269] These precipatory events lead to increased permeability of the colonic bowel wall and allow translocation of enteric bacteria or systemic absorption of endotoxin, or both, possibly initiating an uncontrolled immune response that ends in multisystem organ failure and death. In investigating the effects of malnutrition and endotoxemia on promoting bacterial translocation in a murine model, Deitch and associates[97] showed that a significantly larger number of bacteria translocated to systemic organs in malnourished animals compared to normally nourished mice receiving endotoxin. Glutamine is a preferred fuel source for enterocytes and supports replication and growth of intestinal cells. It has been postulated that a lack of glutamine may be partly responsible for the breakdown in the gut mucosal barrier.[287] It is now well accepted that, when possible, enteric nutritional support is more beneficial for a critically ill patient, because it prevents mucosal atrophy.

Currently, commercially available parenteral solutions do not contain glutamine. However, there is promising evidence that, if added to parenteral nutritional support, glutamine may indeed maintain mucosal integrity. Hwang and associates[169] substituted glutamine for other nonessential amino acids at a dosage of 2 g/dl of parenteral formula and greatly attenuated gut mucosal atrophy. Other investigators, also using a 2% glutamine-enriched parenteral formula, maintained mucosal integrity after massive small bowel resection.[346] Most recently, the ability of glutamine alone to restore gut barrier function has been called into question, and the role of intraluminal fiber has been stressed. Although rapid, appropriate resuscitation and early nutritional support for a critically ill patient are paramount, glutamine supplementation may further augment our ability to modulate the host immune response.[15,245]

CASE STUDIES

PROBLEM: OPEN CHOLECYSTECTOMY

A 45-year-old mother of four is to undergo an open cholecystectomy.

Clinical Presentation

History (Subjective Findings)

The patient's symptoms have been primarily those of recurrent right upper quadrant pain and have not been associated with any extended decrease in food intake or any febrile episodes. She has no history of weight loss and generally eats a balanced diet.

Physical Examination (Objective Findings)

Weight-for-height standards show the patient to be 10% over ideal body weight. On physical examination, the patient is not jaundiced and other than having a slightly obese abdomen is entirely normal.

Diagnostic Studies

Laboratory Studies

The hemogram and white blood cell count are normal. Liver function studies are normal, and the serum albumin is 3.6 g/dl with a total protein of 6.8 g/dl.

Assessment

The patient appears to be an otherwise healthy person with no history of nutritional deficiencies. She has an excess of calorie reserves in the form of adipose tissue. The laboratory data obtained for admission, reviewed from a nutritional perspective, are normal. Based on the expectation of only a minimum postoperative increase in energy expenditure, the finding of no nutritional deficits before surgery, and the likelihood that the patient will be eating in 3 to 5 days after surgery, the patient should require no specialized nutritional support. Some have been enthusiastic about using protein substrates in the postoperative period to mitigate the nitrogen loss, and biochemical difference does result, but the difference appears to be of no practical significance.

Management

The fluid and electrolyte status must be maintained in the postoperative period. Intravenous nutritional support would be needed if the surgery were more extensive than planned or if postoperative complications developed that prevented the gastrointestinal tract from being used as the route for nutritional support.

PROBLEM: ADENOCARCINOMA

A 55-year-old man with adenocarcinoma of the rectum at 10 cm from the anal verge is scheduled for a low anterior resection.

Clinical Presentation

History (Subjective Findings)

The patient has had cramps and diarrhea for the past 3 months. Because of these symptoms, he decreased his total calorie intake, and his weight has declined from 83.25 to 79.75 kg over the past 3 months. He has been receiving no chronic medications and has no significant previous medical history.

Physical Examination (Objective Findings)

The patient weighs 79.5 kg and is 175 cm tall. He has lost 5.4% of his body weight over the past 3 months. His ideal body weight is 68 kg; therefore, he is 117% of ideal body weight and 94.6% of usual adult weight. The results of the examination are normal except for blood in the stool.

Diagnostic Studies

Laboratory Studies

The patient's laboratory values are as follows: serum albumin, 3.2 g/dl; liver function studies: normal; hematocrit: 43%; WBCs: 9600/mm^3 with 23% lymphocytes; absolute lymphocyte count: 2208/mm^3; transferrin: 275 mg/dl; DCH: 14 mm to an intradermal injection of PPD at 24 hours.

Assessment

Although the patient has had a 5% weight loss over the past 3 months, he is still above ideal body weight; this represents a partial loss of excess calories. Given the results of the physical examination and laboratory studies; the expectation that the patient will be on a hypocaloric diet before surgery while receiving mostly a liquid diet and a mechanical and antibiotic bowel preparation; and the fact that he will receive no enteral feedings for 5 to 7 days after surgery, it would be prudent to consider some form of nutritional support. Taking into account that (1) the patient has no preoperative deficits, (2) postoperative hypermetabolism is moderate if no complications develop, and (3) the total period of decreased intake will be 7 to 9 days, a hypocaloric, protein-sparing regimen is reasonable. However, if the patient is not receiving a reasonable enteral diet by 5 to 7 days after surgery, he will benefit most from total intravenous nutritional support to preserve lean body mass.

Management

Using the Long modification of the Harris-Benedict equation, we can estimate the RME expenditure that is likely in the postoperative period. Using an activity factor of 1.2 and an injury factor of 1.35, the patient's RME expenditure is:

$$\text{RME (male)} = [66 + (13.7)(79.5\text{ kg}) + (5)(175\text{ cm}) - (6.8)(55\text{ yr})] \times (1.2) \times (1.35) = 2688\text{ kcal/24 hours}$$

If we were to use a 10% dextrose solution and administer 2.4 L/day with a 4.25% amino acid solution and, in addition, deliver 500 ml of a 10% lipid emulsion, a total of 1747 kcal/24 hours could be delivered. Although this is not balanced support, it does prevent a progressive, unchecked erosion of nutrient stores. This approach provides 840 kcal from dextrose, 550 kcal from fat, and 357 calories from protein. Electrolytes, vitamins, and trace minerals would be added to the dextrose–amino acid solution based on maintenance requirements and supplemental amounts added for extraordinary losses.

PROBLEM: ULCERATIVE COLITIS

A 58-year-old man with ulcerative colitis has undergone an emergency subtotal colectomy with end-ileostomy and mucous fistula for perforated toxic megacolon.

Clinical Presentation

History (Subjective Findings)

The patient has had a long-standing history of ulcerative colitis that has been clinically active over the past 4 months. During this time he has had diarrhea and hematochezia. His weight has gone from 72 to 57 kg. He has had a progressive loss of muscle mass, markedly increased fatigue, and anorexia for the past 3 weeks. For the month before emergency surgery, he basically was on a clear liquid diet with no vitamin or nutrient supplementation and was receiving high-dosage prednisone therapy.

Physical Examination (Objective Findings)

Two days before emergency surgery, the patient weighed 56.8 kg and was 183 cm tall. He had lost 22% of his body weight over a 4-month period. His ideal body weight is 74 kg; therefore, he was 77% of ideal body weight and 78% of usual adult weight.

The morning after surgery, the patient's temperature was 38.8° C (102° F). An abdominal examination showed a right lower quadrant end-ileostomy with no output and a mucous fistula in the midline suprapubically, a long midline incision, and no bowel sounds. The patient appeared emaciated, with an obvious loss of subcutaneous fat and muscle bulk. A clean decubitus ulcer over the right buttock measured 1.5 cm in diameter. The patient was intubated on a ventilator with no effective ventilatory effort. The patient was hemodynamically stable with an adequate urinary output and satisfactory arterial blood gases with an inspired oxygen concentration of 0.5.

Diagnostic Studies

Laboratory Studies

Albumin level: 2.4 g/dl
WBCs: 14,500/mm^3
Hematocrit: 29%
Lymphocytes: 6%
Absolute lymphocyte count: 870/mm^3
Transferrin: 148 mg/dl

DCH testing was not performed because the patient was receiving high-dose methylprednisolone intravenously. A 24-hour urine assay done for creatinine clearance revealed a creatinine excretion of 1100 mg, which represents 65% of predicted creatinine excretion based on the patient's height.

Assessment

The patient suffered a significant loss of nutritional stores before the emergency colectomy. This loss placed him in a deficit state by all measured parameters, with erosion of calorie reserves and protein stores (both somatic and visceral stores); he is now hypermetabolic. Thus the patient with a marked erosion of nutrient stores is now attempting to heal surgical wounds and deal with the bacterial challenge of his colonic perforation. The initial nutritional support must be tailored to the patient's lean body mass, hypermetabolic state, and ability to handle the respiratory consequences of feeding; in all likelihood, the support will not put him in an anabolic state while he is maximally stressed. Over the subsequent days, as he recovers from surgery and the catabolic insult associated with the infectious process, placing him in an anabolic state may be possible.

Management

The patient's RME expenditure was computed with the Long modification of the Harris-Benedict equation, assuming an activity factor of 1.2 and an injury factor of 1.8. The injury factor is a combination of an estimate of the patient's response to surgery, febrile postoperative course, and response to the inflammatory and infectious processes. The injury factor could be further modified by the use of the catabolic index; however, it is unlikely that the patient's BEE is much greater than twice normal.

$$\text{RME (male)} = [66 + (13.7)(56.8\text{ kg}) + (5)(183\text{ cm}) - (6.8)(58\text{ yr})] \times (1.2) \times (1.8) = 2959\text{ kcal/24 hours}$$

Assuming a calorie/nitrogen ratio of 150 kcal/1 g nitrogen, the patient's protein needs would be approximately 20 g of nitrogen daily or 125 g of protein per day. Alternatively, the patient could be assumed to require 1.5 to 2 g/kg LBM of protein per day, which would achieve a similar protein load. Using a 25% dextrose solution and administering 2.3 L/day with 5% amino acids would deliver 2050 kcal and 120 g of protein per day. Additionally, giving 500 ml of a 20% lipid emulsion each day would bring the total calorie intake to 3050 calories/day. The advantage of daily fat administration is that the patient would not receive large amounts of carbohydrates; his calculated tolerance is about 600 g of carbohydrates per day. A large carbohydrate load could have an unfavorable effect on respiratory gas exchange and could increase dependency on mechanical ventilatory support. Macromineral, trace mineral, and vitamin replacements would be added to the amino acid solution to meet maintenance and extraordinary losses. In this individual with a long-standing history of chronic diarrhea, special attention should be given to deficits of magnesium and trace metals, particularly zinc and chromium. Trace metals should be added from the beginning of therapy. If questions exist about the adequacy of replacement, levels should be measured. In most institutions the time needed to obtain such laboratory results makes them interesting but much too late for therapeutic decisions. Because the patient is most likely being given a variety of medications, including steroids, his response to the initiation of nutritional support and subsequent maintenance must be closely monitored.

The first day of therapy would consist of 50 ml/hour of the 25% dextrose–amino acid solution, yielding 1.2 L of fluid. The patient's additional fluid needs must be made up with crystalloid solution given through an alternate access site to maintain the integrity of the alimentation line.

On day 2, if no significant problem with glucose tolerance develops, the infusion could be increased to 77 ml/hour. A rise in the patient's serum glucose to 180 to 200 mg/dl would not be surprising, given his stressed state and the glucocorticoids he is receiving. This does not, in itself, require administration of insulin. If the patient's glucose level rises to the mid to high 200s, he would require insulin, initially given as regular subcutaneous insulin injections based on serum glucose values obtained every 6 hours (sliding scale).

On day 3, the patient's infusion would be increased to 100 ml/hour, the final rate of the 25% dextrose and amino acid solution. If at this time there is a need for continuous insulin replacement, the subcutaneous route can be continued, or two thirds of the total insulin dose of the previous 24 hours given subcutaneously can be placed in the alimentation fluid, resulting in concomitant administration of glucose and insulin along with the amino acids. Although some of the insulin will be bound to the tubing and container, the amino acid mixture will bind an appreciable amount, and incremental amounts of insulin can be added on subsequent days to achieve optimum glucose control. If the patient has significant glycosuria during this period, an apparently adequate urinary output may be inappropriate because of the osmotic effect of the glucose. The osmotic effect of the glucosuria can lead to dehydration.

Administration of the lipid emulsion should begin on day 1 and should be held at a fixed rate, administered over 8 to 10 hours after an initial test infusion shows no hypersensitivity response. Concomitant with the daily increase in the infusion rate of the alimentation fluid would be continual reassessment of the patient's fluid requirements and appropriate reduction in the total non-nutrient fluid given on a daily basis.

After a stable daily infusion rate has been established for 72 hours, a 24-hour urine assay for urea nitrogen should be obtained to assess the adequacy of nitrogen retention. The patient's weight should be monitored daily, with accurate calculation of intake and output and monitoring of urinary glucose. Given the critical nature of the patient's illness, serum electrolyte assays should be done daily. For the first several days calcium and phosphorus levels should be assayed. The magnesium level and coagulation profile should be determined three times a week.

The patient's total calorie and protein needs should be periodically reassessed and adjustments made based on the estimation of ongoing hypercatabolism and degree of stress. As the patient recovers from peritonitis and ileus resolves, enteral feedings should be started. The alimentation fluid can be reduced accordingly as enteral intake increases. Practically speaking, this is best achieved by obtaining daily calorie counts and decreasing the amount of infused nutrients based on the previous day's enteral intake. Once the rate of the hypertonic glucose infusion is 50 ml/hour or less, the infusion can be discontinued after an additional 10- to 12-hour infusion of 5% to 10% glucose to prevent hypoglycemia (Table 9-11).

TABLE 9-11 VARIABLES TO BE MONITORED DURING INTRAVENOUS ALIMENTATION AND SUGGESTED FREQUENCY OF MONITORING

	SUGGESTED MONITORING FREQUENCY	
VARIABLES	FIRST WEEK	LATER
Energy-Fluid Balance		
Weight	Daily	Daily
Metabolic Variables		
Blood measurements		
Plasma electrolytes (Na^+, K^+, Cl^-)	Daily	3 times/wk
Osmolarity*	Daily	3 times/wk
Blood urea nitrogen	3 times/wk	2 times/wk
Plasma total calcium and inorganic phosphorus	3 times/wk	2 times/wk
Blood glucose	Daily	3 times/wk
Plasma transaminases	3 times/wk	2 times/wk
Plasma total protein and fractions	2 times/wk	Weekly
Blood acid-base status	As indicated	As indicated
Hemoglobin	Weekly	Weekly
Ammonia	As indicated	As indicated
Magnesium	2 times/wk	Weekly
Triglycerides	Weekly	Weekly
Urine measurements		
Glucose	4-6 times/day	2 times/day
Specific gravity or osmolarity	Daily	Daily
General measurements		
Volume of infusate	Daily	Daily
Oral intake (if any)	Daily	Daily
Urinary output	Daily	Daily
Prevention and Detection of Infection		
Clinical observations (activity, temperature, symptoms, catheter sites)	Daily	Daily
WBC and differential counts	As indicated	As indicated
Cultures	As indicated	As indicated

*May be predicted from 2 × Na concentration (mEq/L) + [blood glucose (mg/dl) + 18]

ENTERAL ALIMENTATION

Enteral Versus Parenteral Nutrition

The gastrointestinal tract is commonly regarded as an organ system that is involved solely with the digestion and absorption of nutrients. However, recent investigations have demonstrated that this system also regulates and processes metabolic substrates circulating through the splanchnic vasculature and is a major component of host defenses.[340] The gastrointestinal mucosa normally is an efficient barrier that prevents migration of microorganisms and their by-products into the systemic circulation. The intestinal epithelium has approximately one lymphocyte for every five enterocytes. The epithelial cells of the intestinal mucosa are constantly being renewed and thus are markedly affected by nutrient availability, the hormonal environment, and intestinal blood flow.

The most important stimulus for proliferation of mucosal cells is the direct presence of nutrients in the in-

■ Enteral Alimentation section contributed by Mark J. Koruda.

testinal lumen.[175] Bowel rest resulting from starvation or administration of total parenteral nutrition (TPN) leads to villous atrophy,[201] decreased cellularity, and a reduction in intestinal disaccharidase activity.[264] The indirect effects of nutrients on the gastrointestinal (GI) tract are mediated by enterohormones such as gastrin and enteroglucagon, and by nonenteric hormones such as growth hormone and epidermal growth factor.[12]

Intestinal Fuels

Nutrients taken up by enterocytes may enter the intestinal mucosa through the luminal side or the basolateral membrane via the mesenteric arteries. Enterocytes extract glutamine, which is oxidized in preference to glucose, fatty acids, or ketone bodies in the small intestine.[359] Glutamine becomes available to the small intestine from mucosal absorption or systemically as a result of muscle proteolysis. Glutamine is used by the enterocyte as a respiratory fuel generating nitrogen by-products such as ammonia, alanine, and citrulline.

Colonocytes, on the other hand, oxidize the short-chain fatty acid (SCFA) n-butyrate in preference to glutamine, glucose, and ketone bodies.[273] Unlike glutamine, which is synthesized by the body, butyrate is not produced by mammalian tissue and is available to the colonic mucosa only through bacterial fermentation in the colonic lumen. SCFAs, primarily butyrate but also acetate and propionate, are used for energy-consuming cellular processes in the colon, such as sodium absorption and cell proliferation and growth of cells.[272]

In the anaerobic environment of the colon, the best substrates for bacterial fermentation are carbohydrates, which normally reach the cecum in the form of dietary fiber or undigested starch. Intraluminal fermentation of fiber polysaccharides follows a stoichiometric equation[314]:

$$34.4\ C_6H_{12}O_6 \rightarrow 64\ SCFA + 23.75\ CH_4 + 37.23\ CO_2 + 10.5\ H_2O$$

The methane (CH_4) produced is further converted to H_2O and CO_2. The three principal SCFAs—acetate, propionate, and n-butyrate—are produced in a fairly constant ratio of 1:0.3:0.25. These three SCFAs account for approximately 83% of all SCFAs produced.[87] The bacterial flora use less than 10% of the energy available from fiber fermentation for their metabolic activity.[225] The remaining energy is transferred into SCFA, which can be either absorbed or excreted. Based on in vivo perfusion studies, it is estimated that the human colon can absorb up to 540 kcal/day in the form of SCFA.[282]

With the lack of fiber in enteral feeding formulas or with suppression of bacterial flora by administration of antibiotics, SCFA availability may be markedly diminished, which in turn may lead to structural and functional changes within the colon. Additionally, parenteral nutrition formulas lack glutamine and, with their high glucose content, suppress generation of ketone bodies. Current nutritional therapy, therefore, starves the gut. Recent efforts are being directed at tailoring the composition of both enteral and parenteral formulas to meet the specialized needs of gut metabolism (see Nutrients with Potential Special Applications).

Without the physical stimulus of a meal, and with intestinal fuels lacking (e.g., glutamine and n-butyrate), the small intestine[107] and colon[285] atrophy. This atrophy affects not only absorptive cells but also mucus-secreting cells, gut-associated lymphoid tissue (GALT), and brush border enzymes. Brush border enzymes and absorptive cells are essential for nutrient assimilation, and mucus cells and GALT are key components of the intestinal barrier. Bacteria, endotoxins, and other antigenic macromolecules are contained within the intestinal lumen by these barrier functions.

Bacterial Translocation

The upper GI tract is essentially devoid of bacteria as the result of the bactericidal action of hydrochloric acid and the intestinal motility that sweeps any surviving bacteria toward the colon. However, because of the widespread use of antacids, H_2 blockers, and narcotics, bacterial colonization of the upper GI tract is common in critically ill patients. Bacteria exists in the human colon in counts as high as 10^{11}/ml. The homeostasis of these bacteria is closely controlled by the availability of energy substrates, physiochemical conditions of the colonic lumen, and the interactions among microorganisms and the nonmicrobial environment.[164]

Disruption of the intestinal barrier and alteration of the bacterial microflora facilitate translocation of bacteria and absorption of endotoxins from the gut lumen.[37] Bacterial translocation is the process of bacterial migration or invasion across the intestinal mucosa into mesenteric lymph nodes and the portal bloodstream. Bacterial translocation has been studied most extensively in animal models. For example, the translocation of indigenous enteric bacteria into mesenteric lymph nodes occurred in rats following thermal injury, exposure to cold, femoral fracture-amputation, use of oral antibiotics, and with bacterial overgrowth.[93-97,212,213] Even when noxious stimuli are not present, bacterial translocation has been detected in rats receiving TPN.[16]

In one study, intraoperative bacteriologic cultures of portal venous blood were performed in a heterogeneous group of patients undergoing surgery for noninflammatory lesions of the GI tract.[290] In more than 30% of the patients, blood cultures were positive for enteric organisms, demonstrating that bacteria pass from the GI tract to the liver via the portal vein. Life-threatening infections from gut-associated bacteria have been documented in patients with multisystem organ failure syn-

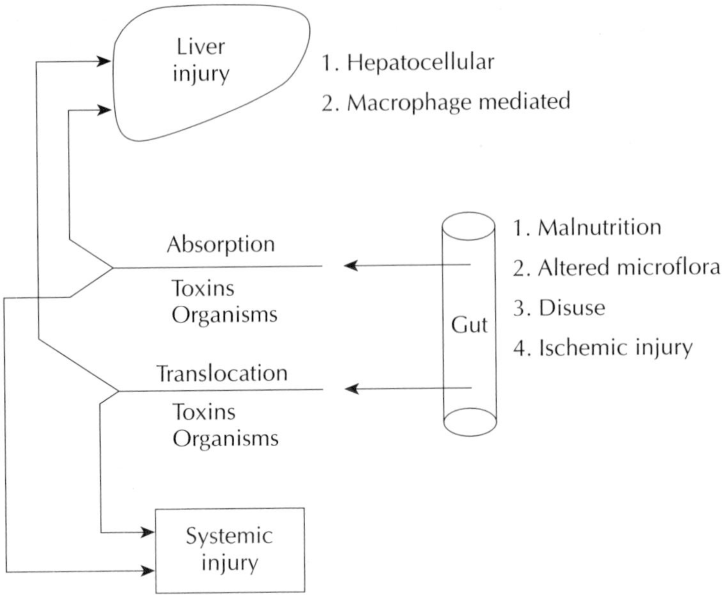

FIGURE 9-5 Hypothesis for the gut's role in the pathogenesis of organ failure syndrome. The mechanisms of bacterial translocation and changes in gut endocrine function are believed to be involved. (From Cerra FB, Holman RT, Bankey PE et al: *Crit Care Med* 18:S154, 1990.)

drome,[217] in those with cancer who have had chemotherapy,[46] and in those who have suffered a major burn injury.[172]

Bacterial endotoxins may also migrate across the gut mucosa. Endotoxins are lipopolysaccharide components of the bacterial cell wall that normally are absorbed in small quantities into the portal bloodstream and usually detoxified by hepatic Kupffer's cells.[241] In rabbits that were given a single dose of endotoxin, underwent temporary occlusion of the superior mesenteric artery, or had a 30% scald burn, fatal endotoxic shock ensued within 12 hours.[149] These injuries were not lethal if the animals were pretreated with antibiotics or if gram-negative bacteria were either absent, or present in reduced amounts in the intestinal tract. Endotoxins given intraperitoneally to mice produce bacterial translocation from the gut to the mesenteric lymph nodes in a dose-dependent manner.[94] The combination of malnutrition with endotoxemia was associated with a significantly higher number of translocated bacteria to systemic organs than was seen in normally nourished animals receiving endotoxin.[97] Conversely, TPN-induced translocation is reduced by adding a dietary fiber.[321] In human subjects, a single intravenous dose of *Escherichia coli* endotoxin significantly increased intestinal permeability.[246] Figure 9-5 outlines the proposed relation between changes in the permeability of the intestinal mucosa and systemic response.

Studies Comparing Enteral and Parenteral Nutrition

Numerous experiments involving animal models have investigated the relative benefits of enteral versus parenteral nutrition. Enterally fed rats demonstrated improved survival after septic challenges[190,192,256] and hemorrhagic hypotension[189] compared with parenterally fed animals. In animals that sustained femoral fractures, lymphocyte responses returned significantly earlier in animals fed enterally compared with the intravenous group.[266] In a rat model, parenteral nutrition and oral elemental diets promoted bacterial translocation from the gut.[16] Finally, enteral feeding, as compared with parenteral nutrition, significantly blunted the hypermetabolic response to burn injury in an animal model.[229]

Border and associates[48] retrospectively examined the effect of enteral feeding on the ICU course of 66 victims of multiple blunt trauma.[48] They reported that enteral protein intake was associated with a reduction in the septic severity score (SSS). Even though patients nourished parenterally received twice the amount of protein that the enterally fed group received, the lack of enteral nutrition resulted in significantly higher septic severity scores (Figure 9-6).

Although an earlier prospective, randomized trial by Adams and associates[6] demonstrated comparable caloric intakes, nitrogen balance, and complication rates between 23 enterally fed trauma patients and 23 patients

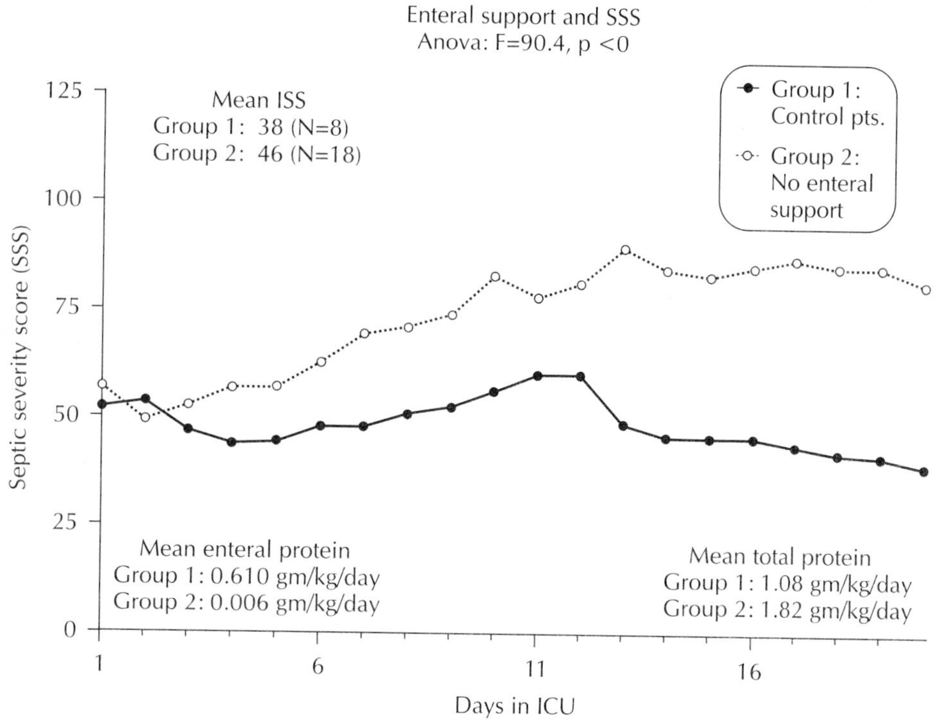

FIGURE 9-6 A comparison of the association between the septic severity score (SSS) and administration of 0.61 g/kg/day of enteral protein (group 1) or no enteral protein intake (group 2). Group 1 had a stable to falling SSS over the 21 days of observation, whereas group 2 had a progressively rising SSS. *ISS,* Injury severity score. (From Border J, Hassett J, LaDuca J: *Ann Surg* 206:427, 1987.)

fed by TPN, recent clincal studies have shown improved outcome with enteral nutrition. Enteral nutrition was associated with reduced morbidity and morality[9] and with improved immune function[19] after burn injury. In prospective, randomized trials, Moore and associates demonstrated reduced septic morbidity[230,231,232] and improved visceral protein synthesis[257] in patients with major abdominal trauma who had received enteral nutrition compared with those managed with TPN. Most recently Kudsk and colleagues[191] randomized 98 patients who suffered major abdominal blunt or penetrating trauma to either immediate postoperative TPN or enteral nutrition. The enteral group had significantly fewer cases of pneumonia, intra-abdominal abscess, and catheter sepsis. They also noted that the most significant changes occurred in the more severely injured patients. It is noteworthy that in the previous studies, the presence of an intestinal anastomosis distal to the site of tube feeding did not preclude early institution of enteral feeding (i.e., within 24 hours of surgery).

Finally, a meta-analysis combined data from eight prospective, randomized trials that compared the nutritional efficacy of early enteral and parenteral nutrition in trauma and other high-risk postoperative general surgical patients.[232] This study demonstrated that early enteral postoperative nutrition resulted in a significant twofold decrease in septic complications compared with patients given TPN.

A variety of evidence, animal and human, suggests that gut translocation of bacteria or bacterial products may occur during critical illness, contributing to the metabolic response, morbidity, and mortality. Evidence is also mounting that current parenteral nutrition regimens contribute to this process by promoting mucosal atrophy and breakdown of the mucosal barrier. It appears that enteral feeding helps maintain gut architecture and function in critically ill patients and ultimately improves outcome by reducing the incidence of gut-origin sepsis.

Implementing Enteral Nutrition

Patient Selection

Generally, the indications for enteral nutrition in a surgical patient are malnutrition, inadequate oral intake, and a functioning GI tract that can be used safely. Appropriate clinical judgment determines whether the gastrointestinal tract is functioning adequately and can be used safely. To establish the need for supplementary feedings, the nutritional assessment should demonstrate that the patient's voluntary intake is insufficient to meet nutritional needs. Specific indications and contraindications for enteral nutrition are listed in the box on the right. Patients with neurologic disorders that prevent satisfactory oral intake and patients with oropharyngeal or esophageal disorders who cannot eat may benefit from enteral nutrition (EN). Patients with burns, short bowel, severe malabsorption, distal enteric or colonic fistulae, ventilator dependence, or obtundation are also candidates for this type of feeding. Additionally, enteric feedings can be used in the transition from TPN to combined parenteral and enteral nutrition to oral intake.

Unfortunately, surgical illnesses are commonly associated with gastrointestinal disorders that may either reduce or preclude the use of enteral nutrition. Diarrhea, gastroparesis, gastroesophageal reflux, and ileus are common in surgical patients. Enteric anastomoses are a relative contraindication to early postoperative administration of enteral nutrition, but several studies have affirmed its safety in the immediate postoperative period.[191,230,233]

INDICATIONS FOR ENTERAL NUTRITION

Considered Routine Care in:

Protein-calorie malnutrition with inadequate oral intake of nutrients for the previous 5 days

Normal nutritional status but less than 50% of required oral nutrients for the previous 7 to 10 days

Severe dysphagia

Major burns

Massive small bowel resection in combination with administration of TPN

Low-output enterocutaneous fistula

Usually Helpful in:

Major trauma

Radiation therapy

Mild chemotherapy

Liver failure and severe renal dysfunction

Contraindicated in:

Complete mechanical intestinal obstruction

High-output intestinal fistula

Shock

Severe diarrhea

Prognosis not warranting aggressive nutritional support

Not desired by the patient or legal guardian and such wish being in accordance with hospital policy and existing law

Access

Enteral nutrition is provided through oral intake, nasoenteric tube, or a tube enterostomy. Nasoenteric tubes are the most common method of access used for gastric feeding. Recent technologic advances have led to the availability of soft nasoenteric tubes that are composed of nonreactive materials such as silicone or polyurethane. These tubes are available in various diameters and are well tolerated by most patients. However, the flexibility of these tubes often makes insertion into critically ill patients difficult as well as dangerous. Useful aids to assist passage of the tube include (1) using stiffeners, either inside (e.g., guide wire or stylet) or outside (e.g., the Cartmill tube) the feeding tube during passage; (2) judicious use of gravity and positioning; and (3) designation of experienced personnel to assist in the task.

A weighted tube may need to be passed through the pylorus into the duodenum if the patient has delayed gastric emptying or is at increased risk of aspiration. Although it is prudent to feed the patient at risk for aspiration into the duodenum or beyond, transpyloric passage of the tube does not eliminate the risk of aspiration.[329] Aspiration is a major complication in patients receiving enteral nutrition, and every effort should be made to reduce the possibility of this untoward event. Important factors in assessing the risk of aspiration include depressed sensorium, gastroesophageal reflux, and a previously documented episode of aspiration. For most patients fed enterally, safety demands that the head be elevated at feeding time and for some period thereafter to prevent regurgitation. Nasogastric intubation, in particular, requires elevation of the head, because the tube may render the upper and lower esophageal sphincters incompetent and liable to reflux. Because many patients are fed continuously over a 24-hour period, this "gold standard" safety measure presents a challenging yet common clinical dilemma. If elevating the patient's head is not possible, an alternative site of nutrient delivery should be considered. Even the presence of a tracheostomy or endotracheal tube does not ensure that regurgitated gastric contents will not be aspirated.

Transpyloric passage of a nasoenteric feeding tube has become a challenge. Use of the gastric prokinetic drug metaclopromide has shown inconsistent results in assisting in transpyloric passage.[83,187,353] Newly developed tubes containing electrodes that permit continuous monitoring of luminal pH may be of benefit in the passage of transpyloric tubes. As the operator places the tube, the pH is monitored, and a sudden rise in pH should indicate the tube's passage into the duodenum. Both fluoroscopy and endoscopy are commonly used to aid in tube placement.[185,261]

Feeding by tube enterostomy is used in patients in need of long-term EN or in patients who have undergone an intra-abdominal operation in which enteral access attained at this initial operation will asssist in postoperative management. These patients typically include trauma victims with multiple injuries, patient (injury severity score [ISS] over 15, especially with a significant head injury), or a patient undergoing a complex proximal gastrointestinal procedure (e.g., pancreaticoduodenectomy).

Tube enterostomy sites include the pharynx, esophagus, stomach, and jejunum (Figure 9-7). Gastrostomies have also been safely placed by means of a percutaneous endoscopic technique even in critically ill patients.[184] Jejunostomy is used as a feeding route for patients who are at increased risk of gastric aspiration or have undergone extensive gastric or duodenal surgery. Recent studies have supported the safe and efficacious use of both the small-caliber (7 French) needle catheter jejunostomy (NCJ)[178,191,230] or the larger bore (16 or 18 French) feeding jejunostomies.[67] Tubes that permit concomitant gastric decompression and jejunal feeding are also available.[274] Even with mild paralytic ileus, low volumes of EN can be given by delivering diet into the duodenum or jejunum while the stomach is decompressed.

In summary, nasoenteric tubes should be selected for patients who need short-term feeding (Figure 9-8). Tube enterostomy is indicated for patients undergoing abdominal surgery who will require nutritional support. Every attempt should be made to feed into the small bowel in critically ill patients with gastroparesis or at significant risk of aspiration.

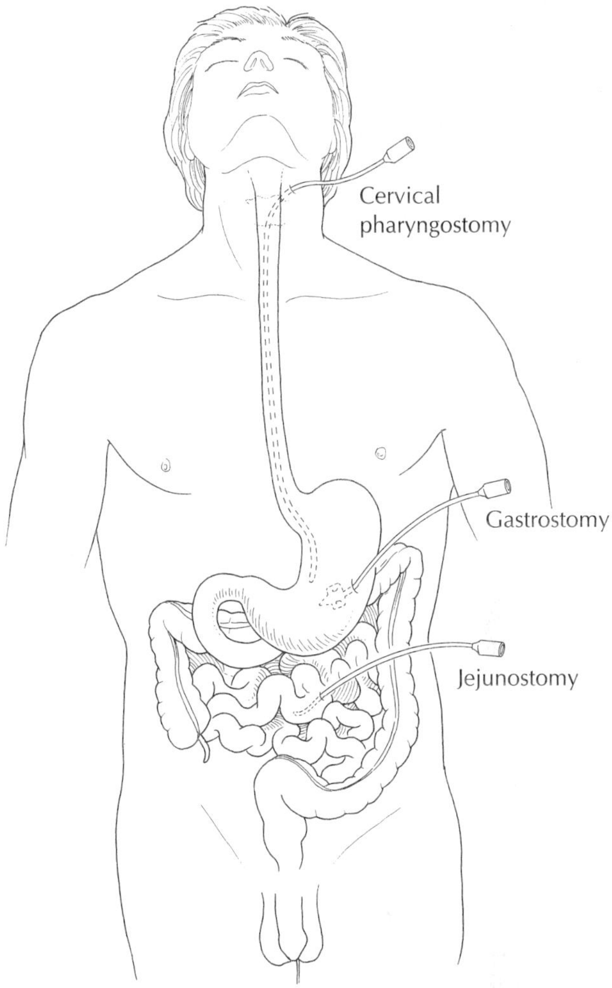

FIGURE 9-7 Sites for tube enterostomy. (Redrawn from Rombeau JL, Caldwell MD: *Clinical Nutrition* 1:276, 1984.)

Enteral Diet Formulas

Once the decision to provide EN is made, the proper formulation should be prescribed. For proper dietary formulation, it is necessary to understand the basic characteristics of diet formulations and to become familiar with the uses and limitations of at least one product in each category.

Several classifications of enteral diet formulations have been proposed.[145,261,309,325] Unfortunately, none is completely satsifactory. The following classifications are based on nutrient composition: (1) polymeric; (2) oligomeric; and (3) modular.

In general, dietary selection for a patient fed enterally is based on the GI tract's ability to digest and absorb major nutrients; on total nutrient requirements; and on fluid-electrolyte restrictions. A typical decision tree for selecting an initial dietary formula is depicted in Figure 9-9.

POLYMERIC DIETS. Polymeric formulas contain 100% of the Recommended Dietary Allowances (RDA) for vitamins and minerals when a total daily prescription of 2 L (on average) is administered. These diets are therefore called "complete" diets. These formulas can be further classified as blenderized whole foods, milk based, and lactose free. This discussion is limited to lactose-free diets, since whole food and mild-based products are rarely prescribed for surgical patients. In polymeric lactose-free formulas, nonprotein carbohydrate calories are provided as oligosaccharides, maltodextrins or polysaccharides, and fat calories as medium-chain triglycerides (MCT) or long-chain triglycerides (LCT) in soy, corn, sunflower, or MCT oil. The nitrogen source is a natural protein (egg, soy, or lactalbumin) that may be intact or partly hydrolyzed. These diets require the ability to digest protein, carbohydrate, and fat. Because polymeric diets are composed of high-molecular-weight compounds, their osmolarity is low. These preparations are relatively more palatable than oligomeric formulas and can be used for oral supplementation or tube feeding. Although more commonly used when feeding into the stomach, polymeric diets also are well tolerated when infused into the jejunum.[165] Most polymeric formulas contain 1 kcal/ml; however, several products have a caloric density of 1.5 to 2 kcal/ml, which is useful when water or sodium restriction is indicated. Polymeric solutions are the least expensive of the enteral formulations. The major disadvantage of these formulas is their fixed nutrient composition. They offer very little flexi-

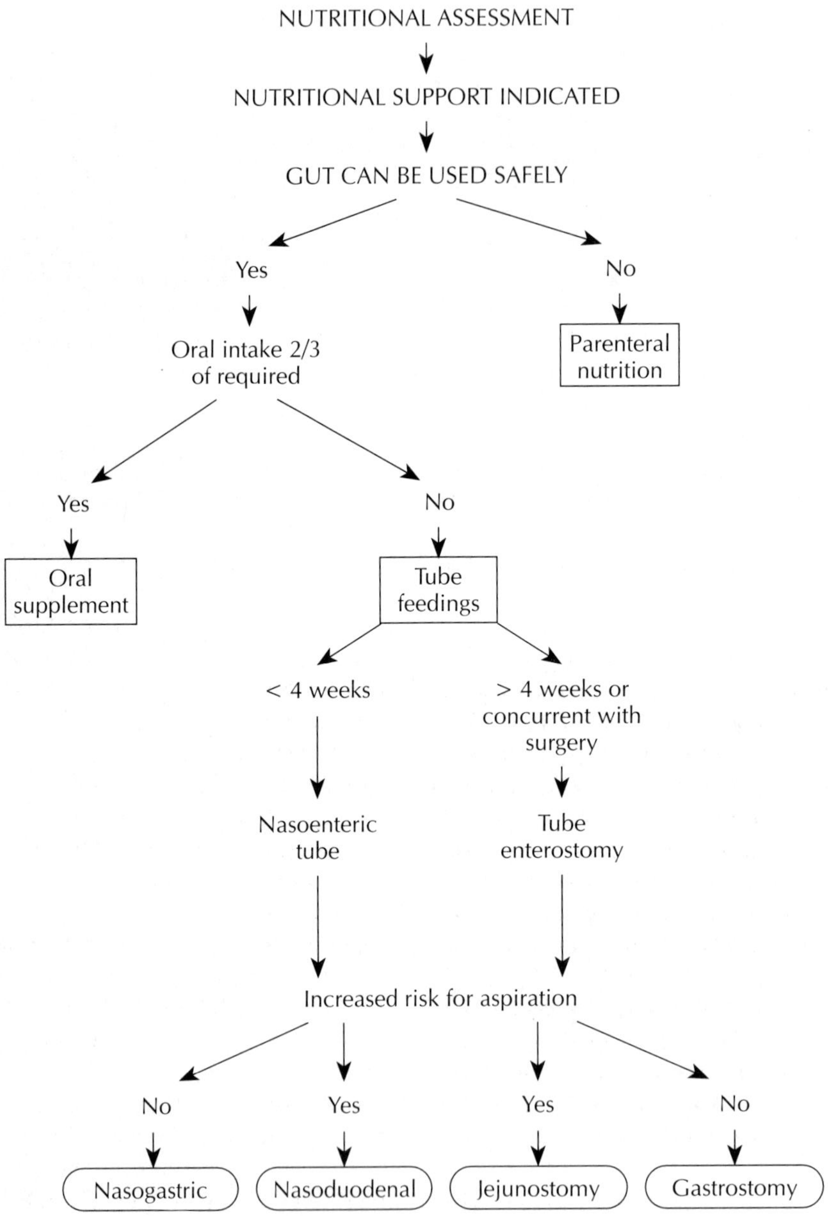

FIGURE 9-8 Decision tree for selecting an enteral nutrition access site. (From Koruda MJ, Geunter P, Rombeau JL: *Critical care clinics,* Philadelphia, 1987, WB Saunders.)

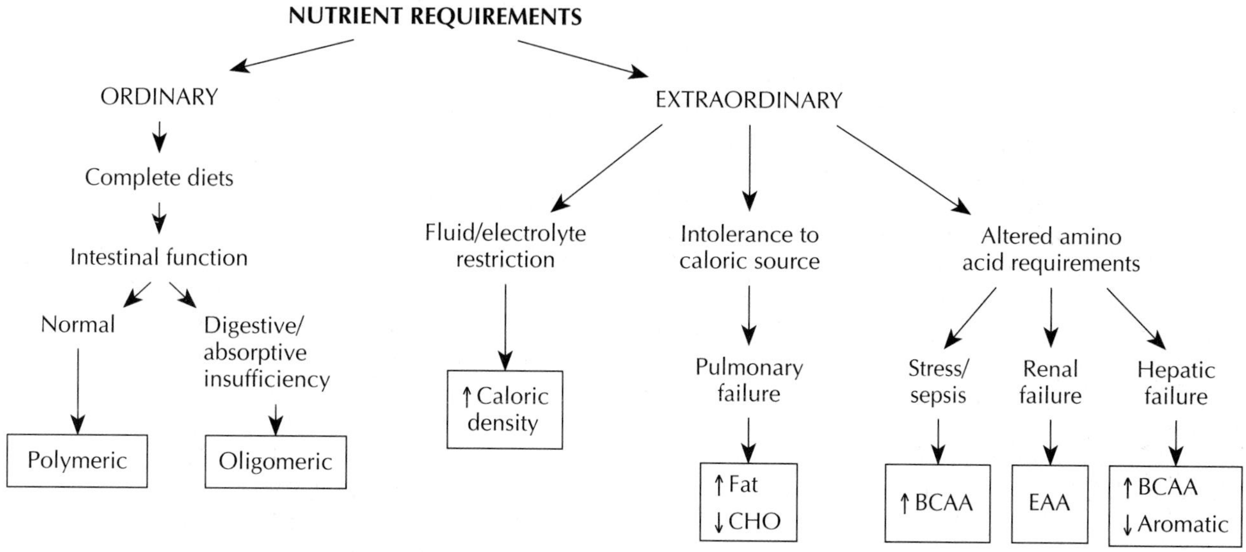

FIGURE 9-9 Decision tree for selecting an enteral diet. *CHO,* Carbohydrate; *BCAA,* branched-chain amino acid; *EEA,* essential amino acid. (From Koruda MJ, Geunter P, Rombeau JL: *Critical care clinics,* Philadelphia, 1987, WB Saunders.)

bility when adapting a formula to individual patient requirements.

A polymeric formula should be the first choice for oral supplementation or tube feeding when gastrointestinal digestion and absorption are intact. Polymeric diets are suitable for most patients.

OLIGOMERIC DIETS. Oligomeric diets are composed of elemental or nearly elemental nutrients that require minimal digestion, are almost completely absorbed, and leave little residue in the colon. These diets are more commonly referred to as "elemental" or "chemically defined" diets. Oligomeric diets contain either crystalline amino acids (elemental) or oligopeptides (dipeptides and tripeptides) and amino acids. The carbohydrate sources are oligosaccharides and disaccharides. The formulas contain variable amounts of fat (1% to 30%) as safflower or MCT oil. All essential minerals and vitamins are included, and they are therefore "complete."

Oligomeric diets require the digestion of both carbohydrate and fat; therefore some pancreatic enzyme activity is needed. Furthermore, mucosal transport systems for glucose, sodium, amino acids, fats, vitamins, and trace elements are necessary for absorption.[262]

The putative advantage of "peptide"-based enteral formulas is the greater ease of absorption of the dipeptide and tripeptide protein moiety. Before absorption, intact protein must be hydrolyzed to peptides or free amino acids. The rate-limiting step of protein assimilation lies in the carrier-specific mucosal absorption of individual amino acids. Dipeptides and tripeptides circumvent this step and are directly absorbed by the enterocyte. Although clinical studies have demonstrated increased absorption of dipeptide and tripeptide solutions,[219,223,311] there is a lack of data from prospective, randomized studies on the suitability and efficacy of enteral products containing oligopeptides.[145,236]

The disadvantages of oligomeric diets are their osmolarity, taste, and cost. As a group, these diets are relatively hyperosmolar, and if delivered too rapidly, osmotic diarrhea can ensue. These formulas are also unpalatable, making flavoring supplements necessary for oral use. Oligomeric diets are also significantly more expensive than their polymeric counterparts. To provide 2000 kcal/day for 10 days as a polymeric formula may cost $40 to $60, whereas to provide it as an oligomeric formula costs $200 to $250.[155]

These formulas are easily delivered by small-bore feeding tube. They may be useful when administered during periods of digestive or absorptive insufficiency, as during the transition stage of gut recovery following peritonitis, prolonged ileus, or major surgery and when polymeric diets are not tolerated.

MODULAR DIETS. Despite the availability of a variety of formulated enteral diets, the standard "fixed-ratio" formulas may not be optimal for some patients. The needs of these patients have spawned the development of modular nutrient systems. A module consists of single or multiple nutrients that can be either combined to produce a nutritionally "complete" diet or supplemented to existing fixed-ratio diets. Modular feeding permits more precise nutrient prescription, allowing the nutritionist to change the ratio of constituent nutrients without affecting the quantity of other constituents. The clinician can select not only the amount of each substrate, mineral, electrolyte, or vitamin component, but also the type of nutrients most appropriate for the patient (e.g., whole protein versus partly hydrolyzed protein versus crystalline amino acids). The major types of modules available for commercial use are carbohydrate, fat, and protein, as well as mineral, electrolyte, and vitamin. Modular feedings are indicated for patients with special nutrient requirements, such as in hepatic failure, renal failure, diabetes, cardiac failure, pulmonary insufficiency, short bowel syndrome, and acid-base or electrolyte disorders. The major disadvantages of modular feeding are increased labor, formula, and monitoring costs. Also, the potential is greater for both deficiency states (if one module is omitted) and metabolic complications. Modular feeding also requires advanced expertise.[208]

SPECIAL DIETS. Special formulas have been designed for use in disease states in which nutrient requirements are specifically altered. In three of these states (hepatic failure, renal failure, and trauma-sepsis), amino acid requirements appear to be altered and in another (pulmonary insufficiency), a particular caloric substrate profile may be indicated. Hence, formulations designed for these disease states can be considered either "special oligomeric" or "special modular" diets. The indications for use of these special formulations are considered in the section on Special Problems and Requirements.

Delivery Methods

Continuous feedings are preferred over bolus feedings in critically ill patients. Critically ill children receiving continuous rather than intermittent feedings show improved weight gain and greater positive nitrogen balance.[250] In adult burn patients, continuous feedings are associated with less stool frequency and a shorter time to achieve nutritional goals.[162] Patients with hemodynamic instability seem to better tolerate the same amount of feedings administered continuously rather than as a bolus. Continuous feedings are required when feeding into the duodenum or jejunum to avoid distention of the bowel, abnormal fluid and electrolyte shifts, and diarrhea.

The use of "starter regimens" when initiating diet administration has been controversial. It is common practice in many institutions for diet formulas to be diluted to one half to one fourth strength at the outset of diet administration. However, studies have repeatedly demonstrated the safe, efficacious use of full-strength isotonic to hypertonic formulas in a variety of patient groups without the use of starter regimens.* In fact, starter regimens have been shown to result in greater gastrointestinal complications and poorer nutritional outcome.[49] A reasonable approach is to start the selected formula at full strength and deliver continuously at 25 ml/hour. Over the first 12 to 24 hours, feeding tolerance is assessed. Poor tolerance is indicated by vomiting, abdominal cramps, abdominal distention, worsening of diarrhea, or gastric residual greater than 50% of the volume administered during the previous 4-hour period. If the feeding is tolerated, the rate is advanced by 25 ml/hour every 12 to 24 hours until the desired volume is attained. Evidence continues to mount that early institution of enteral nutrition in the course of the patient's illness directly improves tolerance.

Monitoring

Patients who receive enteral feedings require the same careful monitoring as those who receive parenteral nutrition. Critically ill patients commonly have overlying or secondary dysfunction of the gastrointestinal tract, which may result in intolerance to enteral diets. Daily evaluation is essential and includes an interview and physical examination, noting the presence of diarrhea, constipation, nausea, abdominal distention, or vomiting. Careful attention to the patient's metabolic status and fluid and electrolyte balance also is especially important. With consistent monitoring, potential complications can be averted in many cases by simple alterations, such as changing the infusion rate, caloric density, or formulation.

Periodic nutritional assessment is required to evaluate the adequacy of the nutritional support. It has been noted that hospitalized patients actually received only 69% to 87% of the calories that had been ordered.[4,110] Therefore, because surgical patients, for a variety of reasons, tend not to receive their prescribed amount of EN, it may need to be supplemented with parenteral feeding until satisfactory, consistent EN is attained.

Unfortunately, there is no optimum way to evaluate the adequacy of a patient's nutritional support. Body weight changes over ensuing weeks is useful. However, in the day-to-day management of a surgical patient, short-term changes in body weight reflect more the variations in fluid status than the direct result of nutritional intervention. Changes in the plasma concentrations of proteins with short half-lives, such as transferrin, retinol-binding protein, and transthyretin (prealbumin), are commonly used to test the adequacy of nutritional intervention. None of these is truly a sensitive or specific

*References 140, 176, 182, 221, 232, 265, and 366.

indicator of nutritional repletion, because each is subject to nonnutritional influences on synthesis and degradation.

Nitrogen balance is considered the most consistent and practical method for estimating the adequacy of nutrition support. A nitrogen balance assessment compares the amount of nitrogen a patient receives (generally 1 g of nitrogen for every 6.25 g of protein) with the amount of nitrogen lost (urine, stool, integument, drainage). Nitrogen intake can be determined readily from the patient's nutrient intake. Nitrogen output is determined from a 24-hour collection of urine that is best done after a patient has been on a stable nutritional regimen for 48 hours or longer. Total urinary nitrogen (TUN) or, more commonly, total urinary urea nitrogen (UUN) is then determined. Urinary urea nitrogen, however, may not be an accurate estimate of TUN in patients receiving nutrition support.[143] Other nitrogen losses (stool, drainage, integument) are then estimated. The calculation is as follows:

$N_{Balance} = N_{In} - N_{Out}$
N_{In} = g of amino acids or protein administered + 6.25
N_{Out} = TUN (g) + X g

Where TUN = UUN + 2 if UUN is measured, and X represents losses from skin and intestinal tract (X = 1 with no oral or enteral feeding and X = 2 with enteral feeding). In most situations the metabolic response to injury creates a hormonal milieu that does not permit attainment of positive nitrogen balance. In the management of most surgical patients, it is more realistic to strive to attain nitrogen equilibrium rather than positive nitrogen balance.

Complications

Complications of EN in the critically ill can be classified as gastrointestinal, metabolic, infectious, aspiration, and mechanical. Complications are common reasons to interrupt enteral feedings. Mechanical problems and gastrointestinal intolerance are the most common reasons for failing to attain desired enteral nutrition delivery.[4,68]

GASTROINTESTINAL COMPLICATIONS. Although gastrointestinal complications may occur in as many as 50% of critically ill patients receiving enteral nutrition, the vast majority of these patients will tolerate sufficient EN.[178]

Nausea and vomiting occur in about 10% to 20% of patients who are tube fed[160]; the causes include formula odor, rapid rate of infusion, formula fat content, lactose intolerance, high osmolality, and delayed gastric emptying.[39] Delayed gastric emptying is very common in surgical patients and is exacerbated by intra-abdominal sepsis, pancreatitis, peptic ulcer disease, skeletal trauma, laparotomy, head injury, myocardial infarction, hepatic coma, hypercalcemia, diabetes mellitus, myxedema, malnutrition, and a variety of medications. Gastric emptying may be improved with metoclopramide, especially in diabetic patients.[187]

Diarrhea is commonly considered a significant problem in the management of tube-fed patients and it is the conception of many that it is the limiting factor in supplying nutrients via the enteral route. As with many popular notions in medicine, the true prevalence of diarrhea in tube-fed patients is not clear. The inconsistency in the definition of diarrhea accounts for the great discrepancies in prevalence rates, ranging from a low of 2% to as high as 68% among critically ill patients.[154,180]

Diarrhea in a tube-fed patient may be caused by any number of agents. In many instances, however, several factors are involved, and it may be impossible to determine the exact cause of the diarrhea.

Bacterial contamination of the enteral products and their delivery systems formerly was a commonly recognized cause of diarrhea.[167,291,296,354] However, recently improved practices for administration of enteral formulas have dramatically lowered the incidence of diarrhea caused by diet contamination.

One commonly held misconception is that hyperosmolar feedings are major offenders predisposing to diarrhea. However, studies have repeatedly demonstrated the safe, efficacious use of full-strength isotonic to hypertonic formulas in a variety of patient groups without the use of starter regimens.*

Medication-related causes of diarrhea include the use of antibiotics, hyperosmolar drug solutions, certain antacids, and other medications that have a direct effect on gastrointestinal function. In a recent study, prospective determinations of the causes of diarrhea in a cohort of patients who were enterally fed were performed. Thirty-two episodes of diarrhea occured in 123 tube-fed patients. A single cause was found in 29 cases. The tube-feeding formula was responsible for diarrhea in only 21% of these cases. Medications were directly responsible in 61%, and *Clostridium difficile* in 17%. Stool osmotic gap correctly distinguished osmotic from non-osmotic diarrhea in all cases.[108] These authors made the eye-opening observation that the elixir medications commonly used in tube-fed patients contain varying amounts of sorbitol, amounts not listed on the package inserts. Theophylline preparations show a particular predilection for producing diarrhea. In a recent review of 20 consecutive patients receiving sorbitol-based theophylline elixer, 15 patients had diarrhea for 2 days or longer.[163] Commonly used medications (acetaminophen, theophylline, cimetidine) contain between 5% and 65% sorbitol in their elixir preparations, certainly enough to cause diarrhea with one dose.[155]

*References 140, 176, 182, 221, 265, and 283.

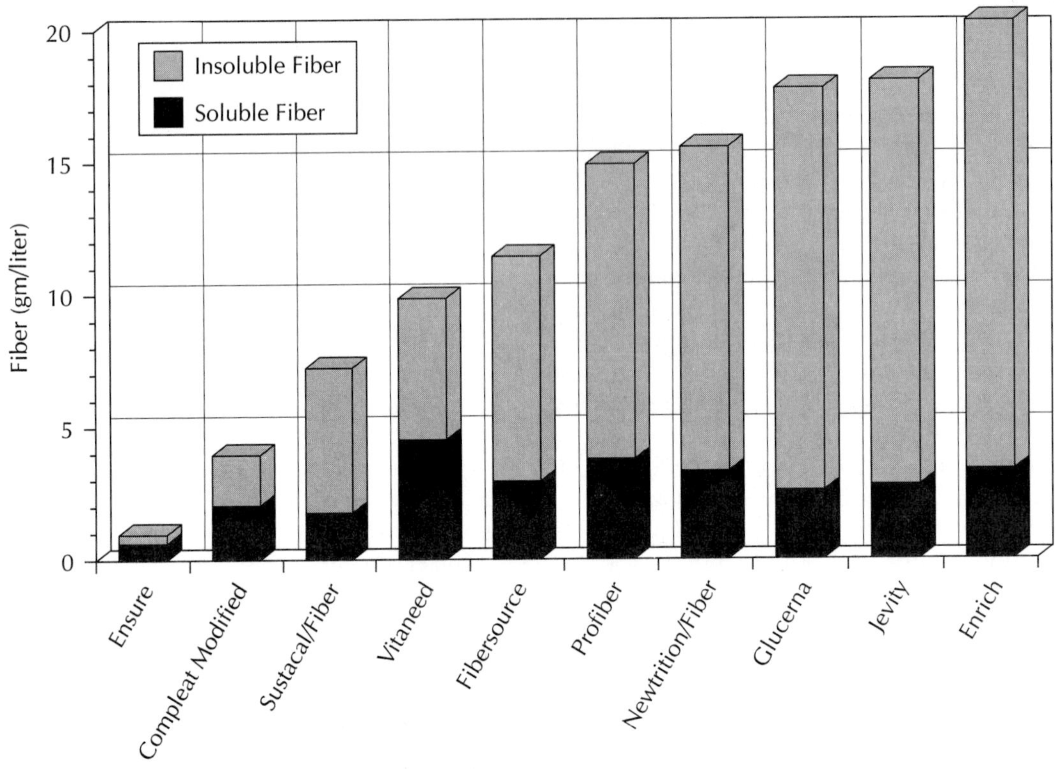

FIGURE 9-10 Soluble and insoluble fiber contents of "fiber-supplemented" enteral feeding formulas. Ensure, a formula that is not fiber supplemented, is included for comparison. (Adapted from Fredstrom S, Baglien K, Lampe J et al: *JPEN* 15:450, 1991.)

Liquid formula diets themselves may induce diarrhea, even in subjects with normal gastrointestinal function.[369] Although most patients have other predisposing factors, diarrhea may subside if EN is discontinued. This effect is particularly common in patients who have not received oral or enteral nutrients for several days. Intestinal atrophy could be the basis for refeeding diarrhea after starvation.[271] The small bowel loses villous height and stops producing brush border enzymes. Support for this concept lies in the widely held observation that enteral feedings are tolerated less well the longer enteral nutrition is delayed in a critically ill patient.[82,140,305]

As the primary site for fecal sodium and water absorption, the colon naturally determines final stool concentration and composition. It has been suggested that in some instances, the diarrhea associated with enteral feeding may result from altered colonic mucosal function. The use of fiber-deficient diets and the prescription of broad-spectrum antibiotics may alter the colonic microflora and hence the production of SCFAs. Diarrhea has also been more prevalent in enterally fed patients receiving antibiotics.[140,144,182] The relatively high incidence of diarrhea in patients undergoing concomitant antibiotic therapy could be due to the detrimental effect on the colonic microflora. A recent study has, in fact, demonstrated diminished fecal SCFA production in patients prescribed broad-spectrum antibiotics.[84] A reduction in SCFA synthesis or a change in their profile may impair sodium/water absorption and predispose to diarrhea. This hypothesis has been tested in a study of normal subjects who were fed, in a cross-over fashion, a fiber-free liquid formula diet with and without supplementation with 1% citrus pectin.[368] The pectin-free diet produced liquid stools with low SCFA content. Pectin supplementation normalized fecal SCFA concentration and stool consistency. However, applying this concept to critically ill patients has not been as successful. Several studies have not been able to demonstrate improvement of the stool output in ICU patients who are fed "fiber"-containing formulas.[100,121,144,153] The lack of demonstrable effect of these diets may result from the type of fiber used. The fiber sources in these studies contained a very small amount of soluble, readily fermentable fiber polysaccharides (Figure 9-10). Hence, with the administration of not readily fermentable fiber sources and the alteration of bacterial flora by the use of broad-spectrum antibiotics, it can be assumed that SCFA production may not have been significant enough to cause a physiologic effect on stool composition.

Hypoalbuminemia is frequently implicated as a cause

TABLE 9-12 CAUSES AND TREATMENT OF DIARRHEA WITH ENTERAL FEEDING

CAUSE	TREATMENT
Infectious	Review potential sources of contamination; treat gastrointestinal pathogens as confirmed
Dietary	
Hyperosmolar solutions	Dilute solutions or decrease volume infused
Lactose deficiency	Change enteral formula to lactose free type
Fat malabsorption	Change enteral formula to low-fat solution; give pancreatic enzymes
Protein malnutrition	Use isotonic solutions—consider oligomeric formula; supplement with parenteal nutrition; use antidiarrheal medication, such as loperamide (Imodium), diphenoxylate (Lomotil), or camphorated opium (Paregoric)
Drugs	Evaluate need for antibiotics
Antibiotics	Use antidiarrheal medication; *avoid* Imodium, Lomotil, Paregoric, and codeine; *use* Kaopectate of cholestyramine
Hyperosmolar electrolyte solutions and medications	Dilute medications; mix with enteral feedings or give parenterally; check for sorbitol-containing elixirs
Other medications (e.g., digoxin, Aldomet)	Antidiarrheal medications (Paregoric, Imodium, Lomotil)
Magnesium-containing antacids	Alternate with magnesium-free antacids

of diarrhea in critically ill patients who receive enteral feedings.[55] Hypoalbuminemia is common in hospitalized patients and usually reflects the degree and duration of hypermetabolism, as well as fluid shifts and plasma losses. The purported mechanism for hypoalbuminemia-induced diarrhea is a decrease in oncotic pressure that produces intestinal edema and either a secretory or a malabsorptive state. The transport of fluids across the capillary wall depends on the difference in hydrostatic and oncotic pressures. Plasma oncotic pressure is between 20 and 25 mm Hg, and albumin accounts for approximately 65% of this effect.

Gottschlich and coworkers[140] extensively investigated the incidence and causes of diarrhea in tube-fed burn patients; the overall incidence of diarrhea in this patient group was 32%. Hypoalbuminemia (less than 2 gm/dl) was present in more patients without diarrhea[21] than in patients with diarrhea[333], although this difference did not reach statistical significance. There is some evidence that correcting hypoalbuminemia with exogenous albumin may improve dietary tolerance in a hypoalbuminemic patient.[119] Several studies have demonstrated success in using peptide-based formulas to avoid diarrhea in tube-fed, hypoalbuminemic, critically ill patients.[55,56] However, in a larger, prospective, randomized study conducted on critically ill, hypoalbuminemic patients, no significant tolerance or nutritional advantage was obtained with a peptide-based formula compared to a standard polymeric formula.[236] The hypothesis of hypoalbuminemia-induced diarrhea in patients still awaits confirmation.

Treatment for diarrhea depends on its cause (Table 9-12). A thorough workup of its possible cause or causes is essential, and should not be automatically discontinued. Nearly 50% of patients with diarrhea associated with EN can be adequately treated by correcting dietary factors.[68]

METABOLIC COMPLICATIONS. The metabolic complications of EN are common in the critically ill and usually can be managed easily when patients are properly monitored. These complications include abnormalities in fluid balance, glucose metabolism, electrolytes, and protein tolerance.[39]

ASPIRATION. A potentially fatal complication of EN, a witnessed episode of aspiration, is an important confirmation of its occurrence. Its prevalence varies from 1% to 44%.* The influence of different feeding methods and sites on aspiration has not been studied in a controlled manner. Standard clinical teaching is that the likelihood of aspiration can be decreased in patients fed beyond the pylorus, but this has not been substantiated in clinical trials. In a recent prospective study of the incidence of aspiration pneumonia among patients receiving enteral nutrition, only 12 of 276 patients (4.4%) experienced aspiration pneumonia.[237] Risk factors for aspiration were determined to be increasing age, and location in the hospital (ICU patients had only a 0.9% rate, compared to 4.9% for medical or surgical wards, $p < 0.05$). Interestingly, there was not statistical difference in the incidence of aspiration among patients with nasoenteric (3.8%), gastrostomy (5.6%), or jejunostomy (5.6%) sites of feeding. This study confirms that aspiration is not an inevitable consequence of severe illness; rather, it can be prevented with adequate nursing care and pulmonary precautions.

Every attempt should be made to have transpyloric feeding tubes passed into the fourth portion of the duodenum to the left of the midline as close to or past the

*References 68, 237, 330, 336, and 360.

ligament of Treitz. Preventive measures to decrease the risk of aspiration include elevating the head of the bed to 30 degrees, periodic measuring of gastric residuals, and inflating endotracheal tube cuffs.[330] Methods for detecting the "silent" aspiration of enteral formulas in intubated patients include checking tracheal aspirates for glucose with glucose-oxidant reagent strips or placing methylene blue dye in the formula and monitoring the tracheal aspirates.[339,360]

MECHANICAL COMPLICATIONS. Any mechanical complications associated with EN are generally related to the tube itself or its anatomic position. Nasoenteric tubes cause nasopharyngeal erosions and discomfort, sinusitis, otitis media, gagging, esophagitis, esophageal reflux, tracheoesophageal fistulae, and rupture of esophageal varices.[39] The tubes can become knotted or clogged. Gastrostomy or jejunostomy tubes can cause obstruction of the pylorus or small bowel. Several recent reports have noted the near-epidemic passage of nasoenteric tubes to anatomic areas outside the gastrointestinal tract, such as the submucosa of the pharynx and the pleural space, with subsequent esophageal perforation, pneumothorax, empyema, pulmonary hemorrhage, and even death.* Risk factors for pulmonary complications related to the passage of nasoenteric feeding tubes include endotracheal intubation or tracheostomy, altered mental status, and the experience of the operator.

Despite these reports, small-bore feeding tubes can be passed safely in most patients. In patients who are at high risk of aspiration or who have undergone previous gastric surgery (such as gastroenterostomy), feeding tubes can be placed distally and more safely with the aid of fluoroscopy or endoscopy.

Special Problems and Requirements

High Branched-Chain Amino Acid (BCAA) Solutions

The hormonal response to stress (trauma, burn, sepsis) promotes early, increased proteolysis and hydrolysis of BCAAs (leucine, isolucine, valine) in skeletal muscle. This process leads to irreversible combustion of BCAAs, which the skeletal muscle oxidizes for energy, making other amino acids (alanine and glutamine) available for gluconeogenesis, enzyme synthesis, wound healing, and immune function.[303] Exogenous administration of BCAAs, as part of total parenteral nutrition or special enteral diets has been proposed to compensate for the altered protein metabolism and blood amino acid levels in a stressed patient; the twin goals are to reduce catabolism of skeletal muscle and increase protein synthesis. Solutions containing 40% to 50% of the branched-chain amino acids are now available.

The enteral diets formulated for use in stressed patients are also high in BCAAs (44% to 50% of total amino acids, compared to 25% to 33% in standard polymeric or oligometric formulas). Nonprotein calories are provided as carbohydrate (maltodextrins) and fat (MCT and soy oil) at a calorie/nitrogen ratio of 80 to 100:1 (compared to about 150:1 for standard formulas). These diets have a caloric density of 1 to 1.2 kcal/ml, are very hyperosmolar (675 to 910 mOsm/kg water), and are expensive.

Numerous clinical studies have examined the effect of administering BCAAs to critically ill patients.[331] The results are controversial. Well-done randomized, prospective, controlled studies have demonstrated that BCAA-enriched formulas improve nitrogen retention, visceral protein status, and glucose homeostasis in moderately to severely stressed patients. No significant improvement in morbidity, length of hospital stay, or mortality has been demonstrated. Therefore, use of these products should be restricted to highly catabolic patients, as documented by markedly negative nitrogen balance, increasing BUN, or intolerance to standard diets.

Acute Renal Failure

Patients with renal failure are unable to excrete the end products of nitrogen metabolism, primarily urea. Urea is generated from dietary amino acids or protein and from endogenous protein. The generation of urea can be partly modulated by nutrient intake: decreasing dietary nitrogen intake decreases urea production, and providing calories limits the breakdown of endogenous protein and hence lowers urea generation. In general, the goal in nutritional management of critically ill patients with renal failure is to optimize energy balance but avoid symptoms of uremia, volume overload, and metabolic complications.

BUN reflects the balance between urea production and excretion and therefore serves as an indicator of the quantity and quality of amino acids that should be given. Obviously, if urea production exceeds its excretion, BUN rises; conversely, when excretion exceeds production, BUN falls. In general, BUN should not be higher than 100 mg/dl. As BUN rises, the quantity of amino acids in the nutrient solution should be reduced.

The specialized amino acid formulas for renal failure contain essential amino acids as the nitrogen source. The enteral diets are lactose free, contain few or no electrolytes or vitamins, and are hyperosmolar. They can be used as oral supplements but are not very palatable.

In theory, by supplying only essential amino acids, urea production is decreased by recycling nitrogen into the synthesis of nonessential amino acids. In clinical trials these products have not shown clinical superiority over products containing essential and nonessential amino acids.[45,103,227] Although these products do not en-

*References 22, 26, 66, 152, 203, 280, 294, and 295.

hance survival or improvement in renal function, dialysis requirements may be reduced. Because of the lack of demonstrable clinical efficacy and the high cost of these formulas, it is recommended that renal failure formulations be used only during the course of *acute* renal failure when attempting to avoid dialysis or to decrease dialysis requirements.

Hepatic Failure and Hepatic Encephalopathy

Hepatic dysfunction in the ICU ranges from the abnormalities seen in liver function test results for a patient with postoperative sepsis to the overt signs of liver failure in a patient with end-stage cirrhosis who has jaundice, ascites, gastrointestinal bleeding, and severe wasting. Most patients with chronic liver disease who are in stable condition can tolerate dietary protein administered at 1 to 1.5 g/kg/day. Anorexia, nausea, and vomiting may preclude enteral feedings in patients who have acute alcoholic hepatitis. In these patients parenteral nutrition has been associated with improved survival.[126]

Protein intake must be altered in patients with advanced hepatic failure and impending encephalopathy. In general, amino acids given intravenously are better tolerated than the equivalent quantity of enteral protein. These patients have elevated blood levels of the aromatic amino acids and low levels of BCAAs.[171] Possible therapeutic approaches in the nutritional management of these patients are to reduce the quantity of dietary amino acids to 20 to 40 g/day or to administer special amino acid solutions designed to correct the altered concentrations of blood amino acids. The specialized formulas for hepatic encephalopathy contain large amounts of BCAAs and small amounts of the aromatic amino acids and methionine. Critical analysis of the prospective, randomized studies evaluating the efficacy of intravenous hepatic formulations in patients with hepatic encephalopathy suggests that these diets have a beneficial effect on the resolution of encephalopathy and nutritional status and perhaps even help improve survival.[78,239,345] It is recommended that these preparations be restricted to patients who exhibit hepatic encephalopathy and that they not be used in those with nonencephalopathic manifestations of liver disease.

Pulmonary Insufficiency

The typical problem-weaning patient is a patient recovering from severe catabolic illness with respiratory failure who is malnourished and shows residual impairment of gas exchange and marginal ventilatory mechanics. Many factors make up the work of breathing and contribute collectively to failure to wean from mechanical ventilation (Figure 9-11).[36] Such patients require optimum nutritional and metabolic attention. For example, untreated metabolic acidosis necessitates a greater minute ventilation, which may exceed the pa-

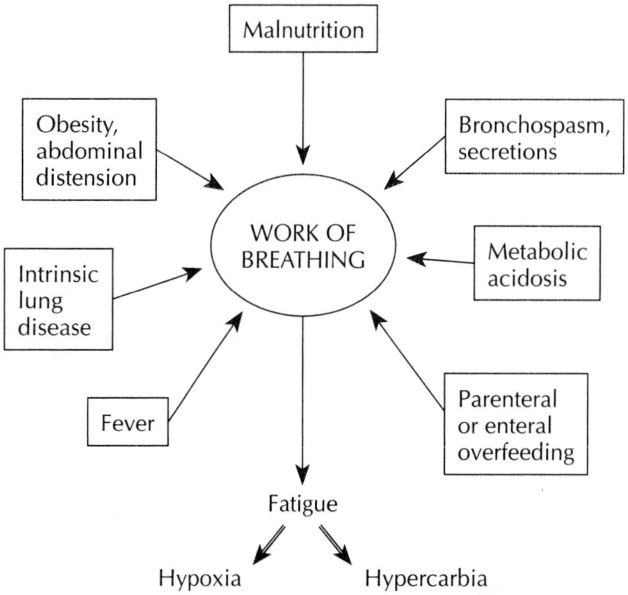

FIGURE 9-11 Summary of the factors that contribute collectively to the work of breathing in a critically ill patient recovering from respiratory failure. (From Benotti P, Bistrian B: *Crit Care Med* 17:181, 1989.)

tient's ventilatory reserve capacity. Metabolic alkalosis reduces oxygen delivery and causes compensatory hypercapnia. Hypophosphatemia and hypomagnesemia are associated with abnormal function of the respiratory muscles.[216,240]

Nutrition is an important consideration for a critically ill patient with respiratory insufficiency, because maintaining nutritional status is associated with enhanced ability to wean patients from ventilatory support.[92,197] High-carbohydrate diets, either parenteral or enteral, and overfeeding have been shown to increase the production of carbon dioxide, oxygen consumption, and ventilatory requirements[24,131,161,343] (Figure 9-12). Glucose infusion rates greater than its maximum oxidation rate (5 to 7 mg/kg/minute) result in net glycogen and fat synthesis and rather dramatic increases in CO_2 production and respiratory quotient (RQ) (Figure 9-13).[60a] In patients with compromised pulmonary function, these sequelae can precipitate respiratory failure or complicate weaning from mechanical ventilation.[24,58] The complete oxidation of fat produces less carbon dioxide than either glucose or protein on a per calorie basis. Replacing carbohydrate calories with fat calories in enteral or parenteral feeding has reduced CO_2 production, oxygen consumption, and minute ventilation.[13,129,161]

Nutritional management of patients with pulmonary compromise should be individualized. Initially, energy requirements should be reassessed to avoid feeding excessive calories; this can be done by providing maintenance or even by reducing calories to provide only 80% to 90% of maintenance. Glucose/carbohydrate dosing should be adjusted to 4 to 5 g/kg/day to prevent carbohydrate-driven increases in RQ. In patients receiving EN, formulas with a high percentage of carbohydrate calories should not be prescribed (e.g., Vivonex TEN [82%]; Precision HN [88%]; Precision LR [89%]; Criticare HN [83%]; Vital [74%]). Most polymeric formulas have about 50% of their total calories as carbohydrates and 30% as fat. For a severely compromised patient being fed enterally, products with a particularly high non-protein-calorie fat/carbohydrate ratio may be beneficial (e.g., Traumacal [49% fat, 51% carbohydrate]; Pulmocare [66% fat, 34% carbohydrate]; Nutrivent [68% fat, 32% carbohydrate]). Alternatively, the caloric distribution of "fixed-ratio" formulas can be modified by adding fat and protein modules.

For patients receiving TPN, providing 60% to 70% of energy requirements as carbohydrate and 30% to 40% as lipid suffices in most cases. In practice, the increment in carbon dioxide output (V_{CO_2}) from an RQ of 0.7 (all fat) to 1 (all carbohydrate) is only 25% and thus is not likely to be of major consequence in the patient to be weaned. More important, it is during *overfeeding*, when the RQ exceeds 1 (net lipogenesis), that substantial increases in V_{CO_2} become clinically important.[351,364]

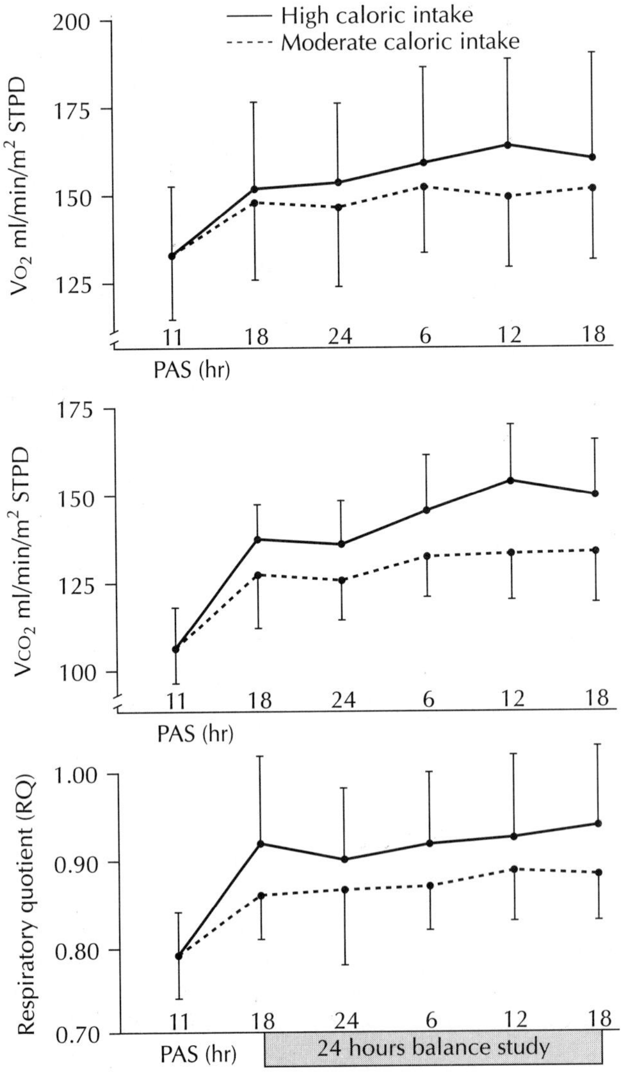

FIGURE 9-12 Volume of oxygen consumed (V_{O_2}), carbon dioxide output (V_{CO_2}), and respiratory quotient (RQ) of nine patients in a postabsorptive state (PAS) during high caloric intake (2 × resting energy expenditure [REE]) and during moderate caloric intake (1.5 × REE). *STPD*, Standard temperature and pressure, dry. (From Van den Berg B, Stam H: *Intensive Care Med* 14:206, 1988.)

Nutrients with Potential Special Applications

Glutamine

Glutamine is classically considered a nonessential amino acid. It is absent from all commercially available parenteral nutrient formulations because of its short shelf life, and it is present as the free amino acid in only a few enteral products. In catabolic states, glutamine concentrations fall rapidly in intracellular pools (mostly skeletal muscle), because glutamine is used for renal ammoniagenesis and serves as an energy substrate for lymphocytes and macrophages.[20] Glutamine is the major source of respiratory fuel for the intestine,[359] and its uptake by the splanchnic bed significantly increases in both animal models and clinical stress states.[220,319] In animal studies, parenteral or enteral supplementation with glutamine stimulated mucosal growth,[169,247,318] enhanced healing of radiation-induced intestinal injury,[188] augmented mucosal immune function,[15,60] and improved survival and reduced bacterial translocation in experimental enteritis.[120]

In clinical studies, glutamine infusions restored the marked fall in muscle glutamine that is associated with injury, and it possibly improves nitrogen balance.[148,326] Wilmore and associates[358] recently reported the effect of glutamine-supplemented parenteral nutrition after bone marrow transplantation.[367] Patients receiving glutamine-supplemented TPN showed improved nitrogen balance, a diminished incidence of clinical infection, and lower rates of microbial colonization and had a shorter hospital stay compared with patients receiving standard TPN.

Further clinical trials are necessary to define the role of glutamine in nutrition support more completely. However, there is mounting evidence that glutamine should be considered a conditionally essential amino acid during certain disease states.[196]

Nutritional Modulation of Immune Function[71]

Although the relationship between malnutrition and susceptibility to infection has been known for decades, short-term, aggressive nutritional repletion has not consistently demonstrated improved clinical outcome. Recent research has not only identified the immunologic deficits that arise as a result of malnutrition, it has also demonstrated that certain components of traditional enteral and parenteral formulations adversely affect immune function, whereas other nutrients may enhance immunologic responses. Specifically, attention currently is focused on the immunostimulatory effects of the amino acid arginine, the omega-3 fatty acid family, and

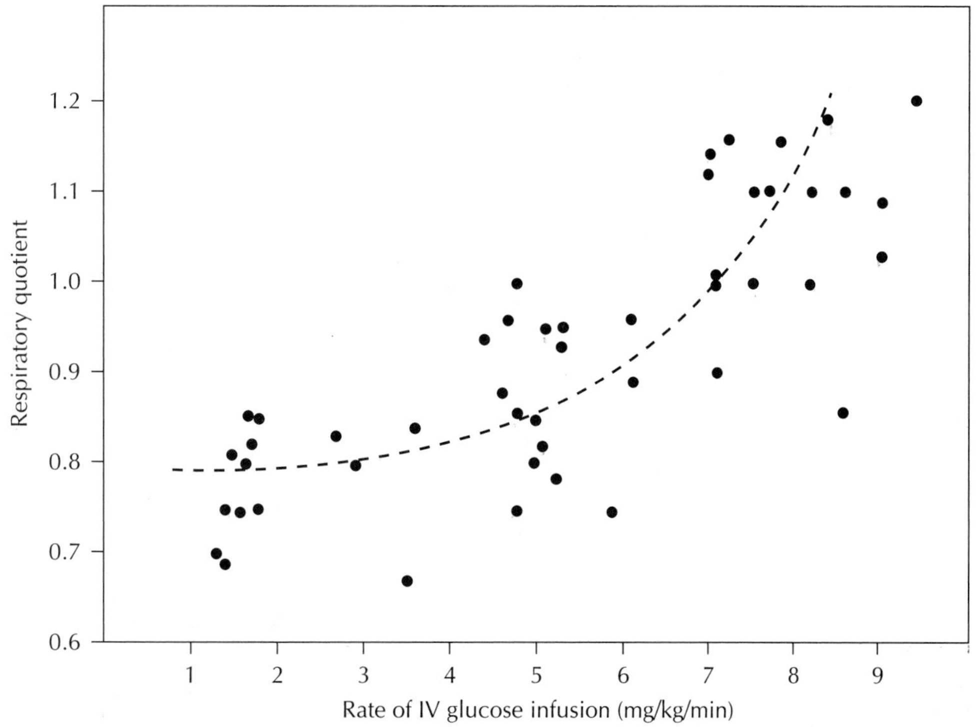

FIGURE 9-13 Respiratory quotient (RQ) as a function of the glucose infusion rate (mg/kg/minute) in 47 observations of 18 severely burned patients. (From Burke J, Wolfe R, Mullany C et al: *Ann Surg* 190:279, 1979.)

ribonucleic acids. Although broadly considered nutrients, these components are more appropriately considered pharmacologic agents for immune stimulation.

Arginine is a semiessential amino acid that is obtained from dietary sources and endogenous synthesis via the urea cycle. It is essential for normal tissue growth, is necessary for collagen synthesis, and has important effects on host defense mechanisms. In animal models, arginine supplementation has promoted wound healing and enhanced T-cell function.[27,29,30,302] In a clinical study, arginine supplementation for postoperative cancer patients enhanced in vitro lymphocyte blastogenesis and increased the percentage of T-helper lymphocytes.[91] In subsequent studies, 30 g of arginine given orally for only 3 days has increased the circulating natural killer (NK) and leukocyte-activated killer (LAK) cells and their respective cytotoxicities in healthy volunteers[249] and women with breast cancer.[57]

Lipids are not only recognized as a caloric source but also as substrates that have profound effects on immune function. Significant components of traditional enteral and parenteral lipid formulations are the omega-6 polyunsaturated fatty acids (PUFA). The omega-6 PUFA are ultimately metabolized to 2-series prostanoids and 4-series leukotrienes. Of the prostanoids, prostaglandin E_2 (PGE_2) may be the most important. High concentrations of PGE_2 are immunosuppressive, inhibiting T-cell mitogenesis, the production of lymphokines, and the generation of cytotoxic cells. On the other hand, omega-3 PUFA are metabolized to 3-series prostanoids and 5-series leukotrienes, which are intrinsically less immunosuppressive.[52] Dietary strategy for lipid supplementation has focused on limiting administration of omega-6 PUFA and replacing them with the less immunosuppressive omega-3 PUFA. A significant reduction in dietary omega-6 PUFA appears to be prudent in the diet of immune-compromised, posttraumatic, postoperative, or infected patients.[183]

Dietary nucleotides are not only important components of DNA and RNA, they are also important regulators of the immune response. Traditional parenteral and enteral nutrition products do not contain nucleotides. Diets lacking nucleotides have resulted in suppression of many aspects of immune function,[193,194,342] which has been reversed with RNA supplementation.[258]

Recently enteral diets designed as immunostimulants have been formulated incorporating some of the above concepts. The Shriner's burn diet is supplemented with 2% arginine, and half of its fat calories are supplied as fish oil (rich in omega-3 fatty acids). This diet has been shown to reduce infections, complications, mortality, and length of hospital stay for burned patients.[8,229] The commercial formula Impact (Sandoz Nutrition, Minneapolis, Minn.) is supplemented with arginine, fish oil, and yeast RNA. A prospective, randomized study of 85 patients who underwent surgery for upper gastrointestinal malignancies suggested that use of Impact improved immunologic, metabolic, and clinical outcomes compared with a standard enteral formula.[89] A third commercially available formula, Immun-Aid (McGaw, Irvine, Calif.), is supplemented not only with arginine, RNA, and omega-3 fatty acids (canola oil), but also glutamine and branched-chain amino acids. This product is currently undergoing clinical trials. Although application of the principles of nutritional immune modulation shows exciting promise in the management of high-risk, critically ill patients, clinical studies substantiating the efficacy of these products are still lacking, and therefore broad application of these regimens cannot be endorsed.

SUMMARY

In the past two decades, nutritional support has rapidly become an integral part of the medical care of hospitalized patients. Parenteral nutrition has been the pri-

ESSENTIALS OF NUTRITIONAL SUPPORT

Five Basic Steps of Nutritional Support

1. Prevent malnutrition.
2. Establish energy goals.
3. Select, establish, and maintain feeding access.
4. Choose and design the optimum formula.
5. Monitor the patient to ensure safe and effective results.[157]

Memory Aids: KCALS and FACE MTV

- K - Keep the patient nourished
- C - Calculate the energy and protein goals
- A - Access
- L - List (or think about) the components of the formula and choose amounts best suited for the patient as follows:
  - F - Fluids: Should fluids be restricted?
  - A - Amino acids/protein: Are special formulas indicated?
  - C - Calories: What are the goals and what is the most appropriate mix of carbohydrate and fat calories?
  - E - Electrolytes: Are there special electrolyte considerations?
  - M - Miscellaneous: Should heparin, insulin, or other substances be added?
  - T - Trace elements: Are standard amounts adequate?
  - V - Vitamins: Are standard amounts adequate?
- S - Special monitoring to ensure safe and effective nutrition support

mary mode of delivering nutrients to these patients, but interest has been renewed in using enteral nutrition in the management of the critically ill. This stems from the improvements in formulas and equipment for nutrient delivery and a better understanding of the importance of maintaining the barrier function of the gastrointestinal epithelium. Malabsorption and ileus, highly prevalent in the critically ill, may restrict the use of enteral nutrition in these patients. Parenteral and enteral nutrition often are given concurrently. Small volumes of enteral diets can be prescribed to patients receiving primarily parenteral nutrition to reduce intestinal atrophy. Parenteral nutrition should supplement an inadequate enteral regimen. Complications should be minimized with careful patient assessment, re-assessment, and monitoring through an established protocol.

In a surgical patient, the issue of total nutrient intake, enteral or parenteral, is crucial. Providing insufficient calories allows excessive catabolism; providing excess calories creates added cardiopulmonary stress. Also, the amounts of carbohydrate, fat, amino acids, or protein needed to meet nutrient requirements are important (see the box at left).

REFERENCES

1 Abel RM, Abbott WM, Fischer JE: Acute renal failure: treatment without dialysis with total parenteral nutrition, *Arch Surg* 103:513, 1972.

2 Abel RM, Abbott WM, Fischer JE: Intravenous essential L-amino acids and hypertonic dextrose in patients with acute renal failure: effects on serum potassium, phosphate, and magnesium, *Am J Surg* 123:632, 1972.

3 Abel RM, Beck CH Jr, Abbott WM et al: Improved renal failure after treatment with intravenous essential L-amino acids and glucose: results of a prospective double-blind study, *N Engl J Med* 288:695, 1973.

4 Abernathy G, Heizer W, Holcombe B et al: Efficacy of tube feeding in supplying energy requirements of hospitalized patients, *JPEN* 13:387, 1989.

5 Abumrad NN, Schneider AJ, Steel DR et al: Aquired molybdenum deficiency, *Clin Res* 27:774A, 1979 (abstract).

6 Adams S, Dellinger EP, Wertz MJ et al: Enteral versus parenteral nutritional support following laparotomy for trauma: a prospective trial, *J Trauma* 26:882, 1986.

7 Aguirre A, Yoshimura N, Westman T et al: Plasma amino acids in dogs with two experimental forms of liver damage, *J Surg Res* 16:339, 1974.

8 Alexander JW, Gottschlich MM: Nutritional immunomodulation in burn patients, *Crit Care Med* 18:S149, 1990.

9 Alexander JW, Macmillan B, Stinnet J: Beneficial effects of aggressive protein feeding in severely burned children, *Surgery* 192:505, 1980.

10 Allardyce DB: Cholestasis caused by lipid emulsions, *Surg Gynecol Obstet* 154:641, 1982.

11 Allen J: The incidence of nosocomial infection in patients receiving total parenteral nutrition. In Johnson IDA, editor: *Advances in parenteral nutrition,* Lancaster, Mich, 1978, MTP Press.

12 Al-Naffusi A, Wright N: The effect of epidermal growth factor (EGF) on cell proliferation of the gastrointestinal mucosa in rodents, *Virchows Arch B Cell Pathol* 40:63, 1982.

13 Al-Saady N, Blackmore C, Bennett E: High-fat, low-carbohydrate, enteral feeding lowers Pa_{CO_2} and reduces the period of ventilation in artificially ventilated patients, *Intensive Care Med* 15:290, 1989.

14 Altay C, Say B, Dogramaci N et al: Nitroblue tetrazolium test in children with malnutrition, *J Pediatr* 81(2):392, 1972.

15 Alverdy JC: Effects of glutamine-supplemented diets on immunology of the gut, *JPEN* 14:185, 1990.

16 Alverdy JC, Aoys E, Moss G: Total parenteral nutrition promotes bacterial translocation from the gut, *Surgery* 104:1988.

17 Amdur MO, Norris LC, Heuser GF: The lipotrophic action of manganese, *J Biol Chem* 164:783, 1946.

18 Anderson GH, Patel DG, Jeejeebhoy KN: Design and evaluation by nitrogen balance and blood aminograms of an amino acid mixture for total parenteral nutrition of adults with gastrointestinal disease, *J Clin Invest* 53:904, 1974.

19 Antonacci A, Cowles S, Reaves L: The role of nutrition in immunologic function, *Infect Surg* 3:590, 1984.

20 Ardawi M: Glutamine and glucose metabolism in human peripheral lymphocytes, *Metabolism* 37:99, 1988.

21 Argov Z, Maris J, Damico L et al: Continuous, graded steady-state muscle work in rats studied by in vivo 31P-NMR, *J Appl Physiol* 63:1428, 1987.

22 Aronchik J, Epstein D, Gefter W: Pneumothorax as a complication of placement of a nasoenteric tube, *JAMA* 252:3207, 1984.

23 Askanazi J, Carpentier YA, Elwyn DH et al: Influence of total parenteral nutrition on fuel utilization in injury and sepsis, *Ann Surg* 191:40, 1980.

24 Askanazi J, Nordenstrom J, Rosenbaum S: Nutrition for the patient with respiratory failure: glucose versus fat, *Anesthesiology* 54:373, 1981.

25 Bagby GJ, Spitzer JA: Lipoprotein lipase activity in rat heart and adipose tissue during endotoxic shock, *Am J Physiol* 238:H325, 1980.

26 Balogh G, Adler S, Vanderwandi J: Pneumothorax as a complication of feeding tube placement, *Am J Roentgenol* 141:1275, 1983.

27 Barbul A: Arginine and immune function, *Nutrition* 6:53, 1990.

28 Barbul A: Arginine biochemistry, physiology, and therapeutic implications, *JPEN* 10:227, 1986.

29 Barbul A, Fishel R, Shimazu S et al: Intravenous hyperalimentation with high arginine levels improves wound healing and immune function, *J Surg Res* 38:328, 1985.

30 Barbul A, Wasserkrug H, Seifter E et al: Immunostimulatory effects of arginine in normal and injured rats, *J Surg Res* 29:228, 1980.

31 Barton RG, Cerra FB: The hypermetabolism organ failure syndrome, *Chest* 95:1153, 1989.

32 Beisel WR: Metabolic response to infection. In Kinney JM, Jeejeebhoy KN, Hill GL, Owen OE, editors: *Nutrition and metabolism in patient care,* Philadelphia, 1988, WB Saunders.

33 Bell LT, Hurley LS: Ultrastructural effects of manganese deficiency in liver, heart, kidney, and pancreas of mice, *Lab Invest* 29:723, 1973.

34 Bell RG, Hazell LA: Influence of dietary protein restriction on immune competence: effect on the capacity of cells from various lymphoid organs to induce graft-vs-host reactions, *J Exp Med* 141:127, 1975.

35 Benditt EP, Wissler RW, Woolridge: Loss of body protein and antibody production by rats on low-protein diets, *Proc Soc Exp Biol Med* 70:240, 1949.

36 Benotti P, Bistrian B: Metabolic and nutritional aspects of weaning from mechanical ventilation, *Crit Care Med* 17:181, 1989.

37 Berg R: Promotion of the translocation of enteric bacilli from the gastrointestinal tracts of mice by oral treatment with peni-

cillin, clindamycin, or metronidazole, *Infect Immun* 33:854, 1981.
38 Bergstrom J et al: Intravenous nutrition with amino acid solutions in patients with chronic uremia, *Acta Med Scand* 191:368, 1972.
39 Bernard M, Forlaw L: Complications and their prevention. In Rombeau J, Caldwell M, editors: *Clinical nutrition.* Vol 1. *Enteral and tube feeding,* Philadelphia, 1984, WB Saunders.
40 Billiar TR, Bankey PE, Svingen BA et al: Fatty acid intake and Kupffer cell function: fish oil alters eicosanoid and monokine production to endotoxin stimulation, *Surgery* 104:343, 1988.
41 Bistrian BR: A simple technique to estimate severity of stress, *Surg Gynecol Obstet* 148:675, 1979.
42 Bivins BA, Bryant PJ, Record KE et al: The effect of ten and twenty percent safflower oil emulsion given as thirty to fifty percent of total calories, *Surg Gynecol Obstet* 156:433, 1983.
43 Black PR, Brooks DC, Bessey PQ et al: Mechanisms of insulin resistance following injury, *Ann Surg* 196:420, 1982.
44 Blackburn GL, Bistrian BR, Maini BS et al: Nutritional and metabolic assessment of the hospitalized patient, *JPEN* 1:11,1977.
45 Blackburn GL, Etter G, Mackenzie T: Criteria for choosing amino acid therapy in acute renal failure, *Am J Clin Nutr* 31:1841, 1978.
46 Bodey G: Antibiotic prophylaxis in cancer patients: regimens of oral, nonabsorbable antibiotics for prevention of infection during induction of remission, *Rev Infect Dis* 3(suppl):S259, 1981.
47 Borah MF, Schoenfeld PY, Gotch FA et al: Nitrogen balance during intermittent dialysis therapy of uremia, *Kidney Int* 14:491, 1978.
48 Border J, Hassett J, LaDuca J: The gut-origin septic states in blunt multiple trauma (ISS 40) in the ICU, *Ann Surg* 206:427, 1987.
49 Borlase BC, Bell SJ: Tolerance to enteral tube feeding diets in hypoalbuminemic critically ill geriatric patients: a prospective, randomized trial, *Surg Gynecol Obstet* 174:181, 1992.
50 Bounous G: Acute necrosis of the intestinal mucosa, *Gastroenterology,* 82:1457, 1982.
51 Bourgeois B, Schmidt BJ, Bourgeois R: Some aspects of catecholamines in undernutrition. In Gardner LI, Amacher P, editors: *Endocrine aspects of malnutrition,* Santa Ynez, Calif, 1973, The KROC Foundation.
52 Bower RH: Nutrition and immune function, *Nutr Clin Pract* 5:189, 1990.
53 Bower RH, Fischer JE: Hepatic indications for parenteral nutrition. In Rombeau JL, Caldwell MD, editors: *Parenteral nutrition,* Philadelphia, 1986, WB Saunders.
54 Bozetti F, Terno G, Bonfanti G et al: Prevention and treatment of central venous catheter sepsis by exchange via a guidewire, *Ann Surg* 198:48, 1983.
55 Brinson R, Curtis W, Singh M: Diarrhea in the intensive care unit: the role of hypoalbuminemia and the response to a chemically defined diet (case reports and review of the literature), *J Am Coll Nutr* 6:517, 1987.
56 Brinson R, Kolts B: Diarrhea associated with severe hypoalbuminemia: a comparison of a peptide-based, chemically defined diet and standard enteral alimentation, *Crit Care Med* 16:130, 1988.
57 Brittenden J, Park K, Hayes P et al: Effect of arginine on natural cytotoxicity in cancer patients and healthy volunteers, *Br J Surg* 79:A442, 1992.
58 Brown R, Heizer W: Nutrition and respiratory disease, *Clin Pharm* 3:152, 1984.
59 Bruce DL, Wingard DW: Anesthesia and the immune response, *Anesthesiology* 34:271, 1971.
60 Burke D, Alverdy J, Aoys E et al: Glutamine-supplemented total parenteral nutrition improves gut immune function, *Arch Surg* 124:1396, 1989.
60a Burke J, Wolfe R, Mullany C et al: Parameters of optimal glucose infusion and possible hepatic and respiratory abnormalities following excessive glucose intake, *Ann Surg* 190:279, 1979.
61 Buse MG, Reid M: Leucine, a possible regulator of protein turnover in muscle, *J Clin Invest* 58:1251, 1975.
62 Buzby GP: Prognostic nutritional index in gastrointestinal surgery, *Am J Surg* 139:160, 1980.
63 Cahill GF: Starvation in man, *N Engl J Med* 282(12):668, 1970.
64 Cannon PR: Antibodies and the protein reserves, *J Immunol* 44:107, 1942.
65 Cannon PR, Humphreys EM, Wissler RW, Frazier LE: Chemical, clinical, and immunological studies on the products of human plasma fractionation: the effects of feeding possible blood substitutes on serum protein regeneration and weight recovery in the hypoproteinemic rat, *J Clin Invest* 23:601, 1944.
66 Carey TS, Holcombe BJ: Endotracheal intubation as a risk factor for complications of nasoenteric tube insertion, *Crit Care Med* 19:427, 1991.
67 Carmon M, Seror R, Udassin R et al: Feeding jejunostomy for postoperative nutritional support, *Clin Nutr* 10:298, 1991.
68 Cataldi-Belcher E, Seltzer M, Slocum B: Complications occurring during enteral nutrition support: a prospective study, *JPEN* 7:546, 1983.
69 Cerra FB: How nutrition intervention changes what getting sick means, *JPEN* 14(5 suppl):164S, 1990.
70 Cerra FB: Hypermetabolism, organ failure, and metabolic support, *Surgery* 101:1, 1987.
71 Cerra FB: Immune system modulation: nutritional and pharmacologic approaches, *Crit Care Med* 18(2 suppl):585, 1990.
72 Cerra FB: Multiple organ failure: clinical trade-offs. In Lumb PD, Shoemaker WC, editors: *Critical care: state of the art,* Fullerton, Calif, 1990, Society of Critical Care Medicine.
73 Cerra FB: Nutrient modulation of inflammatory and immune function, *Am J Surg* 161:230, 1991.
74 Cerra FB: The syndrome of multiple organ failure. In Bihari D, Cerra FB, editors: *New horizon series: cell injury and organ failure,* Fullerton, Calif, 1988, Society of Critical Care Medicine.
75 Cerra FB: The systemic septic response: concepts of pathogenesis, *J Trauma* 30(12 suppl):5169, 1990.
76 Cerra FB, Alden PA, Negro F et al: Clinical sepsis, endogenous and exogenous lipid metabolism, *JPEN* 12:63S, 1988.
77 Cerra FB, Cheung NK, Fischer JE et al: Disease-specific amino acid infusion (F080) in hepatic encephalopathy: a prospective, randomized, double-blind, controlled trial, *JPEN* 9:288, 1985.
78 Cerra FB, Cheung NK, Fischer J: A multicenter trial of branched chain–enriched amino acid infusion (F080) in hepatic encephalopathy, *Hepatology* 2:699, 1982.
79 Cerra FB, Holman RT, Bankey PE et al: n-s PUFA as modulators of cell function in the critically ill, *Pharmacotherapy* 11:71, 1991.
80 Cerra FB, Holman RT, Bankey PE et al: Nutritional pharmacology: its role in the hypermetabolism–organ failure syndrome, *Crit Care Med* 18:S154, 1990.
81 Chazan JA, Boshell BR: Etiological factors in thiazide-induced or aggravated diabetes mellitus, *Diabetes* 14:132, 1965.
82 Chiarelli A, Enzi G, Casadei A et al: Very early nutrition supplementation in burned patients, *Am J Clin Nutr* 51:1035, 1990.
83 Christie D, Ament M: A double-blind cross-over study of metraclopromide vs placebo for facilitating passage of multipurpose biopsy tube, *Gastroenterology* 71:726, 1976.
84 Clausen M, Bonnen H, Tvede M et al: Colonic fermentation to short-chain fatty acids is decreased in antibiotic-associated diarrhea, *Gastroenterology* 101:1497, 1991.
85 Clowes GHA, O'Donnel TF, Blackburn GL et al: Energy metabolism and proteolysis in traumatized and septic man. In Clowes GHA, editor: Response to infection and injury, *Surg Clin North Am* 56:1169, 1976.

86 Cook JA, Halushka PV: Arachidonic acid metabolism in septic shock. In Bihari D, Cerra FB, editors: *New horizons: multiple organ failure,* Fullerton, Calif, 1989, Society of Critical Care Medicine.
87 Cummings J, Branch W: Fermentation and the production of short-chain fatty acids in the human large intestine. In Vahouny G, Kritchevsky D, editors: *Dietary fiber: basic and clinical aspects.* New York, 1986, Plenum.
88 Daly JM, Copeland EM, Dudrick SJ: Intravenous hyperalimentation: effect on immunocompetence in cancer patients, *Ann Surg* 192:587, 1980.
89 Daly JM, Lieberman MD, Goldfine J et al: Enteral nutrition with supplemental arginine, RNA, and omega-3 fatty acids in patients after operation: immunologic, metabolic, and clinical outcome, *Surgery* 112:56, 1992.
90 Daly JM, Reynolds J, Sigal RK et al: Effect of dietary protein and amino acids on immune function, *Crit Care Med* 18:S86, 1990.
91 Daly JM, Reynolds J, Thom AK et al: Immune and metabolic effects of arginine in the surgical patient, *Ann Surg* 208:512, 1988.
92 Deital M, Williams V, Rice T: Nutrition and the patient requiring ventilatory support, *J Am Coll Nutr* 2:25, 1983.
93 Deitch E, Berg R: Bacterial translocation from the gut: a mechanism of infection, *J Burn Care Rehabil* 8:475, 1987.
94 Deitch E, Berg R, Specian R: Endotoxin promotes the translocation of bacteria from the gut, *Arch Surg* 122:185, 1987.
95 Deitch E, Bridges R: Effect of stress and trauma on bacterial translocation from the gut, *J Surg Res* 42:536, 1987.
96 Deitch E, Maejima K, Berg R: Effect of oral antibiotics and bacterial overgrowth on the translocation of the GI tract microflora in burned rats, *J Trauma* 25:385, 1985.
97 Deitch E, Winterton J, Li M: The gut as a portal of entry for bacteremia: role of protein malnutrition, *Ann Surg* 205:681, 1987.
98 Department of Health, Education, and Welfare: The ten state nutrition survey, 1968-1970, Pub no (HSM) 72-8130 to 72-8134, Atlanta, 1972, Centers for Disease Control.
99 Dionigi R, Zonta A, Dominioni L et al: The effects of total parenteral nutrition on immunodepression due to malnutrition, *Ann Surg* 185(4):467, 1977.
100 Dobb G, Towler S: Diarrhoea during enteral feeding in the critically ill: a comparison of feeds with or without fiber, *Intensive Care Med* 16:252, 1990.
101 Doisy EA Jr: Micronutrient controls on biosynthesis of clotting proteins and cholesterol, *Trace Sub Environ Health* 6:193, 1972.
102 Druml W, Widhalm K, Laggner A et al: Fat elimination in acute renal failure, *Clin Nutr* 1:109, 1982.
103 Dudrick SJ, Steiger E, Long J: Renal failure in surgical patients: treatment with intravenous essential amino acids and hypertonic glucose, *Surgery* 68:180, 1970.
104 Dudrick SJ, Vars HM, Rawnsley HM, Rhoads JE: Total parenteral feeding and growth in puppies, *Fed Proc* 25:481, 1966.
105 Dudrick SJ, Wilmore DW, Vars HM, Rhoads JE: Can intravenous feeding as a sole means of nutrition support growth in the child and restore weight loss in an adult? An affirmative answer, *Ann Surg* 169:974, 1969.
106 Durant TM, Long J, Oppenheimer MJ: Pulmonary (venous) air embolism, *Am Heart J* 33:269, 1947.
107 Ecknauer R, Sircar B, Johnson L: Effect of dietary bulk on small intestinal morphology and cell renewal in the rat, *Gastroenterology* 81:781, 1961.
108 Edes T, Walk B, Austin J: Diarrhea in tube-fed patients: feeding formula not necessarily the cause, *Am J Med* 88:91, 1990.
109 Eigler N, Sacca L, Sherwin RS: Synergistic interactions of physiologic investment of glucagon, epinephrine, and cortisol in the dog: a model for stress-induced hyperglycemia, *J Clin Invest* 631:114, 1979.
110 Evans D, DiSipio M, Barot L: Comparison of gastric and jejunal tube feedings, *JPEN* 4:79, 1980.
111 Everson GJ, Shrader RE: Abnormal glucose tolerance in manganese-deficient guinea pigs, *J Nutr* 94:89, 1968.
112 Faintuch J, Machado MCC, Bove P et al: Essential fatty acid deficiency during parenteral hyperalimentation, *Int Surg* 62:243, 1977.
113 Faist E, Mewes A, Baker CC et al: PGE_2-dependent suppression of interleukin in trauma patients, *J Trauma* 27:837, 1987.
114 Feinstein EI: Nutrition in acute renal failure. In Rombeau JL, Caldwell MD, editors: *Parenteral nutrition,* Philadelphia, 1986, WB Saunders.
115 Felig P, Owen OE, Wahren J, Cahill GF: Amino acid metabolism during prolonged starvation, *J Clin Invest* 48:584, 1969.
116 Fernandes G, Nair M, Kazunori O et al: Impairment of cell-mediated immunity functions by dietary zinc deficiency in mice, *Proc Natl Acad Sci* 76:457, 1979.
117 Fiaccadori F, Ghinelli F, Pedretti G et al: Branched chain amino acid–enriched solutions in the treatment of hepatic encephalopathy: a controlled trial. In Capocaccia L, Fischer JE, Rossi-Fanelli F, editors: *Hepatic encephalopathy in chronic liver failure,* New York, 1984, Plenum.
118 Flanagan JP, Gradisar IA, Gross RJ, Kelly TR: Air embolus: a lethal complication of subclavian puncture, *N Engl J Med* 281:488, 1969.
119 Ford E, Jennings M, Andrassy R: Serum albumin (oncotic pressure) correlates with enteral feeding tolerance in the pediatric surgical patient, *J Pediatr Surg* 22:597, 1987.
120 Fox AD, Kripke SA, DePaula J et al: Effect of a glutamine-supplemented enteral diet on methotrexate-induced enterocolitis, *JPEN* 12:325, 1988.
121 Frankenfield D, Beyer P: Soy-polysaccharide fiber: effect on diarrhea in tube-fed, head-injured patients, *Am J Clin Nutr* 50:533, 1989.
122 Fraser CL, Arieff AI: Hepatic encephalopathy, *N Engl J Med* 313:865, 1985.
123 Freund HR: Parenteral nutrition in the septic patient. In Rombeau JL, Caldwell MD, editors: *Clinical nutrition.* Vol 2. *Parenteral nutrition,* Philadelphia, 1986, WB Saunders.
124 Freund HR, Fischer JE: Comparative study of parenteral nutrition in renal failure using essential and nonessential amino acid containing solutions, *Surg Gynecol Obstet* 151:652, 1980.
125 Fulks RM, Li JB, Goldberg AL: Effects of insulin, glucose and amino acids on protein turnover in rat diaphragm, *J Biol Chem* 250:280, 1975.
126 Galambos J, Hersh J, Fulenwider J: Hyperalimentation in alcoholic hepatitis, *Am J Gastroenterol* 72:535, 1979.
127 Gamelli RL, Costanza MC, Foster RS Jr: The effect of protein depletion on bone marrow myeloid cell repopulation, *J Surg Res* 32:264, 1982.
128 Gardner LT, Talbot NB, Cook CD et al: The effect of potassium deficiency on carbohydrate metabolism, *J Lab Clin Med* 35:592, 1950.
129 Garfinkel F, Robinson S, Price C: Replacing carbohydrate calories with fat calories in enteral feeding for patients with impaired respiratory function, *JPEN* 9:106, 1985.
130 Gelfand RA, Hendler RG, Sherwin RS: Dietary carbohydrate and metabolism of ingested protein, *Lancet* 1:65, 1979.
131 Gieseke T, Gurushanthaiah G, Glauser F: Effects of carbohydrates on carbon dioxide excretion in patients with airway disease, *Chest* 71:55, 1977.
132 Giordano C: Use of exogenous and endogenous urea for protein synthesis in normal and uremic subjects, *J Lab Clin Med* 62:231, 1963.
133 Giovanetti S, Maggiore Q: A low-nitrogen diet with proteins of high biological value for severe chronic uremia, *Lancet* 1:1000, 1964.

134 Glazier WB, Silen W: Acute potassium deficit: its relationship to polyuria in the postoperative period, *Arch Surg* 112:1165, 1977.

135 Gluud C, Dejgaard A, Hardt F et al and the Copenhagen Coma Group: Preliminary results of treatment with balanced amino acid infusion in patients with hepatic encephalopathy, *Scand J Gastroenterol Suppl* 18:19, 1983.

136 Gokal R, Millard PR, Weatherall DJ et al: Iron metabolism in haemodialysis patients, *Q J Med* 191:369, 1979.

137 Golden P: Glucose intolerance with hypokalemia, *Diabetes* 22:544, 1973.

138 Goodgame JT, Lowry SF, Brennan MF: Essential fatty acid deficiency in total parenteral nutrition: time course of development and suggestions for therapy, *Surgery* 84:271, 1978.

139 Gordon JE, Scrimshaw NS: Infectious disease in the malnourished, *Med Clin North Am* 54(6):1495, 1970.

140 Gottschlich M, Warden G, Michel M et al: Diarrhea in tube-fed burn patients: incidence, etiology, nutritional impact, and prevention, *JPEN* 12:338, 1988.

141 Grant JP: *Handbook of total parenteral nutrition,* Philadelphia, 1980, WB Saunders.

142 Green R, Charlton RW, Seftel H et al: Body iron excretion in man: a collaborative study, *Am J Med* 45:336, 1968.

143 Grimble G, West M, Acuti A et al: Assessment of automated chemiluminescence nitrogen analyzer for routine use in clinical nutrition, *JPEN* 12:100, 1988.

144 Guenter P, Settle R, Perlmutter S et al: Tube feeding–related diarrhea in acutely ill patients, *JPEN* 15:277, 1991.

145 Guidelines for the scientific review of enteral food products for special medical purposes, *JPEN* 15:137S, 1991.

146 Guidelines for essential trace elements, preparation for parenteral use: a statement by an expert panel, *JAMA* 241(19):2051, 1979.

147 Gump FE, Long CL, Geiger JW et al: The significance of altered gluconeogenesis in surgical catabolism, *J Trauma* 15:704, 1975.

148 Hammarqvist F, Wernermen J, Ali R et al: Addition of glutamine to total parenteral nutrition after elective abdominal surgery spares free glutamine in muscle, counteracts the fall in muscle protein synthesis, and improves nitrogen balance, *Ann Surg* 209:455, 1989.

149 Hammer-Hodges D, Woodruff P, Cuevas P: Role of the intraintestinal gram-negative bacterial flora in response to major injury, *Surg Gynecol Obstet* 138:599, 1974.

150 Harvey KB, Moldawer LL, Bistrian BR et al: Biological measures for the formulation of a hospital prognostic index, *Am J Clin Nutr* 34:2013, 1981.

151 Harris JA, Benedict FG: Biometric studies of basal metabolism in man, Carnegie Institute of Washington, Pub no 279, 1919.

152 Harris MR, Huseby JS: Pulmonary complications from nasoenteral feeding tube insertion in an intensive care unit: incidence and prevention, *Crit Care Med* 17:917, 1989.

153 Hart GK, Dobb GJ: Effect of a fecal bulking agent on diarrhea during enteral feeding in the critically ill, *JPEN* 12:465, 1988.

154 Heimburger D: Diarrhea with enteral feeding: Will the real cause please stand up? *Am J Med* 88:89, 1990.

155 Heimburger D, Weisner R: Guidelines for evaluating and categorizing enteral feeding formulas according to therapeutic equivalence, *JPEN* 9:61, 1985.

156 Heird WC, Winters RW: Total parenteral nutrition: the state of the art, *J Pediatr* 86:2, 1975.

157 Heizer WD, Holcombe B: Approach to the patient requiring nutritional supplementation. In Yamada T, editor: *Textbook of gastroenterology,* Philadelphia, 1991, JB Lippincott.

158 Henriques V, Anderson AC: Uber parenterale Ernahrung durch intravenose injektion, *Hoppe Syeler's Z Physiol Chem* 88:357, 1913.

159 Hensle TE, Blackburn GL, O'Donnell TF et al: Intravenous feeding in hepatic failure, *Surg Forum* 24:388, 1973.

160 Heymsfield S, Bethel R, Ansley J: Enteral hyperalimentation: an alternative to central venous hyperalimentation, *Ann Intern Med* 90:63, 1979.

161 Heymsfield S, Head C, McManus C: Respiratory, cardiovascular, and metabolic effects of enteral hyperalimentation: influence of formula dose and composition, *Am J Clin Nutr* 40:116, 1984.

162 Hiebert J, Brown A, Anderson R et al: Comparison of continuous vs intermittent tube feedings in adult burn patients, *JPEN* 5:73, 1981.

163 Hill D, Henderson L, McClain C: Osmotic diarrhea induced by sugar-free theophylline solution in critically ill patients, *JPEN* 15:332, 1991.

164 Hill M: Factors affecting bacterial metabolism. In Hill M, editor: *Microbial metabolism in the digestive tract,* Boca Raton, Fla, 1986, CRC Press.

165 Hindsdale J, Lipkowitz G, Pollock T: Prolonged enteral nutrition in malnourished patients with nonelemental feeding, *Am J Surg* 149:334, 1985.

166 Hiyama DT, Fischer JE: Nutritional support in hepatic failure: the current role of disease-specific therapy. In Fischer JE, editor: *Total parenteral nutrition,* ed 2, Boston, 1991, Little, Brown.

167 Hosteller C, Lipman T, Geraghty M: Bacterial safety of reconstituted continuous drip tube feeding, *JPEN* 6:232, 1982.

168 Hunt PS, Trotter S: Lymphocyte response after surgery and blood transfusion, *J Surg Res* 21:57, 1976.

169 Hwang TL, O'Dwyer ST, Smith RJ et al: Preservation of small-bowel mucosa using glutamine-enriched parenteral nutrition, *Forum on Fundamental Surgical Problems* 37:56, 1986.

170 Jacobson S, Christenson I, Kager L et al: Utilization and metabolic effects of a conventional and a single-solution regimen in postoperative total parenteral nutrition, *Am J Clin Nutr* 34:1402, 1981.

171 James J, Ziparo V, Jeppsson B: Hyperammonaemia, plasma amino acid imbalance, and blood-brain amino acid transport: a unified theory of portal-systemic encephalopathy, *Lancet* 2:772, 1979.

172 Jarrett F, Balish L, Moylan J: Clinical experience with prophylactic antibiotic bowel suppression in burn patients, *Surgery* 83:523, 1978.

173 Jeejeebhoy KN, Anderson GH, Nakhooda AF et al: Metabolic studies in total parenteral nutrition with lipid in man, *J Clin Invest* 57:125, 1976.

174 Jeejeebhoy KN, Langer B, Tsallas G et al: Total parenteral nutrition at home: studies in patients surviving four months to five years, *Gastroenterology* 71:943, 1976.

175 Johnson L: Regulation of gastrointestinal growth. In Johnson L, editor: *Physiology of the gastrointestinal tract,* New York, 1987, Raven.

176 Jones B, Lees R, Andrews J: Comparison of an elemental and polymeric enteral diet in patients with normal gastrointestinal function, *Gut* 24:78, 1983.

177 Jones IG, Pickens PT: Diabetes mellitus following oral diuretics, *Practitioner* 199:209, 1967.

178 Jones TN, Moore FA, Moore EE: Gastrointestinal symptoms attributed to jejunostomy feeding after major abdominal trauma: a critical analysis, *Crit Care Med* 17:1146, 1989.

179 Juan D: The causes and consequences of hypophosphatemia, *Surg Gynecol Obstet* 153:589, 1981.

180 Kelly T, Patrick M, Hillman K: Study of diarrhea in critically ill patients, *Crit Care Med* 11:7, 1983.

181 Keohane PP, Attrill H, Northover J et al: Effect of catheter tunnelling and a nutrition nurse on catheter sepsis during parenteral nutrition: a controlled trial, *Lancet* 2:1388, 1983.

182 Keohane PP, Attrill H, Love M: Relation between osmolality of diet and gastrointestinal side effects in enteral nutrition, *Br Med J* 288:678, 1984.

183 Kinsella J, Lokesh B: Dietary lipids, eicosanoids, and the immune system, *Crit Care Med* 18:S94, 1990.
184 Kinsella J, Lokesh B, Broughton S et al: Dietary PUFA and eicosanoids: potential effects on the modulation of inflammatory and immune cells: an overview, *Nutrition* 6:42, 1990.
185 Kirby DF, Clifton GL, Turner H et al: Early enteral nutrition after brain injury by percutaneous endoscopic gastrojejunostomy, *JPEN* 15:298, 1991.
186 Kispert PH: Glucocorticoids enhance acute phase protein synthesis in a Kupffer cell–hepatocyte coculture model, *Surg Forum* 42:34, 1991.
187 Kittinger JW, Sandler RS, Heizer WD: Efficacy of metoclopramide as an adjunct to duodenal placement of small-bore feeding tubes: a randomized, placebo-controlled, double-blind study, *JPEN* 11:33, 1987.
188 Klimberg V, Souba W, Dolson D et al: Prophylactic glutamine protects the intestinal mucosa from radiation injury, *Cancer* 66:62, 1990.
189 Knowles R, Prielipp R, Ward K et al: Peptide-based enteral nutrition is superior to parenteral nutrition and elemental enteral nutrition following hemorrhagic hypotension, *Anesthesiology* 71:A164, 1989.
190 Kudsk KA, Carpenter G, Peterson S et al: Effect of enteral and parenteral feeding in malnourished rats with hemoglobin–*E. coli* adjuvant peritonitis, *J Surg Res* 31:105, 1981.
191 Kudsk KA, Croce MA, Fabian TC et al: Enteral versus parenteral feeding: effects on septic morbidity after blunt and penetrating abdominal trauma, *Ann Surg* 215:503, 1992.
192 Kudsk KA, Stone J, Carpenter G et al: Enteral and parenteral feeding influences mortality after hemoglobin–*E. coli* peritonitis in normal rats, *J Trauma* 23:605, 1983.
193 Kulkari S, Bhateley D, Zander A et al: Functional impairment of T lymphocytes in mouse radiation chimeras by a nucleotide-free diet, *Exp Hematol* 12:694, 1984.
194 Kulkarni AD, Fanslow WC, Rudolph FB et al: Modulation of delayed hypersensitivity in mice by dietary nucleotide restriction, *Transplantation* 44:847, 1987.
195 Kulkarni AD, Fanslow WC, Rudolph FB et al: Effect of dietary nucleotides on response to bacterial infections, *JPEN* 10:169, 1986.
196 Lacey JM, Wilmore DW: Is glutamine a conditionally essential amino acid? *Nutr Rev* 48:297, 1990.
197 Larca L, Greenbaum D: Effectiveness of intensive nutritional regimens in patients who fail to wean from mechanical ventilation, *Crit Care Med* 10:297, 1982.
198 LaVia MF, Barker PA, Wissler RW: A study of the correlation of antigen phagocytosis and the splenic histologic reaction with antibody formation in protein-depleted rats, *J Lab Clin Med* 48(2):237, 1956.
199 Law DK, Dudrick SJ, Abdou NI: The effect of dietary protein depletion immunocompetence: the importance of nutritional repletion prior to immunologic induction, *Ann Surg* 179:168, 1974.
200 Leach RM Jr, Liburn MS: Manganese metabolism and its function, *World Rev Nutr Diet* 32:123, 1978.
201 Levine G, Deren J, Steiger E: Role of oral intake in maintenance of gut mass and disaccharide activity, *Gastroenterology* 67:975, 1974.
202 Li S: Acute renal failure. In Fischer JE, editor: *Total parenteral nutrition,* ed 2, Boston, 1991, Little, Brown.
203 Lind LJ, Wallace DH: Submucosal passage of nasogastric tube complicating attempted intubation during anesthesia, *Anesthesiology* 49(2):145, 1978.
204 Long CL: Metabolic response to injury and illness: estimation of energy and protein needs from indirect calorimetry and nitrogen balance, *JPEN* 3:452, 1979.
205 Long CL, Kinney JL, Geiger JW: Nonsuppressibility of gluconeogenesis by glucose in septic patients, *Metabolism* 25:193, 1976.
206 Long JM III, Wilmore DW, Mason AD Jr et al: Effect of carbohydrate and fat intake on nitrogen excretion during total intravenous feeding, *Ann Surg* 185:417, 1977.
207 Lowry SF, Brennan MF: Abnormal liver function during parenteral nutrition: relation to infusion excess, *J Surg Res* 26:300, 1979.
208 Macburney M, Jacobs K, Apelgren K: Modular feeding. In Rombeau J, Caldwell M, editors: *Clinical nutrition.* Vol 1. *Enteral and tube feeding,* Philadelphia, 1984, WB Saunders.
209 MacFadyen BR Jr, Stanley JD, Baquero G et al: Clinical and biological changes in liver function during intravenous hyperalimentation, *JPEN* 3:438, 1979.
210 Madden HP, Breslin RJ, Wasserkrug BA et al: Stimulation of T-cell immunity by arginine enhances survival in peritonitis, *J Surg Res* 44:658, 1988.
211 Madoff RD, Sharpe SM, Fath JJ et al: Prolonged surgical intensive care, *Arch Surg* 120:698, 1985.
212 Maejima K, Deitch E, Berg R: Bacterial translocation from the gastrointestinal tracts of rats receiving thermal injury, *Infect Immun* 43:6, 1984.
213 Maejima K, Deitch E, Berg R: Promotion by burn stress of the translocation of bacteria from the gastrointestinal tracts of mice, *Arch Surg* 119:166, 1984.
214 Maini B, Blackburn GL, Bistrian BR et al: Cyclic hyperalimentation: an optimal technique for preservation of visceral protein, *J Surg Res* 20:515, 1976.
215 Maki DG, Weise CE, Sarafin HW: A semiquantitative culture method for identifying intravenous catheter–related infection, *N Engl J Med* 296:1305, 1977.
216 Malloy D, Dhingra S, Solren F: Hypomagnesemia and respiratory muscle power, *Am Rev Respir Dis* 129:497, 1984.
217 Marshall J, Christou N, Horn R: The microbiology of multiple organ failure, *Arch Surg* 123:309, 1988.
218 Mathur M, Ramalingaswami V, Deo MG: Influence of protein deficiency on 19S antibody-forming cells in rats and mice, *J Nutr* 102:841, 1971.
219 Matthews DM: Memorial lecture: protein absorption—then and now, *Gastroenterology* 73:1267, 1977.
220 McAnena O, Moore F, Moore E et al: Selective uptake of glutamine in the gastrointestinal tract: confirmation in a human study, *Br J Surg* 78:480, 1991.
221 McDonald WS, Claiborne CW, Deitch EA: Immediate enteral feeding in burn patients is safe and effective, *Ann Surg* 213:177, 1991.
222 McFarlane H: Cell-mediated immunity in clinical and experimental protein-calorie malnutrition. In Suskind RM, editor: *Malnutrition and the immune response,* New York, 1977, Raven.
223 Meredith J, Ditesheim J, Zaloga G: Visceral protein levels in trauma patients are greater with peptide diet than with intact protein diet, *J Trauma* 30:825, 1990.
224 Miller SF, Morath MA, Finley RK: Comparison of derived and actual transferrin: a potential source of error in clinical nutritional assessment, *J Trauma* 21(7):548, 1981.
225 Miller T, Wolin M: Fermentations by saccharolytic intestinal bacteria, *Am J Clin Nutr* 32:164, 1976.
226 Millikan WJ Jr, Henderson JM, Warren WD et al: Total parenteral nutrition with F080 in cirrhotics with subclinical encephalopathy, *Ann Surg* 197:294, 1983.
227 Mirtallo JM, Schneider PJ, Mavko K: A comparison of essential and general amino acid infusions in the nutritional support of patients with compromised renal function, *JPEN* 6:109, 1982.
228 Misbin RI, Edgar PJ, Lockwood DH: Influence of adrenergic receptor stimulation on glucose metabolism during starvation in

man: effects on circulating levels of insulin, growth hormone and free fatty acids, *Metabolism* 20:544, 1971.

229 Mochizuki H, Trocki O, Domioni L: Mechanism of prevention of postburn hypermetabolism and catabolism by early enteral feeding, *Ann Surg* 200:297, 1984.

230 Moore E: Early postinjury enteral feeding: attenuated stress response and reduced sepsis, *Contemporary Surgery* 3:43, 1988.

231 Moore E, Jones T: Benefits of immediate jejunostomy feeding after major abdominal trauma: a prospective, randomized study, *J Trauma* 26:874, 1986.

232 Moore F, Feliciano D, Andrassy R et al: Early enteral feeding, compared with parenteral, reduces postoperative septic complications, *Ann Surg* 216:172, 1992.

233 Moore F, Moore E, Jones T et al: TEN versus TPN following major abdominal trauma: reduced septic morbidity, *J Trauma* 29:916, 1989.

234 Moore RS, Cerra FB: Sepsis. In Fischer JE, editor: *Total parenteral nutrition,* ed 2, Boston, 1991, Little, Brown.

235 Morgan A, Filler RM, Moore FE: Surgical nutrition, *Med Clin North Am* 54:1367, 1970.

236 Mowatt-Larssen C, Brown R, Wojtysiak S et al: Comparison of tolerance and nutritional outcome between a peptide and a standard enteral formula in critically ill, hypoalbuminemic patients, *JPEN* 16:20, 1992.

237 Mullan H, Roubenoff RA, Roubenoff R: Risk of pulmonary aspiration among patients receiving enteral nutrition support, *JPEN* 16:160, 1992.

238 Mullen JL, Gertner MH, Buzby GP et al: Implications of malnutrition in the surgical patient, *Arch Surg* 114:121, 1979.

239 Naylor C, O'Rourke K, Detsky A et al: Parenteral nutrition with branched-chain amino acids in hepatic encephalopathy, *Gastroenterology* 97:1033, 1989.

240 Newman J, Neff T, Ziporin P: Acute respiratory failure associated with hypophosphatemia, *N Engl J Med* 296:1101, 1977.

241 Nolan J: The contribution of gut-derived endotoxins to liver injury, *Yale J Biol Med* 52:127, 1979.

242 O'Brien MJ, Gottlieb LS: The liver and the biliary tract. In Robbins SL, Cotran RS, editors: *Pathologic basis of disease,* ed 2, Philadelphia, 1979, WB Saunders.

243 O'Connor LR, Wheeler WS, Bethun JE: Effect of hypophosphatemia on myocardial performance in man, *N Engl J Med* 297:901, 1977.

244 Odessey R, Khairallah EA, Goldberg AL: Origin and possible significance of alanine production by skeletal muscle, *J Biol Chem* 249:7623, 1974.

245 O'Dwyer ST, Scott T, Smith RJ et al: 5FU toxicity on small intestine mucosa but not white blood cell is decreased by glutamine, *Clin Res* 35:369A, 1987 (abstract).

246 O'Dwyer ST, Michie H, Zieglar T et al: A single dose of endotoxin increases intestinal permeability in healthy humans, *Arch Surg* 123:1459, 1988.

247 O'Dwyer ST, Smith R, Hwang T et al: Maintenance of small bowel mucosa with glutamine-enriched parenteral nutrition, *JPEN* 13:579, 1989.

248 Owen OE, Morgan AP, Kemp HG et al: Brain metabolism during fasting, *J Clin Invest* 46:1589, 1967.

249 Park K, Hayes P, Garlick P et al: Stimulation of lymphocyte natural cytotoxicity by L-arginine, *Lancet* 337:645, 1991.

250 Parker P, Stroop S, Green H: A controlled comparison of continuous versus intermittent enteral feeding in the treatment of infants with intestinal disease, *J Pediatr* 99:360, 1981.

251 Parsa MH, Ferrer JM, Habif DV: Long-term indwelling central venous catheters: indications, techniques of placement, precautions, and complications. A scientific exhibit, 58th Annual Clinical Congress, American College of Surgeons, Oct 1972.

252 Parsa MH, Habif DV, Ferrer JM: Techniques for placement of long-term indwelling superior vena cava catheters. New York, 1972, Department of Surgery, Columbia University College of Physicians & Surgeons and the Surgery Service. Harlem Hospital Center (pamphlet).

253 Passwell JH, Steward MW, Soothill JF: The effects of protein malnutrition on macrophage function and the amount and affinity of antibody response, *Clin Exp Immunol* 17:491, 1974.

254 Peaston MJT: A comparison of hydrolyzed L- and synthesized DL-amino acids for complete parenteral nutrition, *Clin Pharmacol Ther* 9:61, 1967.

255 Peters BH, Samaan NA: Hyperglycemia with relative hypoinsulinemia in diphenylhydantoin toxicity, *N Engl J Med* 281:91, 1969.

256 Peterson S, Kudsk K, Carpenter G et al: Malnutrition and immunocompetence: increased mortality following an infectious challenge during hyperalimentation, *J Trauma* 21:528, 1981.

257 Peterson V, Moore E, Jones T et al: Total enteral nutrition versus total parenteral nutrition after major torso injury: attenuation of hepatic protein reprioritization, *Surgery* 104:199, 1988.

258 Pizzini R, Kumar S, Kulkarni A et al: Dietary nucleotides reverse malnutrition and starvation-induced immunosuppression, *Arch Surg* 125:86, 1990.

259 Powell TJ: Skin tunnel for central venous catheter: nonoperative technique, *Br Med J* 1:625, 1978.

260 Powell TJ, Lennard JJ, Lowes J et al: Intravenous feeding in a gastroenterological unit, *J Clin Pathol* 32:349, 1979.

261 Prager R, Laboy V, Venus B et al: Value of fluoroscopic assistance during transpyloric intubation, *Crit Care Med* 14:151, 1986.

262 Randall H: Enteral nutrition: tube feeding in acute and chronic illness, *JPEN* 8:113, 1984.

263 Rappaport MI, Hurd HF: Thiazide-induced glucose intolerance treated with potassium, *Arch Intern Med* 113:405, 1964.

264 Raul F, Norieger R, Doffeol M: Modification of brush border enzyme activities during starvation in the jejunum and ileum of adult rats, *Enzyme* 28:328, 1982.

265 Rees R, Keohane P, Grimble G et al: Tolerance of elemental diet administered without starter regimen, *Br Med J* 290:1869, 1985.

266 Renk C, Owens D, Birkhahn R: Effect of intravenous or oral feeding on immunocompetence in traumatized rats, *JPEN* 4:587, 1985.

267 Reynolds JV, Thom AK, Zhang SM et al: Arginine, protein calorie malnutrition, and cancer, *J Surg Res* 45:513, 1988.

268 Rhoads JE, Alexander CE: Nutritional problems of surgical patients, *Ann N Y Acad Sci* 63:268, 1955.

269 Rhodes RS, Depalma RG, Robinson AV: Intestinal barrier function in hemmorrhagic shock, *J Surg Res* 14:305, 1973.

270 Robin AP, Nordenstrom J, Askanazi J et al: Plasma clearance of fat emulsions in trauma and sepsis: use of a three-stage lipid clearance test, *JPEN* 4:505, 1980.

271 Roediger WEW: Metabolic basis of starvation diarrhoea: implications for treatment, *Lancet* 1:1082, 1986.

272 Roediger WEW: Utilization of nutrients by isolated epithelial cells of the rat colon, *Gastroenterology* 83:424, 1982.

273 Roediger WEW, Rae D: Trophic effect of short chain fatty acids on mucosal handling of ions by the defunctioned colon, *Br J Surg* 69:23, 1982.

274 Rombeau J, Twomey P, McLean G: Experience with a new gastrostomy-jejunal feeding tube, *Surgery* 93:574, 1983.

275 Rose WC, Coon MJ, Lambert GF: The amino acid requirements of man: the role of the caloric intake, *J Biol Chem* 210:331, 1954.

276 Rose WC, Wixom RL: The amino acid requirements in man: XVI. The role of the nitrogen intake, *J Biol Chem* 217:997, 1955.

277 Rosen HM, Yoshimura N, Hodgman JM et al: Plasma amino acid patterns in hepatic encephalopathy of differing etiology, *Gastroenterology* 72:483, 1977.

278 Rossi-Fanelli F, Riggio O, Cangiano C et al: Branched-chain amino acids vs lactulose in the treatment of hepatic coma: a controlled study, *Dig Dis Sci* 27:929, 1982.
279 Rotruck JT, Pope AL, Ganther HE et al: Selenium: biochemical role as a component of glutathione peroxidase, *Science* 179:588, 1973.
280 Roubenoff R, Ravich WJ: Pneumothorax due to nasogastric feeding tubes, *Arch Intern Med* 149:184, 1989.
281 Runyan JW Jr: Influence of thiazide diuretics on carbohydrate metabolism in patients with mild diabetes, *N Engl J Med* 267:541, 1962.
282 Ruppin H, Bar-Meir S, Soergel K: Absorption of short chain fatty acids by the colon, *Gastroenterology* 78:1500, 1980.
283 Ruppin H, Bar-Meir S, Soergel K: Effects of liquid diets on proximal gastrointestinal function, *Gastroenterology* 76:1231, 1979.
284 Rutten P, Blackburn GL, Flatt JP et al: Determination of optimal hyperalimentation infusion rate, *J Surg Res* 18:477, 1975.
285 Ryan G, Dudrick S, Copeland E: Effect of various diets on colonic growth in rats, *Gastroenterology* 77:458, 1979.
286 Ryan JA Jr, Abel RM, Abbott WM et al: Catheter complications in total parenteral nutrition: a prospective study of 200 consecutive patients, *N Engl J Med* 290:757, 1974.
287 Saito H, Trocki O, Alexander JW et al: The effect of route to nutrient administration on the nutritional state, catabolic hormone secretion, and gut mucosal integrity after burn injury, *JPEN* 11:1, 1987.
288 Sanders RA, Sheldon GF: Septic complications of total parenteral nutrition: a five-year experience, *Am J Surg* 132:214, 1976.
289 Sanderson I, Deitel M: Intravenous hyperalimentation without sepsis, *Surg Gynecol Obstet* 136:577, 1973.
290 Schatten W, Desprez J, Holden W: A bacteriologic study of portal vein blood in man, *Arch Surg* 71:404, 1955.
291 Scheimer R, Fitzer H, Gfell M: Environmental contamination of continuous drip feedings, *Pediatrics* 63:232, 1979.
292 Schenker S, Hoyumpa AM Jr: Pathophysiology of hepatic encephalopathy, *Hosp Pract* Sept 1984.
293 Schlichtig R, Ayers SM: *Nutritional support of the critically ill,* Chicago, 1988, Mosby.
294 Scholten DJ, Wood TL, Thompson DR: Pneumothorax from nasoenteric feeding tube insertion: a report of five cases, *Am Surg* 52:381, 1986.
295 Schovlemmer G, Battaglini J: An unusual complication of nasoenteral feeding with small-diameter feeding tubes, *Ann Surg* 199:104, 1984.
296 Schroeder P, Fisher D, Volz M: Microbial contamination of enteral feeding solutions in a community, *JPEN* 7:364, 1983.
297 Scribner BH, Cole JJ, Christopher TG et al: Long-term total parenteral nutrition, *JAMA* 212:457, 1970.
298 Scrimshaw NS, Taylor CE, Gordon JE: Interactions of nutrition and infection. Monograph series 57, Geneva, 1968, World Health Organization.
299 Scrimshaw NS, Taylor CE, Gordon JE: Interactions of nutrition and infection, *Am J Med Sci* 237:367, 1959.
300 Scrimshaw NS, Young VR: The requirements of human nutrition, *Sci Am* 235:51, 1976.
301 Scrutton MC, Utter MF, Mildvan AS: Pyruvate carboxylase. VI. The presence of tightly bound manganese, *J Biol Chem* 241:3480, 1972.
302 Seifter E, Rettura G, Barbul A: Arginine: an essential amino acid for injured rats, *Surgery* 84:224, 1978.
303 Selivanov V, Sheldon G: Enteral nutrition and sepsis. In Rombeau J, Caldwell M, editors: *Clinical nutrition.* Vol 1. *Enteral and tube feeding,* Philadelphia, 1984, WB Saunders.
304 Selvaraj RJ, Bhat KS: Metabolic and bactericidal activities of leukocytes in protein-calorie malnutrition, *Am J Clin Nutr* 25:166, 1972.
305 Seth V, Chandra RK: Opsonic activity, phagocytosis, and bactericidal capacity of polymorphs in undernutrition, *Arch Dis Child* 47:282, 1972.
306 Shapiro AP, Benedek TG, Small JL: Effects of thiazides on carbohydrate metabolism in patients with hypertension, *N Engl J Med* 265:1028, 1961.
307 Sheldon GF, Petersen SR, Sanders R: Hepatic dysfunction during hyperalimentation, *Arch Surg* 113:504, 1978.
308 Shetty PS, Jung RT, Watrasiewicz KE et al: Rapid turnover transport proteins: an index of subclinical protein-energy malnutrition, *Lancet* 2:230, 1979.
309 Shils M, Block A, Chernoff R: *Liquid formulas for oral and tube feeding,* New York, 1979, Memorial Sloan-Kettering Cancer Center.
310 Siegel JH, Cerra FB, Border JR et al: Physiological and metabolic correlations in human sepsis, *Surgery* 86:406, 1979.
311 Silk DBA, Fairclough PD, Clark ML et al: Use of a peptide rather than a free amino acid nitrogen source in chemically defined "elemental" diets, *JPEN* 4:548, 1980.
312 Sirisinha S, Suskind R, Edelman R et al: Complement and C3-proactivator levels in children with protein-calorie malnutrition and effect of dietary treatment, *Lancet* 1:1016, 1973.
313 Smythe PM, Schonland M, Brereton-Stiles GG et al: Thymolymphatic efficiency and depression of cell-mediated immunity in protein-calorie malnutrition, *Lancet* 2:939, 1971.
314 Soergel K: Absorption of fermentation products from the colon. In Kasper H, Goebell H, editors: *Colon and nutrition,* Lancaster, Pa, 1982, MTP.
315 Soeters PB, Fischer JE: Insulin, glucagon, amino acid imbalance and hepatic encephalopathy, *Lancet* 2:880, 1976.
316 Sofio C, Nicora R: High-calorie essential amino acid parenteral therapy in acute renal failure, *Acta Chir Scand (Suppl)* 466:98, 1976.
317 Solomons NW: On the assessment of trace mineral nutrition in patients on total parenteral nutrition, *Nutritional Support Services* 1(3):13, 1981.
318 Souba WW, Smith RJ, Wilmore DW: Glutamine metabolism by the intestinal tract, *JPEN* 9:608, 1985.
319 Souba WW, Wilmore DW: Postoperative alteration of arteriovenous exchange of amino acids across the gastrointestinal tract, *Surgery* 94:342, 1983.
320 Souba WW, Long JM, Dudrick SJ: Energy intake and stress as determinants of nitrogen excretion in rats, *Surg Forum* 29:76, 1978.
321 Spaeth G, Berg R, Specian R et al: Food without fiber promotes bacterial translocation from the gut, 1990.
322 Spitzer JJ, Bagby GJ, Meszaros K, Lang CH: Alterations in lipid and carbohydrate metabolism in sepsis, *JPEN* 12:53S, 1988.
323 Stanford GG, Boyd JL, Chernow B: Middle messenger systems and their alteration in sepsis and multiple organ failure. In Bihari D, Cerra FB, editors: *New horizons: multiple organ failure,* Fullerton, Calif, 1989, Society of Critical Care Medicine.
324 Steffee CH: The relationship of protein depletion to natural resistance, *J Infect Dis* 86:12, 1950.
325 Steffee W, Krey S: Enteral hyperalimentation for patients with head and neck cancer, *Otolaryngol Clin North Am* 13:437, 1980.
326 Stehle P, Zander J, Mertes N et al: Effect of parenteral glutamine peptide supplements on muscle glutamine loss and nitrogen balance after major surgery, *Lancet* 1:231, 1989.
327 Steuhr D, Gross S, Sakuma I et al: Activated murine macrophages secrete a metabolite of arginine with the bioactivity of endothelium-derived relaxing factor and the chemical reactivity of nitrous oxide, *J Exp Med* 169:1011, 1989.
328 Strauss E, Santos WR, DaSilva EC et al: A randomized controlled clinical trial for the evaluation of the efficacy of an enriched

branched chain amino acid solution compared to neomycin in hepatic encephalopathy, *Hepatology* 3:862, 1983.

329 Strong R, Condon S, Solinger M et al: Equal aspiration rates from postpylorus and intragastric-placed small-bore nasoenteric feeding tubes: a randomized, prospective study, *JPEN* 16:59, 1992.

330 Taylor T: Comparison of two methods of nasogastric tube feeding, *Neurol Nurs* 14:49, 1982.

331 Teasley K, Buss R: Do parenteral nutrition solutions with high concentrations of branched-chain amino acids offer significant benefits to stressed patients? *Annals of Pharmacotherapy* 23:411, 1989.

332 Tellado JM, Christou NV: Nutrition and immunity. In Fischer JE, editor: *Total parenteral nutrition,* ed 2, Boston, 1991, Little, Brown.

333 Thomas R: Relationship of albumin to mortality in critically ill respiratory patients, *Am J Clin Nutr* 32:246, 1979.

334 Thomas TG: The intravenous injection of milk as a substitute for the transfusion of blood, *NY Med J* 28:449, 1878.

335 Thonnard-Neumann E: Phenothiazides and diabetes in hospitalized women, *Am J Psychiatry* 124:978, 1968.

336 Toews A, de la Rocha A: Oropharyngeal sepsis with endothoracic spread, *Can J Surg* 23:265, 1980.

337 Toivonen S, Mustala O: Diabetogenic action of furosemide, *Br Med J* 1:920, 1966.

338 Tracey KJ, Fong Y, Hesse DG et al: Cachectin (tumor necrosis factor-alpha) participates in the metabolic derangements induced by gram-negative bacteremia, *Surg Forum* 39:8, 1988.

339 Treloar D, Stechmiller J: Pulmonary aspiration in tube-fed patients with artificial airways, *Heart Lung* 13:67, 1984.

340 Udall J, Walker W: Mucosal defense mechanisms. In Marsh MN, editor: *Immunopathology of the small intestine,* New York, 1987, Wiley & Sons.

341 Vallee BL, Falchuk KH: Zinc and gene expression, *Philos Trans R Soc Lond (Biol)* 294:185, 1981.

342 Van Buren C, Rudolf F, Kulkarni A et al: Reversal of immunosuppression induced by a protein-free diet: comparison of nucleotides, fish oil and arginine, *Crit Care Med* 18:S114, 1990.

343 Van den Berg B, Stam H: Metabolic and respiratory effects of enteral nutrition in patients during mechanical ventilation, *Intensive Care Med* 14:206, 1988.

344 Visocan BJ: Nutritional management of the adult with liver disease. In Skipper A , editor: *Dietician's handbook of enteral and parenteral nutrition,* Gaithersburg, Md, 1989, Aspen.

345 Wahren J, Denis J, Desurmont P: Is intravenous administration of branched chain amino acids effective in the treatment of hepatic encephalopathy? *Hepatology* 3:475, 1983.

346 Wang X, Jacobs DO, O'Dwyer ST et al: Glutamine-enriched parenteral nutrition prevents mucosal atrophy following massive small bowel resection, *Surg Forum* 39:44, 1988.

347 Warnold I, Lundholm K, Schersten T: Energy balance and body composition in cancer patients, *Cancer Res* 38:1801, 1978.

348 Weinsier RL, Butterworth CE Jr: *Handbook of clinical nutrition: clinician's manual for the diagnosis and management of nutritional problems,* St Louis, 1981, Mosby.

349 Weir JB: New methods for calculating metabolic rate with special reference to protein metabolism, *J Physiol* 109:1, 1949.

350 Weisiger RA, Fridovich I: Superoxide dismutase (organelle specificity), *J Biol Chem* 248:3582, 1973.

351 Weissman C, Hyman A: Nutritional care of the critically ill patient with respiratory failure, *Crit Care Clin* 3:185, 1987.

352 Wene JD, Connor WE, denBesten L: The development of essential fatty acid deficiency in healthy men fed fat-free diets intravenously and orally, *J Clin Invest* 56:127, 1975.

353 Whatley K, Turner WW, Dey M et al: When does metoclopramide facilitate transpyloric intubation? *JPEN* 8:679, 1984.

354 White W, Acuff T, Sykes T: Bacterial contamination of enteral nutrient solution: a preliminary report, *JPEN* 3:459, 1979.

355 Wilfson M, Jones MR, Kopple JD: Amino acid losses during hemodialysis with infusion of amino acids and glucose, *Kidney Int* 21:500, 1982.

356 Wilkinson AW: Historical background of intravenous feeding, *Nutr Diet* 5:295, 1963.

357 Wilmore DW: *The metabolic management of the critically ill,* New York, 1977, Plenum.

358 Wilmore DW, Dudrick SJ: Treatment of acute renal failure with intravenous essential L-amino acids, *Arch Surg* 99:669, 1969.

359 Windmueller H, Spaeth A: Uptake and metabolism of plasma glutamine by the small intestine, *J Biol Chem* 249:5070, 1974.

360 Winterbauer R, Durning R, Barron E: Aspirated nasogastric feeding solution detected by glucose strips, *Ann Intern Med* 95:67, 1981.

361 Wissler RW: The effects of protein depletion and subsequent immunization upon the response of animals to pneumococcal infection. II. Experiments with male albino rats, *J Infect Dis* 80:264, 1947.

362 Wissler RW, Woolridge RL, Steffee CH et al: The relationship of the protein reserves to antibody production. II. The influence of protein repletion upon the production of antibody in hypoproteinemic adult white rats, *J Immunol* 52:267, 1946.

363 Wolfe RR, Allsop JR, Burke JF: Glucose metabolism in man: responses to intravenous glucose infusion, *Metabolism* 28:210, 1979.

364 Wolfe RR, O'Donnell T, Stone M: Investigation of factors determining the optimal glucose infusion rate in total parenteral nutrition, *Metabolism* 29:892, 1980.

365 Wunder JA, Stinnet JD, Alexander JW: The effects of malnutrition on variables of host defense in the guinea pig, *Surgery* 84(4):542, 1978.

366 Zarling E, Parmer J, Mobarhan S: Effect of enteral formula infusion rate, osmolality, and chemical composition upon clinical tolerance and carbohydrate absorption in normal subjects, *JPEN* 10:588, 1986.

367 Ziegler TR, Young LS, Benfell K et al: Clinical and metabolic efficacy of glutamine-supplemented parenteral nutrition after bone marrow transplantation, *Ann Intern Med* 116:821, 1992.

368 Zieve L: Hepatic encephalopathy. In Schiff L, Schiff ER, editors: *Diseases of the liver,* Philadelphia, 1987, JB Lippincott.

369 Zimmaro D, Rolandelli R, Koruda M et al: Isotonic tube-feeding formula induces liquid stool in normal subjects: reversal by pectin, *JPEN* 13:117, 1989.

CHAPTER

10

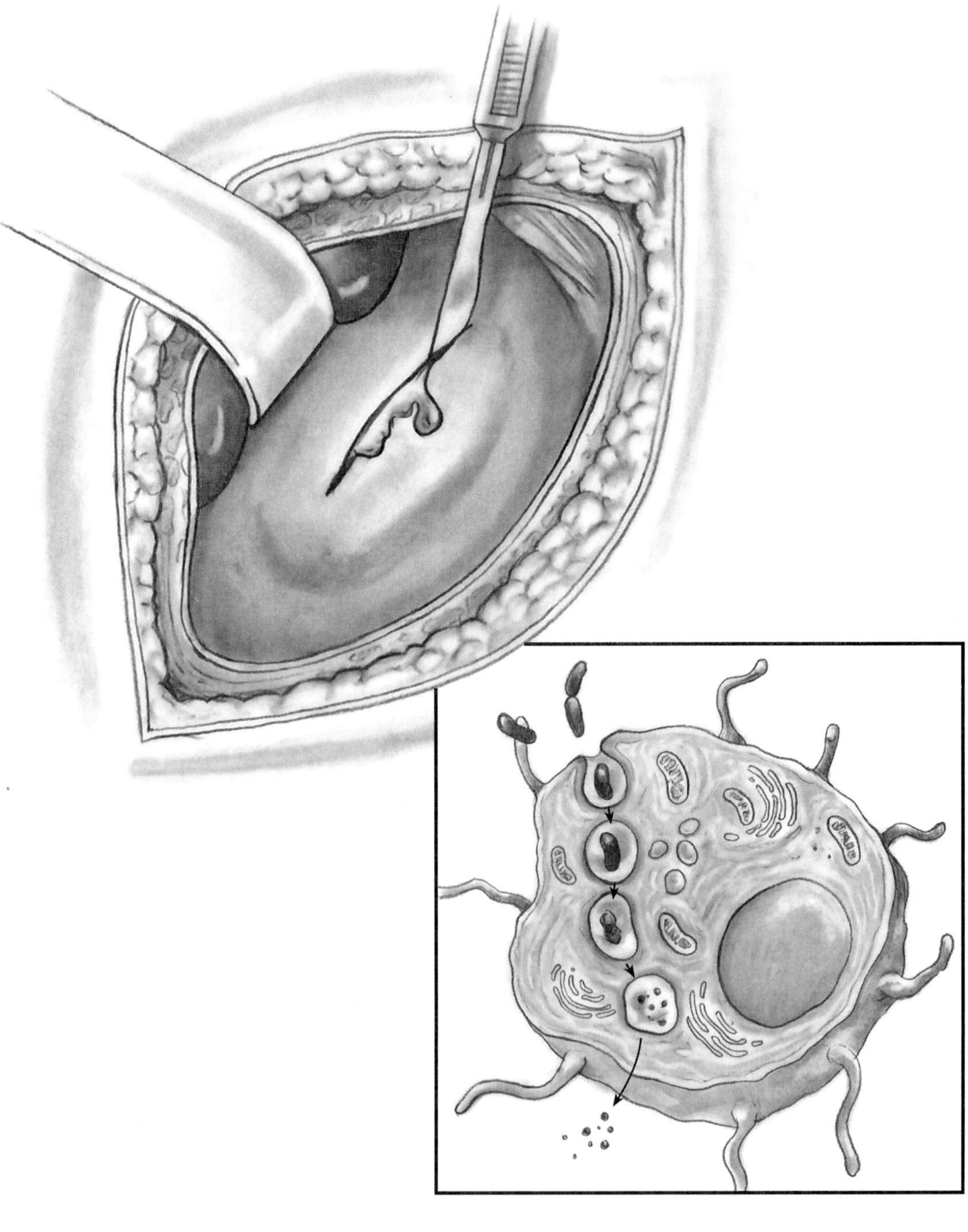

MANAGEMENT OF SURGICAL INFECTION: PATHOGENESIS, DIAGNOSIS, AND TREATMENT

Cleon W. Goodwin • Basil A. Pruitt Jr.

RELATED MATERIAL APPEARS IN CHAPTERS 2, 11, AND 17

Infection is the most frequent source of morbidity in surgical patients and the most common cause of mortality in severely injured patients who can be resuscitated and survive initial surgical intervention.[149] The chance of developing an infection is strongly influenced by both patient and microbial factors as well as the pathophysiologic interactions between host and microorganism. Infection occurs when an imbalance exists between host resistance and microbial invasiveness, and the goal of patient care is the prevention of such an imbalance.

Sepsis is a diagnostic term commonly applied to a patient who manifests the systemic changes and alterations in organ function evoked by an infection. To make a definite diagnosis of sepsis in a surgical patient, the presence of an infection must be objectively confirmed because many of the clinical signs characteristic of sepsis occur in response to injury itself (surgery is a controlled form of injury) in the absence of infection. The clinical diagnosis of sepsis is confounded by the commonality of hyperthermia, tachycardia, hyperventilation, glucose intolerance, leukocytosis, and disorientation as components of the response to both infection and injury.[148] In the early stages of sepsis, before the causative infection has been documented, accentuation of systemic responses to injury or reemergence of the early postinjury pattern of physiologic changes should prompt vigorous diagnostic efforts to confirm the presence of and identify the site of an infection. Because the systemic signs of sepsis are nonspecific, greater reliance must be placed upon local changes and diagnostic technology, such as laboratory tests and radiologic examinations, to confirm the presence of an infection. Early diagnosis of the infection causing sepsis aids in prompt local control and thereby minimizes systemic complications and helps achieve maximum survival.

However, problems of infection still complicate surgery today. The infection rate is 1.5% to 5% in clean procedures,[119] whereas in contaminated wounds the rate is 8.5% to 40%.[42] An estimated 18% to 30% of intraperitoneal procedures involving the colon are followed by abscesses, peritonitis, wound infections, or other infectious processes. The use of nonabsorbable antibiotics for preoperative colon preparation in elective procedures has reduced the rate of postoperative infection to 7% or less,[35] but mortality can reach 30% to 40% in patients who develop fulminating sepsis following trauma or certain types of elective surgery. Immunosuppression from disease or that induced for transplantation is associated with bacterial, fungal, and viral infection and may be lethal. In seriously injured patients who survive acute shock, the primary cause of death, excluding head injuries, is infection resulting in septic shock or progressive multisystem organ failure.[27]

Another significant problem posed by surgical infections, which concerns the public as well as patients and physicians, is the high cost to society. Added hospital expenses and days of productivity lost due to infectious surgical morbidity and mortality result in an annual cost of approximately $10 billion in the United States alone.

Survival or death from invasive infection depends on the dynamic balance between the magnitude of microbial injury and the effectiveness of immunologic defense in conjunction with other organ systems that maintain cellular metabolism and function throughout the body. Prevention of bacterial invasion or proper treatment for established infections necessitates an understanding of the biologic behavior of the invaders and the host's defensive responses.[8] Thus the purpose of this chapter is to relate the typical patterns of surgical infections to the nature of the organisms involved and the damage they cause. Bodily defenses include control of infection by inflammatory and other immunologic reactions accompanied by supportive metabolic and physiologic alterations that preserve life during healing and recovery.

Appreciation of the factors that predispose a surgical patient to infection enables one to match the intensity of microbial surveillance and physiologic monitoring to the relative risk of infection (see box on p. 357). An understanding of the effects of infection on the underlying pathophysiologic response to injury enables one to assess the significance of changes in the patient's status due to infection, to evaluate the results of laboratory tests, and to provide the physiologic support necessary to restore organ function.

PATIENT FACTORS

The severity of injury is the major determinant of the occurrence of infection in the surgical patient. The influence of injury severity on infection rate is well illustrated by burn patients in whom the incidence of burn wound infections is proportional to the extent of burn, being low in patients with burns of less than 30% of the body surface and increasing in a sigmoid dose response fashion as the extent of burn increases above that level. The same relationship holds true in mechanical trauma patients in whom the incidence of postinjury infection is greater in patients with multiple injuries than in those with a single injury.[122] In otherwise uninjured patients, the magnitude of an elective surgical procedure, as indexed by its duration, is also related to the occurrence of infection which increases as operative time increases. The occurrence of infection in surgical patients is also age related. The infection rate following severe

■The authors gratefully acknowledge the contributions of the previous authors of this chapter in the first edition of this text: †George H.A. Clowes Jr., Michael J. Edwards, and Hiram C. Polk Jr.

†Deceased.

HOST FACTORS PREDISPOSING THE SURGICAL PATIENT TO INFECTION

- Severe injury
- Wounds involving colon
- Prolonged injury to treatment interval
- Duration of operation
- Extremes of age
- Inadequacy of local blood supply
  - Shock
  - Technical errors
  - Presence of nonviable tissue
- Preexisting disease
  - Metabolic derangements
    - Diabetes
    - Uremia
    - Increased circulating levels of corticosteroids
    - Obesity
    - Malnutrition
  - Remote infection
  - Immunologic deficiency states
    - Congenital
    - Acquired
- Foreign bodies
  - Debris in wound
    - Trauma related
    - Suture material
  - Invasive monitoring devices
  - Prosthetic material
- Treatment agents
  - Irradiation
  - Steroids
  - Cytotoxic agents
  - Immunosuppressants
  - Sulfonamides
- Immobility
- Time in hospital prior to surgery

injury, such as an extensive burn, is highest in the immunologically immature pediatric age group, lowest in young adults, and somewhat higher in the elderly.

Preexisting disease can predispose a surgical patient to infection. Metabolic diseases, such as diabetes and uremic renal failure as well as conditions characterized by increased circulating levels of corticosteroids, increase the rate of infection following injury or surgery.[20,76,86] Extremes of metabolic activity, as manifested by either obesity or malnutrition, also increase the rate of postoperative wound infections, reported as being 18.1% and 22.4%, respectively, in one frequently cited study.[1] Patients with remote and preexisting infection also experience a higher incidence of postoperative wound infections, presumably the aggregate effect of related changes in the cutaneous flora, therapy-related selection of resistant organisms, and, as described below, the effects of infection on the immune system. Patients with congenital or preexisting acquired immunologic defects, such as complement deficiency states, chronic granulomatous disease and acquired immunodeficiency syndrome, also have increased susceptibility to infections caused by opportunistic organisms.[103,159] The principal effect, means of diagnosis, and current treatment modalities of selected immunodeficiency states are detailed in Appendix 10-1.

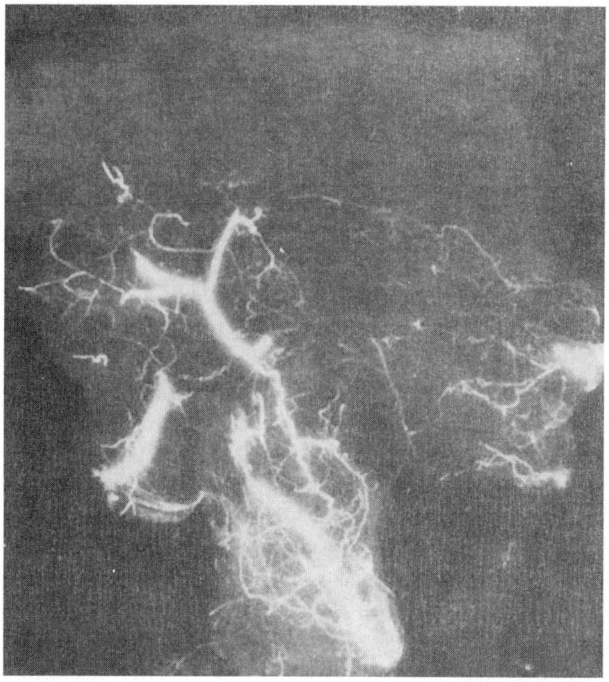

FIGURE 10-1 This radiograph of an autopsy specimen taken from an area of full-thickness burn after arterial injection of radiopaque material confirms the avascular nature of the tissues superficial to the vascular occlusion evident at the base of the eschar.

The adequacy of the circulation plays a key role in the defense of tissue against infection. The ischemic nonviable tissue resulting from a burn or other injury provides a protein rich pabulum that permits unbridled microbial proliferation (Figure 10-1). In addition, the absence of a functioning local blood supply prevents delivery of systemic antibiotics and the cellular components of the host defense system to the site of microbial proliferation.[133] The importance of the local blood supply is reflected by the low incidence of postoperative infections in the well-vascularized scalp, face, and neck and by the relatively high incidence of infections in areas of thick adipose tissue and in the distal areas of extremities. Surgical technique can result in disturbance of the local circulation and increase the risk of infection. Inappropriate placement or tension of ligatures and sutures can produce tissue necrosis. Impairment of the systemic circulation as a consequence of hypovolemia or myocardial dysfunction is associated with an increase in the subsequent incidence of infection in the surgical patient. In burn patients persistent hypovolemic shock, caused by inadequate resuscitation, or shock arising from any cause following resuscitation may result in conversion of a partial-thickness injury or split-thickness skin graft donor site to a full-thickness injury which is much more susceptible to the development of invasive infection.[148]

The interval between injury or insult and treatment also influences the rate of infection. Wound infection rate increases as the injury-to-treatment interval increases due to the combined effect of microbial proliferation and extension of local tissue damage resulting from uncorrected circulatory and ventilatory deficits. Treatment of a traumatic wound should be keyed to the injury-treatment interval. The "golden period," during which traumatic wounds can be primarily closed, previously considered to be 4 to 6 hours, has been extended up to 10 hours or more by the use of prophylactic antibiotics. When the injury-treatment interval has exceeded that limit, delayed primary or secondary closure should be utilized.[151]

The infection enhancing effect of foreign bodies is most evident in patients with traumatic wounds.[198] In such patients the presence of retained soil, clothing, or other debris markedly reduces the number of microorganisms necessary to cause a subsequent infection. Studies by Altemeier and Furste[10] showed that the number of *Clostridium welchii* necessary to cause fatal gas gangrene in an animal model was decreased a millionfold when crushed muscle and sterile dirt were present in the wound. Sutures, surgical implants, and all cannulae and catheters act as foreign bodies and increase the risk of infection by providing a site of attachment for microorganisms and eliciting an inflammatory tissue reaction provoked by the material of which the device is composed and as a result of mechanical trauma. Monofilament sutures have been associated with a lesser occurrence of wound infection than either multifilament or plain catgut sutures. These effects of foreign bodies are eliminated or reduced by prompt irrigation and debridement of traumatic wounds, by the use of tissue compatible suture material, implant material, cannulae and catheters, and by removal of all invasive monitoring and treatment devices at the earliest possible time.

The surgical patient's susceptibility to infection may be increased by a variety of treatment agents. The hematologic and gastroenterologic effects of irradiation contribute to an increased risk of infection. The immunosuppressive effect of radiation is related to both the dose administered and the radiation field. Following 300 rads of whole-body exposure, the number of circulating lymphocytes may fall to levels below 1000/ml and remain at that depressed level for 8 or more weeks. An increase in circulating neutrophils immediately after such an amount of whole-body irradiation is followed by a fall to approximately 4000 neutrophils per milliliter by the tenth postinjury day and a secondary fall to a level of 500/ml or less approximately 30 days after injury.[36] Whole-body irradiation in excess of 1000 rads produces gastrointestinal injury manifested by anorexia, nausea, vomiting, and diarrhea that appear within hours and customarily subside within 48 hours following injury. During a brief latent period, the injured mucosal cells undergo necrosis and subsequent desquamation that is associated with recrudescence of the earlier gastrointestinal symptoms in association with infection and hemorrhage of the denuded intestine.

The risk of infection caused by irradiation is greatest in patients such as those undergoing bone marrow transplantation who receive total body radiation (commonly 1000 to 1400 rads). In patients receiving focal irradiation, the risk of infection is proportional to the exposure of hematopoietically active tissues and the gastrointestinal tract. The risk of exogenously acquired infection is minimized by reducing environmental contamination by the use of a room with laminar air flow and sterilization of all equipment and supplies in that room. Enteral antibiotics and antifungal agents have been used to reduce the microbial density of the enteric contents, and the use of sterilized food eliminates dietary sources of organisms capable of colonizing the gut. The incidence of bacterial and fungal infections increases as the granulocyte count falls below 1500/ml and is particularly great in patients in whom the granulocyte level is below 500/ml. Prophylactic oral antibiotics should be administered to patients with granulocyte counts below 1000/ml, and systemic antibiotics should be given at the first sign of an infection in a profoundly granulocytopenic patient. Granulocyte transfusions have been used to control documented infections and also to correct persistent profound granulocytopenia.[37] Reactivation of latent cytomegalovirus and herpetic infections may also occur as a consequence of postradiation immunosuppression. Systemic antiviral medications should be administered to those patients with reactivated endogenous herpes simplex virus infections.

Cytotoxic agents used in the treatment of various malignancies also exert immunosuppressive effects that are associated with an increased risk of infection. These agents, such as methotrexate, may also cause gastrointestinal mucosal injury that increases the risk of infection due to endogenous enteric microorganisms. Enhancement of infection is also evident in transplant patients

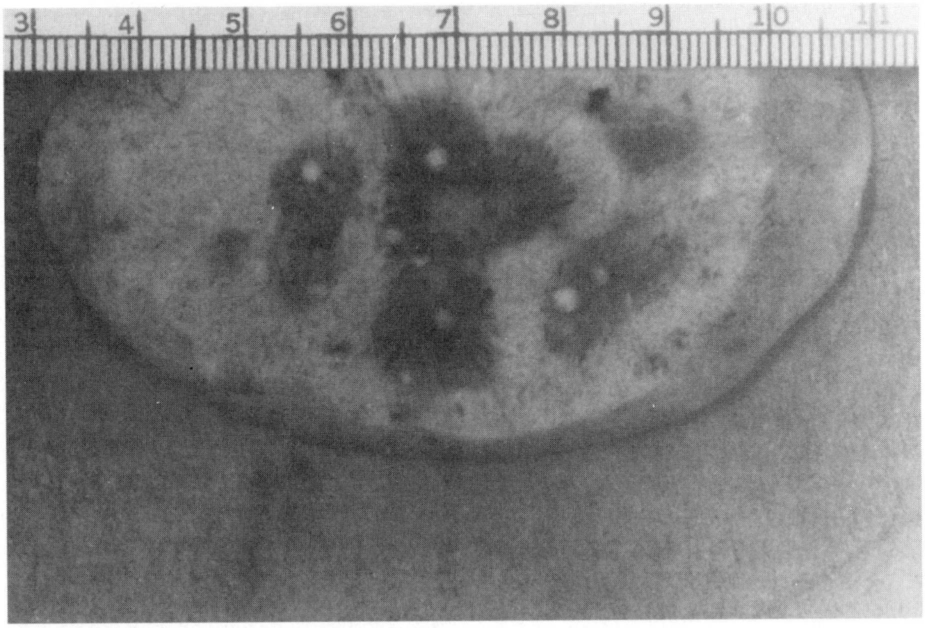

FIGURE 10-2 *Candida* species, the most common nonbacterial burn wound colonizers, infrequently cause invasive burn wound infections in other than severely injured immunocompromised patients. The candidal abscesses evident in this kidney occurred as a result of hematogenous dissemination from a candidal burn wound infection in a 5-year-old child with a 45% burn treated with a topical chemotherapeutic agent containing a sulfonamide.

in whom agents, such as steroids, azathioprine, antithymocyte globulin, and cyclosporin, exert dose-related immunosuppressive effects on various components of the antimicrobial defense system. Although in vitro immunosuppressive effects of antibiotics have been described, they appear to be of little clinical consequence. Sulfonamides, widely used for the topical treatment of burn wounds, have been shown to decrease the candidicidal activity of neutrophils; that action may explain the increase in candidal infections in burn patients that has occurred concomitantly with the use of those agents[98] (Figure 10-2).

Treatment-related immobility increases the risk of both pulmonary and soft tissue infections. Position-dependent atelectasis, particularly in patients requiring mechanical ventilation, plays an important role in the pathogenesis of bronchopneumonia and can be minimized by scheduled endobronchial toilet, position changes, and physical therapy. Frequent position changes, appropriate padding of bony prominences, and the use of air fluidized beds prevent or minimize pressure-induced tissue necrosis and ulceration, sites of which are readily infected by microorganisms from the environment of the patient.

EFFECTS OF INJURY AND SEPSIS ON HOST DEFENSES

Injury impairs the host defense system in proportion to the severity of the injury. The burn patient serves not only as a universal trauma model but also as an infection model in which activity of all components of the immune system is depressed and the risk of infection increased in proportion to the extent of the burn. The wound itself breaches the mechanical barrier of the skin per se in the case of burn injury and the skin and underlying fascial planes in the case of mechanical trauma. Injury activates the complement system primarily via the alternative pathway, resulting in a *consumption opsinopathy*.[69]

Activity of complement components C_1, C_2, C_3, C_4, and C_5 is decreased, and the levels of C_3 cleavage fragments are increased, a configuration consistent with nonspecific complement activation. Circulating levels of the immunoglobulins are initially decreased as a result of hemodilution, enlarged pool size, mechanical leakage (most common in burn patients), and increased catabolism and gradually return to normal levels in the patient who pursues an uncomplicated course. In the early stages of infection, the production of immunoglobulins may actually increase as indicated by the elevated circulating levels of IgM in patients with invasive phycomycosis. Reversion of IgM levels to "normal" has been used as an index of adequate surgical removal of such infected tissue.

The number and function of cell populations of the immune system are altered by both surgery and trauma. Immunologically active cells are affected minimally by elective surgery, moderately by mechanical trauma, and severely by a burn involving more than 50% of the total body surface. Neutrophil number increases immediately following injury but promptly falls to a nadir within 48 hours and thereafter slowly returns to normal or supranormal levels.[57] In the early stages of an infection in a critically ill surgical patient, the neutrophil count may rise, but in patients with severe life threatening infections causing sepsis, a profound neutropenia is commonly observed, particularly when the sepsis is caused by gram-negative organisms. Neutrophil chemotaxis, response to formyl-menthionyl-leucyl-phenylalanine, phagocytic capacity, and bactericidal activity are initially depressed following injury and slowly return to predicted normal levels in the uncomplicated patient.[114] Yurt and associates[197] have recently presented data indicating that extensive injury induces indiscrete neutrophil margination that reduces the number of neutrophils delivered to a wound and increases the susceptibility of that wound to microbial invasion. Neutrophil oxidative activity and glucose utilization are also decreased by injury and even more profoundly impaired by infection.

Chemilumigenic probe methodology permits rapid assessment of both the opsonic capacity of serum and the oxidative activity of neutrophils. Studies using chemiluminescence assays have identified an early postinjury depression of serum opsonic capacity, apparently unrelated to infections, as well as subsequent profound depression of both opsonic capacity and neutrophil oxidative activity in temporal association with sepsis.[9] Persistent depression of neutrophil function commonly accompanies severe infection. The postinjury depression of neutrophil function has been attributed to both intrinsic hypoactivity and humoral depressant factors.[179] Recent studies, however, have provided evidence that such hypofunction is related to early activation that leaves the neutrophil in a state of relative exhaustion.[123]

Injury induces profound changes in lymphocyte populations, that is, a relative decrease in T-cell number and relative increase in B-cell number. In severely injured patients T-suppressor cells have been noted to increase in number late in the first postburn week, and the T-helper and T-suppressor cell ratio has been reported to be decreased at that time.[130] The appearance of T-suppressor effector cells seven days following burn injury has been attributed to an even earlier postinjury generation of suppressor-inducer T cells.[94] Recent studies

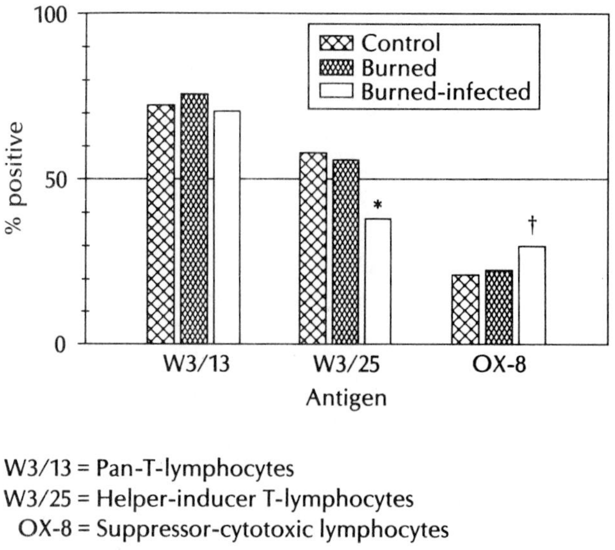

FIGURE 10-3 In a murine model of a 30% burn, the injury itself exerts little effect on lymphocyte populations. Significant changes in helper and suppressor T-cell populations occur only as a result of infection. *Asterisk* (*) equals $p < .01$; *dagger* (†) equals $p < .05$.

have shown that following injury immature, nonlymphocytic cells may contaminate lymphocyte preparations unless narrow gauging is used for sorting of cells by optical means. When such precautions are observed, injury has been found to cause a proportional decrease in helper and suppressor cells, and only when infection supervenes is there a decrease in the helper/suppressor cell ratio, reflecting an increase in suppressor cells and a proportionately greater decrease in helper T-cells[24] (Figure 10-3). The manifestations of lymphocyte impairment following injury include depressed delayed type hypersensitivity reactions to skin test antigens, decreased in vitro responsiveness to mitogens, delayed rejection of cutaneous allografts, and decreased interleukin-2 production.[195]

Macrophage function is also altered following injury. Reduction of T-helper cell activity has been attributed to postinjury impairment of macrophage antigen presentation. A primary macrophage defect has been implicated as the cause of that change, since macrophage antigen presentation activity could be restored in vitro by addition of interleukin-1.[95] In response to sepsis, the macrophage produces increased amounts of interleukin-1, tumor necrosis factor, and complement factor B, all of which influence the systemic response to an infection.[178] Injury and infection exert similar effects on the reticuloendothelial system. Impaired degradation of circulating immunogens, decreased clearance of injected colloidal fat emulsion, and depression of circulating serum fibronectin levels are all indicative of reticuloendothelial system impairment early postinjury, and all can be accentuated or reestablished, following prior resolution, by sepsis.

As previously noted, various therapeutic agents exert deleterious effects on the immune system. Perioperative blood transfusions appear to depress immune function as assessed in vitro, but the clinical significance of those changes is unclear.[70] Sulfonamides present in topical antimicrobial agents applied to burn wounds decrease neutrophil candidicidal activity and may promote multidrug antibiotic resistance in enteric organisms. Radiation depresses the number and function of both neutrophils and lymphocytes. Cytotoxic chemotherapeutic agents may also alter the number and function of both neutrophils and lymphocytes. Steroids should be administered to a surgical patient only on specific indication because they suppress the acute inflammatory response and lymphocyte reactivity to antigens and appear to increase the risk of infection. The clinical relevance of in vitro studies demonstrating that steroids impair neutrophil chemotaxis, phagocytosis, and bactericidal capacity remains undetermined. In laboratory studies a beneficial effect of steroids has been largely confined to models of infection receiving treatment prior to septic challenge.[93,171] Clinical studies purporting to show a beneficial effect of steroid treatment for sepsis have suffered from lack of randomization, imprecise definition of sepsis, and inadequate controls.

INTERACTION OF RESPONSES TO INJURY AND SEPSIS

The interaction between injury and sepsis is complex and incompletely understood. Many physiologic effects attributed to sepsis, such as elevated temperature and heat production, increased catabolism, the hyperdynamic circulatory state, and leukocytosis,[136] are more often responses to wounded tissue. This hypermetabolic state has been documented in humans with uninfected burn injury as being mediated in large part by the beta-adrenergic catecholamines.[191] Further complicating interpretations of the septic physiologic response are inexact descriptions of infection and sepsis. To develop consensus definitions of surgical infection and sepsis, Nance outlined an operationally useful concept.[125] In this definition, the presence of bacteria on a wound does not alone constitute infection. Rather, an infection is characterized by invasion of a host tissue by microorganisms and is associated with a local response to injury (inflammation) and with some degree of systemic response by the host. The term sepsis should be reserved for infections that are accompanied by a major systemic response by the host. A transient bacteremia, while it may produce cardiovascular and other system alterations, is not necessarily sepsis. Endotoxemia not associated with an invasive infection is not sepsis. For a clinical diagnosis of sepsis, microbial invasion must be demonstrated in close proximity to the systemic hemodynamic, immunologic, and metabolic events. However, even when using this definition, with its emphasis on physiologic response, it remains difficult to separate the physiologic changes due to injured tissue from those caused by microbial invasion.

The physiologic effects of injury are related initially to associated loss of intravascular volume. This ebb phase, as described by Cuthbertson,[43] is reversed by adequate resuscitation, and a flow phase characterized by a generalized increased activity of physiologic processes soon follows. The magnitude of tissue injury determines its physiologic impact on its human host (Figure 10-4). Small injuries produce minimal effects, whereas large wounds, represented by massive burns, initiate major alterations in homeostatic responses, surpassing those of other major trauma, peritonitis, and superimposed infection. These hyperdynamic, hypermetabolic processes are driven by a variety of mechanisms, including the systemic beta-adrenergic system described above. The local inflammatory reaction to tissue injury and necrosis plays an important role by initiating the release of various proteolytic enzymes, vasoactive peptides, and pyrogens, all of which have major hemodynamic, immunologic, and metabolic effects. The wound macrophage appears to play a particularly important role in the systemic response to injury. Activated (by local wound factors or endotoxin) macrophages produce interleukin-1, which can cause many of the post-injury metabolic alterations, including proteolysis, increased heat production, and altered thermoregulation.[48] Local factors from wound macrophages appear to be essential signals that result in fibroplasia, angiogenesis, and collagen synthesis in the wounded tissue. On a logistic basis, the local and systemic effects seem to complement each other in promoting prompt and effective wound repair.

When wound closure is delayed, the continued presence of injured tissue invariably is associated with bacterial wound contamination. Such wounds provide a portal for microbial invasion into underlying viable tissue and ultimately for systemic dissemination. Locally released bacterial products, particularly endotoxin, can cause devastating derangements of major physiologic processes. Again the macrophage appears to play an important role in the etiology of the profound cardiovascular collapse and organ failure associated with prolonged sepsis. Macrophages, when activated by endotoxin, produce tumor necrosis factor, a protein which is capable of inducing many of the deleterious effects of endotoxin, including hypotension, metabolic acidosis, hemoconcentration, and death.[180] Further, monoclonal antibodies to tumor necrosis factor protect experimental animals from the lethal effects of endotoxin. Thus the

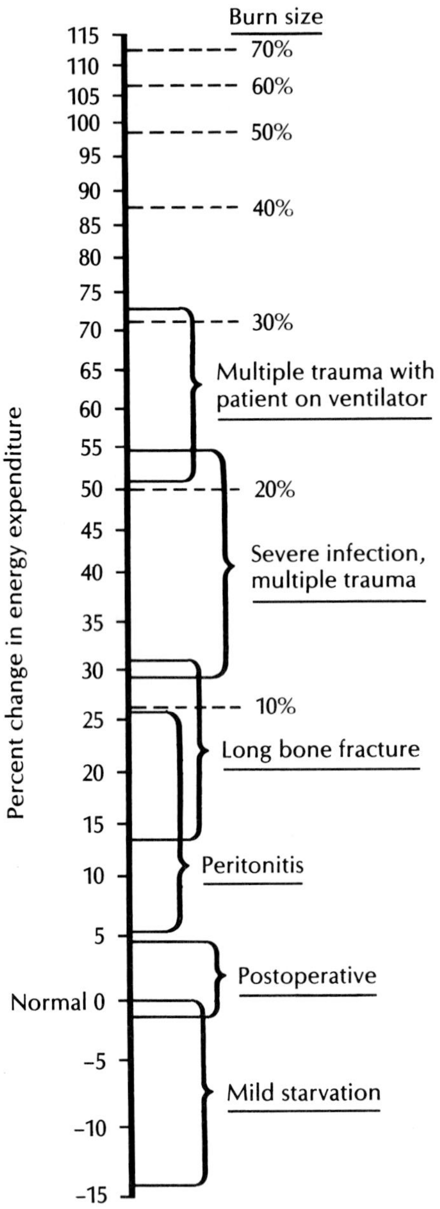

FIGURE 10-4 Injuries of increasing severity cause a similar augmentation of metabolic response. Massive injuries alone often initiate metabolic responses in excess of those associated with infection and sepsis.

initial hyperdynamic presentation of sepsis may be explained by the tissue injury caused by necrotizing infectious processes. With prolonged tissue infection and excess endotoxin production, other factors, such as tumor necrosis, may mitigate the hyperdynamic response, particularly if the patient's previous hypermetabolic response was near the limits of his physiologic reserve. Sepsis in these maximally stimulated patients would not further accentuate the physiologic response to injury and may even suppress it (Table 10-1). This response mimics beta-adrenergic blockade rather than beta stimulation, which sepsis is commonly thought to duplicate. Such data emphasize the major importance of the injury itself and the resulting wound.

Wound Effects

Immediately following injury, local events in the wound are centered on hemostatic mechanisms and the effects of altered capillary permeability. Intravascular fluid, primarily plasma, extravasates into the surrounding interstitial space, and in patients with massive tissue injuries, such as large burns, this edema formation causes profound hypovolemia. In the ensuing days, wound edema is resorbed, and the local inflammatory response initiates wound repair, with collagen synthesis and production of new capillaries. The large granulating wound with its massive vascular bed requires major hemodynamic and metabolic support.

Blood flow to healthy granulating wounds increases massively as angiogenesis proceeds during wound repair and may exceed ten times the blood flow to an equivalent area of uninjured skin.[189] The new vessels are denervated and have no vasoconstrictor tone.[189] These vessels are maximally dilated and thus act as a low resistance shunt. Wound perfusion varies primarily with changes in systemic pressure, and total body blood flow must support the newly added vascular bed by increased cardiac output or by selective diversion of flow from other parts of the body.

The wound uses little or no oxygen for its metabolic processes and appears to be essentially an anaerobic organ.[13,189] Large amounts of glucose are consumed by the wound, and comparable amounts of lactate and pyruvate are produced. Thus the wound preferentially uses anaerobic glycolytic pathways, which are inefficient energy production mechanisms. The increased blood flow to the wound appears to be necessary to provide adequate glucose substrate for the energy requirements of wound healing (Table 10-2). This increased blood flow is not accompanied by concomitant oxygen extraction and is most likely responsible for the systemic decrease in the ratio of arterial to mixed venous oxygen in patients with large inflammatory surfaces. Thus the circulatory and metabolic requirements of the wound in the uninfected injured patient appear to be a major initiator of the hyperdynamic state in such individuals.

Cardiovascular Effects

The response of the cardiovascular system to injury and sepsis varies with time and the institution of therapeutic interventions. Furthermore, cardiac function is strongly influenced by the associated hemodynamic and respiratory responses of the lungs, and overall evaluation of the cardiovascular physiology must consider the inte-

TABLE 10-1 EFFECT OF INJURY AND SEPSIS ON WHOLE BODY, ORGAN BLOOD FLOW, AND OXYGEN UTILIZATION

	NORMAL	NONINFECTED BURN	STABLE BACTEREMIC BURN	SEPTIC BURN
Whole Body				
Blood flow (L/min/m^2)	70-80	82.4	81.9	104.8
Cardiac index (L/min/m^2)	2.5-3.5	8.17	8.79	7.67
A-Vo$_2$ (ml/dl)	4-5	2.8	2.7	3.6
O$_2$ consumption (ml/min/m^2)	125-130	228	283	244
Renal				
Blood flow (L/min/m^2)	.55	.69	1.97	0.45
A-Vo$_2$ (ml/dl)	1.6-1.8	2.41	0.92	0.90
O$_2$ consumption (ml/min/m^2)	9-10	17	18	4
Splanchnic				
Blood flow (L/min/m^2)	.63-.85	1.54	1.74	1.19
A-Vo$_2$ (ml/dl)	4-5	4.6	4.1	6.7
O$_2$ consumption (ml/min/m^2)	34-40	68	66	73

TABLE 10-2 EFFECTS OF INJURY AND SEPSIS ON SUBSTRATE METABOLISM

	INJURY	SEPSIS
Glucose flow	↑	↓
Glucose production	↑	↓
Glucose space	↑	↑↑
Insulinogenic index	No change	↓
Ketogenesis	↓	↓↓
Muscle amino acid release	↑	↑↑
Nitrogen loss	↑	↑↑

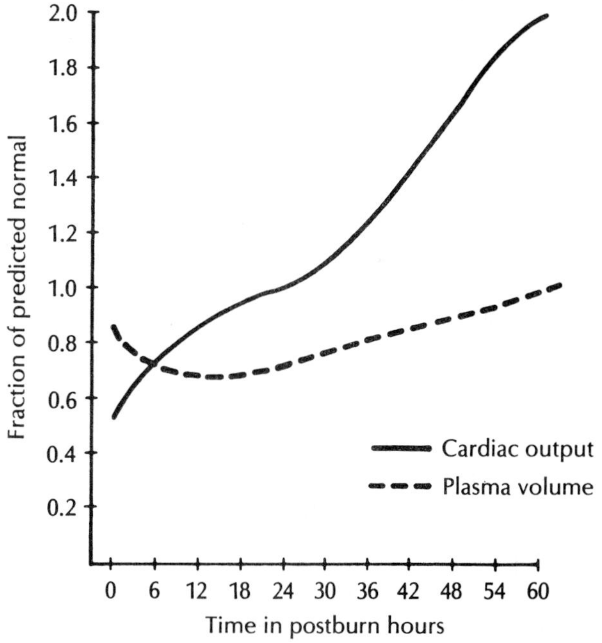

FIGURE 10-5 Changes in cardiac output after major thermal injury. Injuries of lesser severity initiate proportionately smaller elevations in flow.

grated response of these two organs together. The net effect of the circulatory response to injury and sepsis is reflected by the total blood flow as controlled by cardiac output and by distribution of the total flow to the individual organ systems. The partition of flow to the site of injury was described previously.

Hypovolemia usually accompanies a major injury with a reduction of cardiac output and blood pressure. Such responses occur rapidly if the acute injury is associated with rapid blood loss but will occur more slowly, although as profoundly, with a slower but massive loss of intravascular volume, such as occurs with severe thermal injury or multiple trauma. The low cardiac output state associated with acute injury is caused by intravascular volume deficit and not by a primary cardiac defect. Although myocardial depressant factors have been postulated by some investigators, direct studies of myocardial function have demonstrated the opposite circumstance. The mean velocity of left ventricular circumferential fiber shortening was elevated before, during, and after the successful resuscitation of a patient in burn shock, indicating a hypercontractile state following injury, even when cardiac output was depressed.[73] Cardiac output returned to normal with restoration of intravascular volume, demonstrating the major role of hypovolemia as the cause of the initial low output state. Likewise, increased left ventricular contractility is present after major nonburn trauma associated with hemorrhage.[83] This hypercontractility probably arises from the increased levels of circulating en-

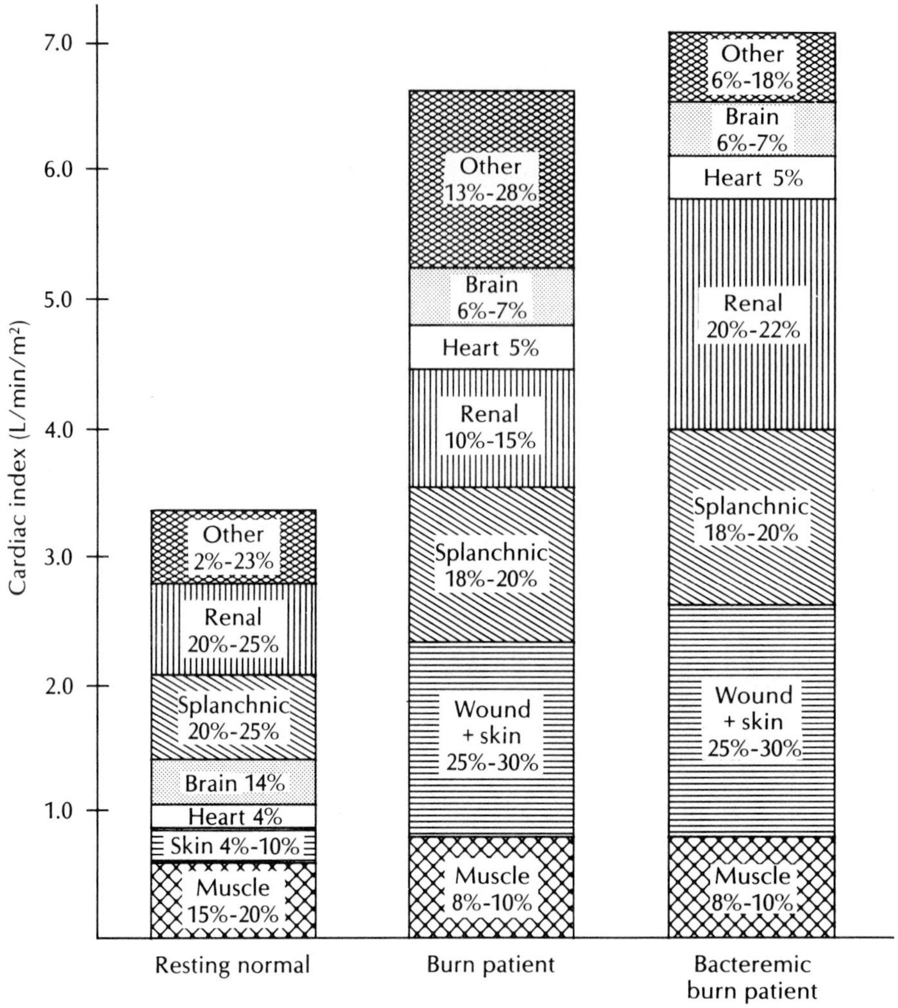

FIGURE 10-6 The distribution of total body blood flow after large burns and the added effect of infection. Flow to the wound is maintained in the hemodynamically stable patient with bacteremia.

dogenous catecholamines and the decreased afterload initiated by a reduced circulating blood volume.

Following successful resuscitation, cardiac output rapidly rises to levels that may exceed twice that of uninjured patients (Figure 10-5). The increased flow roughly matches the demand for oxygen and substrate in the visceral organs and peripheral tissues (Table 10-1). As described previously, the anaerobic wound bed appears to be responsible for the moderate reduction in oxygen extraction in the stable patient. Regional blood flow to the visceral organs generally rises, but this increase is proportional to the overall elevated flow (Figure 10-6). The fractional oxygen extraction of the liver, kidneys, and other abdominal viscera remains approximately unchanged.[190] Blood flow and oxygen consumption by muscle, brain, and presumably other neural tissues remain unchanged following severe injury.[15]

The effects of sepsis on the injured patient depend on the initial extent of tissue involvement. With limited tissue injury, typified by localized chemical peritonitis, the subsequent onset of sepsis is heralded by major physiologic alterations. In patients with large wounds and an associated hypermetabolic state, the early phases of sepsis may be indistinguishable from the already present hyperdynamic state. Generally the onset of sepsis is accompanied by a large increase in cardiac output and a reduction of systemic vascular resistance. The initial vasodilatation may produce a relative hypovolemia because of the increased capacity of the vascular bed, and cardiac output and blood pressure may fall. However, following restoration of intravascular volume, cardiac output rises above normal levels and blood pressure stabilizes. Because of the hyperdynamic flow pattern, oxygen extraction is often reduced, with normal or elevated oxygen use. The importance of this pattern is unclear. Left ventricular contractile function is maintained during normotensive sepsis[25]; however, in comparable groups of traumatized and septic patients, left ventricular ejection fraction was higher in the injured patients.[166] Further, associated ventricular compliance is moderately reduced.

The effect of sepsis on right ventricular function is more pronounced and probably produces major global cardiac dysfunction. Even during the stable phase of sepsis (high cardiac output and low vascular resistance), right ventricular compliance and ejection fraction may be markedly depressed in comparison to concomitant left ventricular function.[187] These manifestations of right ventricular dysfunction may cause similar alterations in left ventricular function by shifting the interventricular septum toward the systemic ventricle.[167] Leftward shift of the septum reduces associated preload and ventricular output. Severe sepsis commonly causes diffuse and global cardiac dysfunction. Contractility is diminished, cardiac output falls, and systemic vascular resistance increases. This phase of terminal or "cold" septic shock closely resembles experimental endotoxic shock, but the direct role of endotoxin in the clinical setting is uncertain.

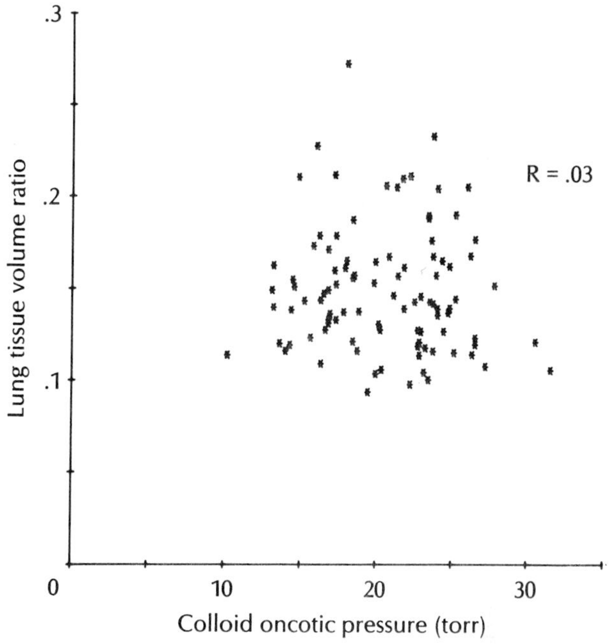

FIGURE 10-7 The relationship of lung water to plasma colloid oncotic pressure. The lung tissue volume ratio normalizes tissue water to lung size so that comparisons can be made among individuals of varying stature. Lung water does not appear to be related to colloid oncotic pressure.

Pulmonary Effects

The initial response of the lung to remote injury is an integral component of the generalized homeostatic mechanisms of the patient. If the injury causes major losses of intravascular volume, pulmonary artery systolic, diastolic, and capillary wedge pressures fall. The pulmonary wedge pressure is a clinically reliable indicator of left ventricle preload as resuscitation is instituted. Fluid resuscitation is most commonly achieved with blood and isotonic crystalloid solutions, depending on the type of fluid loss at the time of injury.[146] Successful resuscitation is reflected by adequate urine output and return of cardiac output to normal. In the absence of pulmonary injury and primary cardiac disease, pulmonary capillary wedge pressure remains in the low range of normal as total body flow is restored.

During and shortly after the resuscitation phase, pulmonary artery pressure may rise in excess of that expected from volume replacement alone. Pulmonary hypertension is particularly pronounced in patients with associated pulmonary injuries, such as inhalation injury, or in those requiring massive fluid replacement. Central venous pressure measurements will be erroneously high and may lead to under resuscitation if misinterpreted. However, elevation of pulmonary vascular resistance may provide protection to the lung during this phase of large fluid volume resuscitation, and the return of these pressures to normal levels 4 to 7 days following injury in the burned patient may explain why pulmonary edema occurs most frequently at this time in patients with inhalation injury. If pulmonary artery hypertension persists or is accentuated, right ventricular dysfunction occurs with a decrease in ejection fraction and an increase in end-diastolic volume index in those patients.[109]

In the absence of pulmonary contusion, inhalation injury, and other direct damage to the lung, airway mechanisms are not affected by remote injury. Pulmonary compliance, resistance, volumes, and dead space remain normal in patients with cutaneous burns alone. Likewise, pulmonary extravascular lung water usually remains unchanged in patients without lung injury. Lung water appears not to correlate with plasma colloid oncoctic pressure (Figure 10-7).

Hyperventilation

Following the onset of postinjury hypermetabolism, ventilation increases to meet the demands for augmented oxygen consumption and carbon dioxide elimination. Clinically, such patients breathe with larger tidal volumes and increased respiratory rates. The work of breathing increases proportionally, but most patients tolerate this situation without incident. However, patients with marginal pulmonary function or with limited cardiovascular reserve may not be able to adapt to this additional workload and will develop respiratory failure requiring mechanical ventilatory support. Infection and sepsis do not appear to play a primary role in this form of pulmonary insufficiency.

Certain groups of patients will hyperventilate out of proportion to the metabolic demands for gas exchange in the lungs and demonstrate prolonged hypocapnia. Patients with large injury surfaces, such as burns or massive intraabdominal injuries, may maintain moderately low PCO_2 in the range of 32 to 35 torr. These patients usually have a long-standing hyperdynamic circulatory state, and the prolonged increase in cardiac output probably explains the hyperpnea in such patients.[186] In addition, beta-adrenergic stimulation also increases ventilation in humans, and catecholamines that mediate the hypermetabolic responses to injury undoubtedly contributed to this situation.[80,191] Other factors, such as elastic loading of the airways, as may occur in intubated patients, increase the ventilatory response and may play a role in post-injury hyperventilation.[44] In burned patients, mafenide acetate, the major topical antimicrobial agent for control of burn wound sepsis, may accentuate hyperventilation as a result of its inhibition of carbonic anhydrase. None of these mechanisms implies the presence of infection or sepsis.

The onset of sepsis in the previously stable patient is commonly heralded by a sudden elevation of ventilation and is particularly evident in those with only a modest increase in metabolic activity. The mechanisms responsible for this hyperventilation are unclear, but most likely the associated increase in cardiac output typifying the early septic response is a major factor. In addition, bacterial endotoxin may cause a marked rise in ventilation through a variety of mechanisms.[85]

Adult Respiratory Distress Syndrome

Respiratory insufficiency frequently occurs in patients with major injuries. Predisposing conditions include direct injury to the lung (contusion, inhalation injury, and aspiration), transfusion reactions, remote fractures, infection, and shock. Although this form of respiratory insufficiency occurs in clinical circumstances that require treatment with large volumes of fluid to restore hemodynamic stability, fluid overload does not appear to be the major cause. This syndrome has been variously labeled shock lung, respirator lung, and DaNang lung, but is now called adult respiratory distress syndrome (ARDS). Adult respiratory distress syndrome results from pulmonary microvascular injury with an increased capillary membrane leak of fluid and protein.[172] Up to a certain point, the lung lymphatic drainage can remove the increased interstital fluid from the alveolar walls and return it to the major circulation. Once the rate of interstitial fluid accumulation exceeds the lymphatic circulation's ability to remove it, alveolar flooding occurs, and gas exchange markedly deteriorates.

While a number of disparate clinical entities predispose the development of ARDS, the common thread uniting these conditions is their ability to cause tissue injury and/or the production of mediators involved in the inflammatory response. These mediators include activated complement components, thromboxane, and fibrinogen fragments.[85,108] Infection and sepsis are the primary inciting events in the majority of episodes of ARDS, and up to 90% of patients have verified sepsis in proximity to onset of ARDS. When patients with large injuries develop sepsis, a rapid increase in lung water can be demonstrated, even before clinical ARDS develops.[181] Gram-negative bacteremia and endotoxemia cause increased lung vascular permeability in experimental models; both of these agents probably release mediators, such as thromboxane, from leukocytes and platelets trapped in the lung.[19,85]

Patients with ARDS have tachypnea and air hunger. Arterial blood gas values demonstrate hypoxemia with respiratory alkalosis. Although pulmonary capillary wedge pressure is normal (less than 15 torr), lung water is increased, indicating interstitial edema. However, the chest radiograph is usually normal or demonstrates a modest increase in the interstitial markings. Compliance may be moderately reduced, as observed clinically by increased peak inflation pressures if the patient is being mechanically ventilated. Pulmonary vascular resistance may exhibit a moderate rise. The ventilation perfusion ratio is elevated and is partially responsible for the hypoxemia. This mismatch is caused in part by the concurrent hyperdynamic state invariably present in patients with early ARDS.[168] At this stage, the respiratory tract is usually sterile.

During the next 24 to 48 hours, the chest radiograph begins to demonstrate bronchopneumonia and widespread atelectasis. Pulmonary vascular resistance now climbs markedly, the functional residual capacity falls, and shunt fraction is elevated more than 30%. At this time, hypoxemia is more pronounced, and carbon dioxide retention becomes evident. Sepsis and hypercarbia promote respiratory muscle fatigue and contribute to ventilatory failure,[84,89] and frank respiratory insufficiency requires mechanical ventilatory support. Pulmonary infection is verified by the presence of bacteria and inflammatory cells in the lung secretions; this complication is often the major cause of death in patients with ARDS. Interstitial fibrosis develops in the few patients who survive the first several weeks.

Metabolic Effects

The metabolic response to injury is characterized by an increase in metabolic expenditure, erosion of lean body mass, altered substrate utilization, augmented heat production, and weight loss. In parallel with the increase in total body blood flow, metabolic rate rises during the flow phase to a level that in severely burned patients may exceed twice that of the uninjured person. The magnitude of this response is proportional to the size of the injury and persists until the tissue injury has resolved. Following injury, heat production is elevated, and patients commonly exhibit elevated core and skin temperatures and higher core-to-skin heat transfer coefficients.[14] Only a small fraction of the hypermetabolic response can be ascribed to the endogenous specific dynamic action of accelerated protein breakdown. The Q_{10} of hyperpyrexia accounts for only a modest fraction of postinjury hypermetabolism, and the elevated heat production after injury is a consequence of an accelerated metabolic state, not of increased heat loss.

Nitrogen loss increases following injury, and 80% to 90% of nitrogen appears in the urine as urea. The amount of nitrogen excreted in the urine is directly proportional to the metabolic rate of the patient. Over a wide range of metabolic responses, varying from that of normal subjects to that of severely injured patients, body protein contributes a constant 15% to 20% of energy required to meet metabolic needs. Alterations in nitrogen economy in regional organ beds are reflected by changes in nitrogen transfer as amino acids.[129] Skeletal muscle is a primary source of nitrogen loss in the urine, and muscle proteolysis is reflected by the increased excretion of creatinine and 3-methylhistidine. This increased nitrogen excretion in the unalimented patient is paralleled by a decrease in lean body mass and weight loss.

Carbohydrates, primarily in the form of glucose, appear to be the best source of nonprotein calories in the injured patient. Certain tissues, including the wound tissue, neural tissues, and the formed elements of blood, use glucose in an obligatory fashion. Provision of glucose to these tissues will occur at the expense of lean body mass if adequate nutrition is not provided. In the unalimented state the major sources of three carbon precursors for new glucose production by the liver are the wound and skeletal muscle. As described earlier, high glucose delivery rate, made possible by the enhanced circulation to the wound, permits the wound to meet its high glucose requirements. In the liver, lactate is extracted and used for new glucose production. Concomitantly, ureagenesis parallels the rise in hepatic glucose output, with the urea ultimately derived from alanine and other glycogenic amino acids released from body protein stores. The mild hyperglycemia characteristically observed in hypermetabolic patients is a consequence of accelerated glucose flow arising primarily from increased hepatic glucose production and not from decreased peripheral utilization.[192]

The onset of sepsis in the injured patient initiates major alterations in glucose, nitrogen, and lipid metabolism at both the visceral and peripheral tissue levels (Tables 10-1 and 10-2). Alteration of glucose metabolism is often the first indication that a patient has an infection. Hyperglycemia in a patient receiving a previously well-tolerated intake of carbohydrates reflects the effect of sepsis on glucose uptake and utilization. Insulin sensitivity of the peripheral tissues, primarily muscle, is reduced in the septic injured patient.[32] The decreased capacity to oxidize glucose observed in patients with sepsis has been attributed to target tissue insulin resistance at both receptor and postreceptor levels.[53] Severe sepsis is associated with a decrease in glucose flow, a decrease in the glucose disappearance proportionality constant, a decrease in the insulin response to a given level of blood glucose, and an increase in the glucose distribution space. The effects of sepsis on hepatic metabolism of carbohydrates include a decreased hepatic extraction of glucose,[112] impaired suppression of endogenous glucose production by exogenous glucose,[18,164] and a decrease in hepatocyte glucose-6-phosphatase activity.[97] Administration of endotoxin, a lipopolysaccharide produced by many gram-negative organisms, results in depletion of liver glycogen content in association with a decrease in glycogen synthase activity. The decrease in hepatocyte adenosine triphosphate content that follows infusion of endotoxin results in a decrease in hepatocyte membrane potential difference and impairs hepatocyte extraction of indocyanine green.[112] Even though the serum levels of gluconeogenic amino acids are increased in patients with sepsis, hepatic glucose production is decreased in response to an intravenous infusion of alanine.[192]

The stage of an infection determines its effect upon protein metabolism. In the early phases of sepsis, the release of acute phase plasma proteins from the liver appears to be increased, resulting in elevated levels of C-reactive protein, fibrinogen, ceruloplasmin, and alpha$_1$ antitrypsin in association with a decrease in circulating levels of transferrin, albumin, and alpha$_2$-macroglobulin.[162] Elevation of C-reactive protein levels has been proposed as a predictor of postoperative sepsis. Laboratory studies have shown that the albumin synthesis rate is increased in septic animals and that the decrease in circulating levels of albumin represents the effects of increased degradation rate and increased distribution space. In the later stages of life-threatening sepsis, even though peripheral release of amino acids is elevated, visceral amino acid clearance is depressed, and hepatic protein synthesis is markedly decreased.[135] In laboratory models of infection, skeletal muscle protein degradation is increased, and amino acid incorporation into protein is decreased.[78,79] Laboratory studies have also shown that injections of endotoxin increase hepatic protein synthesis and decrease muscle protein synthesis.[87]

Sepsis also alters lipid metabolism. The serum concentrations of total cholesterol, high density lipoprotein cholesterol, and apoproteins A and B are decreased and that of triglycerides increased in patients with sepsis. The absence of ketosis in septic patients appears to be related to the effect of sepsis on hepatic metabolic processes. The depression of hepatic ketogenesis by sepsis has been attributed to inhibition of carnitine: acyl CoA transferase I activity by increased hepatic content of malonyl CoA.[182] The respiratory quotient of patients with sepsis is commonly decreased to levels of 0.7 to 0.8, a finding consistent with preferential utilization of lipid as an energy source. An increase in very low density lipoprotein production apparently contributes to the increased serum concentration of triglycerides that serve as ready energy sources in septic patients.[193] The utilization of fat for energy in the presence of sepsis appears to be refractory to the administration of exogenous glucose, insulin, and glucagon.[194] In fact, conversion of glucose to fat is increased in septic patients, and lipid commonly accumulates in the livers of such patients.[184] In laboratory studies, the absolute rate of palmitate oxidation in septic animals was decreased by sympathetic blockade but that change paralleled a decrease in overall metabolic rate.[194] Even though utilization and mobilization of lipids increases following injury, adipocytes exhibit a decreased lipolytic response to epinephrine as a consequence of both altered receptor sensitivity and postreceptor enzymatic activity.[176] This seemingly paradoxic response may represent the effect of prior depletion of adipocyte lipid content, because the adipocytes from the injured animals were smaller than those from uninjured animals.

ALTERATIONS IN HOST DEFENSE IN INJURED PATIENTS

Nonspecific Reactions
- Mechanical barrier loss
- Changes in circulating phagocytes
  - Neutrophils
    - ↓ Chemotaxis
    - ↓ Intracellular killing
      - Degranulation and ↓ lysozyme content
  - Macrophages
    - ↓ Phagocytic activity
    - ↑ Inhibitory function
- Changes in fixed phagocytes (RES)
  - Defective clearance
  - Diminished fibronectin levels
- Activation of the alternate complement pathway

Specific Reactions
- Changes in cell-mediated immunity
  - Prolonged graft survival
  - Cutaneous anergy
    - ↓ Lymphoproliferative response
    - ↓ Lymphokine levels
  - Change in OKT-4 : OKT-8 ratio
    - ↓ Helper function
    - ↑ Suppression
- Changes in humoral immunity
  - Transient immunoglobulin depression
  - Altered antigen responsiveness

Immunologic Consequences

Defects of host defense mechanisms in injured patients have been demonstrated to involve virtually every aspect of the immune response (see the box above). Plasma immunoglobulins (Ig) rapidly fall immediately following injury. IgG demonstrates this response most profoundly and usually requires 3 weeks to regain normal levels. IgM levels generally remain within the normal range throughout the clinical course. As described above immediately following thermal injury, most patients exhibit a marked leukocytosis, with leukocytes being contributed by increased marrow release and peripheral granulocyte demargination. Although the subsequent circulating leukocyte count may remain high, an absolute granulocytopenia results from a depletion of the marginating pool, and 3 to 4 weeks are required to reestablish the marginating pool by increased marrow production. Intervening gram-negative infection will selectively depress the marrow myeloid series, accentuating the granulocytopenia and often producing thrombocytopenia.

After burn injury, the effectiveness of polymorphonuclear leukocyte chemotaxis is inversely related to burn size, and persistent suppression correlates with subsequent mortality. A decrease in leukocyte chemotaxis often heralds systemic sepsis before clinical infection is apparent, but no causal relationship has been established. The cause of this defect seems to be a result of a heat-labile factor deficiency in burn serum, because serum from unburned donors restores chemotactic functions. A similar functional defect involving a heat-stable, nondialyzable chemotactic inhibitor of mononuclear leukocytes has been found in the serum of burned patients. Although the ability of neutrophils to phagocytize bacteria remains normal after injury, subsequent intracellular killing of the bacteria is markedly depressed.[7]

The effect of injury on antibody production appears to be variable. The response to a primary antigen is related inversely to the severity of injury, but the recall response may be intensified. Complement levels fall transiently after injury, but rapidly rebound to often higher than normal concentrations. Lymphocyte function after severe injury appears to affect primarily the T-cell but not B-cell populations.[12] Injury-induced alterations in lymphocyte populations have been described earlier. Injury appears to induce helper cell dysfunction, possibly as a result of decreased interleukin-2 production. Overall, multiple defects in cell-mediated immunity may predispose these patients to subsequent infections. As noted previously in recent animal studies in which narrow gating was used in cytometric analysis, T-cell populations were mildly affected by burn injury per se but markedly affected by sepsis.[24] Although many of the injury-induced changes in immunologic function parallel similar alterations in septic patients, no clear causal connection has been demonstrated between the abnormal immune process and associated infection. Most of the studies of immune function are in vitro assays, and their relevance to clinical situations is unclear. Experiments designed to specifically detect the correlations of leukocyte chemotactic function to susceptibility to infection failed to establish any relationship.[107] Further, current clinical trials of immunomodulators directed toward specific defects in the immune system have not been successful in reducing infectious complications in injured patients.

Effects on Other Organ Systems

Kidney

Renal function after injury reflects intravascular volume and hemodynamic stability. Hypovolemia causes a fall in renal blood flow, which is demonstrated clinically by a fall in urinary output. Conversely, fluid administration restores renal blood flow, and urine output is an available and generally reliable guide to the adequacy of resuscitation after injury. A variety of hormones, including antidiuretic hormone, aldosterone, renin, and angiotensin, fine tune the balance of body salt and water, and normal renal function is usually maintained in the stable infected or injured patient. Oliguric renal failure is unusual during early sepsis if intravascular volume is maintained by vigorous fluid administration. The elevated cardiac output and reduced systemic vascular resistance of early "stable" sepsis allows continued perfusion of the kidney even while being moderately hypotensive. Renal oxygen extraction falls, but oxygen consumption is maintained (Table 10-1). However, renal failure often develops in the face of adequate urinary volume. Creatinine clearance can fall to low levels before blood urea nitrogen and serum creatinine can begin to rise. An inappropriate polyuria often occurs in patients with severe sepsis. In that situation, urine output no longer reflects intravascular status, and fluid infusions must be increased to prevent hypovolemia. The intrarenal distribution of blood flow appears to be undisturbed, and the polyuria may be a consequence of elevated renal blood flow.[39] Urinary sodium falls below 10 mEq/L. Occasionally, it may be difficult to differentiate inappropriate polyuria from mobilization of fluid in the stabilizing patient after resuscitation.

Liver

Splanchnic blood flow rises as the injured patient becomes hypermetabolic (Table 10-1), and this increased perfusion appears appropriate for the metabolic activity of this organ. Unlike the other major organ systems, injury alone may cause varying degrees of hepatic insufficiency, and these abnormalities are often inseparable from the effects of sepsis. Elevations of liver enzymes, particularly serum glutamic-oxaloacetic transaminase (SGOT) and lactic dehydrogenase (LDH), often follow major injury. Not infrequently a picture of intrahepatic cholestasis, with moderate to large rises in serum concentrations of bilirubin and alkaline phosphatase, occurs in the absence of infection. The mechanisms producing the hepatic dysfunction are uncertain and may be related as much to the various treatment modalities required by the injured patient as to the physiologic effects of injury itself. Transfusions, resorption of soft tissue hematomas, and cell death produce large loads of pigment that must be metabolized to bilirubin and excreted. Nutritional support using high concentrations of carbohydrates has been implicated as the cause of cholestatic jaundice.[23] Conversely, starvation produces fatty infiltration of the liver and a similar clinical and biochemical picture. Differentiation from obstructive jaundice is critical because such jaundice usually requires surgical intervention.

Sepsis alone will produce cholestatic jaundice similar in its biochemical and clinical characteristic to that seen in nonseptic states; further, sepsis will accentuate any prior liver abnormalities, often to the point of overt liver failure with falling levels of coagulation factors and refractory hypoglycemia. The effect of sepsis on hepatic metabolic pathways was previously described. The mechanisms by which sepsis causes hepatic dysfunction are the subject of intense investigation. Bacterial endotoxins, either directly or through mediators, such as tumor necrosis factor, are toxic to the hepatocyte and cause a failure of cellular energy production. Complement cleavage products, particularly C5a, may cause hepatocyte damage in sepsis.[170] Hepatic failure usually develops late in the course of sepsis-related multisystem organ failure[64] and usually resolves if the source of sepsis is eliminated and normal function is restored in the other organ systems (especially in the lung and kidney).

Gut

The gastrointestinal tract is a major target organ of the stress response to injury and sepsis. Likewise, the effects of injury alone are difficult to separate from those of sepsis. The immediate gut response to major injury manifests by a reduction in gastrointestinal motility, and ileus is not uncommon after large burns and other remote trauma. If there is no direct injury to the abdominal contents, motility returns soon after successful resuscitation. However, overuse of narcotics, enforced bed rest, and neglect of bowel hygiene (allowing impaction to occur) will retard bowel function and prevent effective use of the gastrointestinal tract for the enteral delivery of nutrients. Conversely, diarrhea and other signs of increased motility occur with overzealous use of the hyperosmolar-defined formula diets required by these injured patients.

The gastrointestinal tract may be the initiator of and the responder to infection and sepsis in critically ill patients. The routine use of antacids and histamine blockers to promote a more neutral pH in the stomach allows overgrowth of predominantly gram-negative bacteria, and aspiration of even small quantities of this enteric flora may lead to florid bacterial pneumonia. Of greater potential concern is the likelihood that the gut may serve as a major source of bacterial flora which is systemically disseminated by translocation through the intact gut wall.[46] Bacterial microflora have been demonstrated in experimental models to cross the intact wall of the gut and to spread to the lymphatic and mesenteric lymph nodes. From those nodes, organisms spread to other visceral organs and the systemic circulation.

The initial response of the gastrointestinal tract to sepsis is a prompt reduction of motility and ileus. As sepsis becomes more pronounced, damage to the gut mucosa occurs, particularly in the stomach and duodenum. These patients demonstrate a breakdown of the gastric mucosal barrier with a diffusion of acid back into the lumen.[92] Although current antacid prophylaxis usually prevents progression of these mucosal lesions, in certain patients the disease progresses and may eventuate in major hemorrhage or perforation. Sepsis is the major coexistent clinical condition associated with these complications of stress ulceration, and resolution of the septic process often reverses these gut lesions, particularly in children.[152] Secondary effects of sepsis on the gastrointestinal tract arise primarily from the inability to use the gut for enteral support during the period of ileus. In such circumstances, mucosal mass is reduced, transport enzyme activity decreased, and gastrointestinal hormones are altered.[100]

Central Nervous System

Central nervous system (CNS) function is usually maintained in the stable, adequately resuscitated injured patient. A decreasing level of consciousness will occur with severe hypovolemia, and the return of consciousness level to normal is a useful guide to resuscitation effectiveness. Blood flow to the central nervous system in the hypermetabolic injured patient is unchanged from that of the uninjured patient and is maintained in the septic patient until late hypodynamic shock ensues. However, mental function is very sensitive to the presence of sepsis; even a mild deterioration of mental status in a previously alert patient frequently signals early sepsis. With prolonged sepsis, a nonfocal severe encephalopathy often develops, resembling a chronic vegetative state. This marked cerebral dysfunction is a result in part of the presence of false neurotransmitters such as octopamine, in septic patients.[61] With elimination of sepsis, CNS status usually returns to the previous state.

MICROBIAL FACTORS

Principal among the microbial factors predisposing the surgical patient to infection is the density of microorganisms present in a wound or other tissue. In an untreated wound the initially sparse microorganisms proliferate and increase in number with time (see the box on p. 371). The occurrence of invasive burn wound sepsis has been correlated with 10^5 or more organisms per gram of burn wound tissue as has the occurrence of infection and graft failure following closure of soft tissue wounds.[155] The detection of bacteria on a specially prepared smear of homogenized biopsy tissue has been equated with a content of more than 10^5 organisms per gram of tissue and likely failure of wound closure.[156] Further wound preparation prior to closure has been recommended when such a smear has been positive. Injury or treatment related immunosuppression and, as previously noted, the presence of foreign bodies all can reduce the microbial density necessary to cause infection. Recent studies, showing that the relationship between microbial density and nonviable tissue and infection in adjacent viable tissue is imprecise and time related, have impugned the reliability of quantitative cultures in diagnosing wound infections. The sloughing of necrotic tissue in a maturing wound occurs as a result of the enzymatic activity of proliferating bacteria and the patient's leukocytes at a time when granulation tissue, developing at the nonviable-viable tissue interface, can protect the patient from microbial invasion. Consequently, high microbial counts can be obtained from a "mature" wound by quantitative culture technique in the absence of infection.

The type of organism present on a wound also changes with time postinjury. The initial flora of a burn or other wound consists of the patient's endogenous flora and those members of the environmental flora deposited on or in the tissues at the time of injury. This largely gram-positive flora is gradually replaced by gram-negative organisms as exemplified by surface culture recovery of gram-negative organisms from 54% of burn wounds 5 days following injury. From the second postinjury week onward gram-negative organisms predominate on burn wounds. This same sequence is observed in other open wounds and even in the tracheobronchial tree following tracheal intubation.

The administration of antimicrobial or other treatment agents can further alter the wound flora. The use of topical burn wound chemotherapy has been associated with an increase in candidal and fungal burn wound infections as has the use of broad spectrum antibiotics

MICROBIAL FACTORS PREDISPOSING THE SURGICAL PATIENT TO INFECTION

- Density of microorganisms
- Microbial synergy
- Antibiotic resistance
  - Intrinsic
  - Mutational
  - Transferrable
- Motility
- Enzyme products
  - Collagenase
  - Elastase
  - Lipase
  - Protease
  - Hemolysin
  - Nuclease
- Metabolic products
  - Extracellular polysaccharides
- Endotoxin
- Exotoxins

in other critically ill patients.[127] True fungal infections, particularly those caused by the Phycomycetes, are most common in patients with acidosis, for example, those with uncontrolled diabetes and those with salicylate toxicity. Lastly, the nonspecific stress of an injury or a surgical procedure can apparently reactivate latent herpes simplex virus and cytomegalovirus.[60,111] The type of organism present in a wound appears to be of less importance than the number of organisms present in terms of failure of secondary wound closure. Streptococci are an exception to that general rule because even small numbers of those organisms can cause rapid lysis of skin grafts and postclosure cellulitis. Fortunately perioperative administration of penicillin or another antistreptococcal antibiotic in patients sensitive to penicillin eliminates the wound complication caused by those organisms.

The increase in the rate of surgical wound infection that accompanies prolonged hospitalization before operation[2] appears to represent the combined effect of severity of disease process that increases the time required to prepare the patient for surgery and the acquisition of the institution's resident flora, some of which may be antibiotic resistant. The resident flora may be acquired from a variety of sources, but convalescent patients represent the most important source of antibiotic resistant organisms, and contact with other patients should be prevented.[117]

Injuries involving the viscera result in peritoneal contamination by enteric flora in which anaerobes and gram-negative aerobes predominate. The role of anaerobes per se in intraabdominal infections is debatable because both aerobes and anaerobes can usually be cultured from the site of infection. The high frequency of anaerobe recovery from intraabdominal infections supports administration of a single antibiotic, the spectrum of which includes anaerobes or multiple antibiotics one of which is active against anaerobes.[74] In wounds confined largely to the surface, such as burn wounds, infections caused by anaerobes are extremely rare. Conversely, in patients with penetrating wounds in which nonviable tissue is present, anaerobic clostridial organisms from the environment can proliferate rapidly and cause gas gangrene. Other anaerobes appear to act synergistically with aerobic organisms to produce infections that burrow along or across tissue planes.[11]

Microorganisms possess genus and strain specific properties that contribute to local cytotoxicity, promote mechanisms that contribute to local cytotoxicity, promote invasion, and evoke systemic responses. Streptococci elicit intense local inflammation that expands by contiguous and lymphatic spread but infrequently invades deep tissues. Staphylococci have a greater propensity to invade deep tissues, but the intensity of the tissue reactions that they elicit commonly results in the formation of a thick inflammatory membrane that limits extension of the abscess but also hinders delivery of systemic antibiotics. Staphylococci also produce toxins capable of evoking systemic responses of variable severity such as the toxic shock syndrome attributed to toxic shock syndrome toxin-1 (TSST-1).[40]

Motility imparted by functioning flagella appears to be an important characteristic of gram-negative bacteria capable of invading through a surface wound such as a burn.[118] Enzymes and metabolic products, such as extracellular polysaccharides, vascular permeability factors, collagenase, elastase, lipase, nucleases, and hemolysins, produced in varying amounts by gram-negative organisms, contribute to local cytotoxicity and promote invasion. Axonemal protein degradation by pseudomonad proteases appears to impair ciliary function and promote tissue destruction within the airway.[82] Endotoxins and exotoxins produced by gram-negative organisms can, by direct or indirect action, cause impaired function of remote organs such as the heart and lungs.

Intrinsic and acquired antibiotic resistance of microorganisms not only influence the likelihood of infection of the patient receiving perioperative antibiotics but make treatment of an established infection more difficult. Acquired resistance is often plasmid mediated, with many plasmids capable of conferring resistance to multiple antibiotics and antimicrobial agents.[115] Antibiotic use results in the selection of resistant organisms from the colonizing or infecting flora and the induction of enzyme production, both of which result in the emergence of resistance during the treatment of an infection.

COMMON PATHOGENS AND THE NATURE OF MICROBIAL INJURY ENCOUNTERED IN SURGERY

Surgeons confront various bacteria in their practice. One important group causes infection in wounds and tissues associated with surgical procedures. Another group of infections requiring drainage, resection of organs, or other procedures induces abscesses, tissue necrosis, and tumefaction. Finally, the group of bacteria causing diseases such as rheumatic fever and endocarditis, which impair organ function, or the viruses of influenza and acquired immunodeficiency syndrome (AIDS), which alter immune reactions, cannot be neglected in the preoperative assessment of surgical risk.

Numerous bacteria, fungi, rickettsia, viruses, and parasites are always present in the atmosphere, ground, or water. Others, such as parasites, live only in certain parts of the world. Many organisms continually reside on the skin or on the membranes of the intestinal tract and other viscera. Food, droplets, dust, or contact may introduce organisms. Although most of these many microbes do not cause human illness, those known as pathogens have the ability, once entry is gained, to invade sterile tissues, to resist destruction by host defenses, to multiply, and to establish an infection.

Pathogenic organisms are generally classified according to the complexity of nuclear and other structures as follows:

1. Viruses contain genetic material but lack much of the cytoplasmic structure. They are capable of multiplying only within living cells of the host.
2. Bacteria, spirochetes, rickettsia, chlamydia, and mycoplasma (procaryotes) have a primitive nucleus.
3. Fungi and protozoa (eucaryotes) have a membrane-bound true nucleus.
4. Parasites such as platyhelminths (flatworms) and nematyhelminths (roundworms), being multicellular organisms, are not truly microbes but can cause serious infections of the intestine, biliary tract, and elsewhere when disseminated.

Pathogenicity and virulence, generally considered synonymous terms, define an organism's ability to resist host defenses and cause disease. Among the more important mechanisms that enable bacteria and fungi to survive within the body are resistance to intracellular killing by phagocytes and elaboration of toxins that cause cellular destruction and permit spread by inhibition of immunologic processes. The number and virulence of microbes versus the effectiveness of the host defense mechanisms at the time of invasion determine the magnitude of an infection. Because space does not permit a discussion of the nature and behavior of each, the characteristics of a few selected organisms typical of important surgical infections are presented to illustrate microbial invasion and injury to the body.

Staphylococci

Staphylococci are gram-positive, facultative aerobes capable of producing lactase and fermenting glucose. *S. aureus,* the staphylococcus with the greatest pathogenicity, produces profuse yellow pus from abscesses and golden-yellow colonies on culture media. The other common member of this genus, *S. epidermidis,* ordinarily is not pathogenic except in debilitated patients with immunodepression, whom it may attack at various sites, including the heart valves or endocardium.

As with other common staphylococci, *S. aureus* is an inhabitant of the skin, especially of moist areas. In the hospital environment, these organisms are transmitted by hand, dust, particles, droplets, and contact. To produce an infection in normal skin takes $7.5 \times 10^6/mn^3$ *S. aureus* organisms, but the presence of a foreign body enhances the infectivity.[56]

In addition to cell surface agents (peptidoglycan, teichoic acid, protein A) that impair phagocytosis and induce cellular necrosis, *S. aureus* elaborates several extracellular pathogenic toxic products. Coagulase-positive organisms are more virulent, but the mechanism responsible for the difference is not clear. Catalase probably protects the organism from the effects of superoxides produced by phagocytes.[106] Food poisoning characterized by vomiting and diarrhea is induced by enterotoxin absorbed from the gut, which temporarily acts on the central nervous system. A pyogenic staphylococcal exotoxin induces the "toxic shock" syndrome, which is similar in many ways to endotoxin shock. Cytolytic factors, alpha- and beta-hemolysins, and leukocidin contribute to pathogenicity.

Phenotype and genotype alterations of staphylococci permit adaptation to conditions within the host and resistance to bacterial killing. Mutation occurs through introduction of extrachromosomal genetic material by phages or by other routes. This mechanism probably plays a role in antibiotic or immunologic resistance. Based on such genetic variations, penicillin-resistant strains of staphylococci have emerged. Therefore treatment of staphylococcal infections may require penicillinase-resistant antibiotics. Although the clinical significance is not clear, structural changes such as the production of L-forms may preserve the organism in a viable state with the capability of returning to normal configuration after long periods of adverse conditions.

Alterations or failure of the host resistance, which are discussed later, obviously affect the illness induced by a staphylococci. Local and systemic reactions of these organisms are characteristically vigorous. Inflammation and abscess formation with yellow pus are typical. Treatment must include drainage and removal of associated foreign substances, such as sutures, splinters, prostheses, dead bone, or other necrotic soft tissue. Dissemination of *S. aureus* in the circulation, as occurs with lung abscess, is serious because of the organism's ability to establish infections at distant sites and in many organs, especially bone, kidney, liver, or brain.

Streptococci

Bacteria of the Streptococcus genus are made up of spheric cells arranged in chains or pairs. They are classified immunologically by serologic identification of cell wall antigens described by Lancefield.[58] The presence or absence of hemolysins, recognized by their ability to destroy red blood cells in culture, further identified these organisms.

S. pyogenes, Lancefield Group A, is usually hemolytic and is often responsible for pyogenic wound infections and severe respiratory tract infection. Lymphangitis and lymphadenopathy may be associated with wounds infected by this organism. Transmittal is by droplet or direct contact. Surgical personnel may be the source of infection and pass the organisms from localized cellulitis or from the flora of the vagina and the respiratory tract.[54] Two hemolysins, O and S, are responsible for some of the deleterious effects of Group A streptococci. Streptolysin O is cardiotoxic and attacks the sterols of cell walls. Proteinases, hyaluronidase, and streptokinase probably contribute to the spread of these organisms within the body. Skin grafts in the presence of beta-hemolytic streptococci will almost certainly fail. Host defenses against streptococci are similar to those against staphylococci. Although M surface protein in Group A streptococci may interfere with osponization, these organisms are rapidly killed after phagocytosis because they contain no catalase to neutralize or inhibit lysosomal enzymes. The propensity to produce pus is explained partly by bacterial or cell wall activation of complement and by local production of C5a, which strongly attracts polymorphonuclear leukocytes and macrophages. Fever and other metabolic changes so apparent with streptococcal infections are related also to release of "pyrogens" from activated macrophages. Group A streptococci also are associated with the nonsupportive complications of glomerulonephritis and rheumatic fever, which are manifestations of immune complex disease.

The pathogenesis of illness caused by Group B streptococci, *S. agalactiae,* which is also hemolytic, is not as clear except that it is prone to bacteremia associated with genitourinary tract infection. The nonhemolytic Group O enterococci, which are inhabitants of the gastrointestinal tract, are prevalent in pelvic and intraabdominal abscesses. The viridians group, which is generally nonpathogenic, is prone to adhere to injured heart valves or endocardium and produce persistent endocarditis. Thus they are of importance in cardiac and vascular surgery.

S. pneumoniae are paired cocci often responsible for pneumonia. The cell wall contains antigens and polysaccharides, to which antibodies are produced. These organisms are important because cellular immunity is partly responsible for defense against them. Thus patients, particularly young children, are prone to fatal pneumonia after splenectomy. Pneumococcal vaccine affords some protection if splenectomy cannot be avoided.

Enteric and Other Gram-Negative Bacteria

Because of the changing population of surgical patients, who at surgery may be older, more debilitated, or more seriously injured than in the past, coliform and other gram-negative organisms have assumed greater importance as causes of illness or death. Important pathogens of this group that cause infections or are surgically significant include the Enterobacteriaceae *(E. coli, Enterobacter, Klebsiella, Proteus, Serratia)*. Pseudomonas and other nonenteric, gram-negative bacteria have certain characteristics resembling those of enteric origin and are often the cause of infections in burns and in patients with depressed phagocytic activity. Other gram-negative enteric organisms that cause diarrhea, abdominal pain, lymph node enlargement, and symptoms difficult to differentiate from an acute surgical abdomen are Salmonella, Shigella, and yersinia. *Y. enterolitica* is important as a cause of mesenteric *adenitis,* which mimics the symptomatology of appendicitis, particularly in young male adults. *Y. pestis* is the agent responsible for bubonic plague, the "Black Death"; it is not an enteric organism but rather is transmitted from rats and other animals by flea bites. Local tissues and lymph nodes become necrotic, infarcted, and inflamed. Progressive toxemia and bacteremia lead to shock and death.

Although *E. coli* and other Enterobacteriaceae may cause diarrhea and are often found in infections throughout the body as well as in intraperitoneal abscesses, most attention has focused on their role in producing 'endotoxin' shock.[105] As normal residents of the gut, particularly the colon, these organisms are introduced into the tissue through perforation of the intestinal wall or by invasive procedures, such as urethral and vascular catheterization.[120] The structure of the bacterial cell wall is closely related to these organisms' pathogenicity and capacity to cause illness. These are aerobic, facultative, non–spore-forming bacteria. Some of these organisms attain mobility with a flagellum that penetrates the outer capsule and carries the H antigen. Motility may be an important feature of ascending infections in the urinary tract. Protruding pili or fimbriae assist in attachment of these organisms to the alimentary, urinary, or respiratory mucosa. The membrane contains endotoxin, a lipopolysaccharide, and the outer layer consists of repetitive O antigen side chains of polysaccharide attached to the lipid A by ketodeoxyoctonate linkages.

Lipid A appears to be responsible for most of the detrimental effects of endotoxin. In small quantities, this agent causes fever by activation of complement through the alternate pathway, which in turn activates macrophages to produce leukocytic endogenous mediator, now called interleukin-1.[49] In experimental doses greater than 1 mg/kg of body weight, endotoxin induces shock and death by a variety of activated endogenous agents, which are discussed later. The O-antigenic substances contribute bacterial resistance to both phagocytosis and the lytic function of complement activated by antigen-antibody complexes. The intermediate layer contains a mucopeptide that may be affected by beta-lactim substances in various antibiotics. The inner layer of the wall consists of the cytoplasmic membrane. Extracellular exotoxins of these bacteria also contribute to invasiveness and pathogenicity. Exotoxins of *E. coli* are responsible for diarrhea, whereas exotoxin A of *Pseudomonas aeruginosa* is a potent inhibitor of protein synthesis that may seriously affect the host's defensive and healing responses.

Anaerobes

Anaerobic bacteria are common in the normal flora throughout the body. Mucosal surfaces are heavily populated with anaerobic organisms, which outnumber aerobic and facultative organisms. Cultures from the gut contain progressively greater proportions of obligate anaerobes from the stomach to colon. Whereas no anaerobes exist in the normal stomach, they constitute 99.9% of the organisms in the colon. The most infectious anaerobic microbes include *Bacteroides fragilis, B. melaninogenicus, Fusobacterium nucleatum,* anaerobic cocci, and *Clostridium perfringens.*[74] Only the clostridia produce spores. Neither *Bacteroides* nor *Fusobacterium* organisms are capable of forming spores and apparently are commensal with man. They are often associated with *E. coli* and other enteric organisms in intraperitoneal infections. Other organs and regions to which anaerobes contribute infections are the appendix; gallbladder; abscesses in the lung, liver, or perirectal spaces; and sebaceous or pilonidal cysts.

Among the more dramatic life-threatening anaerobic infections are gas gangrene, which occurs in devitalized muscle tissue, and postabortal sepsis of pelvic organs. *C. perfringens,* usually in association with other organisms, causes both. Recently improved culture techniques have allowed recognition of *Bacteriodes* and *Fusobacterium* bacteremias, the first originating primarily from the gut and the second from upper respiratory sources. The surgeon should suspect anaerobic infections if the pus or exudate has a foul odor and contains gas. Sulfur granules suggest actinomycosis. Previous treatment with aminoglycosides predisposes to infection by certain anaerobes.

Although the great preponderance of anaerobic infections are of endogenous origin, occasional exogenous infections may be particularly associated with trauma. Impaired blood supply, tissue necrosis, and disruption of mucosal barriers contribute to satisfactory conditions for anaerobes to invade and multiply. Transmission from person to person is rare except in wounds from human bites that contain mixed infections, including anaerobes. Factors that predispose to anaerobic infections are those in which the oxidation-reduction potential is below −200 mV. Conditions such as ischemia, vasoconstriction following injection of epinephrine, shock, and tissue necrosis following trauma or in malignant disease promote anaerobic infections. Also, as in any infection, necrotic tissue and hemorrhage prevent cellular and humoral defense mechanisms from reaching the invading organisms. In short, prevention and treatment depend on adequate debridement of necrotic tissue and open drainage of suspected wounds.

Although most anaerobes are obligate, the more pathogenic are tolerant of air; thus they can survive until conditions become suitable for propagation to establish an infection. The presence of superoxide dismutase activity found in *B. fragilis* correlates with the resistance to oxygen. More than 70% of infections containing anaerobes are mixed. Facultative and aerobic organisms contribute to multiplication of anaerobes by lowering the oxidation-reduction potential or by supplying growth factors.

In addition to the local damage inflicted by anaerobes, exotoxins also cause their systemic effects. Tetanospasmin, the neurotoxin produced by *C. tetani,* induces the muscle spasm of tetanus. This severe disease is caused by implantation of the organism under the skin, usually from earth contaminated by equine feces. While spores may persist in healed wounds for long periods, the average incubation period is 8 days. As many as 25% of patients have no history of injury, and 51% have only a puncture wound. Tetanus is a preventable disease through active immunization with tetanus toxoid; in an emergency involving persons not previously immunized, appropriate wound care combined with tetanus immune globulin should be employed. The efficacy of toxoid immunization is attested to by the absence of tetanus in the U.S. Armed Forces since 1956, compared with as many as 1 million cases annually in developing countries where immunization is not common.[66,67]

Lecithinases (phospholipases) of *C. perfringens* and *C. novyi* damage cell membranes and render capillaries freely permeable to protein and water. Lysis of erythrocytes results in anemia and hemoglobinuria. Collagen barriers, which localize infections within tissues, can be destroyed by the collagenases of *C. perfringens* and

C. histolyticum. These proteolytic processes make amino acids available for bacterial growth. Hyaluronidase released by *C. perfringens* further augments the disruption of tissue and the spread of infection. Other enzymes contained in toxins cause hemolysis and cellular destruction. The enterotoxin of *C. defficile* causes pseudomembranous colitis associated with the alterations of normal colonic flora during antimicrobial therapy. *B. fragilis* produces a heparinase and occasionally intravascular clotting, necessitating increased doses of heparin in septic thrombophlebitis. Various *Bacteroides* species produce fibrinolytic enzymes, phosphatases, proteases, and lipases which complicate the infectious effects of these organisms.

Fungi and Yeasts

Fungi and yeast organisms belong to the group of eucaryotes that have a true nucleus surrounded by a nuclear membrane. Fungi are unicellular organisms that multiply in slender filaments called hyphae, with each cell attached at its end to the next. No cellular differentiation for various functions exists as in higher organisms. Reproduction is by budding. Specialized branches of the hyphae produce conidia, which are the spores representing the infectious particles transmitted by air or by aerosol droplets. In general, fungal disease is not passed from person to person. Certain fungi that grow only as unicellular organisms but reproduce by budding are called yeasts. Many fungi that produce significant infections are "dimorphic"; that is, they may grow either as mycelia or as yeasts, depending on alterations of circumstances such as the lower ambient temperatures in soil or at 37% C in the body. One such fungus is *Histoplasma capsulatum,* the organism responsible for histoplasmosis. Another type of dimorphic fungus is *Coccidioides immitis,* which grows naturally as mycelia but in the tissue as spherules. Proliferation in the body is by rupture of spherules, which release endospores capable of reproducing to form other spherules.

Fungi can invade the mucosa of the respiratory tract following inhalation. In certain parts of the world, fungal pulmonary disease is endemic, especially in rural farming regions. This is primarily because of the nature of the soil and the presence of bird and other droppings in which these molds propagate. Among the more important diseases are histoplasmosis *(H. capsulatum),* blastomycosis *(Blastomyces dermatitidis),* and coccidioidomycosis *(C. immitis)*. Although the pulmonary disease may be mild or transient, the danger lies in dissemination; for example, *H. capsulatum* is rapidly phagocytosed. The lymph nodes are quickly involved, and cellular immunity, the principal defense, develops within two weeks. The disease ultimately resolves by fibrosis and calcification of the foci, both in the lung and elsewhere. Cavities or masses in the lung or mediastinum must be differentiated from cancer or tuberculosis. Diagnosis may require a thoracotomy for resection or biopsy of the mass. The diagnosis of distant lesions in the skin also is made by histologic examination in tissue. Wide dissemination of the fungus usually occurs only in debilitated patients or in those with immunosuppression.

Treatment of the disseminated form of this infection, other than by draining or resecting abscesses, is limited to the use of amphotericin B, a drug with notable toxicity. Pulmonary infections by *B. dermatitidis* or *C. immitis* have many of the same clinical characteristics, as do their complications. The disease they produce is mild except for dissemination in patients with depressed immunocompetence. Skin, bone, and the genitourinary tract become involved, as well as the brain in coccidioidomycosis.

Opportunistic infection by ubiquitous fungi is primarily in debilitated or diabetic patients, in cancer patients undergoing chemotherapy, or in those taking steroids. The genus *Aspergillus* infects the sinuses, ears, and lungs. In the lung, cavities with fungus balls may require resection. Other infections, including mucormycosis, may invade arteries, resulting in infarcts and necrosis. The nasal structures are attacked, requiring debridement. Such organisms may cause serious problems in severe burns.

Candida albicans and other yeasts of this genus, which may be normal inhabitants of the skin and gastrointestinal tract, become invasive in the mouth, vagina, and other organs when overgrowth occurs because of alteration of the normal bacterial flora. Candidiasis becomes invasive with various factors, including malnutrition, steroid or broad-spectrum antibiotic therapy, indwelling catheters, and immunosuppression. Hematogenous infection may be transient or may be responsible for distant abscesses, especially in patients with leukemia or lymphoma. Candidal endocarditis is common in drug addicts and in patients with abnormal heart valves. Despite therapy, the mortality is high (30% to 80%) in such debilitated patients.

Viruses

Viruses are important in surgery because of their ability to induce diseases that require surgical correction, such as congenital malformations or the induction of lesions in normal tissues. For example, hepatitis viruses cause hepatitis and subsequent cirrhosis. The second important feature of viral infection for the surgeon is the ever-present danger of contracting hepatitis by pricking the finger with a contaminated needle or by ingesting material contaminated with feces or other body secretions from patients with hepatitis. Many other viruses can play a major role in tissue destruction and reduction of immunocompetence. The retrovirus of acquired immunodeficiency syndrome poses a potential hazard for surgeons, but documented inoculation of medical personnel by infected patients is extremely rare. This is especially true of patients in whom immunosuppression has been induced following organ transplantation. In this group, cytomegalovirus is an important cause of damage to liver, kidney, lung, and other organs.

Viruses are different from other infectious agents in that they are very small and are obligate intracellular parasites. Their composition and organization are relatively simple. A complete virus particle consists of genetic material encapsulated by a protective coat. Viruses contain either deoxyribonucleic acid (DNA) or ribonucleic acid (RNA), but not both. Having only genetic material but not the mechanism for energy production, viruses must multiply within cells. Subsequently they must be coated before release from the host cell for transport to invade another host cell. A series of steps in this process includes absorption of the virus onto the cell membrane. Then the virus must penetrate the cell by pinocytosis or by fusion of the viral and cell membranes. Enzymatic removal of the viral protein coat leaves bare nucleic acid within the host cell. Viral RNA reproduction occurs within the cytoplasm, whereas viral DNA replication takes place in the nucleus. Protein synthesis of the viral coat, or capsid, follows in the cytoplasm.

DIAGNOSIS OF INFECTION IN THE SURGICAL PATIENT

The patient's history yields important information for detecting infection. A knowledge of the disease process and its mechanisms may suggest the site of infection. Previous injury, particularly if associated with shock requiring massive transfusion therapy and operative treatment, should focus attention on the sites of injury and the operative wound as sites of infection. For example, previous history of blunt abdominal trauma in the seat-belted passenger of a motor vehicle, even if operative intervention was not employed, suggests an intraabdominal source of infection in septic patients. The continued presence of a traumatic wound such as a burn and long term intravascular access sites are frequent causes of infection in severely injured patients. Postinjury treatment with antibiotics can confuse the diagnosis of infection because they may incompletely suppress infection. Because infection can involve any and all organ systems, they all must be evaluated promptly in the infected patient (see the box below).

INFECTIONS IN CRITICALLY ILL SURGICAL PATIENTS

Invasive soft tissue infection
Pneumonia—airborne or hematogenous
Septic thrombophlebitis
Endocarditis
Urinary tract infection—cystitis, pyelonephritis, renal abscess, prostatitis
Intraabdominal sepsis—perforated stress ulcer, acalculous cholecystitis, necrotizing enterocolitis, pancreatitis
Parotitis
Sinusitis
Generalized sepsis—usually arising from other infections listed here

Clinical Signs

Generalized and Local Changes

Fever and chills are hallmark of early response to infection. However, hypermetabolic injured patients are often moderately febrile in the absence of infection (temperatures 38° to 39°C), and, in these patients, a marked change in temperature is a more significant sign of sepsis than is any absolute level. Gram-positive infections tend to elevate body temperature, while gram-negative infection not uncommonly causes hypothermia, especially in hypermetabolic patients. In the early stages of infection, the skin is usually warm and dry until hypovolemia develops. Infected patients often appear plethoric, tachypneic, and anxious.

Local signs depend on the location of the infectious focus. Superficial soft tissue infections involving skin and subcutaneous tissue are more easily detected than are infections involving deeper or intracavitary foci. In deep soft tissue infections, a tender mass with fluctuance can often be detected even when the overlying skin and subcutaneous tissue are erythematous and indurated. Intraperitoneal infection is often associated with abdominal tenderness, guarding, and the other signs of an acute abdomen. Pain and erythema associated with injured tissue suggest infection, although the presence of necrotic tissue alone does not denote infection. Gram-positive organisms tend to produce cellulitis and usually localized tissue damage. The presence of purulent drainage reflects infection, but occasionally no bacteria can be isolated from wound pus (especially if the patient has received antibiotic therapy). Gram-negative infection tends to produce more extensive tissue infarction and necrosis with relatively little pus accumulation. Certain organisms, such as *Pseudomonas aeruginosa,* can produce metastatic infection at sites distant from initial focus.[94] Crepitus accompanies mixed organism and clostridial infections.

Physiologic Signs of Altered Organ Function

Cardiovascular

Tachycardia is usually the first sign of an infectious process. Its predictive accuracy may be obscured in the hypermetabolic injured patient who will demonstrate an increased pulse rate as a manifestation of the injury response. Pulse rate may further increase to maintain cardiac output in the hyperdynamic response to sepsis. Younger individuals tend to increase cardiac output by elevated heart rates, while older persons rely more on the Frank-Starling mechanism (increased preload).[157] Systolic blood pressure tends to be maintained during early sepsis, although it may transiently fall with the initial systemic vasodilatation before restoration of intravascular volume. Later, blood pressure tends to fall, even in the presence of increased cardiac output. Large amounts of fluid are required to maintain total body perfusion, and a sudden increase in fluid requirement may be the presenting sign of systemic infection. In this vasodilated state with a greatly expanded effective blood volume (see Table 10-1), the pulse is full and bounding. In terminal sepsis, blood pressure, pulse rate, and cardiac output fall precipitously.

Renal

Renal function is monitored clinically by urine output. The average-sized adult usually has adequate renal perfusion when hourly outputs are 30 to 50 ml; in children weighing less than 30 kg, 1 ml/kg/hr reflects adequate renal perfusion. Oliguria associated with the early stages of an infection usually reflects an inadequate circulating blood volume and should be treated by fluid infusion and maintenance of the elevated cardiac output. Inappropriate polyuria, as described above may occur in infected patients and may be one of the initial responses to sepsis. A low urine sodium concentration (less than 10 mEq/L) may lead to confusion with the diagnosis of diabetes insipidus. Prolonged sepsis is reflected by a rising blood urea nitrogen and creatinine. The use of nephrotoxic antibiotics, especially the aminoglycosides, may accelerate the course of renal dysfunction in sepsis.

Central Nervous System

A change in mentation is an early but imprecise sign of sepsis, and severely injured patients who are restless, confused, and anxious should be presumed to have sepsis until proven otherwise. However, previous drug abuse and the use of narcotics, cimetidine, and antianxiety drugs alter mental status and confuse interpretation of CNS symptoms in the infected patient.

Gastrointestinal

The most reliable sign of gut failure in sepsis is ileus. In patients previously tolerating enteral feedings, increased gastric or duodenal residual volumes may be the first indications of a reduction in gastrointestinal motility. Prolonged malfunction is seen as abdominal distention and a loss of bowel sounds. Overt bleeding from stress ulceration is now rare, but sepsis may precipitate low grade blood loss thoughout the gastrointestinal tract. Mucosal erosive lesions with slow blood loss is now increasingly recognized in the colon in stressed, predominantly septic patients.[152] Other digestive complications associated with sepsis include pancreatitis, acalculous cholecystitis, and pseudo-obstruction of the colon.

Metabolic

Hyperglycemia, or an increase in insulin requirements in patients already intolerant to glucose, is the most common clinical metabolic derangement induced by infection.[192] Previously tolerated nutritional support often must be discontinued while hyperglycemia is being controlled. Glycosuria with polyuria may accentuate the decrease in intravascular volume in the patient with recent onset of sepsis. Adequacy of fluid loading cannot be accurately guided by urine output during periods of marked hyperglycemia.

Laboratory Tests

Microbiologic Data

Early diagnosis of surgical infection is essential for the successful treatment of the underlying process. The relative nonspecificity of clinical signs of infection has been described, and only direct assessment of microbial involvement can verify that an infection is present. Blood cultures must be obtained in the infected patient at the time of any physiologic deterioration indicating the onset of sepsis. Other cultures, including sputum, urine, wound, and stool, should be obtained on the basis of history and clinical signs and symptoms. Except for blood, positive cultures do not necessarily indicate infection but will reflect the likely organism responsible if infection is present. The distinction between colonization and true tissue infection can only be made in conjunction with clinical and laboratory evidence of a tissue response to infection. In this regard, histologic examination of exudates and biopsy specimens are essential for interpreting culture results. Surveillance cultures are particularly useful for providing an accurate indication of the likely organism responsible for a new infection while identification is being carried out by the microbiology laboratory. With prolonged hospitalization, the organisms recovered from the septic patient will usually be members of the predominant flora in the critical care unit at that point in time.

Surface cultures of the potentially infected wound, even when carried out with quantitative techniques, very often yield erroneous results because the surface flora may not reflect the organisms causing the tissue infection.[153] Even quantitative cultures of biopsy specimens are of limited sensitivity (25% fail to identify any organism) and reliability (bacterial densities agree to within the same $\log_{10}$ in only 38% of paired samples).[196]

Tissue biopsy is the most accurate method of documenting infection and differentiating microbial colonization from invasive infection in accessible wounds and organs. Histologic demonstration of microorganisms in viable tissue is the essential feature of true infection (Figure 10-8). Organisms in overlying necrotic tissue are of little significance; hence it is important that the biopsy specimen include a viable portion of the wound and be representative of the tissue structures involved in the infectious process. Thus when necrotizing fasciitis is suspected, the specimen should include skin, subcutaneous tissue, fascia, and muscle.[147] Histologic examination of the specimen provides early information on the microbial identity (gram-positive or gram-negative bacteria, yeast, fungi, or viruses), which can guide early antimicrobial therapy. Laboratory sensitivity testing to antibiotics is essential for proper selection of these agents. Regular sensitivity testing of the patient's endogenous flora allows identification of emerging antibiotic resistance patterns and dictates alterations in therapy.

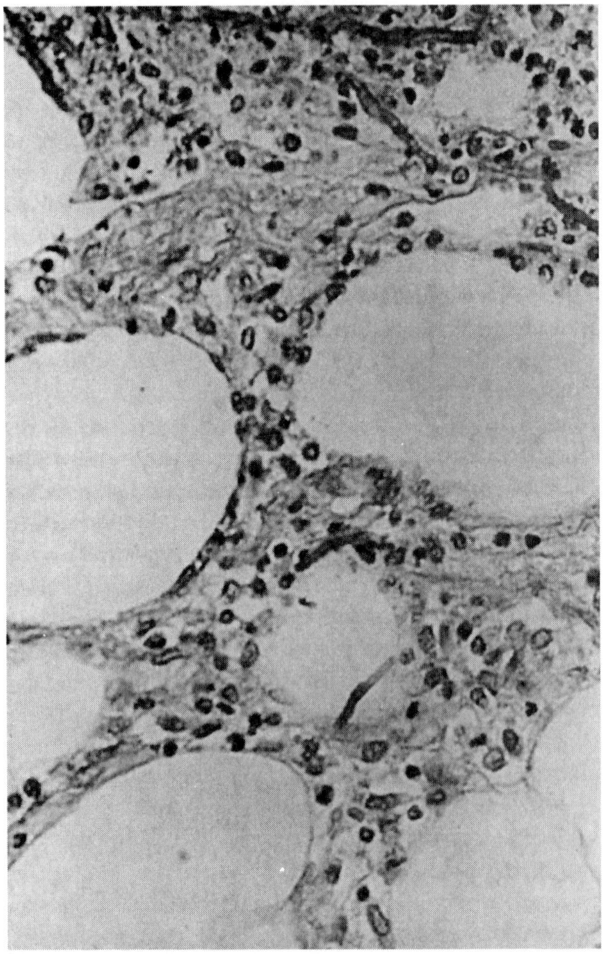

FIGURE 10-8 The identification of microorganisms in viable tissue confirms the diagnosis of infection. This histologic section of a burn wound biopsy shows branching fungal elements characteristic of *Aspergillus* species invading viable tissue.

Acid-Base and Electrolyte Changes

Acid-base changes with infection vary with the progression of sepsis to shock. The onset of sepsis is accompanied by a prompt increase in ventilation. Respiratory alkalosis with a reduced P_{CO_2} and an elevated pH is a regular finding at the early stage of infection. In patients already demonstrating the mild respiratory alkalosis associated with the hypermetabolic state, sepsis further exaggerates these changes. Superimposed on these changes may be those of metabolic alkalosis. The metabolic component usually arises from the antacid therapy necessary for stress ulcer prophylaxis and/or from prolonged gastric drainage after the onset of ileus (which removes potassium, chloride, and acid). As tissue perfusion falls with progression of sepsis, metabolic acidosis occurs, and at the time of death, pH may be below 7.0.

Blood chemistry studies remain normal until organ failure begins. The characteristic changes associated with liver and renal dysfunction are described elsewhere. Electrolyte abnormalities usually are not pronounced with sepsis, since their normality is subject to control by regulating the amount of fluids and electrolytes administered to septic patients. Hyperglycemia is the most sensitive clinical laboratory indicator of the onset of sepsis.

Hematologic Changes

The white blood cell (WBC) count is the most important hematologic indicator of sepsis. While uninfected patients with large areas of injured tissue may demonstrate slight to moderate elevation of WBC count (8000 to 12,000/mm^3), sepsis causes elevations to a higher range (12,000 to 25,000/mm^3). In addition, there are an increased number of immature (band) forms during sepsis-induced leukocytosis. Fulminant gram-negative infection may present with leukopenia, and mortality is correlated with the nadir of the WBC count depression. An even graver indicator of septic deterioration is an associated thrombocytopenia, which in children is a sensitive indicator of severe infection.[38] Thrombocytopenia of sepsis is rarely accompanied by laboratory evidence of disseminated intravascular coagulation (DIC). When prothrombin and partial thromboplastin abnormalities occur, they usually are a result of liver disease and inadequate nutritional supplementation with vitamin K rather than of DIC.

Anemia may develop and persist in patients in whom a large inflammatory surface is present. Periodic blood transfusions may be required until the wound is closed. Frequent blood sampling necessary for the treatment of septic patients accentuates the ongoing transfusion requirement.

Immunologic Assays and Humoral Indicators

At this time, clinically useful diagnostic immunologic assays are limited primarily to fungal and viral infections. Assays based on the antibody response to the presence of a pathogen require time for antibody synthesis and generally are not useful for the immediate diagnosis of an infection caused by a specific pathogen. Further, many individuals have been exposed to these potential pathogens during states of normal health and may already have high antibody titers unrelated to their present illness. Up to 80% of normal adults have complement fixation titers to cytomegalovirus, Epstein-Barr virus, and other viruses and fungi. Therefore, a rise in titer during the period of infection is required to document infection.[101] Immunoglobulin M(IgM) rises in conjunction with phycomycotic infection. The hormonal changes associated with injury, including those of insulin, glucagon, catecholamines, and adrenocorticotropic hormone (ACTH), are indistinguishable from those in patients with early sepsis, and no specific hormonal response is uniquely characteristic of systemic infection.

Radiologic Examinations

Radiographs

Plain radiographs most effectively detect infection when it is located in the chest. The infiltrates characteristic of pneumonia and potentially contaminated or infected fluid collections in the pleural spaces are easily seen. Other aspects of sepsis, such as the early stage of ARDS, can often be detected on chest radiographs. Plain films are less useful for evaluating suspected infection in the abdomen or in the soft tissues. Occasionally, such films will reveal an abdominal air fluid level outside the gastrointestinal tract, displacement of bowel loops or other organs, free air under the diaphragm, or free air in the soft tissues. Clinical studies of abdominal infection have demonstrated that plain radiographs detect less than one third of underlying infectious processes.[71]

Scans

The radiologic procedures most helpful in diagnosing surgical infection (soft tissue infection, fluid collections, and infected masses) are computed tomography (CT), the various radioisotope scans, and ultrasonography. The CT scan is currently considered the most accurate noninvasive technique for identifying septic foci, particularly in the abdomen. The efficiency of the examination is enhanced when it is performed on the basis of clinical information. Fluid collections and abnormal masses can be detected with a sensitivity approaching 100%,[4] but differentiation of an infectious process from other disease states (such as a sterile cyst) is less accurate. Gallium- and indium-labeled leukocytes have a high affinity for infected tissues. Gallium scanning, an older technique now rarely used, requires up to 48 hours to label an infected area, and uninfected inflammatory surfaces cause frequent false positive diagnoses. Indium-leukocyte scans have several advantages over gallium scans: imaging time is shorter, and there are fewer false positive results. However, its relatively low specificity limits its uses as a primary diagnostic tool for infection evaluation, and it is best used in conjunction with CT scans and ultrasonography. The radiolabeled iminodiacetate derivatives are effective agents for evaluating the hepatobiliary tree and identifying conditions associated with biliary tract sepsis. The scanning procedure is rapid and accurate, even in the presence of hyperbilirubinemia. Visualization of labeled material in the gallbladder and in the duodenum indicates the patency of the cystic duct and common bile duct, respectively.[177]

Ultrasonography is easily performed at the bedside, but its accuracy is highly operator dependent. In one study of 52 adult patients who had undergone elective abdominal operations, sonography performed on the seventh postoperative day accurately identified intraabdominal fluid collections.[72] It is particularly helpful in evaluating acute calculous cholecystitis by demonstrating gallbladder dilation, wall thickening, and sludge in the lumen.[134] Likewise, a thickened wall and intracavitary sludge indicates an abscess instead of a simple cyst.

CLINICAL MANIFESTATIONS OF TYPICAL SURGICAL INFECTIONS

Evidence of bacterial and other microbial infection varies widely according to the site and nature of the invading organism. Local inflammation, often accompanied by clinical manifestations of the systemic responses, indicate the presence of infection. Responses include malaise, fever, tachycardia, leukocytosis, respiratory alkalosis, muscle wasting, and accelerated urea excretion.

In general the number of organisms, the extent of cellular damage, and the duration of the infection govern the magnitude of injury inflicted by infection and the responses evoked. This pattern may range from mild symptoms of a localized infection, such as a boil, to widespread sepsis, shock, and even death. Elebute and Stoner[55] devised a scheme for scoring the severity of sepsis based on four effects: (1) local evidence of infection; (2) magnitude and duration of pyrexia; (3) secondary effect, including jaundice, acidosis, system failures, and bleeding diathesis; and (4) laboratory data such as blood cultures or evidence of leukocytosis. Such modes of grading are useful for making comparisons and for estimating the prognosis of individual cases. Others have developed similar methods to assess severity of sepsis to compare the effectiveness of different treatments.[47]

Infection represents successful invasion and proliferation by one or more species of microorganisms anywhere within the body's sterile tissues. Sepsis usually implies a more advanced stage of infection in which microorganisms, having escaped local control by the initial inflammatory reaction, are disseminated to other tissues by direct extension or by bloodstream transmission throughout the body. Inflammation, with its frequently associated suppuration, appears clinically as heat, redness, swelling, pain, and tenderness. These are the visible demonstrations of the complicated immunologic defense by which infection is limited or eliminated. Healing is the process by which deposits of collagen, and in a few instances proliferation of specialized tissue, repair defects caused by wound or disease. In a sense, healing is the end of the inflammatory process. To serve as a framework for the details of injury inflicted by invading bacteria and the defensive immunologic, metabolic, and physiologic responses, this chapter briefly describes the clinical patterns in several typical infectious conditions commonly encountered by the surgeon.

Uneventful Recovery from Major Surgery

For comparison with clinical responses to infection, Figure 10-9 presents data from a series of patients who recovered without complications from major abdominal and thoracic procedures. No tissue necrosis, significant hemorrhage, or infection occurred in these patients. Except for the first 2 days postoperatively, fever was not present and the white blood count rose only an average of 10,200. The metabolic energy expenditure, as measured by oxygen consumption or heat production, was not elevated by more than 10%. This was reflected by the pulse rate, which did not rise above 92 ± 8 beats/min. Cardiac indices, although depressed during anesthesia, rose 25% ±6% above normal during the immediate recovery period. Subsequently, during convalescence, the mean cardiac index was but 9% ± 3% above the normal resting value of 2.8 L/m^2/min. Postoperative pneumonitis was minimal. The estimated mean pulmonary arteriovenous shunt was less than 10% (normal, 33% to 5%). Arterial partial carbon dioxide tension ($PaCO_2$) remained between 32 and 39 mm Hg, with arterial pH values between 7.34 and 7.46. The blood lactate concentration was within the normal range, less than 0.8 mg%. Except during the procedure and the immediate postanesthetic period, no severe metabolic disorders occurred to make demands on organ function or immunologic responses. This benign state of affairs can be attributed to the absence of cellular injury from shock, tissue necrosis, pulmonary dysfunction, or significant infection in any part of the body.

Wound Infection

In a sense, postoperative wound infection represents the simplest form of the surgical infectious process. The time of bacterial entry and the recovery of cultured organisms involved are known, and the infection is usually localized. The swelling, redness, heat, and tenderness of inflammation and pus, when present, are apparent. Systemic responses depend on the magnitude of the infection and include fever up to 39° C (102° F), tachycardia to 100 or more bpm, leukocytosis between 10,000 and 20,000 cells/mm^3 with a shift to more than 85% polymorphonuclear leukocytes, and band forms. Within hours after removing sutures or instituting other measures to drain the subcutaneous tissue as well as deeper layers of the wound, the fever and other systemic manifestations start to subside.

The behavior of the wound and the surrounding tissue reaction varies to some extent with the nature of the invading organism. *Staphylococcus aureus,* present in approximately 19% of wound cultures, usually becomes evident 4 to 6 days postoperatively. Erythema, edema, pain, and tenderness typically precede the formation of creamy yellow pus by one or two days. Infections with hemolytic or other streptococci (3%) proceed more rapidly. Cellulitis (extended red, swollen skin or other surrounding tissue), lymphangitis (red streak ascending along the course of lymphatics above the wound), and bleb (blister) formation are typical. A watery exudate from the wound is common. Wound erysipelas (dermal cellulitis) occurs within 3 days, but this infection is rare today. Gram-negative aerobic organisms found in wound infections are appearing with increasing frequency compared to pyogenic organisms. Included in this group, with their incidence in wound cultures, are *Escherichia* coli, 19%; *Pseudomonas aeruginosa,* 9%; and *Proteus mirabilis* and other *Proteus* species, 9%. Anaerobic streptococci and other enteric organisms such as *Bacteroides* and *Enterobacter* species often accompany these organisms. Development of obvious wound infection by the gram-negative species is usually apparent 1 to 2 weeks postoperatively, being slower than the response to staphylococcal and streptococcal pyogenic organisms. In febrile patients gram-negative bacteremia may be present before inflammation appears in the tissue surrounding the wound. However, gram-negative septic shock is not a common sequelae unless wound drainage is delayed.

Gas gangrene, most often associated with *Clostridium perfringens,* is rare (less than 0.1% of all wounds). Clostridia usually invade ischemic necrotic muscle or other tissue, usually following trauma, in a closed wound with low oxygen tension. Recognition by the presence of severe pain; cellulitis, possibly crepitant; and marked systemic manifestations of fever, hemolysis, and prostration is essential for the prompt treatment necessary for survival. Early opening and debridement of all necrotic fascia and other tissue, with the assistance of antibiotic therapy, can control this type of clostridial infection.

Several factors promote wound infection. Among the more important are inadequate blood supply, whether a result of atherosclerosis, venous congestion, or lymphatic obstruction, and vascular impairment caused by surgery. Traumatic shock or hypovolemic shock causing more than transient arteriolar vasoconstriction may promote infection.[28] Necrotic tissue inevitably becomes seeded by bacteria to produce an infection; this fact emphasizes the importance of gentle tissue handling and the need for debridement of injured tissue.

Diabetic patients are extremely prone to slow healing and infection in extremity wounds. This problem is related both to large vessel atherosclerosis and to microangiopathy. Diabetic neuropathy is associated with loss of sensation leading to frequent trauma of soft tissues with secondary infection. Except for interference with neutrophil function by hyperglycemia, system impairment in diabetic patients exists.

Malnutrition, immunosuppression, uremia, and other conditions contributing to defects of the immunologic system tend to raise the incidence of skin and wound infections.

Septic State

The systemic manifestations of and responses to widespread infection are generally similar regardless of the

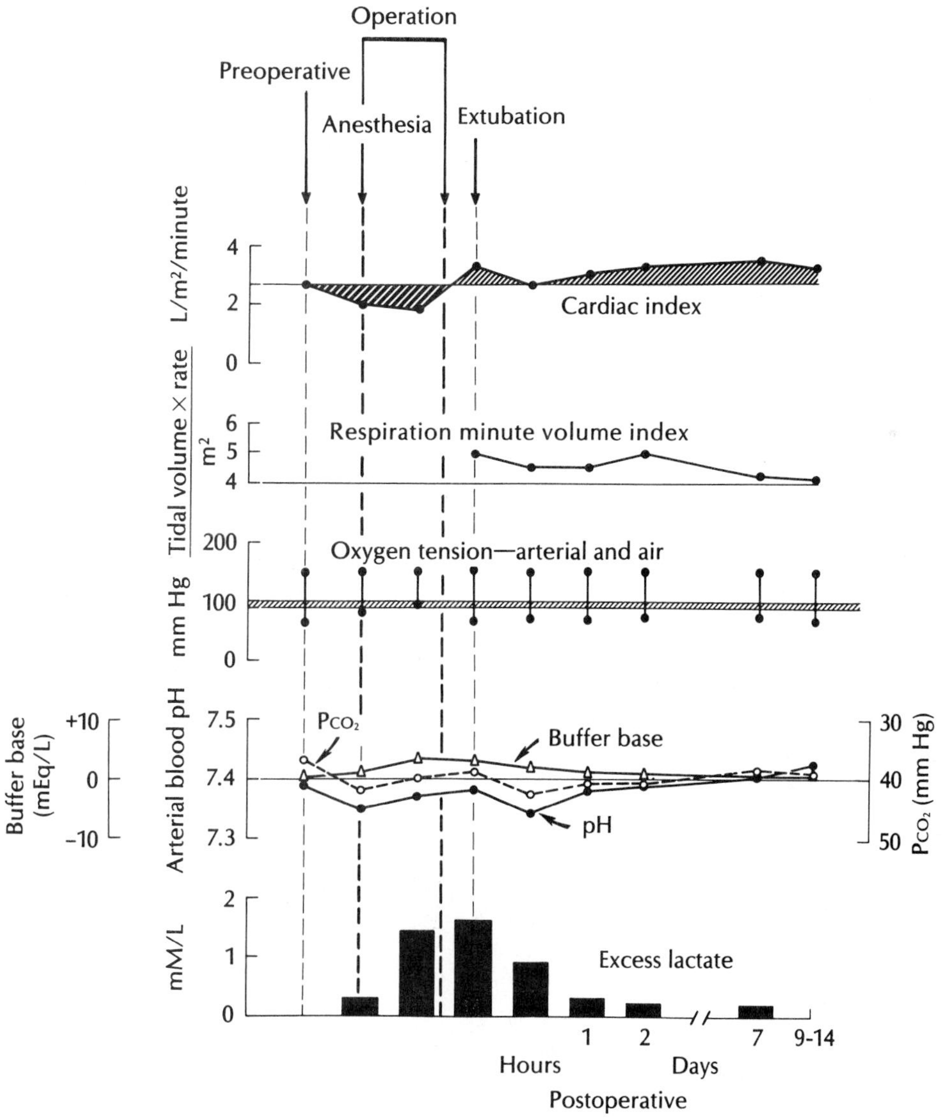

FIGURE 10-9 Circulatory, respiratory, and metabolic data from 30 patients who recovered uneventfully from major surgery. Note that the only acidosis or other alterations of cardiac output and respiration occurred during the procedure and recovery from anesthesia. (From Rubin JW, Clowes GHA Jr: *Surg Clin North Am* 49:489, 1969.)

TABLE 10-3 RESPIRATORY, HEMODYNAMIC, AND METABOLIC RESPONSES IN UNEVENTFUL SURGICAL CONVALESCENCE AND SEPTIC STATES (MEAN VALUES ± STANDARD DEVIATION)

MEASUREMENTS	UNEVENTFUL SURGICAL CONVALESCENCE	SEPSIS: ONSET—DAY 1	SEPSIS: SEPTIC HIGH CARDIAC OUTPUT	SEPSIS: SEPTIC LOW CARDIAC OUTPUT
Respiratory				
Pa_{O_2} (Fi_{O_2}, 0.2) (mm Hg)	76 ± 8	68 ± 26	57 ± 10	52 ± 12
Pa_{O_2} (Fi_{O_2}, 0.4) (mm Hg)	—	102 ± 34	73 ± 24	68 ± 16
Pa_{O_2} (Fi_{O_2}, 1.0) (mm Hg)	388 ± 44	201 ± 45	108 ± 38	106 ± 29
Shunt, estimated	12% ± 8%	21% ± 9%	30% ± 6%	34% ± 8%
Pa_{CO_2} (mm Hg)	36 ± 6	30 ± 6	32 ± 5	35 ± 5
Arterial blood pH	7.39 ± 0.03	7.31 ± 0.07	7.47 ± 0.08	7.22 ± 0.10
Peak inspiratory pressure (cm H_2O)	—	31 ± 4	36 ± 6	41 ± 8
Hemodynamic				
Cardiac index (L/m²/min)	3.6 ± 0.3	3.4 ± 1.9	4.8 ± 1.6	2.0 ± 1.0
Central venous pressure (cm H_2O)	5 ± 3	8 ± 4	10 ± 5	16 ± 6
Pulmonary arterial systolic pressure (mm Hg)	23 ± 4	29 ± 3	36 ± 5	34 ± 6
Pulmonary arterial mean pressure (mm Hg)	19 ± 3	23 ± 4	28 ± 5	29 ± 6
Left atrial (wedge) pressure (mm Hg)	6 ± 2	5 ± 4	11 ± 4	15 ± 3
Mean arterial blood pressure (mm Hg)	86 ± 10	73 ± 16	89 ± 13	65 ± 10
Metabolic				
Basal energy expenditure (kcal/m²/day)	750 ± 56	980 ± 103	950 ± 160	680 ± 169
Body temperature (°F per rectum)	100.2 ± 0.7	101.2 ± 1.1	101.7 ± 1.7	100.1 ± 2.6
Blood glucose (mM/L)	4.2 ± 0.5	6.4 ± 1.2	7.8 ± 1.4	11.3 ± 3.5
Blood free fatty acid (mEq/L)	1.0 ± 0.2	0.8 ± 0.1	0.5 ± 0.2	0.7 ± 0.3
Blood lactate (mM/L)	0.6 ± 0.2	1.3 ± 0.3	1.2 ± 0.2	3.5 ± 0.8
Urinary N excretion (g/m²/day)	6 ± 2	—	9 ± 3	—

body area involved (see Table 10-3 for representative values). Variations depend on impairment of function in one or more organ systems in which cellular damage is caused directly by the local infection or indirectly by an infection in a distant part of the body. Peritonitis, empyema, septic arthritis, gangrene of an extremity, perinephric abscess, or widespread cellulitis qualitatively produce the same set of systemic reactions. Certain specific signs and symptoms, such as localized tenderness or swelling, are related to the tissues involved.

For example, peritonitis usually results from bacterial contamination associated with intestinal disease or injury. Appendicitis, cholecystitis, pancreatitis, and other illnesses in which bacteria from inflamed or gangrenous organs gain entrance to the peritoneum may result in walled-off intraperitoneal infection or general peritonitis. Peritonitis occurs if the process proceeds too rapidly to be isolated by inflammation. Accumulations of blood and bile may be seeded with bacteria and secondarily infected. A foreign body may serve as a nidus around which an infection develops.

Most bacteria require iron to proliferate; thus blood in the peritoneum or other sites fosters infection. Furthermore, bacteria trapped in a clot or in fibrinous adhesions are apparently protected to some extent against antibodies and cellular immune defenses.[3] This concept led to radical debridement of the peritoneum in patients with multiple abscesses following general peritonitis. The results are equivocal because of the effects of secondary bacterial invasion and added trauma.[141] The fulminating course of widespread general peritonitis may lead to a pattern of severe sepsis and possibly fatal septic shock. On the other hand, localization of invading bacteria by inflammation and subsequent formation of one or more intraperitoneal abscesses is typical of a severe but controlled infection. The manifestations of peritonitis also depend on the organs involved, the degree of bacterial contamination, and the period during which the process occurs.

Localized Peritonitis

Intraabdominal infection is preceded by inflammation in a visceral organ (appendicitis, diverticulitis, tuboovarian disease) and is usually accompanied by vague pain, referred to the dermatome from which the organ had its embryonic origin. Signals from the neural pain end organs in the viscera are transmitted via the sympathetic system, which are stimulated by tension or pressure similar to those in the somatic nervous system. As the inflammatory process develops, diffusible agents from the original focus stimulate vasodilation, increased vascular permeability, and the passage of proteins to the surfaces of surrounding viscera. Conversion of fibrinogen to fibrin within the peritoneum produces the yellow plastic adhesions of gut, omentum, and other structures to wall off or isolate the original site of bacterial contamination.

The sensory innervation of the parietal peritoneum accurately localizes pain produced by movement or pressure during peritoneal inflammation. Reflex spasms of the abdominal musculature occur. Subsequently an abscess forms as pus accumulates. Occasionally, if not drained surgically, an abscess may resolve by liquefaction and absorption. More often tissue necrosis evacuates pus and debris along paths of least resistance to the skin surface. Alternately, an intraabdominal abscess may rupture directly into the colon or at the site of an intestinal suture line. If adequately drained naturally or surgically, the abscess collapses and heals by granulation and fibrosis. If not, the abscess may become chronic, with fibrous tissue surrounding it, or may progress to bacteremia and fulminating sepsis.

Septic patients who react appropriately characteristically have continuous fever reaching daily peaks of 38.3° to 39.5° C (101° to 103° F) per rectum, persisting until the site or source of infection is effectively eliminated and pus is prevented from reaccumulating either by antibiotics, resection, or drainage. Tachycardia and an elevation of cardiac output to an average of 56% ± 21% above the normal resting value occur in response to a large decrease in peripheral vascular resistance.[33] Resting energy expenditure (REE) increases 20% or 30% above normal basal metabolic rate. Ileus associated with inflammation and edema of the mesentery and retroperitoneal tissues results in abdominal distention, which necessitates nasogastric drainage. Nutritional intake via the intestinal tract is frequently inhibited. Urinary nitrogen excretion remains elevated, accompanied by muscle wasting and weakness. Fat stores are rapidly depleted unless alimentation is adequate to satisfy both caloric and protein requirements. Leukocytosis greater than 12,000/mm^3 with a shift to the left is characteristic of patients who survive from severe but controlled infection.

General Peritonitis

Following free perforation of the colon, as occasionally occurs during intestinal obstruction and diverticulitis or after a gunshot wound to the cecum, fluid containing bacteria is promptly released into the peritoneum without time for localization by inflammation. Resection or exteriorization of a colonic perforation removes the source of contamination and permits the peritoneal inflammatory reaction to isolate the infection to abscesses within the peritoneum. Characteristically, intraperitoneal abscesses form in both subdiaphragmatic spaces, the gutters, infrahepatic space, pelvis, and most difficult to detect, interloop collections. Most patients require subsequent drainage; this aggressive approach reduces mortality from near 33% to 10% or less.[81,158]

Another example is the secondary infection following the onset of a sterile chemical peritonitis. If not promptly sealed by inflammatory adhesions or dealt with surgically, the acid from a perforated peptic ulcer inflames the peritoneal surfaces. Accumulation of fluid within the peritoneum may serve as an ideal culture medium for growth of intestinal organisms. Preventing these developments requires prompt surgery to close the perforated ulcer. A collection of bile and blood following liver injury with biliary leakage offers a medium favorable for growth of *E. coli* and other enteric organisms.

Patients with general peritonitis promptly manifest acute, diffuse tenderness of the abdominal wall as the parietal peritoneum becomes inflamed. In the early stages, the patients are prone to lie still with shallow respiration and spastic guarding of the abdominal wall. Rigidity follows as the inflammatory process progresses. Nausea and vomiting and absent bowel sounds with ileus occur. Distention is common as intraluminal gas accumulates in the gut.

Initially the patient is alert but irritable and gradually becomes obtunded. Without treatment, evidence of severe dehydration develops; such patients may die of hypovolemia. Hematocrit concentration often rises as much as 20% to 30% above the patient's normal value. Low cardiac output usually responds to rehydration through an infusion of Ringer's lactate solution. Typically the patient enters the "hyperdynamic" state with a significantly elevated cardiac output, in which both organ function and metabolic rates are increased above normal resting values.

PHARMACOLOGY OF ANTIBIOTICS

Once the physician understands the mechanism of antimicrobial action of a given antibiotic, he must consider other factors that determine the success or failure of antimicrobial therapy without significant host toxicity. For an antibiotic to be effective as a prophylactic or therapeutic agent, it must be absorbed and distributed to the site of infection or potential infection. The concentration of antibiotic at that site must be at an effective level and must remain sufficiently high for an adequate period to achieve the desired result. Thus a basic knowledge of pharmacokinetics is required to select the appropriate antibiotic and the proper dosage to combat a given infection. The physician must consider several pharmacokinetics and host factors when making this selection (Figure 10-10).

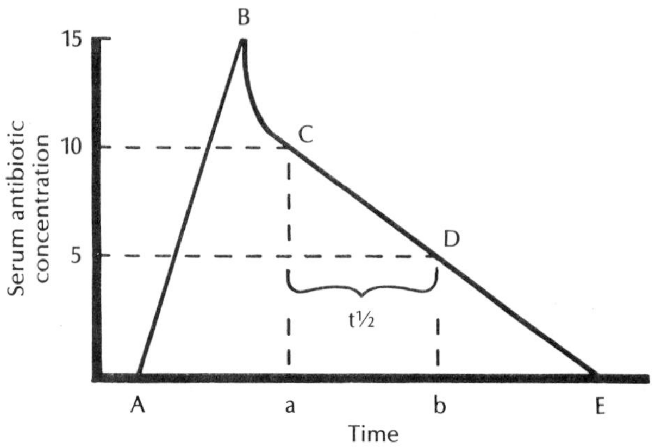

FIGURE 10-10 Segment *AB* represents increasing serum antibiotic concentration with intravenous administration (absorption); point *B* is the peak serum antibiotic concentration; segment *BC* represents the equilibration of the antibiotic to various body compartments (distribution); point *C* represents maximum equilibrated serum antibiotic concentration; segment *CE* represents the elimination of serum antibiotic (excretion); point *D* is one half of the maximum equilibrated serum concentration; segment *ab* is the serum half-life (*t*½) of the antibiotic.

Absorption

The process by which a drug is made available to the fluids of distribution is referred to as absorption. The rate of absorption depends on the method of administration and the physical properties of the drug. The choice of drug and route of administration should be such that the minimum drug concentration achieved at the infected site is at least equal to the minimum inhibitory concentration for the infecting organism. For patients suffering from serious infection, it is necessary to administer the therapeutic agent via the most reliably effective route. Although the pharmacology of gastrointestinal drug absorption is important in considering the gamut of oral medications, surgeons have relatively few occasions for using oral antibiotics in the treatment or prevention of surgical infection. One possible exception is the oral administration of poorly or nonabsorbed antibiotics when preparing patients for colonic surgery. The most reliable route of parenteral administration is usually the method of choice to achieve accurate tissue concentration at the site of infection or potential infection. Intravenous administration may be preferable to intramuscular administration for some agents because fluctuation in tissue levels secondary to erratic absorption is sometimes seen with intramuscular injection. Also, patients receiving therapy over several days via the intramuscular route require painful injections.

Distribution

Once an antibiotic is absorbed, it is distributed throughout the various compartments of body water. Some drugs may penetrate the intracellular compartment, whereas others are excluded; some may penetrate the cerebrospinal fluid, but others may not. When considering the potential limitations in the penetration of various body compartments and cavities of infection by antibiotics, do not expect medicines to substitute for surgery. Abscess cavitities filled with pus or the presence of dead tissue or foreign bodies usually make it impossible for antibiotics to penetrate to sites of infection. Properly selected surgical drainage, excision of dead tissue, and removal of infected protheses are not adjuncts to antibiotic therapy but are essential prerequisites for effective antimicrobial therapy.

The serum levels of the distributed antibiotic are often referred to in the context of presumed efficacy. The inference is that high serum levels mean greater concentrations of antibiotic to kill or inhibit bacteria. However, concentrations in serum may have no therapeutic significance. Peak serum levels are affected by volume of distribution, protein binding, and rapidity of excretion. For example, the cephalosporins have a low concentration in the cerebrospinal fluid but are highly concentrated in human bile. On the other hand, chloramphenicol readily crosses the blood-brain barrier. Thus serum level is of no therapeutic significance; the physician must consider the tissue levels of the antibiotics at the site in question. Tissue concentration of a given antibiotic may vary dramatically from serum levels for a given antibiotic. Likewise the half-life, which is the time required for the maximum equilibrated serum concentration of a drug to decline 50%, must be carefully interpreted in light of the above information. Tissue half-life may be shorter or longer than synchronously determined serum data.[59]

Application

Consideration of various agents used for systemic prophylaxis of wound infection shows the practical applications of pharmacokinetic concepts. The studies of Miles,[121] Burke,[21] and Polk[143] have revealed that the main determinant for supressing infection is the attainment and maintenance of adequate tissue levels of antibiotic during the time the surgical wound is open. Therefore prophylactic therapy requires that the concentrations penetrating the tissues exceed minimum inhibitory concentration for the likely contaminating bacteria before such contamination. This level must be maintained for the duration of the procedure. For example, cefazolin and cephaloridine maintain adequate wound concentrations for a sufficient period of time; on the other hand, cephalothin does not maintain levels consistent with ef-

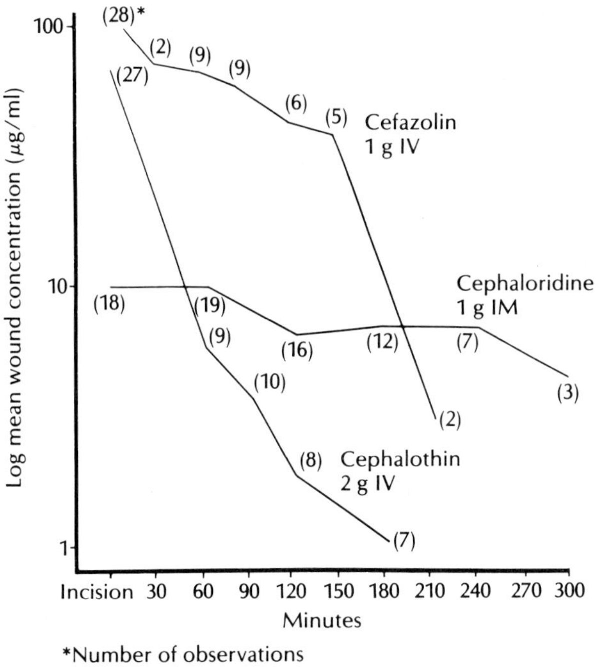

FIGURE 10-11 Cephalosporin wound antibiotic levels. (From Polk HC Jr, Trachtenberg L, Finn MP: *JAMA* 244:1353, 1980.)

fective antimicrobial activity and disappears rapidly from the tissues even when given in doses twice those of cephalothin and cephaloridine. The failure of cephalothin as a systemic prophylactic antibiotic is well documented (Figure 10-11).[34,144]

Consideration of pharmacokinetics in the clinical setting allows the physician to make intelligent decisions concerning not only the choice of agent used but also the dose and interval of administration. The dose of the agent is the most important aspect of pharmacokinetics that relates to the peak serum or tissue level. However, the interval between doses (dosage) is the most important factor in maintaining effective levels. The trough level of antibiotic, or that concentration of antibiotic present just before the following dose, allows the physician to regulate the dosage interval to achieve a constant effective antimicrobial concentration while providing levels below host toxicity. Therefore, although the physician might think that administration of a larger dose of antibiotic will achieve more effective antimicrobial activity, in fact more frequent administration of a lesser dose may be safer and more effective.

Resistance

Although the agent with the appropriate lethal or inhibitory mechanism of action is selected and delivered to the infected or potentially infected tissue, no guarantee exists that infection will be eliminated or prevented. Resistant microbes emerge through chromosomal changes in genetic composition and proliferate through subsequent selection by administrated antibiotics. An organism's genotype dictates the presence of resistance or change in the resistance patterns of a bacterial strain.

Chromosomal resistance develops as the result of spontaneous mutation in a locus that controls susceptibility to a given drug. The drug's presence then serves as a selecting force to promote proliferation of the now-resistant mutant in preference to susceptible microbes. Spontaneous mutation occurs rarely and is an infrequent cause of antibiotic resistance. When it does occur, mutants are commonly resistant by virtue of an altered drug receptor.

Extrachromosomal resistance develops as the result of transfer of circular structures called plasmids. The process of transduction, the bacteriophage-mediated transfer of plasmids, allows resistant bacteria to indirectly confer resistance to susceptible organisms. After the generic material is transferred via the bacteriophage, this locus is then incorporated into the genome of the recipient organism, thus providing the organism and subsequent clones of this bacterial strain with the resistance mechanism.

The most common mechanism of transfer of drug resistance is through conjugation. A protein tube, or pilus, is extended from a resistant organism to a susceptible organism, and the plasmids carrying the genes, which code for the resistant mechanism, are directly transmitted to the recipient. The mechanism of transmitted resistance is commonly the synthesis of enzymes that destroy antimicrobial agents. Other phenotypic expressions of genetically transmitted resistance may take the form of alterations in binding sites at either the cell wall or ribosomal levels.

As the widespread use of antibiotics has continued, successive resistant organisms have been selected for proliferation. Although the gram-positive organisms have maintained relatively stable sensitivity patterns, extensive multiple-resistance patterns have developed in gram-negative organisms. The increased incidence of sexual transfer of bacterial resistance through plasmids seen in gram-negative bacteria is a probable hypothesis for this evolution. The increased prevalence of resultant nosocomial gram-negative pneumonias is clinical evidence of the selection of organisms with the capability to transfer plasmids coded for bacterial resistance. As the synthesis of newer drugs suppresses the present population of infecting gram-negative organisms, formerly commensal organisms have emerged as pathogens. Because of the limited antibiotic arsenal with which to counter the enterococcus, this organism is now being cultured in ever-increasing numbers. Increasing prevalence of vancomycin-resistant enterococcus is a major problem in critical care units.

ANTIBIOTIC PROPHYLAXIS

Antibiotic prophylaxis of surgical infection involves attacking bacterial contamination before the microorganism can induce overt infection. Before the development of animal experiments or controlled clinical trials to validate the concept of antibiotic prophylaxis a wave of initial enthusiasm, such as occurs with any new drug or treatment modality, led to the indiscriminate use of new antibiotics in the futile hope of finally eliminating infection as a surgical complication. Not unexpectedly, this indiscriminate use of antibiotics without scientific basis failed in its goal and led to widespread emergence of resistant organisms and other antibiotic-associated complications. With the development of these side effects, the use of systemic prophylactic antibiotics fell into disrepute. A number of investigations subsequently failed to demonstrate any advantage conferred by antibiotic prophylaxis. Although these studies suffered from conceptual drawbacks in both study design and antibiotic use, researchers believed the use of systemic antibiotic prophylaxis should be abandoned in the face of resultant antibiotic side effects and apparent insignificant prophylactic efficacy.[140]

During this period of disappointment with prophylactic antibiotic efficacy, scientific reevaluation of antibiotic prophylaxis began with studies by Miles and associates[121] and Burke,[22] as they sought to redefine the possible role of antibiotic prophylaxis in the surgical setting. In 1957, Miles noted that a variety of agents could alter the course of a cutaneous infection in a guinea pig model if they were administered within the first few hours of bacterial inoculation of the wound. He labeled this interval of time the "decisive period." Burke's further investigations confirmed that during a definite short period, the antibiotics may suppress the developing staphylococcal dermal or incisional infection. He noted that this effective period begins the moment bacteria gain access to the tissue and ends within three hours. Furthermore, systemic antibiotics have no effect on primary staphylococcal infections if the bacteria have been in the tissue longer than 3 hours before the antibiotics are given. These two animal studies suggest that effective prophylactic antibiotics should be given immediately before surgery and that delaying their administration to the postoperative period will result in loss of efficacy. However, when antibiotics were given within the so-called decisive period, suppression of infection could be demonstrated. The scientific principles for the timing of antimicrobial prophylaxis were thus conclusively established in the animal model, and the stage was set for prospective clinical trials.

Attempting to extrapolate the observations of Miles and Burke from the animal model to the clinical setting, Bernard and Cole[17] conducted the first well-designed clinical studies of prevention of surgical infection by prophylactically administered antibiotics. One hundred forty-five patients undergoing potentially contaminated laparotomy were randomly selected for treatment with a combination of three broad-spectrum antibiotics versus a placebo given preoperatively, intraoperatively, and for 5 days postoperatively. A decreased incidence of infection in the treatment group (8%) was noted as compared with the control group (27%). However, a question of consistency in following protocol and the use of other antibiotics in the postoperative period impaired the acceptance of Bernard and Cole's work.

Benefiting from the recognized deficiencies of previous studies, Polk and Lopez-Mayer[142] conducted a double-blind prospective randomized trial of the effect of 1 g of cephaloridine or a placebo given intramuscularly preoperatively and given at 5 and 11 hours postoperatively to patients who had potentially contaminated emergency operations on the esophagus, stomach, small bowel, or large bowel. All other antimicrobial therapy was withheld for maximum specificity. Patient groups were similar with respect to all recognized clinical determinants of wound infection. This study revealed a reduction in infection rate from 30% in the control group to 7% in antibiotic-treated patients. The statistically significant difference remained when considering any subset of the study, such as gastroduodenal procedures as opposed to colonic procedures. The resultant decreased infection rate in the treatment group correlated directly with serum and wound concentrations. No emergence of resistant organisms was noted during the study; the brief regimen used did not permit sufficient time for the selection of resistant forms.[139]

Since that original trial in 1969, many other parallel observations have been made to offer additional data as to the efficacy of antibiotic prophylaxis; however, not all have fulfilled the rigid criteria necessary to reach significant statistical conclusions. Chodak and Plat[31] found that only 24 of 131 articles regarding antimicrobial prophylaxis between 1960 and 1976 met the criteria of an appropriately designed study; Dipiro[50,51] similarly found only 76 regimens of systemic prophylaxis between 1976 and 1980 that could be evaluated.

In another well-designed clinical trial, Stone and associates[173] demonstrated protection by using systemic prophylactic antibiotic, cefazolin, to 400 patients undergoing gastric, biliary, or colorectal procedures. The study evaluated four treatment categories, with patients receiving antibiotic therapy at the following times:

1. Twelve hours preoperatively
2. Just before operation
3. Postoperatively
4. Not at all

Preoperative prophylaxis decreased the incidence of wound infection versus placebo, whereas postoperative antibiotics afforded no protection. Medication given 1 hour preoperatively provided the same protection as prophylaxis instituted 12 hours before surgery.

Fullen and associates[65] examined patients undergoing procedures for penetrating wounds of the abdomen. They likewise concluded that preoperative initiation of antibiotics offered significant advantages when compared with intraoperative or postoperative initiation of therapy in the prevention of posttraumatic wound or deep infection (Figure 10-12).

These three trials and other well-designed studies have documented the efficacy of systemic preoperative prophylaxis of surgical infection. There has been no increase in resistant organisms when using the same brief regimen of antibiotic prophylaxis.

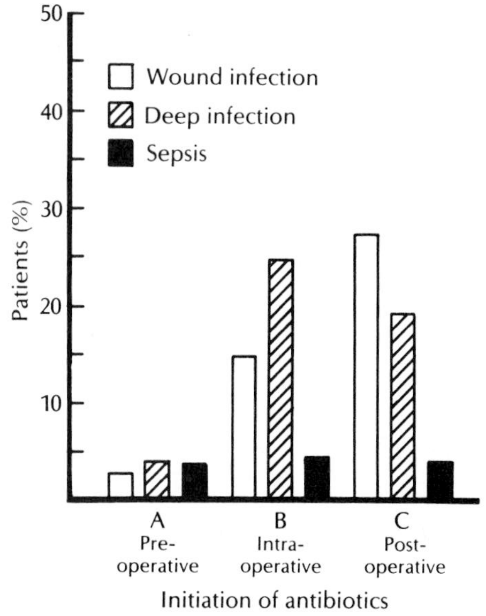

FIGURE 10-12 Distribution of infection rates in patients treated with antibiotics preoperatively, intraoperatively, and postoperatively. (From Fullen WD, Hunt J, Altemeier WA: Prophylactic antibiotics in penetrating wounds of the abdomen, *J Trauma* 12:282, 1972.)

Assessing Risk

Appropriate prophylaxis of surgical infection requires that the patient bear a genuine increased risk of infection after the proposed procedure to justify the risk and cost of administered antibiotics. Such an enhanced risk may be evaluated by considering the frequency or severity of infection or both. For example, infection frequently follows colon surgery and is the source of substantial morbidity but is rarely fatal. Conversely, infection occurs infrequently after replacement of the aortic valve with a prosthetic device but is often fatal when it occurs. Either situation represents a high-risk state in terms of frequency (the colectomy) or severity (the prosthetic aortic valve). Obviously, if either the frequency or severity of associated adverse side effects of the administered antibiotic exceeds the frequency or severity of infection, then preventive measures bear a greater risk than the prevented infection. To adequately assess risk of infection, surgical wounds are categorized according to their susceptibility to infection based on likelihood or presence of contamination at the time of surgery. In conjunction with consideration of various host and operative factors that increase the risk of infection, this categorization serves as a useful adjunct for determining the necessity for prophylaxis. (Table 10-4).

Clean surgical wounds are made under ideal operating room conditions without encountering any inflammatory process and without entry into the gastrointestinal, respiratory, or oropharyngeal tracts. The expected rate of infection in these wounds is 1.5%. As such, no prophylactic antibiotics would be indicated unless the presence of infection would lead to disastrous results, as in the placement of the prosthetic aortic valve described above, or unless other host or operative factors increase the expected infection rate. For example, we know that the numbers of bacteria required to produce overt clinical infection are significantly reduced by the placement of a foreign body. Thus patients undergoing clean procedures, such as prosthetic joint replacement or vascular implants, are given antibiotic prophylaxis because of slightly increased risk of infection and the disastrous consequences of infection. Other factors increasing the risk of infection in clean surgical wounds include uncontrolled diabetes, debilitated nutritional state, extremes of age, and impaired blood supply. For example, an 80-year-old patient with uncontrolled diabetes who undergoes a below-the-knee amputation for ischemic peripheral vascular disease is a candidate for antimicrobial prophylaxis even though the wound is classified as clean.

Distinguishing clean-contaminated wounds from contaminated wounds hinges on assessing the degree of spillage at the time of surgery. Thus both types are considered with regard to antibiotic prophylaxis antibiotic use because the decision to use prophylaxis is made preoperatively, before assessing intraoperative contamination. Clean-contaminated wounds enter the gastrointestinal tract or respiratory tract without significant spillage. Contaminated wounds occur in the gastrointestinal tract with gross spillage, in the genitourinary tract with the presence of infected contents, or in freshly contaminated traumatic wounds. Prophylactic antibiotics are indicated for most clean-contaminated wounds, which have an infection rate of 8%. Prophylactic antibiotics are routinely used for all contaminated wounds, which have an infection rate of 18%. The infection rate in dirty wounds, defined as wounds more than 4 hours old, with the presence of frank pus or associated with perforated

TABLE 10-4 OPERATIVE WOUNDS CLASSIFIED BY RELATIVE CONTAMINATION RESULTING FROM PROCEDURE PERFORMED AND SUBSEQUENT RISK OF INFECTION

CATEGORY	DEFINITION	EXAMPLE	EXPECTED INFECTION RATE (%)
Clean; refined-clean	Elective wound not encountering inflammation made under ideal operating conditions without entering the gastrointestinal, respiratory, or oropharyngeal tract	Inguinal herniorrhaphy Thyroidectomy Vascular surgery Arthroplasty	1.5
Clean-contaminated; potentially contaminated	Wound entering the gastrointestinal or respiratory tract without significant spillage or presence of infection	Prostatectomy in the absence of infected urine Cholecystectomy Colon, gastric resection Pulmonary resection	8
Contaminated	Wounds entering the gastrointestinal tract with gross spillage or entrance of genitourinary tract in the presence of infected contents, or fresh traumatic wounds	Colon resection with spill of feces Choledochotomy with infected bile	18
Dirty	Wound in which a perforated viscus or pus is encountered, or old traumatic wounds	Perforated alimentary tract Abscess with drainage	>40

viscus, exceeds 40%. The purpose of antimicrobial therapy in this population is not only prophylaxis of disseminated infection but also therapy of established infection.[75]

As mentioned earlier, antibiotics are but one tool; they should be regarded as an addition and not an alternative to asepsis, antisepsis, adequate preoperative preparation of the patient, and proper surgical techniques. Furthermore, the phrase prophylactic antibiotic implies that its use is to prevent infection from developing and not to treat an established infection. Failure to differentiate carefully between prophylactic and therapeutic use of antibiotics has frequently led to confusion.

Specific Surgeries

Colorectal Surgery

Infection is the principal complication of colorectal surgery, and the colon's endogenous flora is overwhelmingly the major source of contamination. Mechanisms providing for the reduction of the endogenous colonic microflora are therefore an integral part of any bowel preparation program. Thorough mechanical cleansing of the bowel with laxatives, mannitol, or whole gut irrigation decreases the residual bulk of stool and thereby decreases the number of viable organisms likely to contaminate the operative wound. However, simple mechanical cleansing alone is insufficient to adequately reduce the colonic population of microflora to achieve a significant reduction in wound infection rates. Therefore systemically or orally administered antibiotics have been used in conjunction with mechanical cleansing to provide lower infection rates. In addition, a recent study[52] has shown that injection of a single dose of antibiotic along the site of proposed incision before the procedure also reduces the wound infection rate. Administration of poorly absorbed antimicrobial agents decreases the number of colonic bacteria, providing for a smaller inoculum to the operative wound. Antibiotic agents that are either systemically administered or injected before the incision do not alter the colonic microflora but do assist host defenses in eliminating the inoculum at the time of contamination.

The first controlled prospective, double-blind trial of an oral antibiotic bowel preparation was conducted by Washington and associates[185] in 1974 after more than 25 years of world wide use. This study analyzed three groups of patients. One group received an oral placebo, one group received oral neomycin, and the third group received both neomycin and tetracycline. All patients underwent mechanical cleansing of the bowel. Patients receiving placebo or neomycin had comparable frequencies of wound infection. Among patients receiving neomycin and tetracycline, there was a significant reduction in frequency of wound infection. In prospective randomized, double-blind trials of small numbers of patients, Nichols and Condon[128] have shown that oral antibiotic prophylaxis is helpful in the prevention of wound infections in patients undergoing elective colon procedures. Because of a declining sensitivity pattern of *Bacteroides fragilis* to tetracycline, Nichols and Condon used an erythromycin base in conjunction with neomycin in the antibiotic bowel preparation.

Presently, similarly reduced infection rates are obtained with both methods of oral and systemically administered antibiotics. Obviously, oral bowel preparation cannot be used for the patient with an obstructed or nearly obstructed bowel. Also, in emergency situations time does not allow for orally administered prophylaxis. The complications of superinfection of the gut and enterocolitis are rarely seen with perioperative systemic prophylaxis. Two points remain to be clarified: (1) Will a combination of both oral and systemic prophylaxis lead to a further decrease in the infection rate than either alone? and (2) If so, will the associated side effects remain sufficiently infrequent to justify the benefit? Initial reports suggest that combined oral and systemic prophylaxis does not have additive effects.

Small Bowel Surgery

With the exception of the terminal ileum, the normal small bowel does not harbor resident bacteria. However, in disease states for which surgery is performed, such as obstruction, the small bowel is rapidly populated with the microflora of the colon. In such cases, appropriate antibiotic prophylaxis is indicated.

Appendiceal Surgery

The microflora of the appendix is fecal, and rationale for the use of systemic prophylaxis pertaining to colorectal surgery likewise applies to appendiceal surgery. Common organisms cultured include *B. fragilis, Escherichia coli, Klebsiella pneumonia,* and *Streptococcus faecalis*. The incidence of postoperative wound infection is directly related to the state of the appendix at operation; the possible conditions of the appendix are:

1. Normal
2. Nonperforated
3. Nonperforated but gangrenous
4. Perforated with local peritonitis
5. Perforated with generalized peritonitis

When the appendix is normal or merely inflamed, contamination is present in only 10% to 20% of cases, but this rises sharply to 80% to 90% if the appendix is gangrenous or perforated.[140] With a gangrenous or perforated appendix, the incidence of subcutaneous infection with or without the use of antibiotics is unacceptably high, and the wound should be left open for delayed primary closure. The use of antibiotics in this situation is not prophylactic but therapeutic.

The question arises as to how to approach the patient without gangrene or perforation. Pinto and Sanderson[137] found wound infection rates of 5% in patients with appendicitis without gangrene or perforation treated preoperatively with 1 g of metronidazole per rectum; in patients treated with placebo, the wound infection rate was 7%. Thus no substantial benefit accrued to the metronidazole-treated group. These results are similar to the work of others using metronidazole. However, Busuttil[62] did show a statistical benefit with preoperative cefamandole use when compared with placebo in clinical trials in persons with nonperforated appendicitis. He found no protection by the addition of antianaerobic agents. A seemingly rational policy would be to start all patients scheduled for appendiceal surgery on an appropriate, safe antibiotic and continue the antibiotic therapeutically in the postoperative period if the appendix is found to be gangrenous or perforated at the time of the procedure.

Gastroduodenal Surgery

Stone and associates[173] demonstrated that the administration of a single dose of cefazolin decreased the incidence of wound infection from 27% to 4% in elective gastroduodenal surgery. This study included patients undergoing all gastroduodenal procedures. Since that time, researchers have attempted to identify those patients with particularly increased risk. This selection has been evaluated from both bacteriologic and clinical bases. From a bacteriologic standpoint, the normal stomach contains no resident flora; intraluminal contamination is transient because of the presence of gastric acid. However, in the face of obstruction or antacid prophylaxis, both exogenous and oral endogenous flora proliferate and antibiotic prophylaxis is obviously mandatory.

Gatehouse[68] studied the microflora of both normal patients and patients with gastric ulcer, duodenal ulcer, and gastric carcinoma (Table 10-5). He found that gastric aspirates containing more than 1×10^6 organisms/ml were associated with a wound infection rate of over 90%. With less than 1×10^6 organisms/ml, the rate fell to 16%. Patients with gastric carcinoma and achlorhydria had the highest infection rate (56%), with none of 35 patients having sterile cultures. On the other hand, all cultures from normal volunteers were sterile. Patients with duodenal ulcers and gastric ulcers had infection rates of 17% and 38%, respectively. Quantitative cultures were correlated with gastric pH, with counts of greater than 1×10^6/ml achieved if the pH was above 4. Therefore patients at risk might be identified preoperatively by gastric sampling. Somewhat unexpectedly, patients having duodenal ulcer disease have infection rates from 10% to 18% in the absence of prophylaxis. With the increased levels of acid in duodenal ulcer disease, low quantitative cultures of organisms, and therefore lowered infection rates, would be expected; however, studies have not supported this hypothesis. Perhaps, as some investigators have noted, patients taking cimetidine, which causes relative hypochlorhydria, may be at increased risk of infection. Pollock[145] found that 54% of patients with bleeding duodenal ulcer had significant contamination. The buffering effect of intraluminal blood may be implicated in increased bacterial colonization in these patients. Efforts to identify specific patient populations at increased risk have added to the

TABLE 10-5 ORGANISMS MOST COMMONLY CAUSING POSTOPERATIVE INFECTIONS IN THE GASTROINTESTINAL TRACT

SITE	AEROBES	ANAEROBES
Mouth and esophagus	Streptococci	*Bacteroides* organisms (not *B. fragilis*), peptostreptococci, fusobacteria
Stomach	Enteric gram-negative bacilli, streptococci	*Bacteroides* organisms (not *B. fragilis*), peptostreptococci, fusobacteria
Biliary tract	Enteric gram-negative bacilli, enterococci	*Clostridium* organisms
Distal ileum and colon	Enteric gram-negative bacilli	*B. fragilis*, peptostreptococci, *Clostridium* organisms

From Conte JE, Jacob LS, Polk HC Jr: *Antibiotic prophylaxis in surgery*, New York, 1984, JB Lippincott.

understanding of associated factors involved in wound infection. However, those patients with the lowest risk of infection, undergoing surgery for duodenal ulcer disease have an infection rate of 10% to 18%. Therefore a rational approach would be to use systemic antimicrobial prophylaxis for all procedures that open the stomach or duodenum.

Biliary Surgery

Normal bile is sterile. However, more than 20% of patients undergoing biliary surgery are found to have greater than 1×10^6 organisms/ml in the bile. The most commonly identified organisms include *E. coli, K. aerogenes,* and *S. faecalis.* Chelatin and Elliott[30] identified high-risk groups of patients by retrospective analysis. These groups included patients over 70 years of age, those with acute cholecystitis, and those with common bile duct stones with or without associated jaundice. After preoperative identification as a "high-risk" patient, these patients were given cephaloridine before and after surgery and compared with a placebo-treated control group. Although no reduction in the incidence of positive intraoperative bile cultures was obtained by prophylactic antibiotics, a decreased incidence of wound infection occurred in the treatment group (4%) versus the placebo group (27%). Thus judicious use of prophylactic antibiotics, after proper identification of patients at high risk, allows more specific administration of prophylaxis and minimizes associated antibiotic side effects in the total population. Keighley has identified other groups of patients with increased risk of infection and has suggested that additional high-risk patients may be identified by operative Gram's staining of the bile.[91] McLeish and associates[113] randomly assigned patients to intraoperative treatment with systemic antibiotics, depending on the basis of the intraoperative Gram's stain versus untreated controls. A lower wound infection rate was noted in the treated group. Strachan and associates[175] used cefazolin to study prophylaxis of biliary surgery. They examined three groups of patients. The first group received a single intramuscular preoperative dose. The second group received an identical preoperative dose, with therapy continued for an additional 5 days. The third group received only placebo. Wound infection rates were 3.2%, 5.5%, and 16.9%, respectively, showing that one preoperative dose of cefazolin was as effective as including an additional 5-day course. The method of the intraoperative Gram's stain has been discontinued in the original institution.

Judicious use of prophylaxis seems to dictate that its use be applied only to the high-risk population of patients. In a randomized, prospective trial, Lowery and associates[104] noted that the major influence increasing infection was choledochotomy. Therefore it may be reasoned that all high-risk patients should receive prophylaxis, and in addition, any patient in whom probable choledochotomy may also be required should receive prophylaxis. Obviously, in young patients with preoperatively demonstrated large stones and a normal-size common bile duct, the likelihood of choledochotomy is small and prophylaxis is not indicated.

Vascular Surgery

Infection of a surgical wound is always a costly and distressing problem, and in vascular surgery, the consequences may be particularly devastating, with potential loss of life or limb. In a prospective study of antibiotic prophylaxis in 512 patients undergoing surgery of the abdominal aorta or the lower extremity, Kaiser and associates[90] found that cefazolin given to patients before and after surgery reduced the incidence of postoperative wound infection as compared with a placebo group. Sixteen patients receiving a placebo had wound infections, whereas only two infections occurred in 225 patients receiving cefazolin. Pitt and associates[138] confirmed these findings in a randomized, blind study of cephradine versus a placebo. In ischemic limbs, the thigh area and groins are colonized with bacteria from the patient's bowel. Pitt noted that those incisions involving the groin, as in profundoplasty, femoral embolectomy, and femoral aneurysm repair, were associated with a statistically significant increased risk of infection, which prophylactic antibiotics markedly reduced.

In major elective arterial surgery involving the placement of a prosthesis, postoperative infection is a catastrophe. All patients requiring the placement of a prosthesis should receive antimicrobial prophylaxis. The incidence of infection after procedures on the brachial and carotid arteries that do not involve the placement of prosthetic material is too low to justify the use of prophylactic antibiotics in light of their associated risks.

Cardiothoracic Surgery

Although chest and wound infections occur in patients undergoing cardiac surgery, the primary concern is the infection of a prosthetic heart valve. Endocarditis, which occurs infrequently, is most often secondary to staphylococcal infection. Although the incidence of this complication is low, the effects are devastating, with further surgery required and mortality of approximately 50%. Although controlled trials have not been completed, patients at risk for developing the severe consequences of an infected graft warrant the use of prophylactic antibiotics. Bryan[21] found cefazolin and cefamandole to be equally effective in patients undergoing cardiopulmonary bypass, but no placebo group was included in his study.

Because of transection of the bronchi or lung in pulmonary resections, these wounds are classified as clean-contaminated wounds. Kvale and associates studied 77 patients undergoing pulmonary resection in a prospective double-blind study and found 17 infections in the 34 patients of the placebo group (50%), whereas only 8 infections in the 43 patients of the antibiotic group (19%) were noted.[96] Cefazolin was used in this study, but prophylaxis may be varied, depending on the preoperative sputum culture and sensitivity results.

Urologic Surgery

The design of many studies of the prevention of wound or urinary tract infection following urologic procedures has been unsatisfactory. After three decades of investigation, controversy regarding antimicrobial prophylaxis persists. Obviously, the presence of preoperative bacteriuria requires antimicrobial prophylaxis or therapy. Shah and associates[163] recently reported that short-term antimicrobial prophylaxis reduced postoperative urinary tract infections and other septic complications, indicating the value of prophylaxis in these patients. Urethral instrumentation has been associated with bacteremia in 10% of patients with sterile urine. There have been a number of cases of endocarditis on prosthetic heart valves following genitourinary procedures. Obviously, prophylaxis is mandatory in these cases.

Orthopedic Surgery

Orthopedic prosthetic implants infrequently become infected, but the disastrous consequences of infection outweigh the risk of prophylaxis. Antistaphylococcal drugs decrease the incidence of infection in prosthetic joints after total hip replacement and also decrease postoperative wound infection rates when hip fractures are treated with internal fixation by nail or plate. All procedures involving placement of a prosthesis should include antibiotic prophylaxis. A short preoperative course appears to be as effective as a longer one. Other orthopedic procedures without significant contamination or placement of foreign materials do not require antibiotic prophylaxis.[59]

ANTIBIOTIC SELECTION

Judicious selection of antimicrobial agents is a complex process requiring detailed evaluation of the interaction between the host and the infecting microbe. The number of currently available antibiotics, often evaluated in poorly designed or inconclusive trials, makes thoughtful scientific decisions regarding optimal therapy difficult. When an antimicrobial agent is indicated, a therapeutic or prophylactic goal is set and an agent is chosen that is selective for the likely infecting microorganisms. Several principles must be considered.

First, optimal initiation of therapy requires identification of the infecting microbe. Because therapy may be required before bacteriologic confirmation of the infecting microbe, the physician must begin therapy based on the most likely infecting organism. For example, patients with cholangitis frequently have infection secondary to *E. coli, Klebsiella* organisms, or, less frequently, *Enterococcus* organisms. Therefore appropriate antibiotic therapy may begin while the physician awaits culture identification of the specific organism.

It is common practice for a physician to use a broad-spectrum agent while awaiting specific sensitivity data. However, the physician should always try to maintain the most specific spectrum of therapy to slow the evolution of resistant bacterial strains. For example, a staphylococcal soft-tissue infection, when cultured, demonstrates a pathogen sensitive to both nafcillin and the cephalosporin group. Because nafcillin has no gram-negative coverage, it becomes the antibiotic of choice because of its more specific spectrum.

The additional use of a Gram's stain of infected body fluid narrows the list of potential pathogens and allows the use of more specific therapy. When laboratory findings are available, various agents may be graded as sensitive, intermediate, or resistant to the agent in question. Results may be listed in terms of the minimum inhibitory concentration as defined by the lowest concentration of the antimicrobial agent that will inhibit in vitro growth of the infecting organism. The interpretation of in vitro data requires extrapolation in the in vivo clinical situation. As stated earlier, the pharmacokinetic factors of route of administration, degree of protein binding, volume of distribution to various body compartments, and subsequent tissue levels, as well as other host factors, make interpretation of these in vitro data difficult. As a general rule, however, the antibiotic administered should achieve an in vivo concentration at the site of infection of at least two to four times the minimum inhibitory concentration.

The second consideration in selecting the therapeutic agent is the toxicity of possible antibiotic choices. In general, the drug with the least toxicity should be chosen. Often, the physician sees increasing levels of toxicity associated with increasing efficacy when considering a range of antibiotics to treat a particular infection. In this situation, the physician must assess the risk of potential or existing infection and apply an appropriate antibiotic response. For example, when prophylaxis of colonic surgery is considered, one goal is to prevent postoperative subcutaneous wound infection with moderate morbidity. Therefore a documentably safe agent, such as the first-generation cephalosporin or cefazolin, could be used. On the other hand, when dealing with a synergistic gram-negative infection, more efficacious agents may be indicated, although their use may be associated with more severe or greater frequency of host toxicity. Also, antibiotics with infrequent but inordinately severe complications should be rated a low priority. Obviously, a patient's history of hypersensitivity to a specific antibiotic usually precludes use of that agent.

The route of metabolism of the possible antibiotic choices must be kept in mind. Patients with evidence of either intrinsic renal or hepatic disease should not receive an antibiotic that is dependent on that specific route for excretion if alternative choices are available.

The third consideration regarding selection of a therapeutic agent is the economic impact of antibiotic therapy on health care costs. Approximately one third of the average hospital pharmacy expenditures are for antibiotics. Much of this cost could be avoided with the elimination of antibiotic use in overtly unindicated situations. Studies have revealed that as many as one half of all hospitalized patients who receive antibiotics are being treated inappropriately. Much of this inappropriate antibiotic use stems from a fundamental lack of knowledge concerning the principles of antibiotic prophylaxis. Fry and associates[63] analyzed the use of systemic prophylaxis and found that only 74% of patients received antibiotics preoperatively. However, 79% of patients received prophylaxis for longer than 24 hours postoperatively, with the average period of postoperative prophylaxis being 1 week. This inappropriate use of antibiotics only increases the rate of development of resistant bacterial strains and the incidence of antibiotic side effects. In recent years, with the widespread use of broader-spectrum antibiotics, formerly commensal and rarely infecting organisms have emerged with increased prevalence as infecting agents. Stone and associates[174] noted an increased incidence of systemic candidal infections in the early 1970s. They determined that the prolonged treatment of patients with broad-spectrum antibiotics was the most important predisposing factor in these infections.

Finally, no better evidence exists for the selection of a particular agent than an established, well-documented clinical record of prophylactic or therapeutic efficacy in combination with an established record of infrequent associated side effects. For example, penicillin has an established record in the treatment of streptococcal cellulitis with infrequent associated therapeutic complications. Even though several other agents are effective, penicillin is certainly the drug of choice. However, even penicillin is beginning to be ineffective for some streptococci and pneumococci.

ANTIBIOTIC THERAPY

In concert with the debridement of necrotic tissues, the drainage of abscess cavities, the removal of infected foreign bodies, and the maintenance of adequate nutritional status, antibiotic therapy plays an important role in the eradication of surgical infection. Pharmacokinetic studies have shown that for an agent to be effective, adequate tissue levels must be obtained at the site in question. Therefore the processes of absorption, distribution, and excretion of the selected antimicrobial agent must be considered to provide therapeutic tissue levels for the elimination of sensitive organisms.

Specific Antibiotic Drugs

Penicillins

Since the 1940s, indications for the use of penicillin have undergone considerable modification. Forty years of continued efficacy in the treatment of infections caused by most group A *Streptococcus* and *Pneumococcus* organisms persists to the present. Intravenous administration leads to immediate high serum levels with prompt distribution to most body compartments, making it valuable in management for a variety of infections. Penicillin G is still useful in the treatment of *Clostridium* organisms and group D *Streptococcus* organisms by using large dosage schedules. With the advent of other agents, penicillin now has no role in the therapy of gram-negative infections, with the exception of *Neisseria* organisms.

The vigorous application of penicillin therapy has exerted selection pressures that have generated the proliferation of resistant organisms having the enzyme beta-lactamase. However, the subsequent development of semisynthetic preparations—nafcillin, oxacillin, and methicillin—has provided therapeutic agents to combat many of these resistant microbes. Other alterations have resulted in ampicillin, carbenicillin, ticarcillin, piperacillin, and azlocillin. These derivatives have a broader spectrum of activity with varying degrees of gram-negative efficacy.

Cephalosporins

Like the penicillins, the cephalosporins have as their mechanism of action the inhibition of bacterial cell wall formation. They are customarily grouped into three "generations" of drugs.[62] The first-generation cephalosporins all have a common pattern of antimicrobial activity. These include cephalothin, cephaloridine, cefazolin, and cephradine. The first-generation drugs are effective against most gram-positive cocci and have modest gram-negative coverage. The gram-negative includes only *E. coli, Klebsiella* organisms, and some *Enterobacter* strains. Because of a very low incidence of side effects with a short course of these antibiotics, these agents (with the exception of cephalothin) are of greatest clinical use in infection prophylaxis for patients undergoing various surgical procedures, especially of the gastrointestinal tract. Cephalosporins are often effective for staphylococcal infections also and may be the agents of choice for patients with staphylococcal infections who have penicillin allergy (although cross-allergenicity occurs in 15% of patients).

The second-generation cephalosporins extend the range of gram-negative coverage to include greater activity against *E. coli, Klebsiella* organisms, and *Enterobacter* organisms in addition to activity against *Proteus* and *Bacteroides* organisms. Their best use appears to be in the therapy of established infection when data obtained from sensitivity studies dictate their superior efficacy. Only rarely are the second-generation cephalosporins used as a first-line therapy. It has been said that they are the first therapeutic choice for nothing but the second choice for everything.

The third-generation cephalosporins have increased antimicrobial activity against *Pseudomonas* organisms and *B. fragilis*. Their generation includes moxalactam, cefoperazone, cefotaxime, and cefuroxime. The primary uses of these agents may be in single-drug therapy as a first-line treatment in patients with mixed bacterial infection (e.g., patients with perforated viscus and peritonitis). Prospective controlled trials are underway to determine their ultimate indication and therapeutic efficacy.

Aminoglycosides

The aminoglycosides were the first broad-spectrum antibiotics with major gram-negative coverage. They are presently used in the treatment of aerobic gram-negative enteric bacterial infections and can be used in combination with other microbial agents in the treatment of staphylococcal and enterococcal infections. Although aminoglycosides often provide superior efficacy in the treatment of gram-negative infections, the positive results are not without cost. Nephrotoxicity and ototoxicity, minimized by the careful monitoring of renal function and serum peak and trough levels, still occur in a significant number of cases. In many institutions this class of antibiotic is reserved for specific therapeutic indications. Amikacin appears to maintain in vitro effectiveness in some cases when resistance evolves to both tobramycin and gentamicin. Use of amikacin is therefore reserved for the treatment of gram-negative infections caused by organisms resistant to tobramycin and gentamicin. Increasingly, data seem to indicate that less nephrotoxicity occurs with tobramycin than with gentamicin.

Tetracyclines

The tetracyclines have as their mechanism of action the inhibition of protein synthesis by binding to the 30S ribosomal subunit, interfering with the addition of amino acids to the peptide chain. All tetracyclines have a similar spectrum, with efficacy for most gram-positive and gram-negative enteric bacteria. However, because of sporadic gaps in sensitivity, this class of compounds should be used only when dictated by appropriate laboratory sensitivity data when treating established infection. Tetracycline has been used in prophylaxis of wound infection as an oral preoperative bowel preparation because it is active against *B. fragilis*. Dental problems with young children and rare complications of hepatic toxicity have been noted in previous cases.

Chloramphenicol

Although rarely used because of the infrequent appearances of aplastic anemia noted early in the use of this antibiotic's evolution, chloramphenicol may be a useful antibiotic in seriously ill patients. Scientific reevaluation of this agent has now determined its role in the clinical arsenal. Because of its efficacy in the treatment of *B. fragilis,* chloramphenicol may be used in the treatment of polymicrobial intraabdominal infection. It may also be effective in conjunction with penicillin in the treatment of clostridial infection. The principal complication of chloramphenicol use—bone marrow supression—takes two forms. More commonly it is a dose-related reversible bone marrow depression caused by the inhibition of protein synthesis. Less frequently an idiosyncratic, irreversible, aplastic anemia unrelated to dosage occurs. Because of this infrequent but disastrous complication, use of chloramphenicol is limited to specific indications in seriously ill patients.

Erythromycin

Erythromycin inhibits RNA-dependent protein synthesis by binding to the 50S ribosomal subunit. The spectrum of activity is similar to that of the tetracyclines. Poor absorption of erythromycin base from the gastrointestinal tract provides the basis for its use in oral antibiotic bowel preparation for colon surgery. Although associated with occasional mild gastrointestinal irritation, erythromycin is one of the safest oral antibiotics available today. The local complications of severe pain with intramuscular injection and phlebitis with intravenous administration have prevented its widespread use in parenteral therapy.

Lincosamines

Clindamycin and lincomycin have a broad spectrum of activity against gram-positive cocci and most anaerobic organisms. Gram-negative enteric organisms are resistant to lincosamines. Clindamycin is extremely useful in combination with an aminoglycoside for the treatment of mixed intraabdominal or soft tissue infections. Antibiotic-associated colitis is the major complication. The diarrhea that results usually is caused by an enterotoxin elaborated by *C. difficile*. In severe cases, pseudomembranous enterocolitis may develop. Treatment of this complication consists of discontinuing the lincosamine agent and beginning oral administration of vancomycin or metronidazole.[169]

Vancomycin

Vancomycin is a complex glycopolypeptide unrelated to any other antibiotic. It is effective against most *Staphylococcus* and *streptococcus* organisms. The most important adverse reaction is neurotoxicity as manifested by auditory nerve damage and hearing loss. Its exclusive excretion through the kidney requires monitoring of serum levels in uremic patients to prevent toxic accumulation in the serum. Indications for vancomycin use include treatment of established staphylococcal infection when the infecting organism is resistant to the semisynthetic penicillins and cephalosporins. It may also be used as an orally administered agent in the treatment of pseudomembranous enterocolitis because it has minimum gastrointestinal absorption and is quite effective against intraluminal superinfection caused by *C. difficile*.

Metronidazole

Metronidazole was introduced as an antiparasitic compound for trichomonal infections and amebic infestations. This chemical is poorly absorbed from the gastrointestinal tract and is also effective in the treatment of antibiotic-associated colitis caused by *C. difficile*. Both oral and parenterally administered metronidazole have marked activity against almost all anaerobic bacteria, including *B. fragilis*. As such, this agent has been used as an oral preoperative preparation for patients undergoing elective colon procedures and for patients with *Bacteroides* bacteremia.[169]

Amphotericin B

Amphotericin B, a chemotherapeutic compound, binds the sterols of fungal plasma membranes, which leads to the disruption of electrolyte and fluid balance across the cell membrane, resulting in cell death. Similar effects in the plasma membranes of the host lead to this agent's nephrotoxocity. It should only be used in patients with systemic fungal infections, particularly those caused by *Candida* organisms.

Fungal Infections

Systemic infections caused by fungi are usually acquired through the inhalation of organisms, by direct subcutaneous inoculation, persorption through a grossly intact alimentary tract, or as an opportunistic infection in the immunocompromised host. Fungal diseases that establish infection by a pulmonary route include histoplasmosis, blastomycosis, coccidioidomycosis, and cryptococcal infections. Extrapulmonary manifestations of these infections include the presence of skin or mucosal ulcerations or the erosion of bone at sites of established infection. Thus the possibility of an infection as well as an oncologic cause of a nonhealing ulceration underscores the importance of timely biopsy and appropriate cultures of these lesions. Treatment of these lesions requires measures of local control, including surgical resection or debridement and drainage, whereas amphotericin B is reserved for the treatment of systemic fungal infections.

Sporotrichosis and mycetoma are fungal infections that occur by direct inoculation and are primarily cutaneous and lymphatic infections. A combination of surgical excision and treatment with potassium iodide or amphotericin B provides adequate therapy for sporotrichosis and mycetoma.

In the healthy person who is inoculated, often no established infection occurs because the inoculum is eliminated by intact host defenses. However, a combination of suppression of host defenses and indiscriminate use of broad-spectrum antibiotics provides for the selection of and subsequent invasion by what would otherwise be considered nonpathogenic fungi. Such is often the case with infection by *Aspergillus, Candida,* and *Mucor* fungi. These ubiquitous fungi, under the pressure of selection by administration of broad-spectrum antibiotics, locally or systemically invade the immunosuppressed host.[174] Assorted disease states such as diabetes mellitus, the presence of malnutrition, and the use of steroids provide adequate insults to host defense mechanisms to encourage proliferation of these organisms. Coexisting foreign bodies such as central venous cathethers, bladder catheters, and arterial lines provide portals of inoculation and continuing loci for microscopic proliferation in these foreign bodies. To treat these infectious processes successfully, local foci of infection are removed or treated with topical antifungal agents, and fungemia is treated with appropriate intravenous antibiotics. Amphotericin B is active against a variety of infecting fungal organisms and should only be used in patients with systemic infection. Agents such as nystatin are used for local infection. Diflucon is a useful newer agent with less toxicity.

Useful guidelines for approaching fungal infections in the patient include the following recommendations:

1. Alter predisposing causes, such as removing indwelling foreign bodies, especially central venous lines; control high concentrations of blood carbohydrates by better diabetic management or by termination of intravenous hyperalimentation; and terminate for a specific time all antibacterial chemotherapy in the hope of reestablishing normal flora.
2. Consider altering alimentary fungal status by administering oral antifungal agents such as nystatin.
3. Use systemic parenteral antifungal therapy when the above measures have failed to control the septic state.

Combined Therapy

The simultaneous use of two or more antibiotics requires an understanding of the potential interaction between antimicrobial agents. The primary indications for the clinical use of combination therapy include the following:

1. Treatment of mixed bacterial infections
2. Therapy for severe infections in which a specific cause is unknown
3. Enhancement of antibacterial activity in the treatment of specific infections resistant to single drug therapy

For example, a combination of organisms may cause infection in patients with a perforated abdominal viscus and generalized peritonitis. Therefore a combination of different antibiotics with distinct antimicrobial spectra may be necessary to provide the necessary range of antimicrobial activity. Combination therapy may also be required in patients in whom the causative agent has not been identified. In this situation, two or more drugs may be necessary to select therapy that is efficacious against the range of possible infecting organisms. With some combinations of therapy, one antibiotic may serve to allow greater effectiveness of a second antibiotic than is possible when either agent is used alone. This synergistic effect is best demonstrated by a regimen of penicillin and an aminoglycoside in the treatment of enterococcal infections. With weakening of the cell wall provided by administration of penicillin, the aminoglycoside is allowed to penetrate into the microorganism and may exert its effect through the interference of RNA-mediated transfer of genetic information to the cytoplasm for subsequent protein synthesis. However, superior clinical efficacy of this approach has only rarely been confirmed by controlled clinical trials.

When selecting a combination of agents for therapy, the spectrum of possible infecting microbes should be carefully considered for the most specific combination of agents. The too-commonly practiced philosophy of so-called shotgun therapy, using many agents in large doses, is discouraged. This practice only multiplies the rate of antibiotic-associated complications without increasing therapeutic benefit in the vast majority of patients. Combination therapy, like single-drug therapy, should be specifically directed.

Course and Duration of Therapy

Throughout the course of selected therapy, continual monitoring of various parameters allows the clinician to gauge the patient's response to therapy. After a favorable response is observed, antibiotics are often continued for a time to ensure complete elimination of the infecting microbe. This interval is best determined in the initial treatment plan to prevent excessively long courses of therapy, which lead to increased incidence of antibiotic-associated side effects and the development of resistant bacterial strains. Defining this period is probably the least explained aspect of antimicrobial therapy. No prospective studies have been conducted to see how long therapy should continue. In the past, the general tendency has been to extend therapy longer than is probably necessary to eradicate the infection. Only rarely are extended courses of antibiotics necessary to eradicate infection. Of course, acute infections, such as those involving the urinary tract, require shorter courses of therapy eliminating microbes than do the chronic infections of osteomyelitis and endocarditis. Hepatic abscess is one other example of an infectious process requiring prolonged antibiotic administration in conjunction with surgical drainage for adequate therapy.

Other than the chronicity of infection, factors that effect the duration of therapy include the site and source of infection, the virulence of the infecting organism, and the anticipated host response to microbial challenge. We have noted above that a satisfactory response leads to reassessment of the necessary duration of therapy. However, if prescribed therapy does not attain initial treatment goals, then the patient's lack of progress mandates reassessment of his condition, reevaluation of the possible spectrum of infecting microbes, and possibly additional diagnostic data to enable the physician to make scientific decisions regarding further therapy.

Empiric changes in therapy should not be made without consideration of the potential microbial spectrum. Changes in therapy should be based on the identification of infecting microbes and their sensitivities as determined by Gram's stain and blood culture of excreted body fluids. If the severity of the patient's disease will not be increased by brief cessation of therapy, discontinuance of all antibiotic therapy for a short period of time is beneficial; this allows cultures to be obtained for determining specific therapeutic agents to be used. Also, the physician must not forget that the patients who fail to respond to seemingly appropriate regimens of antibiotic therapy may have surgically correctable causes of infection requiring surgical drainage, excision, or debridement for antimicrobial therapy to be effective.

TREATMENT OF THE SURGICAL PATIENT WITH INFECTIOUS COMPLICATIONS

Treatment of infection in the surgical patient is influenced by both the stage and the location of the infection. Therefore, prompt diagnosis of infection is important, since in the early stages of most infections specific antibiotic therapy and symptomatic treatment may suffice to control the infection. Once microvascular thrombosis and other tissue damage has occurred or an abscess has formed, the effectiveness of antibiotics is reduced, and surgical intervention is required in addition to antibiotic therapy. In the advanced stages of infection, the likelihood of hematogenous dissemination of microorganisms to remote organs increases, as does the risk of the spread of organisms to adjacent tissue via the lymphatics. The severity of the systemic response and the magnitude of organ dysfunction also increase as an infection progresses, necessitating a progressive increase in the intensity of the physiologic support required to maintain organ function.

Infections of surface wounds, such as burns or open soft-tissue wounds resulting from mechanical trauma, particularly those caused by gram-positive organisms, when identified early and treated promptly, commonly respond to antibiotic therapy and local wound care measures. Rapidly spreading soft-tissue infections and those characterized by extensive microvascular injury and tissue necrosis, such as gas gangrene, necrotizing fasciitis, and burn wound infections caused by gram-negative organisms and by invasive true fungi, such as the *Phycomycetes,* require surgical debridement as soon as the diagnosis has been made and the patient has been prepared for surgery. Infections within the vascular tree, such as suppurative thrombophlebitis, similarly require surgical extirpation immediately upon diagnosis.[153] Infections in a closed space, such as a joint, a fascial compartment, cranial sinus, or abscess cavity, or an obstructed hollow viscus such as in the biliary or urinary tract, may show little or only evanescent response to antibiotics and require surgical or some form of percutaneous drainage. In the case of infection associated with obstruction of a hollow viscus, relief of the obstruction is ultimately required.

Spontaneous drainage of a large mature abscess is virtually always inadequate, and adequate drainage should be established by surgical means. If a dense inflammatory membrane has formed around an abscess, debridement of that membrane may be necessary to permit the surrounding tissue to obliterate the abscess cavity. Radiologically guided percutaneous drainage of a favorably sited intraabdominal abscess may be feasible, but multiplicity of abscesses, inaccessibility, loculation, and inadequate response to such drainage are all indications for surgical intervention to establish adequate drainage.[183]

In patients with infections requiring surgical intervention, the timing of surgery should be keyed to the physiologic status of the patient. Organ dysfunction should be corrected as much as possible prior to surgery. If the infection is so advanced that physiologic normality cannot be restored or if the patient shows further physiologic deterioration while being prepared for operation, surgical drainage or excision of the infected tissue in a less than optimally prepared patient may be the only means of arresting such a downhill course. In such patients the compromised physiologic state must be accepted and the attendant increased operative risk balanced against the benefits of eliminating the cause of progressive organ dysfunction and systemic disintegration.

The organisms causing infections within the abdominal cavity and the biliary tract are typically members of the enteric flora, and antimicrobial agents should be selected accordingly. Wound and other nosocomial infections may be caused by members of the patient's endogenous flora but more often are caused by organisms acquired in the hospital. The organisms causing infections in specialized and critical care units change over time and can be viewed as a series of mini-epidemics[153] (Figure 10-13). This continual evolution of opportunistic flora necessitates continuous microbial surveillance so that an appropriate antibiotic can be chosen for initial therapy. When the specific causative organism has been identified and its antibiotic sensitivities determined, the antibiotic regimen can be changed if necessary. Infected burn wounds and other open soft-tissue wounds that are infected should be treated with a topical antimicrobial, preferably one from which the active component can diffuse into the wounds.[116] As illustrated in Table 10-6, the sensitivity of *Pseudomonas* organisms recovered from burn patients to two aminoglycoside antibiotics changed in concert with the level of use of those two agents during the years 1973 to 1980. As the table also shows, a third aminoglycoside antibiotic maintained

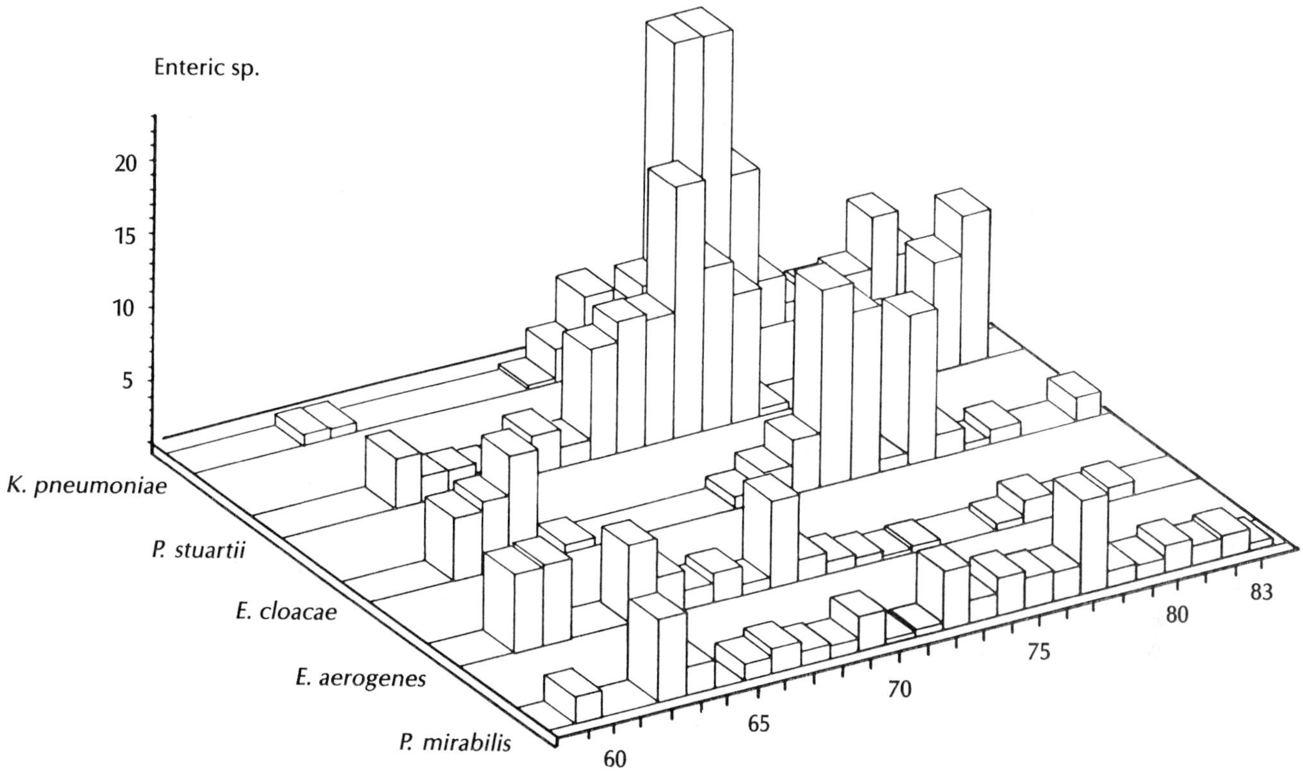

FIGURE 10-13 The recovery of enteric organisms from blood cultures in a burn unit during a 25-year period illustrates the epidemic character of the bacteria causing sepsis in critically ill patients. Note that *Klebsiella pneumoniae* and *Enterobacter cloacae* promptly filled the niche created by the recession of *Providencia stuartii* in the mid and late 1970s.

TABLE 10-6 TEMPORAL CHANGES IN SENSITIVITY OF *PSEUDOMONAS* ORGANISMS RECOVERED FROM BURN PATIENTS TO AMINOGLYCOSIDE ANTIBIOTICS*

ANTIBIOTIC	1973	1974	1975	1976-1977	1978	1979	1980
Gentamicin	84.3	61.8	40.0	19.1	19.7	25.9	70.2
Tobramycin				61.6	17.0	4.0	29.4
Amikacin				98.3	60.0	73.5	74.6

*Percentage of strains inhibited by 12.5 μg/ml.

a high level of effectiveness during a 4-year period of increasing usage and that effectiveness has been maintained to date. The microbial surveillance program must therefore include sensitivity testing to detect resistance in endemic organisms as well as resistance that can be developed in the organism of a given patient during treatment. To ensure adequate antibiotic dosage (the effective half-life of antibiotics may be significantly reduced by increased excretion and serum levels decreased by an increase in distribution space) and minimize side effects, peak and trough levels should be monitored, and the dosage adjusted accordingly in critically ill septic patients.[99,161]

Pneumonia

Pneumonia is the most common life-threatening nosocomial infection and hence cause of sepsis in severely injured and critically ill patients.[77] Pulmonary infection occurs in one of two forms: hematogenous or airborne pneumonia. Airborne pneumonia or bronchopneumonia is the most prevalent.[150] An understanding of the etiologic, pathogenetic, radiographic, and clinical differences between the two forms of pneumonia facilitates early diagnosis and prompt institution of treatment (Table 10-7).

Airborne pneumonia, or bronchopneumonia, occurs in a nonrandom distribution involving mainly the de-

TABLE 10-7 CHARACTERISTICS OF PULMONARY INFECTIONS IN BURN PATIENTS

	AIRBORNE PNEUMONIA OR BRONCHOPNEUMONIA	HEMATOGENOUS PNEUMONIA
DISTRIBUTION	NONRANDOM, IN DEPENDENT AREAS	RANDOM ASSOCIATION WITH PULMONARY CAPILLARIES
Initial lesion	Necrotizing bronchiolitis	Necrotizing alveolar capillaritis
Radiographic presentation	Ill-defined linear infiltrates in lower lobes	Solitary nodular infiltrate in any lobe
Average postburn day of onset	10th	17th
Mortality	34%	92%
Pulmonary infection as primary cause of death	80%	11%

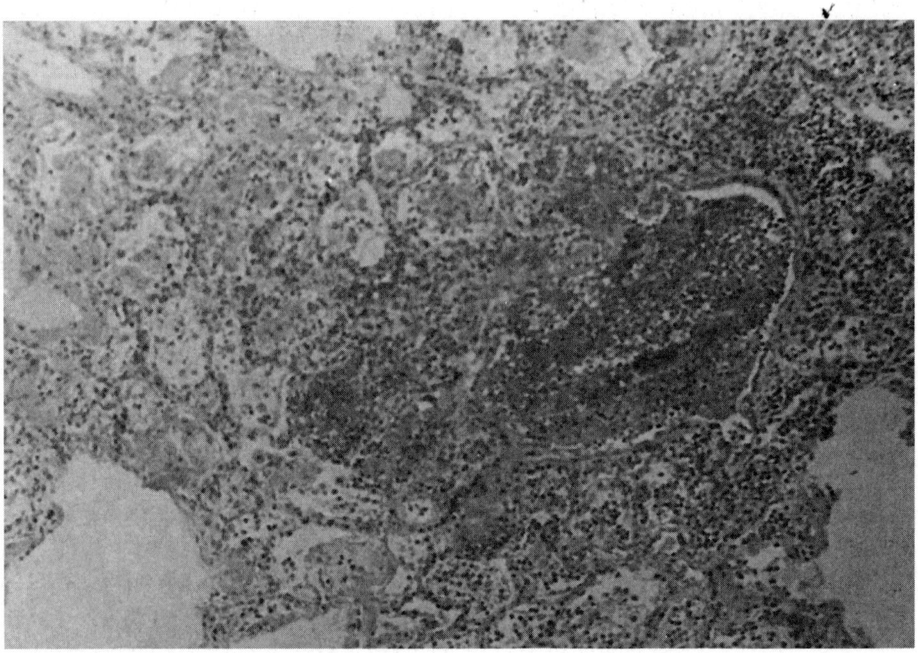

FIGURE 10-14 Hematogenous pneumonia begins as a pulmonary capillaritis following lodgment of blood-borne microorganisms arising in a remote focus of infection. Note the spread of the infection to alveoli adjacent to the involved vessel.

pendent areas of the lung and begins as a bronchiolitis from which the infection spreads to adjacent alveoli. If uncontrolled, the septic process involves progressively greater amounts of pulmonary parenchyma. The emergence of bronchopneumonia as the predominant type of pulmonary infection in severely injured patients is the result of at least two factors. Antimicrobial therapy has decreased wound and other soft-tissue infections that give rise to hematogenous pneumonia, and the more frequent use of mechanical ventilation provides a portal of entry for environmental organisms that then invade airway tissues injured by the endotracheal tube and suction catheters.

Hematogenous pneumonia begins as pulmonary capillaritis secondary to the lodgment of bacteria hematogenously disseminated from a primary site of infection, such as an infected burn or other wound (Figure 10-14). The septic process then spreads to adjacent alveoli, forming a nodular lesion that when large enough will be evident on the chest radiograph. Late in the process, the infection may erode into bronchi supplying that area of the lung. If the primary focus of infection is not controlled, multiple nodular lesions, the distribution of which corresponds to that of the pulmonary vasculature, may appear on sequential chest radiographs.

The diagnosis of pulmonary infection in surgical patients is confounded by the hyperventilatory response to injury, therapeutic agents, and nutritional support. The pulmonary status of the surgical patient must be monitored frequently, and changes in pulmonary function

A

B

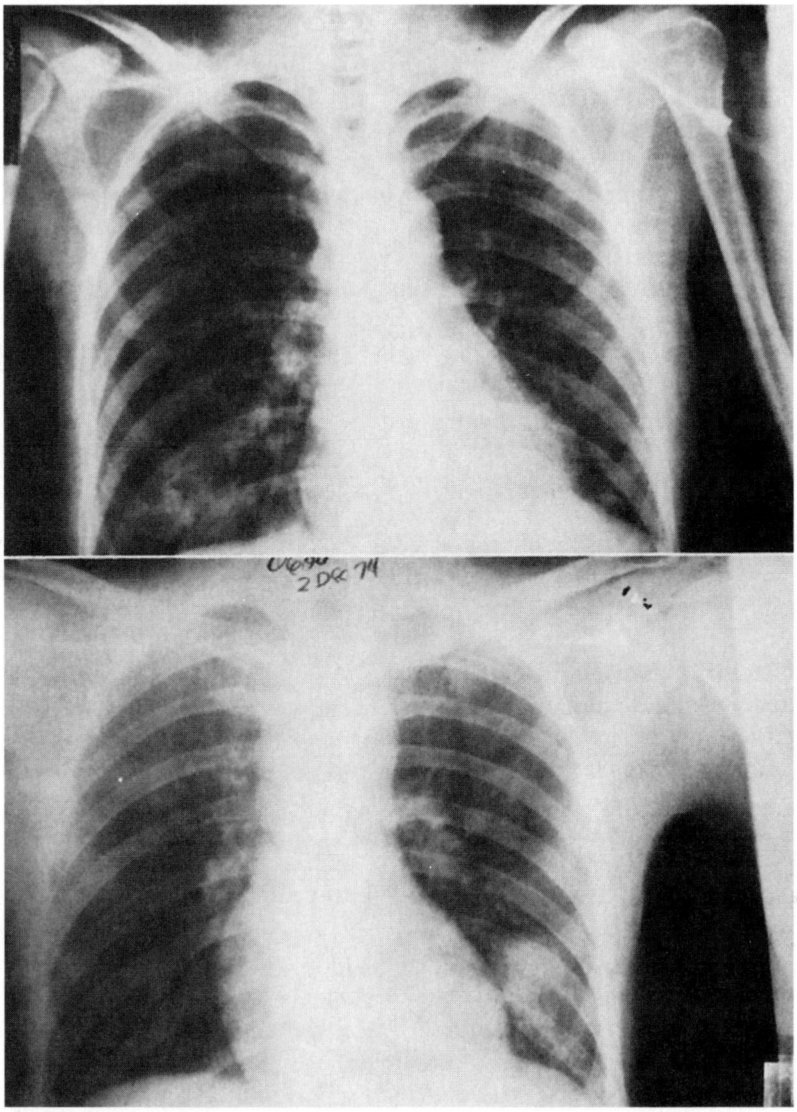

FIGURE 10-15 **A,** The diffuse infiltrate evident in the right lower lobe of this radiograph obtained on the sixteenth postburn day in a 23-year-old patient with a 68% burn is the typical radiographic presentation of airborne or bronchopneumonia. **B,** The solitary nodular infiltrate that was evident on the nineteenth postburn day in this patient who had acute staphylococcal endocarditis is typical of hematogenous pneumonia.

should be correlated with radiographic changes, changes in fluid balance, alterations in nutritional support, and the status of the patient's wounds. The clinical differences between the two forms of pneumonia are helpful in making the proper diagnosis and can be used to guide management; for example, pulmonary infection may be evident prior to the development of sepsis in patients with bronchopneumonia, while sepsis is commonly evident before the pulmonary infection is apparent in patients with hematogenous pneumonia.

Bronchopneumonia occurs relatively early following injury or surgery, usually in the second postinjury week. The initial radiographic presentation is a unifocal or multifocal diffuse infiltrate that, if the disease process is uncontrolled, spreads to involve large areas of pulmonary parenchyma—for example, an entire lobe (Figure 10-15, *A*). The mortality associated with bronchopneumonia is less than that associated with hematogenous pneumonia but, as a reflection of its primary pulmonary origin is often the principal cause of death in the patients who expire.

The secretions of the bronchial tree in a patient suspected of having bronchopneumonia should be sampled for both microscopic and culture examination. The bronchial origin of the sample should be confirmed by the identification of a significant number of granulocytes and a paucity of squamous epithelial cells on a smear stained with methylene blue. The predominant organism should be determined by Gram's stain and cultures used to identify the organism and its sensitivity to antibiotics. Quantitative bacterial cultures are helpful in differentiating microbial colonization of the tracheobronchial tree from pneumonia. A good correlation has been reported between recovery of 10^3 or more organisms per milliliter of specimen obtained by the protected specimen brush technique and histologic evidence of pneumonia.[29] Organisms present in lesser densities are considered to be contaminants. The frequency with which a specific organism causes bronchopneumonia changes across time and in concert with changes in the frequency with which it is recovered from patients and the environment of the treatment facility.[153] Consequently, the initial choice of antibiotic can be based on the results of the treatment facility's microbial surveillance program and later modified on the basis of culture results. Ventilatory support, when required, should be provided.

Hematogenous pneumonia occurs later in a patient's hospital course and is commonly diagnosed in the third post-injury week. The mortality associated with hematogenous pneumonia is greater than that associated with bronchopneumonia but, as a manifestation of its secondary origin from a remote primary focus, hematogenous pneumonia is less commonly the principal cause of death in patients who expire. A solitary nodular pulmonary infiltrate is the initial radiographic presentation of hematogenous pneumonia (Figure 10-15, *B*). If the primary source of infection is not identified and remains untreated, multiple pulmonary infiltrates with random distribution may appear on subsequent chest radiographs. If the pulmonary infection progresses, the multifocal infiltrates may coalesce and be difficult to distinguish from those characteristic of bronchopneumonia. The treatment of hematogenous pneumonia includes ventilatory support and systemic antibiotic therapy. As is the case with bronchopneumonia, the organisms causing hematogenous pneumonia are most commonly the predominant members of the treatment facility's endogenous flora. It is also essential to identify and control the primary septic focus from which the organisms causing the hematogenous pneumonia have spread. The common sources of hematogenous pneumonia that should be considered and dealt with, if identified, include invasive infection of a burn wound, suppurative thrombophlebitis in a previously cannulated vein, peritonitis as a result of visceral perforation, and a soft-tissue infection at a medication injection site.

Suppurative Thrombophlebitis

Intraluminal suppuration can occur in any previously cannulated vein (Figure 10-16). Injury to the vein wall

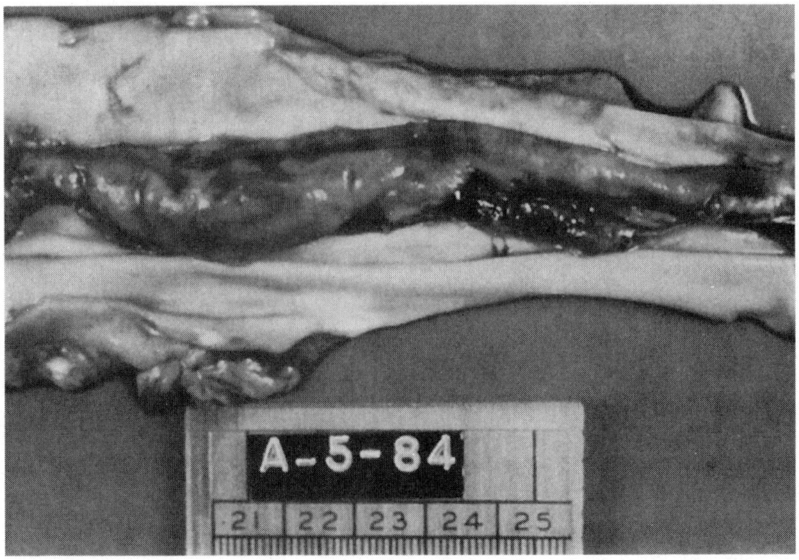

FIGURE 10-16 This large infected clot was noted at autopsy in the inferior vena cava of a 67-year-old patient with a 33% burn who had repeated femoral vein cannulation for fluid and nutrient administration.

where the tip of the cannula lies predisposes that area to the development of infection, the occurrence of which increases with an increasing duration of cannulation.[154] Other etiologic factors include catheter composition and microbial seeding resulting from contamination of the infusion set of episodes of bacteremia.[188] The latter factor may be of particular importance in burn patients. Bacteremia has been documented to occur in association with 20.6% of burn wound debridement procedures, with the incidence of positive blood cultures directly related to the extent of the burn wound and the duration of wound manipulation.[160] Strict limitation of cannula residence within a peripheral or central vein to a maximum of 72 hours has reduced the incidence of suppurative thrombophlebitis from a previous level of 6.9% to 1.4% of burn patients in recent years.[153]

One should consider the diagnosis of suppurative thrombophlebitis in any surgical patient with septicemia in whom there is no other obvious source of infection or in a surgical patient with a pulmonary infiltrate characteristic of hematogenous pneumonia. Since local signs of infection are present in less than half of the patients with suppurative thrombophlebitis, every previously cannulated vein may have to be explored and the site of cannula tip residence examined.[132] A brisk flow of unaltered blood from the proximal end of a vein excludes it from further consideration. If intraluminal pus is identified, the diagnosis of suppurative thrombophlebitis is confirmed. If there is an intraluminal clot present but no pus evident, that section of the vein should be excised and both the vein and the clot subjected to culture and histologic examination. The presence of microorganisms in the clot or the vein wall or a positive culture confirms the diagnosis of intraluminal infection (Figure 10-17).

The treatment of suppurative thrombophlebitis includes the systemic administration of antibiotics active against the infecting organism and, most importantly, surgical removal of the infected vein. The frequency with which multiple areas of intraluminal infection are present proximal to intervening skip areas of relatively normal-appearing vein speaks for excision of the involved vein from the point of cannulation to the point where the vein becomes a tributary of the next larger order of veins (Figure 10-18). Control of this septic process has been achieved in selected cases in which the excision was carried proximally only to that point where the vein wall showed no mural thickening and brisk retrograde flow of unaltered blood was noted. Following excision of the infected vein and grossly involved tributaries, the wound should be loosely packed and covered with an occlusive dressing. Following resolution of the local inflammatory signs, skin grafting or secondary closure can be carried out.

Failure of sepsis to relent following excision of an infected vein may be due to residual infection proximal to the level of excision or suppuration within another vein (Table 10-8). In the former case, the level of excision should be extended proximally, and in the latter the

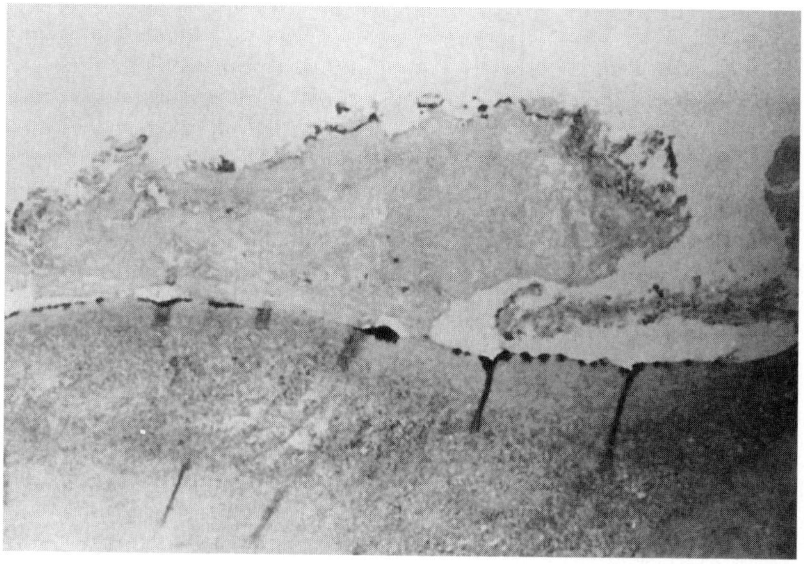

FIGURE 10-17 Histologic section of a vein suspected of harboring suppurative thrombophlebitis reveals a thrombus attached to the vein wall. Note the inflammatory changes of the vein wall at the point of thrombus attachment and the dark-staining masses of bacteria on the surface of the thrombus and at numerous foci on the intimal surface of the vein.

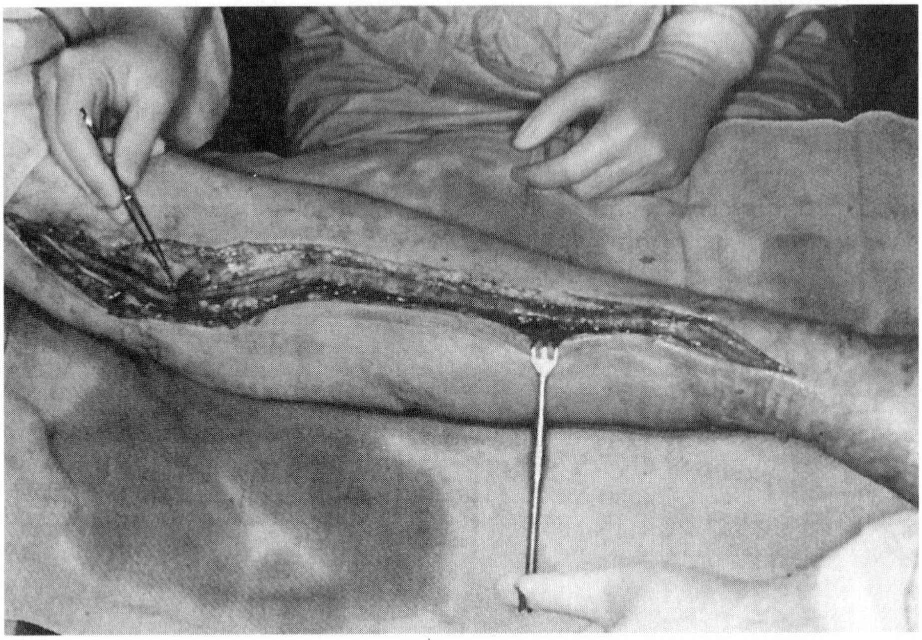

FIGURE 10-18 Suppurative thrombophlebitis caused by *Candida* species developed following cannulation of the cephalic vein in the forearm of this 68-year-old patient with a 33% burn. The length of incision was necessitated by the extent of vein involvement. Note the dark discoloration of the vein just proximal to the wrist, where the infection arose at the site of catheter tip residence. Note also the distension and discoloration of the entire length of exposed vein caused by the infected thrombus.

TABLE 10-8 SUPPURATIVE THROMBOPHLEBITIS—RESULTS OF EXCISION

	NUMBER	PERCENT
Patients treated by vein excision (90 veins excised)	75	
Survivors	30	40%
Causes of treatment failure		
Other disease	20	27%
Hematogenous dissemination of infection	5	7%
Undiagnosed infection in another vein	8	11%
Inadequate excision	12	16%
Total deaths	45	60%

involved vein should be identified and excised. Persistence of the septic state may also be associated with hematogenous pneumonia or acute bacterial endocarditis as a consequence of dissemination prior to excision of the infected vein.

Acute Endocarditis

Acute bacterial or fungal endocarditis can occur in any surgical patient experiencing episodes of bacteremia or fungemia. The high incidence of this cause of sepsis in burn patients (several times that of the general surgical population) has been attributed to the prolonged need for intravenous infusions and the high incidence of suppurative thrombophlebitis.[16] This infectious process is slightly more common on the right side of the heart but may involve either or both sides of the heart (Figure 10-19). Aside from persistent temperature elevation, the clinical findings in surgical patients with acute bacterial endocarditis are inconstant and nonspecific. The appearance and progressive increase in intensity of a heart murmur are pathognomonic, but identification of such a murmur is difficult in patients with a markedly hyperdynamic circulation.[124] In a surgical patient with sepsis in whom no other source of infection can be identified, the recovery of the same organism, particularly coagulase-positive *Staphylococcus aureus*, from two or more blood cultures should contribute to the diagnosis of acute bacterial endocarditis. Two-dimensional echocardiographic examination may confirm the presence of valvular lesions, but small foci of infection may escape echocardiographic detection. The overall accuracy of ultrasonic diagnosis is greatly dependent upon the individual interpreting the test results.

In absence of any other identifiable source of infection, a presumptive diagnosis of acute bacterial endocarditis should be made and systemic antibiotic therapy begun—for example, vancomycin at maximal dosage in patients with staphylococcal endocarditis. If a focus of suppurative thrombophlebitis is identified as the source of the endocarditis, the infected vein should be excised. The adequacy of antibiotic therapy should be monitored and treatment continued for at least 3 weeks or until the blood cultures clear. If antibiotic therapy fails to clear the septicemia or if valvular insufficiency develops, cardiac catheterization should be performed. Documentation of hemodynamically significant valvular insufficiency mandates excision of the infected incompetent valve and insertion of a pulmonary, aortic, or mitral valve prosthesis. The virtually universal mortality associated with valvular incompetence resulting from acute bacterial endocarditis justifies surgical intervention in such patients. Even though two patients so treated later died of other causes, autopsy examination revealed that the endocarditic process had been controlled.

OTHER INFECTION

Other sites of infection that should be considered in a surgical patient with sepsis, with or without positive blood cultures, include the urinary tract and the paranasal sinuses. Significant urinary tract infections are relatively uncommon in critically ill surgical patients, even though urine cultures obtained from catheterized patients are frequently positive for bacteria and yeast. Since clearing of micro-oganisms from the urine following removal of the catheter is the rule, such positive cultures appear to represent either catheter contamination or proliferation of microorganisms in the nonviable bladder mucosa traumatized by the catheter. A prostatic abscess may also serve as the focus of life-threatening infection in patients who require prolonged catheterization. To detect a prostatic infection, prostatic palpation and culture of prostatic secretions should be performed in any patient with otherwise unexplained sepsis.

Suppurative sinusitis may develop in patients who have required prolonged transnasal intubation of the airway or upper gastrointestinal tract.[26] If the diagnosis of sinusitis is confirmed by radiographic studies, systemic antibiotic therapy should be initiated. Surgical drainage of an infected maxillary sinus or other sinus is sometimes necessary. In patients with this complication in whom continued access to the gastrointestinal tract or lower airway is required, consideration should be given to placement of a tracheostomy and/or a gastrostomy to permit removal of the intranasal foreign body.

The recurrent bacteremias associated with repetitive wound manipulation required in the care of burn patients or other surgical patients are particularly hazardous in patients with associated long-bone fractures. Sepsis has been produced by abscesses that have formed in the fracture hematoma of such patients following lodgment of blood-borne organisms. When diagnosed, such abscesses should be immediately drained and systemic antibiotic therapy begun. If the septic process cannot be controlled by such means, amputation may be necessary.

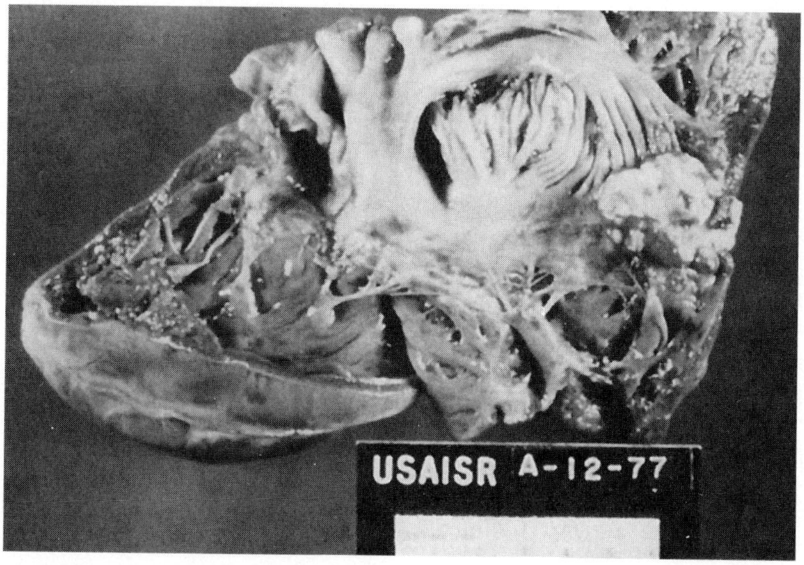

FIGURE 10-19 Autopsy specimen showing a large infected thrombus attached to a leaflet of the tricuspid valve of a 31-year-old patient with a 72% burn who expired with sepsis due to fungal burn wound invasion.

Septicemia

The significance of a positive blood culture depends upon the patient's general condition and the presence of other signs of infection. If a positive blood culture is obtained and *en passant* contamination caused by sampling through contaminated tissue and other sources of contamination can be excluded, no specific source of infection is evident, and the patient's general condition is inconsistent with sepsis, treatment can be delayed but repeat blood cultures should be obtained. If two successive blood cultures are positive for the same organism and exogenous contamination can be excluded, specific systemic antibiotic therapy should be started even if the patient does not appear to be clinically septic. In critically ill burn patients with life-threatening complications and little effective host resistance, multiple organisms may be recovered from a single blood culture or from successive blood cultures.[116a] Such findings should not be regarded as indicative of a technical error, and systemic administration of an antibiotic or antibiotics active against all of the recovered organisms should be started.

The effect of septicemia depends upon the organism recovered.[88] A recent 25-year review of septicemia occurring in patients treated at a referral burn center has shown that gram-negative septicemia and candidemia were associated with a significant increase in burn size-related mortality.[110] Interestingly, gram-positive septicemia exerted no discernible effect on the expected mortality of burn patients treated at that institution.

Viral Infections

Infections resulting from herpes simplex and cytomegalovirus may also cause sepsis in surgical patients, such as those with extensive burns.[60,126] Except for deliberately immunosuppressed transplant patients, clinically significant cytomegalovirus (CMV) infections appear to be uncommon. Even though a significant increase in CMV antibody titer has been reported in 10% of all burn patients and 22% of pediatric burn patients, the clinical significance of the increase is unclear, and it is uncertain whether this represents primary infection, reactivation of latent infection, or the effect of blood transfusion.[101,111] Recognition of prolonged temperature elevation, lymphocytosis in the absence of atypical lymphocytes, and even anicteric hepatitis as the clinical manifestations of CMV infection will forestall the administration of unnecessary antibiotics.[45]

PREVENTION OF SURGICAL INFECTION

Preoperative

Preoperative preparation is directed toward improving resistance to infection, reducing bacterial population sites of potential contamination and infection, and decreasing potential portals of bacterial entry into the interior of the body. If at all possible, remote infections should be eradicated before surgery, because such infections substantially increase the risk of operative wound infection and systemic sepsis. Chronic diseases, such as diabetes mellitus, uremia, cirrhosis, and malnutrition, should be stabilized. Preoperative body hygiene measures reduce infection in the operative wound; an especially effective technique is a preoperative shower or bath with hexachlorophene soap.[41] Major determinants of surgical infection are duration of hospital stay, preparation of the operative site, the use of antibiotics, and surgical technique.

The patient's hospital stay should be as brief as possible. Hospitals, and particularly their critical care units, harbor strains of pathogenic bacteria that are commonly resistant to antibiotics. In the NAS/NRC ultraviolet study, infection rates were twice as great after a two week hospitalization and three times greater after a three week hospitalization when compared with patients admitted only two or three days before surgery.

The goal of preoperative skin preparation is to reduce the skin flora to a level of an insignificant inoculum (because it is impossible to completely sterilize the skin). Removal of body hair is unnecessary for the prevention of infection and may increase wound infections. If hair must be removed, it should be clipped, not shaved, at a time as close to the commencement of the surgical procedure as possible.[6] Hair should never be removed the day before surgery because this technique uniformly results in higher infection rates. Effective degerming agents include iodine compounds, alcohol, chlorhexidine, quaternary ammonium compounds, and hexachlorophene. If used according to manufacturer's instructions, none has demonstrated antibacterial superiority over the others. Before a degerming solution is used, the skin should be defatted by a fat solvent or a nonirritating detergent.

If infection is present before surgery, the responsible organism(s) should be identified, along with its antibiotic sensitivities. Antibiotic selection is based on the bacterial susceptibilities, and therapy should be instituted before the surgical procedure begins (see the section on Prophylactic Antibiotics).

Surgical Technique

Operative technique has a major influence on the rate of surgical infection. Involved are not only the manual skills themselves but also selection of the proper procedure and judgment of how extensive the procedure should be. Clean surgical wounds in elective operations are least likely to become infected, and meticulous care of tissues is essential for maintaining a low infection rate. The surgical wound should be handled gently with instruments whose size and construction are appropriate for the tissue being manipulated. Likewise, sutures and ligatures should be selected so as to leave a minimal amount of foreign material in the wound. Wound closure should be secure but not so tight that the sutures strangulate the wound margins. Finally, infection rate increases with length of time of the procedure, so the operation should be carried out as expeditiously as is safely possible.

Old, potentially infected wounds require a different surgical approach. Foreign bodies and devitalized tissue harbor large numbers of bacteria and increase the probability of infection. Further, this detritus in a sterile wound greatly reduces the bacterial inoculum necessary to produce infection. Wounds in which complete debridement is not possible because of patient instability or proximity of vital structures should not be closed.

The choice of suture material depends on the purpose for which it was intended. Any suture material should excite only a minimal tissue reaction. In general, monofilament sutures are superior to multifilament sutures, and this advantage is particularly evident in contaminated wounds.[5] Hemostasis should be as complete as possible so that fluid collections do not form in the depths of the wound. Approximation of the wound edges along the entire extent is the most effective method to avoid dead spaces and the subsequent formation of seromas or abscesses. However, it is inadvisable to use buried sutures to force portions of the wound surface into apposition, because this technique usually causes additional tissue necrosis and enhances the possibility of infection. Rather, any potential dead space should be evacuated with drains placed in the most dependent portion of the wound. A closed suction drainage system is the most effective method of eliminating dead space and reducing infectious complication.

Invasive Monitoring

The physiologic stability of the patient must be ensured during all phases of medical care. The severely injured and infected patient is particularly susceptible to episodes of hemodynamic decompensation, especially when undergoing a general anesthetic and sizable blood loss.

INFECTION CONTROL MEASURES IN SEVERELY INJURED PATIENTS

- Restricted use of antibiotics according to specific guidelines for the presence of infection
- Separate rooms and nonrecirculating air-exchange system
- Barrier techniques—gloves, aprons, gowns, and masks
- Handwashing
- Control patient and personnel flow from critical care areas to convalescent areas
- Cohorting patients, with disinfection of empty facilities

Invasive monitoring allows careful titration of medications and fluid replacement. Blood pressure measurement with a cuff may be quite inaccurate in the cold, vasoconstricted patient, while intraarterial catheters whose tips lie in a major branch of the aorta provide an accurate pressure reading. The pulmonary capillary wedge pressure reliably reflects the adequacy of intravascular volume and should be used to guide fluid replacement in the unstable patient. Newer devices that measure arterial oxygen saturation by pulse oximetry and monitor end-tidal carbon dioxide concentrations increase the safety of patient care.

Nutritional Support

Malnutrition is associated with a significant increase in surgical infection. Studies have shown that severe malnutrition increases wound infection rates up to three times that of healthy individuals. Specific nutrient deficiencies have been shown to cause abnormalities of immune function and wound healing, and global protein and caloric deficits greatly increase mortality from surgical infection.[131] The metabolic requirements of injured and infected patients may more than double the prior needs. If the patient is markedly hypermetabolic, carbohydrate is the most effective caloric source for preserving lean body mass. Fat in these patients is relatively ineffective in maintaining nitrogen balance and is used primarily to provide essential fatty acids.[102] However, fat does appear to be useful in less ill patients who manifest only a moderate increase in metabolic expenditure. Nitrogen also is essential for maintenance of lean body mass and is best provided in a ratio of 1 g of nitrogen for each 150 kilocalories. Vitamins and minerals are usually provided to critically ill patients, but few studies have defined exact dosage requirements.

Infection Control Measures

With strict adherence to proven infection control measures, infection from exogenous sources can be reduced to minimal levels in injured and surgical patients (see the box at left). The number and types of antibiotics should be restricted, and the criteria for documenting infection should be well defined. Multiple antibiotics for a single infection should be used only if bacteremia continues in spite of therapeutic doses documented by measured plasma antibiotic levels. The indiscriminate use of multiple agents does not improve survival from major injuries and promotes overgrowth of *Candida,* enterococci, and organisms resistant to multiple antibiotics, both in the patient and in the critical care unit. Care is taken not to treat positive cultures in the absence of documented infection, particularly if associated with invasive devices. Gram's staining and microscopic examination of secretions and other body fluids by the physician are essential for differentiating contamination,

APPENDIX 10-A PRINCIPAL EFFECTS, DIAGNOSIS, AND TREATMENT OF SELECTED IMMUNODEFICIENT STATES

DEFECT	PRINCIPAL EFFECT	DIAGNOSTIC TEST	TREATMENT
Humoral Defects			
Complement dysfunction/ deficiency Genetic or acquired	Decrease or absence of complement component	Functional: IgM-sheep red cell hemolysis (classical pathway) Rabbit red cell hemolysis (alternative pathway) Antigenic: C4, C3, factor B quantified by antigen-specific immunoassay	Fresh frozen plasma?
Immunoglobulin deficiency Genetic or acquired	Decrease or absence of immunoglobulin	Quantitative immunoglobulin (IgG, A, M, E) by antigen-specific immunoassay	Globulin replacement (Avoid giving blood products containing IgA to IgA-deficient individual—Administration of IgA can result in severe immune reaction in sensitized individuals)
Cellular Defects			
Lymphocyte dysfunction/ deficiency			
B-cell	Altered antibody production	Functional: Response to antigen challenge Antigenic: Serum immunoglobulins	Globulin replacement
T-cell	Altered cellular immunity or regulatory function	Functional: Skin testing for anergy Mitogen response Enumeration: Flow cytometry with subclass and panmonoclonal antibodies	Specific antibiotic treatment when indicated Steroids and nonsteroidal antiinflammatory agents for associated collagen vascular disease
Large granular lymphocytes (NK; natural killer cells)	Altered response to viral infection; altered tumor surveillance	Functional: Target cell killing Enumeration: Flow cytometry	None
Acquired immunodeficiency syndrome (AIDS)	Virally induced alteration of immune defense; virally induced T-helper defect; decreased production of interferon-α	Antibody titer to HIV Western blot (confirmation) T-lymphocyte helper/suppressor ratio Absolute T helper number	Azidothymidine (investigational)
Neutrophil Defects			
Neutropenia Genetic or acquired	Increased susceptibility to bacterial and fungal infections	Neutrophil count of <1500/ml	Infection surveillance with antibiotic treatment at first sign of infection Transfusion of granulocytes may be effective in young pediatric patients
Oxidase dysfunction/deficiency Genetic: chronic granulomatous disease Acquired: severe trauma	No respiratory burst metabolism; severe impairment of microbicidal action	NBT dye reduction Native, luminol, and lucigenin chemiluminescence Measurement of glucose metabolism by radioisotope tracers Oxidized-reduced difference spectrum of cytochrome b_{245}	Infection surveillance with antibiotic treatment at first sign of infection Transfusion of granulocytes may be effective in young pediatric patients

Continued.

APPENDIX 10-A PRINCIPAL EFFECTS, DIAGNOSIS, AND TREATMENT OF SELECTED IMMUNODEFICIENT STATES—cont'd

DEFECT	PRINCIPAL EFFECT	DIAGNOSTIC TEST	TREATMENT
Myeloperoxidase (MPO) dysfunction Genetic: hereditary MPO deficiency Acquired: drug-induced dysfunction	Decrease or absence of MPO in azurophilic granules	Peroxidase stain of blood smear Oxidized-reduced difference spectrum of myeloperoxidase Luminol-negative: lucigenin-positive chemiluminescence response	Infection surveillance with antibiotic treatment at first sign of infection
Chemotactic/phagocytic dysfunction Genetic: Chédiak-Higashi syndrome (congenital absence of specific granules) Job syndrome Deficiency of Mo_1 surface membrane glycoprotein Acquired: "Down regulation" secondary to in vivo complement activation, drugs, or toxins	Defective chemotaxis/degranulation Impaired phagocytosis Increased susceptibility to bacterial and fungal infections	Chemotactic assays Microscopic detection of morphologic change in response to stimulus Microscopic assessment of granule content Cytometry using anti-Mo_1 antibody	Infection surveillance with antibiotic treatment at first sign of infection Ascorbic acid for Chédiak-Higashi syndrome?

colonization, and true infection. Thus sputum with a few organisms on a stained smear and with no cellular elements is unlikely to represent significant airway infection. Lastly, antibiotic therapy should not be used as a substitute for proper surgical treatment of an infection requiring incision and drainage or excision of the infected wound tissue.

Patients with injuries and infection should be treated in single rooms, isolated from other patients. Although the efficacy of ultrafiltration air exchange has not been conclusively proved, the air-handling system should be of separate, nonrecirculating construction. The single rooms should be closed periodically for extensive decontamination and repainting. Use of barrier techniques, including gloves, aprons, gowns, and masks decreases the cross-contamination of patients. If nothing else, these barrier procedures reinforce the danger of exogenous transfer of infectious agents and constantly remind the staff to wash their hands. Handwashing is the single most effective means of reducing nosocomial infection, and separate sinks in each patient's room are mandatory if handwashing is to be effective. Shared, common sinks serve only to promote crosscontamination. The flow of patients and personnel should be directed away from the critical care unit to the convalescent floor. Patients and staff on step-down units should not return to visit friends and relatives who still remain critically ill, since the convalescent patients are often the major reservoirs for life-threatening nosocomial infections.[165] Only patients experiencing unexpected physiologic instability should be transferred back to the critical care area. Cohorting patients with surgical infection into separate geographic sections of the hospital, although proven effective in controlling burn center epidemics, is too expensive and impractical in most medical centers, where it is not economically feasible to leave large blocks of beds continually unoccupied.

Early Activity and Ambulation

Lack of activity promotes muscle wasting and atrophy, and traction and air-fluidized beds encourage immobility and loss of lean body mass. Such patients have particular difficulty in maintaining adequate pulmonary toilet and often develop respiratory infections. Further, skin breakdown occurs frequently in patients confined to bed, and severe infections may develop in such injured tissue.

Vigorous physical activity promotes preservation of muscle bulk, and supervised activity must be provided continuously on a daily basis to all patients requiring prolonged hospitalization. An adequate number of physical and occupational therapists should be assigned specifically to critical care areas so that each patient participates in a daily program that uses his physical capacity. Patients confined to bed can carry out simple isometric exercises. Critically ill but stable patients often can tolerate moving from bed to specially designed chairs that can constantly vary the sitting positions. Progression from sitting activity to full ambulation is facilitated by sessions on tilt tables, on which upright positioning can be gradually introduced. Walking with assistance from the therapists is begun as soon as the patient tolerates standing. Some patients requiring mechanical ventilation are able to begin ambulation while still connected to the respirator; the ventilator simply is pushed along with the patient.

REFERENCES

1 Ad Hoc Committee of the Committee on Trauma, Division of Medical Sciences, National Research Council Report: Postoperative wound infections: the influence of ultraviolet irradiation of the operating room and the influence of various other factors, *Ann Surg* 160(suppl):53, 1964.

2 Ad Hoc Committee of the Committee on Trauma, Division of Medical Sciences, National Research Council Report: Postoperative wound infections: the influence of ultraviolet irradiation of the operating room and the influence of various other factors, *Ann Surg* 160(suppl):70, 1964.

3 Ahrenholz DH, Simmons RL: Fibrin in peritonitis. I. Beneficial and adverse effects in experimental *E. coli* peritonitis, *Surgery* 130:286, 1980.

4 Alder MI, Willman JL, Haaga JR et al: Role of surgical and percutaneous drainage in the treatment of abdominal abscess, *Arch Surg* 118:273, 1983.

5 Alexander JW, Altemeier WA, Kaplan JZ: Role of suture materials in the development of wound infection, *Ann Surg* 165:192, 1967.

6 Alexander JW, Fischer JE, Boyajian M et al: The influence of hair removal methods on wound infection, *Arch Surg* 118:347, 1983.

7 Alexander JW, Wixon D: Neutrophil dysfunction and sepsis in burn injury, *Surg Gynecol Obstet* 130:431, 1970.

8 Alexander JW: The contributions of infection control to a century of surgical progress, *Ann Surg* 201:423, 1985.

9 Allen RC, Pruitt BA Jr: Humoral-phagocyte axis of immune defense in burn patients, *Arch Surg* 117:133, 1982.

10 Altemeier WA, Furste WL: Gas gangrene, *Surg Gynecol Obstet* 84:507, 1947.

11 Anderson CB, Marr JJ, Ballinger WF: Anaerobic infections in surgery: a clinical review, *Surgery* 78:313, 1976.

12 Antonacci AC, Reaves LE, Calvano SE et al: Flow cytometric analysis of lymphocyte subpopulations after thermal injury in human beings, *Surg Gynecol Obstet* 159:1, 1984.

13 Aulick LH, Baze WB, McLeod CG et al: Control of blood flow in a large surface wound, *Ann Surg* 191:249, 1980.

14 Aulick LH, Hander EH, Wilmore DW et al: The relative significance of thermal and metabolic demands on burn hypermetabolism, *J Trauma* 19:559, 1979.

15 Aulick LH, Wilmore DW, Mason AD Jr et al: Muscle blood flow following thermal injury, *Ann Surg* 188:778, 1978.

16 Baskin TW, Rosenthal A, Pruitt BA Jr: Acute bacterial endocarditis: a silent source of sepsis in the burn patient, *Ann Surg* 184:618, 1976.

17 Bernard HR, Cole WR: The prophylaxis of surgical infection: the effect of prophylactic antimicrobial agents in the incidence of infection following contaminated wounds, *Surgery* 56:151, 1964.

18 Black PR, Brooks DC, Bessey PQ et al: Mechanisms of insulin resistance following injury, *Ann Surg* 196:420, 1982.

19 Brigham KL, Woolverton WC, Blake LH et al: Increased sheep lung vascular permeability caused by *Pseudomonas* bacteremia, *J Clin Invest* 54:792, 1974.

20 Bryan CS, Reynolds KL, Metzger WT: Bacteremia in diabetic patients: comparison of incidence and mortality with nondiabetic patients, *Diabetes Care* 8:244, 1985.

21 Bryan CS, Smith CW Jr, Sutton JP et al: Comparison of cefamandole and cefazolin in cardiopulmonary bypass, *J Thorac Cardiovasc Surg* 86:222, 1983.

22 Burke JF: The effective period of preventive antibiotic action in experimental incision and dermal lesions, *Surgery* 50:161, 1961.

23 Burke JF, Wolfe RR, Mullany CJ et al: Glucose requirements following burn injury, *Ann Surg* 190:274, 1979.

24 Burleson DG, Vaughan GK, Mason AD Jr et al: Flow cytometric measurement of rat lymphocyte subpopulations after burn injury and injury with infection, *Arch Surg* 122:216, 1987.

25 Calvin JE, Driedger AA, Sibbald WJ: An assessment of myocardial function in human sepsis utilizing ECG-gated cardiac scintigraphy, *Chest* 80:579, 1981.

26 Caplan ES, Hoyt NJ: Nosocomial sinusitis, *JAMA* 247:639, 1982.

27 Carrico JC, Meakins JL, Marshall JC, Frye D: Multiple-organ-failure syndrome, *Arch Surg* 121:196, 1986.

28 Chang N, Goodson WH, Gottrup F, Hunt TK: Direct measurement of wound and oxygen tension in postoperative patients, *Ann Surg* 197:470, 1983.

29 Chastre J, Viau F, Brun P: Prospective evaluation of the protected specimen brush for the diagnosis of pulmonary infections in ventilated patients, *Am Rev Respir Dis* 130(5):924, 1984.

30 Chetlin SH, Elliott DW: Preoperative antibiotics in biliary surgery, *Arch Surg* 107:319, 1973.

31 Chodak GW, Plaut ME: Use of systemic antibiotics for prophylaxis in surgery, *Arch Surg* 112:326, 1977.

32 Clemens MG, Chaudry IH, Daigreau N et al: Insulin resistance and depressed gluconeogenic capability during early hyperglycemic sepsis, *J Trauma* 24:701, 1984.

33 Clowes GHA Jr, Vucinic M, Weidner MG: Circulatory and metabolic alterations associated with survival or death in peritonitis—clinical analysis of 25 cases, *Ann Surg* 163:866, 1966.

34 Condon RE, Bartlett JG, Nichols RL et al: Pre-operative prophylactic cephalothin fails to control septic complications of colorectal operations: results of a controlled clinical trial, *Am J Surg* 137:68, 1979.

35 Condon RE, Bartlett JG, Greenlee H et al: Efficacy of oral and systemic antibiotic prophylaxis in colorectal operations, *Arch Surg* 118:496, 1983.

36 Conklin JJ, Kelleher PC, Walker RI: *Medical Bulletin U.S. Army Europe* 40:9, 1983.

37 Conklin JJ, Walker RI, Hirsch EW: Current concepts in the management of radiation injuries and associated trauma, *Surg Gynecol Obstet* 156:809, 1983.

38 Corrigan JJ: Thrombocytopenia: a laboratory sign of septicemia in infants and children, *J Pediatr* 85:219, 1974.

39 Cortez A, Zito J, Lucas CE et al: Mechanisms of inappropriate polyuria in septic patients, *Arch Surg* 112:471, 1977.

40 Crass BA, Bergdoll MS: Toxin involvement in toxic shock syndrome, *J Infect Dis* 153:918, 1986.

41 Cruse PJE, Foord R: A five year prospective study of 23,649 surgical wounds, *Arch Surg* 107:206, 1973.

42 Cruse PJE, Foord R: The epidemiology of wound infection: a ten-year prospective study of 62,939 wounds, *Surg Clin North Am* 60:187, 1980.

43 Cuthbertson DB: The disturbance of metabolism produced by bony and non-bony injury, with notes on certain abnormal conditions of bone, *Biochem J* 24:1244, 1930.

44 Daubenspeck JA: Ventilatory responses to elastic loading at constant Pa_{CO_2} in hypercapneic hyperpnea, *J Appl Physiol* 47:778, 1979.

45 Deep GS Jr, MacMillan BG, Linnemann CC Jr: Unexplained fever

in burn patients due to cytomegalovirus infection, *JAMA* 248:2299, 1982.
46 Deitch EA, Maejima K, Berg R: Effect of antibiotics and bacterial overgrowth on the translocation of the GI tract microflora in burned rats, *J Trauma* 25:385, 1985.
47 Dellinger EP, Wertz MJ, Meakins JL et al: Surgical infection stratification system for intra-abdominal infection: multicenter trial, *Arch Surg,* 120:21, 1985.
48 Dinarello CA: Interleukin 1, *Rev Infect Dis* 6:51, 1984.
49 Dinarello CA, Clowes GHA Jr, Gordon HA et al: Cleavage of human interleukin-1: isolation of a peptide fragment from plasma of febrile humans and activated monocytes, *J Immunol* 133:1332, 1984.
50 DiPiro JT, Record KE, Schanzenbach KS et al: Antimicrobial prophylaxis in surgery. I. *Am J Hosp Pharm* 38:320, 1981.
51 DiPiro JT, Record KE, Schanzenbach KS et al: Antimicrobial prophylaxis in surgery. II. *Am J Hosp Pharm* 38:487, 1981.
52 Dixon JM, Armstrong CP, Duffy SW et al: A randomized prospective trial comparing the value of intravenous and preincisional cefamandole in reducing postoperative sepsis after operations on the gastrointestinal tract, *Surg Gynecol Obstet* 158:303, 1984.
53 Drobny EC, Abramson EC, Baumann G: Insulin receptors in acute infection: a study of factors conferring insulin resistance, *J Clin Endocrinol Metab* 58:710, 1984.
54 Duma RJ, Weinberg AN, Medrek TF, Kunz LJ: Streptococcal infections: a bacteriologic and clinical study of streptococcal bacteremia, *Medicine* (Balt.) 48:87, 1969.
55 Elebute RA, Stoner HB: The grading of sepsis, *Br J Surg* 70:29, 1983.
56 Elek SD, Conen PE: The virulence of *Staphylococcus pyogenes* for man: a study of wound infection, *Br J Exp Pathol* 38:573, 1957.
57 Eurenius K, Brouse RO: Granulocyte kinetics after thermal injury, *Am J Clin Pathol* 60:337, 1973.
58 Facklam RR: A review of microbiological techniques for isolation and identification of streptococci, *Crit Rev Clin Lab Sci* 6:287, 1976.
59 Flint LM, Fry DE: *Surgical infections,* New York, 1982, Medical Examination Publishing.
60 Foley FD, Greenawald KA, Nash G et al: Herpes virus infection in burn patients, *N Engl J Med* 282:652, 1970.
61 Freund H, Atamian S, Holroyde F et al: Plasma amino acids as predictors of the severity and outcome of sepsis, *Ann Surg* 190:571, 1979.
62 Fry DE: The cephalosporin jungle, *Am J Surg* 47:40, 1981.
63 Fry DE, Harbrecht PJ, Polk HC Jr: Systemic antibiotic prophylaxis: need the costs be so high? *Arch Surg* 116:466, 1981.
64 Fry DE, Pearlstein L, Fulton RL: Multiple system failure: the role of uncontrolled infection, *Arch Surg* 115:136, 1980.
65 Fullen WD, Hunt J, Altemeier WA: Prophylactic antibiotics in penetrating wounds of the abdomen, *J Trauma* 12:282, 1972.
66 Furste W: Mechanisms of production of clostridial myositis without a visible wound, *Arch Surg* 119:172, 1984.
67 Furste W, Colon-Figueroa F, Rothstein LB: Tetanus prophylaxis as effected in the United States of America. In Mistico G, Mastroeni P, Pitzurra M, editors: *Proceedings of the Seventh International Conference on Tetanus,* Copanello, Italy, Sept. 10-15, 1984, Rome, 1985, Gangemi Publishing.
68 Gatehouse D, Dimock F, Burdon DW et al: Prediction of wound sepsis following gastric operations, *Br J Surg* 65:551, 1978.
69 Gelfand JA, Donelan M, Burke JF: Preferential activation and depletion of the alternative complement pathway by burn injury, *Ann Surg* 198:58, 1983.
70 George CD, Morello PJ: Immunologic effects of blood transfusion upon renal transplantation, tumor operations, and bacterial infections, *Am J Surg* 152:329, 1986.
71 Glick PL, Pellegrini CA, Stein S et al: Abdominal abscess: a surgical strategy, *Arch Surg* 118:273, 1983.
72 Gold JP, Canizaro P, Kazam E et al: The reliability of the results of ultrasound detection of fluid collections in the early post-ciliotomy period, *Surg Gynecol Obstet* 161:5, 1985.
73 Goodwin CW, Dorethy J, Lam V et al: Randomized trial of efficacy of crystalloid and colloid resuscitation on hemodynamic response and lung water following thermal injury, *Ann Surg* 197:520, 1983.
74 Gorbach SL, Bartlett JG: Anaerobic infections, *N Engl J Med* 290:1177, 1974.
75 Gott JP, Polk HC Jr: Unsuspected intraabdominal infection. In Ballinger WE, editor: *Problems in general surgery,* Philadelphia, 1984, JB Lippincott.
76 Graham BS, Tucker WS Jr: Opportunistic infections in endogenous Cushing's syndrome, *Ann Intern Med* 101:334, 1984.
77 Gross PA, Neu HC, Aswapokee P et al: Deaths from nosocomial infections: experience in a university hospital and a community hospital, *Am J Med* 68:219, 1980.
78 Hasselgren PO, Jagenburg R, Karlstrom L et al: Changes of protein metabolism in liver and skeletal muscle following trauma complicated by sepsis, *J Trauma* 24:224, 1984.
79 Hasselgren PO, Talamini M, James JH et al: Protein metabolism in different types of skeletal muscle during early and late sepsis in rats, *Arch Surg* 121:918, 1986.
80 Heistad DD, Wheeler RC, Mark AL et al: Effects of adrenergic stimulation and ventilation in man, *J Clin Invest* 51:1469, 1972.
81 Hinchey EJ, Schaal PGH, Richards GK: Treatment of perforated diverticular disease of the colon. In Rob C, editor: *Advances in surgery,* St Louis, 1978, Mosby.
82 Hingley ST, Hastie AT, Kueppers F et al: Disruption of respiratory cilia by proteases including those of *Pseudomonas aeruginosa, Infect Immun* 54:379, 1986.
83 Horton JW, Colin D, Mitchell JH: Left ventricular volumes and contractility during hemorrhagic hypotension: dimensional analysis and biplane cinefluorography, *Circ Shock* 11:73, 1983.
84 Hussain SNA, Simkus G, Roussos CJ: Respiratory muscle fatigue: a cause of ventilatory failure in septic shock, *J Appl Physiol* 58:2033, 1985.
85 Hutemeier PC, Watkins WD, Peterson MB et al: Acute pulmonary hypertension and lung thromboxane release after endotoxin infusion in normal and leukopenic sheep, *Circ Res* 50:688, 1982.
86 Huttunen K, Lampainen E, Silvennoinen-Kassinen S et al: The neutrophil function of uremic patients treated by hemodialysis or CAPD, *Scand J Urol Nephrol* 18:167, 1984.
87 Jepson MM, Pell JM, Bates PC et al: The effects of endotoxemia on protein metabolism in skeletal muscle and liver in fed and fasted rats, *Biochem J* 235:329, 1986.
88 Jones WG, Barie PS, Yurt RW et al: Enterococcal burn sepsis: a highly lethal complication in severely burned patients, *Arch Surg* 121:649, 1986.
89 Juan G, Caverly P, Talamo C et al: Effect of carbon dioxide on diaphragmatic function in human beings, *N Engl J Med* 310:874, 1984.
90 Kaiser AB, Clayson KR, Mulherin JL Jr et al: Antibiotic prophylaxis in vascular surgery, *Ann Surg* 188:283, 1978.
91 Keighley MRB, Alexander-Williams J: Multivariate analysis of clinical and operative findings associated with biliary sepsis, *Br J Surg* 63:528, 1976.
92 Kivilaakso E, Silen W: Pathogenesis of experimental gastric mucosal injury, *N Engl J Med* 301:364, 1979.
93 Kopolovic R, Thrailkill KM, Martin DT: A critical comparison of the hematologic, cardiovascular, and pulmonary response to steroids and nonsteroidal antiinflammatory drugs in a model of sepsis and adult respiratory distress syndrome, *Surgery* 100:679, 1986.

94 Kupper TS, Green DR: Immunoregulation after thermal injury: sequential appearance of a I-J, LY-1 T suppressor inducer cells and LY-2 suppressor effector cells following thermal trauma in mice, *J Immunol* 135:3047, 1984.

95 Kupper TS, Green DR, Durums K et al: Defective antigen presentation to a cloned T helper cell by macrophages from burned mice can be restored with interleukin-1, *Surgery* 98:199, 1985.

96 Kvale PA, Ranga V, Kapacz M et al: Pulmonary resection, *South Med J* 70(suppl):64, 1977.

97 LaNoue KF, Mason AD Jr: Carbohydrate metabolism in *Pseudomonas* infection, *Computers Biomed Res* 2:51, 1968.

98 Lehrer RI: Inhibition by sulfonamides of the candidicidal activity of human neutrophils, *J Clin Invest* 50:2498, 1971.

99 Lesar TS, Rotschafer JC, Strand LM et al: Gentamycin dosing errors with four commonly used nomograms, *JAMA* 248:1190, 1982.

100 Levine GM, Deren JJ, Steiger E et al: Role of oral intake in maintenance of gut mass and disaccharide activity, *Gastroenterology* 67:975, 1974.

101 Linnemann CC Jr, BacMillan BC: Viral infections in pediatric burn patients, *Am J Dis Child* 135:750, 1983.

102 Long JM III, Wilmore DW, Mason AD Jr et al: Effect of carbohydrate and fat intake on nitrogen excretion during total intravenous feeding, *Ann Surg* 185:417, 1977.

103 Lopez C, Fitzgerald PA, Siegal FP: Severe acquired immune deficiency syndrome in male homosexuals: diminished capacity to make interferon-a in vitro associated with severe opportunistic infections, *J Infect Dis* 148:962, 1983.

104 Lowrey L, Trachtenberg L, Ray JW et al: Infection complicating cholecystectomy, *Am Surg* 46:386, 1980.

105 Lucas CE, Ledgerwood AM: The cardiopulmonary response to massive doses of steroids in patients with septic shock, *Arch Surg* 119:537, 1984.

106 Mandell GL: Catalase, superoxide dismutase, and virulence of *Staphylococcus aureus:* in vitro and in vivo studies with emphasis on staphylococcal-leukocyte interaction, *J Clin Invest* 55:561, 1975.

107 Manktelou A, Meyer AA: Lack of correlation between decreased chemotaxis and susceptibility to infection in burned rats, *J Trauma* 26:143, 1986.

108 Manwaring D, Curreri PW: Platelet mediation of fragment D-induced respiratory distress syndrome, *Surg Forum* 31:242, 1980.

109 Martyn JAJ, Snider MT, Szyfelbein et al: Right ventricular dysfunction in acute thermal injury, *Ann Surg* 191:346.

110 Mason AD Jr, McManus AT, Pruitt BA Jr: Association of burn mortality and bacteremia, *Arch Surg* 121:1027, 1986.

111 Matthews SCW, Levick PL, Coombes EJ et al: Viral infections in a group of burned patients, *Burns* 6:55, 1979.

112 McDougal WS, Heimburger S, Wilmore DW et al: The effect of exogenous substrate on hepatic metabolism and membrane transport during endotoxemia, *Surgery* 84:55, 1978.

113 McLeish AR, Keighley MRB, Bishop HM et al: Selecting patients requiring antibiotics in biliary surgery by immediate gram stains of bile at operation, *Surgery* 81:473, 1977.

114 McManus AT: Examination of neutrophil function in a rat model of decreased host resistance following burn trauma, *Rev Infect Dis* 5(suppl 5):S898, 1983.

115 McManus AT, Denton CL, Mason AD Jr: Mechanisms of in vitro sensitivity to sulfadiazine silver, *Arch Surg* 118:161, 1983.

116 McManus WF, Goodwin CW Jr, Pruitt BA Jr: Subeschar treatment of burn-wound infection, *Arch Surg* 118:291, 1983.

116a McManus AT, Mason AD Jr, McManus WF et al: Twenty-five year review of *Pseudomonas aeruginosa* bacteremia in a burn center, *European J Clin Microbiol* 4:219, 1985.

117 McManus AT, McManus WF, Mason AD Jr et al: Microbial colonization in a new intensive care burn unit, *Arch Surg* 120:217, 1985.

118 McManus AT, Moody EE, Mason AD Jr: Bacterial motility: a component in experimental *Pseudomonas aeruginosa* burn wound sepsis, *Burns* 6:235, 1980.

119 Mead PB, Pories SE, Hall P, et al: Decreasing the incidence of surgical wound infections, *Arch Surg* 121:458, 1986.

120 Meyers ML, Austin TW, Sibbald WJ: Pulmonary artery catheter infections, a prospective study, *Ann Surg* 201:237, 1985.

121 Miles AA, Miles EM, Burke J: The value and duration of defense reactions of the skin to the primary lodgment of bacteria, *Br J Exp Pathol* 38:79, 1957.

122 Molnar JA, Burke JF: Prevention and management of infection in trauma, *World J Surg* 7:158, 1983.

123 Moore FD Jr, Davis C, Rodrick M et al: Neutrophil activation in thermal injury as assessed by increased expression of complement receptors, 314:948, 1986.

124 Munster AM, DiVincenti FC, Foley FD et al: Cardiac infections in burns, *Am J Surg* 122:524, 1971.

125 Nance FC: Report of the subcommittee to the Scientific Studies Committee of the Surgical Infection Society, April 1986.

126 Nash G, Asch MJ, Foley FD et al: Disseminated cytomegalic inclusion disease in a burned adult, *JAMA* 214:587, 1970.

127 Nash G, Foley FD, Goodwin MN et al: Fungal burn wound infection, *JAMA* 215:1664, 1971.

128 Nichols RL, Broido P, Condon RE et al: Effect of preoperative neomycin-erythromycin intestinal preparation on the incidence of infectious complications following oral administration, *Ann Surg* 178:453, 1973.

129 Odessey R, Khairallah EA, Goldberg AL: Origin and possible significance of alanine production by skeletal muscle, *J Biol Chem* 249:7623, 1974.

130 O'Mahony JB, Palder SB, Wood JJ et al: Depression of cellular immunity after multiple trauma in the absence of sepsis, *J Trauma* 24:869, 1984.

131 O'Neill JA, Caldwell MD, Meng HC: Essential fatty acid deficiency in surgical patients, *Ann Surg* 185:535, 1977.

132 O'Neill JA Jr, Pruitt BA Jr, Foley FD et al: Suppurative thrombophlebitis—a lethal complication of intravenous therapy, *J Trauma* 8:256, 1968.

133 Order SC, Moncrief JA: Vascular destruction and revascularization in severe thermal injuries, *Surg Forum* 15:37, 1964.

134 Orlando R III, Gleason E, Drezner AD: Acute acalculous cholecystitis in the critically ill patient, *Am J Surg* 145:472, 1983.

135 Pearl RH, Clowes GH Jr, Hirsch EW et al: Prognosis and survival is determined by visceral amino acid clearance in severe trauma, *J Trauma* 25:777, 1985.

136 Pepe PE, Hudson LD, Carrico CJ: Early application of positive end-expiratory pressure in patients at risk for the adult respiratory-distress syndrome, *N Engl J Med* 311:281, 1984.

137 Pinto DJ, Sanderson PJ: Rational use of antibiotic therapy after appendicectomy, *Br Med J* 280:275, 1980.

138 Pitt HA, Postier RG, McGowan WAL et al: Prophylactic antibiotics in vascular surgery: topical, systemic or both, *Ann Surg* 192:356, 1980.

139 Polk HC Jr: Diminished surgical infection by systemic antibiotic administration in potentially contaminated operations, *Surgery* 75:312, 1974.

140 Polk HC: *Infection and the surgical patient,* Edinburgh, 1982, Churchill Livingstone.

141 Polk HC, Fry DE: Radical peritoneal debridement for established peritonitis: the results of a prospective randomized clinical trial, *Ann Surg* 192:350, 1980.

142 Polk HC, Lopez-Mayor FJ: Postoperative wound infection: a prospective study of determinant factors and prevention, *Surgery* 66:97, 1969.

143 Polk HC Jr, Miles AA: The decisive period in primary infection of muscle by *Escherichia coli, Br J Exp Pathol* 54:99, 1973.
144 Polk HC, Trachtenberg L, Finn MP: Antibiotic activity in surgical incisions. The basis for prophylaxis in selected operations, *JAMA* 244:1353, 1980.
145 Pollock AV, Arnot RS, Leaper DJ et al: The role of antibacterial preparation of the intestine in the reduction of primary wound sepsis after operations on the colon and rectum, *Surg Gynecol Obstet* 147:909, 1978.
146 Pruitt BA Jr: Advances in fluid therapy in the early care of the burn patient, *World J Surg* 2:139, 1978.
147 Pruitt BA Jr: Biopsy diagnosis of surgical infection, *N Engl J Med* 310:1737, 1984.
148 Pruitt BA Jr: Diagnosis and treatment of infection in the burn patient, *Burns* 11:79, 1984.
149 Pruitt BA Jr: Opportunistic infections in the severely injured patient. In Gruber D, Walker RI, Macvittie TJ, Conklin JJ, editors: *The pathophysiology of combined injury and trauma,* New York, 1987, Academic Press.
150 Pruitt BA Jr, DiVincenti FC, Mason AD Jr et al: The occurrence and significance of pneumonia and other pulmonary complications in burn patients: comparison of conventional and topical treatment, *J Trauma* 10:519, 1970.
151 Pruitt BA Jr, Goodwin CW: Wound care. In Moylan JA, editor: *Trauma surgery,* Philadelphia, 1987, JB Lippincott.
152 Pruitt BA Jr, Goodwin CW Jr: Stress ulcer disease in the burned patient, *World J Surg* 5:209, 1981.
153 Pruitt BA Jr, McManus AT: Opportunistic infections in severely burned patients, *Am J Med* 76(3):146, 1984.
154 Pruitt BA Jr, Stein JM, Foley FD et al: Intravenous therapy in burn patients: suppurative thrombophlebitis and other life threatening complications, *Arch Surg* 100:399, 1970.
155 Raahave D, Friis-Moller A, Bjerre-Jepsen K et al: The infective dose of aerobic and anaerobic bacteria in postoperative wound sepsis, *Arch Surg* 121:924, 1986.
156 Robson MC, Heggers JP: Delayed wound closures based on bacterial counts, *J Surg Oncol* 2:379, 1970.
157 Rodeheffer RJ, Gerstenblith G, Recher LC et al: Exercise cardiac output is maintained with advancing age in healthy human subjects: cardiac dilatation and increased stroke volume compensate for diminished heart rate, *Circulation* 69:203, 1984.
158 Rodkey GV, Welch CE: Colonic diverticular disease with surgical treatments: a study of 338 cases, *Surg Clin North Am* 54:655, 1974.
159 Ross SC, Bensen P: Complement deficiency states in infection: epidemiology, pathogenesis, and consequences of neisserial and other infections and immune deficiency, *Medicine* 63:243, 1984.
160 Sasacki TM, Welch GW, Herndon DN et al: Burn wound manipulation-induced bacteremia, *J Trauma* 19:46, 1979.
161 Sawyers CL, Moore RD, Lerner SA et al: A model for predicting nephrotoxicity in patients treated with aminoglycosides, *J Infect Dis* 153:1062, 1986.
162 Sganga G, Siegel JH, Brown G et al: Reprioritization of hepatic plasma protein release in trauma and sepsis, *Arch Surg* 120:187, 1985.
163 Shah PJR, Williams G, Chaudrey M: Short-term antibiotic prophylaxis and prostatectomy, *Br J Urol* 53:339, 1981.
164 Shaw JHF, Wolfe RR: Response to glucose and lipid infusions in sepsis: a kinetic analysis, *Metabolism* 34:442, 1985.
165 Shirani KZ, McManus AT, Vaughan GM et al: Effect of environment on infection in burn patients, *Arch Surg* 121:31, 1986.
166 Sibbald WF: Myocardial function in the critically ill: factors influencing left and right ventricular performance in patients with sepsis and trauma, *Surg Clin North Am* 65:867, 1985.
167 Sibbald WJ, Driedger AA, Myers ML et al: Biventricular function in the adult respiratory distress syndrome, *Chest* 84:126, 1983.
168 Siegel JH, Giovannini I, Coleman B: Ventilation: perfusion maldistribution secondary to the hyperdynamic cardiovascular state is the major cause of increased pulmonary shunting in human sepsis, *J Trauma* 432, 1979.
169 Simmons RL, Howard RJ: *Surgical infectious diseases,* New York, 1982, Appleton-Century-Crofts.
170 Solomkin JS, Jenkins M, Nelson RD et al: Neutrophil dysfunction in sepsis. II. Evidence for the role of complement activation products in cellular deactivation, *Surgery* 90:319, 1981.
171 Sprung CL, Panagiota MD, Caralis V et al: The effects of high-dose corticosteroids in patients with septic shock: a prospective, controlled study, *N Engl J Med* 311:1137, 1984.
172 Staub NC: Pulmonary edema due to increased microvascular permeability to fluid and protein, *Circ Res* 43:143, 1978.
173 Stone HH, Hooper CA, Kolb LD et al: Antibiotic prophylaxis in gastric, biliary, and colonic surgery, *Ann Surg* 184:443, 1976.
174 Stone HH, Kolb LD, Currie CA et al: *Candida* sepsis: pathogenesis and principles of treatment, *Ann Surg* 179:697, 1974.
175 Strachan CJL, Black J, Powis SJA, et al: Prophylactic use of cephazolin against wound sepsis after cholecystectomy, *Br Med J* 1:1254, 1977.
176 Strome DR, Newman JJ, Goodwin CW Jr et al: Mechanisms of reduced lipolytic response in rat adipocytes following thermal injury, *Surg Forum* 34:103, 1983.
177 Suarez CA, Block F, Bernstein D et al: The role of HIDA/PIPIDA scanning in diagnosing cystic duct obstruction, *Ann Surg* 191:391, 1980.
178 Takemura R, Werb Z: Secretory products of macrophages and their physiological functions, *Am J Physiol* 246:C1, 1984.
179 Tchervenkov JI, Latter DL, Psychogios J et al: Decreased phagocytic cell delivery to inflammatory lesions is due to the host "trauma environment," not to intrinsic cellular defects, *Surg Forum* 37:90, 1986.
180 Tracey KJ, Beutler B, Lowry SF et al: Shock and tissue injury induced by recombinant human cachectin, *Science* 234:470, 1986.
181 Tranbaugh RF, Lewis FR, Christensen JM et al: Lung water changes after thermal injury: the effects of crystalloid resuscitation and sepsis, *Ann Surg* 192:479, 1980.
182 Vary TC, Siegel JH, Nakatani T et al: A biochemical basis for depressed ketogenesis in sepsis, *J Trauma* 26:419, 1986.
183 Walters R, Herman CM, Neff R et al: Percutaneous drainage of abscesses in the postoperative abdomen that is difficult to explore, *Am J Surg* 149:623, 1985.
184 Wannemacher RW Jr, Pace JG, Beall FA et al: Role of liver in regulation of ketone body production during sepsis, *J Clin Invest* 64:1565, 1979.
185 Washington JA, Dearing WH, Judd ES et al: Effect of preoperative antibiotic regimen on development of infection after intestinal surgery, *Ann Surg* 180:557, 1974.
186 Wasserman K, Wipp BJ, Castagna J: Cardiodynamic hyperpnea secondary to cardiac output increase, *J Appl Physiol* 36:457, 1974.
187 Weber KJ, Janiki JS, Schroff S et al: Contractile mechanics and interaction of the left and right ventricles, *Am J Cardiol* 47:686, 1981.
188 Welch GW, McKeel DW Jr, Silverstein P et al: The role of catheter composition in the development of thrombophlebitis, *Surg Gynecol Obstet* 138:421, 1974.
189 Wilmore DW, Aulick LH, Mason AD Jr et al: Influence of the burn wound on local and systemic response to injury, *Ann Surg* 186:444, 1977.
190 Wilmore DW, Goodwin CW, Aulick LH et al: Effect of injury and infection on visceral metabolism and circulation, *Ann Surg* 192:491, 1980.
191 Wilmore DW, Long JM, Mason AD Jr et al: Catecolamines:

mediator of the hypermetabolic response to thermal injury, *Ann Surg* 180:653, 1974.
192 Wilmore DW, Mason AD Jr, Pruitt BA Jr: Impaired glucose flow in burned patients with gram-negative sepsis, *Surg Gynecol Obstet* 143:720, 1976.
193 Wolfe RR, Shaw JHF, Durkot MJ: Effect of sepsis on VLDL kinetics: responses in basal state and during glucose infusion, *Am J Physiol* 248:E732, 1985.
194 Wolfe RR, Shaw JHF: Glucose and FFA kinetics in sepsis: role of glucagon in sympathetic nervous system activity, *Am J Physiol* 248:E236, 1985.
195 Wood JJ, O'Mahony JB, Rodrick ML et al: Abnormalities of antibody production after thermal injury, *Arch Surg* 121:108, 1986.
196 Woolfrey BF, Fox JM, Quall CO: An evaluation of burn wound quantitative microbiology. I. Quantitative eschar cultures, *Am J Clin Pathol* 75:532, 1981.
197 Yurt RW, Pruitt BA Jr: Decreased wound neutrophils and indiscrete margination in the pathogenesis of wound infection, *Surgery* 98:191, 1985.
198 Zimmerli W, Lew PD, Waldfogel FA: Pathogenesis of foreign body infection evidence for local granulocyte defect, *J Clin Invest* 73:1191, 1984.

SUGGESTED READINGS

Aprahamian C, Wittman DH: Operative management of intraabdominal infection, *Infection* 19:453, 1991.
Barber GR, Brown AE: Surgical site infections in the cancer patient, *Infect Med* 11:20, 1994.
Bartels H, Siewert JR: Surgical strategy in septic abdominal complications, *Chir Gastroenterol* 10:20, 1994.
Bellomo R, Tipping P, Boyce N: Continuous venovenous hemofiltration with dialysis removes cytokines from the circulation of septic patients, *Crit Care Med* 21:522, 1993.
Bhatia S, McCullough J, Perry EH et al: Granulocyte transfusions: efficacy in treating fungal infections in neutropenic patients following bone marrow transplantation, *Transfusion* 34:226, 1994.
Clabots CR, Johnson S, Olson MM et al: Acquisition of *Clostridium difficile* by hospitalized patients: evidence for colonized new admissions as a source of infection, *J Infect Dis* 166:561, 1992.
Culver DH, Horan TC, Gaynes RP et al: Surgical wound infection rates by wound class, operative procedure, and patient risk index, *Am J Med* 91 Suppl 3B:152S, 1991.
Dal Nogare AR: Septic shock, *Am J Med Sci* 302:50, 1991.
Deitch EA: The role of intestinal barrier failure and bacterial translocation in the development of systemic infection and multiple organ failure, *Arch Surg* 125:403, 1990.
Deitch EA, Specian RD, Berg RD: Induction of early-phase tolerance to endotoxin-induced mucosal injury, xanthine oxidase activation, and bacterial translocation by pretreatment with endotoxin, *Circ Shock* 36:208, 1992.
File TM Jr, Tan JS: Treatment of bacterial skin and soft tissue infections, *Surg Gynecol Obstet* 172 (suppl):17, 1991.
Freund M, Kleine HD: The role of GM-CSF in infection, *Infection* 20 (suppl 2):S84, 1992.
Gallinaro R, Cheadle WG, Applegate K, Polk HC Jr: The role of the complement system in trauma and infection, *Surg Gynecol Obstet* 174:435, 1992.
Giroir BP: Mediators of septic shock: new approaches for interrupting the endogenous inflammatory cascade, *Crit Care Med* 21:780, 1993.
Glassock RJ, Nast CC, Cohen AH: The renal response to infection, *Adv Exp Med Biol* 252:163, 1990.
Hackford AW, Welch HF: Retroperitoneal infection II: etiology, diagnosis, and treatment, *Complications Surg* 10:46, 1991.
Hart GB: Distinguishing clostridial myonecrosis from other wound infections, *Infect Med* 10:31, 1993.
Herdegen JJ, Casey LC: The role of tumor necrosis factor in infections: pathophysiology and clinical implications, *Infect Med* 10:27, 1993.
Hirn M, Niinikoski J, Lehtonen OP: Effect of hyperbaric oxygen and surgery on experimental multimicrobial gas gangrene, *Eur Surg Res* 25:265, 1993.
Karam GH, Sanders CV, Aldridge KE: Role of newer antimicrobial agents in the treatment of mixed aerobic and anaerobic infections, *Surg Gynecol Obstet* 172 (suppl):57, 1991.
Kroemer G, De Alboran IM, Gonzalo JA, Martinez AC: Immunoregulation by cytokines, *Crit Rev Immunol* 13:163, 1993.
McAfee JG: What is the best method for imaging focal infections? *J Nucl Med* 31:413, 1990.
Molloy RG, Mannick JA, Rodrick ML: Cytokines, sepsis and immunomodulation, *Br J Surg* 80:289, 1993.
Mufson MA: Pneumococcal infection, *Curr Opin Infect Dis* 7:178, 1994.
Nichols RL: Surgical wound infection, *Am J Med* 91 (suppl 3B):54S, 1991.
Nichols RL, Smith JW, Robertson GD et al: Prospective alterations in therapy for penetrating abdominal trauma, *Arch Surg* 128:55, 1993.
Niu MT, Jermano JA, Reichelderfer P, Schnittman SM: Summary of the National Institutes of Health workshop on primary human immunodeficiency virus type 1 infection, *AIDS Res Hum Retroviruses* 9:913, 1993.
Van Deuren M, Dofferhoff ASM, Van der Meer JWM: Cytokines and the response to infection, *J Pathol* 168:349, 1992.
Waydhas C, Nast-Kolb D, Jochum M et al: Inflammatory mediators, infection, sepsis, and multiple organ failure after severe trauma, *Arch Surg* 127:460, 1992.
Wilson SE: A critical analysis of recent innovations in the treatment of intraabdominal infection, *Surg Gynecol Obstet* 177 (suppl):11, 1993.

CHAPTER

11

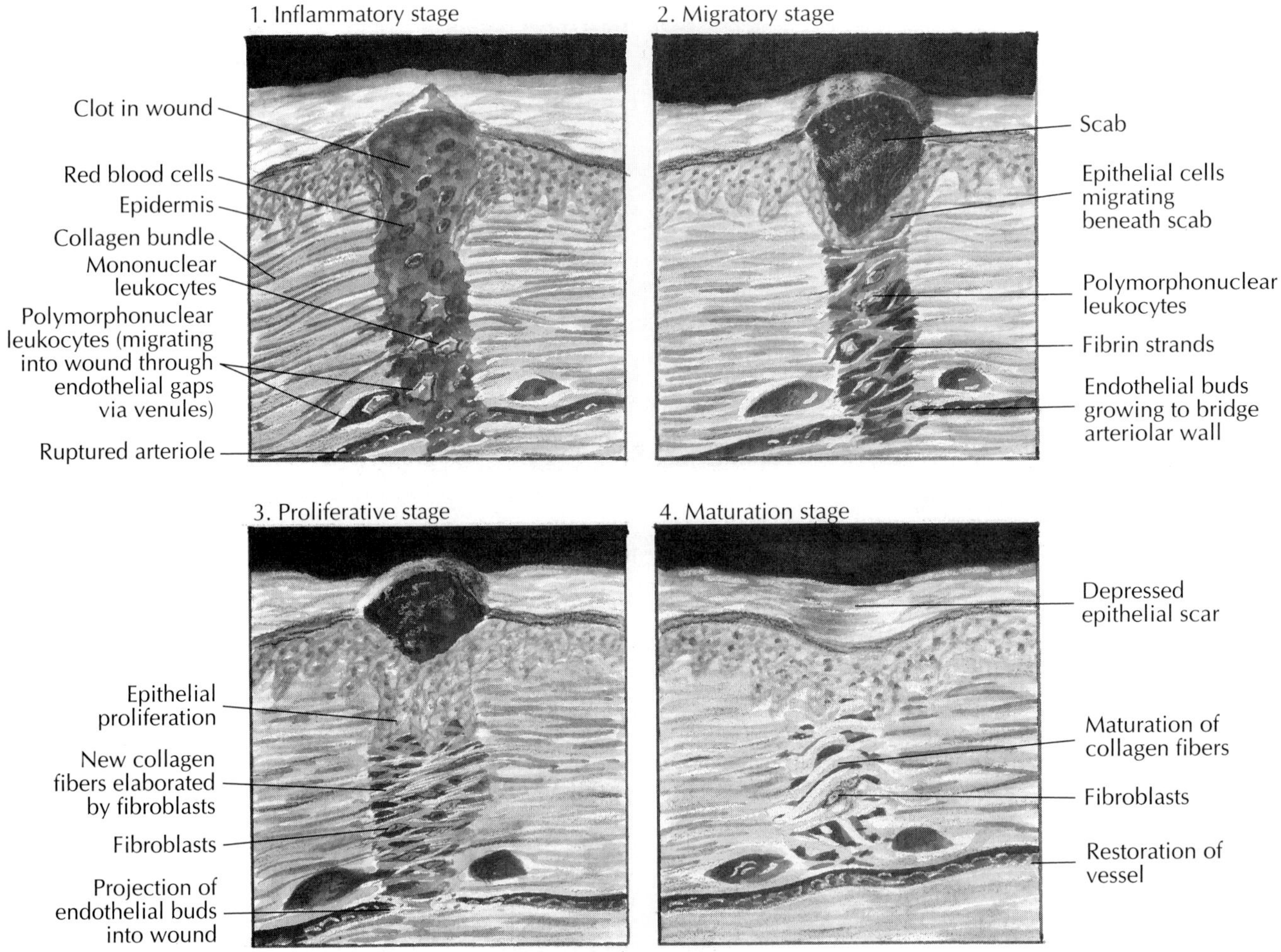

1. Inflammatory stage
2. Migratory stage
3. Proliferative stage
4. Maturation stage
Clot in wound
Red blood cells
Epidermis
Collagen bundle
Mononuclear leukocytes
Polymorphonuclear leukocytes (migrating into wound through endothelial gaps via venules)
Ruptured arteriole
Scab
Epithelial cells migrating beneath scab
Polymorphonuclear leukocytes
Fibrin strands
Endothelial buds growing to bridge arteriolar wall
Epithelial proliferation
New collagen fibers elaborated by fibroblasts
Fibroblasts
Projection of endothelial buds into wound
Depressed epithelial scar
Maturation of collagen fibers
Fibroblasts
Restoration of vessel

After John Craig, M.D.

WOUND HEALING

Stephen J. Mathes • Brent R. W. Moelleken

BIOLOGY OF NORMAL WOUND HEALING

TISSUE RESPONSE TO INJURY

Any type of injury, from blunt trauma to interruption of tissue continuity, alters the homeostatic state of the human organism and triggers a sequence of events that constitutes the acute inflammatory phase. Attracted neutrophils protect the tissue against infection, macrophages remove necrotic debris, chemical mediators are formed, and the stage is set for the subsequent repair phases.

The proliferative phase follows, with fibroblast multiplication, extracellular deposition of collagen and connective tissue matrix, and granulation tissue formation, resulting ultimately in a connective tissue scar. The maturation phase starts gradually as fibroplasia proceeds further; this phase reflects the body's attempt to achieve the best scar to resist tension and shearing forces.

Although wound repair can be divided into these three phases, most processes occur closely in sequence with no clear-cut boundaries.

Vascular Events

Trauma initiates a fairly consistent sequence of vascular events. However, the severing of blood vessels, with subsequent hemorrhage or injury affecting different levels of the microcirculation, may alter this sequence in a way characteristic of the type and severity of injury.

Immediate and transient vasoconstriction, mainly involving arterioles, occurs first. This may result in actual vascular occlusion in an attempt to control hemorrhage. Vasoconstriction lasts from a few seconds in mild injury up to several minutes, as in burns. Active vasodilatation follows, involving the arterioles first, and results in opening of new microvascular beds in the injured area. This fundamental event allows various mediator molecules and inflammatory cells to reach the site of injury. Transudation of protein-poor fluid occurs, without a significant increase in vascular permeability. Increased vascular permeability then takes place, allowing the leakage of protein-rich fluid into the extravascular space. The leakage mainly involves the postcapillary venules and results in slower microcirculation, possibly with stasis.[176] The clinical counterpart of the increased permeability is edema, often observed at the site of injury.

Depending on the type and extent of injury, three permeability patterns can occur separately or in combination. An immediate, transient permeability change usually starts after injury, peaks within 5 to 10 minutes, and phases out within 15 to 30 minutes. It involves exclusively small- to medium-sized venules, leaving the capillaries unaffected, and occurs through gaps formed after contraction of endothelial cells.[176,177] Histamine, serotonin, and bradykinin were shown to induce such a response in an animal model.[176,177] An immediate, sustained response often results from severe injuries and affects all levels of the microcirculation, including venules, capillaries, and arterioles. The mechanism of this permeability change is related to direct damage to local vasculature and lasts from 1 to several days. This pattern often is observed with severe burns. A delayed, prolonged response begins 1 to 2 hours after injury and lasts for several hours or even days.[255] This model is observed in many clinical settings (thermal and mechanical injuries, certain bacterial toxins[232]) and involves both venules and capillaries. Direct injury to the endothelium is believed to occur, although many chemical mediators appear to initiate this permeability change, including the kinins and arachidonic acid metabolites, notably prostaglandins E_1 and E_2.[20]

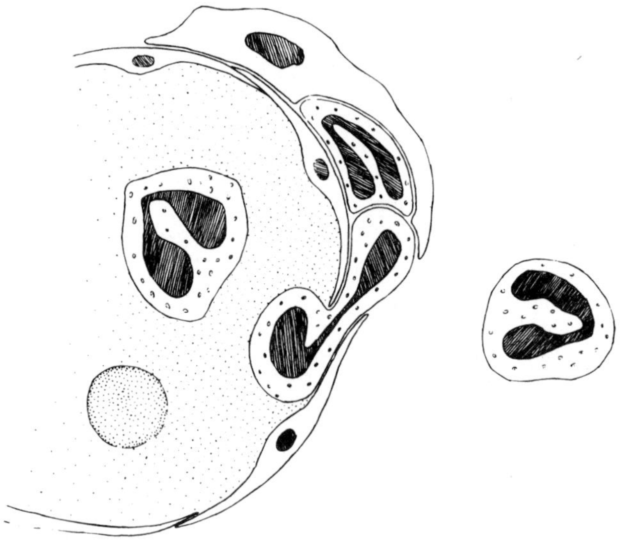

FIGURE 11-1 Migration of polymorphonuclear leukocytes into the perivascular space.

Cellular Events

The various cellular events serve specific purposes during each step of the repair process.

Neutrophils

Concomitant with slowing of the circulation and stasis, neutrophils assume a peripheral orientation within microvessels. Eventually, neutrophils appear to line the endothelium, a phenomenon called *pavementing*. Adherence of neutrophils soon becomes prominent and is followed by their migration to the extravascular space. This migration occurs through junctions between the endothelial cells[178] by an active process of diapedesis (Figure 11-1).

The neutrophils are the first cells to appear at the injury site.[206] By day 2 after injury, macrophages gradually replace neutrophils; differential survival rates probably account for this shift in cell populations.[307] Although wounds of neutropenic animals heal normally,[262] neutrophils assume a major role in protecting against infection, which is deleterious to wound healing. Also, recent evidence suggests that neutrophils are involved in the degree of vasodilatation and increased permeability.[124,168] The neutrophil exerts its functions by releasing a variety of intracellular products (see the box at right).

NEUTROPHIL PRODUCTS WITH A ROLE IN INFLAMMATION

1. Free radicals: damage to endothelium, increase in vascular permeability, production of chemotactic lipids from arachidonic acid
2. Cyclooxygenase products of arachidonic acid: platelet aggregation, contraction of vascular smooth muscle
3. Lipooxygenase products of arachidonic acid: leukocyte chemotaxis, increased vascular permeability
4. Proteases (collagenase, elastase): tissue destruction, release of kinin-like peptide from kininogen (kininogen-activating factor), complement activation
5. Antiproteases ($alpha_1$-antitrypsin, $alpha_2$-macroglobulin): modulation and control of extracellular degradation of structural proteins
6. Band 2 protein (arginine-rich polypeptide): mast cell rupture, increased vascular permeability

Neutrophil function may be modulated by the local wound environment, so that neutrophils are activated and therefore less effective in hypoxic or ischemic wounds.[193]

Macrophages

By day 3 or day 4, mononuclear macrophages have largely replaced the neutrophil leukocytes in the wound space and have become the predominant cells. Their main role once was believed to be exclusively phagocytic. However, current evidence suggests that the macrophage is the most important cell in the healing process. Treatment of guinea pigs with a combination of antimacrophage serum and hydrocortisone results in a significant delay in the histologic appearance of fibroblasts and collagen deposition in the wound site.[155] The fibroblasts that eventually appear are mostly immature, and the amount of collagen laid down is diminished. Macrophage infiltration into the wound always precedes fibroplasia.[237] This sequence further suggests that the macrophage is involved directly in the initiation of fibroplasia.

MACROPHAGE PRODUCTS MEDIATING INFLAMMATION AND REPAIR

1. Neutral proteases: plasminogen activator, collagenase, and elastase
2. Complement factors
3. Reactive oxygen metabolites
4. Growth-promoting factors for fibroblasts and microvessels
5. Arachidonic acid metabolites with vasoactive and chemotactic properties
6. Fibronectin: structural and functional roles
7. Interleukin-1 lymphocyte activator, stimulates collagenase synthesis by fibroblasts
8. Enzyme inhibitors: plasmin and alpha$_2$-macroglobulin

Many experiments provide further proof of the importance of macrophage function. Injection of activated macrophages into rabbit corneas stimulates collagen synthesis by induced fibroblasts.[180] A macrophage-derived growth factor (MDGF) is capable of stimulating mitosis in fibroblasts. Recently, an angiogenesis factor has been extracted from wound fluid that contributes to neovascularization during formation of granulation tissue.[15] The factor is probably a product of activated macrophages bathed in a hypoxic environment.[143] The macrophage also can secrete other products that may act as mediators of inflammation and repair (see the box above).

Lymphocytes

B lymphocytes are not known to exert a significant influence on wound repair. Wounds heal perfectly well in patients receiving large doses of antilymphocytic serum for suppression of immune rejection phenomena after organ transplantation.[212]

T lymphocytes, however, play a significant role in wound modulation. Lymphokines, the products of activated lymphocytes, have numerous effects on fibroblast function and vascular endothelial cells. Gamma-interferon inhibits proliferation of cultured endothelial cells and effects changes in the cytoskeleton.[275] Stimulation with gamma-interferon also has produced a wide range of effects on the antigen expression of vascular endothelial cells.[219] Transforming growth factor type beta (TGF-beta), a lymphokine also secreted by macrophages and platelets, can modulate monocyte chemotaxis and secretion of growth factors, including fibroblast growth factor (FGF).[292] TGF-beta is a potent chemoattractant for fibroblasts.[223] Fibroblast activating factor (FAF) is released by T cells and stimulates fibroblast proliferation in vitro, as well as collagen synthesis.[200] Furthermore, Roberts and colleagues have reported that when gamma-interferon was injected into newborn mice, the formation of granulation tissue increased.[235] Clearly, T cells play an important role in wound healing, albeit one that is not yet fully defined.[17]

Fibroblasts

By day 4 or day 5 fibroblasts are more prominent in the wound, and they become the predominant cells by the end of the first week. These cells originate from local, less-differentiated mesenchymal cells in the perivascular adventitial tissue.[238,272] Once in the wound area, fibroblasts start multiplying and producing collagen[92] and ground substance material. In their active state they appear spindlelike, although they may assume any shape. A series of intracellular changes then occurs, resulting in a characteristic appearance by electron microscopy. The Golgi apparatus is located diffusely throughout the cytoplasm, and mitochondria are large and have irregular cristae. The most prominent feature, however, is the extensively developed and dilated rough endoplasmic reticulum with polysomes attached to its membranes.

The fibroblasts move by forming adhesive contacts with the substratum along a scaffold that probably involves fibrin, fibronectin, and collagen. With this motile activity comes the characteristic polar shape[82] and flattening of the marginal cytoplasm of the advancing edge, resulting in a lamellar appearance. This appearance often is accompanied by "ruffling,"[2] a movement of the front surface of the cell consisting of periodic thickenings in its outermost margin.

As granulation tissue is forming, a "contractile fibroblast" cell, called a myofibroblast, also appears. This cell apparently originates from fibroblasts of normal tissue[80] or from less-differentiated mesenchymal cells. The myofibroblast cell combines the ultrastructural features of the fibroblast and the smooth muscle cell and has a wrinkled nuclear membrane and numerous microfilaments in its cytoplasm. The rough endoplasmic reticulum is prominent, and the cell can produce collagen, mainly type III.[81] The intracellular presence of actin and myosin, correlated with the development of a microfilamentous apparatus, was demonstrated by immunofluorescence.[79,110] Myofibroblasts contribute to wound contraction and are implicated in a variety of human fibrocontractive diseases.[171]

Endothelial Cells

In the normal state endothelial cells perform three important functions. First, as a selective permeability barrier they allow only certain molecules to diffuse into the perivascular space. Second, their monolayer arrangement results in a nonthrombogenic surface that insulates circulating blood elements from highly thrombogenic subendothelial connective tissue. Third, endothelial cells are active in the synthesis and secretion of products

TABLE 11-1 ENDOTHELIAL CELL FUNCTIONS BEFORE AND AFTER INJURY

BEFORE INJURY	AFTER INJURY
1. Acts as a barrier between blood and subendothelial thrombogenic elements 2. Cells' glycocalyx contains anticoagulant (heparin sulfate) and alpha$_2$-macroglobulin (antiprotease, inhibits clotting factors' activation) 3. Synthesizes plasminogen activator, prostacyclin, and antithrombin III	1. Exposes basement membrane materials, activating platelets and clotting factors 2. Releases thromboplastin, activating clotting extrinsic mechanism 3. Synthesizes factor VIII (Von Willebrand's factor) 4. Proliferates and migrates in response to chemical stimuli, with resultant angiogenesis

(Table 11-1) that inhibit hemostasis and thrombosis in the normal state.

Endothelial injury promotes the release of tissue factor (thromboplastin) and factor VIII (von Willebrand's factor), which initiate the extrinsic clotting mechanism and platelet aggregation, respectively. Furthermore, injury disrupts continuity of the thromboresistant monolayer and exposes subendothelial elements that activate platelets and trigger clotting. As hemostasis is achieved after repair of the injury has started, local endothelial cells form new capillaries by a combined process of migration and mitosis.

IMPORTANT PLATELET ACTIVATION PRODUCTS IN TISSUE INJURY

1. ADP: platelet aggregation
2. Thromboxane A_2: platelet aggregation, vasoconstriction
3. Platelet factor 3: activation of factor X, initiation of intrinsic coagulation sequence
4. Serotonin: fibroblast proliferation, collagen synthesis
5. Platelet-derived growth factor: mitogenic for fibroblasts and smooth muscle cells, chemotaxis
6. Platelet factor 4: chemotactic for leukocytes

Platelets

In the normal state platelets maintain microvascular integrity, as evidenced clinically by the bleeding diathesis in thrombocytopenic patients. With endothelial injury, platelets adhere to the subendothelial surface. This activating stimulus is accompanied by shape transformations and followed soon by the external release of platelet granule contents.

Platelets contain two major types of granules: alpha-granules and dense bodies.[257] Alpha-granules contain fibrinogen, fibronectin, platelet-derived growth factor (a mitogen), platelet factor 4 (antiheparin), and platelet-specific proteins. Dense bodies are rich in adenosine diphosphate (ADP) and ionized calcium and contain histamine, serotonin (5-HT), and epinephrine. Platelet aggregation closely follows platelet adherence and activation. Platelet factor 3 becomes activated and, in conjunction with factor V and calcium, activates factor X, triggering the intrinsic pathway of blood clotting. A major contributor to aggregation is thromboxane A_2 (TXA_2), formed by activated platelets. ADP and TXA_2 help in the formation of this "temporary hemostatic plug." Thrombin generated by the clotting sequence, in conjunction with ADP and TXA_2, induces platelet contraction with formation of a definitive "secondary hemostatic plug." Fibrin deposition further stabilizes and consolidates this structure.

The role of platelets in wound repair extends beyond the maintenance of hemostasis (see the box at right). Injection of thrombin-activated platelets into rabbit corneas results in opacification (secondary to collagen deposition) and angiogenesis.[144] Fibroplasia and neovascularization are observed histologically, and collagen synthesis increases to twice control levels.

Mast Cells

The precise role of mast cells in connective tissue repair is not well defined. In the early phases of wound healing, these cells are closely related to newly formed capillaries, but later they become scattered throughout granulation tissue. Recent evidence points to their ability to modulate angiogenesis,[13,75,277] probably through the release of extracellular heparin.

Vasoactive Agents

HISTAMINE. Preformed and stored in granules, histamine is released from mast cells, basophils, and platelets. It is believed to mediate the early vasopermeability response, acting mainly at the precapillary or postcapillary venule level. Histamine can be isolated from early inflammatory exudates, but it disappears within 60 minutes, when local sources largely are depleted. Furthermore, histamine antagonists suppress the early vascular response induced by mild injury, supporting the role of histamine early in inflammation.

SEROTONIN. In humans, serotonin originates mainly from platelets and probably has a negligible effect on vascular permeability. In the rat model, methysergide maleate (serotonin antagonist) does not influence the level of either blood flow or albumin extravasation during inflammation in open granulating wounds.[167]

KININ. The kinins, a series of biologically active peptides, are implicated in local inflammatory vascular responses. A cascade of events (Figure 11-2) begins with the activation of factor XII (Hageman factor) of the clotting system by contact with collagen, basement membrane material, and platelet-derived factors. Activated factor XII (prekallikrein activator, or factor XIIa) is generated and converts plasma prekallikrein into an active proteolytic enzyme called kallikrein. Kallikrein cleaves a plasma glycoprotein precursor, high-molecular-weight kininogen (HMWK), to produce bradykinin. Bradykinin, the vasoactive moiety, is a potent agent that increases vascular permeability and causes blood vessels to dilate. Bradykinin may also induce prostaglandin formation by local cells.[73] Since kallikrein is a potent activator of factor XII, the original stimulus is perpetuated. Kallikrein further demonstrates chemotactic activity and causes aggregation of neutrophils in vitro.[302]

ARACHIDONIC ACID. Mechanical injury and certain chemical mediators (e.g., activated C5 component of complement, or C5a) activate cellular phospholipases through release of arachidonic acid (AA) from cell membranes. This acid is then channeled into one of the two major synthetic pathways (Figure 11-3). The cyclooxygenase pathway eventually leads to the formation of prostaglandins. The lipooxygenase pathway involves the conversion of AA into hydroperoxy derivatives and leukotrienes. Recently, a third mechanism of AA conversion has been discovered—nonenzymatic peroxidation of AA by oxygen-derived free radicals. Highly chemotactic lipids are formed.[228] Prostaglandin E_1 (PGE_1) and prostaglandin E_2 (PGE_2) possess strong vasodilative and vasopermeability-increasing properties. Weeks has suggested that prostaglandins, particularly PGE_1 and PGE_2, are terminal mediators of the acute inflammatory response.[296]

The interactions of prostaglandins and leukotrienes with other mediators of inflammation govern some aspects of vasodilatation and permeability changes.[304] In animal tissues, exogenous prostaglandins are poor inducers of edema.[306] However, adding PGE_1 or PGE_2 markedly potentiates the vasopermeability-increasing property of both histamine and bradykinin.[305]

Synergism in the production of local edema also was observed between PGE_2 and C5a.[303] The permeability-increasing property of C5a largely depends on histamine release. Interestingly, C5a des Arg (C5a decarboxylation product generated by plasma carboxypeptidase B) shows similar synergistic activity in the absence of histamine release.[126] This evidence excludes histamine as a possible mediator of the observed synergism.

Chemotactic Factors

Chemotaxis is a directed movement of cells along a chemical gradient. A chemoattractant diffuses through tissues to establish a gradient and then binds to specific receptors on target cells. Chemotactic events seem to occur in a sequence similar to a cascade,[96] whereby preceding events induce and potentiate those that follow (Figure 11-4).

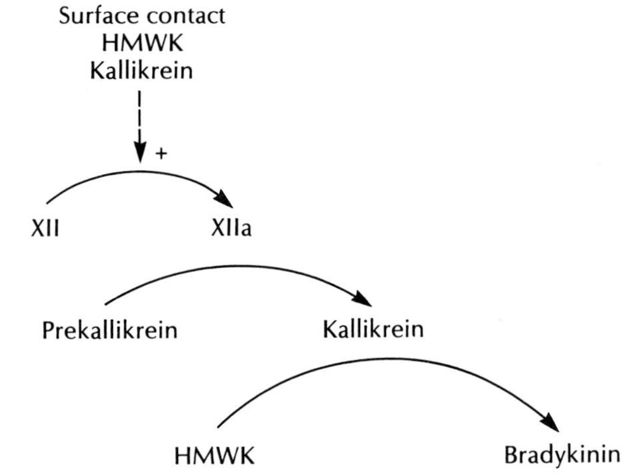

FIGURE 11-2 The plasma kinin cascade system. Kallikrein provides a positive feedback that potentiates the original stimulus. *HMWK,* High-molecular-weight kininogen.

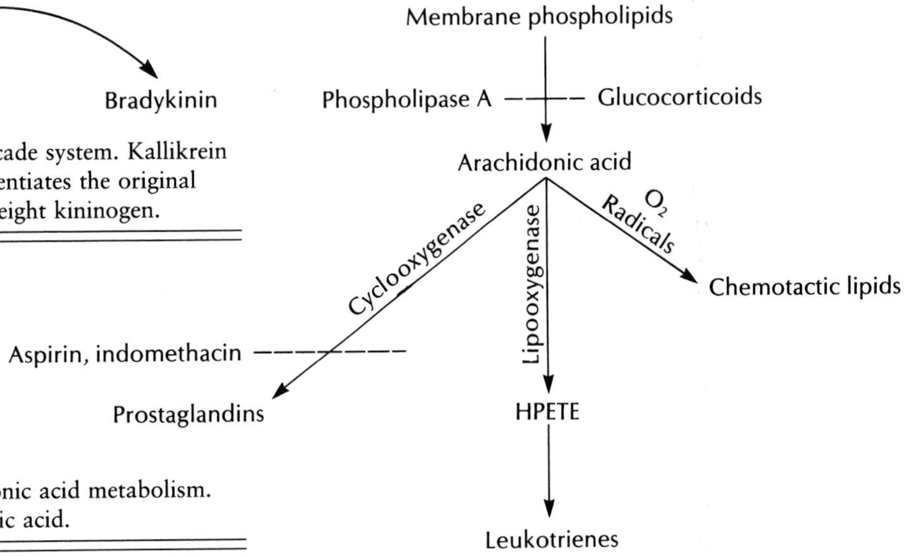

FIGURE 11-3 Pathways of arachidonic acid metabolism. *HPETE,* Hydroperoxyeicosatetraenoic acid.

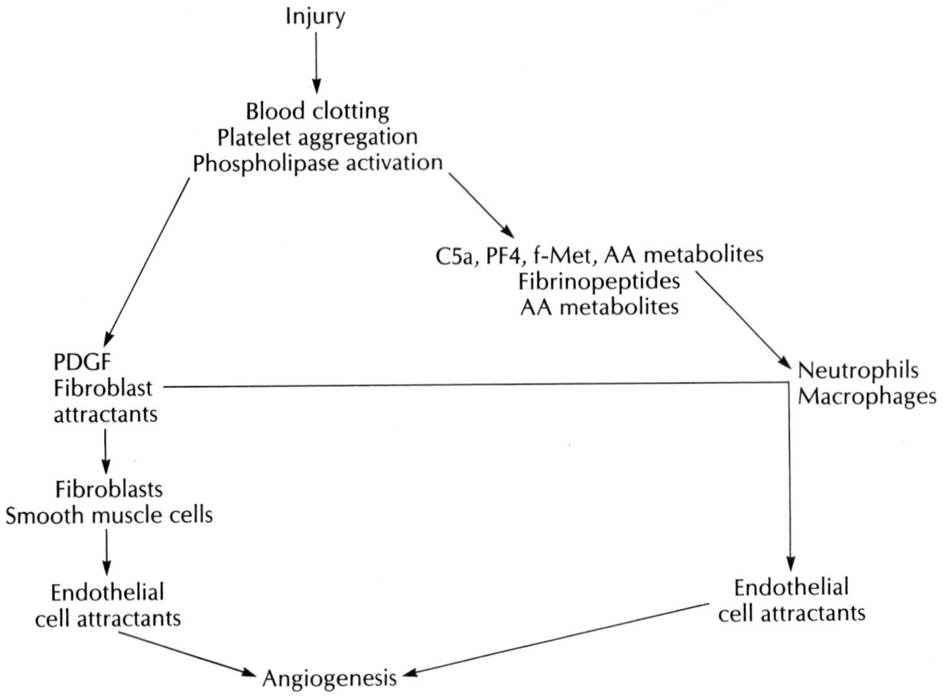

FIGURE 11-4 Sequence of chemotactic events after tissue injury. The consecutive recruitment of various cell populations eventuates an orderly repair process after an injury. *PDGF*, Platelet-derived growth factor. (Modified from Grotendorst GR: *J Trauma* 24(9):S49, Williams & Wilkins, 1984.)

Several products of tissue injury attract leukocytes. Locally released neutral proteases cleave C3 and C5 components of complement, forming C3a and C5a, respectively. As a leukoattractant, C5a is more potent than C3a. Removing the carboxyl terminal arginine from C5a by plasma carboxypeptidase B results in the formation of C5a des Arg, a potent chemotactic factor and perhaps one of the most important leukoattractants. As platelets are activated, they release platelet factor 4 (PF4) and fibrinogen into the medium. PF4 is chemotactic for neutrophils and monocytes.[59] Furthermore, during the conversion of fibrinogen to fibrin, fibrinopeptides are cleaved off. Among these, fibrinopeptide B is chemotactic for both neutrophils and monocytes.[131]

Bacterial products are also chemotactic for leukocytes. Recent attempts to isolate the active fragment from bacterial supernatants have resulted in the synthesis of the chemotactic N-formyl methionyl (N-fMet) peptides. These peptides have specific binding sites on the surface of the neutrophil and are potent chemoattractants.[249] The lipoxygenase pathway of AA metabolism results in the formation of hydroperoxy eicosatetraenoic acid (HPETE), a neutrophil chemoattractant, and leukotriene B_4, a powerful chemotactic agent and aggregator.[209]

Fibroblasts are attracted to collagen, collagen x-alpha chains, and collagenous peptides in vitro.[225] Fibronectin[224] and fibronectin fragments[254] also can attract fibroblasts in vitro. Because of collagen's low solubility and fibronectin's large size and affinity for other tissue matrix components, collagen's role as chemotaxin is being questioned in vivo.[97] Platelet-derived growth factor (PDGF) is a potent attractant for fibroblasts[253] and smooth muscle cells.[98] These cells respond to PDGF by migration and mitosis; in fact, they possess specific PDGF receptors on their cell surface.

Neovascularization is induced by at least two classes of angiogenic factors: those that stimulate only migration of endothelial cells[15] and those that stimulate both migration and mitosis.[113,222] Both activities were demonstrated by activated macrophages in vivo.[115] The angiogenic activity of macrophages is hypoxia dependent,[115] and angiogenesis ceases with better perfusion and oxygenation at the exact site of capillary formation. Thrombin-activated platelets also can induce angiogenesis in vivo.[144] This platelet-derived activity has not yet been attributed to a specific platelet product.

Investigations of the mechanisms of tumor angiogenesis led to the finding that heparin stimulates the migration of capillary endothelial cells in vitro.[13] Later, protamine, a heparin blocking agent, was shown to prevent the neovascularization induced by an inflammatory agent.[277] This finding supports the angiogenic role of heparin in vivo.

Cytokines

Many studies with wound fluid have demonstrated its angiogenic and fibroblastic potential. These activities currently are traced to various cells involved in the repair process, notably the macrophages and platelets.

The release of growth factors from platelets probably produces the growth-promoting activity of normal serum.[239] Clinical experience supports the role of platelets in wound repair in some situations.[144] PDGF has been isolated and partially characterized; it stimulates the growth of fibroblasts and smooth muscle cells after binding to specific cell surface receptors.[105] Endothelial cells do not possess such receptors and show no response to PDGF in vitro.[293]

Epidermal growth factor (EGF, urogastrone) is a heat-stable polypeptide initially purified from the submaxillary glands of mice.[133] It is a 6000 kd single-chain polypeptide.[58] It is found in high concentrations in milk and in Brunner's glands of the small intestine.[204] It stimulates mitosis in epidermal cells[28] and fibroblasts[156] and accelerates human corneal repair.[55] Topical application of EGF stimulates wound healing in rabbits[77] and mice but not in humans.[201] The EGF receptor is found in highest concentration in epithelial cells and fibroblasts.[40] Its most specific action appears to be promoting endothelial cells, epithelial cells, and fibroblasts to continue on in the cell cycle.[99,266] EGF also appears to stimulate fibroblasts to secrete collagenases, which are important in wound remodeling.[29] Transforming growth factor type alpha (TGF-alpha) is related to EGF and exhibits many EGF-like functions. EGF and TGF-alpha are expressed by fibroblasts, skin keratinocytes, vascular endothelial cells, and selected epithelial cells of the gastrointestinal tract. It is synthesized by platelets, keratinocytes, and macrophages. EGF and TGF-alpha have promoted the healing of a variety of skin wounds in a number of experimental systems.[252]

Platelet-derived growth factor is contained in the alpha-granules of platelets. It is released in response to thrombin or fibrillar collagen.[130] PDGF exhibits mitogenic stimuli for smooth muscle cells, fibroblasts, and glial cells.[61] It also plays a role in tissue remodeling by inducing fibroblast secretion of collagenase.[62] It serves as a chemoattractant for neutrophils and can activate neutrophils.[285] In contrast to TGF-beta, PDGF (rPDGF-BB monomer) has been noted to markedly augment fibronectin and glycosaminoglycan deposition in a rabbit ear model. It also greatly increased deposition of collagen.[217] Overall, PDGF appears to act as a potent activator for cells of mesenchymal origin, inducing chemotaxis and proliferation of fibroblasts and macrophages. It also induces new gene expression in monocyte-macrophages and fibroblasts.[105] It increases deposition of extracellular matrix and collagen formation, augmenting the wound breaking strength of incisional and excisional wounds, and has been implicated in initiating a local wound healing cascade via paracrine and autocrine feedback loops to synthesize additional endogenous PDGF.[216]

Fibroblast growth factors (FGFs) are factors bound to heparin and are found in acidic and basic forms. The basic form is more potent. FGF is present in the extracellular matrix bound to heparin sulfate. It exhibits angiogenic properties in the rabbit cornea model[311] and has increased epithelial healing in a number of models. It may act as a mitogen toward capillary endothelial cells, where it is synthesized and stored, and may play an important role in vivo as a promoter of the growth of vascular endothelial cells.[297] Its in vivo safety is currently being investigated.[184]

Insulin-like growth factors (IGFs), also known as somatomedins, are structurally similar to proinsulin. They may play a role in the modulation of fibroblast differentiation during the later stages of wound healing (both IGF-I and IGF-II) in a subcutaneous sponge model as determined by messenger ribonucleic acid (mRNA) semiquantification using polymerase chain reaction (PCR) techniques and 3HdGTP incorporation.[85] Some have theorized that IGF plays a role in the overall growth of an animal, based on circulating hormone, and in paracrine regulation in the local wound environment.[48] IGF acts synergistically with PDGF and FGF by increasing DNA synthesis.[274] The action of IGF seems to be cell-cycle dependent, so that it cannot cause cells in stationary phases to proliferate, but it can augment their division in the presence of PDGF.

Both granulocyte colony-stimulating factor (G-CSF) and granulocyte-macrophage colony-stimulating factor (GM-CSF) induce endothelial cells to proliferate (although less than did basic fibroblast growth factor (bFGF) and migrate (equal to bFGF), but they do not induce endothelial cells to perform many other of their constitutive functions, such as procoagulant activity, platelet activating factor (PAF) activity, expression of leukocyte adhesion molecule-1, or expression of MHC class II antigens.[35]

TGF-beta is a 112-amino acid peptide weighing 25 kilodaltons. It is found in high concentrations in platelet alpha-granules. T lymphocytes also possess TGF-beta. TGF-beta can influence cellular proliferation and is associated with an increase in fibroblasts and collagen deposition in wounds. Its role in extracellular matrix synthesis is still under investigation, but it appears to stimulate the production of elastin and fibronectin.[119,233,234] It may have a role in inducing fibrosis and angiogenesis in newborn mice.[235] It is clear that the influence of these cytokines on wound healing is selective and specialized and involves feedback loops.

TGF-beta is known to increase the vascularity of the dermis of wounds and to enhance the rate of healing

TABLE 11-2 GENERAL FEATURES AND TISSUE DISTRIBUTION OF MAJOR IDENTIFIED COLLAGENS

TYPE	LOCATION	ORIGIN	FEATURES
I	Skin, bone tendon fascia, ligaments; widespread	Fibroblasts	Low in hydroxyproline, broad hybrid of two different chains
II	Hyaline cartilage, humor, nucleus pulposus, notochord	Chondrocytes	High in hydroxyproline, glycosylated, closely associated with cartilage proteoglycans
III	Skin, blood vessels, internal organs, Descemet's membrane	Fibroblasts, smooth muscle cells	High in hydroxyproline, low in hydroxylysine, interchain disulfide bonds
IV	Basement membranes, kidney glomeruli, lens capsule	Epithelial cells	Very high in hydroxylysine, heavily glycosylated, procollagen portions, amorphous
V	Widespread, in association with smooth muscle, placenta	Smooth muscle	High in hydroxylysine, heavily glycosylated, amorphous, may contain procollagen portions

and breaking strength of wounds, partly by increasing the production of other growth factors. It may reverse in part some of the deleterious effects of steroids on wound healing in a rat linear incision model.[10,24]

TGF-beta isoform 1 (TGF-beta-1) has been implicated in scar formation in a fetal wound healing model[162] and in adult wound healing models, in which thicker dermis resulted after skin wounds were treated with TGF-beta. Further research is underway using monoclonal antibodies against TGF-beta-1, with the hopes of inducing a fetal-like scarless state in mature wounds.[125] This goal must be tempered with a study of the loss of strength a wound treated with antibodies against TGF-beta-1 may incur, since the first objective is to heal a wound, whereas the second is to heal it with an acceptable scar. Research continues to uncover the varied individual roles of each growth factor.

Fibrous Proteins

Collagen

Collagen is the ultimate product of fibroblasts, and it gives the healing wound strength. The major structural protein in vertebrates, collagen provides the extracellular framework for all multicellular organisms. Although some tissues contain more of it than others, collagen accounts for approximately 70% of the dry skin weight,[122] achieved through a delicate balance between continuous biosynthesis and degradation in normal tissues.

At least five types of mature collagen currently are recognized (Table 11-2). The difference in their structures and locations and in their interactions with various proteoglycans results in the physical differences among different body tissues.

The fundamental unit, tropocollagen, measures 300 × 1.5 nm and has a molecular weight of 285,000.[229] It consists of three right-handed helical polypeptide chains (alpha chains) assembled into a left-handed superhelix. Collagen molecules are characterized by their high glycine content; glycine occurs on every third residue in a repeating triplet (Gly-X-Y). Furthermore, the molecules contain the unusual hydroxylated amino acids hydroxylysine and 4-hydroxylysine in the Y position.

Electron microscopy has revealed the banded pattern of native collagen with a 680 Å periodicity.[101] Schmitt and colleagues[250] proposed the quarter-stagger arrangement of tropocollagen fibrils because segment–long-spacing (SLS, a form of collagen) aggregates showed the molecular length to be four times the native fibril periodicity (Figure 11-5). The quarter-stagger model was superseded by the Smith pentafibril model,[264] which is more consistent with available data on collagen structure and composition (Figure 11-6).

The biosynthesis of collagen involves two major steps: intracellular synthesis and modification followed by extracellular processing (Table 11-3). Information from different genes is transcribed into mRNA, eventually producing the different collagen types. Cytoplasmic translation of mRNA by ribosomes results in the formation of pro-X chains, which enter the cisternae of the rough endoplasmic reticulum (RER) (Figure 11-7). Signal sequences on the amino terminal are cleaved off, and hydroxylation of proline and lysine residues develops.[104] The hydroxylation reactions require several cofactors—ferrous ions, molecular oxygen, ascorbic acid, and alpha-ketoglutarate. Efficiency in these factors results in a nonhelical protein that is slowly secreted.[104]

As the lysyl residues in the newly formed pro-X chains are hydroxylated, sugar residues (glucose and galactose) are added.[138] The extent of hydroxyproline in mammalian collagens is reasonably constant, but the extent and patterns of lysine hydroxylation and subsequent glycosylation vary considerably among the tissue collagens in any one species.[76] Glycosylation affects the ultimate physical form of the collagen fibrils, because its extent is related inversely to the fibril diameter distribution of a tissue.

Another important step in the intracellular processing of propeptides is the addition of both intrachain and interchain disulfide bonds between cysteine residues in

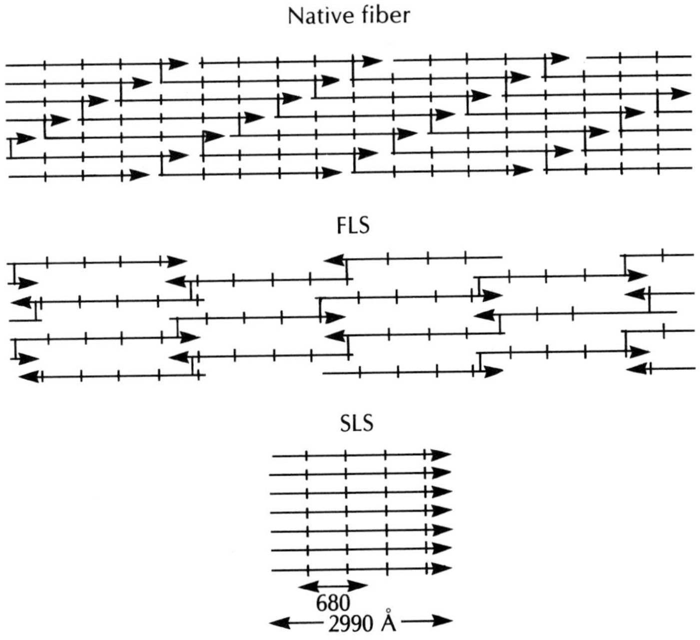

FIGURE 11-5 Schematic representation of the principal forms of tropocollagen aggregation. *Top,* The quarter-stagger, overlapping arrangement of the tropocollagen molecules in the native fiber. Repetition of these overlaps gives rise to the characteristic 680 Å banding seen in electron micrographs of native collagen fibrils. *Middle,* The fibrous–long-spacing (FLS) form of collagen. The same intermolecular cross-links are present as in the native fiber. *Bottom,* The segment–long-spacing (SLS) form of collagen. The tropocollagen molecules are aggregated side to side in parallel array. No fibers are formed, and no intermolecular cross-links are present. (From Peacock EE Jr: *Wound repair,* ed 3, Philadelphia, 1984, WB Saunders.)

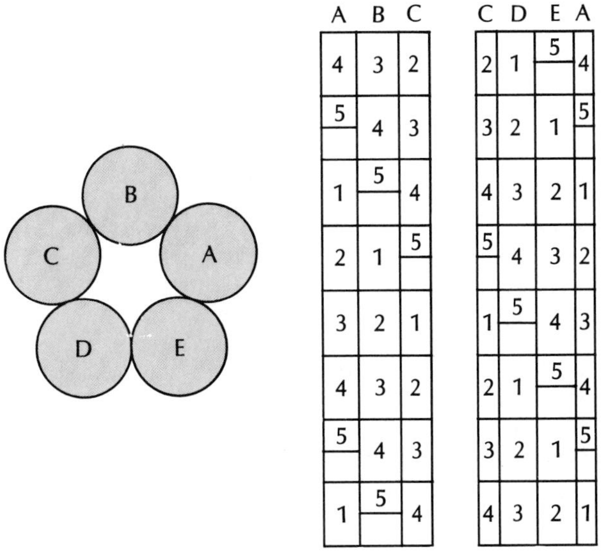

FIGURE 11-6 The Smith model for collagen fibril. In cross-section *(left),* five tropocollagen molecules are shown in a pentagonal arrangement. In the two longitudinal views, the pentafibril is seen from above *(middle),* with fibrils D and E obscured, and below *(right),* with fibrils C and A partially obscured. Intermolecular bonds form between segments 1 and 5 at the overlap zone after a sequential staggering from segments 1 to 4. (From Smith JW: *Nature* 219:157, 1968.)

TABLE 11-3 POSTTRANSLATIONAL MODIFICATIONS IN COLLAGEN BIOSYNTHESIS

PROCESS	ENZYME	BIOLOGIC SIGNIFICANCE
Intracellular Processing		
Hydroxylations of:		
Proline residues	Prolyl 4-hydroxylase Prolyl 3-hydroxylase	4-Hydroxyproline is essential for triple helix formation
Lysine residues	Lysyl hydroxylase	Glycosylation sites; stability of collagen cross-links
Glucosylation of:		
Hydroxylysine	Hydroxylysyl galactosyl transferase	Unknown
Galactolylhydroxylysine (GHL)	GHL glucosyl transferase	Unknown
Triple helix formation	Spontaneous	Formation of functional collagen; can be secreted
Extracellular Processing		
Removal of:		
N-propetides	Procollagen *N*-peptidase	Allow fibril aggregation and ultimate collagen maturation
C-propetides	Procollagen *C*-peptidase	
Fibril aggregation	Spontaneous	Normal collagen fibrils
Oxidative deamination of lysine and hydroxylysine	Lysyl oxidase	Formation of aldehyde groups for collagen cross-links
Covalent cross-links	Spontaneous	Add strength to collagen fibrils; "maturation"

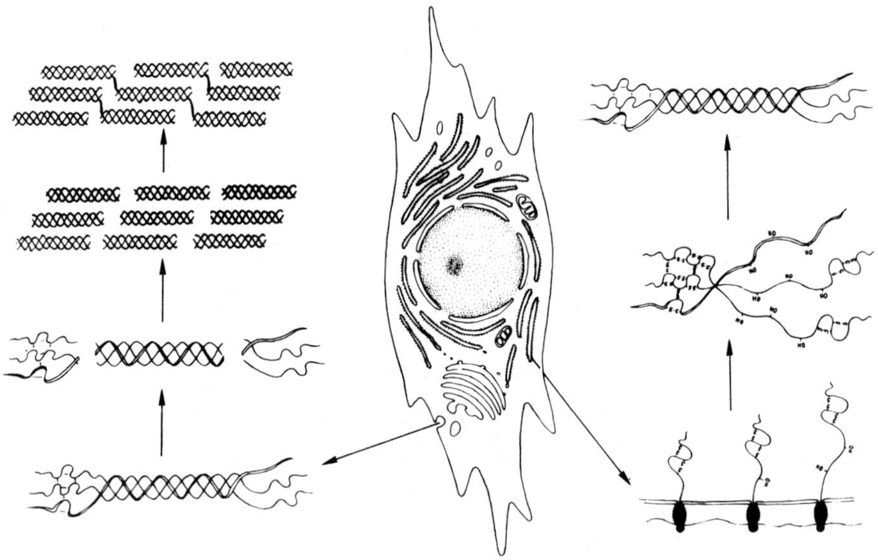

FIGURE 11-7 Schematic diagram showing a fibroblast and the various steps in collagen biosynthesis and modification. Triple helix formation is spontaneous and takes place in the rough endoplasmic reticulum. Extracellularly, cleavage of the nonhelical chains is essential for spontaneous aggregation of collagen fibrils into larger molecules. Note the formation of intermolecular cross-links after fibril aggregation.

the nonhelical domains. Interchain bonds are not synthesized until translation is completed and perhaps not until after the chains are released from the ribosome.[166] Such bonds are among the essential requirements for triple helix formation. If the formation of such bonds is inhibited or the hydroxylation of prolyl residues is prevented, the molecule will not become triple helical and will remain as a nonfunctional protein.[288] Helix formation occurs either in the RER or as the protein leaves it, following release from polysomes.

The newly formed chains possess nonhelical peptide extensions that may facilitate triple helix formation. After assembly in the RER, the protein passes through the Golgi complex for packaging and secretion. If folding

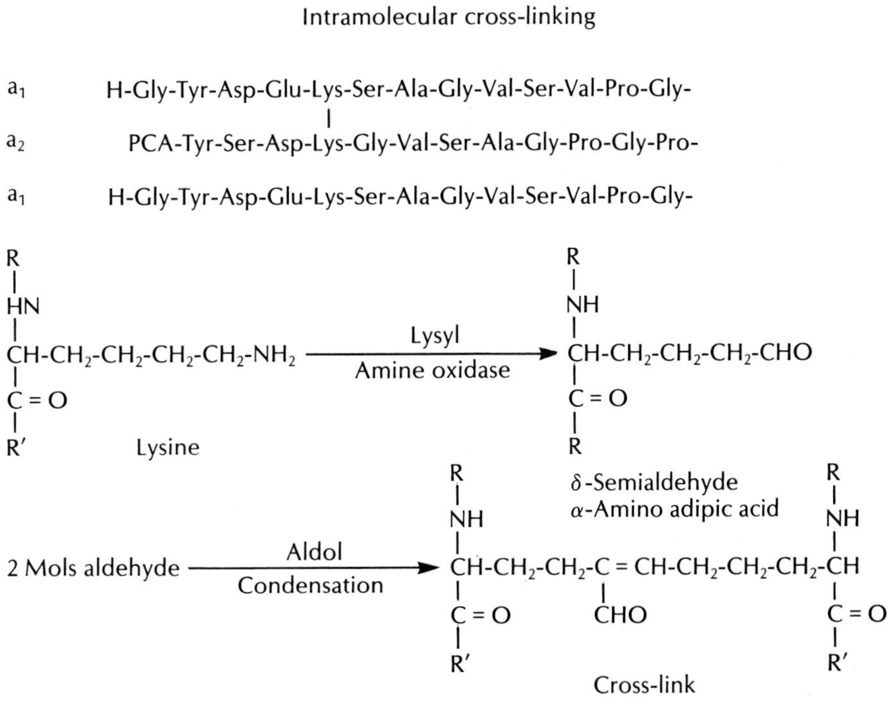

FIGURE 11-8 The postulated formation of intramolecular cross-links. *Top,* A cross-link between lysines in X1 and X2 chains. *Bottom,* A postulated mechanism for such a cross-link. After formation of the cross-link, an aldehyde group is available for further interactions. (From Peacock EE Jr: *Wound repair,* ed 3, Philadelphia, 1984, WB Saunders.)

of pro-X chains into the triple helix conformation is prevented, secretion of the protein is delayed, and the protein tends to accumulate in the cisternae of the RER.[288]

Once extracellular, procollagen molecules are converted to tropocollagen units by enzymatic removal of the globular nonhelical chains from both amino and carboxy terminals by procollagen peptidases. Calcium is required for these reactions. The tropocollagen units then assemble spontaneously into fibrils. Proteoglycan components of connective tissue may influence fibril aggregation and hence their ultimate diameter and three-dimensional orientation.[229] Failure to cleave the extra peptide chains will interfere with aggregation and will result in procollagen molecule accumulation with defective fibrillogenesis. This process occurs in dermatosparaxis, a genetic disorder of cattle.[157] Because dermatosparactic animals lack procollagen peptidase, procollagen molecules accumulate in the skin. Persisting globular chains prevent fibril aggregation and collagen maturation, which results in extreme fragility of the skin and other organs.

After spontaneous formation, the immature fibrils are still "weak" and rely mainly on hydrogen bonds to maintain their arrangement. Interchain covalent bonds are required to provide the necessary tensile strength of the mature collagen fibrils. The first step in the cross-linking process consists of oxidative deamination of the epsilon-amino groups in certain lysyl and hydroxylysyl residues, yielding reactive aldehydes. The enzyme involved, lysyl amino oxidase, is a copper-containing protein that acts preferentially on native collagen fibers.[259] The free aldehyde groups can form two major kinds of cross-links.[276] One is intramolecular and joins two alpha chains in the same molecule through aldol condensation of two aldehyde groups (Figure 11-8). The second is an intermolecular cross-link and involves the condensation between an aldehyde group of a lysine or lysine derivative and an epsilon-amino group of a second lysine or lysine derivative (Figure 11-9). The Schiff base thus formed is the major source of intermolecular cross-links in collagen. Schiff bases, however, are not in themselves stable bonds. The double bond may be reduced, yielding a carbon-to-nitrogen bond, or it may shift in position, yielding a ketone.[14] The change may also involve hydration and oxidation to give a new peptide bond, or it may consist of a more complex rearrangement with additional amino acid side chains in the collagen molecule. If the aldehyde component of the initial Schiff base is derived from hydroxylysine, the cross-link is more stable than if it were from a lysine residue.[14]

As more collagen fibrils aggregate and cross-links are

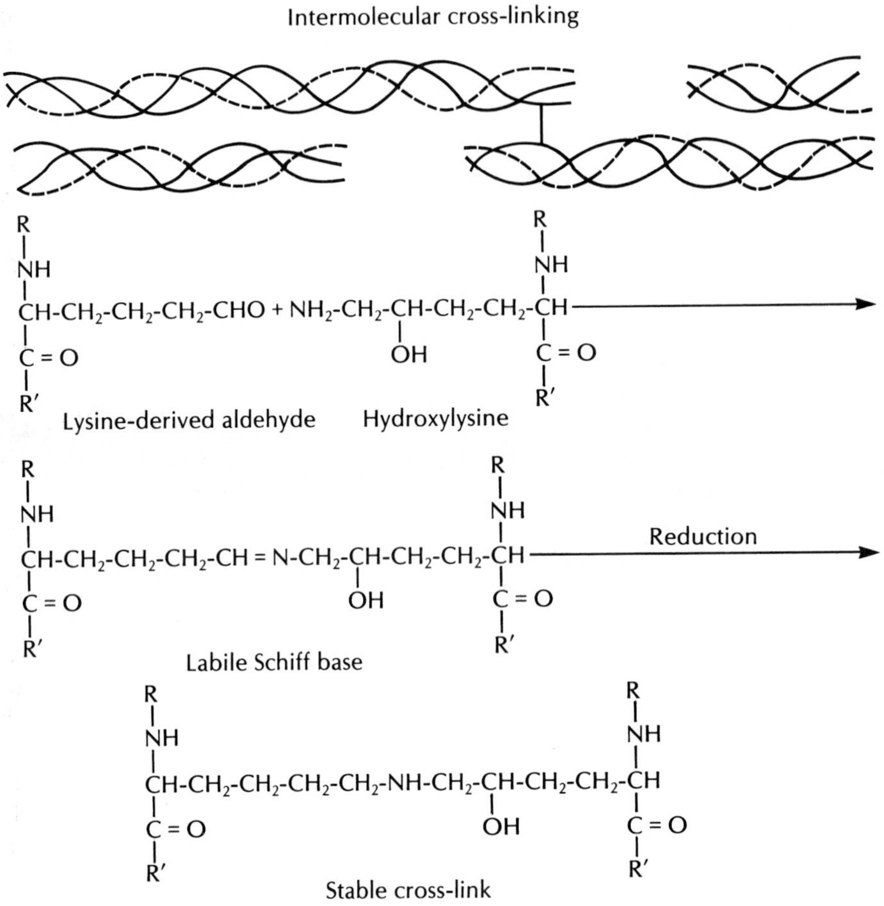

FIGURE 11-9 The postulated formation of intermolecular cross-links. An intermolecular cross-link is shown between tropocollagen molecules. The reactions proposed between lysine-derived molecules involve the formation of a labile Schiff base that stabilizes after reduction, yielding a covalent bond. (From Peacock EE Jr: *Wound repair,* ed 3, Philadelphia, 1984, WB Saunders.)

formed, the solubility of collagen changes accordingly. While tropocollagen is soluble in cold water, early fibrils formed by electrostatic forces can be solubilized in neutral salts. As intramolecular cross-links are formed, collagen loses its salt solubility but can be solubilized in dilute acid. When Schiff bases are further stabilized, collagen becomes insoluble even in acid. These properties are directly relevant to scar mechanics and remodeling.

Elastin

Elastic fibers consist of two protein components—the more common elastin (about 90%), with an amorphous appearance by electron microscopy, and the elastic microfibrils, composed of a specialized glycoprotein. Elastin is the second major fibrous protein in connective tissue. In contrast to collagen, it is in a rather stable state, with a half-life perhaps exceeding the life of an individual.[232] Furthermore, elastin lost with time, as in aging, or through inflammatory processes is not replaced to any significant extent.

Elastin is present in tissues that are under various amounts of stress, adding resiliency and the ability to assume the original contour after distortion. Its structure involves many cross-links, perhaps more widespread than those of collagen, and more lysine residues. Furthermore, most of the cross-links involve three or four peptide chains, thus forming a complex network. The failure to deposit elastin in scar tissue results in stiffness, a major indicator of the imperfect quality of repair.

CONNECTIVE TISSUE

Connective tissue consists mainly of fibrous proteins and other matrix components embedded in ground substance. The role of connective tissue in wound repair is not purely structural. Hyaluronic acid may be involved in angiogenesis, and the scaffold function of fibrous proteins during repair is probably of major importance. The basic biology of various connective tissue components[214,236] is reviewed here as it relates to wound repair.

TABLE 11-4 MUCOPOLYSACCHARIDES OF CONNECTIVE TISSUE AND THEIR LOCATIONS IN THE BODY

	SYNONYMS	DISACCHARIDE REPEATING UNIT	LOCATION
Chondroitin	—	Glucuronic acid + galactosamine	Cornea
Chondroitin-4-sulfate	Chondroitin sulfate A	Glucuronic acid + 4 sulfo-galactosamine	Aorta, cornea, bone
Chondroitin-6-sulfate	Chondroitin sulfate C	Glucuronic acid + 6 sulfo-galactosamine	Tendon, costal cartilage, umbilical cord, nucleus pulposus
Dermatan sulfate	Chondroitin sulfate B	Iduronic acid + 4 sulfo-galactosamine	Skin, heart valves, aorta
Heparan sulfate	Heparitin sulfate	Glucuronic acid + glucosamine	Aorta
Keratan sulfate	Keratosulfate	Galactose + 6 sulfo-glucosamine	Cornea, fetal skeleton
Hyaluronic acid	—	Glucuronic acid + glucosamine	Cartilage

Ground Substance

Ground substance constituents are the glycosaminoglycans (GAGs), glycoproteins, and mucoproteins, in addition to water and electrolytes. Besides their role in the physical makeup of various tissues, current interest in some ground substance components relates to their hypothetical capacity for actively directing tissue repair. This concept evolved from the similarities between wound healing and embryogenesis.[26]

Except for hyaluronic acid (HA), GAGs are not naturally found as isolated polysaccharide chains. They are covalently attached, in varying numbers, to a protein core, resulting in a "bottle brush" structure.[183] GAGs are long-chain polysaccharides composed of repeating disaccharide units (Table 11-4). Each disaccharide consists of a hexosamine linked by a glycosidic bond to a nonnitrogenous sugar. The distinctive feature of GAGs that determines many of their biologic properties is their polyanionic nature, derived from the frequent presence of carbonyl and sulfate groups.

Hyaluronic acid differs from other GAGs in that it is not covalently bound to a protein core, it is unsulfated, and it has a substantially higher molecular weight.[260] Furthermore, hyaluronate is the predominant GAG during early repair, being replaced by sulfated GAG as wounds mature.[47,65] In granulating wounds, HA occurs in higher concentrations at the periphery, suggesting a role for a gradient level. Given hyaluronate's ability to promote cellular migration and proliferation during embryogenesis[281] and the angiogenic property of its lysates, it may indeed mediate cellular migration.

Other Connective Tissue Components

Laminin

Laminin is a large glycoprotein (1 Mdalton) that contains polypeptide chains of 220,000 and 440,000 daltons. An essential component of basement membranes, it is adjacent to the cell membranes, suggesting an interaction with the overlying cells and the underlying collagen molecules, mainly type IV.[181]

Fibronectin

Fibronectin is a ubiquitous, high-molecular-weight glycoprotein (440,000) consisting of two chains held together by disulfide bonds. It is found in plasma and can be associated with cell surfaces, basement membranes, and pericellular matrices. A variety of cells produce it, including fibroblasts, endothelial cells, monocytes, and hepatocytes,[118,197] and it can be found in platelet granules.

Fibronectin can bind some macromolecules, including collagen, fibrin, heparin, and proteoglycans.[243] Since fibronectin forms cross-links to the formed fibrin strands in wounds, it is believed to mediate cell-matrix interactions.[291]

After a wound has occurred, fibronectin is localized in the clot in association with individual strands of fibrin.[94] Cells in the wound space bind to formed collagen after fibronectin is bound to it.[140] Based on this structural role of fibronectin and its chemotactic properties,[23,140] the migration of cells involved in repair results in those cells being related closely to newly formed capillaries, but later they become scattered throughout granulation tissue. Recent evidence points to their ability to modulate angiogenesis,[13,75,277] probably through the release of extracellular heparin.

The relationship between the amount of fibrin deposited in an inflammatory lesion and the extent of subsequent fibrovascular tissue has been previously recognized.[186] Fibrin and fibrin degradation product (FDP) are able to produce leukocytic migration into rabbit corneas with subsequent neovascularization and corneal opacification. However, this occurs after macrophage migration and activation. Thompson and colleagues have shown that low-molecular-weight (50,000) fibrin degradation products induce angiogenesis in the chick chorioallantoic membrane.[278] This induction takes place in the absence of leukocyte infiltration and at a time when DNA synthesis is at its peak. This evidence supports the finding that plasminogen activator plays a role in angiogenesis.[25]

Fibronectins are involved in various biologic processes. In addition to their important functions in cell-to-cell and cell-matrix interactions[291] and as a scaffold for cell migration,[243] fibronectins are capable of accelerating wound repair when applied topically.[74] Fibronectin acts as a cell migration substrate and as a substrate for cell adhesion via integrins.[56] Since digestion products of fibronectin by cathepsin D stimulate DNA synthesis by cultured fibroblasts,[112] one may hypothesize a role for fibronectin in fibrogenesis. The dynamic metabolism of fibronectin during wound repair is in agreement with this proposed function.

SEQUENCE OF EVENTS

The sequence of events leading ultimately to wound repair is well timed. Although this statement may sound like an oversimplification, the sequence itself is the result of complex cell-cell, cell-matrix, and cell-environment interactions. Wound repair occurs in three stages that merge gradually into each other (Figure 11-10).

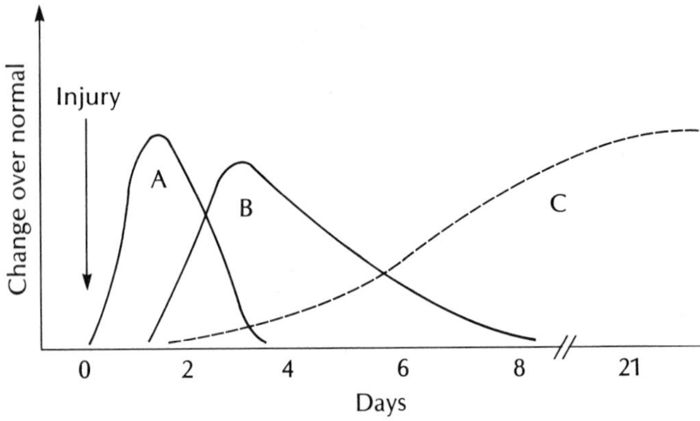

FIGURE 11-10 Schematic diagram of the three phases of wound healing. Curve A represents the inflammatory response; curve B represents fibroblast proliferation and capillary formation; curve C shows the newly deposited collagen and may well be paralleled with collagen maturation. (Modified from Dineen P, Mildich-Smith G: *The surgical wound,* Philadelphia, 1981, Lea & Febiger.)

Inflammation

The inflammatory process is initiated by tissue injury and starts immediately afterward. It peaks for 1 to 2 days, being replaced gradually by day 5 to day 7 by the repair activity proper. Any continuing stimulus may convert acute inflammation into a chronic process with more pronounced tissue destruction and ultimate scarring.

This phase is characterized by vascular changes that allow the exudation of protein-rich plasma and the migration of leukocytes into the wound space. Chemical mediators trigger a cascade of events and invite different cell types sequentially as they are involved (see Figure 11-4).

The epidermis is actively dividing during this phase; in approximated surgical incisions, epidermal continuity is established within 24 to 48 hours. Formation of new blood vessels is also evident in the wound edges. Endothelial cells bud in preexisting capillaries and advance into the wound space, which is filled by now with the fibrin clot. Endothelial migration is helped by plasminogen activator, which is formed by these cells.[170]

Knighton and colleagues[145] described an elegant model to depict the cellular anatomy of repair tissue as related to oxygen tension (Figure 11-11). In this "wound module," macrophages constitute the leading edge, closely accompanied by young fibroblasts. These are followed by replicating fibroblasts clustered around epithelial buds, whereas functioning vessels and mature fibroblasts are at the distant edge. The oxygen pressure (Po_2) in the macrophage layer is low, with an intermediate value (30 to 50 mm Hg) in the area of replicating fibroblasts that peaks over the vessels. Lactate stimulates collagen production by fibroblasts.[151]

By the end of this phase, inflammation has provided the wound spaces with cells essential for debridement of the injured tissue, elimination of bacteria, and mediation of repair.

Fibroplasia

Also referred to as the proliferative phase of repair, fibroplasia usually is established by day 5 after the wound occurs. The duration of this phase varies in different tissues and largely depends on the type of wound. Fibroplasia may last 1 or 2 weeks in incised and sutured wounds and even longer in excised wounds.

Fibroplasia is characterized by the migration of fibroblasts into the wound area and the formation of capillary blood vessels. These events are more florid in open wounds and result in excessive granulation tissue, the "hallmark of healing inflammation."[232]

Once in the wound space, fibroblasts are active in the synthesis and release of collagen and GAG. Collagen fibers deposited early are slender, as shown on light microscopy by silver stain. These argyrophilic fibers, called reticulin fibers, constitute the earliest collagen laid down in wounds. As these fibrils grow larger and thicker, they lose their argyrophilic property. Early capillaries enlarge, endothelial buds acquire a lumen, and both communicate with already established capillaries.

By immunohistochemical staining techniques in dermal granulation tissue, Graham and colleagues showed that the type of collagen deposited at the wound site differs with time.[91] In the open wound model used, the principal collagen type found early is type IV (basement membrane collagen), initially localized to skin appendages, specifically to sites of proliferating epithelium. After 18 hours, type IV and type V collagens are detected

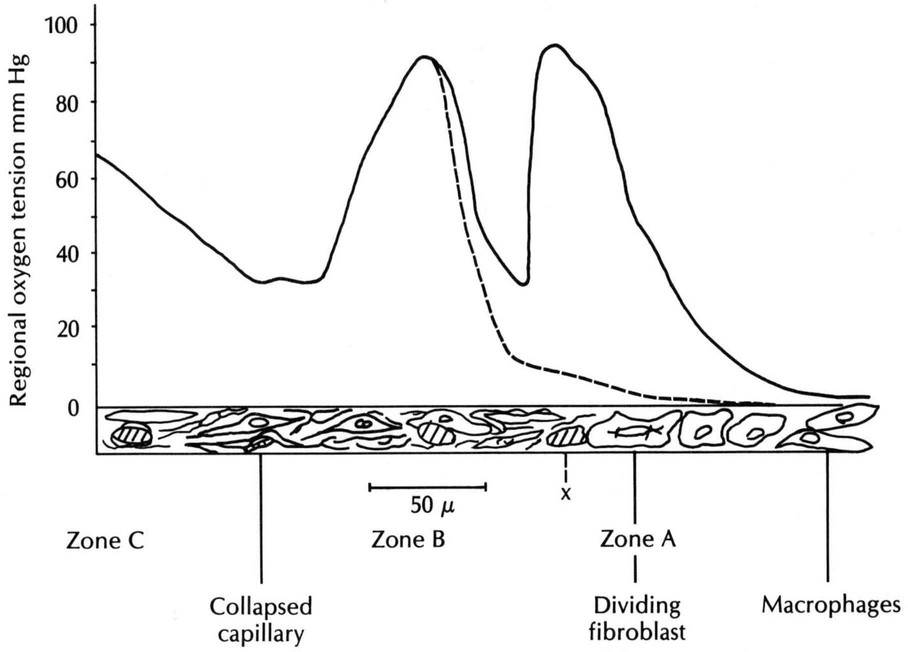

FIGURE 11-11 Cell distribution as related to oxygen tension in the "wound module." These relationships were noted using the rabbit ear chamber model.

in the clot. Type IV collagen found initially at the wound margins subsequently infiltrates the newly formed clot. The deposition of type III collagen (embryonic-type collagen) is noted at 24 hours in the wound margin immediately adjacent to but not within the clot. At 48 hours, type III collagen becomes extensive within the clot and type I collagen (adult type) starts appearing. By 60 hours, type I collagen is predominant and uniformly distributed within the clot, with moderate amounts of type III and type IV still present. Although this pattern of collagen deposition may suggest resumption of a more primitive state by the fibroblast, as in embryogenesis, it may also point to an organizational role of the newly formed matrix. The latter role is in agreement with the early formation of type IV collagen, allowing for subsequent attachment and migration of epithelial cells on the newly formed basement membrane.

By the end of this phase, wounds acquire some tensile strength, which is largely dependent on collagen deposition and cross-linking.

Maturation

Maturation, the last phase of the repair process, also referred to as remodeling, sets in gradually as the fibroblastic activity in the wound diminishes. Its duration is not well defined because of the continuous and dynamic nature of scar remodeling.

Fibroblasts and macrophages decrease in number, with an accompanying decrease in wound vascularity. Scar collagen accumulates and reaches a peak, after which further increase in wound strength is no longer related to further collagen deposition[173] (Figure 11-12). In fact, after peaking, the total scar collagen may even decrease with time and then reach a stable level.

The final mature scar often is noted to decrease in size when compared to the younger early scar. It changes from pink to a pale white, suggesting its avascular nature. Biochemically, the maturation process is directly related to the continuous process of collagen synthesis and breakdown. Blocking collagen synthesis results in the breakdown of old scars because of persisting collagenolysis.

In general, fibers remaining in a scar are those that are oriented along lines of tension. The arrangement of collagen fibers becomes more organized but still quite different from that in uninjured dermis. With further aging of the scar, fibers become more compact, hyaluronic acid is replaced with sulfated GAGs, and water is lost. This compact arrangement enhances further the formation of intermolecular cross-links, with collagen becoming more insoluble and resistant to the action of collagenolytic enzymes.

The factors controlling the dynamic metabolism of collagen in scar tissue are not well understood. The major enzyme responsible for degrading types I, II, and III collagens is a specific collagenase, a neutral metalloproteinase that cleaves the chains of these collagens at a discrete locus across the helix, whether the collagens are polymerized as fibrils or present in solution.[146] Enzymes other than collagenases are required to degrade the var-

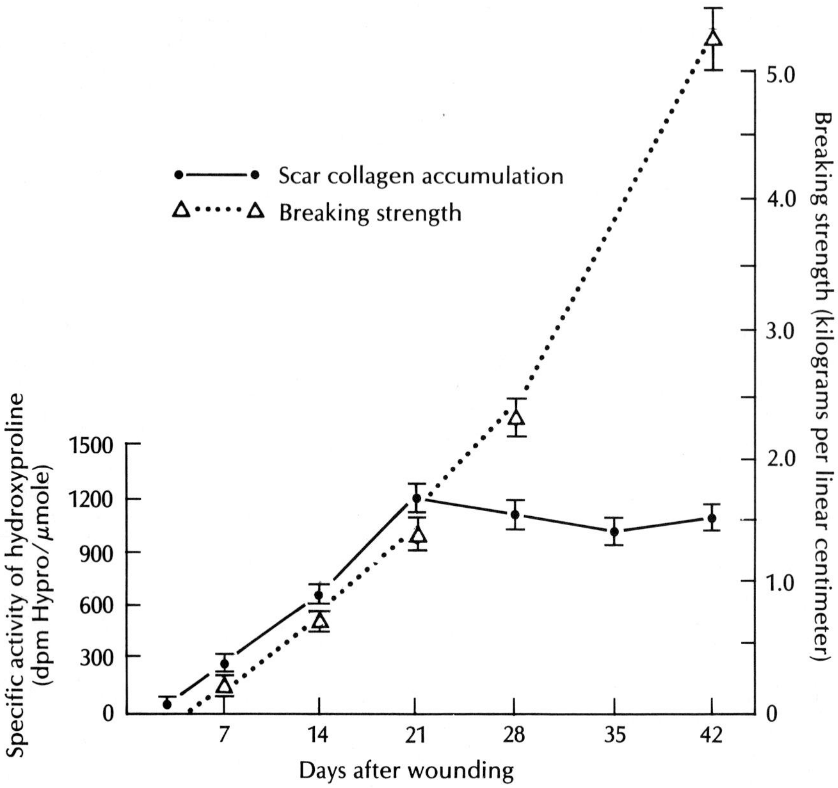

FIGURE 11-12 Breaking strength of rat skin wounds plotted with net collagen deposition in scar tissue. Note that up to 3 weeks after a wound, wound strength correlates well with collagen deposition. After 3 weeks, however, the wound continues to gain strength after net collagen deposition stops. There is no correlation between collagen content and wound strength after 3 weeks. (From Madden JW, Peacock EE Jr: *Ann Surg* 174:511, 1971.)

ious collagen species that generally do not polymerize as typical banded fibrils. Collagen lysis can be regulated at several steps, which may include biosynthesis and secretion of latent collagenase (procollagenase), activation of this latent enzyme, interaction of the active enzyme with collagen substrates, and modulation of enzyme activity by protein inhibitors.

The synthesis and secretion of procollagenase by cells is influenced by interactions with other cells and the surrounding extracellular matrix.[310] Once extracellular, procollagenase can be activated by any of several neutral proteases, such as kallikrein, plasmin, and mast cell proteases.

Binding of active collagenase to collagen fibrils results in their fragmentation at different rates, depending on the source of collagenase and collagen type. Human skin fibroblasts cleave types I and III collagens at a considerably faster rate than type II.[299] Furthermore, fibrils with established intermolecular cross-links are cleaved more slowly than fibrils without such cross-links.

Collagenolysis is probably controlled extracellularly by natural inhibitors of active collagenase.[310] In human serum, the major inhibitory protein is alpha$_2$-macroglobulin. The production of such inhibitors is also another possible regulatory step.

As our understanding of scar physiology and dynamics becomes more extensive, exact control over collagen metabolism will allow alteration of this excess in hypertrophic scars or keloids and its deficiency in weak scars of abnormal structure.

SECONDARY WOUNDS

The faster healing of secondary incisions made over fresh and healing wounds was confirmed experimentally, provided the second wound is made when the proliferative phase of repair has already been established.[66] The advantage for secondarily sutured fascial wounds is greatest at 3 weeks after the initial wound, and little advantage remains after 6 weeks.[66] This fact is evidenced by an accelerated gain in tensile strength at an earlier phase of repair (Figure 11-13).[203]

When the area immediately adjacent to the scar is excised, this phenomenon is no longer observed, proving its local nature.[247] The major difference between primary and secondary wounds is the absence of a "lag phase"

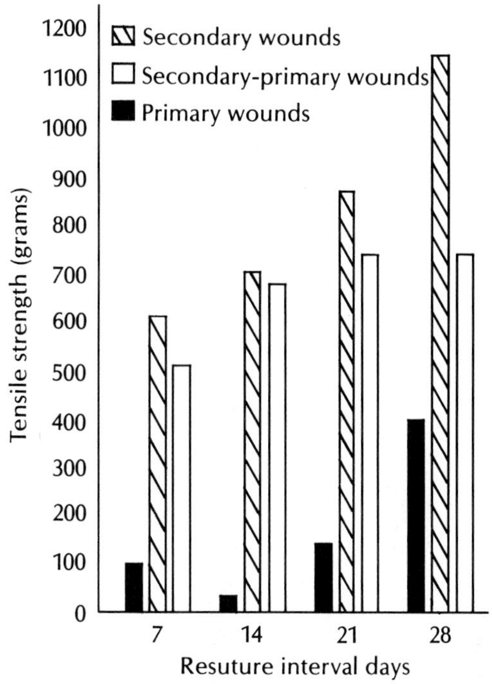

FIGURE 11-13 Tensile strength values in primary and secondary wounds in the skin of rabbits. Clear columns indicate the difference in tensile strength between the secondary and primary wounds. (From Ogilvie RR, Douglas DM: *Brit J Surg* 51:149, 1964.)

(inflammatory) in the latter. Collagen content is the same or sometimes even decreased when compared to primary wounds. Dehiscing and resuturing wounds has no effect on the rate of new collagen deposition per se.[174] Inflammation has already set the stage for repair to take place, and the wound progresses in healing from where it stopped just before separation.

MECHANISMS OF WOUND CLOSURE

In any type of soft-tissue repair, two processes take place in varying proportions: epithelization, when this tissue is originally covered with epithelium, and wound contraction.

In incised and sutured wounds, healing occurs with minimal tissue loss. In such a case, repair occurs by "first intention" or "primary union." The incised space is narrow and fills immediately with a blood-containing fibrin clot. This situation is the one most often encountered in surgical practice. Epidermal continuity is established in 24 to 48 hours, long before the underlying soft-tissue reaction has begun to evolve. In addition, the fibrin clot that fills in the gap constitutes an early barrier between the external environment and the wound space.

A wound left open for a few days and then reapproximated closes by "delayed primary union." If no complications develop, healing progresses as usual, resulting in a good scar identical to a "primary union" scar.

If tissue loss is extensive and not replaced or a surgical policy requires leaving a wound open, the repair process becomes more complicated and prolonged. Such a defect must be filled or covered, but simple regeneration of parenchymal cells cannot completely reconstitute the original architecture. Healing takes place by "secondary union," which differs from primary healing in several respects. Fibrin deposition, necrotic debris, and exudate are more extensive with a more severe inflammatory reaction; healing proper cannot start until inflammation resolves and granulation tissue appears. Furthermore, granulation tissue is more florid and often correlates with the ultimate amount of scarring. Excess granulation may protrude above the wound margins, preventing epithelization. Cauterization with silver nitrate sticks may be helpful in such cases, although surgical excision is frequently required. The phenomenon of wound contraction, which occurs in large surface wounds, is probably the most disturbing feature in this type of repair. Whatever the size of the final scar, it is always smaller than the original tissue defect.

Epithelialization

Skin assumes two important functions in humans. It provides a protective covering against trauma and serves as a selective barrier that controls the exchange of various molecules into and out of our stable internal system. With injury and tissue loss, the epithelium attempts to reestablish its previous integrity and resume its functional and structural roles.

On the basis of their regenerative capacity, epithelial cells are classified as "labile." Under normal conditions they continue to proliferate throughout life, replacing shed or destroyed cells. The basal cells are the major epithelial cells involved in continuous proliferation.

Within 12 hours after a wound occurs (Figure 11-14), many functional and morphologic changes take place in the adjacent epidermis. Basal cells lose their attachment to the underlying dermis and begin to migrate over a collagen-fibronectin scaffold through a process of "contact guidance." The preferential attachment of epithelial cells in culture to type IV collagen and the selective adherence of basal cells to a collagen substrate[223] pinpoint the importance of collagen in guiding epidermal cell migration.

The migrating cells become larger and develop a more flattened appearance than nonmigrating ones. They develop "ruffled borders" in the form of pseudopod-like extensions of their cytoplasm and acquire intracellular actin filaments.[147] This contractile protein is not demonstrable in normal epithelium adjacent to the wound and disappears after healing is over.[83] This phenomenon

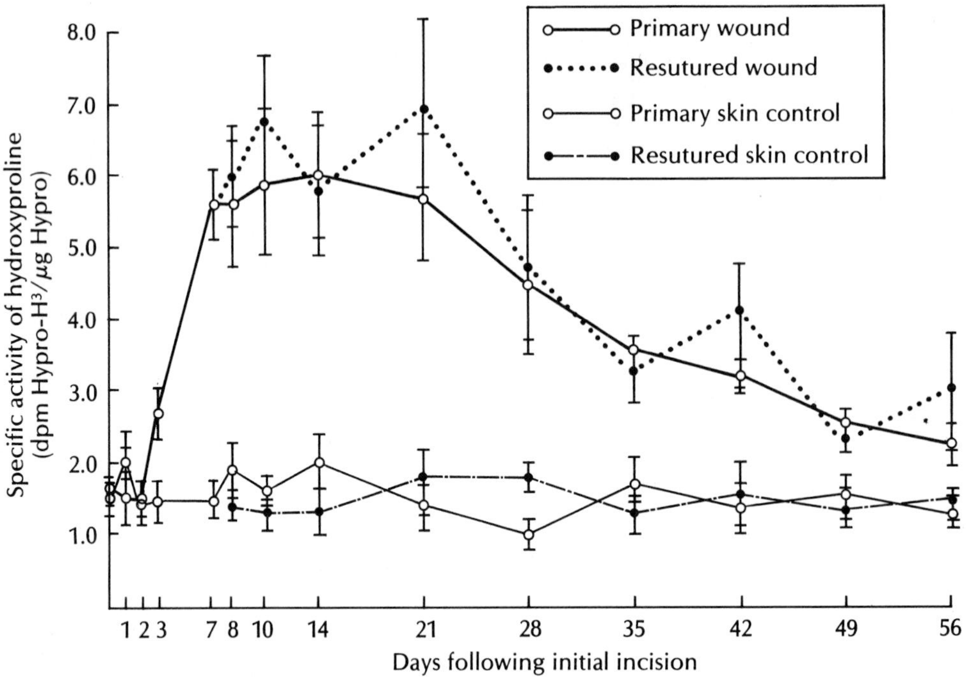

FIGURE 11-14 Rates of new collagen deposition in excised primary wounds and dehisced and resutured wounds in rats. (From Madden JW, Smith HC: *Surg Gynecol Obstet* 130:487, 1970.)

is in agreement with the hypothesis that the contractile apparatus is involved in the migration of epidermal cells. The general belief is that after injury, migration is initiated by a process similar to loss of "contact inhibition" observed in cell cultures.

Cell migration is not limited to the wound edges but also occurs along suture tracts, which behave as "small wounds."[207] These epithelial tracts are normally removed by the inflammatory infiltrate within 10 to 15 days, with possible residual keratinized epithelial pearls. Should these persist for a longer period, the inflammatory reaction becomes severe and often is misinterpreted as a "stitch abscess." Occasionally, entrapment of epithelium occurs, resulting in the formation of inclusion cysts.

As basal cells start migrating, their mitotic rate increases noticeably and peaks in 48 hours after the wound occurs. This increased mitotic activity declines as epithelization is taking place. By the time the latter is complete, mitotic activity has been reduced but is still greater than normal. Epithelial hypertrophy and ongoing mitosis result in epidermal thickening, which resolves gradually with subsequent maturation. The resulting scar epithelium has no appendages, is characteristically thin and fragile, and lacks strong attachments to the underlying dermis. Although epithelization may take place after severe injuries with large skin defects, surgical intervention often is needed to achieve adequate wound coverage (e.g., skin grafts) to accelerate healing and achieve a good functional result.

Wound Contraction

Contraction is the process by which a full-thickness wound is gradually covered by movement of the peripheral skin toward the center of the defect. Hence, an important concept is that preexisting tissue is moved without the formation of new tissue as a primary event. At times wound contraction can achieve complete wound closure with an acceptable result; in experimental animals it could account for 40% to 80% of the closure of excised skin wounds.[3]

The size of the wound does not affect the rate at which it contracts. The amount of available mobile skin determines whether the wound closes completely or not. This fact is best illustrated in lower mammals in whom contraction is the major process by which surface wounds are closed. Their skin moves easily over the underlying fascia because of a prominent layer of loose areolar tissue underlying the panniculus carnosus muscle. Humans have much less dermal mobility because skin attachments to underlying structures are more developed. However, cutaneous laxity may allow for closure of full-thickness defects by a combination of contraction and epithelization. This result is frequently observed in small sacral pressure sores that are managed conservatively. In some areas, however, skin laxity may

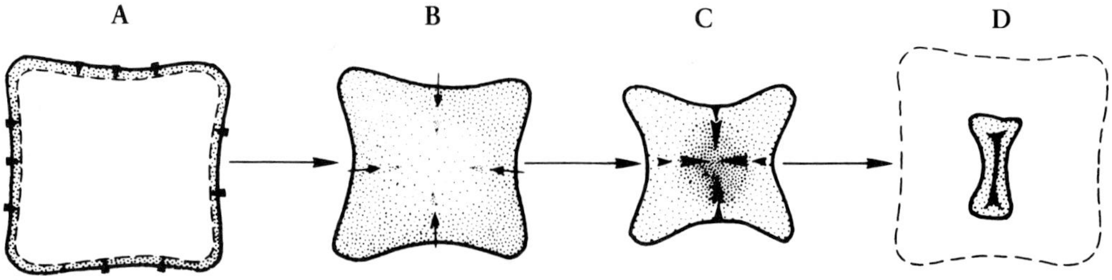

FIGURE 11-15 Suggested mechanisms of wound contraction. **A**, The "purse string" effect, produced by the ingrowing epithelium. **B**, The "picture frame" model, with the force of contraction located in the periphery, pushing tissues inward. **C**, As wound contraction proceeds, myofibroblasts become more uniformly distributed, allowing for a centrally located "pull" mechanism. **D**, Schematic representation of the final appearance of a contracted wound.

be a disadvantage, because contraction may result in a functional deformity, as is observed with eyelid scars and joint contractures. Contraction is limited in such areas as the extremities and anterior chest wall and does not contribute to any significant extent in healing by secondary intention in these locations. Furthermore, contraction does not take place in a symmetric fashion over all wound edges. Wound borders in the direction of maximum skin tension contract less,[248] as do areas more fixed to subcutaneous structures. This results in an irregular scar.

Because contraction involves the movement of tissue located around the wound edges, stretching and tension are expected to result in the surrounding tissue. This induces an "intussusceptive growth,"[127] resulting in epithelial and mesenchymal thickening with restoration of the original tissue architecture. The stimulus involved in stopping the contraction process is not very well understood; a balance between the force of contraction and opposing skin tension is probably a major factor.

The mechanisms of wound contraction are still not very clear, despite the numerous experiments attributing major roles to granulation tissue components. Whereas collagen was shown not to be essential for contraction,[1] myofibroblasts appear to be primarily involved. This assumption is supported by their uniform distribution and temporal quantification with respect to the contraction process.[188] Myofibroblasts in granulation tissue peak in number between 2 and 3 weeks, decreasing in percentage just before wound contraction slows down, and disappearing as contraction is achieved. Furthermore, the inhibition of wound contraction by the topical application of smooth muscle antagonists indicates an important role for this specialized cell in wound contraction.[172]

The force of contraction has been the subject of controversy for many years. Watts and colleagues[294] developed the "picture frame" theory, which purports that the contractile elements (and hence the generated forces of contraction) are located in the wound margins. Excision of that "picture frame" abolishes contraction, but excision of the centrally located core of granulation tissue was of no consequence. Abercrombie and coworkers[4] observed that splinted full-thickness wounds contracted 10 days after injury and removal of the splint. Excision of the central area of granulation tissue just before splint removal reduced the extent of subsequent contraction. This led to the postulation of the "pull" theory, which holds that centrally located myofibroblasts pull the skin periphery inward. This concept is further supported by the finding that myofibroblasts are distributed uniformly throughout granulation tissue[242] instead of being localized in the "picture frame" area. Baur and associates[21] reconciled the previously mentioned models and proposed a role for epithelium (Figure 11-15). They suggested that wound contraction occurs in three sequential steps. An initial contraction force is generated by the advancing epithelial cells joined to form a contractile band ("purse string" effect); this is followed by the contractile action of myofibroblasts that are still located peripherally in the early phases of contraction ("picture frame" concept). As contraction proceeds, myofibroblasts become more uniformly distributed and hence generate the central force of contraction ("pull" concept).

WOUND STRENGTH

The surgeon often is faced with the necessity of achieving the best cosmetic scar. While keeping this need in mind, the surgeon's main concern is the development of wound strength, which is a better guide to proper wound management and closure techniques. The development of wound strength is the preferred measure and objective criterion for evaluating the progress and adequacy of both clinical and experimental repair. The many factors

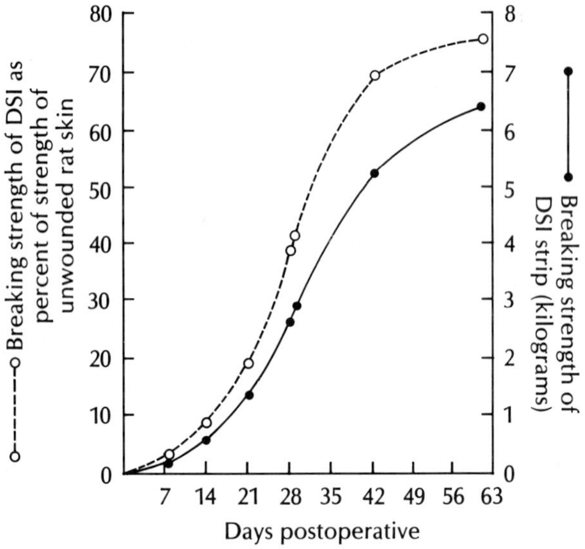

FIGURE 11-16 Increase in breaking strength of a healing wound shown absolutely and as a percentage of the strength of comparable unwounded skin. *DSI,* Dermal skin incision. (From Levenson SM, Geever LV, Crowley JF et al: *Ann Surg* 161:293, 1965.)

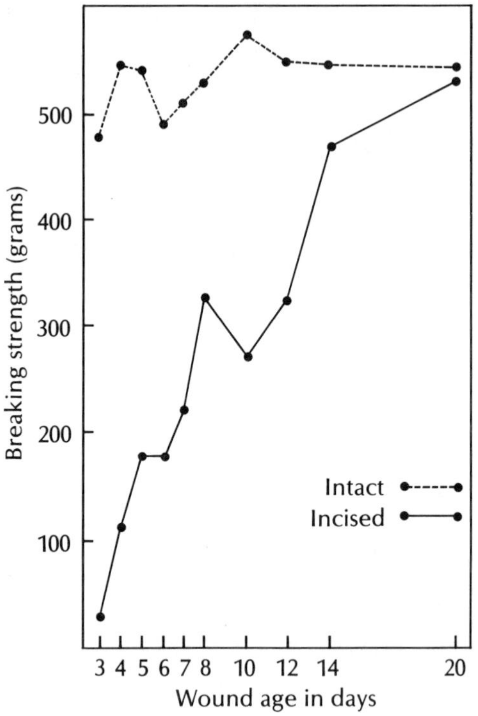

FIGURE 11-17 Breaking strength of epidermal incisions as a function of wound age. The dotted line represents the breaking strength of intact epidermis from animals matched to the experimental group. The early gain in strength between days 3 and 5 is probably explained by epidermal healing, since collagen deposition is not significant yet. (From Rovee DT, Miller CA: *Arch Surg* 96:43, 1968.)

that modulate wound repair can therefore be evaluated according to their influence on the development of wound strength.

The determinations of wound strength and interpretations of such measurements should be carried out with the knowledge of one basic property of skin—viscoelasticity. Stretching forces applied at different rates elicit different elastic skin behavior. A constant force applied rapidly may break the skin with minimal stretching, but the same constant force may stretch the skin without breakage if applied slowly. This property should serve as a guide in detecting the errors inherent in some experimental models.

Breaking Strength and Tensile Strength

The two most commonly used parameters to determine wound strength in nonhollow structures are tensile strength and breaking strength. Tensile strength is defined as the load per unit cross-sectional area at rupture. Breaking strength is the load required to break a wound regardless of any dimension. Tensile strength is more useful when comparing homogeneous structure, because it eliminates a physical variable, that is, thickness, and emphasizes the nature of the material and its tensile property. However, in the clinical situation the surgeon is interested more in the force required to break a wound, regardless of size. Furthermore, estimating cross-sectional areas of tissues often is very difficult, because their constitutive elements may also show individual variations.

A typical breaking strength curve (Figure 11-16) shows a slow rise in wound strength that may be observed as early as day 2 after the wound occurs. Some reports deny any gain in strength that early, illustrating the difficulties inherent in the measurements and the variability of findings among different laboratories.

At this stage the main component contributing to strength is the fibrin clot that fills the wound cavity. Recent evidence suggests a role for cell aggregation centers (CAC) as "initial strength elements."[290] A CAC is a growing cluster of morphologically different cells situated between the wound edges, held together by fibronectin, and embedded in a fibrillar network that progresses to involve larger, more mature collagen bundles. In the beginning, collagen and fibronectin do not bridge the wound and cannot provide strength. However, CAC, fused by collagen and fibronectin interlinks, can provide some tensile strength by bridging the wound edges. Investigating other possibilities, Geever and colleagues[86] suggested that noncollagenous proteins can contribute as early as day 3 to wound strength. In addition, epidermal continuity is established within 24 to 48 hours in well-approximated incisions. The developed epidermal strength is of significant dimensions,[240] the greatest

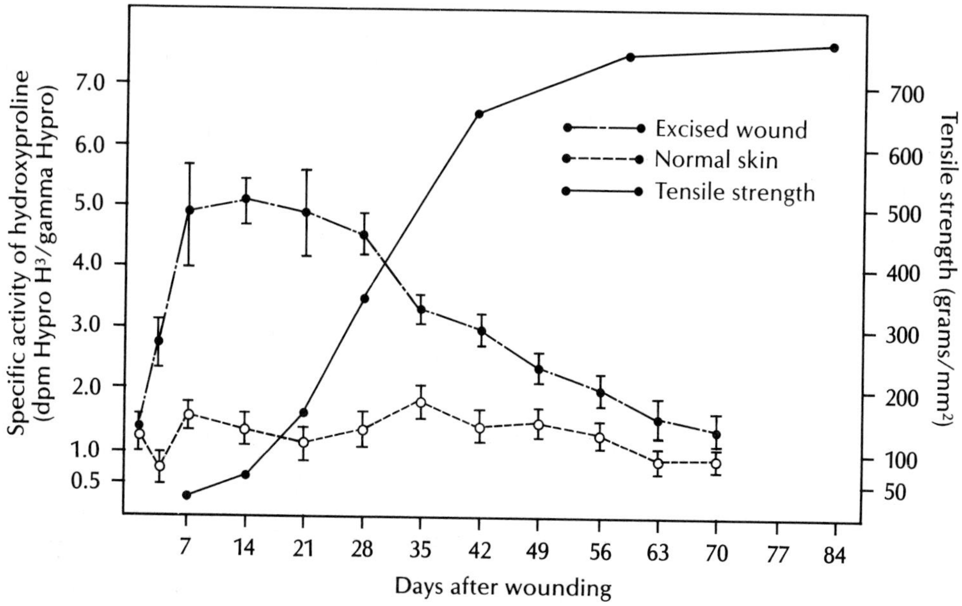

FIGURE 11-18 Relation of the rate of collagen synthesis to the tensile strength of rat skin wounds. (From Madden JW, Peacock EE Jr: *Surgery* 64:288, 1968; tensile strength curve from Levenson M et al: *Ann Surg* 161:293, 1965.)

increase in the rate of strength gain being observed between days 3 and 5 after the wound occurs (Figure 11-17).

With establishment of the fibroblastic phase, collagen is deposited to a greater extent, and the breaking strength increases more rapidly. Three to four weeks after injury, further increase in breaking strength is not paralleled by collagen deposition. In fact, the rate of collagen synthesis decreases as tensile strength is gained (Figure 11-18).

The period of accelerated increase in wound strength lasts from 3 to 6 weeks and is followed by a gradual decrease in strength gain, reaching almost a plateau for that specific wound, a level in the range of 70% to 90% of normal skin strength. However, intestinal wounds may achieve a breaking strength identical to that of normal tissue 1 week after injury.[90]

Bursting Pressure

The mechanical strength of a wound in a hollow viscus can be evaluated by using either of two methods. The breaking strength of an excised strip can be measured, as in skin wounds, or the bursting pressure can be determined. The latter can be done by inflating the viscus, placing it in a water bath, filling it with air, and recording the pressure at the moment of observed rupture. Although this method simulates the clinical setting, it may lead to erroneously above-normal values of bursting pressure in wounded viscera. This occurrence is explained by the established wall tension-pressure relationships existing in hollow structures, according to Laplace's law. In cylindric structures, the law states that $T = PR$ (P = pressure, R = radius of the hollow cylinder, T = wall tension). As pressure is increased, the hollow viscus distends, but to a lesser extent over the healed and probably scarred anastomosis, which is more rigid in structure. Therefore, the developing wall tension is less than in other normal areas, explaining why sometimes viscera burst through normal rather than wounded sites.

To test the mechanical strength of abdominal wounds in vitro, a technique simulating the clinical setting has been developed.[93,287] It consists of measuring the bursting pressure of fascial wounds mounted in a chamber as a diaphragm of tissue. Wound rupture stress is determined by membrane stress analysis, which takes into account the viscoelastic properties of skin.

Despite the availability of many techniques to measure wound strength, most of our information is still based on simple breaking strength measurements.

HEALING OF VARIOUS TISSUES

Fascia

The surgeon often deals with fascia as an essential structure that adds strength to tissues and serves as a versatile element in reconstructive procedures. When fascia is divided during surgical entering of deeper structures for abdominal reconstruction, its healing is crucial to pre-

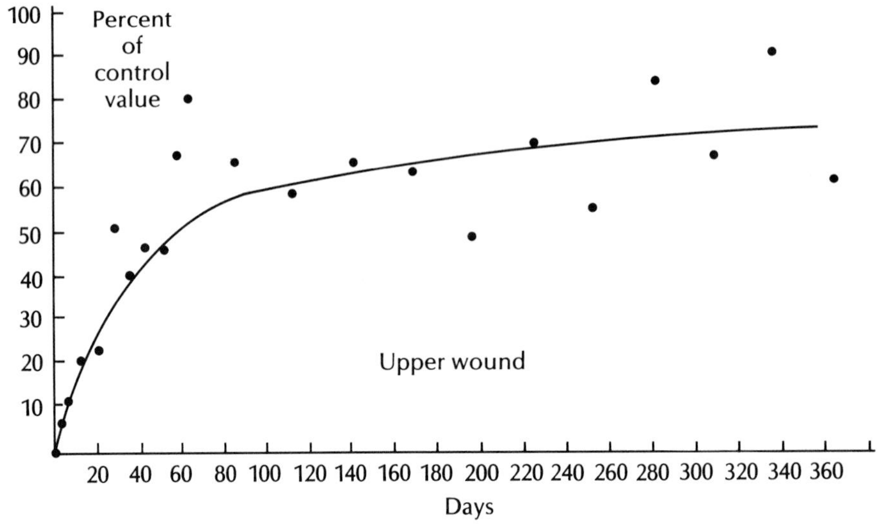

FIGURE 11-19 Tensile strength gain of a wound in the lower dorsal aponeurosis of the rabbit, expressed as a percentage of the tensile strength of unwounded fascia during the same time period. Note that at the end of the 1-year period the wound reaches only about 80% of the control value. (From Douglas DM: *Brit J Surg* 40:79, 1959.)

vent incisional hernias with gaping fascial defects and wound dehiscence.

The healing process in fascia occurs in a way similar to skin repair. However, because fascia is less vascular and has no rapidly growing epithelium, it heals more slowly than skin and achieves a lower maximum breaking strength (Figure 11-19).[66] Furthermore, lost fascia cannot regenerate and must be replaced. Thus synthetic meshes are used as a structural support where fascia is unavailable. Although these features may appear to be disadvantages, fascia usually is a sturdy layer necessary for successful hernia repair and most reconstructive procedures.

Muscle

Skeletal muscle lacerations are frequently encountered in both elective surgery and trauma. Surgeons look skeptically at the possibility of muscle regeneration. However, skeletal muscle regeneration across lacerations has been demonstrated,[39] with little scar tissue separating the muscle segments on either side of the initial laceration.[102] For adequate bridging of fibers across the defect, it is of paramount importance to achieve good apposition of the severed ends, with debridement of any dead or scar tissue that may mechanically hinder regeneration.

The connective tissue framework of muscle is needed to allow adequate regeneration.[43] Regeneration may occur from the outgrowth of fibers on either side of the injury or from satellite cells located within the muscle's connective tissue sheath.[42] The presence of tension is beneficial to the rate and final character of regeneration.[39] Simultaneous denervation of the severed ends does not interfere with regeneration in skeletal muscle,[295] but ultimate restoration of a functional muscle requires an intact motor nerve supply.

The end result of muscle repair and regeneration is recovery of a moderate amount of useful function. With complete transverse lacerations, total recovery often is not possible. In the experimental model, 12 weeks after complete laceration of skeletal muscle, 50% of tension-producing ability and the capacity to contract to 80% of normal were recovered.[84] Heart muscle has no regenerative capacity and thus heals by connective tissue scar formation.

Tendon

Healing of ruptured tendons currently is a challenging area to both surgeon and basic scientist alike. Primary tendon healing occurs from both within and without the tendon itself[132]; the tendon's peculiar anatomy accounts for this duality. Tendons are composed of longitudinally oriented bundles of collagen fibers, each bundle being surrounded by a thin, fibrous, connective tissue structure, the endotenon. The epitenon, a membrane enclosing the bundles, is embedded within a synovial sheath where bending and gliding are prominent. Where a tendon is straight, it usually is surrounded by loose areolar tissue,[210] through a narrow mesotendon constructed in much the same way as a bowel mesentery. Within the tendon and between the fiber bundles are collapsed capillaries and tendon cells, tenocytes. The tenoblast, an immature tenocyte precursor, contributes to intrinsic repair within tendons.[58]

In a healthy, intact tendon, only a scant vascular system can be demonstrated. When a tendon is injured, it becomes extremely vascular and numerous collapsed capillaries can be identified 24 hours after trauma.[58] The inflammatory reaction proceeds as is commonly seen in all healing wounds and is directly related to the size of the wound and the extent of the trauma. Fibroblasts, which may arise from the epitenon, endotenon, or adjacent peritendinous tissues,[159] appear in the wound space in small numbers as early as day 2 or 3 after injury. They become more prominent between days 4 and 7 after division of the tendon, and by day 21, a mass of granulation tissue has formed. The newly formed capillaries arise mostly from the surrounding connective tissue and can be demonstrated by microangiographic techniques.[109]

Collagen synthesis increases sixfold, starting after the first week, and reaches a maximum after about 4 weeks. Even after 3 months, collagen synthesis is about three to four times normal, a situation that probably is related to active remodeling. Fibroblasts and collagen bundles become oriented longitudinally, and by 4 months the newly formed collagen bundles are identical microscopically to those of uninjured tendons.

Since healing depends mainly on the development and ingrowth of fibrovascular tissue from the peritendinous tissues,[226] adhesion formation is unavoidable. Because the wound and surrounding tissues are bathed in the same formed ground substance, adhesions form rapidly.[211] It is believed that early passive motion in a repaired tendon can alter these adhesions, causing them to become nonrestrictive elongated bands.[141]

The development of tensile strength correlates with collagen deposition in the early stages and with remodeling at a later stage, the latter starting probably 3 weeks after injury. However, a diminution in tensile strength characterizes the earliest phase of repair, lasting about 5 days.[182] The tendon becomes soft in the area of repair and if stretched does not hold the sutures properly. This weakness could be attributed to the developing tension on the tendon ends and subsequent ischemia. Although breaking strength is gained continuously with remodeling, Hirsch[108] found that breaking strength did not exceed maximum muscle power until 8 weeks after injury; at 24 weeks, it still was reduced by approximately 50% of preinjury levels.

Bone

In spite of its different structure and consistency, bone behaves very much like other tissues during healing in that repair takes place in three stages: inflammation, proliferation, and remodeling. Of all tissues, bone provides the perfect example of very extensive and essential remodeling to achieve adequate repair.

The process of fracture healing in cortical or compact bone (found in the skull and cortex of long bones) is quite different from that of cancellous or trabecular bone (found in the axial skeleton and metaphyseal regions of long bones). At the moment of fracture in the shaft of a long bone, blood vessels coursing in the canaliculi of haversian systems are torn at the fracture site. If internal fixation is applied with good approximation of bone fragments, bleeding is limited and healing is primary in nature. With external fixation, secondary healing takes place and a larger hematoma results, with blood clotting that extends for a short distance from the fracture site. Simultaneous necrosis of variable bone segments with their associated osteocytes takes place, and formed hematoma bridges the bone gap. A strong inflammatory reaction is induced, which is involved in the removal of necrotic tissue. Osteogenic cells (osteoblasts) from beneath the *periost* and the *endosteum* and undifferentiated mesenchymal cells in the surrounding soft tissues start proliferating. By day 6, a fibrous callus is formed as a result of collagen and glycosaminoglycan deposition and is transformed into a cartilaginous callus. Osteoclasts (multinuclear giant cells involved in bone resorption) gradually remove necrotic bone on either side of the fracture. As capillaries grow into the formed callus, ossification takes place for 1 to 2 weeks, and ultimately trabecular bone is formed. With remodeling taking place, excess callus is removed, and the newly formed bone assumes an architecture similar to that of normal bone. Osteoblasts and osteoclasts are both involved in remodeling, starting very early in fracture healing and becoming intensive 3 to 4 weeks after fracture.

Nervous System

The common belief is that regeneration does not occur in the central nervous system because of an inherent lack of regenerative capability in central neurons.[18] However, this concept currently is being challenged, and central neurons have been shown to be capable of regeneration.[308] The regenerative attempts of central neurons may in fact be blocked by other processes, such as connective tissue formation within the wound.[280] The significance of this finding in the context of repair and regeneration of the central nervous system awaits further investigation.

Peripheral nerves, on the other hand, have the potential for regeneration with accompanying functional recovery. The latter depends on the location, nature, and severity of the injury. Proximal injuries are associated with a poorer prognosis than distal injuries. If structural continuity is preserved and only nerve function is interrupted (neuropraxia), then complete recovery is the rule. Axonal damage with maintained continuity of surrounding mesodermal structures (axonotmesis) is followed by axonal regeneration, usually with complete recovery of function. However, with complete severance of the nerve structure (neurotmesis), the most severe form of injury, recovery often is incomplete.

Nerve transection is followed by a local inflammatory reaction and a series of events characteristic of nerve regeneration. In 24 to 48 hours, the nerve cell loses its dendritic connections, and axonolysis and myelin sheath disintegration occur for a variable distance proximally. Distally, wallerian degeneration is observed, with axonolysis and disintegration of the myelin sheath. Within 3 days, regeneration is already in progress, as evidenced by axonal sprouting and proliferation of Schwann cells. Schwann cells are also phagocytic, removing necrotic debris and establishing a path for the regenerating axons. To the extent that the structural framework of the distal nerve segment is preserved, regeneration is more effective in achieving functional continuity. Fibroblasts from the surrounding nerve sheaths form connective tissue that may prevent axonal progress and entry into the distal nerve segment.

FACTORS THAT MAY MODIFY WOUND HEALING

Clinical experience supported by extensive research has shown clearly that many factors can affect the inflammation-healing sequence. To modify them in favor of adequate healing, the surgeon must understand the effects of such factors and the mechanisms involved.

INJURY

Since the type of injury inflicted determines the amount of tissue necrosis and the degree to which the organism's homeostatic responses are taxed, wound healing may be directly or remotely affected.

Sharp Injuries

The surgeon most commonly is faced with sharp lacerations, best exemplified by surgical incisions and glass injuries. Tissue necrosis is minimal, and the wound often is clean, allowing healing by primary intention. The repair sequence takes place as previously described, and the wound is sealed from the external environment within 24 to 48 hours. The process of epithelization and contraction occurs to a minimum extent, and the best cosmetic result usually is achieved.

Crush Injuries

At the time of impact, appreciable soft-tissue compression accompanies crush injuries. Disruption of tissue continuity requires a large amount of absorbed energy, as opposed to that required by a mechanically shearing force. The consequences are more extensive tissue necrosis and altered architecture in surrounding areas; bacterial contamination is also more significant, this being determined by the circumstances of injury. These factors explain the increased infection rates and suboptimal quality of healing frequently observed in compression injuries.

When skin is involved, the original loss during injury and the subsequent debridement of necrotic tissue determine the ultimate defect. These variables, along with the extent of bacterial inoculation, dictate the method of wound closure, which may be primary, delayed primary, or secondary.

In specialized tissues, such as muscle or nerve, the adequacy of healing following crush injuries is affected largely by the size of the primary defect and the degree to which the connective tissue framework is preserved. When this framework remains intact, regeneration takes place and is more organized and complete, even with necrosis of the constituent fibers. In muscle, if the crush injury is localized, continuity can be restored with minimum scar formation and a variable degree of fiber disorientation.[8] However, poor regeneration and functional deficit result when the tissue defect is large or the connective tissue framework is affected adversely. With nerve injury, the main emphasis is on preserving continuity. When transection results from a compressive force, large segmental losses occur and grafting procedures are needed. Moderate to severe functional loss usually occurs.

Missile Injuries

The effect of projectile missiles—primarily bullets—on living tissue deserves separate mention because of the peculiar mechanisms of injury and their implications for subsequent wound management. Wound ballistics is the study of missile effects on living tissue.

Missile damage to tissues can occur via three mechanisms[208]: crushing and laceration, shock waves, and cavitation effect. Crushing and laceration result from the direct force of the bullet at the time of impact with tissues. A combination of shear and compressive forces results in a rather predictable pattern of injury. With a low-velocity missile, this is the principal mechanism of injury, and the injury usually is confined to the bullet's path. Serious injury results when the bullet actually strikes vital organs, blood vessels, and bone.

With high-velocity bullets (over 1000 m/sec), shock waves are generated in tissue by compressive forces. Such waves, although lasting for 15 to 25 microseconds, generate a high energy that causes little damage to muscle and bone but easily injures gas-filled organs.[106]

Bullets traveling at intermediate (over 330 m/sec) to high velocities can displace tissues in both forward and lateral directions, creating a real cavity. This cavity has a subatmospheric pressure and sucks air into the wound. Its size is determined largely by the bullet energy and the density of the tissue involved. This pulsatile cavity gradually decreases in size until it collapses. The remaining defect is larger in tissues with higher specific gravity. The area of devitalized tissue is even larger than the permanent cavity, reaching 30 to 40 times the diameter of the bullet. Therefore, the management of such wounds should include the excision of this necrotic area, which characteristically does not bleed with incision.

Delay of wound healing in bullet wounds is attributed to tissue necrosis and bacterial contamination. Potentially, pathogenic bacteria may be carried into the wound by the fired bullet and secondary projectiles, such as clothing, gunpowder, and shotgun shell wadding. These foreign bodies should be included in the area of debridement or removed by adequate irrigation.

Thermal Injuries

Burn trauma may influence wound healing by local and systemic mechanisms. Locally, deep dermal and full-thickness burns result in the destruction of cells and connective tissue matrix. Such wounds have been shown to heal much more slowly than excisional skin defects of similar dimensions. However, secondary excision of the necrotic burned tissue accelerates the healing process, which becomes comparable to healing in excisional wounds.[194]

When burns are extensive, many organs are affected in a characteristic fashion, resulting in the "burn syndrome." Initially, tissues such as bone marrow and epidermis show inhibition of cell growth. Rapid recovery follows in the bone marrow, as opposed to a more delayed recovery of epidermal cell growth.[12] Marked impairment of neutrophil[7] and macrophage[165] microbicidal functions also occurs, resulting in a primary delay in wound healing, which may be hindered further by subsequent malnutrition and infection. Infection is the leading cause of death in such patients.

AGE

Clinical experience suggests that wound healing is suboptimal in the elderly. Studies have consistently shown that most wound dehiscences occur in older patients.[189,230] Such patients also have a higher incidence of complications in bowel surgery, as manifested by leakage from or disruption of anastomoses.[123,251] The results of animal experiments are conflicting, probably because of differences in wound behavior between species and the various wound models used. Higher incidences of nutritional deficiency and systemic illnesses such as diabetes, atherosclerosis, uremia, and cirrhosis influence wound healing in the elderly. When such factors are accounted for, or managed perioperatively, surgery probably can be performed with infrequent wound complications in this age group. The main concern is directed to other major complications (pulmonary and cardiovascular) that may adversely affect wound healing.[88]

Fetal Wound Healing

The field of fetal wound healing has become increasingly complex.[5] Fetal wound healing has emerged as a remarkable process in which, in large animal models such as the sheep, virtually scarless healing occurs until the late gestational period, when a transition appears to take place toward adult healing.[164]

The role of the extracellular matrix is important in understanding fetal wound healing. It appears that fibronectin is deposited earlier in fetal wounds than in adult wounds,[161] as is tenascin, an extracellular glycoprotein matrix.[301] Fetal fibroblasts appear unusually proficient in producing collagen, a phenomenon that decreases with subsequent passages of cells in tissue culture.[279] Hyaluronic acid is a high-molecular-weight glycosaminoglycan of the extracellular matrix. It is found in very high concentrations in the embryo and whenever rapid tissue proliferation and regeneration occur.[282] It may play a role in cellular detachment during migration.[284] TGF-beta may be linked with hyaluronic acid–stimulating factor (HASF), which appears to promote the synthesis of only hyaluronic acid and no other extracellular matrix substances.[270] Studies are underway to define the role of hyaluronic acid and hyaluronidase in vivo.

Collagen deposition in a highly organized fashion occurs in fetal wound healing of various animal models, as demonstrated by immunohistochemical studies. Little is known about the mechanism of its organized, scarless deposition.

Fetal fractures created in vivo appear to heal with callus in a highly organized fashion. There are elements of enchondral bone healing, or the development of mature osteocytes from mesenchymal cells or chondroblasts without the usual chondrocyte hypertrophy and death steps. This supports the dedifferentiated state of fetal tissue at the time of injury.[163,192]

Growth factors play a pivotal role in fetal wound healing. Immunohistochemical studies have identified several patterns of growth factor expression in fetal skin over time. TGF-beta and bFGF were present in adult and neonatal wounds but not in fetal wounds. PDGF, however, was present in adult as well as fetal tissues.[300] TGF-beta is not present in significant quantities in tissues at the time when scarless healing occurs. When added to tissues in the fetal milieu, scar formation results.[150] This has led to investigation of the role of TGF-beta-1 involvement in scar formation (see the section on Cytokines). The role of growth factors in fetal wounds continues to be investigated.

MEDICATIONS

A surgical patient often is receiving systemic medication that may accelerate or delay wound healing. The surgeon should be able to make use of such information to maintain the best biologic environment for optimum repair.

Steroids and Vitamin A

Topical corticosteroids have been shown to inhibit epidermal wound healing in animals[309] and humans.[286] Comparisons of steroids of different anti-inflammatory potencies have shown that an intermediate agent (triamcinolone) delays epithelial regeneration, whereas a weaker one (hydrocortisone) has no effect. However, the two demonstrated similar inhibition of dermal collagen biosynthesis.[9] A similar pattern is observed in the healing of full-thickness wounds; a medium-strength steroid (fluocinolone) shows a greater inhibitory effect than a weaker one (hydrocortisone).[179]

Systemic anti-inflammatory steroids decrease the breaking strength of closed wounds,[108] delay reepithelization and angiogenesis,[245] and interfere with wound contraction.[267] These adverse effects are observed mostly when steroids are administered before or within 3 days after the wound occurs,[246] thus implicating their anti-inflammatory property as the principal mode of action. However, the effect on wound contraction still is observed with later administration.

In practice, usual doses of steroids appear to cause only a mild delay in the healing of sutured wounds, a delay that becomes significant only occasionally. When patients are receiving chronic steroid therapy or taking very high doses, healing is more significantly impaired. If administration cannot be delayed until after day 4 following the injury, two alternatives may prove beneficial. The steroid used may be replaced with cortisol, which has a reduced anti-inflammatory action compared with other steroids. The dosage of cortisol also may be transiently reduced during the critical inflammatory phase of healing. Because the anti-inflammatory action of steroids is attributed partly to lysosomal membrane stabilization, concurrent administration of vitamin A may reverse the inhibitory effects of steroids by labilizing such membranes.[298] In fact, vitamin A has been shown to accelerate wound strength gain[70] and reepithelization[114] in steroid-inhibited wounds. Wound contraction[267] and increased susceptibility to infection,[269] however, are not significantly reversed. A daily dose of 25,000 IU appears to benefit such patients. Since vitamin A can restimulate both humoral and cell-mediated immune mechanisms,[49] a topical preparation can be used without affecting any required immunosuppression. In the absence of steroid inhibition, vitamin A has no stimulatory effects on wound healing.[114]

Nonsteroidal Anti-inflammatory Drugs

Commonly used nonsteroidal anti-inflammatory agents (NSAIDs) such as salicylates,[152] and phenylbutazone,[289] have been shown to decrease the tensile strength of healing wounds in the experimental animal. Clinically, therapeutic doses probably have no effect on wound healing. In fact, flurbiprofen was found to improve colonic anastomotic healing with a significant increase in collagen production.[32] Topical NSAIDs reduce inflammation but do not affect the healing process to any significant extent.[9]

Antineoplastic Drugs

Antineoplastic drugs are used frequently as adjuvants to surgical therapy in a combined modality approach to cancer treatment. Since their mode of action is selective inhibition of the most actively dividing cells, such agents may exert adverse effects on wound healing.

Animal experiments, with some conflicting results, provide evidence for the deleterious effects of antineoplastic agents on wound healing.[38,52,60,265] Clinically these findings have little substantial support. Differences in experimental models related to dosage, species-specific dose responses to various agents, and times of administration relative to wounding may explain this discrepancy.

Until further clinical studies support the present experimental findings, the benefit of effective adjuvant chemotherapy appears to outweigh the questionable risk of wound complications in several situations.

Vitamin E

High doses of vitamin E can inhibit collagen synthesis and wound repair. Stabilization of lysosomal membranes has been suggested as a mechanism of action. Vitamin A or anabolic steroids can reverse the inhibitory effects,[71] but in usual doses retardation of wound healing is not likely to be significant.

Phenytoin

Prolonged use of phenytoin commonly results in gingival hyperplasia with occasional cases of retroperitoneal fibrosis, suggesting a stimulatory effect on collagen metabolism. Addition of the drug in tissue cultures enhances proliferation of fibroblasts.[256] Furthermore, phenytoin has been reported to enhance the rate of healing of leg ulcers.[261] The mechanism of action is not completely understood; recent studies tend to support an anticollagenase activity.[20]

Anticoagulants

Anticoagulants predispose to hematoma formation in surgical wounds. This formation predisposes to wound dehiscence and infection and blocks the migration of fibroblasts and other cells into the wound space, preventing the healing process from taking place. Therefore, anticoagulant medications are better avoided in the perioperative period unless the benefit of their use outweighs the risk of hematoma formation. This decision must take into account such factors as prosthetic cardiac values, recent cardiovascular events, ocular surgery, and the patient's coagulation status.

Penicillin G

Penicillamine, a metabolic product of penicillin degradation, blocks collagen cross-links by reacting with free aldehyde groups.[202] This finding led to the suspicion that penicillin G may inhibit wound healing. However, in doses used clinically, penicillin G has no such effect.[220]

Cyclosporin A

Cyclosporin A is an immunosuppressant commonly used in clinical transplantation. In contradistinction to the inhibitory effect of steroids on wound healing, cyclosporin A does not affect collagen synthesis, granulation tissue formation,[6] or wound breaking strength.[72] It has been reported that wound healing is even improved in patients treated with this agent.[258]

HOST DISEASE FACTORS

Malnutrition

Proteins

In the face of surgical stress and the ensuing catabolic state, the patient faces an increase in nutritional requirements to achieve adequate wound healing.[199]

Protein deficiency has long been observed to affect wound healing. The inflammatory phase is prolonged and fibroplasia is impaired during protein depletion.[231] Angiogenesis, connective tissue formation, and wound remodeling also are affected adversely.[221] In open wounds, protein malnutrition results in a significant delay of wound contraction and the formation of granulation tissue.[191] Rats given a protein-free diet experience progressive weight loss and a significant decrease in the breaking strength of sutured skin and abdominal wounds.[121] Healing of intestinal wounds, however, is affected to a much lesser extent.

Methionine and cysteine reverse the prolongation of the inflammatory phase and increase the rate of fibroplasia after protein depletion.[69] Recent evidence suggests that increased arginine levels in intravenous hyperalimentation solutions improve wound healing.[16]

The development of modern nutritional therapy has eliminated many nutritional deficiencies that can delay wound healing. Adequate nutritional assessment and therapy help minimize postoperative wound complications.[123,197] However, there is no evidence to support the routine use of hyperalimentation in uncomplicated surgical procedures.[199]

Vitamin C

The importance of vitamin C in collagen synthesis and wound healing cannot be overemphasized. In the absence of vitamin C, fibroblast function is impaired and lysine residues are not hydroxylated, resulting in a decrease in collagen cross-linking. This is reflected in a poor quality of healing and in capillary fragility. These effects are promptly reversed after administration of vitamin C. Recommended intake is 500 mg a day.

No evidence indicates that supplemental vitamin C accelerates wound healing in a nondeficiency state. However, surgical trauma or serious illness may cause vitamin C deficiency; to prevent wound complications in such cases, administration of vitamin C can be beneficial.

Zinc

Zinc is a constituent of many enzymes; among these RNA and DNA polymerases are involved directly in protein synthesis and subsequently in wound healing. Several studies indicate that wound healing is impaired with low serum zinc levels[44,153]; correcting this deficiency results in normal healing rates. Despite some controversy, zinc supplementation in the absence of a deficiency does not appear to accelerate wound healing above normal rates. The normal level is 120 ± 20 μg/dl (18 ± 3 μmol/L). Recommended daily intake is 15 mg a day.

Anemia, Hypovolemia, and Hypoxia

The effect of anemia on wound healing often is compounded by the associated hypovolemia or hypoxia. When these variables are considered separately, anemia alone has no deleterious effect on wound healing.[107] Clinical studies have shown that hypovolemia is associated with a higher incidence of wound complications.[187] In both situations, the local microcirculation and subsequent tissue oxygenation appear to be the major determinants of normal wound healing. Reducing the inspired-oxygen concentration to 10% results in a significant decrease in wound tensile strength in experimental animals.[268] Interestingly, animals kept on 40% inspired oxygen have increased wound tensile strength compared with control animals kept at 20%. Hyperbaric or 45% oxygen also enhances the healing of open full-thickness skin wounds; this effect occurs only in ischemic wounds.[139] Collagen synthesis is increased above normal in hyperoxia, and its accumulation is related closely to arterial Po_2.[117]

Oxygen also contributes to tissue resistance to infection that may in itself delay wound healing. With higher values of inspired oxygen, leukocyte microbicidal function is improved significantly,[111,142] and susceptibility to infection is decreased markedly.[116]

All this evidence supports the current belief that wound healing can be further stimulated to achieve above-normal rates and quality.

Wound Infection and the Germ-Free State

Surgical wounds frequently are contaminated with bacteria. Local wound factors, such as tissue necrosis, foreign bodies, and hematomas, or systemic impairment of defense mechanisms may allow the bacterial contamination to progress to invasive infection. Bacterial products and the elicited cell-mediated immune responses augment tissue damage[34] and subsequently delay wound healing.

Preventing bacterial infection requires using meticulous aseptic technique, minimizing tissue necrosis, obtaining adequate hemostasis, and eliminating dead space. Using prophylactic antibiotics is also beneficial in some situations.[100]

The effect of microbial flora on wound healing has been studied with conflicting results. Poor formation of granulation tissue and diminished vascular proliferation have been observed in wounds of germ-free guinea pigs compared to conventional animals.[190] However, no differences have been found in the healing rate or histologic characteristics of the wound in germ-free mice compared to conventional mice.[241] Using open-wound contraction as a determinant of wound healing, Donati and colleagues found no apparent differences in the rate of wound contraction when they compared germ-free and conventional wounds.[64] However, conventional wounds demonstrated a more severe, acute inflammatory reaction, more rapid formation of granulation tissue, and more rapid epithelization of the wound margin.

Vascular Diseases

Atherosclerosis

Atherosclerosis is the major cause of arterial insufficiency encountered in surgical wounds. This disease may lead to impaired blood supply and a subsequent decrease in the delivery of oxygen and nutrients to the wound. Wound healing is subsequently delayed and may evolve into a chronic phase of nonhealing.

Atherosclerotic arterial insufficiency also may result in chronic skin ulcers characterized by a black base and minimal granulation tissue. The lesions often are painful and surrounded by thinned skin with no hair.

Incompetent Veins

Loss of competence of the venous valvular system may result from inflammatory conditions, prolonged standing, and pregnancy. The resultant elevation in venous pressure and associated edema interfere with the local capillary blood flow.[149] The subsequent tissue hypoxia and delay in nutrient delivery adversely affect wound healing. Varicose veins are also one of the most common causes of chronic skin ulcers. These are characterized by a significant amount of exudate and granulation tissue, as well as findings of venous insufficiency in the surrounding skin, such as edema, dermatitis, and rusty pigmentation.

Diabetes

Diabetes is often associated with poor wound healing. Granulocytes from diabetic patients demonstrate decreased phagocytic activity[36] and poor chemotaxis.[198] These granulocyte defects and local ischemia secondary to accelerated atherosclerosis and small-vessel disease result in increased susceptibility to infection with mixed pathogens, including anaerobes and gram-negative organisms. All these factors have deleterious effects on wound healing. Other cellular abnormalities attributed to diabetes mellitus include most notably phagocytic, intracellular killing and margination defects by both polymorphonuclear leukocytes (PMNs) and macrophages.[31] Defects in lymphocytic function have also been noted.[218]

Peripheral neuropathy with subsequent loss of pain sensation contributes to the progression of small injuries and limited infection, which are often neglected because of minimal symptomatology. Alterations in the endoneurial vasculature have been noted, as well as a host of other neuronal abnormalities.[283] Peripheral neuropathy in diabetes mellitus differs from that found in ischemia induced by arteriosclerotic disease.

In experimental animals, diabetes mellitus results in decreased accumulation of wound collagen.[198] A decrease in tensile strength of incised wounds has also been reported.[227] In the absence of insulin resistance, insulin improves wound healing only when it is given immediately after injury. Delayed institution of insulin therapy beyond the initial (inflammatory) phase of healing results in no improvement. Hyperglycemia is defined as blood glucose above 200 mg/dl 2 hours after 75 μg glucose challenge. Ideal blood glucose is defined as 140 mg/dl or higher fasting and over 20 mg/dl 2 hours after a 75-mg glucose meal.

A number of microvascular abnormalities have been described in diabetes mellitus. The microangiopathy previously thought to be present as a result of diabetes was described by Goldenberg and coworkers in a retrospective study of amputation specimens.[87] The premise of microangiopathy has subsequently been challenged.[54,154] The ulcers found in diabetics are characterized by tissue and transcutaneous oxygen tensions, which do not differ from those of nondiabetic controls.[313] Local, nonanatomic relative ischemia may result from membrane stiffening on the erythrocyte due to nonenzymatic glycosylation of membrane protein spectrin,[175] a phenomenon that appears to reverse with normoglycemia.[128]

Hyperglycemia itself can induce an increase in glycosylated hemoglobin, causing a deleterious shift in the oxygen-hemoglobin dissociation curve.[169] With the realization that diabetic microangiopathy does not exist as a predominant entity in diabetes mellitus, more aggressive management and reconstructive efforts, even microsurgery, are now offered to diabetic patients.

Jaundice

Jaundiced patients have a significantly higher incidence of wound dehiscence and incisional hernias as compared to anicteric patients.[11] However, clinical and experimental studies have failed to determine whether jaundice alone accounts for the observed effects on wound healing. Clinical jaundice often is associated with poor nutritional status. Nutritional therapy is beneficial in the jaundiced patient and can result in adequate healing. Malignancy, with associated malnutrition, also may be a major cause of impaired healing.[273]

Uremia

Uremia impairs wound healing,[89] and in the absence of significant weight loss, formation of granulation tissue also is delayed.[186] Uremic serum inhibits the growth of fibroblasts in tissue culture.[53] These findings suggest a direct detrimental effect of uremia on wound healing, which adequate dialysis can reverse. Uremia sufficient to inhibit wound healing occurs when the GFR is <2% of normal with sequela of renal failure.

Malignancy

Cancer patients frequently are in a state of protein-calorie malnutrition. The various chemotherapeutic agents also have side effects. Therefore, the cause of the increased incidence of wound complications[230] in such patients is probably multifactorial. However, it appears that malignancy can delay wound healing in the absence of complicating factors. Tumor-bearing rats have a significant decrease in wound tensile strength without experiencing any anorexia or weight loss.[57] In the absence of tumor, greater nutritional deprivation is required to obtain the same degree of impairment in wound breaking strength.[195] A tumor-induced metabolic disturbance has been suggested, because intravenous hyperalimentation restores the quality of wound healing to normal.

Acquired Immune Deficiency Syndrome

Patients with acquired immune deficiency syndrome (AIDS) are prone to systemic and local opportunistic infections. Several cellular abnormalities have been discovered, some of which may affect wound healing. Interleukin-1 (IL-1) coordinates a number of cellular interactions involved with the inflammatory cascade and wound healing. IL-1 production appears to be decreased in AIDS.[312] Anorectal wounds in particular may heal poorly in patients with AIDS, although the results in well-studied groups no longer support the nihilistic attitude of physicians toward anorectal wounds.[244] The breaking strength of wounds and the hydroxyproline content in polyvinyl alcohol sponges is decreased with global T cell depletion.[215] The systematic study of AIDS and wound healing will be a fruitful area of research in the immediate future.

Irradiation

The modern treatment of cancer frequently involves a multidisciplinary approach combining surgery and radiation. The deleterious effects of ionizing radiation on skin and wound healing have been observed clinically and experimentally. Although the mechanism of cell injury is not clear yet, DNA injury by the generated high-energy electrons and free radicals most likely occurs in rapidly dividing cells, which are most sensitive to this type of injury.

Several changes occur in moderately irradiated tissues. In the acute period, within several weeks after radiation therapy, erythema and desquamation of epithelia develop. Vascular and connective tissue damage is still minimal. As the chronic period begins, within 4 to 6 months, the epidermis appears thin and hyperpigmented. A characteristic finding is the decrease in vascular supply secondary to an obliterative endarteritis. Capillaries are progressively fewer in number, with telangiectatic dilatation of the remaining ones. Fibrosis of subcutaneous tissue is also prominent and directly related to the irradiation dose. These chronic changes are irreversible.

The timing of irradiation in relation to a wound is a major factor in determining the severity of adverse effects on healing. Studies on the effect of preoperative irradiation on wound healing show conflicting results. Moore has reported that proper fractionation, over 3 to 5 weeks, of modest radiation doses, given 3 to 6 weeks before surgery, prevents significant impairment of wound healing.[195] However, the benefit of such therapy should be weighed against the risk of injury to vital structures that may be exposed to radiation.

A high incidence of complications accompanies surgery performed on tissues with signs of chronic radiation changes.[127] Fibrosis and diminished vascular supply significantly impair wound healing. Infection is promoted and may result in tissue necrosis, further compounding the original insult. If radiation therapy is started 3 weeks postoperatively, wound healing is generally adequate.[195] However, chronic radiation effects cannot be prevented.

Denervation

Paraplegic patients are susceptible to decubitus ulcers and wound complications. The basic mechanism is believed to be direct pressure over soft tissues, with subsequent ischemia and necrosis. Loss of sensation and physical disability help promote this mechanism of injury. Even without external pressure, wounds below the level of spinal denervation appear to heal poorly.[19]

TECHNICAL FACTORS

Surgical Technique

Surgical technique, an important and controllable factor, has a major influence on wound healing. Expert medical care and an adequate local milieu do not replace the need for a meticulous, aseptic surgical technique.

Tissues should be handled gently to minimize necrosis that may promote infection and delay healing. Adequate hemostasis is required, because hematomas constitute a nidus for infection and prevent migration of fibroblasts and formation of capillaries. Foreign bodies can transform minimal bacterial contamination into overt infection and also can block the progression of normal healing. Careful apposition of wound edges promotes faster healing. Dead space, which may allow collections to form and secondary infection to occur, should be obliterated. Tight sutures and strangulation of tissues by ligatures result in tissue ischemia and necrosis. Electrocoagulation must be used judiciously and precisely. Local anesthetics have been shown to retard wound healing and inhibit collagen and glycosaminoglycan synthesis.[45,196] Use of local anesthetics in nonhealing wounds should be considered carefully, keeping in mind the potential adverse effects on healing.

Suture Materials

Many suture materials have been introduced for use in wound closure. The suture material selected for wound closure has a direct bearing on the quality of subsequent repair. However, as a general rule, suture material does not affect wound collagen synthesis per se.[288]

Sutures can be divided into two categories according to their fate in tissues: absorbable and nonabsorbable (Table 11-5). Tissue enzymes gradually digest absorbable sutures of biologic origin (catgut); hydrolysis principally breaks down those of synthetic origin (polyglycolic acid, polyglactin, polydioxanone). Nonabsorbable sutures (silk, polyamides, polyesters, polypropylene) usually persist within tissues, although silk may disappear after 2 years, and nylon has been reported to degrade slowly.

For wounds requiring long-term support (fascia) or permanent support (vascular prostheses), a nonabsorbable suture is selected. Bacterial contamination may progress to infection in the presence of sutures; absorbable material is preferred in this context. Polyglycolic acid (PGA) sutures serve this purpose well; degradation products of PGA are thought to have a bactericidal action.[67] Polydioxanone (PDS), a new synthetic absorbable suture, has been advocated for use in closure of infected wounds. Compared with other suture material, PDS has been shown to have the least affinity toward both *Staphylococcus aureus* and *Escherichia coli*.[41] However, the superiority of PDS over PGA with enteric wound infection has recently been challenged.[129] In the urinary and biliary tracts, a nonabsorbable foreign material acts as a nidus for stone formation, particularly if bacteria are also present. Because of this, rapidly absorbed sutures are preferred in such locations.

Suture materials can be classified further according to physical configuration. A monofilament suture, made of a single strand, resists bacterial adherence and ties down smoothly. A multifilament suture (braided) consists of several filaments twisted together. Braiding gives better handling and tying qualities but may increase bacterial adherence within suture interstices. Coating braided sutures decreases tissue drag, allows for smooth tying, and may reduce bacterial adherence. In fact, evidence suggests that the coating material may have a more important influence on bacterial adhesion than the physical configuration.[41]

Suture selection should be based on three general principles: the natural strength and healing rates of different tissues, foreign body behavior, and cosmesis. The first principle dictates suture size and the duration of needed mechanical support until healing is achieved. Foreign body behavior of nonabsorbable sutures precludes their use in contaminated or infected wounds and in tissues with a propensity to stone formation. Where wound appearance is important, the smallest inert monofilament suture materials are used; subcuticular closure is also preferred, supported by skin closure tape (e.g., Steri-Strips) where necessary.

Wound Coverage

Wound dressing constitutes a major part of wound care and has a direct influence on the course of healing. Ideally, a dressing should protect wounds against mechanical trauma and bacterial seeding and provide a local milieu considered optimal for wound healing.

Clean wounds closed primarily can be covered with simple dry dressings during the early phases of healing. A nonstick dressing (e.g., Telfa) is preferred. Recently developed synthetic dressings (e.g., OpSite, Tegaderm) have been used to cover sutured wounds and offer several advantages over dry dressings. OpSite is made of a gas-permeable polyurethane adhesive film that allows free passage of oxygen, carbon dioxide, and water vapor while preventing bacteria from entering the wound space. If drainage is minimal, the dressing can be kept

TABLE 11-5 GENERAL FEATURES OF ABSORBABLE (A) AND NONABSORBABLE (NA) SUTURE MATERIALS

SUTURE	RAW MATERIAL	TENSILE STRENGTH (IN VIVO)	TISSUE REACTION	FREQUENT USES
Surgical gut (A) plain	Collagen from sheep or beef intestine	Lost within 7-10 days; faster with severe inflammation; varies with patient characteristics	Moderate	Suture subcutaneous and rapidly healing tissues
Surgical gut (A) chromic	Collagen from sheep or beef intestine; treated to resist digestion	Lost within 21-28 days; varies with patient characteristics	Moderate; less than plain surgical gut	May be used in infected tissues; intended use as an absorbable suture in slowly healing tissues
Polyglactin (A) coated (Vicryl)	Copolymer of lactide and glycolide coated with polyglactin and calcium stearate	Approximately 60% remains at 2 weeks, and 30% at 3 weeks	Mild	Used where an absorbable suture is desired
Polydioxanone (A) (PDS)	Polyester polymer	Approximately 70% remains at 2 weeks, 50% at 4 weeks, and 25% at 6 weeks	Slight	Abdominal and thoracic closure; subcutaneous tissue, colorectal surgery; can be used in infected tissues
Polyglycolic acid (A) (Dexon "S")	Glycolic acid polymer	Approximately 45% remains at 3 weeks	Mild	Peritoneal, fascial, and subcutaneous closures; ligature replaces surgical gut in most applications
Surgical silk (NA)	Protein fiber spun by silkworm	Loses most or all in about 1 year	Moderate	Suturing and ligation; contraindicated in infected tissues; avoid in biliary and urinary tracts
Surgical cotton (NA)	Long-staple cotton fibers	Loses 50% in 6 months, and 70% in 2 years	Minimal	Suturing and ligation in most body tissues; contraindicated in infected tissues
Surgical steel	Alloy of iron-nickel-chromium	Indefinite	Low	Abdominal and sternal closures, retention, tendon repair
Nylon (NA) (Ethilon, Dermalon)	Polyamide polymer	Loses 15%-25% per year	Extremely low	Skin closure, retention, microsurgery, tendon repair, Pull-out suture
Polypropylene (NA) (Prolene, Surgilene)	Polymer of propylene	Indefinite	Minimal	General closure, vascular anastomoses, pull-out suture
Polyethylene terephthalate (NA) (Dacron, Mersilene Ethibond, Ti·Cron)	Polyester polyethylene terephthalate	Indefinite	Minimal	Ti·Cron and Ethibond are coated, supple in handling, and are especially useful in implanting heart valves and vascular prostheses; general closures; retention

in place for up to 7 days. Its transparency allows for easy wound inspection, and the patient can resume normal activities with the dressing in place. OpSite has been successfully used to cover split-thickness graft donor sites, with a significant decrease in patient discomfort and pain.

Draining and infected wounds require dressings that can absorb exudate and remove necrotic tissue remnants after surgical debridement. Wide-mesh cotton gauze applied to the wound surface traps necrotic debris and exudate in its interstices, and those are removed when the dressing is changed. When this layer is dry, adequate mechanical debridement is achieved, with more pain, however, and possible detachment of regenerating epidermal cells. Dampening or wetting this layer allows for easier dressing removal and dilution of the exudate, but debridement becomes less efficient, and the absorptive properties of the dressing are decreased. A second layer of absorbent cotton usually is applied over the cotton gauze. This layer can be moistened with saline or an antibacterial solution to soften necrotic debris, dilute exudate that is drawn into the cotton gauze by capillary action, and provide antibacterial activity. One should be aware, however, of the reported cytotoxicity of several antiseptic agents, with possible deleterious effects on wound healing.[160]

When skin loss is extensive, biologic dressings frequently are helpful in achieving wound coverage and protection against bacterial invasion and excessive evaporative water loss. Human skin (allografts), skin from another species (xenografts), and various skin substitutes have been used. Cutaneous allografts are the most frequently used in many centers and are still the most effective biologic dressings. Compared with gauze dressings, they are less painful, have significantly less bacterial contamination, and may hasten and improve the quality of healing. However, biologic dressings should not be applied to burns before removal of necrotic debris or eschar, or to wounds with a level of bacterial growth of 10^5 or greater per gram of tissue. Totally synthetic composite membranes can be applied to excised wounds or wounds with clean granulation tissue.

MANAGEMENT OF THE CONTAMINATED WOUND

The closure of wounds has been a subject for debate for many centuries. With the advent of aseptic techniques, primary closure of clean wounds has become common practice, with wound infection rates below 5%. However, primary closure of contaminated wounds has consistently resulted in wound infection and dehiscence. Experience with civilian and war wounds, coupled with the elucidation of several principles of wound healing and bacteriology, has allowed for safe delayed primary closure of significantly contaminated wounds.

WOUND PREPARATION

The preparation of a contaminated wound involves eliminating local factors that may promote infection and impair healing. Necrotic tissue should be debrided. Subsequent excision of necrotic tissue may be necessary as it becomes more clearly demarcated. Foreign bodies should be removed by irrigation or included with the debrided tissue.

Irrigation plays a major role in reducing the bacterial population to noninfective levels. Pressure irrigation delivered forcefully with a 35 ml syringe through an 18-gauge needle[271] and pulsating water jet lavage[33,95] have proved more effective than bulb syringe or gravity flow irrigation. Systemic antibiotic prophylaxis is indicated in the closure of moderately and heavily contaminated wounds. Cultures and drug sensitivity testing determine the selection of appropriate antibiotics for chronic wounds. In acutely contaminated wounds, knowledge of local bacterial flora or other likely contaminants would dictate the choice of antibiotic. The role of topical antimicrobials is less defined. Although their benefit in contaminated burn wounds has been established, their necessity is questionable in preparation for delayed primary closure.

TIMING OF WOUND CLOSURE

Initially applied sterile dressings are not changed for 3 to 4 days after surgery. Then, under sterile conditions, the dressing is removed and the wound is inspected. If a suggestion of established infection or incomplete debridement exists, the wound may be cleansed, debrided, and dressed again, with a later attempt at closure. Alternatively, the wound may be allowed to heal by secondary intention. When the tissue defect is extensive, coverage achieved by well-perfused muscle or musculocutaneous flaps may resolve contamination and fight incipient infection. If the wound shows no evidence of infection, it is closed after another 24 hours. It appears that delayed primary closure is best accomplished at 4 to 6 days after debridement.[68,195]

Timing of wound closure can also be adjusted to quantitative wound cultures. When the bacterial count per gram of tissue exceeds 10^5, wound closure is associated with a 100% infection rate.[148] Hence, a more aggressive management can be adopted with periodic debridement monitored by mapping and quantitative culture of contaminated foci.[148] This technique has the double benefit of reducing the incidence of wound infection following delayed primary closure and converting dirty and infected wounds into a more favorable category for closure. The skin is closed with Steri-Strips, and dead space is obliterated with closed-suction drains. Occasionally, in obese patients, closure is more secure and wound edges are better approximated with sutures preplaced at the time of surgery. Minimally reactive sutures (nylon, polypropylene, polydioxanone) are chosen in this situation.

SCAR TISSUE

The imperfection of the wound healing process is seen in the formation of a connective tissue scar that may simply seal wound edges or replace larger skin defects. Scar tissue causes much concern because of the deleterious functional consequences resulting from its formation in several organs of the body. Urethral and esophageal strictures may form after tissue injury and culminate in mechanical obstruction. Peritoneal adhesions frequently have been reported to cause intestinal

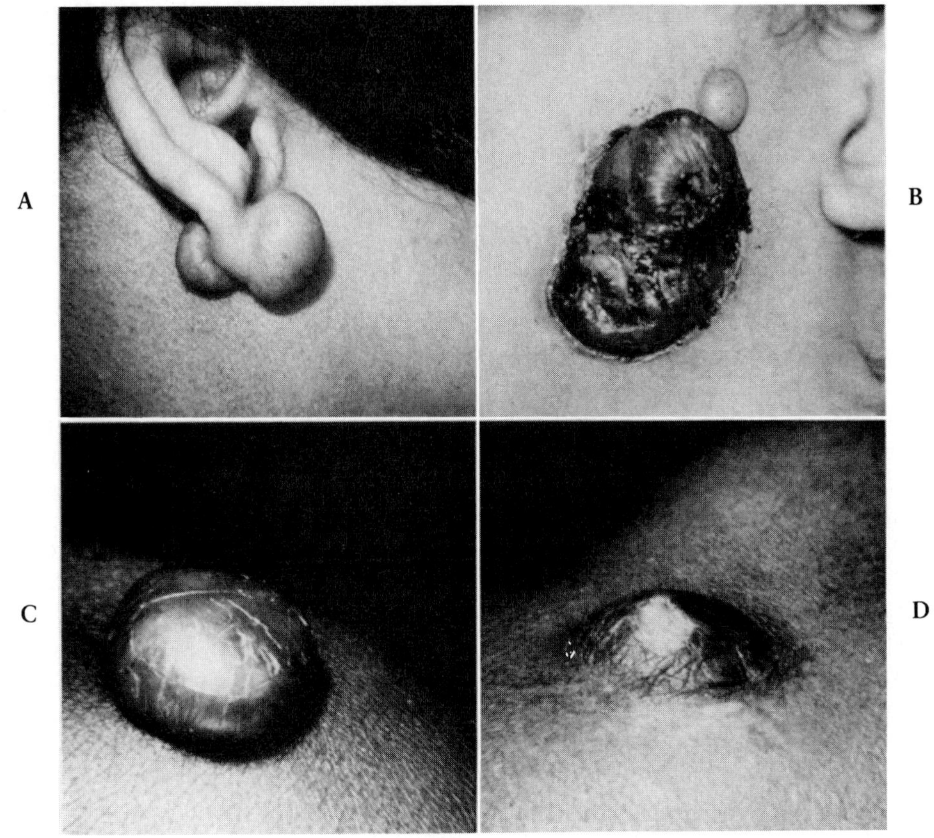

FIGURE 11-20 Keloids. **A,** Pedunculated keloid from ear piercing. **B,** Factitious factors (self-induced scratching) led to keloids. Further injury led to bleeding and the appearance of a pigmented lesion. **C,** Keloid in vaccination scar. **D,** Keloid after triamcinolone injections.

obstruction. Scar tissue surrounding injured or repaired tendons often results in significant limitation of the gliding mechanism. Furthermore, joint contractures, with restricted mobility, can develop from hypertrophic or inappropriately directed scars.

"Surface overhealing," which includes keloids and hypertrophic scars, is often distressing for both patient and surgeon. Because the management of these lesions is still controversial and results often are suboptimal, a separate discussion is in order.

HYPERTROPHIC SCARS AND KELOIDS

Definition

Despite several attempts to differentiate hypertrophic scars from keloids on an etiologic or biochemical basis, the distinction between these lesions is often clinical. Keloids (Figure 11-20) are defined as raised scars that extend beyond the confines of the original wound[213] and invade surrounding tissue, behaving in fact as pseudotumors. Recurrence is the rule after simple excision. Hypertrophic scars (Figure 11-21), although raised, remain within the boundaries of the wound and may regress spontaneously. When persistent, these lesions are treated surgically with successful results. However, in many situations a large hypertrophic scar merges imperceptibly into a keloid, making clinical distinction impossible and

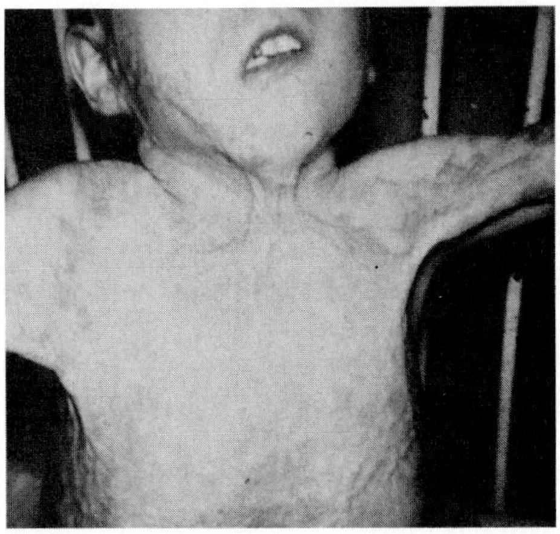

FIGURE 11-21 Hypertrophic scar.

probably unnecessary. Such lesions are better handled as keloids to prevent their recurrence.

Etiology

Keloids and hypertrophic scars are likely to result from a number of factors. Identifying the factors involved may help the clinician decide on their management.

Overabundant scar production has long been noted to occur in areas of increased skin tension. Excised keloids atrophy when grafted into an area of little tension.[37] Furthermore, hypertrophic scars often are treated successfully by surgical maneuvers that tend to reduce skin tension, such as Z-plasty or excision with skin grafting.

Chronic hypoxia is thought to be involved in the development of hypertrophic scars.[135] This theory is supported by observed microvascular occlusion in hypertrophic scars and keloids[137] and by direct measurement of tissue gases.[263] As previously noted, a certain degree of hypoxia induces collagen synthesis by fibroblasts at the wound site. From the therapeutic standpoint, mechanical pressure probably increases hypoxia and results in focal degeneration when applied for long periods (6 to 9 months or longer).

Immune-inflammatory mechanisms have also been implicated in the pathogenesis of keloid scars.[50] Initially suggested by Chylitova and colleagues,[46] this theory was substantiated by the detection of keloid immunoglobulin levels significantly greater than those in normal skin or scar controls.[51,136] However, no differences in serum immunoglobulins could be found among subjects with keloids, hypertrophic scars, mature scars, and normal skin. Hence, quite probably the local immune response may trigger and then sustain a chronic inflammatory reaction with overabundant collagen deposition.

Mast cells frequently have been observed in hypertrophic scars and keloids.[134] Their degranulated appearance suggests active release of histamine, which has established fibroblast-stimulating properties. Elevated histamine levels may also explain the pruritus that often accompanies these lesions.

A familial predilection for keloid formation has been noted. Both autosomal dominant and autosomal recessive patterns have been reported.[30,205] Keloids also are more commonly observed in blacks than in whites. This familial and race-related incidence is observed much less frequently in simple hypertrophic scars.

Biochemically, altered collagen and ground substance kinetics provide intriguing mechanisms of pathologic scar formation, with remarkable therapeutic applications. The basic abnormality is an overabundance of collagen in a ground substance that also has elevated glycosaminoglycan content (mainly chondroitin-6-sulfate). Increased collagen deposition results from enhanced production per fibroblast[50] rather than from an increased number of fibroblasts, each producing a normal amount of collagen. Collagenase activity per tissue dry weight has been found similar in keloid and normal dermal biopsies. However, in tissue culture, collagenase activity has been found to be elevated significantly in keloid compared with normal dermis fibroblast media.[185] The role of glycosaminoglycans in collagenase activity is not yet clear.

CONTROL OF SCAR TISSUE

Local Measures

The mainstay of hypertrophic scar treatment is surgery (Figure 11-22) designed to relieve tension. Such procedures as Z-plasty, excision and grafting, and flap repair often yield good results. The timing of excision is related directly to the maturity of the scar. This may take 6 months to 2 years and is recognized by a change from reddish to pale white discoloration. However, keloids characteristically recur after simple surgical excision and often become larger. Hence, surgery serves mainly to remove excess collagenous tissue; recurrence is prevented by the use of various adjuvant modalities. Intralesional excision of keloids, leaving a tiny rim of keloid scar and a thin surface that does not expose subcutaneous tissue, is advised. This technique allows for splinting of the scar bed and, perhaps more importantly, preservation of the physical integrity of the deepest layer of normal dermis.[212] The collagen kinetics of normal quiescent tissue are not altered, and stimulation of a new keloid formation is avoided.

Local injection of the corticosteroid triamcinolone (9-fluoroacetonide) has become increasing popular in the treatment of keloids. It may be used alone for small

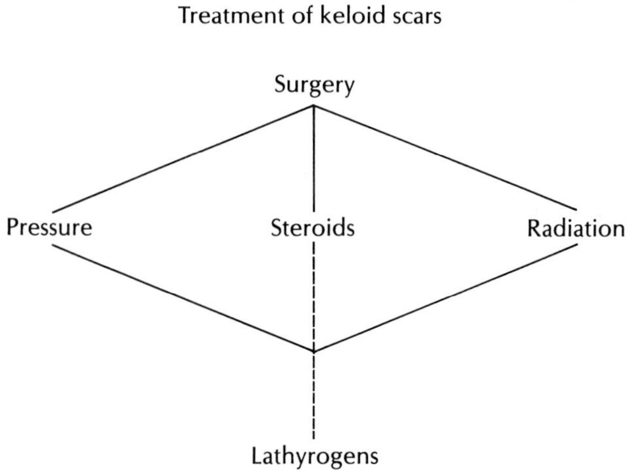

FIGURE 11-22 Therapeutic alternatives in the treatment of keloid scars. In previously established keloids, surgery is always advised to reduce scar collagen load and is combined with one or more of the adjuvant treatments.

lesions or in combination with surgical excision. A 40 mg/ml solution is commonly used, not exceeding a dosage of 80 mg every 6 weeks.[50] Injection of normal skin should be avoided to prevent the complications of skin atrophy and hypopigmentation. The mechanisms of action are probably enhancement of collagenase activity and inhibition of collagen synthesis.

Application of constant pressure has been reported to reduce postburn contracture and hypertrophic scar formation.[22] Custom-made garments can apply an adequate amount of pressure over a wide area. These should be worn at least 12 to 18 hours a day for a minimum of 6 to 9 months. However, this technique often is limited by the heat induced by the tight garment, patient discomfort, and difficulty in design for several areas of the body. A sponge fixation method has been described and found successful in treating early hypertrophic scars and reducing keloid recurrence after excision.[78] Tissue hypoxia and mechanical splinting may be involved, but the exact mechanisms require further investigation.

Radiation has been used successfully to prevent recurrence of keloids after surgical excision.[120,158] Therapy consisting of up to 1800 rad delivered in 300 rad fractions over 1 to 2 weeks has been recommended. Interstitial radiotherapy using a locally implanted ^{192}iridium wire has also been successful.[103] Given the possible risk of carcinogenesis, this modality is better reserved for tenacious keloids found to be refractory to various modes of therapy.

Systemic Anticollagenous Therapy

The purpose of systemic anticollagenous therapy is to correct an abnormal balance between collagen synthesis and degradation in favor of reduced scar formation. Many agents that regulate various steps of collagen metabolism are available.

Proline analogs (*cis*-hydroxyproline, azetidine carboxylic acid) are structurally similar to proline and hence are easily incorporated into newly synthesized collagen molecules. However, because of their abnormal shapes, such analogs prevent triple helix formation. The abnormal collagen is slowly secreted and is much more susceptible to degradation. The role of these drugs is not yet clear in the human situation.

Beta-aminopropionitrile (BAPN) is one of a family of amino nitriles derived from the sweet pea, *Lathyrus odoratus*. These agents, called lathyrogens, can selectively inhibit the enzyme lysyl oxidase. This blocks formation of aldehyde groups, leading to a collagen cross-linking defect. The abnormal molecules are easily solubilized and broken down by tissue enzymes. BAPN is best used before keloids form and after they are excised—at a time when collagen turnover is at its peak. Such a period often extends between days 7 and 28 postoperatively and allows for selective lathyrogen effect on newly synthesized collagen. BAPN does not reduce the total amount of collagen synthesized. It currently is still in the phase of human trials; further study may show it to be a very useful adjuvant to keloid surgery.

Penicillamine, a copper chelator used in the treatment of Wilson's disease, also interferes with lysyl oxidase function. Furthermore, it reacts with formed aldehyde groups, blocking aldol condensation and subsequent cross-linking. Therefore this drug acts very similarly to lathyrogenic agents by preventing collagen maturation. The dose must be adjusted on an individual basis, and tolerance may develop over a 30-day period. Hence, penicillamine is best withheld until approximately 1 month before an excised keloid is expected to reform or just as it is forming.[212]

Colchicine interferes with the secretion of early collagen molecules[63] and has been shown to stimulate collagenase activity.[103] Furthermore, colchicine can interfere with wound contraction.[70] Although this drug is still undergoing clinical trials, it probably will be best used in combination with other agents, allowing for additive effect and reduction of doses to nontoxic levels.

REFERENCES

1 Abercrombie M, Flint MH, James DW: Wound contraction in relation to collagen formation in scorbutic guinea pigs, *J Embryol Exp Morphol* 4:167, 1956.

2 Abercrombie M, Heaysman JEM, Pegrum PM: The locomotion of fibroblasts in culture. II. "Ruffling," *Exp Cell Res* 60:327, 1970.

3 Abercrombie M, Heaysman JEM, Pegrum SM: The locomotion of fibroblasts in culture. IV. Electron microscopy of the leading lamella, *Exp Cell Res* 67:359, 1971.

4 Abercrombie M, James DW, Newcombe JF: Wound contraction in rabbit skin, studied by splinting the wound margins, *J Anat* 94:170, 1960.

5 Adzick NS, Longaker MT, editors: *Fetal wound healing,* New York, 1992, Elsevier Biomedical Press.

6 Ahonen J, Nemlander A, Wiktorowicz K et al: Effect of cyclosporine on wound healing, *Transplant Proc* 15(suppl 1):3092, 1983.

7 Alexander JW, Ogle C, Stinnett JD et al: A sequential prospective analysis of immunologic abnormalities and infection following severe thermal injury, *Ann Surg* 188:809, 1978.

8 Allbrook D, Baker W de C, Kirkaldy-Willis WH: Muscle regeneration in experimental animals and in man, *J Bone Joint Surg (Br)* 48:153, 1966.

9 Alvarez OM, Levendorf KD, Smerbeck RV et al: Effect of topically applied steroidal and nonsteroidal anti-inflammatory agents on skin repair and regeneration, *Fed Proc* 43:2793, 1984.

10 Amento EP, Beck LS: TGF-beta and wound healing, Ciba Foundation Symposium, 157:115, 1991.

11 Armstrong CP, Dixon JM, Duffy SW et al: Wound healing in obstructive jaundice, *Br J Surg* 71:267, 1984.

12 Asko-Seljavaaro S: Altered cell proliferation in burns, *J Trauma* 25:101, 1985.

13 Azizkhan RG, Azizkhan JC, Zetter BR et al: Mast cell heparin stimulates migration of capillary endothelial cells in vitro, *J Exp Med* 152:931, 1980.

14 Bailey AJ, Robins SP, Balian G: Biological significance of the intermolecular cross-links of collagen, *Nature* 251:105, 1974.

15 Banda MJ, Knighton DR, Hunt TK et al: Isolation of a nonmitogenic angiogenesis factor from wound fluid, *Proc Natl Acad Sci USA* 79:7773, 1982.

16 Barbul A, Fischel RS, Shimazu S et al: Intravenous hyperalimentation with high arginine levels improves wound healing and immune function, *J Surg Res* 38:328, 1985.

17 Barbul A, Regan MC: The regulatory role of T lymphocytes in wound healing, *J Trauma* 30(12):S97, 1990.

18 Barnard JW, Carpenter W: Lack of regeneration in spinal cord of rat, *J Neurophysiol* 13:223, 1950.

19 Basson MD, Burney RE: Defective wound healing in patients with paraplegia and quadriplegia, *Surg Gynecol Obstet* 155:9, 1982.

20 Bauer EA, Cooper TW, Tucker DR et al: Diphenylhydantoin therapy of recessive dystrophic epidermolysis bullosa: clinical trials and proposal of mechanisms of action, *Clin Res* 28:563A, 1980.

21 Baur PS Jr, Parks DH, Hudson JD: Epithelial-mediated wound contracture in experimental wounds: the purse string effect, *J Trauma* 24:713, 1984.

22 Baur PS, Parks DM, Larson DL: The healing of burn wounds, *Clin Plast Surg* 4:389, 1977.

23 Baverson JC, Sorgente CV: Chemotactic response of vascular endothelial cells to fibronectin, *J Cell Biol* 87:64a, 1980.

24 Beck LS, Deguzman L, Lee WP et al: TGF-β 1 accelerates wound healing: reversal of steroid-impaired healing in rats and rabbits, *Growth Factors* 5(4):295, 1991.

25 Berman M, Winthrop S, Ausprunk D et al: Plasminogen activator (urokinase) causes vascularization of the cornea, *Invest Ophthalmol Vis Sci* 22:191, 1982.

26 Bertolani CN: Glycosaminoglycan interactions in early wound repair. In Hunt TK, Heppenstall RB, Pines E et al, editors: *Soft and hard tissue repair: biological and clinical aspects,* New York, 1984, Praeger.

27 Billingham RE, Medawar PB: Contracture and intussusceptive growth in healing of extensive wounds in mammalian skin, *J Anat* 89:114, 1955.

28 Birnbaum JE, Sapp TM, Moore JB Jr: Effects of reserpine, epidermal growth factor, and cyclic nucleotide modulators in epidermal mitosis, *J Invest Dermatol* 66:213, 1976.

29 Blay J, Brown KD: Epidermal growth factor promotes the chemotactic migration of cultured rat intestinal cells, *J Cell Physiol* 124:107, 1985.

30 Bloom D: Heredity of keloids: review of the literature and report of a family with multiple keloids in 5 generations, *N Y State J Med* 56:511, 1956.

31 Brayton RG, Stokes PE, Schwartz MS et al: Effect of alcohol and various diseases on leukocyte mobilization, phagocytosis, and intracellular bacterial killing, *N Engl J Med* 282:123, 1970.

32 Brennan SS, Foster ME, Morgan A et al: Prostaglandins in colonic anastomotic healing, *Dis Colon Rectum* 27:723, 1984.

33 Brown LL, Shelton HT, Bornside GH et al: Evaluation of wound irrigation by pulsatile jet in conventional methods, *Ann Surg* 187:170, 1978.

34 Burke JF, Morris PJ, Bondoc CC: The effect of bacterial inflammation on wound healing. In Dunphy JE, Van Winkle W, editors: *Repair and regeneration,* New York, 1969, McGraw-Hill.

35 Bussolino F, Ziche M, Wang JM et al: In vivo and in vitro activation of endothelial cells by colony-stimulating factor, *J Clin Invest* 87(3):986, 1991.

36 Bybee JD, Rogers DE: The phagocytic activity of polymorphonuclear leukocytes obtained from patients with diabetes mellitus, *J Lab Clin Med* 64:1, 1964.

37 Calnan JS, Copenhagen HJ: Autotransplantation of keloids in man, *Br J Surg* 54:330, 1967.

38 Calnan J, Davies A: The effect of methotrexate on wound healing: an experimental study, *Br J Cancer* 19:505, 1965.

39 Carlson BM: The regeneration of skeletal muscle: a review, *Am J Anat* 137:119, 1973.

40 Chabot JG, Walker P, Pelletier G: Distribution of epidermal growth factor binding sites in the adult rat liver, *Am J Physiol* 250:G760, 1986.

41 Chu C, Williams DF: Effects of physical configuration and chemical structure of suture materials on bacterial adhesion: a possible link to wound infection, *Am J Surg* 147:197, 1984.

42 Church JCT: Satellite cells and myogenesis: a study in the fruit bat web, *J Anat* 105:419, 1969.

43 Church JCT, Noronha RFX, Albrook D: Satellite cells and skeletal muscle regeneration, *Br J Surg* 53:638, 1966.

44 Chvapil M: Zinc and wound healing. In Zederfeldt B, editor: *Symposium on zinc,* Lund, Sweden, 1974, AB Tika.

45 Chvapil M, Hameroff SR, O'Dea K et al: Local anesthetics and wound healing, *J Surg Res* 37:367, 1979.

46 Chylitova H, Kulhanek V, Horn V: Experimental production of keloids after immunization with autologous skin, *Acta Chir Plast* 1:72, 1959.

47 Cintron C, Kublin CL: Regeneration of corneal tissue, *Dev Biol* 61:346, 1977.

48 Clemmons DR: Multiple hormones stimulate the production of somatomedin by cultured human fibroblasts, *J Clin Endocrinol Metab* 58:850, 1984.

49 Cohen BE, Cohen IK: Vitamin A: adjuvant and steroid antagonist in the immune response, *J Immunol* 111:1376, 1973.

50 Cohen IK, McCoy BJ: The biology and control of surface overhealing, *World J Surg* 4:289, 1980.

51 Cohen IK, McCoy BJ, Mohanakumar T et al: Immunoglobulin, complement, and histocompatibility antigen studies in keloid patients, *Plast Reconstr Surg* 63:689, 1979.

52 Cohen SC, Gabelnick HL, Johnson RK et al: Effects of antineoplastic agents on wound healing in mice, *Surgery* 78:238, 1975.

53 Colin JF, Elliot P, Ellis H: The effect of uraermia upon wound healing: an experimental study, *Br J Surg* 66:793, 1979.

54 Conrad MC: Large and small artery occlusion in diabetics and nondiabetics with severe vascular disease, *Circulation* 36:83, 1967.

55 Daniele S, Frati L, Fiore C et al: The effect of the epidermal growth factor (EGF) on the corneal epithelium in humans, *Graefes Arch Clin Exp Ophthalmol* 210:159, 1979.

56 Dean DC, Birkenmeier TM, Rosen GD et al: Glycoprotein synthesis and secretion: expression of fibronectin and its cell surface receptors, *Am Rev Respir Dis* 144(3.2):S25, 1991.

57 DeGraaf PW, Zwaveling A: The influence of intravenous hyperalimentation (IVH) on wound healing in tumor-bearing rats, *J Surg Oncol* 24:332, 1983.

58 DeKlerk AJ, Jouch LM: Primary tendon healing: an experimental study, *S Afr Med J* 62(9):276, 1982.

59 Denel TF, Senior RM, Change D et al: Platelet factor 4 is chemotactic for neutrophils and monocytes, *Proc Natl Acad Sci USA* 78:4584, 1981.

60 Desprez JD, Kiehn CL: The effects of Cytoxan (cyclophosphamide) on wound healing, *Plast Reconstr Surg* 26:301, 1960.

61 Deuel TF, Huang JS: Platelet-derived growth factor: purification, properties, and biological activities, *Prog Hematol* 13:201, 1983.

62 Deuel TF, Senior RM, Huang JS et al: Chemotaxis of monocytes and neutrophils to platelet-derived growth factor, *J Clin Invest* 69:1046, 1982.

63 Diegelmann RF, Peterkofsky B: Inhibition of collagen secretion from bone and cultured fibroblasts by microtubular disruptive drugs, *Proc Natl Acad Sci USA* 69:892, 1972.

64 Donati RM, Frank DW, Stromberg LW et al: The effect of the germ-free state on wound healing, *J Surg Res* 11:163, 1971.

65 Dorner RW: Glycosaminoglycans of regenerating tendon, *Arthritis Rheum* 10:275, 1967.

66 Douglas IM: Acceleration of wound healing produced by preliminary wounding, *Br J Surg* 46:401, 1959.
67 Edlich RF, Panek PH, Rodeheaver GT et al: Physical and chemical configuration of sutures in the development of surgical infection, *Ann Surg* 177:679, 1973.
68 Edlich RF, Rogers W, Kasper G et al: Studies in the management of the contaminated wound. I. Optimal time for closure of contaminated open wounds, *Am J Surg* 117:323, 1969.
69 Edwards LC, Dunphy JE: Methionine in wound healing during protein starvation. In Williamson MB, editor: *The healing of wounds,* London, 1957, McGraw-Hill.
70 Ehrlich HP, Hunt TK: Effects of cortisone and vitamin A on wound healing, *Ann Surg* 167:3249, 1968.
71 Ehrlich HP, Tarver H, Hunt TK: Inhibitory effects of vitamin E on collagen synthesis and wound repair, *Ann Surg* 175:235, 1972.
72 Eisinger DR, Sheil AGR: A comparison of the effects of cyclosporin A and standard agents on primary wound healing in the rat, *Surg Gynecol Obstet* 160:135, 1985.
73 Erdos EG: Commentary: the kinins, a status report, *Biochem Pharmacol* 25:1563, 1976.
74 Falcone PA, Banaventuro M, Turner DC et al: The effect of exogenous fibronectin on wound breaking strength, *Plast Reconstr Surg* 74:809, 1984.
75 Folkman J, Shing Y: Control of angiogenesis by heparin and other sulfated polysaccharides, *Adv Exp Med Biol,* 313:355, 1992.
76 Forrest L: Current concepts in soft connective tissue wound healing, *Br J Surg* 70:133, 1983.
77 Franklin JD, Lynch, JB: Effects of topical applications of epidermal growth factor on wound healing, *Plast Reconstr Surg* 64:766, 1979.
78 Fujimori R, Hiramoto M, Ofuji S: Sponge fixation method for treatment of early scars, *Plast Reconstr Surg* 42:322, 1968.
79 Gabbiani G, Chaponnier C, Huttner I: Cytoplasmic filaments and gap junctions in epithelial cells and myofibroblasts during wound healing, *J Cell Biol* 76:561, 1978.
80 Gabbiani G, Hirschel BJ, Ryan GB, et al: Granulation tissue as a contractile organ: a study of structure and function, *J Exp Med* 135:719, 1972.
81 Gabbiani G, LeLous M, Bailey AJ, et al: Collagen and myofibroblasts of granulation tissue: a chemical, ultrastructural and immunologic study, *Virchows Arch [Cell Pathol]* 21:133, 1976.
82 Gabbiani G, Rungger-Brandle E: The fibroblast. In Glynn LE, editor: *Tissue repair and regeneration,* Amsterdam, 1981, North-Holland Biomedical Press.
83 Gabbiani G, Ryna GB: Development of a contractile apparatus in epithelial cells during epidermal and liver regeneration, *J Submicrosc Cytol* 6:143, 1974.
84 Garrett WE Jr, Seaber AV, Boswick J et al: Recovery of skeletal muscle after laceration and repair, *J Hand Surg* 9A:683, 1984.
85 Gartner MH, Bensen JD, Caldwell MD: Insulin-like growth factors I and II expression in the healing wound, *J Surg Res* 52(4):389, 1992.
86 Geever EF, Levenson SM, Manner G: The role of noncollagenous substances in the breaking strength of experimental wounds, *Surgery* 60:343, 1966.
87 Goldenberg SG, Alex M, Joshi RA et al: Nonatheromatous peripheral vascular disease of the lower extremity in diabetes mellitus, *Diabetes* 8:261, 1959.
88 Goodson WH, Hunt TK: Wound healing and aging, *J Invest Dermatol* 73:88, 1979.
89 Goodson WH, Lindenfeld SM, Omachi RS et al: Chronic uremia causes poor healing, *Surg Forum* 33:54, 1982.
90 Gottrup F: Healing of incisional wounds in stomach and duodenum: influence of long-term healing on mechanical strength and collagen distribution, *Acta Chir Scand* 149:57, 1983.
91 Graham MF, Diegelman RF, Linblad WJ et al: Effects of inflammation on wound healing. In Hunt TK, Heppenstall RB, Pines E et al, editors: *Soft and hard tissue repair: biological and clinical aspects,* New York, 1984, Praeger.
92 Grant ME, Prockop DJ: The biosynthesis of collagen, *N Engl J Med* 286:194,242,291, 1972.
93 Greaney MG, Van Noort R, Smythe A et al: Does obstructive jaundice adversely affect wound healing? *Br J Surg* 66:478, 1979.
94 Grinnell F, Billingham RE, Burgess L: Distribution of fibronectin during wound healing in vivo, *J Invest Dermatol* 76:181, 1981.
95 Gross A, Cutright DE, Bhaskar SN: Effectiveness of pulsating water jet lavage in treatment of contaminated crushed wounds, *Am J Surg* 124:373, 1972.
96 Grotendorst GR: Can collagen metabolism be controlled? *J Trauma* 24:9,549, 1984.
97 Grotendorst GR, Pencev D, Martin GR et al: Molecular mediators of tissue repair in soft and hard tissue repair. In Hunt TK, Heppenstall RB, Pines E et al, editors: *Soft and hard tissue repair: biological and clinical aspects,* New York, 1984, Praeger.
98 Grotendorst GR, Seppa MEJ, Kleinman MK et al: Attachment of smooth muscle cells to collagens and their migration toward platelet-derived growth factor, *Proc Natl Acad Sci USA* 78:3669, 1981.
99 Grove RI, Pratt RM: Influence of epidermal growth factor and cyclic AMP on growth and differentiation of palatal epithelial cells in culture, *Dev Biol* 106:427, 1984.
100 Guglielmo BJ, Hohn DC, Koo PJ et al: Antibiotic prophylaxis in surgical procedures: a critical analysis of the literature, *Arch Surg* 118:943, 1983.
101 Hall CE, Jakus MA, Schmitt FO: Electron microscopic observations of collagen, *J Am Chem Soc* 64:1234, 1942.
102 Hall-Craggs ECB: The regeneration in skeletal muscle fibers per continuum, *J Anat* 117:171, 1974.
103 Harris ED, Krane SM: Effects of colchicine on collagenase in cultures of rheumatoid synovium, *Arthritis Rheum* 14:669, 1971.
104 Harwood R, Grant ME, Jackson DS: Collagen biosynthesis: characterization of subcellular fractions from embryonic chick fibroblasts and the intracellular localization of protocollagen prolyl and protocollagen lysyl hydroxylases, *Biochem J* 144:123, 1974.
105 Heldin CA, Westermark B, Wasteson A: Specific receptors for platelet-derived growth factor on cells derived from connective tissue and glia, *Proc Natl Acad Sci USA* 78:3364, 1981.
106 Herrmann JB, Woodward SC, Pulaski EJ: Healing of colonic anastomoses in the rat, *Surg Gynecol Obstet* 119:269, 1964.
107 Heughan C, Grislis G, Hunt TK: The effect of anemia on wound healing, *Ann Surg* 179:163, 1974.
108 Hinshaw DB, Hughes ID, Stafford CE: Effects of cortisone on the healing of disrupted abdominal wounds, *Am J Surg* 101:189, 1961.
109 Hirsch G: Tensile properties during tendon healing, *Acta Orthop Scand* (suppl) 153:13, 1974.
110 Hirschel BJ, Gobbiani G, Ryan GB et al: Fibroblasts of granulation tissue: immunofluorescent staining with anti–smooth muscle serum, *Proc Soc Exp Biol Med* 138:466, 1971.
111 Hohn DC, MacKay RD, Halliday B et al: Effect of oxygen tension on microbicidal function of leukocytes in wounds and in vitro, *Surg Forum* 27:18, 1976.
112 Humphries MJ, Ayad SR: Stimulation of DNA synthesis by cathepsin D digests of fibronectin, *Nature* 305:811, 1983.
113 Hunt TK, Andrews WS, Halliday BJ, et al: Coagulation and macrophage stimulation of angiogenesis and wound healing. In Dineen P, Hildich-Smith G, editors: *The surgical wound,* Philadelphia, 1981, Lea & Febiger.
114 Hunt TK, Ehrlich HP, Garcia JA et al: Effect of vitamin A on reversing the inhibitory effect of cortisone on healing of open wounds in animals and man, *Ann Surg* 170:633, 1969.

115 Hunt TK, Knighton DR, Thakral KK et al: Studies on inflammation and wound healing: angiogenesis and collagen synthesis stimulated in vivo by resident and activated wound macrophages, *Surgery* 96:48, 1984.
116 Hunt TK, Linsey M, Grislis G et al: The effect of differing ambient oxygen tension on wound infection, *Ann Surg* 181:35, 1975.
117 Hunt TK, Pai MP: The effect of varying ambient oxygen tensions on wound metabolism and collagen synthesis, *Surg Gynecol Obstet* 135:561, 1972.
118 Hynes RO, Yamada KM: Fibronectins: multifunctional modular glycoproteins, *J Cell Biol* 95:369, 1982.
119 Ignotz RA, Massague J: Transforming growth factor-beta stimulates the expression of fibronectin and collagen and their incorporation into the extracellular matrix, *J Biol Chem* 261:4337, 1986.
120 Inalsingh CHA: An experience in treating 501 patients with keloids, *Johns Hopkins Med J* 134:284, 1974.
121 Irvin TT: Effects of malnutrition and hyperalimentation on wound healing, *Surg Gynecol Obstet* 146:33, 1978.
122 Irvin TT: *The healing wound: principles and practice,* New York, 1983, Chapman Hall.
123 Irvin TT, Goligher JC: Aetiology of disruption of intestinal anastomoses, *Br J Surg* 60:461, 1973.
124 Issekutz AC: Role of polymorphonuclear leukocytes in the vascular responses of acute inflammation, *Lab Invest* 50:605, 1984 (editorial).
125 Jones SC, Curtsinger LJ, Whalen JD et al: Effect of topical recombinant TGF-beta on healing of partial-thickness injuries, *J Surg Res* 51(4):344, 1991.
126 Jose PJ, Forrest MJ, Williams TJ: Human C5a des Arg increases vascular permeability, *J Immunol* 127:2376, 1981.
127 Joseph DL, Shumrick DL: Risks of head and neck surgery in previously irradiated patients, *Arch Otolaryngol* 97:381, 1973.
128 Juhan L, Bunoacare M, Jouve R et al: Abnormalities of erythrocyte deformability and platelet aggregation in insulin-dependent diabetics corrected by insulin in vivo and in vitro, *Lancet* 1:535, 1982.
129 Kapadia CR, Mann JB, McGeehan D et al: Behavior of synthetic absorbable sutures with and without synergistic enteric infection, *Eur Surg Res* 15:67, 1983.
130 Kaplan KL, Broekman MJ, Chernoff A et al: Platelet alpha-granule products: studies on release and subcellular localization, *Blood* 53:604, 1979.
131 Kay AB, Pepper DS, McKenzie R: The identification of fibrinopeptide B as a chemotactic agent derived from human fibrinogen, *Br J Haematol* 27:669, 1974.
132 Ketchum LD: Primary tendon healing: a review, *J Hand Surg* 2:428, 1977.
133 King LE, Carpenter GF: Epidermal growth factor. In Goldsmith LA, editor: *Biochemistry and physiology of the skin,* New York, 1983, Oxford University Press.
134 Kischer CW, Bunce H, Shetlar MR: Mast cell analysis in hypertrophic scars, hypertrophic scars treated with pressure, and mature scars, *J Invest Dermatol* 70:355, 1978.
135 Kischer CW, Shetlar MR, Shetlar CL: Alterations of hypertrophic scars induced by mechanical pressure, *Arch Dermatol* 111:60, 1975.
136 Kischer CW, Shetlar MR, Shetlar CL et al: Immunoglobulins in hypertrophic scars and keloids, *Plast Reconstr Surg* 71:821, 1983.
137 Kischer CW, Thies AC, Chvapil M: Perivascular myofibroblasts and microvascular occlusion in hypertrophic scars and keloids, *Hum Pathol* 13:819, 1982.
138 Kivirikko KI, Myllyl R: Collagen glycosyltransferases, *Int Rev Connect Tissue Res* 8:23, 1979.
139 Kivisaari J, Ninikoski J: Effects of hyperbaric oxygenation and prolonged hypoxia on the healing of open wounds, *Acta Chir Scand* 141:14, 1975.
140 Klebe RJ: Isolation of a collagen-dependent cell attachment factor, *Nature* 250:248, 1974.
141 Kleinert HE, Kutz JE, Atasoy E et al: Primary repair of flexor tendons, *Orthop Clin North Am* 21:865, 1973.
142 Knighton DR, Hunt TK, Schewenstuhl H et al: Oxygen tension regulates the expression of angiogenesis factor by macrophages, *Science* 221:1283, 1973.
143 Knighton DR, Hunt TK, Schewenstuhl H et al: Oxygen as an antibiotic: the effect of inspired oxygen on infection, *Arch Surg* 119:199, 1984.
144 Knighton DR, Hunt TK, Thakral KK et al: Role of platelets and fibrin in the healing sequence: an in vivo study of angiogenesis and collagen synthesis, *Ann Surg* 196:379, 1982.
145 Knighton DR, Silver IA, Hunt TK: Regulation of wound healing angiogenesis: effect of oxygen gradients and inspired oxygen concentration, *Surgery* 90:262, 1981.
146 Krane SM: The turnover and degradation of collagen. In Fibrosis: CIBA Foundation Symposium 114, London, 1985, Pitman.
147 Krawczyk WS: A pattern of epidermal cell migration during wound healing, *J Cell Biol* 49:247, 1971.
148 Krizek TJ, Robson MC: The evolution of quantitative bacteriology in wound management, *Am J Surg* 130:579, 1975.
149 Krull EA: Chronic cutaneous ulcerations and impaired healing in human skin, *J Am Acad Dermatol* 12:394, 1985.
150 Krummel TM, Nelson JM, Diegelmann RF et al: Fetal response to injury and its modulation with transforming growth factor-beta, *Surg Forum* 38:622, 1987.
151 Laugness U, Udenfriend S: Collagen proline hydroxylase activity and anaerobic metabolism. In Kulonen E, Pikkarainen J, editors: *Biology of fibroblast,* New York, 1973, Academic Press.
152 Lee KH: Studies on the mechanism of action of salicylates. II. Retardation of wound healing by aspirin, *J Pharm Sci* 57:1042, 1968.
153 Lee PW, Green MA, Long WB et al: Zinc in wound healing, *Surg Gynecol Obstet* 143:549, 1976.
154 LeGerfo FW, Coffman JD: Vascular and microvascular disease of the foot in diabetes mellitus: implications for foot care, *N Engl J Med* 311:1615, 1984.
155 Leibovich SJ, Ross R: The role of the macrophage in wound repair: a study with hydrocortisone and antimacrophage serum, *Am J Pathol* 78:71, 1975.
156 Lembach KM: Production of human fibroblast proliferation by epidermal growth factor (EGF): enhancement by an EGF-binding arginine esterase and by ascorbate, *Proc Natl Acad Sci USA* 73:183, 1976.
157 Lenaers A, Ansay M, Nusgens BV et al: Collagen made of extended x-chains, procollagen, in genetically defective desmatosparactic calves, *Eur J Biochem* 23:533, 1971.
158 Levy DS, Salter MM, Roth EE: Postoperative irradiation in the prevention of keloids, *Am J Roentgenol* 127:509, 1976.
159 Lindsay WK, Birch JR: The fibroblast in flexor tendon healing, *Plast Reconstr Surg* 34:223, 1964.
160 Lineaweaver W, Howard R, Soucy D et al: Antimicrobial toxicity, *Arch Surg* 12:267, 1985.
161 Longaker MT, Adzick NS et al: Studies in fetal wound healing. VII. Fetal wound healing may be modulated by elevated hyaluronic acid–stimulating activity in amniotic fluid, *J Pediatr Surg* 25:430, 1990.
162 Longaker MT, Bouhana KS, Roberts AB et al: Regulation of fetal wound healing, *Plast Surg Res Cncl,* Index 38, 145, 1991.
163 Longaker MT, Moelleken BRW, Cheng JC et al: Fetal fracture healing in a lamb model, *Plast Reconstr Surg* 90(2):161, 1992.
164 Longaker MT, Whitby DJ, Adzick NS et al: Studies in fetal wound healing. VI. Second and third trimester fetal wounds demonstrate rapid collagen deposition without scar formation, *J Pediatr Surg* 25:63, 1990.

165 Loose LD, Turinsky J: Macrophage dysfunction after burn injury, *Infect Immun* 26:157, 1979.
166 Lukens LN: Time of occurrence of disulfide linking between procollagen chains, *J Biol Chem* 251:3530, 1976.
167 Lundberg G, Gerdin B: The role of histamine and serotonin in the inflammatory reaction in an experimental model of open wounds in the rat, *Scan J Plast Reconstr Surg* 18:175, 1984.
168 Lundberg G, Lebel L, Gerdin B: The inflammatory reaction in healing wounds: the role of the polymorphonuclear leukocytes, *Int J Tissue React* 6(6):477, 1984.
169 MacDonald MJ, Bleichman M, Bunn HF et al: Functional properties of the glycosylated minor components of human hemoglobin, *J Biol Chem* 254:702, 1979.
170 Maciag T, Kadish T, Wilkin C et al: Organizational behavior of human umbilical vein endothelial cells, *J Cell Biol* 94:511, 1982.
171 Madden JW, Carlson EC: Atypical fibroblasts, wound contraction, and human fibrocontractive diseases. In Proceedings of the International Symposium on Wound Healing, Rotterdam, 1974.
172 Madden JW, Morton D Jr, Peacock EE Jr: Contraction of experimental wounds. I. Inhibiting wound contraction using a smooth muscle antagonist, *Surgery* 76:8, 1974.
173. Madden JW, Peacock EE Jr: Studies on the biology of collagen during wound healing. III. Dynamic metabolism of scar collagen and remodeling of dermal wounds, *Ann Surg* 179:511, 1971.
174 Madden JW, Smith HC: Rate of collagen synthesis and deposition in dehisced and resutured wounds, *Surg Gynecol Obstet* 130:487, 1970.
175 Maeda N, Kon K, Imiazumi I et al: Alteration of rheological properties of human erythrocytes by cross-linking of membrane proteins, *Biochim Biophys Acta* 735:104, 1983.
176 Majno G, Palade GE: Studies of inflammation. I. The effect of histamine and serotonin on vascular permeability: an electron microscopic study, *J Biophys Biochem Cytol* 11:571, 1961.
177 Majno G, Palade GE, Schoefl GI: Studies on inflammation. II. The site of action of histamine and serotonin along the vascular tree: a topographic study, *J Biophys Biochem Cytol* 11:607, 1961.
178 Marchesi VT: The site of leukocyte emigration during inflammation, *Q J Exp Physiol* 46:115, 1961.
179 Marks JG Jr, Carro C, Leitzel K: Inhibition of wound healing by topical steroids, *J Dermatol Surg Oncol* 9:819, 1983.
180 Martin BM, Gimbrone MA Jr, Unanue ER et al: Macrophage-derived growth factor: production by cultured human mononuclear blood cells, *Fed Proc* 40:335, 1981.
181 Martin GR, Kleinman HK, Gauss-Muller V et al: Regulation of tissue structure and repair by collagen and fibronectin. In Dineen P, Hildich-Smith G, editors: *The surgical wound*, Philadelphia, 1981, Lea & Febiger.
182 Mason ML, Allen H: The rate of healing of tendons: an experimental study of tensile strength, *Ann Surg* 113:424, 1941.
183 Mathews MB, Lozaityte I: I. Sodium chondroitin–sulfate protein complexes of cartilage. II. Molecular weight and shape, *Arch Biochem Biophys* 74:158, 1958.
184 Mazue G, Bertolero F, Jacob C et al: Preclinical and clinical studies with recombinant human basic fibroblast growth factor, *Ann N Y Acad Sci* 638:329, 1991.
185 McCoy BJ, Cohen IK: Collagenase in keloid biopsies and fibroblasts, *Connect Tissue Res* 9:181, 1982.
186 McDermott FT, Nayman J, DeBoer WE: Effect of acute renal failure on wound healing: histology and autoradiography in the mouse, *Ann Surg* 168:142, 1968.
187 McGinn FP: Effects of haemorrhage upon surgical operations, *Br J Surg* 63:742, 1976.
188 McGrath MH, Hundahl SA: The spatial and temporal quantification of myofibroblasts, *Plast Reconstr Surg* 69:975, 1982.
189 Mendoza CB, Postlethwait RW, Johnson WD: Incidence of wound disruption following operation, *Arch Surg* 101:396, 1970.
190 Miyakawa M, Isomura N, Shirsawa H et al: Wound healing in germ-free animals, *Acta Pathol Jpn* 8:79, 1958.
191 Modolin M, Bevilacqua RG, Margarido NF et al: The effects of protein malnutrition on wound contraction: an experimental study, *Ann Plast Surg* 12:428, 1984.
192 Moelleken BRW, Longaker MT, Cheng JC et al: Fetal fracture healing: histologic and radiologic correlates, *Surg Forum* 17:668, 1991.
193 Moelleken BRW, Mathes SJ, Amerhauser A et al: An adverse wound environment activates leukocytes prematurely, *Arch Surg* 126(11):225, 1991.
194 Monsaingeon A, Molimard R: Wound healing: comparison of healing rates of burn wounds and of excisional wounds, *Eur Surg Res* 8:337, 1976.
195 Moore MJ: The effect of radiation on connective tissue, *Otolaryngol Clin North Am* 17:389, 1984.
196 Morris T, Appleby R: Retardation of wound healing by procaine, *Br J Surg* 67:391, 1980.
197 Mosher DF: Fibronectin, *Prog Hemost Thromb* 5:111, 1980.
198 Mowat AG, Baum J: Chemotaxis of polymorphonuclear leukocytes from patients with diabetes mellitus, *N Engl J Med* 284:621, 1971.
199 Mullen JL, Getner MH, Buzby GP et al: Implications of malnutrition in the surgical patient, *Arch Surg* 114:121, 1979.
200 Neilson EG, Phillips SM, Jimenez S: Lymphokine modulation of fibroblast proliferation, *J Immunol* 128:1484, 1982.
201 Niall M, Ryan GB, O'Brien B McC: The effect of epidermal growth factor on wound healing in mice, *J Surg Res* 33:164, 1982.
202 Nimini E, Bavetta LA: Collagen defect induced by penicillamine, *Science* 150:905, 1965.
203 Ogilvie RR, Douglas DM: Collagen synthesis and preliminary wounding, *Br J Surg* 51:149, 1964.
204 Olson PS, Poulsen SS, Kirkegaard P: Adrenergic effects on secretion of epidermal growth factor from Brunner's glands, *Gut* 26:920, 1985.
205 Omo-Dare P: Genetic studies on keloid, *J Natl Med Assoc* 67:428, 1975.
206 Ordman LJ, Gillman T: Studies in the healing of cutaneous wounds. I. The healing of incisions through the skin of pigs, *Arch Surg* 93:857, 1966.
207 Ordman LJ, Gillman T: Studies in the healing of cutaneous wounds. II. The healing of epidermal, appendageal, and dermal injuries inflicted by suture needles and by the suture material in the skin of pigs, *Arch Surg* 93:883, 1966.
208 Ordog GI, Waserberger J, Balasubramanium S: Wound ballistics: theory and practice, *Ann Emerg Med* 13:1113, 1984.
209 Palmblad J, Malmsten CI, Uden AM et al: Leukotriene B4 is a potent and sterospecific stimulator of neutrophil chemotaxis and adherence, *Blood* 58:658, 1981.
210 Peacock EE Jr: A study of circulation in normal tendons and healing grafts, *Ann Surg* 149:415, 1959.
211 Peacock EE Jr: Biological principles in the healing of long tendons, *Surg Clin North Am* 45:461, 1965.
212 Peacock EE: *Wound repair*, ed 3, Philadelphia, 1984, WB Saunders.
213 Peacock EE Jr, Madden JW, Trier WC: Biologic basis for the treatment of keloids and hypertrophic scars, *South Med J* 63:755, 1970.
214 Peacock EE, Van Winkle W: *Wound repair*, ed 2, Philadelphia, 1976, WB Saunders.
215 Peterson JM, Barbul A, Breslin RJ et al: Significance of T lymphocytes in wound healing, *Surgery* 102:373, 1989.
216 Pierce GF, Mustoe TA, Altrock BW et al: Role of platelet-derived growth factor in wound healing, *J Cell Biochem* 45(4):319, 1991.
217 Pierce GF, Tarpley JE, Yanagihara D et al: Platelet-derived growth factor (BB homodimer), transforming growth factor beta-1, and basic fibroblast growth factor in dermal wound heal-

ing: neovessel and matrix formation and cessation of repair, *Am J Pathol* 140(6):1375, 1992.

218 Plouffe JF, Silva J, Fekety FR et al: Cell-mediated immunity in diabetes mellitus, *Infect Immun* 21:425, 1978.

219 Pober JS, Bevilacqua MP, Mendrick DL et al: Two distinct monokines, interleukin-1 and tumor necrosis factor, each independently induce biosynthesis and transient expression of the same antigen on the surface of cultured human vascular endothelial cells, *J Immunol* 136:1680, 1986.

220 Pohl R, Hunt TK: Penicillin G and wound healing, *Arch Surg* 101:610, 1970.

221 Pollack SV: Wound healing: a review. III. Nutritional factors affecting wound healing, *J Dermatol Surg Oncol* 5:8, 1979.

222 Polverini PJ, Cotran RS, Gimbrone MA Jr et al: Activated macrophages induced vascular proliferation, *Nature* 269:804, 1977.

223 Postlethwaite AE, Keski-Oja J, Moses HL et al: Stimulation of the chemotactic migration of human fibroblasts by transforming growth factor-β, *J Exp Med* 165:251, 1987.

224 Postlethwaite AE, Keski-Oja J, Balian G et al: Induction of fibroblast chemotaxis by fibronectin: localization of the chemotactic region to a 140,000 molecular weight nongelatin binding fragment, *J Exp Med* 153:494, 1981.

225 Postlethwaite AE, Seyer JM, Kang AM: Chemotactic attraction of human fibroblasts to type I, II, and III collagens and collagen-derived peptides, *Proc Natl Acad Sci* USA 75:871, 1978.

226 Potenza AD: The healing of autogenous tendon grafts within the flexor digital sheath in dogs, *J Bone Joint Surg* 46A:1462, 1964.

227 Prakash A, Pundit PH, Sharma LK: Studies of wound healing in experimental diabetes mellitus, *Int Surg* 59:25, 1974.

228 Prez HD, Weksler BB, Goldstein IM: Generation of chemotactic lipid from arachidonic acid by exposure to a superoxide generating system, *Inflammation* 4:313, 1980.

229 Prockop DJ, Kivirikko K, Tuderman L et al: The biosynthesis of collagen and its disorders, *N Engl J Med* 301:13,77, 1979.

230 Reitamo J, Moller C: Abdominal wound dehiscence, *Acta Chir Scand* 138:170, 1972.

231 Rhoads JE, Fliegelman MT, Paner LM: The mechanism of delayed wound healing in the presence of hypoproteinemia, *JAMA* 118:21, 1942.

232 Robbins SL, Cotran RS, Kumor V: *Pathologic basis of disease,* ed 3, Philadelphia, 1985, WB Saunders.

233 Roberts AB, Anzano MA, Lamb LC et al: Type beta transforming growth factor: a bifunctional regulator of cellular growth, *Proc Natl Acad Sci USA* 83:119, 1985.

234 Roberts CJ, Birkenmeier TM, McQuillan JJ et al: Transforming growth factor beta stimulates the expression of fibronectin and of both subunits of the human fibronectin receptor by cultured human lung fibroblasts, *J Biol Chem* 263:4586, 1988.

235 Roberts AB, Sporn MB, Assoian RK et al: Transforming growth factor type beta: rapid induction of fibrosis and angiogenesis in vivo and stimulation of collagen formation in vitro, *Proc Natl Acad Sci USA* 83:4167, 1986.

236 Ross R: The fibroblast and wound repair, *Biol Rev* 43:51, 1968.

237 Ross R, Benditt EP: Wound healing and collagen formation. I. Sequential changes in components of guinea pig skin wounds observed in the electron microscope, *J Biophys Biochem Cytol* 11:677, 1961.

238 Ross R, Everett NB, Tyler R: Wound healing and collagen formation. VI. The origin of the fibroblast studied in parabiosis, *J Cell Biol* 44:654, 1970.

239 Ross R, Glomset B, Kariya B et al: A platelet-dependent serum factor that stimulates the proliferation of arterial smooth muscle cells in vitro, *Proc Natl Acad Sci USA* 71:1207, 1974.

240 Rovee DT, Miller CA: Epidermal role in the breaking strength of wounds, *Arch Surg* 96:43, 1968.

241 Rovin S, Costich ER, Fleming JE et al: Healing of tongue wounds in germ-free and conventional mice, *Arch Pathol Lab Med* 79:641, 1965.

242 Rudolph R: Location of the force of wound contraction, *Surg Gynecol Obstet* 148:547, 1979.

243 Rusalahti E, Engvall E, Hayman EG: Fibronectin: current concepts of its structure and function, *Coll Relat Res* 1:95, 1981.

244 Safavi A, Gottesman L, Dailey TH: Anorectal surgery in the HIV+ patient: update, *Dis Col Rectum* 34(4):299, 1991.

245 Salmela K, Ahonen J: The effect of methylprednisolone and vitamin A on wound healing. I, *Acta Chir Scand* 147:307, 1981.

246 Sandberg N: Time relationship between administration of cortisone and wound healing in rats, *Acta Chir Scand* 127:446, 1964.

247 Savlov ED, Dunphy JE: The healing of the disrupted and resutured wound, *Surgery* 36:362, 1954.

248 Sawhney CP: The influence of skin tension on the contraction of open wounds and skin grafts in rabbits, *Br J Plast Surg* 30:115, 1977.

249 Schiffmann E, Cororan BA, Aswanikumar V: Molecular events in the response of neutrophils to synthetic *N*-fMet chemotactic peptides: demonstration of a specific receptor. In Gallin TI, Cline PG, editors: *Leukocyte chemotaxis,* New York, 1978, Raven Press.

250 Schmitt FD, Gross T, Highberger JH: Tropocollagen and the properties of fibrous collagen, *Eur Cell Res* (suppl 3):326, 1955.

251 Schrock TR, Deveney OW, Dunphy JE: Factors contributing to leakage of colonic anastomoses, *Ann Surg* 177:513, 1973.

252 Schultz G, Rotatori DS, Clark W: EGF and TGF-alpha in wound healing and repair, *J Cell Biochem* 45(4):346, 1991.

253 Seppa HEJ, Grotendorst GR, Seppa SI et al: The platelet-derived growth factor is a chemoattractant for fibroblasts, *J Cell Biol* 92:584, 1982.

254 Seppa HEJ, Yamade KM, Seppa SI et al: The cell-binding fragment of fibronectin is chemotactic for fibroblasts, *Cell Biol Int Rep* 5:813, 1981.

255 Sevitt S: Early and delayed edema and increase in capillary permeability after a burn of the skin, *J Pathol Bacteriol* 75:27, 1958.

256 Shafer WG: Effect of Dilantin sodium analogues on cell proliferation in tissue culture, *Proc Soc Exp Biol Med* 104:198, 1960.

257 Shattil SJ, Bennett JS: Platelets and their membranes in hemostasis: physiology and pathophysiology, *Ann Intern Med* 96:108, 1980.

258 Sheil AGR: Introduction to clinical studies on other organs. In White DJG, editor: *Cyclosporin A:* proceedings of an international conference on cyclosporin A, Amsterdam, 1982, Elsevier Biomedical Press.

259 Siegel RC, Fu JCC: Collagen cross-linking: purification and substrate specificity of lysyl oxidase, *J Biol Chem* 241:5779, 1976.

260 Silbert JE: Structure and metabolism of proteoglycans and glycosaminoglycans, *J Invest Dermatol* 79(suppl 1):31s, 1982.

261 Simpson G, Kunz E, Slafta J: Use of sodium diphenylhydantoin in treatment of leg ulcers, *N Y State J Med* 65:886, 1965.

262 Simpson DM, Ross R: The neutrophilic leukocyte in wound repair: a study with antineutrophil serum, *J Clin Invest* 51:2009, 1972.

263 Sloan DF, Brown RD, Wells CM: Tissue gases in human hypertrophic burn scars, *Plast Reconstr Surg* 61:431, 1978.

264 Smith JW: Molecular pattern in native collagen, *Nature* 219:157, 1968.

265 Staley CJ, Trippel OM, Preston FW: Influence of 5-fluorouracil on wound healing, *Surgery* 49:450, 1961.

266 Stanulis-Praeger BM, Gilchrest BA: Growth factor responsiveness declines during adulthood for human skin–derived cells, *Mech Ageing Dev* 35:185, 1986.

267 Stephens FO, Dunphy JE, Hunt TK: The effect of delayed administration of corticosteroids on wound contraction, *Ann Surg* 173:214, 1971.

268 Stephens FO, Hunt TK: Effect of changes in inspired oxygen and carbon dioxide tensions on wound tensile strength: an experimental study, *Ann Surg* 175:515, 1971.
269 Stephens FO, Hunt TK, Jawetz E et al: Effect of cortisone and vitamin A on wound healing, *Am J Surg* 121:569, 1971.
270 Stern MG, Longaker MT, Stern R: Hyaluronic acid and its modulation in fetal and adult wounds. In Adzick NS, Longaker MT, editors: *Fetal wound healing,* New York, 1992, Elsevier Biomedical Publishing.
271 Stevenson TR, Thacker JB, Rodheaver GT et al: Cleansing of the traumatic wound by high-pressure syringe irrigation, *JACEP* 5:17, 1976.
272 Steward RJ, Dudley JA, Dewdney J et al: The wound fibroblast and macrophage. II. Their origin studied in a human after bone marrow transplantation, *Br J Surg* 68:129, 1981.
273 Stewart R: Influence of malignant cells on the healing of colonic anastomoses: experimental observations, *Proc R Soc Med* 66:1089, 1973.
274 Stiles CD, Capone GT, Scher CD et al: Dual control of cell growth by somatomedin and platelet-derived growth factor, *Proc Natl Acad Sci USA* 76:1279, 1979.
275 Stolpen AH, Guinan EC, Fiers W et al: Recombinant TNF and immune interferon act singly and in combination to reorganize human vascular endothelial cell monolayers, *Am J Pathol* 123:16, 1986.
276 Tanzer M: Cross-linking. In Ramachandran GN, Reddi AH, editors: *Biochemistry of collagen,* New York, 1976, Plenum Publishing.
277 Taylor S, Folkman J: Protamine is an inhibitor of angiogenesis, *Nature* 297:307, 1982.
278 Thompson WD, Campbell R, Evans T: Fibrin degradation and angiogenesis: quantitative analysis of the angiogenic response in the chick chorioallantoic membrane, *J Pathol* 145:27, 1985.
279 Thomas BL, Krummel TM, Melang M et al: Collagen synthesis and type expression by fetal fibroblasts in vitro, *Surg Forum* 39:642, 1988.
280 Tobin GR, Chvapil M, Gildenberg PL: Collagen biosynthesis in healing wounds of the spinal cord and surrounding membranes, *Surgery* 88:231, 1980.
281 Toole BP: Hyaluronate turnover during chondrogenesis in the developing chick limb and axial skeleton, *Dev Biol* 29:321, 1972.
282 Toole BP: Glycosaminoglycans in morphogenesis. In Hay ED, editor: *Cell biology of the extracellular matrix,* New York, 1982, Plenum Publishing.
283 Tuck RR, Schmelzer JD, Low PA: Endoneural blood flow and oxygen tension in the sciatic nerves of rats with experimental diabetic neuropathy, *Brain* 107:935, 1984.
284 Turley EA, Torrance J: Localization of hyaluronate and hyaluronate-binding protein on motile and nonmotile fibroblasts, *Exp Cell Res* 16:17, 1984.
285 Tzeng DY, Deuel TF, Huang JS et al: Platelet-derived growth factor promotes polymorphonuclear leukocyte activation, *Blood* 64:1123, 1984.
286 Uitto J, Teir H, Mustakallio KK: Corticosteroid-induced inhibition of the biosynthesis of human skin collagen, *Biochem Pharmacol* 21:2161, 1972.
287 Van Noort R, Greaney MG, Black MM et al: A new in vitro method for the measurement of mechanical strength of abdominal wounds in laboratory animals, *Eng Med* 7:217, 1978.
288 Van Winkle W Jr, Hastings JC, Barker E et al: Effect of suture materials on healing skin wounds, *Surg Gynecol Obstet* 140:7, 1975.
289 Velasco M, Guaitero E: A comparative study of some anti-inflammatory drugs in wound healing of the rat, *Experientia* 29:1250, 1973.
290 Viljanto T, Rajamaki A, Reuvall S et al: Cell aggregation centers: initial strength elements in human wound healing, *J Surg Res* 29:414, 1980.
291 Virtanen I, Vartio T, Bradley RA et al: Fibronectin in adhesion, spreading, and cytoskeletal organization of cultured fibroblasts, *Nature* 298:660, 1982.
292 Wahl SM, Hunt DA, Wakefield LM et al: Transforming growth factor type β induces monocyte chemotaxis and growth factor production, *Proc Natl Acad Sci USA* 84:5788, 1987.
293 Wall RT, Harker LA, Quadracci LJ et al: Factors influencing endothelial cell proliferation in vitro, *J Cell Physiol* 96:203, 1978.
294 Watts GT, Grillo HC, Gross J: Studies in wound healing. II. The role of granulation tissue in contraction, *Ann Surg* 148:153, 1958.
295 Webb P: The effect of innervation, denervation, and muscle type on the reunion of skeletal muscle, *Br J Surg* 60:180, 1973.
296 Weeks JR: Prostaglandins, *Annu Rev Pharmacol Toxicol* 12:317, 1972.
297 Weich HA, Iberg N, Klagsbrun M et al: Transcriptional regulation of basic fibroblast growth factor gene expression in capillary endothelial cells, *J Cell Biochem* 47(2):158, 1991.
298 Weissman G, Thomas L: The effects of corticosteroids upon connective tissue and lysosomes, *J Rec Prog Horm Res* 20:215, 1964.
299 Welgus HG, Jeffrey JE, Eisen AZ: The collagen substrate specificity of human skin fibroblast collagenase, *J Biol Chem* 256:9511, 1981.
300 Whitby DJ, Ferguson MW: Immunohistochemical localization of growth factors in fetal wound healing, *Dev Biol* 147(1):207, 1991.
301 Whitby DJ, Longaker MT, Adzick NS et al: Early deposition of tenascin characterizes fetal wound healing, *Plast Surg Res Cncl,* 1988.
302 Wiggins RC, Cochrane CG: Hageman factor and the contact activation system. In Weissman G, Glynn LE, Houch JC, editors: *Chemical messengers of inflammation,* vol 1, *Handbook of inflammation,* Amsterdam, 1979, North-Holland Biomedical Press.
303 Williams TJ: Prostaglandin E2, prostaglandin I2, and the vascular changes of inflammation, *Br J Pharmacol* 65:517, 1979.
304 Williams TJ: Interactions between prostaglandins, leukotrienes, and other mediators of inflammation, *Br Med Bull* 39:239, 1983.
305 Williams TJ, Morley J: Prostaglandins as potent initiators of increased vascular permeability in inflammation, *Nature* 246:215, 1973.
306 Williams TJ, Peck MJ: Role of prostaglandin-mediated vasodilatation of inflammation, *Nature* 270:530, 1977.
307 Willoughby DA: Some views on the pathogenesis of inflammation. In Montagna W, Bentley JP, Dolson R, editors: *The dermis: advances in biology of skin,* vol 10, New York, 1970, Appleton-Century-Crofts.
308 Windle WF: Regeneration of nerves in the vertebrate central nervous system, *Physiol Rev* 36:427, 1970.
309 Winters GD: Epidermal wound healing in corticosteroid-treated skin of the domestic pig: mechanisms of topical corticosteroid activity. In Wilson L, Marks R, editors: *A Glaxo symposium on wound healing,* New York, 1962, Churchill Livingstone.
310 Wolley DE: Mammalian collagenases. In Piez KA, Reddi AH, editors: *Intracellular matrix biochemistry,* New York, 1984, Elsevier Biomedical Press.
311 Woost PG, Jumblatt MM, Eiferman RA et al: Growth factors and corneal endothelial cells. II. Characterization of epidermal growth factor receptor from bovine corneal endothelial cells, *Cornea* 11(1):11, 1992.
312 Wustrow TP: Interactions and biological mechanisms of action of molecular signal peptides, *HNO* 39(8):281, 1991.
313 Wyess CR, Matsen FA, Simmons CW et al: Transcutaneous oxygen tension measurements on limbs of diabetic and nondiabetic patients with peripheral vascular disease, *Surgery* 95:339, 1984.

CHAPTER

12

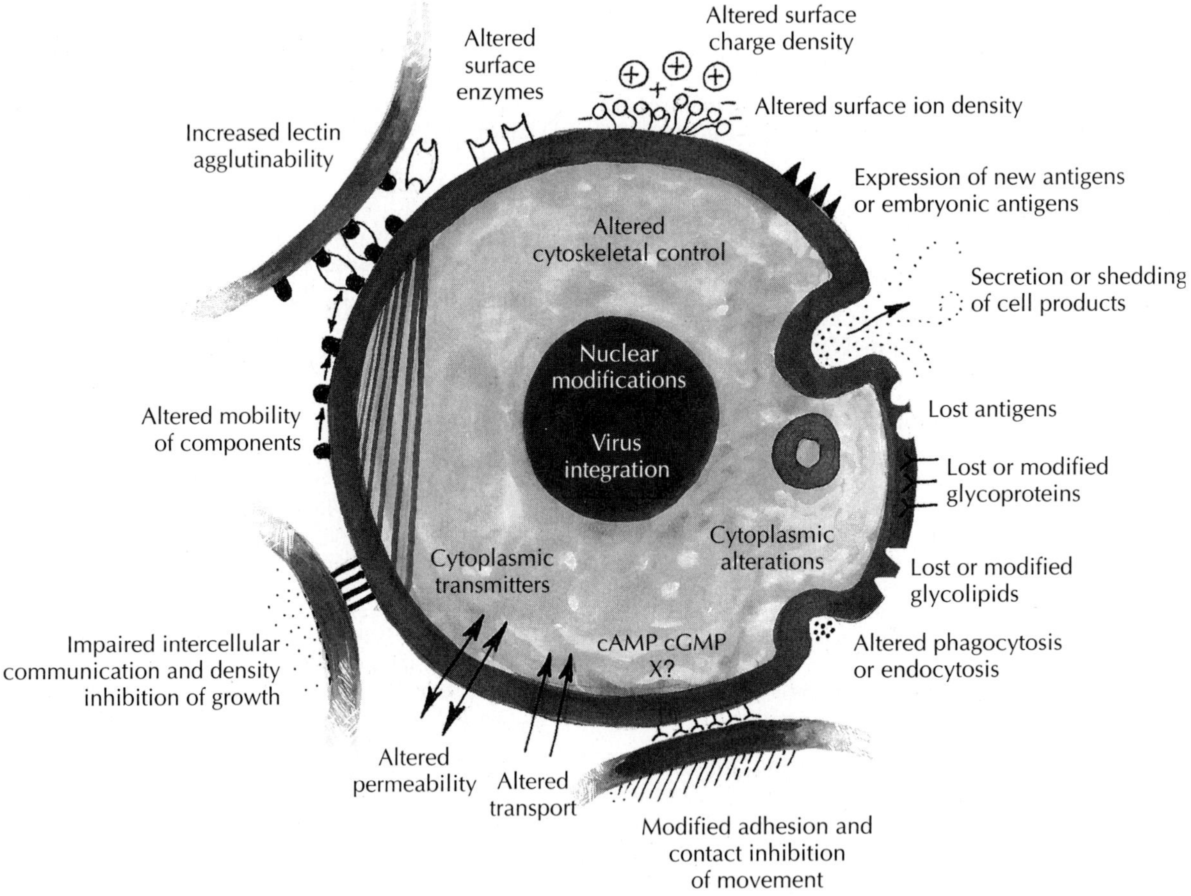

Modified from Nicolson GL: *Biochim Biophys Acta:* 458:1, 1976.

PRINCIPLES OF CANCER BIOLOGY AND CANCER TREATMENT

Roger S. Foster Jr.

This chapter provides an overview of the multidisciplinary concepts important to an understanding of the neoplastic process and its effects on the host. An understanding of the potential contributions of each discipline and collaboration among the disciplines will improve cancer treatment and prevention.

EPIDEMIOLOGY

Cancer epidemiology primarily concerns the patterns of distribution of neoplasia in populations rather than the individual patient. Ultimately, however, the information from epidemiologic studies must be translated into recommendations for the individual. A working knowledge of basic epidemiologic principles is important in understanding the literature related to cancer etiology, risk factors, and detection and the application of this information to the management of the patient.[143,153]

Although most information in this chapter is devoted to treatment, it should be noted that many cancers are preventable and that changes in life-style and other environmental factors can significantly reduce cancer incidence.[72,180] An estimated three fourths of all cancers are caused by extrinsic factors, and at least one fourth are preventable using current knowledge (Table 12-1).[39] Additional cancer deaths can be prevented by effective application of early cancer detection programs for certain cancers.

TABLE 12-1 PROPORTIONS OF CANCER DEATHS IN THE UNITED STATES ATTRIBUTED TO VARIOUS FACTORS

FACTORS OR CLASS OF FACTORS	PERCENTAGE OF ALL CANCER DEATHS: BEST ESTIMATE	PERCENTAGE OF ALL CANCER DEATHS: RANGE OF ESTIMATES
Tobacco	30	25 to 40
Diet	35	10 to 70
Infection	10(?)	1 to ?
Reproductive and sexual behavior	7	1 to 13
Occupation	4	2 to 8
Geophysical factors*	3	2 to 4
Alcohol	3	2 to 4
Pollution	2	<1 to 5
Medicines and medical procedures	1	0.5 to 3
Industrial products	<1	<1 to 2
Food additives	<1	−5† to 2
Unknown	?	?

Modified from Doll R, Peto R: *J Natl Cancer Inst* 66:1191, 1981.

*Geophysical factors cause a much greater proportion of nonfatal cancers (up to 30% of all cancers, depending on ethnic mix and latitude) because of the importance of ultraviolet light in causing the relatively nonfatal basal cell and squamous cell carcinomas of sunlight-exposed skin.

†Allowing for a possible protective effect of antioxidants and other preservatives, additives may have a net anticarcinogenic effect.

Epidemiologic Concepts

The physician must understand the terms that refer to the rates and proportions of conditions occurring in populations. *Prevalence* is the total number of individuals in the population with a given condition at any specified time. *Incidence* is the number of new cases diagnosed during a specified period. *Mortality* is the number of deaths occurring during a specified time. *Cause-specific mortality* is the number of deaths caused by a specific disease during a given period divided by the number of persons with the disease during the same period.

Relative risk of cancer is the probability of cancer development among a group of persons having a particular defined factor(s) divided by cancer probability among an otherwise similar group of persons without the defined factor(s). If the relative risk is more than one, a person with the defined factor is more likely to develop a cancer than a person without this factor. If the relative risk is one, the defined factor and cancer are not associated. If the relative risk is less than one, a person with the defined factor is less likely to develop a cancer than a person without the characteristic. Relative risks are calculated from population data; therefore, it is necessary to have information about the total population from which the cases are drawn. If population data are not available, an estimate of the relative risk may be calculated based on the risk in a control group drawn from the population and calculation of the *odds ratio*, or *relative odds*.

Variables are associated with each other if the occurrence of one is predictive of the likelihood of the other's occurring. Association does not necessarily imply causation; associations can be divided into noncausal (secondary) associations and causal associations. Frequently, associations are believed to be causal when only a secondary association exists. Judging when an association is causally related to a disease may be difficult. A judgment determining that a causal association exists must go beyond mere statistical calculation of significance. Several criteria for deciding when an association may be considered to be causal have been suggested[77,143]:

1. *Strength*. The stronger the association, the more likely it represents a cause-and-effect relationship.
2. *Temporality*. The time sequence is correct; that is, the exposure factor can be measured before onset of the disease.
3. *Specificity*. The exposure factor results in one or only a few diseases.
4. *Consistency*. The association occurs among different groups at different times.
5. *Plausibility*. A plausible biologic mechanism explains the association.
6. *Biologic gradient*. A dose-response relationship

exists (although threshold phenomena may also exist).

7. *Coherence.* The associations lead to theories that correctly predict other associations.
8. *Experimental evidence.* Modification based on the association changes the disease outcome.
9. *Analogy.* The association parallels other known cause-and-effect relationships, particularly when it cannot be explained by any other hypotheses.

Cancer Incidence and Mortality in the United States

In the U.S. population of more than 255 million persons, the total number of new cancer cases in 1992 was estimated at over 1.8 million (Table 12-2).[4] Carcinoma in situ and nonmelanoma skin cancers accounted for approximately 700,000 of the total. The estimated cancer deaths in 1992 were 520,000 with 275,000 male deaths and 245,000 female deaths.[4,5] The age-adjusted mortality rates for most major causes of cancer death, except lung and stomach cancer, have remained relatively stable between 1930 and 1988 (Figure 12-1). The reduction in stomach cancer has been epidemiologically related to changes in the U.S. diet, with a decreased intake of smoked and pickled foods and increased year-round availability of fruits and vegetables. The lung cancer epidemic is related to widespread prevalence of cigarette smoking.[100]

An alternative to examining annual cancer incidence and mortality figures is to calculate the projected risk for an infant born in 1985 of either eventually developing cancer or dying of cancer. This approach is based on the assumption that changes in exposure to carcinogens or anticarcinogens will not occur, nor will changes in survival related to early detection or improved treatment. In addition, one must assume that major changes in the competing causes of death will not occur (Figures 12-2 to 12-5). Clearly the goal is to alter these probabilities; the National Cancer Institute has set a goal of

TABLE 12-2 ESTIMATED NEW CASES AND DEATHS FOR MAJOR SITES OF CANCER—1992*

SITE	CASES	DEATHS
Lung	168,000	146,000
Colon-rectum	156,000	58,300
Breast (female)	181,000	46,300
Prostate	132,000	34,000
Urinary tract	78,100	20,200
Uterus	45,500†	10,000
Oral	30,300	8,000
Pancreas	28,300	25,000
Leukemia	28,200	18,200
Skin (melanoma)	32,000‡	6,700
Ovary	21,000	13,000

From American Cancer Society: *Cancer facts and figures,* 1992.
*Figures rounded to nearest 1,000. Incidence estimates are based on rates from the National Cancer Institute SEER program, 1986-1988.
†If carcinoma in situ is included, cases total over 200,000.
‡Estimated new cases of nonmelanoma over 600,000.

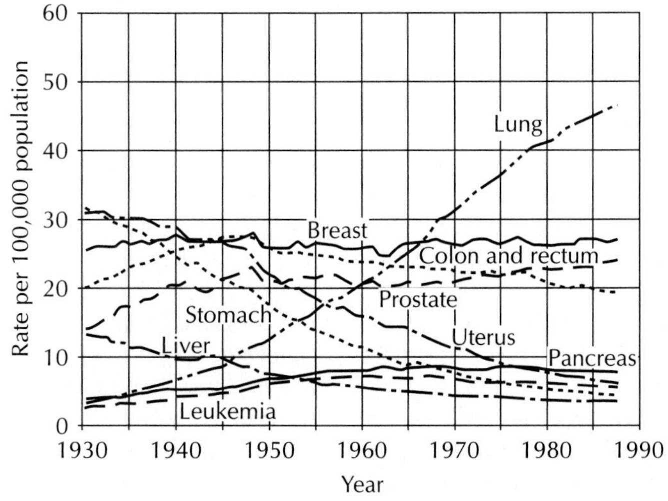

FIGURE 12-1 Cancer death rates by site of origin in the United States from 1930 to 1988. The rate for the population has been standardized for age in the 1970 U.S. population. The rates are for both sexes, except for breast and uterus (female population only) and prostate (male population only). The sources of the data were the National Center for Health Statistics and the U.S. Bureau of the Census. (From the American Cancer Society: *Cancer facts and figures,* 1992.)

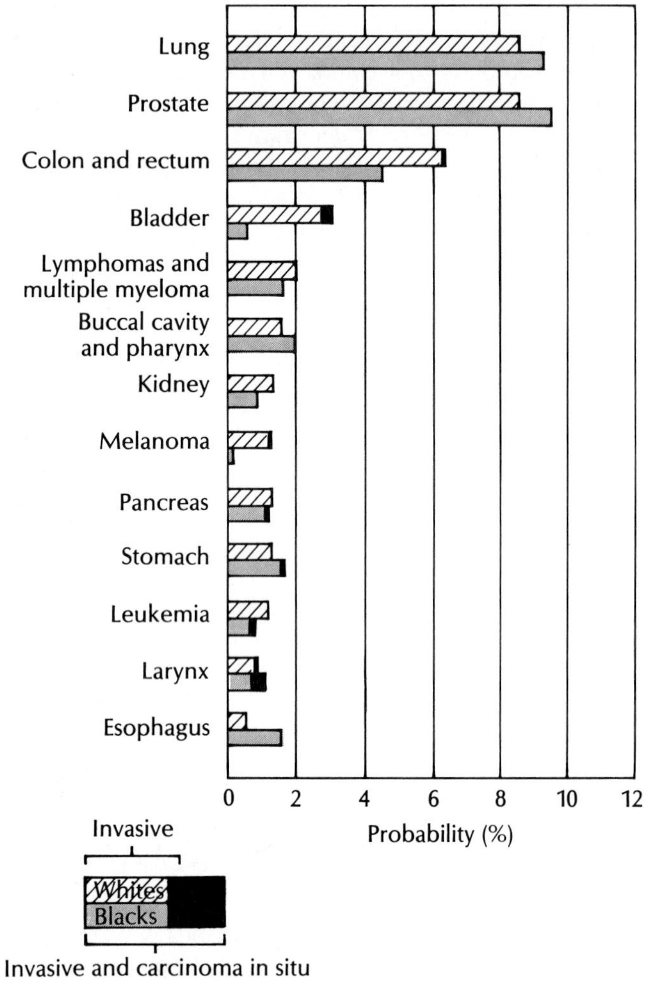

FIGURE 12-2 The probability at birth in 1985 of eventually developing selected types of cancer for white and black males in the United States. (From *CA* 35:1, 19, 1985.)

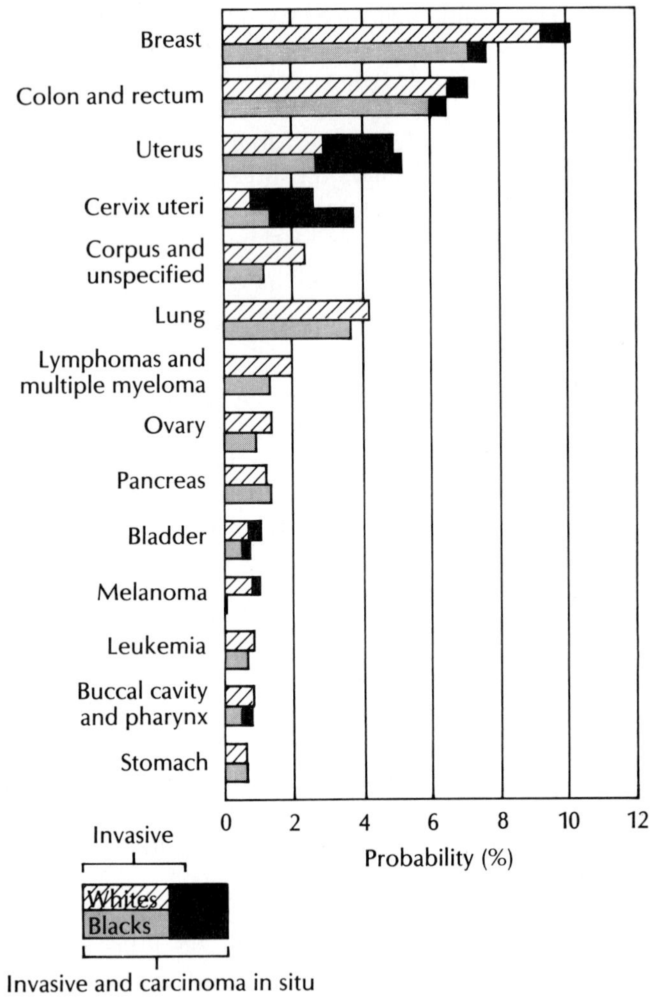

FIGURE 12-3 The probability at birth in 1985 of eventually developing selected types of cancer for white and black females in the United States. (From *CA* 35:1, 19, 1985.)

reducing the age-adjusted cancer death rate by 50% of 1980 levels by the year 2000.[36] If no slowing of the current cancer mortality trends occurs, the estimated number of U.S. cancer deaths in the year 2000 will be 575,000.[37]

ETIOLOGY OF CANCER

A disease is rarely the result of a single causative factor. Cancer results from a combination of genetic inheritance, environmental influences, host responses, and probably some random chance. Many steps occur in the sequence of events from exposure to a cancer-causing factor to the ultimate development of a clinical cancer. Probably not every step in the complex pathway can be known. If one or more necessary steps in the pathway are known and can be interrupted, eliminated, or altered, the resultant cancer can be prevented.

Unfortunately, knowledge of a causative factor is not enough to prevent cancer. For example, tobacco smoke is the leading causative agent of cancer in the United States and is responsible for approximately 30% of all cancer deaths. Tobacco is the sole agent responsible for the continued rise in the age-adjusted death rate from cancer in the U.S. population. Although the incidence of cigarette smoking among physicians has declined from 90% in the 1940s to 7% now, smoking remains a prevalent habit in the general U.S. population (approximately 30% of adults) and is actually increasing among some groups of younger women. The general population knows the causal relationship, but the competing forces of addiction to nicotine, commercial interests of tobacco-based regional economies, and commercial interests of the tobacco manufacturers all contribute to the high rate of exposure to the carcinogens in tobacco smoke.

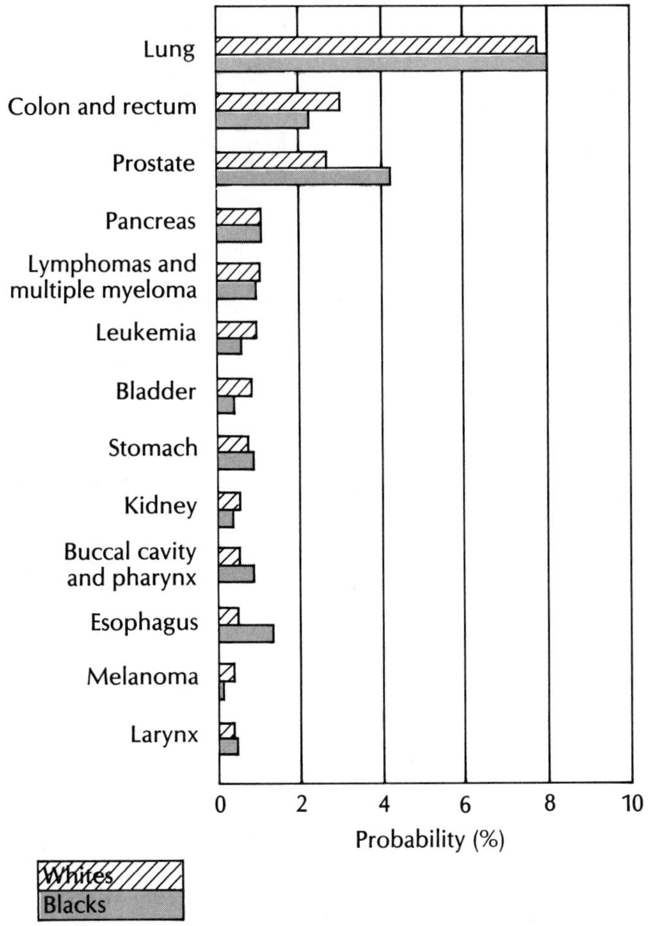

FIGURE 12-4 The probability at birth in 1985 of eventually dying of selected types of cancer for white and black males in the United States. (From *CA* 35:1, 19, 1985.)

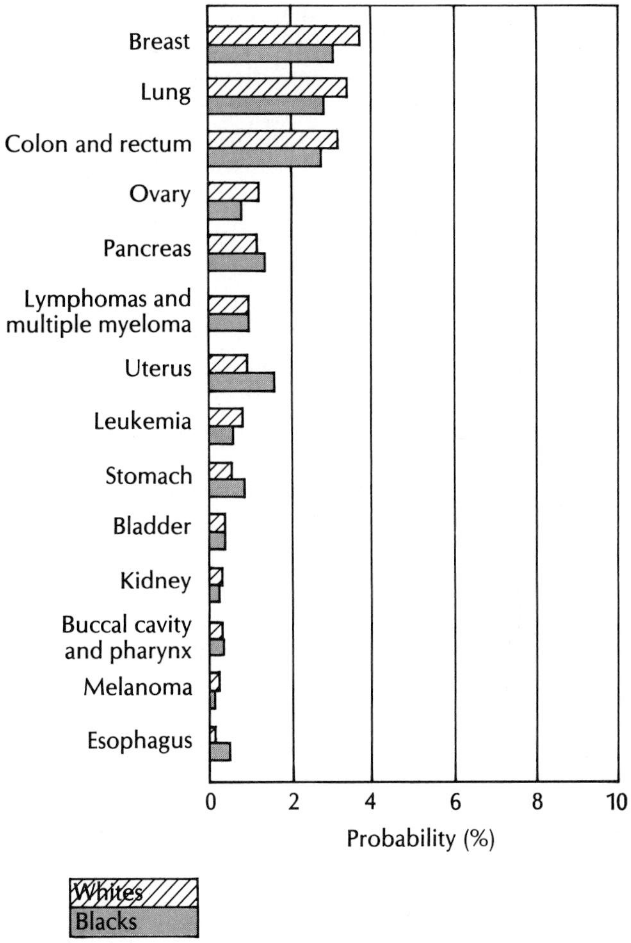

FIGURE 12-5 The probability at birth in 1985 of eventually dying of selected types of cancer for white and black females in the United States. (From *CA* 35:1, 19, 1985.)

Chemical Carcinogenesis

Of the known carcinogenic agents, chemical agents apparently are the most important in the induction of human cancers. Sir Percival Potts, an English surgeon, was the first to recognize chemical carcinogenesis. In 1775 he reported the association between cancer of the scrotum in his patients and their employment as chimney sweeps when they were young boys.[128]

The known chemical carcinogens have a variety of structural formulas and include polycyclic hydrocarbons, azo dyes, nitrosamines, and inorganic compounds such as chromium and nickel (Table 12-3). The important step in the induction of cancer by chemicals appears to be the covalent interaction of the chemical or its metabolite with proteins and other macromolecules, particularly deoxyribonucleic acid (DNA).[107] Many chemical carcinogens are not activated until metabolized by cellular enzyme systems, where they are converted into

TABLE 12-3 SOME CARCINOGENIC CHEMICALS IN HUMANS

CHEMICAL	ORGAN IN WHICH ASSOCIATED NEOPLASM OCCURS
Soots and tars	Skin, lung
Tobacco smoke	Lung, mouth, pharynx, esophagus, bladder
2-Naphthylamine	Urinary bladder
4-Aminobiphenyl	Urinary bladder
Benzidine	Urinary bladder
Nickel compound	Lungs, nasal cavity
Asbestos	Lungs, pleura
Cadmium oxide	Prostate
Diethylstilbestrol (DES)	Vagina
Aflatoxin	Liver
Arsenic	Lungs, skin
Vinylchloride	Liver
Thorotrast	Liver

Partial list adapted from Miller JA: *Cancer Res* 30:559, 1970; and Miller EC: *Cancer Res* 38:1479, 1978.

electrophilic reactants that then exert their biologic effects by interaction with cellular macromolecules, most critically DNA.[108,109] Although interaction with the cellular DNA may be essential, it is not sufficient; cycles of cell proliferation are necessary for initiation of cancer with chemicals.[44]

Various species of animals and various tissues have species-specific and tissue-specific enzyme systems that can markedly alter the sensitivity of a given cell population to a carcinogen. Other factors that can alter a chemical's carcinogenic effect are transportation and concentration in a specific tissue, rate of degradation, and the rate at which a cell is able to repair carcinogen-induced lesions in DNA. Most carcinogens are also either mutagens or can be metabolically converted to mutagens. Persons with an inherited defect in the ability to repair DNA, such as patients with xeroderma pigmentosum, are susceptible to both increased mutagenesis and increased carcinogenesis from chemical and physical carcinogens. The mutagenic and carcinogenic effects of carcinogens appear to be related to the persistence of damage in the cellular DNA.

After exposure to any carcinogen, whether chemical, physical, or viral, an extended period of time often elapses before the neoplasm appears. This period is known as the *latency time.* The length of the latency time is related to the type of carcinogen, its dose, the target cell, and the host animal.

In many circumstances, carcinogenesis can be divided into an initiation phase and a promotion phase (Figure 12-6).[182] An *initiating agent* is a chemical, physical, or biologic agent that can irreversibly alter the DNA of the cell. Change in the DNA, however, is usually not the only requirement for neoplastic transformation; a promoting agent is also needed. A *promoting agent* alters the expression of the cell's genetic information. Promoting agents act through various mechanisms to alter cell functions or to affect the expression of receptors on the cell surface, in the cytoplasm, or in the nucleus, leading ultimately to the progression to cancer.[44] Examples of promoting agents include hormones and drugs that do not act directly with the genetic material.

Promoting agents cannot initiate carcinogenesis, but many (probably most) initiating agents can subsequently serve as promoting agents. Such carcinogens that can both initiate and promote are known as *complete carcinogens.* Agents that can stimulate the process of initiation by a carcinogen are known as *cocarcinogens.* Agents that can inhibit the process of carcinogenesis are *anticarcinogens.* Most cocarcinogens and anticarcinogens act by altering the cellular metabolism, which is important in production of the ultimate carcinogen. Other anticarcinogens, such as retinoids, act as suppressing agents, even after the carcinogenic compound has reacted with its cellular target.[172] Current research on humans is aimed at investigating the possibility that vitamins A, C, and E or their analogs may have anticarcinogenic effects.

FIGURE 12-6 Schematic representation of chemical carcinogenesis. The circles represent cells at various stages in the process of malignant transformation by chemicals. On the left, a normal cell is exposed to procarcinogens. As the carcinogen enters the cell, it may go directly to cytoplasmic (endoplasmic reticulum, *ER*) or nuclear (nuclear membrane, *NM*) sites of constitutive metabolic *(CM)* activity. Alternatively, procarcinogens may complex with a receptor protein *(RP),* form an inducer complex *(IC),* and derepress genes controlling enzymatic activity, leading to induction of metabolism *(IM).* Metabolically activated (electrophilic) ultimate carcinogens may complex with other proteins *(PP)* that prevent immediate degradation or covalent interactions at nearby sites. Ultimate carcinogenic species will interact with a variety of target molecules in the nucleus *(NT),* in the cytoplasm *(CT),* or at the plasma membrane *(PMT).* Carcinogens may also be metabolized in one cell and delivered to other cells in activated form. In both cases, precise interaction with critical cellular targets, possibly DNA, is required for initiation. Several endogenous and exogenous factors will also influence the probability that the carcinogen-cellular interaction will lead to a permanent state of "initiation" of carcinogenesis. Similarly, endogenous and exogenous factors determine the level of preneoplastic progression (→), depicted here for schematic purposes as two cells but representing a series of progressive changes. Each preneoplastic change may be stable for long periods and may even revert (←) to a more dependent stage under the proper conditions. As progression toward malignancy continues, the preneoplastic cell becomes more autonomous (less dependent on exogenous stimulation). Several phenotypic alterations (⇝) become apparent during this prolonged process, and the clone size of preneoplastic cells increases. Ultimately, progression results in a malignant clone with clinical expression of cancer. (From Yuspa SH, Harris CC: Molecular and cellular basis of chemical carcinogenesis. In Schottenfeld D, Fraument JF Jr, editors: *Cancer epidemiology and prevention,* Philadelphia, 1982, WB Saunders.)

Physical Carcinogenesis

Physical agents, including ionizing radiation, ultraviolet radiation, and fibers, can have carcinogenic effects. Within 6 years after their discovery, roentgen rays were suspected to be carcinogenic because of the high frequency of skin cancers on the hands of the early workers using these rays. We now know that all tissues are at risk to cancer induction by ionizing irradiation.

The types of malignancy induced by ionizing radiations depend on several factors, including the dose of radiation, age at the time of exposure, genetic susceptibility, and sex. The risk for development of cancers of the thyroid gland, breast, lung, stomach, and connective tissues is greatest after exposure at young ages.[167] For example, data from populations exposed to radiation from the atomic bomb indicate that female survivors under age 10 years at the time of exposure are now showing a high incidence of breast cancer.[165] The degree of excess risk of breast cancer in the atomic bomb survivors decreases for those exposed after age 20, and women over age 40 at the time of exposure appear to have no increased risk. Solid cancers induced by irradiation tend to appear at the age when the naturally occurring cancer is likely to appear. Women seem to be

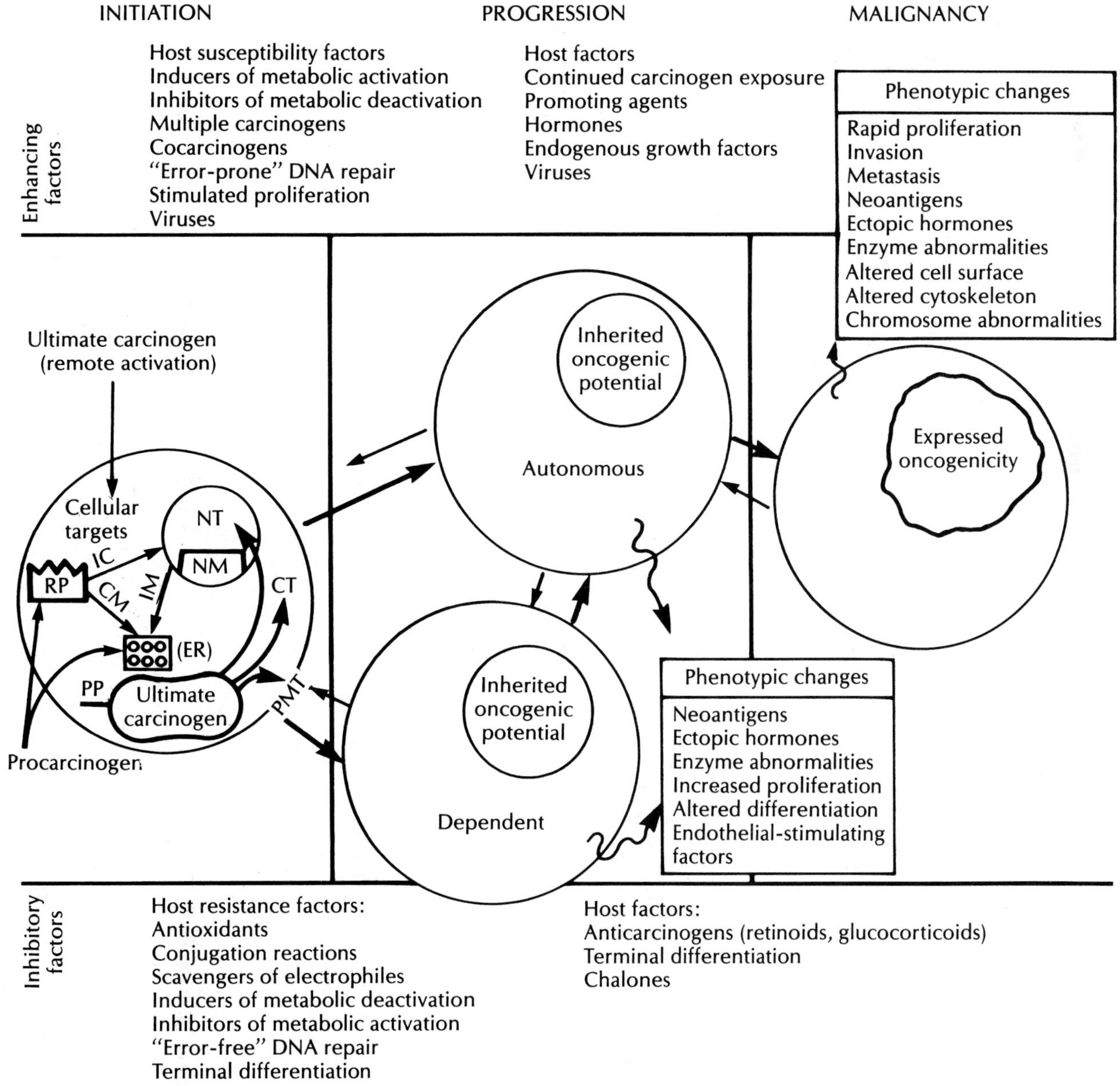

FIGURE 12-6 For legend see opposite page.

30% to 50% more susceptible to irradiation carcinogenesis than men, probably because the breast and thyroid have tissues particularly susceptible to radiation.[80,84]

The mechanism of irradiation carcinogenesis is related to the ability of ionizing radiations to break strong chemical bonds and cause lesions in the chromosomal DNA.[170] Alteration of DNA adjacent to certain oncogenes may be important in malignant transformation. Evidence shows that two or more gene loci may be involved in some malignant transformations. What occurs during the variable but frequently long latency period between radiation exposure and appearance of the malignancy is not well understood, but host factors clearly are important.

Considerable evidence shows that moderate doses of radiation can cause genetic damage that transforms cells, resulting in clinical cancer. The high doses to small volumes that are usually used in clinical therapy tend to sterilize the parenchymal cells and therefore induce fewer tumors despite the higher exposure dose. Although modest doses of radiation to the pelvis are associated with an increase in the incidence of pelvic malignancies, long-term studies of women treated with high doses of radiation for cervical cancer have not indicated an increased occurrence of second pelvic malignancies.[16]

Ultraviolet (UV) radiation is an important cause of skin cancer, by far the most common cancer among whites in North America. Melanin is an important protectant against the effects of UV irradiation, and skin cancers are 70 times more frequent in whites than blacks. Skin cancers tend to occur on those areas of the skin exposed to the sun or other sources of UV light. Changes in life-style and dress and the popular concept that a tan signifies good health have led to a rising incidence of skin cancer, with an incidence in the United States exceeding 600,000 cases annually. Most basal cell carcinomas and squamous cell carcinomas of the skin grow slowly, rarely metastasize when small, and thus are readily curable.

More ominous is the rising incidence of much more lethal melanomas. Ultraviolet light is believed to cause DNA damage primarily through the formation of pyrimidine dimers.[154] Some research suggests that UV irradiation affects the immune mechanisms of the skin, with the induction of suppressor T lymphocytes that interfere with the rejection of tumors.[92] The obvious but not always observed recommendation is to avoid, when possible, exposure to UV radiation. Applying sunscreens to the skin before exposure also offers some protection. Trials are currently under way to determine how administration of the potential anticarcinogens beta-carotene and 13-cisretinoic acid affects the development of skin cancers.

A variety of foreign bodies, including asbestos fibers, talc, and biologic foreign agents such as schistosomal eggs and tubercle bacilli, can act as carcinogens.

Viral Carcinogenesis

Viruses can alter their host cell either independently or by being integrated into the host cell's genetic material. Numerous animal models of viral carcinogenesis exist. Some DNA viruses can be integrated into the genome of a cell and cause malignant transformation. Oncogenic ribonucleic acid (RNA) viruses also exist. In 1970 Baltimore[9] discovered that oncogenic RNA viruses contain an enzyme (reverse transcriptase) that can synthesize DNA from an RNA template. The discovery of reverse transcriptase explained the ability of an RNA virus to incorporate information into the DNA of the host cell, and viruses with these properties have been given the name *retroviruses*. Many recent advances in the understanding of the molecular basis of oncogenesis have come from the study of retroviruses.[184] (See also the following section on Biology and Molecular Biology of Cancer.)

Although a causal role in oncogenesis has not been definitively proved, strong circumstantial evidence implicates both DNA and RNA viruses as etiologic agents in some human tumors. Human malignancies that appear to be etiologically associated with viruses include Burkitt's lymphoma and nasopharyngeal carcinoma (Epstein-Barr virus), cervical cancer (papilloma virus and herpesvirus), hepatoma (hepatitis virus), and adult T-cell leukemia-lymphoma (human T-cell leukemia virus).

The data implicating the Epstein-Barr virus (EBV) as etiologically important in Burkitt's lymphoma are particularly strong. The EBV virus, which is a DNA virus, has been found in cultured Burkitt's cells, and patients with the disease have high titers of antibodies to EBV. EBV antigen has been demonstrated in the cells of Burkitt's lymphoma, and EBV DNA has been demonstrated by molecular hybridization.[133] The evidence linking the herpes simplex virus type 2 as a most important etiologic factor in cervical cancer is similar.

RNA viruses have been the viruses most unambiguously linked with the induction of cancer in experimental animals, and these viruses have been important experimental probes in the study of oncogenes. Only recently has strong evidence shown that retroviruses are probably important etiologic agents in some human cancers. The evidence to date indicates that a family of viruses are T lymphotrophic for human cells and that a subgroup of this family, human T-cell leukemia virus 1, is etiologically associated with a distinct leukemia. Adult T-cell leukemia virus III has been etiologically associated with acquired immune deficiency syndrome (AIDS). In AIDS, the virus has cytopathic effects on the T-cell rather than immortalizing effects.[57]

Immune Surveillance

The precise role of the immune system in the prevention and control of neoplasia is uncertain. In animal models, data indicate that many different immune cell types can participate in the destruction of aberrant cells: T cells, B cells, natural killer (NK) cells, and macrophages. However, animal models of chemical carcinogenesis have failed to show that loss of T cells increases the rate of carcinogenesis. By contrast, decreased cellular immune function does increase susceptibility to viral carcinogenesis.

Patients with immune deficiency and immunosuppressed transplant patients are at increased risk of malignancy. However, only certain types of malignancy are increased in immunosuppressed patients. The types of malignancies that are particularly increased in immunocompromised humans are the lymphoreticular malignancies, squamous cell carcinomas of the skin and cervix, and Kaposi's sarcoma (AIDS patients). Squamous cell carcinoma of the cervix is strongly associated with herpes simplex virus type 2 (HSV 2), and there is speculation that Kaposi's sarcoma is related to a viral agent. The lymphoreticular malignancies may be related to chronic proliferative stimulation of the immune system, a viral agent, or both.

Genetic Factors in Cancer Causation

Heritable genetic factors are related to the development of some cancers. A few, perhaps 1% to 2% of all cancers, have a definite genetic determination, whereas others may occur in persons who have a genetic trait that makes them more susceptible to carcinogens. Examples of cancers related to inheritance of a mendelian dominant trait are colon cancers in patients with familial polyposis, neurofibromatosis and the various cancers associated with it, and the multiple endocrine neoplasia syndrome type II (MEN II).

A second class of hereditary predispositions to cancer results from recessive tumor suppressor genes, with one normal allele being adequate to protect against a particular cancer.[175] Cancers related to recessive genes are retinoblastoma and Wilms' tumor. Knudson[89] has termed these recessive genes *antioncogenes*. (See following section for a discussion of oncogenes and antioncogenes.)

In a child born with the gene for retinoblastoma, the probability that the tumor will develop is 95%, and the average patient will develop three or four retinoblastomas. The risk for retinoblastoma in the carriers of the gene is approximately 100,000-fold greater than for noncarriers. At the cellular level, however, the development of a retinoblastoma from all the millions of retinal cells in each individual is rare.

The genetic trait alone is not sufficient for the development of a tumor. The theoretic model explaining the rarity of cancer development at the cellular level in hereditary cancers is that two or more mutational events must occur before there is oncogenesis. In the inherited cancers, the first mutation is present in all cells derived from the germ line, but an additional somatic mutation must occur before a cancer develops. Part of the evidence supporting the two-mutational model of cancer development is the observation that children with the inherited form of retinoblastoma have a greatly increased risk of developing osteogenic sarcoma after exposure to ionizing radiation.[88]

Some genetically inherited predispositions to cancer appear to be related to either increased chromosomal fragility or defects in the ability to repair damage to the DNA, the so-called chromosomal breakage syndromes.[59] For example, patients with xeroderma pigmentosum have a markedly increased risk of developing skin cancers on exposure to sunlight.[101] The fibroblasts of patients with xeroderma pigmentosum, when studied in vitro, have been found to have deficient DNA repair enzymes; they repair UV-induced DNA damage either very slowly or not at all.

Multifactorial Etiologies and Cancer

The previous discussions of cancer etiology is divided into genetic, chemical, viral, and physical causes. Because it appears that for most malignancies a multistep process must induce a change at two or more sites in the genetic material before a malignancy develops, the cause of a cancer is possibly multifactorial. Although one type of carcinogenic factor may be predominant for some cancers, most cancers are probably the result of multiple interacting carcinogenic and anticarcinogenic effects.

Strong evidence shows shared etiology and even synergism among causative agents for several human cancers. For example, smoking acts synergistically in the production of lung cancer with both ionizing radiation and asbestos.[8,149] Smoking also acts synergistically with alcohol in the etiology of cancer of the oral cavity, pharynx, and esophagus.[76,169] Evidence also suggests that some anticarcinogenic factors may reduce the risk of tumor induction by known carcinogens. For example, increased dietary consumption of beta-carotene may reduce the risk of various cancers, including cancer of the lung in smokers.[14,126]

BIOLOGY AND MOLECULAR BIOLOGY OF CANCER

The development of the adult human being from the fertilized egg is a complex process that depends on multiple interlocking interactions between the genetic material of the gametes and the environment. Most cancers develop from a single cell, and cancers may appropriately be viewed as populations of cells that grow abnormally as a result of abnormalities in the cell's genetic material. The adult person has more than 10^{14} cells, and more than 10^{16} cells are produced in a lifetime. Thus many cells are at risk for the genetic alterations that may lead to a malignancy. In humans, cancer is a relatively common disease; a potentially lethal neoplasm develops in about one fourth of all persons by the time they reach old age. From the perspective of the total cells in the body, however, development of a malignant tumor is relatively rare.

Neoplasms can develop from any normal cell of the body capable of undergoing mitosis. Because tumors are derived from normal cells, they bear some structural and functional resemblance to their cell or tissue of origin. The population of cells in a tumor mass includes not only the malignant cells but also a heterogeneous mixture of stromal, vascular, and lymphohematopoietic cells derived from the host's nonmalignant cell population. Normal tissues are composed of subpopulations of cells capable of dividing and renewing the tissue following cell loss or cell death. Other cells in normal tissue reach a stage of differentiation (terminal differentiation) in which, under usual circumstances, they are incapable of further division. These cells are the functional cells that perform the variety of specialized functions characteristic of vertebrate animals.

Most neoplasms are also composed of both a proliferating or clonogenic population and a population of neoplastic cells incapable of proliferating. Just as the various cells in normal tissue contribute differently to the total function of the tissue or organ, most neoplasms are made up of cells that have diverse characteristics and contribute differently to the behavior and function of the tumor mass ecosystem. In general, cancers behave and progress as populations of cells and not as single cells; however, this concept should not be taken as a denial of the probability that most tumors are derived from a single altered cell or that single cells can metastasize. Recognition of the heterogeneity of cancer cells within a malignant population and the interactions between individual cancer cells and host cells is necessary for an understanding of neoplasia.[74]

Clonal Origin of Cancer

The evidence showing that most cancers originate from a single cell is convincing.[46,123] However, multiple primary tumors may also arise from different cell clones in an individual. Development of multiple primary tumors is particularly likely in those persons with a hereditary predisposition for cancer development. Despite the single-cell clonal origin of most cancers, almost all cancers develop cell populations with considerable heterogeneity of the individual cells within the primary tumor or its metastases. The explanation for this development appears to be related to cancer cells' being genetically more unstable than normal cells; thus subpopulations of cells evolve because of sequential genetic changes. Many of these genetic variants may be nonviable and therefore are eliminated, but those with a selective growth advantage will persist and proliferate. The heterogeneity of advanced tumors is reflected in the problem of drug resistance in patients undergoing chemotherapy.

Neoplasms resemble their tissue of origin to varying degrees. Those that bear the greatest similarity are described as well differentiated and tend to grow more slowly. All neoplasms, however, are capable of transgressing on the structural arrangement of normal tissues in their growth process. Benign neoplasms push aside the normal tissues and may occasionally cause severe symptoms if they occlude the airway, put pressure on important nerves, or secrete hormonal substances. Malignant neoplasms are able to invade and destroy adjacent normal tissue and also may spread to other areas of the body through lymphatic or blood vessels or through the pleural, peritoneal, or dural spaces. The more slowly growing, well-differentiated malignant neoplasms may only grow and compress and destroy the adjacent normal tissue. The less well-differentiated tumors not only have a greater propensity for invading and eroding normal structures, but also a greater capability of metastasizing to distant areas.

Cell Growth Cycle

Knowing the kinetics of cell proliferation is basic to an understanding of cancer and cancer therapy. The cell replication cycle has been conceptually divided into discrete phases (Figure 12-7). After mitosis, the cell enters a period before synthesis of DNA begins known as the G_1 phase. The G_1 phase lasts for varying periods in different proliferating cells. Following G_1, the cells enter the DNA synthetic phase *(S)*. On completion of DNA synthesis, the cells begin the G_2 phase, which precedes mitosis *(M)*. The term G_0, also known as *quiescence,* has been added to the terminology to indicate cells not in the proliferating population but capable of being recruited into this population. Cells recruited from G_0 enter the cycle during the G_1 phase. In the developing organism and in normal tissue, cell proliferation, cell differentiation, and cell death are well balanced. Cell proliferation, varying degrees of differentiation, and cell death also occur in malignant tissue, but the balance has been disrupted in favor of a larger portion of the cells remaining in the proliferating population with incomplete terminal differentiation. Neoplasms may be viewed as caricatures of the normal processes of tissue development and renewal.[144,145]

Because all cells are derived from the common genetic material of the fertilized ovum, selective restriction of the readout of genetic material is necessary for the totipotential ovum to develop into a multicellular organism with specialized functional tissues. In differentiation, a heritable alteration occurs in the pattern of gene readout in one of the two progeny of cells derived from a parent cell. Daughter cells that are structurally and functionally different from the parent cell are thereby pro-

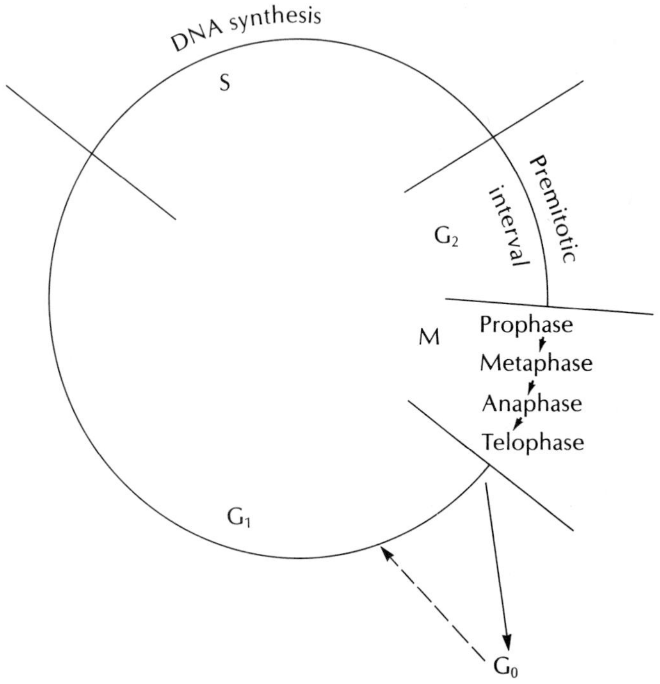

FIGURE 12-7 Schematic representation of the life cycle of cells. G_0 refers to cells that are not in the proliferating population. Some cells in the G_0 population have gone on to terminal differentiation and are presumably no longer capable of proliferation. Other cells in the G_0 population are capable of being recruited back into the proliferative population. G_1 refers to the first growth phase that precedes the S phase of DNA synthesis. G_2, or the second growth phase, is the premitotic interval, and *M* is the mitotic phase.

duced. Many of the exact molecular mechanisms controlling differentiation and cell proliferation are still unknown, but several have been identified. Differentiation and proliferation in normal cells are controlled to varying degrees by both genetic regulation and external stimuli that alter the cell's microenvironment. Abundant evidence indicates that a combination of genetic and environmental factors also controls the proliferative activity and differentiated function of many malignant cells.

A decision point appears to occur early in the G_1 phase of the cell cycle, known as the *restriction point,* during which cells must commit to continuing into the S phase, remain in G_1, or enter the prolonged G_0 quiescent state. Conditions that restrict further proliferation of a normal cell include high cell density and suboptimal concentrations of nutrients or growth factors. Once the cell passes the restriction point and commits to the division process, the cell must continue through the S, G_2, and M phases before returning to the G_1 phase of the cell cycle. If populations of cells that have passed the restriction point are blocked in the S, G_2 or M phase for a time, they tend to die. The mechanism whereby a cell committed to DNA synthesis dies if the process is interrupted is not entirely clear but may be related to the release of lytic enzymes from lysosomes.[146] Malignant cells appear to lose stringent restriction point control and will proceed into the proliferative phase of the cell cycle despite unfavorable growth conditions. Under conditions where normal cells enter a quiescent phase (they have restriction point control), the proliferation of malignant cells may not be restricted (loss of restriction point control). If conditions are sufficiently unfavorable that the malignant cells are unable to complete cell division, they will tend to die, whereas normal cells that have remained in G_1 or G_0 survive.

Flow Cytometry

By flowing suspensions of single cells (or cell nuclei) through a flow chamber that breaks up the stream into microdroplets containing individual fluorescently labeled cells, the individual cells can be analyzed and sorted. Each cell is illuminated by a laser and measured for characteristics such as cell size, granularity, and red or green fluorescence. The cells exhibiting the various characteristics can be both quantified and sorted in the flow cytometer by such parameters as size, density, and electric charge.

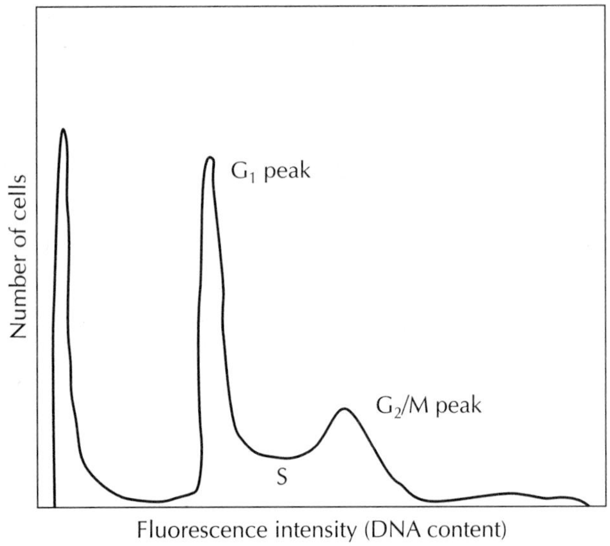

FIGURE 12-8 A flow cytometer histogram of the DNA content of a tumor. The DNA content histogram may be computer analyzed to determine both the proportion of cells that are in the G_1, S, and G_2/M phases of the cell cycle and the degree of aneuploidy.

A widely used clinical application of flow cytometry is to measure the DNA content and estimate the proliferative rate of solid tumors and hematopoietic malignancies (Figure 12-8). Normal resting somatic cells are diploid; normal cells in mitosis are tetraploid, with twice the DNA content of normal resting cells. Normal cells undergoing DNA synthesis have amounts of DNA between that of resting and mitotic cells. Tumor cells may have DNA contents that are normal for their state of proliferation, or they may have grossly abnormal amounts of DNA, which is known as *aneuploidy*. The variations in the DNA content of aneuploid cells are related to gross changes in the structure and number of chromosomes that can be seen when karyotypes are made.

Aneuploidy and increased numbers of cells in S phase are associated with a poorer prognosis. Clinical correlations are being made to determine the extent to which parameters determined by flow cytometry provide prognostic information that augments the traditional histologic prognostic factors such as the number of mitoses, histologic grade, and vascular or lymphatic invasion.

Chromosomal Molecules

The genetic material that stains as chromatin in the nucleus of the cell is organized into long chains of the four nucleotide bases, which can number several billion nucleotides per DNA molecular strand.[45,173,174] The sequence of these four nucleotides determines all the complex genetic information in the cell. Complementary pairs of DNA strands are joined in a double helical arrangement in which nucleotide base pairs of the complementary strands are linked by weak chemical bonds. The complementary strands of the double helix run in opposite directions, and the adenylate nucleotide always pairs with the thymidylate nucleotide, whereas cytidylate always pairs with guanylate.

A variety of important proteins in the chromatin material of the cell nucleus are associated with the double helical DNA and are important in gene transcription. These proteins have been divided into the histone proteins and the nonhistone proteins. The histones are relatively stable, long-lived proteins synthesized primarily during the S phase and are intimately associated with DNA. The histones are believed to be important in packaging the DNA so that in differentiation only a portion of the genetic material is subject to translation by messenger RNA. The chromatin-associated nonhistone proteins tend to have relatively short half-lives and include a diverse group of polypeptides. The nonhistone proteins include DNA and RNA polymerase, proteases, DNA ligase, and phosphoprotein kinase. Alterations occur in the synthesis and turnover of the nonhistone proteins when cells are stimulated to proliferate or are induced by hormones to produce new proteins. Although carcinogenesis is generally attributed to changes in the DNA, carcinogenic agents can possibly bring about changes in gene readout by alteration of the chromatin-associated proteins.

Mammalian DNA has an estimated 50,000 or more genes. As previously discussed, only a small percentage of the DNA in the nucleus of a differentiated cell is available to be transcribed into RNA. Moreover, only a portion of the transcribed nuclear RNA reaches the cytoplasm as messenger RNA to eventually be translated into protein synthesis. Thus, even beyond the point of gene transcription, control mechanisms may be affected and lead to a phenotypically altered cell.

Techniques of Molecular Biology

Over the past several years major technologic advances in molecular biology and genetic engineering have led to rapid progress in the description of some of the molecular events involved in neoplasia.[31,147,161] Detecting the unique sequences of nucleotides in the total DNA of the genome is now theoretically possible by using Southern's transfer analysis.[162] DNA is first digested into fragments by specialized restriction enzymes that cut DNA at specific nucleotide recognition sites. The DNA fragments are then resolved by electrophoresis, transferred to a cellulose membrane, and hybridized with radioisotopically labeled DNA probes. Libraries of specific DNA probes are being developed. A somewhat similar technique for analysis of RNA, called "Northern analysis," has also been developed.[3] The RNA is first digested into

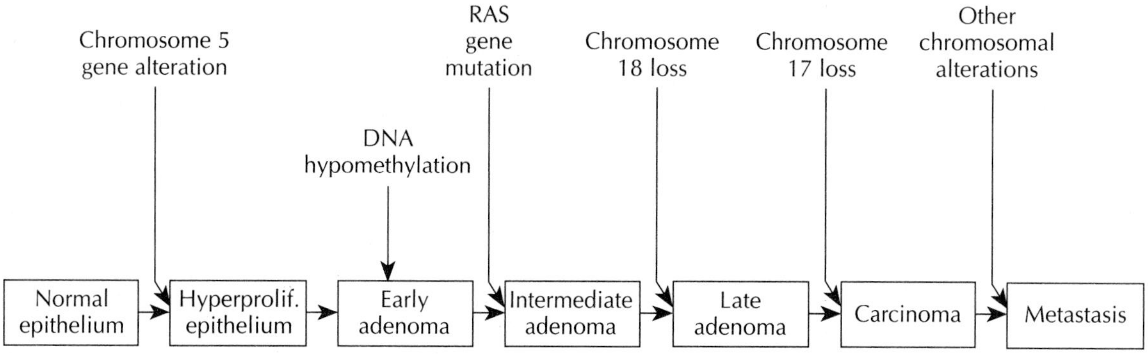

FIGURE 12-9 A multistep genetic model for colorectal tumorigenesis. (Modified from Fearson ER, Vogelstein BA: *Cell* 61:759, 1990.)

fragments and then fractionated electrophoretically. After transfer to a membrane, the specific RNA species can then be identified with isotopically labeled probes.

Another powerful molecular technology leading to greater understanding of cell proliferation and differentiation is recombinant DNA and molecular cloning.[103] Using combinations of restriction enzymes that cleave DNA and DNA ligases that reseal the cut fragments, small fragments of novel DNA can be inserted into the DNA of plasmids. Plasmids are small, circular DNA molecules that replicate as an episome; that is, they replicate autonomously from the chromosomal DNA. In bacteria, plasmids are vectors that can, for example, be responsible for the transfer of antibiotic resistance from one bacterium to another. By inserting multiple DNA fragments into various plasmids and then selectively cloning and identifying the desired recombinants by hybridization with radioactive probes, a vector with a single molecularly cloned DNA fragment can be developed. The plasmid vector can then be injected into new bacteria, where the plasmid multiplies many-fold and can thus be used to grow large quantities of the specifically desired DNA molecule. The large amount of DNA is then available for determining the absolute genetic sequence. Recombinant gene technology is also valuable for the production of large quantities of specific gene products. Similar genetic engineering is being accomplished with mammalian cells and viruses as vectors.

Oncogenes

When the protein product of a gene contributes to tumor formation, the gene is called an *oncogene*. An oncogene may be a mutation of a normal cellular gene, a viral gene introduced into the cell's DNA, or even a normal cellular gene that is present in an excessive number of copies.

Many recent advances in the understanding of oncogenesis have come from using molecular biologic techniques to study retroviruses and oncogenes.[93,162] The retrovirus genome contains RNA rather than DNA. Through the reverse transcriptase enzyme, the RNA information in the viral genome is reverse-transcribed into the host cell DNA, where it is integrated into the host chromosome as a provirus. The integrated provirus is capable of modifying the genetic expression of the region of the host chromosome into which it inserts. Several retroviruses, after a relatively long latent period, are capable of producing lymphoma or leukemia in a variety of species, including human beings.

The study of a second class of retroviruses, the acute transforming retroviruses, led to the discovery of oncogenes. The acute transforming retroviruses contain nucleic acid sequences that were acquired by the virus in the past from normal cellular genes. The corresponding gene regions in normal cells are referred to as *protooncogenes*. A high degree of genetic conservation appears to exist, because extensive cross-species homology occurs in avian species through humans. The normal physiologic function of protooncogenes is uncertain, but in view of their high degree of conservation, they may be essential constituents of the cellular growth regulatory machinery. They may only become oncogenes and cause malignancy after either a quantitative or a qualitative change has affected their expression.

The term *antioncogenes* has been suggested for recessive tumor-suppressor genes that are normally present in the genome.[89,104,175] The concept is that cancer can be produced when both normal alleles of an antioncogene are mutated or lost.

Oncogenes can be grouped, based on the action of the protein produced by the oncogene, into four functional groups: growth factors, protein kinases, G-proteins, and nuclear proteins (see Figure 12-10). The growth-factor oncogenes lead to increased production of growth factors that act as hormonal signals by interacting with membrane receptors that in turn activate intracellular regulatory mechanisms that provide a proliferative signal to the nucleus. Examples of such growth factors encoded by oncogenes are epidermal growth factor, platelet-derived growth factor, and fibroblast growth factor (associated with breast cancer). (See later section for further discussion of growth factors, receptors, and signal transduction.)

Protein kinase oncogenes can lead to increased growth through an increase in the number of protein kinase receptors (due to either increased transcription or gene amplification) or through a mutation that leads to a continuously activated receptor even in the absence of the appropriate growth factor. An example of an oncogene leading to an increase in protein kinase activity is the erbB2 (neu) oncogene, which is often increased in breast cancer.

A family of oncogenes known as *ras* encodes for mutated G-proteins. The ras oncogenes are found particularly in colon, lung, and pancreas cancers. G-proteins are cell membrane signal transducers that activate cyclic adenosine monophosphate (cAMP). Point mutations encoded by the ras oncogenes can lead to G-proteins that cannot become inactivated, which leads to continuous cell stimulation for growth.

Nuclear proteins interact with DNA and RNA to enhance or inhibit transcription and replication. Some oncogenes, such as *myc* and *fos*, produce proteins that interact at the nucleus.

Genetic Changes and Tumor Progression

The development of cancer is a multistep process that may progress through phases of benign neoplasia to low-grade malignancy to high-grade malignancy capable of metastasis. Each step of the process corresponds to the acquisition of a mutation that increases the rate of cell proliferation or delays cell death.[12] The mutations may be either deletion of a tumor suppressor gene or mutation of a protooncogene (a normal gene controlling cell growth) to an oncogene. In general, three to six mutational changes seem to be necessary for the development of carcinoma. Study of the development of colon carcinoma has been an important model (see Figure 12-9).

Growth Factors and Receptors

As noted earlier, the development of a neoplasm can be viewed as a caricature of normal tissue development, differentiation, and renewal.[127,146] In the process of normal tissue differentiation and normal growth and renewal of cell populations, responses to many chemical messengers occur. The chemical messengers associated with proliferation and differentiation include peptide growth factors, steroid hormones, and a diverse set of small molecules called *small effectors*. The chemical messengers that control growth and differentiation work through a set of receptors that lead to mechanisms affecting how genes in the cell are ultimately expressed in the phenotype of the cell.[11] Just as the extracellular and intracellular messengers can have an effect on the control of expression in the phenotype of normal cells, they can also control the expression of specific oncogenes that lead to the malignant phenotype. Thus oncogenes are responsible for the production of specific growth factors, and their expression is controlled by various effector molecules.

Considerable laboratory data and limited clinical data suggest that control of growth factors will lead to new modalities for cancer prevention and therapy that do not necessarily require cell killing for their efficacy. For such therapy to be clinically useful, the malignant cell need not be converted to a cell with a totally normal phenotype. Partial conversion to a benign neoplasm may be adequate. The concept of using therapy that induces differentiation, thereby halting further proliferation, has been applied to several human neoplasms, including neuroblastoma and chronic myelogenous leukemia. Considerable debate surrounds whether therapeutic efforts with "differentiating agents" work by differentiation or by simple cytotoxicity. In principle, however, the concept remains appealing.

The mechanisms by which molecules such as hormones regulate growth and differentiated function can be divided into endocrine, paracrine, and autocrine mechanisms. In the classic endocrine system, hormones produced by one cell are carried through the bloodstream to act at a distance on the specific receptor molecules of other cells. Similarly, in the paracrine system, exogenous hormones produced by one set of cells act on adjacent cells. In the autocrine system, the cell that produces and releases the hormone also has the appropriate receptor on the membrane of its cell surface that can be activated by the endogenously produced hormone (Figure 12-11). The autocrine system of growth factor production by a malignant cell is one mechanism that permits some cells to proliferate independently of exogenous control mechanisms.

The activity of growth and differentiating factors on individual cells depends on the availability of specific receptors either on the cell membrane or in the cell cytoplasm. The receptivity of a particular cell to a chemical signal depends on several receptors, the affinity of the receptors for the various chemical messengers, and how much the cell amplifies the cascade of signals generated by the effector-receptor complex. Examples exist of malignant cells having an increased growth response to growth factors through each of these mechanisms. Steroid hormones form a complex with receptor proteins present in the cytoplasm of the cell, and the complex is then transported to the nucleus, where protein synthesis or cell division is stimulated. Most of the other chemical signals that affect cell growth exert their effect by in-

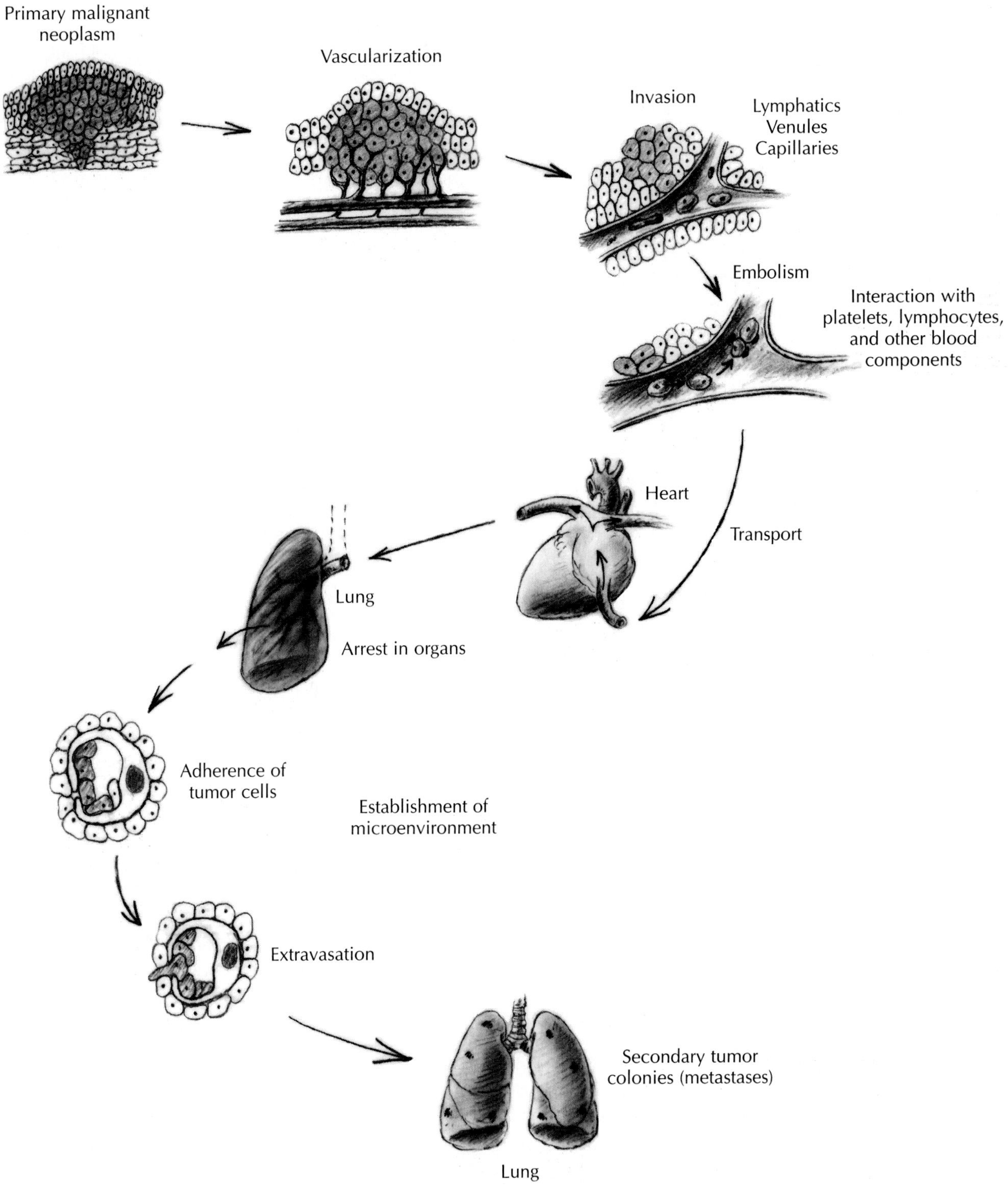

FIGURE 12-16 The sequential steps in metastasis. (Redrawn from Fidler JJ, Poste G: *Hosp Pract* 17:57, 1982.)

TABLE 12-4 COMMON SITES OF METASTASES FOR SOME HUMAN MALIGNANCIES

TYPE OF MALIGNANCY	COMMON SITES OF METASTASES
Breast	Axillary lymph nodes, lung, bone, brain
Colon and rectum	Regional lymph nodes, liver, lung
Esophagus	Direct extension, lymph nodes, liver, lung
Kidney	Lung, liver, bone
Lung	Liver, bone, brain
Melanoma	Lung, liver, bone, brain
Neuroblastoma	Bone, liver, lymph nodes
Oral and pharyngeal	Direct extension, regional lymph nodes, lung, liver, bone
Osteosarcoma	Lung
Ovary	Peritoneum, regional lymph nodes, lung, liver
Pancreas	Liver, adjacent organs, regional lymph nodes
Prostate	Bone, regional lymph nodes
Soft tissue sarcoma	Lung, adjacent organs and tissues
Stomach	Regional lymph nodes, liver, lung
Testis	Regional lymph nodes, lung, liver
Thyroid	Regional lymph nodes, lung, bone, brain
Urinary bladder	Direct extension to adjacent organs, regional lymph nodes, bone, lung, liver
Uterine cervix	Direct extension to adjacent organs, regional lymph nodes, lung, liver, bone
Wilms' tumor	Adjacent organs, regional lymph nodes, liver, lung, bone

of the syndrome can lengthen the duration and improve the quality of life.

Nutritional Effects of Cancer

The nutritional effects of a malignancy on the host are common and may lead to considerable body wasting. Malnutrition can result from mechanical compromise of the gastrointestinal tract, but also may occur for reasons unrelated to simple gastrointestinal obstruction. At times cachexia may be profound and disabling and out of proportion to the expected metabolic demands of the tumor. The body wasting is not simply a result of starvation, but is also related to the metabolic effects of the tumor.[19,113] The cachexia of the cancer patient is in many ways similar to the wasting effects of severe trauma and sepsis: a combination of decreased nutrient intake and altered metabolism occurs.

Decreased nutrient intake is frequently caused by loss of appetite. The causes of anorexia in cancer patients are not well understood but at least partly result from factors released into the bloodstream by the tumor.[112] Psychologic factors[78] and the side effects of treatment may also contribute to loss of taste, anorexia, and nausea.

Alteration of body metabolism in the cancer patient resembles the negative nitrogen balance state that follows such stresses as major surgery or severe trauma. In contrast to simple starvation, in which the metabolic rate falls as a compensatory factor, the metabolic rate in the cancer patient with cachexia either does not fall or decreases to a lesser extent than would be anticipated.[171,181] Tumors can continue to grow and function at a high metabolic rate even when the host is in negative nitrogen balance, as though the tumor tissue and the host tissue were in two separate metabolic compartments.[112] The increased demands on the host's lymphohematopoietic defense system, with the large energy requirements related to the high proliferative rate of the granulocytes, lymphocytes, and monocytes, may further contribute to the metabolic demands. An analogy may be drawn to the burn patient, in whom the hypermetabolic effects are related to the prolonged elevations of catecholamines.[178]

Attempts to force-feed the cancer patient, such as through parenteral nutrition, indicate that some nutritional deficits may be overcome, but usually to a lesser extent than in the malnourished patient without cancer.[121,152] Enteral or parenteral hyperalimentation can improve the host's nutritional status, but probably also frequently enhances the tumor growth rate. Short-term gains from hyperalimentation may be useful in preparing a patient for a surgical procedure. Clinical trials to date have been unconvincing in demonstrating that any increased chemotherapeutic or radiotherapeutic response occurs in patients receiving hyperalimentation.[121,155]

Paraneoplastic Endocrine Syndromes

Various paraneoplastic syndromes produced by ectopic production of polypeptide hormones have been well described (Table 12-5).[15,160] The hormone produced ectopically may be chemically identical to the authentic hormone. In other cases the substance may not be identical but sufficiently similar to produce the biologic effect. Secretion of polypeptide hormones by tumors is usually independent of any response to normal physiologic controls. Some tumors produce polypeptide hormone subunits that are detectable by immunoassay but do not have any detectable biologic effect. Other tumors may produce hormone precursors or prohormones that subsequently become biologically active when metabolized in other areas of the body. More detailed reviews are available in other texts.[23]

Hypercalcemia

Hypercalcemia is particularly common in patients with malignancy and may be the most immediately life-threatening aspect of the malignancy. Hypercalcemia occurs in up to an estimated 10% of patients with cancer. The degree of hypercalcemia frequently represents a condition requiring emergency treatment.[12] Humoral mechanisms responsible for the hypercalcemia of malignancy include production of osteoclast-activating factors, prostaglandin E_2, and parathyroid hormone or parathyroid-like factors. Ectopic production of true parathyroid hormone is probably rare, and most hypercalcemic syndromes caused by tumors without osseous metastases are probably caused by the production of osteolytic humoral factors as yet not well characterized.[118]

Management of the hypercalcemia of malignancy includes administration of sodium-containing fluids and diuretics affecting the loop of Henle or the distal tubule, since reabsorption of calcium in the renal tubules is linked to sodium reabsorption.[117] Additional measures include the administration of corticosteroids, calcitonin, or mithramycin. Longer-term measures to control the tumor should be planned, such as surgical resection, radiotherapy, chemotherapy, or hormonal therapy.

Neurologic Manifestations

Systemic neurologic manifestations of malignancy are those not caused by the direct mechanical effects of metastases. Some may result from cachexia and inanition, but others appear to result from the production of humoral factors that are either toxic or biologically active. The syndromes include cerebellar degeneration, dementia, spinal cord degeneration, peripheral neuropathies, and neuromuscular junction syndromes.[61,73]

Cutaneous Manifestations

Two cutaneous syndromes are usually associated with malignancy, acanthosis nigricans and erythema gyratum repens. Acanthosis nigricans is a hyperkeratosis and pigmentation that occurs most often on the axillae, neck, and anogenital region. Erythema gyratum repens is characterized by rapidly changing and advancing gyrate areas with scaling and pruritus. The rapid increase in size and sudden appearance of multiple keratoses is related to malignancies of the gastrointestinal tract. Further details on cutaneous manifestations of malignancy can be found in specialized texts.[18,69]

CLASSIFICATION AND STAGING OF CANCER

When cancer is suspected, establishing a firm pathologic diagnosis is essential whenever it can be made safely. Although many malignancies have relatively characteristic appearances, these can be deceiving. Inflammatory conditions and benign neoplasms can simulate the appearance of a cancer. An adequate biopsy is the most important procedure in establishing the diagnosis of cancer. If possible, the pathologic diagnosis should be established before an extensive workup is undertaken to plan treatment or to determine prognosis. The pathologic diagnosis defines the cancer's organ or tissue of origin.

After cancer is diagnosed, it is necessary to establish its extent, that is, to stage the disease. The objectives of staging cancer are to:

1. Aid in the planning of treatment
2. Provide a prognosis
3. Assist in the evaluation of treatment results
4. Aid in the continuing investigation of cancer and reporting of results[83]

TABLE 12-5 ECTOPIC HORMONES AND PARANEOPLASTIC HORMONE SYNDROMES

HORMONE OR HORMONE-LIKE SUBSTANCE AND SYNDROME	TUMORS PRODUCING THE SUBSTANCE ECTOPICALLY
Adrenocorticotropic hormone: Cushing's syndrome	Lung (particularly small cell), pancreas, thymus, ovary, thyroid (medullary), cervix, gastric, pheochromocytoma
Antidiuretic hormone: inappropriate diuresis and hyponatremia	Lung (particularly small cell), pancreas, prostate, thymus, lymphoma, ureter
Calcitonin: no evident syndrome	Lung (oat cell), melanoma, breast, bronchial, carcinoids, bladder, pancreas, liver, testis, esophagus, prostate
Erythropoietin: polycythemia	Kidney, liver, cerebellum, uterus, ovary
Insulin-like substances: hypoglycemia	Mesotheliomas, soft tissue sarcomas
Growth hormone: hypertrophic pulmonary osteoarthropathy, acromegaly	Lung, endometrium, gastric, breast, ovary
Human chorionic gonadotrophin: gynecomastia, precocious puberty	Testis, liver, lung, adrenal, breast, stomach, melanoma, ovary
Prolactin: galactorrea, gynecomastia	Kidney, lung
Parathyroid hormone–like substances: hypercalcemia	Lung, kidney, lymphoma, liver, cervix, ovary, testis, breast, pancreas, parotid
Thyroid-stimulating hormone: hyperthyroidism	Choriocarcinoma, testis, breast, lung

TNM System

A system of anatomic classification and staging, the *T*umor, *N*ode, *M*etastasis, or TNM, system, has been widely accepted.[6] The basis of the TNM system is to quantify the extent of disease based on the three modes of malignant spread: T for the degree of the primary tumor's direct extension, N for the extent of lymphatic dissemination, and M for hematogenous dissemination. The extent of disease within each category is defined numerically. Increasing extent of disease at the primary site is defined as T_0, T_{is}, T_1, T_2, T_3, or T_4. Increasing extent of nodal disease is defined as N_0, N_1, N_2, N_3, or N_4. The presence or absence of evidence of extranodal metastasis is indicated by M_0 or M_1 (Table 12-6). For sarcomas, it has been necessary to add an additional designation, G (G_1, G_2, G_3, G_4), for the tumor's histologic grade.

The TNM staging system does not imply a regular or necessarily predictable course of the disease from tumor to nodes and then to distant metastatic sites. Also, evidence of metastasis to the regional lymph nodes does not necessarily imply that the lymph nodes are a way station for cells en route to other organs. More frequently, nodal metastases indicate tumors that are capable of dissemination simultaneously through both lymphatic vessels and blood vessels. Although tumors tend to progress to the higher numeric classifications over time, the extent of disease is also related to the biologic aggressiveness of the malignancy. Some very small primary tumors may have extensive nodal or distant metastases.

TABLE 12-6 TUMOR, NODE, METASTASIS (TNM) SYSTEM OF CANCER STAGING

Tumor		
	T_X	Primary tumor cannot be assessed
	T_0	No evidence of primary tumor
	T_{is}	Carcinoma in situ
	T_1, T_2, T_3, T_4	Increasing size and/or local extent of the primary tumor
Nodes		
	N_X	Regional lymph nodes cannot be assessed
	N_0	No regional lymph node metastases
	N_1, N_2, N_3, N_4	Increasing involvement of regional lymph nodes
Metastasis		
	M_X	Presence of distant metastasis cannot be assessed
	M_0	No distant metastasis
	M_1	Distant metastasis
Histopathology Grade		
	G_X	Grade cannot be assessed
	G_1	Well differentiated
	G_2	Moderately well differentiated
	G_3	Poorly differentiated
	G_4	Undifferentiated

From American Joint Committee on Cancer Staging: *Manual for staging of cancer*, ed 3, Philadelphia, 1988, JB Lippincott.

Stage Groupings

The TNM classification is used to organize groups of patients into stage groupings that have implications for therapy and for prognosis. Typically stages are indicated by using Roman numerals I to IV.

The major agencies responsible for establishing the TNM system are the International Union Against Cancer (UICC) and the American Joint Committee on Cancer Staging (AJC). In the past these two groups used the same symbols with different definitions in many of the sites. More recently they have attempted to make their definitions congruent, but the physician must know which definition of the TNM system is being used. The TNM category of a patient usually refers to the extent of disease at initial diagnosis and staging, but at times TNM staging may define a patient's status later, for example, after a treatment program. The TNM system can be used to refer to the clinical stage (cTNM); the pathologic stage, as defined postoperatively (pTNM); or the postmortem stage, as determined after autopsy (aTNM).

An increasingly bewildering variety of medical imaging procedures is becoming available to aid in identifying the anatomic extent of disease. When combined with fine-needle aspiration cytology, these imaging techniques may define surgically incurable disease and obviate the need for surgical exploration of a major body cavity. Appropriate imaging procedures must be selected judiciously, not indiscriminately. A careful physical examination may detect metastatic disease and make an imaging procedure superfluous. Without symptoms, an imaging procedure may yield results too negligible to make it worthwhile. If surgery and direct visualization of the organ will be carried out no matter what the imaging procedure reveals, the procedure again may be superfluous. If the results of an imaging procedure lead to no clinical action and the patient is not participating in a defined research protocol, a further staging procedure may be pointless. Any staging procedure must be selected because it will provide useful information. If test information will not be used, the test should not be performed.

Tumor Markers

In addition to the anatomic and pathologic classification just discussed, several biochemical products are useful in classifying malignancies further or in following their response to treatment.[43,63,82,96] Examples of clinically useful tumor markers are the progesterone and estrogen receptor proteins in some breast cancers and the elevated

TABLE 12-7 CLINICALLY USEFUL HUMAN TUMOR MARKERS

MARKER	ABBREVIATION	TYPE OF CANCER
Carcinoembryonic antigen	CEA	Colon, lung
Human chorionic gonadotropin	HCG	Choriocarcinoma, testis (germ cell)
M-component immunoglobulin	M-component	Multiple myeloma
Alpha-fetoprotein	AFP	Liver, germ cell
Prostate-specific antigen	PSA	Prostate
Calcitonin	CT	Medullary carcinoma of thyroid

chorionic gonadotropin and alpha-fetoprotein levels in the circulation of some patients with testicular carcinoma. Tumor markers may provide prognostic information at the initial diagnosis or during follow-up, and they may help in the selection of therapy. Tumor markers in the blood may also be useful in following the response to therapy. Most tumor markers detected in the blood are normal biologic products of cells produced either in abnormal amounts or under abnormal circumstances. The surface antigens on cells may serve as biologic markers and are used in the immunologic classification of lymphomas and leukemias. Surface markers on microscopic metastases may also provide a target for radioimmunologic detection or for therapy using radioactively tagged antibodies specific for the surface antigen.

To date tumor markers have not proved useful as blood tests for mass screening for cancer because (1) most tumor markers can also be elevated by nonmalignant conditions (not sufficiently specific), and (2) the assays for many tumor markers are only sufficiently sensitive to detect the marker when it is in the blood in relatively high concentrations (lacks sensitivity).

Two of the most widely used tumor markers are carcinoembryonic antigen[64] and alpha-fetoprotein,[2] which are called *oncofetal proteins*. These proteins are typically produced in high quantities by embryonic cells and then normally disappear by the neonatal period. The oncofetal proteins reappear in elevated quantities when cancers of certain cell types develop. The clinical tumor markers that are currently most useful are shown in Table 12-7. A variety of other tumor markers are being investigated for their clinical value.

A useful role for tumor markers in the blood is the monitoring of the response to therapy.[65] The best examples of tumor markers accurately estimating the response to therapy are in nonseminomatous testicular carcinoma, in choriocarcinoma, and in some patients with carcinoma of the colon and rectum. The concentration of a tumor marker in the blood represents a balance between (1) the kinetics of the product's production rate by the tumor cells; (2) the number of cells producing the product; and (3) the rate of degradation or elimination of the tumor marker. With surgical removal of the tumor mass or complete destruction by radiotherapy or chemotherapy, the concentration of the tumor marker should fall at the rate of its biologic half-life. If only a portion of the tumor has been removed or destroyed, the concentration of the marker will decline at a slower rate than that of its half-life. The direction and rate of change of a tumor marker are more important than its absolute level, unless the level is zero.

PRINCIPLES OF SURGICAL ONCOLOGY

Surgery is the oldest treatment for cancer and has cured more cancers than all other modalities combined. The surgeon plays an important role in the prevention, detection, diagnosis, staging, treatment, and palliation of cancer, and in the rehabilitation of the cancer patient. Because cancer treatment involves the interaction of experts from many disciplines using many therapeutic modalities, the surgeon must interact knowledgeably and cooperatively. In many instances the surgeon coordinates these interactions.

The Surgeon and Cancer Prevention and Detection

The surgeon plays a role in both the primary and the secondary prevention of cancer, that is, the early detection of cancer. The surgeon's advice can be a strong factor in motivating patients to adopt healthy life-styles that reduce carcinogenic risks. This authoritative advice can encourage earlier cancer detection through self-examination of such areas as the skin, breasts, and testes.

In several diseases the risk of cancer development in a nonvital organ is sufficiently high that prophylactic removal of the organ is an appropriate consideration. For example, in patients who have inherited the dominant genetic trait for multiple polyposis of the colon, it is generally recommended that they undergo prophylactic colectomy before age 20. When colectomy is not performed in these patients, approximately one half will have developed colon cancer by age 40 and almost all will have developed colon cancer by age 70.[116] Besides caring for the patient with the disease, the surgeon is also responsible for informing other family members of the hereditary implications. Ulcerative colitis is also associated with a high incidence of colon cancer. When colonic involvement of the disease is total and the ulcerative colitis is chronic, the risk of cancer development is about 2% per year, or 40% after 20 years.[21,81,102]

Family members in multiple endocrine neoplasia syndromes types IIA and IIB have been screened for nonpalpable medullary carcinoma or its precursor, C-cell hyperplasia, using calcium and pentagastrin stimulation tests.[176] If thyrocalcitonin levels are elevated following provocative testing, the patient should have a total thyroidectomy. Genetic testing will soon replace thyrocalcitonin testing.

The role of prophylactic mastectomy in women with strong family histories of breast cancer is more problematic, because a well-established marker is not yet available to indicate whether a given patient has inherited the genetic risk for high susceptibility to breast cancer. This issue is discussed further in Chapter 44.

The Surgeon and Diagnosis and Staging of Cancer: Establishing an Accurate Diagnosis

The surgeon plays a major role in cancer diagnosis and staging. Different neoplasms have very diverse responses to the various therapeutic modalities. An accurate pathologic diagnosis is imperative in planning appropriate management. Material for the pathologist may be obtained from exfoliated cells, blood, effusions, the primary tumor, a lymph node, or a distant metastatic site. Biopsies are obtained by shave biopsy, punch biopsy, fine-needle aspiration (for cytologic examination), core-cutting needle biopsy, incisional biopsy, and excisional biopsy (Figure 12-17). When surgical resection is the appropriate treatment despite what the pathologic process may eventually prove to be, removal of the entire organ may be the most appropriate approach to obtaining a pathologic specimen.

Each technique has its useful role as well as potential pitfalls. In planning the biopsy, the physician must consider the eventual treatment. When surgery is planned, the surgeon should be consulted before obtaining the biopsy whenever the type of biopsy may affect the eventual surgical approach. Once obtained, tissues need to be appropriately handled to preserve the maximum pathologic information. Failure to handle the initial biopsy specimen properly may subject the patient to a second biopsy procedure or compromise subsequent therapy if the initial biopsy removes the major portion of the primary tumor. Fresh specimens may be necessary for touch preparations in the diagnosis of lymphomas. Special preservation may be needed for electron microscopy. Certain biochemical assays, such as estrogen and progesterone receptor assays, may require immediate deep freezing.

Exfoliative Cytologic Examination

Exfoliative cytologic examinations are widely used in the early diagnosis of neoplasia in the uterine cervix and the tracheobronchial area. An obvious exophytic neoplasm indicates the need for a biopsy. Reliance on exfoliative cytology can be particularly misleading when secondary infection of neoplasms exists. The exuberant inflammatory cells mixed with necrotic tumor cells may make accurate diagnosis impossible.

Fine-Needle Aspiration Biopsy

Fine-needle aspiration biopsy techniques use 18- to 27-gauge needles on a syringe; suction is applied as the needle is moved back and forth in the tumor mass with a rotary motion.[87] Individual cells and small clumps of tumor cells are frequently sufficient to permit a highly trained cytopathologist to make a diagnosis. Obtaining specimens by fine-needle aspiration appears so simple that necessary details are often neglected. Inexperienced operators may fail to have the needle in the right tissue, to use adequate suction or adequate rotary motion, or to see that the specimen is immediately fixed so that no drying artifact is present.[94] Some European cytopathologists are trained to read air-dried cytology specimens, but as a rule North American cytopathologists are only experienced in reading cytology specimens that have been fixed immediately in alcohol or with a spray fixative. Cytologic specimens are also used in the diagnosis of exfoliated cancer cells from the uterine cervix, the urinary tract, and occasionally the stomach and esophagus. Cytologic specimens brushed from the bronchi are also useful in diagnosis of lung cancer. When the tumor is subject to secondary infection and inflammation, as with an exophytic cancer of the uterine cervix, oral cavity, colon, or rectum, a cytologic specimen is usually inadequate, and punch biopsy forceps should be used to obtain a specimen for histologic examination.

Core Needle Biopsy

Core-cutting needles of approximately 14 gauge can be used to obtain a core of tissue with its histologic architecture intact. The disposable Tru-Cut needle has proved to be particularly useful. A satisfactory histologic diagnosis of many epithelial malignancies can be made with the core-cutting needle. Bone and soft tissue sarcomas frequently present major difficulties in the interpretation of small biopsy specimens, making core-cutting needle biopsies unsatisfactory.

The Rotex needle has a small auger within a 21-gauge needle.[122] The needle is advanced to the suspect tissue, the auger is screwed into the tissue, and then the sheath of the needle is rotated over the stationary auger to cut a fine microbiopsy. This needle biopsy has proved particularly valuable in the diagnosis of lung lesions.[85,86]

Incisional Versus Excisional Biopsy

Incisional biopsy refers to the surgical removal of a portion of a tumor mass for pathologic examination. Excisional biopsy is surgical removal of the entire tumor mass, usually with little or no margin of normal tissue surrounding the tumor (see Figure 12-18). Excisional biopsies are usually preferred for small lesions when the removal can be accomplished with little cosmetic or functional defect. Incisional biopsy is more appropriate for large tumor masses of the trunk and extremities be-

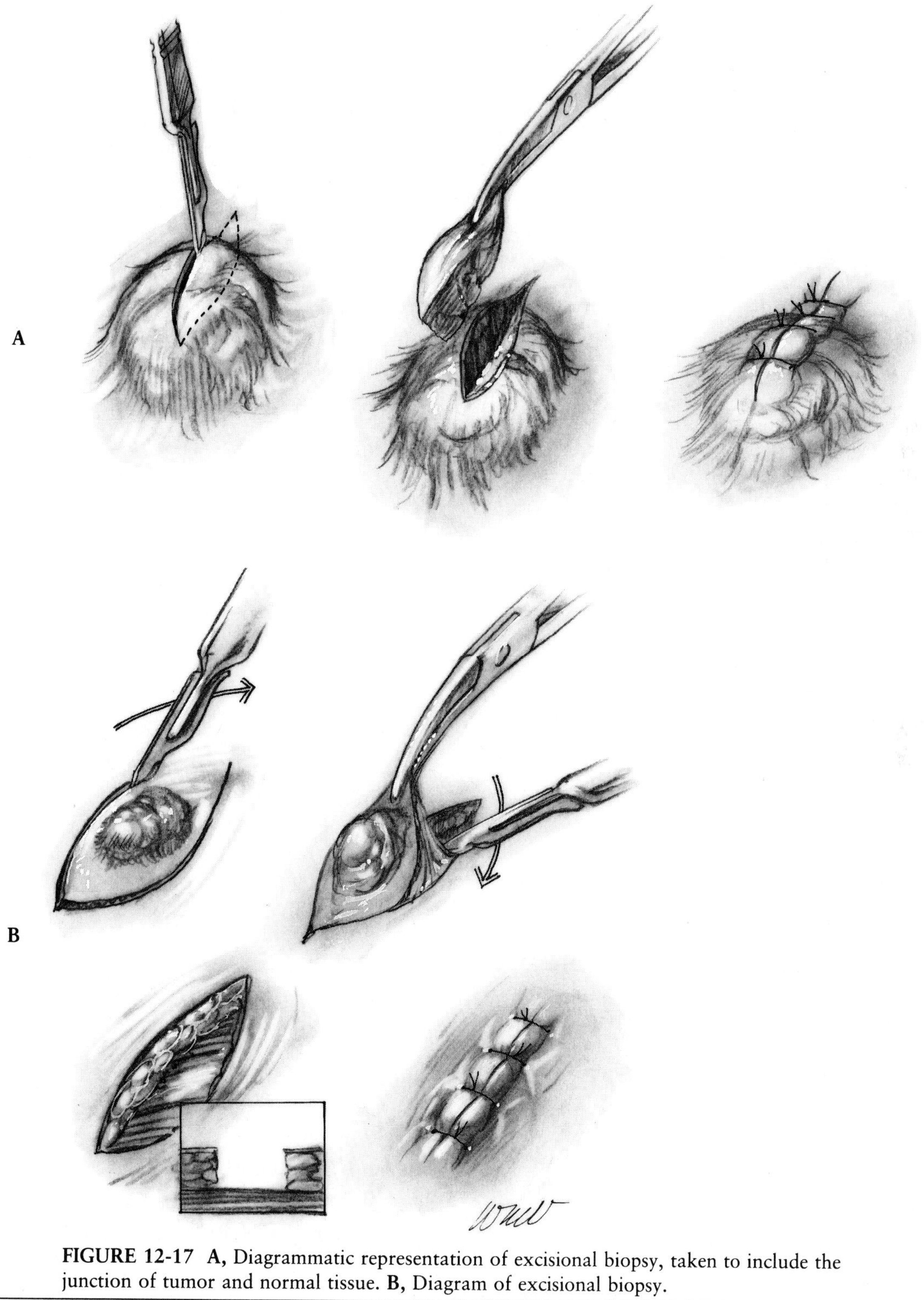

FIGURE 12-17 **A,** Diagrammatic representation of excisional biopsy, taken to include the junction of tumor and normal tissue. **B,** Diagram of excisional biopsy.

cause special planning is needed for the definitive treatment, depending on the pathologic diagnosis.

An important issue in the selection of an incisional or excisional biopsy technique is whether performance of the biopsy procedure will create the risk of contaminating new tissue planes. When a bone or soft tissue sarcoma of the trunk or the extremities is suspected, an incisional biopsy is usually preferred. Incisional biopsy, in contrast to excisional biopsy, decreases the contamination of the tissue planes between muscles at the margins of the tumor mass. Such contamination can compromise the eventual complete wide resection or make resection of surrounding contaminated but otherwise normal tissue more extensive than would have been necessary if an excisional biopsy had not been performed. In other circumstances excision of the tumor mass with an intact capsule or a margin of surrounding normal tissue is important in decreasing the chance of recurrence. For example, the morcellation of tumor contained in lymph nodes during their resection runs the risk of tumor implantation. Incisional biopsy of thyroid and parotid lesions is generally contraindicated because of the risk of tumor implantation in the wound.

Proper placement of biopsy incisions so that they facilitate subsequent treatment is also important. Incisions on the extremities should usually be placed longitudinally. Incisions for a potentially malignant lesion in the breast need to be planned with subsequent surgery in mind.

Instruments used in a biopsy procedure are a potential source of contamination. If they have come in contact with a suspected cancer, they should not be used to take a second biopsy from an uncontaminated area or in new tissue planes.

Little evidence suggests that either incisional or excisional biopsy leads to an increase in hematogenous or lymphatic spread of a malignancy. Several studies have compared the results of preliminary incisional versus excisional biopsy of melanomas and have detected no differences in outcome.[42,90] Studies in breast cancer patients have indicated no adverse effects when a delay of up to several weeks occurs between the initial biopsy and subsequent definitive surgical treatment. Although surgeons have worried about the theoretic possibility that fine-needle aspiration biopsies would contaminate tissue planes, this does not appear to occur with most tumors, except on rare occasions.[30,86] If practical, the surgeon can include excision of the needle tract in the later surgical procedure.

Preliminary Planning

Biopsies frequently require preliminary planning between the surgeon and the pathologist, radiologist, or medical oncologist. The specimen may need to be oriented and preserved properly. Specimens to be examined by electron microscopy, tissue culture techniques, or special biochemical assays can be destroyed by placement in formaldehyde solution.

STAGING. After the diagnosis has been established, it is important to stage the cancer. Proper staging frequently requires the combined efforts of the surgeon, the diagnostic radiologist, the pathologist, the biochemist, the hematologist, the radiotherapist, and the medical oncologist. For some patients, such as those with Hodgkin's disease, the surgeon participates in the diagnosis and staging, whereas the definitive treatment is the radiotherapist's or medical oncologist's responsibility. The staging laparotomy in the patient with Hodgkin's disease is a meticulous inspection for areas of abnormal tissue combined with biopsy of the liver, removal of the spleen, and removal of selected lymph nodes from multiple regions to plan the most effective and least morbid therapy based on the pathologic extent of disease.[27,62]

Proper placement of radiopaque clips may be important in guiding radiotherapy fields. Many radiopaque clips, however, cause artifacts on computed tomography (CT) scans. The use of radiopaque clips should be coordinated with the radiotherapist. Vitallium clips are an alternative because they cause less image distortion.

Another example of adequate pretherapy surgical staging is in the treatment of ovarian cancer.[135] In this case the biologic behavior of the disease is taken into account. Cytologic material is obtained from the peritoneal cavity before any dissection, and the upper abdomen is examined with careful attention to the undersurface of the diaphragm. Biopsies of suspicious lesions of the liver and lesions of the bowel and mesenteric and pelvic surfaces are performed; a portion of the omentum is removed; and aortic nodes may be sampled. These steps are taken in addition to the appropriate pelvic surgery.

In patients with primary operable carcinoma of the breast, prophylactic surgical removal of regional lymph nodes contributes to increased survival by helping identify those patients who may benefit from adjuvant systemic therapy. Further staging information is obtained from biochemical examination of either the primary breast cancer or the metastatic deposits for estrogen and progesterone receptor proteins.

Surgical Treatment of Cancer

Cancers confined to the organ of origin and those with low-grade malignancy can be cured by local resection. Skin cancers such as basal cell carcinomas and well-differentiated squamous cell carcinomas rarely metastasize by hematogenous and lymphatic routes and are readily cured by local excision. Wide local excision is used for malignancies that invade extensively into local structures. Some tumors, such as soft tissue sarcomas,

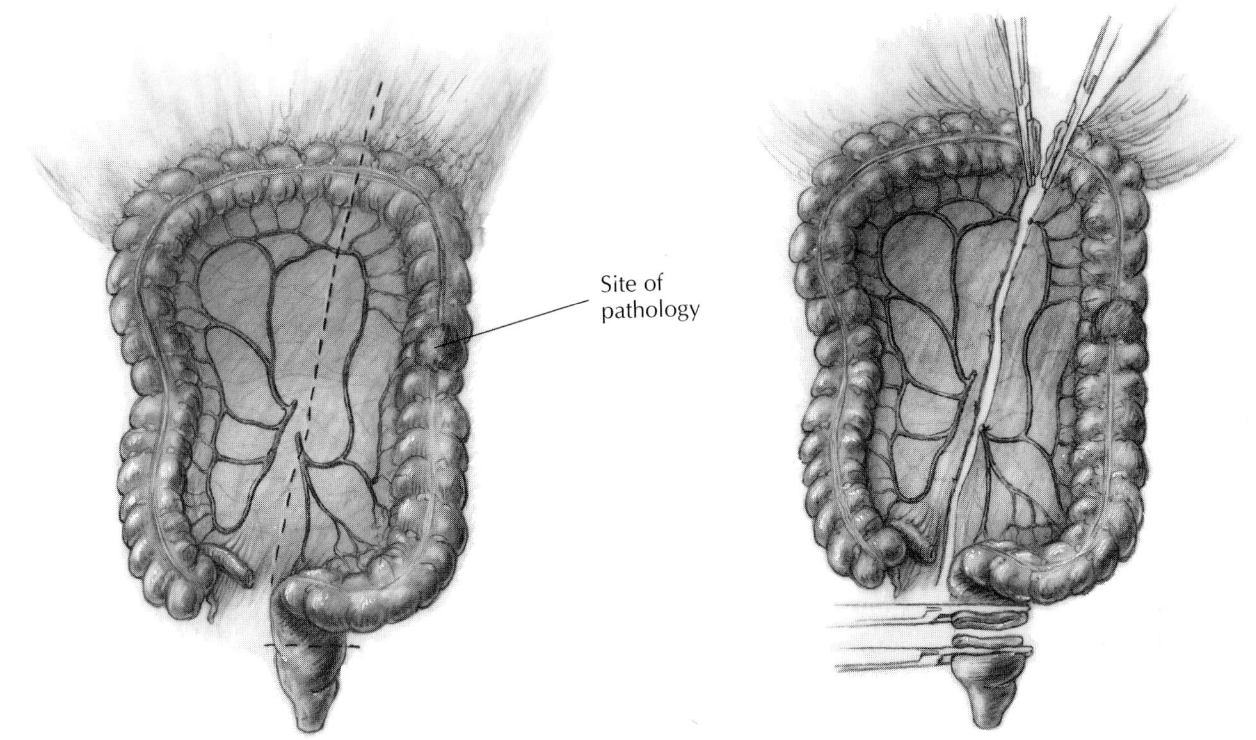

FIGURE 12-18 Diagrammatic representation of en bloc resection of left colon with wide resection of the vasculature and associated lymphatics. (Redrawn from Turnbull RB Jr et al: *Ann Surg* 166:420, 1967.)

have a pseudocapsule; to obtain a wide local excision, the surgeon must be careful to avoid dissecting into this plane.

Tumors that may spread to regional areas are frequently treated by wide excision with en bloc excision of lymphatics (radical resection). Wide, en bloc resections frequently include the organ of origin, any adjacent involved tissues, and the tissues containing the regional lymph node drainage area (Figure 12-18).

Resection of the regional nodal area usually controls progressive tumor growth in that area and cures some cancers. Resection of regional lymph nodes is also called *lymphadenectomy*. If clinical examination demonstrates that the tumor does not appear to involve the lymph nodes, their removal is termed *prophylactic* or *elective lymphadenectomy*. *Therapeutic lymphadenectomy* implies removal of lymph nodes that are believed to contain a tumor. For approximately two thirds of visceral cancers, however, regional nodal spread is accompanied by hematogenous or parietal spread beyond the resectable area, which may not be detectable at the time of surgery. Table 12-8 lists the relative 5-year survival rates for selected cancers for which surgical resection either is or has been the major curative modality.

TABLE 12-8 FIVE-YEAR SURVIVAL RATES (ADJUSTED FOR NORMAL LIFE EXPECTANCY) OF PATIENTS WITH CANCERS FOR WHICH SURGERY IS A MAJOR CURATIVE MODALITY*

	RELATIVE 5-YEAR SURVIVAL RATES (%) ALL STAGES	
TYPE OF CANCER	WHITE	BLACK
Breast	78	63
Colon	58	47
Rectum	55	44
Esophagus	9	6
Stomach	16	17
Pancreas	3	4
Melanoma of skin	82	70
Brain and nervous system	24	33
Thyroid	94	94
Lung and bronchus	13	11
Ovary	39	36
Kidney and renal pelvis	53	52

From American Cancer Society: *Cancer facts and figures,* New York, 1992, American Cancer Society, 1981-1987 patients.

**Curative* is defined as those patients who reach a disease-free survival plateau. Breast and thyroid cancers have not reached a plateau by 5 years.

Because of the frequency of extraregional metastases, the current trend is toward development of therapies adjuvant to the surgical resection. The goals of the adjuvant therapies are both to improve the cure rate and to decrease the morbidity of extensive surgical resections. Local resection of the tumor mass may decrease the morbidity of radiotherapy or chemotherapy by decreasing the amount of treatment necessary. For selected patients with incurable malignancy, surgery may play an important palliative role, as in relieving gastrointestinal tract obstructions.

Extended Resections

Extended resections may be carried out for tumors that infiltrate widely in the local region but have less tendency to form distant metastases. Examples of such procedures include pelvic exenteration, hemipelvectomy, and forequarter amputations.

Local wound seeding and implantation of a tumor is a potential problem when a biopsy is performed or a tumor is entered during the surgical excision. Precautions usually taken to prevent wound seeding are wide local excisions that include any biopsy site or needle tract. If a second body area requires surgery at the time of excision of a malignancy, fresh instruments and gloves are used. For example, if such precautions have not been taken when skin grafts are obtained to cover defects, implantation of a solid neoplasm in the donor site has occurred. Numerous techniques of wound irrigation have been attempted to decrease tumor implantation when contamination has been possible. Wound irrigation solutions have included 0.5% formaldehyde and sterile water to lyse any residual tumor cells. No data confirm the value of such irrigation procedures in clinical practice.

A popular theory to prevent further dissemination of tumors at surgery is the "no touch" approach to tumor excision.[168] This approach includes minimal palpation of the tumor before early ligation of its blood supply. In resection of bowel malignancies, the bowel lumen is occluded with heavy ligatures or clamps proximal and distal to the tumor. Although widely accepted and theoretically attractive, the no touch approach to tumor surgery is frequently impractical, and comparative results do not confirm its importance. The major problem with most visceral malignancies is that metastases have occurred before their diagnosis.

Definitive cancer surgery is rarely an emergency procedure. Patients frequently are anxious to have immediate surgery. Past experience in performing emergent amputations for extremity sarcomas, emergent nephrectomies for Wilms' tumors, and emergent mastectomies for breast cancers has demonstrated no advantage and many disadvantages from hasty surgery. Any clinically evident tumor has been present in the patient for a prolonged period. The exact time at which metastasis occurs in human tumors is not clear, but the process probably begins very early for some minute tumors. In other tumors, significant metastases may not occur until the tumor reaches an enormous size. The disadvantages of a several-week delay between diagnosis of a tumor and definitive surgery are usually far fewer than the disadvantages of proceeding without adequate pathologic diagnosis, staging, and planning of the most appropriate therapy.

In selected patients surgical resection can play an important role in the treatment of isolated metastases to the liver, lung, or brain. Resection of isolated or limited numbers of metastatic foci in these organs, particularly for tumors not particularly responsive to chemotherapy or radiotherapy, has been surprisingly successful.

The lung is a particularly common site for metastases from sarcomas, and resection of pulmonary metastases in patients with soft tissue or bone sarcomas can be followed by apparent cures in more than 25%.[29,131,132] Favorable results in selected cases have been reported following resection of pulmonary metastases in patients with renal cell carcinoma, in testicular carcinoma patients who have failed to respond completely following chemotherapy, in colorectal carcinoma patients, in breast cancer patients, in melanoma patients, and in patients with isolated metastases from the uterine cervix or the head and neck.*

In highly selected patients with limited foci of metastases to the liver (usually from a primary tumor in the colon or rectum) as the only evidence of recurrent or persistent cancer, approximately one fourth appear to be cured by resection. The factors that seem to indicate a more favorable prognosis following resection are solitary versus multiple nodules and relative stability of the metastases during 3 to 6 months of observation.[24,25,53] Current data do not appear to justify liver resection for patients with cancer metastasizing from the lung, breast, pancreas, or stomach.[52,140]

Most patients with malignancies metastasizing to the brain have widespread disease outside the central nervous system, and any radiotherapy is palliative. When a solitary brain metastasis is the only known site of metastatic disease, resection for cure can be considered. One-year survival rates of 22% to 44% have been reported after resection of brain metastases.[56,179] Even when cure is not accomplished, correction of the neurologic deficit may allow the patient to return to fully normal activities. The most common primary tumors metastatic to the brain are lung, breast, and melanoma, and most of these patients have other metastatic disease. Surgery should be considered, particularly for the patient who is relatively young, has a metastasis in a silent area of the brain, and has had a

*References 26, 105, 114, 115, 140, 164, and 177.

tumor-free interval greater than 1 year. Patients with solitary metastases from renal cell carcinomas, melanomas, breast carcinomas, and sarcomas will most likely benefit from surgery. Adjunctive radiotherapy after complete surgical resection of the brain metastasis appears to play a role.[56,145]

Cytoreductive Surgery

The concept of using surgery to reduce the bulk of the tumor even when complete resection cannot be accomplished (cytoreductive surgery) implies that removal of the gross disease will increase the effectiveness of other therapeutic modalities.[157] The idea of cytoreductive surgery has validity, but inappropriate interpretation has also led to misapplication. Cytoreductive surgery is generally valid only when other modalities of therapy are capable of eliminating or at least controlling the residual disease. Moreover, debulking operations before treatment with other modalities are useful only when they succeed in reducing residual tumor to milligram quantities. This surgery appears to be useful in the management of some ovarian cancers.[135] The concept of cytoreductive surgery is also valid in the management of some hormonally active tumors when no other therapeutic modalities are effective.

PRINCIPLES OF RADIATION THERAPY

The basic goal of radiotherapy is to use ionizing radiation to destroy the malignant cells while minimizing the structural or functional injury to the surrounding tissues. To accomplish this goal, either the tumor cells in the treatment field must be more sensitive to the radiation effects or the radiation beam must be focused so that a differential dose occurs between the tumor mass and the surrounding normal tissue. A variation of about 20 to 1 exists between the most radiosensitive tissues in the body and the most radioresistant tissues. In general, tumors arising from radiosensitive tissues tend to be radiosensitive, and tumors arising from radioresistant tissues tend to be less sensitive.

Proliferating cells are more radiosensitive than nonproliferating cells. The proliferating component, or the stem cells, of both normal proliferating tissues and malignancies have similar radiosensitivity. The lymphoid system, the bone marrow, the mucosa of the gut, and the gonads are particularly radiosensitive. Mature bone, cartilage, muscle, and nerves tend to be radioresistant. An important part of the differential effect of radiation therapy on malignant as opposed to normal tissue is the greater capacity of most normal tissues to repair and regenerate.

Biologic Effects of Ionizing Radiation

The biologic effect of ionizing radiation is secondary to a sequence of physical and chemical changes that result from the absorption of the ionizing radiation in the cell.[70] The ionizing radiations, either high-speed subatomic particles or high-energy (short wavelength) electromagnetic radiation, produce activated molecules. The activated molecules from the radiation result from either ionization or excitation.

In ionization, the absorption of the radiation causes the ejection of an orbiting electron, leaving free radicals (molecules with unpaired electrons) and broken chemical bonds. When particulate radiations such as electrons, protons, and alpha particles have sufficient energy, they can directly break chemical bonds and are directly ionizing. Electromagnetic radiations such as x rays and gamma rays are indirectly ionizing and produce their effect by shifting electrons to different orbits, which makes the atoms more unstable. The unstable atoms undergo secondary reactions to produce both stable molecules and chemically reactive free atoms and free radicals. Thus the effects of radiation on biologically important molecules result from either the direct effect of the absorption of energy into the molecule or the indirect effect when the energy initially absorbed by one molecule is being transferred to another.

It is generally believed that the most important effect of the irradiation used in radiotherapy is caused by changes in the nucleic acids with a resultant disruption of the cell's ability to reproduce. Other macromolecules, such as proteins and lipids, are also affected by irradiation, and changes in cell membranes may also play an important role in radiobiologic effects.

Clinical Effects of Radiotherapy

The major clinical effect in the radiotherapy of cancer is its ability to cause dividing cell populations to lose their reproductive capability. The loss of the cell's ability to produce viable progeny capable of sustained reproduction is sometimes called "reproductive death." Cell survival curves illustrate the relationship between radiation dose and reproductive death. The dose-response survival curves for the fraction of cells surviving irradiation at usual therapeutic doses are exponential, or logarithmic, after an initial part of the curve called the "shoulder." The shoulder represents the amount of damage that must accumulate before there is any effect on the cell's ability to replicate (Figure 12-19).

The initial shoulder region is probably the result of the need for a minimum number of targets to be hit before the cell is killed. An important aspect of the exponential part of the dose-response curve in radiotherapy is that it follows first-order kinetics; i.e, for each given increment in dose, a constant proportion of the exposed cells is killed rather than a constant number. The slope of the exponential portion of the dose-response curve varies according to the tissue's radiosensitivity. Lethal radiation damage to a cell is a random

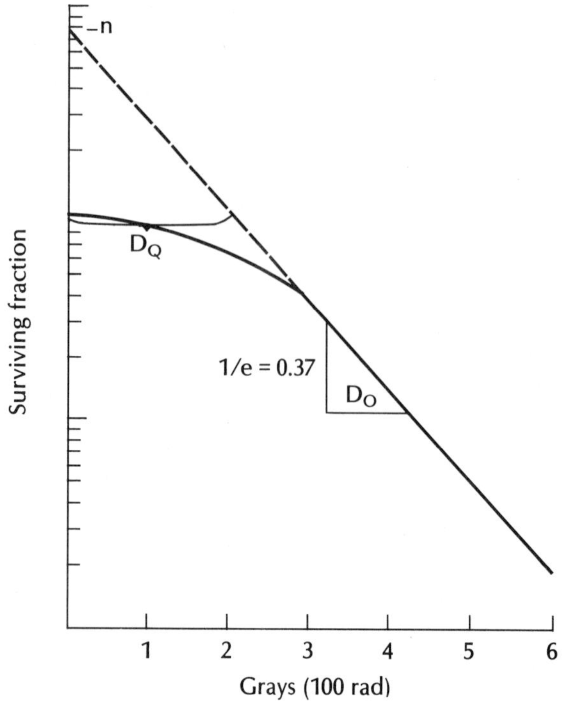

FIGURE 12-19 Idealized radiation survival curve. The shoulder in the low-dose region indicates a reduced efficiency of cell killing. The terminal portion of the radiation kill curve is exponential and is described by the D_0, whereas the initial shoulder region can be described by either the extrapolation number *n* or the D_Q, the quasithreshold dose. The *n* is the number on the ordinate found when the exponential portion is extrapolated to 0 dose, whereas D_Q is the dose in which the straight portion of the survival curve extrapolated backward intersects the line where the survival fraction is unity. (From DeVita DT Jr, Hellman S, Rosenberg SA, editors: *Cancer: principles and practice of oncology,* ed 3, Philadelphia, 1989, JB Lippincott.)

event. If the radiation dose is such that each cell will receive an average of one lethal lesion, random distribution dictates that some cells will receive more than one lethal lesion, some only one, and some less than one. The portion of cells that have no lethal events under these circumstances is e^{-1}, i.e., a survival fraction of 0.37. The dose of radiation needed to reduce the survival fraction to 37% on the exponential portion of the dose-response curve is known as the D_0. The value for D_0 thus represents the slope of the dose-response curve or the radiosensitivity of tissue. For clinical purposes, the dose on the exponential portion of the curve required to reduce the surviving fraction to 10%, i.e, to provide a log kill, may be more useful and is referred to as the D_{10}.

The shoulder portion of the radiation survival curve reflects the amount of damage that must accumulate before lethal damage occurs. The shoulder portion of the radiation curve is described by D_Q, or the quasi-threshold dose. The D_Q is the dose at which the straight portion of the survival curve, when extrapolated backward, is intersected by the survival fraction at unity. The shoulder portion, or D_Q, of the radiation dose-response curve appears to be a measure of cells' ability to repair sublethal damage. When a lapse of several hours or more occurs between radiation doses, the shoulder portion at the initial radiation doses returns (Figure 12-20). Because tissues vary in their D_Q, fractionation of radiation can lead to differential effects on the various tissues in a given radiation field, provided the fractionated doses are large enough to contain a portion of the exponential part of the dose-response curve as well as the shoulder.

The radiosensitivity of cells during the cell division cycle varies considerably. Cells in mitosis are almost always radiosensitive. Cells in the G_2 phase are almost as sensitive. Cells gradually increase in radioresistance as they proceed through the S phase. The G_1 phase is relatively radiosensitive for cells with a short G_1 phase, whereas for cells with a relatively long G_1 phase, a period of radioresistance occurs early in G_1.

The oxygen concentration in tissue being irradiated has an important effect on the biologic outcome of ion-

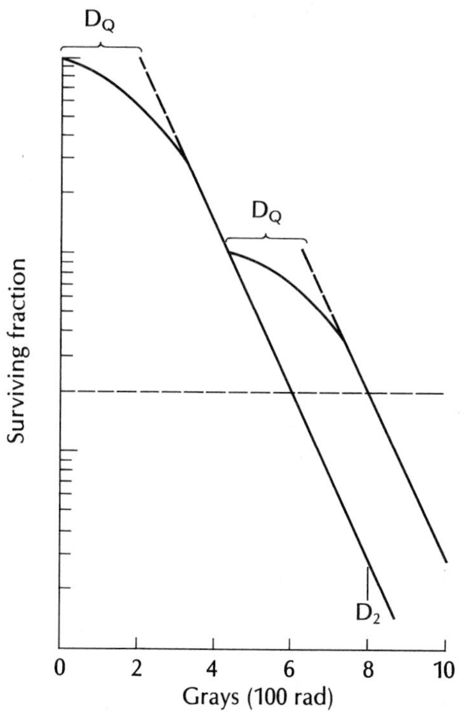

FIGURE 12-20 Two-dose radiation survival curves demonstrating return of the shoulder with fractionation of the radiation dose. (From DeVita DT Jr, Hellman S, Rosenberg SA, editors: *Cancer: principles and practice of oncology,* ed 3, Philadelphia, 1989, JB Lippincott.)

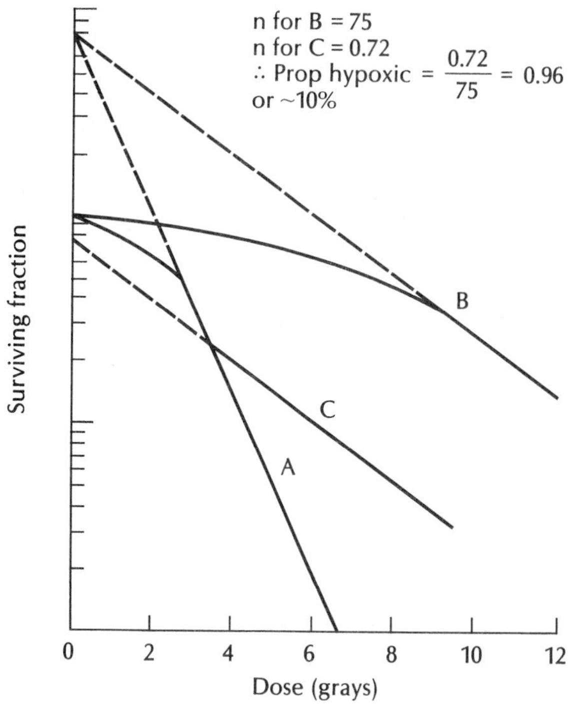

FIGURE 12-21 Idealized survival curves for oxic tumor cells *(A)*, hypoxic tumor cells *(B)*, and a tumor containing both oxic and hypoxic tumor cells *(C)*. This figure demonstrates the effect of different levels of oxygenation on cell kill by radiotherapy. It also shows that different tumor populations have different slopes in the exponential portion of the curve, as well as different shapes in the shoulder portion of the curve. (From DeVita DT Jr, Hellman S, Rosenberg SA, editors: *Cancer: principles and practice of oncology,* ed 3, Philadelphia, 1989, JB Lippincott.)

izing radiation (Figure 12-21). The level of cell killing is directly related to the cellular oxygen tension up to a partial pressure of oxygen of 20 to 30 mm Hg, at which a plateau is reached. The doses required to have the same biologic effect under conditions of complete hypoxia are 2.5 to 3 times higher than the dose required with full oxygenation. Because of loss of blood supply, many tumors have a portion of their cells under hypoxic conditions; thus these cells will have a relative degree of protection. Fractionated doses of radiation to the tumor may be important because more well-oxygenated cells are killed by the initial fractions. With the reduced tumor volume and improved vascularization of tumor cells, later fractions can have more of an effect on the better-oxygenated residuum.

An additional clinical implication is anemia, which can have an effect on the response of a tumor to radiation. The mechanism of the oxygen effect appears related to the length of time the highly reactive free radicals persist; in the absence of oxygen, the free radicals return more rapidly to stable, nonreactive forms. A field of investigative interest is the development of hypoxic-cell–sensitizing drugs that mimic the effects of oxygen.

Variables in the Biologic Response to Radiation

Absorption of radiation energy by tissues depends on several different physical processes, depending on the energy of the radiation. In conventional diagnostic radiology using low-energy radiation, the photoelectric effect is most important. Photoelectric absorption results when the photon gives up all or most of its energy in the process of ejecting a tightly bound orbital electron. The vacancy in the atomic shell is then filled by an electron falling from an outer shell or from outside the atom. An important property of the photoelectric effect is that absorption varies with the cube of the atomic number of the material. Thus material such as calcium (bone) and lead absorb significantly greater amounts of radiation than carbon, hydrogen, and oxygen.

In radiotherapy, where high-energy radiation is used, the Compton effect is the most important absorption process. In the Compton effect, the interaction of the photon is with a distant orbital electron, and only a portion of the photon's energy is given up. A secondary

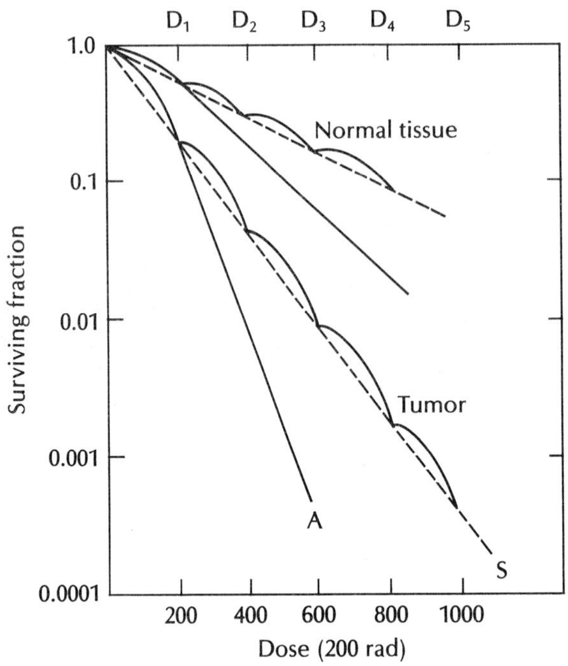

FIGURE 12-22 Cell repair and fractionation effect. Each repeated fractional dose allows for cell repair of sublethal damage and is expressed by the recapitulation of the survival curve's shoulder. If 1000 rad is given as a divided fractional dose (D_1, D_2, D_3, D_4, D_5) of 200 rad daily, it achieves a similar degree of cell kill (*S* on the dashed line) as 600 rad given in one exposure. *A* is the survival curve for single acute exposures of x-rays. This diagram also shows a differential effect on therapeutic ratio between tumor cells and normal cells, which increases with divided or fractional doses of radiation. This is displayed by the increasing differences in the slopes of the solid lines (single dose) and dashed lines (fractional dose). (From Rubin P, Bakemeier RF, Krackov SK, editors: *Clinical oncology for medical students and physicians—a multidisciplinary approach,* ed 6, New York, 1983, American Cancer Society.)

photon of lower energy is given off and scatters in a different direction. The orbital electron that absorbed a portion of the photon's energy (now called a Compton electron) loses this energy through excitation and ionization. Absorption of energy caused by the Compton effect is independent of atomic number and depends more on the electron density of a molecule.

Several quantitative terms are used to describe the amount of energy that is absorbed when radiation interacts with matter. Frequently used units of absorbed dose are *rad* and *gray* (100 rad = 1 gray; 1 rad = 1 centigray or 1 c Gy). One gray refers to the absorption of 1 joule/kilogram. The quantitative term *roentgen* (R) for x rays or gamma rays is based on the ability of radiation to ionize air. At the energies typically used in radiotherapy, 1 R results in an absorbed dose of slightly less than 1 rad (1 c Gy) in soft tissue.

The magnitude of the absorbed radiation dose is not the only important variable in the biologic response to radiation. Equally important is the distribution of the dose over time. As the interval between radiation treatments increases, the total dose to produce the same effect must increase. The varying time-dose relationships appear to occur because cell and tissue recovery occurs during the interval between treatments. In general, normal tissues recover more rapidly than neoplastic tissues, so delivering the total dose over a long time may result in a better therapeutic index. Recovery after irradiation occurs through either cell repair or sublethal damage or by repopulation (Figures 12-22 and 12-23).

The differential between tumor lethal dosage and normal tissue tolerance is exploited in radiotherapy by *fractionation,* in which high-intensity radiotherapy is given over short intervals followed by periods of rest. Another technique for altering the time-dose relationship is *protraction* of the dose, as is used with brachytherapy (use of interstitial or intracavitary radioactive isotopes), in which a low-intensity dosage is given over a prolonged time. A typical daily fraction dosage used clinically in teletherapy is 180 to 250 rad delivered in three to five

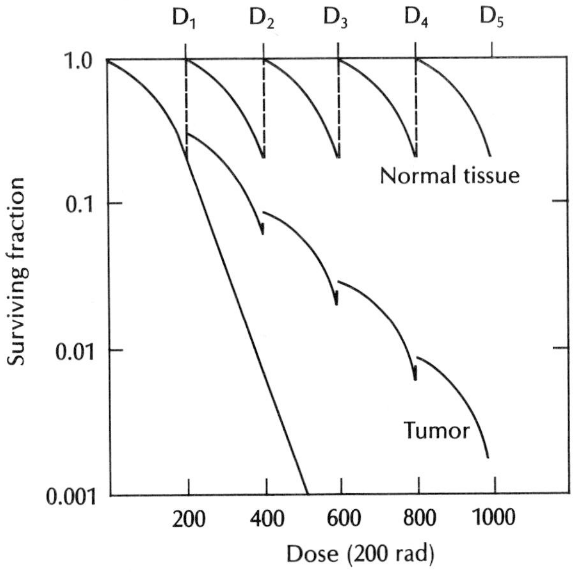

FIGURE 12-23 Repopulation. In a rapid renewal system, repopulation or regeneration of cells within the fractional interval occurs. This figure illustrates that, even if the tumor and normal tissue have the same radiation response, the therapeutic ratio is improved through more rapid regeneration of the normal tissue than that of the tumor. (From Rubin P, Bakemeier RF, Krackov SK, editors: *Clinical oncology for medical students and physicians—a multidisciplinary approach,* ed 6, New York, 1983, American Cancer Society.)

fractions each week. Most tumors treated with curative intent receive doses between 4500 and 7500 rad delivered over 5 to 8 weeks.

Acute and Late Effects of Radiation

The effects of radiation on normal tissues can be divided into acute and late effects. The acute effects are largely on tissues dependent on rapid cell renewal, such as the skin, the oropharyngeal mucosa, the vaginal mucosa, the gastrointestinal mucosa, and the bladder epithelium. These tissues are both very sensitive to radiation and capable of rapid repopulation. The tumor dose fraction that is tolerated in terms of acute effects depends on the volume of tissue being irradiated, the energy of the radiation beam, the type of normal tissue, the age of the patient, and other clinical factors. The radiotherapist attempts to choose fraction doses and time intervals between fractions that provide the greatest differential advantage for the normal tissues relative to proliferation of the clonogenic cells of the malignancy. If excessive acute effects are noted, a small decrease in fraction size or a small delay in treatment interval usually permits the normal tissue to regenerate.

The major dose-limiting factors in radiotherapy are the late effects on the normal tissues. Tolerance doses of various normal tissues for radiotherapy are listed in Table 12-9. The late effects may include fibrosis, necrosis, and nerve damage. The late effects generally are influenced by the total dose and the fraction size; in contrast to the acute effects, these are not particularly related to the treatment interval. It is generally believed that the late effects are predominantly caused by damage to the vasculature and the connective tissue stroma.

Techniques for Delivering Radiotherapy

Radiation therapy techniques are of two general types: brachytherapy and teletherapy. In brachytherapy the radiation source is placed either within or adja target tissue, as with interstitial radiation or intracavitary radiation. Teletherapy uses a radiation source that is at a distance from the patient. The ranges of electromagnetic radiation used in teletherapy are divided into *superficial radiation,* approximately 10 to 125 keV (kiloelectron volts); *orthovoltage radiation,* from 125 to 400 keV; and *supravoltage* or *megavoltage radiation* for energies greater than 400 keV. The important differences in the various types of radiation are related to the relative dose at different depths of penetration. As the energy increases, the penetration of the irradiation increases (Figure 12-24). In modern radiation teletherapy, supravoltage equipment with energies in the range of 2 to 35 meV (million electron volts) is used most often.

In brachytherapy the radiation source is usually close to the target tumor volume, and radiation dosage is related to the inverse square of the distance from the source. Because the dose decreases rapidly as the distance

TABLE 12-9 TOLERANCE DOSES OF RADIATION ON CRITICAL ORGANS AT 200 RAD PER FRACTION

CLASS I ORGANS	INJURY	DOSE FOR 5% INJURY	DOSE FOR 50% INJURY	WHOLE OR PARTIAL ORGAN (FIELD SIZE OR LENGTH)
Bone marrow	Aplasia, pancytopenia	250	450	Whole
		3000	4000	Segmental
Liver	Acute and chronic hepatitis	2500	4000	Whole
		1500	2000	Whole (strip)
Stomach	Perforation, ulcer, hemorrhage	4500	5500	100 cm
Intestine	Ulcer, perforation, hemorrhage	4500	5500	400 cm
		5000	6500	100 cm
Brain	Infarction, necrosis	6000	7000	Whole
		7000	8000	25%
Spinal cord	Infarction, necrosis	4500	5500	10 cm
Heart	Pericarditis and pancarditis	4500	5500	60%
Lung	Acute and chronic pneumonitis	3000	3500	100 cm
		1500	2500	Whole
Kidney	Acute and chronic nephrosclerosis	1500	2000	Whole (strip)
		2000	2500	Whole
Fetus	Death	200	400	Whole

From Phillips TL: Principles of radiobiology and radiation therapy. In Carter SK, Glatstein E, Livingston RB, editors: *Principles of cancer treatment,* New York, 1982, McGraw Hill.

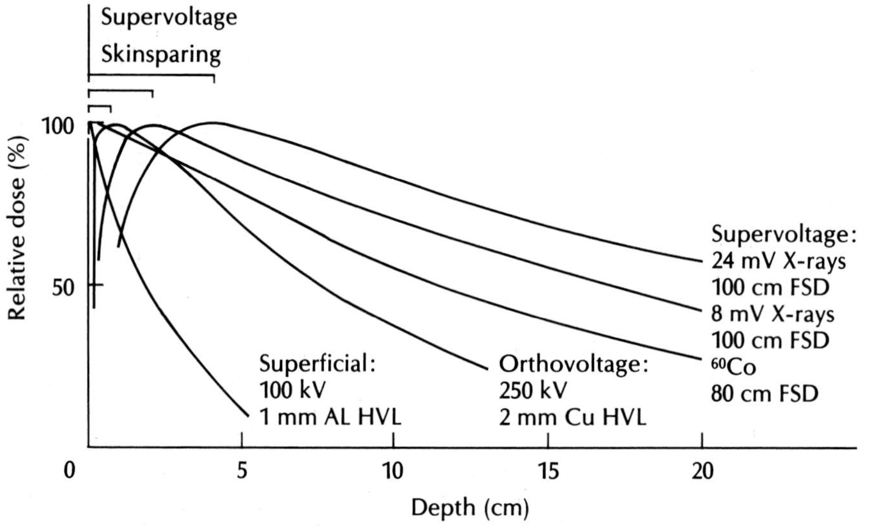

FIGURE 12-24 Relative dose at different depths for various types of ionizing radiation. (From DeVita DT Jr, Hellman S, Rosenberg SA, editors: *Cancer: principles and practice of oncology,* ed 3, Philadelphia, 1989, JB Lippincott.)

from the source increases, the geometry of the source and its placement within the target tissue are important. Thus a therapeutic dose is delivered to the tumor while irradiation of important normal adjacent structures is minimized.

In teletherapy the radiation is from a beam produced by the decay of radioactive isotopes, such as cobalt or cesium, or from various electric machines. The beams are modified by a variety of devices: flattening filters to correct for greater intensity in the center of the beam than on the sides; collimators placed in the head of the machine to vary the exact rectangular beam dimensions; wedges to produce a beam that is more intense on one side than the other. In addition, shielding areas of the patient's body within the treatment field is possible by the construction of blocks designed for each patient.

Before treatment is begun, the target volume must be localized and the dose-limiting normal tissues in the treatment area identified. Localization is accomplished using techniques such as physical examination, radiographs, ultrasound, and CT. The radiotherapist and radiologic physicist design the treatment plan, often using

TABLE 12-10 DOSES OF RADIATION FOR DIFFERENT TUMOR TYPES

DOSE	TUMOR
2000 to 3000 rad	Seminoma, acute lymphocytic leukemia (in central nervous system)
3000 to 4000 rad	Seminoma, Wilms' tumor, neuroblastoma
4000 to 4500 rad	Hodgkin's disease, seminoma, non-Hodgkin's lymphoma, skin cancer (basal and squamous)
5000 to 6000 rad	Lymph nodes (metastatic), squamous cell carcinoma of uterine cervix and head and neck, embryonal cancer, medulloblastoma, retinoblastoma, ovarian cancer, Ewing's tumor, dysgerminomas, breast cancer (after partial mastectomy)
6000 to 6500 rad	Larynx (<1 cm)
7000 to 7500 rad	Oral cavity (<2 cm, 2 to 4 cm), oronasolaryngopharyngeal cancers, bladder cancers, uterine cervical cancer, endometrial cancer, ovarian cancer, lymph nodes (metastatic, 1 to 3 cm), lung cancer (<3 cm)
8000 rad and above	Head and neck cancer (>4 cm), breast cancer (>5 cm), glioblastomas (gliomas), osteogenic sarcomas, melanomas, soft tissue sarcomas (>5 cm), thyroid cancers, lymph nodes (metastatic, >6 cm)

Modified from Rubin P, Siemann D: Principles of radiation oncology and cancer radiotherapy. In Rubin P, Bakemeier RF, Krackov SK, editors: *Clinical oncology for medical students and physicians—a multidisciplinary approach*, ed 6, New York, 1983, American Cancer Society.

a special treatment-planning computer to produce a series of isodose curves, which indicate the doses of radiation in the tumor volume as well as in the adjacent normal tissues. Once a treatment plan has been approved, a special radiation simulator helps correlate the angles and directions of the beam's entry into the patient with the marks placed on the patient's skin. The simulator, designed with a configuration similar to the treatment machines, allows the radiation therapist to select the treatment volume fluoroscopically based on findings from the CT scan or other diagnostic images.

After the treatment volume is localized, the therapist first applies temporary skin marks and then permanent tattoos to the skin. The skin marks are usually drawn on the skin during the first two treatments but then are removed; small, permanent tattoos are made to ensure that each daily treatment is to the proper area. The small tattoos are important for future reference in the event that additional radiotherapy is required later. Often a special immobilization device is built for the patient to ensure exact treatment positioning each day. The patient is positioned under the supervoltage machine each day, and portal films are obtained to ensure that the treatment volume conforms to the computer plan and the setup films done on the simulator.

Electron beam radiation, a specialized type of teletherapy, may be ideal for treating superficial cancers. With electron therapy, in contrast to photon therapy, little sparing of the radiation effects on the skin and superficial tissues occurs, and the maximum penetration is limited to a few centimeters of tissue. Electrons vary greatly in their depth-dose curves, depending on the energy of the electron beam. Electron beams are used primarily as a "boost" or supplemental treatment after photon therapy because of their relative ability to avoid radiation to deeper underlying tissues.

Curative and Palliative Radiotherapy

Radiotherapy may be used with either curative or palliative intent. It can be curative when the therapeutic ratio is favorable, i.e., when all the clonogenic tumor cells can be destroyed without excessive complications of radiotherapy morbidity to the surrounding normal tissue. The dose of radiation capable of providing local tumor control 95% of the time may be termed the *tumor control dose*$_{95}$ *(TCD*$_{95}$*)*. The TCD_{95} varies depending on the tumor's pathologic type and size or distribution. Highly radiocurable tumors have a TCD_{95} in the range of 3500 to 6000 rad; these doses tend to be relatively well tolerated by normal tissues. Examples of highly radiocurable tumors are seminoma, Hodgkin's disease, malignant lymphoma, Wilms' tumor, neuroblastoma, retinoblastoma, Ewing's sarcoma, micrometastases of tumor in lymph nodes, and small laryngeal tumors. Radiocurable tumors with a TCD_{95} between 6000 and 7500 rad, such as moderate to large tumors (T_2 and T_3) of the mouth, pharynx, lung, uterine cervix, and bladder, carry a modest risk of exceeding the tolerance of normal tissues. The least radiocurable tumors have a TCD_{95} of 8000 rad and higher; examples are large (T_3 and T_4) squamous cell carcinomas, adenocarcinomas, and sarcomas. If brachytherapy is applicable in addition to teletherapy, curing the least radiocurable tumors may be possible without exceeding normal tissue tolerance (Tables 12-10 and 12-11).

Palliative radiotherapy plays an important role in controlling distressing symptoms by relieving pain, compression, or obstruction even when cure is not possible. Palliative radiation must be applied judiciously so that the reduction in symptoms exceeds the debility caused by the irradiation. Sometimes palliation can be achieved with lower radiation doses or with total doses delivered in large daily fractions to reduce the treatment

TABLE 12-11 CURATIVE RESULTS IN CANCERS FOR WHICH RADIOTHERAPY IS THE MAJOR TREATMENT MODALITY[93,131,132,159]

TYPE OF CANCER	FIVE-YEAR SURVIVAL RATES (%)
Hodgkin's disease, stages IA and IIA	80
Larynx, stage T_1	80
Lung	
Non–small cell (unresectable)	5
Small cell	5
Prostate, stage B	70 (40 at 10 years)
Seminoma of testis (after orchiectomy)	95
Uterine cervix (combined with surgery)	65
Uterine corpus (combined with surgery) (surgery alone, 60%)	80

period, but often palliative therapy requires doses similar to curative radiation doses.

PRINCIPLES OF CANCER CHEMOTHERAPY

Many parallels exist between chemotherapy for infectious agents and chemotherapy for cancer.[38] The great potential virtue of chemotherapy is that it is a systemic treatment capable of reaching metastases beyond the reach of local and regional treatments such as surgery and radiotherapy. Just as the number of bacteria killed by a given dose of antibiotics is related to first-order kinetics, i.e, a constant percentage rather than an absolute number of bacteria is killed by each dose, so is cancer cell killing by anticancer chemotherapy related to first-order kinetics. A given dose of drug will kill a given percentage of widely different-sized cell populations provided the cells are similarly exposed to the drug and the cells' sensitivity in the differently sized populations is similar.

However, several factors alter the sensitivity and resistance of malignant cells to chemotherapeutic agents and modify the general principle of first-order kinetics. Because proliferating cells are frequently more sensitive to cancer drugs than nonproliferating cells, the cell growth fraction can be important in the response to chemotherapy. The development of drug resistance can lead to subpopulations of cells unaffected by the chemotherapy. Variation in drug distribution in various body areas can lead to lack of efficacious treatment. Despite some similarities between the chemotherapy of bacterial infection and that of malignancy, the effective treatment of cancer with chemotherapy has proved to be much more complex.

Fundamentals of Chemotherapy

Much of the theoretic understanding of the basic principles of anticancer chemotherapy has derived from the work of Skipper[159] and colleagues, using rodent models. Skipper experimentally demonstrated the principle of first-order kinetic killing of cancer cells (Figure 12-25). A dose of chemotherapy that reduces the number of cancer cells by five logarithms will leave a single cancer cell if the initial population is 100,000 cells. If a billion cells are present when the dose is given and all other factors are the same, the surviving cells would number 1000. Thus the chance of eradicating the last colonogenic cell in a cancer will be greater if the population size is small.

An additional factor that affects the ability of anticancer chemotherapy to have a greater effect on smaller tumor populations is that the growth fraction tends to be higher in small tumor masses than in large ones. As tumors grow, an ever-increasing fraction of the daughter cells tends to enter a nonproliferating state, G_0. Because many anticancer drugs are selectively toxic for proliferating cells, large tumors tend to be less affected by chemotherapy as the nonproliferating component of the tumor cell population becomes larger.[99] A portion of the tumor cells in the G_0 state can theoretically be recruited back into the cell cycle if the total tumor cell population is reduced, such as by partial surgical resection or chemotherapy. This theoretic concept is applied in therapy when the grossly evident primary tumor is removed surgically and then chemotherapy is used to treat residual micrometastatic disease.

The relationship between tumor burden and the efficacy of chemotherapy is only partly explained by differences in growth kinetics. The development of drug resistance also appears to be related to the size of the tumor population. The spontaneous mutation rate within a population of cancer cells is in the range of one cell per million (10^6) or higher. Thus by the time a population of cancer cells is large enough to become clinically apparent (10^6 or larger), a high possibility exists of a mutant subpopulation resistant to a particular drug or several drugs.[66] Moreover, exposure to anticancer drugs apparently may increase not only the rate of development of resistance to the given drug but also the development of subpopulations resistant to drugs never used on the tumor.[33]

The clinical implication of these concepts is that the success of chemotherapeutic treatment will be greatest when the smallest population of tumor cells is to be eliminated. The greatest opportunity for chemotherapeutic cure occurs with the initial course of treatment before further cell division leads to spontaneous development of resistance or the induction of resistance by the mutational effect of the chemotherapeutic agents. Failure to give chemotherapy in full doses may lead to inadequate cell kill and development of resistant cells during tumor cell repopulation. The use of combination chemotherapy rather than single agents is in part related to the concept of overcoming any resistance already pres-

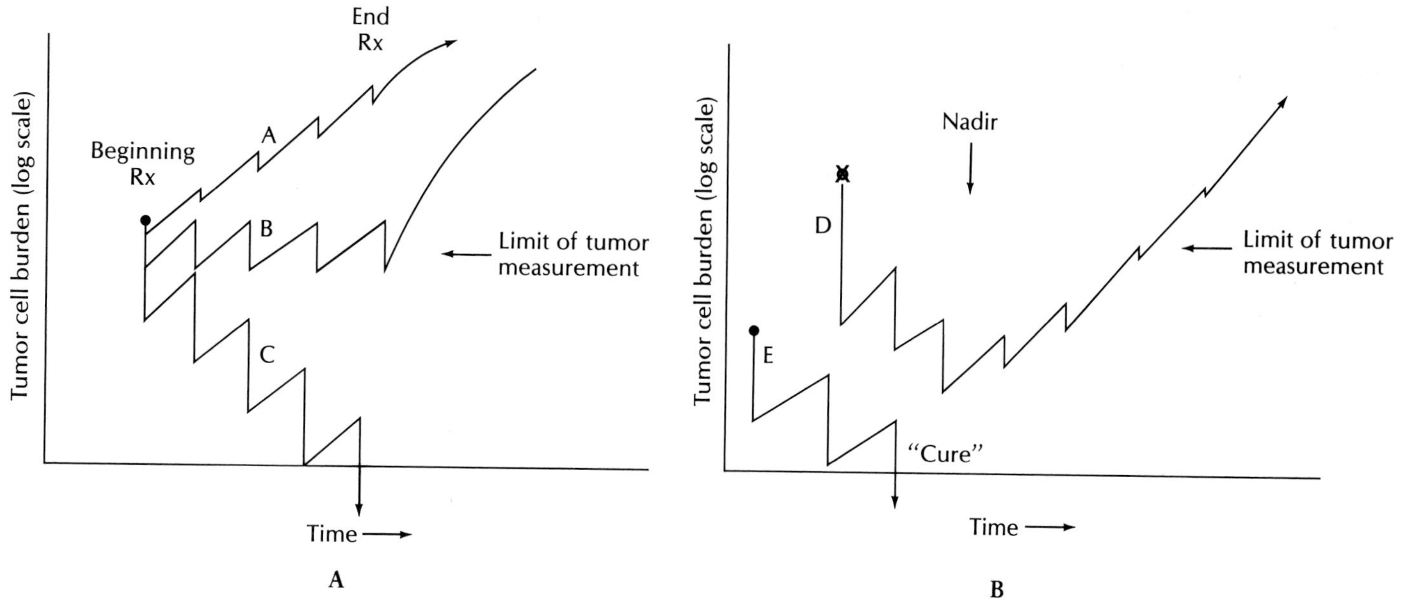

FIGURE 12-25 **A,** Idealized patterns of tumor cell population behavior associated with chemotherapeutic success and failure. *Curve A,* Tumor cell repopulation is greater than tumor cell kill per dose. *Curve B,* A "stay even" situation, which cannot be maintained indefinitely because of eventual selection of drug-resistant tumor cells or cumulative drug toxicity. *Curve C,* The tumor cell kill per dose is greater than the tumor cell repopulation in the intervals between doses for long enough to eradicate all viable tumor cells, with or without immune assistance. This can be achieved only if selection and overgrowth of the permanently drug-resistant neoplastic cells do not occur. **B,** *Curve D,* Remission followed by relapse during undiminished treatment with the same drug(s). The successive repetitive doses do not kill the same fraction of the total neoplastic cells as the first dose, even though the sensitive tumor cell kill per dose may remain the same. *Curve E,* The tumor cell burden at initiation of chemotherapy contained no tumor cells that were permanently resistant to the drug(s), and the dose levels were adequate, thus "cure." This radiotherapy left a relatively small residual of viable tumor cells. (From Skipper HE: *Cancer chemotherapy,* vol 1, Ann Arbor, Mich, 1978, University Microfilms International.)

ent and decreasing the opportunity for the development of resistance if repeated single-drug treatment is used.

The efficacy of anticancer chemotherapy is also related to the occurrence of some selective killing of cancer cells over normal cells. Selective killing occurs partly because the resting cells not in DNA synthesis are refractory to many anticancer drugs. A direct relationship exists between cell kill and the growth fraction of both the tumor and the normal tissues. Whereas individual cancer cells do not generally proliferate faster than the cells of their tissue of origin, the fraction of cells in DNA synthesis is usually higher. Rapidly repopulating tissues such as the bone marrow and gastrointestinal mucosa have a proliferating progenitor cell population sensitive to many chemotherapeutic drugs and also a stem cell population that is in a resting phase unless called to repopulate the progenitor cell population. In the experimental treatment of certain lymphomas, the differential kill between the lymphoma and the normal hematopoietic cells may reach 10,000-fold.[22]

The differential toxicity between the effects of anticancer chemotherapy on the tumor cells and the host's cells is relative. Unwanted effects of chemotherapy on the host can be numerous and may limit the dose levels of chemotherapy that can be administered. Dose-limiting toxicities of chemotherapy can be thought of as either *acute* or *chronic* (repeated dose) dose-limiting toxicities. For example, the acute dose-limiting toxicity of bleomycin is mucositis, and for doxorubicin it is myelosuppression. The chronic dose-limiting toxicity caused by the effect of cumulative doses of bleomycin is pulmonary damage, and for doxorubicin, cardiac damage.

Chemotherapy is usually given in repeated courses with a period allowed for the recovery of the normal tissues, particularly the gastrointestinal mucosa and the bone marrow. If the rate of regrowth of the tumor cell population during the rest period is low enough that tumor repopulation is only partial by the time normal tissues have recovered, then repeated courses may lead to cure, provided resistant cell populations do not

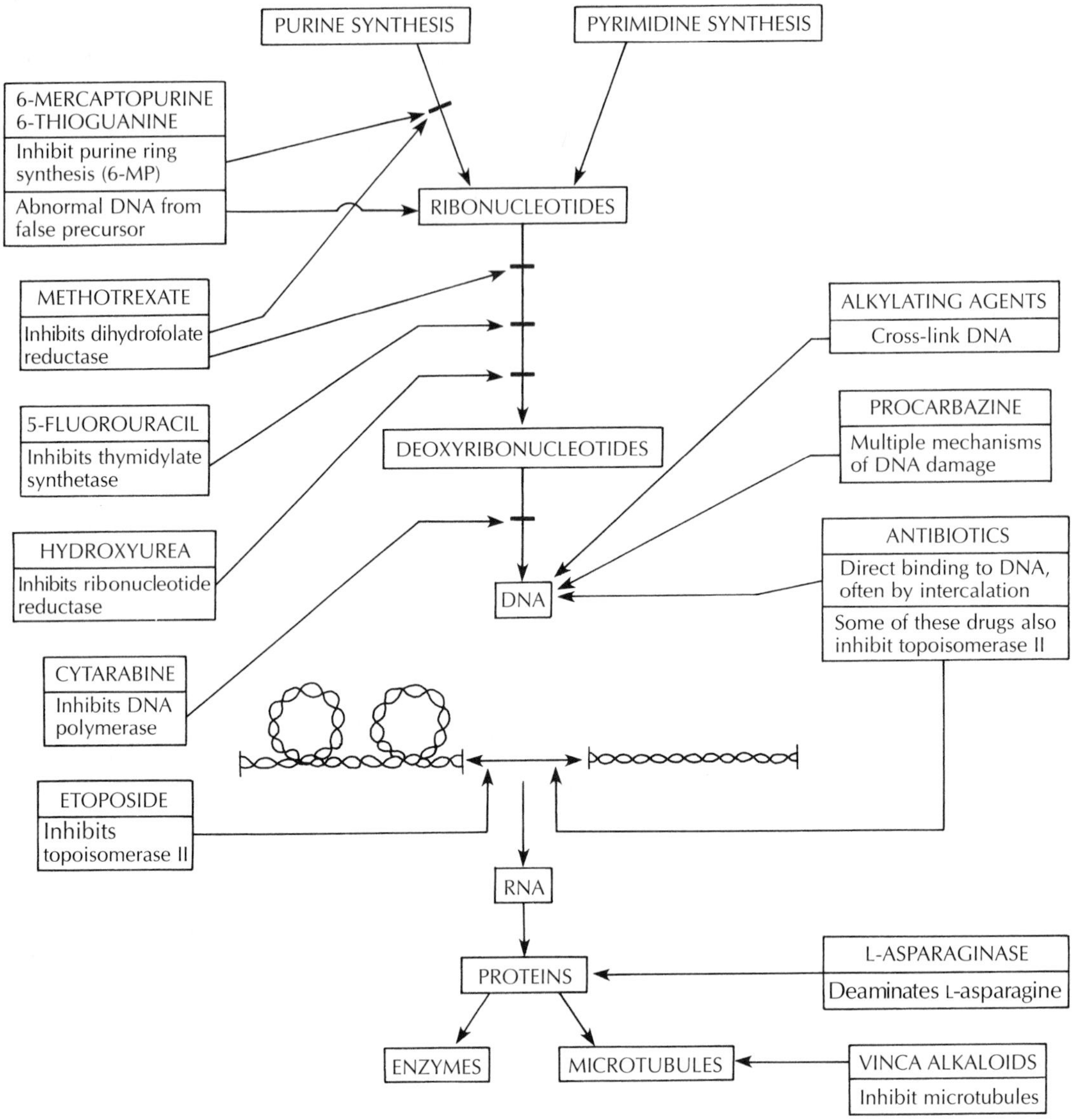

FIGURE 12-26 Major mechanisms of action of selected anticancer drugs. Isomeric forms of DNA are shown as the site of action of drugs that inhibit topoisomerase II. (Modified from Haskell CM, editor: *Cancer treatment*, ed 3, Philadelphia, 1990, WB Saunders. Redrawn from Glisson BS, Ross WE: *Pharmacol Ther* 32:89, 1987.)

emerge. The pattern of recovery of the normal tissues is relatively consistent from patient to patient. The life span of mature blood cells and the storage compartment in the bone marrow is such that after chemotherapeutic toxicity to the progenitor cell population, the nadir of platelets and leukocytes is between 14 and 18 days after treatment. Recovery is usually apparent by 21 days and is usually complete by 28 days. The pattern of bone marrow recovery has led to the frequent adoption of a 4-week period between courses of chemotherapy.

In some chemotherapy protocols, a second dose is given on day 8 in the cycle before the onset of the leukopenia and the recruitment of repopulating stem cells. Second doses in a course of chemotherapy given during days 14 to 21 may be particularly toxic to the recovering bone marrow. Whereas this approach is theoretically sound for many tumors, tumors with very rapid proliferative rates that would regrow excessively between treatment courses require additional strategies. One approach is to use a non-marrow-toxic agent between the courses of the marrow-toxic agents.

The general mechanism of most anticancer drugs at the molecular level is that they interfere with either DNA synthesis or DNA function (Figure 12-26). The past practice of developing anticancer drugs almost exclusively for their effects on DNA may have been too limited an approach, and current investigations are seeking to exploit the selective effect of drugs on the cancer cell membrane.[166] A few agents take advantage of special metabolic characteristics of some cancer cells.

The effects of anticancer drugs, whether therapeutic or toxic, are related both to the concentration of the drug and the period when there is an effective concentration of the drug.[28] Over a considerable range of doses, cytotoxicity is equal to concentration (C) multiplied by the time (T) of exposure ($C \times T$). As in all drug therapies, the absorption, distribution, biotransformation, and excretion of the anticancer drugs are important in their biologic effects. Between different individuals and even between species, the relative doses to produce similar effects are related to the surface area.[55] Doses expressed in milligrams per square meter (mg/m^2) of surface area are more accurate than doses expressed in milligrams per kilogram (mg/kg) of body weight. The dose-response curve for most anticancer drugs is relatively steep. For example, a twofold increase in drug dose may lead to a tenfold or one logarithmic increase in cell kill.

These pharmacokinetic and dose-dependency principles have important therapeutic implications. Small reductions in the doses of cytotoxic agents may result in large reductions in the efficacy of the drug therapy. In tumors with rapid growth rates, the *dose rate,* or the length of the intervals between cycles of treatment, may have a profound influence on the likelihood of a response. Administration of chemotherapy in situations in which the physician is not equipped to manage the complications of marrow toxicity or in which ill-advised attempts are made to spare the patient certain side effects may lead to a failure of response and doom the patient because of the opportunity for drug resistance. These principles are most important when the chemotherapy program has been shown to have the potential for cure as opposed to palliation.

For most cancers, the practice of continuing patients on anticancer drug therapy for extended periods, so-called maintenance therapy, has not proved beneficial. Most current multidrug chemotherapy programs involve repeated cycles of chemotherapy for 3 to 12 months. However, for most malignancies, when cytotoxic chemotherapy is used the optimal dose and duration of therapy is unknown. Current clinical trials are investigating the concept of escalating the initial doses of treatment and shortening the duration.

Anticancer Drugs

The safe use of cytotoxic anticancer drugs requires a thorough understanding of their actions, pharmacokinetics, and toxicities. The following brief review of the selected aspects of anticancer drugs in Table 12-12 presents the general principles of treatment with the various drugs. Physicians involved in supervising the administration of these agents should consult more detailed texts.[28,68] Table 12-13 lists the established and putatively possible cure rates for selected malignancies for which chemotherapy is now the major therapeutic modality.

Chemotherapy also offers the potential of worthwhile palliation for several other malignancies. Advanced malignancies for which currently standard chemotherapeutic agents offer so little benefit to the patient that they should usually not be used include the following:[68]

- Carcinoma of the stomach
- Bronchogenic carcinoma other than small cell
- Head and neck carcinoma
- Carcinoma of the cervix
- Renal carcinoma
- Pancreatic, liver, and bile duct carcinomas
- Thyroid carcinoma

For these advanced malignancies, most patients are better served by participating in controlled investigations of new therapies or by being given compassionate, symptomatic care only.

Alkylating Agents

Alkylating agents form carbonium ions that react with nucleic acids, causing breakage of DNA strands and abnormal base-pairing of the nucleotides in DNA. Some types of alkylating agents cause DNA cross-linking. In addition to reacting with nucleic acids, the alkylating agents also react with proteins, sulfhydryls, and amino acids, resulting in multiple lesions in both dividing and nondividing cells. Thus alkylating agents are cell-cycle-nonspecific agents, although rapidly proliferating tissues are somewhat more sensitive to their effects. Guanine is particularly susceptible to alkylation, and many of the lethal effects as well as mutagenic effects of the alkylating agents are probably related to binding with guanine. The various alkylating agents differ in their metabolism, pharmacokinetics, chemical reactivity, and transport mechanism into cells. Because of these differences, tumors differ in their spectrum of response and resistance to alkylating agents.

Nitrogen mustard has been useful in the treatment of Hodgkin's lymphoma, particularly in combination with other agents. Cyclophosphamide has been used in the treatment of lymphomas, neuroblastomas, breast and ovarian carcinomas, small cell lung carcinoma, chronic lymphocytic leukemias, and acute leukemias. Phenylalanine mustard, or melphalan (Alkeran, L-PAM), is typically used to treat multiple myeloma and has been used for carcinoma of the breast and ovary. Chlorambucil (Leukeran) has been used in the treatment of chronic lymphatic leukemia, multiple myeloma, and nodular lymphomas. The nitrosoureas have found use in the treatment of Hodgkin's disease and other lymphomas.

Antimetabolites

The antimetabolites are drugs that bear structural similarities to important cellular molecules and serve as fraudulent substrates.

TABLE 12-12 MAJOR CYTOTOXIC ANTICANCER DRUGS: DOSES, TOXICITIES, AND MAJOR CLINICAL INDICATIONS

AGENT	ROUTE*	REPRESENTATIVE DOSES† (mg/m²)	SCHEDULE
Alkylating Agents			
Cyclophosphamide (Cytoxan)	IV	400	qd × 5 (daily for 5 days)
	PO	50-100	qd × 14
Melphalan (L-Pam, Alkeran)	IV	4	qd × 5
	IV	8	q4w
	PO	8	qd × 5
	PO	4	qd
Chlorambucil	PO	1-3	qd
Busulfan (Myleran)	PO	2-6	qd
Ifosfamide plus	IV	1800-2400	qd × 5
mesna	IV	1800-2400	qd × 5
Nitrosoureas			
BCNU (carmustine)	IV	150-225	q6w
CCNU (lomustine)	PO	100-150	q6w
Streptozotocin	IV	500	qd × 5, q3-4w
Antimetabolites			
Methotrexate (MTX)	IV	25	2 × weekly
	IM	25	2 × weekly
	IV	1500 (high dose with leucovorin rescue)	q3w
5-Fluorouracil (5-FU)	IV	500	qw or qd × 5
	IV	800-1200	24h × 5, q 3-4 wk
	IA	800-1200	24h, qd × 14-21
Cytarabine (Cytarabine HCI, arabinosyl cytosine, ara-C; Cytosar)	IV	100	q12h × 5-10d
	IV	2000-3000	q12h × 6d
6-Thioguanine	IV	100	qd × 5
Vinca Alkaloids			
Vincristine sulfate (Oncovin)	IV	1.0	qw
Vinblastine sulfate (Velban)	IV	6.0	qw
		2.0	24h x5d, q 3 wk
	IV	86	2d qwk
VP-16 (Etoposide)	PO	200	2d qwk
VP-26	IV	67	qwk
Antibiotics			
Dactinomycin (actinomycin D)	IV	0.6	qd × 5
Doxorubicin (Adriamycin)	IV	75	q3w
	IV	20	qw
Mithramycin	IV	1.75	qod to toxicity
for high Ca^{++}	IV	0.75	qd × 3-4
Bleomycin	IV	10	qw
	IM	10	qw
Daunorubicin	IV	30	qd × 3, q3w
Mitomycin C	IV	2.0	qd × 3, q3w
Other Agents			
Cisplatin	IV	50-100	q3-4w
	IV	20	qd × 5
Carboplatin	IV	300	qd × 5
Dacarbazine (DTIC)	IV	375	qd × 5
Mitoxantrone	IV	14	q3w
Mitotane (o,p'-DDD)	PO	5000	qd

Modified from Chabner BA, Myers CE: Clinical pharmacology of cancer chemotherapy. In DeVita VT Jr, Hellman S, Rosenberg SA, editors: *Cancer: Principles and practice of oncology,* ed 3, Philadelphia, 1989, JB Lippincott.

**IV,* Intravenous; *PO,* oral; *IM,* intramuscular; *IA,* intraarterial.

†Representative doses are given to provide the reader with a general concept of the dose range. Often patients are treated simultaneously with multiple chemotherapeutic agents at doses and schedules different from those indicated here.

MAJOR TOXICITIES‡	MAJOR CLINICAL INDICATIONS
Myelosuppression, alopecia, cystitis	Hodgkin's and non-Hodgkin's lymphomas, multiple myeloma, lymphocytic leukemia, many solid tumors
Myelosuppression	Multiple myeloma, breast and ovarian cancer
Myelosuppression	Hodgkin's disease; locally for malignant effusions
Myelosuppression, pulmonary toxicity	Chronic granulocytic leukemia
Myelosuppression, cystitis	Testicular carcinoma
Myelosuppression, leukemia, pulmonary fibrosis, renal (for both BCNU and CCNU elevation)	Intracranial tumors, melanoma
	Lymphomas, lung cancer
Renal failure, hyperglycemia, hepatic enzymes	Islet cell carcinomas, gastrinomas, glucagonomas
Oral and gastrointestinal ulcers, myelosuppression, hepatotoxicity	Choriocarcinoma, acute lymphocytic leukemia, carcinoma of cervix and head and neck
Myelosuppression, stomatitis, diarrhea	Carcinoma of breast, ovary, and large bowel
Bone marrow depression	Acute leukemia
Myelosuppression	Acute leukemia
Mild myelosuppression, neuropathy, constipation	Acute leukemia, Hodgkin's disease, lymphomas and solid tumors
Alopecia, neuropathy, myelosuppression	Hodgkin's disease, miscellaneous solid tumors
Myelosuppression, neuropathy	Small cell carcinomas of lung, testis
Myelosuppression, alopecia, gastrointestinal ulcers	Wilms' tumor, sarcoma, testicular carcinomas
Myelosuppression, alopecia, cardiomyopathy	Wide variety of carcinomas, soft tissue sarcomas, leukemia, lymphomas
Myelosuppression, hypocalcemia, renal, hepatic	Embryonal carcinoma of testis
	Hypercalcemia
Pulmonary fibrosis, alopecia, stomatitis, edema	Hodgkin's and non-Hodgkin's lymphomas, cancer of head and neck, testicular carcinoma
Myelosuppression, alopecia, cardiomyopathy	Acute leukemia
Fever, pulmonary fibrosis, allergic reactions	Adenocarcinomas, stomach, pancreas, colon, breast, chronic myelogenous leukemia
Myelosuppression, renal failure, Mg^{++} wasting, neuropathy	Testicular and ovarian carcinoma; bladder, osteocarcinoma, small-cell lung
Myelosuppression	Similar to cisplatin
Myelosuppression, flulike syndrome	Melanoma, sarcomas
Myelosuppression, cholestasis, cardiomyopathy (limited risk)	Spectrum of clinical activity appears similar to doxorubicin
Gastrointestinal, CNS, adrenal insufficiency	Adrenal carcinoma

‡For many anticancer drugs, usual therapeutic doses cause depression of peripheral white blood cell counts and platelets. The maximum effect of bone marrow toxicity occurs 2 to 3 weeks after last dose for melphalan, cyclophosphamide, chlorambucil, methotrexate, 5-fluorouracil, 6-thioguanine, and doxorubicin. For the nitrosoureas, it occurs at 6 to 8 weeks. Cyclophosphamide can cause alopecia and hemorrhagic cystitis. The alkylating agents have relatively high carcinogenic potential compared to the antimetabolites.

TABLE 12-13 CANCERS FOR WHICH CHEMOTHERAPY AS THE MAJOR MODALITY OF THERAPY IS POTENTIALLY CURATIVE*

TYPE OF CANCER	CURABILITY (%) ESTABLISHED	PUTATIVE
Hodgkin's, stages III and IV	40	80
Lymphoma, diffuse histiocytic	40	65
Lymphoma, Burkitt's[186]	50	70
Lymphoma, lymphoblastic	40	70
Gestational choriocarcinoma	>60	>80
Acute lymphatic leukemia, pediatric	50	80
Acute lymphatic leukemia, adult	20	40
Acute myeloid leukemia, pediatric	20	40
Acute myeloid leukemia, adult	10	20

Modified from Frei E III: *Cancer Res* 45:6523, 1985.
**Curative* is defined as the portion of patients who reach a disease-free survival plateau.

5-Fluorouracil (5-FU) is useful in treatment of carcinoma of the breast and colon; ovarian, pancreatic, and gastric carcinomas show some limited response. 5-FU acts as a fraudulent uracil, which after suitable intracellular transformation is converted into various fluorinated nucleotides. The primary cytotoxic action of 5-FU is to block the thymidylate synthase reaction and thus inhibit DNA synthesis. 5-FU is not itself incorporated into DNA. It also has an important effect on RNA processing and function because it is incorporated into the various types of RNA. 5-FU is rapidly metabolized in many tissues, including the liver. Metabolism of 5-FU is sufficiently rapid that during infusion into the liver for the treatment of metastases less than 50% of the drug reaches the systemic circulation. The major toxic effects of 5-FU are on the bone marrow and gastrointestinal mucosa. 5-FU may cause conjunctivitis and also reversible neurotoxicity, which is usually manifested as cerebellar dysfunction.

Of the antifolates, the most important in clinical use to date is methotrexate. Methotrexate is used in the treatment of breast carcinoma and head and neck carcinomas. It is also used in the treatment of acute lymphocytic leukemia, gestational choriocarcinoma, lymphomas, and sarcomas. Methotrexate inhibits the enzyme dihydrofolate reductase, which is responsible for maintaining the intracellular pool of folates in the reduced (active) state. Inhibition of dihydrofolate reductase leads to a deficiency of tetrahydrofolic acid. Tetrahydrofolic acid is critically important in the metabolic transfer of one-carbon units in various biochemical reactions, including the synthesis of thymidylic acid (needed for DNA) and inosinic acid (needed for RNA).

The biochemical effects of methotrexate can be reversed by administration of the reduced folate leucovorin. Even after otherwise lethal doses of methotrexate, leucovorin "rescue" can prevent severe gastrointestinal and hematologic toxicity if it is given within 36 hours. Methotrexate is primarily excreted by the kidneys, and thus decreased renal function leads to an increased risk of toxicity. Methotrexate distributes slowly into third-space accumulations of fluid such as ascites and pleural effusions. Methotrexate also exits slowly from third-space accumulations, and drug reentry into the systemic circulation may lead to unexpected toxicity. In patients with ascites or large pleural effusions, the effusions should be evacuated or the blood levels of methotrexate monitored. Toxicities of methotrexate include its effect on the rapidly replicating cells of the bone marrow and gastrointestinal tract. Methotrexate can also cause acute and chronic hepatic injury, as well as renal toxicity at high doses. Intrathecal methotrexate, which is used in the treatment of carcinomatous meningitis and in central nervous system prophylaxis for patients with acute lymphocytic leukemia, can cause a variety of acute and chronic neurotoxicities.

Tumor cells can develop resistance to methotrexate through several different mechanisms, such as an increase in the dihydrofolate reductase enzyme. The increased enzyme is a result of amplification of the gene coding for the enzyme.[33,151] Cells can also be resistant if they have an absent or altered transport mechanism for methotrexate or develop an altered enzyme that fails to bind to methotrexate.

Cytosine arabinoside (ara-C, cytarabine) is an analog of deoxycytidine. It has found particular use in inducing remissions in patients with acute nonlymphocytic leukemias. Ara-C has several mechanisms of action, including incorporation into DNA. After biochemical conversion, it also can result in a nucleotide that acts as an inhibitor of DNA polymerase. In addition to the cytotoxic effects at high doses, relatively low doses of ara-C have been used clinically, based on the concept that the drug may be capable of inducing terminal differentiation in some myeloid leukemia cells.[136]

The major toxic effects of ara-C are on the bone marrow and the gastrointestinal mucosa. High doses can cause neurotoxicity.

Purine analogs are formed by the substitution of a thiol group into the purine nucleus in place of the 6-hydroxyl group, producing the purine analogs 6-mercaptopurine (6-MP) and 6-thioguanine (6-TG). In their native state, both 6-MP and 6-TG are inactive and require activation to the nucleotide level by the enzyme hypoxanthine-guanine phosphoribosyl transferase

(HGPRTase). As monophosphate nucleotides, these analogs inhibit de novo purine synthesis, and as triphosphates, they are incorporated into DNA. Azathioprine, which has been widely used clinically for its ability to suppress cell-mediated immunity, is metabolized to 6-MP by the liver. 6-MP is used in the treatment of acute lymphoblastic and myeloblastic leukemias. Biochemical resistance to purine analog occurs in cells that lack the activating enzyme HGPRTase. The primary toxicities of the thiopurines are on the bone marrow, with lesser toxicity on the oral and gastrointestinal mucosa. Hepatic dysfunction, which is usually reversible, may occur occasionally.

Various adenosine analogs have been developed that have antitumor and antiviral effects as well as immunosuppressive effects. Adenosine arabinoside (ara-A), which is used clinically in the treatment of infections with DNA viruses, inhibits DNA polymerase. Administering doses of ara-A that are cytotoxic is difficult because of its limited aqueous solubility and its rapid deamination by adenosine deaminase. Drug researchers are currently trying to develop agents resistant to deamination (e.g., 2-fluoro-ara-A) and to combine adenosine analogs with inhibitors of adenosine deaminase (e.g., 2′-deoxycoformycin).

Antitumor Antibiotics

The anthracyclines, which are clinically useful in the treatment of breast carcinomas, sarcomas, lymphomas, and acute leukemia, are fermentation products of *Streptomyces* species. Daunorubicin (daunomycin) is one of the most effective chemotherapeutic agents against acute leukemia. Doxorubicin (Adriamycin) is used to treat a variety of solid tumors, including cancers of the breast, lung, and ovary as well as soft tissue sarcomas. At high doses the anthracyclines are cytotoxic, and at low doses they can alter the function of the cell membrane.

The exact mechanism of the cytotoxic effect of the anthracyclines is uncertain. However, the planar structure of daunorubicin and doxorubicin allows them to intercalate between the base pairs of DNA, with resultant inhibition of DNA, RNA, and ultimately protein synthesis. The liver is the main site of metabolism. Acute toxicity is related to myelosuppression and mucositis. The anthracyclines almost always cause alopecia, which is reversible once treatment is discontinued. The most serious toxicity of the anthracyclines is cardiac toxicity, as manifested by a cardiomyopathy with decreased contractility and congestive heart failure. The cardiac toxicity is dose dependent and for daunorubicin occurs at an increasing rate in patients treated with cumulative doses of more than 550 mg/m^2 of body surface. Current drug development efforts are aimed at dissociating the cardiac toxicities of the anthracyclines from their therapeutic effects.

The anthracyclines are administered intravenously, and great care must be taken to reduce possible extravasation. Extravasation can lead to severe local reactions, progressing to deep ulcerations that may require debridement and grafting to heal.

Bleomycin is a mixture of small-molecular-weight peptides isolated from the fungus *Streptomyces verticillus*. Bleomycin is widely used in the treatment of squamous cell carcinoma of the head and neck, lymphomas, and testicular cancer. It binds to DNA, causing single- and double-strand breaks. Bleomycin can be administered by intravenous, intramuscular, or subcutaneous injection. Because it is primarily eliminated in the urine, bleomycin pharmacokinetics are markedly altered in patients with abnormal renal function. In contrast to most other antitumor cytotoxic agents, bleomycin has limited hematopoietic toxicity. Its most important toxicity is progressive pulmonary interstitial fibrosis. Pulmonary toxicity is initially manifested by cough, dyspnea, and bibasilar infiltrates on chest radiograph. Toxicity will most likely occur in patients with underlying pulmonary disease or in those over age 70 and when total cumulative doses over 250 mg/m^2 are administered. Lung biopsy may be necessary to distinguish bleomycin toxicity from infiltrates caused by infection or tumor.

Actinomycin D has been effective in the treatment of Wilms' tumor, Ewing's sarcoma, embryonal rhabdomyosarcoma, and gestational choriocarcinoma. The antibiotic intercalates with DNA and inhibits DNA and RNA synthesis. The major dose-limiting toxicity of actinomycin D is myelosuppression, but gastrointestinal toxicity is also significant. Actinomycin D also enhances x-irradiation toxicity.

Mitomycin C has some activity in gastric, pancreatic, and breast cancers and is generally used with other agents. Mitomycin C appears to inhibit DNA through alkylation and cross-linking and also has intercalation properties. The major dose-limiting toxicity of mitomycin C is myelosuppression. The nadir of leukocytes and platelets occurs at 4 to 6 weeks.

Mithramycin is an important agent because its hypocalcemic effect can be valuable in the treatment of patients with severe hypercalcemia. It binds to DNA and interferes with RNA synthesis. Side effects include acute nausea and vomiting, hepatic and renal toxicity, and depression of platelets. The hypocalcemic effect of mithramycin is related to inhibition of osteoclast function. In patients with hypercalcemic crises of either malignant or nonmalignant origin, brief courses of mithramycin can lower the serum calcium for 7 to 10 days.

Cisplatin and Carboplatin

Cisplatin has proved to be highly effective in the treatment of carcinomas of the head and neck, testis, and ovary. Cisplatin induces DNA cross-links that lead to changes in DNA conformation and inhibition of DNA synthesis. The process of cross-link formation continues for hours after the exposure to the drug and is opposed by the cell's repair processes, which excise and rebuild damaged DNA segments. Cisplatin is administered intravenously with vigorous hydration and diuresis to minimize renal toxicity. Without adequate hydration, nephrotoxicity is common. With vigorous diuresis, most patients are able to tolerate repeated doses without renal dysfunction. Nausea and vomiting are fairly severe after cisplatin administration and are only partly relieved by standard antiemetic agents. Hypomagnesemia is common, and although the patient is usually asymptomatic, occasionally tetany may occur. Myelosuppression is moderate in most patients at usual therapeutic doses of cisplatin.

Carboplatin has a spectrum of activity similar to cisplatin but a different spectrum of drug toxicity. The dose-limiting toxicity of carboplatin is myelotoxicity. Nephrotoxicity, neurotoxicity, and ototoxicity are less common than with cisplatin.

Plant Alkaloids

Screening of plant extracts has produced two therapeutically useful anticancer classes of drugs, the Vinca alkaloids and the podophyllotoxins.

The *Vinca* alkaloids, vincristine and vinblastine, are derived from an ornamental shrub, *Vinca rosea,* or periwinkle. Vincristine has been used effectively in the treatment of acute lymphocytic leukemia, Hodgkin's disease, non-Hodgkin's lymphomas, Ewing's sarcoma, neuroblastoma, Wilms' tumor, breast carcinoma, and sarcomas. Vinblastine is useful in the treatment of Hodgkin's disease, non-Hodgkin's lymphomas, breast and testicular carcinomas, and methotrexate-resistant choriocarcinoma. The *Vinca* alkaloids bind to tubulin, the intracellular protein that forms the microtubular apparatus important in maintaining cell structure and forming the mitotic spindle. Both vincristine and vinblastine are metabolized in the liver and excreted in the bile, with very little excretion in the urine. In patients with hepatic dysfunction, doses of the *Vinca* alkaloids must be reduced, but no dose reduction is required for renal dysfunction. The toxicity of vincristine is mainly caused by its neuropathic effects. Patients typically have mild sensory impairment and paresthesia as well as constipation from autonomic nerve dysfunction; moderate symptoms are not regarded as dose-limiting toxicities. More severe neurotoxicity, such as severe paresthesia, ataxia, footdrop, and muscle wasting are to be avoided and are dose limiting. Vinblastine causes myelosuppression and occasionally neurologic toxicity that is similar but generally less severe than that following vincristine.

The podophyllotoxins, VP-16 etoposide and VP-26, were derived from the mandrake plant and have antitumor activity against lymphomas, small cell carcinomas of the lung, and testicular carcinomas. They cause DNA strand breakage by inhibiting topoisomerase II. The dose-limiting toxicity is usually leukopenia. A mild peripheral neuropathy may occur after administration of these drugs. Neuropathy may be severe in patients previously treated with vincristine.

Procarbazine

Procarbazine is used in the treatment of Hodgkin's disease and carcinoma of the lung. After metabolic activation, the various products derived from procarbazine appear to act as alkylating agents, affecting nucleic acids, phospholipids, and proteins. Myelosuppression, which may be delayed for several weeks, is the usual dose-limiting toxicity. Other adverse reactions include nausea, vomiting, and central nervous system depression. Procarbazine is a monoamine oxidase inhibitor (MAOI), and thus other MAOIs should be avoided during treatment, and patients should be advised to avoid foods containing tyramine, such as bananas, cheese, yogurt, and wine. Procarbazine may also have effects similar to those after disulfiram (Antabuse) administration, leading to sweating, flushing, and headache after alcohol ingestion. Procarbazine is both a potent immunosuppressant and a potent mutagen.

Hexamethylmelamine

Hexamethylmelamine is active against breast cancer, ovarian cancer, small cell lung cancer, and the lymphomas. Its mechanism of action is uncertain. The nausea and vomiting produced by hexamethylmelamine are frequently severe and are often dose limiting. In addition, it causes neurotoxicity, with mood alterations, hallucinations, and peripheral neuropathy.

L-Asparaginase

L-Asparagine is a nonessential amino acid for normal cells, but some tumor cells lack the enzyme L-asparagine synthetase. Tumor cells lacking this enzyme must obtain asparagine from the extracellular pool. L-Asparaginase depletes the extracellular pool by degrading asparagine, which leads to selective toxicity of tumor cells lacking the synthetic enzyme. The drug has been useful in some patients with acute lymphocytic leukemia. Gastrointestinal toxicities of L-asparaginase have included anorexia, nausea, vomiting, hepatic dysfunction, and pancreatitis. Neurologic toxicities have included lethargy, somnolence, seizures, and coma.

Mitotane

Mitotane, or o,p′-DDD, is a derivative of the insecticide DDT and has been used for the treatment of unresectable adrenocortical carcinoma. Mitotane inhibits cortisol production by the tumor and can cause tumor regression in some patients. When treated with therapeutic doses of o,p′-DDD, most patients have gastrointestinal and neurologic toxicity.

Streptozocin

Streptozocin is particularly useful in the treatment of unresectable islet cell carcinoma and malignant carcinoid. The drug has an inhibitory effect on DNA synthesis and also on the key enzymes in gluconeogenesis, which may lead to hypoglycemia. Gastrointestinal toxicity includes nausea and vomiting as well as transient and usually mild changes in liver function. Renal toxicity may be manifest as renal tubular acidosis, glucosuria, aminoaciduria, or azotemia. Leukopenia and anemia may also occur.

Dacarbazine

Dacarbazine (DTIC, dimethyl-triazeno-imidazole-carboxamide) has been used in the treatment of malignant melanoma, Hodgkin's disease, and soft tissue sarcomas. DTIC appears to function as an alkylating agent. Myelosuppression is the usual dose-limiting toxicity.

PRINCIPLES OF HORMONAL THERAPY

Hormonal therapy of cancer usually refers to (1) the manipulation of steroid hormones by administration of the hormone or an antagonist of the hormone; or (2) the manipulation of the hormone by surgical or radiotherapeutic ablation of the gland(s) controlling its secretion. When the available cytotoxic chemotherapy provides only palliative effects and does not cure the tumor, endocrine manipulations in hormonally responsive tumors frequently provide longer durations of palliation with fewer adverse effects than with cytotoxic chemotherapy.

Hormones function by binding to specific receptors on the cell membrane, within the cytoplasm, or within the cell nucleus. The general mechanism of action of steroid hormones is that they first bind to a cytosolic receptor. The hormone-receptor complex is then translocated to the nucleus of the cell, where it binds to an acceptor site on the chromatin. The nuclear binding then influences the transcription of messenger RNA, with its ultimate effects on protein synthesis and cell replication. Assay for the level of receptor proteins in the tumor predicts likelihood of response to a particular hormonal therapy. Refer to the section on receptors and growth factors earlier in this chapter and in Chapter 44.

Oophorectomy to treat metastatic breast cancer was one of the earliest effective systemic treatments for cancer, and it remains a first-line therapy for selected premenopausal patients. Effective ovarian ablation can also be accomplished with radiotherapy. The formerly useful procedures of adrenalectomy and hypophysectomy in the treatment of metastatic breast cancer have now been supplanted by pharmacologic agents that block the effects of estrogens at the cellular level (antiestrogens such as tamoxifen)[79,106] or that block secretion of estrogens from the adrenal gland (medical adrenalectomy with aminoglutethimide plus a glucocorticoid to block ACTH secretion by the pituitary).[148]

Orchiectomy has been used extensively for the palliative treatment of metastatic prostatic carcinoma. Estrogens have also been useful in the palliation of prostatic cancer, as have antiandrogens.[58] Analogs of luteinizing hormone-releasing hormone (LHRH) that reduce testosterone to castration levels are being evaluated as an alternative to orchiectomy.[125]

The major antitumor hormonal agents used in current clinical practice are summarized in Table 12-14.

PRINCIPLES OF TUMOR IMMUNOLOGY AND IMMUNOTHERAPY

The principles of human tumor immunology are based on an understanding of the immune response and its regulation. This section can provide only a brief outline of this subject. More extensive reviews are available in other texts.[71,75]

Antigens are the chemical structures that can be recognized by the cellular or the humoral immune response. The aim in tumor immunology is to discover unique antigens associated with tumors that might provide a target for either immunodiagnosis or immunotherapy. In human beings, most antigens identified to date are tumor-associated antigens (TAA) rather than the tumor-specific-transplantation antigens (TSTA) that have been identified in some experimental tumors. Examples of TAA in human beings are (1) the oncofetal antigens, such as carcinoembryonic antigen and alpha-fetoprotein; (2) antigens specific for a certain cell lineage, such as the CA-125 antigen, which is associated with ovarian cancer and other tumors derived from the celomic epithelium; and (3) antigens related to the degree of differentiation, such as the T-cell phenotypic markers T1, T3, T4, and T8. Evidence that TSTAs occur in human cancers is equivocal. Data suggest, however, that TSTAs exist in melanoma, osteosarcoma, neuroblastoma, and Burkitt's lymphoma. Gestational choriocarcinomas are unique in that they possess paternal histocompatibility antigens. It has been suggested that the ready curability of gestational choriocarcinomas by chemotherapy is related to the participation of the patient's immune response against the paternal antigens.

The potential mechanisms for the killing of tumor cells include T-cell–mediated cytotoxicity, macrophage-mediated cytotoxicity, natural killer cell activity, and antibody-dependent tumor cell killing. The mechanism of T-cell–mediated cytotoxicity has been extensively

TABLE 12-14 MAJOR ANTITUMOR HORMONAL AGENTS: DOSES, TOXICITIES, AND MAJOR CLINICAL INDICATIONS

AGENT	USUAL DOSE	MAJOR CLINICAL INDICATION	TOXICITIES
Estrogen			
Diethylstilbesterol (DES)	1-3 mg po qd 5 mg po tid	Prostate cancer Postmenopausal breast cancer	Fluid retention, gastrointestinal upset, uterine bleeding, hypercalcemia (if bone metastases), risk of death from cardiovascular disease
Antiestrogen			
Tamoxifen	10 mg po bid	Breast cancer	Hypercalcemia, hot flashes, transient thrombocytopenia, abnormal uterine bleeding
Progestins			
Hydroxyprogesterone caproate (Delalutin)	1 g IM biw	Breast, endometrial cancers	Fluid retention, hypercalcemia
Medroxyprogesterone acetate (Provera)	200-600 mg IM biw 100-200 mg po qd	Breast, endometrial, renal cancers	
Megestrol acetate (Megace)	40 mg qid 40-320 mg qd	Breast cancer Endometrial cancer	
Androgens			Virilization, fluid retention, hypercalcemia, cholestatic jaundice
Fluoxymesterone (Halotestin)	10-40 mg qd (divided doses) 40-320 mg qd	Breast cancer	
Corticosteroids			
Prednisone	40 mg/m_2 qd	Lymphomas, leukemia, multiple myeloma, breast cancer	Fluid retention, hypokalemia, diabetes mellitus, euphoric state, osteoporosis, immunosuppression, Cushing's syndrome
Dexamethasone (Decadron)	2-10 mg/m^2	Cerebral edema	
Aminoglutethimide (Elipten, Cytadren)	250 mg po qid (with hydrocortisone)	Breast cancer	Adrenal suppression, rash, ataxia, somnolence
Thyroid hormone			
L-Thyroxine	2 μg/kg qd	Thyroid cancer	Hyperthyroidism, osteoporosis
Somatostatin analog			
Octreotide acetate (Sandostatin)	100-600 μg qd	Carcinoids, VIPomas	Gastrointestinal upset, cholelithiasis, hypothyroidism, steatorrhea

studied in vitro. Direct contact between T cells and the tumor cell membrane antigen produces lethal membrane damage. Natural killer (NK) cell activity is associated morphologically with large granular lymphocytes (LGL). NK cells have the property of selectively killing tumor cells rather than nonmalignant cells. NK cell activity can be augmented by a variety of factors, including interleukin-2, interferon, and immunostimulants such as Calmette-Guérin bacillus (BCG) and *Corynebacterium parvum*. Another population of killer cells distinct from the NK cells is lymphokine-activated killer (LAK) cells. LAK cells have a broad cytotoxicity against tumor cells. LAK cells are generated in the presence of interleukin-2 in vitro, and it is thus possible to expand the LAK cell population in vitro and then to infuse these cells into the host to obtain an enhanced antitumor effect.[139]

Macrophages, after they have been activated by various factors, develop tumoricidal or tumorostatic activity. Macrophage activators include a lymphokine from T cells, gamma-interferon, and endotoxins. In addition to tumor inhibitory factors, under some circumstances macrophages produce factors that can stimulate tumor growth and suppress T-cell-mediated immunity.

The binding of antibody to antigenic sites on the tumor cell membrane can lead to tumor cell destruction through either humoral or cellular mechanisms. In complement-dependent cytotoxicity, tumor cell lysis depends on activation of the complement cascade by the antibody. In antibody-dependent cell-mediated cytotoxicity (ADCC), the IgG antibodies bind to the specific tumor-associated antigens. The IgG antibody then serves as a bridge between the tumor cell and the various effector cells that bear an Fc fragment receptor. Effector cells for ADCC include lymphocytes, activated macrophages, and polymorphonuclear cells.

Despite the wide variety of potential antitumor immunologic mechanisms just outlined, many tumor cells evidently survive and continue to proliferate. A tumor may evade recognition and destruction by the immune system through several mechanisms. The tumor cell surface may not have a unique antigen because the entire tumor or a subpopulation of cells may fail to express the tumor antigen. It has also been shown that tumor-associated antigens may be modulated. After contact with a specific antibody directed against the cell surface antigen, the antigen disappears from the cell surface and is not expressed again until the excess antigen in the environment disappears. Some tumor antigens are only recognized if histocompatibility antigens are also present on the same cell surface, and thus tumor cells that fail to express the normal histocompatibility antigens will then fail to elicit an immune response. Even when potentially immunogenic, tumor-associated antigens are present on the cell, a deficiency in antigen-presenting cell mechanisms may lead to a lack of immune response. With large tumor volumes, sufficient excess tumor-associated antigen may be shed into the circulation to inhibit the immune response. Circulating tumor antigen may also complex with antibodies to form antigen-antibody complexes (circulating immune complexes) that are capable of inhibiting the function of the various effector cells required for ADCC.

A variety of specific and nonspecific suppressor mechanisms may inhibit the immune response to a tumor. Antigen presentation by the intravenous route, which may bypass certain antigen-presenting cells, leads preferentially to the development of specific suppressor cells. Nonspecific suppression of the immune response may occur because of inhibitory factors produced by a tumor, malnutrition, or treatment, particularly chemotherapy and radiation. After surgery and anesthesia, depression of both T-cell and B-cell function occurs for up to several weeks, depending on the amount of operative trauma and the length of the procedure.

Biologic Response Modification

Attempts at therapy through the manipulation of the overall biologic response of the host to a tumor have been termed biologic response modification. Although many biologic response modifiers affect the immune system, this effect is not directed against a specific antigenic determinant. To date, immunotherapy and biologic response modification have had only very limited clinical efficacy and remain investigational therapies. Attempts have been made to augment the immune response with nonspecific stimulants such as BCG, *Corynebacterium parvum,* interferon, lymphokines, and chemicals such as levamisol. The interaction of activator and suppressor mechanisms in the immune system is so complex that identifying appropriate timing and doses of the nonspecific agents in the clinical situation generally has proved impossible. It is anticipated that more specific immune modulation with cell populations such as lymphokine-activated killer cells and tumor infiltrating lymphocytes (TIL cells) with specific lymphokines,[139] and with monoclonal antibodies directed at highly specific antigens on particular tumors will prove more efficacious. Administration of interferons has had some limited success, and further therapeutic trials are under way.[17]

Hematopoietic Growth Factors

Hematopoiesis is controlled by a series of glycoprotein growth factors that act on stem cells and precursor cells. With the advent of recombinant DNA technology, these factors are now becoming available in large quantities for clinical use and especially in cancer therapy. The biology of these factors was initially worked out in tissue culture; thus many of the names relate to their in vitro function. Granulocyte colony stimulating factor (G-CSF) stimulates the production of neutrophilic granulocytes. Granulocyte-macrophage colony stimulating factor (GM-CSF) stimulates the proliferation of a more immature precursor cell that gives rise to macrophages, neutrophils, and eosinophils. Macrophage colony stimulating factor (M-CSF) stimulates the growth of macrophage and monocyte precursor cells. Erythropoietin stimulates the red cell precursors. In addition to increasing the growth rates of progenitor cells, many of the colony stimulating factors can "prime" the target cells to enhance their physiologic function related to bacteria, parasites, and tumor cells. Many other factors, including interleukins 1, 4, 5, 6, and 7, stimulate the production of the colony stimulating factors and/or modify the growth and function of hematopoietic cells.

The hematopoietic growth factors are being used in cancer therapy to minimize (shorten the duration of) chemotherapy-induced neutropenia and thrombocytopenia, to treat anemias and granulcytopenias, and to increase the number of precursor cells in peripheral blood.

Gene Therapy

Gene therapy is a technique in which a functioning gene is inserted into the cells of a patient to provide a new function to the cells or to correct an inborn genetic error. The principal technology is to transfer genes into cells using a replication-incompetent retrovirus. The replication-incompetent retroviruses can infect cells and carry with them the potentially therapeutic genes, but are not capable of forming new virus. The cells to be transduced are removed from the body and manipulated in tissue culture. Lymphocytes, particularly the subpopulation of tumor infiltrating lymphocytes (TILs), are particularly good candidates for the development of anticancer therapy. Scientists are attempting to insert genes that enhance the immune recognition of tumor cells by the lymphocytes or that increase the ability of the lymphocytes to produce antitumor lymphokines, such as tumor necrosis factor. Another approach is to resect a portion of the tumor and then introduce genes that increase the immunogenicity of the tumor, in hopes that the enhanced immune response will attack both the gene-modified tumor cells and unmodified tumor cells.[7,139]

Monoclonal Antibodies

Development of the technology to hybridize a myeloma cell with a lymphocyte creating a specific antibody, thus producing an immortalized cell line that elaborates a specific monoclonal antibody, has provided a powerful technology for diagnosis that also has a great potential for therapy.[110,142] The presence of tumor-associated antigens on the surface of cancer cells presents potential targets for monoclonal antibodies. Studies in animal models, particularly heterografts in the nude mouse, have demonstrated that monoclonal antibodies administered systemically can localize at the tumor site. Moreover, monoclonal antibodies conjugated with radioisotopes, toxins, and drugs also localize at the tumor site with the appropriate antigen of their surface.

Preliminary clinical trials of monoclonal antibodies have suggested their potential efficacy in diagnosis. For example, bone marrow aspirates of some newly diagnosed breast and bowel cancer patients have been found to have cells that are positive for a cancer-associated antigen to which a monoclonal antibody has been made. The incidence of putative metastatic cancer cells identified by the monoclonal antibodies correlates with the clinical stage of the cancer, but further follow-up is necessary to confirm the prognostic significance of these observations relative to the biology of breast or bowel cancer. In vivo studies in human beings are currently being carried out to study the value of radioconjugated monoclonal antibiotics for tumor imaging.

Therapeutic trials with monoclonal antibodies directed against leukemic cells and lymphomas have had some limited therapeutic effects.[110] One of the problems with monoclonal antibody treatment is that tumor cells are capable of modulating their cell surface antigens so that the antigens disappear within minutes to hours of exposure to the antibody. Tumor cells are also heterogeneous in the expression of tumor-associated antigens on their cell surface, and tumor cell clones lacking the antigen may rapidly appear after treatment with monospecific antisera. Despite problems in the therapeutic use of monoclonal antibodies, many predict that conjugates of antibodies, particularly with radioisotopes, will be important tools to help detect and treat cancer.[95]

HYPERTHERMIA

Hyperthermia as cancer therapy is undergoing clinical investigation because of the observation that tumor tissue is more sensitive to hyperthermia than normal tissue.[60] Several common factors in malignancies that seem to render them more sensitive to heat include elevated rates of glycolysis and lactic acid production and decreased adenosine triphosphate (ATP) substrate. These factors appear to be related to decreased blood supply and loss of normal growth controls. Because not all tumor cells reside in poorly perfused, acidic, or nutrient-deprived microenvironments, cells at the tumor margin will probably have thermal sensitivities similar to their corresponding normal tissue cells. Thus the most effective use of hyperthermia probably will be in conjunction with either radiotherapy or chemotherapy. Evidence does suggest a synergism between hyperthermia and both radiotherapy and chemotherapy, although the synergism apparently is no greater for tumor tissue than for normal tissue. Partly because of the lack of differential synergism, most protocols separate the application of hyperthermia and other modalities by at least a few hours or longer. Three lines of research in hyperthermia are being pursued:

1. The possibility of enhancing the thermal sensitivity of tumors compared to normal tissue by increasing the differences in pH and energy supply
2. The possibility of fractionating hyperthermia treatments to take advantage of differences in the heat decay in tumors relative to normal tissue
3. The development of noninvasive tools to measure blood flow, heat decay, pH, and energy levels

MULTIMODALITY THERAPY

The previous discussions have outlined the biologic behavior of malignancies and the basic principles of treatment with the various modalities. The history of cancer therapy has provided repeated demonstrations that many patients with apparently localized disease relapse eventually at distant sites even though the locoregional therapy is effective. There are also numerous examples of systemic therapies for disseminated malignancies capable of causing complete regression of all clinical evidence of disease for a period, only to have the disease recur at the site of the bulkiest original disease or in sanctuaries not reached by the systemic therapy.

The biologic basis for therapeutic failures after initially effective systemic treatment of disseminated malignancies varies.[152] Some systemic therapies may fail because the drug does not penetrate into pharmacologic sanctuaries. For example, in the treatment of acute lymphatic leukemia of childhood with chemotherapy, the central nervous system pharmacologic sanctuary has been treated with radiotherapy or with intrathecal drug injection. The recurrence after systemic therapy frequently is caused by drug resistance. As the cells in a tumor mass increase, the likelihood of resistant cell lines increases; by the time a tumor contains 10^9 cells, resis-

TABLE 12-15 CANCERS FOR WHICH ADJUVANT CHEMOTHERAPY POTENTIALLY FACILITATES CURABILITY AFTER LOCOREGIONAL TREATMENT WITH SURGERY AND/OR RADIOTHERAPY[55]

TYPE OF CANCER	LOCOREGIONAL MODALITIES (CURE WITH SURG + OR − RADIO ONLY)*	MULTIMODAL THERAPY, PERCENTAGE CURABILITY† (OR 5-YEAR SURVIVAL FOR BREAST CANCER AND 3.5 YEAR SURVIVAL FOR COLON CANCER)	
		ESTABLISHED	PUTATIVE
Wilms' tumor	Surg + or − radio (30)	80	90
Osteosarcoma[140]	Surg + or − radio (20)	50	80
Rhabdomyosarcoma	Surg + or − radio (30)	50	80
Ewing's tumor	Surg + or − radio (10)	50	80
Neuroblastoma[139]	Surg + or − radio (30)	30	60
Testicular, nonseminomatous	Surg + or − radio (60)	70	90
Lung, small cell[100]			
Limited	Surg and/or radio (5)	10	20
Advanced	Radio (0)	0	5
Breast, stage II‡			
Premenopausal	Surg + or − radio (70)	(80)	(85)
Postmenopausal	Surg + or − radio (60)	(70)	(75)
Ovarian, stages III and IV[121]	Surg + or − radio (10)	10	20
Gastric, stage I[41]	Surg + or − radio (30)	30	45
Colon, stage III §[113]	Surgery	(70)	—

Modified from Frei E III: *Cancer Res* 45:6523, 1985.
**Surg + or − radio*, surgery with or without radiotherapy.
†Curability is defined as the portion of patients who reach a disease-free survival plateau, usually within 5 years. For primary breast cancer, a significant risk continues after 5 years, and although decreasing with time, continues beyond 15 years.
‡Primary operable breast cancer with histologic evidence of axillary node metastases.
§Colon carcinoma with regional node metastases (Dukes' C).

tant cells probably are already present, even before the first administration of chemotherapy. Because the primary tumor contains the cells present for the longest period, it is more likely to contain cells that have spontaneously developed drug resistance.[38,67] The successful locoregional control of the bulky primary tumor mass may have an important influence on the efficacy of systemic therapy by removing cells that (1) have developed genetic resistance; or (2) are resistant because of decreased growth fraction in large tumors relative to micrometastases.

The biologic basis of the eventual appearance of systemic metastases despite effective surgical or radiotherapeutic control is presumably caused by micrometastases that were undetectable at the initial therapy. The addition of "adjuvant" systemic therapy at the initial ablation of the locoregional tumor has so far proved to benefit survival in the treatment of breast carcinoma, colon carcinoma, Wilms' tumor, testicular cancer, soft tissue sarcomas of childhood, and osteosarcoma. Systemic adjuvant therapy attempts for head and neck, uterine, gastric, and kidney cancers as well as melanoma have not yet proved effective.

On the basis of experimental animal studies, Schabel[150] has summarized the use of adjuvant systemic therapy after surgical resection in murine tumor systems. Many of these principles are being tested in human beings. Schabel observed that (1) surgical cure rates decreased as the size of the primary tumor mass at surgery increased; (2) grossly evident "primary" tumors were not curable by drug treatment alone; (3) surgical adjuvant chemotherapy with appropriate agents could increase the cure rate after surgical resection; and (4) the effectiveness of chemotherapy was directly related to drug dose and inversely related to the body burden of metastatic tumor at the time of treatment. The most effective drugs in the adjuvant setting were those with proven efficacy in the treatment of advanced disease. Lack of response of advanced disease to a drug, however, did not preclude the possibility of response to that drug in the adjuvant setting. Examples for which systemic adjuvant chemotherapy is potentially additive to locoregional therapy to improve the curability of human cancers are shown in Table 12-15.

The availability of effective systemic therapy has affected the necessary extent of local therapy for some tumors. For example, the high cure rate of gestational choriocarcinoma by chemotherapy has eliminated the need for hysterectomy, which was formerly the only available, albeit frequently ineffective, therapy. In testicular cancer, combination chemotherapy has been sufficiently efficacious to reduce the need for radical surgery or radiotherapy to the retroperitoneal lymph nodes for nonseminomatous tumors.[41] Systemic adjuvant therapy of breast cancer has reduced both the incidence of systemic and locoregional recurrence. In patients treated by partial mastectomy and radiotherapy to the residual breast tissue, systemic chemotherapy has decreased further occurrence of cancer in the ipsilateral breast.

Combined modality therapy has its risks. If no increased therapeutic efficacy occurs, the patient is unnecessarily subjected to the additional toxicities of new therapies. When radiotherapy is combined with chemotherapy in the treatment of Hodgkin's disease, for example, the risk of secondary malignancies, particularly acute myelogenous leukemia, is greatly increased over that of either modality alone. Current approaches reserve combined chemotherapy and radiotherapy treatments to selected patients with Hodgkin's disease. Most of these patients are treated selectively with one or the other modality. Surgical staging of Hodgkin's disease patients is frequently used in the selection of the appropriate treatment modality.[32,141]

One of the oldest and best studied uses of combined modality treatment has been in children with Wilms' tumors. In the first quarter of this century, the 2-year survival rate after surgical treatment was less than 10%. With improvements in surgical and anesthetic technique, the 2-year survival rate had increased to 30% by 1932. The addition of radiotherapy appeared to increase 2-year survival to 40% by the 1940s. The addition of adjuvant chemotherapy in the 1950s and 1960s approximately doubled the rate to about 80%.[34] A series of randomized clinical trials by the U.S. Wilms' Tumor Study Group has led to further refinement in therapy, with current 2-year survival rates of approximately 90%.[20] As a result of the cooperative group studies, the extent of therapy and the number of modalities used are now tailored to the stage of disease at presentation. Many patients can now be treated with surgery and chemotherapy, omitting the radiotherapy, which has long-term effects on skeletal growth and development.

The challenge in the modern therapy of cancer is to integrate and tailor the different treatments so that each patient receives optimal benefit. Further refinement of cancer therapy will require careful clinical trials with extensive interdisciplinary cooperation.

CANCER RESEARCH AND CLINICAL TRIALS

Most clinicians are aware of the carefully controlled scientific methodology that lies behind the laboratory research that is rapidly increasing our knowledge of cancer biology. Many clinicians are unfortunately less familiar with the application of scientific methodology to clinical problem solving. In an era of rapidly proliferating medical technology, many may not recognize that one of the greatest medical advances during this century has been the introduction of the controlled clinical trial into clinical medicine. Medical school teaching at the clinical level has tended to emphasize the student's role as an individual problem solver. Patterns of care and patient management tend to be learned from preceptors or authorities and are modified by the physician's most recent experiences. As a result, alternative therapies are often the subject of debate and anecdotal reports rather than controlled scientific investigation. The historic approach to medical education and communication has tended to promote the waxing and waning of fashionable medical therapies without a specific relationship to scientific data. Controlled clinical trials have gained increasing acceptance in the development of cancer therapies and have been particularly important in the recent rapid advances in cancer treatment.

When no proven effective treatment exists and the relative merits of competing therapies are uncertain, the most appropriate approach for both patient and physician may be participation in a clinical trial. Some clinicians are concerned that if they admit to patients that the optimal therapy for their condition is uncertain and can only be determined through a clinical study, their authoritarian position will be undermined and cause patients to lose confidence in them. Some clinicians recognize correctly that participation in a clinical trial leads to scrutiny of their clinical care and requires increased effort in patient explanation and data recording. With proper explanation, most patients, even when faced with serious illness, are willing to participate in clinical trials; they recognize that even if they do not benefit, the knowledge gained will be beneficial to others.

In addition to the specific answers derived from the results of the clinical trial, frequently both patient and physician receive other benefits. The clinical trial should be the result of a carefully designed protocol that represents the considered opinion of a group of "experts" in the area. Through participation in the trial, the patient is in effect receiving the benefit of multiple "second opinions." Physicians, through their participation, receive the stimulation of interaction with others at the forefront of therapeutic advances and often find that their medical education is advanced in other areas, both directly and indirectly related to the clinical trial.

Clinical trials in cancer therapy have been divided into three types, or phases:

1. Phase I studies are conducted on small groups of patients to determine the toxicity of a therapy and the maximally tolerated dose level. Any therapeutic effects are of interest but are the secondary end point of a phase I trial.
2. Phase II studies are carried out to determine the tumor types for which the new therapy appears to be promising.
3. Phase III studies compare the new therapy to an alternative therapy or to the natural history of the disease in an untreated or placebo-treated popu-

lation. The phase III trial is particularly important in determining whether any toxic effects are tolerable in the context of the observed therapeutic effect and the toxicity and efficacy of any alternative therapies.

Phase I and II studies are usually carried out on patients for whom no effective standard therapy is available. It is important to distinguish "standard therapy" from effective standard therapy. Because of side effects, some "standard therapies" have such limited chance of being beneficial that trying them before offering a patient participation in a phase I or II clinical trial is usually pointless.

Other texts should be sought for details of the design, conduct, and appropriate interpretation of controlled clinical trials.[134,158] Intuition, hunches, deductive reasoning, compassion, and communication skills all play a role in the art of clinical practice; but the evaluation of the efficacy of most therapies requires an experimental evaluation. An experimental evaluation requires that a planned intervention be administered to a defined patient population under controlled conditions so that well-defined medical questions may be answered.

Physicians have a responsibility not only to provide care to their patients but also to recognize when further debate is fruitless and when further knowledge is needed. Sir Austin Bradford Hill[77] has emphasized that, when possible, clinical care should be based on strong scientific evidence, but that this does not imply crossing every 't', and swords with every critic, before we act. All scientific work is incomplete, whether it be observational or experimental. All scientific work is liable to be upset or modified by advancing knowledge. That does not confer upon us a freedom to ignore the knowledge we already have, or to postpone the action that it appears to demand at a given time.

REFERENCES

1 Aaronson SA: Growth factors and cancer, *Science* 254:1146, 1991.

2 Albert ME, Uriel J, de Nechaud B: Alpha-fetoglobulins in the diagnosis of human hepatoma, *N Engl J Med* 278:984, 1968.

3 Alwine JC, Kemp DJ, Stark GR: Method for detection of methyl-specific RNAs in agarose gels by transfer to diazobenzyloxymethyl-paper and hybridization with DNA probes, *Proc Natl Acad Sci USA* 74:5350, 1977.

4 *American Cancer Society: cancer facts and figures,* 1992, New York, American Cancer Society.

5 American Cancer Society: Cancer statistics, 1992, *CA* 42:1, 1992.

6 American Joint Committee on Cancer Staging: *Manual for staging of cancer,* ed 3, Philadelphia, 1988, JB Lippincott.

7 Anderson WF: Human gene therapy, *Science* 256:808, 1992.

8 Archer VE, Gillam JD, Wagoner JD: Respiratory disease mortality among uranium miners, *Ann NY Acad Sci* 271:280, 1976.

9 Baltimore D: Viral RNA dependent DNA polymerase, *Nature* 226:1209, 1970.

10 Barker BE, Sanford KK: Cytologic manifestations of neoplastic transformation *in vitro, J Natl Cancer Inst* 44:39, 1970.

11 Berridge MJ: The molecular basis of communication within the cell, *Sci Am* 253:142, 1985.

12 Bilezekian JP: Management of acute hypercalcemia, *N Engl J Med* 326:1196, 1992.

13 Bishop JM: Molecular themes in oncogenesis, *Cell* 64:235, 1991.

14 Bjelke E: Dietary vitamin A and human lung cancer, *Int J Cancer* 15:561, 1975.

15 Blackman MR, Rosen SW, Weintraub BD: Ectopic hormones, *Adv Intern Med* 23:85, 1978.

16 Boice JD Jr, Day NE, Anderson A et al: Cancer risk following radiotherapy of cervical cancer: a preliminary report. In Boice JD Jr, Fraumeni JF Jr, editors: *Radiation carcinogenesis: epidemiology and biological significance,* New York, 1984, Raven Press.

17 Borden EC: Interferons—expanding therapeutic roles, *N Engl J Med* 326:1491, 1992.

18 Braverman IM: *Skin signs of systemic disease,* ed 2, Philadelphia, 1981, WB Saunders.

19 Brennan MF: Uncomplicated starvation versus cancer cachexia, *Cancer Res* 37:2359, 1977.

20 Breslow N, Churchill G, Beckwith JB et al: Prognosis for Wilms' tumor patients with nonmetastatic disease at diagnosis—results of the second national Wilms' tumor study, *J Clin Oncol* 3:521, 1985.

21 Brooke BN: Ulcerative colitis and carcinoma of the colon, *J R Coll Surg Edinb* 14:274, 1969.

22 Bruce WR, Meeker BE, Valeriote FA: Comparison of the sensitivity of normal hematopoietic and transplanted lymphoma colony-forming cells to chemotherapeutic agents administered in vivo, *Natl Cancer Inst* 37:233, 1966.

23 Bunn PA: Paraneoplastic syndromes. In Devita VT Jr, Hellman S, Rosenberg SA, editors: *Cancer: principles and practice of oncology,* ed 3, Philadelphia, 1989, JB Lippincott.

24 Cady B, McDermott WV: Major hepatic resection for metachronous metastases from colon cancer, *Ann Surg* 201:204, 1985.

25 Cady B, Monson DO, Swinton NW: Survival of patients after colonic resection for carcinoma with simultaneous liver metastases, *Surg Gynecol Obstet* 131:697, 1970.

26 Cahan WG: Excision of melanoma metastases to lung: problems in diagnosis and management, *Ann Surg* 178:703, 1973.

27 Cannon WB, Nelsen TS: Staging of Hodgkin's disease: a surgical perspective, *Am J Surg* 132:224, 1976.

28 Chabner BA, Myers CE: Clinical pharmacology of cancer chemotherapy. In Devita VT Jr, Hellman S, Rosenberg SA, editors: *Cancer: principles and practice of oncology,* ed 3, Philadelphia, 1989, JB Lippincott.

29 Creagen ET, Fleming TR, Edmonson JH et al: Pulmonary resection for metastatic nonosteogenic sarcoma, *Cancer* 44:1908, 1979.

30 Crile G Jr, Vickery AL: Special uses of the Silverman biopsy needle in office practice and at operation, *Am J Surg* 83:83, 1952.

31 Cross M, Dexter TM: Growth factors in development, transformation, and tumorigenesis, *Cell* 64:271, 1991.

32 Crowther D, Wagstaff J, Deakin D et al: A randomized study comparing chemotherapy alone with chemotherapy followed by radiotherapy in patients with pathologically staged IIIA Hodgkin's disease, *J Clin Oncol* 2(8):892, 1984.

33 Curt GA, Clendeninn NJ, Chabner BA: Drug resistance in cancer, *Cancer Treat Rep* 68(1):87, 1984.

34 D'Angio GJ, Evans A, Breslow N et al: Biology and management of Wilms' tumor. In Levine AS, editor: *Cancer in the young,* New York, 1981, Masson Publishing USA, Inc.

35 DeVita VT Jr: Principles of chemotherapy. In DeVita VT Jr, Hellman S, Rosenberg SA, editors: *Cancer principles and practice*

of oncology, ed 3, Philadelphia, 1989, JB Lippincott.
36 DeVita VT Jr: U.S. House Appropriations Hearings on DHHS, NIH, NCI: Statement by Vincent T. DeVita, Jr., Director, National Cancer Institute, March 7, 1984. Year 2000 goals, House Committee Report #98-911, fiscal year 1985.
37 DeVita VT Jr: Testimony before United States House of Representatives Committee on Appropriations, March 1984.
38 DeVita VT Jr: The relationship between tumor mass and resistance to chemotherapy: implications for surgical adjuvant treatment of cancer, *Cancer* 51:1209, 1983.
39 Doll R, Peto R: The causes of cancer: quantitative estimates of avoidable risks of cancer in the United States today, *J Natl Cancer Inst* 66:119, 1981.
40 Douglass HO, The Gastrointestinal Tumor Study Group: Controlled trial of adjuvant chemotherapy following curative resection for gastric cancer, *Cancer* 49:1116, 1982.
41 Einhorn LH, Crawford ED, Shipley WV et al: Cancer of the testis. In DeVita VT Jr, Hellman S, Rosenberg SA, editors: *Cancer: principles and practice of oncology,* ed 3, Philadelphia, 1989, JB Lippincott.
42 Epstein E, Bragg K, Linden G: Biopsy and prognosis of malignant melanoma, *JAMA* 208:1369, 1969.
43 Ewing HP, Newsom BD, Hardy JD: Tumor markers, *Curr Probl Surg* 19(2):53, 1982.
44 Farber E: Cellular biochemistry of the stepwise development of cancer with chemicals: G.H.A. Clowes Memorial Lecture, *Cancer Res* 44:5463, 1984.
45 Felsenfeld G: DNA, *Sci Am* 253:58, 1985.
46 Fialkow PJ: The origin and development of human tumors studied with cell markers, *N Engl J Med* 291:26, 1974.
47 Fidler JJ: Tumor heterogeneity and the biology of cancer invasion and metastasis, *Cancer Res* 38:2651, 1978.
48 Fidler JJ, Poste G: The biologic diversity of cancer metastases, *Hosp Pract* 17(7):52, 1982.
49 Fisher ER, Fisher B: Recent observations on concept of metastasis, *Arch Pathol* 83:321, 1967.
50 Folkman J: The vascularization of tumors, *Sci Am* 234:59, 1976.
51 Folkman J: Tumor angiogenesis. In Klein G, Weinhouse S, editors: *Advances in cancer research,* Orlando, Fla, 1985, Academic Press, Inc.
52 Foster JH: Survival after liver resection for secondary tumors, *Am J Surg* 135:389, 1978.
53 Foster JH, Lundy J: Liver metastases, *Curr Probl Surg* 18(3):161, 1981.
54 Frei E, III: Curative cancer chemotherapy, *Cancer Res* 45:6523, 1985.
55 Freireich EJ, Gehan EA, Rall DP et al: Quantitative comparison of toxicity of anticancer agents in mouse, rat, hamster, dog, monkey, and man, *Cancer Chemother Rep* 50:219, 1966.
56 Galicich JH, Sundaresan N, Thaler HT: Surgical treatment of single brain metastases: evaluation of results by computerized tomography scanning, *J Neurosurg* 53:63, 1980.
57 Gallo RC, Wong-Staal F: Current thoughts on the viral etiology of certain human cancers: the Richard and Hinda Rosenthal Foundation Award Lecture, *Cancer Res* 44:2743, 1984.
58 Geller J, Vazakas G, Fruchtman B et al: The effect of cyproterone acetate on advanced carcinoma of the prostate, *Surg Gynecol Obstet* 127:748, 1968.
59 German J: Genes which increase chromosomal instability in somatic cells and predispose to cancer, *Prog Med Genet* 8:61, 1972.
60 Gerweck LE: Hyperthermia in cancer therapy: the biological basis and unresolved questions, *Cancer Res* 45:3408, 1985.
61 Glaser GH, Pincus JH: Neurologic complications of internal disease. In Baker AB, Baker LH, editors: *Clinical neurology,* vol 4, Philadelphia, 1984, Harper & Row.
62 Glatstein E, Guernsey JM, Rosenberg SA et al: The value of laparotomy and splenectomy in the staging of Hodgkin's disease, *Cancer* 24:709, 1969.
63 Go VLW, Zamcheck N: The role of tumor markers in the management of colorectal cancer, *Cancer* 50:2618, 1982.
64 Gold P, Freedman SO: Specific carcinoembryonic antigens of the human digestive system, *J Exp Med* 122:467, 1965.
65 Goldenberg DM, Neville AM, Carter AC et al: Carcinoembryonic antigen: its role as a marker in the management of cancer—National Institute of Health Consensus Development Conference Statement, *Cancer Res* 41:2017, 1981.
66 Goldie JH, Coldman AJ: A mathematical model for relating the drug sensitivity of tumors to their spontaneous mutation rate, *Cancer Treat Rep* 63:1727, 1979.
67 Goldie JH, Coldman AJ: The genetic origin of drug resistance in neoplasms: implications for systemic therapy, *Cancer Res* 44:3643, 1984.
68 Haskell CM, editor: *Cancer treatment,* ed 3, Philadelphia, 1990, WB Saunders.
69 Haynes HA, McLean DI: Cutaneous aspects of internal malignant disease. In Fitzpatrick TB, Eisen AZ, Wolff K et al, editors: *Dermatology in general medicine,* ed 3, New York, 1983, McGraw-Hill.
70 Hellman S: Principles of radiation therapy. In DeVita VT Jr, Hellman S, Rosenberg SA, editors: *Cancer: principles and practice of oncology,* ed 3, Philadelphia, 1989, JB Lippincott.
71 Hellstrom HK, Hellstrom I: Possibilities for active immunotherapy of human cancer, *Cancer Invest* 10:285, 1992.
72 Henderson BE, Ross RK, Pike MC: Toward the primary prevention of cancer, *Science* 254:1131, 1991.
73 Hensen RA, Urich H: *Cancer and the nervous system,* Oxford, 1982, Blackwell Scientific Publications.
74 Heppner GH: Tumor heterogeneity, *Cancer Res* 44:2259, 1984.
75 Herberman RB, editor: *Basic and clinical tumor immunology,* Boston, 1983, Martinus Nijhoff.
76 Herity B, Moriarty M, Bourke GJ, Daly L: A case-control study of head and neck cancer in the Republic of Ireland, *Br J Cancer* 43:177, 1981.
77 Hill AB: The environment and disease: association or causation? *Proc R Soc Med* 58:295, 1965.
78 Holland JCB, Rowland J, Plum M: Psychological aspects of anorexia in cancer patients, *Cancer Res* 37:2425, 1977.
79 Horwitz KB, McGuire WL: Antiestrogens: mechanism of action and effects in breast cancer. In McGuire WL, editor: *Breast cancer, advances in research and treatment,* vol II, New York, 1978, Plenum Press.
80 Howe GR: Epidemiology of radiogenic breast cancer. In Boice JD Jr, Fraumeni JF Jr, editors: *Radiation carcinogenesis: epidemiology and biological significance,* New York, 1984, Raven Press.
81 Hughes RG, Hall TJ, Block GE et al: The prognosis of carcinoma of the colon and rectum complicating ulcerative colitis, *Surg Gynecol Obstet* 146:46, 1978.
82 Hurwitz M, Sawicki M, Samara G, Passaro P Jr: Diagnostic and prognostic molecular markers in cancer, *Am J Surg* 164:299, 1992.
83 International Union Against Cancer (UICC): TNM classification of malignant tumors, Geneva, 1978, Committee of Clinical Oncology, UICC.
84 Jablon S: Epidemiologic perspectives in radiation carcinogenesis. In Boice JD Jr, Fraumeni JF Jr, editors: *Radiation carcinogenesis: epidemology and biological significance,* New York, 1984, Raven Press.
85 Jackson R, Coffin LH, DeMeules JE et al: Percutaneous needle biopsy of pulmonary lesions, *Am J Surg* 139:586, 1980.
86 Johnson RD, Gobien RP, Valicenti JF Jr: Current status of radio-

logically directed pulmonary thin needle aspiration biopsy: an analysis of 200 consecutive biopsies and review of the literature, *Ann Clin Lab Sci* 13:225, 1983.
87 Kline TS: *Handbook of fine needle aspiration biopsy cytology,* St Louis, 1981, Mosby.
88 Knudson AG Jr: Genetic predisposition to cancer. In Hiatt HH, Watson JD, Winsten JA, editors: *Origins of human cancer, Book A,* Cold Spring Harbor, NY, 1977, Cold Spring Harbor Laboratory.
89 Knudson AG Jr: Hereditary cancer, oncogenes, and antioncogenes, *Cancer Res* 45:1437, 1985.
90 Knutson CO, Hori JM, Spratt JS Jr: Melanoma, *Curr Probl Surg* 8(12):1, 1971.
91 Kramer S, Hanks GE, Diamond JJ et al: The study of the patterns of clinical care in radiation therapy in the United States, *CA* 34(2):75, 1984.
92 Krioke ML: Immunologic mechanisms in UV radiation carcinogenesis. In Weinhouse S, Klein G, editors: *Advances in cancer research,* vol 34, New York, 1981, Academic Press.
93 Land H, Parada LF, Weinberg RA: Cellular oncogenes and multistep carcinogenesis, *Science* 222:771, 1983.
94 Lee KR, Foster RS Jr, Papillo JL: Fine needle aspiration of the breast: its usefulness is dependent upon the proficiency of the aspirator, *Acta Cytolog* 31:281, 1987.
95 Levy R: Biologicals for cancer treatment: monoclonal antibodies, *Hosp Pract* November 1985, p 67.
96 Liotta L: Cancer cell invasion and metastatis, *Sci Am* February 1992, 266:54.
97 Liotta LA, Hart IR: Tumor invasion and metastases—role of the extracellular matrix: Rhoads Memorial Award Lecture, *Cancer Res* 46:1, 1986.
98 Livingston RB: Small cell carcinoma of the lung, *Blood* 56:575, 1980.
99 Lloyd HH: Estimation of tumor cell kill from Gompertz growth curves, *Cancer Chemother Rep* 59:267, 1975.
100 Loeb LA, Ernster VL, Warner KE et al: Smoking and lung cancer: an overview, *Cancer Res* 44:5940, 1984.
101 Lynch HT, Fusaro RM, editors: *Cancer associated genodermatoses,* New York, 1982, Van Nostrand Reinhold.
102 MacDougall IPM: The cancer risk in ulcerative colitis, *Lancet* 2:655, 1964.
103 Maniatis T, Fritsch EF, Sambrook J: *Molecular cloning: a laboratory manual,* Cold Spring Harbor, NY, 1989, Cold Spring Harbor Laboratory.
104 Marshall CJ: Tumor supressor genes, *Cell* 64:313, 1991.
105 McCormack PM, Bains MS, Beattie EJ et al: Pulmonary resection in metastatic carcinoma, *Chest* 73:163, 1978.
106 McGuire WL: Physiologic principles underlying endocrine therapy of breast cancer. In McGuire WL, editor: *Breast cancer, advances in research and treatment,* vol I, New York, 1977, Plenum Press.
107 Miller EC: Studies on the formation of protein-bound derivatives of 3, 4-benzpyrene in the epidermal fraction of mouse skin, *Cancer Res* 11:100, 1951.
108 Miller EC: Some current perspectives on chemical carcinogenesis in humans and experimental animals: presidential address, *Cancer Res* 38:1479, 1978.
109 Miller JA: Carcinogenesis by chemicals: an overview—G.H.A. Clowes Memorial Lecture, *Cancer Res* 30:559, 1970.
110 Miller RA, Maloney DG, Warnke R et al: Treatment of B cell lymphoma with monoclonal anti-idiotype antibody, *N Engl J Med* 306:517, 1982.
111 Moertel CG, Fleming TR, MacDonald JS et al: Levamisole and fluorouracil for adjuvant therapy of resected colon carcinoma, *N Engl J Med* 322:352, 1990.
112 Morrison SD: Partition of energy expenditure between host and tumor, *Cancer Res* 31:98, 1971.
113 Morrison SD: Origins of anorexia in neoplastic disease, *Am J Clin Nutr* 31:1104, 1978.
114 Morrow CE, Vassilopoulos PP, Grage TB: Surgical resection for metastatic neoplasms of the lung, *Cancer* 45:2981, 1980.
115 Mountain CF, Khalil KG, Hermes KE et al: The contribution of surgery to the management of carcinomatous pulmonary metastases, *Cancer* 41:833, 1978.
116 Mulvihill JJ: Cancer control through genetics. In Arrighi FE, Rao PN, Stubblefield E, editors: *Genes, chromosomes, and neoplasia,* New York, 1981, Raven Press.
117 Mundy GR, Ibbotson KJ, D'Souza SM et al: The hypercalcemia of cancer: clinical implications and pathologic mechanisms, *N Engl J Med* 310:1718, 1984.
118 Mundy GR, Martin TJ: The hypercalcemia of malignancy: pathogenesis and management, *Metabolism* 31(12):1247, 1982.
119 Neijt JP, Van Der Burg MEL, Vreisendorp R.: Randomised trial comparing two combination chemotherapy regimens (HEXA-CAF vs CHAP-5) in advanced ovarian carcinoma, *Lancet* 9:594, 1984.
120 Nicolson GL: Trans-membrane control of the receptors on normal and tumor cells. II. Surface changes associated with transformation and malignancy, *Biochim Biophys Acta* 458:1, 1976.
121 Nixon DW, Lawson DH, Kutner M et al: Hyperalimentation of the cancer patient with protein-calorie undernutrition, *Cancer Res* 41:2038, 1981.
122 Nordenstrom B: New instruments for biopsy, *Radiology* 117:474, 1975.
123 Nowell PC: The clonal evolution of tumor cell populations, *Science* 194:23, 1976.
124 Old LJ: Cancer immunology: the search for specificity—G.H.A. Clowes Memorial Lecture, *Cancer Res* 41:361, 1981.
125 Parmar H, Phillips RH, Lightman SL et al: Randomized controlled study of orchidectomy vs. long-acting D-TRP-6-LHRH microcapsules in advanced prostatic carcinoma, *Lancet* 1:1201, 1985.
126 Peto R, Doll R, Buckley JD et al: Can dietary beta-carotene materially reduce human cancer rates? *Nature* 290:201, 1981.
127 Pierce GB, Shikes R, Fink LM: *Cancer, a problem of developmental biology,* Englewood Cliffs, NJ, 1978, Prentice-Hall.
128 Potts P: *Chirurgical observations relative to the cataract, the polypus of the nose, the cancer of the scrotum, the different kinds of ruptures and the mortification of the toes and feet,* London, 1775, Hawkes, Clarke & Collins.
129 Prosnitz LR, Kapp DS, Weissberg JB: Radiotherapy (first of two parts), *N Engl J Med* 309:771, 1983.
130 Prosnitz LR, Kapp DS, Weissberg JB: Radiotherapy (second of two parts), *N Engl J Med* 309:834, 1983.
131 Putnam JB, Roth JA, Wesley MN et al: Survival following aggressive resection of pulmonary metastases from osteogenic sarcoma: analysis of prognostic factors, *Ann Thorac Surg* 36:516, 1983.
132 Putnam JB, Roth JA, Wesley MN et al: Analysis of prognostic factors in patients undergoing resection of pulmonary metastases from soft tissue sarcomas, *J Thorac Cardiovasc Surg* 87:260, 1984.
133 Rapp F: The challenge of herpesviruses, *Cancer Res* 44:1309, 1984.
134 Redmond C, Fisher B: Design of the controlled clinical trial. In Pilch YH, editor: *Surgical oncology,* New York, 1984, McGraw-Hill.
135 Richardson GS, Scully RE, Nikrui N et al: Common epithelial cancer of the ovary, *N Engl J Med* 212:415, 474, 1985.
136 Roberts JD, Ershler WB, Tindle BH, Stewart JA: Low-dose cytosine arabinoside in the myelodysplastic syndromes and acute myelogenous leukemia, *Cancer* 56:1001, 1985.
137 Rosen EM, Cassady JR, Frantz CN et al: Neuroblastoma: the

Joint Center for Radiation Therapy/Dana-Farber Cancer Institute/Children's Hospital experience, *J Clin Oncol* 2(7):719, 1984.

138 Rosen G, Marcove RC, Huvos AG et al: Primary osteogenic sarcoma: eight-year experience with adjuvant chemotherapy, *J Cancer Res Clin Oncol* 106(suppl):55, 1983.

139 Rosenberg SA: The immunotherapy and gene therapy of cancer, *J Clin Oncol* 10:180, 1992.

140 Rosenberg SA, editor: *Surgical treatment of metastatic cancer,* Philadelphia, 1987, JB Lippincott.

141 Rosenberg SA, Kaplan HS: The evolution and summary results of the Stanford randomized clinical trials of the management of Hodgkin's disease: 1962-1984, *Int J Radiat Oncol Biol Phys* 11:5, 1985.

142 Rosenberg SA, Longo DL, Lotze MT: Principles and applications of biologic therapy. In DeVita VT Jr, Hellman S, Rosenberg SA, editors: *Cancer: principles and practice of oncology,* ed 3, Philadelphia, 1989, JB Lippincott.

143 Rothman KJ: Causation and causal inference. In Schottenfeld D, Fraumeni JF Jr, editors: *Cancer epidemiology and prevention,* Philadelphia, 1982, WB Saunders.

144 Rubin H: Cancer as a dynamic development disorder, *Cancer Res* 45:2935, 1985.

145 Rubin P, Siemann D: Principles of radiation oncology and cancer radiotherapy. In Rubin P, Bakemeier RF, Krackov SK, editors: *Clinical oncology for medical students and physicians—a multidisciplinary approach,* ed 6, New York, 1983, American Cancer Society.

146 Ruddon RW: *Cancer biology,* New York, 1987, Oxford University Press.

147 Samara G, Hurwitz M, Sawacke M, Passaro E Jr: Molecular mechanisms of tumor formation, *Am J Surg* 164:389, 1992.

148 Santen RJ, Samojlik E, Lipton A et al: Kinetic, hormonal and clinical studies with aminoglutethimide in breast cancer, *Cancer* 39:2948, 1977.

149 Saracci R: Asbestos and lung cancer: an analysis of the epidemiological evidence on the asbestos-smoking interaction, *Int J Cancer* 20:323, 1977.

150 Schabel FM Jr: Surgical adjuvant chemotherapy of metastatic murine tumors, *Cancer* 40:558, 1977.

151 Schimke RT: Gene amplification, drug resistance, and cancer, *Cancer Res* 44:1735, 1984.

152 Schirrmacher V: Cancer metastasis: experimental approaches, theoretical concepts, and impacts for treatment strategies. In Klein G, Weinhouse S, editors: *Advances in cancer research,* Orlando, Fla, 1985, Academic Press.

153 Schottenfeld D, Fraumeni JR Jr, editors: *Cancer epidemiology and prevention,* Philadelphia, 1982, WB Saunders.

154 Setlow JK, Setlow RB: Nature of the photoreactable ultraviolet lesion in deoxiribonucleic acid, *Nature* 197:560, 1963.

155 Shamberger RC, Brennan MF, Goodgame JT Jr et al: A prospective, randomized study of adjuvant parenteral nutrition in the treatment of sarcomas: results of metabolic and survival studies, *Surgery* 96:1, 1984.

156 Sherman DM, Weichseibaum R, Hellman S: The characteristics of long-term survivors of lung cancer treated with radiation, *Cancer* 47:2575, 1981.

157 Silberman AW: Surgical debulking of tumors, *Surg Gynecol Obstet* 155:577, 1982.

158 Simon RM: Design and conduct of clinical trials. In DeVita VT Jr, Hellman S, Rosenberg SA, editors: *Cancer: principles and practice of oncology,* ed 3, Philadelphia, 1989, JB Lippincott.

159 Skipper HE: *Cancer chemotherapy,* vol 1, Ann Arbor, Mich, 1978, University Microfilms International.

160 Smith LH: Ectopic hormone production, *Surg Gynecol Obstet* 141:443, 1975.

161 Solomon E, Borrow J, Goddard AD: Chromosome aberrations and cancers, *Science* 254:1153, 1991.

162 Southern EM: Detection of specific sequences among DNA fragments separated by gel electrophoresis, *J Mol Biol* 98:503, 1975.

163 Stiles CD: The biological role of oncogenes—insights from platelet derived growth factor: Rhoads Memorial Award Lecture, *Cancer Res* 45:5215, 1985.

164 Takita H, Edgerton F, Karakousis C et al: Surgical management of metastases to the lung, *Surg Gynecol Obstet* 152:191, 1981.

165 Tokunaga M, Land CE, Yamamoto T et al: Breast cancer among atomic bomb survivors. In Boice JD Jr, Fraumeni JF Jr, editors: *Radiation carcinogenesis: epidemiology and biological significance,* New York, 1984, Raven Press.

166 Tritton TR, Hickman JA: Cell surface membranes as a chemotherapeutic target. In Muggia FM, editor: *Experimental and clinical progress in cancer chemotherapy,* Boston, 1985, Martinus Nijhoff.

167 Tucker MA, Meadows AT, Boice JD Jr et al: Cancer risk following treatment of childhood cancer. In Boice JD Jr, Fraumeni JF Jr, editors: *Radiation carcinogenesis: epidemiology and biological significance,* New York, 1984, Raven Press.

168 Turnbull RB Jr, Kyle K, Watson FR et al: Cancer of the colon: the influence of the no-touch isolation technic on survival rates, *Ann Surg* 166:420, 1967.

169 Tuyns AJ: Alcohol. In Schottenfeld D, Fraumeni JF Jr, editors: *Cancer epidemiology and prevention,* Philadelphia, 1982, WB Saunders.

170 Upton AC: Biological aspects of radiation carcinogenesis. In Boice JD Jr, Fraumeni JF Jr, editors: *Radiation carcinogenesis: epidemiology and biological significance,* New York, 1984, Raven Press.

171 Waterhouse C: How tumors affect host metabolism, *Ann NY Acad Sci* 230:86, 1974.

172 Wattenberg LW: Chemoprevention of cancer, *Cancer Res* 45:1, 1985.

173 Weinberg RA: The molecules of life, *Sci Am* 253:48, 1985.

174 Weinberg RA: The action of oncogenes in the cytoplasm and nucleus, *Science* 230:770, 1985.

175 Weinberg RA: Tumor supressor genes, *Science* 254:1138, 1991.

176 Wells SA, Baylin SB, Linehan WM et al: Provocative agents and the diagnosis of medullary carcinoma of the thyroid gland, *Ann Surg* 188:139, 1978.

177 Wilkins EW Jr: The status of pulmonary resection of metastases: experience at Massachusetts General Hospital. In Weiss L, Gilbert HA, editors: *Pulmonary metastasis,* Boston, 1978, GK Hall.

178 Wilmore DW, Long JM, Mason AD et al: Catecholamines: mediator of the hypermetabolic response to thermal injury, *Ann Surg* 180(4):653, 1974.

179 Winston KR, Walsh JW, Fischer EG: Results of operative treatment of intracranial metastatic tumors, *Cancer* 435:2639, 1980.

180 World Health Organization: *Prevention of cancer, technical report series* 276, Geneva, 1964, World Health Organization.

181 Young VR: Energy metabolism and requirements in the cancer patient, *Cancer Res* 37:2336, 1977.

182 Yuspa SH, Harris CC: Molecular and cellular basis of chemical carcinogenesis. In Schottenfeld D, Fraumeni JF Jr, editors: *Cancer epidemiology and prevention,* Philadelphia, 1982, WB Saunders.

183 Ziegler JL: Burkitt's lymphoma, *N Engl J Med* 305:735, 1981.

184 Zur Hausen H: Viruses in human cancers, *Science* 254:1167, 1991.

CHAPTER

13

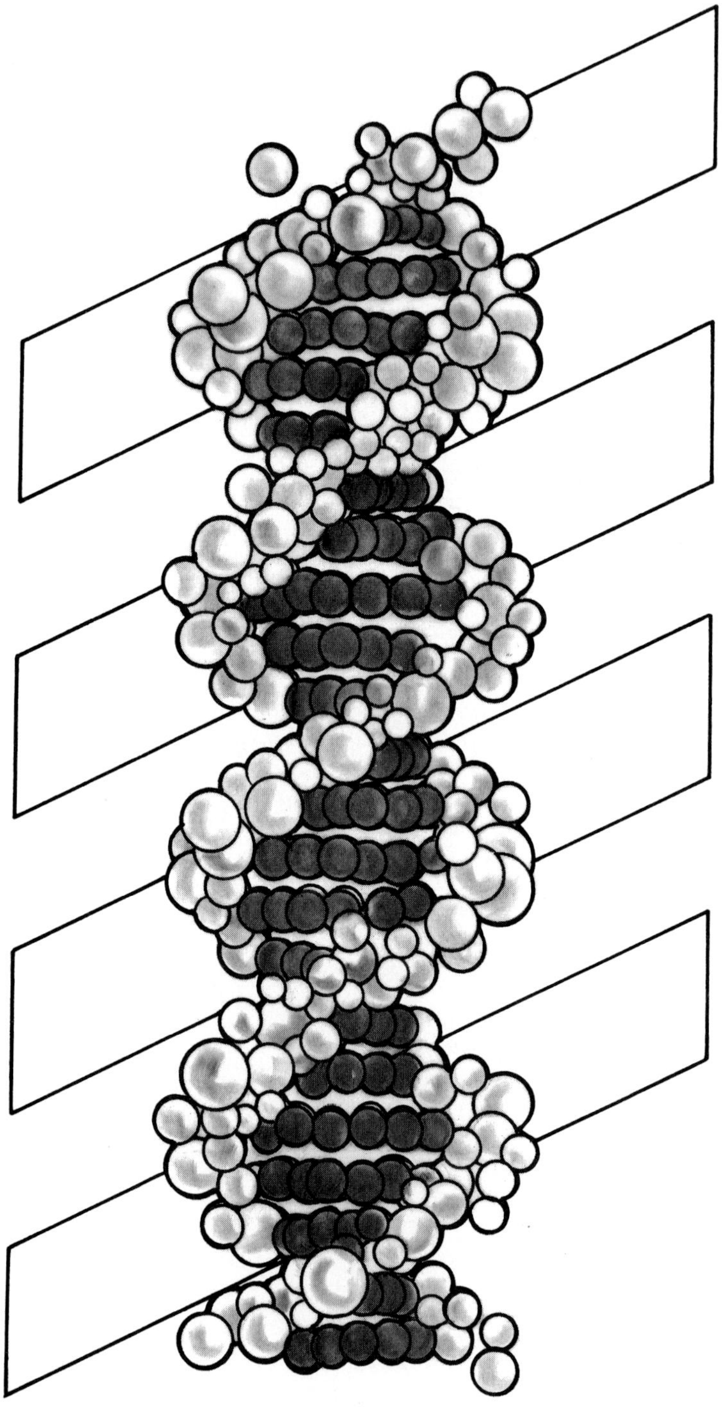

MOLECULAR BIOLOGY FOR SURGEONS

Carl E. Haisch • Sally A. Huber • Nicholas H. Heintz • Patricia A. Lodge • Chen Feng Qi

Molecular biology traces its beginnings to the work of Gregor Mendel who showed in 1866 that certain traits in flowers were transmitted by specific factors in either a dominant or recessive manner. Fleming subsequently identified chromosomes, which Sutton later established to be Mendel's "factors." Fleming also demonstrated segregation of the chromosomes during gamete formation and deduced the presence of genes on chromosomes. This discovery was followed in 1941 by the work of Tatum, Beadle, and Lederberg who demonstrated that each gene regulated the production of a specific protein, which later led to the concept of "one gene, one protein."

Genes are made up of DNA, a concept suggested by Avery and later proven by Hershey in 1952. DNA is comprised of a sequential arrangement of four nucleotides with a base (adenine, guanine, cytosine, or thymine) attached to a sugar and phosphate backbone. DNA is the information repository of all organisms encoding all the information required for the growth, differentiation, and development of an organism. The advances in molecular biology have provided, for the first time, detailed descriptions of the mechanisms that handle information flow in biologic systems.[41,58]

The era of recombinant DNA technology is of recent origin. Berg and colleagues successfully inserted genes of the simian virus 40 into a gamma-bacteriophage in 1971, studies which ultimately led to cloning techniques that allowed insertion of large quantities of foreign DNA into bacteria and other organisms or cells. When provided with the appropriate DNA sequences, prokaryotic cells can produce large amounts of foreign proteins. Other technology allows the elaboration of large foreign DNA fragments, permitting one to physically map regions of chromosomes important in human disease. In 1987 Mullis described the technique of amplifying a specific segment length of DNA many fold in vitro, a procedure called the polymerase chain reaction (PCR). PCR has revolutionized genetic analysis of tissue specimens and has led to new diagnostic procedures of ever increasing value.[41] Using highly radioactive nucleic acid probes, in situ hybridization has allowed localization of specific genes of interest in tissue specimens. All of these developments in molecular biology have provided the basis for exciting developments that continue almost daily.

SIGNIFICANCE TO SURGEONS

DNA is responsible for the function of cells, interactions between cells, tissue repair, and regeneration. Specific mutations in genes have been associated with errors in growth regulation and tumor formation. Other alterations at the molecular level may result in atherosclerosis, thrombotic abnormalities, and other diseases of interest to surgeons. Careful evaluation of tissues removed at surgery using molecular techniques could provide a wealth of new information on the pathogenesis of these diseases. The surgeon plays a crucial role in medical research and the development of future therapies. At the very least, such studies could benefit the surgeon by ultimately improving our comprehension of the disease process.

RELATIONSHIP OF DNA, RNA, AND PROTEIN

DNA, RNA, and proteins dictate the structure of cells and are responsible in large part for the function of the cell. The basic genetic information of the cell is contained in the DNA of the cell nucleus. It is estimated that 100,000 genes are contained in the 3 billion nucleotide base pairs of the human genome.[60] Not all the DNA is used to directly code for proteins, as DNA sequences are used to regulate gene expression and DNA replication. Simple replication sequences such as those found in centromeres may serve a structural role. Additionally, the organization of genes often includes segments of DNA (called introns) that are not used to code for protein.

Watson and Crick first demonstrated that DNA exists as two complementary strands that form a double helix. The basic structure of the DNA consists of a backbone of sugar and phosphate groups. Attached to the sugar-phosphate backbone are bases, either guanine, cytosine, thymine, or adenine. A phosphate group connects the 5′ carbon atom of one sugar to the 3′ carbon atom of the next. The bases that encode information are attached to the sugar part of the backbone (Figure 13-1). In the double helix the guanine on one strand of DNA pairs with the cytosine on the other strand; thymine pairs with adenine.[19,58] The sugar is ribose in RNA and deoxyribose in DNA. Ribose has a hydroxyl (OH) group attached at the 2′ position of the sugar ring; the deoxyribose has a hydrogen atom. This unique structure allows the RNA to be chemically less stable than DNA, a fact that has been confirmed by showing that an aqueous solution of RNA undergoes hydrolytic cleavage at a much faster rate than DNA. Thus DNA is better suited to the function of maintaining information over a long time.[15]

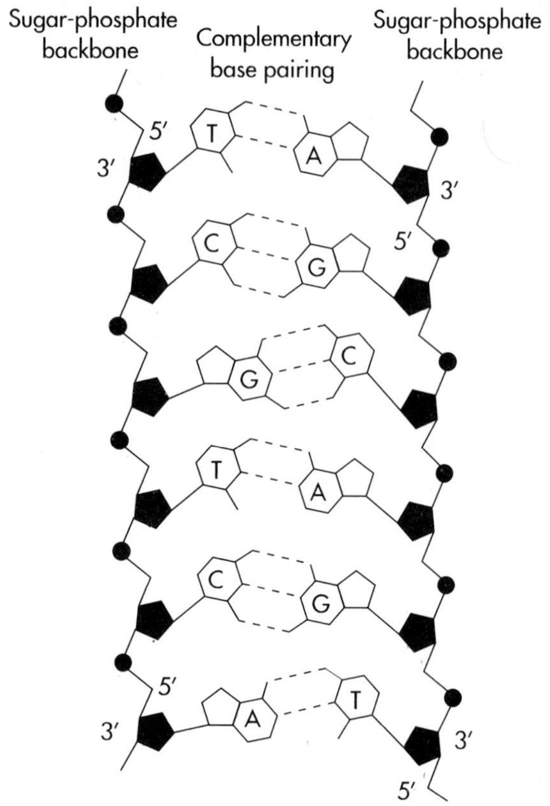

FIGURE 13-1 The basic structure of DNA, with adenine pairing with thymine and guanine pairing with cytosine. The purine or pyrimidine is bound to the sugar (hexagon), which in turn is bound to a phosphate. This pattern is repeating. (From Watson JD, Gilman M, Witkowski J, Zoller M: *Recombinant DNA*, ed 2, New York, 1992, Scientific American Books, WH Freeman.)

DNA is a double helix; RNA is a single strand. In contrast to DNA, thymine is not used in RNA but is replaced by the base uracil. RNA is synthesized on a DNA template by a process called transcription. In transcription, the DNA is selectively copied to produce an RNA precursor that encompasses the information encoded by genes. This precursor is then processed to produce messenger RNA, which acts as a template for a series of amino acids to be placed in a specific order, thereby producing a protein. This basic process is central to the formation of structural and regulatory proteins and therefore is the central mechanism of the cell for executing its individual processes.

The sequence of DNA is preserved with a very high order of specificity during replication, with errors occurring at a rate of one mistake per 10 million base pairs, to as few as one in 10 billion base pairs.[59] This specificity is possible because of three mechanisms that maintain high fidelity of the DNA replication process. The first process involves selecting which of the four nucleotides is added to the emerging strand. The second mechanism uses a proofreading process that checks the most recently added nucleotide, excising those that are not correct. The last process takes place after synthesis and corrects the errors which the first two processes have missed. It relies on the resulting synthesized structure and checks for conformational changes from the original DNA.[7,20]

DNA Replication

DNA polymerases are the key to DNA replication. These enzymes allow accurate replication of the DNA strand. DNA strands always grow in a 5′ to 3′ direction. The simplest replication mechanism would have been for the strands to unravel as a zipper, and two enzymes to replicate the missing strands using each of the original

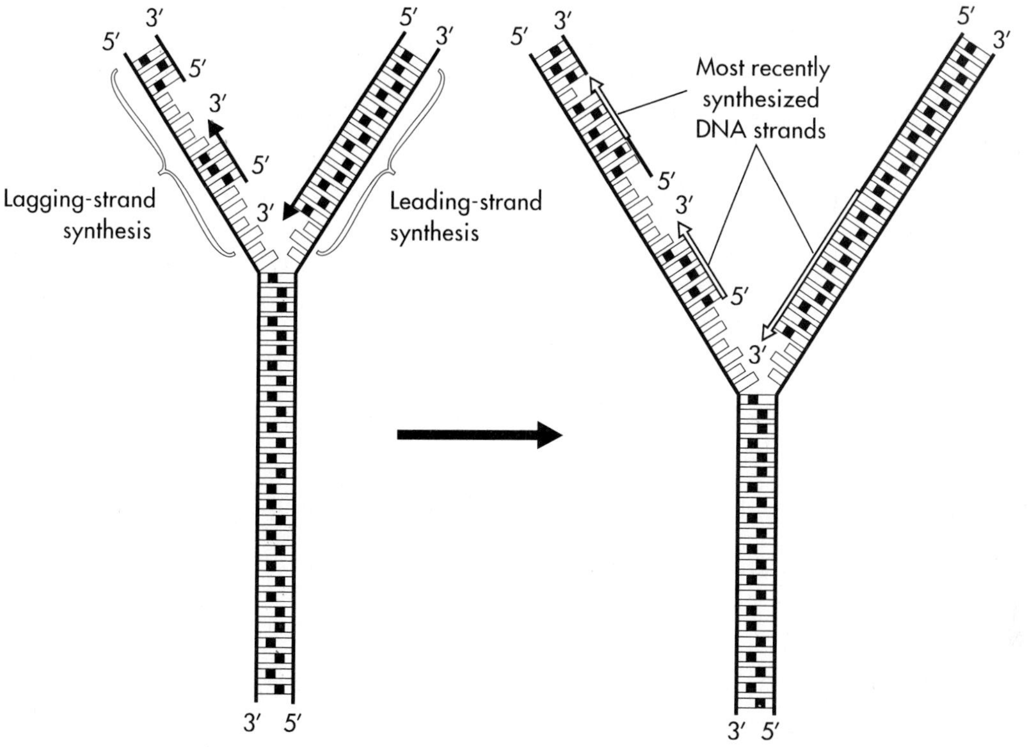

FIGURE 13-2 The basic structure of DNA during replication. There is a leading strand and a lagging strand. DNA synthesis occurs only in a 5′ to 3′ direction. Thus the lagging strand has small segments of DNA called *Okazaki fragments.* These fragments are sealed together with a DNA ligase. (From Alberts B, Bray D, Lewis J et al: *Molecular biology of the cell,* ed 2, New York, 1989, Garland Publishing.)

strands as a template. This means there would have to be a 5′ to 3′ DNA polymerase enzyme as well as a 3′ to 5′ DNA polymerase. However, no 3′ to 5′ DNA polymerase has been discovered. Thus there must be another means of replication for the strand to be synthesized in the 3′ to 5′ direction.[27]

The solution to this problem occurred in the late 1960s with the discovery of pieces of DNA that were 1000 to 2000 nucleotides long, called *Okazaki fragments* at the growing fork. These fragments were synthesized in the 5′ to 3′ direction and joined together after their synthesis to create long DNA chains using the DNA ligase enzyme, which seals single-stranded nicks during DNA replication and repair[38] (Figure 13-2).

Because of asymmetric synthesis, the DNA daughter strands are synthesized by two enzymes, DNA polymerases alpha and delta. The strand synthesized continuously by polymerase delta is the leading strand. The synthesis slightly proceeds the other daughter strand, which is known as the lagging strand. After exposure of the lagging template strand, Okazaki fragments are synthesized by polymerase alpha. The short spaces between the Okazaki fragments are sealed using DNA ligase. Thus the synthesis of the lagging strand is a discontinuous backstitching mechanism; only 5′ to 3′ DNA polymerases are needed for DNA replication.[38] DNA replication begins at the replication origin, which is where the two strands of the DNA have separated and serve as templates for synthesis. Replication origins can be as long as 300 to 1000 nucleotides. An initiator protein binds to origin sequences and directs the assembly replication complexes that move away from the origin of replication in opposite directions, until all the DNA template downstream has been replicated.[17]

RNA Synthesis

RNA occurs in the cell in multiple forms: messenger RNA (mRNA), ribosomal RNA (rRNA), small nuclear RNA (snRNA), and transfer RNA (tRNA).[36] Transcription is the process of synthesizing a complementary copy of RNA from a DNA template.[15,31] To transcribe RNA a specific enzyme in the nucleus, called an RNA polymerase, binds tightly to predetermined sites on DNA called promoters. The RNA polymerase and associated proteins unravel a short segment of the DNA double helix, thus exposing the nucleotides on both

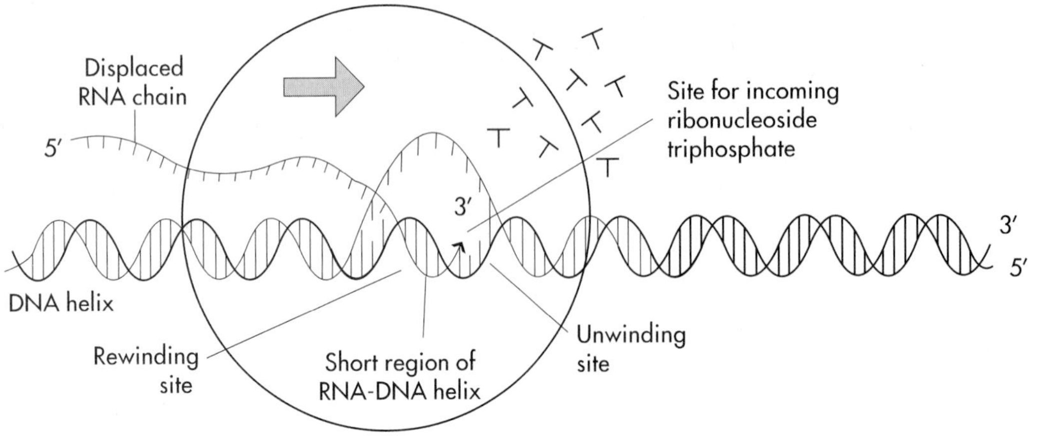

FIGURE 13-3 The RNA polymerase moving along the DNA helix to give a messenger RNA, which will be the template for protein construction. (From Alberts B, Bray D, Lewis J et al: *Molecular biology of the cell*, ed 2, New York, 1989, Garland Publishing.)

DNA strands. Which DNA strand is transcribed depends on the orientation of the promoter sequences.[25] As for DNA, RNA is synthesized 5′ to 3′ and thus is reading the DNA sequence of nucleotides 3′ to 5′. By convention the promoter region is called the 5′ end of the transcription unit. Transcription continues along the DNA in a 5′ to 3′ direction until a termination signal releases the RNA from the DNA template (Figure 13-3).

Three different polymerases direct the synthesis of RNA: RNA polymerase II transcribes structural genes composed of introns and exons; RNA polymerase I directs the synthesis of ribosomal RNAs, structural components of ribosomes used for protein synthesis; and polymerase III transcribes tRNA and snRNAs. Each RNA polymerase is able to recognize the appropriate class of promoter elements due to regulatory sequences located in the promoter. For polymerase II genes, the amount of mRNA for a specific gene product is often controlled during development and in specific tissues by proteins called *transcription factors*. These proteins bind to promoter elements and modulate the frequency of the transcription event.

For structural genes encoding proteins, transcription duplicates the entire portion of DNA, including both introns and exons. Exons are portions of the genetic code that are represented in the final processed mRNA. Introns are intervening segments of genetic material that will be spliced out of the mRNA before translation of the proteins. The mRNA, which can range from 70 to greater than 10,000 nucleotides long, then migrates to the cytoplasm.[15]

Transfer RNA (tRNA), snRNA, and rRNA are transcribed from DNA using separate RNA polymerases.[48] The tRNA consists of 70 to 90 nucleotides that fold into a specific tertiary structure. A loop in the middle of the tRNA molecule contains a complementary recognition codon for a specific amino acid. The specific amino acid attaches to the 3′ end of the tRNA chain. Matching nucleotide sequences in the mRNA with complementary sequences in the tRNA allows the amino acids to assemble according to a specific sequence[15] (Figure 13-4).

The tRNA becomes bound to its particular amino acid through its specific enzyme, an aminoacyl-tRNA synthetase. Twenty of these enzymes are specific for each amino acid. They covalently link the amino acid to the tRNA.[47] It must be noted that the number of possible nucleotide combinations with four nucleotides is 64. Three of these codes are for termination of a polypeptide chain and are known as stop codons. Of the 61 remaining codons only two are specific for one amino acid, methionine and tryptophan. All other amino acids have more than one codon.[13] Like tRNA, snRNA is transcribed by RNA polymerase II. SnRNA is a critical component of the splicing machinery that excises introns during mRNA processing.

In the cytoplasm the mRNA goes to the ribosomes. The ribosome consists of RNA and protein organized into a small and large subunit. The small subunit allows interaction between the codons on the mRNA and tRNA, and peptide formation proceeds on the large subunit. The rRNA gives the ribosome its grooved structure, which enables it to accommodate an mRNA and a protein simultaneously.[33,37]

The ribosome contains binding sites for the growth of a polypeptide. There is a peptidyl-tRNA binding site (P-site), which holds the tRNA molecule that is linked to the growing end of the polypeptide chain. A second site is the aminoacyl-tRNA binding site (A-site),

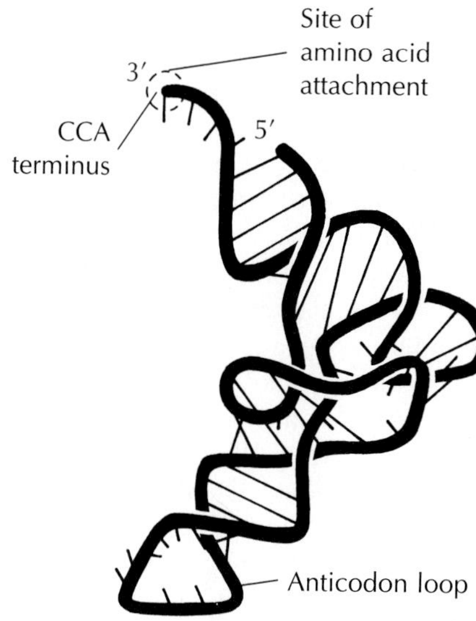

FIGURE 13-4 The looped structure of transfer RNA. The amino acid attaches to the 3′ end of the structure, and the anticodon portion at the base of the loop encodes for the messenger RNA. (From Watson JD, Gilman M, Witkowski J, Zoller M: *Recombinant DNA,* ed 2, New York, 1992, Scientific American Books, WH Freeman.)

which holds the incoming tRNA molecule with an attached amino acid. The polypeptide chain grows by a stepwise addition of amino acids to the carboxyl-terminal end.[10,57]

Any one of the three stop codons (UAA, UAG or UGA) in the mRNA molecule will halt the translation process. When a stop codon is reached a molecule of water is added to the peptidyl-tRNA.[9,12]

It is obvious that there are three possible reading frames on the RNA. Untranslated reader sequences on the 5′ end of the mRNA intersect with the ribosome to determine the precise start point. This process depends upon a number of protein initiation factors, and the small ribosomal subunits which help the initiator tRNA molecule to find a special AUG codon (the start codon) on the mRNA molecule.[26,39]

Recombinant DNA Technology

Molecular biology has revolutionized medical care. It allows one to isolate, alter or manufacture genes, and place them into either cells or germ lines of animals. Because of this it has allowed the manufacture of previously unavailable hormones and production of animals which have unique characteristics.

Recombinant DNA technology utilizes a number of procedures. The most important is cleavage of DNA by restriction endonucleases and subsequent[52] sequencing of nucleotides in the individual DNA segments. DNA cloning is performed by identifying, isolating, and inserting a specific DNA fragment into a self-replicating genetic element (a plasmid or viral DNA called the vector) so that both the vector and the foreign DNA are reproduced. Lastly, genetic engineering allows introduction of genes or their modified versions into cells or organisms.

A brief description of recombinant DNA techniques follows. The cell containing the DNA of interest is lysed with detergents, and cellular proteins are digested by proteases. The DNA is precipitated from the lipids and proteins in the cell fluid. This then results in long DNA molecules that can be characterized by restriction enzyme analysis.[2]

Restriction endonucleases are usually derived from bacteria and protect these procaryotes from viral infection by destroying the viral DNA. These enzymes cut the DNA at specific nucleotide sequences called recognition sites, which are four to eight base pairs long. This process results in pieces of DNA of defined length called restriction fragments.[52] Restriction fragments can be rapidly separated into different sizes by gel electrophoresis. A sample of digested DNA is placed at one end of an agarose gel slab along with appropriate size standards as controls. An electrical charge is placed across the gel. The phosphate backbone of the DNA has a negative charge, which results in the DNA fragments moving in a straight line toward the positive electrode. The length of the fragment determines its rate of migration in the gel; shorter fragments move farther down the lane. If the gel is soaked in ethidium bromide and then illuminated with ultraviolet light, the DNA fragments can be visualized.[2] DNA fragments that have been separated on gels can be transferred to solid membrane supports to produce what is called a *Southern blot.* The Southern blot can be hybridized to the specific probe to identify specific DNA fragments.[53]

DNA probes, which are homologous to a specific gene in a DNA segment, are often used to identify a DNA fragment carrying a gene that has been isolated either by cleavage with restriction enzymes or by amplification by PCR. Because sensitivity of DNA probes is excellent, these probes can identify a specific DNA fragment among millions of unrelated DNA pieces. Much of the sensitivity of this procedure is derived from labeling the probe to high specific activity with radioactive phosphorus (^{32}P), which facilitates detection of the bound radioactive material by radioautography. A gene can be detected even when only one DNA copy per cell is present.[6,16]

The DNA probe may represent a sequence complementary to the mRNA specified by the gene, hence the designation cDNA (complementary DNA). The steps in producing a cDNA probe involve identifying a tissue or a cell line that expresses the gene and subsequent extraction of the relevant mRNA. Incubation of the mRNA with retroviral reverse transcriptase and the appropriate nucleotides (adenine, cytosine, guanine and thymidine) results in the synthesis of a cDNA from the mRNA template. Incubation is a major technique for obtaining DNA for PCR. Generally, one or more of the nucleotides used in the synthesis of the cDNA is radiolabeled. This cDNA is then cloned in a vector or may be directly amplified using PCR, which will be discussed later.[24]

With some probes, specificity of binding can be a problem. Because all DNA is composed of the same four nucleotides, hybridizing the probe to cellular DNA at low temperatures may result in nonperfect matches and nonspecific binding. Hybridizing at 60°C rather than at 37°C results in more stringent binding (specific). Under stringent conditions, one can be more certain that the probe binds to the appropriate portion of the cellular DNA. Because the probe is labeled with ^{32}P, its presence can be detected using radioautography.[1]

The procedure to detect DNA by filter hybridization is called a Southern blot analysis. The DNA probe can also be used to detect mRNA by Northern blot analysis. While Southern blots demonstrate the presence of a gene in a cell, a Northern blot indicates whether the gene is "active" or is transcribed into mRNA and presumably translated into protein. Thus simple questions can be answered using probes: Is a gene present? How much of the gene is present? Is the gene expressed? How much gene expression is present in a specific tissue?

Clinical Uses of Recombinant DNA Techniques

Recombinant DNA techniques have become increasingly important in the production of numerous biologic substances including insulin and human growth hormone. The first protein produced by recombinant DNA technology was somatostatin.[28] The gene was synthesized and cloned into a plasmid vector for expression in *Escherichia coli.* These advances were possible because of success in a number of areas of molecular biology including oligonucleotide synthesis, isolation of enzymes that join and cleave DNA, characterization of bacterial plasmids, and an understanding of gene expression. Because of these advances, new treatments are emerging for numerous conditions including cancer, allergies, autoimmune disease, neurologic disorders, heart disease, blood disorders, infections, and genetic diseases.

Insulin was first produced by introducing the genes for A and B chains into separate colonies of *E. coli.* The chains were then produced separately and the A and B chains purified from the *E. coli.* The chains were then mixed to form the active recombinant insulin. Because human genes were used, it obviated the production of antibodies, which was an impediment when pig insulin was used in the past. Similarly, bacteria have been used to produce human growth hormone (hGH). The bacteria could be engineered to secrete hGH, which can be subsequently purified. The purification required many steps when produced intracellularly. Thus secretion of the protein was a major advance and helped to increase the utility of the hormone.[21,22]

Because mammalian cells process their proteins differently than do prokaryotes, mammalian cells have been used both to study the proteins that are active in a mammalian cell and to produce new protein drugs. The steps required to isolate mammalian genes and express them in mammalian cells are similar to those used for bacterial systems. First the gene must be isolated by cloning; second the gene must be able to be manipulated in a test tube; finally the gene must be able to be returned to the cell to determine how it functions.

The problem of getting the gene into the cell called for some unique solutions. The first technique injected the DNA into the cell. Microinjection is useful and very effective for a small number of cells (a few hundred cells per experiment). The DNA is introduced into the nucleus of the cell using a fine glass needle. This technique is still used today for certain experiments.[8]

The problem remained of getting genes into a series of cells en masse. The first method used an inert carbohydrate polymer (dextran) and DEAE (diethylaminoethyl). DNA stuck to the polymer; the large polymer stuck to the cell surface and was taken into the cell by endocytosis. Some of the DNA was incorporated into the nucleus and the cell recognized it as its own DNA. This method was inefficient and has largely been replaced by using DNA precipitated with calcium phosphate. This technique gives a much higher yield efficiency of transfections. Lipofection, another method for transfection, packages DNA into liposomes. This technique allows the lipid vesicle package to fuse with the cell membrane and to deliver the DNA contents into the cytoplasm. The cells can also be rendered permeable to DNA by an electrical pulse. A cell suspension, at a high density, is mixed with the DNA to be delivered. It is placed in a small chamber and a brief electric pulse applied, rendering the cells permeable to the DNA. The cells are then plated in fresh medium and later checked for DNA incorporation. This technique is called electroporation.[49]

Another method of introducing DNA into cells involves viral infection. Presently, retroviruses are used to provide stable gene transfers. The viral DNA is integrated into the host genome and is replicated along with the host DNA. This last technique is used frequently and is discussed later in this chapter.[18]

A major protein that has been produced using a vector and mammalian cell culture is the tissue plasminogen activator (tPA). Tissue plasminogen activator is produced from a mammalian cell line carrying an integrated vector. The result is protein, which can be used for heart attack patients by breaking up blood clots. Another protein of interest is the clotting protein factor VIII. Because of its size and complexity, factor VIII can only be produced in mammalian cell culture. This will prevent hemophiliacs from contracting the HIV virus because factor VIII will no longer need to be isolated from human blood.

TRANSGENIC ANIMALS

The formation of a transgenic mouse can be accomplished using the same technology as described earlier. These animals are useful for determining what effects a particular gene has in the production of a human disease condition, such as cancer. Early attempts to insert foreign genes into recipient mice used a virus. The mice were mated and the fertilized egg was removed from the oviducts with the two pronuclei present. The gene of interest was injected into a pronucleus, and the fertilized eggs were implanted into pseudopregnant mice. The number of mice that may have the gene integrated into their chromosomes is between a few percent and 40%.

A different technique using embryonic stem cells to carry the foreign gene into the animal is also being used. In this technique the DNA can be introduced into embryonic stem cells and then placed in the developing embryo. Mice are mated and the blastocyst isolated. The blastocyst has the innermost cell layer transferred to a Petri dish. These cells are the embryonic stem cells. At this stage the desired DNA can be introduced into the stem cells by transfection, retroviral infection, or electroporation. These selected cells can then be injected into a blastocyst and placed into a pseudopregnant mouse. The presence of the gene can be determined by performing a Southern blot on the cells before they are injected into the blastocyst. This procedure results in a model that can be manipulated much more easily and with greater accuracy than previous techniques.[23,44]

When two mice that result from these manipulations are bred, one-fourth of the offspring will be homozygous for the gene of interest. This result allows study of the animal with a normal gene that has had an abnormal gene added.[40,56] There is also technology to produce mice that have a specific gene missing, called "knockout mice." Some of these mice have major histocompatibility complex (MHC) class II missing or have the β_2-microglobulin gene missing, rendering the animals effectively MHC class I or class II deficient.

This model with the added gene or altered gene allows study of various diseases such as a disease that causes destruction of the myelin-producing cells in the brain. Patients with this disease also have a deficiency in their immune system. Transgenic mice with myelin deficiency similar to that in human patients can be developed using genetic material from papovavirus called JC. This procedure results in animals with similar myelin deficiency in their brains and therefore can be used to study the disease process.[50]

Other diseases that can be studied are retinoblastoma and osteogenesis imperfecta. Mice have been manipulated genetically to produce transgenic animals that at about 5 months of age develop eye tumors. Studies with these mice have resulted in a better understanding of the genetic basis for human retinoblastoma. Osteogenesis imperfecta can be introduced into animals using a mutant gene resulting in a mouse that dies soon after birth and that has similar defects to that seen in humans with this disease.[55]

POLYMERASE CHAIN REACTION

One of the major breakthroughs in molecular biology is the advent of DNA amplification by PCR. This procedure allows the DNA from a selected region of a genome to be amplified more than a millionfold. Briefly the process is summarized as denaturation of the original DNA, annealing of the primer to the target portion of DNA, and extension of the primer. The process requires a primer, the four deoxyribonucleotide triphosphates, a DNA sample, and a heat-stable Taq DNA polymerase. The reaction is performed in a thermal cycler that is programmed for precise temperatures at timed intervals.

The basic procedure of PCR is to briefly heat (90°C) the DNA to separate the two strands of the DNA double helix in a thermal cycler. This mixture is subsequently cooled (46°C) with a large excess of DNA nucleotides in the presence of the DNA polymerase enzyme from the bacteria *Thermus aquaticus* (Taq) along with two primers usually 50 to 2000 base pairs long. Next the combination is heated to 70°C, which is the optimal temperature for the *T. aquaticus* DNA polymerase. The polymerase then uses the DNA, which is present as a single strand, and the free nucleotides to make two complementary strands to the DNA. The machine then heats the mixture to 90°C and all the DNA strands separate. This procedure is repeated multiple times and the copies of the original gene are markedly increased. The amplified DNA can then be run on a gel, blotted, and checked with an appropriate DNA probe. Clinical uses of PCR are described later.[3]

This technology can also be used to study gene expression. Messenger RNA can be detected and quantified using reverse transcriptase. The retroviral enzyme reverse transcriptase can make DNA from an RNA template. After cDNA synthesis, the small amount of DNA can be amplified using PCR.

USES OF MOLECULAR BIOLOGY

One of the major interests of surgeons using molecular biology has been in understanding the basic cellular changes in cancer. A variety of mechanisms can explain the cellular abnormalities seen in cancer. The involvement of virus in the genesis of cancer was suggested by Rous in the early 1900s. He demonstrated that filtered cell-free extracts from chicken tumors could cause new tumors when inoculated into healthy chickens. This transmitted factor was later shown to be a virus.

The largest of these cellular alterations is in the chromosome. Cytogenetic studies indicated a correlation in chromosomal alterations and malignancies. Both deletions and insertions can occur and lead to phenotypic alterations. For example a meningioma is associated with the deletion of chromosome 22. A deletion on the long arm of chromosome 18 is associated with changes in cellular contact inhibition, which have been implicated in colon tumor formation.

Insertions can also cause changes in cellular growth. For example trisomy 7 is associated with epithelial tumors. This trisomy results in twofold or higher rate of proliferation thus increasing cellular activity. This enhanced proliferation is then responsible for the increases in cellular growth.[46]

Viral agents are responsible for a number of cancers causing an estimated 15% to 20% of all cancers. Cervical and hepatocellular carcinoma account for approximately 80% of all virally linked cancers. Determining how these viruses induce cancer illustrates the usefulness and power of DNA technology.

Tumor viruses may be either DNA or RNA viruses. These viruses carry genetic elements called oncogenes that give the viruses the ability to transform cells. A large number of oncogenes have been identified. The oncogenes encode proteins called oncoproteins, which bring about oncogenic transformations. The exact working mechanism of oncogenes is still being studied because a thorough understanding of their mechanism is not available.

The oncogenes of RNA tumor viruses or retroviruses originate from the cellular DNA. The Rous sarcoma virus (RSV) has DNA that is very closely related to cellular DNA. These sequences of the RSV are related not only to the chicken but also to vertebrates including humans. Thus the oncogene from the RSV is a derivative of a normal cellular gene called proto-oncogene. More than 25 distinct cellular proto-oncogenes have been identified. These oncogenes encode a number of proteins that can induce generation of rapidly growing tumors within a few weeks of inoculation.[51]

Some retroviruses cause tumors that take a long time to develop. Some of the tumors that are induced are linked to DNA sequences from an adjoining cellular gene. Thus the tumor is caused either by additional genetic material or by a novel version of the normal cellular message.

The study of bladder cancer demonstrated the importance of a point mutation in the development of a tumor. In early work with the EJ bladder carcinoma cell line, DNA was isolated and studied in detail. A number of laboratories developed DNA libraries from tumors that reacted with retroviral oncogenes. These were then used to study the DNA from cell cultures transformed by human tumor DNA. This work led to the conclusion that the oncogene in the human tumor is the cellular counterpart of the transforming genes of the retrovirus. Preliminary comparison showed no major differences between the retroviral transforming gene and the cellular oncogenes. However, additional analysis of the gene showed that the guanine within the normal gene had been converted to a thymine in the oncogene. This analysis demonstrated the importance of point mutations in the production of human cancer.[14]

The preceding examples illustrate that an understanding of the genetic basis of cancer is possible. However, understanding all of the genetic abnormalities in all tumors will require additional investigation.

Gene therapy is a possible use of molecular biology to aid in therapy for cancer. Rosenberg[45] recently published two case reports. The first patient had tumor infiltrating lymphocytes isolated from a tumor. These cells then had the neomycin phosphotransferase (Neo) gene inserted into the cells to be used as a tracer. The cells were then injected back into the patient, and then peripheral blood samples and biopsies of several tumors were obtained. Polymerase chain reaction analyses of the patient's peripheral blood and results of several tumor biopsies showed the presence of the tracer gene; thus the tumor-infiltrating lymphocytes were homing back to the original tumors. A second patient with multiple melanoma had tumor-infiltrating lymphocytes isolated. These cells were genetically engineered for production of tumor necrosis factor. The hope was that administration of these genetically engineered cells would home to the tumor and then be able to kill portions of the tumor by secreting tumor necrosis factor. This therapy resulted in almost complete regression of multiple melanoma nodules with little or no viable tumor remaining. Thus it can be shown that gene therapy may have an active role in cancer therapy in the near future.

Use of Polymerase Chain Reactions

PCR has been used in the diagnosis of genetic diseases such as sickle cell anemia because the mutations could be studied directly. PCR can also be used to detect the virus for AIDS. PCR can detect dormant viruses and viruses that cannot be cultured. The clinical applications of PCR for the diagnosis of viral infections include the detection of neonatal infection, early infection, resolution of indeterminate serologies, viral typing, and detection of new agents.[61]

PCR also has a place in a number of bacterial infections, especially slow-growing organisms. The first reports showed the usefulness of this technique in the diagnosis of pathogens such as mycobacteria, *Chlamydia trachomatis, Legionella pneumophila,* and Lyme disease.[4,30] Some of the tests for mycobacteria use a probe that is specific for the species of interest after the genes for the mycobacterium have been isolated. Many bacterial diagnoses can be made using PCR, including *Mycobacterium tuberculosis, Mycobacterium leprae, Chlamydia trachomatis, Borrelia burgdorferi* (Lyme disease), *Mycoplasma pneumoniae, Legionella pneumophila, Rickettsia rickettsii, Clostridium difficile,* and *Treponema pallidum.*[5,29]

Antibiotic susceptibility can also be determined using PCR. One can detect conserved gene sequences or those specifying specific enzymes such as beta-lactamase. This sort of data would be most useful in pathogens resistant to certain agents such as methicillin in the case of *Staphylococcus aureus.* Because of the speed with which PCR can be performed, antibiotic resistance can be determined much more quickly compared to culture techniques.[11]

Because of the time required for fungal culture, PCR can help in the rapid diagnosis of a number of fungal and parasitic diseases. PCR can be used in the diagnosis and identification of *Cryptococcus neoformans* and *Pneumocystic carinii.* With the development of pathogen-specific probes, rapid and sensitive diagnosis of fungal sepsis and pulmonary disease is possible.[61]

PCR holds the promise of rapid and more accurate diagnosis. It also may surpass the present gold standard of culture and sensitivity for bacterial, viral, and fungal identification.

Use of Genetically Modified Vascular Endothelial Cells

The endothelium is an excellent target for gene transfer. Gene transfer has been undertaken in bone marrow cells of mice, dogs, primates, and humans. However, there is a variable ability to express certain genes in these cells. Other cell types have been considered including fibroblasts, lymphocytes, human keratinocytes, and hepatocytes. Because of its proximity to the bloodstream, however, the vascular endothelial cell is an attractive target to deliver functional genes in vivo. Zwiebel and associates[63] have described the use of a retrovirus that contains the neomycin resistance gene along with either the adenosine deaminase gene or the rat growth hormone (rGH) gene. The authors used this gene to infect rabbit endothelial cells and demonstrated that the endothelial cells expressed the gene. They also demonstrated that the cells would secrete the rGH when the cells were seeded onto a 4 mm Corvita vascular graft. The rGH continued to be secreted into the tissue culture media for at least 4 weeks. This experiment has shown that vascular endothelial cells can be used to carry genes and secrete the proteins for which these genes are encoded in vitro; however, the development of an in vivo model is important.[63]

The same sort of model has been carried a step further in vivo by Wilson and colleagues.[62] These authors infected endothelial cells with a retrovirus containing a marker gene, beta galactosidase, and then implanted the grafts with the infected vascular endothelial cells into dogs. The grafts were then removed and divided for analysis. The cells did not change their classical endothelial cell markers, but the gene was shown to be functional. This sort of therapy could be useful in the therapy of atherosclerosis and the design of new drug delivery systems. In the latter they would be ideal because of their proximity to the vascular system.[62]

This concept has been applied in the repair of denuded portions of iliofemoral arteries in pigs. The denuding of the endothelium was accomplished by partially inflating a balloon catheter within the vessel and then passing the balloon through the vessel. This area of denuded vessel was then seeded with genetically altered endothelial cells that contained the beta-galactosidase gene. Approximately 2% to 11% of the cells adhered to the denuded blood vessel. Light microscopy showed the presence of beta-galactosidase staining primarily in the endothelial cells of the intima in experimentally seeded vessels.[35] These three experiments indicate that the vascular endothelial cell can be used to carry genetic information and that it may have a place in therapy for various diseases.

Several authors have indicated their concern about the presence of a retrovirus in the animal recipient. No retrovirus was detectable in the cell lines after numerous passages in vitro. The other concern is the longevity of the recombinant genes in vivo. The expression of beta-galactosidase appeared to be constant in the vessels examined up to 4 weeks after surgery. These experiments demonstrated the feasibility of introducing genetically altered endothelial cells in vivo and having them function. This technique could be useful after performing a balloon angioplasty and placing cells in the injured area to prevent thrombosis.

These three studies have demonstrated that genetically altered cells may have a place in vascular surgery. They could be altered to produce additional tPA to prevent thrombosis in small artificial grafts for distal bypass.[42] The cells could also be used to prevent further damage in atherosclerotic areas or to introduce a drug to a very specific area of the body.

Use of Retrovirus to Alter Hepatocytes

Liver transplantation is still necessary to treat liver failure even though other therapeutic modalities are being investigated. Hepatocyte transfer has been considered for both liver insufficiency and replacement of inherited liver metabolic defects. Hepatocyte transplantation still requires more refinement and there is still interest in the development of an artificial liver. However, it may be possible to correct hepatic metabolic defects using retroviral gene technology.

Moscioni and colleagues[34] used a retroviral gene vector to transfer a gene for beta-galactosidase and of hygromycin B phosphotransferase to groups of rats. One group of animals underwent a partial hepatectomy followed 24 hours later by introduction of the retrovirus. Two other groups of animals were used, one that had retrovirus introduced and then partial hepatectomy and a third group that had retrovirus introduced and no hepatectomy performed. Those animals that had successful uptake of retrovirus had undergone partial hepatectomy and later retroviral introduction. Previous attempts to introduce genes into mammalian cells were conducted in cultured rat and rabbit hepatocytes, but this study demonstrated that gene introduction can occur in vivo. It should be noted that the timing of the hepatectomy and later retroviral introduction was crucial. Partial hepatectomy results in peak DNA synthesis 24 hours after surgery, thus this is the optimal time for retroviral gene transfer into the hepatocytes. The authors hope to repeat the study in another animal model using hepatocyte mitogens before retroviral infusion.

This model demonstrates that there may be clinical applicability for introducing retroviral vectors that carry corrected genes to hepatocytes. This procedure may result in the correction of inherited metabolic liver defects, thereby preventing the need for whole organ liver transplantation in some patients.

SUMMARY

The possibility of using genetically altered cells is now available. This technology holds promise for multiple uses that include cancer therapy, drug delivery, and vascular surgery. Molecular biology will also provide increased understanding of cancer and immunology problems that have not been solved with previous technology. All these areas are extremely important to the surgeon who must have a basic knowledge of molecular biology to understand the papers and concepts as this field continues to expand rapidly.

GLOSSARY

base A purine (adenine or guanine) or a pyrimidine (uracil, cytosine, thymine) used in DNA or RNA.

centromere The narrowed region of the chromosome, which defines long and short arms.

double helix The twisted shape assumed by DNA when it is double stranded.

eucaryote Cells that have a nucleus with DNA that is surrounded by a double-layered membrane.

exons Portions of the genetic code that are represented in the final mRNA.

genome All of the genetic material of an organism, defined in terms of DNA.

initiator protein Binds to the origin sequence for DNA replication and directs the assembly of new DNA.

introns Intervening segment of genetic material that will be spliced out of the mRNA before translation into proteins.

messenger RNA (mRNA) A single-stranded copy of RNA, which is translated into protein.

Northern blot The analysis of size-separated RNA fragments onto nitrocellulose.

nucleotide One of the building blocks that makes DNA or RNA and is made up of a phosphate, a sugar, and a base.

Okazaki fragments Fragments of DNA 1000 to 2000 nucleotides long that are present in DNA replication. They are used to replicate the lagging daughter strand.

oncogene A cancer-inducing gene.

polymerase chain reaction (PCR) A rapid way to increase the amount of DNA in a test tube.

procaryote Cells without nuclei such as bacteria.

promoter A portion of DNA that signals expression of a gene. It is at the beginning of a gene and controls the expression of the particular gene.

proto-oncogene A normal gene that may become an oncogene.

recognition codon The end of the tRNA that is coded for a nucleotide sequence of a specific amino acid in the mRNA.

restriction endonuclease An enzyme from bacteria that cuts DNA at specific nucleotide sequences.

restriction sites A series of nucleotides at which a restriction enzyme will cut a portion of DNA.

ribosomal RNA (rRNA) Structural component of ribosomes for protein synthesis.

RNA polymerase The enzyme that binds to the promoter, unravels a portion of DNA, and is responsible for the production of mRNA.

small nuclear RNA Excises intron during mRNA processing.

Southern blot Analysis of size-separated DNA on nitrocellulose.

stop codon A combination of nucleotides which signal the end of transcription.

termination signal A series of nucleotides that signal the RNA to be released from the DNA template.

transcription Process by which a complementary copy of RNA is formed from DNA.

transfer RNA (tRNA) Nucleotides 70 to 80 nucleotides long that are encoded for a specific amino acid, which is brought to the site of protein synthesis in the cell.

vector A construct such as a virus into which a specific portion of DNA or RNA is introduced. This construct is then used to infect a cell or procaryote and introduce its own genetic code into the cell or procaryote.

Western blot The protein of interest is separated and transferred from an SDS-polyacrylamide gel.

REFERENCES

1 Abelson J, Butz E, editors: Recombinant DNA, *Science* 209:1317, 1980.

2 Ausobel FM, Brent R, Kingston RE et al, editors: *Current protocols in molecular biology,* New York, 1989, John Wiley & Sons.

3 Bloch W: A biochemical perspective of the polymerase chain reaction, *Biochemistry* 30:2735, 1991.

4 Bobo L, Coutlee F, Yolkin RH et al: Diagnosis of *Chlamydia trachomatis* in cervical infection by detection of amplified DNA with an enzyme immunoassay, *J Clin Microbiol* 28:1968, 1990.

5 Brisson-Noel A, Lecossier D, Nassif X et al: Rapid diagnosis of

tuberculosis by amplification of mycobacteria DNA in clinical samples, *Lancet* 2:1069, 1989.
6 Brown JM, Harken AH, Sharefkin JB: Recombinant DNA and surgery, *Ann Surg* 212:178, 1990.
7 Brutlag D, Kornberg A: Enzymatic synthesis of deoxyribonucleic acid: a proofreading function for the 3′ to 5′ exonuclease activity in DNA polymerases, *J Biol Chem* 247:241, 1972.
8 Capecchi M: High efficiency transformation by direct microinjection into cultured mammalian cells, *Cell* 22:479, 1980.
9 Caskey CT: Peptide chain termination, *Trends Biochem Sci* 5:234, 1980.
10 Clark B: The elongation step of protein biosynthesis, *Trends Biochem Sci* 5:207, 1980.
11 Courvalin P: Genotypic approach of bacterial resistance to antibiotics, *Antimicrob Agents Chemother* 35:1019, 1991.
12 Craigen WJ, Caskey CT: The function, structure, and regulation of *E. coli* peptide chain release factors, *Biochemie* 69:1031, 1987.
13 Crick FHC: The genetic code III, *Sci Am* 215(4):55, 1966.
14 Dalgleish AG: Viruses and cancer, *Br Med Bull* 47:21, 1991.
15 Darnell JE Jr: RNA in the molecules of life. *Readings from Scientific American,* New York, 1985, WH Freeman.
16 Davis LG, Dibner MD, Battey JF: *Basic methods in molecular biology*, New York, 1986, Elsevier.
17 Dodson M, Echols H, Wickner S et al: Specialized nucleoprotein structures at the origin of replication of bacteriophage lambda: localized unwinding of duplex DNA by a six-protein reaction, *Proc Natl Acad Sci USA* 83:7638, 1986.
18 Eglitis MA, Anderson WF: Retroviral vectors for introduction of genes into mammalian cells, *Biotechniques* 6:608, 1988.
19 Felsenfeld G: DNA in the molecules of life. *Readings from Scientific American,* New York, 1985, WH Freeman.
20 Fersht AR: Enzymatic editing mechanisms in protein synthesis and DNA replication, *Trends Biochem Sci* 5:262, 1980.
21 Goeddel DV, Heyneker HL, Hozumi T et al: Direct expression in *Escherichia coli* of a DNA sequence coding for human growth hormone, *Nature* 281:544, 1979.
22 Goeddel DV, Kleid DG, Bolivar F et al: Expression of chemically synthesized genes for human insulin, *Proc Natl Acad Sci USA* 76:106, 1979.
23 Gordon JW, Ruddle FH: Integration and stable germ line transmission of genes injected into mouse pronuclei, *Science* 214:1244, 1981.
24 Grunstein M, Hogness DS: Colony hybridization: a method for the isolation of cloned DNAs that contain a specific gene, *Proc Natl Acad Sci USA* 72:3961, 1975.
25 Hawley DK, McClure WR: Compilation and analysis of *Escherichia coli* promoter DNA sequences, *Nucleic Acids Res* 11:2237, 1983.
26 Hunt T: The initiation of protein synthesis, *Trends Biochem Sci* 5:178, 1980.
27 Inman RB, Schnos M: Structure of branch points in replicating DNA: presence of single-stranded connection in lambda DNA branch parts, *J Mol Biol* 56:319, 1971.
28 Itakura K, Hirose T, Crea R et al: Expression in *E. coli* of a chemically synthesized gene for the hormone somatostatin, *Science* 198:1056, 1977.
29 Kato N, Ou C-Y, Dato H et al: Identification of toxigenic *Clostridium difficile* by the polymerase chain reaction, *J Clin Microbiol* 29:33, 1991.
30 Malloy DC, Nauman RK, Paxton H: Detection of *Borrelia burgdorferi* using the polymerase chain reaction, *J Clin Microbiol* 28:1089, 1990.
31 McClure W: Mechanism and control of transcription initiation in prokaryotes, *Annu Rev Biochem* 54:171, 1985.
32 Modrich P: DNA mismatch correction, *Annu Rev Biochem* 56:435, 1987.
33 Moore PB: The ribosome returns, *Nature* 331:223, 1988.
34 Moscioni AD, Rozga J, Neuzil DF et al: In vivo regional delivery of retrovirally mediated foreign genes to rat liver cells: need for partial hepatectomy for successful foreign gene expression, *Surgery* 113:304, 1993.
35 Nabel EG, Plautz G, Boyce FM et al: Recombinant gene expression in vivo within endothelial cells of the arterial wall, *Science* 244:1342, 1989.
36 Noller HF: Structure of ribosomal RNA, *Annu Rev Biochem* 53:119, 1984.
37 Noller HF: Structure of ribosomal RNA, *Annu Rev Biochem* 53:119, 1984.
38 Ogawa T, Okazaki T: Discontinuous DNA replication, *Annu Rev Biochem* 49:421, 1980.
39 Pain VM: Initiation of protein synthesis in mammalian cells, *Biochem J* 235:625, 1986.
40 Palmiter RD, Brinster RL: Germ line transformation of mice, *Annu Rev Genet* 20:465, 1986.
41 Passaro E Jr, Hurwitz M, Samara G, Sawicki M: Molecular biology: an overview, *Am J Surg* 164:146, 1992.
42 Podrazik RM, Whitehill RA, Ekhterae D et al: High-level expression of recombinant human tPA in cultivated canine endothelial cells under varying conditions of retroviral gene transfer, *Ann Surg* 216:446, 1992.
43 Radman M, Wagner R: The high fidelity of DNA duplication, *Sci Am* 259 (2):40, 1988.
44 Robertson E, Bradley A, Kuehn M, Evans M: Germline transmission of genes introduced into cultured pluripotential cells by retroviral vector, *Nature* 323:445, 1986.
45 Rosenberg SA: Gene therapy for cancer, *JAMA* 268:2416, 1992.
46 Samara G, Hurwitz M, Sawicki M, Passaro E: Molecular mechanisms of tumor formation, *Am J Surg* 164:389, 1992.
47 Schimmel PR: Aminoacyl tRNA synthetases: general scheme of structure-function relationships in the polypeptides and recognition of transfer RNAs, *Annu Rev Biochem* 56:125, 1987.
48 Schimmel PR, Soll D, Abelson JN, editors: *Transfer RNA: structure, properties and recognition, and biological aspects* (2 vol), Cold Spring Harbor, NY, 1980, Cold Spring Harbor Laboratory.
49. Shigekawa I, Dower WJ: Electroporation of eukaryotes and prokaryotes: a general approach to the introduction of macromolecules into cells, *Biotechniques* 6:742, 1988.
50 Small JA, Scangos GA, Cork L et al: The early region of human papovavirus JC induces dysmyelination in transgenic mice, *Cell* 46:13, 1986.
51 Smith AE, Smith R, Paucha E: Characterization of different tumor antigens present in cells transformed by simian virus 40, *Cell* 18:335, 1979.
52 Smith HO: Nucleotide sequence specificity of restriction endonucleases, *Science* 205:455, 1979.
53 Southern EM: Detection of specific sequences among DNA fragments separated by gel electrophoresis, *J Mol Biol* 98:503, 1975.
54 Spradling AC, Rubin GM: Transposition of cloned P elements into Drosophila germ line chromosomes, *Science* 218:341, 1982.
55 Stacey A, Bateman J, Choi T et al: Perinatal lethal osteogenesis imperfecta in transgenic mice bearing an engineered mutant pro-α1(I) collagen gene, *Nature* 332:131, 1988.
56 Thomas KR, Capecchi MR: Site-directed mutagenesis by gene targeting in mouse embryo-derived stem cells, *Cell* 51:503, 1987.
57 Watson JD: The involvement of RNA in the synthesis of proteins, *Science* 140:17, 1963.
58 Watson JD, Crick FHC: Molecular structure of nucleic acid. Structure for deoxyribose nucleic acid, *Nature* 171:737, 1953.

59 Watson JD, Gilman M, Witkowski J, Zoller M: *Recombinant DNA,* New York, 1992, Scientific American Books, WH Freeman.
60 Weinberg RA: *The molecules of life: readings from Scientific American,* New York, 1985, WH Freeman.
61 White TJ, Madej R, Persing DH: The polymerase chain reaction: clinical applications, *Adv Clin Chem* 29:161, 1992.
62 Wilson JM, Birinyi LK, Salomon RN et al: Implantation of vascular grafts lined with genetically modified endothelial cells, *Science* 244:1344, 1989.
63 Zwiebel JA, Freeman SM, Kantoff PW et al: High-level recombinant gene expression in rabbit endothelial cells transduced by retroviral vectors, *Science* 243:220, 1989.

Trauma remains the leading cause of death in children and in adults throughout their working years. The "neglected disease of modern society," traumatic injury is a problem of epidemic proportions. However, care of the trauma patient has often been overlooked in medical education and deprived of the emphasis it deserves, even though traumatic injury involves an immeasurable loss in human potential and an enormous financial burden for the victims, their families, and society. We have provided a separate section on trauma to put this topic in proper perspective—and, more important, because any physician, regardless of specialty, may be called upon to aid a trauma victim. Part Two is a general source of information on the management of trauma resulting from various causes.

PART TWO

MANAGEMENT OF CRITICALLY ILL OR INJURED PATIENTS

CHAPTER

14

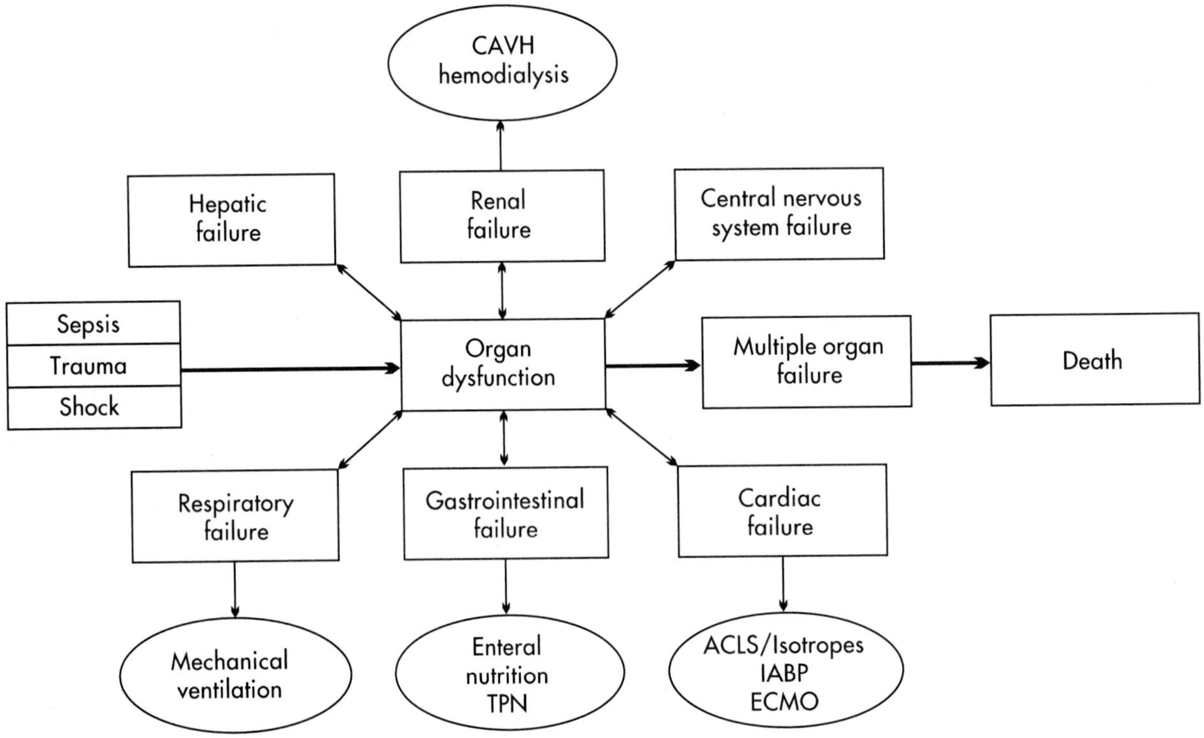

CAVH = Continuous arteriovenous hemofiltration
TPN = Total parenteral nutrition
ACLS = Advanced cardiac life support
IABP = Intraaortic balloon pump
ECMO = Extracorporeal membrane oxygenation

CRITICAL CARE

Steven R. Shackford • Frederick B. Rogers • Krista L. Kaups

The creation of specialized care units has spawned a medical discipline that has become known as "critical care." Critical care medicine focuses on the treatment of patients with severe illness and on prevention or early recognition of severe illness in high-risk patients. A busy surgeon cannot be at the bedside of a severely ill patient to manage firsthand each of the myriad of problems that can accompany critical surgical illness. Nevertheless, the surgeon should direct the consultative care provided by others to a surgical patient in the intensive care unit (ICU).

Because of its history and evolution, surgical critical care has embraced relatively complex technologies capable of measuring and calculating a host of physiologic parameters. The use of computers with these technologies allows derivation of a vast number of variables, available at a keystroke. Understandably, such "high-tech" medicine can lead to an arcane discipline that may intimidate the "nonintensivist" practitioner. Furthermore, the rapid availability of volumes of data on a critically ill patient can lead to information overload. The purpose of this chapter is to lessen the complexity and esoterism of surgical critical care, enabling the busy practitioner to decide when ICU care is useful, to understand recent changes in the discipline, and to focus on parameters relevant to the care of critically ill patients.

HISTORY

The surgeon's involvement in specialized care units began more than 100 years ago, when areas were created specifically for patients to recover from the effects of surgery. Such recovery rooms, immediately adjacent to the operating theater, were direct antecendents of today's specialized units.[23] As the complexity of surgical procedures increased and general anesthesia was developed, the specialized recovery areas evolved into comprehensive monitoring facilities with a specialized nursing staff. Initially, the medical management of patients in these units was directed by the operating surgeon. Later, anesthesiologists began to share this responsibility with surgeons, and the units became known as postanesthetic care units.[44] By 1940 the physicians and nurses staffing these units had become highly competent in the management of postoperative complications, to the extent that patients treated in the specialized units had significantly lower postoperative morbidity and mortality rates than patients not similarly treated.[44]

The application of temporary physiologic monitoring and support to nonsurgical patients was furthered by two events that occurred almost simultaneously: the development of positive pressure ventilation with endotracheal intubation, and the 1952 worldwide poliomyelitis epidemic. It became efficient to sequester and treat patients with acute and chronic respiratory failure in specialized respiratory care units. Respiratory units for the management of acute and chronic pulmonary failure were developed and refined. Care improved even further with the introduction of electrodes to measure blood gases.[46] The success of these units led to the creation of similar units to manage myocardial infarction, shock, and trauma. The acuity of illness and the severity of the physiologic derangements noted in these patients drove improvements in technology and accelerated the application of monitoring devices, which previously had been used only in the laboratory.[55] Examples of the improved technology included the development of portable hemodialysis systems and refinements in mechanical ventilators. Advances in cardiac surgery spawned a generation of systems to support the heart and lungs, and these soon found a ready application in the ICU.

Today the ICU and its staff can maintain or sustain failing organs to a degree not dreamed possible a decade ago. This degree of sophistication has evolved because of parallel developments in medicine and industry, which are likely to continue.

SERVICES ESSENTIAL TO AN INTENSIVE CARE UNIT

- Cardiopulmonary resuscitation
- Airway management (including endotracheal intubation and mechanical ventilation)
- Oxygen delivery systems and qualified respiratory therapists or registered nurses
- Emergency temporary cardiac pacing
- Continuous ECG monitoring
- Comprehensive laboratory service
- Nutritional support services
- Specialized physiologic monitoring equipment
- Portable life support equipment for use in patient transport

From Task Force on Guidelines, Society of Critical Care Medicine: *Crit Care Med* 16:808, 1988.

FUNCTION OF THE ICU

The functions of the ICU are determined primarily by the type of patient in need of care, the goals of treatment, and the therapies provided. The Society of Critical Care Medicine has published guidelines defining the patient in need of critical care.[56] These patients are divided into two categories: individuals who *are* physiologically unstable and therefore require continuous and coordinated physician, nursing, and respiratory care for constant surveillance and titration of therapy; and patients who *are at risk* for physiologic decompensation and thus require constant monitoring to prevent adverse occurrences. The first category comprises patients whose illness or injury poses an immediate threat to survival (e.g., hypothermic patients, coagulopathic victims of multiple trauma, or a patient who develops pneumonia and respiratory failure in the postoperative period). The second category includes patients with significant pre-existing disease (e.g., cardiac, pulmonary, or renal) who are at risk for exacerbation of underlying problems in the postoperative period, and patients at risk for postoperative physiologic perturbations because of the surgical procedure they underwent (e.g., craniotomy, aortic aneurysmectomy). It is estimated that as many as 45% of all ICU patients are admitted because they are at risk for medical or postoperative complications.[22]

One of the goals of ICU care is to ensure the immediate availability of physician, nursing, and respiratory personnel who have specific training and interest in the problems and therapies of critical illness. These personnel generally are physically located in the ICU and do not have responsibilities to other areas of the hospital. Because of the greater staffing demands of the critically ill, the patient-to-nurse ratio often ranges from 3 : 1 to 1 : 1, depending on the acuity of illness and the patient's status.

The ICU also provides continuous physiologic monitoring and therapies not available in other areas of the hospital. The range of technologies and interventions provided varies significantly with the size and type of unit, but continuous electrocardiographic (ECG) monitoring, pulse oximetry, invasive arterial monitoring, and mechanical ventilation are considered essential in most units. The Society of Critical Care Medicine has issued recommendations for the types of services available in a critical care setting (see the box above).

ICU Admission and Discharge Criteria

The admission and discharge criteria, priorities for the triage of patients to the ICU, should be established. For example, a patient who is critically ill or unstable and needs continuous monitoring or intensive treatment (e.g., ventilator support or continuous vasoactive drug infusion) should have a higher priority than a patient who is not critically ill but whose condition *may* deteriorate to the point that immediate intensive treatment may be needed. Lower priority patients are those who currently are stable but who could benefit from intensive monitoring and early detection of an adverse event (e.g., a patient with new-onset cardiac arrhythmia who may have had a myocardial infarction). The lowest priority patients are those who are critically ill or unstable but whose previous state of health, underlying disease, or acute illness severely reduces the likelihood of recovery or benefit from ICU treatment. When ICU beds are limited, high-priority patients are admitted in preference to lower priority patients. Discharge from the ICU is appropriate when the reason for admission no longer exists and the patient no longer requires intensive monitoring or therapy. Discharge may also be appropriate if the patient's condition has worsened or failed to improve, and there is no anticipated benefit from further intensive therapy.

Organization of the ICU

The design of an ICU is both a physical and an administrative issue. The physical structure should allow patients to be gathered in a single geographic area so that monitoring and interventional equipment can be used most efficiently. Individual patient rooms provide privacy and allow isolation, to reduce the spread of infection. The rooms must be large enough to allow for bulky life support equipment, such as ventilators, dialysis machines, and intra-aortic balloon pumps. Frequently needed supplies and sinks for handwashing should be available in the patient's room. A centralized nurses' station, where every patient can be observed at all times either directly or by closed-circuit camera, is essential. Monitored data should be relayed to a centralized station. Classrooms, a lounge area, a locker-room for staff members, and a waiting area for the patients' families are also essential.

The ICU director should be responsible for patient care, administration of the ICU, and education of the staff. Administrative responsibilities include triage and bed allocation, discharge planning, development of unit policies, participation in quality improvement activities, and interaction with other departments to facilitate smooth operation of the ICU. To be effective in unit management, the ICU director must have the authority to control admissions, discharges, and bed allocation and to intervene, when appropriate, in patient care.

Intensive care in a tertiary care center often is provided by a team directed by an intensivist. In addition to the physicians and nurses, team members may include a respiratory therapist, a pharmacist, and a nutritionist. ICUs that use the team approach have shown an improved outcome, especially when the team is directed by an intensivist with formal education in critical care.[8]

COSTS RELATED TO ICU PATIENT CATEGORY

"Low cost" ICU patients
- Monitoring only; generally leave ICU in 1 or 2 days
- Intensive short-term conventional therapy

"Higher cost" ICU patients
- Extensive ICU therapies; die within a few days
- Typical ICU patients

"Highest cost" ICU patients
- Extensive ICU therapies; spend weeks in ICU
- Probability of hospital mortality in moderate range
- Outcome opposite that predicted at the time of ICU admission
- Transferred from another hospital
- Multiple admissions to the ICU
- Delayed admission to the ICU
- Multiple organ system failure

From Rippe JM, Irwin RS, Alpert JS, Fink MP: *Intensive care medicine,* Boston, 1991, Little, Brown.

ICU Charges

Critical care services consume 15% to 20% ($20 billion to $30 billion) of the health care dollars directed toward hospital care; this equates to 4% of the gross national product of the United States.[7] It is little wonder that the ICU is sometimes referred to as the "expensive care unit." Along with the growing realization of the cost of critical care is the realization that its benefits have not been proven.

Currently 50% to 80% of ICU direct costs are for personnel.[22] Patients hospitalized in an ICU receive approximately three times as much nursing care (nurse-to-patient ratios 1:1 or 1:2) as ward patients (1:6 or more). In addition to the personnel costs, it is estimated that a minimum of $10,000 per year in capital expense is required to support each critical care bed.[7] Thus a day in the ICU costs three to four times as much as a hospital day on a general floor.

A large portion of the critical care resources are used by a small portion of the patients. For example, only 5.8% of ICU patients receive prolonged mechanical ventilation (longer than 7 days), yet they consume 37% of all ICU resources.[39] Furthermore, it has been estimated that 65% of the total annual resources encumbered by the delivery of critical care is expended for the support of patients who are not likely to survive (see the box above). In fact, nonsurvivors consume more ICU days per patient than do survivors, and ICU charges constitute a greater proportion of the total hospital charges for nonsurvivors than for survivors.

Clearly, the allocation of resources for critical care will change in the future; we simply cannot afford the current system. One proposed solution is that the ICU designate a physician who is uninvolved in patient care but who will serve as a resource allocator or gatekeeper and triage patients accordingly.[39] Greater emphasis also will be placed on assessing the usefulness of technologies before their widespread use; this was not done previously with many of the devices now indigenous to the ICU. For example, flow-directed pulmonary artery catheters became the standard of care before their efficacy in improving outcome was established. Limited resources most likely will reduce the number of critical care beds. This may not necessarily portend an adverse situation, however, because we already have a higher percentage of critical care beds than any other country. For example, approximately 1.5% of hospital beds in New Zealand are allocated to intensive care, compared to the approximately 6% to 10% so allocated in the United States.[28] In Japan, 2% of hospital beds are committed to critical care, whereas in most European countries 2% to 4% of beds are designated to critical care.[49]

MONITORING

The word "monitor" comes from the Latin *monitus,* meaning "to warn." The purpose of closely monitoring critically ill patients is to detect physiologic derangement as early as possible, allowing timely intervention. However, the benefits of advanced monitoring systems can be derived only if the individuals using them understand the indications for their use and the limitations of the technology. Furthermore, the use of monitoring systems is no substitute for frequent physical assessment.

Arterial Catheter

Indications

Arterial catheters are inserted to continuously measure arterial blood pressure and to provide access to arterial blood for the purpose of determining oxygen and carbon dioxide tensions (blood gas analysis). There are no absolute indications of the use of arterial catheters. Because sphygmomanometry frequently underestimates the blood pressure in patients in shock[10] and overestimates blood pressure in hypertensive patients with severe atherosclerosis,[34] these patients should have an arterial pressure monitor inserted. Patients receiving a vasoactive drug, or any patient requiring arterial puncture three or more times a day for blood gas analysis, should also have an arterial catheter. The most commonly used arteries are the radial, dorsalis pedis, femoral, axillary, brachial, and temporal arteries.

Complications

Thrombosis and infection are the two major complications of arterial catheters. The size of the cannula and the duration of monitoring are the factors that most influence the rate of thrombosis. Catheters larger than 20 gauge[12] and catheters left in place for longer than 3 days[6] increase the rate of thrombosis. For example, radial artery cannulation with a 20-gauge catheter for 1 to 3 days produced an arterial occlusion rate of 11%, whereas those in place for 4 to 10 days had an occlusion rate of 29% ($p < 0.05$).[6] Only 10% of the patients with occluded radial arteries developed ischemic necrosis of the skin in the affected hand. Distal embolization or hand ischemia following radial catheterization is extremely rare. Most radial arteries eventually recanalize after removal of the catheter.

The risk of life-threatening septicemia from arterial catheters is less than that associated with intravenous devices. Two factors that have been reported to increase the incidence of arterial catheter infections are duration longer than 4 days and insertion via cutdown.[3] Site (e.g., radial artery, femoral artery) does not appear to affect infection rates.

Pitfalls of Arterial Monitoring

Damping of the waveform may produce a discrepancy between the actual intravascular pressure and the recorded pressure. Both overdamping and underdamping are possible. An overdamped system can be caused by air bubbles in the fluid-filled system, by overly compliant tubing connecting the cannula to the transducer, or by the presence of injection ports between the patient and the transducer. The result is a widened, slurred pressure with the systolic and diastolic pressures converging toward the mean arterial pressure. This results in an erroneously low systolic and erroneously high diastolic pressure. An underdamped system usually is caused by excessive tubing length (longer than 3 feet) but can also

TABLE 14-1 MEASURED HEMODYNAMIC PARAMETERS OBTAINABLE FROM A PULMONARY ARTERY CATHETER

PARAMETER	ABBREVIATION	NORMAL VALUE
Central venous pressure	CVP	2-8 mm Hg
Right atrial pressure	RAP	2-8 mm Hg
Pulmonary artery pressure	PAP	Diastole: 5-12 mm Hg Systole: 15-30 mm Hg Mean: 5-10 mm Hg
Pulmonary capillary wedge pressure	PCWP	2-12 mm Hg
Cardiac output	CO	3-7 L/min
Mixed venous oxygen saturation	SvO_2	75%
Core temperature	T	37° C (98.6° F)

be seen in patients with tachycardia and a high systemic vascular resistance. The result is a narrow, peaked waveform where the systolic and diastolic pressures diverge from the mean arterial pressure, resulting in an erroneously high systolic and an erroneously low diastolic pressure. Because of the problems encountered with damping artifact, it is more accurate to follow the mean arterial pressure, since it is minimally affected by either overdamping or underdamping.

Positive pressure ventilation may affect the arterial waveform in a biphasic manner. In early inspiration, the systolic blood pressure increases, and in late inspiration and early expiration, the systolic blood pressure decreases. The decrease in systolic blood pressure with mechanical ventilation is more pronounced during hypovolemia (so-called cycling with the ventilator). The mean arterial pressure will remain accurate and should be the parameter monitored during positive pressure ventilation.

Pulmonary Artery Catheter

Indications

Since the pulmonary artery catheter (PAC) was introduced into clinical practice in 1970,[55] it has become a common resource in the management of the critically ill. The PAC can provide directly measured data (Table 14-1) and derived variables (Table 14-2).

The pulmonary capillary wedge pressure (PCWP) is one of the most important parameters measured with the PAC. Because there are no valves between the left atrium and pulmonary artery, inflation of the balloon and occlusion of flow in the pulmonary artery allows back pressure from the left atrium to be measured at the tip of the catheter. Thus the PCWP is an approximation of the left ventricular end-diastolic pressure and can be used to judge the adequacy of the left ventricular filling pressure (preload). Monitoring left ventricular function is important, because the function of the ventricles may be disparate in critically ill patients. As such, a patient may be in frank left ventricular failure and manifest normal right heart filling pressures (i.e., have a normal central venous pressure [CVP]). The PCWP also gives information about the pulmonary microvascular pressure. A high PCWP (over 18 mm Hg) implies an elevated pulmonary capillary hydrostatic pressure. A PCWP below 25 mm Hg, secondary to left heart failure or fluid overload, usually results in fluid translocation out of the capillaries into the pulmonary interstitium, producing pulmonary edema. If a patient has clinical manifestations of interstitial or alveolar edema (e.g., as seen in chest radiograph or arterial blood gases), without an elevation in the PCWP, an increase in the microvascular permeability (such as seen in sepsis) should be suspected. The distinction between edema caused by cardiac failure and edema caused by a permeability defect is critical, because the treatment approaches are radically different.

Cardiac output (CO) can be measured by thermodilution using the Fick principle.[14] The cardiac index (CI) normalizes the CO to a patient's body surface area (BSA). A low CI can be seen in hypovolemia or heart failure. Septic shock is usually characterized by a high CI.

The systemic vascular resistance (SVR) is a derived value that attempts to quantify the peripheral vascular tone, or "afterload." The SVR of the peripheral vascular bed is influenced by nervous, hormonal, chemical, and physical stimuli. For example, hypovolemia causes the release of vasoactive mediators, which produce vasoconstriction and an abnormally high SVR. The hemodynamic profile of some commonly encountered physiologic perturbations are shown in Table 14-3.

Mixed venous blood, sampled from the pulmonary

TABLE 14-2 DERIVED HEMODYNAMIC PARAMETERS OBTAINABLE FROM A PULMONARY ARTERY CATHETER

PARAMETER	ABBREVIATION	FORMULA FOR CALCULATION	NORMAL VALUE
Cardiac index	CI	$\frac{\text{Cardiac output (CO)}}{\text{Body surface area (BSA)}}$	2.5-4 L/min/m^2
Stroke volume	SV	$\frac{\text{Cardiac output}}{\text{Heart rate (HR)}}$	60 ml/beat
Systemic vascular resistance	SVR	$\frac{\text{(Mean arterial pressure [MAP]} - \text{CVP)80}}{\text{CO}}$	800-1200 dynes/sec/cm^{-5}
Pulmonary vascular resistance	PVR	$\frac{\text{(PAP} - \text{PCWP)80}}{\text{CO}}$	150-250 dynes/sec/cm^{-5}
Left ventricular stroke work index	LVSWI	SVRI*(MAP − CVP)(0.0136)	43-61 g/m/m^2
Arterial oxygen content	CaO_2	1.36(Hgb)(SaO_2†) + 0.003 PaO_2	20 ml O_2/dl
Mixed venous oxygen O_2/dl content	CVO_2	1.36(Hgb)(SvO_2‡) + 0.003 PaO_2	5 ml
Oxygen delivery	DO_2	CO (CaO_2)	800-1200 ml/min
Oxygen consumption	VO_2	CO (CaO_2 − CvO_2)	225-275 ml/min

* SVRI: Systemic vascular resistance index
†SaO_2: Arterial hemoglobin saturation (%)
‡SvO_2: Venous hemoglobin saturation (%)

TABLE 14-3 CHARACTERISTIC HEMODYNAMIC PROFILES OF DISEASES COMMONLY ENCOUNTERED IN THE ICU

	PCWP	CI	SVR
Hypovolemia	↓	↓	↑
Cardiac failure	↑	↓	↑
Early sepsis	↔	↑↑	↓

CI, Cardiac index; *PCWP,* pulmonary capillary wedge pressure; *SVR,* systemic vascular resistance.

artery through the distal port of the PAC, is useful in determining the adequacy of oxygen delivery. A low mixed venous partial pressure of oxygen (Po_2) (normal: 40 mm Hg, 75% saturation) indicates increased extraction by the peripheral tissues, suggesting compensation for reduced flow (decreased perfusion). A high mixed venous Po_2 indicates decreased extraction, suggesting high flows (increased perfusion), a peripheral arteriovenous shunt, or uncoupling of oxidative phosphorylation—as may occur in tissue death. If the catheter is improperly positioned and blood is obtained from the superior vena cava (i.e., not true mixed venous blood), it may have a falsely elevated Po_2 because it doesn't include venous blood from the cardiac circulation (which is markedly desaturated). Blood from the right atrium may have a falsely low Po_2 if the sample is taken too close to the coronary sinus. Blood from the inferior vena cava may have a relatively high venous oxygen saturation, because it contains the venous effluent from the kidney, which extracts little oxygen and receives approximately 20% of the cardiac output.

When making clinical decisions using the mixed venous blood, the physician should rely more on the hemoglobin saturation in the mixed venous blood than on the actual Po_2. The Po_2 of mixed venous blood lies on the steep portion of the oxyhemoglobin dissociation curve, and a minor error in measuring the partial pressure can produce a major error when calculating saturation. Catheters are now commercially available that are equipped with an oximeter at the tip that can continuously measure mixed venous O_2 saturation (Svo_2) by means of spectrophotometry. The benefit of continuous Svo_2 monitoring is that an abrupt drop in saturation may be an early indicator of deranged cardiopulmonary function. Continuous Svo_2 monitoring may not only result in improved patient care,[2] but also decrease the number of arterial blood gas (ABG), cardiac output, and hemoglobin determinations that need to be monitored, thus decreasing cost.[20]

Optimal hemodynamic function is best assessed by measuring tissue perfusion. Currently tissue perfusion cannot be measured directly. However, it can be assessed indirectly from the derived variables of oxygen delivery (Do_2) and oxygen consumption (Vo_2). Because oxygen is not stored in the tissues, metabolism depends on oxygen delivery by the blood. The amount of oxygen uptake by tissues, or oxygen consumption, depends on metabolic demand. Usually an excess of oxygen is delivered to make up for any increase in metabolic demand. When Do_2 falls below a critical threshold (approximately 300 to 330 ml/min/m^2), oxygen consumption is decreased because of reduced oxygen availability, and a tissue oxygen debt arises. This results in anaerobic metabolism, with production of lactic acid and a metabolic acidosis. This indicates reduced perfusion, even though other parameters of hemodynamic function, such as CI or CVP, may be normal. Thus it is necessary to measure CI and calculate Do_2 and Vo_2 to determine the adequacy of tissue perfusion in critically ill patients.

Core temperature, which can be measured with the thermistor at the tip of a PAC, is less likely to be influenced by transient changes in the ambient temperature of the surrounding environment; therefore it is a more accurate reflection of body temperature than peripherally determined values.

Several types of clinical situations can arise in which the catheter is helpful in decision making: (1) cardiac function compromised by myocardial infarction; (2) severe pulmonary disorders that require mechanical ventilatory support *and* positive end-expiratory pressure (PEEP) of 15 cm H_2O or higher; (3) cardiac dysfunction requiring two or more vasoactive drugs or aortic balloon counterpulsation to maintain perfusion; (4) multiple organ failure with sepsis and cardiac dysfunction; and (5) elective surgical procedures in patients with significant underlying myocardial disease who are at high risk for perioperative myocardial dysfunction.

Insertion

Pulmonary artery catheters are manufactured in a variety of sizes and lengths to fit each patient's needs. The most widely used is a No. 7 French (Fr), 110 cm long, four-lumen catheter (Figure 14-1). At the tip is a balloon, which is connected to a balloon inflation port. A port to measure pulmonary artery pressure and, when the balloon is inflated, pulmonary capillary wedge pressure is also located at the tip of the catheter. A thermistor port, close to the tip, is connected by insulated wires to a plug, which can be plugged into a computer that can calculate the CO by thermal dilution. The most proximal port is used to measure CVP and to inject cold saline for CO determinations. Newer generation catheters have additional lumens for a fiberoptic oximetry system to continuously monitor mixed venous oxygen saturation and for drug infusion.

The PAC usually is inserted under sterile conditions, commonly via the subclavian or internal jugular vein. After all lines are flushed, the balloon is checked to ensure that it is functional, and the proximal and distal

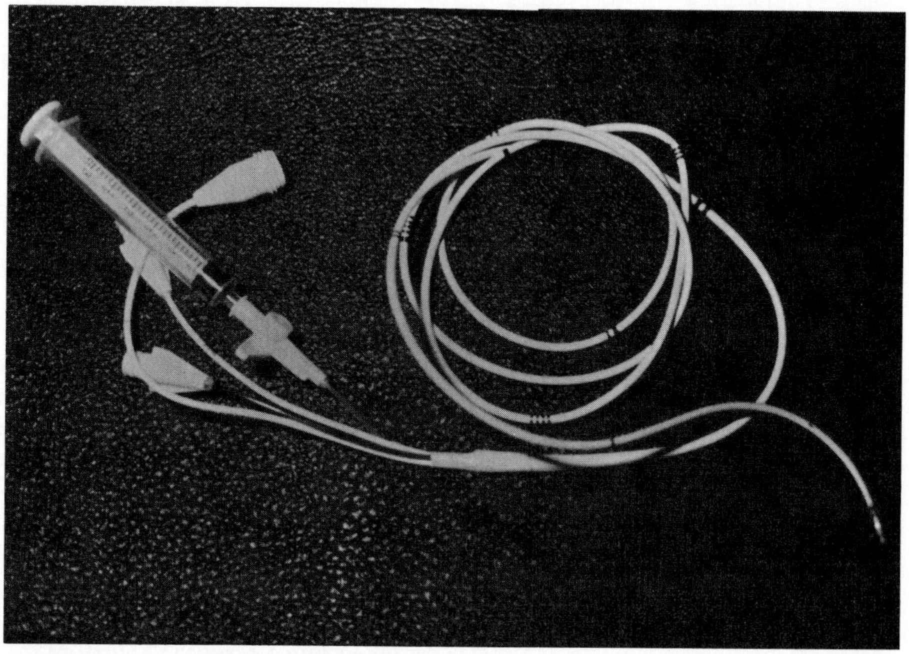

FIGURE 14-1 Pulmonary artery catheter. Note the syringe connected to the balloon inflation port. Also note the marks along the catheter, which indicate the distance in centimeters from the tip (1 mark = 10 cm). (From Voyce SJ, Urbach D, Rippe JM: Atlas of procedures in the intensive care unit. In Rippe JM, editor: *Intensive care medicine,* ed 2, Boston, 1991, Little, Brown.)

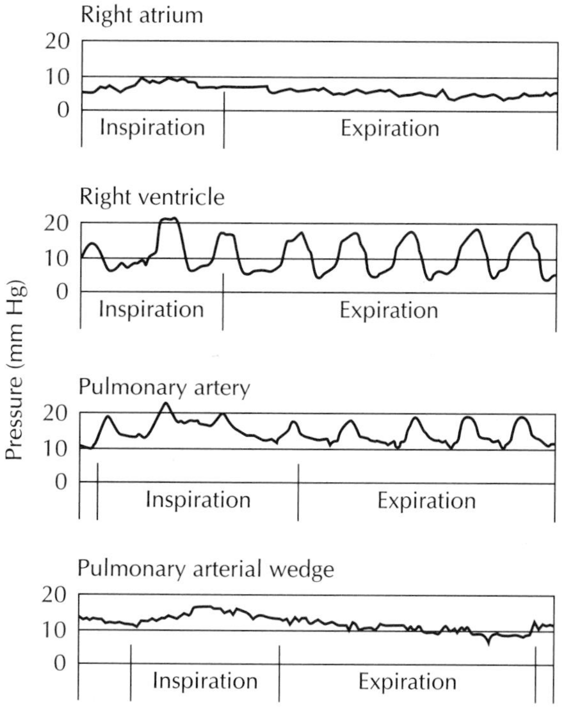

FIGURE 14-2 Pressure tracings commonly seen during insertion of a pulmonary artery catheter through the right atrium, right ventricle, and pulmonary artery. With balloon inflation the catheter will "float" into the "wedge" position. (From Abrams JH, Cerra F, Holcroft JW: Care in the ICU: cardiopulmonary monitoring. In Erhlich N, editor: *Care of the surgical patient,* New York, 1989, Scientific American Medicine.)

ports are connected to pressure transducers attached to continuous pressure display monitors. After the catheter is inserted into the vein, it is advanced approximately 15 cm, where variation in pressure is seen on the monitor, with respiration confirming that the PAC is in the thorax (Figure 14-2). The balloon is then inflated and the catheter advanced, directed by flow through the right atrium, right ventricle, and pulmonary outflow tract and into the pulmonary artery (Figure 14-2). Once entry into the pulmonary artery has been confirmed, the catheter is advanced until a wedge tracing appears (seen as a dampening of the pulmonary artery waveform). The balloon is then deflated, and the pulmonary artery waveform should return. Reinflation of the balloon should produce a wedge tracing. The catheter is secured in place with the balloon in a deflated position. A chest radiograph should be done to confirm the position of the catheter. The tip of the catheter should be just distal to the right or left main pulmonary artery in the right or left lower lung fields.

Complications

Ventricular arrhythmia, which has been reported in as many as 60% of patients undergoing right heart catheterization,[53] is one of the most common complications of the PAC. Therefore monitoring of the ECG is essential while the PAC is being inserted and while it is in place. Using prophylactic lidocaine and fully inflating the balloon (so that the catheter tip does not protrude into the wall of the ventricle) may decrease ectopy during insertion. If ectopy occurs, the catheter tip must be withdrawn from the ventricle.

Two of the most significant complications of the PAC are pulmonary infarction and rupture of the pulmonary artery. A catheter that is advanced too far peripherally can occlude the blood supply to a segment of lung, resulting in a wedge-shaped infiltrate or infarct. If the balloon is overinflated, the pulmonary artery can rupture. This complication is rare (occurs in 0.2% of catheterizations), but it can lead to massive exsanguinating hemoptysis.[32] Less significant complications include rupture of the balloon and infection at the insertion site. Balloon rupture is another of those complications that become more likely the longer the catheter is in place. Other than losing monitoring capability, the complication is self-limited. However, air embolism could occur if repeated attempts are made to inflate a ruptured balloon. Infection rates are low if the catheter is removed within 72 hours. The catheter sepsis rate associated with the PAC is less than 1%.[35] There have been reports of right-sided septic endocarditis following insertion of a PAC, but this is rare.[21]

Pitfalls of PAC Monitoring

The PCWP measurement will be erroneous if the PAC is located in a branch of the pulmonary artery where blood flow is decreased. Because flow is decreased, the hydrostatic pressure in the capillary will be low, and the pressure measured by the PAC will be more a reflection of alveolar pressure than the PCWP. Thus, for a PAC to reflect an accurate PCWP, it should not be located in arteries of the pulmonary apex where blood flow is relatively low compared to the lung base. Because the catheter is flow directed, it usually goes to the regions or zones where blood flow is greatest.

The PCWP may be erroneously elevated during positive pressure ventilation, especially if PEEP is being used. Positive pressure ventilation increases intra-alveolar pressure during inflation of the lungs, and that increase is transmitted directly to the intrathoracic vessels. The effect of positive pressure ventilation on the PCWP can be exaggerated during hypovolemia, because pulmonary blood flow is reduced. In such cases the PCWP will be more a reflection of the alveolar pressure (which will be high because of the positive pressure) than the capillary hydrostatic pressure (which will be low as a result of hypovolemia). Therefore, to accurately assess cardiac filling pressures in such patients, the PCWP should be measured between ventilatory cycles at end expiration.

Mitral regurgitation can lead to the erroneous assumption that the PAC will not "wedge." Mitral regurgitation produces large "V" waves on the PCWP tracing as a result of regurgitation of blood from the left ventricle into the left atrium and pulmonary veins during systole. These large "V" waves can easily be mistaken for a PAP waveform. However, the "V" wave occurs *after* the "T" wave on the ECG, whereas the PAP wave occurs *before* the "T" wave. Attempts to push the catheter more distally to "wedge" it poses the risk of lung infarction or rupture of the pulmonary artery.

Pulse Oximetry

Pulse oximetry assesses hemoglobin saturation by sensing the difference in light absorption between reduced (red) and unreduced (blue) hemoglobin. The transmitter light is received by a photodiode placed on the skin overlying a superficial capillary bed (e.g., nail bed, ear, nose), which is programmed to calculate the oxygen saturation in each pulse by the ratio of the wave lengths of the reduced and unreduced hemoglobin.

Indications

Pulse oximetry is useful in clinical situations in which hypoxemia may be common, such as during intubation or immediately after surgery.[51] It provides a dynamic assessment of oxygen saturation, which is useful in determining the efficacy of interventions intended to improve or prevent hypoxemia (e.g., intubation, increased inspired oxygen concentration). Pulse oximetry also aids in weaning from mechanical ventilation and can decrease the number of blood gas determinations.

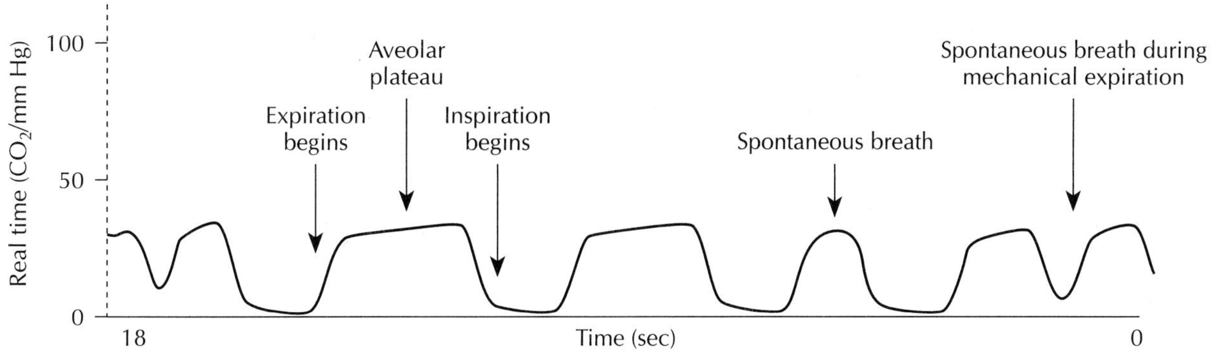

FIGURE 14-3 End-tidal carbon dioxide ($ETCO_2$) tracing (capnogram) during mechanical and spontaneous ventilation. The CO_2 concentration, in millimeters of mercury (mm Hg), is located on the ordinate, and the time, in seconds, is on the abscissa. CO_2 concentration is increased in the exhaled breath. (From Carlon GC, Cole R, Miodownik S et al: *Crit Care Med* 16:551, 1988.)

Pitfalls of Pulse Oximetry Monitoring

Any disruption of the interface between the sensing probe and the skin (e.g., wetness, edema, motion) interferes with the absorption of transmitted light and will invalidate the reading. Local factors such as temperature or vasoconstriction may also affect the measurement.[41] The earlobe is thought to be the best site for the pulse oximeter, because it is the least affected by vasoconstriction artifact. Factors that can cause a falsely low saturation reading include (1) nail polish; (2) dark skin; (3) intravascular methylene blue; and (4) hyperlipidemia. Conditions that can produce elevated saturation reading include (1) hypothermia; (2) carbon monoxide poisoning; and (3) hyperbilirubinemia.

End-Tidal Carbon Dioxide Monitoring (Capnography)

Capnography measures the carbon dioxide (CO_2) concentration in the exhaled breath by infrared spectrometry. The waveform shows variations in the amount of CO_2 throughout the respiratory cycle and is called a capnogram (Figure 14-3). Capnography is becoming routine in the intensive care unit for determining the presence or absence of tidal ventilation.

Indications

Capnography is useful for detecting esophageal intubation, airway obstruction, or unintentional extubation. It is extremely valuable in emergency airway management.[37] Attempts have been made to use end-tidal CO_2 ($ETCO_2$) monitoring as an alternative to arterial blood gas determination when weaning patients from mechanical ventilation.[24] However, because significant changes in the arterial partial pressure of carbon dioxide ($PaCO_2$) correlate poorly with changes in $ETCO_2$, capnography is not recommended for this purpose. Continuous monitoring of the $ETCO_2$ during CPR has been used to predict the outcome. Resuscitation was more likely to be successful in patients who showed an abrupt increase in $ETCO_2$.[15]

Pitfalls of $ETCO_2$ Monitoring

In healthy individuals, the difference between $ETCO_2$ and arterial CO_2 is approximately ± 1.5 mm Hg. This differential is due to a combination of dead space ventilation and intrapulmonary shunt. Conditions that lower the $ETCO_2$ relative to the PCO_2 (increased dead space ventilation) include pulmonary embolism, atelectasis, pulmonary edema, pneumothorax, or chronic obstructive pulmonary disease.

Conditions such as trauma and sepsis in which the metabolic rate is increased will increase the absolute $ETCO_2$. In these circumstances the $ETCO_2$ is an accurate reflection of the PCO_2. Any condition that causes a decreased metabolic rate, such as hypothermia, general anesthesia, or hypothyroidism, will correspondingly decrease CO_2 production and lower the $ETCO_2$.

Central Venous Pressure Monitoring

Indications

Central venous pressure (CVP) can be used as an assessment of right heart function, and when combined with the PCWP can be used to calculate pulmonary vascular resistance.

Insertion

The common sites of insertion of CVP catheters are the subclavian, internal jugular, external jugular, and antecubital veins. The internal jugular and subclavian sites are the two most commonly used. The subclavian site generally is more comfortable for the patient and easier to maintain.

Complications

Early complications are related to insertion. Pneumothorax occurs in 1% to 5% of cases and is more frequently encountered with the subclavian approach.[13] Bleeding, which occurs in up to 5% of cases, usually can be stopped by applying pressure. If the subclavian artery is punctured, the bleeding can be controlled by applying pressure above and below the clavicle. If a puncture of the artery is not recognized and the artery is inadvertently cannulated, significant bleeding can occur. Arterial puncture can also result in arteriovenous fistula or pseudoaneurysm. Other complications associated with insertion of a CVP catheter are air embolism, retained catheter fragment, nerve injury (phrenic, brachial plexus, recurrent laryngeal nerve, or sympathetic trunk), tracheal injury, and injury to the thoracic duct, producing a chylous pleural effusion.

Thrombosis and infection are late complications. Thrombosis often is clinically occult, with the diagnosis being suspected in fewer than 10% of vessels demonstrated to be thrombosed by venography. The risk of infection increases geometrically if the catheter has been in place for 3 days or longer.[33] Studies of risk factors for nosocomial infection, as determined by multivariate analysis of prospectively collected data, show that catheters left in place for longer than 3 days have an increased risk of catheter sepsis that is 1.8 times that of those left in less than 3 days.[33] Triple-lumen catheters are thought to present the highest risk of infection because of the increased number of ports for intravenous access. However, several studies have shown that the infection rate of triple-lumen catheters is comparable to that for single-lumen catheters when the former are properly maintained.[36] The practice of changing a CVP catheter over a guide wire is logical in the evaluation of a febrile patient with no obvious source of infection. If the catheter is identified as the source of infection, the CVP access is changed to a new site.

MONITORING EQUIPMENT

Pitfalls

An inadequate dynamic response can lead to inaccuracies in the pressure reading. The dynamic response of a system is determined by its resonant frequency and damping coefficient. When the frequency of the pressure waveform approaches the resonant frequency (3 to 5 hertz [Hz] in arterial lines), amplification of the signal, or "ringing," occurs. To prevent ringing, monitoring systems have a resonant frequency above 20 Hz. The system component most likely to cause amplification of the pressure is noncompliant tubing between the patient and the transducer. The damping coefficient is a measure of how quickly an oscillating system comes to rest. For example, compliant tubing has a high damping coefficient and absorbs energy, resulting in a decreased transmitted waveform. A system with noncompliant tubing has a low damping coefficient and causes an increased pressure waveform. A quick bedside test of the efficiency of the transducing system is called a flash-flush. The pigtail of the continuous flush device is pulled and quickly released, which should generate a characteristic square waveform. Over-damped signals are usually due to air bubbles, kinking, or compliant tubing; underdamping can be due to tubing that is too long (Figure 14-4).

CARDIAC RESUSCITATION

Initial Management

Cardiac arrest in the ICU is usually a witnessed event, because the patients are continuously monitored. Initiation of cardiopulmonary resusciatation (CPR) has sev-

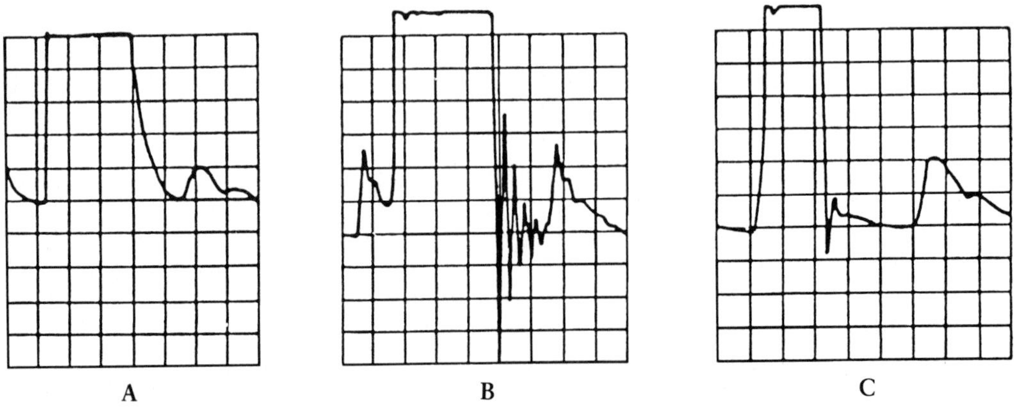

FIGURE 14-4 Flash-flush test. **A,** Overdamped system. **B,** Underdamped system. **C,** Optimal damping. (From Seneff M. In Rippe JM, editor: *Intensive care medicine,* ed 2, Boston, 1991, Little, Brown.)

eral components, the first ones being the "ABCs" of basic life support and simultaneous summoning of help. The ABCs consist of airway management, breathing, and circulation. If the patient has not been intubated, the airway is opened with either a chin-lift or jaw-thrust maneuver to clear the upper airway. The practitioner must assess whether spontaneous respirations are present. If not, bag-mask ventilation is begun. The airway should be secured by means of tracheal intubation to lessen the risk of aspiration, to increase the fraction of inspired oxygen (FiO_2), and to provide more efficient tidal ventilation. The presence of a blood pressure is confirmed by a pulse check of the carotid artery. If no pulse is present, closed chest cardiac compressions are begun after the patient has been placed on a back board. Cardiac compressions should be done at a rate of 80 to 100/minute, and the adequacy of compressions should be assessed by searching for a palpable pulse in the femoral or carotid artery. If the patient has an arterial cannula, the adequacy of compressions can be gauged by observing the pressure tracing on the monitor. During CPR the mean arterial pressure seldom exceeds 40 mm Hg and coronary artery blood flow ceases, worsening the cardiac ischemia. Intravenous access, if not previously available, should be obtained, preferably in a central venous location to permit direct cardiac administration of drugs. If not already in place, cardiac monitoring electrodes should be placed to assess the underlying cardiac rhythm. The ABCs of basic life support serve only to temporize until the therapies of defibrillation and drugs can be given.

Ventricular Fibrillation

Successful resuscitation of a patient with ventricular fibrillation requires rapid electrical defibrillation (Figure 14-5).

Electromechanical Dissociation

Electromechanical dissociation (EMD) is a condition in which an electrical complex is present on the monitor, but the patient has no effective pulse. This can be caused by cardiac tamponade, hypovolemia, tension pneumothorax, and pulmonary embolism. When the diagnosis of EMD is made and the patient has either tamponade or hypovolemia, preparation should begin for left thoracotomy, aortic cross-clamping, and open chest massage.

Asystole

Asystole, or cardiac standstill, should be confirmed in two leads of the ECG. The practitioner must be sure that fine ventricular fibrillation is not being interpreted as a "flat-line ECG." The mainstays of therapy are epinephrine, bicarbonate, atropine, and pacing (Figure 14-6).

Ventricular Tachycardia

Once ventricular tachycardia has been confirmed, a decision regarding the stability of patient's condition is essential. If the condition is stable, intravenous antiarrhythmic drugs are the treatment of choice. If the patient's condition is unstable, electrical cardioversion is indicated (Figure 14-7).

MECHANICAL SUPPORT FOR FAILING ORGANS

Of all the technologies that seem to dissociate or differentiate the ICU from the rest of the hospital, the "hardware" for supporting failing organs is the most noticeable. The most common of these devices are ventilators and hemodialysis machines. Specialized ICUs also have machines to support the heart (balloon pumps) and both the heart and lungs (extracorporeal oxygenation and carbon dioxide removal).

Mechanical Ventilation

Mechanical ventilation is indicated whenever the cardiopulmonary unit (heart, lungs, and respiratory muscles) is incapacitated so that it can no longer sufficiently supply oxygen to or remove carbon dioxide from the blood. Three of the most common indications for mechanical ventilation are (1) respiratory distress (from any cause, as indicated by dyspnea, increased respiratory rate, and hypoxemia or hypercarbia); (2) shock (as indicated by inadequate oxygen delivery to meet metabolic need); and (3) paralysis affecting the muscles of respiration (diaphragm and intercostals).

Mechanical ventilators have two primary functions: oxygenation (increasing the saturation of hemoglobin with oxygen) and ventilation (removal of carbon dioxide). One or both functions may be needed, depending on the indication for mechanical ventilation. Oxygenation is primarily controlled by enriching the inspired gases with oxygen. This is done with an oxygen blender situated in the inspiratory limb of the ventilator circuit. The FiO_2 can range from ambient (approximately 20%, or 0.2) to 100% (FiO_2 = 1). Oxygenation can also be improved by applying PEEP, which can increase the functional residual capacity of the lung by recruiting perfused but not ventilated alveoli. Ventilation is controlled primarily by setting the ventilator rate and the tidal volume, the product of which determines the minute ventilation. Minute ventilation does not necessarily mean alveolar ventilation, especially in patients with increased dead space (lung or airway volume that is ventilated but not perfused). Thus the volume of dead space ventilation must be subtracted from the minute ventilation to obtain the alveolar ventilation. Alveolar ventilation is inversely related in a linear fashion to the carbon dioxide tension in the arterial blood ($PaCO_2$).

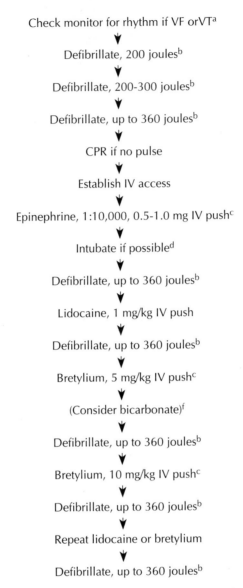

Check monitor for rhythm if VF orVT[a]

↓

Defibrillate, 200 joules[b]

↓

Defibrillate, 200-300 joules[b]

↓

Defibrillate, up to 360 joules[b]

↓

CPR if no pulse

↓

Establish IV access

↓

Epinephrine, 1:10,000, 0.5-1.0 mg IV push[c]

↓

Intubate if possible[d]

↓

Defibrillate, up to 360 joules[b]

↓

Lidocaine, 1 mg/kg IV push

↓

Defibrillate, up to 360 joules[b]

↓

Bretylium, 5 mg/kg IV push[c]

↓

(Consider bicarbonate)[f]

↓

Defibrillate, up to 360 joules[b]

↓

Bretylium, 10 mg/kg IV push[c]

↓

Defibrillate, up to 360 joules[b]

↓

Repeat lidocaine or bretylium

↓

Defibrillate, up to 360 joules[b]

FIGURE 14-5 Ventricular fibrillation (and pulseless ventricular tachycardia).[a] This sequence was developed to assist in teaching how to treat a broad range of patients with ventricular fibrillation (VF) or pulseless ventricular tachycardia (VT). Since some patients may require care not specified herein, this algorithm should not be construed as prohibiting flexibility. The flow of the algorithm presumes that VF is continuing.

[a]Pulseless VT should be treated identically to VF.

[b]Check pulse and rhythm after each shock. If VF recurs after transiently converting (rather than persists without ever converting), use whatever energy level has previously been successful for defibrillation.

[c]Epinephrine should be repeated every 5 minutes.

[d]Intubation is preferable; if it can be accomplished simultaneously with other techniques, the earlier the better. However, defibrillation and epinephrine are important initially if the patient can be ventilated without intubation.

[e]Some may prefer repeated doses of lidocaine, which can be given in boluses of 0.5 mg/kg every 8 minutes, to a total dosage of 3 mg/kg.

[f]The value of sodium bicarbonate is questionable during cardiac arrest, and it is not recommended for a routine cardiac arrest sequence. Consideration of its use in a dose of 1 mEq/kg is appropriate at this point. Half of the original dose may be repeated every 10 minutes if it is used. (From *Textbook of advanced cardiac life support* [#70-1043], Dallas, 1987, 1990, The American Heart Association.)

If rhythm is unclear and ventricular fibrillation
is possible, defibrillate as for VF. If asystole is present[a]

↓

Continue CPR

↓

Establish IV access

↓

Epinephrine, 1:10,000, 0.5-1.0 mg IV push[b]

↓

Intubate when possible[c]

↓

Atropine, 1.0 mg IV push (repeated in 5 min)

↓

(Consider bicarbonate)[d]

↓

Consider pacing

FIGURE 14-6 Asystole (cardiac standstill). This sequence was developed to assist in teaching how to treat a broad range of patients with asystole. Some patients may require care not specified herein. This algorithm should not be construed to prohibit such flexibility. The flow of the algorithm presumes that asystole is continuing.

[a]Asystole should be confirmed in two leads.

[b]Epinephrine should be repeated every 5 minutes.

[c]Intubation is preferable; if it can be accomplished simultaneously with other techniques, the earlier the better. However, cardiopulmonary resuscitation (CPR) and use of epinephrine are more important initially if the patient can be ventilated without intubation (endotracheal epinephrine may be used).

[d]The value of sodium bicarbonate is questionable during cardiac arrest, and it is not recommended for a routine cardiac arrest sequence. Consideration of its use in a dose of 1 mEq/kg is appropriate at this point. Half of the original dose may be repeated every 10 minutes if it is used. (From *Textbook of advanced cardiac life support* [#70-1043], Dallas, 1987, 1990, The American Heart Association.)

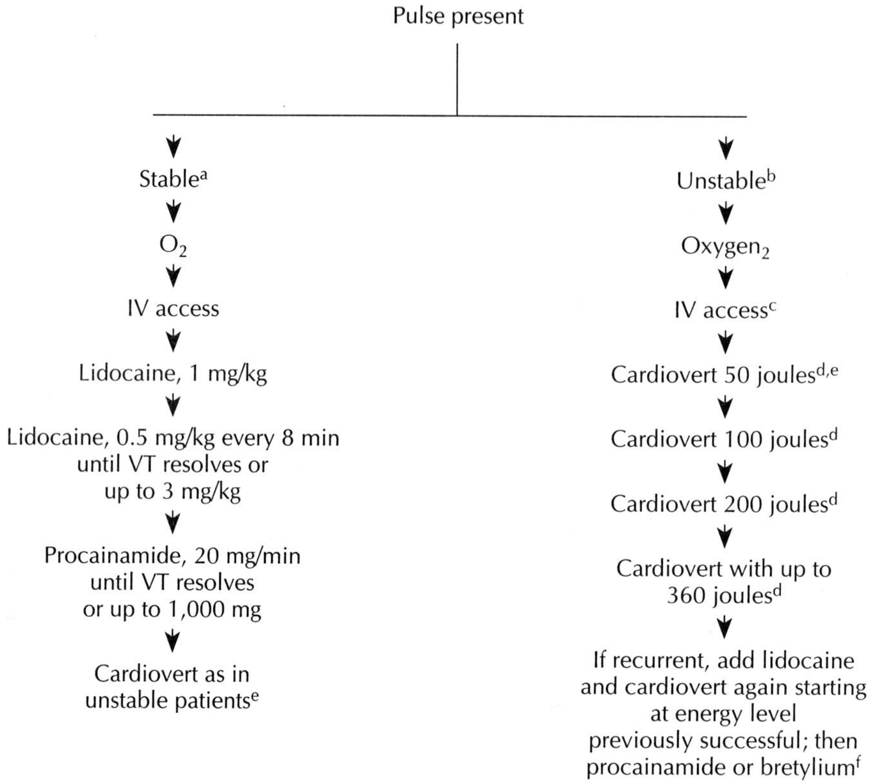

FIGURE 14-7 Sustained ventricular tachycardia (VT). This sequence was developed to assist in teaching how to treat a broad range of patients with sustained VT. Since some patients may require care not specified herein, this algorithm should not be construed as prohibiting flexibility. The flow of the algorithm presumes that VT is continuing.

[a]If the patient becomes unstable (see footnote *b* for definition) at any time, move to "Unstable" arm of algorithm.

[b]*Unstable* indicates symptoms (e.g., chest pain or dyspnea), hypotension (systolic blood pressure <90 mm Hg), congestive heart failure, ischemia, or infarction.

[c]Use central intravenous access if possible.

[d]If hypotension or pulmonary edema is present or the patient is unconscious, unsynchronized cardioversion should be performed to avoid delay associated with synchronization.

[e]In the absence of hypotension, pulmonary edema, or unconsciousness, a precordial thump may be tried before cardioversion.

[f]Once VT has resolved, begin intravenous infusion of an antiarrhythmic agent that has aided resolution of VT. If hypotension or pulmonary edema is present or the patient is unconscious, use lidocaine if cardioversion alone is unsuccessful, followed by bretylium. In all other patients, the recommended order of therapy is lidocaine, procainamide, and then bretylium. (From *Textbook of advanced cardiac life support* [#70-1043], Dallas, 1987, 1990, The American Heart Association.)

That is, doubling the alveolar ventilation should result in a 50% reduction in the $PaCO_2$, all other things being equal.

Mechanical ventilators are not inherently complex. A ventilator is simply a combination of a power source, an air source with an oxygen blender, and an injector or a piston to drive the gases into the airway. However, refinements on this basic theme can be complex. Space does not allow an in-depth review of these refinements, many of which are covered elsewhere,[4] but some basic features of mechanical ventilators are worthy of review.

Controlling the Minute Ventilation

Tidal volume can be controlled in a number of ways by adjusting the inspiratory flow rate and the duration of the inspiratory cycle. Termination of the inspiratory phase can be determined by a preset volume (volume cycled), pressure (pressure cycled), duration (time cycled), or flow rate (flow cycled). Most ventilators are volume cycled but pressure limited. This means that the tidal volume can be present and delivered as long as a preset pressure is not exceeded. If the preset pressure is exceeded, an alarm sounds and no further volume is delivered. The usual tidal volume for an adult is 12 to 15 ml/kg. Smaller tidal volumes have been shown to lead to atelectasis. After the tidal volume is set, the respiratory rate should be set. In an adult, the initial ventilator rate should be set at 8 to 10 breaths/minute. At a setting of 10 breaths, each respiratory cycle will last 6 seconds.

Controlling Oxygenation

The goal of oxygen therapy should be to keep the hemoglobin saturation above 90%, well above the steep part of the oxyhemoglobin dissociation curve, rather than to achieve a specific PaO_2. The lowest possible FiO_2 necessary to achieve this goal should be selected, because exposure to high levels of oxygen for prolonged periods can lead to oxygen toxicity and pulmonary fibrosis. An FiO_2 above 0.5 is considered toxic. If an FiO_2 above 0.5 is needed to keep the hemoglobin saturation above 90%, PEEP should be added to the system. PEEP usually is added in increments of 5 cm H_2O until the desired oxygen saturation is achieved.

Troubleshooting

Occasionally ventilators malfunction, and occasionally patients deteriorate or become disconnected from the ventilator. In each case a ventilator alarm may sound or light up to indicate that a preset parameter is not being fulfilled. The physician or nurse must determine whether the problem is with the patient or the ventilator. If the patient develops distress or hemodynamic instability and the ventilator appears to be malfunctioning, it is imperative to apply bag ventilation to the airway and switch ventilators. Although a myriad of problems can occur, only a few are frequent and severe enough to review here.

The pressure alarm may be set off because the patient coughed during the inspiratory phase, thus increasing the airway pressure, or because the patient's pulmonary compliance has deteriorated. Compliance is a measure of the "flexibility" or distensibility of the lungs, respiratory muscles, and chest wall. It can be calculated by dividing the tidal volume by the peak airway pressure. Healthy lungs are highly compliant, whereas diseased lungs are stiff and have low compliance. It is important to monitor the delivered tidal volume and the peak airway pressure frequently, because when a patient's condition is deteriorating, changes in compliance often precede changes in blood gases. Causes of decreased compliance include tension pneumothorax, pulmonary edema, atelectasis, and hydrothorax or hemothorax.

Ventilator Modes

Mechanical ventilators can be configured in various ways to provide adequate oxygenation and ventilation. These configurations are known as ventilatory modes, and they differ primarily in the amount of work done on the lung by the ventilator and the amount of work done on the lung by the patient.

CONTROLLED MECHANICAL VENTILATION. With controlled mechanical ventilation (CMV), all the work on the lung is done by the ventilator. The rate, tidal volume, and FiO_2 are set, and the patient does not breathe spontaneously. As a result, the mean airway pressure is always positive. High CMV rates delivered to poorly compliant lungs can result in high peak airway pressures and impaired cardiac function. Cardiac function is compromised because the increased airway pressures lead to increased pulmonary vascular resistance and diminished venous return. The CMV mode is indicated in heavily narcotized, sedated, or paralyzed patients. Once the patient is less narcotized, change to another mode is preferable to allow the patient to assume some of the work of breathing. Furthermore, if the patient does not use the muscles of respiration, they will atrophy, and weaning from the ventilator can be prolonged while the muscles regain their tone and strength.

INTERMITTENT MANDATORY VENTILATION. The intermittent mandatory ventilation (IMV) mode allows the patient to breath spontaneously between ventilator breaths from a second respiratory circuit in parallel with the ventilator. The patient gradually takes over the work of breathing from the ventilator as the number of IMV breaths is decreased. Obvious advantages of this mode include a reduction in the mean airway pressure (since some of the breaths are spontaneous), improved cardiac function (lowered pulmonary vascular resistance), and intermittent use of the respiratory muscles, ensuring that they maintain their tone.

SYNCHRONIZED INTERMITTENT MANDATORY VENTILATION. Synchronized intermittent mandatory ventilation (SIMV) is a hybrid of IMV and CMV, since spontaneous breaths are assisted by the ventilator between controlled breaths. The initiation of the ventilator breath is synchronized to the patient's inspiratory effort. SIMV does not appear to offer any physiologic advantages over IMV with regard to cardiac function or mean airway pressure.

PRESSURE SUPPORT VENTILATION. Pressure support ventilation is a form of ventilator support in which flow is provided to the patient until a predetermined pressure is reached during inspiration. Because no mandatory breaths are provided by the ventilator, the patient must have some spontaneous ventilatory effort, and because no flow occurs during exhalation, no PEEP is generated. This mode is useful in weaning patients from the ventilator by gradually reducing the pressure support so that the patient slowly assumes more of the work of breathing.

REVERSED INSPIRATORY TO EXPIRATORY RATIO. During spontaneous ventilation, the expiratory phase normally is longer than the inspiratory phase. The same is true for mechanically ventilated breaths—the inspiratory phase is driven by the positive pressure generated by the ventilator, and the expiratory phase is passive, generated by the elastic recoil of the lungs, chest wall, and respiratory muscles. As such, complete exhalation usually takes twice as long as inhalation; thus the ratio between inhalation and exhalation (I/E ratio) normally varies between 1:2 and 1:4. When pulmonary compliance decreases and airway resistance increases, high flow rates during inspiration can cause turbulance in the airways. This increases the relative airway resistance and airway pressure and produces uneven distribution of the tidal volume. Reducing the flow rate but maintaining the same tidal volume can be accomplished by increasing the duration of the inspiratory phase, thus altering the I/E ratio. Reverse I/E ratio has been shown to reduce the peak airway pressure and improve oxygenation in patients with severe adult respiratory distress syndrome (ARDS) when compared to CMV and IMV. However, the test of its efficacy awaits a prospective randomized trial.

HIGH-FREQUENCY VENTILATION. Conventional respiratory support, as previously outlined, is based on the concept of a high tidal volume and a relatively low ventilator rate to deliver the minute ventilation. High-frequency ventilation (HFV) reverses this relationship, using a low tidal volume and a high ventilator rate. The major proposed advantage of this mode is reducing airway pressure, thus preventing cardiac depression and pulmonary barotrauma.[27] High-frequency ventilation uses rates above 60 breaths/minute with a tidal volume only slightly greater than the respiratory dead space. To accommodate the high rate, flow must be very high, usually above 100 L/minute. Because HFV lowers the airway pressure, it has been useful in the management of bronchopleural fistulae. It can also be used during procedures on the airway, such as bronchoscopy and laryngoscopy. Potential complications with this mode include inspissated respiratory secretions from a lack of humidification and tracheal mucosal damage, because the high flow rate may create a surface shear. Because the high flow rate and high ventilator rate may be insufficient to allow adequate elimination of carbon dioxide, this mode frequently is used with a conventional IMV mode set at a low rate.

Intra-Aortic Balloon Pump

The intra-aortic balloon pump (IABP) was developed in the 1960s as a circulatory assist device to reduce the mortality from refractory cardiogenic shock after myocardial infarction. The balloon-tipped catheter functions on the principle of counterpulsation. The balloon is quickly inflated with either CO_2 or helium during diastole to occlude the distal aorta, thus increasing proximal aortic presure and improving coronary and cerebral perfusion. The balloon is deflated during systole, decreasing afterload and allowing unimpeded blood flow. The IABP cycle is coordinated with the patient's ECG or pressure wave from an arterial line. The IABP has been shown to increase diastolic pressure and cardiac output and decrease lactate production by the failing myocardium.[45] The IABP improves cardiac function in 80% to 85% of patients in cardiogenic shock.[45]

Unfortunately, when more than 40% of the left ventricle is infarcted, any improvement with IABP counterpulsation is only temporary, and the patient eventually will succumb when the device is removed unless an adjunctive procedure, such as a heart transplant, is performed.[40] Occasionally an area of infarction is surrounded by a zone of viable ischemic tissue, and it is possible that the IABP can be used to support marginally a viable myocardium until the patient undergoes thrombolytic therapy, angioplasty, or coronary artery bypass. The balloon pump has also been used in weaning patients from cardiopulmonary bypass,[9] in patients with severe myocardial contusions with cardiogenic shock,[52] and for perioperative support of the heart in noncardiac surgery, such as resection of an aortic aneurysm.[25]

Insertion

The IABP is programmed so that the balloon will trigger on the R wave of the ECG and inflation occurs at the peak of the T wave. Deflation occurs just before the QRS complex. Counterpulsation usually is set at a 1:2 assist ratio (1 balloon inflation for every 2 systoles), and the effects of augmentation, timing, and balloon volume are adjusted. A good arterial waveform with a sharp upstroke and pulse pressure of at least 40 mm Hg is necessary for reliable triggering of the IABP (Figure 14-8).

Weaning from the IABP begins by reducing the counterpulsation ratios. Hemodynamic parameters (especially CI) must be assessed at every ratio change. Several hours should elapse between each ratio change, because rapid weaning from counterpulsation can result in cardiac decompensation.

Extracorporeal Membrane Oxygenation and Carbon Dioxide Removal

The mortality rate for acute respiratory failure remains 30% to 70%, despite improvements in respiratory therapy, fluid management, and nutritional support.[18] Ultimately, it is the inability to provide oxygen to the patient that results in death. Providing oxygen to patients with poorly compliant lungs using conventional ventilators requires high airway pressures, high levels of PEEP, and an increased FiO_2. However, these measures may actually enhance the pulmonary injury by increasing the risk of barotrauma and oxygen toxicity in the unaffected pulmonary parenchyma.

The use of extracorporeal oxygenation initially was proposed as a means of providing oxygen to patients in whom the native lung was no longer capable of this function. The patients were placed on an extracorporeal membrane oxygenator (ECMO) with a roller pump to provide flow through the oxygenator. Carbon dioxide was removed by the native lung. Treatment with ECMO required systemic anticoagulation, which often led to hemorrhagic complications. Unfortunately, the mortality rate of patients given ECMO therapy was 90%, no different from patients treated with conventional ventilators.[38] On the other hand, ECMO was found to be very successful in managing neonatal respiratory failure, especially in cases of congenital diaphragmatic hernia.[48]

Recent modifications in the procedure and advances in technology have rekindled interest in the use of ECMO in adults. Gattinoni and colleagues have emphasized the importance of extracorporeal CO_2 removal and the use of venovenous (rather than venoarterial) access.[19] Extracorporeal oxygenation and CO_2 removal allow low inflation pressures and low FiO_2, thus avoiding the injurious aspects of conventional ventilation. Venovenous access maintains normal pulmonary nutrient flow and avoids arterial embolization of white cells and platelets, which is known to occur with the membrane oxygenator. Heparinization is still required, but hemorrhagic complications appear to be decreasing. Early trials in adults have been promising, with 50% to 70% survival in patients with established ARDS.[1,19]

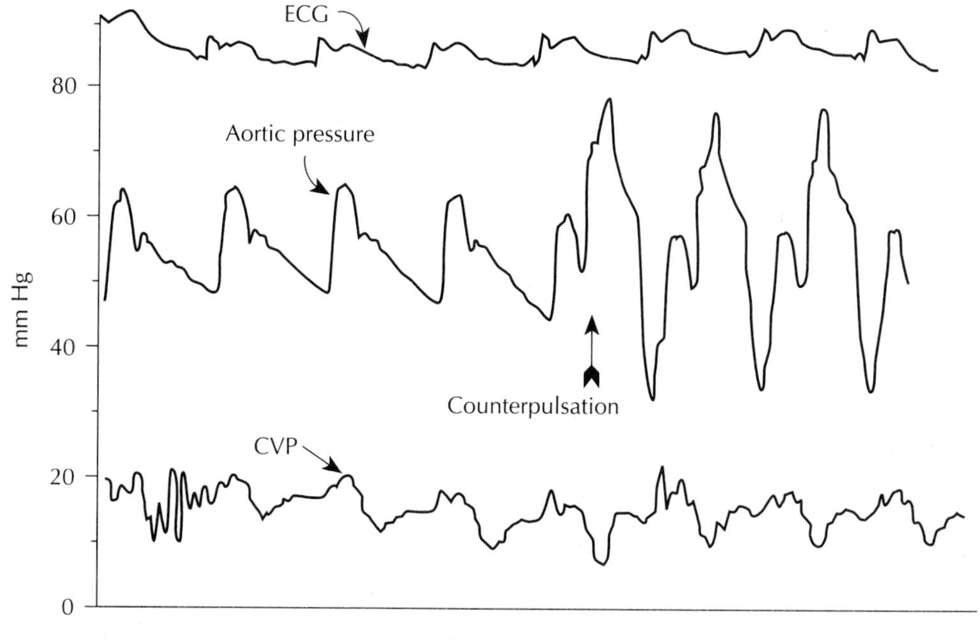

FIGURE 14-8 Aortic tracing during counterpulsation. Initiation of intra-aortic counterpulsation (IACP) decreases the systolic blood pressure and significantly increases the diastolic (coronary perfusion) pressure. *CVP,* Central venous pressure. (From Mueller HS: Management of acute myocardial infarction. In Shoemaker WC, editor: *Critical care,* ed 2, Philadelphia, 1989, WB Saunders.)

Continuous Arteriovenous Hemofiltration

The mortality rate of acute renal failure in the ICU is reported to be 50% to 90%.[18] Treatment consists of maintaining solute removal and acid-base balance, correcting electrolyte abnormalities, treating volume overload, and providing nutritional support. Hemodialysis and continuous arteriovenous hemofiltration (CAVH) may provide these life-sustaining functions to allow sufficient time for recovery of renal function.

Hemodialysis is based on the diffusion of solutes and water through a semipermeable membrane separating two fluids (blood and the dialysate). The dialysate removes excess sodium and potassium, provides buffers, and maintains appropriate levels of chloride, magnesium, and calcium. Excess water is removed by ultrafiltration, using positive pressure applied to the blood and negative pressure applied to the dialysate. Hemodialysis has several disadvantages, including the intermittent nature of the treatment, the hemodynamic instability it tends to induce, and the equipment and staffing required.

Continuous arteriovenous hemofiltration was developed in 1977.[5] Blood (from either an artery or a vein) is passed through a hemofilter and then returned to the patient. The filter consists of thousands of hollow fibres in a plastic casing. Vascular access generally is via femoral cannulae, with heparin often given on one side of the system to prevent clotting. Access ports are present on the filter to allow administration of replacement fluids. With the filter in place, extracellular fluid is removed at a rate independent of blood flow and on the net pressure difference across the membranes. As blood enters the hemofilter, the transmembrane pressure gradient favors the movement of fluid and particles across the membrane. As ultrafiltrate is removed, the plasma proteins become more concentrated, the oncotic pressure increases and, eventually, ultrafiltration stops. The ultrafiltrate consists of plasma water and non-protein-bound low- and mid-molecular-weight solutes and is formed at approximately 5 to 10 ml/minute and 12 to 15 L over 24 hours.

CAVH may also be enhanced by applying negative pressure on the ultrafiltrate side to increase the ultrafiltration rate and solute clearance. The disadvantages of adding negative pressure are that the circuit becomes more complex, fluid shifts are greater, and more replacement fluid is required.

Indications

Several factors can indicate a need to dialyze an ICU patient (see the box at right). The advantages of CAVH are that it is a continuous rather than an intermittent therapy and that fluid balance can be more easily managed. It is a particularly helpful technique in patients with renal failure who require administration or removal of large volumes of fluid. CAVH is also useful in patients with refractory congestive heart failure who would be particularly susceptible to the hemodynamic instability associated with hemodialysis. No specific contraindications to CAVH are known, although systemic heparinization, which is recommended, may be contraindicated in some patients.

INDICATIONS FOR DIALYSIS IN THE INTENSIVE CARE UNIT

- Uremia
- Fluid overload and pulmonary edema or hypertension
- Electrolyte disturbances
  - Hyponatremia
  - Hyperkalemia
  - Hypercalcemia
- Acid-base disturbances
- Uremic pericarditis
- Uremic coagulopathy
- Drug overdose

From Rippe JM, Irwin RS, Alpert JS, Fink MP: *Intensive care medicine*, Boston, 1991, Little, Brown.

ICU COMPLICATIONS

Complications of ICU patients are additional physiologic derangements of homeostasis superimposed on an underlying disease. Complications in severely ill patients usually occur because normal defense mechanisms are overcome or bypassed. These complications may provide the "second hit," which pushes a tenuous patient into the syndrome of multiple organ failure (MOF). Therefore preventing complications is extremely important.

Nosocomial Pneumonia

Pneumonia is a common complication in the ICU. In ventilated patients, the normal respiratory tract barriers to infection (i.e., nasal mechanisms, cough and gag reflexes, and cilial clearance) have been overcome, and colonization of the lower respiratory tract with pathogens occurs in virtually 100% of patients by day 7 of intubation. The risk of pneumonia is greatest in the first 10 days of mechanical ventilation; 90% of cases occur during this time.[30] The causative organisms for ICU-acquired pneumonia differ considerably from community-acquired pathogens and most often are gram-negative organisms. The mortality rate of patients with nosocomial pneumonia occurring in the ICU is 10% to 25%.

Respiratory tract colonization in the ICU occurs through hematogenous spread from another source of infection, spread from equipment and caregivers, and contamination through aspiration from the gastrointestinal tract. Although contaminated respiratory care equipment has been implicated in outbreaks of pneumonia in the past, it is now an infrequent cause. Scrupulous cleaning of equipment, meticulous handwashing by caregivers, and disposable suction materials have contributed to this reduced incidence. Blood-borne infection from another site is also thought to be rare, although bacterial translocation through ischemic gastrointestinal mucosa is being implicated with increasing frequency. A recent review of ICU patients showed that the patients who developed pneumonia were also those who had evidence of loss of gastric mucosal integrity, suggesting that the onset of pneumonia was a result of bacterial translocation from the stomach into the bloodstream.[17]

Currently, aspiration of gastric contents around the endotracheal tube cuff probably is the most common cause of respiratory tract colonization. Although the stomach normally is sterile, several factors contribute to bacterial overgrowth and subsequent aspiration. Among these are the use of antacids and histamine antagonists, which change the normally sterile environment of the stomach to a more alkaline one. Also, the use of broad-spectrum antibiotics and gastric ileus lead to rapid bacterial overgrowth in the proximal gastrointestinal tract.

Numerous antibiotic regimens have been proposed to "decontaminate" the stomach.[54] Using a decontamination regimen reduced oral and tracheal colonization with gram-negative organisms from 50% to 85% to 5% to 15%.[42] Although the incidence of pneumonia was lower and the therapy had few side effects, no decrease has been shown in the length of stay in the ICU or in the overall mortality rate.

Preventing aspiration is important. The stomach should remain decompressed at all times. If possible, the head of the bed should be kept elevated. The mouth, oropharynx, and trachea should be suctioned frequently, especially whenever the endotracheal tube cuff is being deflated. Obviously, extubation, as early as possible, is the cornerstone of prevention.

Stress Gastritis

In the past, upper gastrointestinal bleeding was common in critically ill patients, occurring in up to 50% of patients during their stay in the ICU. In most cases the cause was stress gastritis. Available treatment was limited and consisted of surgical intervention, with an attendant high mortality rate.

Bleeding in stress gastritis usually comes from superficial erosions caused by a breakdown of the normal protective mechanisms of the mucosa.[50] One of the most important contributing factors in the development of stress gastritis is the occurrence of ischemia and resultant loss of mucosal integrity. Improvements in monitoring, resuscitation, antacid therapy, and nutrition in the ICU have lessened the incidence of this complication. Surveillance endoscopic studies of ICU patients have shown that essentially all ICU patients have some disruption of gastric mucosa, but only 10% to 15% of patients have visible bleeding, and still fewer require blood replacement and surgical intervention. Those at risk for significant bleeding include patients with major trauma, sepsis, or MOF (see the box above).

RISK FACTORS FOR THE DEVELOPMENT OF STRESS BLEEDING

- Burns (>35% body surface area)
- Sepsis
- Shock
- Multiple trauma
- Coagulopathy
- Head injury
- Multiple organ system failure
- Renal failure
- Respiratory failure
- Hepatic failure

From Durham RM, Shapiro MJ: *Intensive Care Med* 6:260, 1991.

Because gastric acid is essential for the occurrence of stress gastritis, initial efforts at reducing this complication have been directed at manipulating the gastric pH. Generally, a pH of 3.5 or higher lessens the risk of bleeding, and a pH of 7 or higher appears to prevent this complication entirely. Antacids administered at regular intervals (usually 30 to 60 ml every 1 to 2 hours), either by mouth or via a nasogastric tube, are a common means of prophylaxis. Antacids reduce the incidence of bleeding, have relatively minor side effects, and are relatively inexpensive.

Numerous studies have documented the benefits of histamine (H_2) receptor blockade in reducing bleeding caused by stress gastritis in critically ill patients. They are as effective as antacids in reducing clinically significant bleeding. If gastric pH cannot be adequately controlled with H_2 blockers alone, antacids may be added. H_2 blockers offer the advantage of potentially continuous pH control and a lesser requirement for nursing intervention than with antacids. Disadvantages include medication-related side effects, including confusion, altered metabolism of other medications, and bone marrow depression. These problems occur most often with cimetidine, which is the original drug in the class.

Sucralfate is a mucosal protective agent that binds to the gastric mucosa and increases the secretion of mucus and bicarbonate. Sucralfate should not be given in conjunction with either H_2 blockers or antacids, because it is most effective in an acid environment. It is given either by mouth or as a slurry via a nasogastric tube. The effectiveness of sucralfate appears to be comparable to that of either antacids or H_2 blockers, and its side effects consist of reduced gastric absorption of some medications and hypophosphatemia resulting from binding to the aluminum salt.

Although routine use of prophylaxis against stress gastritis has been beneficial in reducing the incidence of bleeding, concerns have been raised that these therapies actually increase the incidence of nosocomial pneumonia. The normally low pH of the stomach produces an environment that is essentially sterile. This environment is further maintained by normal peristalsis, which serves to keep bacteria in the less acidic duodenum and small bowel, away from the stomach. As mentioned previously, when these mechanisms are altered by ileus, obstruction, or acid-reducing therapies, bacterial overgrowth occurs. It is this colonization that is thought to be the cause of most cases of pneumonia in the ICU, either by direct spread through a disrupted gastric barrier (translocation) or by aspiration of gastric contents into the respiratory tract.[54]

Currently, sucralfate appears to offer the benefits of bleeding prophylaxis without bacterial overgrowth.

Sinusitis

Normal mucociliary action in the sinus mucosa, as well as drainage via the ostia, ensures that the sinuses are sterile in a healthy individual. When drainage is impeded (by nasotracheal or nasogastric tubes), sinusitis can occur. Sinusitis and sinus infections in an ICU patient can be a focus of occult sepsis. The infections usually are caused by several organisms, the most prevalent being *Staphylococcus aureus* and gram-negative organisms. Antibiotic resistance is common, because many patients in the ICU are already receiving broad-spectrum antibiotics.

The incidence of sinusitis depends on how the condition is defined. Some authors have defined it as fluid within the sinus (rather than the presence of an actual pathogen) associated with systemic signs of infection. Almost all patients who are nasotracheally intubated for longer than 7 days have fluid in the sinus.[16] If fever, leukocytosis, and sinus tenderness are added to the radiographic signs to make the diagnosis, sinusitis occurs in 1% to 5% of ICU patients.[11,26]

The diagnosis can be made from symptoms of facial pain and purulent nasal discharge, combined with radiographs revealing sinus opacification, air fluid levels, or mucosal thickening. A comatose patient is unable to complain of discomfort, and purulent nasal discharge may not be evident. Furthermore, obtaining adequate radiographic studies may be impossible in these patients, who cannot be positioned and are transported with difficulty. Ultrasonography to detect fluid in the sinuses is a noninvasive method, performed at bedside, that can be used in conjunction with clinical criteria to make the diagnosis. The definitive diagnostic test is antral tap which, although highly sensitive and specific, is an invasive procedure and impractical as a screening measure.

RISK FACTORS FOR COGNITIVE IMPAIRMENT IN THE ICU

Age ≥60 years
Addiction to alcohol, drugs, or both
Cerebral injury or disease
Chronic cardiac, renal, or hepatic disease
Visual or auditory impairment
Preoperative depression
History of delirium or functional psychosis
Family history of psychosis

From Monks R: Cognitive and sensory defects. In Wilmore DW, Brennon MF, Harlen AH, editors: *Care of the surgical patient,* New York, 1988-1992, Scientific American Books.

Complications of acute sinusitis include bacteremia, meningitis, orbital cellulitis and abscess, cavernous sinus thrombosis, epidural abscess, and osteomyelitis of the skull. Although rare, these severe complications can be rapidly fatal and serve to emphasize the need for prompt recognition of sinusitis in an ICU patient.

Treatment of acute sinusitis involves removing all impediments to sinus drainage. Nasotracheal tubes should be changed to orotracheal tubes or tracheostomy at the earliest opportunity. The head of the bed should be elevated to promote ostial drainage. Antihistamines to reduce mucosal edema and antibiotics appropriate for the causative organism should be given. If the condition does not respond to these measures, surgical drainage should be undertaken.

Delirium and Agitation

Approximately 10% to 15% of all ICU patients show changes in mental status at some time during their ICU admission.[31] Delirium refers to an acute confusional state with widespread impairment of cognitive functions, altered consciousness, and disturbance of cerebral metabolism. Common symptoms include rapid fluctuations in the level of consciousness, difficulty sustaining attention, easy distractibility, and consistent lack of orientation in all three spheres. Prodromal findings include restlessness, anxiety, irritability, and sleep disruption. Some patients may be recognized as having delirium because of hypervigilance and restlessness, but other patients will be somnolent and lethargic.

Because delirium often goes unrecognized, its incidence is difficult to ascertain. Known risk factors include increasing age, pre-existing drug or alcohol abuse, and previous impairment of mental status (see the box above). Potential causes of delirium include underlying cerebral disease, drug or alcohol withdrawal, and medication (see the box on p. 551). The specific pathophysiology of delirium has not been defined, but it has

COMMON DELIRIUM-INDUCING DRUGS USED IN THE ICU

Atropine sulfate
Cimetidine
Diphenhydramine hydrochloride
Lidocaine
Meperidine hydrochloride
Mexiletine
Morphine sulfate
Penicillin
Pentazocine
Procainamide hydrochloride
Promethazine hydrochloride
Propranolol hydrochloride
Quinidine sulfate
Ranitidine
Rifampin

Adapted from Tesar GE, Stern TA: Evaluation and treatment of agitation in the intensive care unit, *J Intensive Care Med* 1:137, 1986.

been suggested that it is caused by a depletion or excess of central neurotransmitters.

The diagnosis of delirium is made on a clinical basis, although laboratory tests, such as electrolytes and glucose levels, blood counts, ammonia levels, and blood gases, may be helpful in excluding other causes. A history may be difficult to obtain from the patient, but reviewing the patient's chart and talking with the patient's family may often reveal evidence of risk factors. A review of the patient's current medications, as well as prehospital use of medications, is essential. A mental status examination often reveals surprising lapses in orientation and reasoning, and memory impairment.

Prompt recognition of delirium and appropriate treatment are important to prevent injury to the patient and the ICU staff. All nonessential medications should be discontinued and underlying causes treated. Benzodiazepines have proven highly effective in the treatment of alcohol withdrawal, with chlordiazepoxide and lorazepam used most frequently. Efforts to orient the patient to his surroundings are helpful and are aided by providing the patient with eyeglasses and hearing aids. At times, the presence of a family member is of great help in calming and orienting an agitated patient. Because pain is a frequent cause of agitation in a postoperative patient, the patient must be given pain medications as needed. If these conservative measures fail, administration of haloperidol, as an antipsychotic and sedating agent, is recommended. This drug has been used extensively for this purpose and has been found to have minimal effects on blood pressure, pulmonary artery pressure, heart rate, and respiratory status, and it is well tolerated in critical illness.

Pressure Sores

As with most other ICU complications, pressure sores are a serious but largely preventable problem. (The frequently used term "decubitus ulcer" is less correct and probably should be discarded.) The incidence of pressure sores is 3% to 4% during acute hospitalizations, with most developing during the initial 2 weeks of hospitalization, the time when a patient may well require intensive care. An estimated 90% to 95% of pressure sores involve the sacral and coccygeal regions, ischial tuberosities, and greater trochanters. In a critically ill patient who may be neurologically impaired or who may be receiving muscle relaxants, pressure sores may also be seen on the back of the head, over the spinous processes, and on the prominences of the elbows and the heels.

Pressure sores are ischemic ulcerations of the skin over weight-bearing areas. The critical elements in the development of ischemic necrosis are the amount of pressure applied and the time of application. As little as 70 mm Hg applied for 2 hours has been demonstrated to cause irreversible necrosis. Relieving pressure for even 5 minutes every 2 hours significantly reduces ischemia.[29] Moisture from sweat, urine, and wound drainage can cause maceration of the skin, which increases the risk of skin breakdown by a factor of five.[43] It is widely recognized that patients with altered mental states or spinal cord injuries or those who require prolonged immobilization (e.g., traction) are at far greater risk for the development of pressure sores. Any factor that impairs wound healing, such as malnutrition or diabetes, also predisposes to skin breakdown.

A pressure sore is a full-thickness injury of the skin. It is quite common for the subcutaneous injury to be much larger than the apparent skin lesion—a pathologic "tip of the iceberg." The grading system developed by Shea is widely used and allows objective description of the degree of injury.[47] In stage I, the skin is erythematous or blistered but intact. This is rapidly reversible when pressure is relieved. In stage II, the full thickness of the skin is involved to the subcutaneous fat, and drainage and pain may be present. Stage III involves the skin and subcutaneous fat with undermining of the tissues; an ulcer or eschar or necrotic tissue may be seen in the wound. In stage IV lesions, the injury extends into the muscle and muscle fascia and may penetrate to the bone, with resultant osteomyelitis.

Pressure sores can be prevented by removing the inciting factors. Good nursing practice dictates that an immobile patient be turned every 2 hours. Pillows and padding can be used as adjuncts to relieve pressure, but padding should **not** be placed over bony prominences, because this only exacerbates the pressure problem. Other adjunctive measures include using egg crate and gel mattresses, which allow more even distribution of weight. The development of specialized beds, such as the air-fluidized bed and the "air-pillow" bed (in which individual air-filled cushions can be selectively inflated or deflated to provide even distribution of pressure) has aided the management of this difficult problem.

Despite meticulous care, skin breakdown may still occur. In early stages, recognizing the problem and relieving pressure are sufficient therapy. In more advanced cases, necrotic tissue must be debrided and infection controlled. Enzymatic debridement may be useful in a superficial lesion, but a deeper pressure sore requires surgical debridement. Although often used, wet-to-dry dressings are harmful, because they contribute to wound dessication and reinjure the wound with each dressing change. Many commonly used antimicrobial agents, such as iodine or hydrogen peroxide, have deleterious effects on wound healing and should be avoided. Once the wound has been adequately debrided, occlusive dressings provide protection.

Infection of a pressure sore may be difficult to ascertain but cannot be overlooked in a febrile patient. Suspicion of infection should be heightened in an immunocompromised patient who is unable to manifest fever or leukocytosis. A quantitative culture of the wound is more accurate in diagnosing infection, because wound swabs reflect surface colonization rather than invasive infection. After the wound has been cleaned, a 1 g specimen of tissue is sent for culture. Growth of more than 10^{56} colonies indicates an invasive infection. Topical antibiotics, combined with debridement, may be helpful in treating a superficially colonized pressure sore, but systemic infection requires the addition of systemic antibiotics. Complications of untreated pressure sores include bacteremia, sepsis, and osteomyelitis.

REFERENCES

1 Anderson HL III, Delius RE, Sinard JM et al: Early experience with adult extracorporeal membrane oxygenation in the modern era, *Ann Thorac Surg* 53:553, 1992.
2 Baek PL, McMichan JC, Marsh HM et al: Continuous monitoring of mixed venous oxygen saturation in critically ill patients, *Anesth Analg* 61:513, 1982.
3 Band J, Make D: Infections caused by arterial catheters used for hemodynamic monitoring, *Am J Med* 67:735, 1979.
4 Banner MJ, Smith RA: Mechanical ventilation. In Civetta JM, Taylor RW, Kirby RR, editors: *Critical care,* ed 2, Philadelphia, 1988, JB Lippincott.
5 Bartlett RH, Bosch J, Geronemus R et al: Continuous arteriovenous hemofiltration for acute renal failure, *ASAIO Proc* 11:67, 1988.
6 Bedford RF: Long-term radial artery cannulation: effects on subsequent vessel function, *Crit Care Med* 6:64, 1988.
7 Birnbaum ML: Cost containment in critical care, *Crit Care Med* 14:1068, 1986.
8 Brown JJ, Sullivan G: Effect on ICU mortality of a full-time critical care specialist, *Chest* 96:127, 1989.
9 Buckley MJ, Craven JM, Gould HK et al: Intra-aortic balloon pump assist for cardiogenic shock after cardiopulmonary bypass, *Circulation* 48 (suppl 3):90, 1973.
10 Cohn J: Blood pressure measurement in shock: mechanism of inaccuracy in auscultatory and palpatory methods, *JAMA* 199:972, 1967.
11 Deutschman CS, Wilton P, Snow J et al: Paranasal sinusitis associated with nasotracheal intubation: a frequently unrecognized and treatable source of sepsis, *Crit Care Med* 14:111, 1986.
12 Downs JB, Chapman R, Hawkins I: Prolonged radial artery catheterization, *Arch Surg* 108:671, 1974.
13 Eerola R, Kaukinen L, Kaukinen S: Analysis of 13,800 subclavian catheterizations, *Acta Anaesthesiol Scand* 29:293, 1985.
14 Ellis RJ, Gold J, Rees JR et al: Computerized monitoring of cardiac output by thermal dilution, *JAMA* 220:507, 1972.
15 Falk JL, Rackow EC, Weil MJ: End-tidal carbon dioxide concentration during cardiopulmonary resuscitation, *N Engl J Med* 318:607, 1988.
16 Fassoulaki A, Pamouhtsoglou P: Prolonged nasotracheal intubation and its association with inflammation of paranasal sinuses, *Anesth Analg* 69:50, 1989.
17 Fiddian-Green RG, Baker S: Nosocomial pneumonia in the critically ill: product of aspiration or translocation? *Crit Care Med* 19:763, 1991.
18 Fry DE, Pearlstein L, Fulton RL et al: Multiple system organ failure: the role of uncontrolled infection, *Arch Surg* 115:136, 1980.
19 Gattinoni L, Pesenti A, Mascheroni D et al: Low-frequency positive-pressure ventilation with extracorporeal CO_2 removal in severe acute respiratory failure, *JAMA* 256:881, 1986.
20 Gore JM, Sloan K: Use of continuous monitoring of mixed venous saturation in the coronary care unit, *Chest* 86:757, 1984.
21 Greene JF, Fitzwater JE, Clemner TP: Septic endocarditis and indwelling pulmonary artery catheters, *JAMA* 233:891, 1975.
22 Henning RJ, McClish D, Daly B et al: Clinical characteristics and resource utilization of ICU patients: implications for organization of intensive care units, *Crit Care Med* 15:264, 1987.
23 Hilberman M: The evolution of the intensive care unit, *Crit Care Med* 3:159, 1975.
24 Hoffman RA, Krieger BP, Kramer MR et al: End-tidal carbon dioxide in critically ill patients during changes in mechanical ventilation, *Am Rev Respir Dis* 140:1265, 1989.
25 Hollier LH, Pitell JA, Puga FJ: Intra-aortic balloon counterpulsation as adjunct to aneurysmectomy in high-risk patients, *Mayo Clin Proc* 56:565, 1981.
26 Kaups KL, Cohn SM, Lavelle WG et al: Maxillary sinusitis is rare in the ICU: a prospective study, *Chest* 98:1345, 1990.
27 Klain M: High-frequency ventilation. In Shoemaker WC, Ayers S, Grenvik A et al, editors: *Textbook of critical care,* Philadelphia, 1989, WB Saunders.
28 Knaus WA, Wagner DP, Draper EA: The APACHE III prognostic system, *Chest* 100:1619, 1991.
29 Kosiak M, Kubicek WG, Olson M et al: Etiology and pathology of ischemic ulcers, *Arch Phys Med Rehabil* 39:623, 1958.
30 Langer M, Mosconi P, Cigada M et al: Long-term respiratory support and risk of pneumonia in critically ill patients, *Am Rev Resp Dis* 140:302, 1989.
31 Lipowski ZJ: Delirium (acute confusional states), *JAMA* 258:1789, 1987.
32 McDaniel D, Stone J, Flatas A et al: Catheter-induced pulmonary artery hemorrhage, *J Thorac Cardiovasc Surg* 82:1, 1981.
33 Maki DG: Nosocomial bacteremia: an epidemiologic overview, *Am J Med* 70:719, 1981.
34 Messerli F, Ventura H, Amodeo D: Osler's maneuver and pseudohypertension, *N Engl J Med* 312:1548, 1985.
35 Michel L, Marsh HM, McMichan JC et al: Infections of pulmonary artery catheters in critically ill patients, *JAMA* 245:1032, 1981.
36 Miller JJ, Venus B, Mathru M: Comparison of the sterility of long-term central venous catheterization using single-lumen and triple-lumen pulmonary artery catheters, *Crit Care Med* 12:634, 1984.

37 Murray IP, Modell JM: Early detection of endotracheal tube accidents by monitoring of carbon dioxide concentrations in respiratory gas, *Anesthesiology* 59:344, 1983.

38 National Heart, Lung and Blood Institute-NIH: Extracorporeal support for respiratory insufficiency, Bethesda, Md, DHEW, 1980.

39 Osborne ML: Physician decisions regarding life support in the intensive care unit, *Chest* 101:217, 1992.

40 Page DL, Caulfield JB, Kastor JA et al: Myocardial changes associated with cardiogenic shock, *N Engl J Med* 285:133, 1971.

41 Palve H, Vuori A: Pulse oximetry during low cardiac output and hypothermia states immediately after open heart surgery, *Crit Care Med* 17:66, 1989.

42 Poole GV, Muakkassa FF, Griswold JA: Pneumonia, selective decontamination, and multiple organ failure, *Surgery* 111:1, 1992.

43 Reuler JB, Cooney TG: The pressure sore: pathophysiology and principles of management, *Ann Intern Med* 94:661, 1981.

44 Ruth HS, Hawgen FP, Grave DD: Anesthesia Study Commission of the Philadelphia County Medical Society: findings of eleven years' activity, *JAMA* 135:881, 1947.

45 Scheidt S, Wilner G, Mueller H et al: Intra-aortic balloon counterpulsation in cardiogenic shock: report of a cooperative clinical trial, *N Engl J Med* 288:979, 1973.

46 Severinghaus JW, Bradley AF: Electrodes for blood PO_2 and PCO_2 determinations, *J Appl Physiol* 13:515, 1958.

47 Shea JD: Pressure sores: classification and management, *Clin Orthop* 112:89, 1975.

48 Short BL, Anderson KD: Extracorporeal membrane oxygenation in neonates. In Shoemaker WC, Ayres S, Grenvik A et al, editors: *Textbook of critical care,* Philadelphia, 1989, WB Saunders.

49 Sirio CA, Tajimi K, Tase C et al: An initial comparison of intensive care in Japan and the United States, *Crit Care Med* 20:1207, 1992.

50 Skillman JJ, Gould SA, Chung RSK et al: The gastric mucosal barrier: clinical and experimental studies in critically ill and normal man, and in the rabbit, *Ann Surg* 172:564, 1970.

51 Smith DC, Canning JJ, Crul JF: Pulse oximetry in the recovery room, *Anaesthesia* 44:345, 1989.

52 Snow N, Lucas AE, Richardson JD: Intra-aortic balloon counterpulsation for cardiogenic shock from cardiac contusion, *J Trauma* 23:426, 1982.

53 Sprung C, Poxen R, Rozanski J et al: Advanced ventricular arrhythmias during bedside pulmonary artery catheterization, *Am J Med* 72:203, 1982.

54 Stoutenbeek CP, Van Saene HKF: Infection prevention in intensive care by selective decontamination of the digestive tract, *J Crit Care Med* 5:137, 1990.

55 Swan HJC, Ganz W, Forrester J et al: Catheterization of the heart in man with use of a flow-directed balloon-tipped catheter, *N Engl J Med* 283:447, 1970.

56 Task Force on Guidelines, Society of Critical Care Medicine: Recommendations for services and personnel for delivery of care in a critical care setting, *Crit Care Med* 16:809, 1988.

CHAPTER

15

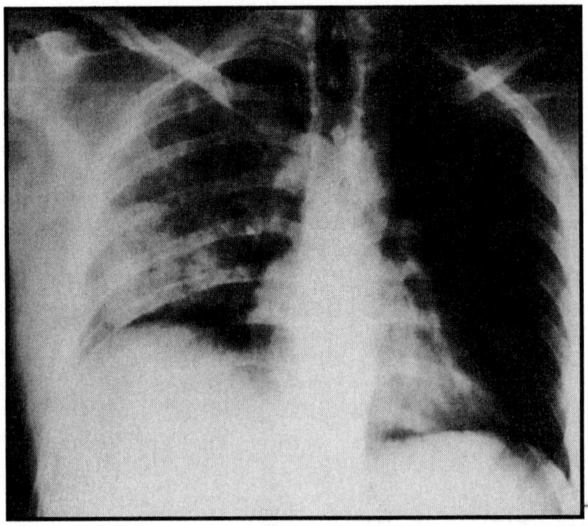

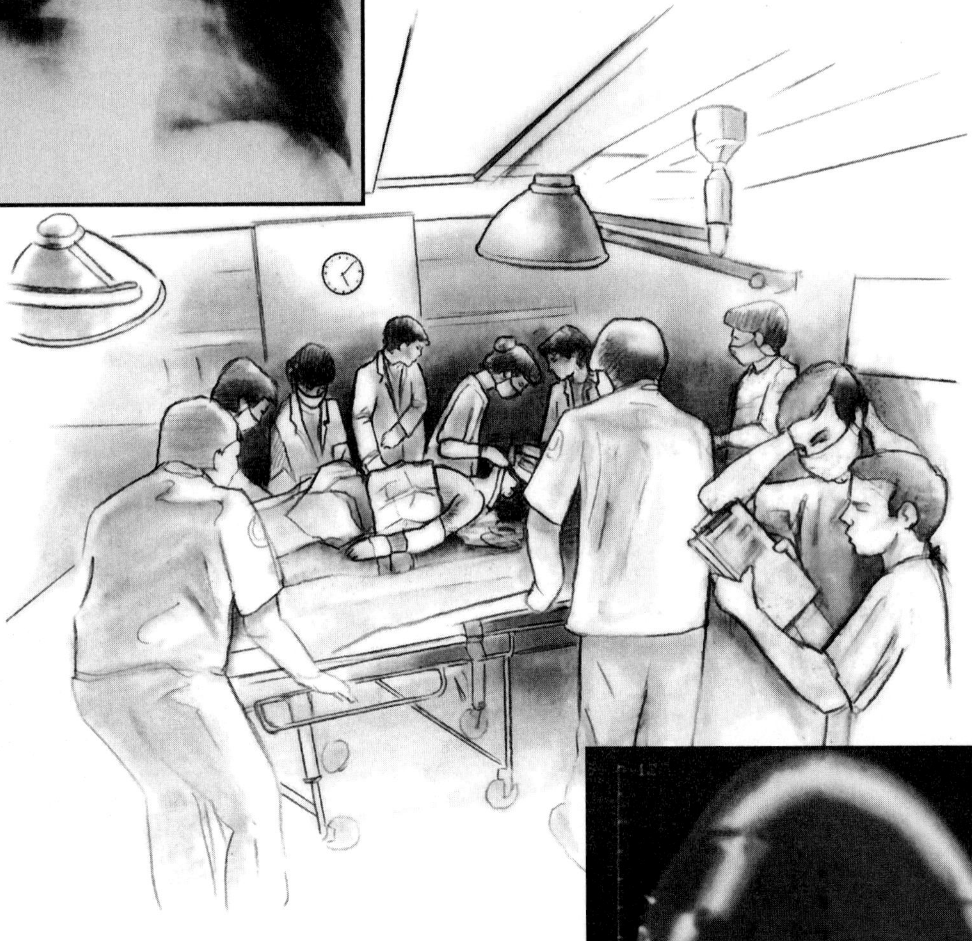

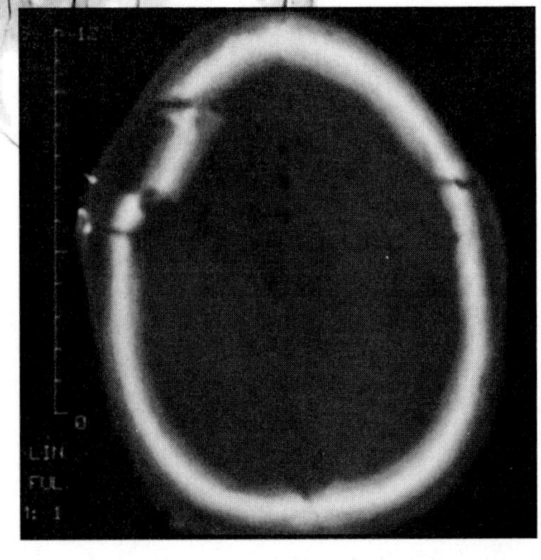

EARLY CARE OF MULTISYSTEM TRAUMA

Robert A. Read • Ernest E. Moore • Frederick A. Moore

A favorable outcome for a critically injured patient demands an integrated, multidisciplinary team effort from the injury scene through rehabilitation. The team comprises emergency medical technicians (EMTs), emergency department (ED) personnel, trauma surgeons, and a myriad of ancillary supportive and consulting services. Initial treatment is dictated by the patient's immediate physiologic requirements for survival (i.e., the ABCs: *a*irway, *b*reathing, and *c*irculation), and it is often begun before specific diagnoses have been established. Trauma patients frequently have multiple life-threatening injuries requiring rapid triage with simultaneous diagnostic and therapeutic interventions. The trauma surgeon must assume ultimate responsibility for the injured patient, assimilating key diagnostic results and orchestrating specific interventions implemented by trauma team members. This chapter deals with resuscitation and early definitive care within the first 24 hours after injury; Chapters 4 and 5 provide more detail on postoperative care and rehabilitation.

PREHOSPITAL CARE

Evaluation and resuscitation of an injured patient begins at the scene of injury. The U.S. Department of Transportation requires all ambulance attendants to have emergency medical technician (EMT) training. The EMT ambulance (EMT-A, or basic) can (1) provide airway assistance; (2) tamponade external bleeding; (3) immobilize fractured extremities; (4) apply the pneumatic antishock garment (PASG); and (5) perform closed-chest cardiopulmonary resuscitation. In most metropolitan regions, ambulance paramedics and helicopter flight nurses have advanced EMT skills. The EMT paramedic (EMT-P) can also (1) perform endotracheal intubation, (2) place peripheral intravenous (IV) cannulae, and (3) vent the chest for pneumothorax. In cases of prolonged transport time, flight nurses may also perform cricothyrostomy and tube thoracostomy, and insert central venous catheters.

Emergency transportation in the United States usually is obtained through the 911 Emergency Medical System (EMS). A central communications dispatcher receives the 911 call, activates the prehospital team, and alerts the potential receiving hospital. In most urban systems this prehospital response is multitiered, with first responders (e.g., firefighters and police officers) providing rapid, basic EMT care, followed by paramedics and flight nurses with advanced EMT skills. Pre-established field protocol manuals, radio communication with a physician at the base hospital, and routine trip audits ensure appropriate medical supervision.[214]

Prehospital care of a critically injured patient differs considerably from care of a medical arrest victim. For patients in cardiac arrest, providing advanced cardiac life support in the field clearly improves survival[45,56,217,264]; however, in prehospital trauma care, the primary objective is to deliver the patient safely to a trauma center with definitive surgical capabilities. The goals of the prehospital trauma team are to (1) ascertain the need for emergency care; (2) avoid further injury; (3) initiate treatment according to protocol; (4) establish radio communication with the base hospital; and (5) provide rapid transportation to the appropriate trauma facility. The treatment priorities at the scene are to (1) control external hemorrhage with direct pressure; (2) extricate the injured patient; (3) establish and maintain a patent airway and assist ventilation when needed; (4) protect the spine following blunt trauma; and (5) stabilize pelvic and long-bone fractures with the PASG and splints. The role of intravenous fluid administration remains controversial, but IV fluids may be indicated with prolonged transport time. Hypertonic saline solutions may significantly augment the circulating blood volume during prehospital transport.[305,323] The techniques used to achieve these initial goals depend on the patient's condition, the training and experience of the prehospital personnel, and the distance to the hospital.[40,118]

Advance notification of the receiving emergency department facilitates organization of the trauma team and ensures that ancillary services are available. The box below lists important prehospital information. The most valuable factors are mechanism of injury, level of consciousness, ventilatory status, systolic blood pressure, heart rate, and arrival time. Preparation for a hypotensive patient with a mediastinal gunshot wound is clearly different from that for an alert, normotensive victim of a vehicular accident. As a rule, with critical injuries, the shorter the distance to the hospital, the more succinct the verbal report. Assessment by more systematic injury scores may be appropriate for field triage in regionalized trauma systems, but to date these scoring systems have lacked specificity.

PREHOSPITAL INFORMATION NEEDED FOR ACUTE TRAUMA VICTIMS

- Patient's age and sex
- Mechanism of injury
- Time of injury
- Level of consciousness
- Systolic blood pressure
- Heart rate
- Respiratory rate
- Overt and suspected injuries
- Treatment initiated
- Estimated time of arrival
- Revised trauma score

REGIONALIZED TRAUMA SYSTEM

Optimum care of an injured patient requires a system that delivers the right patient to the right hospital in the shortest possible time. The American College of Surgeons' (ACS) Committee on Trauma has developed criteria to stratify hospitals into level I, II, III, or IV according to their capability for managing the acutely injured, providing education programs, and conducting trauma research.[39] The trauma center designation also depends on geographic constraints and population density, as well as regional hospital capabilities. Level I trauma centers are best prepared to treat critically injured patients with multisystem injuries; however, the prehospital trauma scores devised to select these high-risk patients are currently unsatisfactory. Moreover, in the United States, because of geographic limitations, much of the acute trauma is treated in level II facilities, and in many rural areas level III hospitals serve as trauma centers. Thus cost-effective and optimum trauma care may require federally subsidized state regulation defining comprehensive regionalized trauma systems such as that existing in Germany.[247,313]

The type of prehospital transportation depends on the patient's condition, the distance to the regional trauma facility, the weather, and accessibility to the scene. In urban regions, ground transportation with ambulances provides efficient access to capable trauma centers. The exception may be problems with traffic congestion or natural barriers, such as rivers. In rural areas, however, transport time becomes problematic for a se-

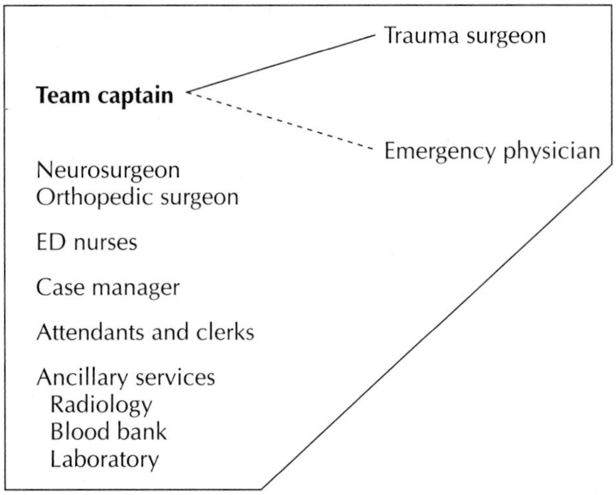

FIGURE 15-1 The emergency department (ED) trauma team consists of a team captain, consultants, ED nurses, and ancillary services. Successful trauma resuscitation requires the coordinated efforts of this team.

verely injured patient requiring advanced surgical care. For distances less than 25 miles, ambulance is preferred. When the distance is greater than 25 miles, aircraft may be more efficient. In general, the helicopter is optimal up to a distance of 100 miles, and fixed-wing aircraft become useful for longer distances.

EMERGENCY DEPARTMENT ORGANIZATION

The emergency department (ED) trauma team varies from hospital to hospital but generically consists of physicians, nurses, and attendants (Figure 15-1). Organizing the team with a predetermined captain is essential to achieve optimum use of individual talents. Upon notification from prehospital personnel en route, the resuscitation team begins assembling in the ED. Although most in-hospital trauma alert protocols use a paging system, we have found that a trauma light panel, activated in the ED and simultaneously displayed in the operating room and anesthesia and surgery departments, is a valuable adjunct.[196]

Team Captain

The team captain directs resuscitation and evaluation of the injured patient. An experienced trauma surgeon is best qualified for this position, although in most hospitals emergency physicians assume this role until a qualified surgeon arrives. The team captain's responsibilities are to (1) ensure continuous assessment of the patient by collecting information from team members and assimilating this with personal observations; (2) determine the need for therapeutic and diagnostic procedures; (3) coordinate the activities of ancillary services and surgical consultants; and (4) make triage decisions. Team captains must divorce themselves from technical procedures so that they can continue to review vital data and begin diagnostic and therapeutic efforts in the proper sequence. If resuscitation demands surgical expertise (e.g. cricothyrostomy or exigent thoracotomy), the trauma surgeon should relinquish the leadership position to another physician until this resuscitative procedure is completed.

Trauma Team Members

Competent and collegial physician team members are indispensable for efficient ED resuscitation. In urban teaching institutions, general surgery and emergency medicine residents provide ample staff. In smaller rural hospitals, however, primary care physicians with varied trauma experience are often the basic team members until a surgeon arrives. The physician's fundamental role, regardless of training, is to execute therapeutic and diagnostic procedures ordered by the team captain. Physicians may offer the team captain valuable clinical information but should resist independent decision making. This admonition is particularly germane to surgical consults, where multiple or conflicting orders may cause confusion. Conversely, it is essential to integrate the recommendations of the neurosurgeon if head injury is a factor or of the orthopedic surgeon if a major pelvic fracture exists.

The ED nurses are also invaluable in trauma care. A central function of the nurses is to obtain and report vital signs to the team captain. Abrupt changes and overall trends in vital signs frequently affect triage decisions; this information should be recorded temporally on an ED flow sheet, together with other resuscitation data. A large flow sheet or chalkboard, strategically located in the resuscitation room, can be helpful. Computer-assisted monitoring may provide an additional means to accomplish both meticulous record keeping and rapid visual display. The ED nurses also organize equipment and supplies for invasive procedures. Nursing priorities must be established so that nurses do not become entangled in technical procedures that may distract them from primary responsibilities. Major trauma facilities have added an additional nursing function—case manager. The case manager helps coordinate the treatment of trauma patients throughout their hospital stay, and this team member can be particularly helpful in the early phase of trauma care, which requires multispecialty involvement.

Ancillary personnel are also crucial for trauma diagnosis and efficient resuscitation. Radiology technicians are called upon for cervical spine, chest, and pelvic radiographs. Major clinical decisions frequently are based on these screening films, and adequate quality is essential. Blood bank technicians screen blood and prepare for occasional extraordinary demands of multiple blood-component therapy. Occasionally O-negative blood is required for immediate resuscitation, and type-specific blood should be available within 15 minutes. In urban EMS systems, paramedics often obtain blood samples en route to the hospital to minimize the blood type and cross-match delay.

Successful trauma resuscitation requires an integrated, multidisciplinary effort. The trauma team is a coordinated group of specialists dedicated to specific roles and priorities in the treatment of a critically injured patient, and their expertise is optimized by the leadership of a trauma surgeon.

INITIAL EVALUATION AND RESUSCITATION

Triage at the ED entrance is an important component of early trauma management, requiring the sound judgment of an experienced individual, often the ED charge nurse or emergency physician. Initial management of a critically injured patient demands simultaneous evaluation and treatment. Vital functions are quickly assessed while an empiric sequence of lifesaving therapeutic and diagnostic procedures is begun, dictated by the patient's physiologic status (Figure 15-2). The ACS Committee on Trauma emphasizes primary versus secondary survey in their Advanced Trauma Life Support (ATLS) course.[38]

Primary Survey (Life-Sustaining Priorities)

The patient's physiologic requirements govern initial resuscitation. The fundamental goal is to re-establish adequate oxygen supply to vital organs. Tissue oxygen delivery is largely determined by blood oxygen content, circulating blood volume, and cardiac output. The first priorities are to secure a patent airway and to optimize ventilation. In victims of blunt trauma, the cervical spine must be immobilized while a patent airway is established. The pleural space may need to be evacuated of blood and air to facilitate ventilation. For patients in persistent shock, tube thoracostomies are inserted before a chest radiograph is obtained (Figure 15-3). Blood from the thorax should be collected in sterile containers with isotonic saline for later autotransfusion.[126]

After a secure airway has been established, the next priority is to enhance cardiovascular performance. Initially, hypotension is assumed to be the result of acute blood loss and is treated with rapid volume infusion. External hemorrhage is controlled with manual pressure over bleeding sites to prevent further blood loss. Blind clamping is ill advised because of the risk of injury to adjacent structures, particularly nerves. Tourniquets generally are not indicated for extremity trauma, because splinting and compression usually control even arterial bleeding. The scalp is highly vascular and may be the source of significant blood loss; temporary mass sutures or Rainey clips may be needed to control scalp bleeding.

Intravascular volume restitution is started with administration of crystalloid via large-bore peripheral IV catheters. Refractory hypotension despite rapid crystalloid infusion suggests active bleeding or myocardial dysfunction. Cardiogenic shock is further characterized by distended neck veins or a persistently elevated central venous pressure (CVP) over 15 cm H_2O. However, in patients with mixed pathologic conditions, cardiac dysfunction may be masked until hypovolemia is corrected. Tension pneumothorax is the most common source of cardiogenic shock after injury. The next most common causes are myocardial contusion following blunt trauma, and pericardial tamponade after penetrating thoracic wounds.

Secondary Survey (Triage Decision Making)

The second echelon of ED management encompasses detailed assessment of the patient's overall condition and identification of potential life-threatening injuries (see Figure 15-2). EMTs and flight nurses often note important clues suggesting occult injury and should be queried before leaving the ED. In blunt trauma cases, the type of impact, vehicular damage, use of restraining devices, and condition of the other victims are helpful observations. For penetrating wounds, a description of the weapon and the amount of blood lost at the scene may be useful.

A rapid but systematic physical examination is essential and must be documented in the medical record. Patients are completely disrobed, examined for spinal injuries, and then rolled for inspection of the flanks and back. Important but frequently neglected aspects of the physical examination include detailed neurologic function, peripheral pulses, rectal examination for blood and sphincter tone, and inspection of the perineum, back, and axillae. A lateral cervical spine radiograph is obtained following major blunt trauma to the upper torso, neck, or head. The cervical spine is assumed to be unstable until all seven cervical and first thoracic vertebral bodies are visualized and a reliable, nontender physical examination is obtained. Splinting long-bone fractures decreases pain and minimizes additional soft tissue damage and blood loss. Prompt insertion of a nasogastric tube decompresses the stomach. With midfacial fractures, the tube should be placed orally to minimize the risk of passage into the cranial vault.[79] Blood in the gastric aspirate may be the only sign of an otherwise

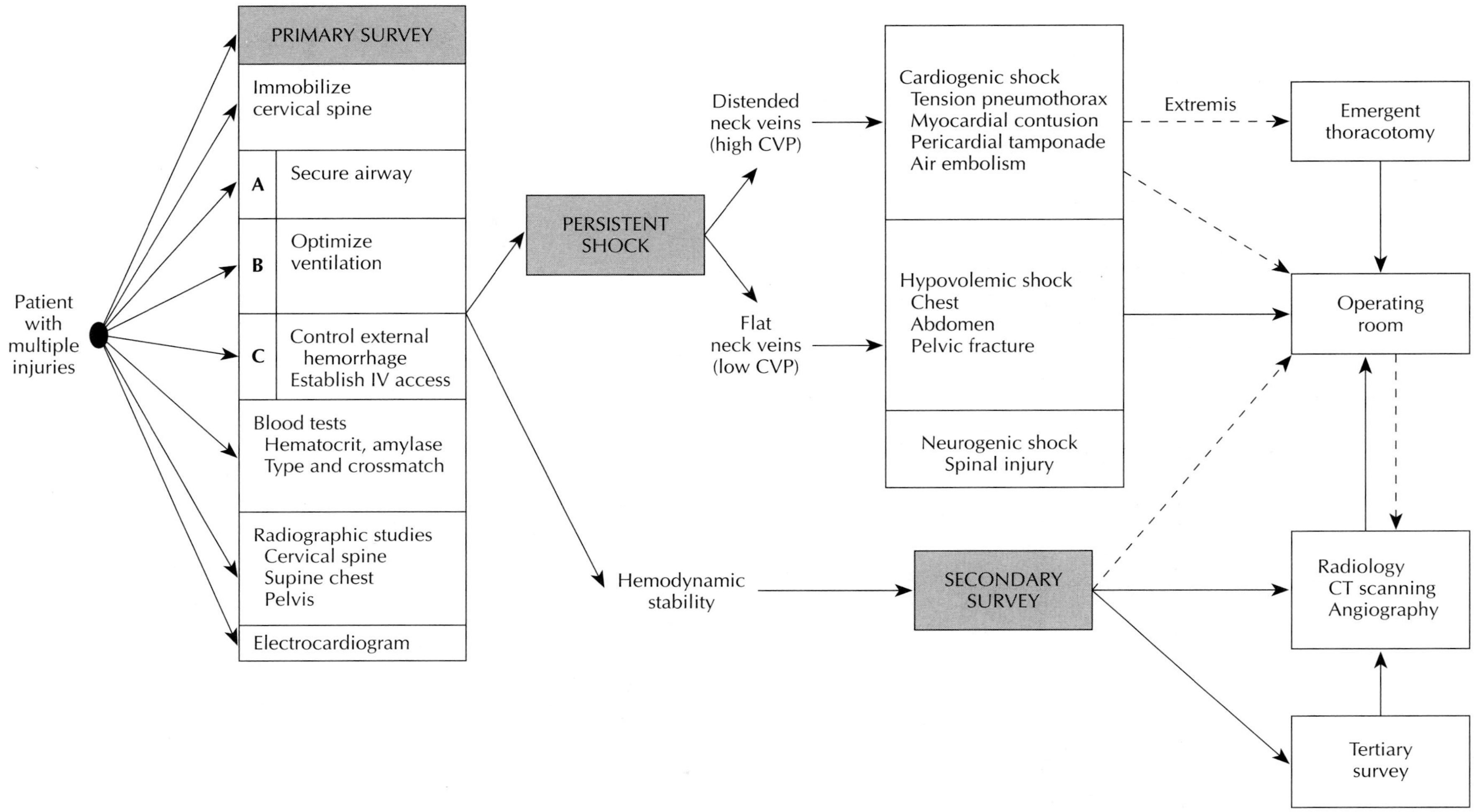

FIGURE 15-2 Initial ED trauma evaluation and resuscitation involve a sequence of simultaneous diagnostic and therapeutic procedures dictated by the patient's injuries and physiologic status.

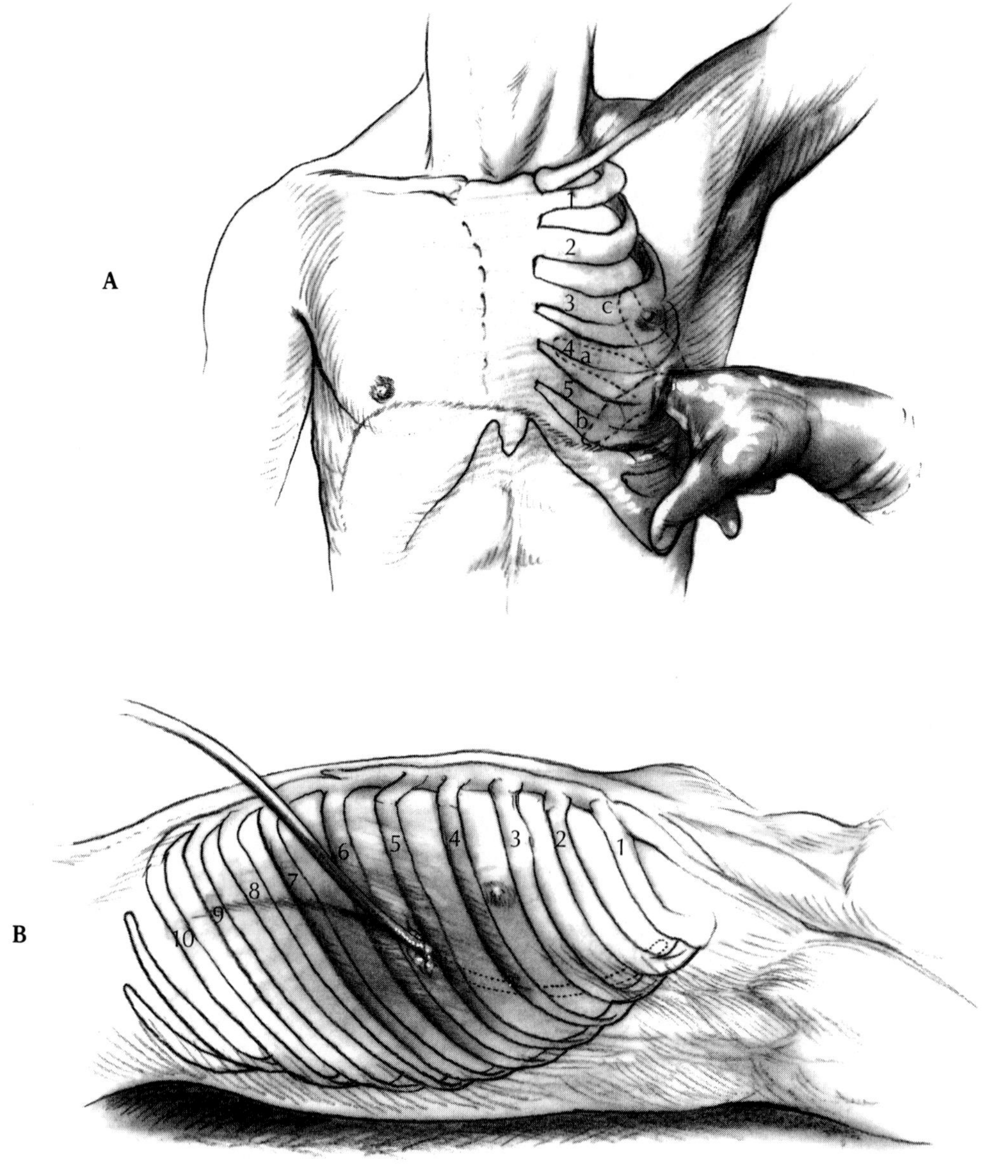

FIGURE 15-3 Air and blood are evacuated from the pleural space by tube thoracostomy in the fourth or fifth intercostal space. The tubes are placed after pneumohemothoraces have been verified by chest radiograph (or empirically for patients in persistent shock). Before a thoracostomy tube is placed, a gloved finger is inserted to verify intrapleural positioning of the tube and to prevent injury to the diaphragm. (Figures 15-3, 15-4, 15-5, 15-6, 15-8, 15-9, 15-17, 15-24, 15-25, 15-26, 15-27, 15-28, and 15-29 are redrawn from Moore EE, Eiseman B, Van Way C: *Critical decisions in trauma,* St Louis, 1985, Mosby.)

occult injury to the stomach or duodenum. A Foley catheter empties the bladder, may demonstrate hematuria, and permits monitoring of urinary output.

Occult regions of major hemorrhage include the pleural spaces, abdomen, retroperitoneum, and skeletal fractures. A chest radiograph is the most reliable screen for thoracic fractures and mediastinal and intrathoracic bleeding. The chest film also helps confirm the positions of the central venous catheter and endotracheal, nasogastric, and thoracostomy tubes. In a patient with multisystem injuries, the initial abdominal examination is notoriously unreliable in detecting acute intraperitoneal hemorrhage or visceral perforation. Intoxication, head injury, or pain from associated fractures often masks peritoneal irritation, resulting in a false negative examination in 20% to 50% of acutely injured patients.[163] Diagnostic peritoneal lavage (DPL) is still the most expedient and reliable method of identifying significant intraperitoneal hemorrhage,[202,256] although ED ultrasonography is becoming an alternative.[111,301] The sensitivity of DPL for significant intraperitoneal blood loss exceeds 98%.[72] Plain abdominal radiographs are primarily helpful in mapping bullet trajectories or characterizing pelvic fractures after blunt trauma.

An electrocardiogram (ECG) is routinely obtained after significant blunt chest trauma, whereas arterial blood gas (ABG) determinations are obtained in selected patients to confirm adequate ventilation and monitor intrapulmonary shunting. A blood sample for group typing should be sent promptly to the blood bank if the patient manifests signs suggesting hypovolemia. Tetanus prophylaxis is mandatory unless the patient's current immunization status is known, but systemic antibiotics should be withheld unless a specific indication arises. Routine laboratory tests for acute trauma include a complete blood count (CBC) and urinalysis for hematuria.[290]

Tertiary Survey (Reevaluation and Disposition)

The third echelon in the management of trauma patients consists of a compulsive and systematic reevaluation after all life- and limb-threatening injuries have been cared for and toxic or metabolic derrangements have been corrected. This survey frequently is done 12 to 24 hours after admission. Patients are systematically re-examined for occult injuries not evident on presentation because of other urgent, life-threatening conditions and changes in consciousness caused by pain, injury, or intoxicants. Persistent or newly discovered neck pain suggests a cervical spine fracture; confusion or subtle neurologic signs may be due to a cerebral contusion or hematoma; tachypnea associated with decreased breath sounds may indicate a delayed pneumothorax; increasing abdominal pain and tenderness suggest an occult bowel perforation; and swelling, pain, and ecchymoses of extremities may be caused by underlying fractures. Indeed, the most commonly overlooked injuries are fractures, which may include unstable cervical injuries. The signs and symptoms of significant occult injuries are at times difficult to discern amid the distracting pain of strains, contusions, and abrasions.

After a detailed re-examination and a survey of pertinent diagnostic studies (e.g., repeat hematocrit, serum amylase, chest radiograph), plans are made for appropriate disposition and follow-up. These measures may include physical therapy and rehabilitation, further diagnostic studies, alcohol detoxification, or simply a return visit to the primary physician's office.

Airway Management

Establishing a patent airway and ensuring adequate ventilation are the utmost priorities in a critically injured patient. Early signs of hypoxia include anxiety, restlessness, and confusion. The principal causes of hypoxia in trauma patients are airway obstruction and hypoventilation. Airway obstruction may be caused by (1) loss of protective reflexes in a comatose patient; (2) foreign bodies, including blood, secretions, teeth, or bony fragments; (3) extensive swelling or collapse of pharyngeal soft tissues following midfacial injuries; or (4) direct trauma to tracheolaryngeal structures. Signs of impending airway obstruction include hoarseness, stridor, nasal alar flaring, snoring, or accessory muscle breathing. Hypoventilation occurs with (1) blunted ventilatory drive resulting from intracranial injury; (2) impaired pulmonary mechanics caused by hemopneumothorax, flail chest, an open thoracic wound, a diaphragmatic tear, or a bronchopleural fistula; or (3) respiratory muscle weakness caused by spinal cord trauma. Clinical evidence of inadequate ventilation includes poor air exchange at the nose and mouth, diminished breath sounds, and decreased chest wall excursion.

Airway management in an injured patient usually can be accomplished with simple techniques, but occasionally it may be extremely challenging. The first maneuver is to clear the airway manually of debris and to suction secretions from the oropharynx. In an unconscious or obtunded patient, elevating the angle of the mandible and placing an oropharyngeal airway may maintain airway patency. Supplemental oxygen is given by nasal cannula or oxygen mask. Nasal prongs provide 40% oxygen concentration at 6 L/minute, whereas a reservoir mask can deliver 90% concentration at 12 L/minute.

In blunt trauma cases, airway control must proceed on the assumption that the cervical spine is unstable. Significant instability of the cervical spine is present in 12% of patients with major head injuries, more than 20% of accident fatalities, and 60% of patients with fatal head injuries.[43] The dominant mechanism for cervical spine injury is hyperextension from direct impact on the head within the vehicle, although axial loading,

A

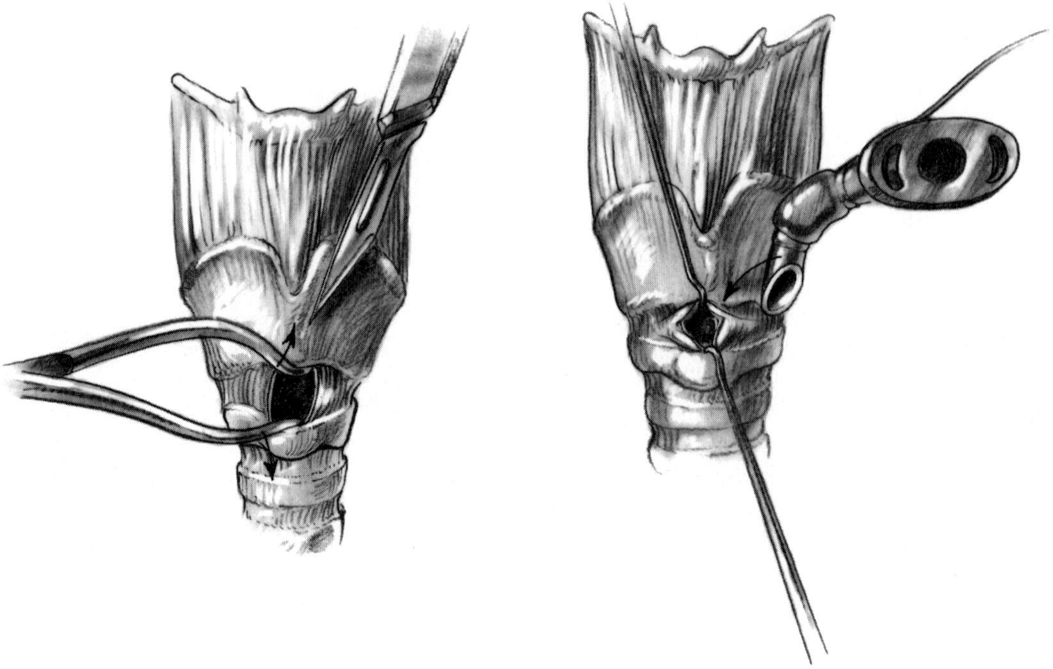

B

FIGURE 15-4 **A,** Through a vertical skin incision, the cricothyroid membrane is incised horizontally. **B,** The thyroid cartilage is retracted superiorly with a tracheal hook to facilitate placement of the cricothyrostomy tube. The cricothyroid space in an adult usually will accept a 6 mm tube.

hyperflexion, and violent rotation are contributing forces. Neck injuries associated with neurologic deficits in adults most often occur at the C5-6 and C6-7 levels.[50] A quality cross-table, lateral cervical spine (CTLCS) radiograph will delineate the vast majority of unstable cervical spine fractures. The most common radiographic errors are inadequate visualization of C7-T1 and poor definition of the occiput, C1, and C2 components. Although anteroposterior, oblique, and open-mouth views should be obtained eventually,[269] initial airway management is based on clinical judgment in light of the CTLCS film and physical and neurologic examination.

The timing of active airway management is crucial. Premature attempts at endotracheal intubation frequently are difficult and may precipitate urgent surgical intervention. Conversely, undue delay may compromise the patient and preclude simple means of airway access. Bag-mask ventilation performed by an experienced person is an effective temporizing measure, particularly when adequate oxygenation is continuously verified with pulse oximetry. However, prolonged bag-mask ventilation has disadvantages: it consumes the full attention of a skilled trauma team member, it may insufflate air into the stomach, and it is resisted by patients breathing spontaneously. Patients with persistent airway obstruction, signs of inadequate ventilation, expanding cervical hematomas, or deteriorating vital signs require intervention. Patients with major head injuries are intubated promptly to facilitate hyperventilation for reducing intracranial pressure (ICP).[232]

The method of airway management used depends on (1) whether the patient has maxillary facial trauma; (2) whether cervical spine injury is suspected; (3) the patient's overall condition; and (4) the physician's expertise. Patients in respiratory distress with severe facial injury require prompt percutaneous or surgical cricothyrostomy with placement of a tube with a 6 mm inner diameter (ID) (Figure 15-4).[174] The rare exception is the patient with direct laryngeal trauma or tracheal disruption; these injuries require emergency tracheostomy.[83,284] Percutaneous transtracheal ventilation (PTV) may be an acceptable alternative to either of these surgical airway procedures, particularly in children.[124,215] A large-bore angiocatheter is placed through the cricothyroid membrane and attached to an oxygen source. This technique entrains a relatively low volume of highly concentrated oxygen into the lungs and may temporize patients by providing reasonable oxygenation. Extended PTV, however, is limited by ventilation (carbon dioxide [CO_2] exchange) and is contraindicated with airway obstruction unless the high-frequency ventilation technique is used.[123]

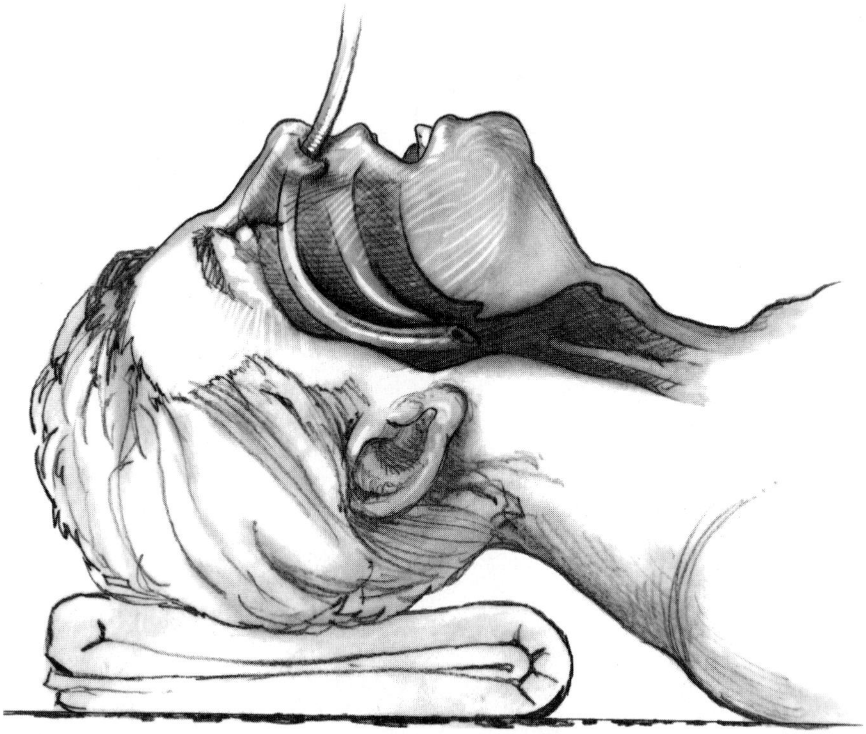

FIGURE 15-5 Blind nasotracheal intubation requires spontaneous ventilation. Airflow noise is used as a guide as the tube is gently advanced into the larynx during inspiration.

Nasotracheal intubation (Figure 15-5) is a safe method for establishing an airway in nonapneic patients who may have a cervical spine injury. Although this is a "blind" procedure, the success rate exceeds 90% in experienced hands in the acute setting.[42] Careful technique minimizes the principal complications, nasal bleeding and retropharyngeal tears.[296] An important advantage of the nasotracheal route is that intubation can be performed in an alert patient without need for excessive sedation or muscle relaxation; thus repeat attempts can be made without precipitating a "crash intubation" scenario. If the nasotracheal approach is unsuccessful, standard orotracheal intubation should be done. In most awake, critically injured patients, muscle relaxation is necessary to facilitate mouth and head positioning during orotracheal intubation. Either nondepolarizing agents (atracurium and vecuronium) or succinylcholine (1.5 mg/kg) are used because of their rapid onset and relatively brief duration.[246,292] Muscle fasciculations and transient elevations in ICP are attenuated by pretreatment with small doses of nondepolarizing drugs. Despite favorable pharmacokinetics, muscle relaxation with succinylcholine may precipitate the need for a surgical airway procedure should the orotracheal route fail. Trauma team members must anticipate and prepare for this before any muscle relaxant is administered. Experienced personnel, oximetric monitoring, and equipment for bag-mask ventilation, suctioning, and cricothyrostomy must be available.

For an unconscious patient, orotracheal intubation with in-line cervical traction is the preferred airway access.[156] It can be performed quickly, safely, and with greatest security because the larynx and trachea are visualized. Moreover, the larger endotracheal tube facilitates ventilation, pulmonary suctioning, and bronchoscopy when indicated. The most common error is advancing the tube into the right mainstem bronchus. Auscultation of the chest usually reveals this complication, but radiographic confirmation of the tube's final position should be obtained as soon as possible.

Circulation

With ventilation optimized, the next priority is to improve oxygen transport to vital organs. Postinjury shock occurs because of inadequate circulating blood volume (cardiac preload), impaired myocardial function (diastolic filling or contractility), altered vascular resistance (ventricular afterload), or a combination of these.[288] Acute blood loss resulting in hypovolemia is the most common cause of shock in a patient with multisystem trauma.[309] Although passive leg raises,[88] Trendelenburg's position,[272] and use of the PASG[88,244] have been recommended to improve venous return, the mainstay of initial therapy is rapid IV volume infusion.[318] Crystalloid

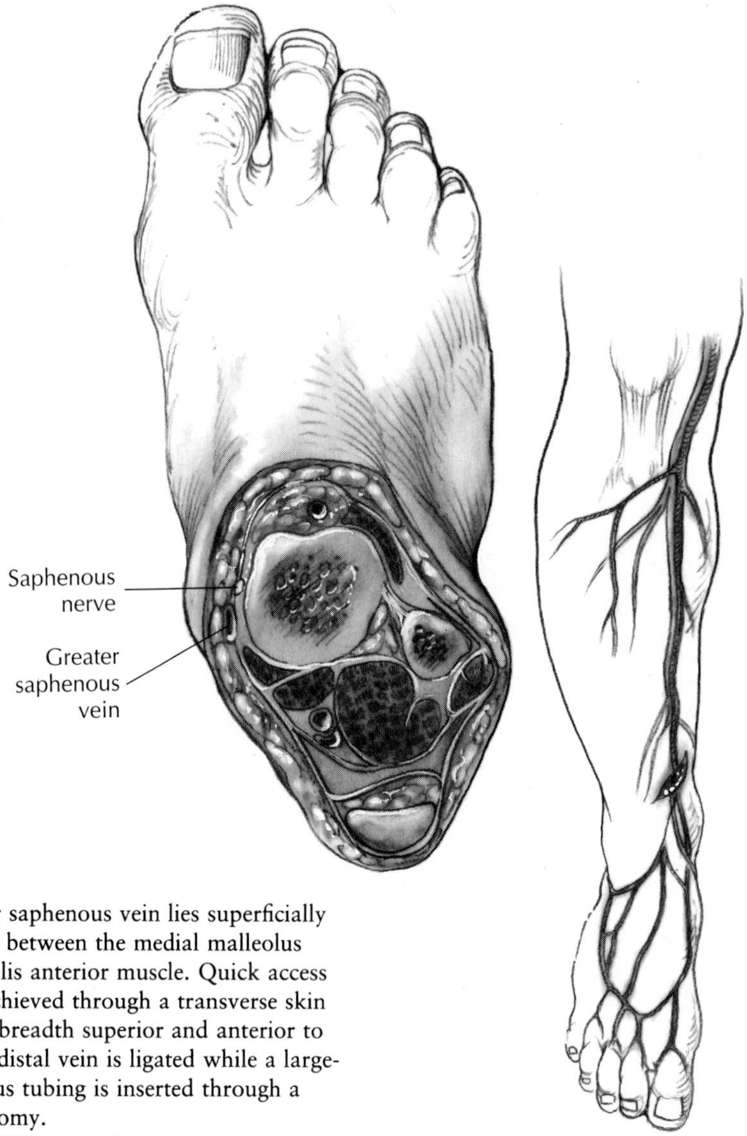

FIGURE 15-6 The greater saphenous vein lies superficially on the anterior periosteum between the medial malleolus and the tendon of the tibialis anterior muscle. Quick access to the saphenous vein is achieved through a transverse skin incision made one finger's breadth superior and anterior to the medial malleolus. The distal vein is ligated while a large-bore catheter or intravenous tubing is inserted through a proximal transverse veinotomy.

solutions are preferred for early resuscitation.[262] Colloid solutions have not proved to be more effective in restoring tissue perfusion,[58,207] are costly, and may aggravate post-traumatic complications, including respiratory distress syndrome[154] and renal dysfunction.[153] Lactated Ringer's solution has a theoretic advantage over normal saline, because it provides a better buffer for the metabolic acidosis of protracted shock.[27,41,297] Renewed interest is being shown in hypertonic saline solutions, which can significantly expand circulating blood volume.[323]

The route of venous access for fluid administration depends on the patient's hemodynamic status and the skill of the trauma team. In most patients, short, 14-gauge catheters can be readily inserted into the antecubital veins. This percutaneous route is quick, simple, and free of complications. In most prehospital systems, these catheters are placed while the patient is being transported to the hospital. When vascular collapse precludes percutaneous access in the arm, the practical alternatives are subclavian, internal jugular, femoral, or saphenous vein catheterization.

Although the central venous route is safe in hypovolemic patients, line placement at this site interferes with other life-sustaining procedures.[275] For this reason we prefer short, 10-gauge catheters or direct IV extension tubing into the greater saphenous vein through an ankle cutdown (Figure 15-6). A transverse incision is made between the medial malleolus and the tibialis anterior tendon. This cutdown site is remote from other resuscitative maneuvers and does not interfere with concurrent use of the PASG device. Percutaneous femoral vein cannulation with 8.5 French (Fr) introducers is our alternative if the patient demands rapid transport to the operating room (OR).[95] The argument against using venous access in the leg with abdominal trauma is that extravasation may occur via an injured vena cava, but this argument has not been substantiated.[243] In such a patient, however, central venous introducers should be secured as secondary IV routes after thoracic assessment has been completed.

In adults, crystalloid solution is infused as quickly as possible until blood pressure and heart rate respond satisfactorily.[27] Patients with free intraperitoneal or intrathoracic bleeding should be transported to the OR immediately, without awaiting normalization of vital signs.[159] As a general rule, the carotid pulse is palpable at a systolic blood pressure (SBP) of 60 mm Hg, the femoral pulse at 70 mm Hg, and the radial pulse at 80 mm Hg.[38] With massive hemorrhage, the equivalent crystalloid replacement for blood loss may approach a ratio of 8 : 1 because of the progressive fall in plasma oncotic pressure and intracellular sequestration of sodium.[29] The systemic blood pressure, heart rate, urinary output (should be over 0.5 ml/kg/hour in adults) and overall appearance of the patient are the practical guidelines to follow in the initial treatment of profound hypovolemia.[276] The CVP reflects right ventricular dyastolic filling and is most helpful in distinguishing persistent hypovolemic shock from cardiogenic shock. As with interpretation of other vital signs, isolated readings may be misleading, and trends should be analyzed in conjunction with the volume of fluid given. A CVP that remains below 5 cm H_2O implies hypovolemia. On the other hand, a CVP above 15 cm H_2O may be falsely elevated because of rapid fluid infusion, a sudden increase in thoracic pressure from patient straining or agitation, or a malpositioned catheter.

Acute whole blood loss can be replaced initially with crystalloid because, given in sufficient quantity, (1) this solution effectively repletes extracellular as well as intracellular deficits; (2) hemodilution may enhance distal perfusion by decreasing blood viscosity; and (3) compensatory increases in cardiac output and peripheral oxygen extraction improve tissue oxygenation.[200,310] The role of hypertonic saline, particularly with head injury, currently is under investigation.[323] Blood should be added to the resuscitation when crystalloid infusion exceeds 50 ml/kg (3.5 L for a 70 kg adult).[9] Un-cross-matched, type-specific whole blood is rarely associated with complications[94] and is available within 15 minutes in most hospitals. If type-specific blood is unavailable, reconstituted type O-negative packed red blood cells should be used. In the future red cell substitutes or recombinant hemoglobin may serve as temporizing agents in cases of profound blood loss.[99] Although micropore filters generally are placed in the infusion line for banked blood, they impede the infusion rate and their value in removing microaggregates is questionable.[53,257]

The most devastating complication of massive blood and fluid resuscitation is a refractory coagulopathy.[57,129] Paradoxically, clotting is accelerated at the capillary level as a result of shock and tissue damage,[108] but the circulating blood becomes hypocoagulable. A number of factors are responsible for this. Banked blood is deficient in factors V, VIII, and platelets, and replete with fibrin-split products and vasoactive substances. These features generally become important when more than 15 units have been given acutely.[36,179] Autotransfused blood generally is safe,[167] but in large quantities it can also adversely affect the coagulation cascade.[193,274] Timely replacement with fresh frozen plasma and platelets minimizes the risk of coagulopathy during massive transfusion.[90] Although blood components are not usually indicated in the early resuscitation phase, anticipated needs should be conveyed promptly to the blood bank. Sequential coagulation profiles consisting of prothrombin time, activated partial thromboplastin time, and platelet counts are obtained to confirm adequate component therapy. We prefer to maintain the platelet count above 50,000/mm^3. If a coagulopathy ensues, further analysis is carried out with fibrinogen level, template bleeding time, and heparin-corrected thrombin times.[90] When nonmechanical bleeding persists despite normalization of the coagulation profiles, fresh whole blood is administered.

In the initial period of massive blood transfusion, potential complications include hypocalcemia, acidosis, and hypothermia. Hypocalcemia, from citrate binding, does not usually occur until the blood transfusion rate exceeds 1 unit/5 minutes. Moreover, decreased serum-ionized calcium depresses myocardial function before impairing coagulation.[286,300] Calcium gluconate (10 mg/kg intravenously) should be reserved for ST interval prolongation on the ECG or unexplained hypotension during massive transfusion. The protective role of calcium blockers during reperfusion in experimental shock emphasizes the rationale for selective calcium supplementation.[314]

Hypothermia has been associated with decreased survival in experimental hemorrhagic shock and appears to be an adverse factor clinically.[57,125,129] Moderate hypothermia (32° C [90° F]) causes platelet sequestration and inhibits release of platelet factors important in the intrinsic clotting pathway. On the other hand, modest hypothermia may be protective during resuscitation by reducing oxygen demands. The core temperature of injured patients often falls insidiously because of environmental exposure at the scene and in the emergency department and as a result of administration of cold resuscitation fluids. Lactated Ringer's solution should be prewarmed to 40° C (104° F) in incubators in the ED, and blood should always be infused via warming devices. A very simple method of preventing hypothermia involves heating and aerosolizing oxygen for a ventilated patient. In cases of severe hypothermia (temperature below 32° C [59.6° F]), we use closed thoracic lavage[12,226] and femoral arteriovenus rewarming with the level I rapid infusion device.[93]

Administration of bicarbonate for systemic acidosis remains controversial. Moderate acidosis (pH 7.2) may impair coagulation,[51,108] myocardial contractility,[32,45] and oxidative metabolism.[80] In a trauma patient, acidosis usually is caused by anaerobic production of lactic acid.[91] Although administering sodium bicarbonate corrects systemic acidosis, secondary alkalosis potentially increases hemoglobin affinity for oxygen and thereby impairs tissue oxygenation. Also, sodium bicarbonate may exacerbate intracellular acidosis by increasing CO_2 clearance.[49] Consequently, bicarbonate infusion should be limited to cases of protracted shock. Mixed venous pH levels, obtained from a CVP line, may be used to estimate the systemic arterial pH.[190] Blood gases should be corrected for core body temperature (increased pH 0.015/1° C drop).

Emergency Department Thoracotomy

ED thoracotomy is an integral part of the initial management of a trauma patient who arrives in extremis or who deteriorates into cardiac arrest.[11,34,263] Continued external cardiac compression may be ineffective in a hypotensive patient,[265] and irreversible cortical damage can be a permanent sequela of prolonged resuscitation.[54,117] The basic goal of emergency thoracotomy is to re-establish perfusion to critical organs (i.e., the brain and heart). The specific objectives are to (1) release pericardial tamponade; (2) control intrathoracic blood loss; (3) control transpulmonary air embolism; (4) initiate internal cardiac massage; and (5) cross-clamp the descending thoracic aorta to enhance coronary and cerebral perfusion and decrease subdiaphragmatic bleeding.[52,144,180,188]

The chest is opened via a left anterolateral thoracotomy through the fourth or fifth intercostal space (Figure 15-7, *A*). This exposure gives quick access to the heart, descending thoracic aorta, and left lung. The incision should be extended across the sternum into the right pleural cavity (Figure 15-7, *B*) for penetrating wounds in the right chest or superior mediastinum. The heart is exposed via a generous incision in the pericardium anterior to the phrenic nerve, and the thoracic aorta is clamped just inferior to the left pulmonary hilum (Figure 15-7, *C*). Protracted hemorrhagic shock may induce idioventricular arrhythmias refractory to conventional drug therapy.[315] In such a patient, temporary cardiac pacing may be needed until the metabolic environment of the myocardium improves.[184]

The mechanism of injury largely determines whether the patient survives after an ED thoracotomy. The greatest success is achieved with penetrating cardiac wounds; particularly stab injuries to the right side of the heart, where pericardial tamponade is the predominant cause of hemodynamic demise.[11] Survival with intact neurologic function, on the other hand, is rare in a patient who undergoes cardiac arrest as a result of exsanguinating blunt trauma.[11,34,61] Adding laparotomy in the ED for definitive control of abdominal hemorrhage has not improved this dismal outcome.[164]

Cardiogenic Shock

Cardiac dysfunction must be considered in patients who remain hypotensive despite adequate ventilatory support and volume loading. The most common causes of cardiogenic shock after injury are (1) tension pneumothorax; (2) pericardial tamponade; (3) myocardial contusion or infarction;[46] and (4) air embolism.

Tension Pneumothorax

Tension pneumothorax develops when a pleural or bronchial tear serves as a one-way valve leading to progressive increase of intrapleural air and positive pressure. The ipsilateral lung collapses, and with increasing pleural pressure, the mediastinum shifts to the contralateral side. Restricted air exchange and ventilation-perfusion mismatch cause hypoxemia. Cardiac performance is further compromised as venous return becomes impaired because of rising intrathoracic pressure. Physical signs of tension pneumothorax are tracheal deviation away from the affected hemithorax and increased thoracic resonance to percussion with diminished breath sounds on the involved side. Patients in persistent shock after a penetrating thoracic wound or blunt chest trauma should have the injured hemithorax vented empirically without waiting for radiographic confirmation of a pneumo/hemothorax. Although inserting a large-bore needle into the anterior second intercostal space may be appropriate as a temporary measure in the field, it is no substitute for placing a large chest tube (36 Fr in adults) via the lateral fifth intercostal space[185] (see Figure 15-3). Persistent, massive air leakage following tube thoracostomy suggests a major bronchial tear. Treatment of this injury involves early bronchoscopy and thoracotomy to repair significant tears.[16,103] Mechanical ventilation of these patients with large bronchopleural fistulae may require intubation with a double-lumen tube and independent lung ventilation.

Pericardial Tamponade

Traumatic cardiac tamponade is caused by acute accumulation of blood or air in the pericardial sac. A patient with chronic pericardial disease can tolerate a gradual accumulation of more than a liter of fluid; in

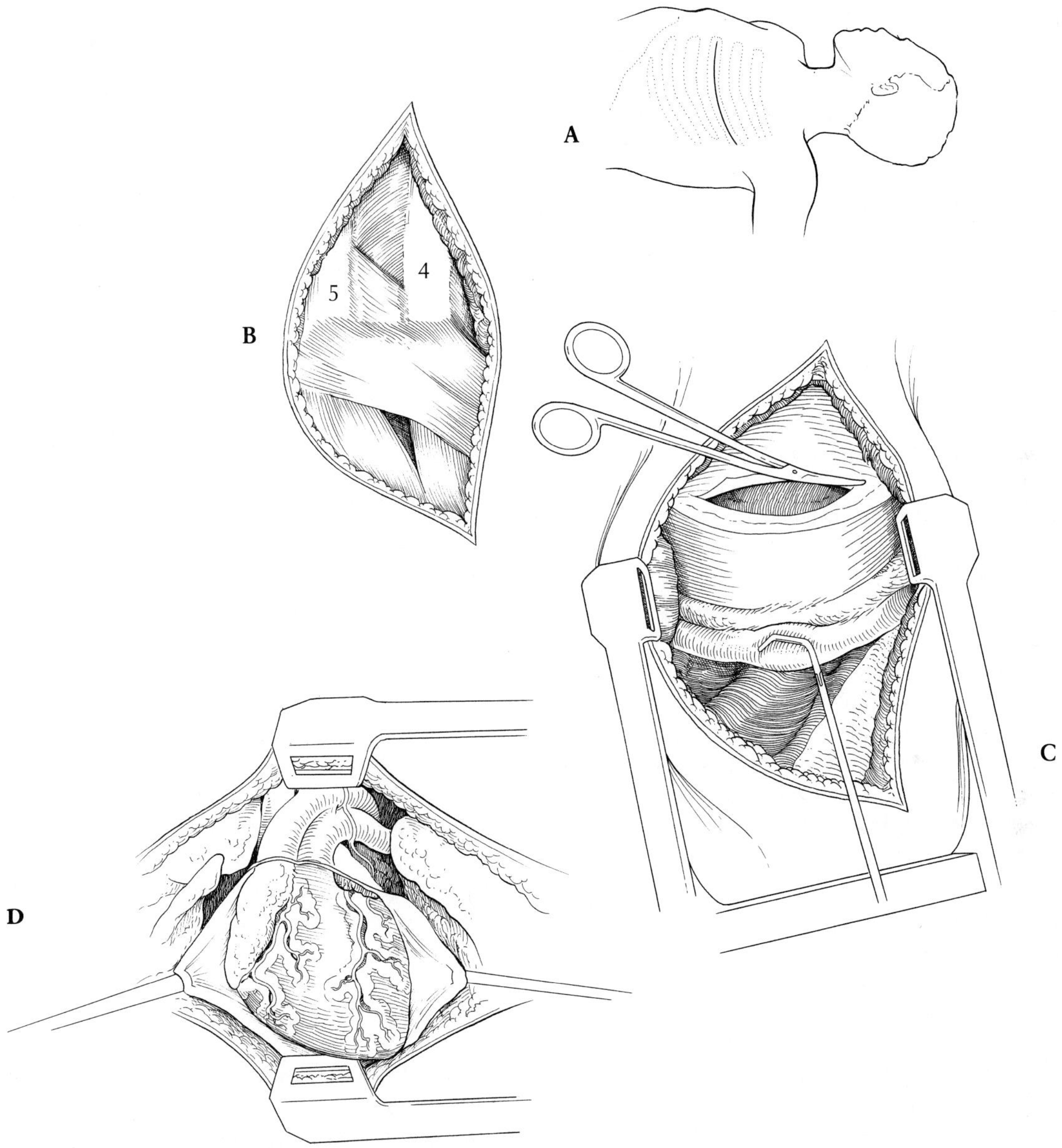

FIGURE 15-7 A, Resuscitative anterolateral thoracotomy is performed through an incision in the left fifth intercostal space. The skin, lateral pectoralis major muscle, and serratus anterior muscle are divided, exposing the ribs and intercostal muscles. The chest is entered through the fifth intercostal space, with care taken not to injure the underlying lung. **B,** Bilateral anterolateral thoracotomy provides access to both thoracic cavities and to the pulmonary hila, heart, and proximal great vessels. **C,** The lung is reflected superomedially, exposing the descending thoracic aorta, which is controlled with a Satinsky vascular clamp or digital pressure. A pericardiotomy is performed with scissors anterior to the phrenic nerve. **D,** The heart is delivered from the pericardium for repair of cardiac wounds and internal cardiac compression.

contrast, acute collection of 150 ml of blood may precipitate profound hemodynamic instability. The pathophysiology of this condition is dominated initially by impaired diastolic ventricular filling, caused by an increase in intrapericardial pressure.[78] This situation is later aggravated by depressed contractility arising from myocardial ischemia.[310]

Physical signs of acute cardiac tamponade may be subtle, particularly with hypovolemia. Beck's triad (arterial hypotension, central venous hypertension, and distant heart sounds) is absent in more than one third of patients with postinjury tamponade,[62] and classic pulsus paradoxus is rarely discernible.[26] Early recognition depends on a high index of suspicion. Pericardial tamponade most often occurs with penetrating heart wounds,[18,62,299] but it also can result from blunt cardiac rupture.[160] Tearing of low-pressure atria may be particularly insidious because blood loss into the pericardium often is small and clotted blood may temporarily seal these injuries. Pericardial tamponade must be assumed in all patients with central penetrating chest injuries. On the other hand, cardiac wounds occur via remote entrance sites in 20% of patients.[18,299] Axillary, back, supraclavicular, and subxiphoid wounds can be associated with pericardial violation.

Diagnosis of acute pericardial tamponade most often is based on (1) the presence of a high-risk wound, (2) systemic hypotension, and (3) distended neck veins with persistent CVP readings above 15 cm H_2O. Portable chest radiographs, ECGs, and tube thoracostomy drainage are rarely decisive factors in confirming tamponade, although emergency department echocardiography may be helpful.[119] Diagnostic testing and management of pericardial tamponade in the ED depend on (1) the patient's hemodynamic status; (2) the skills and experience of the resuscitation team; and (3) the availability of an operating room. Definitive treatment of a normotensive patient is best rendered in the OR, where illumination of the field, operating instruments, and surgical assistance are optimal. On the other hand, a patient who remains hypotensive despite an elevated CVP is in a precarious condition because small additional increments of hemopericardium will precipitate dramatic hemodynamic deterioration. Pericardial aspiration of as little as 15 ml of blood can improve cardiac performance enough to allow the patient to be transported safely to the OR. Moreover, significant subendocardial ischemia may occur despite a normal systemic blood pressure.

Pericardiocentesis can be performed by several routes. In the emergency setting, an 18-gauge, polyethylene catheter can be introduced via the left xiphoid-costal angle and directed toward the posterior aspect of the left shoulder (Figure 15-8). Although ECG monitoring or ultrasound guidance is desirable for elective diagnostic pericardiocentesis, it usually is not practical when acute therapeutic drainage is needed. Pericardial aspiration for acute hemopericardium is falsely negative in 15% of patients because the blood is clotted.[62,299] In this situation a subxiphoid window may be an alternative temporizing measure,[168,299] but it does not provide access to the cardiac wound if bleeding is reactivated. If the patient is in extremis, an emergency left anterior thoracotomy[11] (see Figure 15-7) should be carried out promptly, the pericardium opened widely anterior to the phrenic nerve, and cardiorrhaphy accomplished with pledgeted sutures (or skin staples for more extensive lesions).[166,270] The patient should then be transferred to the OR for definitive cardiorrhaphy and closure of the thoracotomy.

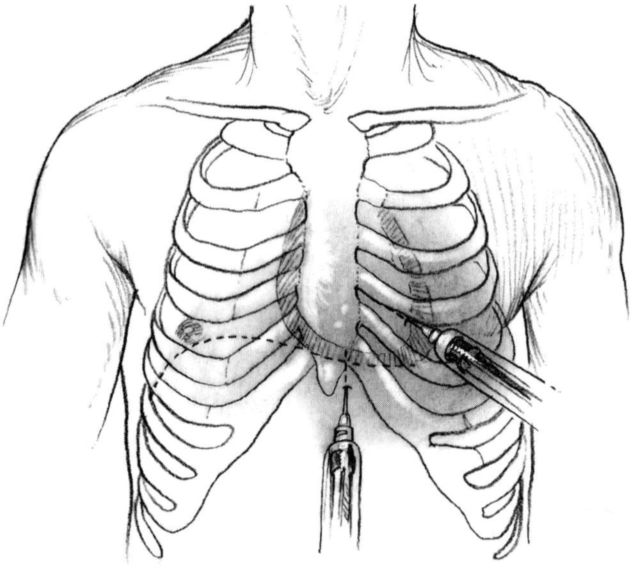

FIGURE 15-8 Pericardiocentesis is performed to decompress pericardial tamponade. A large-bore needle is advanced blindly into the pericardial sac from a subxyphoid approach. Removing even a small amount of pericardial fluid may improve cardiac function dramatically. After the initial aspiration, the needle can be exchanged for a pigtail catheter to facilitate additional pericardial drainage en route to the operating room.

Myocardial Contusion or Infarction

Cardiogenic shock may be caused by direct myocardial injury, ischemia caused by protracted shock or myocardial infarction caused by acute coronary thrombosis.[46] Myocardial contusion is present in 15% to 40% of patients admitted to the intensive care unit with blunt chest trauma.[46] The right ventricle is most often contused, presumably because of its greater exposure to an anterior chest impact. Cardiac pump failure and ventricular arrhythmias are the major acute complications.

Most life-threatening arrhythmias occur within 6 hours of injury.

Initial treatment for cardiac contusion is similar to that for acute myocardial infarction. Fundamental principles include adequate ventilation, judicious fluid administration, monitoring of serum electrolytes, and pharmacologic suppression of life-threatening arrhythmias. Right ventricular distension may compromise left ventricular filling volume and thus decrease cardiac output.[287] If the patient remains in refractory shock, emergency intra-aortic balloon counterpulsation may be used to increase cardiac output, reduce myocardial work, and augment coronary perfusion.[2,224,278] The percutaneous approach via the common femoral artery allows insertion of the balloon device in the ED.

Air Embolism

Air embolism is an uncommon but quickly lethal complication of pulmonary injury. Although most cases are described following penetrating trauma,[101,131,224,291] air emboli may also be produced by blunt pulmonary lacerations. In either situation, the typical clinical scenario follows intubation of a hypovolemic patient with thoracic trauma. Positive airway pressure introduces air emboli into pulmonary veins from terminal bronchi; the emboli traverse the left heart into the coronary circulation causing cardiac standstill. Resuscitation consists of emergency thoracotomy (see Figure 15-7), pulmonary hilar cross-clamping, air aspiration from the left ventricle, and open cardiac massage. Indeed, hypertension is advocated to clear intracoronary air. Pulmonary lobectomy often is required but should be performed after transfer to the OR.

Hypovolemic Shock

Acute blood loss is the most common cause of posttraumatic shock seen in the ED. Although external sources of blood loss usually are obvious, significant and occasionally exsanguinating occult bleeding can occur into the pleural cavities, abdomen, retroperitoneum, and pelvis. Patients in profound shock are quickly intubated and volume loaded; chest tubes are placed empirically. Recalcitrant, profound shock may warrant ED resuscitation thoracotomy and aortic cross-clamping. Patients who are in shock but who respond to initial volume infusion require rapid assessment of their chest, abdomen, and pelvis for occult injuries. A normal supine chest radiograph effectively rules out significant intrathoracic hemorrhage. Conversely, large collections of intrathoracic blood require prompt placement of large-bore thoracostomy tubes. Continuous, large-volume thoracic blood loss requires expedient operating room thoracotomy.[157] Similarly, a rapid diagnostic peritoneal lavage (DPL) is performed on victims of blunt trauma to rule out an abdominal source. However, patients in unstable condition with penetrating abdominal wounds should be transferred immediately to the operating room without DPL confirmation.

Pelvic and retroperitoneal injuries pose unique diagnostic and triage challenges to the trauma team. Supine and inlet views on pelvic radiographs frequently demonstrate pelvic fractures, but they may not accurately portray the magnitude of the pelvic disruption and thus the risk of associated vascular injuries. These patients require a multidisciplinary approach involving trauma surgery, orthopedics, and radiology. Initial therapeutic procedures include careful physiologic monitoring, presumptive blood component therapy, and PASG for continuing hypovolemia.

Diagnostic Adjuncts

Diagnostic Peritoneal Lavage (DPL)

In cases of multisystem trauma, the initial physical examination of the abdomen often fails to detect significant intraabdominal injury. Delay in diagnosis increases morbidity and mortality, prolongs hospitalization, and ultimately increases health care costs. The introduction of diagnostic peritoneal lavage by Root and colleagues in 1965 provided a safe, inexpensive way to quickly identify life-threatening intraperitoneal injuries.[256] Despite the widespread popularity of CT scanning in the United States and of ultrasonography in Europe and Japan, we believe DPL remains an integral part of the evaluation of a critically injured patient.

There are three fundamental methods of introducing the DPL catheter into the peritoneal cavity: the closed approach, the open approach, and the semi-open approach. With the closed approach, the catheter is inserted in a blind percutaneous fashion. The major problem is uncontrolled depth of penetration, which puts the underlying intraperitoneal or retroperitoneal structures at risk of perforation. Unfortunately, the currently available Seldinger wire techniques in adults have proved suboptimal because of inadequate lavage return. The open procedure, in which the abdominal wall is traversed under direct visualization, is safer but more time-consuming, and it introduces air into the peritoneal cavity.

We prefer the semi-open technique, performed at the infraumbilical ring, as a compromise. This approach is quick, easy, and extremely reliable, and it can be used in a patient with a major pelvic fracture because the enlarging anterior hematoma is limited by the infraumbilical ring. Before the DPL catheter is introduced, the stomach and bladder are decompressed with a nasogastric tube and a Foley catheter, respectively. The periumbilical area is shaved, prepped with povidone-iodide solution, and draped sterilely. The area is infiltrated generously with a local anesthetic (1% Xylocaine without epinephrine). A gently curved incision is made to one

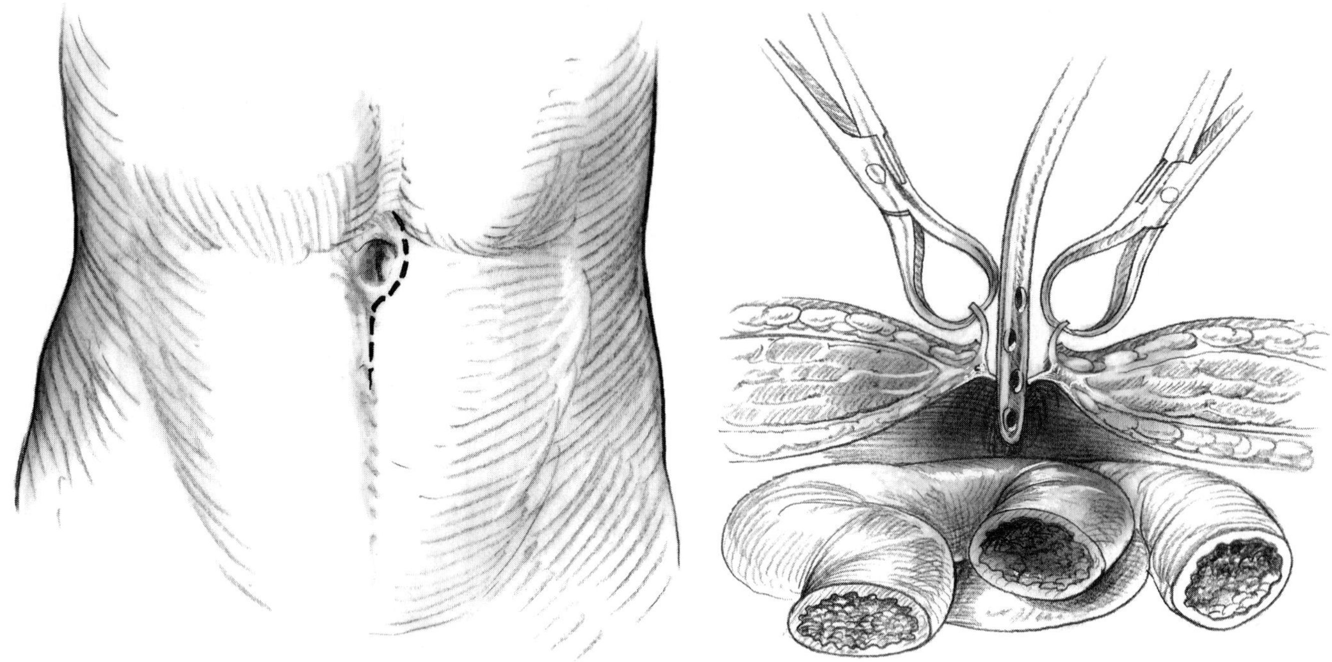

FIGURE 15-9 **A,** Semi-open diagnostic peritoneal lavage is performed through a gently curved periumbilical incision, which allows access to the inferior portion of the umbilical ring. **B,** The free edges of the incised midline fascia are elevated with towel clips to minimize injury to the underlying viscera during introduction of the lavage catheter. (After Fritzler.)

side of the umbilicus, at the level of the infraumbilical ring (Figure 15-9, *A*). The advantages of this site are relative avascularity, a paucity of preperitoneal fat, and greater adherence of the peritoneum as a result of obliteration of the umbilical arteries and urachus. The incision is carried down to the linea alba, ensuring meticulous hemostasis. A 5 mm incision is made in the linea alba, and the free edges are grasped with towel clips. While the abdominal wall is elevated by traction on the towel clips, a standard dialysis catheter with its trocar is inserted into the peritoneal cavity toward the pelvis (Figure 15-9, *B*). Once the peritoneum is entered, the trocar is withdrawn and the catheter is directed toward the pelvic floor. The tap is considered positive if more than 10 ml of gross blood is aspirated. Otherwise, 1 L (15 ml/kg in children) of warmed 0.9% sodium chloride is infused. If the clinical condition permits, the patient is rolled from side to side to enhance intraperitoneal sampling. The saline bag is then lowered to the floor for the return of lavage fluid by siphonage. A minimum 75% recovery of lavage effluent is required for the test to be considered valid. The fluid is sent for laboratory analysis of red blood cell (RBC) and white blood cell (WBC) counts, lavage amylase (LAM) and lavage alkaline phosphatase (LAP) levels, and examination for the presence of bile.

The criteria for a positive DPL result are outlined in Table 15-1. In cases of blunt abdominal trauma, significant visceral damage is found in more than 90% of patients with an RBC count above 100,000/mm^3, but in fewer than 2% of those with a count under 20,000/mm^3. However, RBC counts between 20,000 and 100,000/mm^3 may reflect serious injury in 15% of 35% of cases, and such counts merit further diagnostic evaluation—our current preference is abdominal computed tomography (CT) scanning or intraoperative laparoscopy. Occasionally, an elevated WBC count (over 500/mm^3), LAM, or LAP will signal an otherwise occult intestinal injury.[1] The contents of a perforated viscus evoke a migration of leukocytes into the peritoneal cavity, but this response may be delayed for at least 3 hours after injury. Conversely, an isolated WBC count over 500/mm^3 in a DPL done promptly after injury often is nonspecific. We repeat the DPL in 4 hours if the initial WBC count is elevated and perform a laparotomy if the count is still elevated. A LAP above 3 IU/L is more

TABLE 15-1 CRITERIA FOR A POSITIVE RESULT ON DIAGNOSTIC PERITONEAL LAVAGE FOLLOWING BLUNT ABDOMINAL TRAUMA

INDEX	POSITIVE	EQUIVOCAL
Aspirate		
Blood	>10 ml	—
Fluid	Enteric contents	—
Lavage		
Red blood cells	>100,000/mm^3	>20,000/mm^3
White blood cells	—	>500/mm^3
Enzymes	Amylase >20 IU/L and alkaline phosphatase >3 IU/L	Amylase >20 IU/L or alkaline phosphatase >3 IU/L
Bile	Confirmed biochemically	—

accurate than a lavage WBC count in detecting small bowel injury. From a series of nearly 2000 DPLs performed over a 4-year period, we found that, despite otherwise negative DPL findings, an LAM above 20 IU/L combined with a LAP above 3 IU/L was 97% specific for small bowel perforation.[161,162] Serial or repeat DPLs are also valuable in patients with multisystem injuries who develop signs of hypovolemia or unexplained blood loss during extensive diagnostic or therapeutic interventions such as CT head scans, aortography, or pelvic angiography.

Diagnostic peritoneal lavage does have inherent limitations and a morbidity rate of about 1%. The serious complications, which most often occur when the closed technique is used, include perforations of the small bowel, mesentery, bladder, and retroperitoneal vascular structures. Previous abdominal surgery, a gravid uterus, and massive obesity are relative contraindications for DPL, but the only absolute one is an existing indication for laparotomy. In patients with previous midline abdominal incisions, DPL can be performed through a left lower quadrant transverse incision, although this is technically more challenging. Moreover, intraabdominal adhesions can loculate both the lavage fluid and free blood, increasing the risk of a false negative study. Thus, in a patient with previous extensive abdominal surgery, only a positive DPL result is useful. Finally, DPL does not sample an intact retroperitoneum and may not adequately reflect isolated hollow viscus or diaphragmatic perforation.

Computed Tomography

Computed tomography (CT) plays an important role as a diagnostic adjunct in early evaluation of abdominal and pelvic injuries.[67] The limitations of this diagnostic modality center on its timely completion, the availability of experienced radiologists, equipment variability, patient cooperation, the need for oral and intravenous contrast enhancement agents, and cost. Indeed, several studies have confirmed these concerns by prospectively comparing CT to DPL in acutely injured patients. Davis and colleagues found DPL to be 100% accurate in five patients requiring surgery, whereas CT failed to detect four injuries in three of these same five patients.[59] Our prospective study of 100 patients yielded similar results. DPL was sensitive for each of five actively bleeding, solid-organ injuries following blunt trauma, whereas CT was positive in only one. Moreover, CT scans missed hemoperitoneum in excess of 500 ml in four patients.

The same conclusions can be drawn from the more recent investigation by Fabian and colleagues[63] of 91 patients admitted for blunt abdominal trauma who underwent both CT and DPL examinations. On the other hand, CT has the unquestionable virtue of injury specificity. Clearly, select patients with isolated, self-limiting injury to the liver or spleen can be treated expectantly primarily on the basis of CT scanning.[66]

We believe CT should complement DPL in the evaluation of blunt abdominal trauma. Four groups of patients are particularly suitable for CT scanning: (1) patients with delayed presentation (over 12 hours) who are hemodynamically stable and do not have overt signs of peritonitis; (2) patients in whom DPL results are equivocal and repeated physical examination is unreliable or untenable (e.g., those who required prolonged general anesthesia for neurosurgical or orthopedic procedures; patients with altered mental status caused by head injury, drugs, or alcohol; or patients with spinal cord injury); (3) patients in whom DPL is difficult to perform (e.g., morbid obesity, portal hypertension, or previous laparotomies); and (4) patients at high risk for retroperitoneal injuries in whom DPL results are unremarkable (e.g., the unrestrained, intoxicated driver who strikes the steering column or a patient with postinjury hyperamylasemia). CT is also valuable for defining the extent and configuration of complex pelvic fractures. However, it must be emphasized that CT scanning may not demonstrate blunt pancreatic fractures in the first 6 hours after injury, and it cannot be relied on for early detection of hollow viscus perforation.

Diagnostic Ultrasound

Quality ultrasound machines have become portable, and their role in the initial evaluation of blunt abdominal trauma is expanding. Indeed, diagnostic ultrasound currently is used routinely in emergency departments in Japan and Germany.[87] Ultrasonography can demonstrate the presence of free intraperitoneal fluid and locate solid-organ hematomas.[301] The procedure is particularly appealing for an injured patient who is pregnant because of the relatively limited hazard from radiation or contrast media. However, ultrasonography has limited value in the assessment of solid-organ fractures and is relatively poor at detecting acute hollow visceral perforation. Moreover, the accuracy of ultrasonography is operator dependent and can be compromised by lower rib fractures, extensive soft tissue injuries, or dressings.[111] In one comparative study, Gruessner and colleagues[104] found DPL superior to ultrasonography and concluded that CT studies should be viewed as complementary rather than competitive. However, with more sophisticated equipment (and resolution of territorial dispute with radiology), ultrasonography could largely supplant DPL in the emergency evaluation of the critically injured. For example, work is under way to generate three-dimensional computer reconstructions of ultrasound images.

Laparoscopy

With the advent and development of new technology, diagnostic laparoscopy will no doubt have a role in evaluation, as well as definitive treatment, of the acutely injured. In the past, laparoscopy was limited by the time required to perform the examination and the need for specialized equipment and general anesthesia. Several studies have confirmed the utility of laparoscopy done with local anesthesia in the ED to identify diaphragmatic injuries and quantitate the amount of intraperitoneal blood.[116,148,324] Currently, however, the major limitation is inability to perform a comprehensive examination of the entire abdomen and pelvis, particularly the posterior recesses and retroperitoneum. Nevertheless, enthusiasm for laparoscopy will continue with the advent of more sophisticated equipment and the potential for therapeutic intervention.

PRINCIPLES OF INITIAL MANAGEMENT

A detailed physical examination of the patient should be done in the ED as soon as lifesaving priorities and treatment have been established and begun. One efficient method is to examine the patient systematically, literally from head to toe. The patient must be completely disrobed and, once spinal injury has been excluded, rolled from side to side so that the back and flanks can be inspected. The mechanism of injury, as well as the patient's response to initial resuscitation, governs the speed and detail of the initial physical examination.

Details of the patient's medical history, as well as those related to the injury, are crucial to ED triage decisions. The prehospital team can provide valuable information about hemodynamic stability and the mechanism of injury. For example, a history of high-deceleration vehicular impact may be the persuasive factor in a decision to perform thoracic aortography despite a normal chest radiograph. Review of the patient's past medical history should include (1) pre-existing medical illness; (2) current medications, including recent drug ingestion; (3) allergies; (4) tetanus immunization; and (5) time of last meal.

Initial laboratory testing generally is limited but includes a baseline hematocrit (Hct), white blood cell (WBC) count, serum amylase, and urinalysis. Testing of blood ethanol levels and toxicologic analysis should be done when appropriate. Blood typing should be performed immediately on patients with signs of hypovolemic shock, and formal cross-matching should be individualized according to the response to fluid administration.

Head and Spinal Injuries

The scalp should be inspected for continuous blood loss or underlying fractures, and direct pressure should be applied to active bleeding sites. Application of Rainey clips or temporary mass suturing may be needed to achieve hemostasis of large wounds. Scalp avulsions should be preserved in sterile dressings for potential reimplantation.[211] Hemotympanum, ecchymosis over the mastoid process (Battle's sign), or periorbital ecchymosis (raccoon eyes) suggests basilar skull fracture. Accompanying otorrhea or rhinorrhea indicates leakage of cerebrospinal fluid (CSF) from an underlying dural tear. Midfacial or maxillary instability also is associated with anterior basilar skull fractures. In such patients the gastric tube should be inserted via the mouth to prevent transcranial placement, which could occur with insertion through the nose.[79]

A neurologic examination should be performed and repeated regularly to identify changes in function. The initial neurologic examination should assess (1) level of consciousness; (2) pupilary size and responsitivity; and (3) best motor response. This examination, which can be performed quickly and repeated often, is sensitive for traumatic neurologic dysfunction. The character and evolution of neurologic dysfunction is helpful in differentiating acute neurosurgical emergencies. For example, a patient with a deteriorating level of consciousness, expanding pupil, and contralateral hemiparesis is considered to have an expanding intercerebral mass lesion until proven otherwise. This patient requires emergency CT scanning and craniotomy to survive. In contrast, an obtunded patient without focal neurologic deficits has global cerebral dysfunction. Traditionally, the Glasgow Coma Scale (GCS) has been used to document neurologic function (Table 15-2). However, this scale is based on an assessment of cerebral cortical function and therefore is of limited value in an obtunded or unconscious patient. A GCS score below 9 indicates serious head injury, although responsiveness to stimuli may be falsely depressed by intoxicants or postinjury shock.

TABLE 15-2 GLASGOW COMA SCALE (GCS)

SCORE	EYE	VERBAL	MOTOR
1	No response	No response	No response
2	Open to pain	Incomprehensible	Extensor (decerebrate)
3	Open to command	Inappropriate	Flexor (decorticate)
4	Spontaneous	Confused	Nonspecific movement
5		Converses	Localizes to pain
6		Alert	Obeys commands

The initial management of a patient with a serious head injury is directed at maintaining cerebral oxygen delivery, limiting intracranial pressure, and quickly diagnosing and treating intracranial mass lesions.[255] This is accomplished with (1) intubation and hyperventilation to control ICP (partial pressure of carbon dioxide [P_{CO_2}] is kept between 25 and 30 mm Hg); (2) cardiopulmonary support and timely blood transfusions to optimize cerebral oxygen delivery; (3) limitation of sodium and free-water infusions to minimize cerebral edema; (4) osmotic diuresis (mannitol) to decrease interstitial fluid (cerebral edema); and (5) ICP monitoring, cranial imaging (CT) and, when necessary, prompt craniotomy. Skull radiographs are primarily indicated to detect fractures over the middle meningeal artery or transverse sinus and to establish the trajectory of a projectile with penetrating wounds. Air-fluid levels in the sphenoid or frontal sinuses occasionally call attention to otherwise occult basilar skull fractures. When possible, CT scans of the head should be obtained before an emergency laparotomy or thoracotomy so that a multiteam approach can be used in the OR. Mortality increases threefold when evacuation of an acute subdural hematoma is delayed for longer than 4 hours.[268] On the other hand, a patient who remains in shock with a grossly positive peritoneal aspirate requires immediate laparotomy while an ICP monitor is placed or a craniotomy is performed simultaneously.

The cervical, thoracic, and lumbar spine should be palpated for deformity and tenderness. Flaccid paralysis with loss of extremity reflexes and anal tone is diagnostic of a spinal cord injury. Priapism is a corroborative but frequently absent sign. With blunt trauma, the cervical spine is assumed to be unstable until the clinician obtains (1) high quality radiographs demonstrating the vertebral bodies and processes of C1 through T1; and (2) a reliable, nontender physical examination.[20] Cervical immobilization is crucial to protect a possibly unstable spine. Soft collars are grossly inadequate for this purpose, and even hard collars, as well as the four-part brace, permit a substantial degree of cervical motion.[5,120,241] If cervical spine injury is strongly suspected or has been verified, bilateral sandbags and a Philadelphia collar with wide tape across the forehead are secure methods of acute stabilization.[115] Fractures of the cervical spine with significant malalignment are treated in the ED with axial traction. Gardner-Wells tongs or a halo ring is secured to the outer table of the cranium and attached to a traction device. Five to 10 pounds of traction is applied, and cervical alignment is verified with repeat radiographs. Spinal injuries with neurologic deficits are currently treated acutely in the ED with cervical immobilization, realignment when appropriate, and high-dose infusion of steroids. Intravenous Solu-Medrol is administered as a 30 mg/kg bolus and continued at a rate of 5.4 mg/kg/hour over the ensuing 23 hours.

Blunt Cervical Trauma

Laryngotracheal Disruption

Blunt laryngotracheal disruption is uncommon but can be quickly fatal if mistreated.[83,107] The injury usually occurs when the aerodigestive structures are compressed between the steering wheel or dashboard and the vertebral column, or when a patient is clotheslined by a wire fence while riding a snowmobile, trail bike, or sled.[281] Acute signs include airway distress, dysphonia, dysphagia, stridor, hoarseness, and hemoptysis. Supporting physical findings are cervical contusion, subcutaneous emphysema, crepitus, and distorted laryngeal landmarks. Securing the airway and providing adequate ventilation are the foremost priorities, but these efforts must be tempered by the realization that active airway management may be extremely difficult. Premature efforts at intubation may obscure or extend the injury or, more importantly, may precipitate airway decompensation. Emergency cricothyrostomy proximal to a tracheal injury may worsen ventilation by breaching the deep cervical fascia, and tracheostomy in the ED may be challenging if the distal trachea retracts into the superior mediastinum. For these reasons, unless the patient shows life-threatening airway distress, assessment and airway intervention are best achieved in the OR with optimum lighting, equipment, and personnel.[107] A systemic approach should be pursued, starting with indirect laryngoscopy and complete evaluation for associated pharyngoesophageal tears and possible recurrent laryngeal nerve damage.

Carotid and Vertebral Artery Injury

Blunt carotid or vertebral injuries are rare and typically delayed in presentation.[19,81,139] The mechanism of injury comprises both direct compression and stretch from cervical hyperextension. The characteristic injury is an intimal disruption with associated dissection and thrombosis.[233] Patients show a range of clinical signs referrable to their vascular injury, including neck hematomas, neurologic deficits, Horner's syndrome and, in an alert patient, isolated limb paresis.[141] Timely diagnosis depends largely on clinical suspicion and is confirmed with angiography.

The treatment of patients with carotid injuries is controversial but can be stratified by the degree of neurologic deficit and the presence or absence of arterial flow.[204] Patients who have no neurologic deficits or moderate deficits with prograde arterial flow and localized lesions are candidates for surgical repair or bypass. Patients manifesting profound neurologic deficits and coma with diminished but present prograde arterial flow probably benefit from repair; however, these patients show significant morbidity and mortality.[145,253] Asymptomatic patients with arterial dissections extending into the carotid sinus can be managed expectantly, although the role of systemic anticoagulation remains unsettled. Patients with high carotid artery occlusions and evolving neurologic deficits may be candidates for extracranial-intracranial bypass.[3,96,143]

Penetrating Neck Wounds

Active airway management is imperative in a patient with a serious penetrating neck wound. Procrastination may allow a cervical hematoma to expand, precluding simple airway management and precipitating emergency surgical airway control, a potential bloody catastrophe. Neurologic deficits from penetrating spinal injuries are uncommon and rarely result in significant spinal instability. Therefore the clinician should not hesitate to use oral intubation in a neurologically intact patient requiring prompt airway control. Massive oropharyngeal bleeding may necessitate emergency cricothyrostomy; however, this procedure may release the tamponade provided by the deep cervical fascia. External bleeding should be controlled with digital compression. Clamps should not be blindly inserted into the neck to achieve hemostasis.

The indications for diagnostic testing and surgical neck exploration are controversial.[98,264] Selective neck exploration is supported by clinical studies from trauma facilities with substantial experience managing penetrating cervical trauma.[73,213] If the staff has limited experience, however, the safest policy is to explore all anterior zone II injuries (in the midneck) when the platysma muscle has been violated. Clinical signs requiring formal exploration or extensive diagnostic testing include the following: (1) *vascular:* expanding hematoma, external hemorrhage, and diminished carotid pulse; (2) *visceral:* subcutaneous air, hemoptysis, and dysphagia; (3) *airway:* stridor, hoarseness, and dysphonia; (4) *neurologic:* cortical, cranial, and brachial plexus dysfunction. Angiography before surgery is indicated in a hemodynamically stable patient with multiple wounds or zone I injuries (caudad to the cricoid cartilage) to identify lesions involving the thoracic outlet vessels, which may require sternotomy for proximal control.[266] Selective arterial embolization may be definitive for zone III injuries (cephalad to the angle of the mandible). Symptomatic, isolated zone II injuries generally are explored without the aid of arteriography. Endoscopy of the pharynx, trachea, and esophagus is performed during surgery to detect suspected injuries.[127,158,213]

Blunt Chest Trauma

Pulmonary contusions, blunt cardiac trauma, and disruptions of the trachea, bronchi, or great vessels[219,222] are the principal life-threatening, nonpenetrating chest injuries.[146] These lesions are usually caused by rapid deceleration following high-speed vehicular impact or falls from great heights, but they occasionally occur with direct blows to the chest. The typical patient suffers multisystem trauma that may obscure these life-threatening injuries. Although flail chest or fractures of the first rib,[251] sternum, and scapula, suggest intrathoracic injury, the key to timely diagnosis is a high index of suspicion based on the circumstances of the accident and the patient's overall appearance.[298]

Pulmonary Contusion

Pulmonary contusion occurs in 35% to 65% of severely injured patients[15] and is almost invariably a component of multisystem trauma.[319] The pathophysiology includes alveolar overdistention, shearing of low-density alveolar tissue versus heavier hilar structures, and tissue disruption caused by shock waves at air-fluid interfaces. The net result is impaired alveolar gas exchange from altered capillary membrane integrity, edema formation, local hemorrhage, and increased pulmonary vascular resistance.

The first clinical signs are those of acute hypoxemia, including agitation, confusion, tachycardia, and air hunger. Nearly three fourths of these patients have some element of flail chest. The initial chest radiograph may be deceptively benign, with perhaps only a small, localized infiltrate. Radiographic evidence of overt consolidation typically evolves during the first 24 to 36 hours,[15] and the clinical course often deteriorates over this same period. Hemopneumothorax complicates the initial presentation in 25% to 50% of patients, and occasionally secondary hemoptysis compromises ventilation. Pulmonary laceration, hematoma, and bronchopleural fistulae may further confuse the diagnosis.

ED management of pulmonary contusion consists primarily of maintaining effective ventilation and oxygenation while preventing fluid overload. Tube thoracostomies are placed to treat hemopneumothoraces, and patients are monitored expectantly with pulse oximetry and serial ABG determinations. Aggressive pulmonary physiotherapy, including intercostal nerve blocks and epidural anesthesia to alleviate chest wall pain, obviates the need for endotracheal intubation in most patients.[298] When mechanical ventilation is required, early use of positive end-expiratory pressure (PEEP) may be beneficial.[225,312] Adult respiratory distress syndrome (ARDS), pneumonia,[15] and pneumatocele or pulmonary abscess are sequelae of severe lung contusion.

Tracheobronchial Disruption

The mechanism of intrathoracic tracheal or bronchial disruption from blunt trauma is thought to involve a sudden rise of intraluminal pressure against a closed glottis, combined with shearing forces as the airway is compressed against the spine.[103] Tears most often occur in the mainstem bronchi within 2.5 cm. of the carina and vary from small perforations of the membranous portion to total avulsions. These injuries are classified by the relationship between the site of injury and the mediastinal pleura. Intrapleural rupture of the right main or distal left bronchus beyond the parietal pleural reflection into the pleural cavity manifests as a pneumothorax with a persistent bronchopleural fistula. Intramediastinal rupture in the trachea or proximal bronchus produces mediastinal and deep cervical emphysema. Either variant may be associated with hemoptysis and inadequate ventilation. Early bronchoscopy is necessary if tracheobronchial injury is suspected. Although minor tears may be treated without surgery, major disruptions require immediate thoracotomy.[135]

Ruptured Thoracic Aorta

A ruptured thoracic aorta is highly lethal and accounts for a significant number of motor vehicle fatalities.[102,217] Nearly 85% of victims who suffer this injury will die at the scene of the accident.[229] The remaining 15% reach the hospital alive because the aortic adventitia and surrounding mediastinal tissue prevent free intrathoracic bleeding. The mechanism for aortic tear probably involves a number of factors. With sudden horizontal deceleration, the heart and aorta move forward and twist on the relatively fixed descending aorta at a time when intraluminal aortic pressure is markedly increased. In more than 90% of the patients who survive to reach the ED, the aortic disruption is located in the isthmus just distal to the left subclavian artery.[321] Abrupt vertical deceleration from falls or airplane crashes, on the other hand, creates an axial stress, resulting in a higher proportion of tears in the ascending aortic root. Aortic injury may also occur in the middle and distal descending aorta, as well as in the major arch branches.[133,320] Multiple aortic lesions have been noted in 20% of victims who die in automobile wrecks,[102] but they are rare in patients who survive.[30]

A person with a contained aortic disruption may have deceptively little physical evidence of this catastrophic injury. Early recognition is crucial; of those surviving 1 hour after the injury, 15% rupture into the thorax within 6 hours and 25% within 24 hours.[229] Most of these patients have multisystem trauma that masks the subtle signs of aortic injury. Retrosternal or interscapular pain from mediastinal blood dissection is the most common complaint and is reported to occur in one fourth of the patients. Other symptoms include hoarseness caused by recurrent laryngeal nerve pressure, dysphagia from esophageal compression, and ischemic complaints from vascular impairment in the spinal cord or extremities.[176] Generalized hypertension probably is the most common sign of occult aortic injury; it is attributed to the stretching of the sympathetic nerves around the aortic isthmus and has been observed in as many as half of these patients.[77] Upper extremity hypertension "pseudocoarctation," caused by subadventitial aortic dissection, may be identified in one third of patients, and a precordial or interscapular systolic murmur may be heard in one fourth. Additional physical findings include blood extravasation in the base of the neck and signs of vascular ischemia in the spinal cord or extremities. Unfortunately, these clinical signs and symptoms often are subtle and, more importantly, are not pathognomonic for disruption of the thoracic aorta.

Most thoracic tears are first suspected because of abnormalities on the initial chest radiograph (see the box below). Widening of the superior mediastinum is the most specific sign. Although the strict definition of this is width greater than 8 cm on a 100 cm supine radiograph, the mere subjective impression of widening is more accurate.[106] Furthermore, interpretation of the chest radiograph is most reliable when the radiograph is performed in a posteroanterior projection with the patient erect. Most mediastinal widening is due to venous bleeding, and fewer than one fifth of patients with mediastinal bleeding have an aortic injury.[106] Conversely, as many as one fourth of patients with acute tears of the thoracic aorta may have a normal mediastinal shadow on an initial chest radiograph.[4]

CHEST RADIOGRAPHIC SIGNS OF DISRUPTION OF THE DESCENDING THORACIC AORTA

Widened superior mediastinum
Ill-defined aortic knob
Obliterated aortopulmonary window
Left pleural apical cap
Rightward deviation of the nasogastric tube
Tracheal deviation to the right
Downward displacement of the left mainstem bronchus
Abnormal contour of the descending aorta
Obliterated paraspinous strip
Left hemothorax

The other suggestive signs on plain chest radiographs are far less sensitive and specific.[237] For these reasons, radiographic confirmation (angiography, transesophageal echocardiography, or intravascular ultrasonography) is imperative before thoracotomy. Also, with an ascending aortic tear, cardiopulmonary bypass is warranted. Dynamic CT scanning has proved useful in the evaluation of chronic dissections of the thoracic aorta but thus far has not been uniformly reliable for acute injury because of the inability to identify the site and source of mediastinal blood. However, CT scanning may be a reliable screening test for angiography. Intra-arterial ultrasonography is a relatively new diagnostic modality that may prove useful in critically injured patients with multisystem trauma.[245] An ultrasound probe is inserted through an introducer (size 6 Fr) via the femoral artery and advanced under fluoroscopic guidance into the descending aorta. This can be done in the ED, OR, or ICU as other lifesaving procedures or resuscitations are underway. Transesophageal echocardiography may also be valuable in this scenario.

A problem with thoracic aortography is the time required to complete the study. One critical triage decision in the ED is what to do with a patient who has major head injury, widened mediastinum on chest radiograph, and a grossly positive result on a peritoneal tap.[17,134] In a hemodynamically unstable patient without ongoing intrathoracic hemorrhage and a positive peritoneal aspirate, we believe laparotomy should be performed first because intraperitoneal hemorrhage is the most likely cause of instability. In a patient in stable condition, however, we prefer CT scanning of the head and arteriography before laparotomy, which allows a team approach during surgery. The aortic isthmus can be approached via a left posterolateral thoracotomy while a second team explores the abdomen.[321]

Penetrating Thoracic Wounds

Fewer than 15% of patients with penetrating chest injuries require thoracotomy.[232,252] Indications for immediate exploration are cardiac tamponade, persistent hemorrhage, and air embolism.[16] Specific surgical criteria for unrelenting bleeding, however, must be tempered by the patient's clinical status.[157,223]

Practical guidelines for prompt thoracotomy include initial chest tube drainage of more than 25% of the patient's estimated blood volume (1200 to 1500 ml in adults) or more than 5% (250 ml/hour) for 3 consecutive hours. Success with simple tube thoracostomy depends on tamponade of the injured lung against the rigid chest wall, facilitated by the relatively low pulmonary vascular pressure. The initial chest tube output, therefore, is not as critical as the rate of continuous bleeding once the lung has been re-expanded. The clinical setting and the patient's hemodynamic status are equally important factors. Initial chest drainage of 1200 ml of blood does not require thoracotomy in a stable patient, particularly if some delay since injury has occurred. On the other hand, thoracostomy output may be deceptively small in a patient with a malfunctioning tube in the midst of a clotted hemothorax. Serial chest radiographs are essential. Cardiac, great vessel, or pulmonary hilar wounds usually are characterized by refractory shock. A patient in stable condition who requires thoracotomy for persistent, moderate hemorrhage most often has an internal mammary, intercostal arterial, or peripheral lung injury. Finally, a stable patient with a transmediastinal wound may be managed selectively with the aid of angiography, esophagoscopy, and esophagography.[6]

Abdominal visceral injury may also occur with penetrating wounds of the lower thorax, because the diaphragm rises to the midchest with full expiration.[6,203] The lower thorax is defined superiorly by the nipple line (fourth intercostal space) anteriorly, the tip of the scapula posteriorly, and the costal margins inferiorly. The incidence of thoracoabdominal injury in this region is 15% for stab wounds and nearly 50% for gunshot wounds.[203] As would be expected by anatomic proximity, the liver, colon, spleen, and stomach are the usual sites of visceral injuries. Isolated diaphragmatic defects can be serious because over time the persistent negative pleuroperitoneal pressure gradient encourages visceral herniation into the pleural cavity, frequently resulting in strangulated gut.[307] Physical examination is notoriously inaccurate for detecting thoracoabdominal trauma and may miss as many as a third of the serious injuries.[203] Diagnostic peritoneal lavage therefore is recommended for evaluation of all penetrating wounds of the lower thorax. Because blood loss may be minimal after perforation of the diaphragm, the RBC threshold for laparotomy is lowered to $5000/mm^3$ to identify these isolated injuries.[293] Thoracoscopy or laparoscopy may prove beneficial in the evaluation, as well as the treatment, of diaphragmatic injuries.[116]

Blunt Abdominal Trauma

Our management plan for patients with significant abdominal trauma is outlined in Figure 15-10.[76] Patients with overt peritonitis or massive hemoperitoneum are intubated, volume loaded, and transferred emergently to the operating room for abdominal exploration.[44] Patients with a high-energy transfer injury, particularly when intoxicated or with a concurrent head injury, undergo prompt diagnostic peritoneal lavage during their initial evaluation. A positive DPL result in these high-risk patients requires emergency abdominal exploration. Hemodynamically stable patients who have equivocal DPL results (20,000 to 100,000 $RBCs/mm^3$) undergo abdominal CT scanning to rule out major solid-organ injury. Major spleen and liver injuries (above grade III)

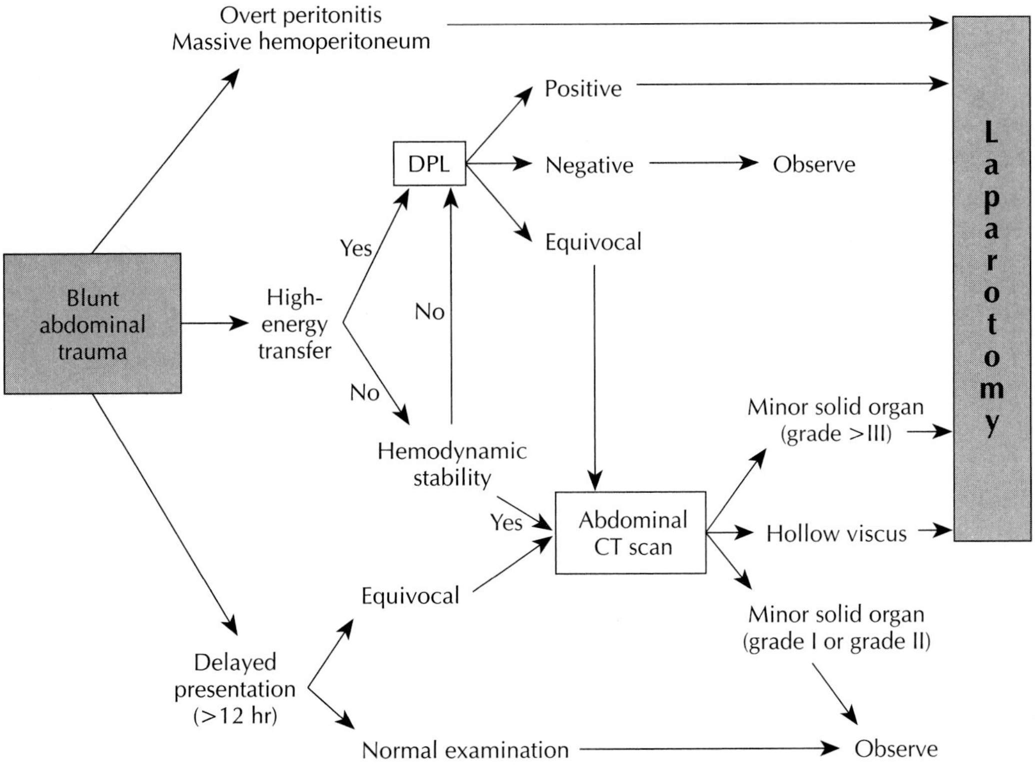

FIGURE 15-10 Decision algorithm for initial evaluation of blunt abdominal trauma in an adult. Diagnostic peritoneal lavage plays a central role in the evaluation of these severely injured patients. A computed tomography (CT) scan is a valuable adjunct with relatively low-risk patients.

in adult patients are explored, whereas lesser injuries are observed. Patients who are hemodynamically stable following low-energy transfer are evaluated by abdominal CT scanning and observed if solid-viscera injuries below grade III are confirmed. Alternatively, if the CT scan is not available or if there are several patients, DPL is used as the initial screening test, and patients with positive results undergo CT scanning. Patients who seek medical help more than 12 hours after trauma are either observed or evaluated with an abdominal CT scan, depending on their initial physical examination and associated injuries. This diagnostic algorithm provides a general guideline for initial evaluation; as more information becomes available, the algorithm is modified to include additional diagnostic studies or therapeutic interventions. These might include (1) radiographic studies of the spine, chest, and pelvis; (2) CT scan of the head; (3) intravenous pyelography;[105] (4) retrograde cystourethrography; (5) contrast duodenography; or (6) diagnostic or therapeutic angiography.

The decision algorithm is also modified for pregnant patients or children. Pregnancy alters both the susceptibility to blunt injury and the physiologic response to injury.[21,260] The gravid uterus occupies the pelvis and lower abdomen and, hence, is vulnerable to a variety of insults from direct blows or seat belt injuries.[47] These insults result in a spectrum of injuries ranging from minor soft tissue contusions to disruption of the uterine wall or placental abruption and possibly exsanguination, as well as fetal loss. The significance of relatively minor injuries, thus, requires an aggressive approach to the early evaluation of these patients. We routinely use DPL (open technique) in pregnant patients while simultaneously evaluating the gravid uterus with ultrasound, noninvasive fetal monitoring, or amniocentesis.[60,216] Hemodynamic instability, rupture of the uterus, placental abruption, fetal distress, and a bloody result on amniocentesis are indications for emergency abdominal exploration and uterine evacuation, with the rare possibility of hysterectomy.

Evaluation of trauma in pediatric patients poses special challenges to the clinician because of the size and unique physiology of children. The elasticity of the lower rib cage and the relatively large size of the abdominal cavity increase the child's susceptibility to intraabdominal injury. On the other hand, the injury pattern en-

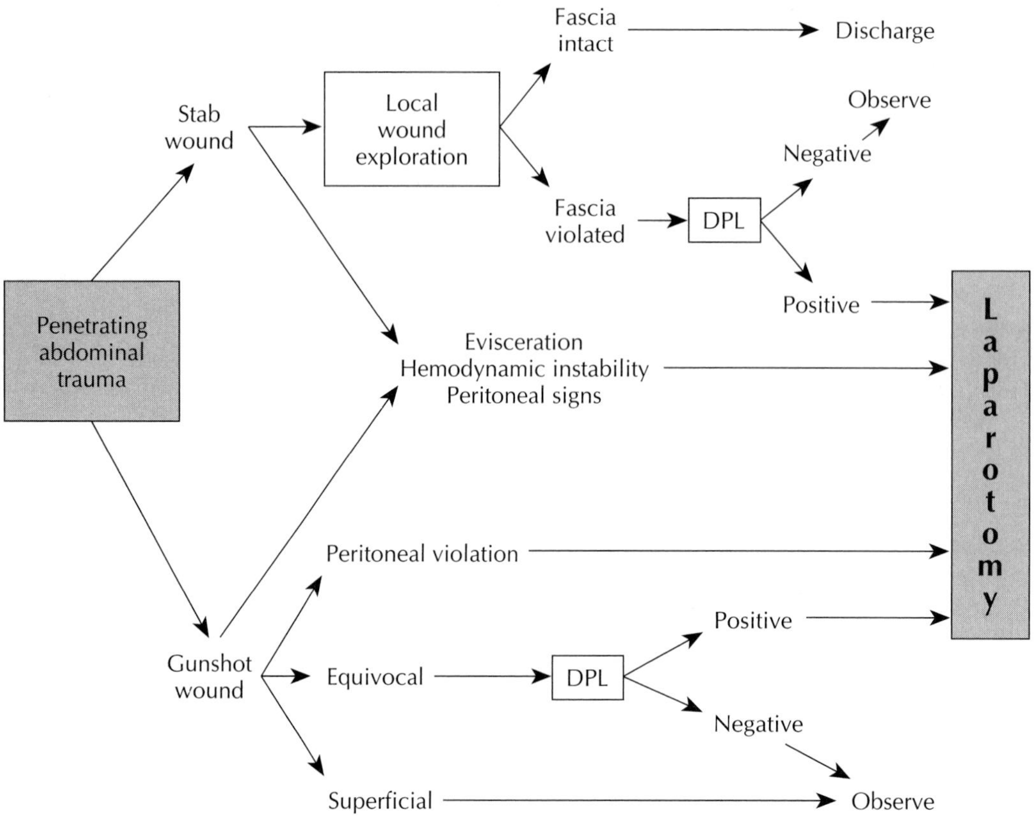

FIGURE 15-11 Decision algorithm for evaluating penetrating abdominal trauma in an adult.

countered in children and the greater potential for spontaneous hemostasis warrants a more selective approach. Liver and spleen injuries are common and frequently amenable to nonsurgical management, whereas significant pancreatic fractures and intestinal perforations are uncommon.[221] Despite these facts, we maintain an aggressive attitude toward abdominal evaluation because of the child's limited physiologic reserve. Grossly positive results from DPL in hemodynamically stable children are further evaluated by CT scan to verify solid-organ injury that may be managed expectantly. However, early abdominal exploration is performed in cases of hemodynamic instability, a need for continuous blood transfusions, or a peritoneal lavage result positive by enzymes.

Penetrating Abdominal Wounds

Initial management of patients with penetrating abdominal trauma can be simplified to (1) aggressive resuscitation; (2) directed physical examination; and (3) related diagnostic studies and therapeutic interventions (Figure 15-11). Hemodynamic stability, the nature of the penetrating object, and the location of wounds are key factors in the decision algorithm. Patients with massive hemoperitoneum or persistent hemodynamic instability are promptly intubated, volume loaded, and transported emergently to the operating room for abdominal exploration. Hemodynamically stable patients, on the other hand, are managed according to the mechanism of injury.

Civilian (low-energy) gunshot wounds to the anterior abdomen enter the peritoneal cavity in 80% of patients, resulting in significant visceral injury in 95%. Thus laparotomy is performed for gunshot wounds that violate the peritoneum, as determined by physical examination and corroborated by biplanar abdominal radiographs demonstrating the missile trajectory.[194] Bullets entering the upper abdomen may penetrate the chest, causing concomitant intrathoracic injuries. Similarly, bullets may traverse the abdomen and enter the retroperitoneal space, endangering major abdominal vessels, bowel, and kidneys. When no exit site appears on the patient and the bullet cannot be seen on torso radiographs, transvascular embolization should be considered. If the bullet tract is tangential and appears superficial in the abdominal wall, patients can be managed individually based on diagnostic peritoneal lavage or laparoscopy.[293]

Stab wounds to the anterior abdomen are managed

selectively.[170,295] Patients with significant hemodynamic instability or obviously life-threatening wounds are promptly transported to the operating room for abdominal exploration. The remaining patients, who are hemodynamically stable, initially are evaluated in the ED. Although two thirds of these patients have wounds that enter the peritoneum, fewer than half of these wounds result in visceral injury requiring surgical repair. Except in cases of evisceration, violation of the peritoneum cannot be ascertained by the gross appearance of the wound site, and blind probing may be misleading. Formal wound exploration using local anesthesia in the ED is the most reliable means to establish the depth of penetration and hence the need for further evaluation. DPL is performed in all patients with suspected or proven penetration of the peritoneal cavity.[69] Although there is some disagreement over the crucial RBC count, most authorities agree that 100,000 RBCs/mm^3 is an indication for laparotomy. Because of the proportionally higher number of isolated gastrointestinal perforations following a stab wound, however, peritoneal lavage has a 5% false negative rate. Thus all patients with a negative lavage result are admitted for at least 24 hours of observation and undergo prompt exploration if signs of peritoneal irritation ensue. Fortunately, most injuries missed by the initial DPL involve the stomach or small bowel. These usually are recognized within 6 to 12 hours and are associated with little excess morbidity.

Penetrating flank wounds pose unique diagnostic problems. These wounds are associated with retroperitoneal injury to the colon, duodenum, kidneys, and major vascular structures. Accordingly, life-threatening injuries may exist despite hemodynamic stability and a negative DPL result. The triple-contrast (oral/intravenous/rectal) CT scan has been useful in this situation, and most surgeons maintain a low threshold for early abdominal exploration if the scan shows the wound track to be near a significant retroperitoneal structure.

Preoperative administration of broad-spectrum antibiotics is indicated for penetrating abdominal wounds because of the relatively high incidence of distal ileal or colonic perforation.[198] The optimum antimicrobial agent has not been established, but a number of single agents provide effective activity against anaerobic as well as aerobic bacteria.[23,85] Tetanus prophylaxis should be administered according to standard guidelines established for contaminated wounds.

Pelvic Trauma

Major pelvic fractures are some of the most challenging injuries (Figure 15-12). Life-threatening pelvic hemorrhage can be difficult to control because of extensive interconnecting pelvic vascular channels that are difficult to ligate or tamponade.[74,206,259] These injuries typically are the result of high-energy transfer, such as automobile-pedestrian and motorcycle accidents, or falls. Patients often have multisystem trauma and thus a combination of potentially serious injuries. Major pelvic fractures should be categorized according to the mechanism of injury as well as the fracture geography. Anteroposterior impact fractures often are associated with symphyseal diastasis and sacroiliac disruption. Similarly, the vertical shear injury results in displacement of the posterior column. Both of these injury patterns are associated with major blood loss and, because of the force encountered, multiple associated injuries. On the other hand, lateral compression fractures typically encountered in side-impact motor vehicle accidents are not as often associated with major pelvic blood loss because the posterior elements usually are stable.

The initial physical examination should include manual compression of the bony pelvis and inspection of the perineum, rectum, and vagina for ecchymosis or open wounds. Plain radiographs of the pelvis are a priority in a patient suspected of having a fracture, although the anteroposterior view may not reflect the full magnitude of bony instability. Massive hemorrhage most often occurs with crush, vertical shear, or Malgaigne's (hemipelvis) fractures. Initial management of major pelvic injuries demands a multidisciplinary approach. Early orthopedic and interventional radiologic consultation is particularly important with posterior column involvement. Mechanical tamponade should be attempted promptly with a pneumatic antishock garment or placement of an external pelvis fixator in the ED if hypovolemia persists.[277] These maneuvers help align and compress pelvic bone fragments and reduce the volume of the pelvic space.

With significant blood loss, early recognition of a source outside the pelvis is imperative. Thus DPL is an integral part of the initial evaluation.[97] This is done at the infraumbilical ring to avoid the dissecting pelvic hematoma, and the catheter is left in place to facilitate serial lavages as other diagnostic procedures are completed. A grossly negative lavage reliably excludes life-threatening intraperitoneal blood loss. However, a grossly positive aspirate, particularly in a hemodynamically unstable patient, requires emergency abdominal exploration because aspiration of more than 20 ml of gross blood is associated with a 95% chance of active splenic, hepatic, or mesenteric hemorrhage. A grossly negative but cell count–positive lavage must be interpreted cautiously, because as many as 20% are positive merely from a ruptured pelvic hematoma or trivial hepatic or splenic injury. In a patient in stable condition, CT scanning in conjunction with serial lavage should be used to clarify the source of bleeding after the primary problems have been addressed.

A patient with continuous hemorrhage, despite the PASG, requires a critical triage decision. An individual

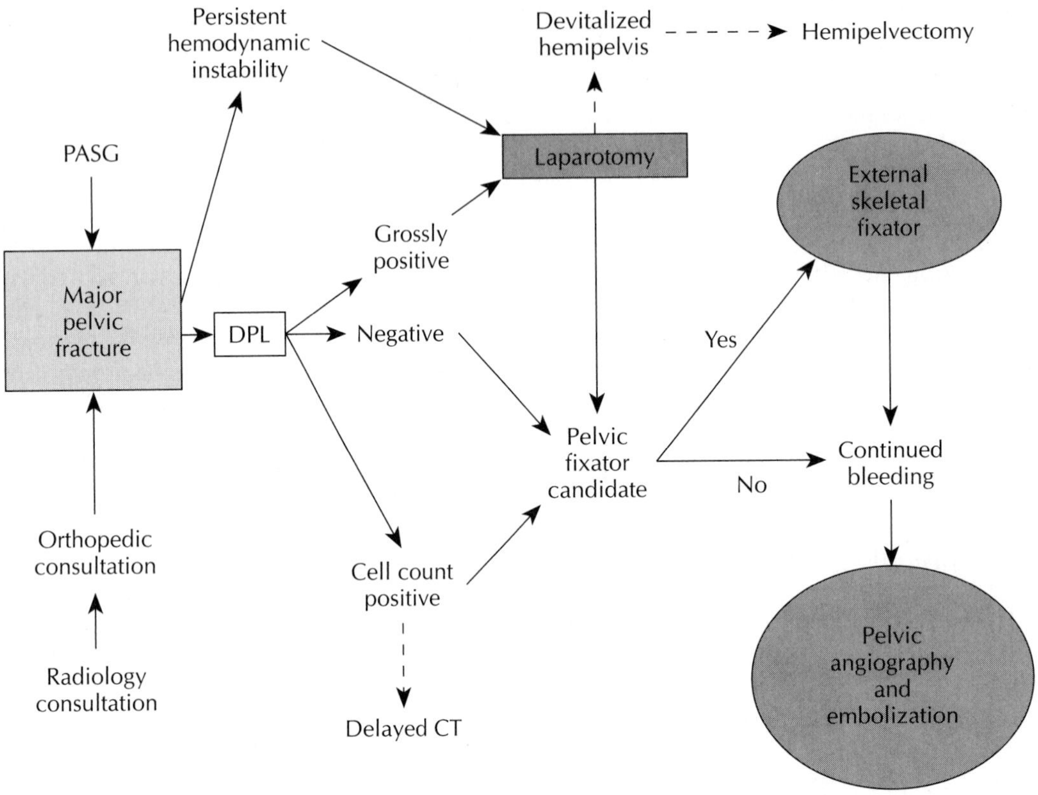

FIGURE 15-12 Decision algorithm for evaluating major pelvic fractures in an adult. Evaluation and treatment of these complex injuries requires consultation with orthopedic and radiologic specialists.

in unstable condition with a grossly positive DPL should undergo laparotomy because of the high probability of solid visceral or major vascular injury. But a patient with a positive lavage by RBC count should have the pelvic bleeding managed first. The key decision is whether to use skeletal fixation or selective embolization, and thus orthopedic and interventional radiology consultation should be obtained early. External skeletal fixation is appropriate if the primary fracture is an open-book disruption of the anterior ligaments of the sacroiliac joint, whereas persistent bleeding from a massively crushed pelvis should be approached by embolization. Unfortunately, the fracture geography often is between these extremes, so the decision is not straightforward.

Rectal and genitourinary injuries must be excluded in patients with major pelvic fractures.[261] Digital rectal examination may identify bony fragment penetration or reveal blood. A displaced prostate suggests urethral injury, which may also be manifested by gross blood at the urethral meatus. Pelvic fractures usually cause posterior urethral tears (above the urogenital diaphragm), whereas anterior lesions typically are associated with perineal straddle trauma. If urethral disruption is suspected, insertion of a Foley catheter should be deferred until a retrograde urethrogram can be obtained. ED management of complete urethral disruption calls for transcutaneous suprapubic cystostomy. Displaced pelvic rami fractures may also perforate the extraperitoneal bladder. Hematuria is absent in more than 10% of such patients, and the ability to void does not exclude the injury. Gravity flow cystography with 250 ml of contrast material and postvoiding views should be performed in patients with displaced anterior pelvic fractures.

Extremity Injuries

A rapid, complete neurovascular assessment of all four extremities should be done while the patient is in the ED and carefully documented in the medical records. Although definitive treatment of limb trauma usually is a lower priority (unless open, free hemorrhage is present), early identification facilitates a multiteam approach in the OR once life-threatening injuries have been controlled elsewhere. In addition to quantitating pulses and observing gross motor function, the clinician should inspect the limb for deformity, swelling, ecchymosis, and skin perforations.

Vascular Injuries

An expanding pulsatile hematoma or spurting, bright red blood indicates arterial injury. Manual pressure will control most bleeding, and blind clamping should be avoided. Limb-threatening vascular injury must be considered with a fracture or penetrating wound close to major arteries or with a proximal major joint dislocation. Classic signs of ischemia are pain, pallor, paresthesia, paralysis, and pulselessness. Palpable pulses may be present initially in more than one fourth of patients with major proximal arterial lesions. Shock and hypothermia, on the other hand, may induce peripheral vasoconstriction that mimics arterial insufficiency, underscoring the importance of comparing findings in one limb with those in the contralateral extremity. A thrill or bruit suggests traumatic arteriovenous fistula.

Prompt recognition of vascular compromise is crucial for functional limb salvage. Although 6 hours usually is considered a safe warm ischemic period, this amount of time may not be tolerated when arterial occlusion is complicated by protracted hemorrhagic shock, increased compartment pressure from soft tissue damage, disrupted collateral vessels, and associated venous impairment. Popliteal arterial disruption is particularly hazardous because of sparse collateral circulation around the knee and concomitant venous injury; the amputation rate may be as high as 20% with blunt dislocation or close-range shotgun wounds. Crushing injuries to the trifurcation vessels in the lower leg also have a poor prognosis because of the small caliber of these vessels and the surrounding soft tissue damage. Isolated extremity injuries resulting in obvious arterial bleeding, limb-threatening ischemia, or rapidly expanding hematomas are best managed by immediated exposure, control, and radiographic evaluation when necessary in the operating room.

Exclusion angiography is indicated for an injured extremity with (1) a pulse index below 0.95 compared to the contralateral limb following penetrating wounds near major vessels or high-risk blunt fractures (e.g., suprachondylar, knee dislocation); (2) shotgun injuries or multiple penetrating wounds; (3) potential arteriovenous fistula; and (4) question of bullet embolization.[165] Formal arteriograms generally are performed in the radiology department by experienced interventional radiologists; however, simple single-plane exclusion angiograms can be obtained expeditiously in the ED. Also, arterial Doppler studies may reduce the need for formal extremity runoff angiograms. Digital subtraction angiography should be used to evaluate injuries in children because of the relatively high complication rate of arterial cannulation in this age group.

Limb Replantation

Limb replantation has advanced immensely with the development of microvascular surgery and should be considered with an acute, clean amputation. Guillotine-type injuries have a better prognosis than avulsions, and upper extremities are rehabilitated more successfully than lower.[267] Warm ischemia that lasts longer than 8 hours generally limits replantation, but with proper cooling, the safe period may be extended to 24 hours. Amputated parts should be placed in a plastic bag and immersed in ice water. The decision for replantation should be discussed with the reconstruction team as soon as possible, and clearly tempered by associated injuries and the patient's personal needs.

SURGICAL MANAGEMENT OF SPECIFIC INJURIES

The decision to perform urgent surgery is a pivotal ED triage decision made by the trauma surgeon. The OR in many hospitals is not immediately adjacent to the ED and may be farther removed if the patient must undergo evaluation in the radiology department. Thus the timing of patient transport to the OR is crucial and depends on the mechanism of injury, the patient's physiologic status and response to resuscitation, the result of critical diagnostic studies and appropriate consultation, and the availability of an operating room. The ED stay for a patient in refractory shock with an abdominal gunshot wound is brief (e.g., 10 to 15 minutes), whereas a patient in stable condition with multisystem blunt trauma may remain in the ED or radiology department for some time. Premature triage to the OR may lead to an unnecessary laparotomy and delayed evaluation of life- or limb-threatening extra-abdominal injuries. However, an undue delay in the ED may result in physiologic deterioration leading to irreversible shock and coagulopathy. Transfer to the OR should be done by experienced personnel prepared to manage acute emergencies en route. Common errors include inadequate airway management, insecure lines and tubes, and insufficient monitoring of the patient. Each hospital should establish protocols to ensure timely, efficient, and safe patient transport from the ED resuscitation suite to the OR.

Organization of the Trauma Operating Room

Although organization of the OR generally is the prerogative of anesthesiologists, the trauma surgeon is ultimately responsible for the patient and should assist in creating the optimum environment for ongoing resuscitation and definitive surgical treatment. A specific OR suite should be designated for trauma. The unique features of this room should include ample space to accommodate special equipment and additional personnel, supplementary cabinet space for trauma instruments, auxiliary lighting for multiteam operations, large writing boards to record key laboratory data, and speaker telephones to facilitate communication with the laboratory, blood bank, and consultants.

Adequate monitoring is critical for a patient in persistent shock who is undergoing emergency surgery. A CVP catheter should be placed for serial readings and a Swan-Ganz catheter inserted as soon as feasible in patients with extensive injuries. An arterial cannula provides constant blood pressure readings, as well as access for blood gas determinations to ascertain acid-base, ventilatory, and oxygen transport status. Core temperature should be monitored continuously, and hypothermia should be minimized by infusing all fluids via warmers and heating gases from the ventilator. The ECG should be displayed and the pulse rate made audible. Urinary output and thoracostomy drainage should be channeled into receptacles that indicate the volume accumulated. All these indices are important in the continuous assessment of the patient; the more visible and accessible these data are to the surgeon and anesthesiologist, the better the team effort.

Head and Spinal Trauma

Surgical management of intracranial trauma is rarely started without the diagnostic aid of CT scanning. With a closed injury, urgent craniotomy usually is performed to decompress and evacuate an expanding mass lesion (epidural, subdural, or intracerebral hematoma) or to elevate a depressed skull fracture.[268] With major penetrating wounds, craniotomy usually is required for depressed bone fragments, dural lacerations, and extruded brain.[132] Preoperative CT scanning is important to identify associated intracranial bleeding and cerebral contusion. The specifics of surgical treatment for both open and closed head injuries are detailed in Chapter 26.

The role of emergency surgical intervention for acute spinal injuries is controversial.[258] Although some authorities advocate aggressive spinal cord decompression, most believe this should be reserved for a patient with deteriorating neurologic function who has vertebral malalignment or spinal cord compression.[50,220] CT scanning and magnetic resonance imaging (MRI) have been valuable in planning the acute surgical approach. Surgical management of unstable spinal fractures is discussed in Chapter 26.

Cervical Trauma

Carotid and Vertebral Artery Injuries

The anterior aspect of the chest and both sides of the neck should be prepped and draped widely. The carotid artery is exposed via an oblique incision along the anterior border of the sternocleidomastoid muscle. The incision can be extended cephalad to the mastoid process and combined with mandibular subluxation or resection for high carotid lesions at the base of the skull. Conversely, carotid injuries extending into the thoracic outlet or involving the aortic arch and great vessels are exposed with a combination of neck and median sternotomy incisions. Temporary carotid shunting is reserved for a patent internal carotid artery with a stump pressure below 50 mm Hg or for known occlusion of the contralateral carotid artery.[7,55] Systemic heparin is desirable when a shunt is in place and should be given routinely, unless contraindicated by associated injuries. Distal carotid thrombectomy is accomplished by manually extracting clots from the internal carotid artery with forceps until back-bleeding is established. Fogarty catheters should not be used to clear internal carotid occlusions that extend into the carotid sinus because of the potential for cerebral embolization. Proximal carotid thrombectomy is facilitated by the patient's arterial pressure and occasionally by gentle use of a Fogarty catheter. Most intimal tears require only simple suture repair. More extensive injuries can be reconstructed with transposition of the ipsilateral external carotid artery or interposition bypass grafting with saphenous vein or synthetic material.[147] Completion angiography routinely is performed to evaluate the repair and exclude residual thrombi or arterial injury.

Vertebral artery injury is reported infrequently, most likely because of the vessel's deep location and the usual tolerance to occlusion.[175,248] Although the vertebral arteries carry 10% of the cerebral circulation, the contralateral vessel provides adequate flow unless it is hypoplastic or atherosclerotic. Thus ligation is the preferred treatment for acute vertebral injury unless there is angiographic evidence of contralateral disease or the vessel is a major extracranial branch to the cervical spinal cord, which is rare.

Pharyngoesophageal Injuries

Blunt pharyngoesophageal injury is rare, and most injuries are caused by gunshot wounds. The diagnosis usually is established by endoscopy or oral contrast studies, but neither is uniformly reliable. Endoscopy during surgery with methylene blue or air insufflation may be necessary to identify small injuries. Small pharyngeal tears have been treated successfully without surgery, but the safest policy is to explore all injuries promptly. Full-thickness lacerations are closed with a single layer of interrupted sutures reinforced with a pleural patch when possible. The prevertebral space is drained with soft drains because of the high incidence of small esophageal leaks. These drains should be separated from the suture line with viable tissue to prevent erosion and breakdown of the surgical repair.

Laryngotracheal Injuries

Blunt trauma of the cervical airway, caused by anterior compression of the neck against the spine, may include fracture, avulsion, or dislocation of laryngotracheal structures and is often complicated by swelling and damage in intraluminal soft tissue. Airway management is a primary concern, but if ventilation is adequate, invasive measures should be deferred until the patient is in the OR.[83,107,280] If the patient is not in respiratory distress, indirect laryngoscopy is undertaken immediately. Vocal cord mobility is assessed, and the area is checked for tears, hematomas, or distortion. If major injury is confirmed, a tracheostomy should be performed using local anesthesia. Proximal tracheal injury, when conveniently located, may be converted to a tracheostomy. General anesthesia is induced once airway control has been accomplished. Exploration of the neck for blunt trauma usually is performed via a collar incision at the level of injury, whereas an oblique peristernocleidomastoid incision is used on the side of a penetrating wound. Tracheal tears are repaired primarily with absorbable suture. Significant laryngeal disruption requires open exploration with placement of an intraluminal stent. The specifics of surgical treatment are reviewed in Chapter 27.

Chest Trauma

Cardiac Wounds

In a patient with pericardial tamponade, a preliminary subxiphoid window may be a useful temporizing measure.[299] If the patient is in extremis, however, left anterolateral thoracotomy (see Figure 15-7) should be performed immediately to evacuate the pericardium and digitally control the bleeding site. When exposure is suboptimal, the incision can be carried across the sternum into the right side of the chest. Median sternotomy is otherwise preferred for a hemodynamically stable patient with a cardiac wound. The pericardium is opened widely anterior to the phrenic nerve, and the contained blood is rapidly evacuated to identify the bleeding sites. Wounds of the vena cava and atria are controlled with a partially occluding vascular clamp, and those of the ventricle are controlled with direct finger occlusion. Low-pressure venous injuries are repaired by running sutures, and those of the myocardium are closed with interrupted mattress sutures reinforced with pledgets.[62,270] Sutures must be placed deep to the coronary arteries when near them. Temporary occlusion of inflow may be required to repair large ventricular defects,[299] but cardiopulmonary bypass is rarely necessary for initial surgical management. Transected coronary arteries are ligated, and immediate reconstruction is done only if severe cardiac dysfunction ensues.[59] Valvular and septal injuries generally are treated later if the patient is hemodynamically stable.[59] Performing cardiac auscultation and determining chamber oxygen saturation during surgery may reveal these complications (frequently these lesions extend and become symptomatic postoperatively).[65]

Most patients who survive blunt cardiac rupture have pericardial tamponade, and median sternotomy is preferred for individuals who can be stabilized hemodynamically with pericardiocentesis.[146] Most salvageable lesions are atrial tears, and approximately two thirds of these are on the right side.[160,231] Bleeding usually can be controlled with a vascular clamp, but balloon catheters occasionally are helpful in the resuscitation phase. As with penetrating injuries, simple suture repair is adequate for most lacerations, but sutures must be placed carefully near the atrioventricular groove to avoid compromising the coronary arteries.[231] Traumatic rupture of the pericardium has been reported without associated cardiac involvement.[31] These injuries should be treated surgically to prevent herniation of the heart or of abdominal viscera in the event of an adjacent diaphragmatic tear.

Great Vessel Injuries

Penetrating wounds to the thoracic great vessels are frequently lethal because of immediate exsanguination into the chest. Paradoxically, in patients who survive to reach the OR, the bleeding is often contained within the mediastinum. The surgical approach is similar for blunt and penetrating trauma: median sternotomy with neck extention for right-sided injuries, and high left anterolateral thoracotomy continued cephalad via the sternum and into the neck (trapdoor incision) for left-sided injuries.[101,320] The most versatile incision for moribund patients is a bilateral anterior thoracotomy across the sternum (see Figure 15-7, *B*). Free intrathoracic bleeding should be controlled digitally and partial-occlusion vascular clamps applied when feasible. Hematomas should not be entered until proximal and distal arterial isolation has been established, and dissection of the superior mediastinum and thoracic outlet must be done with thorough knowledge of the busy regional anatomy. Cardiopulmonary bypass may be required for ascending aortic lesions. Lateral arteriorrhaphy is preferred, but more than half of injuries of the thoracic great vessels require interposition grafting.[101] For injuries of the proximal innominate artery, the graft may be placed in the aortic root to bypass the lesion before the hematoma is opened.

In 95% of aortic disruptions in patients who survive rapid deceleration injury, the disruptions occur in the descending thoracic aorta just distal to the left subclavian artery.[133,134,321] A standard left posterolateral thoracotomy provides optimum exposure to the distal arch and descending thoracic aorta. Preparation for surgery includes insertion of a double-lumen endotracheal tube for single-lung ventilation, arterial pressure monitoring, and placement of a Swan-Ganz catheter to assess and optimize oxygen transport during surgery. Blunt aortic tears vary from small lacerations to circumferential separation. The most controversial issue in their repair is whether distal aortic perfusion is needed during cross-clamping and repair. For the typical isthmus injury, recommendations range from partial cardiopulmonary bypass with anticoagulation to no protective measures.[4] Although the clamp-and-sew technique may be appropriate for small tears that can be repaired in less than 30 minutes, we favor partial left heart bypass using a heparin-less centrifugal pump (Figure 15-13). This technique reduces the risk of decompensation of the frequently contused myocardium while maintaining distal aortic perfusion pressure, reducing the incidence of paraplegia and splanchnic reperfusion injury. Injury to the ascending aorta, which is more common with vertical deceleration, is best approached via medial sternotomy with cardiopulmonary bypass. For innominate arterial injury, the median sternotomy is extended across the sternoclavicular joint into the right side of the neck[101,320]; for proximal left subclavian injury, the trapdoor incision is preferred.

Esophageal Perforation

Blunt rupture of the esophagus is rare,[177,285] is often accompanied by tracheal injury,[285] and usually occurs longitudinally above the pulmonary hilum, whereas penetrating injuries occur throughout the esophagus. Exposure is obtained with a left thoracotomy for injuries involving the lower third of the esophagus, but a right-sided thoracotomy is preferred for higher lesions. Acute esophageal injuries are repaired primarily. Most authorities recommend that the repair be reinforced with a parietal pleural flap[177,289] or muscle flap. A nasogastric tube is inserted through the injured segment into the stomach for early enteral feeding.[197] For extensive injuries, a gastrostomy (for decompression) and needle catheter jejunostomy are done.

Treatment of an esophageal wound becomes more complex if the diagnosis is delayed. Urschel and colleagues[304] devised the concept of esophageal exclusion and diversion in continuity. During the initial thoracotomy, the esophageal wound is sutured, mediastinal and pleural drainage is established, and the esophagus distal to the injury is ligated to prevent reflux of gastric contents. Large-caliber chromic sutures, which lyse spontaneously in approximately 2 weeks, are used for temporary ligation. A gastrostomy is done for postoperative enteral feeding.[189] Diversion is completed with a cervical esophagostomy to allow egress of oral secretions. Numerous modifications of this approach exist, including esophageal transection with later reconstruction. The most important principle is adequate mediastinal drainage because esophageal breakdown, with resultant fistula, is the rule with delayed recognition.

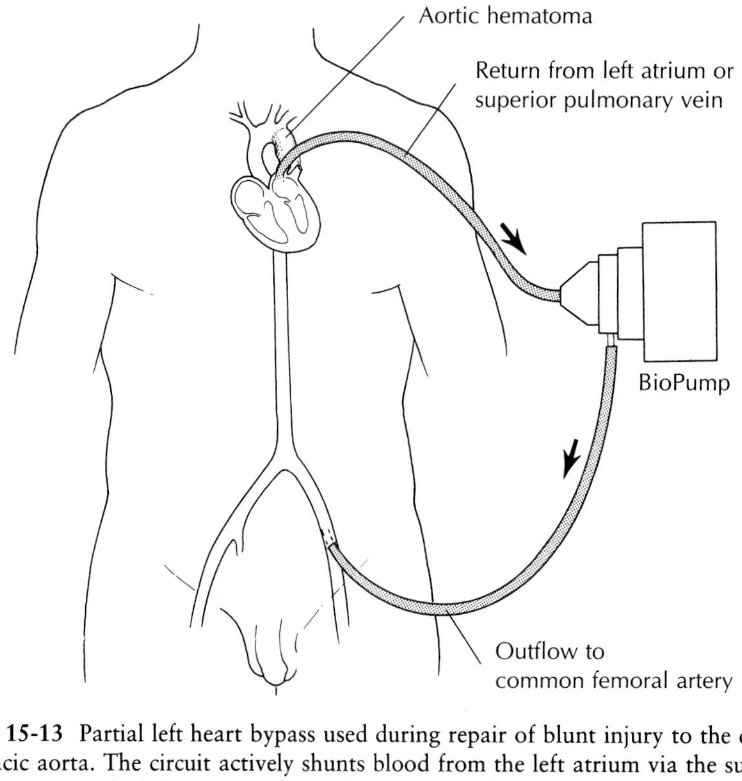

FIGURE 15-13 Partial left heart bypass used during repair of blunt injury to the descending thoracic aorta. The circuit actively shunts blood from the left atrium via the superior pulmonary vein to the left common femoral artery using the BioPump centrifugal pump system (Bio-Medicus, Inc, Minneapolis, Minn).

Lung Injuries

Early thoracotomy for noncardiac penetrating wounds usually is done for unrelenting bleeding,[100,157,273] massive air leak, or air ambolus. Surgical exposure is best achieved via a posterolateral thoracotomy on the injured side, but anterolateral thoracotomy with transsternal extention is used for patients in extremis. For active parenchymal bleeding or air leakage, simple pneumorrhaphy with running absorbable sutures should suffice in most patients. Segmental debridement with staple closure occasionally is required, but formal lobectomy is rarely necessary and should be reserved for massive tissue disruption or hilar vascular injury.

Tracheobronchial Injuries

Tracheobronchial disruption from closed trauma is most likely to involve the main bronchi within 2.5 cm of the carina.[103,122] Early and repeated bronchoscopy is helpful for diagnosing and treating persistent air leaks and lobar atelectasis. Although minor tears may be managed without surgery, major disruptions require immediate thoracotomy.[122,135] Exposure is achieved via a posterolateral thoracotomy in the fifth intercostal space on the side of the injury. If a standard endotracheal tube has been inserted, it can be advanced beyond the injury into the uninvolved bronchus. However, a split-function endotracheal tube may be useful for extensive injuries. Primary suture repair or reimplantation is usually feasible in the acute setting, although extensive damage may require pulmonary resection.[48,103,122,175] Surgical management of injuries recognized late is complex and often complicated by delayed bronchial stricture (see Chapter 27).

Abdominal Trauma

Hepatic Injuries

The liver is the most frequently injured intra-abdominal organ, but more than 85% of hepatic wounds can be managed by simple hemostatic techniques.[308] Gauze packing will terminate active hemorrhage from most superficial hepatic wounds. For continued surface bleeding, electrocautery and topical hemostatic agents generally are effective.[152] Prophylactic perihepatic drainage is not necessary for these minor parenchymal lacerations.[187,279]

The first priority with severe hepatic bleeding is to resuscitate the patient. Pringle's maneuver (temporary occlusion of the porta hepatis, that is, the portal vein, hepatic artery, and common bile duct) and tight liver packing are critical maneuvers to attenuate blood loss. Although the human liver's tolerance to warm ischemia was traditionally considered to be minutes, the safe period now is considered to be in excess of an hour.[114] If Pringle's maneuver fails to slow bleeding, the reason is a hepatic vein–retrohepatic vena caval tear or an aberrant derivation of the lobar hepatic artery.[212] In Michels' anatomic study, a left hepatic artery arose from the left gastric artery in 25% of patients and was the primary artery for the left lobe in 12%. Similarly, a right hepatic artery originated from the superior mesenteric artery in 17% of patients and was the principal lobar artery in 12%. Such accessory hepatic arteries do not lie within the porta hepatis and therefore must be occluded separately.[178] If hepatic vascular inflow occlusion is successful, the liver should then be mobilized to allow adequate inspection of the extent of injury. The fracture sites are then systematically explored by tractotomy,[227] with individual ligation of the divided intrahepatic blood vessels and bile ducts.

If inflow occlusion, individual vessel ligation, and packing do not achieve adequate hemostasis, selective hepatic artery ligation (SHAL) should be considered.[169] This procedure is usually safe, because the lobar portal vein provides sufficient oxygen to the dearterialized hepatic tissue until collaterals are functional. SHAL failure after an effective Pringle's maneuver implies portal or hepatic vein injury. If bleeding persists, the choice is whether to proceed with hepatic resection or to use abdominal packing. Packing is clearly preferred with refractory coagulopathy, hypothermia, extensive bilobar injuries, other life-threatening injuries, or lack of blood bank support.[68] Reoperation is planned within 24 hours for removal of the packs and additional hepatic debridement. Packs should be removed early because they increase intraabdominal pressure, which may compromise splanchnic and renal perfusion, and the collected blood is a good medium for bacterial proliferation.

Hepatic lobectomy following trauma is formidable, with a mortality rate exceeding 50%. Liver anatomy varies, and the surgeon must be familiar with the prevalent anomalies of the hepatic arteries and veins and the biliary duct system[109,136] (Figure 15-14). Drainage of the common bile duct via a T-tube is not beneficial following major hepatic resection,[155,242] but drainage of the perihepatic area is important because of the high incidence of postoperative bile leaks.[71]

Retrohepatic vena caval injury is rare and constitutes the only immediate indication for hepatic lobectomy in an adult. Injury of the vena cava from blunt trauma usually occurs at its junction with a major hepatic vein. The typical clue to such an injury is failure of Pringle's maneuver corroborated by outpouring of desaturated blood with mobilization of the liver. Most authorities recommend hepatic vascular exclusion by placing a retrohepatic vena caval shunt.[140] We prefer a balloon shunt introduced via the saphenofemoral junction for this purpose (Figure 15-15).[239] Despite these adjuncts, the mortality rate continues to exceed 80% in adults. In a child, neither a shunt nor hepatic lobectomy is necessary because the confluence of the major hepatic veins and vena

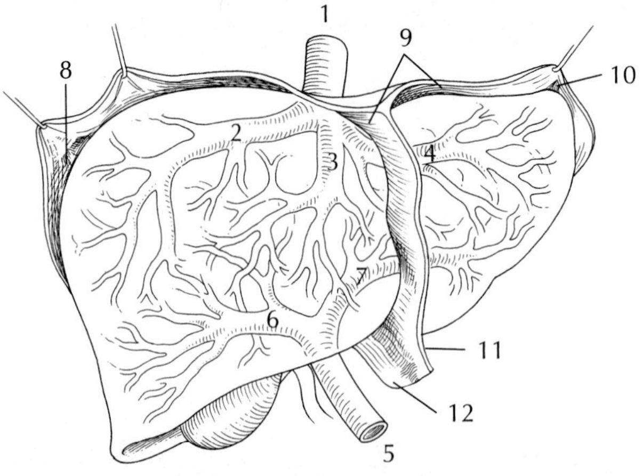

FIGURE 15-14 Surgical anatomy of the liver: *1,* Inferior vena cava; *2,* right hepatic vein; *3,* middle hepatic vein; *4,* left hepatic vein; *5,* portal vein; *6,* right branch of portal vein; *7,* left branch of portal vein; *8,* right triangular ligament; *9,* coronary ligament; *10,* left triangular ligament; *11,* falciform ligament; *12,* round ligament of the liver (ligamentum teres).

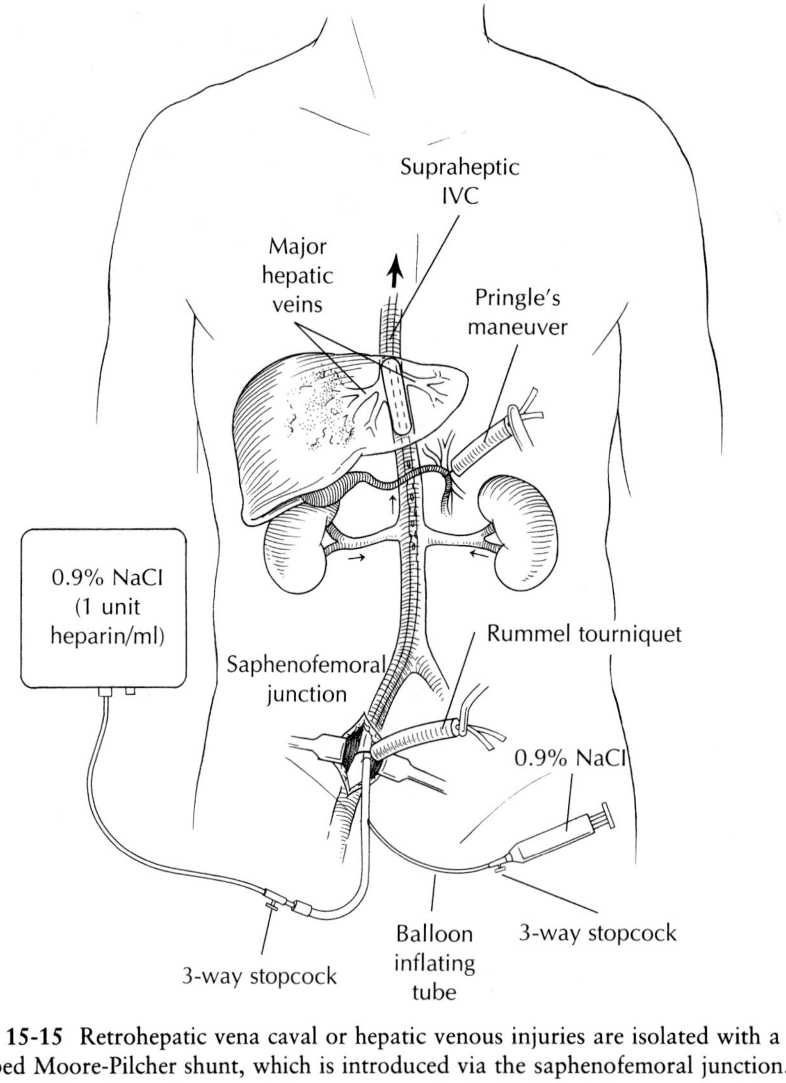

FIGURE 15-15 Retrohepatic vena caval or hepatic venous injuries are isolated with a balloon-tipped Moore-Pilcher shunt, which is introduced via the saphenofemoral junction. Hepatic arterial and portal venous inflow are controlled with Pringle's maneuver. The balloon is inflated with saline in the retrohepatic vena cava at the level of the hepatic veins.

cava is more extrahepatic; consequently, repair can be done by direct exposure, and patient salvage is greater.[37]

Splenic Injuries

Surgical management of an injured spleen has changed radically over the past decade.[238] Once regarded as *mysterii pleni organon,* the spleen is now considered an important immunologic factory as well as a reticuloendothelial filter. Although the risk of postsplenectomy sepsis is greatest in a child under 2 years of age, an asplenic adult is clearly vulnerable.[303] This danger of overwhelming sepsis has prompted the current enthusiasm for splenic salvage procedures. The risk of complications from splenorrhaphy, however, must not exceed the risk of total splenectomy.[199] Repair of the spleen is attempted only if (1) the patient is hemodynamically stable and has no other immediate life-threatening injuries; (2) the spleen is amenable to repair; and (3) the surgeon is familiar with salvage techniques.[182,238]

The most important feature of splenorrhaphy is mobilization. The spleen must be freed by incision of its superior (phrenicolienal) and lateral (lienorenal) peritoneal attachments. These ligaments are essentially avascular and can be divided without direct visualization. The inferior (lienocolic) ligament may contain sizable blood vessels and therefore should be divided and ligated to facilitate splenic mobility. A plane is then developed posterior to the pancreas with blunt finger dissection. Once mobile, the spleen is rotated medially into the abdominal wound for complete inspection.

Small capsular avulsions are controlled with electrocautery and topical hemostatic agents are applied to the denuded parenchyma. Argon beam coagulation offers a significant advantage in achieving effective hemostasis of splenic tissue. Deep parenchymal lacerations require individual vessel ligation; if bleeding persists, interlocking mattress sutures are placed. The thickened capsule in a child permits direct suturing, whereas bolsters usually are needed in an adult (Figure 15-16). Major splenic fractures should be managed by anatomic resection. The spleen is composed of autonomous vascular compartments based on secondary divisions of splenic artery. In 85% of patients, the splenic artery bifurcates into two primary branches, supplying the superior and inferior lobes. The lobar arteries further divide into cephalic and caudal segments. Segmental arterial ligation produces demarcation at the avascular intersegmental plane, permitting amputation of the ischemic portion (Figure 15-17).[25,218] Hemostasis of the cut end of viable spleen is then achieved with sutures and topical agents. Occasionally splenic artery ligation is necessary to control bleeding, but this maneuver carries an immunologic penalty.

Splenectomy remains the optimum management technique when the spleen is pulverized or the patient has other life-threatening injuries. The splenic artery and vein should be ligated individually. Reimplantation of the splenic tissue restores some of the immune function lost with splenectomy.[112,230] We section the removed spleen into five fragments (40 × 40 × 3 mm) and enclose them in greater omental pouches. The left upper quadrant is not drained following splenorrhaphy or splenectomy unless for a concurrent pancreatic injury. Because of the risk of overwhelming pneumococcal sepsis, all patients undergoing loss of more than 50% of the spleen should be given polypneumococcal vaccine after surgery.

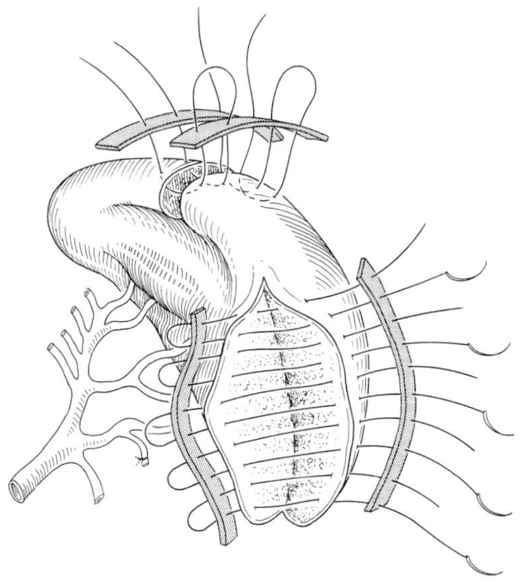

FIGURE 15-16 A damaged spleen can be repaired by using mattress sutures over Teflon pledgets.

Stomach and Small Bowel Wounds

With penetrating abdominal trauma, stomach and small bowel perforations are the second most common type of wounds, after liver injuries. Although blunt gastric rupture is rare,[322] proximal jejunal and distal ileal disruptions occur after abrupt deceleration, particularly with lap belt restraints.[317] The most important feature of surgical management is complete inspection of the gastrointestinal tract and adjacent mesentery. Failure to visualize the posterior aspect of the stomach or duodenum with an anterior gastric wound is a common oversight and may lead to serious complications from a missed perforation. In general, a gunshot wound leaves an even number of perforations; an odd number suggests a missed exit wound, although occasionally the bullet comes to rest within the gut lumen or makes a tangential wound. When a hematoma is present, the mesenteric border of the bowel must be exposed to exclude perforation.

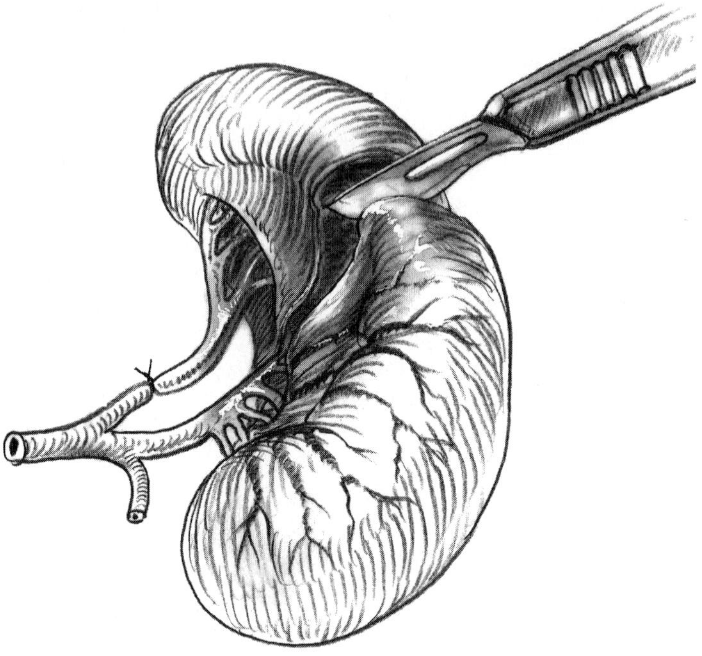

FIGURE 15-17 After ligation of the splenic vessels of the superior pole, ischemic tissue is clearly demarcated, allowing anatomic resection. (After Giddings.)

Primary repair of the stomach and small bowel is usually safe because of the rich blood supply and relatively modest bacterial content of these areas. All defects in the gut should be identified before repair of an apparently isolated injury is begun. Intestinal wounds should be sealed with noncrushing clamps while awaiting formal closure to prevent further peritoneal contamination. Simple perforations of the stomach and small bowel should be closed with standard techniques in either one or two layers. Two adjacent holes are usually connected, and the bowel is closed transversely to avoid narrowing the lumen. Minimal debridement is required after stab injuries and low-energy gunshot wounds, but devitalized tissue from high-energy injuries must be removed. Mesenteric bleeding should be controlled by ligating individual vessels as close to the bowel as possible. If questionable areas of viability or multiple perforations are found in a short segment of small bowel, the segment should be resected and the ends anastomosed. In rare cases of extensive ischemic gut caused by injury to the proximal superior mesenteric artery, the remaining viable bowel ends can be brought out as temporary enterostomies.

Duodenum/Pancreas Injuries

The anatomic and physiologic complexities of the duodenum and pancreas (Figure 15-18) have given rise to a variety of surgical techniques for treating these structures. Injuries overlooked or underestimated may lead to disastrous complications; on the other hand, inappropriately aggressive management can result in permanent morbidity or death during surgery. Blunt duodenal injury is usually caused by abrupt deceleration, which crushes the retroperitoneal duodenum against the spine or causes a blowout of the air-filled, closed duodenal loop.[151] The most common site for nonpenetrating pancreatic disruption is the area overlying the vertebral column. Prompt recognition is essential for successful treatment of pancreaticoduodenal injuries. These structures must be examined completely during celiotomy if any of the following pertain: (1) a history of rapid deceleration; (2) blood is the nasogastric aspirate; (3) blood or bile staining the midline retroperitoneum; or (4) wounds penetrating the upper midabdomen. A generous Kocher maneuver is performed to expose the pancreatic head and first two portions of the duodenum, and the lesser sac is opened widely through the gastrocolic omentum to allow examination of the body and tail of the pancreas and third portion of the duodenum. The fourth portion of the duodenum can be seen better if the ligament of Treitz is divided.

Limited duodenal contusions discovered during laparotomy are best left alone; most hematomas reabsorb within 1 to 2 weeks. Placement of a gastrostomy and feeding jejunostomy should be considered for extensive contusions when delayed resolution of the hematoma is expected.[86] Limited perforations and simple lacerations of the duodenum are closed primarily using standard

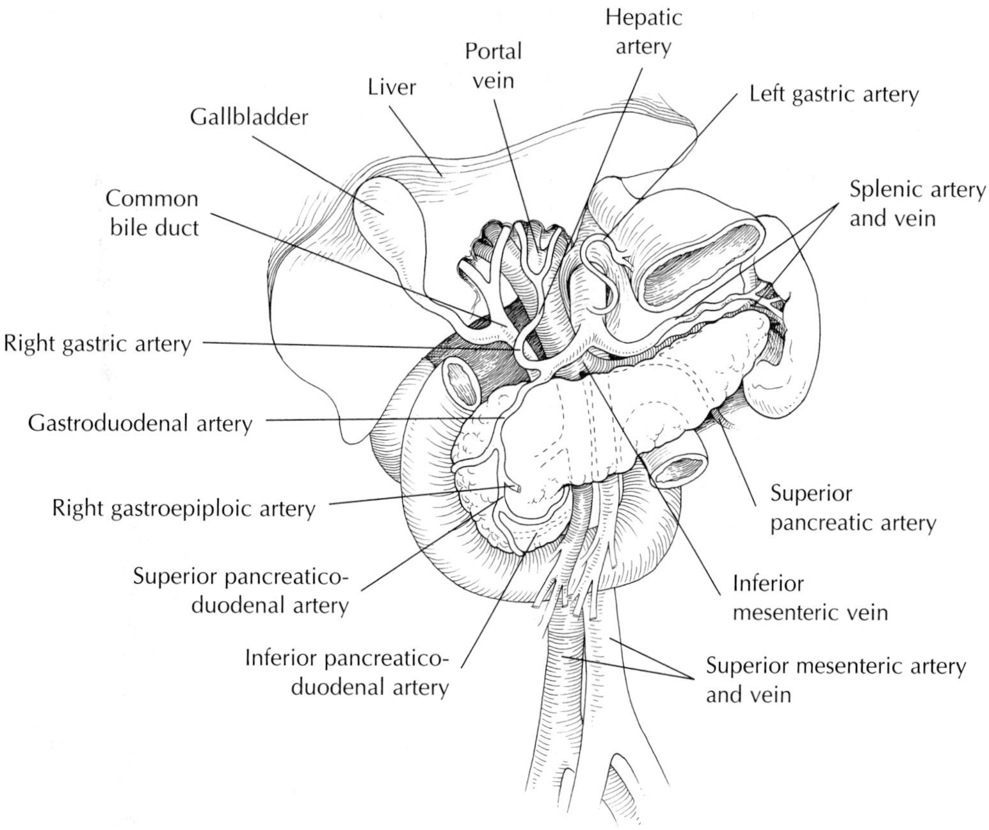

FIGURE 15-18 Anatomic relationships of the pancreas and duodenum, showing adjacent organs and important nearby vascular structures.

suture techniques. Presumptive drainage is not used for these minor defects. Extensive duodenal injuries may require one of a variety of patch bypass procedures for safe closure. These include serosal patch procedures, resection with duodenojejunostomy, and Roux-en-Y reconstruction (Figure 15-19).[18,128] Extensive resectional procedures that are necessary (e.g., pancreaticoduodenectomy) are performed only for massive combined pancreaticoduodenal injuries. Management of complex duodenal injuries, particularly when such injuries are recognized late, is controversial.[201] Some authorities believe suction decompression of the duodenum is important and can be done by transpyloric nasogastric tube, tube duodenostomy, or retrograde tube jejunostomy. We favor exclusion for precarious duodenal injuries.[13,306] A gastrotomy is made on the greater curvature of the antrum, through which the pylorus is closed with a 2-0 polypropylene purse-string suture. A side-to-side gastrojejunostomy is then completed using the gastrotomy (Figure 15-20). Specific indications for these protective measures include: (1) free perforation, with delay of surgery for more than 24 hours; (2) injury involving more than 75% of the wall in the first or second portion of the duodenum; and (3) associated injuries of the pancreatic head or distal common bile duct. A needle catheter jejunostomy should be placed for early postoperative enteral feedings in patients with high-risk duodenal wounds.[191,192,195]

Surgical decisions for pancreatic trauma are based on the injury site and the status of the ductal system.[33,110,121] Most injuries are superficial contusions and lacerations, and the integrity of the main duct is not in question.[283] Peripancreatic drainage is routine for such minor lesions because disruption of the parenchyma and peripheral ducts may produce fistula. Closed-suction catheters are effective for removing pancreatic juice, and fistulae usually resolve with adequate drainage. Location dictates the management of deep fractures or penetrating wounds with suspected ductal violation. Major injuries in the body and tail of the pancreas warrant distal resection.[35] Removal of this portion of the gland is not associated with endocrine deficiency, and the spleen can be preserved with little additional effort. Roux-en-Y internal drainage of the distal pancreas is frequently complicated by the formation of a fistula and secondary infection. Surgery for injuries to the right side of the

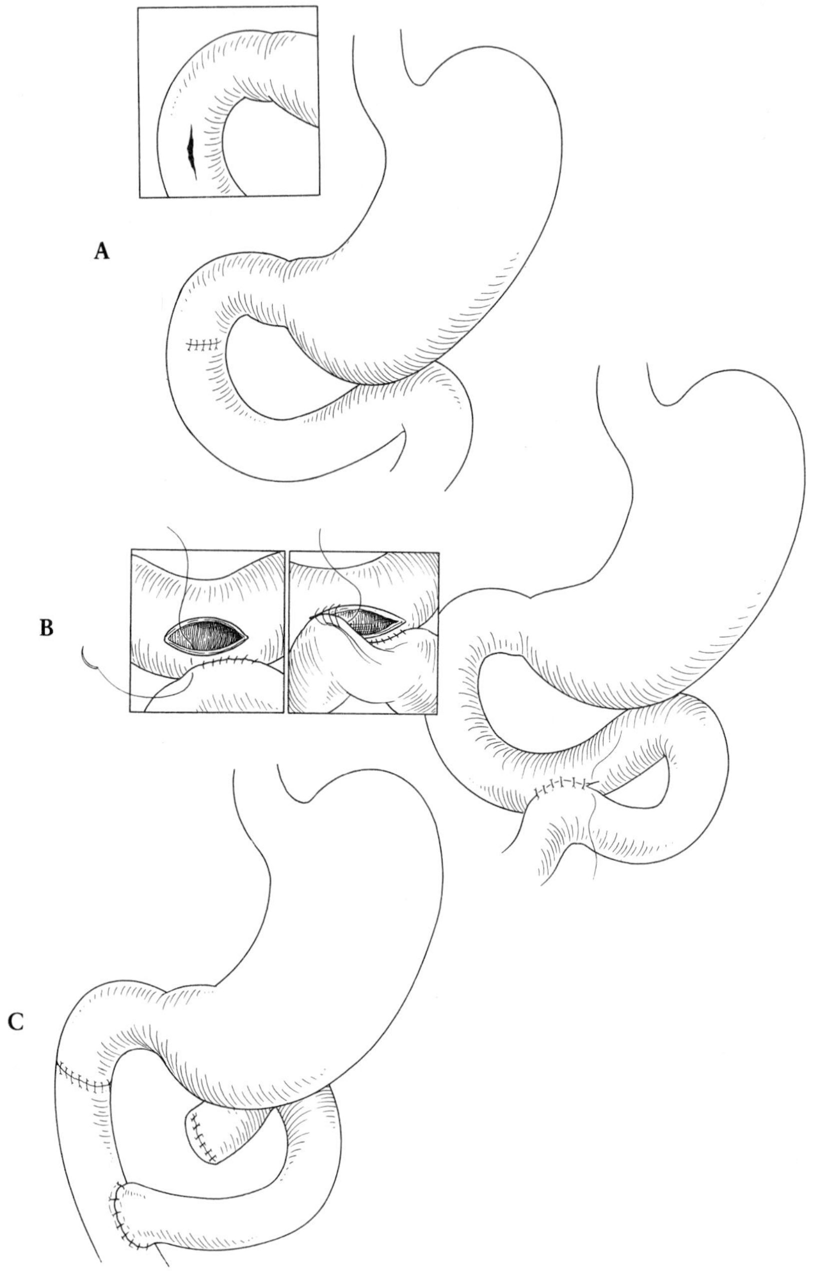

FIGURE 15-19 Procedures used to treat duodenal injuries. **A,** Most duodenal injuries require only simple primary repair using one- or two-layer suture techniques. **B,** More extensive duodendal injuries that preclude primary repair but show no significant narrowing of the lumen can be managed with the serosal patch technique. This involves suturing the serosa of a loop of jejunum to the edges of the duodenal defect, which is subsequently resurfaced with intestinal mucosa. **C,** Extensive disruptions of the duodenum can be repaired with a variety of resection and reconstruction techniques, including end-to-end Roux-en-Y duodenojejunostomy.

superior mesenteric vein generally is conservative. Because ductal integrity is the critical factor, pancreatography may be used during surgery to define the status of the duct.[14] Options for trauma of the pancreatic head with ductal involvement include anterior Roux-en-Y pancreaticojejunostomy, pancreatic division with Roux-en-Y drainage of both segments, pancreaticoduodenectomy,[149] or external drainage. The last approach is preferred for most injuries, despite the risk of pancreatic fistula formation. Early postoperative nutrition via jejunostomy is an important adjunct; jejunal administration of a defined, elemental, low-fat diet with neutral pH has little stimulatory effect on the pancreas.

Colonic Wounds

The most common type of colon injuries are penetrating wounds. However, blunt disruptions and hemorrhagic contusions can result from high-energy transfer. Surgical management of colon perforation has changed dramatically over the last 25 years.[209,282] The practice of mandatory colostomy, adopted from military experience, has given way to a selective policy of primary colon repair. The intraperitoneal colon can be safely closed primarily in at least 70% of patients in the civilian setting.[271] The criteria for primary repair are (1) injury less than 6 hours old; (2) no or only one associated intraperitoneal injury; (3) absence of hemorrhagic shock; and (4) a patient who is otherwise in stable condition. Although some suggest that right-sided colon injuries can be treated more aggressively than left-sided ones, this theory has not been substantiated.[294] Exteriorization of the sutured colon is a viable alternative to colostomy when the factors listed previously preclude safe intraperitoneal repair. The exteriorized segment will heal in 75% of patients, sparing the added morbidity of colostomy closure. The success of exteriorization is enhanced by attention to technical details, such as (1) debriding adequately and suturing meticulously, using resection when injury is extensive; (2) using wide mobilization of the involved colon segment to prevent obstruction and tension on the suture line; (3) maintaining the repair in a moist environment; and (4) delaying intraperitoneal return of the colon until at least the seventh postoperative day.

If the surgeon believes primary repair or exteriorization is ill-advised for clinical or technical reasons, colostomy is appropriate.[22] The colostomy and nonfunctional mucous fistula should exit close to each other on the abdominal wall to facilitate subsequent takedown and closure. When the colonic wound permits, a loop colostomy is considered adequate. If the colon must be divided for technical reasons, the distal colon can be simply stapled rather than fashioning a mucous fistula, especially if the distal colon is too short to bring out. The skin and subcutaneous tissue should be left open after the fascia is closed to reduce the risk of infection.

A

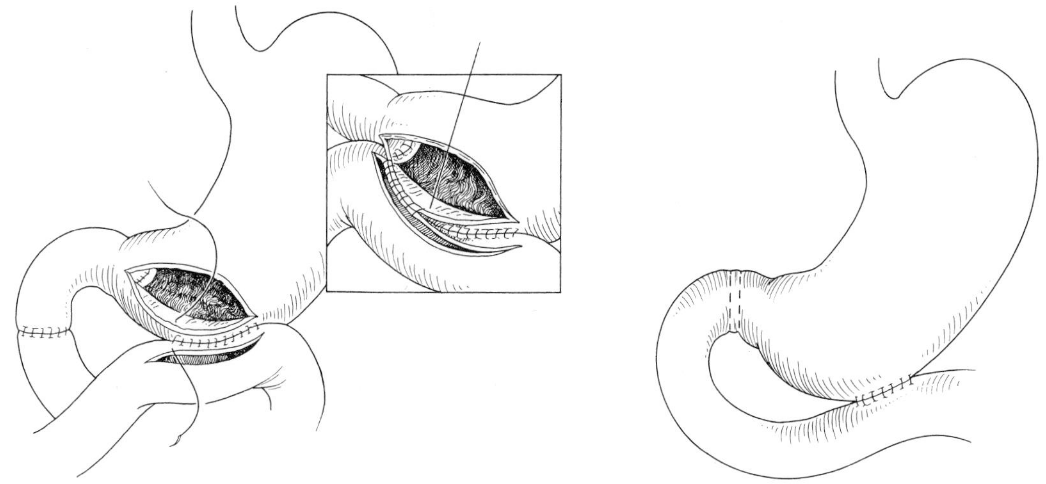

B

FIGURE 15-20 **A,** Pyloric exclusion and gastrojejunostomy are done to protect severe duodenal injuries that have been closed primarily. The pylorus is sutured closed through a dependent distal gastrotomy. A gastrojejunostomy is then fashioned to a proximal loop of jejunum. **B,** An alternative method of pyloric exclusion uses an intestinal stapling device to occlude the proximal duodenum. A gastrojejunostomy is then performed between the dependent stomach and the proximal jejunum.

Rectal Injuries

Rectal injury is usually caused by gunshot wounds or bone fragmentation from major pelvic fractures.[113] These injuries are at high risk of septic complications because of the heavy bacterial load contaminating a hematoma in the poorly vascularized soft tissue of the pelvis. Fecal diversion with a proximal colostomy is mandatory for all full-thickness rectal defects.

The patient should be placed in the lithotomy position on the operating table to provide adequate exposure of the perineum and abdomen. The abdomen is explored through a midline laparotomy and associated intraperitoneal injuries managed as indicated. Before any significant pelvic hematoma is entered, proximal vascular isolation of the distal aortal or common iliac vessels is obtained. The retrorectal space is opened to the level of the coccyx, and devitalized tissue is debrided. Ideally the rectal wound is closed, although most unrepaired rectal injuries deep in the pelvis heal adequately. Retrograde injection of methylene blue or rectosigmoidoscopy during surgery may help identify lesions difficult to visualize directly. Adequate drainage of these wounds is critical, using sump or Penrose drains placed in the presacral space and brought out through the perineum anterior to the tip of the coccyx. Fecal diversion is established with a proximal colostomy. When possible a loop sigmoid colostomy is constructed, with a distal limb stapled (Figure 15-21). A large Foley catheter is then placed through a small temporary colotomy in the distal limb to facilitate evacuation of colonic and rectal contents by copious irrigation with saline and antibiotic solution.

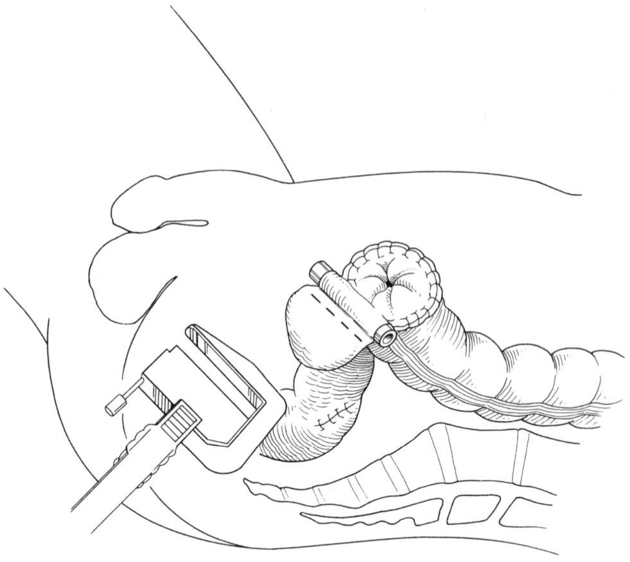

FIGURE 15-21 Sigmoid loop colostomy is performed for rectal injury. Staple closure of the distal limb ensures complete fecal diversion.

Major Abdominal Vascular Injuries

Vascular trauma is responsible for most deaths caused by penetrating abdominal wounds. The most lethal injuries are those in the retrohepatic vena cava,[129,236] visceral aorta,[181] and main portal vein.[228,236] Blunt trauma usually involves the venous system; the abdominal aorta is rarely disrupted, and injury here may dissect later.[142] Although the diagnosis of major abdominal vascular injury is occasionally subtle because of retroperitoneal tamponade, these patients typically arrive at the hospital in shock. Successful treatment demands quick recognition and prompt resuscitation with adequate volume replacement, including blood, followed by ample vascular exposure so that the hemorrhage can be controlled quickly.

Preparation of the patient for surgery includes the chest and upper legs to facilitate access for proximal and distal vascular control, and sterile equipment should include a variety of vascular clamps, tourniquets, and shunts that allow temporary, nontraumatic occlusion of vessels. Visceral rotation is valuable for surgical exposure of major intra-abdominal vascular wounds.[10] Left peritoneal reflection is carried out for midline and left-sided supramesocolic hematomas. Mobilization of the left aspect of the colon, spleen, stomach, and distal pancreas in a plane deep to the pancreas provides optimum exposure of the suprarenal aorta, celiac axis, proximal superior mesenteric artery, and left renal vessels (Figure 15-22). For right-sided supramesocolic hematomas, reflection of the ascending colon, duodenum, and pancreatic head provides a wide view of the infrahepatic vena cava, portal venous system, and right renal vessels (Figure 15-23). Proximal vascular control of inframesocolic or pelvic bleeding is better obtained with right visceral rotation because of the position of the vena cava and iliac veins. Anterior penetrating vascular wounds usually have a posterior component that may be temporarily tamponaded by adjacent soft tissue; thus both sides must be inspected for entrance and exit sites.

Abdominal Aortic Injuries

Abdominal aortic injuries should be closed by lateral arteriorrhaphy when possible. For large-caliber gunshot wounds, autogenous vein patching may be appropriate, but for complete transection, synthetic graft interposition is used. Extraanatomic bypass is not warranted for intestinal contamination. Extensive damage to the celiac trunk usually can be treated by ligation because of the rich collateral circulation. However, occlusion of the superior mesenteric artery (SMA) proximal to the middle colic branch requires reconstruction.[84,150] Autogenous grafting of the saphenous vein may be necessary either as an interposition or in the form of a bypass from the

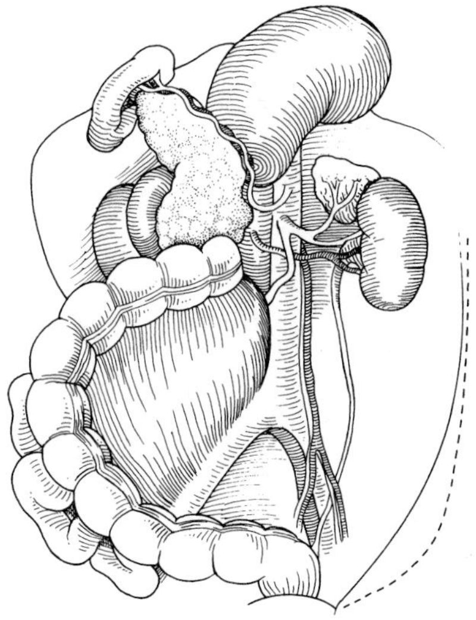

FIGURE 15-22 Left medial visceral rotation exposes the left-sided retroperitoneal structures, including the left kidney, aorta, and major visceral vessels.

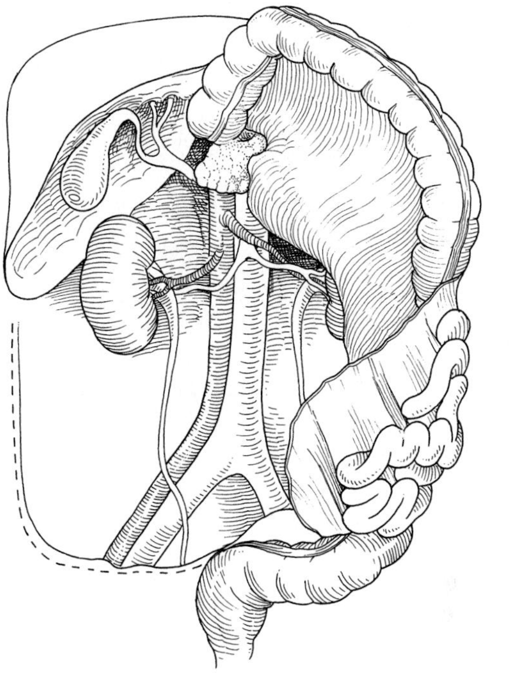

FIGURE 15-23 Right medial visceral rotation exposes the right kidney, infrahepatic vena cava, and distal aorta.

aorta to the SMA; a second-look procedure is recommended for most cases.

Inferior Vena Cava Wounds

Vena caval injuries should be repaired primarily, even if luminal diameter is compromised, although a vein patch may be necessary for extensive injuries.[183,185] The fear that pulmonary emboli will develop after repair has not been confirmed.[249] For massive tissue loss, the infrarenal cava can be ligated with little hemodynamic change; careful postoperative treatment minimizes long-term sequelae. However, abrupt occlusion of the suprarenal cava may have serious consequences, including renal impairment from venous hypertension. Reconstruction can be accomplished by panel saphenous vein interposition or synthetic grafting.[257]

Portal Vein Injuries

Portal vein bleeding can be temporarily controlled by digital pressure, but definitive repair at the confluence of the superior mesenteric and splenic veins may require division of the pancreas (Figure 15-24). With severe injuries, portal vein ligation is a reasonable alternative and is tolerated in more than 80% of patients.[24,228,236] A second-look procedure should be done 24 hours later and portosystemic shunting performed if bowel viability is jeopardized.

Iliac Artery and Vein Injuries

Iliac arterial and venous injury caused by penetrating wounds or blunt injury, including pelvic fractures, is serious because of the lack of tamponade in the pelvis and extensive interconnecting collaterals.[186] The common and external iliac arteries should be repaired; the proximal hypogastric artery may be transposed to the external iliac for reconstruction. Although venorrhaphy is preferred, iliac veins are generally ligated if major injury has caused a loss of substance.[249,250] Temporary packing may be needed for presacral and deep pelvic venous bleeding. Occasionally bilateral internal iliac arteriography may be used to localize a major point of bleeding, which can then be controlled by surgical ligation or embolization through the catheter.

Urologic Trauma

Renal Trauma

Surgical management of renal parenchymal trauma is limited. Minor injuries (contusions and shallow parenchymal fractures without contrast extravasation) represent 70% of blunt renal injuries and require no surgical intervention. Intermediate injuries (parenchymal laceration through the corticomedullary junction with contrast extravasation) account for 20% of blunt trauma. Although somewhat controversial, kidney salvage appears greatest with initial nonsurgical care of these lesions.[234,256] Major injuries (shattered kidneys, renal artery occlusion) require prompt exploration. Similar classification and management decisions pertain to penetrating wounds. Although penetrating renal injuries

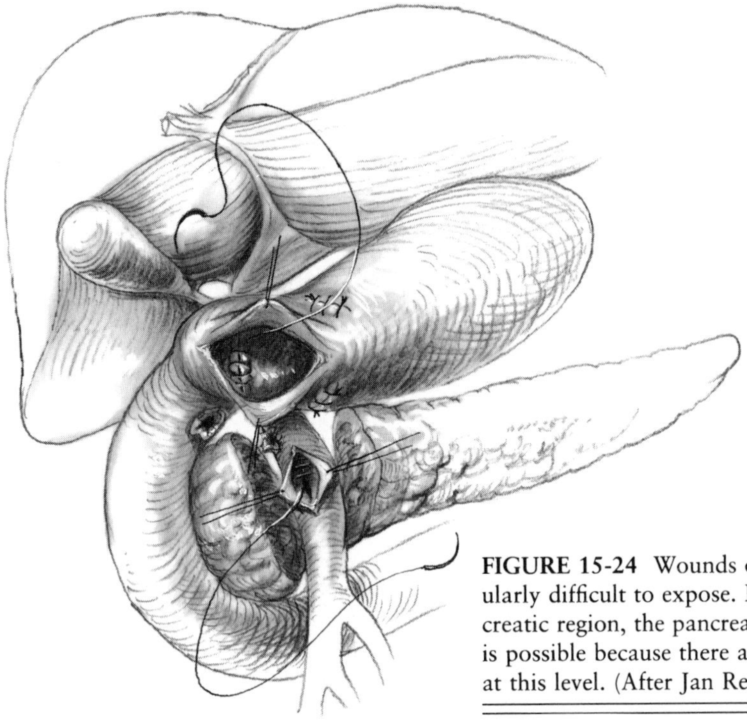

FIGURE 15-24 Wounds of the main portal vein are particularly difficult to expose. For such injuries in the retropancreatic region, the pancreas should be divided sharply; this is possible because there are no anterior venous tributaries at this level. (After Jan Reddin.)

are usually more severe than those with blunt trauma, nearly 60% can be treated without surgery.[316] Contrast extravasation, if confined within Gerota's (renal) fascia, does not warrant immediate surgery (see Chapter 38).

Renovascular Trauma

Renovascular trauma is uncommon, and kidney salvage is poor following complete occlusion of the renal artery.[8,302] On the other hand, revascularization has been successful 12 to 19 hours after injury, supporting an aggressive attempt despite late recognition.[172,302] Renal artery thrombectomy alone often results in early thrombosis. The damaged vessel should be resected and a reanastomosis performed or an aortic-renal bypass graft inserted (see Chapter 42). The right renal vein should be reconstructed, whereas the left vein usually can be ligated if this is done medial to the entrance of the gonadal vein.[173,235]

Ureteral Disruption

Ureteral disruption usually occurs with penetrating wounds but occasionally may result from blunt avulsion.[26,240] Suspected ureteral injury may be evaluated during surgery with a 5 ml intravenous injection of indigo carmine or methylene blue, with the physician observing the area for leakage of bluish urine. Ureteral contusion may also be caused by gunshot wounds. Despite an innocuous appearance, contusions pose a small risk of subsequent necrosis and formation of a urinary fistula.[28] Ureteral repair is accomplished by various techniques, depending on the level of injury (i.e., upper, middle, or lower third)[240] (see Chapter 38).

Bladder Perforations

Bladder perforations may be either intraperitoneal or extraperitoneal.[254] The less common intraperitoneal rupture usually occurs at the dome, where the bladder is weakest. These injuries usually are explored transperitoneally, repaired in two layers, and drained by a suprapubic cystostomy (see Chapter 38). Most extraperitoneal bladder injuries are due to pelvic fracture,[311] and the smaller lesions are treated by urethral drainage alone.[254]

Urethral Tears

Although definitive management is a low priority, these injuries frequently are debilitating because they produce secondary impotence, incontinence, and stricture formation.[205] Posterior urethral injury usually is associated with pelvic fracture, whereas anterior tears most often are caused by straddle injury falls. Suprapubic cystostomy is performed initially for all major urethral injuries. Primary reconstruction is advocated for anterior tears, but delayed repair is generally preferred for posterior lesions.[171] The secondary urethroplasty, if needed, is done after 3 to 6 months (see Chapter 38).

Gynecologic Trauma

Injury to the normal female reproductive organs is rare and usually is caused by penetrating wounds. Most injuries to the uterus and adnexa can be treated with simple suture repair. Hysterectomy is occasionally necessary for lower segment injuries complicated by major hemorrhage.

Unfortunately, trauma during pregnancy is not rare.[60,215] The mother must take priority over the fetus in surgical decision making, and the best insurance for saving the fetus is maternal survival. If the mother is hemodynamically stable, preoperative real-time sonography is valuable for identifying placental separation and for determining the physiologic status of the fetus. Hysterectomy is usually unnecessary but is justified for uncontrolled uterine hemorrhage or if the gravid uterus interferes with surgical treatment of associated injuries. The decision-making process for emergency cesarean delivery is discussed in Chapter 39.

Peripheral Vascular Injuries

Minimizing the time lag from vascular injury to definitive repair is a primary goal in the surgical treatment of an ischemic limb. Protracted shock, increased compartment pressure, disrupted collateral vessels, and venous occlusion may shorten the usual warm ischemic tolerance of 6 hours. The formation of thrombi in the distal arterial tree over time may further compromise revascularization efforts.

Planning the Surgical Approach

Important decisions in planning the surgical approach include (1) the need for preoperative angiography;[64] (2) the timing of bony stabilization in the event of long-bone fracture; (3) the position of the patient on the operating table and the selection of an incision that ensures adequate proximal and distal vascular control; and (4) the need for fasciotomy. In general, preoperative angiography is appropriate in a threatened limb only if the site of injury is in question, as with multiple gunshot wounds or crush injury.[82,186] Bony stabilization is usually done before revascularization. Although external skeletal fixation is preferred, open internal plating may be necessary (see Chapter 42). If limb ischemia has been prolonged and a time-consuming stabilization procedure is expected, the arterial injury should be explored first and a temporary shunt inserted before bone fixation.

Fasciotomy for compartment hypertension is required much more often in the leg than in the arm. In the lower leg, all four compartments (anterior, lateral, superficial posterior, and deep posterior) should be widely decompressed (Figure 15-25). Indications for immediate lower leg, four-compartment fasciotomy (Figure 15-26) include: (1) ischemic limb, with a delay of more than 6 hours between injury and definitive repair; (2) crush injuries; (3) combined arterial and venous injuries at the popliteal level; and (4) compartment hypertension documented by direct measurement (see Chapter 42).

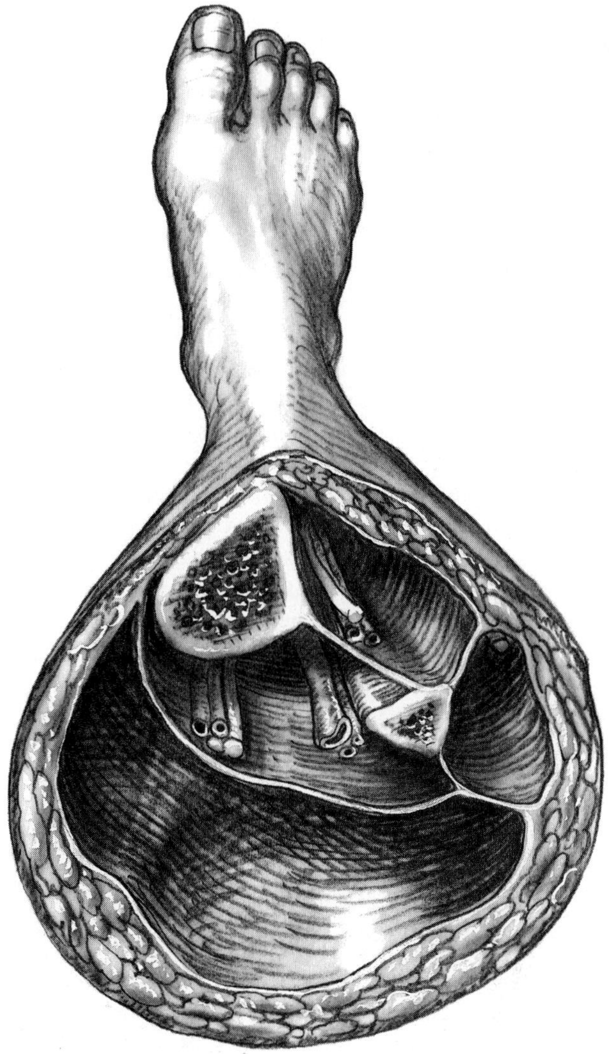

FIGURE 15-25 The four compartments of the lower leg are the anterior compartment, the lateral compartment, the deep compartment, and the superficial posterior compartment. Usually all four require decompression for compartment syndrome following peripheral vascular injury. (After Strawn.)

OR preparation of a patient with peripheral vascular injury follows the general guidelines outlined for torso trauma; resuscitation must be prompt and complete, and appropriate monitoring should be established. The entire extremity should be prepared, including the hand or foot, to allow assessment of distal perfusion during surgery. A variety of vascular clamps and embolectomy catheters should be immediately available. Systemic heparinization is generally not advised; rather, a diluted heparin solution is infused into the distal arterial tree to achieve regional anticoagulation.

The surgical incision for exploration of vascular

trauma is made via conventional approaches used for elective vascular procedures and in most cases parallels the course of the vessel (see Chapter 42). The incision may require some modification if additional surgical access is required for bony fixation.

Control of the proximal artery is the first maneuver; vascular tapes are preferred to prevent clamp injury to a normal vessel. The intact distal artery should then be isolated and controlled before the traumatic hematoma is unroofed. If free bleeding ensues despite occlusion of the proximal and distal arteries, digital pressure should be applied to tamponade the bleeding until the source can be identified. Such bleeding is usually caused by associated venous disruption or arises from arterial branches between the tapes. Blind clamping is avoided because of the risk of nerve damage and further vascular injury. Once hemostasis has been achieved, an appropriate-size Fogarty catheter is inserted into the distal tree for retrieving clots and infusing heparin solution. The same process is then performed in the proximal segment. The latter maneuver may reopen important collateral channels that will function during the vascular repair.

Arterial repair is accomplished with standard vascular technique (see Chapter 42). Contusions must be explored and the underlying intima debrided back to a clean surface. Lateral arteriorrhaphy or venous patching is preferred, but their feasibility depends on the mechanism of injury and the location of the arterial wound. In addition, if the adequacy of the lumen is in question, the vessel should be transected and an end-to-end anastomosis completed. When the vessel is freely mobile, it can be rotated for suturing (Figure 15-27). Arteries less than 6 mm in diameter should be spatulated and at least their corner sutures placed in an interrupted fashion (Figure 15-28). Interposition grafting should be used for segmental loss, eliminating tension on the suture line. Although most authorities recommend autogenous vein for contaminated wounds, polytetrafluoroethylene (PTFE) is probably an acceptable substitute in vessels larger than 4 mm in diameter.[70] Associated venous injury is repaired when practical, although the cost/benefit ratio of lengthy reconstruction is debatable.[210] The surgical management of traumatic arteriovenous fistulae,[138] particularly with delayed presentation, involves several unique features, which are reviewed in Chapter 42.

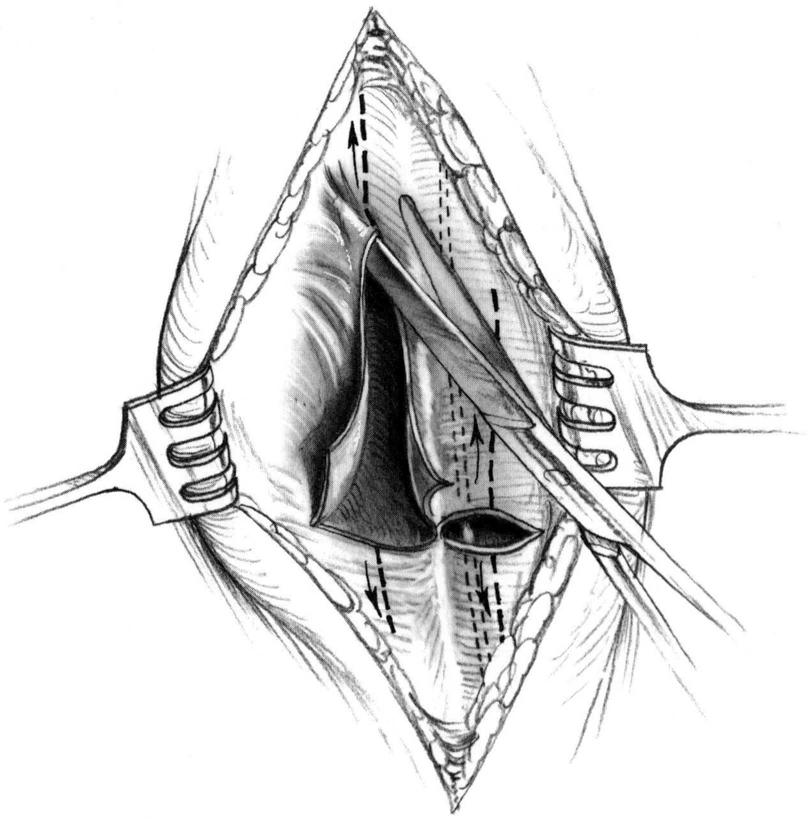

FIGURE 15-26 Compartment syndrome of the lower leg can be managed by wide release of all four compartments. These wounds are generally left open until the swelling has resolved.

Upper Extremity Vascular Trauma

AXILLARY ARTERY TRAUMA. Because of their proximity, the axillary vein or brachial plexus is involved in approximately one half of patients with axillary arterial trauma. Surgical exposure is achieved with a transverse infraclavicular incision, curved across the axilla and extended parallel to the proximal brachial artery in the medial upper arm.[100] For proximal injuries, fibers of the pectoralis major muscle are separated bluntly and the pectoralis minor muscle is retracted laterally. The pectoralis major tendon may be divided if quick, wide exposure is required. The pectoralis minor muscle may also need to be divided for access to the middle segment of the axillary artery. The axillary artery should not be mobilized extensively because of the numerous sizable collateral branches. Consequently, roughly half of these injuries require interposition grafting.

BRACHIAL ARTERY TRAUMA. Ischemia caused by brachial artery trauma depends on the level of occlusion and, particularly, the status of the profundus branch. The median nerve is adjacent to the brachial artery throughout its course in the upper arm and is involved with the injury in one third of patients.[17,92] The surgical

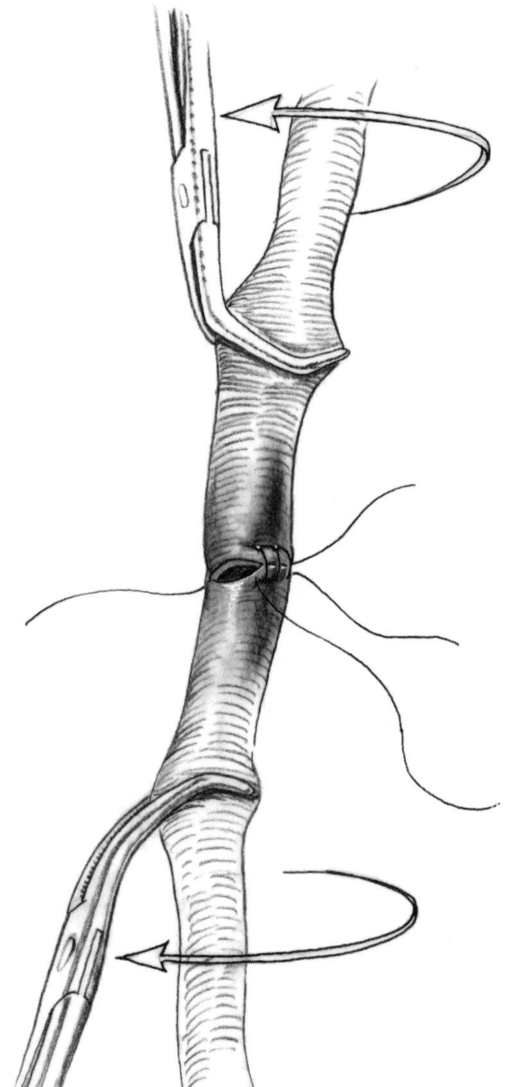

FIGURE 15-27 Arteriorrhaphy can be accomplished in a mobile artery by rotating the vessel 180 degrees to expose the posterior defect. (After Giddings.)

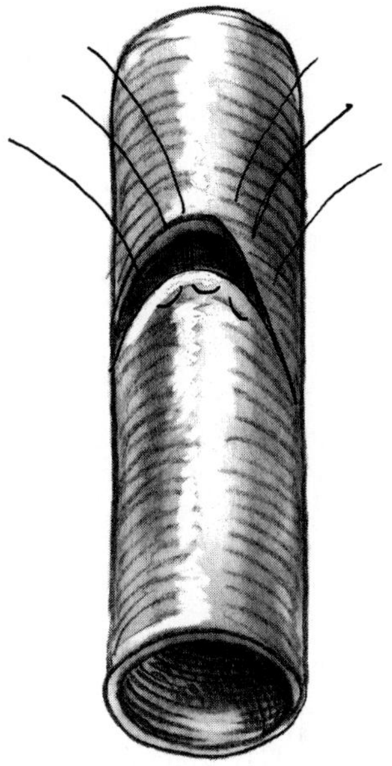

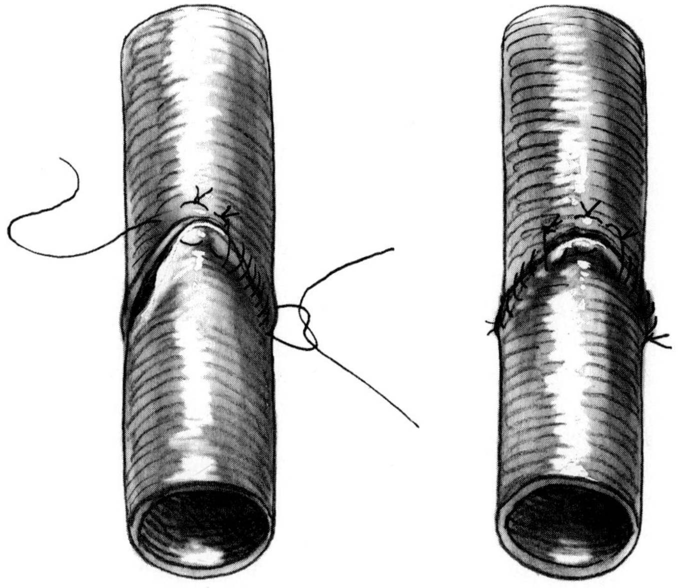

FIGURE 15-28 A number of techniques can be used to achieve optimum results when repairing small vessels. In this technique, the anastomosis is secured with mattress sutures, and the repair is completed with running sutures. (After Fritzler.)

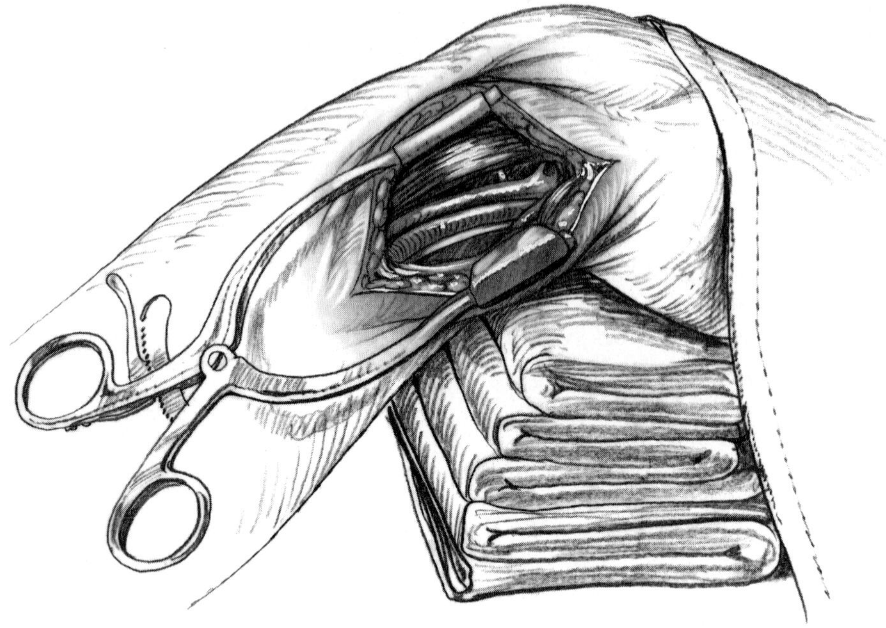

FIGURE 15-29 Exposure of the popliteal vessels is typically achieved through a medial leg incision extending between the sartorius and vastus lateralis muscles. The deep fascia is incised, exposing the neurovascular structures. (After Fritzler.)

incision parallels the brachial artery in the medial upper arm and is extended transversely across the antecubital fossa for distal exposure. Brachial artery trauma is usually not amenable to lateral arteriorrhaphy, but the vessel can be mobilized in most cases to achieve end-to-end anastomosis.

RADIAL AND ULNAR ARTERY TRAUMA. The Allen test is helpful in evaluating injuries to the radial and ulnar arteries. Success with these injuries is limited primarily by concomitant nerve trauma, which accompanies these injuries in nearly two thirds of patients. The ulnar artery is the larger of the two and is usually the origin of the common interosseous artery. The surgical incision parallels the artery on its respective sides of the forearm's volar aspect. Repair should be done by interrupted suture technique with simple magnification assistance. Although ligation of an isolated radial or ulnar injury is tempting with apparently adequate collateral flow, it is not always safe. The deep palmar arch is absent in 10% of the normal population; in 80%, the principal artery of the thumb is the first major branch of the deep radial arch.[92,228] Thus thumb ischemia is a risk with radial artery ligation. On the other hand, a radial or ulnar repair may not remain patent if its counterpart is intact with ample collateral circulation.[228]

Lower Extremity Vascular Trauma

FEMORAL ARTERY TRAUMA. The common femoral artery and bifurcation into the superficial and profunda arteries are approached via a longitudinal incision in the upper thigh. A proximal extension across the inguinal ligament may be necessary for high lesions. The distal profunda femoris artery can be approached through a lateral incision. The superficial femoral artery is exposed by the standard medial thigh incision along the anterior border of the sartorius muscle. Arterial reconstruction requires an interposition graft in approximately one half of patients, and we prefer an autogenous vein harvested from the contralateral limb. The proximal profunda femoris artery should be repaired, whereas more distal lesions may be ligated without concern.

POPLITEAL ARTERY TRAUMA. Politeal artery disruption is perhaps the most challenging peripheral vascular injury. Despite prompt recognition, amputation rates for blunt trauma continue to approach 20%. Performing angiography in the OR through the femoral artery can minimize preoperative delay. Four-compartment fasciotomy (see Figure 15-26) should be done immediately if there is any question of compartmental hypertension. Although its use is controversial, we recommend systemic heparinization unless associated injuries preclude it. External bony fixation is preferred before vascular repair, but a temporary arterial shunt may be indicated when ischemia has been prolonged. Vascular access may be obtained through a posterior or medial approach, although the latter is preferred (Figure 15-29). After vascular control has been established, catheter thrombectomy is performed on the proximal and distal segments. Distal removal of emboli should be done as thoroughly as possible in the trifurcation vessels. The contused popliteal artery must be debrided adequately. Saphenous vein interposition is required in most full-thickness injuries; completion arteriography is essential to detect technical errors, other distal lesions, and residual emboli. Finally, concomitant venous injury should be repaired. Perhaps no other region shows such compelling reason to reconstruct associated venous trauma.

INFRAPOPLITEAL TRIFURCATION VESSEL TRAUMA. Injuries to the infrapopliteal trifurcation vessels are usually caused by severe blunt trauma, and the magnitude of soft tissue and associated bone or nerve damage generally determines their outcome.[130] Surgical treatment of bone and soft tissue is reviewed in Chapters 19 and 20; surgery for nerve injury is discussed in Chapter 26.

Preoperative angiography is mandatory for infrapopliteal artery trauma because of the region's complex anatomy. Normally the anterior tibial artery bifurcates from the popliteal trunk first, and the peroneal artery then divides from the posterior tibial artery. Although it has not been established conclusively, it appears that a patent anterior or posterior tibial artery is sufficient to maintain a viable foot. Under these circumstances, fasciotomy may be the only procedure necessary. Exploration is generally not done for primary neurorrhaphy in a threatened limb.[137] When arterial reconstruction is deemed essential, the standard vascular incisions are used (see Chapter 42). For proximal injuries, the medial knee incision (see Figure 15-29) provides optimum access to the trifurcation region for proximal vascular control and catheter embolectomy. The more distal tibial arteries are explored directly over their anatomic course. As with small vessels in the forearm, simple magnification should be used during the vascular repair. The role of postoperative anticoagulation is controversial, but it often is used for a threatened lower leg.

REFERENCES

1 Alyono D, Perry JF: Value of quantitative cell count and amylase activity of peritoneal lavage fluid, *J Trauma* 21:345, 1981.

2 Ammons MA, Moore EE, Moore FA, Hopeman AR: Intra-aortic ballon pump for combined myocardial contusion and thoracic aortic rupture, *J Trauma* 30:1606, 1990.

3 Anson J, Crowell RM: Review article: cervicocranial arterial dissection, *Neurosurgery* 29:89,1991.

4 Applebaum A, Karp RB, Kirklin JW: Surgical treatment for closed thoracic aortic injuries, *J Thorac Cardiovasc Surg* 71:458, 1976.

5 Aprahamian C, Thompson BM, Finger WA et al: Experimental cervical spine injury model: evaluation of airway management and splinting techniques, *Ann Emerg Med* 13:584, 1984.

6 Aronoff RJ, Reynolds J, Thal ER: Evaluation of diaphragmatic injuries, *Am J Surg* 144:671, 1982.

7 Baker WH, Littooy FN, Hayes AC et al: Carotid endarterectomy without a shunt: the control series, *J Vasc Surg* 1:50, 1984.

8 Barlow B, Gandhi R: Renal artery thrombosis following blunt trauma, *J Trauma* 20:614, 1980.

9 Barnes A, Allen TE: Transfusions subsequent to administration of universal donor blood in Vietnam, *JAMA* 204:695, 1968.

10 Bascaglia LC, Blaisdell WF, Lim RC: Penetrating abdominal vascular injuries, *Arch Surg* 99:764, 1969.

11 Baxter BT, Moore EE, Cleveland HC et al: Emergency departmental thoracotomy following injury: critical determinants for survival, *World J Surg* 12:671, 1988.

12 Baxter BT, Moore EE, McCroskey BL, Moore FA: Chest tube irrigation for postinjury hypothermia, *Ann Emerg Med* 17:196, 1988.

13 Berne CJ, Donovan AJ, White EF et al: Duodenal diverticulization for duodenal and pancreatic injury, *Ann J Surg* 127:503, 1974.

14 Berni GA, Bandyk DF, Oreskovich MR et al: Role of intraoperative pancreatography in patients with injury to the pancreas, *Am J Surg* 143:602, 1982.

15 Blair E, Cemalettin T, Davis JH: Delayed or missed diagnosis in blunt chest trauma, *J Trauma* 11:129, 1971.

16 Borlase B, Metcalf RK, Moore EE: Indications for emergent operation following penetrating thoracic wounds, *Am J Surg* 1986.

17 Borman KR, Aurbakken CM, Weigelt JA: Treatment priorities of combined blunt abdominal and aortic trauma, *Am J Surg* 144:728, 1982.

18 Breaux EP, Dupont JB, Albert HM et al: Cardiac tamponade following penetrating mediastinal injuries: improved survival with early pericardiocentesis, *J Trauma* 19:461, 1979.

19 Brown MF, Graham JM, Feliciano DV et al: Carotid artery injuries, *Am J Surg* 144:748, 1982.

20 Bucholz RW, Burkhead WZ, Graham W et al: Occult cervical spine injuries in fatal traffic accidents, *J Trauma* 19:768, 1979.

21 Buchsbaum HJ: Accidental injury complicating pregnancy, *Am J Obstet Gynecol* 102:752, 1968.

22 Burch JM, Feliciano DV, Mattox KL: Colostomy and drainage for civilian rectal injuries: is that all? *Ann Surg* 209:600, 1988.

23 Burke JF: The effective period of preventive antibiotics in penetrating wounds of the abdomen, *Surgery* 50:161, 1961.

24 Busuttil RW, Kitahama A, Cerise E et al: Management of blunt and penetrating injuries to the porta hepatis, *Ann Surg* 191:641, 1980.

25 Campos Christo M: Segmental resections of the spleen, *O Hospital* (Rio) 62:187, 1961.

26 Carlton CE, Scott RJ, Guthrie AG: The initial management of ureteral injuries, *J Urol* 105:335, 1971.

27 Carrico CJ, Canizaro PC, Shires GT: Fluid resuscitation following injury: rationale for use of balanced salt solution, *Crit Care Med* 4:46, 1976.

28 Cass AS: Ureteral contusion with gunshot wounds, *J Trauma* 24:59, 1984.

29 Cervera AL, Moss G: Progressive hypovolemia leading to shock after continuous hemorrhage and 3:1 crystalloid replacement, *Am J Surg* 129:670, 1975.

30 Cimochowski GE, Barcia PJ, DeMeester TR et al: Multiple transections of the thoracic aorta secondary to blunt trauma, *Ann Thorac Surg* 15:536, 1973.

31 Clark DE, Wiles CS, Lim MK et al: Traumatic rupture of the pericardium, *Surgery* 93:495, 1983.

32 Clowes GHA, Sabga GH, Konitaxis A et al: Effects of acidosis on cardiovascular function in surgical patients, *Ann Surg* 154:524, 1961.

33 Cogbill TH, Moore EE, Kashuk JL: Changing trends in the management of pancreatic trauma, *Arch Surg* 177:722, 1982.

34 Cogbill TH, Moore EE, Millikan JS et al: Rationale for selective application of emergency department thoracotomy in trauma, *J Trauma* 123:453, 1983.

35 Cogbill TH, Moore EE, Morris JA Jr et al: Distal pancreatectomy for trauma: a multicenter experience, *J Trauma* 31:1600, 1991.

36 Collins JA: Problems associated with the massive transfusion of stored blood, *Surgery* 75:274, 1974.

37 Coln D, Crighton J, Schorn L: Successful management of hepatic vein injury from blunt trauma in children, *Am J Surg* 140:858, 1980.

38 Committee on Trauma, American College of Surgeons: *Advanced trauma life support program,* Chicago, 1992, ACS.
39 Committee on Trauma, American College of Surgeons: Hospital and prehospital resources for optimal care of the injured patient, *Bull Am Coll Surg* 68:11, 1983.
40 Copass MK, Oreskovich MR, Baldergroen MR et al: Prehospital cardiopulmonary resuscitation of the critically injured patient, *Am J Surg* 148:20, 1984.
41 Coran AG, Ballantine TV, Horwitz DL et al: The effect of crystalloid resuscitation in hemorrhagic shock on acid-base balance: a comparison between normal saline and Ringer's lactate solution, *Surgery* 69:874, 1971.
42 Danzl DF, Thomas DM: Nasotracheal intubations in the emergency department, *Crit Care Med* 8:677, 1980.
43 Davis D, Bohlman H, Walker E et al: The pathological findings in fatal craniospinal injuries, *J Neurosurg* 34:603, 1971.
44 Davis JJ, Cohn I, Nance FC: Diagnosis and management of blunt abdominal trauma, *Ann Surg* 183:672, 1976.
45 DeBard ML: Cardiopulmonary resuscitation: analysis of six years' experience and review of the literature, *Ann Emerg Med* 10:408, 1981.
46 DeGroot M, Prewitt RM: Right ventricular contusion: experimental pathophysiology and treatment in an open-chest canine preparation, *J Trauma* 24:721, 1984.
47 Denis R, Allad M, Atlas H et al: Changing trends with abdominal injury in seat belt wearers, *J Trauma* 23:1007, 1983.
48 Deslauriers J, Beaulieu M, Archambault G et al: Diagnosis and long-term follow-up of major bronchial disruptions due to nonpenetrating trauma, *Ann Thorac Surg* 33:32, 1982.
49 Douglas ME, Downs JB, Mantini EL et al: Alternation of oxygen tension and oxyhemoglobin saturation: a hazard of sodium bicarbonate administration, *Arch Surg* 114:326, 1979.
50 Ducker TB, Russo GL, Bellegarrique R et al: Complete sensorimotor paralysis after cord injury: mortality, recovery, and therapeutic implications, *J Trauma* 19:837, 1979.
51 Dunn EL, Moore EE, Breslich DJ et al: Acidosis-induced coagulopathy, *Surg Forum* 30:471, 1979.
52 Dunn EL, Moore EE, Moore JB: Hemodynamic effects of aortic occlusion during hemorrhagic shock, *Ann Emerg Med* 12:238, 1982.
53 Dutschi MB, Haisch CE, Reynolds L et al: Effect of micropore filtration on pulmonary function after massive transfusion, *Am J Surg* 138:8, 1979.
54 Earnest MP, Breckenridge JC, Yarnell PR et al: Quality of survival after out-of-hospital cardiac arrest: predictive value of early neurologic evaluation, *Neurology* 29:56, 1984.
55 Ehrenfeld WK, Stoney RJ, Wylie EJ: Relation of carotid stump pressure to safety of carotid artery ligation, *Surgery* 93:229, 1983.
56 Eisenberg M, Hallstrom A, Bergner L: Cardiac resuscitation in the community: importance of rapid provision and implications for program planning, *JAMA* 241:1905, 1979.
57 Elerding SC, Aragon GE, Moore EE: Fatal hepatic hemorrhage after trauma, *Am J Surg* 138:883, 1979.
58 Erstad BL, Gales BJ, Rappaport WD: The use of albumin in clinical practice, *Arch Intern Med* 151:901, 1991.
59 Espada R, Whisennand HH, Mattox KL et al: Surgical management of penetrating injuries to the coronary arteries, *Surgery* 78:755, 1975.
60 Esposito TJ, Gens DR, Smith LG et al: Trauma during pregnancy: a review of 79 cases, *Arch Surg* 126:1073, 1991.
61 Esposito TJ, Jurkovich GJ, Rice CL et al: Reappraisal of emergency room thoracotomy in a changing environment, *J Trauma* 31:881, 1991.
62 Evans J, Gray LA, Rayner A et al: Principles for the management of penetrating cardiac wounds, *Ann Surg* 189:777, 1979.
63 Fabian TC, Mangiante EC, White TJ et al: A prospective study of 91 patients undergoing both computed tomography and peritoneal lavage following blunt abdominal trauma, *J Trauma* 26:602, 1986.
64 Fabian TC, Reiter CB, Gold RE et al: Digital venous angiography: a prospective evaluation in peripheral arterial trauma, *Ann Surg* 199:710, 1984.
65 Fallahnejad M, Kutty ACK, Wallace HW: Secondary lesions of penetrating cardiac injuries: a frequent complication, *Ann Surg* 191:228, 1980.
66 Federico JA, Horner WR, Clark DE, Isler RJ: Blunt hepatic trauma: nonoperative management in adults, *Arch Surg* 125:905, 1990.
67 Federle MP, Crass RA, Jeffrey B et al: Computed tomography in blunt abdominal trauma, *Arch Surg* 117:645, 1982.
68 Feliciano DV, Mattox KL, Jordan GL: Intra-abdominal packing for control of hemorrhage: a reappraisal, *J Trauma* 21:285, 1981.
69 Feliciano DV, Bitondo CG, Steed G et al: 500 open taps on lavages in patients with abdominal stab wounds, *Am J Surg* 148:772, 1985.
70 Feliciano DB, Mattox KL, Graham JM et al: Five-year experience with PTFE grafts in vascular wounds, *J Trauma* 25:71, 1985.
71 Fisher RP, O'Farrell KA, Perry JK: The value of peritoneal drains in the treatment of liver injuries, *J Trauma* 18:393, 1978.
72 Fisher RP, Berverlin BC, Engrav LH et al: Diagnostic peritoneal lavage: fourteen years and 2,586 patients later, *Am J Surg* 136:701, 1978.
73 Flax RL, Fletcher HS, Joseph WL: Management of penetrating injuries of the neck, *Am Surg* 39:148, 1973.
74 Flint LM, Brown A, Richardson JD et al: Definitive control of bleeding from severe pelvic fractures, *Ann Surg* 189:709, 1979.
75 Flint LM, McCoy M, Richardson JD et al: Duodenal injury: analysis of common misconceptions in diagnosis and treatment, *Ann Surg* 191:697, 1980.
76 Foley RW, Harris LS, Pilcher DB: Abdominal injuries in automobile accidents: review of care of fatally injured patients, *J Trauma* 17:611, 1977.
77 Fox S, Pierce WS, Waldhausen JA: Acute hypertension: its significance in traumatic aortic rupture, *J Thorac Cardiovasc Surg* 77:622, 1970.
78 Frank MJ, Nadimi M, Lesniak JL et al: Effects of cardiac tamponade on myocardial performance, blood flow and metabolism, *Am J Physiol* 220:179, 1971.
79 Frenstad JD, Martin SH: Lethal complication from insertion of nasogastric tube after severe baseline skull fracture, *J Trauma* 22:190, 1982.
80 Fry DE, Ratciffe DJ, Yates JR: The effects of acidosis on canine hepatic and renal oxidative phosphorylation, *Surgery* 88:296, 1980.
81 Fry DE, Fry WJ: Extracranial carotid artery injuries, *Surgery* 88:581, 1980.
82 Frykberg ER, Crump JM, Vines FS et al: A reassessment of the role of arteriography in penetrating proximity-extremity trauma: a prospective study, *J Trauma* 29:1041, 1989.
83 Fuhrman GM, Stieg FH, Buerk CA: Blunt laryngeal trauma: classification and management protocol, *J Trauma* 30:87, 1990.
84 Fullen WD, Hunt J, Altemeier WA: The clinical spectrum of penetrating injury to the superior mesenteric arterial circulation, *J Trauma* 12:656, 1972.
85 Fullen WD, Hunt J, Altemeier WA: Prophylactic antibiotics in penetrating wounds of the abdomen, *J Trauma* 12:282, 1972.
86 Fullen WD, Selle JG, Whitely DH et al: Intramural duodenal hematoma, *Ann Surg* 179:549, 1974.
87 Furtschegger A, Egender G, Jaske G: The value of sonography in the diagnosis and follow-up of patients with blunt abdominal trauma, *Br J Urol* 62:110, 1988.

88 Gaffney FA, Bastian BC, Thal ER et al: Passive leg raising does not produce a significant or sustained autotransfusion effect, *J Trauma* 22:190, 1982.
89 Gaffney FA, Thal ER, Taylor WF et al: Hemodynamic effects of medical anti-shock trousers (MAST garment), *J Trauma* 21:391, 1981.
90 Galloway WB: Coagulation problems in the trauma patient. In Moore EE, Eiseman B, Van Way CW, editors: *Critical decisions in trauma,* St Louis, 1984, Mosby.
91 Garrison HG, Hansen AR, Cross RE et al: Effects of ethanol on lactic acidosis in experimental hemorrhagic shock, *Ann Emerg Med* 13:26, 1984.
92 Gelberman RH, Nunley JA, Koman LA et al: The results of radial and ulnar arterial repair in the forearm, *J Bone Joint Surg* 64A:383, 1982.
93 Gentilello LM, Cobean RA, Offner PJ et al: Continuous arteriovenous rewarming: rapid reversal of hypothermia in critically ill patients, *J Trauma* 32:316, 1992.
94 Gervin AS, Fischer RP: Resuscitation of trauma patients with type-specific uncross-matched blood, *J Trauma* 24:327, 1984.
95 Getzer LC, Pollak EW: Short-term femoral vein catheterization: a safe alternative access, *Am J Surg* 138:875, 1979.
96 Gewertz BL, Samson DS, Ditmore QM: Management of penetrating injuries of the internal carotid artery at the base of the skull utilizing extracranial-intracranial bypass, *J Trauma* 20:365, 1980.
97 Gilliland MG, Ward RE, Flynn TC et al: Peritoneal lavage and angiography in the management of patients with pelvic fracture, *Am J Surg* 144:744, 1982.
98 Golueke PJ, Goldstein AS, Sclafani SJA et al: Routine versus selective exploration of neck injuries: a randomized, prospective study, *J Trauma* 12:1010, 1984.
99 Gould SA, Rosen AL, Sehgal LR et al: Red cell substitutes: hemoglobin solution or fluorocarbon? *J Trauma* 22:736, 1982.
100 Graham JM, Feliciano DV, Mattox KL et al: Management of subclavian vascular injuries, *J Trauma* 20:537, 1980.
101 Graham JM, Mattox KL, Beal AC: Penetrating trauma of the lung, *J Trauma* 19:665, 1979.
102 Greendyke RM: Traumatic rupture of the aorta: special reference to automobile accidents, *JAMA* 195:527, 1966.
103 Grover FL, Ellestad C, Avom KV et al: Diagnosis and management of major tracheobronchial injuries, *Ann Thorac Surg* 328:384, 1979.
104 Gruessner R, Mentges B, Duber C et al: Sonography vs peritoneal lavage in blunt abdominal trauma, *J Trauma* 29:242, 1989.
105 Guice K, Oldham K, Eide B et al: Hematuria after blunt trauma: when is pyelography useful? *J Trauma* 23:305, 1983.
106 Gundry SR, Williams S, Burney RE et al: Indications for aortography in blunt thoracic trauma: a reassessment, *J Trauma* 22:664, 1982.
107 Gussack GS, Jurkovich GJ: Treatment dilemmas in laryngotracheal trauma, *J Trauma* 28:1439, 1988.
108 Hardaway RM, Chun B, Rutherford RB: Coagulation in shock in various species, including man, *Acta Chir Scand* 130:157, 1965.
109 Healey JE, Schroy PC: Anatomy of the biliary ducts within the human liver, *Arch Surg* 66:599, 1953.
110 Heitsch RC, Knutson CW, Fulton RL et al: Delineation of critical factors in the treatment of pancreatic trauma, *Surgery* 80:523, 1976.
111 Hoffmann R, Nerlich M, Muggia-Sullam M et al: Blunt abdominal trauma in cases of multiple trauma evaluated by ultrasonography: a prospective analysis of 291 patients, *J Trauma* 32:452, 1992.
112 Horton J, Orden ME, Williams S, Coln D: The importance of splenic blood flow in clearing pneumococcal organisms, *Ann Surg* 195:172, 1982.
113 Howell HS, Bartizal JF, Freeark RJ: Blunt trauma involving the colon and rectum, *J Trauma* 16:624, 1976.
114 Huguet C, Nordlinger B, Block P, Conard J: Tolerance of the human liver to prolonged normothermic ischemia, *Arch Surg* 113:1448, 1978.
115 Hulke DF, Mondelsohn RA, States JD et al: Cervical fractures and fracture-dislocation sustained without head impact, *J Trauma* 18:533, 1978.
116 Ivatury RR, Simon RJ, Weksler B et al: Laparoscopy in the evaluation of the intrathoracic abdomen after penetrating injury, *J Trauma* 33:101, 1992.
117 Jackson RE, Joyce K, Danosi SF et al: Blood flow in the cerebral cortex during cardiac resuscitation in dogs, *Ann Emerg Med* 13:657, 1984.
118 Jacobs LW, Sinclair A, Beiser A et al: Prehospital advanced life support: benefits in trauma, *J Trauma* 24:8, 1984.
119 Jimenez E, Martin M, Krukenkamp I, Barnett J: Subxiphoid pericardotomy versus echocardiography: a prospective evaluation of the diagnosis of occult, penetrating cardiac injury, *Surgery* 108:676, 1992.
120 Johnson RM, Hart DL, Simmons EF et al: Cervical orthoses: a study comparing their effectiveness in restricting cervical motion in normal subjects, *J Bone Joint Surg* 59A:332, 1977.
121 Jones RC: Management of pancreatic trauma, *Ann Surg* 187:555, 1978.
122 Jones WS, Mavroudis C, Richardson JD et al: Management of tracheobronchial disruption resulting from blunt trauma, *Surgery* 95:319, 1983.
123 Jorden RC, Moore EE, Marx JH: A comparison of percutaneous transtracheal ventilation and endotracheal ventilation in an acute trauma model, *J Trauma* 25:978, 1985.
124 Jorden RC, Moore EE, Marx JH et al: Percutaneous transtracheal ventilation in a canine shock model, *Ann Emerg Med* 13:22, 1984.
125 Jurkovich GJ, Greiser WB, Luterman A, Curreri PW: Hypothermia in trauma victims: an ominous predictor of survival, *J Trauma* 27:1019, 1987.
126 Jurkovich GJ, Moore EE, Medina G: Autotransfusion in trauma: a pragmatic analysis, *Am J Surg* 148:782, 1984.
127 Jurkovich GJ, Zingarelli W, Wallace J, Curreri PW: Penetrating neck trauma: diagnostic studies in the asymptomatic patient, *J Trauma* 25:819, 1985.
128 Kashuk JL, Moore EE, Cogbill TH: Management of the intermediate-severity duodenal injury, *Surgery* 92:758, 1982.
129 Kashuk JL, Moore EE, Millikan JS et al: Major abdominal vascular trauma: a unified approach, *J Trauma* 22:672, 1982.
130 Keely SB, Snyder WH, Weigelt JA: Arterial injuries below the knee: 51 patients with 82 injuries, *J Trauma* 23:285, 1983.
131 King MW, Aitchison JM, Nel JP: Fatal air embolism following penetrating lung trauma: an autopsy study, *J Trauma* 24:753, 1984.
132 Kirkpatrick JB, Di Maio V: Civilian gunshot wounds of the brain, *J Neurosurg* 49:185, 1978.
133 Kirsh MM, Orringer MB, Behrendt DM: Management of unusual traumatic ruptures of the aorta, *Surg Gynecol Obstet* 146:365, 1978.
134 Kirsh MM, Behrendt DM, Orringer MB et al: The treatment of acute traumatic rupture of the aorta: a 10-year experience, *Ann Surg* 184:308, 1976.
135 Kirsh MM, Orringer MB, Behrendt DM et al: Management of tracheobronchial disruption secondary to nonpenetrating trauma, *Ann Thorac Surg* 22:93, 1976.
136 Kitahama A, Elliot LF, Overby JL et al: The extrahepatic biliary tract injury: perspectives in diagnosis and treatment, *Ann Surg* 196:536, 1982.
137 Kline DG, Hackett ER: Reappraisal of timing for exploration of civilian peripheral nerve injuries, *Surgery* 78:54, 1975.

138 Kollmeyer KR, Hunt JL, Ellman BA et al: Acute and chronic traumatic arteriovenous fistulae in civilians, *Arch Surg* 116:697, 1981.

139 Krajewski LP, Hertzer NR: Blunt carotid artery trauma: report of two cases and review of the literature, *Ann Surg* 191:341, 1979.

140 Kudsk KA, Sheldon GF, Lim RC: Atrial-caval shunting (ACS) after trauma, *J Trauma* 22:81, 1982.

141 Landolt AM, Millikan CH: Pathogenesis of cerebral infarction secondary to mechanical carotid artery occlusion, *Stroke* 1:52, 1970.

142 Lassonde J, Laurendeau F: Blunt injury of the abdominal aorta, *Ann Surg* 194:745, 1981.

143 LeBlanc KA, Benzel EC: Trauma to the high cervical carotid artery, *J Trauma* 24:992, 1984.

144 Ledgerwood AM, Kazmers M, Lucas CE: The role of thoracic aortic occlusion for massive hemoperitoneum, *J Trauma* 16:610, 1976.

145 Ledgerwood AM, Mullins RJ, Lucas CE: Primary repair versus ligation for carotid artery injuries, *Arch Surg* 115:488, 1980.

146 Liedtke AJ, Allen RP, Nellis SH: Effects of blunt cardiac trauma on coronary vasomotion, perfusion, myocardial mechanics, and metabolism, *J Trauma* 20:777, 1980.

147 Liekweg WG, Greenfield LJ: Management of penetrating carotid arterial injury, *Ann Surg* 188:587, 1978.

148 Livingston DH, Tortella BJ, Machiedo GW, Rush BJ: The role of laparoscopy in abdominal trauma, *J Trauma* 33:471, 1992.

149 Lowe RJ, Saletta JD, Moss GS: Pancreaticoduodenectomy for penetrating pancreatic trauma, *J Trauma* 17:731, 1977.

150 Lucas CE, Richardson JD, Flint LM et al: Traumatic injury of the proximal superior mesenteric artery, *Ann Surg* 193:30, 1981.

151 Lucas CE, Ledgerwood AM: Factors influencing outcome after blunt duodenal injury, *J Trauma* 15:839, 1975.

152 Lucas CE, Ledgerwood AM: Prospective evaluation of hemostatic techniques for liver injuries, *J Trauma* 16:422, 1976.

153 Lucas CE, Ledgerwood AM, Higgins RF: Impaired salt and water excretion after albumin resuscitation for hypovolemic shock, *Surgery* 86:541, 1979.

154 Lucas CE, Ledgerwood AM, Higgins RF et al: Impaired pulmonary function after albumin resuscitation from shock, *J Trauma* 20:446, 1980.

155 Lucas CE, Walt AJ, Analysis of randomized biliary drainage for liver trauma in 189 patients, *J Trauma* 12:925, 1972.

156 Majernick TG, Bienick R, Houston JB, Hughes HG: Cervical spine movement during orotracheal intubation, *Ann Emerg Med* 15:417, 1986.

157 Mansour MA, Moore EE, Moore FA, Read RA: Exigent postinjury thoracotomy: analysis of blunt versus penetrating trauma, *Surg Gynecol Obstet* 175:97, 1992.

158 Mansour MA, Moore EE, Moore FA, Whitehill TA: Conservative management of penetrating neck wounds: a 12-year prospective analysis, *Am J Surg* 162:517, 1991.

159 Martin RR, Bickell WH, Pepe PE et al: Prospective evaluation of preoperative fluid resuscitation in hypotensive patients with penetrating truncal injury: a preliminary report, *J Trauma* 33:1, 1991.

160 Martin TD, Flynn TC, Rowlands BJ et al: Blunt cardiac rupture, *J Trauma* 24:287, 1984.

161 Marx JA, Bar-Or D, Moore EE et al: Lavage alkaline phosphatase in the detection of small bowel injury, *Ann Emerg Med* 12:68, 1983.

162 Marx JA, Moore EE, Bar-Or D: Peritoneal lavage in small bowel and colon injuries: the value of enzyme determination, *Ann Emerg Med* 12:68, 1983.

163 Marx JA, Moore EE, Jorden RC et al: Limitations of CT scanning in the evaluation of acute abdominal trauma: a prospective comparison with peritoneal lavage, *J Trauma* 25:933, 1985.

164 Mattox KL, Allen MK, Feliciano DV: Laparotomy in the emergency department, *JACEP* 8:180, 1979.

165 Mattox KL, Beall AC, Ennix CL et al: Intravascular migratory bullets, *Am J Surg* 137:192, 1978.

166 Mattox KL, Feliciano DV: Role of external cardiac compression in truncal trauma, *J Trauma* 22:934, 1982.

167 Mattox KL, Walker LD, Beall AC et al: Blood availability for the trauma patient: autotransfusion, *J Trauma* 15:663, 1975.

168 Mayor-Davis JA, Brite RS: Subxiphoid pericardial window: helpful in selected cases, *J Trauma* 30:1399, 1990.

169 Mays ET: Lobar dearterialization for exsanguinating wounds of the liver, *J Trauma* 12:397, 1972.

170 McAlvanah MJ, Shaftan GW: Selective conservation in penetrating abdominal wounds: a continuing reappraisal, *J Trauma* 18:206, 1978.

171 McAninch JW: Traumatic injuries to the urethra, *J Trauma* 21:291, 1981.

172 McAninch JW, Carroll PR: Renal trauma—kidney preservation through improved vascular control: a refined approach, *J Trauma* 22:285, 1982.

173 McCombs PR, De Laurentis DH: Division of the left renal vein: guidelines and consequences, *Am J Surg* 138:257, 1979.

174 McGill J, Clinton JE: Cricothyrotomy in the emergency department, *Ann Emerg Med* 11:361, 1982.

175 Meier DE, Brink BE, Fry WJ: Vertebral artery trauma: acute recognition and treatment, *Arch Surg* 116:236, 1981.

176 Merrill WH, Lee RB, Hammon JW et al: Surgical treatment of acute traumatic tear of the thoracic aorta, *Ann Surg* 207:699, 1988.

177 Michael L, Grillo HC, Malt RA: Esophageal perforation, *Ann Thorac Surg* 33:203, 1982.

178 Michels NL: Newer anatomy of liver—variant blood supply and collateral circulation, *JAMA* 172:125, 1960.

179 Miller RD, Robbins TO, Tong MJ et al: Coagulation defects associated with massive blood transfusions, *Ann Surg* 174:794, 1971.

180 Millikan JS, Moore EE: Outcome of resuscitative thoracotomy and descending aortic occlusion performed in the operating room, *J Trauma* 24:387, 1984.

181 Millikan JS, Moore EE: Abdominal aortic trauma: critical factors in determining mortality, *Surg Gynecol Obstet* 160:313, 1985.

182 Millikan JS, Moore EE, Moore GE, Stevens RE: Alternatives to splenectomy in adults after trauma, *Am J Surg* 144:711, 1982.

183 Millikan JS, Moore EE, Cogbill TH et al: Inferior vena cava injuries: a continuing challenge, *J Trauma* 23:207, 1983.

184 Millikan JS, Moore EE, Dunn EIL et al: Temporary cardiac pacing in traumatic arrest victims, *Ann Emerg Med* 9:591, 1980.

185 Millikan JS, Moore EE, Steiner E et al: Complications of tube thoracostomy for acute trauma, *Am J Surg* 140:738, 1980.

186 Millikan JS, Moore EE, Van Way CW et al: Vascular trauma in the groin: contrast between iliac and femoral injuries, *Am J Surg* 142:695, 1981.

187 Moore EE: Critical decision making in management of acute hepatic injury, *Am J Surg* 148:712, 1984.

188 Moore EE: Emergency thoracotomy and descending thoracic aortic cross-clamping. In Moore EE, Eiseman B, Van Way CW, editors: *Critical decisions in trauma,* St Louis, 1984, Mosby.

189 Moore EE, Dunn EL, Jones TN: Immediate jejunostomy feeding: its use after major abdominal trauma, *Arch Surg* 116:681, 1981.

190 Moore EE, Good JT: Mixed venous and arterial pH: a comparison during hemorrhagic shock and hypothermia, *Ann Emerg Med* 11:300, 1982.

191 Moore EE, Jones TN: Nutritional assessment and preliminary report on early support of the trauma patient, *J Am Coll Nutr* 2:45, 1981.

192 Moore EE, Jones TN: Benefits of immediate jejunostomy feeding after major abdominal trauma: a prospective, randomized study, *J Trauma* 26:987, 1986.

193 Moore EE, Dunn EL, Breslich DJ et al: Platelet abnormalities associated with massive autotransfusion, *J Trauma* 20:1052, 1980.
194 Moore EE, Moore JB, Van Duzer-Moore S et al: Mandatory laparotomy for gunshot wounds penetrating the abdomen, *Am J Surg* 140:847, 1980.
195 Moore EE, Moore FA: Immediate enteral nutrition following multisystem trauma: a decade of experience, *J Am Coll Nutr* 10:633, 1991.
196 Moore EE, Moore FA, Pons PT, Markovchick V: Technical note—trauma team activation: the sequential light panel, *J Trauma* 33:904, 1992.
197 Moore FA, Feliciano DV, Andrassy RJ et al: Early enteral feeding compared with parenteral reduces postoperative septic complications: the results of a meta-analysis, *Ann Surg* 216:172, 1992.
198 Moore FA, Moore EE, Mill MR: Preoperative antibiotics for abdominal gunshot wounds: a prospective, randomized study, *Am J Surg* 146:762, 1983.
199 Moore FA, Moore EE, Moore GE et al: Risk of splenic salvage in the adult following trauma: analysis of 200 adults, *Am J Surg* 148:800, 1984.
200 Moore FD, Dagher FJ, Boyden CM et al: Hemorrhage in normal man. I. Distribution and dispersal of saline infusions following acute blood loss: clinical kinetics of blood volume support, *Ann Surg* 163:485, 1966.
201 Moore JB, Moore EE: Changing trends in the management of combined pancreaticoduodenal injuries, *World J Surg* 8:791, 1984.
202 Moore JB, Moore EE, Markovchick VC et al: Diagnostic peritoneal lavage for abdominal trauma: superiority of the open technique at the infraumbilical ring, *J Trauma* 21:570, 1981.
203 Moore JB, Moore EE, Thompson JS: Abdominal injuries associated with penetrating trauma in the lower chest, *Am J Surg* 140:724, 1980.
204 Moore OS, Karlan M, Siglar L: Factors influencing the safety of carotid ligation, *Am J Surg* 118:666, 1969.
205 Morehouse DD, MacKinnon KJ: Management of prostatomembranous urethral disruption: thirteen years' experience, *J Urol* 123:173, 1980.
206 Moreno C, Moore EE, Rosenberg A et al: Hemorrhage associated with major pelvic fractures: a multispecialty challenge, *J Trauma* 96:987, 1986.
207 Moss GS, Lowe RJ, Jilek J et al: Colloid or crystalloid in the resuscitation of hemorrhagic shock: a controlled clinical trial, *Surgery* 89:434, 1981.
208 Mucha P: Pelvic fractures. In Moore EE, Mattox KL, Feliciano DV, editors: *Trauma*, Norwalk, Conn, 1991, Appleton & Lange.
209 Mulherin JL, Sawyers JL: Evaluation of three methods for managing penetrating colon injuries, *J Trauma* 15:580, 1975.
210 Mullins RJ, Lucas CE, Ledgerwood AM: The natural history following venous ligation for civilian injuries, *J Trauma* 20:737, 1980.
211 Nahai F, Hester TR, Jurkiewicz MJ: Microsurgical replantation of scalp, *J Trauma* 1986.
212 Nakamura S, Tsuzuki T: Surgical anatomy of the hepatic veins and the inferior vena cava, *Surg Gynecol Obstet* 152:43, 1981.
213 Narrod JA, Moore EE: Selective management of penetrating neck wounds: a prospective study, *Arch Surg* 119:574, 1984.
214 National Research Council: Accidental death and disability: the neglected disease of modern society, Washington, DC, 1966, National Academy of Science.
215 Neff CC, Pfister RC, Sonnenberg EC: Percutaneous transtracheal ventilation: experimental and practical aspects, *J Trauma* 23:84, 1983.
216 Neufield JDG, Moore EE, Marx JA, Rosen P: Trauma in pregnancy, *Emerg Med Clinics North Am* 5:623, 1987.
217 Neuman TS, Bockman MA, Moody P et al: An autopsy study of traumatic deaths: San Diego, 1979, *Am J Surg* 144:722, 1982.
218 Nguyen Huu H, Person H, Hong R et al: Anatomical approach to vascular segmentation of the spleen (Lien) based on controlled experimental partial splenectomies, *Anat Clin* 4:265, 1982.
219 Nichols GG, De Muth WE: Blunt cardiac trauma: the effect of alcohol on survival and metabolic function, *J Trauma* 20:58, 1980.
220 O'Brien PJ, Schweigel JF, Thompson WJ: Dislocations of the lower cervical spine, *J Trauma* 22:710, 1982.
221 Oldham KT, Guice KS, Ryckman F et al: Blunt liver injury in childhood: evolution of therapy and current perspective, *Surgery* 100:542, 1986.
222 O'Neal BJ, McDonald JC: The risk of sepsis in the asplenic adult, *Ann Surg* 194:775, 1981.
223 Oparah S, Mandal AK: Penetrating stab wounds of the chest: experience with 200 consecutive cases, *J Trauma* 16:868, 1976.
224 Orlando R, Drezner AD: Intra-aortic balloon counterpulsation in blunt cardiac injury, *J Trauma* 23:424, 1983.
225 O'Rourke PP, Crone RK: High-frequency ventilation: a new approach to respiratory support, *JAMA* 250:1845, 1983.
226 Otto RJ, Metzler MH: Rewarming from experimental hypothermia: comparison of heated aerosol inhalation, peritoneal lavage, and pleural lavage, *Crit Care Med* 16:869, 1988.
227 Pachter HL, Spencer FC, Jofstetter SR, Coppa GF: Experience with the finger fracture technique to achieve intrahepatic hemostasis in 75 patients with severe injuries of the liver, *Ann Surg* 197:771, 1983.
228 Parks BJ, Arbelaez J, Horner RL: Medical and surgical importance of the arterial blood supply of the thumb, *J Hand Surg* 3:383, 1978.
229 Parmley LF, Mattingly TW, Maneon WC: Nonpenetrating traumatic injury of the aorta, *Circulation* 17:1089, 1958.
230 Patel J, Williams JS, Shmigel B, Hinshaw JR: Preservation of splenic function by autotransplantation of traumatized spleen in man, *Surgery* 90:683, 1981.
231 Patton AS, Guyton SW, Lawson DW et al: Treatment of severe atrial injuries, *Am J Surg* 141:465, 1982.
232 Paul RL, Polanco O, Turney SA et al: Intracranial pressure response to alterations in arterial carbon dioxide pressures in patients with head injuries, *J Neurosurg* 36:714, 1972.
233 Perry MO, Snyder WH, Thal ER: Carotid artery injuries caused by blunt trauma, *Ann Surg* 192:74, 1980.
234 Peterson NE: Intermediate-degree blunt renal trauma, *J Trauma* 17:425, 1977.
235 Peterson NE, Millikan JS, Moore EE: Combined renal and caval trauma: a review of personal and recorded experience, *J Urol* 33:567, 1985.
236 Peterson SR, Sheldon GF, Lim RC: Management of portal vein injuries, *J Trauma* 19:616, 1979.
237 Phillips EA, Rogens WF, Gasper MR: First rib fractures: incidence of vascular injury and indication for aortography, *Surgery* 89:42, 1981.
238 Pickhardt B, Moore EE, Moore FA et al: Operative splenic salvage in the adult: a decade perspective, *J Trauma* 29:1386, 1989.
239 Pilcher DB, Harman PK, Moore EE: Retrohepatic vena cava balloon injuries: a continuing challenge, *J Trauma* 17:837, 1977.
240 Pitts JC, Peterson NE: Penetrating injuries of the ureter, *J Trauma* 21:978, 1981.
241 Podolsky S, Baraff LJ, Simon RR et al: Efficacy of cervical spine immobilization methods, *J Trauma* 23:461, 1983.
242 Posner M, Moore EE: Extrahepatic biliary tract injury: operative management, *J Trauma* 25:833, 1985.
243 Posner MC, Moore EE, Greenholz SK et al: Natural history of inferior vena cava injuries: nonoperative management in a swine model, *J Trauma* 26:698, 1986.

244 Pricolo VE, Burchard KW, Singh AK et al: Trendelenburg versus PASG application: hemodynamic responses in man, *J Trauma* 26:718, 1986.
245 Read RA, Moore EE, Moore FA et al: Intravascular ultrasound (IVUS) for the diagnosis of traumatic aortic disruption: a case report, *Surgery* 114:624, 1993.
246 Redan JA, Livingston DH, Tortella B, Rush B: The value of intubating and paralyzing patients with suspected head injury in the emergency department, *J Trauma* 31:371, 1991.
247 Rehn J, Müller-Fäber J: Our experience with the changes in the care of the multiple trauma patient over the past twenty years, *World J Surg* 7:173, 1983.
248 Reid JDS, Weigelt JA: Forty-three cases of vertebral artery trauma, *J Trauma* 28:1007, 1988.
249 Rich NM, Hughes CW, Baugh JH: Management of venous injuries, *Ann Surg* 171:724, 1970.
250 Rich NM, Collins GJ, Anderson CA et al: Venous trauma: successful venous reconstruction remains an interesting challenge, *Am J Surg* 134:226, 1977.
251 Richardson JD, McEhein RB, Trinkle JK: First rib fracture: a hallmark for severe trauma, *Ann Surg* 181:251, 1975.
252 Richardson JD, Flint LM, Snow NJ et al: Management of transmediastinal gunshot wounds, *Surgery* 90:671, 1981.
253 Richardson JD, Simpson C, Miller FB: Management of carotid artery trauma, *Surgery* 104:673, 1988.
254 Richardson JD, Leadbetter GW: Nonoperative treatment of the ruptured bladder, *J Urol* 114:213, 1975.
255 Roberts B, Hardesty WH, Holling HE et al: Studies on extracerebral blood flow, *Surgery* 56:827, 1964.
256 Root HD, Hauser CW, McKinley CR et al: Diagnostic peritoneal lavage, *Surgery* 57:633, 1965.
257 Rosaria MD, Rumsey EW, Arakalki G et al: Blood microaggregation and ultrafilters, *J Trauma* 18:498, 1978.
258 Rosenthal RE, Lowery ER: Unstable fracture—dislocation of the thoracoabdominal spine: results of surgical treatment, *J Trauma* 20:485, 1980.
259 Rothenberger D, Fischer R, Strate R et al: The mortality associated with pelvic fractures, *Surgery* 84:356, 1978.
260 Rothenberger D, Quattlebaum FW, Perry JF et al: Blunt maternal trauma: a review of 103 cases, *J Trauma* 18:173, 1978.
261 Rothenberger D, Velasco R, Strate R et al: Open pelvic fracture: a lethal injury, *J Trauma* 18:184, 1978.
262 Rush BF, Richardson JD, Bosomworth P et al: Limitation of blood replacement with electrolyte solutions: a controlled clinical study, *Arch Surg* 98:49, 1969.
263 Safar P: Resuscitation from clinical death: pathophysiologic limits and therapeutic potentials, *Crit Care Med* 16:923, 1988.
264 Saletta JD, Lowe RJ, Lim LT et al: Penetrating trauma of the neck, *J Trauma* 16:579, 1976.
265 Sanders AB, Kern KB, Ewy GH et al: Improved resuscitation from cardiac arrest with open-chest massage, *Ann Emerg Med* 13:672, 1984.
266 Schaff AV, Brawley RK: Operative management of penetrating vascular injuries of the thoracic outlet, *Surgery* 82:182, 1977.
267 Scott FA, Howar JW, Boswick JA: Recovery of function following replantation and revascularization of amputated hand parts, *J Trauma* 21:204, 1981.
268 Seelig JM, Becker DP, Miller JD et al: Traumatic acute subdural hematoma: major mortality reduction in comatose patients treated within four hours, *N Engl J Med* 304:1511, 1981.
269 Shaffer MA, Doris PE: Limitations of the cross-table lateral view in detecting cervical spine injuries: a retrospective analysis, *Ann Emerg Med* 10:508, 1981.
270 Shamoun JM, Barraza KR, Jurkovich GJ, Salley RR: In extremis use of staples of cardiorrhaphy in penetrating cardiac trauma: case report, *J Trauma* 29:1589, 1989.
271 Shannon FL, Moore EE: Primary colon repair: a safe alternative, *Surgery* 95:851, 1985.
272 Sibbald WJ, Paterson NAM, Holliday RL et al: The Trendelenburg position: hemodynamic and normotensive patients, *Crit Care Med* 7:218, 1979.
273 Siemens R, Polk HC, Gray LA et al: Indications for thoracotomy following penetrating thoracic injury, *J Trauma* 17:493, 1977.
274 Silva R, Moore EE, Bar-Or D et al: The risk-benefit of autotransfusion: a comparison to banked blood in a canine model, *J Trauma* 24:557, 1984.
275 Simpson ET, Aitchison JM: Percutaneous infraclavicular subclavian vein catheterization in shocked patients: a prospective study in 172 patients, *J Trauma* 22:781, 1982.
276 Skillman JJ, Hedley-Whyte J, Pallotta JA: Cardiorespiratory, metabolic, and endocrine changes after hemorrhage in man, *Ann Surg* 174:911, 1971.
277 Slatis P, Karaharju FW: External fixation of unstable pelvic fractures, *Clin Orthop* 151:73, 1980.
278 Snow N, Richardson JD, Flint LM: Myocardial contusion: implications for patients with multiple traumatic injuries, *Surgery* 92:744, 1982.
279 Soderstrom CA, Maekawa K, DuPriest RW et al: Gallbladder injuries resulting from blunt abdominal trauma, *Ann Surg* 193:60, 1981.
280 Sofferman RA: Management of laryngotracheal trauma, *Am J Surg* 141:412, 1961.
281 Stanley RB: Value of computed tomography in management of acute laryngeal injury, *J Trauma* 24:359, 1984.
282 Stone HH, Fabian TC: Management of perforating colon trauma: randomization between primary closure and exteriorization, *Ann Surg* 190:430, 1979.
283 Stone HH, Fabian TC, Satiani B et al: Experiences in the management of pancreatic trauma, *J Trauma* 21:257, 1981.
284 Støren G, Bugge-Asperheim B, Geiran OR, Dodgson MS: Rupture of the cervical trachea following blunt trauma, *J Trauma* 20:93, 1980.
285 Stothert JC, Buttorff J, Kaminski DL: Thoracic esophageal and tracheal injury following blunt trauma, *J Trauma* 20:992, 1980.
286 Stulz PM, Scheidegger D, Drop CJ et al: Ventricular pump performance during hypocalcemia: clinical and experimental studies, *J Thorac Cardiovasc Surg* 78:185, 1979.
287 Sturm JA, Lewis FR, Trentz O et al: Cardiopulmonary parameters and prognosis after severe multiple trauma, *J Trauma* 19:305, 1979.
288 Swan KG, Vidaver RM, La Vigne JE et al: Acute alcoholism, minor trauma, and shock, *J Trauma* 17:215, 1977.
289 Symbas PN, Hatcher CR, Vlasis SE: Esophageal gunshot injuries, *Ann Surg* 191:703, 1980.
290 Takahashi M, Maemura K, Sawada Y et al: Hyperamylasemia in critically injured patients, *J Trauma* 20:951, 1980.
291 Thomas AN, Stephens BG: Air embolism: a cause of morbidity and death after penetrating chest trauma, *J Trauma* 14:633, 1978.
292 Thompson JD, Fish S, Ruiz R: Succinylcholine for endotracheal intubation, *Ann Emerg Med* 11:526, 1982.
293 Thompson JS, Moore EE: Peritoneal lavage in the evaluation of penetrating abdominal trauma, *Surg Gynecol Obstet* 153:861, 1981.
294 Thompson JS, Moore EE, Moore JB: Comparison of penetrating injuries of the right and left colon, *Ann Surg* 193:414, 1981.
295 Thompson JS, Moore EE, Van Duzer-Moore S et al: The evaluation of abdominal stab wound management, *J Trauma* 20:478, 1980.
296 Tintinalli JE, Claffey J: Complications of nasotracheal intubation, *Ann Emerg Med* 10:142, 1981.
297 Trinkle JK, Rush BF, Eiseman B: Metabolism of lactate following major blood loss, *Surgery* 63:782, 1968.

298 Trinkle JK, Richardson JD, Franz JL et al: Management of flail chest without mechanical ventilation, *Ann Thorac Surg* 19:335, 1975.
299 Trinkle JK, Toon RS, Franz JL et al: Affairs of the wounded heart: penetrating cardiac wounds, *J Trauma* 19:467, 1979.
300 Trunkey D, Holcroft J, Carpenter MA: Calcium flux during hemorrhagic shock in baboons, *J Trauma* 16:633, 1978.
301 Tso P, Rodriguez A, Cooper C et al: Sonography in blunt abdominal trauma: a preliminary progress report, *J Trauma* 33:39, 1992.
302 Turner WW, Snyder WH, Fry WJ: Mortality and renal salvage after renovascular trauma: a review of 94 patients treated in a 20-year period, *Am J Surg* 146:848, 1983.
303 Upadhyaya P, Simpson JS: Splenic trauma in children, *Surg Gynecol Obstet* 127:781, 1968.
304 Urschel HC, Razzuk MA, Wood RE et al: Improved management of esophageal perforation: exclusion and diversion in continuity, *Ann Surg* 179:587, 1974.
305 Vassar MJ, Perry CA, Gannaway WL, Holcroft JW: 7.5% sodium chloride dextran for resuscitation of trauma patients undergoing helicopter transport, *Arch Surg* 126:1065, 1991.
306 Vaughan GD, Frazier OH, Graham DY et al: The use of pyloric exclusion in the management of severe duodenal injuries, *Am J Surg* 134:785, 1977.
307 Waldschmidt ML, Laws HL: Injuries of the diaphragm, *J Trauma* 20:587, 1980.
308 Walt AJ, The mythology of hepatic trauma—or, Babel revisited, *Am J Surg* 135:12, 1978.
309 Watkins GM, Rabelo A, Bevilacqua RG et al: Bodily changes in repeated hemorrhage, *Surg Gynecol Obstet* 139:162, 1974.
310 Wechsler AS, Auerback BJ, Graham TC et al: Distribution of intramyocardial blood flow during pericardial tamponade: correlation with microscopic anatomy and intrinsic myocardial contractility, *J Thorac Cardiovasc Surg* 68:847, 1974.
311 Weems WL: Management of genitourinary injuries in patients with pelvic fractures, *Ann Surg* 189:717, 1979.
312 Weigelt JA, Mitchell RA, Snyder WH: Early positive end-expiratory pressure in adult respiratory distress syndrome, *Arch Surg* 114:497, 1979.
313 West J, Trunkey DD, Lim RC: Systems of trauma care: a study of two countries, *Arch Surg* 114:455, 1979.
314 White BC, Godzinski DS, Hoehner PJ et al: Effect of flunarizine on canine cerebral cortical blood flow and vascular resistance post cardiac arrest, *Ann Emerg Med* 11:119, 1982.
315 White BC, Hoehner PJ, Petinga TJ et al: The electrocardiographic characterization of terminal arrhythmias of hemorrhagic shock in dogs, *JACEP* 8:298, 1979.
316 Whitney RF, Peterson NE: Penetrating renal injuries, *Urology* 7:7, 1976.
317 Williams JS, Kirkpatrick JR: The nature of seat belt injuries, *J Trauma* 11:207, 1971.
318 Wilson JN, Marshall SB, Beresford V et al: Experimental hemorrhage on survival and a comparative evaluation of plasma volume changes, *Ann Surg* 144:696, 1958.
319 Wilson RF, Gibson DB, Antoneko D: Shock and acute respiratory failure after chest trauma, *J Trauma* 17:697, 1977.
320 Woelfel GE, Moore EE, Cogbill TH et al: Severe thoracic and abdominal injuries associated with a lap-harness seat belt, *J Trauma* 24:166, 1984.
321 Woodring JH: The normal mediastinum in blunt traumatic rupture of the thoracic aorta and brachiocephalic arteries, *J Emerg Med* 8:467, 1990.
322 Yajko RD, Seydel F, Trimble C: Rupture of the stomach from blunt abdominal trauma, *J Trauma* 15:177, 1975.
323 Younes RN, Ann F, Accioly CQ et al: Hypertonic solutions in the treatment of hypovolemic shock: a prospective, randomized study in patients admitted to the emergency room, *Surgery* 111:380, 1992.
324 Zantut LF, Rodrigues AJ, Birolini D: Laparoscopy as a diagnostic tool in the evaluation of trauma, *Panam J Trauma* 2:6, 1990.

CHAPTER

16

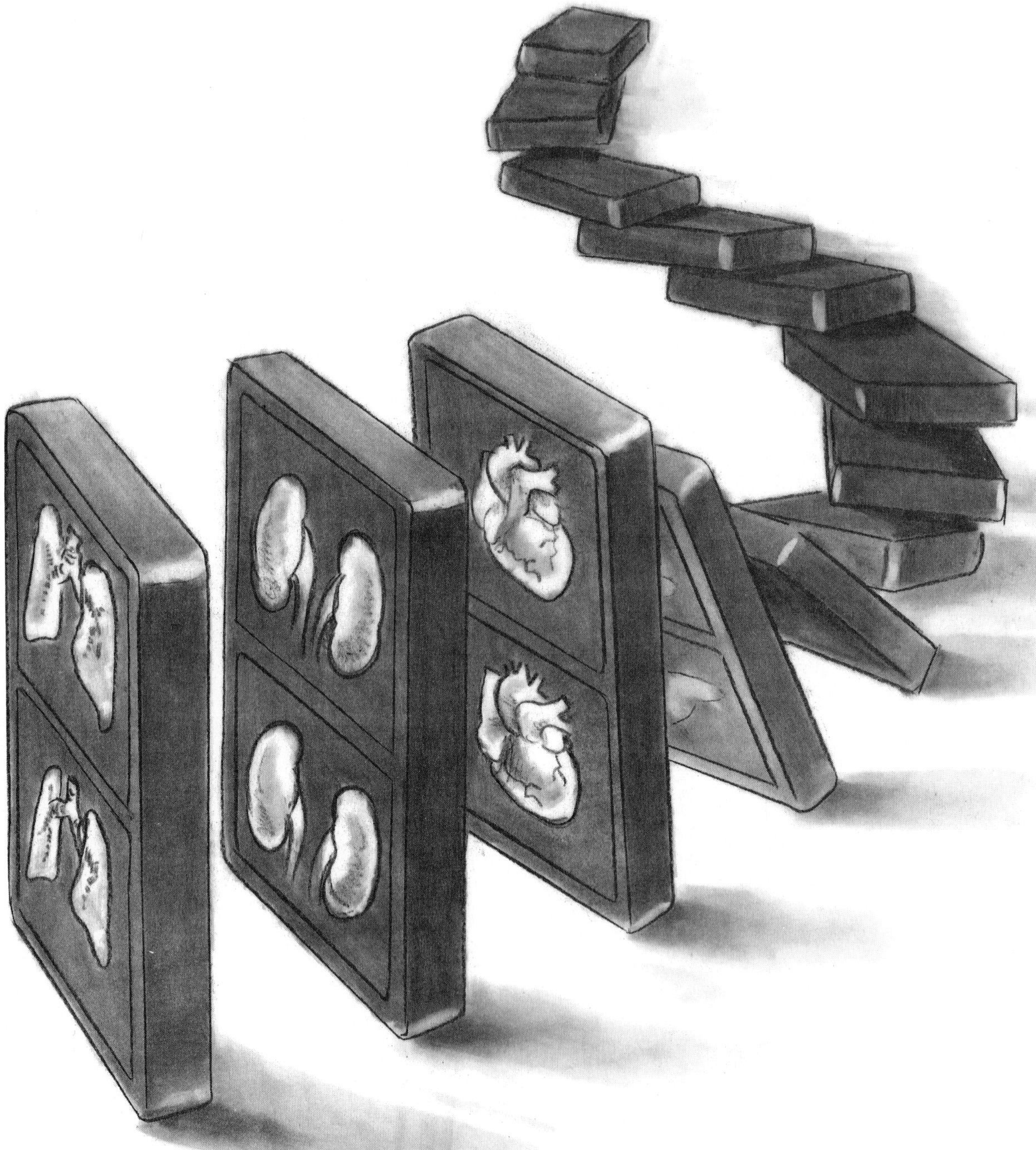

MULTIPLE ORGAN FAILURE

Edwin A. Deitch

Multiple organ failure has reached epidemic proportions in most intensive care units and is fast replacing single organ failure as the leading cause of death in these patients. Multiple organ failure is not limited to any one group of patients, nor is it the province of any one medical specialty. It occurs in patients of all ages, in patients with medical as well as surgical diseases, and in all parts of the world.

The ubiquitous and significant nature of multiple organ failure (MOF) syndrome is clearly illustrated by the followings facts: (1) MOF is responsible for 50% to 80% of all deaths in surgical intensive care units; (2) the costs engendered by the condition exceed $150,000 per patient; and (3) the mortality rates of patients with established MOF have not appreciably improved since the syndrome's initial description approximately 20 years ago.[18,61,82]

There are two primary reasons for the current inability to save many patients with MOF: treatment options are primarily supportive, and the basic pathophysiology of this syndrome has not been fully elucidated. Consequently, once the syndrome is fully manifest, even the best attempts at therapy are all too often fruitless. Thus, at a time when spectacular advances in the field of organ transplantation have revolutionized the treatment of patients with end-stage chronic single organ failure, our inability to successfully treat patients with acute organ failure remains the major unsolved problem in critically ill postoperative or injured patients. However, although specific therapeutic interventions are not yet available to consistently prevent or halt the progression of organ dysfunction, progress is being made. This chapter reviews our current understanding of this complex syndrome and integrates evolving concepts that are likely to influence current and future therapy.

HISTORICAL PERSPECTIVE

Multiple organ failure syndrome was recognized as a distinct clinical entity only relatively recently, in the mid-1970s. The idea that a severe physiologic insult could lead to the failure of several organs was first proposed by Tilney and colleagues in 1973,[199] when they described the postoperative course of a group of patients with ruptured aortic aneurysms. The researchers observed that massive acute blood loss and shock could lead to postoperative failure of initially uninvolved organs. This concept, that a severe physiologic insult could result in damage to distant organs, was formalized in a classic editorial by Baue[17] titled, "Multiple, progressive, or sequential systems organ failure: a syndrome for the '70s." Shortly afterward, Eiseman and colleagues[68] and Fry and coworkers[81] coined the terms "multiple organ failure" and "multiple system organ failure," respectively, to describe this syndrome. Since then, MOF has emerged as the leading cause of death in the surgical intensive care unit.

In many respects MOF can be viewed as a syndrome of surgical progress, a testimony to our increasing ability to keep patients with heretofore rapidly lethal medical problems alive for longer and longer periods. It is no coincidence that the emergence and recognition of MOF coincided with major advances in the metabolic and physiologic care of critically ill or injured patients. Thus it should come as no surprise that as we have improved our ability to support organ function and prolong survival in patients with highly lethal conditions, we have uncovered new and unexpected clinical problems, such as MOF, for which no definitive therapeutic answers are initially available. As recently reviewed by Baue,[16] this concept is not new, that strengthening one weak link in the physiologic chain leads to the uncovering of a second and previously unsuspected weak link. A brief review of the evolution of trauma care during the twentieth century illustrates this important concept.

This history begins with World War I, when "wound" shock syndrome was identified. Because the role of blood volume in controlling cardiac output was not appreciated at this time, wound shock was not recognized as a manifestation of blood and fluid loss. Various causes of this mysterious shock syndrome were proposed, including vasomotor exhaustion, adrenal failure, and traumatic toxemia. Because physicians were unaware of the causal relationship between acute blood loss and irreversible wound shock, wound shock remained a common cause of death throughout the war. After the war, animal studies were performed to investigate the physiology of wound shock. These studies established the role of acute blood loss in the development of wound shock syndrome. Consequently, during the latter half of World War II, blood was used liberally to prevent and treat shock, and the previously common syndrome of irreversible wound shock was largely eliminated. However, despite this improved early survival, many of these patients later died of acute renal failure. Thus, by the end of World War II, the weak link had become the kidney.

Progress in preventing acute renal failure during the Korean War was hampered by the prevailing concept that an injured patient did not need saline, because the body was actively conserving sodium through increased release of aldosterone. Also, it was current practice to limit salt administration to injured or postoperative patients to prevent edema. Thus, during the Korean War, acute renal failure remained the most common cause of delayed death in successfully resuscitated patients, and the term "post-traumatic renal insufficiency" was used for the first time. Studies by Shires and coworkers[184] during the 1960s helped clarify why volume resuscitation with just blood did not prevent renal failure. These studies documented that injury, shock, and acute blood loss were also associated with the movement of sodium and water from the intravascular to the intracellular space. As a result of these studies and the work of many others, it became clear that optimal resuscitation of injured patients involved not just restoring blood volume with plasma and red blood cells, but also administering adequate amounts of salt-containing solutions to maintain renal perfusion. Thus, studies of the physiology of post-traumatic renal insufficiency eventually led to the realization that injury-induced renal failure could be largely prevented by resuscitating these patients with blood plus sufficiently large amounts of crystalloids to maintain an effective circulating intravascular volume. Because of this better understanding of the physiology of injury and the need for acute volume resuscitation, acute renal failure was largely prevented in the Vietnam War.

However, although improved resuscitation regimens limited acute circulatory and subsequent renal failure during the Vietnam War, a new syndrome (weak link) involving the lungs emerged as more severely injured patients survived for longer periods. This new syndrome of pulmonary failure, now called *acute respiratory distress syndrome* (ARDS), was known then by many names, including Da Nang lung, wet lung syndrome, and post-traumatic pulmonary insufficiency. Thus, in the 1970s the organ system limiting survival had shifted from the kidneys to the lungs.[10] Currently the mortality rate of patients with ARDS remains high, but improvements in the ventilatory and physiologic management of these patients have shifted the cause of death from impaired gas exchange to multiple organ failure. More than 75% of patients with ARDS who ultimately die now die of MOF and end-stage systemic hemodynamic instability.[148] Viewed in this context, MOF clearly represents the most recent, but surely not the last, obstacle that must be overcome to improve survival in critically ill surgical patients.

This brief review illustrates the importance of mechanistically based therapy directed at the underlying physiologic disturbances. Because MOF, at its most basic level, is a cellular disease mediated by protein and lipid molecules, therapy must not only include organ-based supportive therapy, it also must extend to the cellular and molecular levels. For example, it is now clear that in MOF, organ injury is not directly due to exogenous factors, such as bacteria or toxins, but rather is largely a consequence of the patient's own endogenously produced mediators. Because we have expanded our understanding of the basic biology of injury, inflammation, and immunology, we are in the exciting position of integrating these basic scientific advances into everyday clinical practice.

THE CLINICAL SYNDROME

Epidemiology and Diagnosis of Organ Failure

Although initially associated with occult or uncontrolled infection,[81,166] MOF has now been documented to occur after a number of diverse clinical conditions, including mechanical and thermal trauma,[1,73,135] pancreatitis,[6] and shock.[100] Although infection and shock are the two most common clinical predisposing factors, processes that induce a major inflammatory response (e.g., severe tissue injury or pancreatitis) appear capable of initiating a cascade of events that culminates in MOF. Thus, MOF is not a specific disease entity but instead reflects the body's response to a severe insult that disrupts the homeostatic mechanisms. The major predisposing factors for the development of MOF and the patient groups at highest risk are summarized in Table 16-1.

The risk of MOF varies according to the criteria used to define organ failure and the patient group studied. Nonetheless, if one examines high-risk patient groups, the frequency of MOF (defined as failure of two or more organs) is relatively constant and ranges from about 7% to 8% in victims of multiple trauma[73] or patients undergoing emergency surgery[81] to almost 11% among patients in intensive care units (ICUs).[119] Not surprisingly, the incidence of single organ failure is threefold to fourfold higher than MOF among ICU patients (Figure 16–1).

Although any organ system can fail, the systems that have been studied most extensively are those that can be monitored clinically. The initial studies on MOF focused primarily on the pulmonary, hepatic, renal, and gastrointestinal systems. In these studies the indicators of organ failure were considered to be: a need for prolonged ventilatory support (longer than 5 days); a doubling of serum liver enzyme levels, associated with a bilirubin value over 2 mg/dl; a serum creatinine above 2 mg/dl; or upper gastrointestinal stress bleeding requiring transfusion with 2 or more units of blood. However, the diagnosis of organ failure has become increasingly confusing for two reasons. First, the criteria used to define organ failure, or even which or how many organs should be evaluated, vary from series to series. Second, the definition of organ failure has been expanded to include organ dysfunction. Table 16-2 is a synthesis of the current literature in which the degree of organ failure has been stratified into organ dysfunction (early) and advanced failure (late) stages.

TABLE 16-1 EPIDEMIOLOGY OF MULTIPLE ORGAN FAILURE

PREDISPOSING FACTORS	HIGH-RISK PATIENT GROUPS
Shock	Victims of multiple trauma
Infection	Burn patients
Massive blood therapy	Pancreatitis
Cardiovascular instability, pre-existing organ disease	Patients requiring emergency abdominal surgery or postoperative patients with major complications
Pre-existing organ disease	Patients in intensive care units

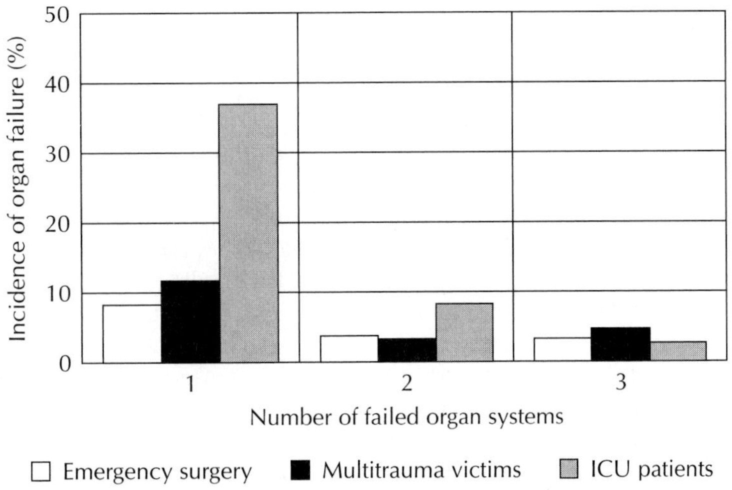

FIGURE 16-1 Demographic information on the incidence of multiple organ failure after emergency surgery (in trauma victims and in the intensive care unit).

TABLE 16-2 CRITERIA FOR DIAGNOSIS OF ORGAN DYSFUNCTION AND FAILURE

ORGAN OR SYSTEM	DYSFUNCTION	ADVANCED FAILURE
Pulmonary	Hypoxia requiring respirator-assisted ventilation for at least 3-5 days	Progressive ARDS requiring PEEP >10 cm/H_2O and FIO_2 >0.5
Hepatic	Serum bilirubin ≥2-3 mg/dl or liver function values twice normal or higher	Clinical jaundice with bilirubin ≥8-10 mg/dl
Renal	Oliguria ≤479 ml/24 hr or rising creatinine (≥2-3 mg/dl)	Renal dialysis
Intestinal	Ileus with intolerance to enteral feeding for longer than 5 days	Stress ulcers requiring transfusion; acalculus cholecystitis
Hematologic	PT and PTT ↑ >25% or platelets <50,000-80,000	Disseminated intravascular coagulation
Central nervous system	Confusion, mild disorientation	Progressive coma
Cardiovascular	Decreased ejection fraction or capillary-leak syndrome	Hypodynamic response refractory to inotropic support

PEEP, Positive end-expiratory pressure; *FIO_2*, fraction of inspired air in oxygen; *PT*, prothrombin time; *PTT*, partial thromboplastin time.
From Deitch EA: *Ann Surg* 216:117, 1992.

Natural History

Regardless of the cause, the syndrome of MOF generally follows a predictable course, beginning with the lungs and followed by hepatic, intestinal, and renal failure in that order. Hematologic and myocardial failure usually are later manifestations of MOF, whereas central nervous system (CNS) alterations can develop either early or late. Physiologically, these patients are hypermetabolic and have a hyperdynamic circulation, which is characterized by increased cardiac output and decreased systemic vascular resistance. This sequence of organ failure can run a rapid course, with full manifestation of the syndrome occurring over several days, or it can take weeks to evolve. In the most common temporal sequence, evidence of pulmonary failure is present by 2 to 3 days after the initiating event. Over the subsequent week, signs of liver and intestinal failure become apparent, and by the second week after the physiologic insult, evidence of progressive renal failure is present.

However, this typical sequential pattern may be modified by pre-existing disease or by the nature of the precipitating clinical event. For example, renal failure may precede hepatic or even pulmonary failure in patients with intrinsic renal disease or those who have sustained prolonged periods of shock. Hepatic or myocardial failure may be an early or even the first manifestation of the syndrome in a patient with cirrhosis or preexisting heart disease. These clinical exceptions illustrate an important biologic principle: although the systemic responses are similar among patients developing MOF, the exact sequence of organ failure can be influenced by the patient's acute disease processes or physiologic reserve, or both. In addition, the temporal pattern of organ failure can be helpful clinically. For example, intra-abdominal infection is much more likely when clinical sepsis precedes the onset of pulmonary failure than when clinical sepsis develops after pulmonary failure.[81,148]

As previously mentioned, the criteria of organ failure or dysfunction vary from series to series, and this variability makes comparisons between different clinical reports difficult. Nonetheless, in almost all series the prognosis is related more to the number of organs that have failed than to any other variable, including the underlying process that initiated MOF syndrome (Figure 16-2). For example, in Fry and coworkers' original clinical report,[81] as the number of organs that failed increased from one to four, the mortality rate progressively increased from 30% to 100%. This concept was verified and expanded in a prospective multi-institutional study on acute organ failure involving 5677 patients in medical and surgical intensive care units.[119] This study not only documented a direct relationship between mortality and the number of organs that failed, it also showed the correlation between mortality and the length of time the patient was in organ failure. Thus, the prognosis appears to be directly related to both the number of organs that fail and the length of time the patient is in organ failure.

Despite these prognostic and epidemiologic studies, problems still exist in the early identification of which high-risk patients will develop MOF and in comparing the results of therapeutic studies from different institutions. Because fewer than 10% of high-risk patients develop MOF, one major clinical challenge has been to identify and accurately categorize patients at increased risk of MOF before organ failure develops. A second challenge has been to develop a system for quantitating the severity of MOF in this heterogeneous group of patients. Until these two challenges are met, it will remain

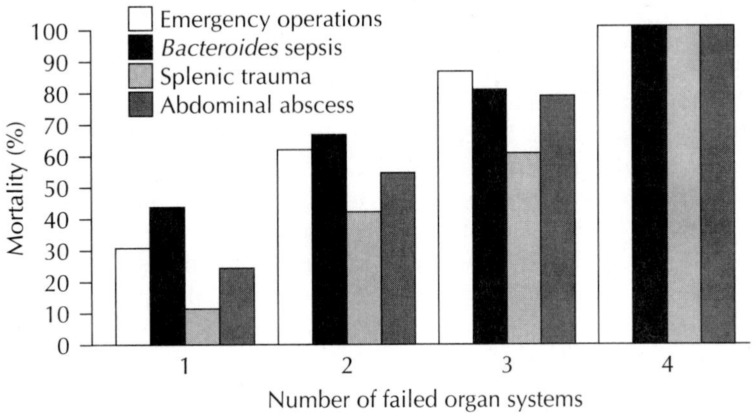

FIGURE 16-2 Mortality rate among four different groups of patients, illustrating that the mortality rate appears to be linearly related to the number of organ systems involved. (From Fry DE: *Multiple system organ failure,* St Louis, 1992, Mosby.)

difficult, if not impossible, to critically evaluate the potential efficacy of therapeutic and prophylactic treatment regimens carried out at different institutions, and to identify the patient for whom further therapy is not warranted. For these reasons, many investigators are attempting to develop clinically accurate scoring systems that can be used to identify or categorize patients with MOF. Although no scoring system currently exists that is accurate enough to be used in individual patients, progress is being made.[47,64] Hopefully, such a system will become available over the next several years. Until then, the current lack of an objective, reproducible system for identifying and categorizing patients for inclusion in potential clinical trials is a major factor limiting the evaluation of prophylactic and therapeutic agents.

CLINICAL PARADOXES IN MULTIPLE ORGAN FAILURE

1. Organs that fail are frequently not directly injured in the initial insult.
2. There is a lag period of days to weeks between the initial insult and the development of organ failure.
3. Not all patients with clinical sepsis with MOF have microbiologic evidence of infection (septic state).
4. No septic focus can be identified clinically or at autopsy in more than 30% of bacteremic patients who die of clinical sepsis and MOF.
5. Identification and treatment of suppurative infections in patients with MOF may not improve survival.

From Deitch EA: *Ann Surg* 216:117, 1992.

PATHOPHYSIOLOGY

General Concepts

MOF has been the focus of extensive clinical and laboratory studies over the past decade. These studies have generated several distinct and often conflicting hypotheses to explain the mechanisms responsible for developing and perpetuating acute organ failure. In evaluating any of the current hypotheses, several clinical facts must be considered. First, organ failure in this syndrome is unique in that the organs that fail usually are not directly injured or involved in the primary disease. Second, there is a lag phase of days to weeks between the initial or subsequent inciting events and the development of distant organ failure. Although it is clear that an untreated focus of infection can induce MOF, it is equally clear that not all patients who die of MOF have untreated infections.[6,87] Furthermore, identification and treatment of an occult septic focus in patients with established MOF have not consistently improved survival. These clinical paradoxes are summarized in the box above. They indicate that MOF is a systemic process mediated by an endogenous or exogenous circulating factor or factors whose effects are not immediately apparent after the initiating physiologic insult.

When evaluating the role of putative systemic mediators and the potential accuracy of proposed mechanisms of MOF, it is important to keep certain clinical observations in mind. First, infection is only one of several pathologic conditions that seems able to initiate the cascade of events that culminate in MOF; others include endotoxemia, trauma with retained necrotic or injured tissue, and shock. Second, although the systemic clinical manifestations of MOF (fever, leukocytosis, hypermetabolism, and a hyperdynamic circulatory state) are all typical of the septic response observed with gram-negative infections, the septic response is not diagnostic of infection; the septic response can be induced by severe perfusion deficits as well as by the continued presence of dead and injured tissue. Based on these clinical observations and the host's limited repertoire of effector molecules, it would be expected that the same or similar mediator systems are involved in the pathogenesis of organ injury even when the initiating events are different.

A major conceptual advance in understanding the biology of MOF has been the realization that the host is not an innocent bystander whose tissues are being directly damaged by invading bacteria or products of injured tissue; rather, it is an active participant in this destructive process. For example, until relatively recently it was believed that bacteria or their products, such as endotoxin, were directly responsible for the pathophysiologic manifestations of the septic response. However, it is now clear that cytokines and other mediators produced by the host in response to invading bacteria or their products are the direct mediators of the septic response, organ dysfunction, and MOF. This shift in thought has major implications. For example, if the body is an innocent bystander that is being directly injured by invading bacteria, one primary goal of therapy would be to increase the inflammatory and immune responses and thereby bolster the body's ability to fight infection. In contrast, if the paradigm of MOF is modified to take into account that the body is being injured by an excessive or uncontrolled inflammatory response to the invading bacteria and not by the bacteria themselves, then therapy would focus on ways to modulate the body's immunoinflammatory response and thereby limit tissue injury. As is discussed in more detail later, the realization that the body is destroying itself rather than being destroyed by bacteria has led to a shift in research from attempts to understand and bolster a failing immune system to attempts to understand and selectively limit the body's uncontrolled or excessive inflammatory response. Finally, in attempting to understand the physiology of MOF, it is important to realize that the septic (hypermetabolic) response, ARDS, and MOF are not unrelated distinct entities but appear to represent a physiologic continuum of progressively increasing severity.

Role of Infection

In the initial publications of Eiseman and colleagues[68] and Polk and Shields,[166] uncontrolled or occult infection was implicated as the common denominator in the development of MOF in these otherwise heterogeneous patients. Because clinical sepsis preceded organ failure in these patients and an association between an untreated septic focus and the development of MOF had been documented by several investigators, it was logical at that time to propose that MOF was the external expression of an occult septic focus.[17,81,166] Today, although it is clear that an untreated or inadequately treated focus of infection is a common cause of MOF, it has become equally clear that not all septic-appearing patients who develop or die of MOF have untreated infections.[87] Currently, uncontrolled infection is the initiating cause of MOF in about half of the patients. In the remainder, MOF occurs either without a clinically identifiable focus of infection or infection develops as a preterminal event and is of no apparent prognostic importance.

The reason for this initial error in equating MOF with systemic infection is that the systemic clinical manifestations of MOF (fever, leukocytosis, hypermetabolism, and a hyperdynamic circulatory state) are characteristic of gram-negative sepsis. Recognition that a similar response can be induced by other microorganisms, including gram-positive bacteria, viruses, and fungi, as well as by stimuli that lead to an excessive and prolonged inflammatory response (e.g., pancreatitis, major thermal injuries, and polytrauma) has led to a reappraisal of the relationship of the septic response to infection. As a result, it is now generally accepted that (1) not all septic-appearing patients have an underlying infection; (2) large amounts of dead or injured tissue can replace bacteria as the stimulus for the septic response; and (3) it frequently is impossible to differentiate clinically the patient with systemic infection from the patient who appears septic but does not have microbiologic evidence of systemic infection. Thus, one point that deserves special emphasis is the fact that remarkable physiologic similarities exist between systemic infection (classic sepsis), MOF, and a septic state in which there is no microbial evidence of infection. The similarities include altered intermediary metabolism, a hyperdynamic circulation, and systemic signs of inflammation. Therefore, it is likely that the mediators responsible for the external expression of these three clinical syndromes are similar. This assumption is supported by the fact that a classic septic response can be induced in normal human volunteers by injecting inflammatory agents,[213] endotoxin,[102,170] or cytokines, such as tumor necrosis factor.[144,193]

One major recent conceptual advance is the recognition that sepsis and infection are not synonymous and that the septic state can occur without infection. For these reasons, investigators and clinicians have begun using the terms "sepsis syndrome," "septic state," or "systemic inflammatory response syndrome (SIRS)" to describe this phenomenon.[25,26,33,87] In fact, dissatisfaction

Steps	Promoting factors
Colonization of oropharynx/stomach with potential pathogens	Antibiotic therapy Gastric acid neutralization
↓ Aspiration of oropharyngeal/gastric secretions	Depressed consciousness Presence of endotracheal tube Presence of nasogastric tube
↓ Impaired local defenses	Impaired ability to clear secretions Impaired mucociliary mechanism Atelectasis
↓ Impaired systemic immune defenses	Immune suppression
↓ Pneumonia	

FIGURE 16-3 Pathogenic factors that contribute to the development of nosocomial pneumonia.

with the ambiguous nature of the term "sepsis" has engendered a number of position papers as well as editorials whose goal is to redefine and clarify the terms used to describe the septic-appearing patient.[25,26,30,188,192] Although consensus has not yet been reached on the definition of sepsis, it is clear that sepsis does not equal infection and that classic infection is present in fewer than 50% of clinically septic patients.[192]

When infection does appear to directly cause ARDS or MOF, the origin is equally likely to be pleuropulmonary as intra-abdominal. Furthermore, many patients with intra-abdominal infections ultimately develop secondary pulmonary infections during their hospital course.[171] This predisposition for secondary pulmonary infections in patients with abdominal infections appears to involve a number of factors. Patients with intra-abdominal infections are immunosuppressed, their pulmonary bacterial clearance mechanisms are impaired, and the therapy these patients receive (Figure 16-3) potentiates the risk of nosocomial pneumonia. Consequently, patients with intra-abdominal infection are as likely to die of intercurrent pulmonary sepsis as they are from the original intra-abdominal infectious process.[110] Although gram-negative enteric bacilli are most commonly associated with ARDS, MOF, and septic shock, other microorganisms, including *Enterococcus, Bacteroides fragilis, Candida,* and even viral pathogens have been documented as playing a role in the pathogenesis of MOF.[61]

Endotoxin as a Mediator of MOF

A discussion of the biology of endotoxin is warranted, because gram-negative infections or bacteremias are relatively common in patients with MOF, because endotoxin mimics many of the pathophysiologic changes observed with gram-negative infections, and because endotoxin is likely to be a proximal mediator in MOF.

Numerous studies have documented that many of the effects observed when endotoxin is injected into experimental animals are similar to those observed in septic humans. For example, both septic humans and animals given endotoxin develop fever, hypotension, systemic acidosis, arterial hypoxia, disseminated intravascular coagulation (DIC), and similar changes in intermediary metabolism. Endotoxin appears to exert most of its toxic effects by triggering overproduction and release of endogenous factors, and endotoxic shock appears to be caused by activation of endogenous host systems and cells, especially macrophages. As Thomas[197] stated, the lethal effects of endotoxin appear to be due to the fact that "our arsenals for fighting off bacteria are so powerful and involve so many defense mechanisms, that we are more in danger from them than from the invaders."

Endotoxin activates both the classic and alternate pathways of complement, resulting in the production of the anaphylatoxins C3a and C5a, which have vasodilatory and immunomodulatory properties, including activation of neutrophils and macrophages. Clinical and experimental endotoxemia is associated with activation of the coagulation system and the resultant development of systemic microvascular thrombosis, which can lead to organ ischemia and injury. Endotoxin can activate the coagulation system directly via factor XII (Hageman's factor) or indirectly by several mechanisms, including stimulating macrophages to produce tissue procoagulation factor. Also, endotoxin exerts a direct procoagulant effect on endothelial cells.

Arachidonic acid metabolites produced by endotoxin-activated macrophages also appear to play a role in endotoxin-mediated disease. Endotoxin can elicit the production of prostaglandins and leukotrienes, and inhibitors or antagonists of these metabolites can modulate some of the deleterious physiologic effects of endotoxin. Other macrophage products have been shown to be induced by endotoxin, including interleukin-1, tumor necrosis factor, colony-stimulating factors, and interferons. Each of these factors, alone or in combination, can have profound effects on several homeostatic systems and organs. Another potential mediator of endotoxin-induced tissue injury and shock is platelet activating factor (PAF). PAF is produced by many cells, including macrophages, neutrophils, platelets, and endothelial cells. Its biologic activities include increased vascular permeability, hypotension, and death. Furthermore, endotoxin-induced hypotension is associated with detectable levels of PAF, and PAF antagonists reverse endotoxin-induced shock. Finally, endotoxin can induce the release of tissue-destructive products, such as oxidants and lysosomal enzymes, from activated neutrophils and macrophages. The difficulty in determining the exact role of these endotoxin-induced secondary mediators in tissue injury, organ failure, and shock is compounded by the fact that these mediators appear to interact synergistically.

Despite endotoxin's deleterious effects, under most clinical circumstances the immune response to a bacterial or endotoxin challenge is beneficial. B cells are activated to produce antibodies, macrophages are activated to become more efficient phagocytes, neutrophils are released from the bone marrow, and the reticuloendothelial system (RES) is primed to clear more efficiently the circulation of blood-borne bacteria and debris. Thus endotoxin has a wide range of activities. On the positive side, endotoxin stimulates B cell proliferation, activates macrophages, primes the RES, induces granulocytosis, increases serum complement levels, and promotes an inflammatory response. On the other hand, when excessive, the interaction of endotoxin with these same components of the immunoinflammatory systems can result in profound systemic changes and can potentiate the development of organ injury.

Macrophage Hypothesis of MOF

Dissatisfaction with infection as an explanation for the development of MOF, coupled with advances in molecular biology and a better understanding of the basic biology of injury and inflammation, led to the macrophage hypothesis of MOF. In this hypothesis, organ injury and MOF are related to the uncontrolled production and liberation of cytokines and other products by activated macrophages.[33,77] Support for this hypothesis is based on the recognition that activation of macrophages and release of cytokines can produce a syndrome practically indistinguishable from the systemic response to severe infection.

This hypothesis has several attractive features. It clarifies the clinical paradox of why infection is not found in a relatively large percentage of septic-appearing patients with MOF. The concept of an uncontrolled inflammatory response that leads to MOF provides a mechanism by which noninfectious causes of MOF (e.g., pancreatitis, thermal injury, or polytrauma) result in distant organ injury. It also explains the clinical observation that large amounts of dead or injured tissue can replace bacteria as the stimulus for the septic response. Similarly, if the same mediators were involved in inflammatory as well as infectious disease processes, it would explain why it is frequently impossible to clinically differentiate a patient with systemic infection from a patient who appears septic but does not have microbiologic evidence of infection.

The clinical correlate of the macrophage hypothesis of MOF is the uncontrolled inflammatory response. Normally, inflammation operates within a restricted environment to contain and eradicate infecting organisms and to clear damaged tissues of cell debris or foreign materials. Although overproduction of cytokines and activation of macrophages can have profound detrimental effects, cytokines also have beneficial effects. Both cytokines and macrophages are essential for normal antimicrobial and immune activity, wound healing, and optimal substrate mobilization (Table 16-3).[78]

Nonetheless, since inflammatory processes are intrinsically destructive to the surrounding tissues, if the inflammatory response escapes local control and becomes systemic, it could result in distant organ injury. In the same fashion that endotoxin exerts profound effects on several humoral and cellular inflammatory and immune effector systems, so, too, can the products of activated macrophages. In addition, through this uncontrolled intravascular inflammatory response, the vascular endothelium may be damaged, thereby further potentiating distant organ injury. Ultimately, systemic inflammation may become self-perpetuating because of the continued "leak" or "spill-over" of locally or systemically produced inflammatory mediators into the circulation and because of the body's inadequate regulation of the inflammatory response. Thus, although inflammation aids the body at the local tissue level, systemic activation represents a major potential liability. This hypothesis, that MOF and distant organ injury are related to an uncontrolled or persistent systemic inflammatory state, is consistent with the autopsy study of Nuytinck and coworkers,[157] who found an association between the presence of ARDS or MOF and histologic evidence of organ inflammation. Furthermore, elevated circulat-

TABLE 16-3 CONSEQUENCES OF CYTOKINE INSUFFICIENCY OR EXCESS

CYTOKINE INSUFFICIENCY	CYTOKINE EXCESS
• Impaired wound healing • Increased susceptibility and decreased resistance to infection • Impaired metabolic response to injury	• Local tissue destruction • Microvascular injury (capillary leak) • Excessive hypermetabolism (cachexia) • Hemodynamic insufficiency culminating in a refractory shock state

From Deitch EA: *Ann Surg* 216:117, 1992.

ing levels of several cytokines have been detected in the serum of patients with infectious conditions,* and tumor necrosis factor and interleukin-6 have been detected in infected and noninfected burn patients.[93,134,155] Elevated cytokine levels have also been documented in inflammatory and noninflammatory states in the absence of infection.†

The cytokine family of proteins includes interleukins (ILs), interferons (INFs), colony-stimulating factors (CSFs), and tumor necrosis factor (TNF). Special attention is due the proinflammatory cytokines (IL-1, IL-6, TNF-alpha, and INF-gamma), because these cytokines are involved or associated with infection, inflammation, and the evolution of MOF. These four cytokines share many common effects and when injected into animals or humans recreate many of the systemic, immunologic, and metabolic signs associated with the septic response.‡ For example, they activate macrophages, neutrophils, and endothelial cells, induce fever and an acute phase response, and modulate both the metabolic response and wound healing. TNF rather than IL-1 or IL-6 appears to be the key messenger that initiates and orchestrates the septic response,§ because (1) after an endotoxin (human) or bacterial challenge (primate), TNF levels rise and peak well before other potential mediators, including IL-1 or IL-6; (2) administering monoclonal antibodies against TNF improves survival and attenuates the expected increase in IL-1 and IL-6 in a lethal bacteremic model; (3) administering TNF and endotoxin induces similar metabolic responses in humans; and (4) TNF administration mimics the response to injury. In fact, TNF is capable of inducing a whole cascade of secondary factors, a partial list of which includes other cytokines, growth factors, endocrine hormones, acute phase proteins, eicosanoids, and endothelial factors.[202]

Although attractive, the macrophage hypothesis of MOF has yet to be verified. It has been difficult to draw definitive clinical or mechanistic conclusions on the exact role of cytokines in organ failure or outcome, because the frequency of cytokine detection and the clinical significance of cytokinemia have varied from series to series.* This failure to consistently and reproducibly identify elevated cytokine levels in critically ill, infected, or septic-appearing patients has been one of the major factors limiting acceptance of the macrophage hypothesis of MOF. Furthermore, the fact that most cytokines are pleiotropic and have several diverse biologic activities has further confounded the interpretation of data.[7,77] For example, depending on the cell type of the target cell or the environment in which the cytokine is acting, a single cytokine may act as either a positive or a negative signal. Thus, understanding cytokine effects is complicated, because the precise biologic effect of a cytokine can vary depending on the exact clinical or experimental circumstances in which it is measured.

There are several potential physiologic explanations for these inconsistent clinical results.† First, since the half-lives of TNF and the other cytokines in the circulation is very short (minutes), random blood sampling may miss the peaks of activity. Second, since TNF is present in the circulation only briefly during the earliest phase of the critical illness or infection, samples taken once the disease process is established may be too late. Third, circulating levels of cytokines, especially TNF and IL-1-alpha, may be misleading and not reflect their tissue levels or biologic activity; that is, cytokines are usually produced and exert their biologic effects locally within organs and tissues and thereby function primarily as paracrine (cell-cell) or autocrine (self-stimulating) mediators rather than endocrine mediators. Consistent with this observation is the recent discovery of cell-associated forms of TNF and IL-1-alpha that may differ from those found in the circulation.[7,77,78] Thus, although most clinical studies investigating the role of cytokines in injury and infection have measured circulating cytokine levels, the concentrations of these proteins in the tissues are more likely to be of clinical and biologic importance. Also, the toxicity of TNF, as well as other cytokines, is synergistically enhanced by other factors.[202] For example, IL-1 by itself, even when administered in high doses, is minimally toxic, yet when co-administered with normally nontoxic doses of TNF, the combination is lethal.

*References 38, 51-53, 86, 95, 99, 211, and 212.
†References 108, 124, 136, 137, 182, and 205.
‡References 12, 77, 78, 144, 157, and 192.
§References 79, 102, 144, 145, 192, and 201.

*References 38, 51-53, 86, 93, 95, 99, 134, 155, 211, and 212.
†References 77, 79, 102, 144, 145, 193, and 201.

Endotoxin also potentiates the toxicity of TNF such that simultaneous administration of individually innocuous doses of endotoxin plus TNF induces a rapidly fatal shock syndrome. Other cytokines, such as PAF, IL-6, and INF-gamma increase TNF toxicity, whereas TGF-beta (transforming growth factor type beta) attenuates TNF toxicity.[202] These complex cytokine interactions further limit the clinical usefulness of random measurements of blood cytokine levels.

Undoubtedly, as more basic and clinical information on macrophage and cytokine biology emerges, their precise role in critically ill patients will be better defined. Nonetheless, it seems clear that cytokines in conjunction with the neuroendocrine axis play a major role in the metabolic response to injury and in the transition from hypermetabolism to organ dysfunction and MOF. Consequently, if MOF represents the terminal phase of the hypermetabolic response, as proposed by Cerra and others,[42] then it should be possible to reduce the incidence of MOF by limiting the development of an uncontrolled systemic inflammatory-hypermetabolic state. The elegant clinical studies of multitrauma patients carried out by Border and colleagues,[32] Seibel and coworkers,[179] and other researchers[24,88,115] indicate that early surgical fixation of long-bone fractures, rather than traction fixation, reduces the incidence of ARDS and MOF and shortens the number of days the patient spends on the ventilator and in the ICU. These clinical studies on the early and definitive fixation of fractures support the hypothesis that, by preventing progressive macrophage activation (and thereby limiting the systemic inflammatory response), early and complete successful management of major trauma improves outcome. Thus, although originally it was believed that the cytokines' primary role was in immunologic homeostasis, it is now clear that certain cytokines also have profound effects on intermediary metabolism, substrate mobilization, wound healing, and the cardiovascular system.[7,12,77,78]

Microcirculatory Hypothesis of MOF

Impaired microcirculatory blood flow, with its sequela of cellular and organ dysfunction, has been proposed as one of the primary factors responsible for initiating or perpetuating MOF. As outlined in the box, this hypothesis is consistent with a number of clinical observations.* Although the mechanisms may vary depending on the clinical circumstance, the net result of impaired microcirculatory blood flow is a reduction in nutrient blood flow and focal ischemia. The mechanisms by which microcirculatory failure can lead to injury include inadequate oxygen delivery to tissues and cells,[37,185,200] ischemia-reperfusion phenomenon,[90,169] and tissue injury resulting from endothelial-leukocyte interactions.[159,163] There are many points where the microcirculatory and macrophage[84,85] or endotoxin-mediated[37,200] hypotheses of organ failure overlap and interact.[163,164] For example, clinical and experimental observations clearly document that systemic inflammation adversely affects the microcirculation, whereas ischemia activates neutrophils and primes macrophages and can thereby exaggerate the body's inflammatory response to subsequent stimuli.

*References 13, 16, 23, 40, 73, 96, and 157.

MICROCIRCULATORY HYPOTHESIS OF MOF: CLINICAL OBSERVATIONS

1. Circulatory shock and tissue hypoxia are associated with increased organ injury and MOF.
2. Circulatory shock is associated with adverse changes in the microcirculation (vascular congestion, microthrombi, and increased capillary permeability).
3. Autopsy evidence of diffuse microvascular injury is frequently seen in patients with MOF.
4. The pulmonary microcirculation of patients with ARDS contains neutrophils, platelets, and fibrin.
5. Hemodynamic studies in patients with ARDS or MOF indicate that microvascular nutrient blood flow to the liver, gut, and kidneys is inadequate.
6. Disseminated intravascular coagulation (DIC) and microcirculatory thrombosis are common occurrences in septic patients and in patients with MOF.

The role of inadequate oxygen availability in the pathogenesis of tissue and cellular injury during periods of prolonged hypotension or organ ischemia is well established. However, because the contributions of reperfusion-mediated injury and leukocyte-endothelial interactions to this process of microcirculatory failure and organ injury are only now being elucidated, these two areas are discussed in more detail.

Ischemia-Reperfusion Injury

As is illustrated in Figure 16-4, the re-establishment of blood flow after ischemia can itself cause tissue injury.[90,169] During the period of ischemia, energy stores are depleted by the continuing energetic demands to maintain cellular homeostasis and because the capacity to regenerate adenosine triphosphate (ATP) is reduced by oxidative phosphorylation. If the period of ischemia is sufficiently prolonged, ischemia-induced tissue hypoxia can lead to irreversible tissue injury. However, in many circumstances and in a number of tissues, most of the tissue damage occurs after oxygenation is restored rather than during the period of ischemia. The mediators of tissue and endothelial cell injury appear to be xanthine oxidase–generated oxidants and the products of activated neutrophils. Support for the role of reperfusion-mediated injury comes from studies documenting that both postischemic microvascular and tissue injury can

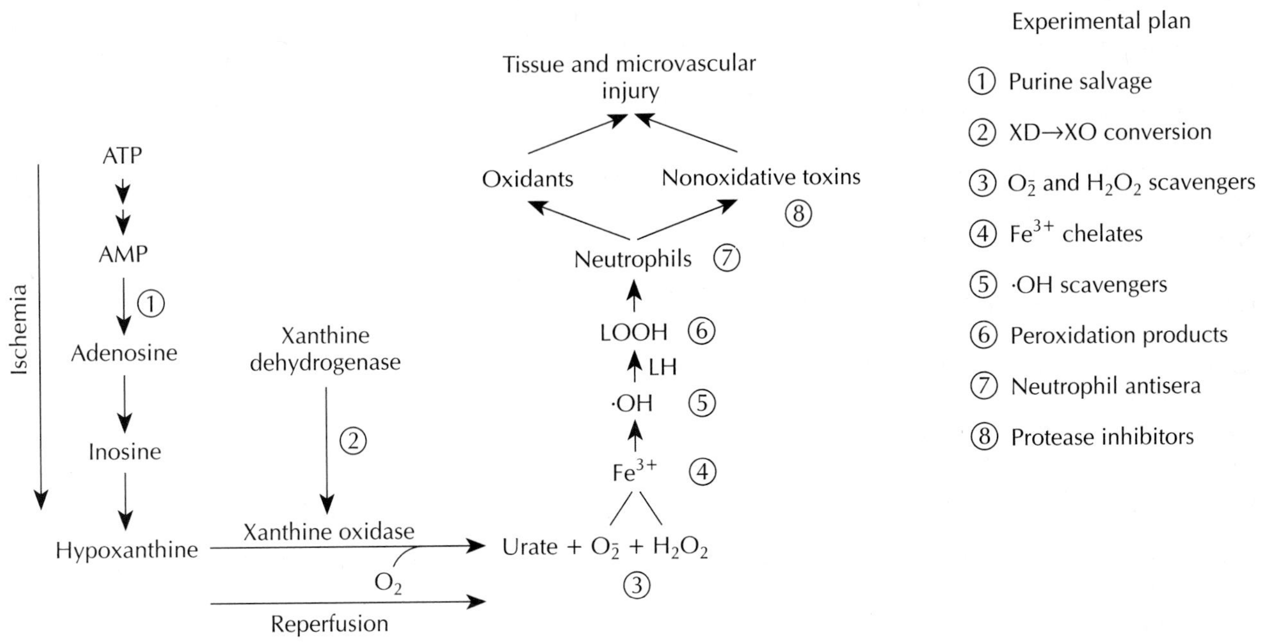

FIGURE 16-4 Schematic illustration of the proposed pathway by which ischemia-reperfusion results in microvascular and tissue injury. The process begins with tissue ischemia, with the consequent production of hypoxanthine from adenosine triphosphate (ATP) and the conversion of xanthine dehydrogenase to xanthine oxidase. Upon reperfusion, oxygen radicals are formed from O_2 by the enzymatic action of xanthine oxidase. These oxidants, in combination with recruited neutrophils, cause endothelial and tissue injury. Potential points of therapeutic intervention are illustrated in the side panel.

be prevented or ameliorated by pharmacologic agents that interrupt this pathway. These agents include inhibitors of xanthine oxidase activation, antioxidants, iron chelators, hydroxyl radical scavengers, and various monoclonal antibodies directed at specific neutrophil and endothelial surface antigens. Consequently, although reperfusion is necessary to restore metabolic activity, it can induce or aggravate the extent of ischemic tissue injury. In this context, hemorrhagic shock or any disease process that causes systemic hypotension can be viewed as causing a global ischemia-reperfusion syndrome.

Since 1981, when ischemia-reperfusion–mediated tissue injury was first shown to occur in the feline intestine, this phenomenon has been documented to occur in essentially every tissue and organ. Although there are several important biologic sources of oxygen radicals, xanthine oxidase and leukocytes appear to be the major sources in clinical disease states.[90,169] Although unproven, the fact that the conversion of xanthine dehydrogenase to xanthine oxidase takes only 10 seconds in intestinal tissue, 8 minutes in cardiac muscle, and about 30 minutes in the liver, spleen, kidneys, and lungs[139] may help to explain the differential relative susceptibility of these organs to ischemia-reperfusion–mediated tissue injury.

Role of Leukocyte-Endothelial Interactions

Although the role of neutrophils in endothelial cell and tissue injury has been appreciated for some time, the recognition that endothelial cells actively participate in the regulation of blood flow,[206] coagulation, and inflammation[159,163,164] is more recent. Endothelial-leukocyte interactions resulting in tissue injury appear to be a common pathway by which a diverse number of initiating factors, including bacteria, endotoxin, cytokines, and ischemia can lead to tissue injury, organ failure, and MOF. For example, endotoxin, TNF, IL-1, and, to a lesser extent, other cytokines induce a change in endothelial phenotype from a noninflammatory to a proinflammatory, procoagulant phenotype.[164] These activated proinflammatory endothelial cells have lost their anticoagulant properties and now express tissue factor and acquire the capacity to bind factor VIIa, and thus activate the extrinsic clotting pathway. Also, these proinflammatory endothelial cells now express surface receptors (endothelial-leukocyte adhesion molecule [ELAM-1] and intracellular cell adhesion molecule [ICAM-1]), which promote leukocyte adherence and secrete leukocyte activating factors such as IL-1, PAF, and IL-8. This shift in endothelial phenotype contributes to the development of focal microvascular thrombosis and leukocyte-mediated endothelial injury. If widespread, this phenomenon can progress to tissue ischemia and ultimately organ failure.

Although the theory is as yet untested clinically, experimental studies using monoclonal antibodies directed at neutrophil (CD 18/CD 11) or endothelial cell (ICAM-1, ELAM-1) adhesion molecules* indicate that shock or ischemia-reperfusion–mediated endothelial cell and organ injury can be ameliorated by preventing neutrophil adhesion to endothelial cells. Thus the experimental evidence generated to date is consistent with the concept that systemic processes, such as ischemia and inflammatory or infectious insults, which injure or activate endothelial cells, can ultimately lead to microvascular-mediated organ injury. However, the clinical efficacy and safety of a therapeutic strategy directed at preventing neutrophil-endothelial adhesion is difficult to determine because the induction of a proinflammatory endothelial cell phenotype is of distinct benefit to the body in controlling and eradicating bacterial invaders. For example, at foci of bacterial invasion, endotoxin or inflammatory cytokines induce expression of endothelial cell ELAM-1, which binds to circulating neutrophils and thus recruits them to the inflammatory site. In this situation blockading activation of endothelial cells and the recruitment of neutrophils may potentiate infection.

Gut Hypothesis of MOF

Although the previously described hypotheses of MOF explain many aspects of this complex syndrome, none explain the clinical paradox of why no infectious focus can be identified either clinically or at autopsy in more than one third of *bacteremic* patients who die of MOF.[87] This clinical observation, plus the recognition that intestinal bacteria can escape from the gut and cause systemic or peritoneal infections, led to the development of the gut hypothesis of MOF[32,63,142] (Figure 16-5). The general phenomenon of loss of the intestinal barrier function, leading to the systemic spread of bacteria and/or endotoxin, has been called *bacterial translocation*.[19,54] Several major lines of evidence support the potential clinical relevance of bacterial translocation. These include (1) a large body of experimental data documenting that intestinal bacteria can escape from the gut and induce both lethal and nonlethal systemic infectious syndromes[4,57,175,217]; (2) clinical studies indicating that loss of the intestinal mucosal barrier to bacteria contributes to the development of systemic infections or MOF, or both[32,83,87,113]; and (3) recent human studies documenting that intestinal permeability is increased during sepsis,[224] shortly after thermal injury,[60] and in healthy volunteers receiving a single dose of endotoxin.[158] Conflicting data are available on whether intestinal barrier function is[174] or is not[149] lost in trauma victims.

*References 14, 39, 101, 146, 153, and 207.

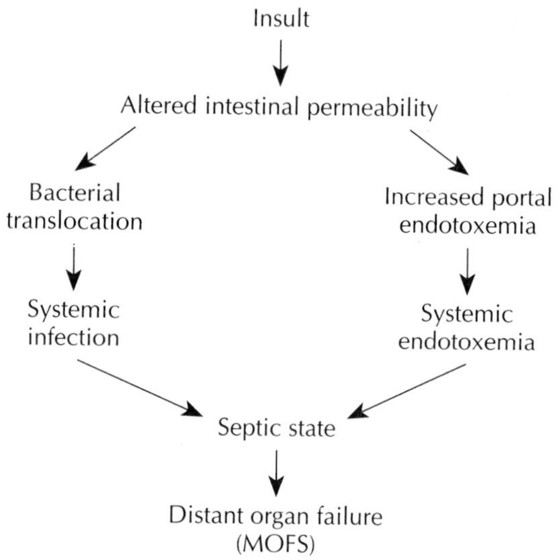

FIGURE 16-5 Schematic illustration of the gut hypothesis of multiple organ failure, in which intestinally derived bacteria or endotoxin or both contribute to organ failure.

In this light the phenomenon of bacterial translocation helps to explain the apparent paradox of why no septic focus can be identified clinically or at autopsy in more than 30% of bacteremic patients, including those who die of clinical sepsis and MOF.[32,87] Furthermore, gut-derived portal or systemic endotoxemia, or both, may serve as a signal that triggers or exacerbates the hypermetabolic and immunoinflammatory responses and thereby contributes to the development of the septic state, even in patients without microbiologic evidence of infection. Thus the general phenomenon of bacterial translocation supplies a mechanism by which patients can develop enteric bacteremias without an identifiable focus of infection or can develop a septic state without microbiologic evidence of infection.

Experimental studies on the pathophysiology of bacterial translocation and gut barrier failure indicate that one or more of three basic pathophysiologic conditions appear to be necessary for bacterial translocation to occur.[57] These are (1) disruption of the ecologic balance of the normal indigenous microflora, resulting in bacterial overgrowth with gram-negative enteric bacilli; (2) impaired immune defenses; and (3) physical or functional loss of the mucosal barrier. These conditions are commonly observed in critically ill or injured patients at risk of developing enteric bacteremias or MOF. These patients frequently have experienced major blood loss or a hypotensive episode, which may injure the gut mucosa; they frequently are immunocompromised, and the antibiotic regimens they receive may disrupt the normal ecology of the gut flora, resulting in impaired resistance to colonization and leading to subsequent colonization with exogenous pathogens.[204] In addition, therapeutic regimens, such as neutralization of gastric acid as prophylaxis for stress ulcer, may result in colonization of the stomach and distal intestine with potential pathogens.[67] Hyperosmolar enteral or parenteral feedings may not only disrupt the normal bacterial ecology of the gut, but may also result in mucosal atrophy and altered intestinal mechanical defenses.[191,219] The hypoalbuminemia and capillary leak syndrome that commonly occur in these patients can result in intestinal edema, impaired jejunoileal peristalsis, intestinal stasis, bacterial overgrowth, and increased intestinal permeability. Thus these and other changes can easily be seen to theoretically promote the failure of the gut barrier to bacteria and endotoxin.

Based on the concept that life-threatening infections can originate from the gut, several groups of investigators have attempted to reduce the incidence of systemic infections in high-risk patients. This was accomplished by oral administration of nonabsorbable antibiotics (most recently in combination with systemic antibiotics) directed against gram-negative, enteric bacilli and *Candida* organisms. This process is called "selective gut decontamination."[194] In selective gut decontamination, the anaerobic intestinal flora is preserved, since loss of the anaerobes is associated with intestinal overgrowth by gram-negative, enteric bacilli, *Pseudomonas* species, and *Candida* organisms. In one regard, the results of these clinical trials are encouraging, since selective gut decontamination reduced the incidence of pneumonia, primary bacteremias, and other infectious complications by about 50%.[168] However, the clinical efficacy of selective decontamination in high-risk patients remains controversial, because most studies have not documented an improvement in survival despite this major reduction in the rate of infection.[168] The failure of selective gut decontamination to improve survival has raised questions about the clinical relevance of gut-origin infections to the outcome in critically ill ICU patients.

One explanation for the failure of selective gut decontamination to improve survival is that this therapy does not address the primary intestinal problem, which is loss of intestinal barrier function. This explanation is based on experimental studies indicating that after hemorrhagic shock, burns, or endotoxin challenge, the physical barrier function of the intestinal mucosa appears to be of primary importance in preventing or limiting the escape of bacteria or endotoxin.[55,56,129] Thus, control of the gut microflora is unlikely to be fully effective in preventing gut-origin septic states in patients with a damaged intestinal mucosa and an activated immunoinflammatory system. The failure of selective gut decontamination to improve survival highlights the complexity and potential interrelationships of the physiologic systems involved in the development of MOF. For example, the observations that burn, shock, and endotoxin-induced mucosal injury and bacterial translocation can be prevented by blocking xanthine oxidase–generated oxidants[55,56,129] illustrates the potential reciprocal relationships between gut barrier failure and microcirculatory failure and helps to explain why therapy directed at just the gut flora may not be fully effective.

Gut-Liver Axis in MOF

There is increasing evidence of a clinically important relationship between the state of intestinal barrier function, Kupffer cell function, the hypermetabolic response, and distant organ injury.[22,42,147,218] Because the hepatic reticuloendothelial system (Kupffer's cells) appears to play a role in the clearance of translocating bacteria or endotoxin from the portal blood, impaired hepatic RES activity could potentiate the systemic effects of gut barrier failure by allowing gut-derived bacteria or endotoxin to reach the systemic circulation. Also, the presence of bacteria and endotoxin in the portal circulation would promote hepatic macrophages to secrete various factors, including cytokines, oxidants, and proteases. These macrophage-derived products may directly injure or alter hepatocyte function and, in concert with other soluble or cellular factors, exacerbate the septic state and lead to impaired functioning of distant organs. In this manner the gut-liver axis may promote or potentiate the development or progression of MOF.

Clinically, the development of established MOF is preceded by a phase of persistent hypermetabolism, which is usually associated with some degree of respiratory dysfunction.[42] Progression of this syndrome is characterized first by a rising bilirubin level and clinical evidence of liver dysfunction, followed by a rising creatinine level and progressive renal failure. The hypothesis that loss of intestinal barrier function and the escape of bacteria and endotoxin induces a hypermetabolic response is consistent with experimental observations that endotoxin infused through the portal vein induces a hypermetabolic response[9] and that immediate enteral feeding blunts the hypermetabolic response after thermal injury.[147] Because immediate enteral feeding also maintains gut mass and prevents the excessive secretion of catabolic hormones, it appears that immediate enteral feeding prevents the expected hypermetabolic response by maintaining intestinal barrier function and consequently preventing the translocation of bacteria or endotoxin into the portal or systemic circulations.[147] Although further studies are needed to verify these findings, loss of intestinal barrier function apparently can induce a hypermetabolic state.

Thus, there is evidence to suggest that changes in intestinal barrier function that lead to excessive portal endotoxemia or bacteremia may contribute to hepatic dysfunction. Similarly, impaired hepatic dysfunction that results in decreased bile flow and systemic endotoxemia could further compromise intestinal barrier function, leading to a further leak of bacteria and endotoxin from the gut. In this way, dysfunction of various aspects of the gut-liver axis could initiate a vicious cycle of hepatic injury and bacterial (endotoxin) translocation. Furthermore, in conditions where RES activity is impaired, intestinal and other antigens may spill over into the systemic circulation. For example, portal and systemic endotoxemia are relatively common in patients with obstructive jaundice, cirrhosis, and acute or chronic liver disease. Also, Border and colleagues[32] have documented the fact that, in victims of blunt trauma, gut-origin bacteremia appears only after clinical evidence of liver dysfunction is apparent. In this fashion, the presence of bacteria and endotoxin in the portal circulation would promote hepatic macrophages to secrete various factors into the systemic circulation that may further impair distant organ function.

Two-Hit Phenomenon in MOF

In some patients the development of MOF can be clearly traced to a single, major, clinically definable insult, but in many patients this is not the case. Instead, the development of MOF follows a series of smaller and occasionally unrecognized clinical events. One way these relatively modest clinical insults could ultimately lead to MOF is if one insult could prime the body's immunoinflammatory systems such that the physiologic response to a subsequent insult is exaggerated. The phrase "two-hit phenomenon in MOF" is used to describe such a biologic phenomenon.

An example of this phenomenon would be a patient who sustains an episode of hypotension. By decreasing blood flow to various organs, this hypotensive episode could lead to a mild (clinically undetectable) focal or global ischemia-reperfusion injury, induce tissue inflammation, and prime resident macrophages and neutrophils. A subsequent insult, such as infection or endotoxemia, would then lead to an amplified tissue response manifest as increased macrophage cytokine production, neutrophil oxidant release, and microcirculatory failure. Because the gut appears to be particularly sensitive to ischemia-reperfusion–mediated injury, early failure of intestinal barrier function may further contribute to this process by amplifying the magnitude of the systemic inflammatory signal. In this light it appears that an inflammatory stimulus may not need to be overwhelming, just persistently greater than the body's ability to clear it, to promote MOF.

In this paradigm, shock leading to tissue ischemia primes the body for an exaggerated response to subsequent insults such as bacteria or endotoxin. Other potential physiologic primers besides tissue ischemia include significant tissue injury or bacteria that induce a systemic inflammatory state. Also, the same factors that prime the body can also serve as secondary or subsequent signals. Since the magnitude of an insult required to prime macrophages or neutrophils is only one tenth to one hundredth the magnitude necessary to activate these cells,[48] it becomes apparent how modest or even mild insults can predispose to MOF. Although unproven clinically, this two-hit hypothesis is consistent with experimental studies. For example, it is well documented experimentally that a large number of physiologic insults, such as shock, mechanical trauma, or burn injury, prime the body to the extent that otherwise nonlethal bacterial or endotoxin challenges become lethal.[62]

A Unifying Approach to the Pathophysiology of MOF

Over the past two decades, several hypotheses have been proposed, rejected, and revised to explain specific aspects of the development of MOF. Although components of many of these hypotheses originally were contradictory, as new insights into the biology of inflammation were generated, it became clear that the gut, macrophage, microcirculatory, and infectious hypotheses of MOF clearly overlap. For example, endotoxin and bacteria, whether tissue-or gut-derived, efficiently induce cytokine secretion by resident tissue macrophages, promote a proinflammatory endothelial cell phenotype, stimulate neutrophil protease and oxidant production, and activate several humoral protein cascades, including the complement and coagulation systems. It is time to begin constructing an integrated picture in which all these systems interact to produce the pathophysiologic processes involved in the evolution of organ injury.

The basic elements of this integrated scheme are an uncontrolled or persistent immunoinflammatory response and tissue hypoxia. A simplified version of this complex process is illustrated in Figure 16-6. The process begins with an initiating clinical event that affects several homeostatic and effector systems. These altered, normally well-controlled homeostatic systems interact to amplify or modulate each other. This integrated hypothesis is illustrated using shock as the initiating insult and gut-derived endotoxin or bacteria as the trigger that initiates the cascade of events that culminates in organ injury.

During periods of shock or tissue hypoperfusion, oxygen delivery to the gut is impaired, resulting in intestinal injury[44] and increased intestinal permeability.[55] Increased permeability of the gut subsequently results in luminal bacteria and endotoxin reaching the portal and systemic circulations,[55,175] where they activate resident macrophages[22,195] and circulating neutrophils,[94,151] as well as several humoral plasma protein cascades.[152] The

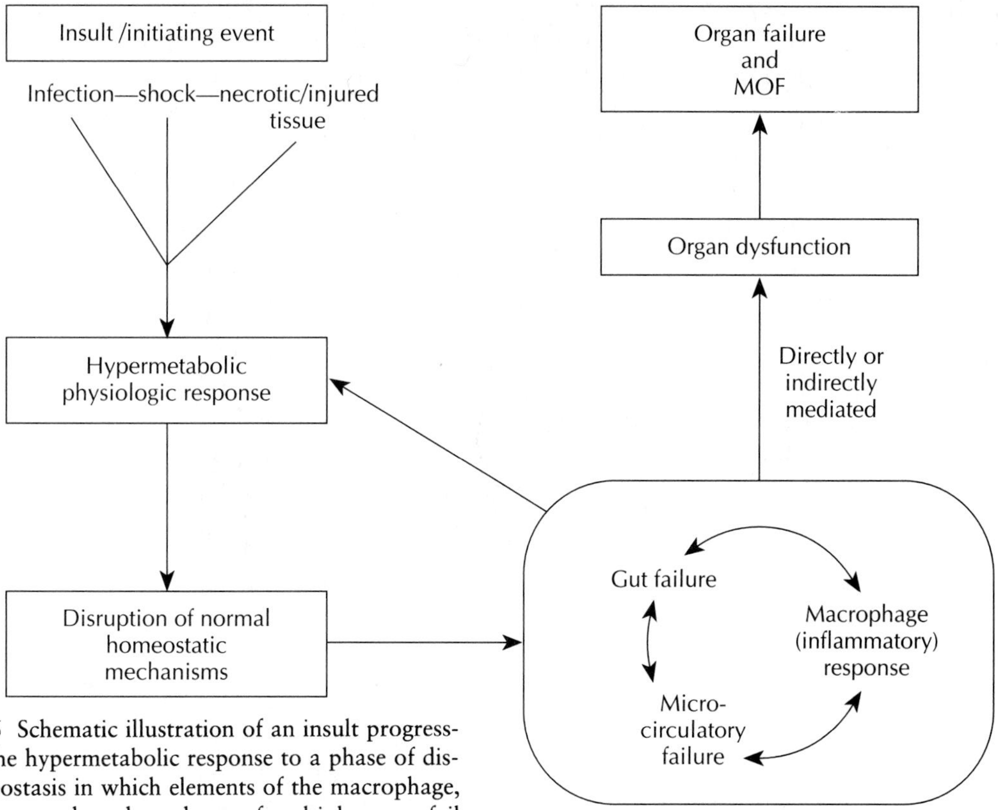

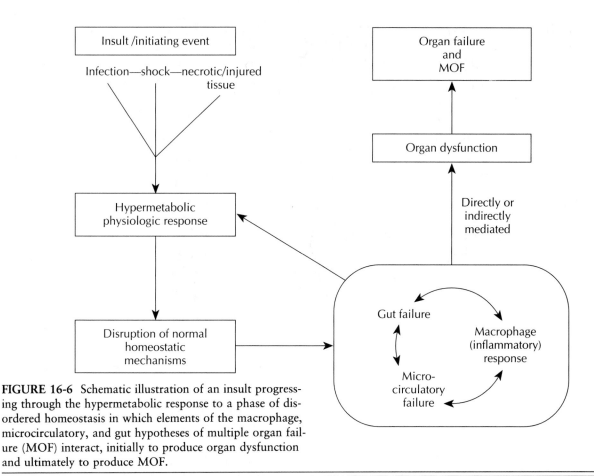

FIGURE 16-6 Schematic illustration of an insult progressing through the hypermetabolic response to a phase of disordered homeostasis in which elements of the macrophage, microcirculatory, and gut hypotheses of multiple organ failure (MOF) interact, initially to produce organ dysfunction and ultimately to produce MOF.

products of these activated leukocytes and protein cascades may in turn further impair oxygen delivery by their effects on the microcirculation,[140,159,165] as well as potentiate the continued translocation of bacteria or their products from the gut by increasing the degree of intestinal permeability.[56,196] Once this cycle is initiated, it can theoretically become self-sustaining. A similar cycle can be initiated in which the initial trigger is at the macrophage or microcirculatory level rather than the gut. For example, infectious or inflammatory states, by activating endogenous inflammatory mediators, can impair tissue oxygen delivery[37,196] and increase intestinal permeability.[130] Therefore, it appears that under the right conditions, the cumulative disruption of several interacting systems may ultimately result in distant organ injury. An important corollary of this multifactorial hypothesis of MOF is that preventing and treating MOF must be both multimodal and directed at the cellular processes involved in organ injury.

THERAPY

The treatment of MOF includes general supportive measures, organ-specific therapy, and therapy directed at the underlying biology of this disease process.

General Supportive Therapy

Prevention

The best treatment for MOF and its potential sequelae is prevention. As early as 1977 it was apparent that intraoperative and postoperative errors in technique or judgment were major contributing factors in more than half of the patients who developed MOF.[68] This observation illustrated the physiologic importance of good surgical technique and mature clinical judgment. Debriding necrotic tissue, controlling bacterial contamination, and preventing the development of postoperative fluid collections (seromas and hematomas) reduce the local environment in which bacteria multiply and improve delivery of the body's antibacterial defense factors to the sites of injury or infection. Early, definitive primary or reoperative surgery to remove necrotic tissue, drain abscesses, or control peritoneal soilage may bolster the body's defenses by reducing the circulating levels of inflammatory mediators and limiting the period of stress.

Prevention takes different forms in different patients. Because infection, shock (inadequate tissue perfusion), or a persistent hyperdynamic, inflammatory state are the major risk factors associated with the development or progression of MOF, it seems clear that our initial therapeutic efforts should be directed at their early treatment or prevention. Nowhere are these concepts more clearly illustrated than in the treatment of the trauma victim. In these patients a policy of aggressive resuscitation and cardiovascular stabilization, plus early fixation of femoral fractures and other injuries, has been documented to reduce the incidence of ARDS and MOF and to shorten the number of days on the ventilator and the time in the ICU.[24,88,115,179] The prevailing physiologic explanation for why immediate treatment of all treatable injuries, including long-bone fractures, prevents the development or progression of pulmonary failure and subsequent MOF is that this approach is the best way to shut down or limit the inflammatory response and thereby restore a more normal physiologic state. In this regard, immediate treatment of all injuries in the trauma patient is similar to the early definitive surgical approach described above for nontrauma patients. Furthermore, in both patient groups this approach not only enhances the body's systemic defenses and limits the hypermetabolic response, it may also limit the incidence or magnitude of gut barrier failure. In this fashion, treatment can prevent development of a vicious cycle of gut failure leading to the translocation of bacteria or endotoxin from the gut to the portal and systemic circulations, where they can fuel the septic response.

In addition to good clinical judgment and immediate surgical treatment of injuries and complications, other factors appear to be important in preventing or limiting distant organ dysfunction. These include optimizing oxygen delivery, providing aggressive nutritional support, and ensuring early diagnosis and treatment of infectious complications (see the box).

PREVENTION OF MULTIPLE ORGAN FAILURE

1. Avoid intraoperative and postoperative errors in technique or judgment.
2. Ensure early, definitive treatment of all treatable injuries.
3. Provide rapid cardiovascular resuscitation.
4. Optimize oxygen delivery.
5. Provide aggressive nutritional support.
6. Ensure early diagnosis and treatment of infectious complications.

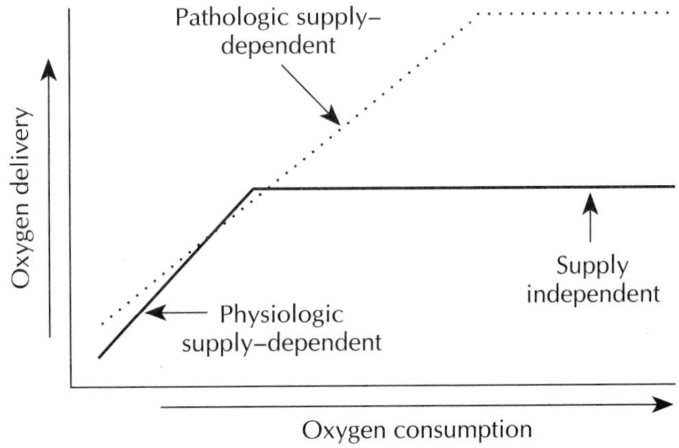

FIGURE 16-7 Under normal physiologic conditions, increases in the rate of oxygen consumption at the tissue level do not depend on increases in oxygen delivery. However, in patients with sepsis, adult respiratory distress syndrome, or multiple organ failure, increases in oxygen consumption become dependent on increases in oxygen delivery. The condition in which supranormal levels of oxygen delivery are required to meet tissue oxygen demands is called *pathologic supply–dependent oxygen consumption.*

Oxygen Delivery

Increasing evidence indicates that inadequate oxygen delivery may play a role in the development or perpetuation of organ dysfunction, injury, or failure.[11,21,186,221] Furthermore, it recently has become clear that a normal or even increased cardiac output does not ensure that sufficient oxygen is being delivered to the tissues to meet their metabolic needs.[11,21,186,221]

Because oxygen is not stored in the tissues, oxidative metabolism depends on a continuous delivery of adequate amounts of oxygen to the tissues. Because oxygen delivery to the tissues ordinarily greatly exceeds oxygen demands, tissue oxygen uptake increases as metabolic demands increase. Under normal circumstances even moderate decreases in oxygen delivery can be compensated for by an increase in the amount of oxygen extracted from the blood (Figure 16-7). Consequently, oxygen delivery must be significantly reduced to become a limiting factor in tissue metabolism. Thus, during periods of hypermetabolism, when tissue oxygen demands increase, the amount of oxygen extracted increases concomitantly to match the higher level of metabolic demand. The term "supply-independent oxygen consumption" is used to describe this normal physiologic relationship, in which oxygen consumption is independent of oxygen delivery. However, a point is reached where the maximum ability of the tissues to extract oxygen from the bloodstream is exceeded. At this point, further increases in tissue oxygen consumption become dependent on an increase in oxygen delivery, and oxygen delivery is now "supply dependent." If oxygen delivery does not increase sufficiently to meet the increased oxygen demands, a shift from oxidative to anaerobic metabolism occurs, resulting in lactic acidosis. Prolonged failure to meet the oxygen needs of the tissue eventually leads to cellular death and organ dysfunction. Although under most conditions oxygen consumption is not supply dependent, there is evidence that this physiologic situation changes at some point in patients who develop ARDS or MOF.

A common clinical example of the physiology of supply-dependent oxygen delivery is hemorrhagic shock, in which the loss of intravascular volume leads to decreased cardiac output and hence inadequate tissue perfusion. Although less obvious clinically, oxygen delivery appears to be supply dependent in patients with sepsis, ARDS, or MOF, even when cardiac output and total body oxygen delivery are above normal.[11,21,186,221] This relative failure of oxygen delivery is called "pathologic supply-dependent oxygen delivery" (see Figure 16-7). The mechanisms explaining why these hypermetabolic patients develop pathologic supply-dependent oxygen delivery are both poorly understood and controversial. However, most of the evidence suggests that this relative failure of oxygen delivery is due to a maldistribution of perfusion at both the organ and microcirculatory levels.[37,177] In this situation, even though the patient has a hyperdynamic circulatory response (increased cardiac output), some tissues are overperfused while others are underperfused, with the net result being patchy areas of organ injury. Although most investigators accept this hypothesis as being the most likely explanation for pathologic supply-dependent oxygen delivery, some contradictory evidence suggests that organ dysfunction is not due to impaired oxygen delivery and cellular hypoxia per se but, instead, is due to an uncoupling of mitochondrial oxidative phosphorylation, leading to impaired ATP production and hence cellular injury.[143,189]

Nonetheless, since most of the evidence indicates that oxygen delivery becomes supply dependent at some point in patients with ARDS or MOF[11,96,221] and that, in this situation, the delivery of supranormal amounts of oxygen improves survival,[21,96,185,186] it appears wise to optimize oxygen delivery in all high-risk patients. The best way to ensure that oxygen consumption is not supply dependent is to take serial measurements of oxygen consumption as oxygen delivery is increased.[60,130,140] Extensive studies in high-risk surgical patients show that survival can be improved by maintaining the cardiac index at or above 4.5 L/min/m^2, oxygen delivery at 600 ml/min/m^2, and oxygen consumption at 170 ml/min/m^2.[21,185,186] Methods of improving oxygen delivery are discussed in greater detail later in this chapter.

Nutritional Support

The role of total body and organ-specific nutritional support in preventing and treating MOF has received increasing attention over the past decade. It is now well recognized that septic or MOF patients pass through a continuum of metabolic alterations as they progress from uncomplicated trauma through the sepsis syndrome to frank MOF, with the end result being a hyperglycemic, hypermetabolic, immunocompromised catabolic patient with marked muscle wasting and organ failure. In contrast to an unstressed individual whose intermediary metabolism is primarily under neuroendocrine control, a septic patient has a hypermetabolic response whose mediators include proinflammatory factors, such as the macrophage products IL-1, IL-6, and TNF, as well as the traditional neuroendocrine mediators.[118] One practical consequence of this metabolic information is the realization that the appropriate nutritional approach to a patient with sepsis or MOF must differ from that for healthy individuals.

To provide optimal nutritional support, it is necessary to calculate the patient's estimated nutritional needs, to document the amount of nutritional support being administered, and to verify that the level of calculated nutritional support is meeting the patient's actual requirements.[20] Although controversy still exists over the optimal nutrient mix for the individual patient, it is clear that patients with or at risk of developing MOF require higher levels of energetic substrates (calories) and protein. Although both the amount of calories and protein required to meet the metabolic demands of these patients are increased, relatively more protein than calories is required.[20] Thus, the optimal nonprotein calorie/nitrogen ratio is lower in a critically ill patient (100:1) than in a healthy individual (150:1), and the amount of protein administered daily is higher (1.5 to 2.5 g/kg versus 1 g/kg).

The route of nutrient delivery also seems to be important, because clinical and experimental evidence indicates that enteral alimentation is physiologically superior to parenteral alimentation. This beneficial role of enteral feeding has received increasing attention since it was first shown that animals fed enterally survive a septic insult better than animals fed an identical diet parenterally.[120] Also, early enteral feeding has been experimentally documented to bolster antibacterial body defenses,[120] blunt the hypermetabolic response to trauma, [147] maintain mucosal mass and barrier function, and limit or prevent disruption of the normal gut microflora.[58,191,219]

Clinically, the ability of high-protein enteral feedings to improve survival was conclusively shown in a prospective, randomized trial of burned children.[5] In this study, burned children were randomized to receive their nutritional support either parenterally or enterally. The enterally fed children had less impairment of their systemic immune defenses, fewer infections, and an increased survival rate compared to the parenterally fed children. Similarly, two prospective, randomized clinical trials have documented that enterally fed trauma victims had fewer infectious complications than parenterally fed patients.[121,150] The results of one of these studies is illustrated in Table 16-4. In contrast to these clinical trials, Cerra and coworkers[41] did not find that enteral feeding prevented MOF in patients with sepsis. However, be-

TABLE 16-4 SEPTIC MORBIDITY

SEPSIS	ENTERAL FEEDING	TOTAL PARENTERAL NUTRITION	LEVEL OF STATISTICAL SIGNIFICANCE
Pneumonia	6/51 (11.8%)	14/45 (31%)	<.02
Intra-abdominal abscess	1/51 (1.9%)	6/45 (13.3%)	<.04
Empyema	1/51 (1.9%)	4/45 (9%)	NS
Line sepsis	1/51 (1.9%)	6/45 (13.3%)	<.05
Fasciitis/dehiscence	3/51 (5.9%)	4/45 (8.9%)	NS
Abscesses (intra-abdominal and/or empyema)	2/51 (3.9%)	8/45 (17.8%)	<.03
Pneumonia and/or abscesses	8/51 (13.7%)	17/45 (37.8%)	<.02
Pneumonia, abscesses, and/or line sepsis	9/51 (15.7%)	18/45 (40%)	<.02

From Kudsk KA et al: *Ann Surg* 215:503, 1992.

cause the patients in this study did not receive enteral feedings until an average of 5 days after the onset of their illness, the enteral feedings appeared to have been started too late to be effective.

The exact reasons why enteral feedings appear physiologically superior to parenteral feedings in maintaining intestinal barrier function, mucosal mass, and body immune function are not fully known. However, it appears that maintaining mucosal mass and perhaps mucosal integrity requires specific nutrients, such as glutamine,[148,190] as well as the presence of intraluminal bulk fiber.[191] Wilmore and colleagues[219] and Souba and coworkers,[190] as well as others, have stressed the importance of glutamine as the major respiratory fuel of intestinal enterocytes and have documented that administering glutamine protects the intestinal mucosa from injury in a number of experimental models. Thus, gut barrier failure may occur in critically ill patients at least partly because current methods of parenteral nutrition do not fully support intestinal growth, structure, and function. In fact, it has recently been documented that parenterally fed human volunteers manifest a greater splanchnic and systemic cytokine and metabolic response to parenteral endotoxin than enterally fed volunteers.[80] The results of this study and the previously described human and animal studies indicate that the route by which patients are fed may influence the immunoinflammatory and metabolic response to injury, as well as the incidence of infectious complications, and may modulate clinical outcome. Thus, one hypothesis to explain the observation that enteral feeding appears clinically superior to parenteral feeding is that parenteral feeding predisposes to an exaggerated cytokine response due to the loss of intestinal barrier function.

Although it frequently is impossible to administer all the required nutrients enterally, the gut should be used to deliver at least a portion of the patient's needs whenever possible. Practically, this means that most critically ill patients, at some time, will be receiving nutrients by both enteral and parenteral routes. Although the optimal means of enteral feeding is not known, it currently is my practice to administer 60 ml of a high-protein enteral diet every 2 hours to all high-risk patients.[141] Because gastric motility may be impaired in these patients, the stomach is aspirated every 2 hours just before the enteral feeding. In this way, the risk of aspiration of gastric contents is significantly reduced. The enteral feedings are begun in nonoperative patients as soon as they have been stabilized and in postoperative patients in the immediate postoperative period. Using this approach, the presence of an ileus is not an absolute contraindication to enteral feeding, and stress ulcer prophylaxis is not necessary.[141]

In summary, since loss of intestinal barrier function can lead to the translocation of bacteria and endotoxin which can fuel the septic response, ways are needed to prevent, limit, or speed the repair of acquired intestinal mucosal injury that frequently occurs after shock, sepsis, or trauma. For this reason investigations are underway to test the ability of specific nutrients, such as glutamine[190,219] or short-chain fatty acids,[172] growth factors,[112] trophic gut hormones,[71,123] and intraluminal bulk,[191] as well as immediate enteral feeding, to prevent or limit gut atrophy or injury. Thus, in the future, the optimal therapy to maintain or restore intestinal mucosal structure and function may be a combination of specific enterally administered nutrients and mucosal trophic factors. Also, since growth hormone has been documented to preserve lean body mass in both healthy volunteers and postoperative patients fed hypocaloric diets,[114,133] its use may improve total body nitrogen balance in a hypermetabolic patient. In fact, as we learn more about the basic biology of the metabolic response to injury, it appears more likely that specific nutrients will be used to modulate the inflammatory and immune systems to the advantage of the patient.[43,220] Until then, although it frequently is impossible to administer all the required nutrients enterally, the gut should be used as soon as possible to deliver at least a portion of the patient's nutritional needs.[141]

Infection and the Body

Because infection appears to be a primary predisposing factor in up to two thirds of the patients who develop ARDS or MOF, this is an area of major importance. The development of infection requires both a susceptible host and the presence of a bacterial or fungal pathogen. Thus, therapeutic maneuvers must be directed not just toward eradicating invading microorganisms, but also toward mechanisms to increase the body's resistance to infection. Thus immunomodulation begins in the emergency room by restoring intravascular volume and improving oxygen delivery to the tissues; moves to the operating room, where the injuries or disease processes are definitively treated and necrotic tissue is removed; and continues in the critical care unit with aggressive nutritional and organ-directed support.

Although the immune state of the individual patient can be significantly modified by factors such as age, nutritional state, and premorbid physiologic status, it is now generally accepted that the extent of injury is directly related to the magnitude of immunosuppression.[59] This concept is best illustrated in burn and trauma victims, where (1) the risk of infectious complications increases as the magnitude of the injury increases; and (2) the ability to survive an infectious complication is inversely related to the magnitude of the insult. For many years it has been known that patients who sustain major injuries develop multiple defects in their immune systems. These include alterations in immunoglobulin levels, changes in the concentrations and activities of components of both the classic and alternate complement pathways, reduced circulating plasma fibronectin, depressed serum opsonic activity, and impairment or dysregulation of macrophage, lymphocyte, and neutrophil function, as well as reduced RES activity.[59]

Although injury is clearly associated with multiple defects in the humoral and cellular components of the nonspecific inflammatory and the specific immune systems, no consensus has been reached on the prognostic or clinical significance of many of these immune defects. This confusion is compounded by the fact that different laboratories employ different methods to measure specific immune parameters in patients often treated with different clinical regimens. Perhaps of greater significance is the fact that, in many studies, only one immunologic variable is measured. Since immune defects do not occur in isolation, it is difficult to determine whether a particular abnormality is a primary event of clinical importance or is secondary to another, unmeasured, abnormality. The profile on which many of the immunologic predictors of infection and death have been based is schematically illustrated in Figure 16-8. It can be seen that the immunologic parameter measured initially decreases post injury or insult. In patients who do not survive, it remains depressed, whereas in survivors it returns to normal or supranormal levels. However, studies of this kind represent only associations and should not be interpreted as showing cause-and-effect relationships.

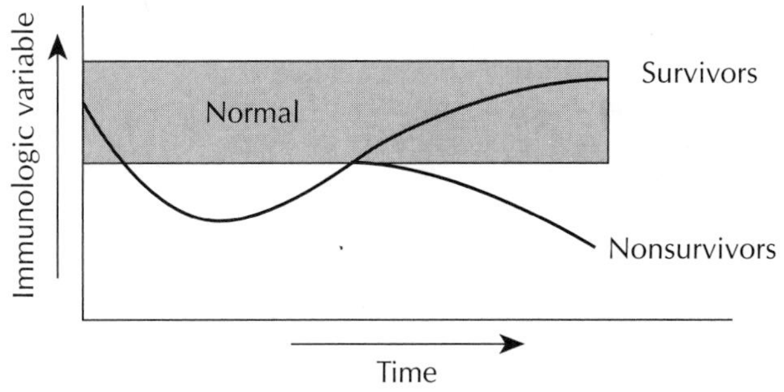

FIGURE 16-8 Schematic illustration of the biphasic nature of many of the elements of the host's immune and antibacterial defense systems, in which an initial decrease in function is followed by recovery in survivors or persistant or recurrent depression in patients who do not survive.

The extensive observations that the immune system is depressed in critically ill patients have led to interest in developing immunotherapeutic approaches to bolster the body's antibacterial defense systems. The use of agents to prevent infections has a long history, the most famous of these early studies being the use of cowpox as a vaccine by Jenner in 1798 to prevent the development of smallpox. Although active immunization with vaccines has been effective in preventing certain infections, such as tetanus, rabies, and polio, the use of vaccines directed against common pathogens, such as the enteric bacilli or *Pseudomonas* organisms, has been largely unsuccessful in critically ill patients. The reason for this lack of success is the antigenic diversity of these microorganisms and the need for the body to be able to respond immunologically to the administered antigen. Likewise, based on the results of a controlled, double-blind prospective study of the passive administration of intravenous gamma-globulins to burn patients,[215] nonspecific passive immunization also does not appear to prevent infection. In contrast to these studies, administration of an antibody made in humans to the mutant J5 strain of *Escherichia coli* was found to reduce the mortality rate of patients with severe gram-negative infections.[222] Similar results were found in burn patients, where the use of hyperimmune anti-*Pseudomonas* gamma-globulin reduced the mortality rate from *Pseudomonas* infections.[116] Although these early and two subsequent clinical trials using anti-endotoxin monoclonal antibodies were encouraging,[92,223] their clinical efficacy remains unproved.

Interest also has focused on other modalities, such as use of immunologically active compounds, known as biologic response modifiers. Compounds altering immune responses were formerly called immunoadjuvants, immunopotentiators, or immunomodulators. These

TABLE 16-5 BIOLOGIC RESPONSE MODIFIERS (BRMs)

BRM*	ACTIONS
Interleukin-1	T cell activator
Interleukin-2	Augments T cell proliferation and natural killer (NK) cell cytoxicity
Interleukin-6	B cell growth factor and hepatocyte stimulator
Interferons	Augment PMN, macrophage, and B and T cell function
Colony-stimulating factors	Augment differentiation and function of PMNs and macrophages
Thymopentin	Stimulates T cell proliferation and activates NK cells
Levamisole	Enhances PMN, macrophage, and T cell function
Glucan	Activates PMNs, macrophages, and T cells
Corynebacterium parvum	Stimulates PMNs, macrophages, and T cells
Muramyl dipeptide	Activates PMN, macrophages, B cells, and NK cells

*This is only a partial list of BRMs, and only selected major actions of each are listed.

terms have been replaced by the more descriptive term *biologic response modifier* (BRM). A partial list of these compounds and their mechanisms of action are outlined in Table 16-5. Because almost all of these compounds have several diverse immunologic effects, they may function as stimulatory or suppressive agents, based on the dosage of the agent administered and the exact immune function measured. Although these BRMs have all been documented to be effective in experimental models, the results of published clinical series have not been as encouraging. For example, although thymopentin (TP-5) reduced infectious mortality in animal studies, a controlled clinical trial of TP-5 in seriously burned patients failed to show any benefit.[216] The explanation for the failure of TP-5 may be that TP-5's primary effect is on cell-mediated immunity, and cell-mediated immunity is not critical in controlling acute bacterial infections. Instead, cell-mediated immunity is important in infections caused by slow-growing intracellular bacteria, fungi, and viruses, infective agents that are not commonly seen in these patients.

Human and animal studies have documented a clear association between impaired neutrophil and RES function and infection. Because these phagocytic defenses are the body's primary defense against the bacteria that commonly cause infections in these patients, agents that bolster these systems are more likely to reduce the incidence of infection than agents that primarily affect cell-mediated immunity. In this regard, BRMs, such as the colony-stimulating factors or glucan, which increase macrophage and neutrophil bactericidal activity, appear to be potentially beneficial agents. Currently, human clinical trials with these agents are in progress.

Another option under investigation is the combined use of BRMs with antibiotics, the concept being that the BRM will function synergistically with the antibiotic by bolstering the body's intrinsic antibacterial defense systems. However, the administration of BRMs in a patient with endotoxemia or an uncontrolled inflammatory state is not without risk because, experimentally, certain BRMs have been documented to predispose the body to endotoxic shock. Thus the usefulness of this approach must await clinical studies.

One of the most difficult decisions to make in a patient with MOF is whether and when to begin antibiotic therapy. This decision is made more difficult by the fact that only some of the patients who appear clinically septic do in fact have infections. Thus the first step in the patient suspected of being infected is a thorough search for the focus of infection and an attempt to obtain microbiologic verification of an underlying infectious process. When an infection is found, many of these patients require drainage or surgery, in addition to antibiotics, to control the infectious process. Examples of patients requiring mechanical treatment of their infections range from an intubated patient with suppurative sinusitis to a patient with a perforated viscus or leaking anastomosis. When a site of infection is found, the initial empiric antibiotic regimen chosen is based on the results of a Gram's stain.

If there is no definitive microbiologic evidence of infection, the decision on when and which antibiotics to use must be made on a patient-by-patient basis. If antibiotics are used, the choice of agents is based primarily on the patient's clinical status, specific disease processes, and the suspected pathogens. Depending on the patient's clinical response and the results of cultures, the empirically chosen antibiotic regimen may be left unchanged or modified.

Optimal antibiotic therapy requires not just that the antibiotics chosen be effective against the invading bacteria, but also that the tissue and serum levels be high enough. To achieve effective antibiotic levels, administration of higher than normal doses of antibiotics may be required for two reasons.[125] First, the volume of antibiotic distribution may be greatly increased as a result of increased capillary permeability. Second, because these patients are hypermetabolic, the half-life of the administered antibiotics frequently is reduced.

Prospective, randomized studies have made it clear that certain therapeutic modalities are not beneficial in the treatment of patients with severe infections or septic shock. These include the opioid antagonist naloxone,[65] plasma fibronectin repletion,[132] and steroids.[27,208] Not only are steroids not indicated in the treatment of septic shock, because they do not improve survival, in some patient subgroups (those with renal failure), steroid therapy actually increases mortality.

In summary, despite the development of successive

generations of more powerful antibiotics, infection remains a common cause of death. This fact is not surprising, because it is of little importance which organism is causing the infection if the patient's intrinsic antibacterial defenses cannot respond. Realization of the limits of antibiotic therapy has prompted the study of the effects of injury on the body's immune and inflammatory systems and the search for ways to bolster these failing systems, thereby improving survival.

Role of Empiric Laparotomy in Patients with MOF

A question that continues to plague clinicians is the role of empiric laparotomy in a patient with MOF. The concept that MOF is the external expression of an occult infectious focus led to a general belief that the presence of MOF without an identifiable focus of infection is an indication for an empiric laparotomy. However, as more patients with MOF without clinical or radiographic evidence of intra-abdominal sepsis were empirically explored, it became obvious that a large number of these patients did not have an intra-abdominal infectious process.[35,104] The beneficial role of empiric laparotomy was further called into question by clinical studies documenting that identification and treatment of occult intra-abdominal septic foci in patients with *established* MOF did not consistently improve survival.[35,104,156] Thus, with the development of more sophisticated and reliable noninvasive imaging techniques, MOF does not require laparotomy if there is no clinical or radiographic evidence suggesting intra-abdominal disease. This is especially true when an alternative focus of infection has been identified, such as pneumonia.

Nonetheless, in certain patient groups intra-abdominal infectious processes are especially likely to be the cause of MOF. These include patients who have undergone elective or emergency abdominal surgery, especially when "sepsis" precedes pulmonary failure and/or MOF syndrome evolves very rapidly.[68,81,148] In contrast, when ARDS is the first manifestation of MOF and precedes the septic response, occult intra-abdominal infection is less common. The decision whether to operate is even more difficult in a patient with a gram-negative enteric bacteremia without an identifiable focus of infection. Although bacteremia in this circumstance clearly points to the gut microflora as the source of invading bacteria, it has become clear that in some circumstances bacteremia actually may be an expression of failed body defenses rather than infection in the traditional sense. The realization that loss of intestinal barrier function and the subsequent escape (translocation) of bacteria from the gut to the systemic circulation can occur[63] has helped explain the apparent paradox of why no septic focus could be identified clinically or at autopsy in more than 30% of bacteremic patients, including those who died of clinical sepsis and MOF.[32,87]

Organ-Directed Therapy

One of the difficulties in treating patients with MOF is that dysfunction of one organ frequently contributes to the failure of other organs. Although the pathophysiologic assessment and treatment of specific organ systems is discussed individually in this section, in reality none of the organ systems function in isolation. Because injury to one organ may result in injury to or dysfunction of other organs, supporting one organ may help to prevent or mitigate the failure of other organ systems.

Cardiovascular System

Because a hyperdynamic circulation with increased cardiac output is one characteristic of MOF, less attention has been focused on the heart than other organs. However, it is now recognized that normal or even increased cardiac output does not ensure that oxygen delivery to the individual organs is sufficient to meet their metabolic requirements. That is, restoring cardiovascular (microcirculatory) function to normal levels may not be enough to achieve optimal microcirculatory nutrient organ blood flow and oxygen delivery. As previously discussed (see Figure 16-7), this failure is related at least partly to the fact that oxygen consumption becomes supply dependent in patients with MOF. Consequently, therapy directed at increasing oxygen delivery to supranormal levels to optimize oxygen consumption at the tissue level is of major clinical importance.

The three major factors that influence oxygen delivery are cardiac output, arterial oxygen saturation, and the level of hemoglobin. Therefore each of these variables should be optimized in high-risk patients and patients with established MOF (see the box on p. 630). Consequently, sufficient fluids should be administered to maintain a clinically optimal preload and hence cardiac output. When cardiac output cannot be maintained at sufficient levels with fluid therapy, cardiotonic drugs are added to increase contractility. In a volume-resuscitated patient, dobutamine currently is generally used as the initial drug of choice. If dobutamine is not effective, norepinephrine may be tried. However, because of their peripheral vasoconstrictive effects, norepinephrine or high-dose dobutamine may impair mesenteric and renal blood flow. Consequently, low-dose dopamine should be administered concomitantly with these vasoactive agents to maintain renal and mesenteric perfusion. It is important to prevent arterial hypoxemia and to maintain arterial oxygen saturation (PaO_2) at 90% or higher, and mechanical ventilation may be required to achieve this. Because the increased shunting of blood across the pulmonary circulation secondary to ventilation-perfusion mismatches is a major cause of hypoxia in patients with ARDS or MOF, continuous positive airway pressure (CPAP) or positive end-expiratory pressure (PEEP) frequently is used to recruit collapsed alveoli and thereby increase the functional residual capacity of the lungs and

REGIMEN FOR IMPROVING OR MAINTAINING OXYGEN DELIVERY

Oxygen delivery = (Cardiac output) × (Oxygen saturation) × (Oxygen-carrying capacity)
Cardiac output
- Provide fluids to maintain optimal preload (PAWP 15 to 18 mm Hg)
- Administer inotropic agents dobutamine or norepinephrine when required to maintain cardiac index ≥4.5 L/min/m²*

Oxygen saturation (Pa_{O_2})
- Maintain arterial oxygen saturation at 90% or higher (Pa_{O_2} ≥60 torr)
- Administer supplemental oxygen via mask or ventilator
- Use CPAP or PEEP to decrease ventilation-perfusion (V/P) mismatches

Oxygen-carrying capacity
- Maintain hemoglobin at 10-12 g/dl

PAWP, Pulmonary artery wedge pressure; *CPAP*, continuous positive airway pressure; *PEEP*, positive end-expiratory pressure.
*Concomitant low-dose dopamine therapy may be required to maintain renal and mesenteric perfusion.

reduce the shunt fraction. Also, since oxygen-carrying capacity is directly related to the hemoglobin level, hemoglobin levels should be maintained at 10 to 12 g/dl. It is important to remember that *once oxygen consumption becomes supply dependent, a decrease in any one of these three variables must be compensated for by an increase in the other two.* For example, a 25% decrease in the oxygen saturation or hemoglobin level requires a compensatory 25% increase in the cardiac output.

The only way to verify that oxygen consumption is not supply dependent is to take serial direct measurements of oxygen consumption as oxygen delivery is increased.[11,96,221] Extensive studies in high-risk surgical patients have demonstrated that survival can be improved by maintaining the cardiac index at or above 4.5 L/min/m^2, oxygen delivery at 600 ml/min/m^2, and oxygen consumption at 170 ml/min/m^2.[21,185,186] The physiologic reason that these supranormal levels of cardiac output and oxygen delivery are required to optimize tissue oxygen consumption appears to be related to the fact that the ability of the tissues to extract oxygen is decreased at a time when the metabolic demands are increased. Finally, it is important to note that the patient's increased oxygen demands can be met by maneuvers directed at decreasing oxygen needs as well as by therapy aimed at increasing oxygen delivery. For example, by decreasing the work of breathing, controlling fever, and preventing overfeeding, oxygen demands can be reduced, thereby improving the relationship between oxygen delivery and oxygen consumption.

Pulmonary System

Increased microvascular permeability that results in hypoxia, atelectasis, and increased pulmonary shunting are the principal pathophysiologic hallmarks of ARDS.[66] Since Ashbaugh and colleagues[10] first described ARDS in a small group of patients in 1967, this syndrome has grown to become one of the commonest clinical problems in the ICU. Currently the mortality rate of patients with ARDS is 50% to 60%, and reaches 90% with underlying disease, sepsis, or other organ failure. With few exceptions ARDS appears to be a pulmonary response to a systemic inflammatory or septic state, which is initiated and perpetuated by inflammatory mediators.[66] The triggers that induce this systemic state are not limited to infection and include the same factors that initiate MOF. Because the exact mediators responsible for lung injury and the development of ARDS are not known, therapy in a patient at increased risk of developing ARDS is directed primarily toward preventing or limiting pulmonary injury. Once ARDS has occurred, therapy is principally supportive. Therefore prevention is a key therapeutic goal. This strategy has been successful in reducing the incidence of ARDS and improving survival in victims of multiple trauma.[32] In these patients, prophylactic therapy includes early, definitive treatment of all injuries, with surgical stabilization of unstable bony injuries; assisted mechanical ventilation with PEEP before respiratory failure occurs; early enteral nutritional support; early ambulation; and limited use of sedatives.

Once ARDS is established, therapeutic options are limited to continuing prophylactic measures plus therapy directed at supporting pulmonary function, as well as a search for treatable pulmonary or nonpulmonary contributing factors, such as infection.[173] Unfortunately, the survival rate of patients with *established* ARDS has not improved during the past 20 years despite numerous technical advances in ventilatory support. Currently the mortality rate of this patient group remains above 50%,[66,148] a value essentially unchanged from Ashbaugh and coworkers' original report.[10] Nonetheless, if a hypoxic patient cannot be adequately ventilated with standard ventilator settings plus PEEP, high-frequency jet ventilation[111] or pressure-controlled inverse ratio ventilation[162] may be helpful. Although modified techniques of ventilatory management have been used to minimize pulmonary damage from increased levels of PEEP and high concentrations of inspired oxygen, neither high-frequency positive pressure ventilation nor high-frequency jet ventilation have been documented as superior to conventional ventilatory techniques.[107,214] Whether the use of pressure-controlled inverse ratio ventilation to limit pulmonary barotrauma will be associated with improved survival has yet to be established.[162] Similarly, although initial studies suggested that extracorporeal membrane oxygenation (ECMO) improved survival in patients dying of refractory ARDS,[85] subsequent studies have not verified its clinical usefulness.[103]

A number of vasoactive agents have been demonstrated to improve pulmonary function in experimental models of lung injury[66]; however, with the exception of prostaglandin E_1 (PGE_1), limited experience with these agents is available in humans. In two prospective, randomized trials, PGE_1 was documented to improve pulmonary function[106,187] and in one study to improve survival.[106] However, a recent multi-institutional trial has called into question the ultimate clinical effectiveness of PGE_1, because although it improved pulmonary function and oxygen delivery in patients with established ARDS, it did not improve survival.[28] More information is required, especially in patients with early ARDS, to determine the role of PGE_1 in routine clinical care. PGE_1 appears to exert its beneficial physiologic effects by selectively vasodilating the vasoconstricted pulmonary circulation, thereby improving arterial oxygenation, cardiac output, and hence oxygen delivery.

The decision on when to use empiric antibiotic therapy in patients with ARDS who are suspected of having pulmonary or systemic infections is both complicated and controversial. Because ARDS and pneumonitis frequently are radiographically indistinguishable, and because the upper airways of patients with ARDS frequently are colonized with potential pathogens, it often is difficult to accurately diagnose a pulmonary infectious process in an ARDS patient. Currently the best approach to this difficult problem is to obtain a bronchoscopically directed culture and to treat the patient according to the results of the Gram's stain and culture.

Gastrointestinal and Hepatic Systems

The transition from clinical hypermetabolism to frank MOF is accompanied by failure of hepatic metabolic function[42] and is associated with disturbances in normal intestinal functions. Gut failure can take many forms in these patients, including stress ulcers, ileus, intolerance to enteral feeding, and loss of barrier function. Once liver dysfunction or gut failure has occurred, no specific agents are available that can selectively restore function in these organs to normal. Therefore therapy must be directed at preventing or limiting organ dysfunction or injury. The principles of organ support that were discussed previously (rapid hemodynamic stabilization, optimizing oxygen delivery, nutritional support, and early treatment of injuries and infection) apply to the gut-liver axis as well as other organs.

Gastrointestinal bleeding and ileus are well-recognized complications in critically ill patients. Traditionally, therapeutic goals have centered on preventing stress-induced bleeding. However, the gastrointestinal tract is now recognized to have important endocrine, immunologic, metabolic, and barrier functions in addition to its traditional role in digestion and nutrient absorption. Therefore gastrointestinal-directed therapy must include more than prophylaxis of stress bleeding and nasogastric decompression during periods of ileus. This concept is supported by several studies documenting that, despite their ability to reduce the incidence of stress bleeding, antacids and histamine (H_2) blockers have not improved survival.[49] For example, in one study of 200 patients on ventilators,[50] the mortality rate of patients treated prophylactically with cimetidine was significantly higher than those who did not receive cimetidine. Antacids and H_2 blockers do not improve survival in intubated patients apparently because they promote the development of nosocomial pneumonia; that is, by alkalinizing the stomach, these drugs allow gastric and upper aerodigestive bacterial colonization with potential pathogens, thereby promoting the development of pneumonia. Consequently, the realization that using these drugs to prevent stress-induced bleeding is associated with an increased incidence of pneumonia in ventilator-dependent patients has resulted in a re-evaluation of the risk-benefit ratio of gastric alkalinization.

Since sucralfate prevents stress bleeding and does not impair the gastric acid barrier or promote bacterial overgrowth of the upper gastrointestinal tract, its use should not predispose to the development of pneumonia. This assumption is supported by several prospective, randomized trials, which documented that sucralfate is as effective as antacids or H_2 blockers in preventing stress-induced bleeding while minimizing the risk of pneumonia.[67,203] Thus, at this time, if stress ulcer prophylaxis is used, sucralfate appears to be the drug of choice. However, there is evidence that stress ulcer prophylaxis can be achieved without drugs if the gut is fed.[141] Furthermore, as was discussed earlier, feeding the gut enterally may also improve intestinal barrier function and maintain a more normal intestinal microflora.

The use of enterally administered and hypopharyngeally applied nonabsorbable antibiotics to reduce the incidence of nosocomial pneumonia and gut-origin bacteremias has been an intense area of interest since 1984, when Stoutenbeek and colleagues[194] documented that this approach reduced the incidence of infections in trauma victims. Since then, selective antibiotic gut decontamination has been prospectively tested and documented to reduce the incidence of nosocomial infections by about 50% in several patient groups.[97] However, although this antibiotic regimen reduces the incidence of infections and even septic mortality, it has not been documented to increase survival.[97] Consequently, routine clinical use appears premature.

Because of the potential relationship between loss of intestinal barrier function and the subsequent systemic spread of intestinal bacteria or endotoxin, or both, preserving intestinal structure and function may be important in preventing the development or progression of MOF. Although currently there is no established therapy to maintain or augment barrier function, future options involve development of therapeutic approaches to prevent, limit, or speed the repair of intestinal mucosal injury that may occur after shock, sepsis, or trauma. These future options also include enteral delivery of nutrients, administration of growth factors, and use of agents to prevent oxidant-mediated intestinal injury. Nonintestinal factors may also impair gut function and lead to intestinally mediated distant organ dysfunction. Hypotension, hemodynamic instability, or vasoactive agents that decrease intestinal perfusion may promote bacterial translocation or systemic endotoxemia by increasing intestinal permeability. Systemic insults or drugs that decrease intestinal motility may be deleterious, since ileus is associated with bacterial overgrowth and loss of resistance to colonization. Uncontrolled distant infections, such as pneumonia, or endotoxemia may alter intestinal permeability and promote translocation of bacteria or endotoxin from the gut. Thus, attention should be paid to systemic factors that may influence intestinal function as well as factors that directly affect the gut.

Renal System

The mortality rate of acute renal failure has not changed over the past decade and remains at about 50%.[45] Renal failure may occur before or after other organs have failed. When renal failure occurs before other organs fail, it is almost always a consequence of inadequate volume resuscitation or severe, prolonged shock. In contrast, renal failure that develops after other organs have failed may be due to ischemia, microemboli, or nephrotoxic drugs, such as the aminoglycosides, or it may be a manifestation of uncontrolled infection or endotoxemia. Although the exact pathophysiologic mechanisms of acute renal failure at the cellular level have yet to be elucidated, it is clear that a decrease in effective renal blood flow is a common cause of renal injury. In this circumstance, as renal vascular resistance increases, renal blood flow decreases and blood is shunted from the renal cortex to the juxtamedullary and medullary regions in an attempt to maintain an adequate glomerular filtration rate (GFR). However, at some point renal vascular resistance increases such that renal perfusion falls below a level sufficient to maintain an adequate GFR. This decrease in GFR is generally manifest as oliguria and an increasing serum creatinine concentration.

Because under normal circumstances the kidneys receive 20% to 30% of the cardiac output, decreasing renal blood flow increases the proportion of the cardiac output available to perfuse more oxygen-dependent organs, such as the brain and heart. Although decreased renal blood flow may be beneficial in the short term, acute renal failure will occur unless effective renal perfusion can be restored. Therefore a major goal of therapy is to prevent acute renal failure by restoring or maintaining effective renal blood flow. It is not always possible to prevent acute renal failure. Therefore, since the mortality rate of oliguric renal failure (50%) is about twice that of nonoliguric or high-output renal failure (25%), a second major therapeutic goal is to convert oliguric to nonoliguric renal failure.

Prevention of renal failure is based on avoiding renal ischemia and maintaining effective renal perfusion and oxygen delivery. Consequently, therapy is directed toward maintaining an adequate circulating blood volume by ensuring adequate fluid resuscitation and cardiovascular function and by avoiding hypoxia. In some patients this requires the use of a Swan-Ganz catheter to ensure that cardiovascular hemodynamics are optimal. As was discussed in the section on the cardiovascular system, it may be necessary to administer low-dose dopamine to maintain renal perfusion when other vasoactive drugs are used. It is also important to avoid nephrotoxic renal injury by monitoring levels of aminoglycosides and ensuring that endogenously produced nephrotoxic substances, such as myoglobin, are effectively cleared.[167] Because the mortality rate associated with nonoliguric renal failure is about half that of oliguric renal failure, it is important to attempt to convert oliguric to nonoliguric renal failure. If oliguria develops that is not responsive to volume administration or improvements in oxygen delivery, a trial of furosemide and mannitol appears warranted, because this drug combination has been documented to convert oliguric to nonoliguric renal failure in about two thirds of patients.[69,128] Although not fully proven, some clinical evidence indicates that low-dose dopamine (2 to 5 μg/kg/min) also may be beneficial in converting oliguric to nonoliguric renal failure.[91] Other potential options that have been shown experimentally to prevent or limit the development of ischemia-mediated acute tubular necrosis include the use of oxygen free radical scavengers,[161] inhibiting thromboxane synthesis,[117] or even epidermal growth factor to enhance regeneration and repair of renal tubular cells.[109]

Once renal failure is established, dialysis may be required to maintain fluid and electrolyte balance and to treat uremia. Nutritional support should not be reduced in these patients, even if this increases the need for or frequency of dialysis. The complications associated with hemodialysis in an acutely ill patient, especially cardiovascular instability, have given rise to new approaches to maintaining fluid balance and/or urea clearance. These techniques, called *extracorporeal continuous arteriovenous hemofiltration* (CAVH)[122,160] and *continu-*

ous arteriovenous hemodialysis (CAVHD),[210] are based on the technique of ultrafiltration. This involves using the patient's own arterial pressure to drive the blood through an ultrafiltration cartridge containing filters that are permeable to water, electrolytes, and small and medium-sized molecules. Because the arterial-to-venous blood pressure of the patient determines the rate of blood flow, hemodynamic instability and dialysis-induced shock are obviated.

Recently, a modification of these extracorporeal support techniques in which plasmapheresis was added has been documented to improve survival in a small group of patients with MOF.[15] The concept behind this approach is that by adding plasmapheresis to CAVHD, it would be possible to remove endotoxin and other potential mediators from the bloodstream and thereby reduce the septic response. Clearly, these results must be verified before this technique can be fully recommended. Nonetheless, the concept of removing circulating mediators, including endotoxin,[36] is an attractive one and has been extended to the treatment of patients with ARDS.[84]

Cellular- and Molecular-Based Therapy

Treatments such as artificial ventilation or hemodialysis are important in prolonging survival in MOF patients with established end-stage organ failure. However, these therapeutic efforts are largely palliative and do little to improve survival or reverse the underlying processes leading to or perpetuating organ failure. For these reasons it is important to focus on potential therapeutic approaches directed against the potential initiators, systemic mediators, potentiators, and effectors of organ and cellular injury in this syndrome.

As was previously discussed, four major and to some extent overlapping hypotheses have been proposed to explain various aspects of the pathophysiology of MOF: (1) the infection hypothesis; (2) the macrophage-cytokine hypothesis; (3) the microcirculatory hypothesis; and (4) the gut hypothesis. Based on the pathophysiology that underlies these hypotheses, there are multiple potential sites at which intervention to modulate the system in favor of the host is possible. For example, this process theoretically can be controlled at the initiator, systemic mediator, effector, tissue, or cellular levels (Table 16-6). Although this concept will be illustrated using the example of bacteria and/or endotoxin as the initiators or perpetuators of MOF, many of the same strategies can be applied to cytokine-mediated or microcirculatory-induced organ injury.

Therapy directed against endotoxin, as the biologic initiator of the inflammatory cascade that ultimately leads to organ injury, is physiologically attractive for several reasons. First, endotoxin is capable of initiating the cascade of physiologic events that culminate in organ failure. Second, in some clinical series[138,209] the presence of endotoxemia was a more accurate indicator of sepsis, ARDS, or septic shock than positive blood cultures. Third, clinical[180] and experimental[181] studies document that plasma endotoxin levels can rise significantly after systemic administration of antibiotics as a result of the release of endotoxin from bacterial cells. In this context, it is possible that antibiotic-mediated bacterial lysis may liberate larger amounts of circulating endotoxin than can be rapidly cleared by the liver, resulting in exacerbation of the inflammatory response. Because survival in bacteremic or infected patients with ARDS or MOF often is not improved despite adequate antimicrobial therapy, it is possible that anti-endotoxin therapy in conjunction with antimicrobial agents may improve survival in some patients with gram-negative sepsis by shutting down or controlling the septic response. Several

TABLE 16-6 CELLULAR-BASED POTENTIAL THERAPEUTIC STRATEGIES

LEVEL OF INTERVENTION	FACTOR	STRATEGY
Initiator	Endotoxin	Antibody-mediated neutralization
Mediator	TNF	Antibody-mediated neutralization
	IL-1	Target cell receptor blockade
	Phospholipids	PAF-antagonists
		Thromboxane receptor antagonists
		Cyclooxygenase inhibitors
		Lipoxygenase inhibitors
Effector	Neutrophils	Anti-adherence (CD 11/18) monoclonal antibodies
		Antioxidants
		Inhibitors of activation/degranulation
	XO-generated oxidants	Antioxidants
		Inhibitors/inactivators of XO
Tissue level	Endothelial cell	Anti–ELAM-1 or Anti–ICAM-1 antibodies
Cellular level	Calcium	Calcium channel blockers

XO, Xanthine oxidase.

clinical trials have been carried out to test this hypothesis. Most recently, two prospective, randomized trials using two different monoclonal antibodies against endotoxin have been published documenting that survival can be improved to a limited extent in subgroups of patients with sepsis.[92,223]

A second potential site of therapeutic intervention would be at the level of the cytokine cascade. Since TNF and IL-1 appear to be the major proximal mediators of the septic response, use of specific antibodies to block or neutralize these substances would appear to be preferable to blocking the cascade of mediators released in turn by these two cytokines. As was previously discussed, administering antibodies against TNF-alpha improves survival in primates and other mammalian species challenged with otherwise lethal doses of bacteria or endotoxin.[105,201,202] The results of a phase 1 study in which 14 patients with septic shock received recombinant anti-TNF have been reported.[72] Although too few patients were studied to reach any conclusions on survival, anti-TNF therapy did improve arterial blood pressure, and no adverse drug-related reactions were observed. One advantage of anti-TNF antibodies over anti-endotoxin antibodies is that the former are likely to be effective in patients with gram-positive infections or nonbacterial inflammatory states associated with macrophage overactivity as well as in patients with gram-negative infections. Unfortunately, the ultimate clinical usefulness of anti-TNF antibodies is likely to be limited, because in experimental studies, anti-TNF antibodies must be given either before or shortly (minutes) after the insult to be effective.

A second cytokine-based therapeutic strategy is to block the receptor on the target cells to which the cytokine binds. Based on experimental studies with a newly discovered and recently cloned member of the IL-1 cytokine family, called IL-1 receptor antagonist (IL-1ra),[2,8,75] this approach appears feasible. IL-1ra binds to the IL-1 receptor on various target cells, but because it has no agonist activity, this cytokine functions as a naturally occurring specific receptor antagonist. The use of a receptor blocker is appealing, because it is likely to be effective in dampening the body's response during both infectious and inflammatory states. However, one major potential problem with using antibodies directed against these two cytokines, as well as other proinflammatory mediators, is that under normal physiologic conditions, both TNF and IL-1 play important roles in eradicating invading bacteria, in wound healing, and in metabolic homeostasis.[7,12,77,78] This concern is verified by recent studies documenting that, when given at low or moderate doses, TNF and IL-1 improve survival after endotoxin or bacterial challenge.[3,89,183] Thus, although administration of large doses of cytokines is deleterious, at physiologic levels these same cytokines exert important beneficial effects. Because controlled clinical trials using anti-TNF antibodies or the recombinant IL-1ra currently are underway in patients with sepsis, more information on their clinical usefulness should be forthcoming in the near future.

Also, a number of other cytokine- or mediator- based adjuvant therapies, including cyclooxgenase blockade,[70,98] platelet activating factor (PAF) antagonists[76] and immunomodulators such as INF-gamma[126,127] granulocyte-macrophage colony-stimulating factor (GM-CSF),[46] or thymopentin,[74] currently are in various stages of investigation, but to date these agents have either not been adequately tested clinically or the results of clinical trials are controversial.

The rationale for using drugs to inhibit or block phospholipid mediators is based largely on the results of animal models of sepsis.[31] These studies documented an association between increased levels of phospholipid mediators, such as PAF, thromboxane A_2, or the leukotrienes, and increased organ injury or death. Furthermore, the use of antagonists and blockers of these phospholipid mediators improved survival. However, because the phospholipid mediators appear later in the inflammatory cascade, at a time when many other cellular and humoral mediator systems have been activated, it is questionable whether selective blockade or neutralization of individual phospholipid mediators will be of significant clinical benefit.

As was discussed under the section on infection, the rationale for using immunomodulators, such as INF-gamma, GM-CSF, or thymopentin, is to bolster the body's immune system and thereby reduce the incidence of, or mortality from, bacterial infections. However, the safety of administering these immunomodulatory agents in a patient with endotoxemia or an uncontrolled inflammatory state is questionable, because experimentally immune stimulants have been documented to predispose the patient to endotoxic shock. Thus the clinical usefulness of this approach may vary from patient to patient and may be based on whether the major threat to the patient is infection or an excessive inflammatory response.

At the microvascular and tissue levels, therapy directed at specific effectors of tissue injury, such as neutrophil oxidants and proteases or xanthine oxidase–generated oxidants, is potentially feasible, as is therapy directed at preventing or limiting neutrophil-endothelial interactions.* The concept of anti-adhesion therapy, in which neutrophil-endothelial interactions are blocked, is based on the observation that damage to the vascular system is a common and major component of sepsis and MOF. One strategy to prevent or limit neutrophil-mediated endothelial damage is to prevent neutrophils from binding to the endothelium by blocking either the neu-

*References 14, 39, 55, 101, 146, 153, and 207.

trophil (CD 11/CD 18) or endothelial (ICAM-1, ELAM-1) adhesion molecules with monoclonal antibodies. A second strategy is to prevent neutrophil activation or degranulation, or both, and thereby decrease both neutrophil adhesion to the endothelium and the amount of tissue destructive products released by the neutrophils that do adhere. The most promising agent in this regard is pentoxifylline. Pentoxifylline not only decreases neutrophil adhesion to endothelial cells, it also inhibits cytokine-mediated neutrophil activation and degranulation, decreases TNF production by macrophages, and decreases platelet aggregation.[29] Although no human information is available on the effectiveness of pentoxifylline in septic states, this drug has been documented to increase survival in several animal models of sepsis.[176,178] Nonetheless, although a misguided neutrophil that becomes activated at the wrong time or place can damage healthy tissue, inhibiting neutrophil function is not without the potential risk of increasing the patient's susceptibility to infection.

A large body of information exists linking intracellular calcium overload to cellular damage and death after ischemic as well as septic insults.[131] In fact, calcium has been removed from advanced cardiac support regimens because of its potentially harmful effects during ischemia.[198] Because free intracellular calcium levels are elevated in conditions associated with MOF and calcium channel antagonists have been documented to minimize cellular damage after ischemic insults[154] or endotoxin challenge,[34] the role of the slow calcium channel blockers, such as verapamil or nifedipine, in the treatment of sepsis is conceptually appealing.

Thus, based on our knowledge of the biology of the sepsis syndrome and the preliminary results of clinical trials using various agents to block specific mediators involved in the septic response, it is not unlikely that, in the future, treatment of a septic patient will be similar to that of a patient with cancer, where several agents with different actions are combined to produce the desired biologic effect. However, the successful development of this strategy will require ways of blocking the deleterious effects of cytokines and other mediators of the inflammatory response while maintaining their beneficial effects.

CONCLUSION

The goal of this chapter has been to summarize and put into perspective a portion of the enormous amount of clinical and experimental information generated during the past decade on the pathophysiology and potential treatment of MOF. Although many facets of MOF remain shrouded in mystery, confusion, or controversy, progress is being made. Testable hypotheses on the cause and pathophysiologic features of organ failure have been generated, and a consensus has been reached on several aspects of the care of these patients. As we continue to expand our understanding of the basic mechanisms involved in this syndrome, we undoubtedly will develop new and effective therapeutic strategies, to the benefit of our patients.

REFERENCES

1 Aikowa N, Shinozawa Y, Ishibiki K et al: Clinical analysis of multiple organ failure in burned patients, *Burns* 13:103, 1987.
2 Alexander HR, Doherty GM, Bruesh CM et al: A recombinant human receptor antagonist to interleukin-1 improves survival after lethal endotoxemia in mice, *J Exp Med* 173:1029, 1991.
3 Alexander HR, Doherty GM, Fraker DL et al: Human recombinant interleukin-1: protection against lethality of endotoxin and experimental sepsis in mice, *J Surg Res* 50:421, 1991.
4 Alexander JW, Boyce ST, Babcock GF et al: The process of microbial translocation, *Ann Surg* 212:496, 1990.
5 Alexander JW, MacMillan JC, Stinnet JD et al: Beneficial effects of aggressive protein feeding in severely burned children, *Ann Surg* 192:505, 1980.
6 Allardyce DB: Incidence of necrotizing pancreatitis and factors related to mortality, *Am J Surg* 154:295, 1987.
7 Arai K, Lee F, Miyajima A et al: Cytokines: coordinators of immune and inflammatory responses, *Annu Rev Biochem* 59:783, 1990.
8 Arend WP: Interleukin-1 receptor antagonist: a new member of the interleukin-1 family, *J Clin Invest* 88:1445, 1991.
9 Arita H, Ogle CK, Alexander JW et al: Induction of hypermetabolism in guinea pigs by endotoxin infused through the portal vein, *Arch Surg* 123:1420, 1988.
10 Ashbaugh DG, Bigelow DB, Petty TL et al: Acute respiratory distress in adults, *Lancet* 2:319, 1967.
11 Astiz ME, Rackow EC, Falk JL et al: Oxygen delivery and consumption in patients with hyperdynamic septic shock, *Crit Care Med* 15:26, 1987.
12 Balkwill FR, Burke F: The cytokine network, *Immunol Today* 10:299, 1989.
13 Barroso-Aranda J, Schmid-Schonbein GW, Zweifach BW et al: Granulocytes and no-reflow phenomenon in irreversible hemorrhagic shock, *Circ Res* 63:437, 1988.
14 Barton RW, Rothlein R, Ksiazek J et al: The effect of anti-intercellular adhesion molecule-1 on phorbol ester–induced rabbit lung inflammation, *J Immunol* 143:1278, 1989.
15 Barzilay E, Kessler D, Berlot G et al: Use of extracorporeal supportive techniques as additional treatment for septic-induced multiple organ failure patients, *Crit Care Med* 17:634, 1989.
16 Baue AE: Historical perspective. In Deitch EA, editor: *Multiple organ failure: pathophysiology and basic concepts of therapy,* New York, 1990, Thieme Medical Publishers.
17 Baue AE: Multiple, progressive, or sequential system failure: a syndrome for the '70s, *Arch Surg* 110:779, 1975.
18 Baue AE: Multiple organ failure: patient care and prevention, St Louis, 1990, Mosby.
19 Berg RD, Garlington AW: Translocation of certain indigenous bacteria from the gastrointestinal tract to the mesenteric lymph nodes and other organs in a gnotobiotic mouse model, *Infect Immun* 23:403, 1979.
20 Bessey PQ: Nutritional support in critical illness. In Deitch EA, editor: *Multiple organ failure: pathophysiology and basic concepts of therapy,* New York, 1990, Thieme Medical Publishers.
21 Bihari D, Smithies M, Gimson A et al: The effects of vasodilatation with prostacyclin on oxygen delivery and uptake in critically ill patients, *N Engl J Med* 317:397, 1987.
22 Billiar TR, Maddaus MA, West MA et al: The role of the intes-

tinal flora on the interactions between nonparenchymal cells and hepatocytes in coculture, *J Surg Res* 44:397, 1988.
23 Blaisdell FW: Pathophysiology of the respiratory distress syndrome, *Arch Surg* 108:44, 1974.
24 Bone L, Johnson K, Weigelt J et al: Early versus delayed stabilization of femoral fractures: a prospective, randomized study, *J Bone Joint Surg* 71:336, 1989.
25 Bone RC, Fisher CJ, Clemmer TP et al: Sepsis syndrome: a valid clinical entity, *Crit Care Med* 17:389, 1989.
26 Bone RC, Balk RA, Cerra FB et al: Definitions for sepsis and organ failure and guidelines for the use of innovative therapies in sepsis, *Crit Care Med* 20:864, 1992.
27 Bone RC, Fischer CJ, Clemmer TP et al: The Methylprednisolone Severe Sepsis Study Group: a controlled clinical trial of high-dose methylprednisolone in the treatment of severe sepsis and septic shock, *N Engl J Med* 317:653, 1987.
28 Bone RC, Slotman G, Maunder A et al: Randomized, double-blind, multicenter study of prostaglandin E_1 in patients with adult respiratory distress syndrome, *Chest* 96:114, 1989.
29 Bone RC: Inhibitors of complement and neutrophils: a critical evaluation of their role in the treatment of sepsis, *Crit Care Med* 20:891, 1992.
30 Bone RC: Let's agree on terminology: definitions of sepsis, *Crit Care Med* 19:973, 1991.
31 Bone RC: Phospholipids and their inhibitors: a critical evaluation of their role in the treatment of sepsis, *Crit Care Med* 20:884, 1992.
32 Border JR, Hasset JM, LaDuca J et al: Gut origin septic states in blunt multiple trauma (ISS = 40) in the ICU, *Ann Surg* 206:427, 1987.
33 Border JR: Hypothesis: sepsis, multiple organ failure, and the macrophage, *Arch Surg* 123:285, 1988.
34 Bosson S, Kuenzig M, Scwartz SI: Verapamil improves cardiac function and improves survival in canine *E. coli* endotoxin shock, *Circ Shock* 16:307, 1985.
35 Bunt TJ: Nondirected relaparotomy for intra-abdominal sepsis: a futile procedure, *Am Surg* 52:294, 1986.
36 Bysani GK, Shenep JL, Hildner WK et al: Detoxification of plasma containing lipopolysaccharide by adsorption, *Crit Care Med* 18:67, 1990.
37 Cain SM, Curtis SE: Experimental models of pathologic oxygen supply dependency, *Crit Care Med* 19:603, 1991.
38 Cannon JG, Tompkins RG, Gelfand JA et al: Circulating interleukin-1 and tumor necrosis factor in septic shock and experimental endotoxin fever, *J Infect Dis* 161:79, 1990.
39 Carlos TM, Harlan JM: Membrane proteins involved in phagocyte adherence to endothelium, *Immunol Rev* 114:5, 1990.
40 Carrico CJ, Meakins JL, Marshall JC et al: Multiple-organ-failure syndrome, *Arch Surg* 121:196, 1986.
41 Cerra FB, McPherson JP, Konstantinides FN et al: Enteral nutrition does not prevent multiple organ failure syndrome after sepsis, *Surgery* 104:727, 1988.
42 Cerra FB: Hypermetabolism, organ failure, and metabolic support, *Surgery* 101:1, 1987.
43 Cerra FB: Nutrient modulation of inflammatory and immune function, *Am J Surg* 161:230, 1991.
44 Chiu CJ, McArdle A, Brown R et al: Intestinal mucosal lesions in low-flow states, *Arch Surg* 101:478, 1970.
45 Cioffi GW, Ashikaga T, Gamelli RL: Probability of surviving postoperative acute renal failure: development of a prognostic index, *Ann Surg* 200:2, 1984.
46 Cioffi WG, Burleson DG, Jordan DG et al: Effects of granulocyte-macrophage colony-stimulating factor in burn patients, *Arch Surg* 126:74, 1991.
47 Civetta JM, Hudson-Civetta JA, Nelson LD: Evaluation of APACHE II for cost containment and quality assurance, *Ann Surg* 212:266, 1990.
48 Cochrane CG: The enhancement of inflammatory injury, *Am Rev Respir Dis* 136:1, 1987.
49 Cook DJ, Witt LG, Cook RJ et al: Stress ulcer prophylaxis in the critically ill: a meta-analysis, *Am J Med* 91:519, 1991.
50 Craven DE, Kunches LM, Kilinsky V et al: Risk factors for pneumonia and fatality in patients receiving continuous mechanical ventilation, *Am Rev Resp Dis* 133:792, 1986.
51 Damas P, Reuter A, Gysen P et al: Tumor necrosis factor and interleukin-1 serum levels during severe sepsis in humans, *Crit Care Med* 17:975, 1989.
52 de Groote MA, Martin MA, Densen P et al: Plasma tumor necrosis factor levels in patients with presumed sepsis, *JAMA* 262:249, 1989.
53 Debets JM, Kampmeijer R, Linden MP et al: Plasma tumor necrosis factor and mortality in critically ill septic patients, *Crit Care Med* 17:489, 1989.
54 Deitch EA, Maejima K, Berg RD: Effect of oral antibiotics and bacterial overgrowth on the translocation of the GI tract microflora in burned rats, *J Trauma* 25:385, 1985.
55 Deitch EA, Bridges W, Baker J et al: Hemorrhagic shock–induced bacterial translocation is reduced by xanthine oxidase inhibition or inactivation, *Surgery* 104:191, 1988.
56 Deitch EA, Ma L, Ma WJ et al: Inhibition of endotoxin-induced bacterial translocation in mice, *J Clin Invest* 84:36, 1989.
57 Deitch EA: Bacterial translocation of the gut flora, *J Trauma* 30:s184, 1990.
58 Deitch EA: Gut failure: its role in multiple organ failure syndrome. In Deitch EA, editor: *Multiple organ failure: pathophysiology and basic concepts in therapy,* New York, 1990, Thieme Medical Publishers.
59 Deitch EA: Infection in the compromised host, *Surg Clinic North Am* 68:181, 1988.
60 Deitch EA: Intestinal permeability is increased in burn patients shortly after injury, *Surgery* 107:411, 1990.
61 Deitch EA: *Multiple organ failure: pathophysiology and basic concepts of therapy,* New York, 1990, Thieme Medical Publishers.
62 Deitch EA: Review of the effect of stress and trauma on plasma fibronectin and the reticuloendothelial system, *JBCR* 4:344, 1983.
63 Deitch EA: The role of intestinal barrier failure and bacterial translocation in the development of systemic infection and multiple organ failure, *Arch Surg* 125:403, 1990.
64 Dellinger EP: Use of scoring systems to assess patients with surgical sepsis, *Surg Clin North Am* 68:123, 1988.
65 Demaria A, Heffernan JJ, Grindlinger GA et al: Naloxone versus placebo in the treatment of septic shock, *Lancet* 1:1363, 1985.
66 Demling RH: Current concepts on the adult respiratory distress syndrome, *Circ Shock* 30:297, 1990.
67 Driks MR, Craven DE, Celli BR et al: Nosocomial pneumonia in intubated patients given sucralfate as compared with antacids or histamine type 2 blockers: the role of gastric colonization, *N Engl J Med* 317:1378, 1987.
68 Eiseman B, Beart R, Norton L: Multiple organ failure, *Surg Gynecol Obstet* 144:323, 1977.
69 Eliahou HE: Mannitol therapy in oliguria of acute onset, *Br Med J* 1:807, 1964.
70 Evans DA, Jacobs DO, Revhaug A et al: The effects of tumor necrosis factor and their selective inhibition by ibuprofen, *Ann Surg* 209:312, 1989.
71 Evers BM, Izukura M, Townsend CM et al: Differential effects of gut hormones on pancreatic and intestinal growth during administration of an elemental diet, *Ann Surg* 211:630, 1990.
72 Exley AR, Cohen J, Buurman W et al: Monoclonal antibody to TNF in severe septic shock, *Lancet* 335:1275, 1990.
73 Faist E, Baue AE, Dittmer H et al: Multiple organ failure in polytrauma patients, *J Trauma* 23:775, 1983.

74 Faist E, Markewitz A, Fuchs D et al: Immunomodulatory therapy with thymopentin and indomethacin, *Ann Surg* 214:264, 1991.
75 Fasano SB, Cousart S, Neal S et al: Increased expression of the interleukin-1 receptor on blood neutrophils of humans with the sepsis syndrome, *J Clin Invest* 88:1452, 1991.
76 Fletcher JR, Earnest MA, DiSimone AG et al: Platelet activating factor receptor antagonist improves survival and attenuates eicosanoid release in severe endotoxemia, *Ann Surg* 211:312, 1990.
77 Fong Y, Lowry SF: Cytokines and the cellular response to injury and infection. In Wilmore DW, Brennan M, Harken A et al, editors: *Care of the surgical patient,* New York, 1990, Scientific American Books.
78 Fong Y, Moldawer LL, Shires GT et al: The biologic characteristics of cytokines and their implications in surgical injury, *Surg Gynecol Obstet* 170:363, 1990.
79 Fong Y, Tracey KJ, Moldawer LL et al: Antibodies to cachectin/tumor necrosis factor reduce interleukin-1β and interleukin-6 appearance during lethal bacteremia, *J Exp Med* 170:1627, 1989.
80 Fong Y, Marano MA, Moldawer LL et al: The acute splanchnic and peripheral tissue metabolic response to endotoxin in man, *J Clin Invest* 85:1896, 1990.
81 Fry DE, Pearlstein L, Fulton RL et al: Multiple system organ failure: the role of uncontrolled infection, *Arch Surg* 115:136, 1980.
82 Fry DE: *Multiple system organ failure,* St Louis, 1992, Mosby.
83 Garrison RN, Fry DE, Berborich S et al: Enterococcal bacteremia: clinical implications and determinants of death, *Ann Surg* 196:43, 1982.
84 Garzia F, Todor R, Scalea T: Continuous arteriovenous hemofiltration countercurrent dialysis (CAVH-D) in acute respiratory failure, *J Trauma* 31:1277, 1991.
85 Gattinoni L, Pesenti A, Mesheroni D et al: Low-frequency positive-pressure ventilation with extracorporeal carbon dioxide removal in severe acute respiratory failure, *JAMA* 256:881, 1986.
86 Giardin E, Grau GE, Dayer JM et al: Tumor necrosis factor and interleukin-1 in the serum of children with severe infectious purpura, *N Engl J Med* 319:397, 1988.
87 Goris RJ, Beokhorst PA, Nuytinck KS: Multiple organ failure: generalized autodestructive inflammation, *Arch Surg* 120:1109, 1985.
88 Goris RJ, Gimbrere JS, Van Niekerk JL et al: Early osteosynthesis and prophylactic mechanical ventilation in the multitrauma patient, *J Trauma* 22:895, 1982.
89 Gough DB, Moss NM, Jordan A et al: Recombinant interleukin-2 improves immune response and host resistance to septic challenge in thermally injured mice, *Surgery* 104:292, 1988.
90 Granger DN: Role of xanthine oxidase and granulocytes in ischemia-reperfusion injury, *Am J Physiol* 24:H1269, 1988.
91 Graziani G, Cantaluppi A: Dopamine and furosemide in oliguric renal failure, *Nephron* 37:39, 1984.
92 Greenman RL, Schein RM, Martin MA et al: A controlled clinical trial of E5 murine monoclonal IgM antibody to endotoxin in the treatment of gram-negative sepsis, *JAMA* 266:1097, 1991.
93 Guo Y, Dickerson C, Chrest FJ et al: Increased levels of circulating interleukin-6 in burn patients, *Clin Immunol Immunopathol* 54:361, 1990.
94 Guthrie LA, McPhail PM, Johnson PB: Priming of neutrophils for enhanced release of oxygen metabolites by bacterial lipopolysaccharide, *J Exp Med* 160:1656, 1984.
95 Hack CE, de Groot ER, Felt-Bersma RJ et al: Increased plasma interleukin-6 in sepsis, *Blood* 74:1704, 1989.
96 Harkema JM, Chaudry IH: Oxygen delivery and multiple organ failure. In Deitch EA, editor: *Multiple organ failure: pathophysiology and basic concepts of therapy,* New York, 1990, Thieme Medical Publishers.
97 Hartenauer U, Thulig B, Diemer W et al: Effect of selective flora suppression on colonization, infection, and mortality in critically ill patients: a 1-year prospective study, *Crit Care Med* 19:463, 1991.
98 Haupt MT, Jastremski MS, Clemmer TP et al: Effect of ibuprofen in patients with severe sepsis: a randomized, double-blind, multicenter study, *Crit Care Med* 19:1339, 1991.
99 Helfgott DC, Tatter SB, Santhanam U et al: Multiple forms of INF-beta-2/IL-6 in serum and body fluids during acute bacterial infection, *J Immunol* 142:948, 1989.
100 Henao FR, Daes JE, Dennis RJ: Risk factors for multiorgan failure: a case control study, *J Trauma* 31:74, 1991.
101 Hernandez L, Grisham M, Twohig B et al: Role of neutrophils in ischemia-reperfusion–induced microvascular injury, *Am J Physiol* 253:H699, 1987.
102 Hesse DG, Tracey KJ, Fong Y et al: Cytokine appearance in human endotoxemia and primate bacteremia, *Surg Gynecol Obstet* 166:147, 1988.
103 Hickling KG: Extracorporeal carbon dioxide removal in severe acute respiratory failure, *Anaesth Intensive Care* 14:46, 1986.
104 Hinsdale JG, Jaffe BM: Re-operation for intra-abdominal sepsis: indications and results in the modern critical care setting, *Ann Surg* 199:31, 1984.
105 Hinshaw LB, Tekamp-Olsen P, Chang AC et al: Survival of primates in LD_{100} septic shock following therapy with antibody to tumor necrosis factor, *Circ Shock* 30:279, 1990.
106 Holcroft JW, Vassar MJ, Weber CJ: Prostaglandin E_1 and survival in patients with adult respiratory distress syndrome, *Ann Surg* 203:371, 1986.
107 Holzapfel L, Perrin RF, Gaussorgues P et al: Comparison of high-frequency jet ventilation to conventional ventilation in adults with respiratory distress syndrome, *Intensive Care Med* 13:100, 1987.
108 Hooks JJ, Moutsopoulos HM, Geis SA et al: Immune interferon in the circulation of patients with autoimmune disease, *N Engl J Med* 301:5, 1979.
109 Humes HD, Cieslinski DA, Coimbra TM et al: Epidermal growth factor enhances renal tubular regeneration and repair and accelerates the recovery of renal function in postischemic acute renal failure, *J Clin Invest* 84:1757, 1989.
110 Hunt JL: Generalized peritonitis: to irrigate or not to irrigate the abdominal cavity? *Arch Surg* 117:209, 1982.
111 Hurst JM, Dehaven CB: Adult respiratory distress syndrome: improved oxygenation during high-frequency jet ventilation/continuous positive airway pressure, *Surgery* 96:764, 1984.
112 Jacobs DO, Evans DA, Mealy K et al: Combined effects of glutamine and epidermal growth factor on the rat intestine, *Surgery* 104:358, 1988.
113 Jarret F, Balish L, Moylan JA et al: Clinical experience with prophylactic antibiotic suppression in burn patients, *Surgery* 83:523, 1978.
114 Jiang ZM, He GZ, Zhang XR et al: Low-dose growth hormone and hypocaloric nutrition attenuate the protein catabolic response following a major operation, *Ann Surg* 210:513, 1989.
115 Johnson K, Cadambi A, Seibert G: Incidence of adult respiratory distress syndrome in patients with multiple musculoskeletal injuries: effect of early operative stabilization of fractures, *J Trauma* 25:375, 1985.
116 Jones CE, Alexander JW, Fisher MW: Clinical evaluation of *Pseudomonas* hyperimmune globulin, *J Surg Res* 14:87, 1973.
117 Kaufman RP, Klausner JM, Anner H et al: Inhibition of thromboxane synthesis by free radical scavengers, *J Trauma* 28:458, 1988.
118 Kispert P, Caldwell MD: Metabolic changes in sepsis and multiple organ failure. In Deitch EA, editor: *Multiple organ failure: pathophysiology and basic concepts of therapy,* New York, 1990, Thieme Medical Publishers.

119 Knaus WA, Draper EA, Wagner DP et al: Prognosis in acute organ sytem failure, *Ann Surg* 202:685, 1985.
120 Kudsk KA, Stone JM, Carpenter G et al: Enteral and parenteral feeding influences mortality after hemoglobin *E. coli* peritonitis in normal rats, *J Trauma* 23:605, 1983.
121 Kudsk KA, Croce MA, Fabian TC et al: Enteral versus parenteral feeding: effects of septic morbidity after blunt and penetrating abdominal trauma, *Ann Surg* 215:503, 1992.
122 Lauer A, Saccaggi A, Ronco C et al: Continuous arteriovenous hemofiltration in the critically ill patient, *Ann Intern Med* 99:455, 1983.
123 Lehy T, Puccio F, Chariot J et al: Stimulating effect of bombesin on the growth of gastrointestinal tract and pancreas in suckling rats, *Gastroenterology* 90:1942, 1986.
124 Levine B, Kalman J, Mayer L et al: Elevated circulating levels of tumor necrosis factor in severe chronic heart failure, *N Engl J Med* 323:236, 1990.
125 Livingston DH, Shumate CR, Polk HC Jr et al: More is better: antibiotic management after hemorrhagic shock, *Ann Surg* 208:451, 1988.
126 Livingston DH, Malangoni MA: Interferon-gamma restores immune competence after hemorrhagic shock, *J Surg Res* 45:37, 1988.
127 Livingston DH, Appel SH, Wellhauser SR et al: Depressed interferon-gamma production and monocyte HLA-DR expression after severe injury, *Arch Surg* 123:287, 1988.
128 Luke RG, Briggs JD, Allison ME et al: Factors determining the response to mannitol in acute renal failure, *Am J Med Sci* 259:168, 1970.
129 Ma L, Ma JW, Deitch EA et al: Genetic susceptibility to mucosal damage leads to bacterial translocation in a murine burn model, *J Trauma* 29:1245, 1989.
130 Mainous MR, Tso P, Berg RD et al: Studies of the route, magnitude, and time course of bacterial translocation in a model of systemic inflammation, *Arch Surg* 126:33, 1991.
131 Malcolm DS, Holaday JW, Chernow B et al: Calcium and calcium antagonists in shock and ischemia. In Chernow B, Holaday JW, Zaloga GP, editors: *Pharmacologic approach to the critically ill patient,* ed 2, Baltimore, 1988, Williams & Wilkins.
132 Mansberger AR, Doran JE, Treat R et al: The influence of fibronectin administration on the incidence of sepsis and septic mortality in severely injured patients, *Ann Surg* 210:297, 1989.
133 Manson JM, Wilmore DW: Positive nitrogen balance with human growth hormone and hypocaloric intravenous feeding, *Surgery* 100:188, 1986.
134 Marano MA, Fong Y, Moldawer LL et al: Serum cachectin/tumor necrosis factor in critically ill patients with burns correlates with infection and mortality, *Surg Gynecol Obstet* 170:32, 1990.
135 Marshall WG, Dimick AR: Natural history of major burns with multiple subsystem failure, *J Trauma* 23:102, 1983.
136 Maury CP, Teppo AM: Raised serum levels of cachectic/tumor necrosis factor-alpha in renal allograft rejection, *J Exp Med* 166:1132, 1987.
137 Maury CP, Salo E, Pelkonen P: Circulating interleukin-1β in patients with Kawasaki disease, *N Engl J Med* 318:1670, 1988.
138 McCartney AC, Banks JG, Clements GB et al: Endotoxemia in septic shock: clinical and postmortem correlations, *Intensive Care Med* 9:117, 1983.
139 McCord JM: Oxygen-derived free radicals in postischemic tissue injury, *N Engl J Med* 312:159, 1985.
140 McCord JM: Oxygen-derived radicals: a link between reperfusion injury and inflammation, *Fed Proc* 46:2402, 1987.
141 McDonald WS, Sharp CV, Deitch EA: Immediate enteral feeding in burn patients is safe and effective, *Ann Surg* 213:177, 1991.
142 Meakins JL, Marshal JC: The gastrointestinal tract: the "motor" of MOF, *Arch Surg* 121:197, 1986.
143 Mela L, Bacalzo LV, Miller LD: Defective oxidative metabolism of rat liver mitochondria in hemorrhagic and endotoxin shock, *Am J Physiol* 220:571, 1971.
144 Michie HR, Spriggs DR, Mangue KR et al: Tumor necrosis factor and endotoxin induce similar metabolic responses in human beings, *Surgery* 104:280, 1988.
145 Michie HR, Manogue KR, Spriggs DR et al: Detection of circulating tumor necrosis factor after endotoxin administration, *N Engl J Med* 318:1481, 1988.
146 Mileski W, Winn R, Vedder NB et al: Inhibition of neutrophil adherence with the monoclonal antibody 60.3 during resuscitation from hemorrhagic shock in primates, *Surgery* 108:206, 1990.
147 Mochiuzuki H, Trocki O, Dominioni L et al: Mechanism of prevention of postburn hypermetabolism and catabolism by early enteral feeding, *Ann Surg* 200:297, 1984.
148 Montgomery AB, Stager MA, Carrico CJ et al: Causes of mortality in patients with adult respiratory distress syndrome, *Am Rev Respir Dis* 132:485, 1985.
149 Moore FA, Moore EE, Poggetti R et al: Gut bacterial translocation via the portal vein: a clinical perspective with major torso trauma, *J Trauma* 31:629, 1991.
150 Moore FA, Moore EE, Jones TN et al: TEN versus TPN following major torso trauma: reduced septic morbidity, *J Trauma* 29:916, 1989.
151 Moore FD Jr, Moss NA, Revhaug A et al: A single dose of endotoxin activates neutrophils without activating complement, *Surgery* 102:200, 1987.
152 Morrison DC, Ryan JL: Endotoxins and disease mechanisms, *Annu Rev Med* 38:417, 1987.

153 Mulligan MS, Varani J, Dame MK et al: Role of endothelial-leukocyte adhesion molecule-1 (ELAM-1) in neutrophil-mediated lung injury in rats, *J Clin Invest* 88:1396, 1991.
154 Nayler WG, Ferrari R, Williams A: Protective effect of pretreatment with verapamil, nifedipine, and propranolol on mitochondrial function in the ischemic and reperfused myocardium, *Am J Cardiol* 46:242, 1980.
155 Nijsten MW, Hack CE, Duis HH et al: Interleukin-6 and its relation to the humoral immune response and clinical parameters in burned patients, *Surgery* 109:761, 1991.
156 Norton LW: Does drainage of intra-abdominal pus reverse multiple organ failure? *Am J Surg* 149:347, 1985.
157 Nuytinck HK, Xavier JM, Offermans W et al: Whole body inflammation in trauma patients: an autopsy study, *Arch Surg* 123:1519, 1988.
158 O'Dwyer ST, Mitchie HR, Ziegler TR et al: A single dose of endotoxin increases intestinal permeability in healthy humans, *Arch Surg* 123:1459, 1988.
159 Osborn L: Leukocyte adhesion to endothelium in inflammation, *Cell* 62:3, 1990.
160 Ossenkoppele GJ, Meulen J, Bronsveld W et al: Continuous arteriovenous hemofiltration as an adjunctive therapy for septic shock, *Crit Care Med* 13:102, 1985.
161 Paller MS, Hoidal JR, Ferris TF: Oxygen free radicals in ischemic acute renal failure in the rat, *J Clin Invest* 74:1156, 1984.
162 Papadakos PJ, Halloran W, Hessney JI et al: The use of pressure-controlled inverse ratio ventilation in the surgical intensive care unit, *J Trauma* 31:1211, 1991.
163 Pober JS, Cotran RS: The role of endothelial cells in inflammation, *Transplantation* 50:537, 1990.
164 Pober JS, Cotran RS: Cytokines and endothelial cell biology, *Physiol Rev* 70:427, 1990.
165 Pober JS: Cytokine-mediated activation of vascular endothelium: physiology and pathology, *Am J Pathol* 133:426, 1988.
166 Polk HC, Shields CL: Remote organ failure: a valid sign of occult intra-abdominal infection, *Surgery* 81:310, 1977.
167 Reed RL, Wu AH, Crotchett PM et al: Pharmacokinetic monitoring of nephrotoxic antibiotics in surgical intensive care patients, *J Trauma* 29:1462, 1989.
168 Reidy JJ, Ramsay G: Clinical trials of selective decontamination of the digestive tract: review, *Crit Care Med* 18:1449, 1990.
169 Reilly PM, Schiller HJ, Bulkley GB: Pharmacologic approach to tissue injury mediated by free radicals and other oxygen metabolites, *Am J Surg* 161:488, 1991.
170 Revhaug A, Michie HR, Manson JM et al: Inhibition of cyclooxygenase attenuates the metabolic response to endotoxin in humans, *Arch Surg* 123:162, 1988.
171 Richardson JD, DeCamp MM, Garrison RN et al: Pulmonary infection complicating intra-abdominal sepsis: clinical and experimental observations, *Ann Surg* 195:732, 1982.
172 Rolandelli RH, Koruda MJ, Settle RG et al: Effect of intraluminal short-chain fatty acids on healing of colonic anastamosis in the rat, *Surgery* 100:198, 1986.
173 Runcie C, Ramsay G: Intra-abdominal infection: pulmonary infection, *World J Surg* 14:196, 1990.
174 Rush BF, Sori AJ, Murphy TF et al: Endotoxemia and bacteremia during hemorrhagic shock, *Ann Surg* 207:549, 1988.
175 Rush BF: Irreversibility in hemorrhagic shock is caused by sepsis, *Am J Surg* 55:204, 1989.
176 Schade UF: Pentoxifylline increases survival in murine endotoxin shock and decreases formation of tumor necrosis factor, *Circ Shock* 31:171, 1990.
177 Schirmer WJ, Fry DE: Microcirculatory arrest. In Fry DE, editor: *Multiple organ failure,* St Louis, 1992, Mosby.
178 Schonharting MM, Schade UF: The effect of pentoxifylline in septic shock: new pharmacologic aspects of an established drug, *J Med* 20:97, 1989.
179 Seibel R, Laduca J, Hassett JM et al: Blunt multiple trauma (ISS = 36), femur traction, and the pulmonary failure-septic state, *Ann Surg* 202:283, 1985.
180 Shenep JL, Flynn PM, Barrett FF et al: Serial quantitation of endotoxemia and bacteremia during therapy for gram-negative bacterial sepsis, *J Infect Dis* 157:565, 1988.
181 Shenep JL, Morgan KA: Kinetics of endotoxin release during antibiotic therapy for experimental gram-negative bacterial sepsis, *J Infect Dis* 150:380, 1984.
182 Shenkin A, Fraser WD, Series J et al: The serum interleukin-6 response to elective surgery, *Lymphokine Res* 8:123, 1989.
183 Sheppard BC, Fraker DL, Norton JA: Prevention and treatment of endotoxin and sepsis lethality with recombinant tumor necrosis factor, *Surgery* 106:156, 1989.
184 Shires GT, Cunningham JN, Baker CR et al: Alterations in cellular membrane function during hemorrhagic shock in primates, *Ann Surg* 176:288, 1972.
185 Shoemaker WC, Kram HB, Appel PL et al: The efficacy of central venous and pulmonary artery catheters and therapy based upon them in reducing mortality and morbidity, *Arch Surg* 125:1332, 1990.
186 Shoemaker WC, Appel PL, Kram HB et al: Prospective trial of supranormal values of survivors as therapeutic goals in high-risk surgical patients, *Chest* 84:1176, 1988.
187 Shoemaker WC, Appel PL: Effects of prostaglandin E_1 in adult respiratory distress syndrome, *Surgery* 99:275, 1986.
188 Sibbald WJ, McCormack D, Marshall J et al: "Sepsis": clarity of existing terminology. . .or more confusion? *Crit Care Med* 19:996, 1991.

189 Siegel JH, Cerra FB, Coleman B et al: Physiologic and metabolic correlations in human sepsis, *Surgery* 86:163, 1979.

190 Souba WW, Smith RJ, Wilmore DW: Glutamine metabolism by the intestinal tract, *J Parenter Enteral Nutr* 9:608, 1985.

191 Speath G, Berg RD, Specian RD et al: Food without fiber promotes bacterial translocation from the gut, *Surgery* 108:240, 1990.

192 Sprung CL: Definitions of sepsis: have we reached a consensus? *Crit Care Med* 19:849, 1991.

193 Starnes HF, Warren RS, Jeevanandam M et al: Tumor necrosis factor and the acute metabolic response to tissue injury in man, *J Clin Invest* 82:1321, 1988.

194 Stoutenbeek CP, van Saene HK, Miranda DR et al: The effect of selective decontamination of the digestive tract on colonisation and infection rate in multiple trauma patients, *Intensive Care Med* 10:185, 1984.

195 Sullivan BJ, Swallow CJ, Girotti MJ et al: Bacterial translocation induces procoagulant activity in tissue macrophages: a potential mechanism for end-organ dysfunction, *Arch Surg* 126:586, 1991.

196 Sun X, Hsueh W: Bowel necrosis induced by tumor necrosis factor in rats is mediated by platelet activating factor, *J Clin Invest* 81:1328, 1988.

197 Thomas L: *The lives of a cell: notes of a biology watcher,* New York, 1974, Viking Press.

198 Thompson BM, Steuven HS, Tonsfeldt DJ et al: Calcium: limited indications, some danger, *Circulation* 74(suppl 4):90, 1986.

199 Tilney NL, Bailey GL, Morgan AP: Sequential system failure after rupture of abdominal aortic aneurysms: an unsolved problem in postoperative care, *Ann Surg* 178:117, 1973.

200 Townsend MC, Hampton WW, Haybron DM et al: Effective organ blood flow and bioenergy status in murine peritonitis, *Surgery* 100:205, 1986.

201 Tracey KJ, Fong Y, Hesse D et al: Anti-cachectin/TNF monoclonal antibodies prevent septic shock during lethal bacteremia, *Nature* 330:662, 1987.

202 Tracey KJ: Tumor necrosis factor (cachectin) in the biology of septic shock syndrome, *Circ Shock* 35:123, 1991.

203 Tryba M: Risk of acute stress bleeding and nosocomial pneumonia in ventilated intensive care patients: sucralfate versus antacids, *Am J Med* 83(suppl 3B):117, 1987.

204 Van der Waaij D, Berghuis-de Vries JM, Lekkerkerk-van der Wees JE: Colonization resistance of the digestive tract in conventional and antibiotic-treated mice, *H Hyg* 69:405, 1971.

205 Van Oers MH, Hayden AA, Aarden LA: Interleukin-6 in serum and urine of renal transplant recipients, *Clin Exp Immunol* 71:314, 1988.

206 Vane JR, Anggard EE, Botting RM: Regulatory functions of the vascular endothelium, *N Engl J Med* 323:27, 1990.

207 Vedder NB, Winn RK, Rice CL et al: A monoclonal antibody to the adherence-promoting leukocyte glycoprotein, CD-18, reduces organ injury and improves survival from hemorrhagic shock and resuscitation in rabbits, *J Clin Invest* 81:939, 1988.

208 Veterans Administration Systemic Sepsis Cooperative Study Group: Effect of high-dose glucocorticoid therapy on mortality in patients with clinical signs of severe sepsis, *N Engl J Med* 317:659, 1987.
209 Vijaykumar E, Raziuddin S, Wardle EN: Plasma endotoxin in patients with trauma, sepsis, and severe hemorrhage, *Clin Intensive Care* 2:4, 1991.
210 Voerman HJ, Schijndel RJM, Thijs LG: Continuous arterial-venous hemodialfiltration in critically ill patients, *Crit Care Med* 18:911, 1990.
211 Waage A, Halstensen A, Espevik T: Association between tumor necrosis factor in serum and fatal outcome in patients with meningococcal disease, *Lancet* 1:355, 1987.
212 Waage A, Brandtzaeg P, Halstensen A et al: The complex pattern of cytokines in serum from patients with meningococcal septic shock: association between interleukin-6, interleukin-1, and fatal outcome, *J Exp Med* 169:333, 1989.
213 Watters JM, Bessey PQ, Dinarello CA et al: Both inflammatory and endocrine mediators stimulate host response to sepsis, *Arch Surg* 121:179, 1986.
214 Wattwill LM, Sjostrand UM, Borg UR: Comparative studies of IPPV and HFPPV and PEEP in critical care patients: a clinical evaluation, *Crit Care Med* 11:30, 1983.
215 Waymack JP, Jenkins M, Alexander JW et al: A prospective trial of prophylactic intravenous immune globulin for the prevention of infections in severely burned patients, *Burns* 15:71, 1989.
216 Waymack JP, Jenkins M, Warden GD et al: A prospective study of thymopentin in severely burned patients, *Surg Gynecol Obstet* 164:423, 1987.
217 Wells CL, Rotstein OR, Pruett TL et al: Intestinal bacteria translocate into experimental intra-abdominal abscesses, *Arch Surg* 121:102, 1986.
218 West MA, Keller GA, Cerra FB et al: Killed *E. coli* stimulate macrophage-mediated alterations in hepatocellular function during in vitro coculture, *Infect Immun* 49:563, 1985.
219 Wilmore DW, Smith RJ, O'Dwyer ST et al: The gut: a central organ after surgical stress, *Surgery* 104:917, 1988.
220 Wilmore DW: Catabolic illness: strategies for enhancing recovery, *N Engl J Med* 325:695, 1991.
221 Wolf YG, Corter S, Perel A: Dependence of oxygen consumption on cardiac output in sepsis, *Crit Care Med* 15:198, 1987.
222 Ziegler EJ, McCutchan JA, Fierer J et al: Treatment of gram-negative bacteremia and shock with human antiserum to a mutant *Escherichia coli, N Engl J Med* 307:1225, 1982.
223 Ziegler EJ, Fisher CJ, Sprung CL et al: Treatment of gram-negative bacteremia and septic shock with HA-1A human monoclonal antibody against endotoxin, *N Engl J Med* 324:429, 1991.
224 Ziegler TR, Smith RJ, O'Dwyer ST et al: Increased intestinal permeability associated with infection in burn patients, *Arch Surg* 123:1313, 1988.

CHAPTER

17

"Rule of nines"

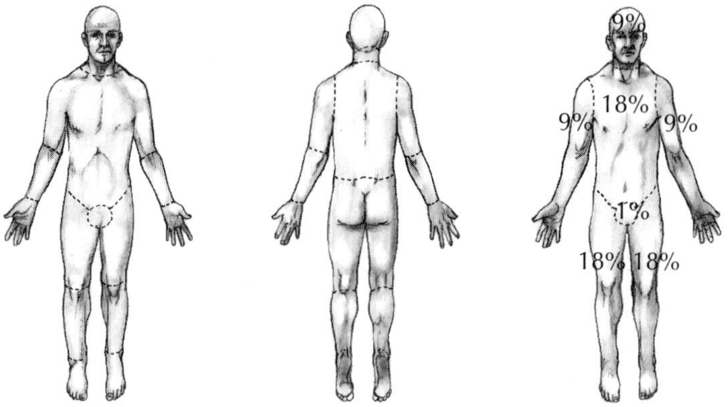

Burn estimate and diagram
age versus area

Area	Birth-1 year	1-4 years	5-9 years	10-14 years	15 years	Adult
Head	19	17	13	11	9	7
Neck	2	2	2	2	2	2
Anterior trunk	13	13	13	13	13	13
Posterior trunk	13	13	13	13	13	13
Right buttock	2.5	2.5	2.5	2.5	2.5	2.5
Left buttock	2.5	2.5	2.5	2.5	2.5	2.5
Genitalia	1	1	1	1	1	1
Right upper arm	4	4	4	4	4	4
Left upper arm	4	4	4	4	4	4
Right lower arm	3	3	3	3	3	3
Left lower arm	3	3	3	3	3	3
Right hand	2.5	2.5	2.5	2.5	2.5	2.5
Left hand	2.5	2.5	2.5	2.5	2.5	2.5
Right thigh	5.5	6.5	8	8.5	9	9.5
Left thigh	5.5	6.5	8	8.5	9	9.5
Right leg	5	5	5.5	6	6.5	7
Left leg	5	5	5.5	6	6.5	7
Right foot	3.5	3.5	3.5	3.5	3.5	3.5
Left foot	3.5	3.5	3.5	3.5	3.5	3.5

THERMAL INJURIES

Basil A. Pruitt Jr. • Cleon W. Goodwin • William G. Cioffi Jr.

DEFINITION OF THE PROBLEM

The precise incidence of burn injury is unknown, but based on several regional surveys burns are estimated to affect more than 1.4 million persons in the United States annually.[20] Most of those injuries are minor and can be cared for on an outpatient basis because more than 80% of burns involve less than 20% of the total body surface.[163] However, approximately 54,000 burn patients per year require in-hospital care because of the extent or anatomic location of their burns or other complicating features, such as the extremes of age, associated injury, or preexisting disease.

In recent years, burns have resulted in approximately 5,000 deaths annually, although this figure does not include deaths due to arson or suspicious circumstances (estimated at 300/year) or those from suicidal intent (estimated at 150/year). In addition to the loss of human life, the lifetime cost of all fire and burn injuries is enormous and was estimated in 1985 at $3.8 billion.[248] House fires cause greater then 70% of all deaths, with three fourths of these attributable to smoke and fumes and only 20% to burns themselves. However, house fires account for only a small fraction of all burn admissions (4%), with scald injuries the most predominant. The multisystem effects of an extensive burn injury necessitate multispecialty medical care, intensive nursing care, and high-volume laboratory support for these patients, who are best cared for in a specialized treatment facility.

Local Changes

The degree of cell injury caused by thermal energy is determined by the temperature and duration of the heat exposure. A heat source of less than 45°C (113°F) results in no injury even with prolonged exposure.[263] As the temperature increases above that level, the duration of exposure causing tissue damage decreases, so that exposure to water at 54°C (129.2°F) for 30 seconds causes a partial-thickness burn, and exposure to a radiant heat source, delivering 4.8 kcal/cm^2 in 0.54 seconds, causes a full-thickness skin burn.[90] Heat sufficient to cause protein coagulation and cell death, if applied for sufficient time, produces full-thickness necrosis of the skin, whereas application of less thermal energy produces only partial-thickness injury, with variable damage to cells from which they may recover.

The area of cell death resulting from burn injury is called the *zone of coagulation;* areas of lesser cell injury are called the *zone of stasis* and the *zone of hyperemia.*[129] The zone of coagulation extends through the entire thickness of the dermis in a full-thickness, or third-degree, burn but only through a portion of the dermis in a partial-thickness, or second-degree, burn (Figure 17-1). In the zone of stasis, initially attenuated blood flow is restored with time, whereas in the zone of hyperemia blood flow is increased, and an inflammatory response is evident shortly after injury. If blood flow is not reestablished to the zone of stasis because of the inflammatory response, the tissue may die. Attempts to decrease the inflammatory response and restore blood flow using monoclonal antibodies directed against neutrophil and endothelial cell adhesion molecules have shown promise in animal models. In an area of partial-thickness burn, the zone of stasis takes the form of a concentric hemispheroid mass of tissue surrounding the zone of coagulation and involving a variable depth of dermis.

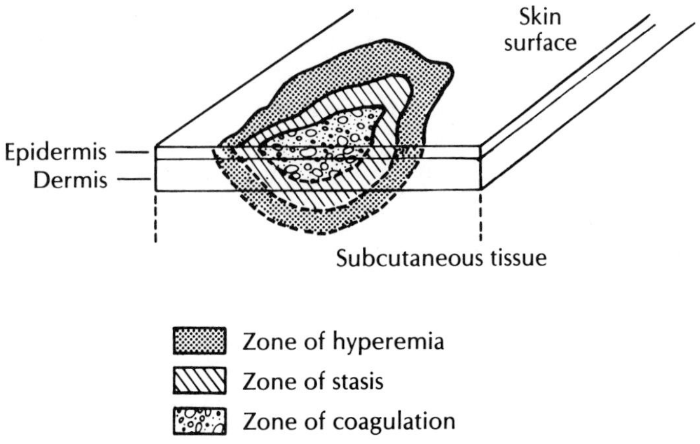

FIGURE 17-1 Thermal energy produces concentric zones of decreasingly severe tissue injury. In full-thickness, or third-degree burns, the zone of coagulation involves the entire thickness of the dermis, but in partial-thickness, or second-degree burns (as shown here), the zone of coagulation involves only a portion of the dermis.

The zone of hyperemia is evident as yet another concentric hemispheroid mass of tissue surrounding the zone of stasis or is present by itself in superficial injuries, such as a sunburn.

In addition to permanent or temporary interruption of the local blood supply, thermal injury results in the rapid formation of edema in burned tissues. The cellular injury caused by heat liberates cellular enzymes and substances such as histamine, serotonin, kinins, prostaglandins, leukotrienes, and interleukin I, as well as the activation of complement, all of which may alter transcapillary fluid movement and exert hemodynamic, metabolic, and immunologic effects both locally and systemically.* The development of edema, although partially dependent on the volume of resuscitation fluids infused, is rapid, with several studies documenting a doubling of tissue water content within 1 hour of injury. The mechanism responsible for such a rapid increase is poorly understood. Net capillary exchange depends on the capillary filtration coefficient (CFC) and the net filtration pressure. Although Pitt and colleagues[216] and Arturson and Mellander[11] have reported a 100% to 300% increase in CFC, this rise is insufficient to account for the magnitude of tissue edema.

Net filtration pressure is determined by capillary and interstitial hydrostatic pressures, the plasma and interstitial colloid osmotic pressure, and the capillary reflection coefficient. The local hemodynamic effects of the aforementioned liberated substances result in a modest increase in capillary hydrostatic pressure, which contributes to tissue edema. Recently, Lund and colleagues[157,158] have measured interstitial hydrostatic pressure immediately after thermal injury and have noted a large decrease in pressure from −11 mm Hg to −150 mm Hg. The magnitude of change is sufficient to account for the initial rapid edema formation that has been measured. The interstitial colloid osmotic pressure also increases secondary to changes in the capillary reflection coefficient, an index of capillary permeability that indicates how easily plasma protein can enter the interstitial space. In general, burn injury decreases the reflection coefficient, which permits proteins of up to 108 A° to pass into the interstitium.

The aggregate local response is one of initial rapid increase in extravascular volume in the burned area, associated with an initial local increase in lymph flow.[11] The continued accumulation of edema fluid in the burn-injured tissue has been considered a manifestation of increased vascular permeability. Subsequent diminution and even cessation of lymph flow from the burned area has been attributed to obstruction of the lymphatic vessels by serum proteins that have leaked through the walls of damaged capillaries.[12]

Studies by Brown and associates[35] in a murine model of burn injury have revealed that water and albumin content of the burn wound were at a maximum 24 hours postburn. The water and albumin content of the injured tissues remained markedly elevated, and the rate of entry of albumin into the burn wound was increased throughout the first 6 days postburn. Stability of the total albumin pool size between 24 and 72 hours postburn indicates that the quantity of albumin transferred out of the wound equaled that entering the wound, and that a state of dynamic equilibrium had been established between the burn wound and plasma albumin pools. Those changes, and the observation that postburn treatment

* References 3, 31, 99, 116, 137, and 264.

of the burned animals with hyaluronidase was associated with a lesser increase in the albumin and water content of the burn wound, provide evidence that changes in water and albumin content of the burn wound are related to changes in the interstitial tissue.

On the basis of studies using various-sized dextrans, Arturson[10] has concluded that in patients with burns of more than 25% of the total body surface, there is a generalized increase in capillary permeability that accounts for the formation of edema in unburned areas. Other investigators[75,161] have suggested that the edema in unburned tissue represents the combined volume and oncotic pressure effects of the administration of large volumes of colloid-free resuscitation fluid. Both mechanisms may be operative in patients with extensive burns, and edema formation in uninjured tissue may be quite extensive.

Systemic Changes

In a very real sense the burn patient is truly the universal trauma model.[226] The systemic response to burn injury involves all organ systems in the stereotypic biphasic pattern of early hypofunction and later hyperfunction that characterizes the multisystem response to any injury. Changes in central nervous system function occur in reverse order as they do in the immune system (Table 17-1). The incidence, magnitude, and duration of these changes are proportional to the extent of burn, reaching an apparent physiologic maximum in patients with burns over 50% of the total body surface (Figure 17-2). The magnitude of physiologic alteration changes over time, with the maximum perturbation seen in the first 2 weeks postburn, followed by slow return toward normal as the burn wound is closed by healing or grafting.[226]

Cardiovascular Changes

The initial hemodynamic response to a significant burn is a decrease in cardiac output, associated with a marked increase in peripheral vascular resistance as a result of the immediate neurohormonal response to the injury.[238] Without treatment, hypovolemia caused by progressive loss of fluid through the burn-injured capillaries reduces cardiac filling and further decreases cardiac output, resulting in diminished blood flow to the kidneys and other organs. This decrease in cardiac output elicits a generalized vasoconstrictive response, which maintains the elevation of peripheral resistance. The hypovolemia and decrease in cardiac output that occur in the early postburn period are associated with a redistribution of blood flow such that a greater fraction of cardiac output is supplied to the viscera and a lesser fraction to the carcass, although the absolute amount of perfusion may be inadequate.[16,17] The distribution of cardiac output is returned toward normal with fluid resuscitation (Table 17-2).

Some investigators[25] have proposed that a myocardial depressant factor is the cause of unresponsiveness to fluid resuscitation in patients, particularly the elderly, with extensive burns. However, a specific burn-related myocardial depressant factor has been neither identified nor characterized. Studies by Dorethy and associates[81] have shown that patients with a lower-than-predicted cardiac output in the first 24 hours postburn actually had a hyperdynamic myocardium with increased left ventricular ejection fraction and velocity of myocardial fiber shortening as measured by echocardiography. In those study patients, a decrease in left ventricular end diastolic volume was consistent with a persistent functional hypovolemia, indicating a need for the administration of additional resuscitation fluid (Table 17-3). In

TABLE 17-1 BIPHASIC ORGAN SYSTEM RESPONSE TO BURN INJURY

ORGAN SYSTEM	EARLY CHANGE (PHASE ONE)	LATER RESPONSE (PHASE TWO)
Cardiovascular	Hypovolemia	Hyperdynamic state
Pulmonary	Hypoventilation	Hyperventilation
Central nervous	Agitation	Obtundation*
Endocrine	Catabolic effects	Anabolic effects
Gastrointestinal	Ileus	Hypermotility
Urinary	Oliguria	Diuresis
Skin	Hypoperfusion	Hyperemia

* Usually associated with septic or metabolic complications.

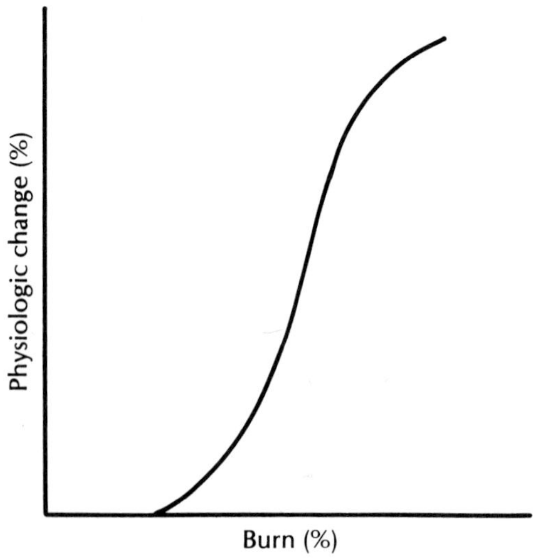

FIGURE 17-2 The occurrence, magnitude, and duration of pathophysiologic changes are related in sigmoid dose-response fashion to the extent of burn injury.

TABLE 17-2 EFFECT OF INJURY AND RESUSCITATION ON DISTRIBUTION OF CARDIAC OUTPUT FOLLOWING A 40% BURN INJURY IN A CANINE MODEL

PARAMETER	PREBURN	1 HOUR POSTBURN (NO RESUSCITATION)	5 HOURS POSTBURN (4 HOURS OF BROOKE-FORMULA RESUSCITATION)
Cardiac index L/min/m²	5.77	3.78	5.68
Organ blood flow (% of cardiac output)	42.0	48.0	44.0
Carcass blood flow (% of cardiac output)	58.0	52.0	56.0

TABLE 17-3 ECHOCARDIOGRAPHIC ASSESSMENT OF CARDIAC FUNCTION IN BURN PATIENTS 12 TO 24 HOURS POSTBURN

CARDIAC FUNCTION	PATIENTS WITH DECREASED CARDIAC OUTPUT	PATIENTS WITH "NORMAL" CARDIAC OUTPUT
Stroke index (ml/m²)	27 ± 11*	43 ± 11
Ejection fraction	0.74 ± 0.07	0.73 ± 0.07
Velocity of circumferential fiber shortening (circ/sec)	1.73 ± 0.14	1.89 ± 0.80
Left ventricular end diastolic volume index (ml/m²)	37 ± 16*	16 ± 16

* $P < 0.001$.

a rodent model, Cioffi and associates[54] reported that postburn papillary muscle dysfunction could be completely reversed by adequate fluid resuscitation.

Cardiac output in patients receiving adequate resuscitation returns to predicted normal levels in the latter half of the first 24 hours postburn. With repletion of the plasma volume by continued fluid resuscitation in the second 24 hours postburn, cardiac output rises to supranormal levels (the earliest manifestation of postburn hypermetabolism), where it remains until the burns are closed.[238]

Pulmonary Changes

The response of the pulmonary vasculature to burn injury is similar to that of the peripheral circulation. However, the elevation of pulmonary vascular resistance is higher and lasts longer than that of peripheral vascular resistance.[15] Lymph flow in the lung increases, but the lymph/plasma protein ratio changes little, indicating that pulmonary capillary permeability is largely unaffected by burn injury per se.[77]

Minute ventilation may be unchanged or even decreased early following burn injury in patients without inhalation injury who develop hypovolemia. Following resuscitation, minute ventilation increases in proportion to burn size.[230] This hyperventilation is the result of an increase in both respiratory rate and tidal volume and characteristically is not associated with hypoxemia. The hyperventilation usually peaks early in the second postinjury week and then gradually recedes. In patients showing this postburn hyperventilation in the absence of inhalation injury, true shunt has been insignificant, carbon monoxide diffusing capacity unimpaired, and the lung clearance index uniform and normal. Pulmonary resistance appears to be unaffected. Static and dynamic compliance are modestly decreased, and pressure volume work of breathing is increased commensurate with the decrease in compliance, but these changes are not striking and appear to be disproportionately small in relation to the marked increase in minute ventilation. In the absence of significant parenchymal change, this increase in minute ventilation appears to be a manifestation of postburn hypermetabolism that relents as the burn wound heals or is closed by grafting. This postburn hyperventilation can be accentuated by the use of topical mafenide acetate on the burn wound (mafenide is an inhibitor of carbonic anhydrase),[214] sepsis, supervening pulmonary parenchymal disease, acute intraabdominal disease, fever, and anemia.[215]

Renal Changes

The response of the kidney to burn injury is also biphasic and reflects the previously noted hemodynamic changes. Early postburn diminution of renal plasma flow and glomerular filtration rate result in oliguria in association with decreased free water osmolar and endogenous creatinine clearance.[206] If resuscitation is inordinately delayed and the hypovolemia progresses, acute renal failure may occur.

Following resuscitation, the burn-related edema fluid is resorbed and cardiac output rises to supranormal levels, both of which increase renal blood flow and promote postinjury diuresis. This diuresis is often modest in amount and duration because of both slow mobilization of the edema and the marked increase in evaporative water loss from the burn surface. The marked elevation of cardiac output and renal blood flow documented after resuscitation and the eventual diuresis of the salt and water administered during resuscitation necessitates adjustment in dosage of drugs excreted primarily by the kidney. Following resuscitation, excessive administration of carbohydrate or protein-containing nutrients may affect urinary output by inducing an osmotic diuresis. Alteration of the nutritional regimen or administration of insulin may be necessary to reduce the osmotic load presented to the kidney.

During the postresuscitative phase, plasma renin and antidiuretic hormone (ADH) levels remain elevated in the milieu of a hyperdynamic circulation, suggesting a resetting of the hormonal control mechanisms.[270] Cioffi and colleagues[59] documented a significant decrement in renal free water clearance with a significant elevation of the urine K+ /Na+, ratio indicating that the kidney is sensitive to the hormonal changes. They also found that blood volume was 80% of predicted value. These findings indicate that the hormonal changes are appropriate and suggest that a paradoxical dissociation between blood volume and flow exists in these patients.[59]

Gastrointestinal Changes

Cessation of propulsive activity is the initial response of the gastrointestinal tract to burn injury.[222] The resulting ileus that precludes effective oral resuscitation and necessitates nasogastric intubation to prevent aspiration in patients with extensive burns is the net effect of hypovolemia and the neurologic and endocrine response to the injury. Studies by Asch and colleagues,[16] using radiolabeled microspheres in a canine model of burn injury, showed that total gastric blood flow was little affected in the first 5 hours postburn, but more recent studies[149] have identified significant shock-related diminution of gastric mucosal blood flow. Histologically, the ischemic changes of the upper gastrointestinal tract appear to be focal and result in mucosal cell injury, as manifested by superficial erosions in the stomach and duodenum[70] (Figure 17-3). These mucosal lesions may progress to frank ulceration if the upper gastrointestinal tract is not protected by administration of antacids or H_2 histamine-receptor antagonists.[167]

The translocation of bacteria and bacterial products such as endotoxin to mesenteric lymph nodes and the hepatic portal system has been documented following thermal injury and other traumatic insults in a variety of animal models. In rodent models following burn injury, gut mucosal atrophy and increased mucosal permeability have been reversed by IGF-1 therapy.[125] The relevance of this interesting phenomenon in human beings remains to be documented. However, LeVoyer and colleagues[152] reported a significant increase in intestinal permeability on post burn day (PBD) 2 to the

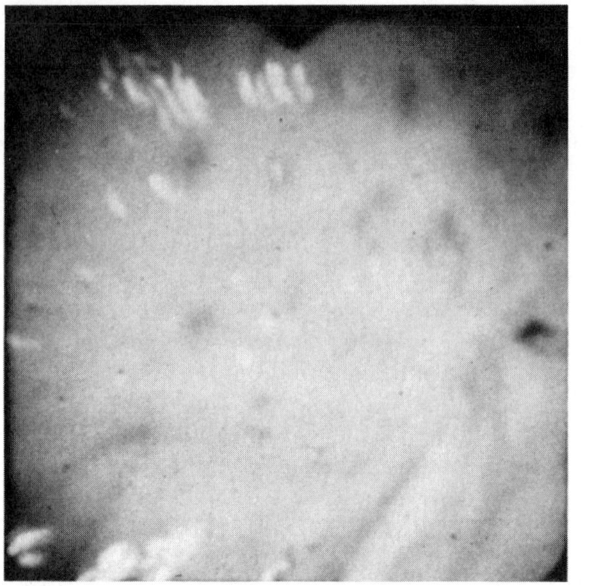

FIGURE 17-3 Punctate hemorrhagic erosions of the gastric mucosa are evident on endoscopic examination as early as 5 hours after burn injury in 86% of patients with burns involving more than 35% of the total body surface.

monosaccharide lactulose in thermally injured patients who ultimately developed an infection. Whether this finding was merely an epiphenomenon or causally related to the development of infection remains to be proven.

Following resuscitation, gastrointestinal motility returns, at which time nasogastric drainage can be stopped and oral feeding resumed. Later in the postburn course, gastrointestinal hyperactivity and diarrhea may occur as a result of the combined effect of increased gastrointestinal blood flow and excessive nutrient administration. Administration of lactose-based nutritional regimens and intestinal bacterial overgrowth secondary to broad-spectrum antibiotic administration are additional causes of diarrhea in burn patients.

Neuroendocrine Changes

The central nervous system response to severe injury is closely related to both the hemodynamic and metabolic status of the individual patient. In those patients in whom mild to moderate hypovolemia or hypoxemia occur in the immediate postburn period, agitation may be noted. If the volume and oxygen deficits become significant, obtundation may supervene. In the immediate post-injury period, assessment of the central nervous system status may be confounded by the neurologic effects of toxic materials present in the fire environment or drugs present in the circulation at the time of injury. In the postresuscitation state, sympathetic outflow is increased in association with the hypermetabolic response, and neurologic hyperactivity may be evident.[296] In patients who develop septic and metabolic complications, obtundation may be evident and clear only when the complication is effectively treated. Inappropriate drug administration and the effect of sensory deprivation common in the critical care environment may also alter the patient's mental status.

The early hypovolemia-associated decrease in metabolic rate is transient, and as resuscitation fluids are administered, a catabolic hormonal pattern is established characterized by elevated catecholamine, cortisol, and glucagon levels and depressed triiodothyronine and insulin levels.[233] These neuroendocrine changes result in an increase in metabolic rate that is proportional to burn size and associated with an increase in glucose flow and a negative nitrogen balance.[299] In the uncomplicated burn patient, these circulating hormone levels return toward normal as the wounds heal or are grafted, after which convalescence begins and reconstitution of body mass occurs. Sepsis and other complications, in their early stages, cause an exaggeration of the neuroendocrine changes, when they occur early postinjury, or a reversion to the early postinjury pattern, when they occur later.[298] Conversely, in the end-stages of life-threatening complications, the injury pattern of endocrine change may be attenuated in a manner consistent with endocrine exhaustion.

IMMUNOLOGIC EFFECTS OF BURN INJURY

I. Destruction of mechanical barrier of skin
II. Humoral factors
  - IgG depression
  - IgM depression
  - Decreased levels of fibronectin
  - Complement activity decreased—C_1, C_2, C_3, and C_4
III. Cellular changes
  - Lymphocytes
    - T cells increased relative to B cells
    - Decreased response to phytohemagglutinin
    - Decreased mixed lymphocyte culture response
    - Depressed delayed-type hypersensitivity reaction to skin test antigens
    - Decreased interleukin II production
    - Sequential emergence suppressor-inducer and suppressor-effector T cells
    - Delayed allograft rejection
  - Neutrophils
    - Impaired chemotaxis
    - Decreased phagocytic capacity
    - Decreased bactericidal activity
    - Decreased chemoluminescent response to stimuli
    - Decreased glucose utilization
IV. Reticuloendothelial system
  - Impaired clearance of colloidal fat
  - Decreased monocyte responsiveness

Hematologic Changes

The formed elements of the hematologic system are also affected in direct proportion to the extent of the burn. Immediate red cell destruction is evident histologically as coagulated masses of erythrocytes within the microvasculature in areas of full-thickness burn. During the first 5 to 7 days postburn, a continuing loss of red cells occurs, approximating 8% to 12% of the circulating red cell mass per day. This loss presumably results from the reticuloendothelial clearance of damaged cells and blood sampling for clinical management.[238] Although higher loss rates have been reported, elution of the radiolabeled red cell tag may have influenced those results.[153]

In successfully resuscitated burn patients, an early increase in fibrin-split product levels, accompanied by a marked depression of platelet and fibrinogen levels, is succeeded by an elevation of platelet fibrinogen, factor V, and factor VIII levels.[66,69] Secondary depression of clotting factors occurs in association with either sepsis or intravascular coagulation. Because fibrinogen appears to be little affected by sepsis per se, fibrinogen levels may be helpful in differentiating between sepsis and disseminated intravascular coagulation.[174]

Immunologic Changes

Burn injury causes global impairment of the immune system, as outlined in the box at left. The cutaneous barrier to invading organisms is destroyed, circulating levels of the immunoglobulins are depressed, and the cellular components are altered in terms of both number and subpopulations. Activation and depletion of the alternative complement pathway and an initial depression and secondary elevation of fibronectin levels have also been identified after burn injury.[99,142] Several immunosuppressive factors have been identified in the serum of patients after burn injury. The incriminated factors include an immunosuppressive polypeptide of approximately 10,000 daltons molecular weight,[63] complement degradation products that impair phagocytosis,[4] fragments of immunoglobulins, breakdown products of the coagulation and fibrinolytic systems,[209] prostaglandins, and endotoxin.[289]

An early postburn leukopenia is commonly followed by leukocytosis, with the initial depression representing mainly margination of circulating leukocytes.[169] The relatively low density of polymorphonuclear leukocytes present in extensive burn wounds is considered to be indicative of burn size-related indiscrete margination and explains in part the greater susceptibility to infection of patients with more extensive burns.[304,305] Depression of neutrophil chemotactic,[290] phagocytic,[108] and bacterial activity[5] have all been identified following burn injury. More recently, increased CR3 receptor expression,[188] cytosolic oxidative activity,[51] and actin polymerization[40] have been noted in granulocytes from burn patients, indicating a generalized activation of circulating granulocytes. Compounds potentially causing this indiscriminant activation include complement products, endotoxin, platelet activating factor (PAF), and other cytokines.[52] The perturbations which affect granulocyte function following thermal injury are diverse and indicate a more complex problem than just simple hypofunction. Thus, therapy directed toward nonspecific activation of granulocyte oxidative function may be unwise.

Burn size-related alterations of lymphocyte populations have also been described, that is, depression of helper cells[205] and generation of suppressor inducer T cells followed by emergence of suppressor effector T cells.[139] Reduced helper T-cell activity has been related to impairment of macrophage antigen presentation reversible by addition of interleukin I.[140] Other investigators[302] have described a burn size-related suppression of interleukin-2 production by lymphocytes in burn patients which they have related to infection susceptibility. Other studies have demonstrated marked impairment of IL-2 receptor expression and have proposed that the receptors present are nonfunctional.[97] Increased levels of soluble IL-2 receptors have been identified in the serum of burn patients.[280] Those circulating soluble receptors may inhibit immune responses that are dependent on IL-2 by binding IL-2.

Meticulous identification of cell populations by careful gating has shown that burn injury per se produces proportionate decreases in all lymphocyte populations, and only when the burn wounds become infected are a relative decrease in helper T cells and a decrease in the helper/suppressor ratio noted.[42] Recent studies have shown that immediately after injury there is a depression in the number of specific receptors on T-helper cells, which returns to normal in the second or third postburn week. Conversely, receptors on the suppressor T cells show a much more transient depression and are actually increased in the second and third week postburn. These alterations in receptor number are consistent with the peak incidence of infection that occurs in the second and third week after injury.

In addition to the reduction in IL-2 production noted earlier, alterations in the circulating levels of other cytokines in burn patients have also been reported. Positive correlation between levels of IL1B, TNF2, and IL-6 have been reported.[85] IL-6 and TNF2 levels were significantly elevated in infected patients, suggesting that these cytokines play a role in the response to infection in burned patients.[84]

Impairment of reticuloendothelial system (RES) function after burn injury has also been reported. Depressed clearance of colloidal suspensions from the blood have been reported in both animal models and burn patients with fatal injuries.[112] An early postburn increase in antibody-forming cells has been attributed to impaired RES ability to degrade immunogens released from the burn wound.[245] Studies by others[142] suggest that the initial impairment of RES function may be related to the decrease in circulating levels of fibronectin.

These changes in the aggregate result in depression of the immune response as demonstrated by prolonged cutaneous allograft survival in burn patients and impaired delayed hypersensitivity[168] as well as an increase in susceptibility to infection and sepsis.

A variety of therapeutic interventions to enhance immune competence in burn patients have been evaluated. The intravenous administration of immunoglobulin G promptly normalized circulating serum levels, but was associated with no change in incidence of infection or mortality.[269] The administration of IL-2 in animal models of infection following burn injury has prolonged survival and improved resistance to a secondary septic challenge.[106] The administration of granulocyte macrophage colony stimulating factor, which elicited no clinically significant side effects in burn patients, increased the number of circulating neutrophils and the superoxide production of those cells in response to challenge.[50] The clinical effectiveness of such hemopoietic growth factors remains to be defined. The multiplicity of immunologic impairments speaks against the universal effectiveness of a single agent and in favor of multimodal therapy to address the deficit in concert.

ELECTRIC INJURY

Pathophysiology

Electric current damages tissue by the conversion of electric energy into heat. The effects of electricity depend on current voltage, type of current (direct or alternating), pathway of the current, and duration of contact. Any voltage above 40 volts is potentially dangerous, and voltage above 1000 volts has been arbitrarily defined as high-tension. Alternating current is considered more dangerous than direct current because of its likelihood of producing cardiac and/or pulmonary arrest and its tetanic effect, which may "lock" the patient to the source of electricity. An alternating current frequency of 60 cycles/second is extremely dangerous to the heart and respiratory center, whereas current frequencies above that level are less injurious to tissue. Passage of current through the heart or respiratory center is most apt to be associated with sudden death.

Differences in the conductivity of various tissues (e.g., nerve greatest and bone least) are of essentially no importance when the injury is produced by high-voltage electricity. All body tissues and fluids are conductive, and hence the body acts as a volume conductor of electricity. Heat is produced as a function of current density, that is, the voltage drop and current flow per unit cross-sectional area.[126] As a consequence, severe injury is common when a digit or an extremity comes in contact with high-tension electricity, and major injury to the trunk is rare.

Electric injury is most severe at contact points where current density is highest and causes charring of the skin and at sites of current arcing (commonly the flexor surface of joints), where charring also occurs (Figure 17-4). At voltages below 1000, resistance at a site of charring rises rapidly and limits subsequent current passage and tissue heating. Above 1000 volts relatively constant levels of current are maintained, and intense arcing is associated with greater tissue destruction.[261] After cessation of current flow, the involved body part acts as a volume radiator. The superficial tissues that cool more rapidly are less liable to be severely injured than the deeper tissues that cool more slowly. Low-voltage direct current, such as that produced by automobile batteries or electrosurgical devices, may produce tissue injury usually of limited extent.[146]

The characteristics of electric injury frequently necessitate modification of the treatment used for patients with conventional thermal injury. Cardiopulmonary arrest often occurs in patients who have sustained high-voltage electric injuries and must be treated promptly by cardiopulmonary resuscitation. Cardiac arrhythmias may also occur during and even after resuscitation. Patients who have sustained a cardiac arrest should undergo continuous electrocardiographic (ECG) monitoring for at least 48 hours after the last evidence of dysrhythmia.[274]

The risk of acute renal failure is relatively high in patients with electric injury.[80] Renal failure occurs as a result of underestimation of fluid needs that lead to administration of inadequate amounts of resuscitation fluid and the liberation of myoglobin from injured muscle. This myoglobin may precipitate in the renal tubules unless a brisk urinary output is maintained. Extensive tissue destruction may also cause release of potassium, and the resulting hyperkalemia may reach sufficient levels to interfere with cardiac function. Edema of tissues beneath the investing fascia of a limb injured by high voltage electricity may impair nutrient blood flow to those deep tissues and blood flow to distal unburned tissue, necessitating performance of a fasciotomy to reduce the tissue pressure within a muscle compartment and restore cir-

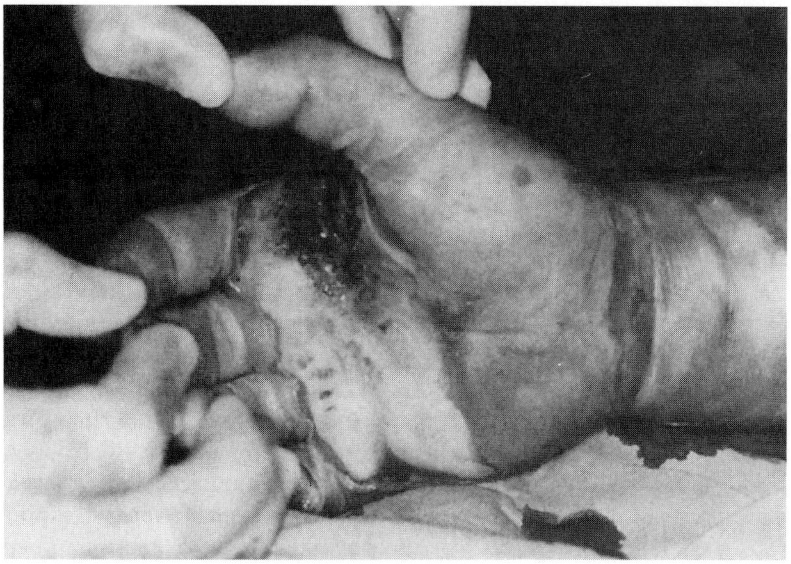

FIGURE 17-4 Charring is evident on the palmar aspect of the first web space in this patient, whose right hand made contact with a high-tension line. Note the full-thickness burn of the flexor surface of the wrist due to arcing of the current. Typical flexion deformity of all digits required forcible extension to expose the palmar burns.

culation. Electric injury has also been reported to cause intestinal perforation, focal pancreatic necrosis, focal gallbladder necrosis, and hepatic injury; but such injuries of remote organs are rare.[201] One author has reported a marked increase in cholelithiasis following high-voltage electric injury, but that finding has not been confirmed by others.[23]

Deficits of peripheral nerve, spinal cord, cerebellar, and cerebral function may be present immediately following injury or may be of delayed onset.[221] A thorough neurologic examination should be performed on admission and at scheduled intervals thereafter to identify and record any nerve deficit. After direct nerve injury return of function is uncommon, but resolution of early deficits in function of nerves not directly injured is common.[293] Sensory nerves appear to be less sensitive to current injury than motor nerves. Late-appearing functional deficits of nerves far removed from the points of contact may be part of a polyneuritic syndrome. Immediate spinal cord deficits resulting from direct neuronal damage are more commonly transient than are later-appearing spinal cord deficits, presenting as quadriplegia, hemiplegia, transverse myelitis (an amyotrophic lateral sclerosis-like syndrome), or localized nerve deficits with signs of ascending paralysis.[151]

Damage of cells can also be caused by what is termed electroporation, a mechanism by which transmembrane potentials of as little as 100 to 500 mv increase the size of the pores in cell membranes.[143] Those changes in pore size are associated with alterations in cell function that may be sufficiently severe to cause cell death. Electroporation may occur even when tissue heat is less than that required to produce coagulation necrosis and has been implicated as the cause of rhabdomyolysis and as an etiologic factor of otherwise inexplicable persistent neurologic signs and symptoms following electric injury. The clinical significance of electroporation and the role of nonionic surfactant treatment that has been proposed by some remain uncertain.

Moderate to large blood vessels subjected to high-voltage electric current may be the site of delayed hemorrhage. Although some reports[218] have suggested that such hemorrhage is caused by an electric injury-specific arteritis, hemorrhage from such vessels seems to occur only when wound debridement has been inadequate or a vessel exposed by debridement has undergone exposure-related desiccation and necrosis.

Compression fractures of vertebral bodies may be produced by the tetanic contractions of the paraspinous muscles, and long bone fractures may be caused by falls occurring at the time of the injury.[187] Appropriate radiographic studies should be obtained to identify such fractures.

Cataract formation is a common sequel of high-voltage electric injury, particularly in patients with a contact point on the head or neck.[258] Such cataracts may be evident within a day or two of the time of injury or may first present 3 or more years after the electric injury.

Management

In many patients who have come in contact with high-voltage electricity, the majority of the cutaneous burn has been produced by the ignition of clothing as a result of arcing. The cutaneous damage caused by the electric injury may be of limited extent at the sites of contact or at sites of arcing across the flexor surfaces of a limb. In either instance, deep tissue injury may be initially inapparent and lead to underestimation of fluid needs. If one uses a standard formula to estimate resuscitation needs in such patients, the resulting inadequate resuscitation may permit the development of oliguria. If oliguria does occur, additional fluids should be empirically administered until the desired hourly urinary output has been achieved. In patients with significant urinary hemochromogen concentrations (a dark red or brown urine) fluids should be administered to obtain an hourly urinary output of 75 to 100 ml. Administration of sodium bicarbonate solution in an attempt to alkalinize the urine has been reported to decrease pigment precipitation in the renal tubules. If the patient does not respond to the administration of more than the estimated volume of resuscitation fluids, or if the hemochromogens do not promptly clear from the urine, 12.5 g of mannitol should be added to each liter of intravenous fluid until the pigment has cleared from the urine. The treatment of hyperkalemia is guided by the severity of the electrolyte disturbance, using infusion of hypertonic glucose, insulin, and calcium salts; the enteric administration of ion exchange resins; or hemodialysis as indicated.

A need for fasciotomy of an electrically injured limb is indicated by cyanosis and impaired capillary refilling of distal unburned skin or nail beds, stony hardness of a muscle compartment, absence of or progressively diminished pulsatile flow in distal arteries as assessed with the ultrasonic flowmeter, and an intramuscular compartment pressure of more than 30 mm Hg measured by a wick catheter.[124] If those indications are present, a fasciotomy should be performed in the operating room as soon as the patient is hemodynamically stable.

Although both the tissue "wash-out" of ^{133}Xenon and the tissue uptake of technetium-99m pyrophosphate have been used to assess muscle viability, the clinical reliability, accuracy, and usefulness of those diagnostic modalities remain to be confirmed.[60,127] At operation the viability of the deep muscles and vital structures in the limb must be assessed because nonviable perosseous muscle may underlie more superficial viable muscle. All necrotic tissue is debrided to eliminate the principal source of hyperkalemia and reduce the risk of infection. In patients with extensive tissue damage and destruction of vital structures, amputation should be carried out at a level proximal to the area of tissue death. Following debridement the operative wounds should be dressed and the patient rescheduled for a second wound exploration 24 to 72 hours later. At that time, residual necrotic tissue is debrided as necessary or, if no further debridement is required, the wound can be closed by approximation of the skin edges or by skin grafting.

Children, usually those younger than 3 years, may sustain house current electric burns of the mouth as a consequence of biting or sucking on a live extension cord. The burn often involves the oral commissure and characteristically has the appearance of an avascular full-thickness burn. The frequency of bleeding from the labial artery justifies the in-hospital care of these patients. Because the final results seem little influenced by early surgical excision,[208] we treat all such injuries conservatively with periodic debridement of only grossly nonviable tissue. What initially appeared to be severe lesions have, with such treatment, healed with a minimum of cosmetic defects (Figure 17-5). Following spontaneous healing, elective repair of any functional or cosmetic defect can be carried out.

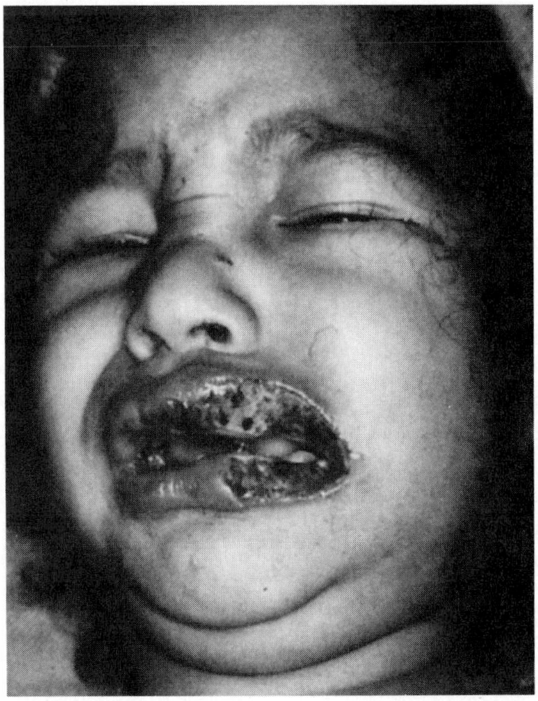

FIGURE 17-5 These apparently disfiguring burns of the lips due to house current healed uneventfully with such minor deformity that no reconstructive surgery was required.

Cutaneous burns in patients with electric injury are best treated with Sulfamylon burn cream. The active constituent (mafenide acetate) can diffuse into underlying nonviable tissue to control the microbial density.

Lightning Injury

A lightning bolt has currents ranging from 12,000 to 2,000,000 Å and is characteristically of brief duration.[8] Because lightning may induce either asystole or fibrillation, cardiopulmonary resuscitation is often required for patients struck by lightning. Even though late signs of acute myocardial damage have been reported, persistent or recurrent ECG abnormalities are rare.[6] Neurologic deficits and coma are common immediately following lightning injury, but usually resolve in a matter of hours. Skin burns produced by lightning typically have a splashed-on spidery, or arborescent, character and are commonly superficial and heal without the need for grafting (Figure 17-6). The immediate institution of cardiopulmonary resuscitation and the early recognition and prompt treatment of the complications of lightning injury permit salvage of fully two thirds of lightning-injured patients.[73a]

CHEMICAL INJURY

Chemical injuries are caused by the thermal energy produced when strong acids and strong alkalis react with tissue. The severity of the injury, like other thermal injuries, is related to the duration of exposure and the concentration of the injurious agent. Because alkalis bind more avidly to tissues and thus are more difficult to remove, they cause more severe damage than acids. Tissue injury is minimized if the chemical agent is removed from contact with exposed body surfaces. All clothing, including shoes, that contains the chemical should also be removed rapidly, and copious water lavage instituted. While acids usually can be removed by 30 to 60 minutes of water irrigation, alkali burns may require hours of lavage. Unfortunately, even prolonged lavage often fails to prevent deep tissue injuries following contact with strongly basic chemicals. Neutralizing agents should be avoided, because the intense exothermic reactions occurring with their use cause further thermal damage. Chemical burns appear deceptively superficial during the first 24 hours after injury, and failure to recognize the true extent of damage may lead to underestimation of resuscitation fluid needs.

Specific treatment medications are required in patients injured by certain chemicals. Alkali powders, such as anhydrous ammonia or lime, should be brushed away from the skin before lavage. If water is applied to the dry powder, the strongly alkaline solution produced will cause extensive tissue damage. Metallic sodium may ex-

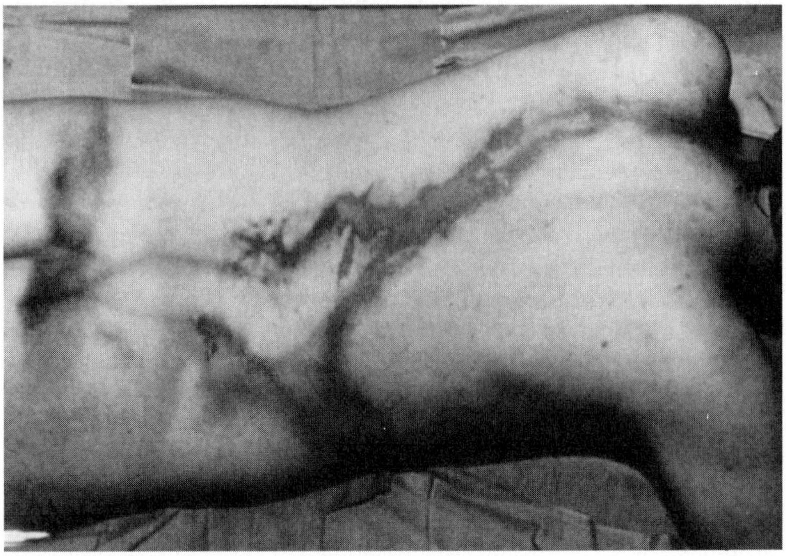

FIGURE 17-6 These serpiginous burns, typical of lightning injury, healed spontaneously.

plode when coming in contact with water and should be removed with instruments before any diluting agent is applied. Phenol has limited solubility in water and is best removed with solvents, such as glycerol, polyethylene glycol, or propylene glycol.[210] Continuous water lavage of acute phenol burns should be initiated if these solvents are not available. The metabolic inhibitory effect of phenol may induce hypothermia, necessitating use of external warming devices.

White phosphorus burns are particularly dangerous injuries, not only to the patient but also to treatment personnel. Exposure of retained phosphorus particles to air causes ignition and additional thermal injury to the patient or nearby medical staff. Copper sulfate solutions have been used to bathe white phosphorus burns; this solution forms a blue-gray cupric phosphide coating over the retained particles, impeding ignition and facilitating their identification. However, copper absorbed from the solution may cause hemolysis and acute renal failure.[221] The safer approach to the treatment of white phosphorus burns is the continuous application of water-soaked dressings until the particles are surgically removed. Ignition of retained particles is prevented by dressings kept wet with water or saline, and the particles can be identified by an ultraviolet light in the operating room. The phosphorus particles are then debrided and placed in water to prevent ignition.

Hydrofluoric acid may cause progressive tissue destruction after removal of surface contamination. Severe and continuous deep tissue pain indicates further chemical injury of the underlying subcutaneous tissue and muscle. Initial local treatment consists of water lavage, zephirin soaks, and application of calcium gel. Local or regional arterial injection of calcium gluconate has provided dramatic relief in isolated cases, but the effectiveness of such treatment has not been confirmed in clinical trials. If local measures are ineffective in relieving deep tissue involvement, excision and immediate grafting remove the injured tissue and relieve the pain.[137] Petroleum distillates and solvents damage tissue and cells by the process of delipdation. Tissue injury and the occurrence of systemic toxicity due to transcutaneous absorption are related to duration of exposure.

Immediate and copious lavage of chemically injured eyes with water or saline is essential to retain vision and minimize damage to the globe and surrounding structures. Extended irrigation is necessary in patients with injuries caused by strong alkalis, and a small cannula sutured to the conjunctival sulcus or a scleral contact lens with an irrigating side arm facilitates lavage. Lavage should be continued until the pH returns to normal. A cycloplegic agent, such as 1% atropine, in combination with a miotic agent, is administered to reduce the effects of iritis. Surveillance cultures dictate the choice of ophthalmic antibiotics.

The subconjunctival injection of autologous serum, the local application of eidetic acid or cysteine, and mucosal grafts have been recommended to reduce scar formation, but such interventions have had only limited success.[147] Symblepharon adhesions should be lysed before dense scarring forms between the globe and the eyelid, and xerophthalmia is treated with tear solutions.

Alkali injuries often cause devastating scar formation on the cornea and deeper ocular structures, and corneal transplants have been generally unsuccessful in restoring vision.

HISTORICAL BACKGROUND

Before 1900, burn care was largely empiric and focused on applying materials of varying toxicity to the burn wound. Little attention was given to the prevention or correction of hypovolemia or the other systemic effects of thermal injury. In the first decade of the twentieth century, Parascondolo in Italy reported the successful resuscitation of burn patients using intravenously administered saline.[184] A few years later, in the same decade, Sneve[273] in the United States recommended the use of saline given intravenously, by clysis, or by enema to prevent and correct burn shock. The first formula to estimate the resuscitation fluid needs of burn patients was proposed at a 1942 meeting of the National Research Council and was based on laboratory studies carried out by Harkins.[65] Since then, various burn-patient fluid-resuscitation formulas have been developed and used successfully to prevent or correct the development of burn shock, restore blood flow to the vital organs, and reduce the occurrence of acute renal failure.

The deleterious effect of many of the agents used for burn-wound care led to their abandonment in the first three decades of the twentieth century.[219] The recognition of the importance of maintaining a clean, dry burn wound resulted in the introduction of the exposure technique of burn-wound care by Wallace in the 1940s.[288] Description of the pathogenesis of invasive burn-wound infection led to the contemporaneous development in the 1960s of mafenide acetate burn cream by Moncrief and associates[186] and 0.5% silver nitrate soaks by Moyer and associates[189] to control bacterial density in the burn wound.[282] Effective topical chemotherapy of the burn wound has significantly reduced the occurrence of invasive burn-wound infection and materially contributed to an increase in survival of burn patients. Since then, early excision of the burned tissue has had a renaissance and is now widely used. Burn-wound excision has, in turn, focused attention on the use of biologic dressings and the development of skin substitutes and even culture-derived epidermal tissue to effect early closure of the excised wounds.

EPIDEMIOLOGY OF BURN INJURY

The epidemiology of burn injuries has remained relatively constant over the last decade. The most important factors influencing the rate of thermal injuries are age, sex, occupation, and economic status. In most published series, the highest peak incidence occurs in children less than 5 years of age (Figure 17-7); this observation is

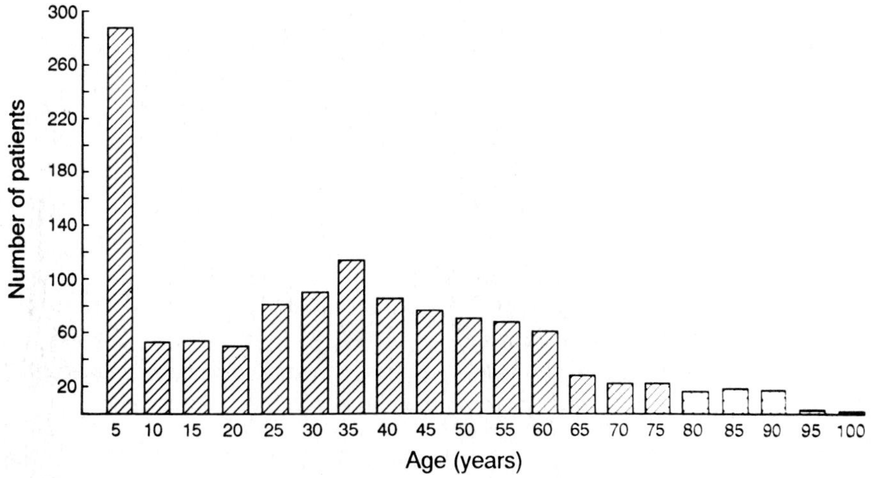

FIGURE 17-7 The age distribution of 1220 patients admitted in 1993 to the New York Hospital—Cornell University Medical College Burn Center. The largest population in most burn facilities comprises small children and infants, a result in part of admission criteria for extremes of age and for social circumstances.

true not only for hospitalized burn patients but also for all patients seeking care for burn injury.[48,93] Although the vast majority of the burns in the pediatric age group are caused by scalds (approximately 45% of all scalds), most fatal injuries are a result of flame injuries. Children account for a disparate number of deaths from flame injury, presumably secondary to their difficulty in escaping from burning buildings. In addition, about 10% of residential fire deaths can be attributed to children playing with matches, a scenario most commonly seen in young boys. Overall, burns in this age group occur with equal frequency in both sexes, and nearly all children are burned in homes. Inflicted immersion scald injury is a major cause for hospitalization in children less than 5 years of age. Because of the predominance of child abuse as a cause of burn injury in children, this etiology should be considered in any child presenting with a thermal injury.

The incidence of burn injuries declines in late childhood and adolescence until this population begins regular employment. At that time, a large increase in the rate of thermal injuries occurs that is related to occupational injuries. The youngest employed workers (ages 15 to 24) sustain the highest number of work-related burns; with increasing training and experience, the number of burn injuries decreases. Over one half of occupational thermal injuries occur in heavy industry, whereas the smallest incidence take place in service-related professions.[2] As opposed to early childhood burns, males are much more likely to sustain job-related burn injuries, reflecting in part the predominance of male employment in heavy industrial jobs. In the 15- to 24-year age group, the largest number of burn admissions are due to automobiles, including injury from crash-related fires, radiator scalds, and flash burns secondary to priming the car's carburetor with a volatile substance. Isolated burn injuries related to professional activities are unusual in the military populations, and when they occur, the burn is often only one component of a multiple injury incident.[29] The combination of burns with other trauma results in a much higher mortality rate than can be accounted for by the separate effects of each individual injury.

The economically disadvantaged are at greatest risk for injury and death from fire presumably secondary to their living conditions, which may contain many unsafe or fireprone conditions. In New York State, the nonwhite population is involved with serious burns nearly three times more often than the white population (66 per million versus 23 per million).[93] The relationship between median family income and burn rates is strong and linear: In this study, for every $1000 decrease in family income, the burn rate increased by 4.9 burns per 10,000 person-years. Other factors, such as dense urban environments and cultural practices, also influence the incidence of serious thermal injuries.

A large number of burn injuries are preventable. Cigarettes and faulty heating equipment, accounting for 28% and 15% of deaths, respectively, represent obvious areas in which prevention is possible. Clothing ignition, which accounts for 3% of all deaths and is most common in the elderly age group, could be decreased by extension of flammability standards, which have been applied to children's sleepwear and other clothing. The greatest potential for preventing tap water scalds lies in modifying hot water systems to prevent discharge of water at a temperature greater than 120°F.

HIERARCHICAL ORGANIZATION OF BURN CARE

First-Responder Burn Care

First-responder care for burn patients includes that needed by any injured patient as well as that which is burn specific. The burning process should be stopped as rapidly as possible by extinguishing the flames, diluting and washing away offending chemicals, or removing the patient from contact with an electric current. The rescuer must take every precaution to avoid becoming part of the circuit when trying to break contact between a patient and a source of electricity. Cardiopulmonary resuscitation should be instituted as indicated and is most often necessary in patients who have sustained high-voltage electric injury. Subsequent ventilatory support depends on both the patient's general condition and pulmonary status. If the patient was burned in a closed space, some degree of carbon monoxide poisoning should be assumed, and 100% oxygen should be administered by a tight-fitting nonrebreathing face mask. If the patient has impaired ventilatory exchange because of obtundation or some other reason, an endotracheal tube should be placed and mechanical ventilatory support provided.

The burn wounds should be covered with a clean sheet or dressing to prevent further contamination of the wound surface and reduce the pain in areas of partial-thickness burn. The patient should then be covered with a clean blanket to conserve body heat and minimize the risk of hypothermia. If the patient's hemodynamic status permits, burned extremities should be elevated.

Following the described field resuscitation, patients with moderate and major burn injuries should be promptly transported to a hospital for definitive care. If the patient has only burns, and transport to the hospital will require no more than 30 to 45 minutes, intravenous fluids need not be started in the field. If transportation to a definitive treatment facility requires more than 45 minutes, or if the patient has experienced blood loss caused by associated mechanical injuries, a physiologic salt solution should be administered through as large a cannula as can be readily inserted into a peripheral vein. Transportation should not be delayed by prolonged unsuccessful efforts to establish intravenous access.

The use of cold water soaks or ice packs will rapidly reduce the pain present in areas of partial-thickness burns and may also reduce the extent of tissue damage in those patients in whom such treatment can be initiated within 10 to 15 minutes of the time of injury.[74] If more time has elapsed, radiative loss of heat and heat transfer by the circulation at the periphery of the burn will have returned tissue temperature to essentially normal levels, and tissue injury will be little influenced by such treatment. If cold soaks or ice packs are used, their application should be limited to the time necessary to achieve pain relief or tissue euthermia to avoid the induction of total body hypothermia, which can cause cardiac arrhythmia and even death.

Emergency Room Burn Care

Emergency room care for the burn patient who has received no prehospital care parallels that previously described and represents an extension of prehospital care for those patients who have received such care. Intravenous access should be obtained by insertion of the largest cannula that will fit in the largest available vein. Ideally, a vein underlying unburned skin should be used but, if such a site is unavailable, the cannula can be placed through a burn wound. If, because of the depth and location of the burns, no other intravenous access site is available, cannulation of a central vein is acceptable. Resuscitation should be begun by infusion of a physiologic salt solution.

A brief history of the circumstances surrounding the injury should be obtained, with particular attention given to the causative agent; whether the injury occurred in a closed space; associated mechanical trauma; and in patients with electric injury, the voltage of the current in order to assess the risk of systemic toxicity, inhalation injury, associated visceral and osseous injuries, and the likelihood of deep tissue injury, respectively. The presence of preexisting diseases and medication intake should also be determined with special reference to insulin dosage in diabetics, anticonvulsant therapy in patients with seizure disorders, and cardiovascular or pulmonary medications in patients with significant cardiovascular and pulmonary diseases.

The extent and depth of the burn injury should then be estimated as described later, resuscitation fluid needs estimated, and infusion of fluids adjusted as necessary. The amount and type of fluids administered should be accurately recorded. An indwelling urethral catheter should be placed and the hourly urinary output used as a guide to the adequacy of resuscitation.

The ventilatory status must also be assessed. The administration of 100% oxygen should be continued in all patients with carbon monoxide poisoining. In addition to the indications that pertain to all surgical patients, burn-related edema of the upper airway, significant inhalation injury (as defined later), and carbon monoxide poisoning in the presence of obtundation are indications for mechanical ventilation in the burn patient. A nasogastric tube should be placed in all patients with postinjury ileus, with the tube placed to provide suction to prevent emesis and aspiration.

Electrocardiographic monitoring should be instituted in patients with high-voltage electric injury and continued for 24 hours beyond the last evidence of dysrhythmia. ECG monitoring is also indicated in patients who sustained associated myocardial trauma at the time of the burn and patients with preexisting cardiac disease. As described later in greater detail, the circulatory status of burned extremities, particularly those with circumferential burns, should be monitored on a regularly scheduled basis to determine the need for escharotomy and/or fasciotomy.

The need for analgesia in burn patients is inversely proportional to the depth of the burn. Full-thickness burns, in which the cutaneous nerve endings have been coagulated, are generally insensate, whereas partial-thickness burns, particularly superficial partial-thickness burns, may be exquisitely painful. Pain control is most safely achieved by the intravenous administration of a narcotic, using the smallest dose sufficient to control pain. During the immediate postburn period of systemic hypovolemia and edema formation, intramuscular or subcutaneous administration of analgesics is ineffective in relieving pain because of impaired mobilization and absorption of the injectate. The persistence of pain in that situation commonly leads to repeated administration of narcotics by those routes and subsequent respiratory depression when fluid resuscitation restores circulation to the injection site and results in the simultaneous mobilization of multiple doses of narcotic.

BURN PATIENT TRIAGE

Initial burn-wound care, except in the case of patients with chemical injury, should be delayed until resuscitation has been initiated and some degree of hemodynamic and pulmonary stability achieved. At that point, the burn wounds should be cleansed with any available surgical detergent disinfectant, all body hair shaved from the wound and a generous margin of unburned skin at the periphery of all burns, and all nonviable tissue debrided. Bullae larger than 2 cm in diameter should be excised because they are easily ruptured, following which the nonviable epidermis collapses over the protein-rich blister fluid in which colonizing organisms readily proliferate to serve as a nidus of infection. Bullae less than 2 cm in diameter can be left intact.

The regionalized hierarchical organization of burn care in the United States, in which burn center density corresponds to population density, reflects the proportional relationship between burn size and physiologic change and the necessity to provide high-intensity nursing care and multispecialty medical care for patients with extensive burns. The American Burn Association has established criteria defining those burn patients who are best treated in a burn center where the global pathophysiologic changes and life-threatening complications of severe burn injury can be best monitored and treated.[247]

Burn patients who should be referred to a burn center include those with the following: (1) partial and full-thickness burns of more than 10% of the body surface when less than 10 or greater than 50 years of age; (2) partial and full-thickness burns of more than 20% of the body surface area when 10 to 50 years of age; (3) significant partial and full-thickness burns that involve the face, hands, feet, genitalia, or perineum or those that involve the skin overlying major joints; (4) full-thickness burns of more than 5% at any age; (5) significant electric or lighting injury; (6) significant chemical burns; (7) significant inhalation injury; (8) lesser burns in association with preexisting illness that could complicate management, prolong recovery, or enhance mortality; (9) lesser burns in association with concomitant trauma sufficient to influence outcome; and (10) lesser burns associated with a need for special social, emotional, or long-term rehabilitation support or when abuse or neglect is suspected.

Those patients with uncomplicated lesser burns can receive definitive care in a general hospital from medical personnel having experience and expertise in the care of such patients. That subset of patients with minor burns, that is, partial-thickness burns of less than 5% or full-thickness burns of less than 1% of the body surface can be treated, at least initially, in a physician's office or a hospital emergency room.

BURN PATIENT TRANSFER

The transfer of a burn patient must be coordinated between the referring and receiving physicians.[57,276] The physicians involved should review the resuscitative care received by the patient (i.e., fluids infused, medications given, pertinent laboratory values, and the patient's current hemodynamic and pulmonary status) to assess patient stability and optimize patient safety during transfer (Figure 17-8). Needed alterations in treatment should be identified by the burn center physician and recommendations made for the treatment alteration before patient movement. In general, burn patients best tolerate transfer as soon as resuscitative therapy has achieved hemodynamic and pulmonary stability. If there is any question about the adequacy of resuscitation, transfer should be delayed until such concerns have been addressed.

Continuity and safety during the transfer of a severely burned patient are optimized if a physician can accompany the patient. If such escort is not possible, an appropriately trained and credentialed nurse should accompany the patient. Ground transportation, rotary wing aircraft, and fixed wing aircraft can all be used for the transfer of burn patients, depending on the distance involved. Pretransfer stability is particularly important in patients who are to be transferred by helicopter, wherein limited space, poor lighting, noise, and vibration make anything but the simplest of monitoring procedures exceedingly difficult.[231]

The physician who is directing the aeromedical transfer team should assess the patient to be transferred while still in the referring hospital and make any necessary adjustments in treatment at that time. In 124 aeromedical transfers involving 148 burn patients, the treatment modifications most commonly required before patient movement could be undertaken were placement or change in placement of cannulae and catheters, alteration of pulmonary management, alteration of fluid therapy, and restoration of impaired blood flow in an extremity by the performance of escharotomy.[284] In-flight management adjustments paralleled those necessary before patient movement, that is, alterations of fluid therapy and ventilator adjustments.

Contraindications to burn-patient movement are most frequently encountered when aeromedical transfer is considered later in the postburn course and consist of hypoxemia despite administration of oxygen, congestive heart failure, cardiac arrhythmias, active hemorrhage, and systemic sepsis.[193] Such problems should be addressed and the underlying process brought under control before transfer requiring more than 30 to 60 minutes is undertaken. All pertinent records or copies thereof should accompany the patient.

DURATION OF HOSPITAL CARE

Duration of hospital care of burn patients is related to burn depth, burn extent, preexisting disease, presence of associated injuries, and occurrence of complications. Partial-thickness burns that are other than deep dermal in character and remain uninfected characteristically heal within 3 weeks. Full-thickness burns require skin

U.S. ARMY INSTITUTE OF SURGICAL RESEARCH

PATIENT TRANSFER INFORMATION SHEET

Date and time of call ______
Referring MD ______ Telephone ______
Hospital ______ City ______ State ______
Means of transportation ______ Accompanying personnel ______

PATIENT INFORMATION

Name ______ ______ Status: Active duty ______
Retired ______
Age ______ Sex ______ Preburn weight ______ Dependent ______
VAB/BEC ______
Date of burn: ______ Cause ______ Civilian ______

Extent of burn: ______ Third degree ______
Areas burned: ______
Inhalation injury: ______ Associated injuries: ______
Preexisting diseases: ______ Allergies: ______

TREATMENT CHECKLIST (Advise diplomatically when indicated)

Resuscitation: Calculated need (2 ml/kg% TBS) ______
Fluid in ______ Urine output ______
Airway ______ Blood gases ______ Tracheostomy ______
Medications: Analgesics or sedatives ______ Tetanus ______
Antibiotics ______ Other medications ______
Escharotomies: Arms ______ Legs ______ Chest ______
Wound care: Wash and debride ______ Topical agent ______
Lab tests: HCT ______ Electrolytes ______ BS ______ BUN ______
Request: Insert NG tube—Avoid general anesthesia or
IM medications—Keep I and O

INFORMATION FOR FLIGHT PLAN

Burn team ______ Family to accompany patient ______
Location of nearest airport with jet traffic ______
ETA at destination ______ Transportation for team at destination ______
Instructions to referring MD ______
Information from air evacuation personnel ______

FIGURE 17-8 Review of a checklist such as this with the referring physician facilitates identification of treatment changes needed before transfer and ensures continuity of care and patient safety during transport.

grafting for closure, and staged excision and grafting will be necessary in patients with extensive full-thickness injuries. Most burn injuries are of varying depth, with intermixed areas of partial-thickness and full-thickness skin damage. In patients with burns of more than 20% of the body surface, one can in general anticipate that the hospital stay will be equal in days to the extent of the burn expressed as a percentage of the total body surface (e.g., 40 hospital days for a patient with a 40% burn). This "average" comprises patients with massive burns or burns complicated by associated injury who die early postburn and those whose hospital stay far exceeds the average because of associated injury or supervening complications.

BURN PATIENT MORTALITY

Because of the many variables, such as age, associated injury, and supervening complications that affect burn-related mortality, raw mortality is of little value and in fact may be misleading when trying to assess treatment outcome. A technique of data transformation (probit or logit transformations are commonly used) is necessary to transform the sigmoid dose-response relationship between burn size and mortality to a straight line relationship to generate an error term that will permit comparison of outcomes.[68,240] To assess burn-specific mortality, patients with associated injury should be excluded from burn mortality analyses. Outcome analyses should be limited to those patients received at the burn treatment facility within the first 10 days postburn because the death rate of burn patients is relatively high in the first 10 days postburn and significantly lower thereafter (unpublished data). Because burn injury outcome is influenced by age, either patient groups must be stratified by age (0 to 14 years, 15 to 49 years, and over 50 years are commonly used strata) or, preferably, the analysis should incorporate a continuous curvilinear function of age.[37,162,240]

Inhalation injury and infection both exert enhancing effects on the mortality rate in burn patients.[2,162,308] Recent data have shown the mortality effects of those disease processes to be independent, additive, and age and burn-size related.[268] Consequently it is important to determine the comparability of presence of inhalation injury and pneumonia in burn patient populations that are being compared, and the distribution of those comorbid factors by age and burn size within each population, to evaluate the clinical importance of any observed difference in outcome. It is also important to consider the distribution of burn size within the total population of burn patients being analyzed because a mortality curve only for patients with small burns can be unwarrantedly biased in an upward direction. To avoid such an error, a separate outcome analysis should be made on that subset of patients in the population being analyzed who had burns of more than 40% of the body surface.

The conventional statistic for assessment and comparison of burn patient mortality is the LA_{50} (i.e., the extent of burn that is associated with death in 50% of the patients having burns of that extent). Probit analysis of burn patient mortality in the mid-1940s showed that the LA_{50} of pediatric burn patients was 51% of the body surface, the LA_{50} of young adults was 43% of the body surface, and the LA_{50} of older adults was 23% of the body surface.[38] Analysis of the outcome of burn patients without associated injury admitted within 4 days of injury and treated at the United States Army Institute of Surgical Research during the 5-year period 1985 to 1989 reveals an LA_{50} for children of 0 to 14 years of 53.4% of the body surface, an LA_{50} for young adults of 75.6%, and an LA_{50} for patients over 40 years of 44% (unpublished data) (Table 17-4). The improvement in survival reflects the effects of physiologically based resuscitation, control of burn wound infection, improved pulmonary care, and other improvements in wound care, as well as the improvements in general supportive care that have occurred during the last five decades.

TABLE 17-4 IMPROVEMENT IN BURN PATIENT SURVIVAL: 1945-1989

	LA_{50}	
AGE GROUP	1945-1947	1985-1989
Pediatric	51%	53.4%
Young adults	43%	75.6%
Older adults	23%	44%

OBJECTIVE FINDINGS

Physical Examination

The adequacy of ventilation of any burn patient should be assessed immediately on admission. Respiratory arrest may occur in the immediate postburn period as a consequence of high-voltage electric injury or drug overdose and must be treated by intubation and mechanical ventilatory support. The presence of inhalation injury should be documented at the time of initial examination. Ninety percent of patients with inhalation injury have significant head and neck burns, but many patients with head and neck burns do not have inhalation injury.[81] Singeing of the nasal vibrissae is so common in patients with face burns that it is not a reliable indication of inhalation injury. The mucosa of the oral pharynx should be inspected, and the presence of inflammatory mucosal changes confirms the presence of upper airway inhalation injury.

The detection of turbulent air flow in the upper airway, wheezing, bronchorrhea, a brassy cough, and hoarseness are all indicative of airway edema caused by inhalation injury. Clinical progression of those signs, particularly in patients with a PaO_2 of less than 70 torr, is an indication for endotracheal intubation and mechanical ventilation. Massive intraoral and pharyngeal edema can form rapidly following imbibition or involuntary instillation of boiling liquids and can be of such magnitude that endotracheal intubation is necessary (Figure 17-9). Later in the postburn course, pulmonary edema as a consequence of excessive resuscitation, pneu-

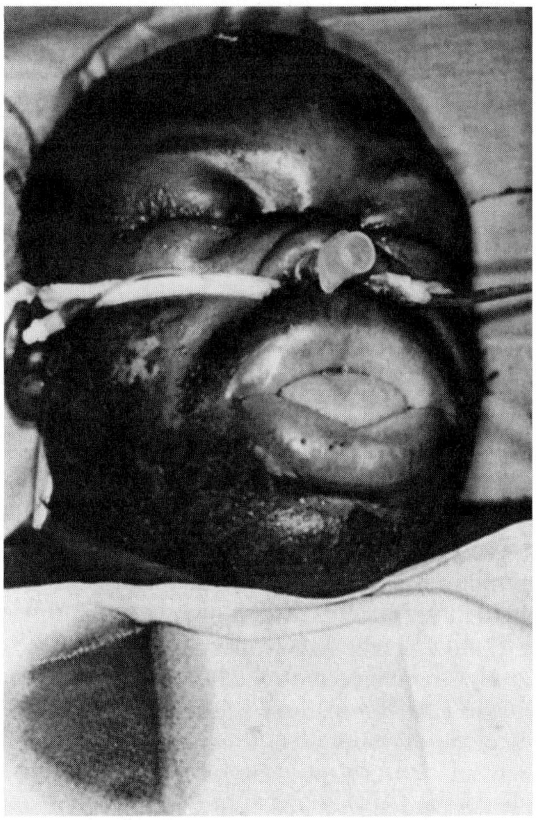

FIGURE 17-9 Instillation of boiling water caused edema of the lips and tongue of this patient. Swelling of pharyngeal tissues necessitated nasotracheal intubation to maintain a patent airway.

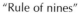

"Rule of nines"

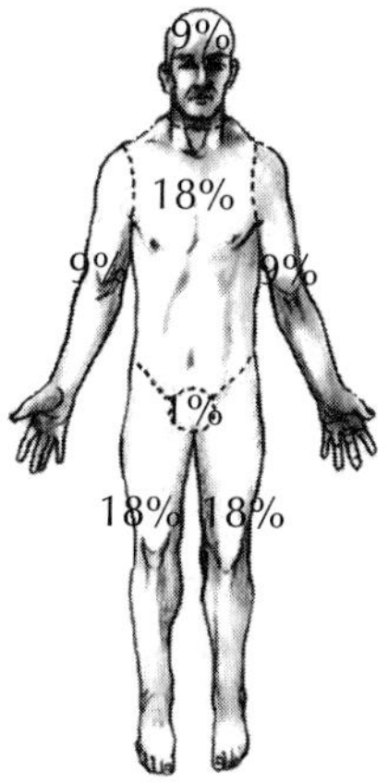

FIGURE 17-10 The "rule of nines" can be used to estimate the extent of injury in burned adults.

monia, pulmonary embolus, and all of the disease entities causing respiratory insufficiency in other patients may cause pulmonary insufficiency in the burn patient. The ventilatory management of such respiratory insufficiency is dictated by the severity of insufficiency and the underlying disease.

Hemodynamic Status

Immediately after a burn, before significant transvascular plasma loss has occurred, the pulse rate is commonly elevated and the blood pressure is either normal or slightly elevated as a result of the increased circulating levels of catecholamines. In the absence of treatment, plasma loss is progressive and associated with a further increase in pulse rate and a progressive fall in blood pressure. Because of the increased circulating levels of vasoactive hormones, the pulse rate may remain elevated as resuscitation proceeds and is not a reliable guide to the adequacy of fluid therapy.

Urinary Output

Even though urinary output does not bear a constant relationship to blood volume and cardiac output, the hourly urinary volume is the most readily available and generally reliable guide to the adequacy of fluid resuscitation. An indwelling urethral catheter should be placed and connected to a closed drainage system. The hourly urinary volume should be recorded, and the infusion of resuscitation fluids modified according to those hourly measurements.

Extent of Burn

The severity of burn injury is related to both the depth and extent of the wound, with the latter factor being the predominant determinant of the magnitude of pathophysiologic change and fluid needs. To estimate fluid needs, one must determine the percentage of the total body surface that has been injured (first-degree burns are not included in this calculation). This calculation is performed using the "rule of nines," which expresses the fact that the surface area of various anatomic regions represents 9% or a multiple thereof of the total body surface; that is, the head and neck are 9%, each upper extremity is 9%, the anterior and posterior trunk 18% each, each lower extremity 18%, and the genitalia and perineum 1% (Figure 17-10). The distribution of surface area by body part is quite different in infants, in whom the head and neck represent a considerably greater percentage and each lower extremity a lesser percentage of the total surface area than in the adult. Those percentages decrease and increase, respectively, with age and assume adult proportions by age 16. For precise estimation of burn extent, one should use a burn diagram in which the percentage of total body surface represented

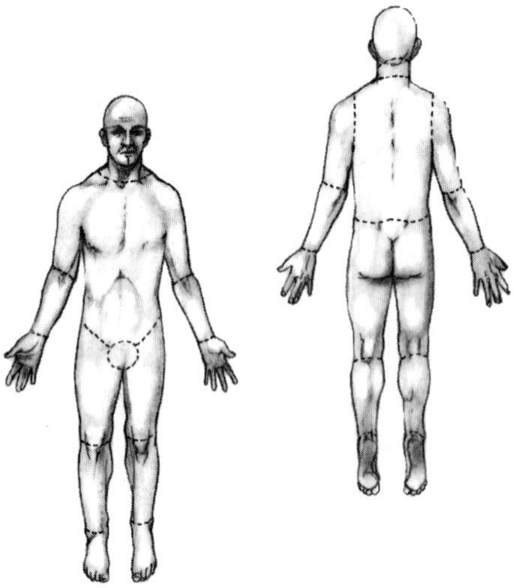

Burn estimate and diagram
age versus area

Area	Birth-1 year	1-4 years	5-9 years	10-14 years	15 years	Adult
Head	19	17	13	11	9	7
Neck	2	2	2	2	2	2
Anterior trunk	13	13	13	13	13	13
Posterior trunk	13	13	13	13	13	13
Right buttock	2.5	2.5	2.5	2.5	2.5	2.5
Left buttock	2.5	2.5	2.5	2.5	2.5	2.5
Genitalia	1	1	1	1	1	1
Right upper arm	4	4	4	4	4	4
Left upper arm	4	4	4	4	4	4
Right lower arm	3	3	3	3	3	3
Left lower arm	3	3	3	3	3	3
Right hand	2.5	2.5	2.5	2.5	2.5	2.5
Left hand	2.5	2.5	2.5	2.5	2.5	2.5
Right thigh	5.5	6.5	8	8.5	9	9.5
Left thigh	5.5	6.5	8	8.5	9	9.5
Right leg	5	5	5.5	6	6.5	7
Left leg	5	5	5.5	6	6.5	7
Right foot	3.5	3.5	3.5	3.5	3.5	3.5
Left foot	3.5	3.5	3.5	3.5	3.5	3.5

FIGURE 17-11 The use of a burn diagram permits a precise estimation of the extent of burn. Note how the percentage of the total body surface area represented by the head and lower extremities changes with age.

by anatomic parts at various ages is displayed, as shown in Figure 17-11. In determining the extent of small, irregularly disposed burns, one can utilize the fact that one surface of the patient's hand represents approximately 1% of the total body surface and estimate how many "hands" would be required to cover the burns.

Depth of Burn

The depth of the burn wound determines the type of wound care required, the time required for healing, the need for skin grafting, and the ultimate functional and cosmetic results (Table 17-5). The most superficial burn has been termed a *first-degree* burn and is exemplified by a sunburn in which the skin is pink or light red in color, dry with no or small blisters, painful to the touch, and heals within 3 to 6 days. Most patients with first-degree burns do not require hospital care, unless it is of such extent as to cause postural hypotension that is best treated by application of cool compresses, which may also provide some pain relief. A severe sunburn may be followed by exfoliation of the superficial epidermis. The pruritus elicited by the exfoliation may be so severe, particularly in young children, that symptomatic treatment is required.

Second-degree, or partial-thickness, burns may be further subdivided into superficial and deep dermal injuries. Superficial partial-thickness burns are produced by brief contact with hot liquids, flashes of flame, and brief exposure to flames. They are typically bright red or mottled red in color and have a moist surface, and show exquisite sensitivity to stimuli (even a current of air). If protected from infection, these burns heal within 10 to 21 days.

TABLE 17-5 CLINICAL CHARACTERISTICS OF PARTIAL-THICKNESS AND FULL-THICKNESS BURN WOUNDS

	PARTIAL-THICKNESS BURNS		
	SECOND-DEGREE BURNS		
FIRST-DEGREE BURNS	SUPERFICIAL	DEEP DERMAL	FULL-THICKNESS OR THIRD-DEGREE BURNS
Cause*			
Sun Minor flash	Hot liquids Flashes of flame Brief exposure to dilute chemicals	Hot liquids Flashes of flame Brief exposure to dilute chemicals	Flame High-voltage electricity Exposure to concentrated chemicals Contact with hot metal
Color*			
Pink or light red	Bright red or mottled red	Dark red or yellow-white	Pearly white or charred Translucent and parchmentlike
Surface*			
Dry or small blisters	Variably sized bullae Moist and weeping	Large bullae often ruptured Slightly moist	Dry with shreds of nonviable epidermis Thrombosed vessels visible
Texture*			
Soft with minimal edema and later superficial exfoliation	Thickened by edema but pliable	Moderate edema with decreased pliability	Inelastic and leathery
Sensation*			
Hypersensitive	Hypersensitive	Decreased pinprick sensation Intact deep-pressure sensation	Hypalgesic
Healing*			
3 to 6 days	10 to 21 days	>21 days	Grafting required

* These criteria apply to all categories of burns.

Deep dermal burns caused by immersion in hot liquids and longer exposure to flame are characteristically dark red or yellow-white in color, have a slightly moist surface, and show decreased pinprick sensation with intact deep pressure sensation. These burns require more than 3 weeks for spontaneous healing and, when healed, are often the site of marked hypertrophic scar formation.

Third-degree, or full-thickness, burns are caused by exposure to concentrated chemicals, high-voltage electricity, flame, and prolonged contact with hot objects. These burns may be pearly white, charred, or parchmentlike in appearance, with thrombosed superficial veins visible through the translucent eschar. These wounds are characteristically dry and insensate. Grafting is required for wound closure.

Laboratory Findings

Admission laboratory studies are necessary to define the patient's baseline conditions at the onset of injury and to determine the presence of any preexisting illnesses. Omission of important blood measurements is minimized by laboratory admission protocols. Blood chemistries should include major electrolytes, including the divalent cations, liver and renal status panels, and glucose. Many causes of mental status alteration can be evaluated by these measurements. Toxicology screening, including assays for opiates and other psychoactive drugs, anticonvulsants, and alcohol, is useful for deducing causes leading to the injury and for guiding treatment in the hospital. Acute drug overdose or abrupt cessation of antiseizure medications and subsequent collapse onto an exposed heat source is a particularly common cause of burn injuries. Screening for the major blood-borne contagious diseases, hepatitis and sexually transmitted disease, allows the burn center staff to take proper isolation precautions. Surveillance microbial cultures are obtained on admission to detect preclinical infections or the introduction of dangerous nosocomial agents.

In the absence of prior disease or hemodynamic stability, arterial blood gas and pH levels usually are within normal ranges on admission. The pH reliably reflects tissue perfusion following thermal injury, and acidosis reflects underresuscitation of the new patient. With adequate volume replacement, pH returns to the normal range. Hypoxemia on admission indicates inhalation injury so severe that death during the resuscitation phase is likely. Carboxyhemoglobin determination is the most critical measurement to be obtained after arrival to the burn center. Optimal salvage from carbon monoxide intoxication depends on early diagnosis and treatment. Because removal from the intoxicating environment and oxygen administration rapidly lowers blood concentration of carbon monoxide, early measurement is necessary to detect true severity of poisoning. On some city emergency medical services, carboxyhemoglobin measurement is made at the scene of the injury. Arterial Po_2 levels in the presence of carbon monoxide-bound hemoglobin give no indication of the oxygen-carrying capacity of the blood, or the lack of it, and blood gas measurement without simultaneous carboxyhemoglobin measurement is almost without value.

Radiologic studies usually provide normal baseline data. Chest radiographs, even in patients with inhalation injury, detect no abnormalities unless the patient has prior (and usually known) thoracic disease. Occasionally, patients will have a pneumothorax from the blast effect of an explosion or a recently placed central venous cannula. The chest radiograph is useful for verifying the positions of central venous cannulas, nasogastric tubes, and endotracheal tubes inserted during the admission work-up. Angiography is useful primarily for the evaluation of concomitant injuries, such as a comminuted knee fracture, a widened mediastinum, or a penetrating wound in proximity of major vessels. Hematuria in patients who sustain burns in a blast environment or who were forced to jump from high elevations should be evaluated with an intravenous pyelogram.

ASSESSMENT OF FACTORS THAT INFLUENCE TREATMENT

The extent of the burn injury expressed as a percentage of the total body surface determines the occurrence, magnitude, and duration of the multisystem pathophysiologic changes that occur after burn injury and the patient's response to resuscitation. As part of the initial assessment of any burn patient, the extent of the burn should be calculated to estimate fluid needs and plan other aspects of the resuscitation regimen, including initiation of necessary physiologic monitoring. Because fluid needs are also body-size and in turn body-weight dependent, the patient should be weighed on admission. If the patient cannot be weighed, an estimate of preburn weight should be obtained from the patient or a reliable family member.

Age also exerts an influence on fluid resuscitation requirements and other treatment needs. Burn patients in the young adult age range of 15 to 40 years are the most resistant to fluid overload, organ failure, and later complications and are the patients least likely to require invasive physiologic monitoring. Children younger than 5 years require greater amounts of resuscitation fluid because of their greater body surface area per unit of body mass.[107,220] Such patients, particularly children younger than 2 years, should be monitored meticulously because their cardiopulmonary reserve may be limited, as is the case in the elderly. The limited cardiovascular reserve of the very young, the very old, and patients with preexisting heart disease necessitates close monitoring of the hemodynamic response to injury and resuscitation in such patients and modification of the resuscitation regimen as indicated by the monitoring data.[237]

The time interval between injury and initiation of treatment also appears to influence the resuscitation fluid needs of burn patients. In patients in whom the infusion of resuscitation fluids is inordinately delayed (i.e., an interval of more than 2 hours), more than the estimated amount of resuscitation fluid is commonly needed, and it is in these patients, as well as in patients with inhalation injury, that additional fluids may be required to achieve the desired physiologic endpoints of resuscitation.

RESUSCITATION

Several formulas have been proposed for estimating burn patient fluid resuscitation needs (Table 17-6).* Even though the amount and composition of the fluids recommended by the various formulas differ markedly, each formula has been used successfully to resuscitate large numbers of burn patients. The success of the different formulas speaks for the physiologic reserve of burn patients and against unique precision of any one formula in preventing or correcting the hemodynamic changes that occur in burn patients.

After calculation of fluid requirements, the rate of volume infusion is regulated so that one half of the required volume will be infused during the first 8 hours postburn, the period during which capillary permeability is greatest and intravascular volume decreases most rapidly. During the subsequent 16 hours of the first postburn day, the remaining half of the estimated resuscitation volume should be administered. The volume of fluid actually infused should be guided by physiologic monitoring of the patient's response to the burn injury and treatment.

Capillary permeability returns toward normal during

*References 26, 65, 81, 91, 183, 219, 220, 237, and 246.

TABLE 17-6 FORMULAS USED TO ESTIMATE RESUSCITATION FLUIDS FOR BURN PATIENTS

FORMULA	ELECTROLYTE-CONTAINING SOLUTION	COLLOID-CONTAINING FLUID EQUIVALENT TO PLASMA	GLUCOSE IN WATER
First 24 Hours Postburn			
Burn budget of Moore and Cope	Lactated Ringer's—1000-4000 ml 0.5 normal saline—1200 ml	7.5% of body weight	1500-5000 ml
Evans	Normal saline—1 ml/kg/% burn	1 ml/kg/% burn	2000 ml
Brooke	Lactated Ringer's—1.5 ml/kg/% burn	0.5% ml/kg/% burn	2000 ml
Parkland	Lactated Ringer's—4 ml/kg/% burn	—	—
Hypertonic sodium solution	Volume of fluid containing 250 mEq of sodium/L to maintain hourly urinary output of 30 ml	—	—
Modified Brooke	Lactated Ringer's—2 ml/kg/% burn	—	—
Second 24 Hours Postburn			
Burn budget of Moore and Cope	Lactated Ringer's—1000-4000 ml 0.5 normal saline—1200 ml	2.5% of body weight	1500-5000 ml
Evans	50% of first 24 hr requirement	50% of first 24 hr requirement	2000 ml
Brooke	50% to 75% of first 24 hr requirement	50% to 75% of first 24 hr requirement	2000 ml
Parkland	—	20% to 60% of calculated plasma volume	As necessary to maintain urinary output
Hypertonic sodium solution	33% isotonic salt solution orally up to 3500 ml limit	—	—
Modified Brooke	—	0.3 to 0.5 ml/kg/% burn*	As necessary to maintain urinary output

*Administered as a plasma equivalent (e.g., albumin diluted to physiologic concentration in 0.9% sodium chloride solution).

the latter half of the first postburn day, and functional capillary integrity is essentially restored during the second 24 hours postburn[236] (Figure 17-12). Consequently, the volume of infused fluid required to maintain blood volume in the second postburn day is less than in the first postburn day, and colloid-containing fluids can be used to keep the volume of administered fluids at a minimum. All of the formulas recognize the time-related change in transcapillary fluid movement and recommend infusion of a lesser volume of fluid during the second postburn day.

Physiologic Response to Resuscitation

Patients in whom resuscitation is based on the Brooke formula experience an early modest (approximately 20%) decrement in blood and plasma volume, with subsequent restoration of plasma volume to predicted normal levels during the latter part of the second 24 hours postburn.[238] Cardiac output is initially depressed but increases to predicted normal levels between the twelfth and eighteenth hours postburn during a time when there is a modest progressive decrease in blood and plasma volume (Figure 17-13). As plasma volume returns toward normal during the second postburn day, cardiac output rises to supranormal levels of 2 to 2½ times predicted normal and slowly returns to normal as the burn wound is closed. The hyperdynamic cardiac response, which in part is mediated by catecholamines, is characterized by tachycardia and increased myocardial O_2 requirements. Although the increased cardiac output appears to be a beneficial adaptive response to injury, the often marked increase in cardiac work may be detrimental. Minifee and colleagues[180] documented a significant decrease in myocardial work as assessed by rate pressure product in a group of adolescent burn patients treated with IV propranolol (Inderal) without affecting O_2 delivery and consumption. Unfortunately, further studies revealed a significant increase in protein catabolism using this approach, which was thought to be mediated by a reduction in beta-adrenergic stimulated lipolysis.[118] Trials using cardiac selective beta blockers are now under way. It should be stressed that artificially limiting the available cardiac reserve may be detrimental, especially if the patient is additionally stressed by cold exposure or sepsis.

Most of the formulas recommend the administration

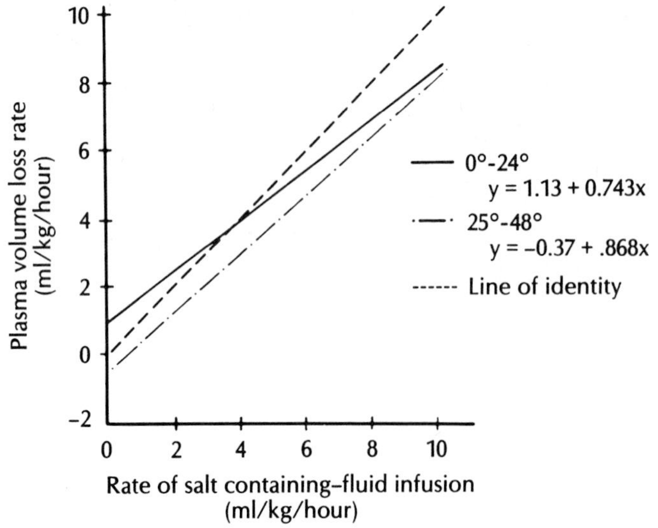

FIGURE 17-12 Regression curves relating plasma volume loss rate of infusion of salt-containing fluids in 10 extensively burned patients in the first and second 24 hours postburn. The obligatory plasma volume loss at zero infusion rate indicated by the positive Y intercept of the first 24-hour curve is a manifestation of increased capillary permeability. The negative Y intercept of the curve for the second 24 hours indicates restoration of capillary integrity and edema resorption with spontaneous plasma volume increase at zero infusion rate. Note that it required a 4.4 ml/kg/hr infusion rate to maintain plasma volume in the first 24 hours postburn and that plasma volume was increased at all infusion rates in the second 24 hours postburn.

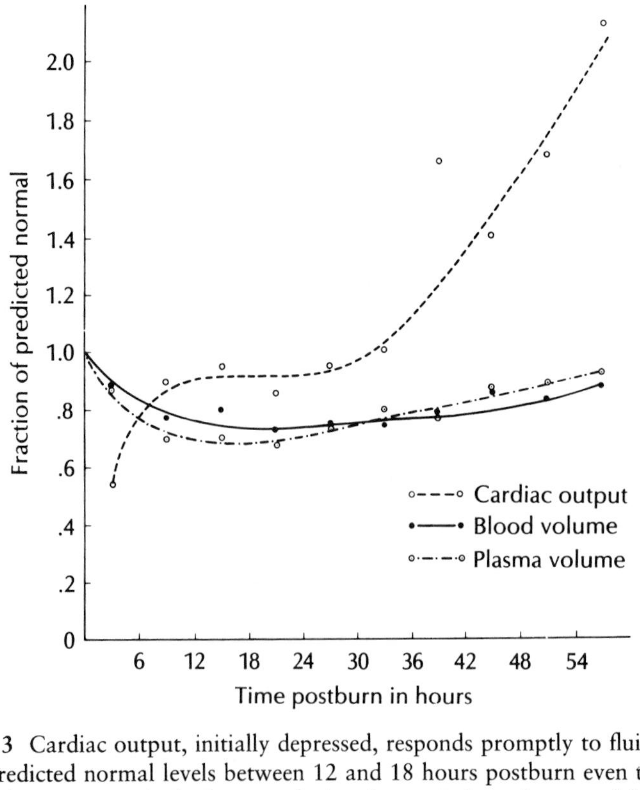

FIGURE 17-13 Cardiac output, initially depressed, responds promptly to fluid therapy and rises to predicted normal levels between 12 and 18 hours postburn even though blood and plasma volume progressively decrease during that period. In the second 24 hours, as continued resuscitation restores plasma volume to predicted normal levels, cardiac output rises to supranormal levels.

of a total resuscitation volume (crystalloid and colloid-containing fluids) of approximately 2 ml/kg body weight/% burn during the first 24 hours. One formula that was originally proposed for use in patients (usually older patients and those with extensive burns) who did not respond in the anticipated manner to resuscitation with a lesser volume recommends a total volume dose of 4 ml/kg body weight/% burn. The impaired cardiac response to fluid infusion in such patients was attributed to a circulating myocardial depressant factor, but, as noted previously in a study of burn patients with depressed cardiac output during the first postburn day, the myocardium was found to be hyperdynamic.[24,82]

Effects of Resuscitation Fluid Composition

Resuscitation fluid composition appears to be less important in the first 24 hours postburn than in the second 24 hours postburn. Calculations of transcapillary fluid movement during the first 24 hours postburn indicate that colloid-containing fluids are retained within the vascular tree to no greater extent than an equal volume of crystalloid fluid.[236] In the second 24 hours postburn, when functional capillary integrity has been restored, colloid-containing fluids augment intravascular volume to a greater extent than do crystalloid fluids. Some laboratory studies[33] have shown that a colloid effect is evident as early as the latter half of the first 24 hours postburn. All of the formulas provide merely a first approximation of fluid needs, and regardless of the formula used, one should add or withhold fluid in accordance with the individual patient's response.

Hypotension, tissue hypoxia, and acute organ failure (particularly renal failure)—the complications of delayed and inadequate fluid replacement—are seldom encountered today in burn patients in whom formula-based resuscitation is promptly initiated. Conversely, the complications of excessive fluid administration (i.e., pulmonary and cerebral edema) have become more common. Pulmonary edema is infrequent in the first 48 hours postburn, even when amounts of resuscitation fluid far in excess of formula estimates are infused. The immediate postburn elevation of pulmonary vascular resistance, which exceeds in magnitude and duration that of peripheral vascular resistance, appears to protect the lung during the resuscitation phase.[15] The consequences of administration of excessive amounts of resuscitation fluid may only become evident when pulmonary vascular resistance returns to normal, and the edema in the burned tissues is resorbed and expands intravascular volume; that is, pulmonary edema in burn patients is most commonly observed 3 to 6 days postburn.

Although the predominant or even exclusive use of crystalloid fluids as recommended by currently popular resuscitation regimens has been incriminated as a cause of pulmonary edema, studies by Goodwin and associates[103] and Tranbaugh and associates[283] have indicated that lung water is little changed during the first 24 hours postburn and is little affected by the observed changes in plasma colloid oncotic pressure. A modest increase in extravascular lung water occurs after resuscitation in association with an increase in pulmonary capillary blood flow as the circulating blood volume is expanded by edema resorption.

In a controlled randomized study,[103] there was no increase in lung water during the first 7 days postburn in patients who received only crystalloid-containing fluid in the first 24 hours, but a progressive rise in extravascular lung water occurred over the first week postburn in patients who received colloid-containing fluids in the first 24 hours postburn (Table 17-7). The infusion of colloid-containing fluids in the first 24 hours postburn exerted no protective effect on the lung in patients who received such fluids, and they had a higher incidence of

TABLE 17-7 POSTBURN CHANGES IN LUNG WATER AND CARDIAC OUTPUT AS RELATED TO COMPOSITION OF RESUSCITATION FLUIDS

	LUNG WATER ml/ml OF ALVEOLAR VOLUME		CARDIAC OUTPUT (L/min)	
POSTBURN DAY	CRYSTALLOID RESUSCITATION	COLLOID RESUSCITATION	CRYSTALLOID RESUSCITATION	COLLOID RESUSCITATION
0.5	0.130	0.130	4.07	4.30
1.0	0.122	0.125	4.55	5.28
1.5	0.124	0.120	4.29	4.51
2.0	0.137	0.123	4.89	4.65
2.5	0.138	0.141	5.45	5.30
3.0	0.139	0.144	6.83	6.74
5.0	0.149	0.167	8.28	7.70
7.0	0.137	0.173	9.19	10.20

pulmonary edema and a higher mortality rate than patients who received only crystalloid fluid in the first 24 hours postburn.

Hypertonic Saline Resuscitation

To reduce the amount of fluid administered during resuscitation, the use of hypertonic saline solutions has been advocated, particularly in those patients considered to be volume sensitive (i.e., the very old, the very young, and those with preexisting cardipulmonary disease).[41, 183] The use of hypertonic resuscitation has been credited with inducing higher urinary outputs, minimizing the fractional retention of the administered sodium dose, reducing the need for escharotomy, and decreasing the occurrence of ileus. Natriuresis and mild kaluresis are observed following infusion of hypertonic saline solutions, but laboratory studies[195] have failed to confirm a significant diuretic effect of hypertonic salt solution. In these studies using a canine model of a 40% burn, the animals receiving hypertonic salt solution resuscitation retained a lesser percentage of the administered sodium than those animals resuscitated with lactated Ringer's solution. Animals receiving one half of the fluids estimated by the original Brooke formula retained a smaller total amount of sodium (they received a much lower total sodium dose) (Table 17-8). Because organ failure was not evident in the animals receiving one half of the fluids estimated by the Brooke formula and they were adequately resuscitated as judged by all clinical indices, infusion of the least volume and sodium doses that protect organ function appears to be a desirable endpoint of resuscitation.

A minimum fluid volume appears to be necessary even when infusing hypertonic salt solution in order to deliver the contained sodium to the site where water is osmotically transferred; for example, animals receiving concentrated hypertonic salt solution (1200 mEq of sodium/L) experienced a more profound decrease and slower recovery of both plasma volume and cardiac output than animals receiving solutions containing 300 mEq of sodium/L or less.[194]

Human studies[266] have shown that when the serum sodium concentration is increased above 165 mEq/L as a result of hypertonic salt infusion, a marked drop in urinary output occurs, necessitating infusion of more dilute solutions to continue resuscitation. Moreover, the depletion of intracellular water by more than 15% has been associated with impairment of cell function, and hypertonically induced transfer of greater volumes of intracellular water should be avoided. The physiologic tolerance of burn patients to hypertonic resuscitation appears to be defined by those limits of serum sodium elevation and cellular dehydration.

In the vast majority of uncomplicated burn patients, any of the cited formulas can be used to guide resuscitation, but in volume-sensitive patients with limited cardiopulmonary reserve, hypertonic resuscitation may be advantageous. Laboratory studies[192] have shown that the restorative effect on cardiac output of 1 mEq of sodium is equal to that of 13 ml of salt-free noncolloid fluid.[192] Substitution of salt dose for volume dose in that ratio can be used to reduce the volume of resuscitation fluid given to patients lacking in physiologic reserve. Postresuscitation fluid management in patients treated this way must be rigorously monitored because they experience thirst and, if unrestricted, avidly imbibe water and develop delayed-onset edema. Conversely, in patients in whom a large volume of fluid is required because of delay in initiation of resuscitation, the salt content can be reduced to minimize expansion of the exchangeable sodium mass and simplify postresuscitation fluid management.

Burn injury destroys the water vapor barrier of the skin, and evaporative water loss from the burn wound

TABLE 17-8 EFFECT OF SODIUM AND VOLUME DOSAGE OF RESUSCITATION FLUIDS ON SODIUM BALANCE AND URINARY OUTPUT IN A CANINE 40% BURN MODEL

FORMULA	VOLUME DOSE (ml/kg)	SODIUM DOSE (mEq/kg)	MEAN URINARY SODIUM CONCENTRATION (mEq/L)	MEAN URINARY OUTPUT (ml/hr)	SODIUM RETAINED: % OF ADMINISTERED DOSE	SODIUM RETAINED: mEq/kg
No resuscitation	0	0	25.2	9.4	0	−0.62
One-half Brooke formula	90	5.44	16.1	15.1	91.8	4.99
Brooke formula	130	10.88	39.7	18.0	94.03	10.22
Hypertonic lactated saline ([Na] = 300 mEq/L)	40	12.0	226.2	11.1	64.33	7.72
Concentrated hypertonic lactated saline ([Na] = 1200 mEq/L)	10	12.0	236.2	12.2	52.01	6.28

is prodigious after resuscitation.[301] In addition, circulating levels of renin, angiotensin, and aldosterone limit renal salt excretion.[271] These factors complicate postresuscitation fluid management of patients who have received hypertonic salt solutions by limiting the ability of the burn patient to excrete the administered salt and promoting the development of hypernatremia.[220,291] Many of the advocates of hypertonic resuscitation also use 0.5% silver nitrate soaks as topical burn wound therapy, and such hypotonic soaks induce transeschar leeching of large quantities of sodium. Resuscitation with hypertonic salt solutions appears to offer no particular advantage for the majority of even extensively burned patients and is best reserved for those patients with limited cardiopulmonary reserve.

Modified Brooke Formula

The clinical and laboratory studies referred to here lead to the conclusion that the goal of burn patient resuscitation is to maintain vital organ function and minimize both the immediate and delayed physiologic cost of inadequate or excessive fluid and salt administration. A modification of the Brooke formula, omitting the infusion of both colloid-containing fluid and electrolyte-free water in the first 24 hours, is presently used to minimize the amounts of fluid and sodium infused during the resuscitation period.

Estimation of fluid needs for the first 24 hours after burn injury are as follows: adults, 2 ml lactated Ringer's solution/kg body weight/% burn; children, 3 ml lactated Ringer's solution/kg body weight/% burn.[107] One half of the fluid volume is scheduled for infusion in the first 8 hours postburn.

An estimation of fluid needs for the second 24 hours postburn injury for adults and children is presented in the box below. Restoration of capillary integrity in the second 24 hours permits use of colloid-containing fluid (an albumin solution) to minimize the fluid volume administered. In the adult burn patient, no salt-containing fluid other than that used to dilute the albumin to physiologic concentration is infused in the second 24 hours postburn, and electrolyte-free fluid is administered to maintain urinary output and minimize salt loading. In burned children, salt loading is reduced in similar fashion, but solutions of 5% dextrose in 50% normal saline in the very young, or 5% dextrose in 25% normal saline in older children, may be required to prevent the induction of symptomatic hyponatremia.

Flow diagrams for the management of fluid resuscitation in adult burn patients are presented in algorithms I and II at the end of this chapter.

ESTIMATION OF FLUID NEEDS FOR SECOND 24 HOURS POSTBURN

Colloid-Containing Fluids*

Adults and children: amount proportional to extent of burn

30% to 50% burn: 0.3 ml/kg body weight/% burn

50% to 70% burn: 0.4 ml/kg body weight/% burn

>70% burn: 0.5 ml/kg body weight/% burn

Electrolyte-Free Water

Adults: 5% dextrose in water to maintain adequate urinary output

Children: 5% dextrose in 50% to 25% normal saline as needed to maintain adequate urinary output and avoid symptomatic hyponatremia

* Given as albumin diluted to physiologic concentration in normal saline.

MONITORING RESUSCITATION

Frequent, scheduled monitoring of the patient's general condition and hemodynamic status is mandatory to avoid the complications of inadequate or excessive resuscitation. The hourly urinary output is a generally reliable and readily available index of resuscitation adequacy. An indwelling urethral catheter should be placed and the rate of fluid infusion regulated to obtain 30 to 50 ml of urine per hour in the adult and 1 mg/kg/hour in patients weighing less than 30 kg. Adjustment of the rate of fluid administration is necessary if the hourly urinary output falls below or exceeds the desired urine output range by more than 33%.

Invasive monitoring of cardiac function is not required in the vast majority of burn patients and is reserved for those patients who do not respond to resuscitation in the anticipated manner and in whom the value of the hemodynamic information obtained outweighs the mechanical and infection-related risks posed by invasive monitoring. If it is necessary to administer more than three times the estimated resuscitation volume during the first 12 hours postburn and on into the latter half of the first postburn day, colloid-containing fluid should be administered to reduce the infused volume. Placement of a Swan-Ganz catheter to measure pulmonary capillary wedge pressure is indicated in such patients to assess intravascular volume status and myocardial function. Persistent oliguria in the presence of a pulmonary capillary wedge pressure within or above the physiologic range has been used as an indication for the administration of dopamine or another inotropic agent.[1]

Oliguria is most often caused by hypovolemic depression of cardiac output as a consequence of inadequate fluid resuscitation. If oliguria persists even after fluid loading, and cardiac insufficiency can be ruled out, a diuretic can be administered to promote urinary output.

Whether such forced urine output protects against acute renal failure is controversial. Administration of a diuretic obviates further use of the hourly urinary output as an index of resuscitation adequacy, and other indices must be monitored thereafter. The patients who most often require a diuretic are those with (1) high-voltage electric injury; (2) associated mechanical injury involving muscle; and (3) extensive burns and a delay in institution of fluid therapy.

The compensatory elevation of systemic vascular resistance, commonly observed in underresuscitated patients, characteristically responds to increased fluid infusion. Occasionally, elevation of systemic vascular resistance may persist or recur, even in patients who have received more than estimated fluid needs and appear to be adequately resuscitated but have persistent oliguria.[238] A continuous infusion of nitroglycerin, labetolol, or sodium nitroprusside may allow precise control of afterload reduction. Such treatment should be used only in patients who have received adequate fluid loading to avoid the further depression of cardiac output that occur in hypovolemic patients after afterload reduction.

During the second 24 hours postburn, the total resuscitation fluid volume can be minimized by a planned 25% to 50% reduction in the rate of fluid administration. If the hourly urinary output is maintained at desired levels for the subsequent 3 hours, further stepwise reduction of the fluid infusion rate can be made.

Changes in the patient's general condition can provide early evidence that the patient's physiologic needs are not being met. Anxiety and restlessness are early signs of hypoxemia and hypovolemia that should be corrected by appropriate therapeutic manipulation. Sphygmomanometric monitoring of blood pressure, particularly in a burned limb with progressive edema formation, can mislead the unwary. As edema develops beneath the burn wound, the auditory blood pressure signal may become progressively attenuated, prompting administration of even more fluid, which produces even more edema and further impairs accurate assessment of blood pressure. Massive fluid overloading can result from such monitoring. Monitoring of the blood pressure by the use of peripheral intravascular cannulae may even be inaccurate in patients with massive burns in whom severe vasospasm is caused by elevated circulating levels of catecholamines and other vasoactive materials.

Serum chemistries and arterial blood gases should be measured at least daily during the resuscitation and postresuscitation diuretic phases and as indicated thereafter. Patients with preexisting cardiovascular disease and patients with high-voltage electric injury should undergo ECG monitoring. A chest radiograph should be obtained daily throughout the resuscitation and edema resorption periods and thereafter as frequently as required by the patient's respiratory status.

MAINTENANCE OF THE PERIPHERAL CIRCULATION

Third-degree burns involving the entire circumference of an extremity may restrict the blood flow to underlying or distal unburned tissue. Tissue pressure progressively increases as edema forms beneath the inelastic eschar. As transcapillary extravasation of fluid further increases, tissue pressure will exceed venous pressure and approach arteriolar pressure. When tissue pressure reaches those levels, nutrient blood flow to unburned tissue may be sufficiently limited to cause tissue hypoxia and cell death. Extensive partial-thickness burns of a limb seldom cause vascular impairment themselves, but exaggerated edema formation resulting from infusion of excessive amounts of resuscitation fluid may compromise the blood flow in tissues beneath circumferential deep dermal limb burns. Edema formation in a burned limb can be minimized and the need for escharotomy reduced by constant elevation of the limb and active exercise of the entire extremity for 5 minutes every hour.[259]

Swelling and coolness to the touch, normal accompaniments of thermal injury, are not signs of circulatory compromise in a burned limb. Cyanosis of distal unburned skin, impaired capillary refilling, and neurologic changes, particularly unrelenting deep tissue pain and progressive paresthesias, are all imprecise signs of circulatory embarrassment in a burned limb. Use of the Doppler ultrasonic flowmeter to detect pulsatile flow in the distal palmar arch vessels in the upper limb or the posterior tibial artery in the lower limb, is the most reliable means of identifying those patients requiring escharotomy to maintain or restore blood flow to unburned tissues in a burned limb.[191] Blood flow in individual digital vessels of the fingers or toes can also be evaluated by flowmeter examination. Escharotomy is indicated if there is absence of pulsatile flow in the examined vessel or if serial examination reveals progressive diminution of the flow signal.

Other findings that have been reported to be indicative of compartment pressures that threaten nutrient blood flow include a decrease in perception of the vibrations generated by a 250 cycles/second tuning fork, a muscle blood flow of less than 1.5 ml/min/100 g of muscle as reflected by delayed washout of intramuscularly injected xenon 133, and elevated muscle compartment pressures ($>$30 mm Hg) as measured by either a wick or slit catheter. The uncertain correlation of those assessments and the need for escharotomy and fasciotomy, the complexity of the isotope measurements, and the risk of infection associated with the invasive techniques support the use of the ultrasonic evaluation of peripheral flow.

Escharotomy can be performed as a ward procedure because the incisions are placed in insensate full-thick-

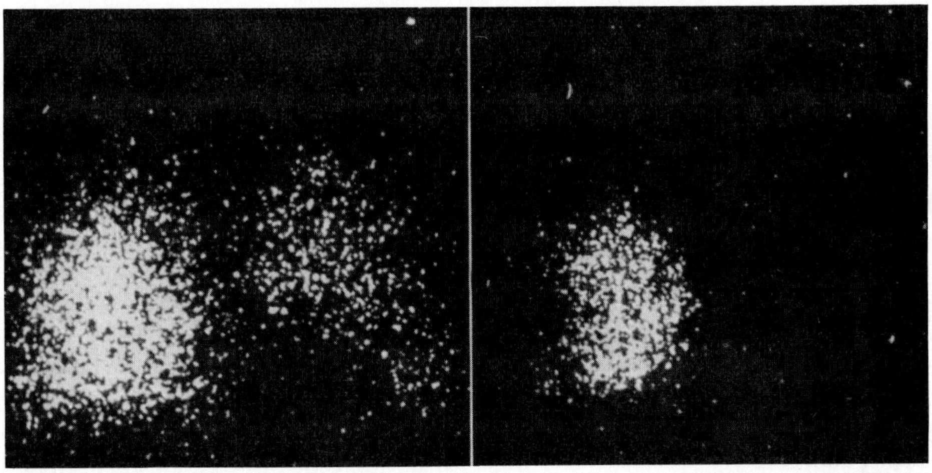

FIGURE 17-16 Xenon pulmonary scintiphotograms of a patient with severe inhalation injury of the right lung. Scintiphotograph on left shows inequality of isotope retention at 90 seconds. Later, at 120 seconds, all isotope has washed out except for the area of severe injury in right lung. In the absence of injury, only sparse background radiation should be visible 60 seconds after injection.

positive scintigrams occur in patients who are heavy cigarette smokers or who have other forms of chronic lung disease.

Although the true incidence of inhalation injury is unknown, approximately 25% of patients admitted to burn centers are diagnosed with this comorbid injury. Between 1985 and 1990, 330 of 1256 patients admitted to the United States Army Institute of Surgical Research (USAISR) were documented to have concomitant inhalation injury.[257] The utility of obtaining both ^{133}Xenon and bronchoscopic studies is outlined in Table 17-9. Similar to our previous review of inhalation injury, patients who have had a positive xenon scan and a positive bronchoscopic examination (severe injury) have a significantly greater morbidity and mortality than those patients with positive scans but negative bronchoscopsy (mild injury).

For the otherwise stable patient with a mild injury, humidified air and oxygen may be the only treatment necessary. Prophylactic antibiotics, given either parenterally or intratracheally, have been shown in clinical trials to be of no value in preventing later pulmonary infection.[150] Further, such prophylactic therapy promotes the emergence of later infections with organisms resistant to multiple antibiotics. Likewise, the prophylactic administration of steroids has no effect on the course of inhalation injury and increases infectious complications.[292]

Recent animal studies have indicated that after smoke exposure, a cascade of proinflammatory mediators such as platelet activating factor is liberated, which results in further airway damage by endogenous release of various oxidants.[128] This endogenous mediated injury is the target of current investigations seeking to limit the degree of tissue injury. As an example, postinjury treatment with pentoxifylline has shown promising results in an ovine model.[204]

Despite an increased understanding of the pathophysiologic mechanisms initiated after smoke inhalation, the current treatment of severe injury remains entirely supportive. Such therapy is tailored to meet ven-

TABLE 17-9 INHALATION INJURY PATIENTS

	XENON (+)	BRONCHOSCOPY (+)
N	85	245
Age (mean ± sem)	33.5 ± 1.9 yr	35.6 ± 1.3 yr
TBSA burn (mean ± sem)	26.2 ± 1.8%	46.1% ± 1.6%*
Intubation frequency	24.7% (21)	97.5% (239)*
Pneumonia frequency	13.1% (11)	46.9% (115)*
Mortality	3.6% (3)	38.3% (94)*
Predicted mortality (1980-1984 predictor)	15.7% (14)	50.2% (123)
95% conf. intervals	(10.5 – 21.5%)	(45.6 – 55.1%)

*$P < 0.0001$

tilatory support requirements, to treat intervening pulmonary infection, and to provide meticulous fluid management to limit the consequences of the noncardiogenic pulmonary edema that may occur.

The incidence of pneumonia has been reported to increase mortality of thermally injured patients by as much as 40%. Unfortunately, the incidence of pneumonia is increased nearly fivefold in patients with inhalation injury compared to those without injury. The reason for the increased incidence of infection is multifactorial but includes impaired mucociliary clearance mechanisms, defective alveolar macrophage function, distal airway obstruction and subsequent alveolar collapse, and the increased requirement for airway intubation and ventilatory support.

If pneumonia develops, antibiotic therapy is based on verification of infection and isolation of the offending organism. Surveillance respiratory cultures are quite valuable in allowing proper selection of antibiotics while awaiting definitive culture results. However, antibiotic treatment of positive respiratory tract cultures without clinical evidence of infection is rarely justified. Meticulous pulmonary toilet must accompany antibiotic therapy, and frequent bronchoscopic irrigation and suctioning are valuable adjuncts.

Pulmonary edema is treated by meticulous fluid management and respiratory support as needed. This complication most often occurs when edema in the burn wound is being mobilized during the first week after the burn. If pulmonary edema in burn patients with inhalation injury does not respond to maximum fluid restriction consistent with adequate intravascular volume maintenance (normal serum sodium and graded weight loss), compromised respiratory function must be treated with assisted ventilation. Diuretics should be used with caution and excessive diuresis avoided because of the high incidence of hypovolemia and hypernatremia. Most patients respond to mechanical ventilation with positive end-expiratory pressure and can be weaned from the ventilator during the second week after the burn. However, if pulmonary infection supervenes, a prolonged course of sepsis and respiratory failure is the rule, and the endotracheal tube should be replaced by tracheostomy in patients requiring intubation for longer than 2 weeks.[156]

In patients with more severe injury, mechanical ventilatory support is frequently required. In our previously referenced series of patients, 97% of bronchoscopically positive patients required at least short-term ventilatory support compared to only 24.7% of patients with inhalation injury whose bronchoscopic examination was normal. The increased severity of the insult was documented by a 3.5-fold increase in the incidence of pneumonia (46.9% vs 13.1%) and an 11-fold increase in mortality (38.3% vs 3.6%). This increased requirement for ventilatory support is expected, as a manifestation of the dose-related changes in Va/Qc (ventilation-perfusion ratio) mismatching secondary to acute inflammatory occlusion of small airways identified in an ovine model.[267]

The institution of conventional volume limited mechanical ventilatory support, although required for maintenance of physiologic stability, may further increase the damage to the airway. This concept led to a clinical trial of high-frequency flow interruption (HFFI) in a series of patients with inhalation injury. The need for intubation and mechanical ventilation in the study patients was defined by the usual criteria. Compared to historical controls, a significant decrease in the incidence of pneumonia and a decrease in mortality anticipated by the currently used mortality predictor at the USAISR was documented in the first 54 patients.[58] Further comparisons to concomitant conventionally treated patients demonstrated a real and significant decrease in the mortality in those patients treated with HFFI.

The hypothesis that ventilator mode-induced pulmonary damage is decreased by the use of HFFI compared to volume-limited conventional ventilation was confirmed in a primate smoke inhalation model.[53] Primates receiving a moderate smoke injury were random-

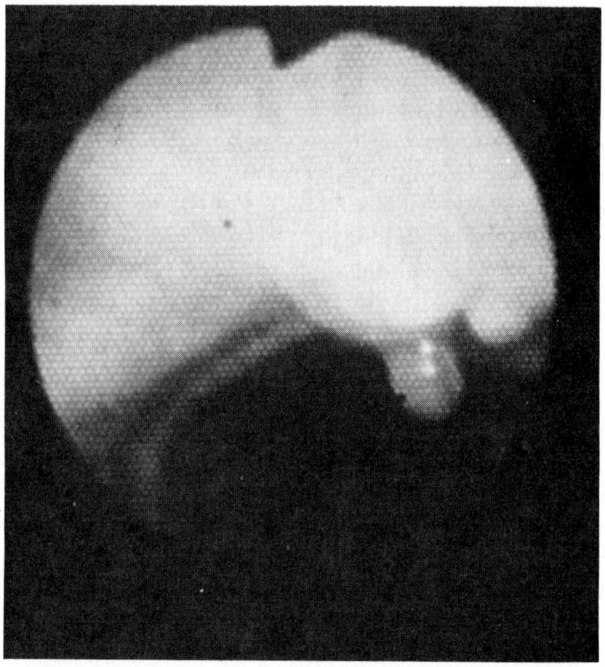

FIGURE 17-17 Large inflammatory granuloma at the site of a tracheostomy stoma. The lesions may be sufficiently large to require excision.

ized to a 7-day trial of three modes of ventilatory support: volume limited conventional ventilation, high frequency flow interruption, and high frequency oscillatory ventilation. The animals supported with HFFI had significantly less pulmonary damage at sacrifice than the other two groups. The findings of these studies have led to the use of HFFI in our institution on all patients with inhalation injury who require ventilatory support.

The long-term morbidity in patients surviving inhalation injury is related primarily to treatment, particularly to the use of invasive airway devices necessary to preserve respiratory function. Sequelae are generally more common and more severe after tracheotomy than after translaryngeal intubation, but the duration of tube placement appears to be the most important etiologic factor in permanent damage.[156] Tracheal stenosis and granuloma formation are the most frequently observed lesions (Figure 17-17). Follow-up fiberoptic bronchoscopy to document any airway lesions should be performed in all patients in whom the duration of intubation exceeds 10 days and who demonstrate signs of airway compromise. Xeroradiograms may provide additional information about the degree of tracheal stenosis. Although somewhat insensitive, spirometry, including assessment of flow-volume loops, may be useful as a noninvasive screening method to identify patients with significant narrowing of the airway.[213]

POSTRESUSCITATION FLUID AND ELECTROLYTE MANAGEMENT

Administration of the intravenous fluids required for resuscitation of patients with extensive burns commonly produces a 15% to 20% increase in body weight. Even when amounts far in excess of estimated resuscitation fluid volumes have been administered, acute pulmonary edema is rare in the first 48 hours postburn, except in those patients with limited myocardial reserve. Even in those patients, pulmonary edema is much more common after resuscitation, when edema resorption expands the intravascular volume. Whenever pulmonary edema occurs in a burn patient, fluid administration should be reduced, pulmonary function supported as necessary, and cardiac function evaluated by extensive monitoring. Administration of a diuretic may be necessary, depending on the severity of the pulmonary fluid overload.

The administration of resuscitation fluids expands both total body water and the exchangeable sodium mass[220] (Table 17-10). Destruction of the water vapor barrier function of the skin by the burn injury acounts for the prodigiously increased evaporative water loss from the wounds of patients with extensive burns; and the previously mentioned elevated circulating levels of renin, angiotensin, and aldosterone account for the avid retention of sodium after resuscitation. Previous reports have suggested that secretion of these hormones is altered after thermal injury by resetting of neural control mechanisms, which is not sodium or volume dependent.

TABLE 17-10 RETENTION OF FLUID AND SODIUM ADMINISTERED DURING RESUSCITATION OF 8 EXTENSIVELY BURNED PATIENTS*

PARAMETER	EXCHANGEABLE SODIUM MASS (PERCENTAGE OF PREDICTED)	EXTRACELLULAR FLUID VOLUME (INCREASE ABOVE PREDICTED)
Fifth postburn day	145%	153%
Twelfth postburn day	121%	128%

*Mean extent of burn was 47.6% (range was 34.0% to 57.2%).

Cioffi and colleagues[59] have identified a significantly depressed total blood volume in postresuscitative thermally injured patients despite a markedly elevated cardiac index and renal plasma flow. Plasma renin activity and antidiuretic hormone levels were elevated and altered in the direction expected from the blood volume measurements. This paradoxical dissociation of blood volume and flow indicates that in burn patients, increased blood flow does not entirely depend on increased blood volume. Knowledge of these physiologic changes characteristic of the burn patient aids the management of postresuscitation fluid therapy and electrolyte abnormalities.

After resuscitation further administration of salt-containing fluids should be confined to the correction of documented deficits. The diuresis of retained resuscitation fluid, which characteristically begins late in the second or during the third postburn day, parallels edema resorption. The diuresis may be surprisingly modest in patients with extensive burns in whom evaporative water loss is markedly elevated. If diuresis does occur, the urinary output should not be volumetrically replaced, and fluid therapy should provide that amount of electrolyte-free water necessary to avoid both hyponatremia and hypernatremia while permitting a 10% weight loss per day of the weight gained during resuscitation so the patient will return to preburn weight by the seventh to tenth postburn day.

Hyponatremia

Mild hyponatremia, as manifested by a serum sodium concentration approximating that of lactated Ringer's solution (i.e., 130 mEq/L), is commonly observed at the completion of resuscitation. Such mild hyponatremia infrequently causes symptoms and is corrected by reducing the fluid infusion rate.

Burn wound care can affect sodium balance following resuscitation. Transeschar salt losses are modest in patients treated by the exposure technique, but up to 300 mEq of sodium/day has been recovered from dressings of patients treated by the occlusive dressing technique.[22] The leeching of sodium from the eschar into hypotonic 0.5% silver nitrate soaks can cause the rapid development of pronounced hyponatremia. In patients with burns of up to 50% of the total body surface, oral administration of 10 g of sodium chloride and 30 to 50 ml of molar sodium lactate per day is recommended. In patients with more extensive burns, 15 to 30 g of sodium chloride and 50 to 80 ml of molar sodium lactate per day is recommended to prevent the development of hyponatremia in patients treated with 0.5% silver nitrate soaks.[189]

Later in the postburn course, reduction of evaporative water loss from a previously exposed burn wound by application of occlusive dressings, biologic dressings, or cutaneous autografts can result in hyponatremia if the administration of electrolyte-free fluid is not correspondingly reduced. Hyponatremia may also occur in burn patients with sepsis. Reduction of glomerular filtration rate in association with elevation of true renal plasma flow may reduce free water clearance early in the course of an infection.[30] The source of infection in such patients should be identified and the septic process controlled.

Symptomatic hyponatremia occurs most commonly in burn patients in whom the administration of electrolyte-free fluid has depressed the serum sodium concentration to 120 mEq/L or less. Rapid lowering of the serum sodium concentration may evoke symptoms of hyponatremia even when the serum sodium concentration is greater than 120 mEq/L. Hypotonic fluids should be cautiously administered to burned children because their relatively small fluid compartments make them particularly susceptible to rapid changes in serum sodium concentration and the development of symptomatic hyponatremia. Hyponatremia was found to be the most common cause of seizures in a group of 36 burned children who had one or more convulsive episodes.[177] In the 22 patients in whom the convulsive activity was related to hyponatremia, the seizures occurred in 15 children when the serum sodium was 125 mEq/L or less, and in 7 when those children were receiving 5% dextrose in water. The presence of cerebral edema in such patients is confirmed by CT evidence of reduction of ventricular volume and obliteration of the subdural space. The occurrence of hyponatremia in the burned child can be minimized by carefully regulating the infusion rate and salt concentration of administered fluids or by combining electrolyte-containing and electrolyte-free fluids before administration.

The clinical manifestations of hyponatremia determine the necessary treatment. Mild hyponatremia can be treated by discontinuing the infusion of hypotonic fluid and restricting total fluid intake to permit the elevated water losses of the burn patient to restore a normal sodium concentration. Symptomatic hyponatremia should be treated by the administration of a diuretic and hypertonic salt solutions, with anticonvulsive mediation given if seizures occur.

Hyponatremia has also been reported as a manifestation of the *sick cell* syndrome, in which a cellular energy deficit impairs the ability of the cell to exclude sodium.[123] The increase in red cell sodium concentration noted in burn patients receiving inadequate nutritional support can be corrected by administration of sufficient calories.[69] Other studies[122] have shown that the sick cell syndrome can be corrected by intravenous administration of insulin and glucose, as well as by blood transfusions.

Hypernatremia

Hypernatremia is the most common electrolyte abnormality following the edema resorption phase in patients with extensive burns. The most frequent cause of hypernatremia is the inadequate replacement of evaporative water losses, the total of which ranges from 2.0 to 3.1 ml/kg body weight/%burn/day.[114] Such losses may be exacerbated by the use of air-fluidized beds.[178]

Underestimation of insensible water loss (predominantly transeschar water loss), the most common cause of hypernatremia in burn patients, was identified in 61% of the 51 patients in whom a serum sodium concentration of 146 mEq/L or higher was documented during a 1-year period[291] (Table 17-11). Insensible water loss in burn patients can be estimated according to the formula:

$$\text{Insensible water loss (ml/hr)} = (25 + \%\text{ of body surface burned}) \times \text{Total body surface area in m}^2$$

TABLE 17-11 CAUSES OF HYPERNATREMIA IN BURN PATIENTS TREATED DURING AN 18-MONTH PERIOD

CAUSE	NUMBER OF PATIENTS
Inadequate replacement of insensible water loss	31
Sepsis	16
Osmotic diuresis associated with diabetes mellitus or hypermetabolism	2
Defect in osmotic regulation (diabetes insipidus)	2
Total patients with hypernatremia	51*

*10.9% of 468 admissions.

This formula estimates the insensible water loss at the lower end of the range of observed losses. The adequacy of hydration should be closely monitored by daily measurements of body weight, serum osmolality, and serum sodium concentration and the administration of fluids adjusted accordingly.

An elevated urinary glucose concentration, caused by either preexisting diabetes mellitus or administration of excessive glucose, as well as an elevated urinary nitrogen concentration, can induce an osmotic diuresis that results in hypernatremia. The increased urinary water loss in such patients can be eliminated by the administration of insulin and/or reduction in the amount of carbohydrate-containing and nitrogen-containing nutrients administered to the burn patient. The increase in ventilatory rate and body temperature and the increase in renal blood flow noted in some patients early in the course of infection contribute to increased water loss that may cause hypernatremia in septic burn patients. Identification of the septic process and its control by surgical excision and administration of appropriate antimicrobial agents will reduce sepsis-related water losses. Defects in the regulation of water balance only rarely cause hypernatremia. The diagnosis of central diabetes insipidus should be made only after all other causes have been excluded in a patient in whom polyuria and hypernatremia are unresponsive to fluid administration and are corrected by the intramuscular administration of 10 units of vasopressin every 6 hours. Nephrogenic diabetes insipidus may occur after systemic amphotericin therapy in patients with fungal infections.

DISTURBANCES OF POTASSIUM BALANCE

Potassium should not be added to the resuscitation fluids given to a burn patient because modest hyperkalemia is commonly produced by the release of potassium from red cells and other tissues injured by the burn. This hyperkalemia may be accentuated if inadequate resuscitation permits the development of acidosis as a result of impaired tissue perfusion. If the acidosis is corrected by rapid fluid infusion, the serum potassium level concomitantly recedes. If the serum potassium elevation causes cardiac dysfunction, it should be treated by administration of ion exchange resins or, in severe cases, infusion of calcium gluconate, sodium bicarbonate, glucose, and insulin.

Hypokalemia, as a consequence of increased potassium losses, may occur after resuscitation. The postresuscitation elevation of renal potassium loss can be further increased by alkalosis secondary to hyperventilation and the kaluretic effect of mafenide acetate burn cream.[294] The transeschar loss of potassium, up to 275 mEq/m^2 of burn surface per day, predisposes patients treated with 0.5% silver nitrate soak therapy to develop hypokalemia.[189] Potassium losses can be further increased if diarrhea is induced by enteral feedings or by enteric bacteria. Potassium supplements should be administered to prevent or correct potassium deficits as assessed by monitoring serum levels and urinary losses.

OTHER ELECTROLYTE ABNORMALITIES

In patients with burns on more than 30% of the body surface, mild depression of serum calcium levels is common. Some investigators[154] have identified low levels of ionized calcium in the early postinjury period in association with low levels of phosphate, and they have attributed those changes to increased circulating levels of calcitonin and catecholamines. In our experience, ionized calcium levels appear little influenced by burn injury, and the decrease in total serum calcium is consistent with the decrease observed in calcium-binding proteins. Transeschar leeching of calcium by 0.5% silver nitrate soak topical therapy may further depress serum calcium to symptomatic levels, necessitating intravenous administration of calcium salts.[12] Hypophosphatemia is often identified following resuscitation and is presumed to be dilutional. However, dilutional hypophosphatemia may be accentuated by administering large volumes of phosphate binding antacids for prophylaxis against gastric stress ulcerations and by initiating enteral feeding early in the postburn course leading to refeeding induced hypophosphatemia. Reduction of the antacid dose and phosphate replacement may be necessary.

Anorexia in the early postburn period and impaired wound healing later in the postburn course have been attributed to depression of serum zinc levels.[61,144] Documented zinc deficiency appears to be uncommon in burn patients in whom a regular diet customarily maintains zinc levels within the normal range. Muscle cramps and psychiatric signs such as hallucinations have been attributed to depression of serum magnesium to levels below 1.4 mEq/L.[32] In burn patients with symptomatic hypomagnesemia, the clinical signs responded to the administration of magnesium salts. In our experience, adequate nutrition has prevented the development of hypomagnesemia.

BURN WOUND CARE

Initial Wound Management

In the absence of chemical injury that requires immediate removal of the offending agent and lavage of the wound, attention is directed to the burn wound only after the patient is stabilized. After maintenance of airway, restoration of intravascular volume, and adequacy of peripheral circulation are verified, the patient may be safely removed to a bed or treatment room. This environment should be warm to reduce patient discomfort and prevent hypothermia. The burn should be gently bathed with a nonirritating detergent and copiously irrigated. Loose necrotic tissue is debrided, including intact bullae. Any hair is shaved from the burn wound and a 3- to 4-inch margin of unburned skin. Removal of body hair often reveals additional burn injury that would have otherwise remained undetected, especially on the scalp. General anesthesia is not required for initial wound debridement and is contraindicated in most patients. Profound cardiovascular collapse with cardiac arrest is an extremely common event following general anesthesia in the early resuscitation phase. Small doses of intravenous analgesics to provide adequate pain relief are safely tolerated once fluid resuscitation has been successfully instituted. After thorough debridement, the patient is weighed, and mapping of the burn on injury diagrams is accomplished most accurately at this time. Finally, a topical antimbicrobial agent is applied to the wound.

Topical Antimicrobial Therapy

The primary goal of wound care in the burned patient is control of infection until spontaneous healing or surgical closure occurs. The injured and nonviable tissue predisposes the burn wound to microbial colonization and subsequent invasion of organisms into viable tissue, and the incidence of wound infection increases as burn size increases.[222] Immediately after injury, bacterial density in the wound is low and is confined to surface contaminants, usually gram-positive cocci. In the untreated burn, bacterial density increases with time; gram-negative bacteria soon predominate and begin to penetrate the eschar, commonly migrating along viable sweat glands and hair follicles. The avascular nature of the wound prevents the delivery of the blood-borne components of the host defense system and systemically administered antibiotics to the burn, and bacterial proliferation may progress in an unrestrained fashion.[207] If bacterial density at the junction of the eschar with underlying viable tissue rises to 10^5/gram of tissue or higher, wound infection and subsequent systemic dissemination are likely to occur.[185] The most effective method for controlling bacterial proliferation in the burn eschar is the use of topical antimicrobial agents that are active against the flora populating the wound.

The cause of burn wound infection has changed over the past several decades and may be related to the proliferation of broad-spectrum antibiotics. Before the introduction of effective antimicrobial agents in the late 1940s, streptococcal wound sepsis was the major cause of death from infection in thermally injured patients. Patients developed infection early, and the clinical course was one of rapid deterioration and death. With the introduction and gradual widespread use of first-generation penicillins between 1945 and 1965, the incidence of serious streptococcal burn sepsis fell dramatically, whereas that for staphylococcal infection increased. These latter infections occurred later in the course after burn injury and were paralleled by a slower rise in the staphylococcal bacterial count in the burn wound. Most staphylococcal burn infections were caused by hospital-acquired organisms, tended to occur in epidemics, and were often resistant to early penicillins. Staphylococcal infections were partially controlled, but not eliminated, by the advent of penicillinase-resistant antibiotics. By the early 1960s, *Pseudomonas aeruginosa* burn wound infection and its consequences were the most frequent cause of death in major burn centers.[228,286] From the 1970s, other nosocomial, gram-negative bacterial and fungal organisms joined *P. aeruginosa* as major causes of infection and mortality. Successful control of burn wound infection was first demonstrated for two topically applied agents, mafenide acetate burn cream and 0.5% silver nitrate soaks, and such treatment rapidly became the established method for limiting bacterial proliferation in the eschar.[186,189] The use of these topical preparations has been associated with a marked increase in survival of patients with burns involving 30% to 60% of the total body surface.[228] A third topical agent, silver sulfadiazine burn cream, has also been shown to be effective in controlling burn wound flora when applied early in the course after burn injury.[96] Other topical agents have been used for burn wound therapy, but none have been shown in clinical trials to be effective in preventing burn wound infection.

Each of the three currently used topical agents have unique advantages and limitations (Table 17-12). Sulfamylon burn cream is an 11.1% water-soluble suspension of mafenide acetate. It is bacteriostatic for both gram-positive and gram-negative organisms and is uniquely effective against the latter group, particularly against *P. aeruginosa* and *Clostridia* organisms. The high solubility of mafenide acetate allows it to diffuse through the eschar and makes it the agent of choice for the treatment of wounds in which bacteria have penetrated and proliferated. The major disadvantages of mafenide acetate are transient pain following application on partial-thickness burns and carbonic anhydrase inhibition. Small doses of analgesics administered shortly before applying mafenide to a second-degree burn effectively attenuate patient discomfort, and any residual pain resolves within half an hour. Carbonic anhydrase inhibition causes renal bicarbonate wasting and contraction of total body buffer base. In addition, mafenide accentuates hyperventilation after burn injury. The combined renal and respiratory effects predispose the patient to a compensated meta-

TABLE 17-12 TOPICAL CHEMOTHERAPEUTIC AGENTS FOR BURN WOUND CARE

	MAFENIDE ACETATE	SILVER NITRATE	SILVER SULFADIAZINE
Active component concentration	11.1% in water-miscible base	0.5% in aqueous solution	1.0% in water-miscible base
Spectrum of antibacterial activity	Gram-negative—good Gram-positive—good Yeasts—minimal	Gram-negative—good Gram-positive—good Yeasts—good	Gram-negative—selectively good Yeasts—good
Method of wound care	Exposure	Occlusive dressings	Exposure or single-layer dressings
Advantages	Penetrates eschar Wound appearance readily monitored Joint motion unrestricted No gram-negative resistance	Painless No hypersensitivity reactions No gram-negative resistance Dressings reduce evaporative heat loss Greater effectiveness against yeasts	Painless Wound appearance readily monitored when exposure method used Easily applied Joint motion unrestricted when exposure method used Greater effectiveness against yeasts
Disadvantages	Painful on partial-thickness burns Acidosis as a result of inhibition of carbonic anhydrase Hypersensitivity reactions in 7% of patients	Deficits of sodium, potassium, calcium, and chloride No eschar penetration Limitation of joint motion by dressings Methemoglobinemia—rare Argyria—rare Staining of environment and equipment	Neutropenia Hypersensitivity—infrequent Limited eschar penetration Resistance of certain gram-negative bacteria, clostridia

bolic acidosis, which may become uncompensated if pulmonary complications occur. With continued use of mafenide, these physiologic alterations ameliorate and acid-base balance is maintained in the stable patient.

Silvadene burn cream is a 1% suspension of silver sulfadiazine in a water-soluble base. Unlike mafenide, silver sulfadiazine is poorly soluble and has only limited ability to penetrate into the burn wound. As such, it is relatively ineffective in controlling bacterial proliferation in the eschar once high bacterial densities have occurred. Silver sulfadiazine is painless on application (and is often soothing) and causes no acid-base abnormalities. The major limitations of this topical agent are depression of myeloid elements in blood and resistance exhibited by certain gram-negative bacteria. Silver sulfadiazine myeloid toxicity presents typically as granulocytopenia within the first 5 days after injury; temporary cessation of this agent usually allows prompt return of neutrophil count to previous values. However, when severe thrombocytopenia accompanies neutropenia, a fulminant septic course often follows. Nearly all *Enterobacter cloacae* and certain *Pseudomonas* strains develop resistance to silver sulfadiazine. McManus and associates[170] have shown sulfadiazine resistance in gram-negative organisms to be mediated by plasmids that confer resistance not only to the sulfonamide but also to other antibiotics and antimicrobial agents. The exclusive use of silver sulfadiazine may be responsible for epidemics of infection caused by bacterial species resistant to multiple antibiotics.

Silver nitrate is applied as a 0.5% solution in saturated multilayered dressings. Although the solution is painless, the dressings may be uncomfortable and will decrease patient mobility. Silver nitrate solution has a broad antibacterial spectrum. It precipitates on contact with tissue and does not penetrate the eschar. Therefore silver nitrate therapy must be initiated before significant wound colonization takes place. Electrolyte abnormalities, alkalosis, and water loading are common and result from the transeschar absorption of water from the hypotonic soak solutions and from loss of sodium, potassium, chloride, and calcium into the dressings. Hyponatremia may develop with surprising speed, and judicious sodium supplementation should accompany use of silver nitrate soaks.

Burns of sufficient severity to require hospitalization should be treated with topical antimicrobial agents. The burn creams, mafenide and silver sulfadiazine, most commonly are used by the exposure method or with occlusive dressings, whereas silver nitrate must be used with dressings. The exposure method appears to be the best approach for patients with large burns. This technique allows continuous observation of the burn and facilitates early recognition of wound deterioration and infection, and patient activity and compliance with early rehabilitation programs are enhanced. These advantages are usually not realized when occlusive dressings are used. In addition to limiting patient activity, dressings are painful when changed. Further dressings promote microbial proliferation by maintaining a warm, moist environment and elevate body temperature by their insulative effect. Following daily cleansing and debridement, mafenide or silver sulfadiazine is applied to the burn with a gloved hand or a sterile spatula in a thickness of approximately 3 to 4 mm. Additional agent is applied whenever portions are inadvertently wiped off the wound. In burns particularly prone to infection, mafenide cream is applied after the morning wound care, and silver sulfadiazine is applied 12 hours later to minimize the side effects of the two agents and to take advantage of the broader activity of mafenide acetate against gram-negative bacteria and the superior activity of silver sulfadiazine against candidal species. Silver nitrate soaks should be used for topical therapy in patients allergic to sulfonamides.

Monitoring the Burn Wound

At least once a day, topical agents and wound exudate should be cleansed away so that the entire burn wound is exposed. At this time, the surgeon inspects the wound for changes in the eschar's appearance over time. Particularly important is hands-on palpation of all portions of the wound to detect any subeschar purulence; these collections should be unroofed before extension into deeper viable tissue occurs. Any alterations indicative of wound infection should be evaluated by prompt biopsy of the involved areas. An increase of 10^2 or greater of bacterial density in surveillance biopsies dictates a reevaluation of topical therapy. In most cases, mafenide should be added to or substituted for currently used topical therapy. Finally, daily evaluations allow timely decisions for surgical closure of deep dermal and full-thickness wounds. The exposure method of burn care makes continuous wound observation possible throughout the remainder of the hospital day.

DIAGNOSIS AND TREATMENT OF BURN WOUND INFECTIONS

The use of topical burn wound chemotherapeutic agents has significantly reduced the incidence of invasive burn wound infections, but the protection provided by such therapy is imperfect.[55,241] Topical antimicrobial agents do not sterilize burn wounds, but retard proliferation of the microorganisms that invariably colonize burn wounds and maintain the microbial density at levels against which even an immunocompromised host can defend.[185] If topical therapy fails to limit microbial proliferation and host defense capabilities are exceeded, invasive bacterial, fungal, and even viral burn wound infection will develop. This complication of burn injury occurs most commonly in patients with burns of more than 30% of the body surface, particularly in burned children.[228] A flow diagram outlining burn wound treatment is presented in algorithm III at the end of this chapter.

Diagnosis

Hypothermia, tachycardia, tachypnea, disorientation, glucose intolerance, and changes in white cell numbers are of little assistance in diagnosing infection in the burn patient because similar changes are commonly elicited by burn injury per se in the absence of infection.[227] The unreliability of systemic signs as indicators of infection necessitates at least daily examination of the entire burn wound of each patient to identify an invasive infection before local extension or systemic spread precludes successful therapeutic intervention.

The most common wound change characteristic of invasive wound infection is focal, dark red, brown, or black discoloration of the eschar; but such tinctorial changes are nonspecific because minor trauma, causing intraeschar hemorrhage, may produce similar changes in the eschar.[224] The rapid conversion of an area of partial-thickness injury to full-thickness skin necrosis is the most reliable sign of invasive burn wound infection (Figure 17-18). Invasive fungal infections, particularly those caused by *Phycomycetes* species are characterized by extension of necrosis with surprising velocity and magnitude.[225] Unexpectedly rapid separation of the eschar is another clinical sign of invasive wound infection, most often seen in association with fungal infection, but such separation may occur in the absence of infection when the burn injury has been of sufficient depth to cause liquefaction of the underlying subcutaneous fat. Other clinical signs of invasive burn wound infection are listed in the box on page 683.

The imprecision and unreliability of local signs and symptoms necessitate use of other methods to diagnose burn wound infections. Surface culture techniques may be used for epidemiologic monitoring and to characterize the microbial flora of the burn wounds of an individual patient, but even quantitative culture techniques are inaccurate in diagnosing burn wound infection. Falsely high quantitative culture results can be produced by culture of pooled secretions or exudates; culture of an eschar at the time of sloughing, which occurs as a result of bacterial lysis of denatured collagen; or by delay

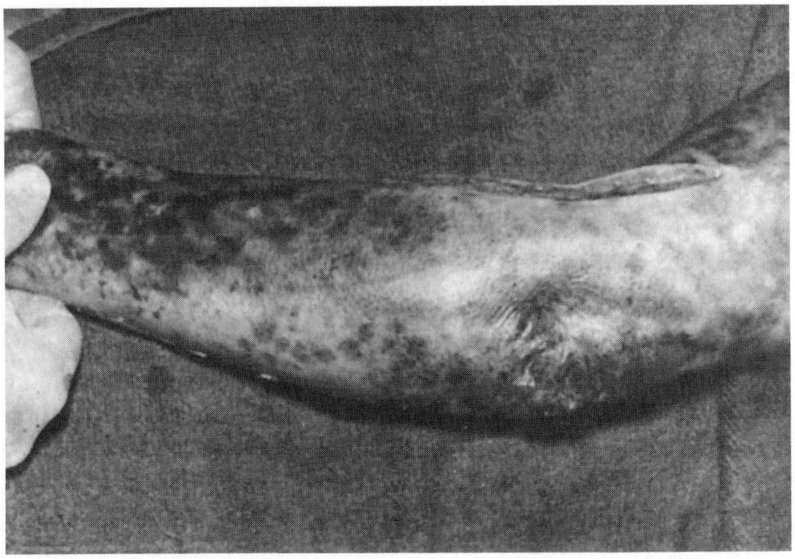

FIGURE 17-18 The multiple areas of dark discoloration in the full-thickness burns on the arm of this patient appeared on the sixth postburn day. Invasive burn wound infection was confirmed by histologic examination of the tissue obtained by subsequent biopsy of one of the black areas of necrosis on the extensor surface of the lower third of forearm. Note the six focal areas of faint discoloration in curvilinear distribution on the ulnar aspect of the mid-forearm.

CLINICAL SIGNS OF INVASIVE BURN WOUND INFECTION

Focal areas of dark red, brown, or black eschar discoloration
Conversions of partial-thickness injury to full-thickness necrosis
Hemorrhagic discoloration of subeschar tissue
Green pigment visible in subcutaneous fat*
Erythematous necrotic lesions (ecthyma gangrenosum) in unburned skin*
Edema and/or violaceous discoloration of unburned skin at wound margin
Accelerated separation of eschar†
Rapid centrifugal expansion of subcutaneous edema with central necrosis†
Vesicular lesions in healing or healed partial-thickness burns‡
Crusted serrated margins of partial-thickness burns of the face‡

* Characteristic of *Pseudomonas* infection.
† Characteristic of fungal infection.
‡ Characteristic of herpes simplex infection.

in specimen transport, permitting microbial proliferation. Conversely, falsely low quantitative culture counts are produced by culture of a nonrepresentative desiccated area of the wound, culture of residual topical agent, storage or transport conditions that permit desiccation of the specimen, and inability of surface culture techniques to sample the nonviable–viable tissue interface where infection first occurs. The reliability of quantitative culture results is further impugned by the discordance of microbial density in paired samples of burn wound biopsy specimens.[303] The correlation between negative burn wound biopsy histologic evidence and low quantitative culture counts of a wound biopsy is generally good, but there is very poor correlation between quantitative culture counts of more than 10^5 organisms/gram of tissue and histologic evidence of invasive burn wound infection.[172]

The histologic examination of a burn wound biopsy is the most reliable means of differentiating colonization of nonviable tissue from invasive infection of viable tissue.[232] The burn wound biopsy should be obtained from that area of the wound where the changes indicative of infection are most prominent (Figure 17-19, *A*). If a local anesthetic is deemed necessary, it should be injected at the periphery of the biopsy site to avoid distortion of the specimen's morphologic structure. At the time of biopsy, the specimen should be inspected because the

A 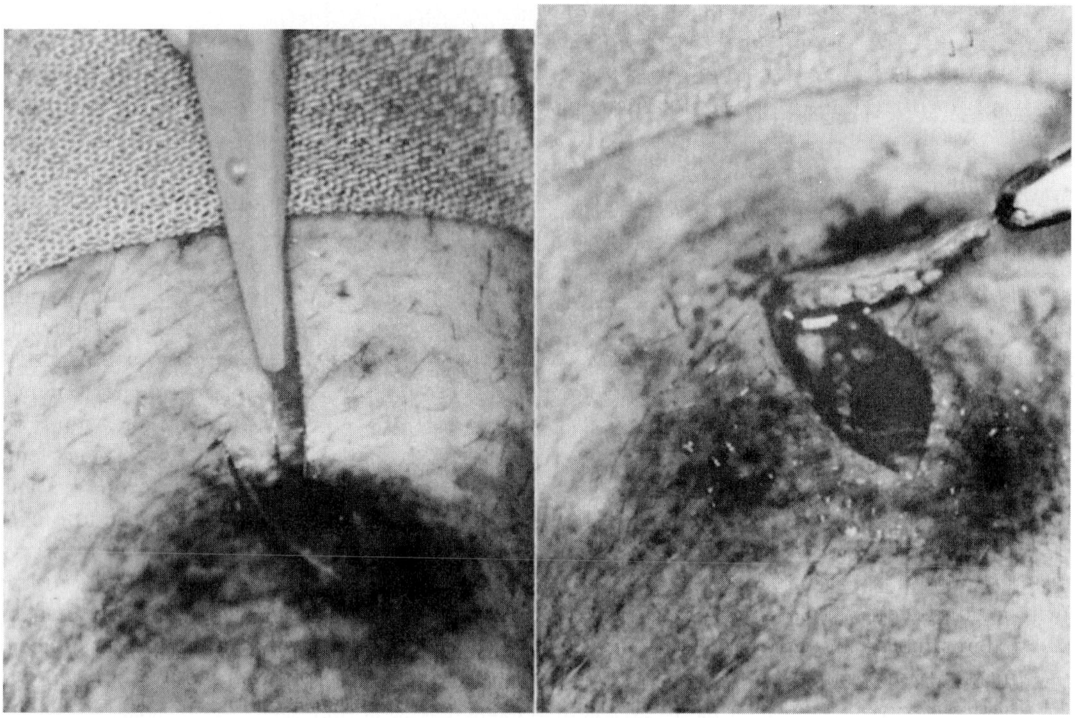 B

FIGURE 17-19 **A,** The area of dark discoloration in this burn wound prompted a biopsy using a scalpel as shown here. **B,** Elevation of the elliptical biopsy sample reveals the presence of unburned subcutaneous tissue that must be included in the specimen.

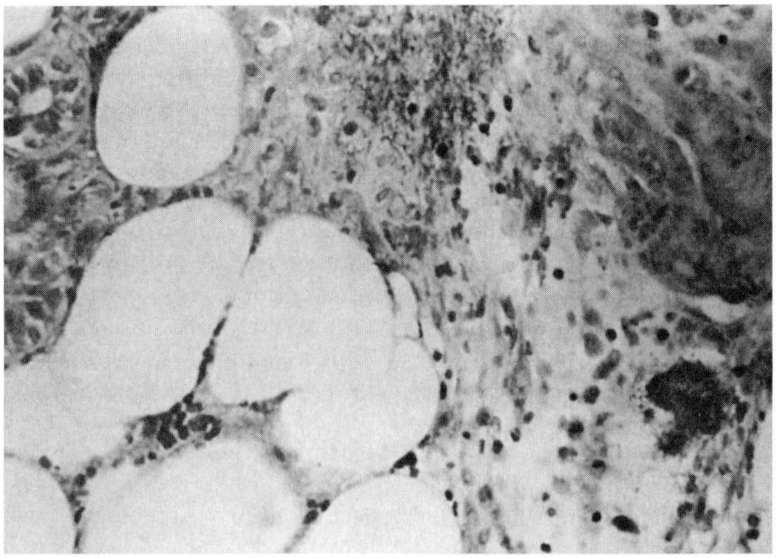

FIGURE 17-20 Photomicrograph of a histologic section from a burn wound biopsy showing dark-staining bacillary organisms in viable subcutaneous tissues at the 12 o'clock position. Note the dense nodular focus of the bacteria at the 4 o'clock position.

HISTOLOGIC CRITERIA OF BURN WOUND INFECTION

Microorganisms present in unburned tissue
Heightened inflammatory reaction in unburned tissue
Hemorrhage present in viable subeschar tissue
Small-vessel thrombosis and ischemic necrosis in unburned tissue
Dense microbial growth along hair follicles and sweat glands*
Intense microbial proliferation in subeschar space*
Intracellular viral inclusions

*Characteristic of deep colonization.

TABLE 17-13 HISTOLOGIC STAGING OF THE MICROBIAL STATUS OF BURN WOUNDS

STAGE	CHARACTERISTICS
I. Colonization	
A. Superficial	Microorganisms present on wound surface
B. Penetration	Microorganisms present in variable thickness of eschar
C. Proliferation	Multiplication of microorganisms in subeschar space
II. Invasion	
A. Microinvasion	Microscopic foci of microorganisms in viable tissue adjacent to subeschar space
B. Generalized	Multifocal or widespread penetration of microorganisms deep into viable subcutaneous tissue
C. Microvascular	Involvement of small blood vessels and lymphatics

presence of extensive hemorrhagic discoloration of the subcutaneous tissue is consistent with invasive infection. Using a scalpel, a 500 mg lenticular tissue sample that includes underlying or adjacent unburned tissue as well as the eschar is obtained (Figure 17-19, *B*). To identify and determine the antibiotic sensitivities of the organisms present, a portion of the specimen is sent in the unfixed state to the microbiology laboratory. The remainder of the biopsy sample is sent to the pathology laboratory, where it is processed using either a rapid section technique requiring 3 to 4 hours or a frozen section technique by which slides can be prepared for histologic examination within 30 minutes.[135,136]

Identification of bacteria, fungi, or viruses in viable tissue in a histologic section prepared from a burn wound biopsy confirms the diagnosis of invasive burn wound infection (Figure 17-20). The other histologic criteria indicative of burn wound infection are listed in the box above. False-negative histologic readings can occur as a result of erroneous histologic interpretation or by examination of a biopsy specimen that has been harvested from a nonrepresentative area of the wound. The frozen section method of biopsy specimen preparation is associated with a false-negative rate of 3.6%, which can be corrected by subsequent review of the permanent sections prepared from the specimen. A false-positive histologic reading can result from erroneous histologic interpretation or by examination of a biopsy specimen that includes only colonized eschar. The results of the histologic examination of a biopsy specimen must always be interpreted in light of the burn patient's general condition. When the histologic examination of a biopsy from a patient with systemic sepsis is reported as negative, a repeat biopsy should be obtained. If the repeat biopsy is also negative, an infection in a site other than the burn wound should be sought.

The microbial status of the burn wound can be classified on the basis of the density and depth of penetration of microorganisms according to the staging system described in Table 17-13 and Figure 17-21. A histologic classification of stage II confirms the presence of invasive burn wound infection. The likelihood of systemic spread of infection and a fatal outcome increases as the infection progresses beyond stage IIA (microinvasion) and becomes stage IIB (generalized). The microvasculature of each histologic section prepared from a burn wound biopsy should be carefully examined because microbial invasion of such vessels is associated with a high incidence of hematogenous dissemination to remote tissues and organs. Even if histologic examination of a wound biopsy reveals only colonization, stage I, the density and depth of penetration of microorganisms in that biopsy should be compared with that of prior and subsequent biopsies. A progressive increase in the number of organisms and in depth of penetration evident in serial biopsies is indicative of inadequate control of the microbial population of the burn wound. When such progression is noted, wound care should be altered by discontinuing application of a topical agent with limited diffusibility and the institution of mafenide acetate topical therapy.

Treatment

Histologic confirmation of invasive burn wound infection requires change in both local and systemic therapy. If another topical agent is being used, it should be stopped and mafenide acetate burn cream applied to the wounds twice a day. General supportive measures necessary to maintain or restore cardiac output and pulmonary and metabolic function should be instituted. Systemic antibiotic therapy should be initiated by ad-

A

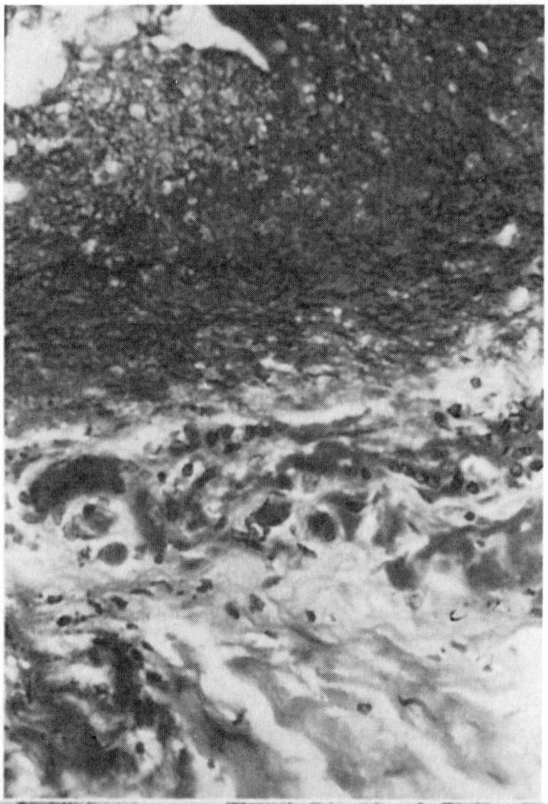

B

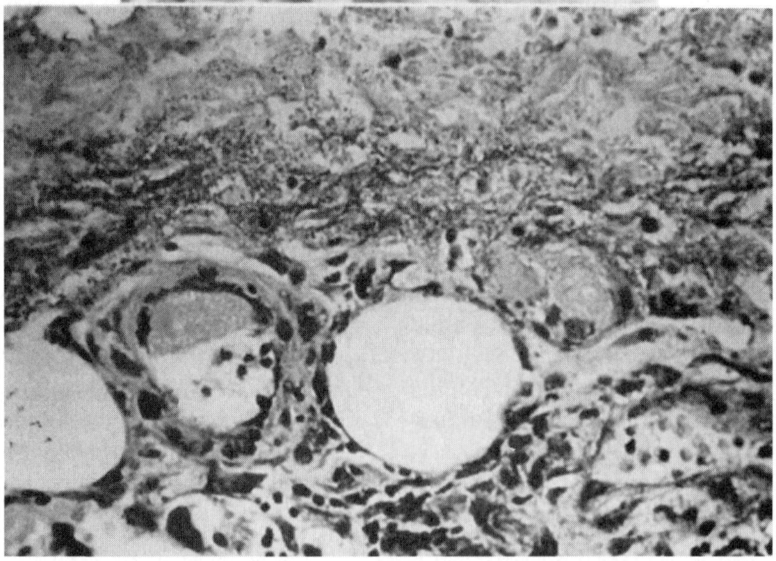

FIGURE 17-21 **A,** Photomicrograph of a biopsy specimen showing proliferation of bacillary organisms at the viable/nonviable tissue interface without involvement of viable tissue—stage Ic. **B,** Photomicrograph of a biopsy specimen showing dark-staining bacilli present in unburned tissue in the center of the field just beneath the burned tissue occupying the upper half of the field. The presence of inflammatory cells in the area of infection reflects an intact local circulation and indicates that the infected tissue was unburned—stage IIa.

ministration of antibiotics selected on the basis of organism prevalence and antibiotic sensitivity as determined by the institution's microbial surveillance program. The results of culture and sensitivity testing of the organisms recovered from the biopsy material are used to adjust the antibiotic therapy as indicated.

The local care required to treat a burn wound infection is determined by the characteristics of the septic process caused by the infecting organism. Streptococcal burn wound infections typically occur in the early postburn period but are infrequent. Streptococcal organisms have little tendency to invade deep tissues but may evoke an intense, local inflammatory reaction characterized by edema, rapidly expanding erythema of unburned skin at the periphery of the wound, and lymphangitis. Streptococcal wound infections respond promptly to the administration of penicillin or another antibiotic if the patient is allergic to penicillin. Staphylococcal infections

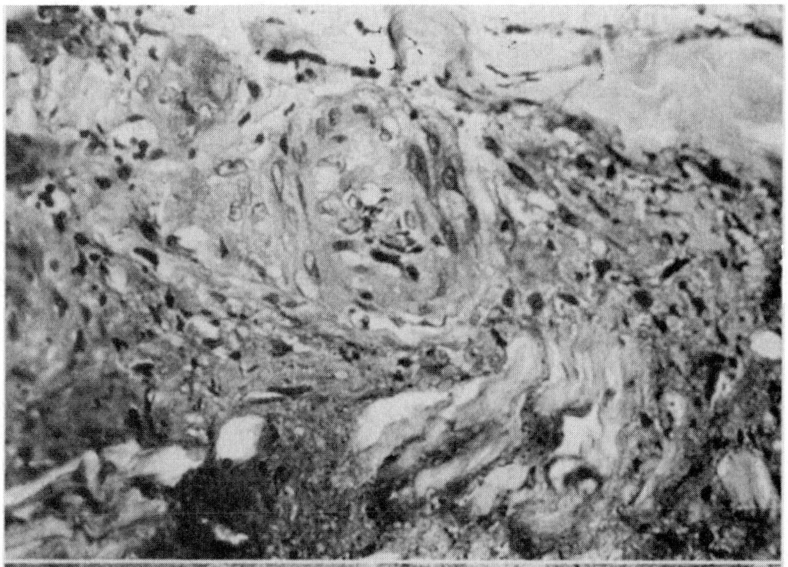
C

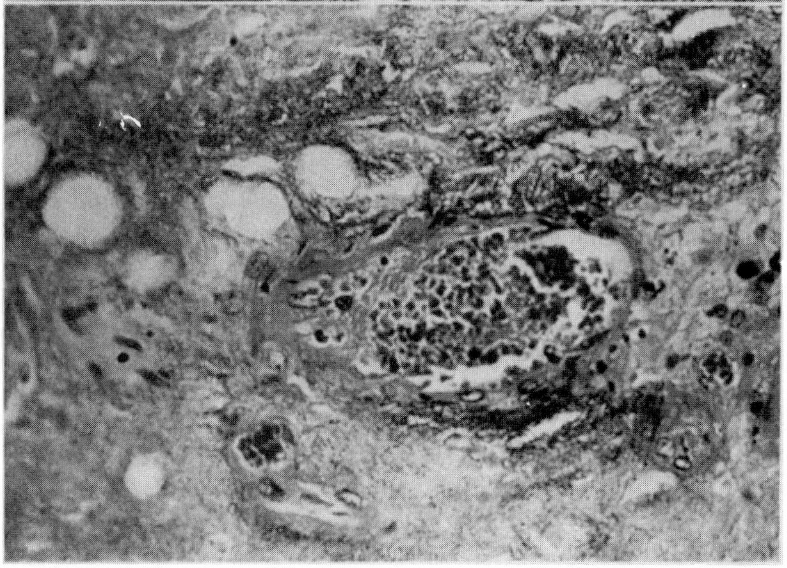
D

FIGURE 17-21 cont'd **C,** Photomicrograph of a biopsy specimen showing extensive invasion with dense concentration of bacillary organisms deep within unburned tissue at the 6 o'clock position—stage IIb. **D,** Photomicrograph of a biopsy specimen showing extensive invasion of unburned tissue with microvascular involvement. Note the dense dark-staining masses of organisms invading the vessel wall at the 12 o'clock and 6 o'clock positions in the center of the field—stage IIc.

are more likely to involve deep tissues, but the intensity of the inflammatory reaction often leads to formation of a thick inflammatory membrane that not only retards extension of the abscess but also limits the effectiveness of parenteral antibiotic therapy. Systemic effects of variable severity may also be elicited by staphylococcal toxins such as toxic shock syndrome toxin-1 (TSST-1).

Invasive burn wound infections, although rare, are most commonly caused by gram-negative bacteria, especially *Pseudomonas* organisms. Burn wound infections caused by gram-negative organisms spread rapidly in viable tissue and may disseminate both regionally and systemically via the lymphatic and vascular systems.[281] The cytotoxic metabolic products and enzymes (e.g., endotoxins, exotoxins, slime, vascular permeability factors, collagenase, elastase, lipase, nucleases, and hemolysins) liberated in variable amounts by gram-negative organisms facilitate spread of infection caused by those organisms and may even cause dysfunction of remote organs.[223] All tissue infected by gram-negative organisms should be excised as soon as the patient's general condition permits. An antibiotic-containing solution should be infused into the area of infection and the immediately surrounding subcutaneous tissues 6 hours before and immediately before excision to minimize the hematogenous dissemination of infecting bacteria and their metabolic products during excision.[175] A solution of 150 ml of saline containing 10 g of a broad-spectrum penicillin should be injected into the infected areas of the wound using a No. 20 spinal needle to keep the number of injection sites to a minimum. Subeschar antibiotic infusions administered twice a day are continued in patients whose general condition will not permit surgical debridement of the infected tissue. In a small number of patients with focal and even multifocal *Pseudomonas* organism burn wound infection of very limited extent, the subeschar infusion of antibiotics alone has arrested the septic process as indexed by containment of the infection and subsequent desiccation and spontaneous slough of the necrotic tissue.

After excision, if one is confident that all infected tissue has been removed, the wound should be covered with a biologic dressing or skin substitute to prevent desiccation of the exposed tissue and formation of a new eschar. If the adequacy of the excision is uncertain, 0.5% silver nitrate or 5% mafenide acetate soak dressings should be applied and the patient returned to the operating room 24 to 48 hours later, where further debridement is carried out if necessary. The wounds are closed by skin grafting only when it is certain that the wound infection has been controlled.

The mortality rate of patients with generalized burn wound infection, particularly those with systemic dissemination, is discouragingly high. The importance of diagnosing invasive wound infection early in the septic process (when it is amenable to control) has been demonstrated in a group of 19 extensively burned patients with histologically verified *Pseudomonas* burn wound infection treated by subeschar antibiotic infusion and, when possible, surgical excision of the infected tissue.[176] Nine of the 19 patients died with uncontrolled infection. In 10 patients the wound infection was controlled, but five of those patients later died from other causes. In the five surviving patients, all blood cultures obtained before excision of the infected tissue were negative, indicating that the diagnosis of invasive burn wound infection had been made before the septic process gained access to the general circulation.

Fungal Infections

Nonbacterial organisms may also cause invasive burn wound infections. *Candida* species infrequently cause invasive wound infections, but are the nonbacterial organisms that most frequently colonize burn wounds.[36] The frequency of recovery of *Candida* species increases as the extent of the burn increases. Although the topical application of antifungal agents such as clotrimazole may clear a burn wound of *Candida* organisms, such treatment does not appear to alter patient outcome. *Aspergillus* species are the filamentous fungi that most often cause burn wound infections and are most frequently recovered from burn wound biopsies[32] (Table 17-14 and Figure 17-22). The infections caused by those organisms, characteristically localized and superficial to the investing fascia, can in most instances be adequately treated by local excision.[224]

Phycomycotic burn wound infections occur most commonly in the presence of acidosis, such as occurs in uncontrolled diabetes mellitus.[89] Infections caused by the *Phycomycetes* organisms, which have a propensity to

TABLE 17-14 YEAST AND FUNGI RECOVERED FROM BURN WOUND BIOPSIES (1990-1993)

ORGANISM	NUMBER OF PATIENTS WITH POSITIVE BIOPSY CULTURE	NUMBER OF ISOLATES
Yeasts	35	79
Aspergillus sp.	50	185
Cladosporium sp.	27	29
Fusarium sp.	14	20
Penicillium sp.	12	14
Alternaria sp.	7	9
Phycomycetes (*Mucor* sp.)	2	3
Acremonium sp.	2	2
Other	74	224

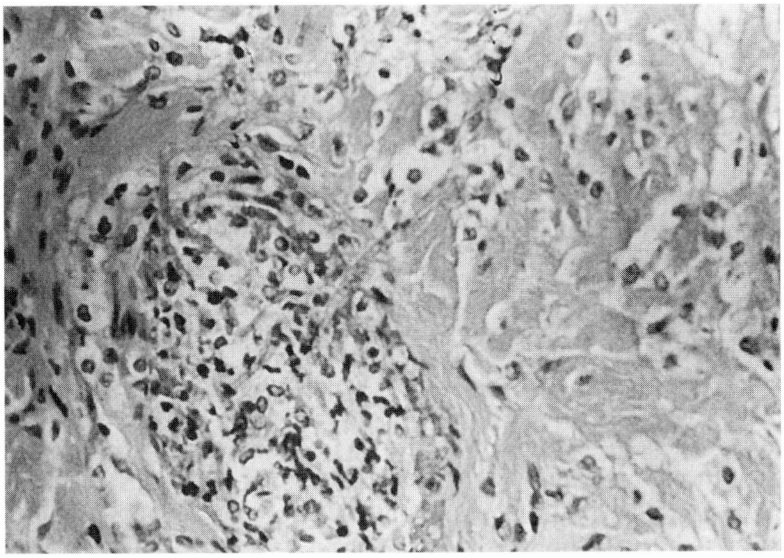

FIGURE 17-22 Photomicrograph of a wound biopsy specimen from a patient with invasive fungal burn-wound infection. Note the inflammatory reaction and the microvascular penetration by *Aspergillus* species.

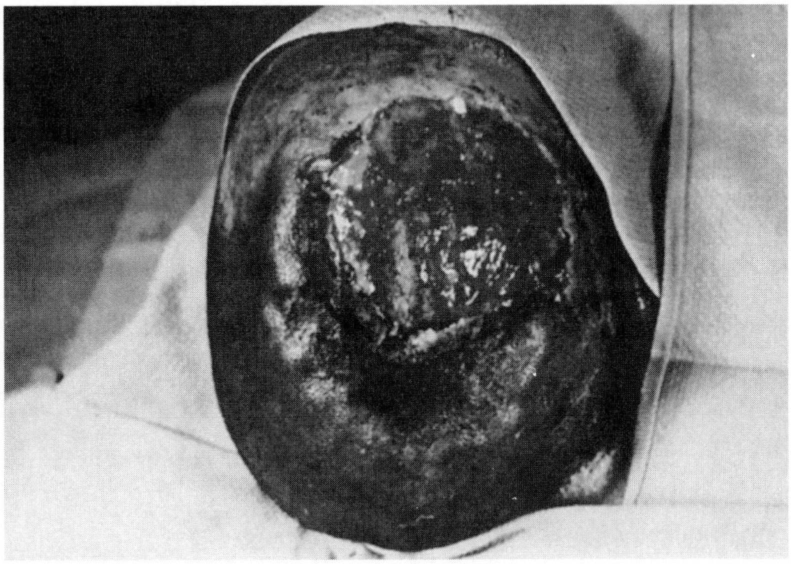

FIGURE 17-23 Rapid centrifugal expansion of ischemic necrosis is characteristic of phycomycotic burn-wound infection. The extent of the invasion of the microorganisms along the galea is indexed by the ridge of edema in the scalp peripheral to the area of ischemic change.

invade the microvasculature, are characterized by rapid centrifugal spread of ischemic necrosis and extension along and across fascial planes (Figure 17-23). Radical excision is required to control phycomycotic wound infection, and amputation may even be necessary to encompass all infected tissue on a limb.[225] Systemic antifungal therapy consisting of amphotericin B in combination with 5-fluorocytosine is indicated in patients with evidence of progressive local extension, blood cultures positive for fungi, or evidence of systemic dissemination of fungal infection. Currently available clinical data provide little support for the use of fluconozole in this type of patient.

Viral Infections

Viral burn wound infections are most frequently caused by herpes simplex virus.[95] These infections most commonly present as vesicles in healing or recently healed partial-thickness burns, particularly those of the nasolabial area[134] (Figure 17-24). Microscopic examination of a lesion biopsy or lesion scrapings is the most reliable means of diagnosing cutaneous viral infections in the burn patient (Figure 17-25). The vesicular lesions are easily ruptured and readily colonized by bacteria from adjacent burn wounds, which may obscure the light microscopic findings characteristic of hepatic infection. Electron microscopic examination of the biopsy material may then be necessary to identify intracellular virions.

Specific treatment is not required for cutaneous herpes simplex infections. Systemic herpetic infections involving the liver, spleen, bone marrow, and adrenals have been reported in burn patients, as have infections involving the lower respiratory tract.[200] Adenine arabinoside, acyclovir, or gangcyclovir given parenterally have all been recommended for such patients but the effectiveness of those agents is unverified.

BURN WOUND EXCISION

Timing of Excision

Once the burn depth is determined to be deep partial-thickness or full-thickness, wound excision (and closure) should be initiated. The first surgical procedure should occur once the patient has stabilized, resuscitation is complete, and fluid mobilization is in progress. Burn wound sepsis at any time requires immediate surgical excision of the infected wound. Associated complications, such as inhalation injury and respiratory failure, should not delay excisional therapy, particularly in patients with massive or deteriorating burns. Because the burn is the underlying cause for the exaggerated physiologic response and concomitant clinical derangements after injury, most associated complications will not resolve until the eschar is removed and the wound closed.

Total excision of a large burn in an adult patient in a single procedure is associated with massive blood loss and no improvement in survival.[44,120] Although early total excision has been shown to abrogate the hypermetabolic response in a rodent model, partial excision and wound closure does not effectively reduce the hyper-

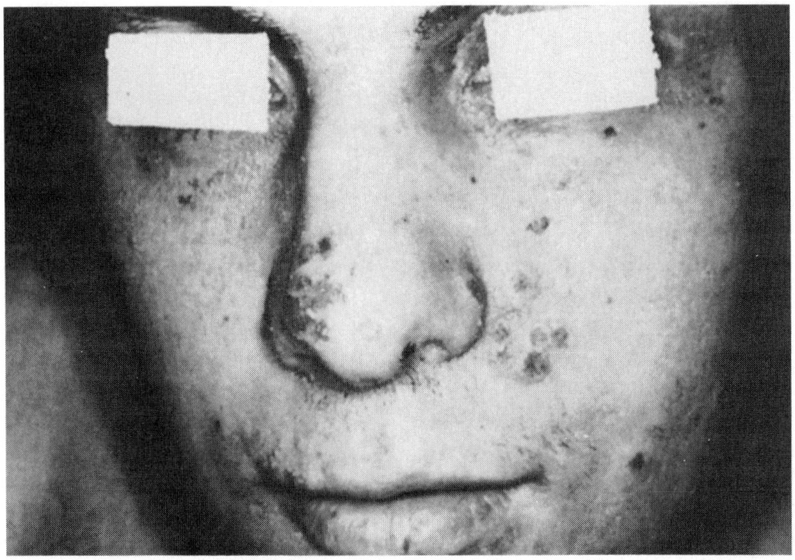

FIGURE 17-24 The rounded lesions in the recently healed superficial partial-thickness burns in the nasolabial area of this patient are characteristic of herpetic burn-wound infection. Note the typical crusting of the base of the ruptured vesicles.

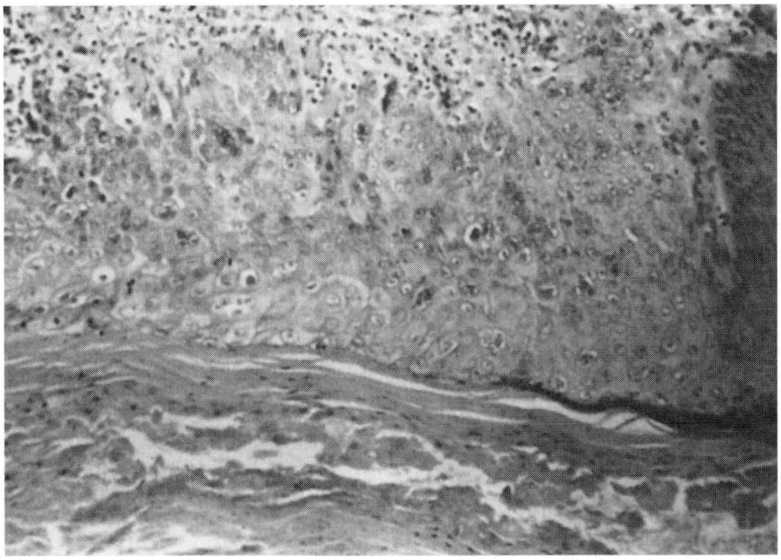

FIGURE 17-25 Photomicrograph of a burn-wound biopsy specimen showing the type A Cowdry bodies pathognomonic of herpes simplex virus infection.

metabolic state.[75,141] Length of stay may be reduced with early excision of small burns (less than 10% of body surface area), but this advantage in patients with larger burns has not been established. In patients with uninfected wounds, the extent of each surgical excision is limited to 20% of the total body surface, blood loss equivalent to the patient's blood volume, or 2 hours of operative time, whichever occurs first. However, if the wound is invaded, all of the infected burn must be excised if the patient is to survive. In such situations, more extensive excisions will be necessary. With the limited source of autograft in patients with large burns, the use of excisional therapy requires ready availability of effective substitute biologic dressings to close the open wound. The particular method of excision is determined by the depth of injury and the stability of the patient.

Tangential Excision

Tangential excision is best used for burns that are deep dermal in depth or extend into the superficial portions of the subcutaneous fat.[40,129,132] Using a guarded dermatome, burn eschar is serially excised down to the level of viable tissue represented by brisk capillary bleeding (deep dermal burn) or glistening, bright yellow subcutaneous fat (full-thickness burn). Blood loss is large, especially in wounds excised more than 1 week after injury. Often the burn wound varies in depth, and a major advantage of tangential excision is the maximal salvage of uninjured tissue. After hemostasis is achieved, the excised wound should be covered with a biologic dressing, preferably autograft. Moistened gauze dressings can be used to protect temporarily the newly excised wound bed, but closure with a viable biologic dressing should be carried out within 24 to 48 hours to prevent neoeschar formation over the excised site. Graft take in adequately excised wounds is highly successful. Following tangential excision, if the viability or bacterial density of the underlying tissue is uncertain, the wound should be excised further to the level of the investing fascia.

Excision to Fascia

Removal of the burn at the level of the investing fascia is indicated for deep third-degree burns characterized by a charred, rigid eschar and thrombosed vessels, and for any deteriorating burn with which retention of infected tissue is a possibility. The main advantages of this technique are the rapidity with which it can be completed and the relatively small loss of blood compared to the more commonly used technique of tangential excision. Operative bleeding occurs from large vessels perforating the muscular fascia into the subcutaneous tissue. These vessels are easily visualized and secured before division. If the burn wound is infected (as indicated by preoperative biopsy), it should be closed temporarily with cutaneous allografts. An uninfected wound bed should be covered by cutaneous autografts, which take readily on healthy fascia. The step-off defects and loss of subcutaneous fat mass following fascial excision cause marked cosmetic deformity in the first weeks after surgery; however, these defects are much less apparent after 1 year.

BURN WOUND CLOSURE

A full-thickness burn wound can be closed by split-thickness skin grafting after surgical removal of all nonviable tissue. The clinical assessment of the readiness of a wound for closure is generally sufficient, but if any doubt exists, laboratory confirmation of the clinical assessment is provided by the presence of fewer than 10^5 organisms per gram of tissue in a biopsy obtained from the wound bed.[253] Uniform adherence of a biologic dressing to the burn wound indicates that an excellent take of autograft skin will occur.

Closure of as much area of the burn wound as possible by grafting broad planar areas of the body surface to reduce the level of physiologic stress and the risk of infection takes precedence in patients with extensive burns. In patients with burns of less than 50% of the total body surface, early coverage of functionally important areas (e.g., hands, feet, and joints) takes priority. In patients with extensive burns, thin split-thickness skin grafts should be used to ensure optimal take and permit early reharvest of available donor sites, whereas in patients with limited burns, thicker split-thickness skin grafts can be used to optimize functional and cosmetic results. In patients with extensive burns, the use of mesh autografts, which permit up to a ninefold expansion of a skin graft, partially overcomes the shortage of available donor sites.[79]

The length of time required for epithelization of the interstices of sixfold-expanded or ninefold-expanded mesh grafts is so long that such grafts are seldom used; a threefold or fourfold expansion is most commonly used (Figure 17-26). To prevent desiccation of the wound bed exposed in the interstices of a mesh graft, occlusive dressings are applied until the interstices are closed by epithelial spread. Widely expanded autograft may also be covered by allograft skin as a means of preventing desiccation. The allograft will separate from the wound when epithelization is complete. Finally, some investigators have suggested that sheets of allogenic or autologous cultured keratinocytes placed over widely expanded autografts will hasten wound closure.

Biologic Dressings

A biologic dressing can be used for temporary coverage of a burn wound for which cutaneous autografts are not available. Viable cutaneous allograft that derives a blood supply from the underlying wound bed is the most frequently used and effective biologic dressing[239] (Figure

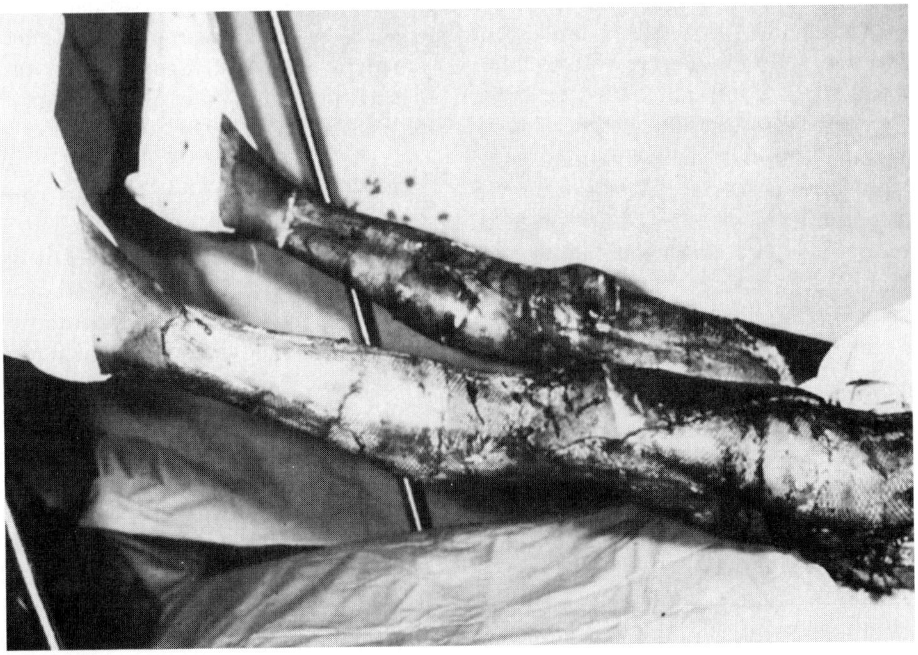

FIGURE 17-26 The investing fascia exposed by scalpel excision of the full-thickness burns of the legs of this patient has been covered with meshed autografts expanded in a 3 : 1 ratio. Note the blood-stained, dark-appearing fine mesh gauze used to dress the skin graft donor site on the anterior aspect of the left thigh.

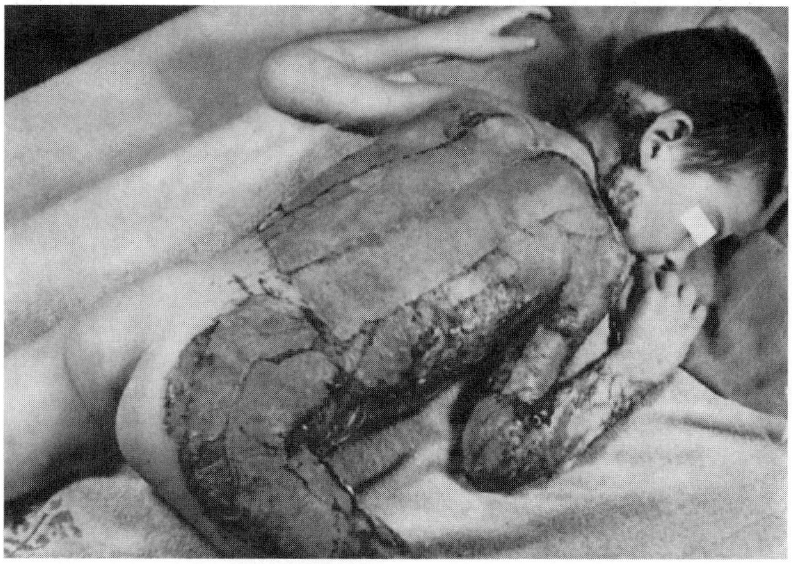

FIGURE 17-27 Allograft skin has been used to provide temporary coverage of the full-thickness burns of the posterior trunk and posterolateral aspect of the right thigh of this patient. The grafts are securely adherent throughout and well vascularized, indicating readiness of the wound for autografting.

17-27). Xenograft skin and amnion, less effective biologic dressings, do not derive a blood supply from the host and are attached to the wound bed by ingrowth of granulation tissue.[62,272] The application of a biologic dressing to a burn wound limits the growth and proliferation of the bacteria present on the wound surface, prevents wound desiccation, and reduces evaporative water and heat loss from the wound. Biologic dressings also decrease exudative protein and red cell loss from the wound surface, reduce wound pain, facilitate the motion of involved joints, and promote granulation tissue angiogenesis[92] (see box below).

The application of biologic dressings has been reported to accelerate the healing of both superficial and deep partial-thickness burns and improve the quality of healing of superficial partial-thickness burns, as indicated by less wound edema and the more orderly regeneration of collagen.[179] Biologic dressings have also been used to effect debridement of residual nonviable tissue after excision or eschar separation, provide immediate coverage of viable tissue after burn wound excision, and protect granulation tissue between repeated harvesting of cutaneous autografts in patients with extensive burns (Figure 17-28). As previously noted, a biologic dressing can also be used as test material to determine the readiness of a burn wound for autografting.

BENEFICIAL EFFECTS OF BIOLOGIC DRESSINGS

Reduction of evaporative water and heat loss
Prevention of wound desiccation
Protection of exposed tendons, vessels, and nerves
Promotion of granulation tissue angiogenesis
Limitation of bacterial growth and proliferation
Reduction of exudative protein loss
Reduction of red blood cell loss from wound
Reduction of wound pain
Facilitation of movement of involved tissues

Skin Substitutes

Skin substitutes have been developed to surmount the limitations of biologic dressings, which include possible disease transmission, complex storage requirements, finite shelf life, and the difficulty of matching supply with demand. All unilamellar membranes have been ineffective as skin substitutes, and a bilaminate structure mimicking the morphologic design of skin appears necessary for a membrane to function effectively as a skin substitute.[235] The dermal analog, or inner layer, should contain pores of sufficient size to permit biologic union by the ingrowth of fibrovascular tissue, and the epidermal analog, or outer layer, should have pores that permit passage of water vapor but are sufficiently small to prevent microbial invasion. Other desirable properties of a skin substitute include tissue compatibility, absence of anti-

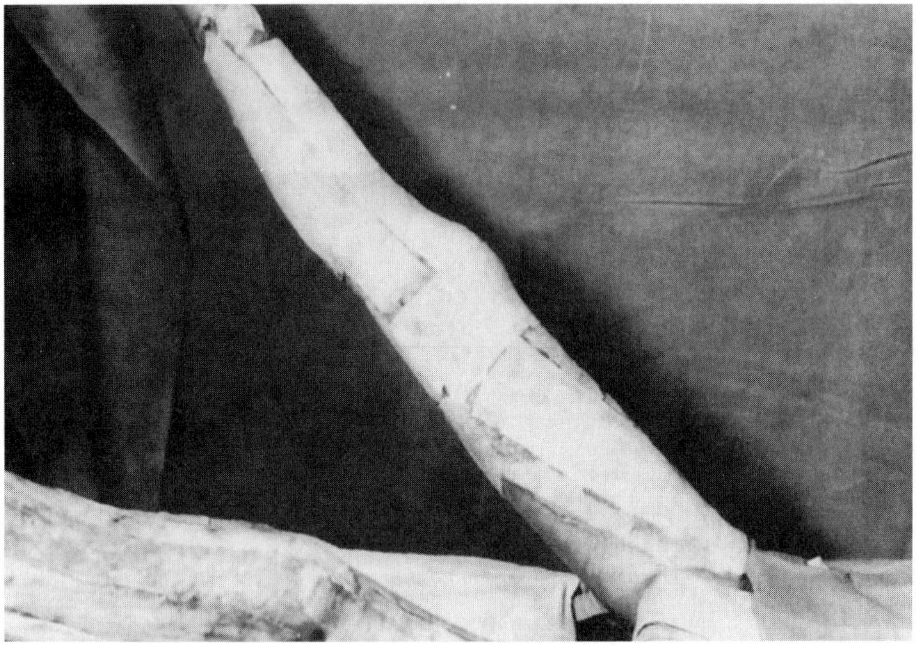

FIGURE 17-28 A paucity of donor sites in this patient necessitated the use of porcine cutaneous xenografts to cover the leg burns until previously used donor sites could be reharvested.

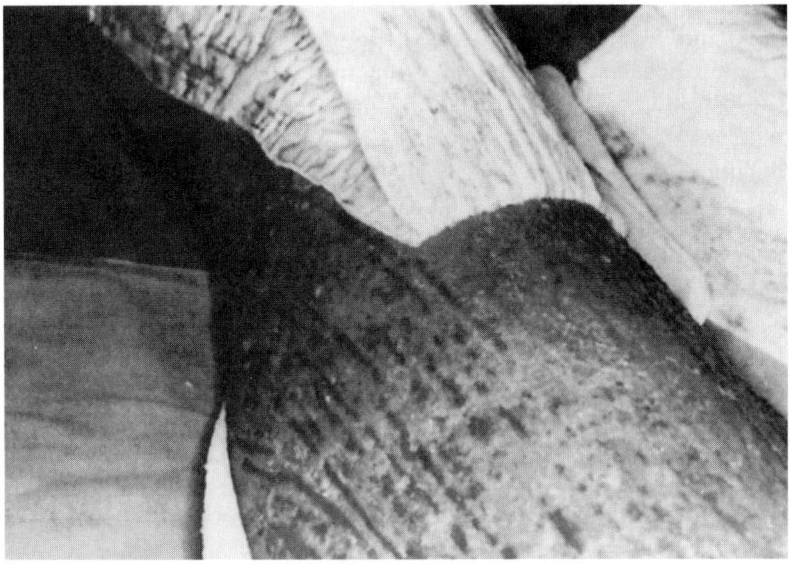

FIGURE 17-29 A totally synthetic bilaminate skin substitute used as a temporary wound cover in a patient with limited donor sites is removed before grafting. Note the healthy granulation tissue covering the wound and the absence of membrane fragment retention in the wound bed.

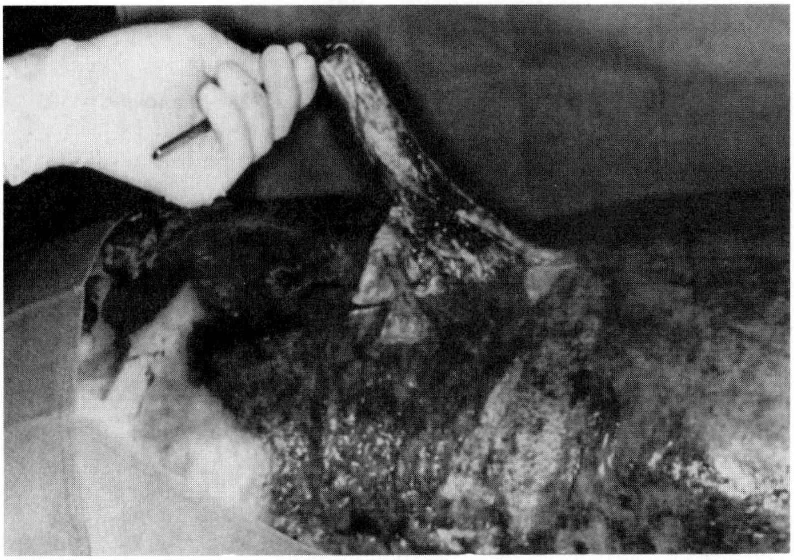

FIGURE 17-30 A bilaminate skin substitute composed of a collagen gel dermal analog and a Silastic epidermal analog has been used to cover the wounds on the back of this patient after excision of the burn tissue. The membrane is removed as shown at the time of autografting. Note that the wound bed is clearly visible through the intact membrane on the upper back. Note also the tensile strength and integrity of the portion of the membrane being removed and the excellent appearance of the wound bed exposed by removal of the membrane.

genicity and toxicity, sufficient elasticity and drapeability to permit close apposition and conformity to minute irregularities of the wound surface, sufficient tensile strength to resist linear and sheer stress, low cost, minimum of storage requirements, and an indefinite shelf life (Figure 17-29). None of the presently available skin substitutes satisfy all of these requirements.

Several collagen-based bilaminate temporary skin substitutes have been used clinically. In terms of submembrane formation of granulation tissue, submembrane suppuration, wound adherence, conformation to the wound surface, and membrane pliability, Biobrane, which consists of a collagen gel dermal analog and a Silastic epidermal analog, is indistinguishable from porcine cutaneous xenograft when applied to a freshly excised burn wound[253] (Figure 17-30).

Several skin substitutes are being developed as permanent dermal analogs to be used after full-thickness excision. One such substitute, consisting of a dermal analog of collagen enriched with chrondroitin 6 sulfate and a Silastic epidermal analog, has been developed by Burke and associates.[39] When granulation tissue ingrowth has produced adequate vascularization of the dermal analog of that skin substitute, the Silastic membrane is removed and the wound closed by direct application of a thin split-thickness skin graft to the underlying vascularized collagen of the dermal analog. The exogenous collagen is apparently gradually replaced by host tissue. A multicenter trial using this material was published in 1988.[115] The authors reported effective immediate closure of the burn wound in some patients. Delayed vascularization, problems with conformability, and submembrane suppuration led to failure of the product in other patients. Currently this material has not been released for general clinical use. Other investigators have developed a living tissue analog that is composed of human neonatal fibroblasts, which are cultivated on a polygalactin acid vicryl mesh to function as a dermal replacement. Such products have undergone limited clinical trials with variable success.

Culture-Derived Tissue

Epidermal sheets produced by the culture of autogenous or allogeneic keratinocytes have also been used in lieu of split-thickness skin grafts to close wounds after excision of burned tissue.[98,159] The initial enthusiasm surrounding the ability to achieve geometric expansion of a 2 × 2 cm skin biopsy to 1 to 2 m^2 of confluent cultured epithelial sheets has been replaced by guarded optimism. Anecdotal reports of isolated patient success led to larger, more closely scrutinized series. Our own trial in 16 patients in whom cultured autologous keratinocytes were applied to an average of 15.7% of the body surface revealed an overall 47% engraftment rate.[256] However, successful engraftment was considerably less in patients with burns greater than 70% total body surface area (TBSA) (30% engraftment) and those in whom burn wound excision had been at the level of the fascia (32.5% engraftment). Thus the technique is least successful in those patients who might benefit the most. Of equal concern is the lack of long-term durability in those patients with successful engraftment.[78] The 3 to 4 weeks required for the culture growth of epidermal sheets, the susceptibility of such tissue to microbial lysis, the tissue's lack of resistance to minor trauma, and the late occurrence of contraction and scar formation at present limit the clinical usefulness of autogenous epidermal sheets. Development of techniques to shorten the time required for culture growth and the development of an artificial dermis would significantly increase the usefulness of such culture-derived material. Several groups are currently working on composite skin replacements which use cultured human keratinocytes with a dermal matrix that has been seeded with human fibroblasts.[64]

Treatment of Split-Thickness Skin Graft Donor Sites

The time required for the healing of split-thickness skin graft donor sites is directly related to the thickness of the skin graft that has been harvested. Topical antimicrobial agents need not be applied to donor sites, and fine mesh gauze is the simplest, most inexpensive donor site dressing. The fine mesh gauze should be applied and trimmed to conform to the donor site immediately after graft harvest. Hemostasis can be achieved by the prompt application of warm saline-soaked laparotomy pads, which are removed at the completion of the operation. The donor sites should then be exposed to radiant heat until they dry. If the donor sites are thereafter kept clean and dry, the fine mesh gauze will separate as reepithelialization of the donor site occurs.

In areas where the skin surface moves with body motion, an inelastic fine mesh gauze dressing may cause discomfort. Use of donor site dressings possessing elasticity may reduce such local discomfort. Application of a bilaminate membrane composed of an outer layer of polyurethane foam and an inner layer of hydrocolloid polymer complex to split-thickness skin graft donor sites has been reported to decrease donor site pain and accelerate healing of the underlying donor site.[251] Acceleration of skin graft donor site healing is desirable in patients with extensive burns in whom repeated use of limited donor sites is required, but the cost of the necessarily frequent replacement of the membrane during the first 24 to 48 hours following graft harvest is a detracting feature of such treatment. Other synthetic biologic dressings may achieve the same results but with considerable cost compared to fine mesh gauze.

In patients with extensive burns, the scalp is an excellent donor site that customarily heals rapidly without hypertrophic scar formation, although allopecia may be a problem, especially in young children.[279] Donor sites on the medial aspect of the thighs and the medial aspect of the upper arms should be avoided if possible because the difficulty in drying such donor sites increases the risk of maceration and infection. If a donor site should become infected, the donor site dressing should be removed after application of warm saline soaks, after which the donor site should be treated as any other partial-thickness wound.

Pharmacologic treatment of donor sites with various growth factors has been relatively unrewarding. Brown and colleagues[34] reported an open label trial of topical epidermal growth factor (EGF) administration in elderly patients requiring split-thickness skin grafting. Patient donor sites were treated with silver sulfadiazine or silver sulfadiazine containing EGF. The donor sites receiving EGF healed on average 1.5 days faster than the controls, a difference which was statistically significant but of questionable clinical importance. Other investigators have failed to show that EGF therapy is beneficial. The successful application of biologic mediators to stimulate wound healing will require a more thorough understanding of the regulatory events involved in normal wound healing.

TREATMENT OF BURNS OF SPECIAL AREAS

Ears

Following burns to the ears, better cosmetic and functional results are obtained by delaying surgical therapy to obtain as much spontaneous healing as possible. Early excision sacrifices viable tissue at the margins of the injury and results in increased deformity. When infection occurs, it involves primarily the auricular cartilage and presents with edema and painful swelling. Because *P. aeruginosa* is nearly always the etiologic organism, mafenide acetate, with its unique ability to penetrate deep tissues, is the agent of choice for preventing auricular chondritis after burn injury. Even when other topical agents are being used for burns in other locations, topical mafenide is continuously applied until the ear has healed completely. If localized chondritis develops the focus of infection should be unroofed, all necrotic cartilage excised, and the wound loosely packed open. The wound is closed when control of the infection is certain. If extensive chondritis develops, the overlying skin is bivalved in the longitudinal plane of the ear and infected cartilage removed.[83] The wound flaps are packed open with gauze until all evidence of infection is resolved. At that time, the two skin remnants are allowed to adhere and heal. All viable skin should be retained and can be used in later reconstruction with prosthetic inserts.

Eyelids

The unique anatomy and function of the eyelids make them particularly susceptible to major complications. Eyelid skin is redundant and loosely attached to underlying conjunctiva and tarsal plate, and healing burns in this location often lead to marked contracture and ectropion formation. As the lid surface shortens, the cornea becomes increasingly exposed and susceptible to injury. Initially, the eye surface is protected by Bell's phenomenon, in which the globe spontaneously rotates upward and behind the shortened lid when the patient sleeps. Operative correction of the ectropion is indicated when conjunctivitis, keratitis, or corneal ulceration develops.[13] The release incision is placed at the lid margin just behind the lashes and is carried down to the tarsal plate. The resulting defect is closed with a split-thickness skin graft for a large defect; a full-thickness skin graft can be used in more limited releases. Secretions from eyes with corneal defects should be cultured. Ophthalmic ointment containing an antibiotic active against both gram-positive and gram-negative species, including *Pseudomonas,* is applied until the corneal injury has healed.[181]

Bone

Fractures and direct thermal injury to bone are the major skeletal complications in burned patients. Plaster casting as a method of immobilization prevents the use of topical antimicrobial chemotherapy on burns overlying sites of fracture, leading to an increased risk of infection. Traditional management relied on skeletal traction in an effort to reduce the risk of orthopedic hardware infection. Use of effective topical chemotherapy and early burn wound excision that reduces the bacterial density of the wound has altered the current treatment of long bone fractures in thermally injured patients. Operative intervention to include the use of external and internal fixation can be used safely when tailored to the specific needs of individual patients. Such treatment should allow earlier mobilization of the patient and hopefully decrease pulmonary complications.

Direct heat injury to the periosteum and bone often is not evident until the overlying damaged skin has sloughed or is excised. Once all nonviable tissue has been removed to the level of the cortex, two options are available for wound closure. If local soft tissue flaps are available, they may be rotated to close the defect even if the cortex is nonviable. In patients with smaller burns, in whom local tissue is not available for transfer, a microvascular free flap is another alternative. In patients with extensive burns, or those in which no tissue is available for transfer, the exposed cortical bone should be removed with an osteotome or by a rotary burr until viable bone is encountered.[14] The debrided bone is then treated with serial dressing changes until a thick bed of granulation tissue forms. A split-thickness skin graft is placed on the granulation tissue, closing the wound. Thermal injury to the skull is caused most commonly by electrical injuries. Necrotic calvarium is removed by a rotary burr in much the same fashion as described above. Decortication is carried out in the area of deepest injury to a level of bleeding cancellous bone. The peripheral areas of necrosis are subsequently encompassed in the debridement until the necrotic bone has been removed. If the inner table is nonviable, debridement is deepened until the dura identified by its surface vessels can be visualized. A layer of inner table bone, so thin that it can be indented with an instrument, is left over the dura to prevent desiccation until a layer of granulation tissue forms. The wound is temporarily covered by allograft until it is ready for closure with autograft. Full-thickness defects of the skull are repaired electively with bone grafts during convalescence.

METABOLIC CHANGES IN NUTRITIONAL SUPPORT

The metabolic response to severe injury characteristically manifests as a biphasic reaction.[66] The ebb phase immediately follows injury and is characterized by circulatory instability and poor tissue perfusion. With successful resuscitation, the ebb phase gives way to the flow phase, which is characterized by increased total body blood flow and metabolic activity. Although major trauma and infection can cause substantial elevations of metabolic expenditure, large thermal injuries cause the greatest degree of hypermetabolism, which may approach twice resting levels and may exceed the limits of the injured patient's physiologic reserve[296] (Figure 17-31). The clinical manifestations of marked hypermetabolism are increased energy expenditure and erosion of body mass and must be compensated by intensive nutritional support. Provision of nutrients by enteral techniques is safest and most practical in the majority of burned patients, but complications associated with burn injury occasionally may preclude use of the gut and dictate reliance on parenteral techniques.

Postburn alterations in water and electrolyte requirements must be integrated into the planning of parenteral nutrition formulations; the increased water requirement actually may facilitate the administration of the in-

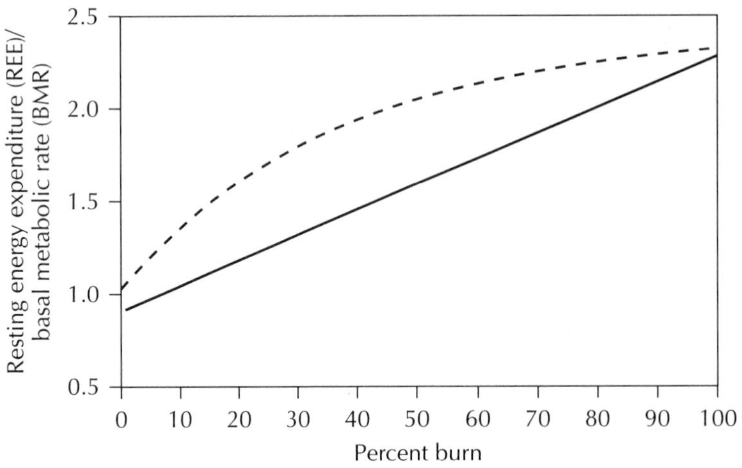

FIGURE 17-31 Metabolic response, as measured by indirect calorimetry, is related to extent of burn. The solid line represents the current linear relationship between REE and burn size. The dashed line depicts a curvilinear function generated from data collected on patients cared for in 1972 to 1973. Note the significant difference between the two curves.

creased nutrients required by burned patients. The use of parenteral nutrition is associated with a number of complications, most of which can be avoided with the use of rigorous monitoring protocols and experienced personnel.

Altered Thermoregulation

With the onset of postburn hypermetabolism, heat production is elevated and burned patients commonly exhibit elevated core and skin temperatures and higher core-to-skin heat transfer coefficients.[296] Central thermoregulation appears to be altered in burned patients, with an upward shift of the temperature of maximal comfort and least metabolic expenditure. The patients seem to be internally warm and not externally cold.[300] The hypermetabolic response can be decreased only moderately (about 10%) but not eliminated by external heating of burn patients to temperatures above thermoneutral level. Because thermal injury abolishes the water vapor barrier function of skin, evaporative water loss through the burn wound has been suggested as the cause of the hypermetabolic response.[254] However, Zawacki and colleagues[307] demonstrated that coverage of the burn wound with water-impermeable dressings under environmentally controlled conditions reduced evaporative water loss but produced only a modest reduction in metabolic rate. Although animal studies indicate that caloric intake increases metabolic response over that expected from the specific dynamic action of the nutrients, such findings have not been demonstrated in burned patients.

Only a small fraction of the hypermetabolic response can be ascribed to the endogenous specific dynamic action of accelerated protein breakdown.[110] The Q^{10} effect of hyperpyrexia accounts for only a modest fraction of postburn hypermetabolism, and the augmented heat production after injury is a consequence of an elevated metabolic state, not of increased thermoregulatory drives.[19] Current techniques of burn wound and general care appear to have reduced the magnitude of hypermetabolism evoked by a burn.[47]

Neurohormonal Changes

Catecholamines appear to be the major mediators of the hypermetabolic response to thermal injury. Adrenergic activity is related to the extent of burn injury and to total body blood flow and oxygen consumption. In burned patients adrenergic blockade of beta, but not of alpha, receptors blunts many of the manifestations of hypermetabolism, including the rises in metabolic rate, ventilation, pulse rate, and free fatty acids. Conversely, many of the metabolic changes in burned patients can be reproduced by administering beta-adrenergic agonists to normal subjects. Increased thyroid hormone activity does not appear to explain the higher metabolic response to patients with large burns. Although levels of total T^3 and T^4 may be depressed and of reverse T^3 elevated after injury, the unbound metabolically active forms ("free" T^3 and T^4) are normal in stable, hypermetabolically burned patients.[28] These free fractions fall only when the patient becomes septic and clinically deteriorates. That adequate thyroid function may be necessary to facilitate physiologic adaptation by the severely burned patient to postinjury metabolic demands is demonstrated by the apparent relationships among plasma levels of T^3, T^4, and catecholamines.[27] Burn injury alters adrenal activity by abolishing the normal diurnal variations in glucocorticoid concentration, but these hormones do not appear to influence metabolic activity directly and play only a permissive role in relation to the catecholamines.[287]

Substrate Availability after Injury

Nitrogen loss increases after thermal injury, and 80% to 90% of the nitrogen appears in the urine as urea, which may exceed 40 g/day in fed patients with severe burns.[295] Losses of nitrogen through the burn wound may account for 20% to 25% of total daily nitrogen loss.[275] Over a wide range of metabolic responses, varying from those of normal uninjured subjects to those of severely burned patients, body protein contributes a constant 15% to 20% of the energy required to meet metabolic needs.[86] Alterations in nitrogen economy in regional organ beds are reflected by changes in nitrogen transfer as amino acids. Following severe burns, peripheral amino acids, principally alanine and glutamine, are released in increased quantities into the circulation.[18] Alanine appears to act as a carrier of nitrogen from muscle to liver and is derived from the transamination of pyruvate from branched-chain amino acids.[203] Skeletal muscle is the primary source of the nitrogen excreted in the urine, and muscle proteolysis is reflected by the increased excretion of urea, creatinine, and 3-methylhistidine. This catabolic response is prolonged and persists even into the convalescent phase, although the switch from net protein catabolism to net protein anabolism occurs during convalescence despite an elevated rate of protein breakdown.[131]

The major sources of three-carbon precursors for new glucose production by the liver are the wound and skeletal muscle. The wound uses glucose principally by anaerobic glycolytic pathways, producing large amounts of lactate as an end product. The wound meets its high glucose requirements through high glucose delivery rates, which arise from the enhanced circulation to the wound. In the liver, lactate is extracted and is used for synthesis of glucose via the Cori cycle.[94] Concomitantly, alanine and other glycogenic amino acids also contribute to increased gluconeogenesis.[298] Increased ureagenesis parallels the rise in hepatic glucose output. Peripheral amino acids and wound lactate account for approximately one half to two thirds of the new glucose produced by the liver. The mild hyperglycemia characteristically observed in the hypermetabolic burned patient is a consequence of accelerated glucose flow arising from increased hepatic glucose production, not from decreased peripheral use.[298]

Because glucose obtained by gluconeogenic pathways is ultimately derived from protein stores, depletion of body protein during periods of starvation leads to energy deficits and malfunctioning of glucose-dependent energetic processes at the cellular level. Hepatic clearance of indocyanine green, an energy-dependent active transport process, is decreased in severely injured patients when energy that is normally supplied as glucose is replaced by an isocaloric glucose-free source.[166] Active transport mechanisms responsible for maintaining transmembrane ionic gradients in erythrocytes are deranged in catabolic, thermally injured patients.[69] The abnormal sodium-potassium gradients in red blood cells can be reversed by providing high levels of carbohydrate (glucose). Glucose-insulin solutions correct the "sick cell syndrome" in burned patients, who exhibit a prompt natriuresis and nonosmotic diuresis when metabolic requirements for energy are met by glucose.

Effect of Nutritional Support

In order to preserve body integrity following large burns, increased quantities of calories and nitrogen are necessary to match elevated energy expenditure and nitrogen losses. Although the intake of nitrogen alone partially preserves body protein and improves nitrogen balance after injury, the addition of nonprotein calories to the source of nitrogen further improves nitrogen balance. Following parenteral administration, nitrogen balance on a fixed amino acid formulation is determined by energy content; conversely, nitrogen content determines nitrogen balance on a fixed energy formulation.[165]

After injury, the individual effects of glucose and amino acids on nitrogen equilibrium appear to be mediated by at least two different mechanisms.[182] Amino acid administration accelerates synthesis of visceral and muscle protein without affecting the rate of protein breakdown. Glucose reduces whole-body protein catabolism and decreases the total amino acid pool, exerting little effect on protein synthesis. Both mechanisms improve nitrogen balance, and both glucose and nitrogen should be components of the nutritional regimen for severely injured, catabolic patients. Studies in animal models have suggested that the use of branched-chain amino acid solutions following major surgery and trauma leads to improved nitrogen conservation and decreased muscle catabolism, but the efficacy of these formulations in burned patients has never been demonstrated.

The role of fat as a source of nonprotein calories depends on the extent of injury and associated metabolic response. When hypercaloric diets not containing nitrogen are administered, carbohydrate is more effective than fat in sparing body protein when each calorie source is used alone. The reduction in nitrogen excretion by parenteral fat emulsions is accounted for by the glycerol content of the fat emulsions.[298] In patients with small burns, fat and carbohydrate are equally effective in maintaining nitrogen balance. However, in a study of severely hypermetabolic patients with large burns receiving constant doses of amino acid (11.7 g/m^2/day), carbohydrate decreased nitrogen excretion, but equicaloric doses of fat (as lipid emulsions) failed to exert a similar effect.[69] The small improvement in nitrogen balance was caused by the free glycerol present in the emulsion. The administration of insulin to this group of patients further decreased nitrogen loss. In contrast to the response of starvation-adapted patients, the signals that increase skeletal muscle proteolysis and gluconeogenesis in hypermetabolic patients override the ability to adapt to starvation by developing ketosis, decreasing nitrogen excretion, reducing energy expenditure, and using lipid substrates.[166]

Estimation of Nutrient Needs

Several methods are available for estimating calorie requirements. Many formulas, including the frequently used Harris-Benedict equation, predict basal energy expenditure on the basis of body size and age. The equations are then adjusted by a numeric factor related to size of injury to predict energy requirements in burned patients. Current formulas, including our own recently revised formula, predict caloric requirements that are significantly less than the formulas derived in the late 1970s and early 1980s.[47] This decrement in resting energy expenditure (REE) is hypothesized to be secondary to effective topical wound care and the increased use of burn wound excision, which decrease the bacterial load of the wound compared to techniques that relied on spontaneous wound separation.

The goal of nutritional support is to provide sufficient calories to meet energy expenditure and maintain lean body mass. Although supranormal caloric support is achievable in burned patients, overfeeding may be as deleterious as underfeeding. Excess carbohydrate administration may initiate lipogenesis leading to hepatic steatosis as well as increased CO_2 production, which may affect weaning from ventilatory support. Because the metabolic rate of a burn patient changes with time and can be influenced by infection and sepsis as well as the effects of surgery, indirect calorimetry should be used to measure metabolic rate serially to identify necessary adjustments in the level of metabolic support in patients with extensive burns. For difficult-to-manage patients, indirect calorimetry is helpful in determining actual energy requirements.

Nitrogen requirements of burned patients exceed those of uninjured subjects, but specific guidelines are less precise for nitrogen than for calories. The proportion of nitrogen to energy intake (nitrogen/calorie ratio, g/kcal) needed to achieve nitrogen equilibrium is lower in critically ill patients. Injured hypermetabolic patients demonstrate inefficient use of administered protein and have an effective nitrogen/calorie ratio between 1:100 and 1:200, with an optimum around 1:150. Higher concentrations of nitrogen in animal diets improve nitrogen balance but have no effect on body weight.[182] Further, higher nitrogen intake does not improve survival and may cause fatty infiltration of the liver following thermal injury. Thus a nitrogen/calorie ratio of 1:150 appears to be a satisfactory guideline for determining nitrogen requirements in hypermetabolic patients and can be conveniently estimated for patients with large burns as 15 g/m^2 of body surface area.

Vitamin requirements in critically ill hypermetabolic patients remain poorly defined. The fat-soluble vitamins (A, D, E, and K) are stored in fat deposits and are slowly depleted with parenteral feeding. The water-soluble vitamins (B complex and C) are not stored in appreciable amounts and are depleted rapidly. Care must be taken to ensure that all vitamins are supplemented. The dosage guidelines recommended by the Nutritional Advisory Group of the American Medical Association (NAG/AMA) are reasonable for burned patients unless symptoms of deficiency occur.[265] Ascorbic acid plays an essential role in wound repair, and plasma levels are frequently depressed in burned patients.[154] Therefore it seems prudent to supplement the NAG/AMA formulation with 250 to 500 mg of vitamin C daily. Larger doses may cause diarrhea and renal stone formation and will interfere with certain laboratory tests. Excessive doses of vitamins A and D produce toxic symptoms, and monitoring of serum levels is misleading if the concentrations of the vitamin carrier proteins are decreased, as commonly occurs in critically ill patients.

Even less is known about trace mineral requirements following thermal injury. Zinc is an important cofactor in wound repair, and zinc deficiency has been documented in burned patients. Periodic measurements of zinc, copper, manganese, and chromium levels provide the best guidelines for replacement dosages. Trace elements are present in varying concentrations as contaminants in parenteral amino acid solutions.

As discussed previously, fat appears to be an ineffective calorie source for the maintenance of nitrogen equilibrium and lean body mass in hypermetabolic patients with large burns. Patients with only moderate elevations of metabolic rate can use lipid calories more efficiently; however, such individuals usually tolerate enteral diets, and table food or defined formula diets contain all necessary fat nutrients. When fat is omitted from nutritional solutions for patients receiving total parenteral nutrition for prolonged periods, essential fatty acid deficiency may develop.[116] This deficiency manifests as dermatitis, hemolytic anemia, thrombocytopenia, impaired wound healing, loss of hair, and early death. Although no exact requirement is known, 2% to 4% of daily energy requirement should consist of linoleic acid.[250] A triene/tetraene ratio in tissue fats greater than 0.4 indicates essential fatty acid deficiency, but such determinations may not be clinically practical. The administration of 1 liter of the commercially available lipid emulsions twice a week will provide adequate replacement of essential fatty acids.

Administration of Nutrients

Whenever possible, nutrients should be administered by the gastrointestinal route; parenteral nutrition should be reserved only for those patients with an inoperative gut. In patients with smaller burns (less than 30% of the body surface) and no other complicating diseases, the gastrointestinal tract returns to functional status quickly after burn injury. When evidence of gut function such as the passage of stool or flatus is present, enteral feedings (either orally or by tube) can be instituted and quickly progressed to full requirements.

Spontaneous oral intake is the safest and best tolerated method of nutritional intake. This technique is quite successful in patients with smaller burns and no complicating diseases. However, most patients will eat little more than their usual level of intake before injury, and patients with larger thermal injuries and the accompanying high energy requirements rarely are able to meet caloric goals by oral intake. Such patients who do not meet nutritional requirements should have a narrow-caliber, soft feeding tube inserted into the distal duodenum or proximal jejunum to ensure adequate dietary intake.

Enteral feeding offers several advantages over parenteral feeding and is associated with a significantly lower complication rate. Enteral nutrients appear to maintain the integrity of the gastrointestinal tract by an as yet undefined trophic mechanism. An oral diet preserves gut mucosal mass and maintains digestive enzyme content, whereas parenteral feeding results in a decrease in mucosal cell turnover.[87] Other studies have verified that oral feeding stimulates the gut to elaborate trophic hormones, particularly gastrin. Enteral calories initiate greater insulin release when compared with parenteral nutrition, and insulin appears to promote anabolism.[121] Enteral feedings, when administered via a properly placed nasogastric tube may be safely continued even during operations. Although several studies have suggested a benefit to the use of enteral formulas enriched with glutamine, omega-3 fatty acids, RNA nucleotides, arginine, and fiber, convincing clinical data are lacking.

Total parenteral nutrition should be instituted when the gastrointestinal tract proves inadequate to supply caloric requirements. Prolonged postresuscitation ileus, overuse of narcotics, and constipation are frequent causes of failure of successful enteral alimentation. Hypertonic solutions are administered by infusion pumps beginning at relatively slow infusion rates (1 L/24 hr). Gradually, the infusion rate is increased to the maximal levels of fluid and energy requirements. The speed with which the infusion rate can be increased is determined by the patient's glucose tolerance. With each increment, small doses of insulin may be administered subcutaneously or added to the infusion to maintain normoglycemia. Later, as the patient's endogenous insulin production increases, exogenous insulin may be decreased or eliminated.

Monitoring Nutritional Status

Systematic monitoring protocols facilitate assessment of nutritional status and any metabolic derangements. The patient's nutrient and fluid needs must be reviewed daily and correlated with laboratory data. The best measures for assessing the adequacy of nutritional support in burned patients are body weight, nitrogen balance, and calorie counts. Tests of immunocompetence, although useful in chronically ill patients, have not yet been demonstrated to predict nutritional status in burned patients. The use of serum visceral protein levels as an index of nitrogen balance is of little benefit in thermally injured patients.[46] Standard anthropometric measurements such as triceps skinfold thickness, arm-muscle circumference, and creatinine/height index are valuable for patients with chronic diseases but often are unusable in burned patients who have extensive skin wounds and, frequently, amputations.

Change in body weight is the most easily quantified index of metabolic balance. The magnitude and duration of weight loss are related directly to the extent of burn injury. Weight loss is not obligatory and can be reversed with vigorous nutritional support. Rapid changes in weight almost always arise from alterations in body water balance. An increase in weight exceeding 0.4 kg/day in an adult indicates water accumulation. Comparison of intake and output records with weight changes allow accurate estimates of lean body mass alteration in most situations. Long-term trends are most useful.

Nitrogen balance studies reflect alterations in body protein stores. Nitrogen balance is the algebraic sum of daily intake and loss of nitrogen. Intake is easily quantified, but nitrogen loss is difficult to determine in burned patients because of the difficulty of measuring losses through the burn wound. Calorie counts are carried out by the dietitian and dietary technicians working with the nutrition support team. When calorie counts are combined with daily weight determinations and nitrogen

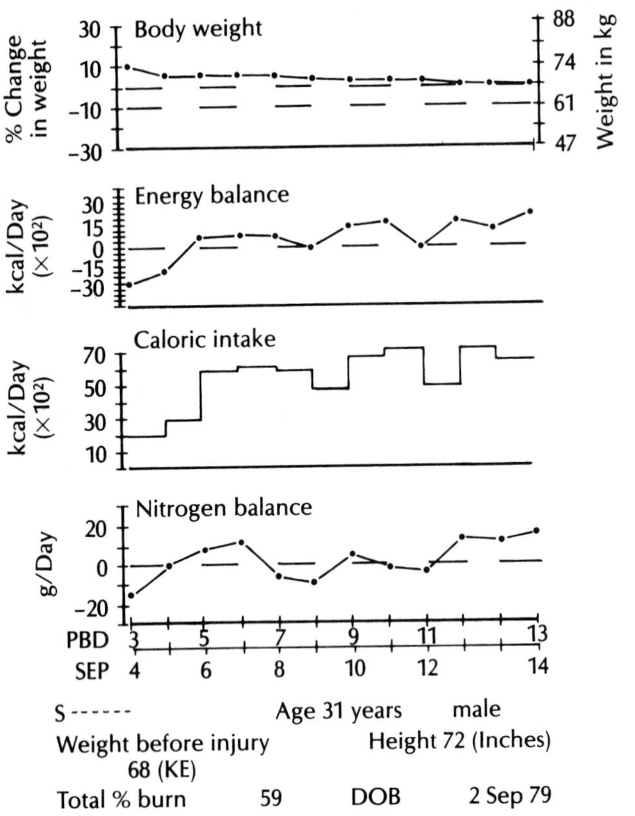

FIGURE 17-32 Computer graphic record of nutritional status in a patient with a 59% body surface burn. These records are posted by each patient's bed and promote staff awareness and patient compliance with nutritional support programs. The initial large weight gain, evident on day 4 after burn injury, was caused by initial fluid resuscitation; wound edema has been fully mobilized and excreted by day 10.

balance studies, the overall effectiveness of nutritional support in preserving or restoring body mass can be assessed on a continuous basis. Computer monitoring of nutritional support provides a means for accurate record-keeping and for quality control and evaluation of techniques and diets (Figure 17-32). The data files store information about each nutrient, laboratory data, patient condition, and associated complications.

Other Aspects of Nutritional Support

Metabolic expenditure can be minimized by blunting a variety of stressful stimuli. Thermally injured patients, particularly children, have difficulty maintaining body temperature in cold environments. Because of an apparent change in the hypothalamic set point, burned patients require higher ambient temperatures for comfort. The temperature of thermal neutrality in severely burned patients is 30° to 31°C (86° to 88° F), approximately 4°C higher than that in normal subjects.[297] Warming burned patients to this level decreases metabolic rate and corresponding energy requirements. Thermal blankets, radiation reflectors, and heat lamps may be required to maintain the patient's temperature above 37°C (98.6°F).

Pain accompanies wound manipulation and other care procedures. Such pain accentuates metabolic expenditure, and controlled administration of narcotics will reduce metabolic rate in such patients. Adequate analgesics and sedation should be provided so that the patient will have periods of uninterrupted rest.

Because hypovolemia, dehydration, and sepsis are potent stimuli of catecholamine secretion, appropriate volume replacement and antibiotic administration should be used as indicated. Systemic infection accentuates erosion of body mass, and additional calories must be supplied to maintain nitrogen balance at the same level obtained on lower caloric intake before infection.[298]

Pharmacologic attempts to limit hypermetabolism and catabolism and promote anabolism have thus far been disappointing. Human growth hormone administration has been shown to increase nitrogen retention when administered to thermally injured patients.[299] Limitations of growth hormone therapy include promotion of insulin resistance as well as salt and water retention.[105] In children this therapy decreases the time required for donor site wound healing and hospital stay, although no effect on catabolism was noted.[119] Part of the effect of growth hormone is thought to be mediated via hepatic production of insulin-like growth factor 1. Adult burn patients, when administered growth hormone, do not demonstrate a consistent IGF-1 response, and the clinical benefit noted in children has not been documented in the older age group.

Preliminary studies of direct IGF-1 infusion appear promising as a method to decrease catabolism.[49] Exogenous IGF-1 administration to thermally injured rodents decreased significantly the hypermetabolic response and promoted an increase in lean body mass.[278] Short-term IGF-1 administration to burned humans resulted in a decrease in protein oxidation but did not alter resting energy expenditure.[49] Pharmacologic promotion of anabolism has also been attempted by administration of β_2-adrenergic agonists in animal models of thermal injury with some success,[160] although human trials have not been undertaken.

Lack of activity promotes muscle wasting and atrophy. Vigorous physical therapy promotes preservation of muscle bulk, and supervised activity must be provided continuously on a daily basis to all patients requiring prolonged hospitalization. Skeletal traction and air-fluidized beds encourage immobility and loss of lean body mass. Most of these patients are usually capable of simple isometric exercises. Meticulous wound care and expeditious wound closure are the most effective measures of limiting the injury and its associated metabolic sequelae.

DIAGNOSIS AND TREATMENT OF COMPLICATIONS

Septic Complications

Infection remains the most frequent cause of morbidity and mortality in burn patients, even though the incidence of invasive burn wound sepsis has been significantly reduced by the use of topical antimicrobial therapy.[224] In general, the enhancement of infection control practices by single bed isolation and other measures also appears to have significantly reduced the incidence and severity of infection-related complications[171] (Table 17-15). This persistence of infection in sites other than the burn wound results from the aggregate effect of the polymicrobial flora colonizing burn wounds and the burn size-related global immunosuppression that predisposes the burn patient to infection. The use of topical burn wound chemotherapy has been associated not only with the emergence of pneumonia as the most common cause of life-threatening sepsis but also with a significant change in the type of pneumonia prevalent in burn patients.

Airborne pneumonia, or bronchopneumonia, has replaced hematogenous pneumonia as the prevalent form of pulmonary infection in burn patients.[244] The decrease in the occurrence of invasive burn wound infection as a result of effective topical chemotherapy has been associated with a decrease in hematogenous pneumonia. The emergence of bronchopneumonia as the predominant type of pulmonary infection also reflects the effect of improved ventilatory management of patients with inhalation injury, which reduces early mortality and permits the later development of infection in a severely damaged airway.

The diagnosis of pulmonary infection in burn patients is confounded by the hyperventilatory response to thermal injury and by the ventilatory effects of inhalation injury, therapeutic agents, and nutritional support. The pulmonary status of a burn patient must be monitored frequently, and changes in pulmonary function should be correlated with radiographic changes, changes in fluid balance, alterations in nutritional support, and the status of the burn wound.

Hematogenous pneumonia represents systemic dissemination of microorganisms from a remote primary focus of infection. The sudden appearance of a solitary nodular pulmonary infiltrate, which is characteristic of hematogenous pneumonia, should prompt a search for the primary source of infection, which is most commonly an infected burn wound, a focus of suppurative thrombophlebitis, peritonitis secondary to visceral perforation, or an inapparent soft tissue infection.[243] The diagnosis and treatment of bronchopneumonia and hematogenous pneumonia are presented in Chapter 10.

TABLE 17-15 CAUSES OF DEATH IN BURN PATIENTS (1987-1991)

PRINCIPAL CAUSE OF DEATH	NUMBER OF DEATHS (%)
Infection	39 (42)
Resuscitation failure	12 (13)
Cardiovascular disease	10 (11)
Inhalation injury	10 (11)
Neurologic disease	7 (7)
Other	15 (16)

Infections can occur in literally any organ or tissue in the immunosuppressed patient with extensive burns. Commonly encountered processes, discussed in greater detail in Chapter 10, include suppurative thrombophlebitis,[242] acute endocarditis,[21] suppurative sinusitis,[45] and prostatic abscesses. Life-threatening abscesses have also formed following lodgement of blood-borne organisms in the fracture hematomas of patients with associated long bone fractures. When diagnosed, such abscesses should be immediately drained and systemic antibiotic therapy initiated. If the septic process cannot be controlled by such means, amputation is necessary.

Septicemia

The significance of a positive blood culture depends on the patient's general condition and the presence of other signs of infection. If a positive blood culture is obtained from a patient whose general condition is inconsistent with sepsis and no specific source of infection is evident, treatment can be delayed while repeat blood cultures are obtained. If two successive blood cultures are positive for the same organism, and exogenous contamination (such as that caused en passant by sampling through the burn wound) can be excluded, specific systemic antibody therapy should be started even if the patient does not appear to be clinically septic. In critically ill burn patients with life-threatening complications and little effective host resistance, multiple organisms may be recovered from a single blood culture or from successive blood cultures.[173] Such findings should not be regarded as indicative of a technical error, and systemic administration of maximum doses of an antibiotic or antibiotics active against all of the recovered organisms should be initiated.

The impact of septicemia on the burn patient depends on the organism recovered.[133] A recent 24-year review of septicemia occurring in patients treated at a referral burn center has shown that gram-negative septicemia and candidemia were associated with a significant increase in burn-size related mortality.[162] Interestingly, gram-positive septicemia exerted no discernible effect on the expected mortality of burn patients treated at that institution.

Renal Failure

The use of large volumes of electrolyte-containing fluids to restore intravascular volume has nearly eliminated renal failure during the resuscitation phase of burn care. Oliguria during the first 24 postburn hours usually reflects inadequate fluid volume replacement and is treated by additional fluid administration.

Renal failure that occurs later in the postburn course is almost always a component of sepsis and multisystem organ failure. The use of nephrotoxic drugs, particularly the aminoglycoside antibiotics, may contribute to renal dysfunction. Toxicity can be minimized by frequent monitoring of plasma drug concentrations and adjusting dosages to provide maximum safe therapeutic levels. Subtherapeutic dosages of potentially nephrotoxic antibiotics or less toxic but less therapeutically effective agents inadequately treat the underlying septic process and accelerate the course of renal and other organ system failure. Maintenance of adequate intravascular volume, total body blood flow, and ventilation will minimize the incidence of renal failure. The detection and eradication of the primary septic process is of paramount importance. When renal failure does occur it is treated as in other patients. If dialysis is required the magnitude of hypermetabolism evoked by the burn typically renders peritoneal dialysis ineffective and mandates hemodialysis.

Gastrointestinal Complications

The digestive tract is a major target organ of the pathophysiologic response to burn injury. Complications associated with severe burns include stress ulceration of the stomach and duodenum (Curling's ulcer), acalculous cholecystitis, superior mesenteric artery syndrome, acute pancreatitis, nonocclusive ischemic enterocolitis, pseudoobstruction of the colon, and hepatic dysfunction.

Curling's ulcers present as a spectrum of lesions in the stomach and duodenum. Serial endoscopic examinations have shown that punctate hemorrhages and shallow mucosal erosions occur soon after burn injury in up to 90% of patients with burns exceeding 35% of body surface.[71] With current prophylactic measures, these lesions heal after successful resuscitation and initiation of enteral feedings.[72] The presence of gastric acid is required for the progression of the early erosions to more extensive ulcers, but concentrations of acid and gastrin often lie within the normal range in patients with active ulceration.[255] Controlled randomized trials of antacids and placebo have definitively demonstrated the beneficial effects of continuous gastric acid neutralization in preventing upper gastrointestinal hemorrhage and perforation of stress ulcers.[164]

Following admission, 30 ml of antacid is administered each hour through the nasogastric tube to maintain the gastric pH above 5. The dosage is increased to 60 ml/hr if gastric acidity persists below this level. Cimetidine is equally effective in preventing Curling's ulcers, and in patients who cannot tolerate antacids, administration of cimetidine, 400 mg intravenously every 4 hours, is an acceptable alternative to antacids.[149] Thrombocytopenia and alterations in mental status may be associated with the use of cimetidine therapy in burned patients and can be confused with the clinical presentation of sepsis.

In the rare patient who requires operative intervention for hemorrhage or perforation of Curling's ulcer, vagotomy and gastric resection has produced the best immediate and long-term survival rates.[234] Recent studies have suggested that acid-buffering therapy as a method for stress ulcer prophylaxis promotes bacterial overgrowth in the stomach.[285] It is hypothesized that the subclinical aspiration of colonized gastric contents, which occurs in almost all critically ill patients, then leads to nosocomial pneumonia. Nonacid-buffering prophylaxis using sucralfate has been promoted as a means to reduce the gastric bacterial overgrowth and thus reduce the incidence of nosocomial pneumonia. Although a recent study in burn patients demonstrated that such therapy was efficacious in terms of stress ulcer prophylaxis, there was no reduction in the incidence of gram-negative pneumonia, and the sucralfate patient group actually had a higher incidence of gram-positive bacterial pneumonia.[56]

Acute acalculous cholecystitis, although uncommon in burn patients, occurs as two distinct clinical syndromes. In one form, the gallbladder is infected by hematogenous seeding from a primary source in the septic patient, usually from the invaded burn wound.[198] The other form occurs in critically ill patients who have developed marked dehydration, ileus, or pancreatitis. The gallbladder and bile in this latter presentation are often sterile. Physical examination is difficult in these patients, who may be obtunded and have painful abdominal burn wounds. Jaundice and complaints of abdominal pain in conscious patients suggest acalculous cholecystitis, and such patients should be evaluated by ultrasonography and CT. Once the diagnosis is made, cholecystectomy is indicated.

Superior mesenteric artery syndrome may develop in burned patients who experience marked weight loss. The superior mesenteric artery obstructs the transverse portion of the duodenum, and oral alimentation becomes

the burned part is splinted in an antideformity position. In addition, almost continuous use of a splint may be necessary for rapidly contracting scars, particularly in children. Splints are extraordinarily useful for immobilizing a newly grafted burn wound until total adherence occurs. The splint is molded in the operating room to fit the grafted wound and its dressings. Three days later the dressings are changed and the splint reapplied. Successive daily changes continue for 2 to 3 more days.

Prevention and Treatment of Hypertrophic Scarring

Hypertrophic scar formation in burned patients can be minimized by timely resurfacing of the wound and by adequate excision of early scar tissue in wounds closed later during hospitalization. Scar hypertrophy is particularly severe in children and young adults and in deep dermal burns that are allowed to close spontaneously more than 2 weeks after injury. Hypertrophic scar may also occur on donor sites in thin-skinned patients, particularly if it was necessary to harvest that site on multiple occasions.

Burn scar hypertrophy follows a predictable natural course in the adult. Generally, healed burns are flat and pliable at the time of discharge. During the next 2 to 6 months, hypertrophy becomes pronounced and presents as raised, erythematous immature scar tissue. During the next 6 months, the thickened scar gradually thins out, loses its reddish coloration, and takes on the appearance of mature scar more closely resembling adjacent uninjured tissue. In children, this process may require 2 to 3 years. When possible, surgical reconstruction should not be carried out when the burn scar is immature; continuation of the remodeling process at this stage often obliterates the effect of the corrective procedure.

External pressure applied immediately after burn wound closure is widely used to reduce scar formation.[142] Although there is some controversy about the influence of pressure on the long-term course of burn scar maturation, clinical experience indicates that continuous application of pressure during the first months after injury, when such scars begin to enlarge rapidly, significantly reduces much of the bulk of the immature scar. Furthermore, cessation of therapy at this time results in marked raising of the scar tissue within days, and this process can be reversed if pressure therapy is reinstituted. The elastic pressure garments are tailored to the individual patient and must be replaced periodically as the garment loses its elasticity or the child grows. The garment must be worn at all times except when bathing. Additional pressure can be distributed to difficult-to-reach areas, such as joints, by custom-made foam inserts placed under the compression garments. The face is especially difficult to treat with elastic masks; rigid plastic masks molded from impressions of the patient's face are effective alternatives. The application of silicone gel sheets has been reported to exert similar preventive and ameliorative effects on postburn scarring.[262]

Burn Scar Carcinoma

Burn scar carcinoma, or Marjolin's ulcer, is a rare neoplasm that occurs in unstable scar of a full-thickness burn. Often the burn was originally allowed to heal by scar formation or was covered by a thin split-thickness autograft that only partially survived. The resulting areas of thin epithelium are quite susceptible to trauma and continually break down and heal. Eventually, a carcinoma occurs in these areas of intense epithelial activity. The latent period ranges from 1 to 75 years, with a mean of approximately 35 years.[9,100] Although basal cell carcinomas have occurred in old burn scars, they are exceedingly rare, and most of Marjolin's ulcers are squamous cell carcinomas. These tumors are highly invasive, and regional node metastases were present in 35% of 46 cases reported by Novick et al.[202]

Metastases are more frequent in primary tumors located on the extremities than in those on the trunk. All ulcerative lesions in burn scars should be biopsied. If no tumor is found, the ulcerated area with a 2 cm margin of skin is excised and the defect closed with a skin graft. If carcinoma is found, extirpation of the tumor must include all involved tissue as verified by histologic examinations of wound margins. In many cases of burn scar carcinoma on the extremities, amputation is necessary. Novick and associates[202] recommend prophylactic regional node dissection of burn scar carcinomas of the lower extremities because of the poor prognosis associated with metastases in such patients.

Psychosocial Support

Burned patients display a variety of psychologic reactions to their injury, including withdrawal, denial, regression, anxiety, and depression. Withdrawal and regression are especially evident in children, who will often refuse to acknowledge parents and will not cooperate with nutritional support or rehabilitation programs. A more pervasive disorder has been concretely defined in burned patients by Perry et al.[212]: the posttraumatic stress disorder. This disorder is characterized by recurrent and intrusive recollections of the initial injury, avoidance of circumstances that refresh memories of the event, loss of interest in daily activities, feelings of isolation, hyperalertness, memory impairment, and sleep disturbances.

Noncompliance with burn therapy is a serious outward manifestation of the patient's attempt to avoid recollections of the traumatic event. These authors dem-

Text continued on p. 714.

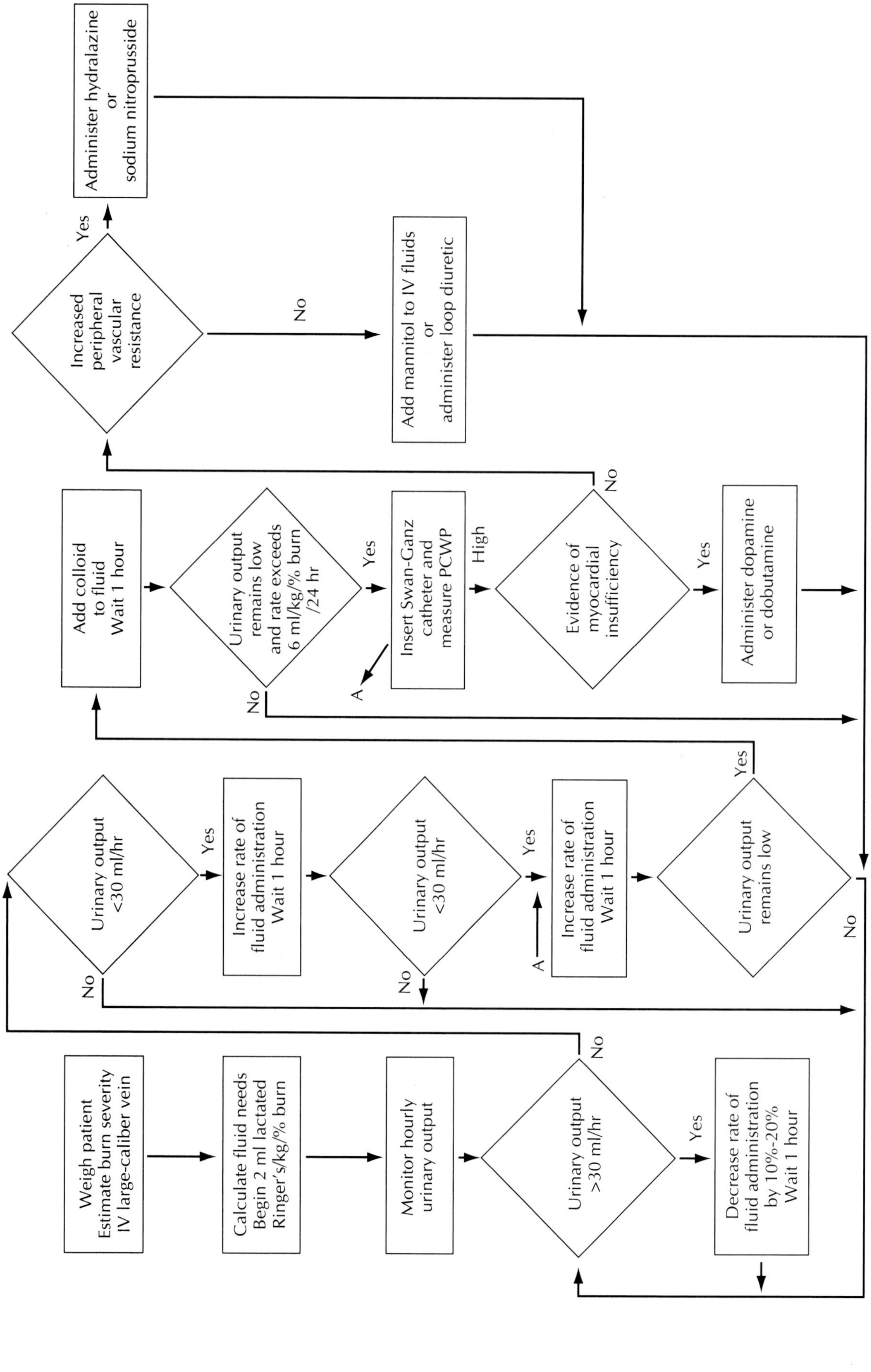

ALGORITHM I: FLUID THERAPY FOR THE FIRST 24 HOURS

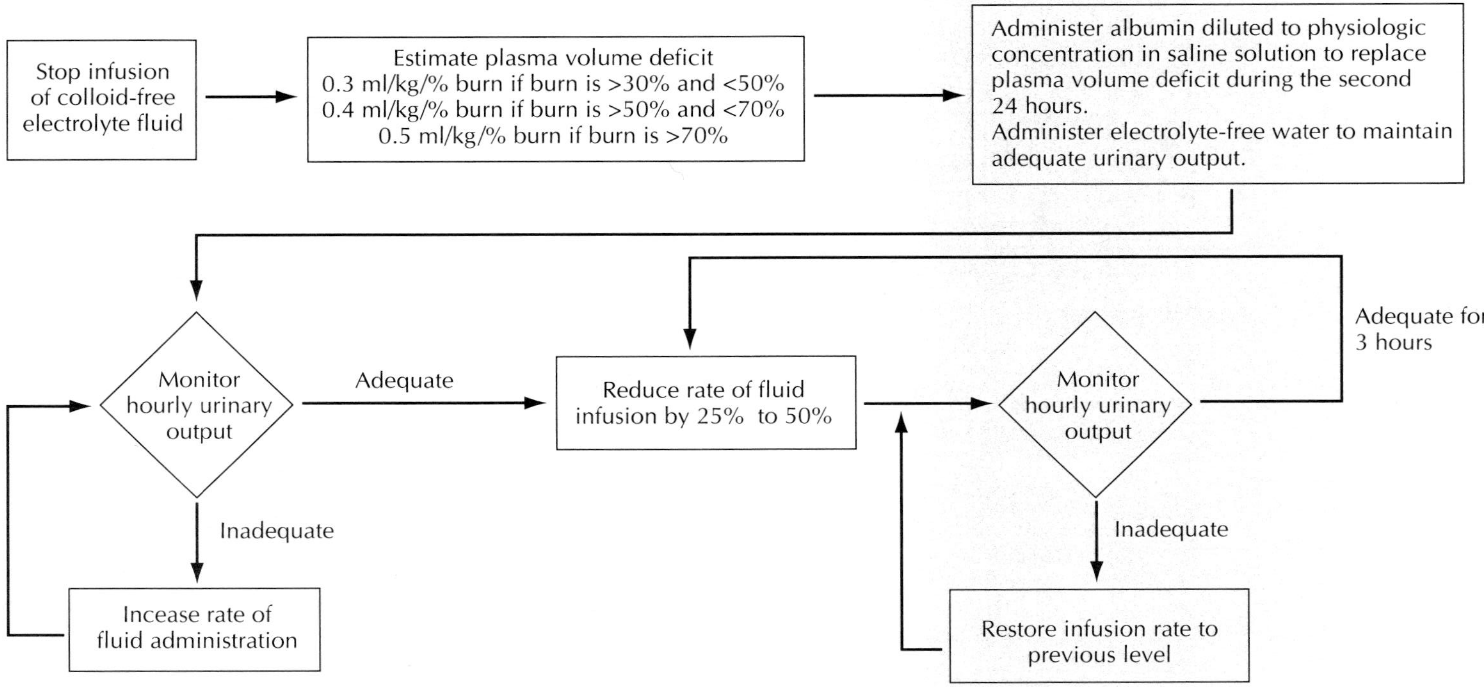

ALGORITHM II: FLUID THERAPY FOR THE SECOND 24 HOURS

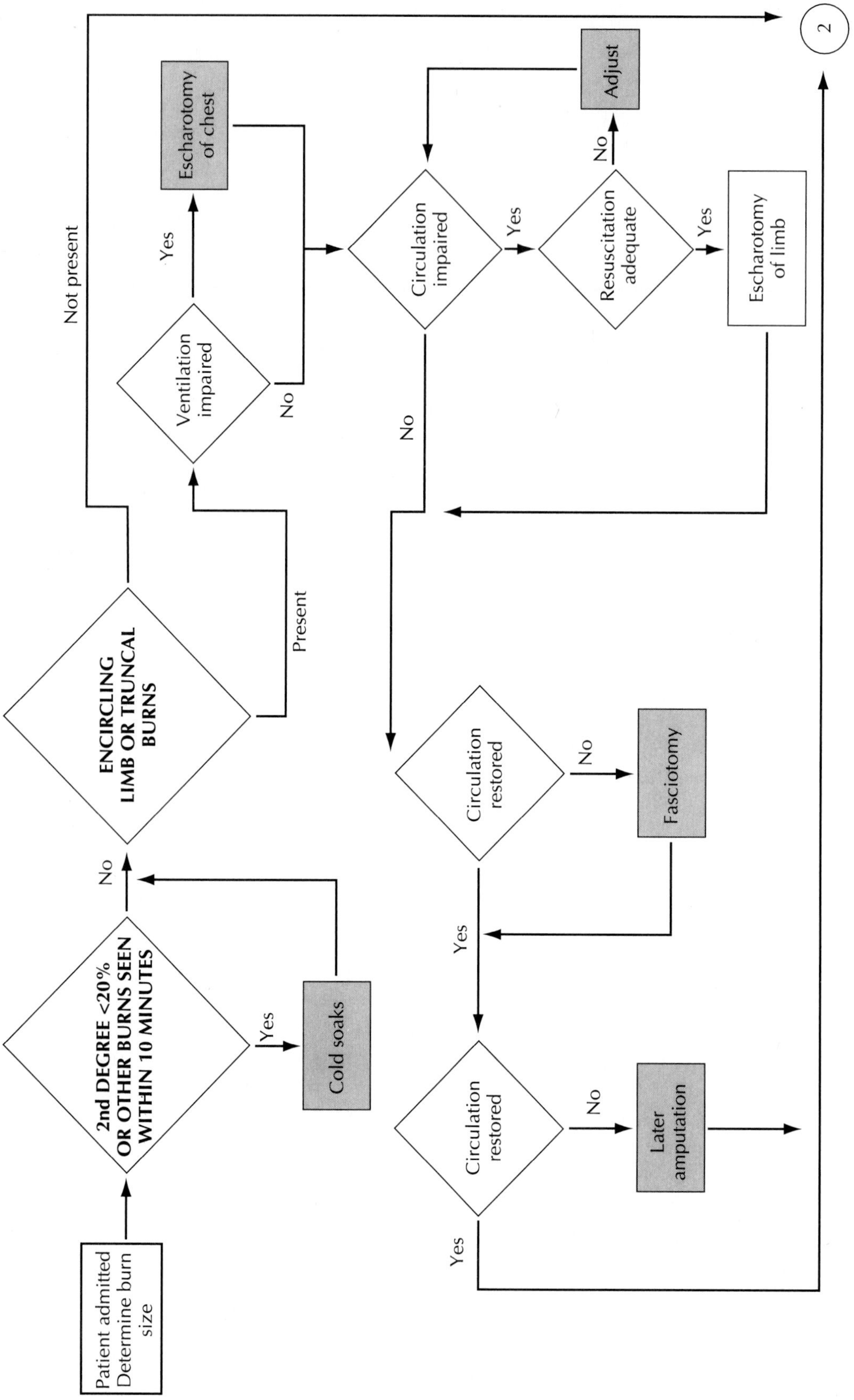

ALGORITHM III A: BURN WOUND TREATMENT

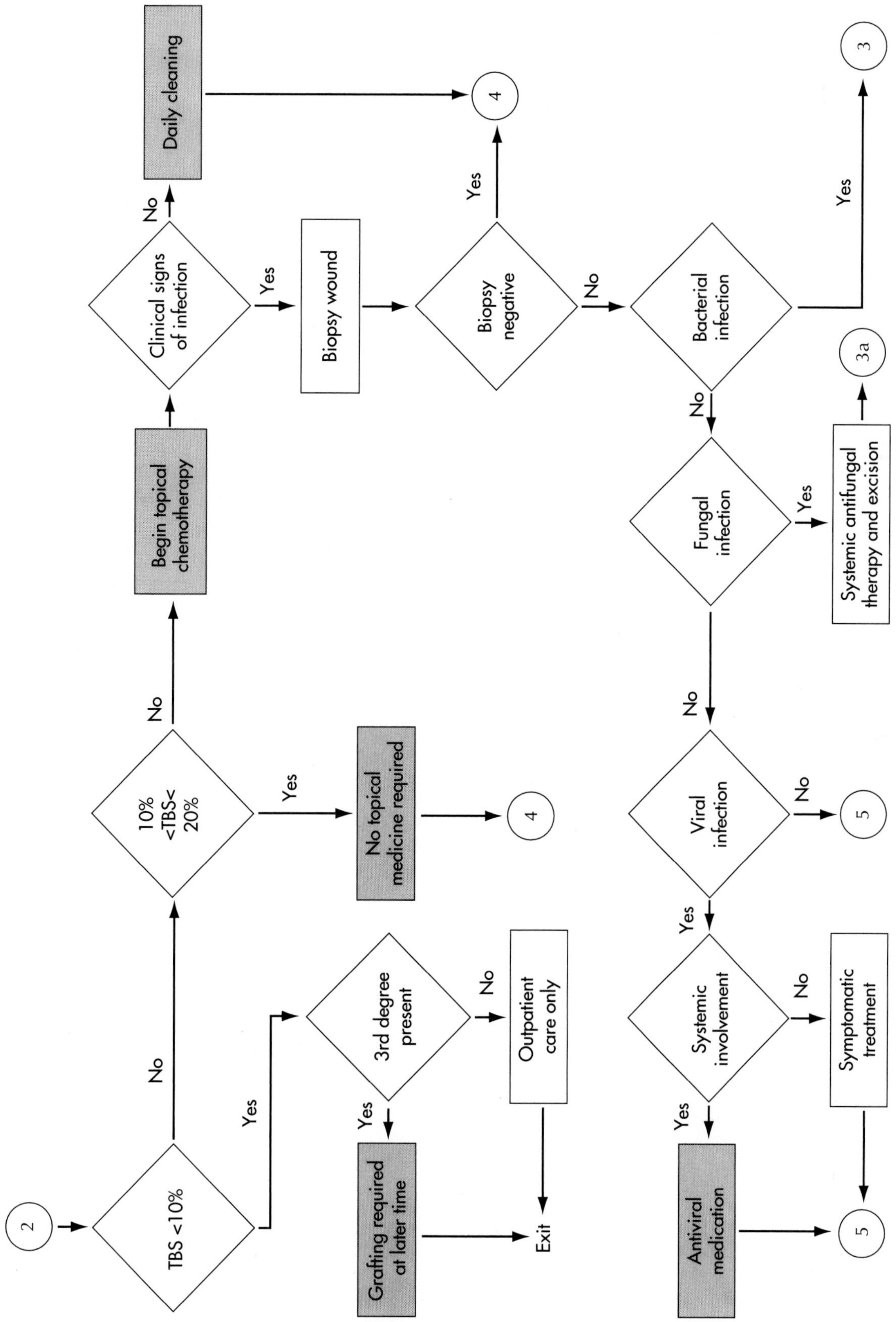

ALGORITHM III B: BURN WOUND TREATMENT

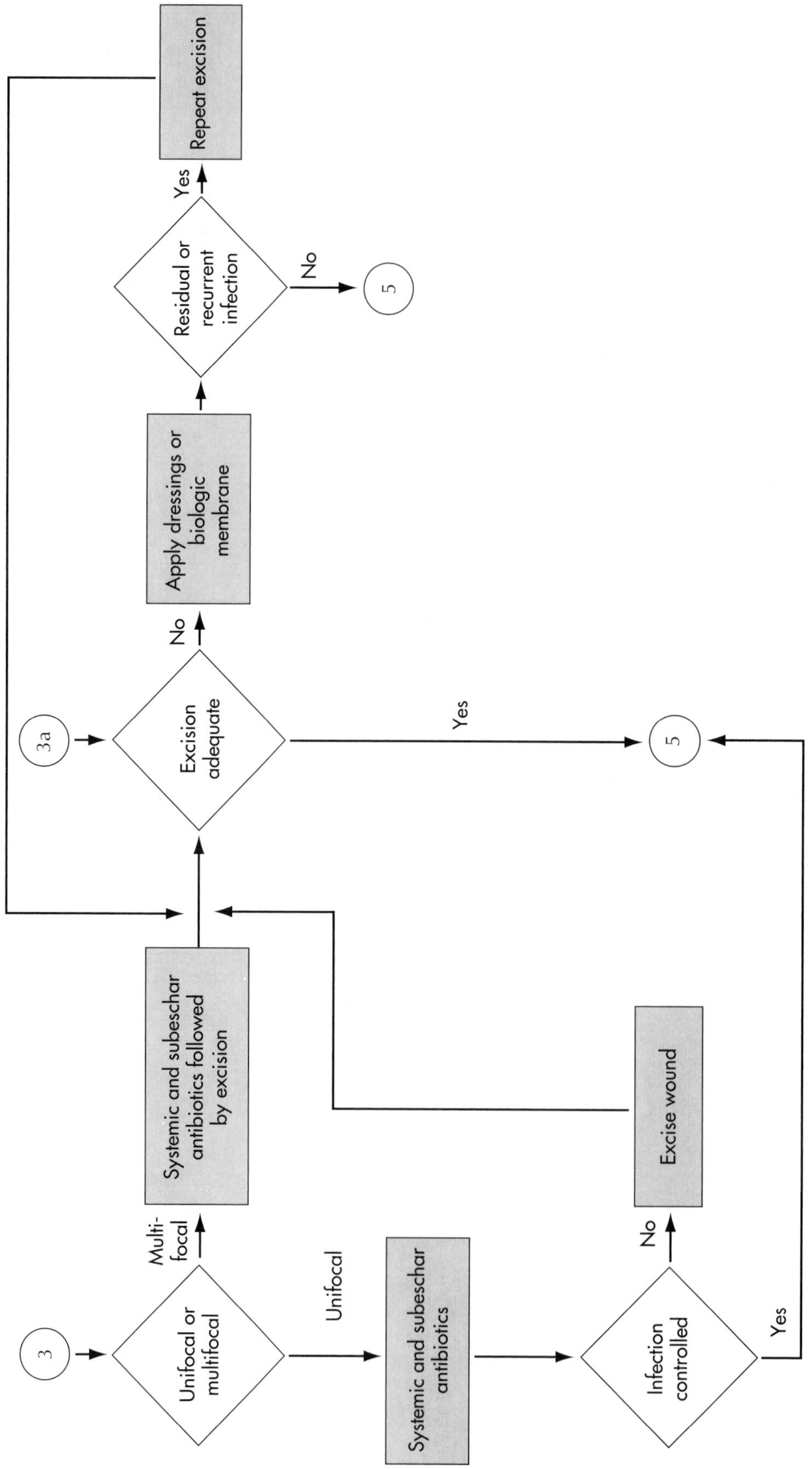

ALGORITHM III C: BURN WOUND TREATMENT

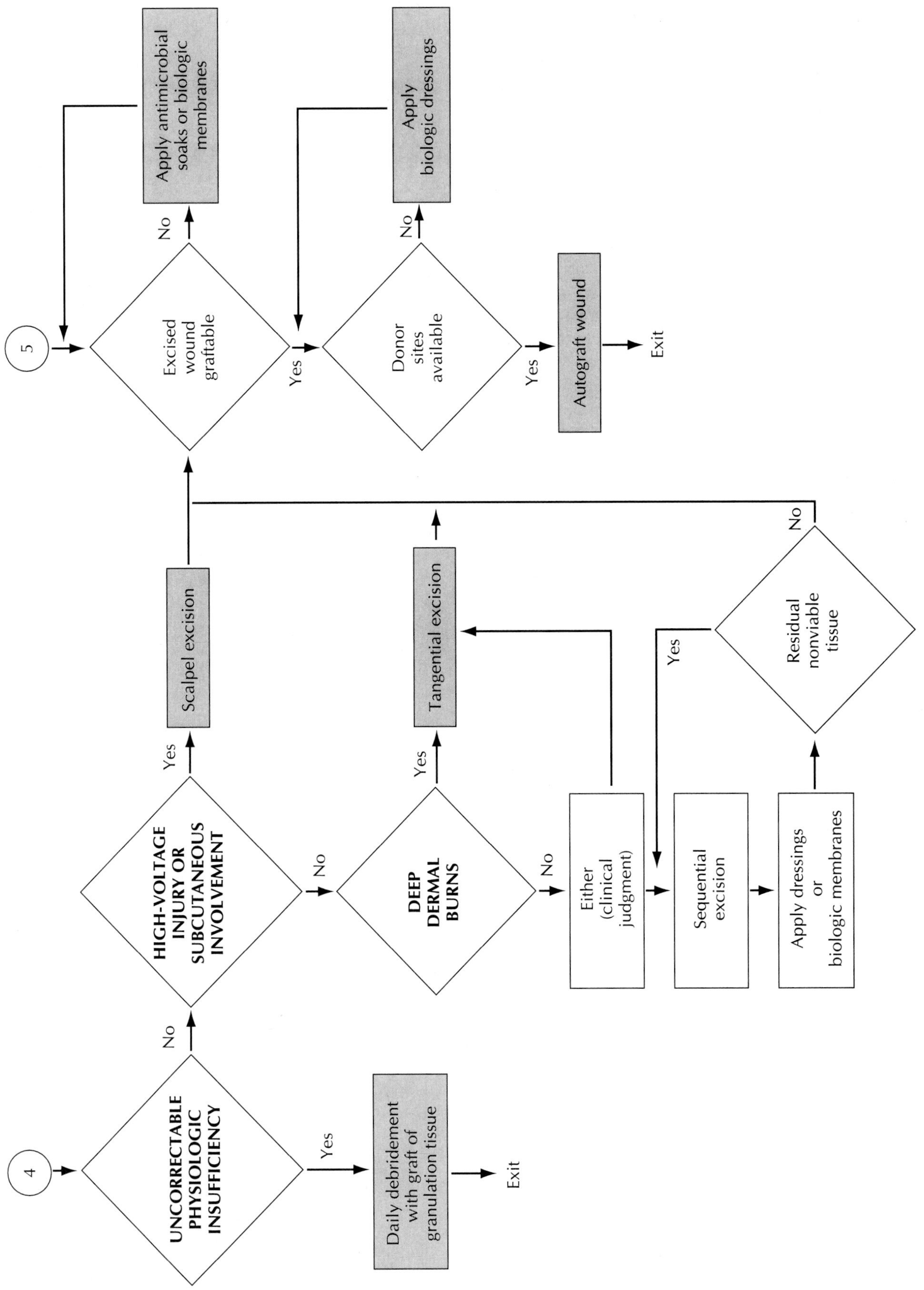

ALGORITHM III D: BURN WOUND TREATMENT

onstrated that the presence of symptoms of the posttraumatic stress disorder occurring during the acute hospitalization correlate with a psychologic impairment during convalescence.[211] Both short-term and long-term psychotherapeutic support is frequently necessary in burned patients, and a full-time psychiatrist is an essential member of the burn team.

Medication therapy is used sparingly for psychiatric problems in burned patients, and the major therapeutic approach relies on direct patient contact with the psychiatrist and other medical personnel. Psychotic episodes and major hallucinations are treated pharmacologically only if patients become dangerous to others or themselves or if their actions compromise their medical care. Small doses of antipsychotic drugs, such as haloperidol, are carefully titrated to mitigate the major manifestations of this disorder. Occasionally, prolonged anxiety or depression requires medication to promote patient cooperation with medical care. Burns in adults are frequently associated with alcohol abuse, and major withdrawal syndromes, including delirium tremens, occur early in the postburn course. Treatment is most effective if begun early. The patient should be treated with thiamine hydrochloride (intravenously while on parenteral fluids and orally after gut function has returned). Benzodiazepines appear to be effective and safe for prophylaxis of the alcohol withdrawal syndrome; however, levels of this class of drug may rise to very high levels in burned patients, and administration should be titrated to avoid oversedation. Central nervous system alpha blockade using clonidine may also be used.

Aftercare and Follow-Up

Burn injury should be viewed as a chronic disease in which initial care or hospitalization is only the initial event. Because wound maturation continues for many months to several years after injury, constant reassessment is necessary to prevent delayed loss of function or acceleration of disfigurement. Depression, loss of housing, and physical disability hinder successful reincorporation into society and require that a multidisciplinary team of medical personnel, occupational and physical therapists, and social workers be available to the patient after leaving the hospital. Initial follow-up visits should be scheduled every several weeks. As the patient adapts to wound treatment requirements and rehabilitation programs, the interval between outpatient visits may increase. Severe itching, vague neuritic pain, and follicular infections in the healed burn are common complaints during the first year after injury. Printed explanations of burn care and detailed treatment procedures are quite effective in allaying patient anxiety and ameliorating patient discomfort.

REFERENCES

1 Agarwal N, Petro J, Salisbury RE: Physiologic profile monitoring in burned patients, *J Trauma* 23:577, 1983.

2 Agee RN, Long JM, Hunt JL et al: Use of ^{133}Xenon in early diagnosis of inhalation injury, *J Trauma* 16:218, 1976.

3 Alexander F, Mathieson M, Teoh KHT et al: Arachidonic acid metabolites mediate early burn edema, *J Trauma* 24:709, 1984.

4 Alexander JW: Alteration of opsonin activity after burn injury. In *Proceedings of the 40th anniversary symposium,* Fort Sam Houston, Texas, 1989, US Army Institute of Surgical Research.

5 Alexander JW, Wixson DP: Neutrophil dysfunction in sepsis in burn injury, *Surg Gynecol Obstet* 130:431, 1970.

6 Amy BW et al: Lightning injury with survival in five patients, *JAMA* 253:243, 1985.

7 Andes WA, Hunt JL: Myocardial infarction in the thermally injured patient, *Proc Am Burn Assn* 6:24, 1974.

8 Apfelberg DB, Masters FW, Robinson DW: Pathophysiology and treatment of lightning injuries, *J Trauma* 14:453, 1974.

9 Arons MS et al: Scar tissue carcinoma: part I. A clinical study with special reference to burn scar carcinoma, *Ann Surg* 161:170, 1965.

10 Arturson G: Capillary permeability in burned and non-burned areas in dogs, *Acta Chir Scand* (Suppl) 274:55, 1961.

11 Arturson G, Mellander S: Acute changes in capillary filtration and diffusion in experimental burn injury, *Acta Physiol Scand* 62:457, 1964.

12 Arturson G, Saeda S: Changes in transcapillary leakage during healing of experimental burns, *Acta Chir Scand* 133:609, 1967.

13 Asch MJ, Moylan JA, Bruck HM et al: Ocular complications associated with burns: review of a five-year experience including 104 patients, *J Trauma* 11:857, 1971.

14 Asch MJ, Curreri PW, Pruitt BA Jr: Thermal injury involving bone: report of 32 cases, *J Trauma* 12:135, 1972.

15 Asch MJ, Feldman RJ, Wallser HL et al: Systemic and pulmonary hemodynamic changes accompanying thermal injury, *Ann Surg* 178:218, 1973.

16 Asch MJ, Meserol PM, Mason AD et al: Regional blood flow in the burned unanaesthetized dog, *Surg Forum* 22:55, 1971.

17 Aulick LH, Goodwin CW Jr, Becker RC et al: Visceral blood flow following thermal injury, *Ann Surg* 193:112, 1981.

18 Aulick LH, Wilmore DW: Increased peripheral amino acid release following burn injury, *Surgery* 85:560, 1979.

19 Aulick LH, Hander EH, Wilmore DW et al: The relative significance of thermal and metabolic demands on burn hypermetabolism, *J Trauma* 19:559, 1979.

20 Baker SP, Ginsburg MJ, O'Neill B, Li G: *The injury fact book,* ed 2, New York, 1992, Oxford University Press.

21 Baskin TW, Rosenthal A, Pruitt BA Jr: Acute bacterial endocarditis: a silent source of sepsis in the burn patient, *Ann Surg* 184:618, 1976.

22 Batchelor AD, Sutherland AB, Colver C: Sodium balance studies following thermal injury, *Br J Plast Surg* 18:130, 1965.

23 Baxter CR: Present concepts in the management of major electrical injury, *Surg Clin North Am* 50:1401, 1970.

24 Baxter CR: Fluid volume and electrolyte changes in the early postburn period, *Clin Plast Surg* 1:693, 1974.

25 Baxter CR, Cook WA, Shires GT: Serum myocardial depressant factor of burn shock, *Surg Forum* 17:1, 1966.

26 Baxter CR, Shires T: Physiologic response to crystalloid resuscitation of severe burns, *Ann NY Acad Sci* 150:874, 1968.

27 Becker RA, Vaughan GM, Goodwin CW Jr et al: Interactions of thyroid hormones and catecholamines in severely burned patients, *Rev Infect Dis* 5:908, 1983.

28 Becker RA, Wilmore DW, Goodwin CW Jr et al: Free T4, free T3, and reverse T3 in critically ill, thermally injured patients, *J Trauma* 20:713, 1980.

29 Bellamy RF: The causes of death in conventional land warfare: implications in combat casualty care research, *Milit Med* 149:55, 1984.
30 Bilbrey GL, Beisel WR: Depression of free water clearance during pneumococcal bacteremia, *Ann Surg* 177:112, 1973.
31 Bjornson AB, Bjornson HS, Knippenberg RW: Temporal relationships among immunologic alterations in a guinea pig model of thermal injury, *J Infect Dis* 153:1098, 1986.
32 Broughton A, Anderson IRM, Bowden CH: Magnesium-deficiency syndrome in burns, *Lancet* 2:1156, 1968.
33 Brouhard BH, Carvajal HF, Linares HA: Burn edema and protein leakage in the rat. I. Relationship to time of injury, *Microvasc Res* 15:221, 1978.
34 Brown GL, Manney LB, Griffen J et al: Enhancement of wound healing by topical treatment with epidermal growth factor, *N Engl J Med* 321(2):76, 1989.
35 Brown WL, Bowler EG, Mason AD Jr: Studies of disturbances of protein turnover in burned troops: use of an animal model. In *Annual Research Progress Report,* Fort Sam Houston, TX, 1981, US Army Institute of Surgical Research, pp 233-259.
36 Bruck HM, Nash G, Stein JM et al: Studies on the occurrence and significance of yeast and fungi in the burn wound, *Ann Surg* 176:108, 1972.
37 Bull JP: Revised analysis of mortality due to burns, *Lancet* 2:1133, 1971.
38 Bull JP, Squire JR: A study of mortality in a burns unit: standards for the evaluation of alternative methods of treatment, *Ann Surg* 130:160, 1949.
39 Burke JF, Yannas IV, Quinby WC et al: Successful use of a physiologically acceptable artificial skin in the treatment of extensive burn injury, *Ann Surg* 194:413, 1981.
40 Burke JF, Bondoc CC, Quinby WC: Primary burn excision and immediate grafting: a method shortening illness, *J Trauma* 14:389, 1974.
41 Burleson DG, Drost AC, Cioffi WG et al: Cellular host defense function after thermal injury: assessment by flow cytometry on peripheral blood cells. In Pruitt BA, editor: *The US Army Institute of Surgical Research Annual Research Progress Report for Fiscal Year 1991.* San Antonio, US Government Printing Office.
42 Burleson DG, Vaughn GK, Mason AD Jr et al: Use of light scatter in flow cytometry measurements of rat lymphocyte subpopulation after burn injury with infection, *Arch Surg,* 122:216, 1987.
43 Caldwell FT, Bowser BH: Critical evaluation of hypertonic and hypotonic solutions to resuscitate severely burned children: a prospective study, *Ann Surg* 189:546, 1979.
44 Canizaro PC, Sawyer RB, Switzer WE: Blood loss during excision of third-degree burns, *Arch Surg* 88:800, 1964.
45 Caplan ES, Hoyt NJ: Nosocomial sinusitis, *JAMA* 247:639, 1982.
46 Carlson DE, Cioffi WG, Mason AD et al: Evaluation of serum visceral protein levels as indicators of nitrogen balance in the thermally injured patient, *JPEN* 15(4):440, 1991.
47 Carlson DE, Cioffi WG, Mason AD Jr et al: Resting energy expenditure in thermally injured patients, *Surg Gynecol Obstet* 174:270, 1992.
48 Chatterjee BF, Barancik JI, Fratianne RB et al: Northeastern Ohio trauma study. V. Burn injury, *J Trauma* 26:844, 1986.
49 Cioffi WG: Short-term anabolic effect of recombinant human insulin-like growth factor in thermally injured patients. In Pruitt BA, editor: *The US Army Institute of Surgical Research Annual Research Progress Report for Fiscal Year 1991.* San Antonio, US Government Printing Office.
50 Cioffi WG, Burleson DG, Jordan BS et al: Granulocyte-macrophage colony stimulating factor in burn patients, *Arch Surg* 126:74, 1991.
51 Cioffi WG, Burleson DG, Jordan BS et al: Granulocyte oxidative activity following thermal injury, *Surgery* 112(5):860, 1992.
52 Cioffi WG, Burleson DG, Pruitt WG Jr: Leukocyte responses to injury, *Arch Surg* 128:1260, 1993.
53 Cioffi WG, deLemos RA, Coalson JJ et al: Decreased pulmonary damage in primates with inhalation injury treated with high frequency ventilation, *Ann Surg* 218(3):328, 1993.
54 Cioffi WG, DeMules JE, Gamelli RL: The effects of burn injury and fluid resuscitation on cardiac function in vitro, *J Trauma* 26:844, 1986.
55 Cioffi WG, Kim SH, Pruitt BA Jr: Cause of mortality in thermally injured patients. In Lorenz S, Zellner PR, editors: *Die Infektion Beim Brandverletzten,* Proceedings of the "Infektionsprophylaxe und Infectionsbekampfung beim Brandverletzten" International Symposium, Darmstadt Germany, 1993, Dr. Dietrich Steinkopff Verlag, GmbH & Co.
56 Cioffi WG, McManus A, Rue LW III et al: Comparison of acid neutralizing with non-acid neutralizing stress ulcer prophylaxis in thermally injured patients, *J Trauma* 36:541, 1994.
57 Cioffi WG, Pruitt BA Jr: Aeromedical transport of the thermally injured patient, *Med Corps Int* 4(3):23, 1989.
58 Cioffi WG, Rue LW, Graves TA et al: Prophylactic use of high frequency ventilators in patients with inhalation injury, *Ann Surg* 213(6):575, 1991.
59 Cioffi WG, Vaughan GM, Heironimus JD et al: Dissociation of blood volume and flow in regulation of salt and water balance in burn patients, *Ann Surg* 214(3):213, 1991.
60 Clayton JM, Hayes AC, Hammel J et al: Xenon-133 determination of muscle blood flow in electrical injury, *J Trauma* 17:293, 1977.
61 Cohen IK, Scheckter PJ, Henkin RI: Hypogeusia, anorexia and altered zinc metabolism following thermal burn, *JAMA* 223:914, 1972.
62 Colocho G, Graham WP III, Greene AE et al: Human amniotic membrane as a physiologic wound dressing, *Arch Surg* 109:370, 1974.
63 Constantian MB: Association of sepsis with an immunosuppressive polypeptide in the serum of burn patients, *Ann Surg* 188:209, 1978.
64 Cooper ML, Hansbrough JF, Spielvogel RL et al: In vivo optimization of a living dermal substitute employing cultured human fibroblasts on a biodegradable polyglycolic acid or polyglactin mesh, *Biomaterials* 12(2):243, 1991.
65 Cope O, Moore FD: The redistribution of body water in the fluid therapy of the burn patient, *Ann Surg* 126:1010, 1947.
66 Cuthbertson DP, Tilstone WJ: Metabolism during the postinjury period, *Adv Clin Chem* 12:1, 1969.
67 Curreri PW, Katz AJ, Dotin LN et al: Coagulation abnormalities in the thermally injured patient, *Curr Top Surg Res* 2:401, 1970.
68 Curreri PW, Luterman A, Braun DW Jr et al: Burn injury: analysis of survival and hospitalization time for 937 patients, *Ann Surg* 192:472, 1980.
69 Curreri PW, Wilmore DW, Mason AD Jr et al: Intracellular cation alterations following major trauma: effect of supranormal caloric intake, *J Trauma* 11:390, 1971.
70 Curreri PW, Wilterdink ME, Baxter CR: Characterization of elevated fibrin split products following thermal injury, *Ann Surg* 191:157, 1975.
71 Czaja AJ, McAlhany JC, Pruitt BA Jr: Acute gastroduodenal disease after thermal injury: endoscopic evaluation of incidence and natural history, *N Engl J Med* 291:925, 1974.
72 Czaja AJ, McAlhany JC, Pruitt BA Jr: Gastric acid secretion and acute gastroduodenal disease after burns, *Arch Surg* 111:243, 1976.

73 Czaja AJ, Rizzo TA, Smith WR et al: Acute liver disease cutaneous thermal injury, *J Trauma* 15:887, 1975.
73a Death by lightning (editorial), *Lancet* 1:230, 1977.
74 DeCamara DL, Raine T, Robson MC: Ultrastructural aspects of cooled thermal injury, *J Trauma* 21:911, 1981.
75 Demling RH, Lalonde C: Effect of partial burn excision and closure on postburn oxygen consumption, *Surgery* 104:846, 1988.
76 Demling RH, Kramer GC, Gunther R et al: Effect of non-protein colloid on postburn edema formation in soft tissues and lungs, *Surgery* 95:593, 1984.
77 Demling RH, Wong C, Jin LJ et al: Early lung dysfunction after major burns: role of edema and vasoactive mediators, *J Trauma* 25:959, 1985.
78 Desai MH, Mlakar JM, McCauley RL et al: Lack of long-term durability of cultured keratinocyte burn-wound coverage: a case report, *J Burn Care Rehabil* 12(6):540, 1991.
79 DiVincenti FC, Curreri PW, Pruitt BA Jr: Use of mesh skin autografts in the burn patient, *Plast Reconstr Surg* 44:464, 1969.
80 DiVincenti FC, Moncrief JA, Pruitt BA Jr: Electrical injuries: a review of 65 cases, *J Trauma* 9:497, 1969.
81 DiVincenti FC, Pruitt BA Jr, Reckler JM: Inhalation injuries, *J Trauma* 11:109, 1971.
82 Dorethy JW, Welch GW, Treat RC et al: The hemodynamic response to thermal injury in burned soldiers. I. Sequential hemodynamic alterations in severe thermal injury in the military population: colloid-crystalloid vs. crystalloid fluid resuscitation. In *Annual Research Progress Report,* Fort Sam Houston, TX, 1977, US Army Institute of Surgical Research, pp 120-138.
83 Dowling JA, Foley FD, Moncrief JA: Chondritis in the burned ear, *Plast Reconstr Surg* 42:115, 1968.
84 Drost A, Burleson DG, Cioffi WG et al: Plasma cytokines following thermal injury and their relationship with patient mortality, burn size, and time post burn, *J Trauma* 35(3):335, 1993.
85 Drost A, Burleson DG, Cioffi WG et al: Plasma cytokines following thermal injury and their relationship to infection, *Ann Surg* 218(1):74, 1993.
86 Duke JH, Jorgensen SB, Broell JR et al: Contribution of protein to caloric expenditure following injury, *Surgery* 68:168, 1970.
87 Eastwood GL: Small bowel morphology and epithelial proliferation in intravenously alimented rabbits, *Surgery* 82:613, 1977.
88 Reference deleted in proofs.
89 Espinosa CG, Halkias DG: Pulmonary mucormycosis as a complication of chronic salicylate poisoning, *Am J Clin Pathol* 80:508, 1983.
90 Evans EI, Brooks JW, Schmidt FH et al: Flash burn studies on human volunteers, *Surgery* 37:280, 1955.
91 Evans EI, Purnell OJ, Robinette PW et al: Fluid and electrolyte requirements in severe burns, *Ann Surg* 135:804, 1952.
92 Faulk WP, Matthews R, Stevens PJ et al: Human amnion as an adjunct in wound healing, *Lancet* 1:1156, 1980.
93 Feck G, Baptiste MS: The epidemiology of burn injury in New York, *Public Health Rep* 94:312, 1979.
94 Felig P: The glucose-alanine cycle, *Metabolism* 22:179, 1973.
95 Foley FD, Greenwald KA, Nash G et al: Herpesvirus infection in burned patients, *N Engl J Med* 282:652, 1970.
96 Fox CL Jr, Rappole BW, Stanford W: control of *Pseudomonas* infection in burns by silver sulfadiazine, *Surg Gynecol Obstet* 128:1021, 1969.
97 Gadd MA, Hansbrough JF, Hoyt DB et al: Defective T-cell surface antigen expression after mitogen stimulation: an index of lymphocyte dysfunction after controlled murine injury, *Ann Surg* 209:112, 1989.
98 Gallico GG III, O'Connor NE, Compton CC: Permanent coverage of large burn wounds with autologous cultured epithelium, *N Engl J Med* 311:448, 1984.
99 Gelfand JA, Donelan M, Burke JF: Preferential activation and depletion of the alternative complement pathway by burn injury, *Ann Surg* 198:58, 1983.
100 Geyer RP: "Bloodless" rats through the use of artificial blood substitutes, *Fed Proc* 34:1499, 1975.
101 Giblin T, Pichrell K, Pitts W et al: Malignant degeneration in burn scars: Marjolin's ulcer, *Ann Surg* 162:291, 1965.
102 Goodwin CW, Pruitt BA Jr: The massive burn with sepsis and Curling's ulcer. In Hardy JD, editor: *Critical surgical illness,* ed 2, Philadelphia, 1980, WB Saunders.
103 Goodwin CW, Lam V, Mason AD Jr et al: Colloid and crystalloid have same effect on lung water after thermal injury, *Surg Forum* 32:294, 1981.
104 Goodwin CW, Dorethy J, Lam V et al: Randomized trial of efficacy of crystalloid and colloid resuscitation on hemodynamic response and lung water following thermal injury, *Ann Surg* 197:520, 1983.
105 Gore DC, Honeycutt D, Jahoor F et al: Effect of exogenous growth hormone on glucose utilization in burn patients, *J Surg Res* 51:518, 1991.
106 Gough DB, Moss HM, Jordan A et al: Recombinant interleukin-2 (rIL-2) improves immune response and host resistance to septic challange in thermally injured mice, *Surgery* 104(2):292, 1988.
107 Graves TA, Cioffi WG, McManus WF et al: Fluid resuscitation of infants and children with massive thermal injury, *J Trauma* 28(12):1656, 1988.
108 Grogan JB: Altered neutrophil phagocytic function in burn patients, *J Trauma* 16:734, 1976.
109 Grube BJ, Marvin JA, Heimbach DM: Therapeutic hyperbaric oxygen: help or hindrence in burn patients with carbon monoxide poisoning? *J Burn Care Rehabil* 9(3):249, 1988.
110 Gusberg RJ, Scholz PM, Gump FE, Kinney JM: Can protein breakdown explain the increased calorie expenditure in injury and sepsis? *Surg Forum* 24:79, 1973.
111 Halebian P, Robinson N, Barie P et al: Whole body oxygen utilization during carbon monoxide poisoning and isocapnic nitrogen hypoxia, *J Trauma* 26:110, 1986.
112 Hanback LD, Rittenbury MS: Response of the reticuloendothelial system in thermal injury, *Surg Forum* 16:47, 1965.
113 Hansborough JR, Piancentine JG, Eiseman B: Immunosuppression by hyperbaric oxygen, *Surgery* 87:662, 1980.
114 Harrison HN, Moncrief JA, Duckett JW et al: The relationship between energy metabolism and water loss from vaporization in severely burned patients, *Surgery* 56:203, 1964.
115 Heimbach D, Luterman A, Burke J et al: Artificial dermis for major burns: a multicenter randomized clinical trial, *Ann Surg* 208(3):313, 1988.
116 Helmkamp GM, Wilmore DW, Johnson AA et al: Essential fatty acid deficiency in red cells after thermal injury: correction with intravenous fat therapy, *Am J Clin Nutr* 26:1331, 1973.
117 Herndon DN, Abston S, Stein MD: Increased thromboxane B_2 levels in the plasma of burned and septic burned patients, *Surg Gynecol Obstet* 159:210, 1984.
118 Herndon DN, Barrow RE, Rutan TC et al: Effect of propranolol administration on hemodynamic and metabolic responses of burned pediatric patients, *Ann Surg* 208(4):484, 1988.
119 Herndon DN, Barrow RE, Kunkel KR et al: Effects of recombinant human growth hormone on donor-site healing in severely burned children, *Ann Surg* 212(4):424, 1990.
120 Herndon DN, Parks DH: Comparison of serial debridement and autografting and early massive excision with cadaver skin overlay in the treatment of large burns in children, *J Trauma* 26:149, 1986.

121 Heymsfield SB, Bethel RA, Ansley JD et al: Enteral hyperalimentation: an alternative to central venous hyperalimentation, *Ann Intern Med* 90:63, 1979.
122 Hinton P, Allison SP, Littlejohn S et al: Insulin and glucose to reduce catabolic response to injury in burn patients, *Lancet* 1:767, 1971.
123 Hinton P, Allison SP, Littlejohn S et al: Electrolyte changes after burn injury and effect of treatment, *Lancet* 2:218, 1973.
124 Holliman CJ, Saffle JR, Kravitz M et al: Early surgical decompression in the management of electrical injuries, *Am J Surg* 144:733, 1982.
125 Huang KF, Chung DH, Herndon DN: Insulinlike growth factor 1 (IGF-1) reduces gut atrophy and bacterial translocation after severe burn injury, *Arch Surg* 128:47, 1993.
126 Hunt JL, Mason AD Jr, Masterson TS et al: The pathophysiology of acute electric injuries, *J Trauma* 16:335, 1976.
127 Hunt JL, Sato RM, Baxter CR: Acute electric burns: current diagnostic and therapeutic approaches to management, *Arch Surg* 115:434, 1980.
128 Ikeuchi H, Sakano T, Sanchez J et al: The effects of platelet-activating factor (PAF) and a PAF antagonist (CV-3988) on smoke inhalation injury in an ovine model, *J Trauma* 32(3):344, 1992.
129 Jackson BM, Stone PA: Tangential excision and grafting of burns: the method and report of 50 consecutive cases, *Br J Plast Surg* 25:416, 1972.
130 Jackson DM: Second thoughts on the burn wound, *J Trauma* 9:839, 1969.
131 Jahoor F, Desai M, Herndon DN, Wolfe RR: Dynamics of the protein metabolic response to burn injury, *Metabolism* 37(4):330, 1988.
132 Janzekovic Z: Present clinical aspects of burns: a symposium, *Mlachinska Lrygia* 99:99, 1968.
133 Jones WG, Barie PS, Yurt RW et al: Enterococcal burn sepsis: a highly lethal complication in severely burned patients, *Arch Surg* 121:649, 1986.
134 Kagan RJ, Naraqui S, Matsuda T et al: Herpes simplex virus and cytomegalovirus infections in burn patients, *J Trauma* 25:40, 1985.
135 Kim SH et al: Frozen section technique to evaluate early burn wound biopsy: a comparison with the rapid section technique, *J Trauma* 25:1134, 1985.
136 Kim SH, Hubbard GB, Wurley BL et al: A rapid section technique for burn wound biopsy, *J Burn Care Rehabil* 6:433, 1985.
137 Kohnlein HE, Merkle P, Springorum HW: Hydrogen fluoride burns: experiments and treatment, *Surg Forum* 24:50, 1973.
138 Kupper TS, Deitch EA, Baker CC et al: the human burnwound as a primary source of interleukin-I activity, *Surgery* 100:409, 1986.
139 Kupper TS, Green DR: Immunoregulation after thermal injury: sequential appearance of I-J$^+$, Ly-1 T-suppressor inducer cells and Ly-2 T-suppressor effector cells following thermal trauma in mice, *J Immunol* 133:3047, 1984.
140 Kupper TS, Green DR, Durum SK et al: Defective antigen presentation to a cloned T-helper cell by macrophages from burned mice can be restored with interleukin-I, *Surgery* 98:199, 1985.
141 LaLonde C, Demling R: The effect of complete burn wound excision and closure on postburn oxygen consumption, *Surgery* 102:862, 1987.
142 Lanser ME, Saba TM: Correction of serum opsonic defects after burn and sepsis by opsonic fibronectin administration, *Arch Surg* 118:338, 1983.
143 Larson DL, Baur P, Lenares HA et al: Mechanisms of hypertrophic scar and contracture formation in burns, *Burns* 1:119, 1975.
144 Larson DL, Maxwell R, Abston S et al: Zinc deficiency in burned children, *Plast Reconstr Surg* 46:13, 1970.
145 Lee RC, Gottlieb LJ, Krizek TJ: Pathophysiology and clinical manifestations of tissue injury in electrical trauma, *Adv Plastic Reconstr Surg* 8:9, 1992.
146 Leeming MN, Ray C Jr, Howland WS: Low voltage direct current burns, *JAMA* 214:1681, 1970.
147 Lemp MA: Cornea and sclera, *Arch Ophthalmol* 92:158, 1974.
148 Lescher TJ, Teejarden DK, Pruitt BA Jr: Acute pseudo-obstruction of the colon in thermally injured patients, *Dis Colon Rectum* 21:618, 1978.
149 Levine BA, Schwesinger WH, Sirinek KR et al: Cimetidine prevents reduction in gastric mucosal blood flow during shock, *Surgery* 84:113, 1978.
150 Levine BA, Petroff PA, Slade CL et al: Prospective trials of dexamethasone and aerosolized gentamicin in the burned patient, *J Trauma* 18:118, 1978.
151 Levine NS, Atkins A, McKeel D et al: Spinal cord injury following electrical accidents: case reports, *J Trauma* 15:459, 1975.
152 LeVoyer T, Cioffi WG, Pratt L et al: Alterations in intestinal permeability following thermal injury, *Arch Surg* 127(1):26, 1992.
153 Loebl EC, Baxter CR, Curreri PW: The mechanism of erythrocyte destruction in the early postburn period, *Ann Surg* 178:681, 1973.
154 Loven L, Nordstrom H, Lennquist S: Changes in calcium and phosphate and their regulating hormones in patients with severe burn injuries, *Scand J Plast Reconstr Surg* 18:49, 1984.
155 Lund CC, Levenson SM, Green RW: Ascorbic acid, thiamine, riboflavin, and nicotinic acid in relation to acute burns in man, *Arch Surg* 55:557, 1947.
156 Lund R, Goodwin CW, McManus WF et al: Upper airway sequelae in burn patients requiring endotracheal intubation or tracheostomy, *Ann Surg* 201:374, 1985.
157 Lund T, Bert JL, Onarheim H et al: Microvascular exchange during burn injury. I: A review, *Circ Shock* 28:179, 1989.
158 Lund T, Wiig H, Reed RK, Aukland K: A "new" mechanism for oedema generation: strongly negative interstitial fluid pressure causes rapid fluid flow into thermally injured skin, *Acta Physiol Scand* 129:433, 1987.
159 Madden MR, Finkelstein JL, Stianocoieko L: Grafting of cultured allogeneic epidermis on second and third-degree burn wounds in 23 patients, *J Trauma* 26:955-962, 1986.
160 Martineau L, Little RA, Rothwell NJ, Fisher MI: Clenbuterol, a β_2-adrenergic agonist, reverses muscle wasting due to scald injury in the rat. *Burns* 19(1):26, 1993.
161 Mason AD Jr: The mathematics of resuscitation, *J Trauma* 20:1015, 1980.
162 Mason AD Jr, McManus AT, Pruitt BA Jr: Association of burn mortality and bacteremia: a 25 year review, *Arch Surg* 121:1027, 1986.
163 Mason AD Jr, Pruitt BA Jr: Epidemiology of burn injury. Paper presented at the Fifth International Congress on Burn Injuries, Stockholm, Sweden, June 19, 1978.
164 McAlhany JC, Czaja AJ, Pruitt BA Jr: Antacid control of complications from acute gastroduodenal disease after burns, *J Trauma* 16:645, 1976.
165 McDougal WS, Wilmore DW, Pruitt BA Jr: Effect of intravenous near isosmotic nutrient infusions on nitrogen balance in critically injured patients, *Surg Gynecol Obstet* 145:408, 1977.
166 McDougal WS, Wilmore DW, Pruitt BA Jr: Glucose-dependent hepatic membrane transport in nonbacteremic thermally injured patients, *J Surg Res* 22:697, 1977.
167 McElwee HP, Sirinek KR, Levine BA: Cimetidine affords pro-

tection equal to antacids in prevention of stress ulceration following thermal injury, *Surgery* 86:620, 1979.

168 McIrvine AJ, O'Mahony JB, Saporoschetz I et al: Depressed immune response in burn patients: use of monoclonal antibodies and functional assays to define the role of suppressor cells, *Ann Surg* 196:297, 1982.

169 McManus AT: Examination of neutrophil function in a rat model of decreased host resistance following burn trauma, *Rev Infect Dis* 5(suppl 5):898, 1983.

170 McManus AT, Denton CL, Mason AD Jr: Mechanisms of in vitro sensitivity to sulfadiazine silver, *Arch Surg* 118:161, 1983.

171 McManus AT, Mason AD Jr, McManus WF et al: Control of *Pseudomonas aeruginosa* infections in burned patients, *Surg Res Comm* 127:61, 1992.

172 McManus AT, Kim SH, Mason AD Jr et al: A comparison of quantitative microbiology and histopathology in divided burn wound biopsies, *Arch Surg* 122:74, 1987.

173 McManus AT, Mason AD Jr, McManus WF et al: Twenty-five year review of *Pseudomonas aeruginosa* bacteremia in a burn center, *Eur J Clin Microbiol* 4:219, 1985.

174 McManus WF, Eurenius K, Pruitt BA Jr: Disseminated intravascular coagulation in burned patients, *J Trauma* 13:416, 1973.

175 McManus WF, Goodwin CW, Mason AD Jr et al: Burn wound infection, *J Trauma* 21:753, 1981.

176 McManus WF, Goodwin CW Jr, Pruitt BA Jr: Subeschar treatment of burn wound infection, *Arch Surg* 118:291, 1983.

177 McManus WF, Hunt JL, Pruitt BA Jr: Postburn convulsive disorders in children, *J Trauma* 14:396, 1975.

178 McNabb LJ, Hyatt J: Effect of an air-fluidized bed on insensible water loss, *Crit Care Med* 15(2):161, 1987.

179 Miller TA, Switzer WE, Foley ED et al: Early homografting of second-degree burns, *Plast Reconstr Surg* 40:117, 1967.

180 Minifee PK, Barrow RE, Abston S et al: Improved myocardial oxygen utilization following propranolol infusion in adolescents with postburn hypermetabolism, *J Pediatr Surg* 24(8):806, 1989.

181 Mitchell WH, Parson BJ, Weiner LJ: *Pseudomonas* ulceration of the cornea following major total body burn: a clinical study, *J Trauma* 16:317, 1976.

182 Moldawer LL, O'Keefe SJD, Bothe A et al: In vivo demonstration of nitrogen-sparing mechanisms for glucose and amino acids in the injured rat, *Metabolism* 29:173, 1980.

183 Monafo WW: The treatment of burn shock by the intravenous and oral administration of hypertonic lactated saline solution, *J Trauma* 10:575, 1970.

184 Monafo WW: *The treatment of burns,* St Louis, 1970, Warren H Green.

185 Moncrief JA, Lindberg RB, Switzer WE et al: Use of topical antibacterial therapy in the treatment of the burn wound, *Arch Surg* 92:558, 1966.

186 Moncrief JA, Lindberg RB, Switzer WE et al: The use of a topical sulfonamide in the control of burn wound sepsis, *J Trauma* 6:407, 1946.

187 Moncrief JA, Pruitt BA Jr: Electric injury, *Postgrad Med* 48:189, 1970.

188 Moore FD Jr, Davis C, Rodrick M et al: Neutrophil activation in thermal injury as assessed by increased expression of complement receptors, *N Engl J Med* 314:948, 1986.

189 Moyer CA, Brentano L, Gravens DL et al: Treatment of large human burns with 0.5% silver nitrate solution, *Arch Surg* 90:812, 1965.

190 Moylan JA, Adib K, Burnbaum M: Fiberoptic bronchoscopy following thermal injury, *Surg Gynecol Obstet* 140:541, 1975.

191 Moylan JA, Inge WW Jr, Pruitt BA Jr: Circulatory changes following circumferential extremity burns evaluated by the ultrasonic flowmeter: an analysis of 60 thermally injured limbs, *J Trauma* 11:763, 1971.

192 Moylan JA, Mason AD Jr, Rogers PW et al: Postburn shock: a critical evaluation of resuscitation, *J Trauma* 13:354, 1973.

193 Moylan JA Jr, Pruitt BA Jr: Aeromedical transportation, *JAMA* 224:1271, 1973.

194 Moylan JA Jr, Reckler JM, Mason AD Jr: Hypertonic lactate saline resuscitation in thermal injury, *Surg Forum* 22:49, 1971.

195 Moylan JA Jr, Reckler JM, Mason AD Jr: Resuscitation with hypertonic lactate saline in thermal injury, *Am J Surg* 125:580, 1973.

196 Moylan JA, Wilmore DW, Mouton DE et al: Early diagnosis of inhalation injury using xenon lung scan, *Ann Surg* 176:477, 1972.

197 Munster AM, Goodwin MN, Pruitt BA Jr: Acalculous cholecystitis in burned patients, *Am J Surg* 122:591, 1971.

198 Nadel E, Kozerefski PM: Rehabilitation of the critically ill burn patient, *Crit Care Q* 7:19, 1984.

199 Naraizzi LR: Computerized tomographic correlate of carbon monoxide poisoning, *Arch Neurol* 36:38, 1979.

200 Nash G, Foley FD: Herpetic infection of the middle and lower respiratory tract, *Am J Clin Pathol* 54:857, 1970.

201 Newsome TW, Curreri PW, Eurenius K: Visceral injuries: an unusual complication of an electric burn, *Arch Surg* 105:494, 1972.

202 Novick M, Gard DA, Hardy SB et al: Burn scar carcinoma: a review and analysis of 46 cases, *J Trauma* 17:809, 1977.

203 Odessey R, Khairallah EA, Goldberg AL: Origin and possible significance of alanine production by skeletal muscle, *J Biol Chem* 249:7623, 1974.

204 Ogura H, Cioffi WG, Okerberg CV et al: The effects of pentoxifylline on pulmonary function following smoke inhalation, *J Surg Res* 56:242, 1994.

205 O'Mahony JB et al: Changes in T-lymphocyte subsets following injury: assessment by flow cytometry and relationship to sepsis, *Ann Surg* 202:580, 1985.

206 O'Neill JA Jr, Pruitt BA Jr, Moncrief JA: Studies of renal function during the early postburn period. In Matter P, Barclay TL, Konickova Z, editors: *Research in burns,* Bern, 1971, Hans Huber Publishers.

207 Order SE, Moncrief JA: Vascular destruction and revascularization in severe thermal injury, *Surg Forum* 15:37, 1964.

208 Orgel MG, Brown HC, Woolhouse FM: Electrical burns of the mouth in children: a method for assessing results, *J Trauma* 15:285, 1975.

209 Ozkan AN, Hoyt DB, Ninnemann JL: Generation and activity of suppressor peptides following traumatic injury, *J Burn Care Rehabil* 8:527, 1987.

210 Pardoe R, Minami RT, Sato RM et al: Phenol burns *Burns* 3:29, 1976.

211 Perry S, Blank K: Delirium in burn patients, *J Burn Care Rehabil* 5:210, 1984.

212 Perry S, Frances A, Clarkin JA: *DSM-III casebook of differential therapeutics: a clinical guide to treatment selection,* New York, 1985, Brunner/Mazel.

213 Petroff PA, Hander EW, Clavton WH et al: Pulmonary function studied after smoke inhalation, *Am J Surg* 132:346, 1976.

214 Petroff PA, Hander EW, Mason AD Jr: Ventilatory patterns following burn injury and effect of Sulfamylon®, *J Trauma* 15:650, 1975.

215 Petroff PA, Pruitt BA Jr: Pulmonary disease in the burn patient. In Artz CP, Moncrief JA, Pruitt BA Jr, editors: *Burns: a team approach,* Philadelphia, 1979, WB Saunders.

216 Pitt RM, Parker JC, Jurkovich GJ et al: Analysis of altered capillary pressure and permeability after thermal injury, *J Surg Res* 42:693, 1987.

217 Plum F, Posner J, Raymond FH: Delayed neurological deterioration after anoxia, *Arch Intern Med* 110:18, 1962.

218 Ponten B, Erikson V, Johansson SH et al: New observations on tissue changes along the pathway of the current in an electrical injury, *Scand J Plast Reconstr Surg* 4:75, 1970.
219 Pruitt BA Jr: Multidisciplinary care and research for burn injury, *J Trauma* 17:263, 1977.
220 Pruitt BA Jr: Advances in fluid therapy and the early care of the burn patient, *World J Surg* 2:139, 1978.
221 Pruitt BA Jr: The burn patient. I. Initial care, *Curr Probl Surg* 16(4):43, 1979.
222 Pruitt BA Jr: The burn patient. II. Later care and complications of thermal injury, *Curr Probl Surg* 16(5):10, 1979.
223 Pruitt BA Jr: Infections of burns and other wounds caused by *Pseudomonas aeruginosa.* In Sabbath LD, editor: *Pseudomonas aeruginosa: the organism, diseases it causes and their treatment,* Bern, 1980, Hans Huber Publishers.
224 Pruitt BA Jr: The diagnosis and treatment of infection in the burn patient, *Burns* 11:79, 1984.
225 Pruitt BA Jr: Phycomycotic infections. In Alexander JW, editor: *Problems in general surgery,* Philadelphia, 1984, JB Lippincott.
226 Pruitt BA Jr: The universal trauma model, *Bull Am Coll Surg* 70(10):2, 1985.
227 Pruitt BA Jr: Host-opportunist interactions in surgical infection, *Arch Surg* 121:13, 1986.
228 Pruitt BA Jr, Curreri PW: The burn wound and its care, *Arch Surg* 103:461, 1971.
229 Pruitt BA Jr, Dowling JA, Moncrief JA: Escharotomy in early burn care, *Arch Surg* 96:502, 1963.
230 Pruitt BA Jr, Erickson DR, Morris A: Progressive pulmonary insufficiency and other pulmonary complications of thermal injury, *J Trauma* 15:369, 1975.
231 Pruitt BA Jr, Fitzgerald BE: A military perspective. In *Emergency medical services: measures to improve care,* Port Washington, NY, 1980, Independent Publishers Group.
232 Pruitt BA Jr, Foley FD: The use of biopsies in burn patient care, *Surgery* 73:887, 1973.
233 Pruitt BA Jr, Goodwin CW Jr: Nutritional management of the seriously ill burned patient. In Winters RW, editor: *Nutritional support of the seriously ill patient,* New York, 1983, Academic Press.
234 Pruitt BA Jr, Goodwin CW Jr: Stress ulcer disease in the burned patient, *World J Surg* 5:209, 1981.
235 Pruitt BA Jr, Levine NS: Characteristics and uses of biologic dressings and skin substitutes, *Arch Surg* 119:312, 1984.
236 Pruitt BA Jr, Mason AD Jr: Hemodynamic studies of burned patients during resuscitation. In Matter P, Barclay TL, Konickova Z, editors: *Research in burns,* Bern, 1971, Hans Huber Publishers.
237 Pruitt BA Jr, Mason AD Jr, Hunt JL: Burn injury in the aged or high risk patient. In Siegel JH, Chodoff PD, editors: *The aged and high risk surgical patient,* New York, 1976, Grune & Stratton.
238 Pruitt BA Jr, Mason AD Jr, Moncrief JA: Hemodynamic changes in the early postburn patient: the influence of fluid administration and of a vasodilator (Hydralazine), *J Trauma* 11:36, 1971.
239 Pruitt BA Jr, Silverstein P: Methods of resurfacing denuded skin areas, *Transplant Proc* 3:1537, 1971.
240 Pruitt BA Jr, Tumbusch WT, Mason AD Jr et al: Mortality in 1100 consecutive burns treated at a burns unit, *Ann Surg* 159:396, 1964.
241 Pruitt BA Jr, O'Neill JA Jr, Moncrief JA et al: Successful control of burn wound sepsis, *JAMA* 203:1054, 1968.
242 Pruitt BA Jr, Stein JM, Foley FD et al: Intravenous therapy in burn patients: suppurative thrombophlebitis and other life threatening complications, *Arch Surg* 100:399, 1970.
243 Pruitt BA Jr, DiVincenti FC, Mason AD et al: The occurrence and significance of pneumonia and other pulmonary complications in burn patients: comparison of conventional and topical treatment, *J Trauma* 10:519, 1970.
244 Pruitt BA Jr, Flemma RJ, DiVincenti FC et al: Pulmonary complications in burn patients: a comparative study of 697 patients, *J Thorac Cardiovasc Surg* 59:7, 1970.
245 Rapaport FD, Bachvaroff RJ: Kinetics of humoral responsiveness in severe thermal injury, *Ann Surg* 184:51, 1976.
246 Reiss E, Stirman JA, Artz CP et al: Fluid and electrolyte in burns, *JAMA* 152:1309, 1953.
247 Resources for optimal care of patients with burn injury. In *Resources for optimal care of the injured patient,* Chicago, IL, 1990, American College of Surgeons, p 55.
248 Rice DP, MacKenzie EJ et al: *Cost of injury in the United States: a report to Congress,* San Francisco, 1989, Institute for Health and Aging, University of California and Injury Prevention Center, The Johns Hopkins University.
249 Richardson JC, Chambers RA, Heywood PM: Encephalopathies of anoxia and hypoglycemia, *Arch Neurol* 1:178, 1959.
250 Rivers JPW, Frankel TL: Essential fatty acid deficiency, *Br Med Bull* 37:59, 1981.
251 Roberts LW, McManus WF, Mason AD Jr et al: Duoderm in the management of skin graft donor sites. In Hall CW, editor: *Surgical research recent developments,* New York, 1985, Pergamon Press.
252 Roberts LW, McManus WF, Shirani KZ et al: Biobrane® and porcine xenograft—a comparative study. Presented at the 17th Annual Meeting of the American Burn Association, Orlando, Florida, March 29, 1985.
253 Robson MC, Heggars JP: Delayed closures based on bacterial counts, *J Surg Oncol* 2:379, 1970.
254 Roe FC, Kinney JM, Blair C: Water and heat exchange in third degree burns, *Surgery* 56:212, 1964.
255 Rosenthal A, Czaja AJ, Pruitt BA Jr: Gastrin levels and gastric acidity in the pathogenesis of acute gastroduodenal disease after burns, *Surg Gynecol Obstet* 144:232, 1977.
256 Rue LW, Cioffi WG, McManus WF, Pruitt BA Jr: Wound closure and outcome in extensively burned patients treated with cultured autologous keratinocytes, *J Trauma* 34(5):662, 1993.
257 Rue LW III, Cioffi WG, McManus WF, Pruitt BA Jr: Improved survival of burn patients with inhalation injury, *Arch Surg* 128:772, 1993.
258 Saffle JR, Crandall A, Warden GD: Cataracts: a long-term complication of electrical injury, *J Trauma* 25:17, 1985.
259 Salisbury RE et al: Postburn edema of the upper extremity: evaluation of present treatment, *J Trauma* 13:857, 1973.
260 Salisbury RE, McKeel DW, Mason AD Jr: Ischemic necrosis of the intrinsic muscles of the hand after thermal injury, *J Bone Joint Surg* 56A:1701, 1974.
261 Sances A Jr, Mvklebust JB, Larson SJ et al: Experimental electrical injury studies, *J Trauma* 21:589, 1981.
262 Sang TA, Monafo WW, Mustoe TA: Topical silicone gel: a new treatment of hypertrophic scars, *Surgery* 106:781, 1989.
263 Savitt S: *Burns, pathology and therapeutic applications,* London, 1957, Butterworth.
264 Shea SM, Caulfield JB, Burke JF: Microvascular ultrastructure in thermal injury: a reconsideration of the role of mediators, *Microvasc Res* 5:87, 1973.
265 Shils MD: Parenteral multivitamins: time for changes, *Bull Parenter Drug Assoc* 30:226, 1976.
266 Shimazaki S, Yoshioka T, Tanaka N et al: Body fluid changes during hypertonic lactated saline solution therapy for burn shock, *J Trauma* 17:38, 1977.
267 Shimazu T, Yukioka T, Hubbard GB et al: A dose-responsive model of smoke inhalation injury. Severity related alteration in cardiopulmonary function, *Ann Surg* 206(1):89, 1987.

268 Shirani KZ, Pruitt BA Jr, Mason AD Jr: The influence of inhalation injury and pneumonia on burn mortality, *Ann Surg* 205:927, 1987.
269 Shirani KZ, Vaughn GM, McManus AT et al: Replacement with modified immunoglobulin G in burn patients: preliminary kinetic studies, *Am J Med* 76(suppl 3a):175, 1984.
270 Shirani KZ, Vaughn GM, Robertson GL et al: Inappropriate vasopressin secretion (SIADH) in burned patients, *J Trauma* 23(3):217, 1983.
271 Shirani KZ, Vaughan GM, Mason AD Jr et al: Elevation of plasma renin activity, angiotensins I and II, and aldosterone in burn patients: Na^+/volume-responsive but not volume-dependent, *Surg Forum* 35:62, 1984.
272 Silverstein P, Curreri PW, Munster AM: Evaluation of fresh viable porcine cutaneous xenografts as a temporary burn wound cover, *Annual Research Progress Report.* Brooke Army Medical Center, Fort Sam Houston, TX, June 30, 1971, US Army Surgical Research Unit.
273 Sneve H: The treatment of burns and skin grafting, *JAMA* 45:1, 1905.
274 Solem L, Fischer RP, Strate RG: The natural history of electrical injury, *J Trauma* 17:487, 1977.
275 Soroff HS, Pearson E, Artz CP: An estimation of the nitrogen requirements for equilibrium in burned patients, *Surg Gynecol Obstet* 112:159, 1961.
276 Stein JM, Stein ED: Safe transfer of civilian burn casualties, *JAMA* 237:489, 1977.
277 Stewart RD: The effect of carbon monoxide on humans, *Ann Rev Pharmacol* 15:409, 1975.
278 Strock LL, Singh H, Abdullah A et al: The effect of insulin-like growth factor I on postburn hypermetabolism, *Surgery* 108:161, 1990.
279 Taylor JW et al: Scalp as a donor site, *Am J Surg* 133:218, 1977.
280 Teodorczyk-Injeyan JA, Sparkes BG, Mills GB et al: Impaired expression of interleukin-2 receptor in the immunosuppressed burn patient: reversal by exogenous IL-2, *J Trauma* 27:180, 1987.
281 Teplitz C: Pathogenesis of *Pseudomonas* vasculitis in septic lesions, *Arch Pathol* 80:297, 1965.
282 Teplitz C, Davis D, Mason AD Jr et al: *Pseudomonas* burn wound sepsis. I. Pathogenesis of experimental *Pseudomonas* burn wound sepsis, *J Surg Res* 4:200, 1964.
283 Tranbaugh RF, Lewis FR, Christensen JM et al: Lung water changes after thermal injury: the effects of crystalloid resuscitation and sepsis, *Ann Surg* 192:479, 1980.
284 Treat RC, Sirinek KR, Levine BA et al: Air evacuation of thermally injured patients: principles of treatment and results, *J Trauma* 20:275, 1980.
285 Tryba M: Risk of acute stress bleeding and nosocomial pneumonia in ventilated intensive care unit patients: sucralfate vs antacids, *Am J Med* 83(Suppl 3B):117, 1987.
286 Tumbusch WT, Vogel EH Jr, Buthiewicz JV et al: Septicemia in burn injury, *J Trauma* 1:22, 1961.
287 Vaughan GM, Becker RA, Allen JP et al: Cortisol and corticotrophin in burned patients, *J Trauma* 2:263, 1982.
288 Wallace AB: Treatment of burns: a return to basic principles, *Br J Plast Surg* 1:232, 1948.
289 Warden GD: Burn-related humoral immunosuppressants. In *Proceedings of the 40th anniversary symposium,* Fort Sam Houston, Texas, 1989, US Army Institute of Surgical Research.
290 Warden GD, Mason AD Jr, Pruitt BA Jr: Evaluation of leukocyte chemotaxis in vitro in thermally injured patients, *J Clin Invest* 54:1001, 1974.
291 Warden GD, Wilmore DW, Rogers PW et al: Hypernatremic state in hypermetabolic burn patients, *Arch Surg* 106:420, 1973.
292 Welch GW, Lull RJ, Petroff PA et al: The use of steroids in inhalation injury, *Surg Gynecol Obstet* 145:539, 1977.
293 White JW, Deitch EA, Gillespie TE et al: Cerebellar ataxia after an electric injury: report of a case and review of the literature, *J Burn Care Rehabil* 4:191, 1983.
294 White MG, Asch MJ: Acid-base effects of topical mafenide acetate in the burned patient, *N Engl J Med* 284:1281, 1971.
295 Wilmore DW: Nutrition and metabolism following thermal injury, *Clin Plast Surg* 1:603, 1979.
296 Wilmore DW, Long JM, Mason AD Jr et al: Catecholamines: mediator of the hypermetabolic response to thermal injury, *Ann Surg* 180:653, 1974.
297 Wilmore DW, Mason AD Jr, Johnson DW et al: Effect of ambient temperature on heat production and heat loss in burn patients, *J Appl Physiol* 38:593, 1975.
298 Wilmore DW, Mason AD Jr, Pruitt BA Jr: Impaired glucose flow in burn patients with gram-negative sepsis, *Surg Gynecol Obstet* 143:720, 1976.
299 Wilmore DW, Mason AD Jr, Pruitt BA Jr: Insulin response to glucose in hypermetabolic burn patients, *Ann Surg* 183:314, 1976.
300 Wilmore DW, Orcutt TW, Mason AD Jr et al: Alterations in hypothalamic function following thermal injury, *J Trauma* 15:697, 1975.
301 Wilson JS, Moncrief JA: Vapor pressure of normal and burned skin, *Ann Surg* 162:130, 1965.
302 Wood JJ, O'Mahony JB, Rodrick ML et al: Abnormalities of antibody production after thermal injury, *Arch Surg* 121:108, 1986.
303 Woolfrey BF, Fox JM, Quall CO: An evaluation of burn wound quantitative microbiology. I. Quantitative eschar cultures, *Am J Clin Pathol* 75:532, 1981.
304 Yurt RW, McManus AT, Mason AD Jr et al: Increased susceptibility to infection related to extent of burn injury, *Arch Surg* 119:183, 1984.
305 Yurt RW, Pruitt BA Jr: Decreased wound neutrophils and indiscrete margination in the pathogenesis of wound infection, *Surgery* 98:191,1985.
306 Zarem HA, Rattenborg CC, Harmel MH: Carbon monoxide toxicity in human fire victims, *Arch Surg* 107:851, 1973.
307 Zawacki BE, Spitzer DW, Mason AD Jr et al: Does increased evaporative water loss change hypermetabolism in burned patients? *Ann Surg* 171:236, 1970.
308 Zawacki BE, Azen SP, Imbus SH et al: Multifactorial probit analysis of mortality in burned patients, *Ann Surg* 189:1, 1979.

CHAPTER

18

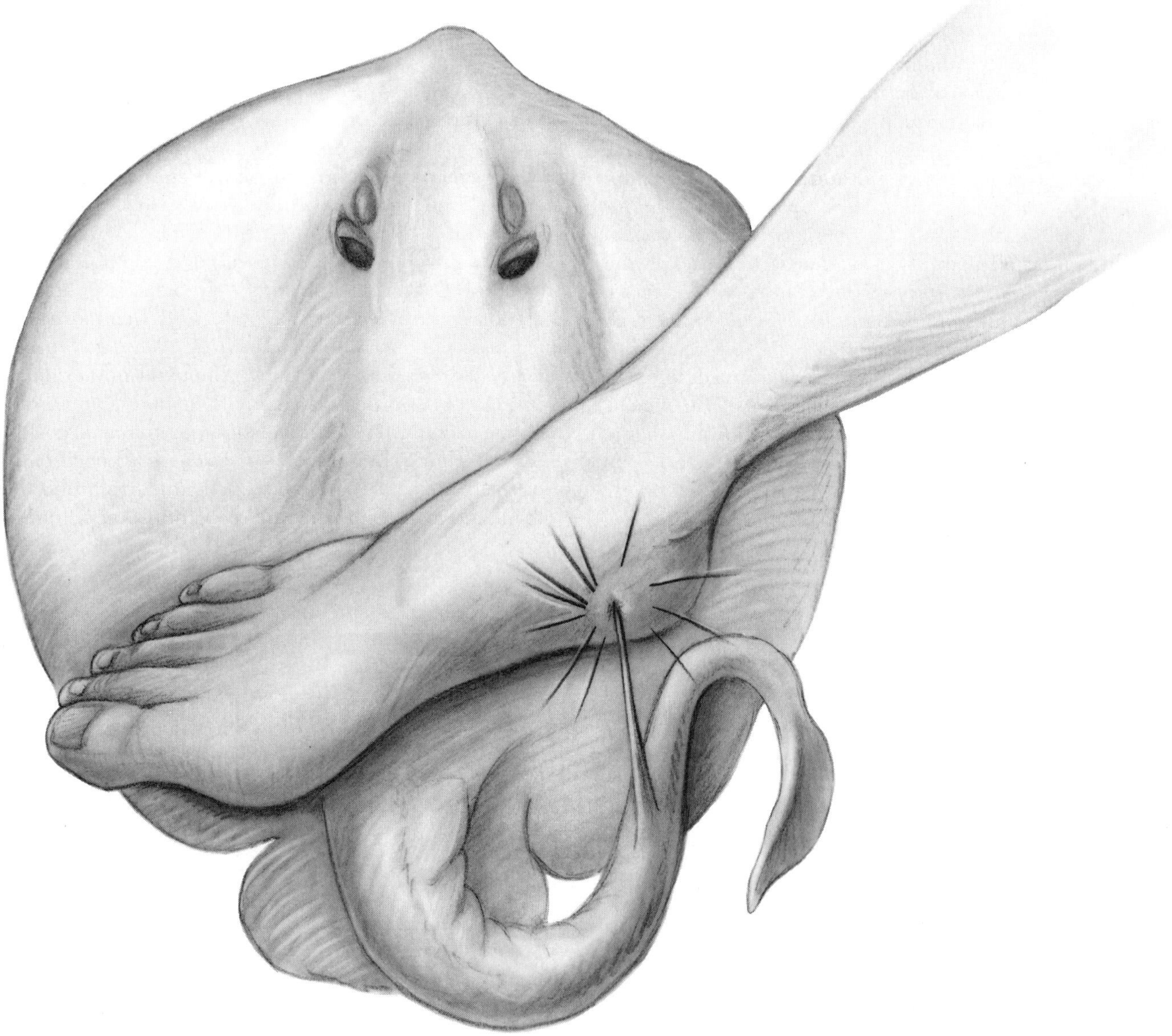

ENVIRONMENTAL INJURIES

Paul S. Auerbach • Rachel L. Chin • Rebecca Smith-Coggins

People who vacation, explore, preserve, and harvest encounter the natural environment. Although humans continue to devise intricate shelters and methods to escape animals, insects, and natural meteorologic forces, at times our surroundings still have the upper hand. This chapter highlights special situations related to the natural environment that might lead a victim to require a surgeon's care. Because a proper operating theater is an infrequent luxury in the wilderness, each discussion includes instructions for emergency field care.

SNAKE BITES

In the United States approximately 7000 envenomations, with 10 to 20 deaths, are reported each year.[199] Of the more than 3000 species of snakes worldwide, only about 300 are dangerous to humans.[273] Roughly 20 of the 120 species of snakes found in the United States are venomous. Indigenous venomous snakes are found in every state except Hawaii, Alaska, and Maine.[82] Indigenous venomous reptiles include members of the families Crotalidae (pit vipers) and Elapidae (coral snakes). Exotic snakes—Viperidae (true vipers), Colubridae ("hind-fang" snakes), and Hydrophidae (sea snakes)—are frequently imported to the United States for legal public and illegal private collections (the "underground zoo"), which contributes to the perplexities of identification and treatment.[118,245,257] Appendix 18-A offers a list of poisonous snakes a physician may encounter in the United States and Canada.

The management of venomous snake bites is frequently controversial and varies regionally. This section offers an approach that balances medical and surgical considerations.

Natural History

Snakes do not attack humans except in self-defense. A snake can strike accurately at a distance of one half its body length, with a striking speed estimated to exceed 2.4 m per second.[274] Snakes can strike in any direction; thus approaching them from the rear is not necessarily safe. If appropriately provoked, a snake may strike repeatedly. Venom mass may be released in increasing amounts with each bite.[185] *Snake Venom Poisoning,* by F.E. Russell, presents a superlative review of the subject.[226] Rattlesnake bites in humans are associated with massive venom release (20%), partial venom expulsion (60%), or no venom release (20%).

Pit Vipers

Members of the family Crotalidae, pit vipers include rattlesnakes, cottonmouths (water moccasins), and copperheads. A crotalid has two elongated, canaliculate maxillary teeth (to allow passage of venom from specialized venom glands), which it can fold against the roof of its mouth (Figure 18-1). Crotalids have vertically elliptic pupils, a depressed facial pit (heat receptor) between the eye and the nostril, a triangular head, and a single subcaudal row of belly scales leading up to the tail. Nonvenomous snakes and coral snakes, in contrast, do not have elongated fangs, and have a double row of subcaudal scales. Rattlesnakes have a distinctive rattle attached to the tail; however, this may be absent, because the rattle sometimes breaks off. Coloring is a difficult criterion for amateurs to use for identification.

Coral Snakes

Members of the family Elapidae, coral snakes have two elongated, canaliculate maxillary fangs somewhat shorter than those of the pit vipers. Most elapids have round pupils and no facial heat-sensory pits. Coral snakes have a black head, and the body has bands of red and black separated by rings of white or yellow. In general, the apposition of red on yellow (or white) indicates a venomous species; red apposed on black indicates lack of venom. Thus the rule, "Red on yellow, kill a fellow; red on black, venom lack." In the United States, the smaller western (Sonoran) coral snake *Micruroides euryxanthus euryxanthus),* which measures less than 50 cm, is found in Arizona and New Mexico. The larger eastern coral snake *(Micrurus fulvius fulvius),* which can grow to 0.9 m, is found in the Southeast and Gulf Coast states. The Texas coral snake *(M. fulvius tenere)* is found in the Mississippi basin and westward through central Texas. Other members of the family Elapidae include certain cobras, kraits, and sea snakes.

Colubrid Snakes

Some members of the family Colubridae ("hindfang" snakes) have fixed fangs and larger rear teeth. The family contains both venomous and nonvenomous species. In general, colubrid envenomations are less severe than those of crotalids or elapids. Typical rear-fanged snakes include the night snake *(Hypsiglena torquata),* the Sonora lyre snake *(Trimorphodon lambda),* the California lyre snake *(T. vandenburghi),* the Texas lyre snake *(T. vilkonsoni),* the red neck keelback *(Rhabdophis subminatus),* and the wandering garter snake *(Thamnophis elegans vagrans).**

Venom

Snakes produce venom in modified salivary glands located below the eyes in the soft tissue of the maxilla. Muscles aid the glands by forcing the liquid product into ducts and then into the hollow fangs.

Snake venoms are mixtures of peptide and nonpeptide toxins and enzymatic proteins of high and low (less than 30,000) molecular weight. Purified toxin fractions are highly active and linked to specific chemical and physiologic receptor sites. The enzymes present include hyaluronidase; transaminase; L-arginine-ester hydrolase; collagenase; lactic dehydrogenase; ribonuclease (RNase); deoxyribonuclease (DNase); acetylcholinesterase; 5'-nucleotidase; phosphodiesterase; phosphomonoesterase; alkaline phosphatase; acid phosphatase; nicotinamide-adenine dinucleotidase; phospholipase A, B, C, and D; various endonucleases; and assorted proteinases.[226] Crotalid venoms contain more than 40 different proteins, polypeptides, and peptides, with significant cross-antigenicity among species.

Procoagulant esterases act on fibrinogen to alter coagulation. Although platelet levels or platelet function, or both, may be normal, clotting time may be prolonged with defibrination, hypofibrinogenemia, and diffuse bleeding.[179, 232, 261, 271] In other instances, platelet aggregation and red cell lysis may result in microangiopathic hemolytic anemia and thrombocytopenia.[120] L-arginine-ester hydrolase releases bradykinin from plasma kininogen, causing vasodilatation and hypotension. Hyaluronidase cleaves glycoside bonds in acid mucopolysaccharides and facilitates the spread of venom. Other proteins contribute to severe organ system derangement and local tissue reactions.

Labeling the venom of a particular snake species a *neurotoxin* or a *cardiotoxin* is misleading because each component of venom exerts profound effects on many physiologic systems.[141] Thus in a particular victim, a predominantly neurotoxic venom may produce profound illnesses totally unrelated to the nervous system. For this reason, a victim of a venomous snakebite requires careful monitoring of all physiologic parameters.

*References 43, 161, 163, 226, 236, and 263.

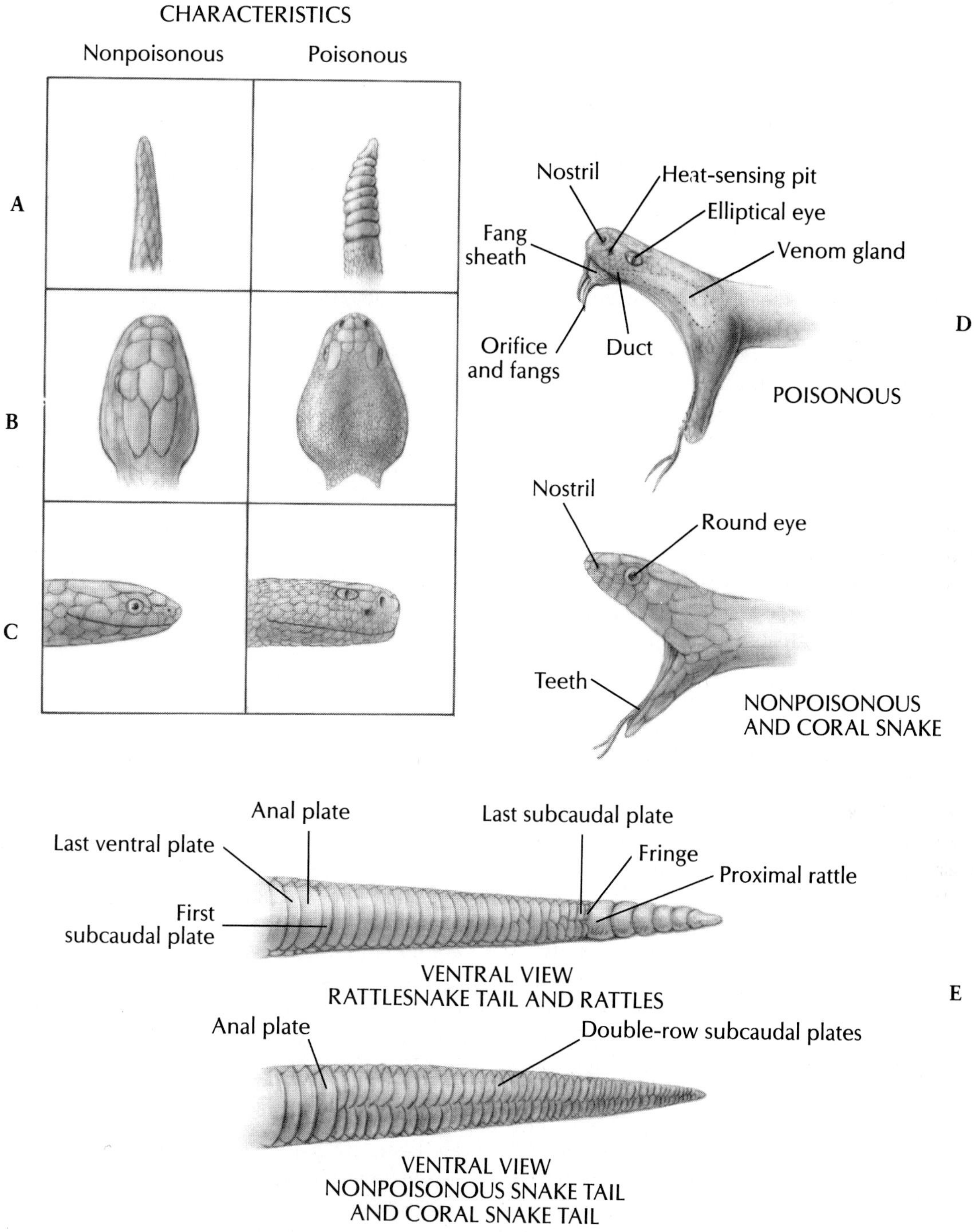

FIGURE 18-1 Characteristics of venomous crotalids. Many species have two hinged fangs that can be folded against the roof of the mouth. **A,** Tail rattles (may be absent) in rattlesnakes. **B,** Triangular head. **C,** Heat-sensing facial pit between the eye and the nostril. **D,** Well-developed venom glands, duct, and fangs. **E,** Single subcaudal row of belly scales leading up to the tail.

Clinical Presentation

The severity of a snake envenomation depends on the nature of the venom (species variation), the amount of venom (size and age of the snake), the number and location of the bites, and the victim's age, size, and underlying health.

Local Tissue Reaction

A pit viper bite generally induces tissue swelling within 5 to 10 minutes. This swelling initially surrounds the fang marks and progresses to involve the extremity (most bites occur on the legs and hands), usually over the course of 10 to 36 hours. The bite of the eastern diamondback rattlesnake produces the most severe pain and swelling (an entire extremity may be involved within 1 to 2 hours), followed in decreasing order of severity by the western diamondback, prairie, timber, red, Pacific, and black-tailed rattlesnakes and the sidewinder. Swelling may be minimal from the bite of the pygmy rattlesnake, massasauga, or copperhead. It is particularly noteworthy that the bite of the Mojave rattlesnake produces no severe local reactions; however, the venom is a potent systemic toxin.

Swelling usually is confined to the skin and rarely extends below external muscle fascia. Arterial circulation is rarely compromised, although claims have been made to the contrary.[122,158] Rare cases of muscle compartment syndromes have been documented.

Within several hours of the bite, local discoloration of the skin, bruising, and vesiculation may occur. Within 24 hours of the bite, petechiae and hemorrhagic blisters may be noted. Untreated, the local skin reaction can proceed to tissue sloughing, limb necrosis, and indolent infection. The bite of the coral snake generally is minimally painful, with little local tissue reaction. Fang marks may be difficult to identify.

Systemic Venom Effects

As previously noted, venom contains numerous enzymes and toxins that have at times been labeled *neurotoxins, cardiotoxins,* and *myotoxins.* These wreak havoc on several organ systems in a relatively predictable fashion, depending on the species and size of the snake. Problems encountered include nausea, vomiting, weakness, paresthesiae, hypotension, prolonged bleeding (epistaxis, petechiae, ecchymoses, hemoptysis, hematuria, hematochezia), hemolysis, pulmonary edema, acute tubular necrosis, renal failure, muscle necrosis, myocardial ischemia, paralysis, respiratory failure, and seizures. Immediate collapse, hypotension, arrhythmias, and coagulopathy may indicate intravascular envenomation, as a fang enters directly into a vein.

Signs of Envenomation

With crotalid envenomations, symptoms include diaphoresis; nausea; metallic, minty, or rubbery taste; pain; focal or diffuse weakness; paresthesiae; altered mental status (secondary to shock or hypoxia); and blurred vision. In order of decreasing frequency, signs include fang marks, swelling, blood pressure changes, ecchymosis, vesiculation, swollen lymph nodes, fasciculations, necrosis, hypersalivation, cyanosis, and bleeding disorders. In most cases of significant envenomation (with the exception of that caused by the Mojave rattlesnake), local tissue effects are noted within 15 minutes of the bite.[119] Immediate paresthesiae, anxiety, diaphoresis, and nausea (less than 5 minutes after the bite) can sometimes be attributed to fright and hyperventilation.

In the case of coral snake envenomation, pain at the site of the bite is minimal to moderate. Numbness and local weakness follow within 60 to 90 minutes. In a few hours the patient may develop systemic symptoms, including tremors, altered mental status (euphoria is common), ptosis, dysphagia, and hypersalivation. If the envenomation is severe (as with the bite of the eastern coral snake), the victim suffers dysarthria, diplopia, dysphagia, and dyspnea, reflecting cranial nerve and bulbar paralysis. In extreme cases this evolves to complete muscular and respiratory paralysis.

Emergency Field Care

In caring for a snakebite victim in the field, proper identification of the snake is helpful, because it allows the physician to anticipate signs and symptoms.[183] If positive identification of the live animal cannot be made at the scene of the accident, an extremely careful attempt should be made to capture the snake by striking it behind the head with a long stick, taking care to remain out of the snake's striking range (generally three quarters of the body length). Second or third strikes may cause severe envenomation. Decapitated head reactions may occur for an hour after death, so the seemingly dead snake must be carried in a container impenetrable by the snake or at a distance from the rescuer (on a long stick). If one does not know how to handle snakes, it is best to leave the animal at the scene.

Incision and suction should be used only under these conditions: (1) the victim is seen within 5 minutes of the bite; (2) the victim is elderly or chronically ill; (3) the victim weighs less than 31.5 kg; (4) the snake is positively identified as venomous; (5) clear puncture wounds are noted; *and* (6) antivenin is unavailable for at least 2 hours.

Two longitudinal, parallel incisions should be made directly through the fang marks for a length of 5 mm to a depth of 5 to 10 mm. Crisscross incisions are contraindicated. It is probably far superior to apply suction with The Extracter (Sawyer Products, Safety Harbor, Fla.) and to use the mouth only as a last resort, because introducing mouth flora into the wound creates a contaminated human bite. Suction with The Extracter should be applied for 1 hour. If oral suction is used, a rescuer with denuded intraoral mucous membranes should take care to quickly spit out the mixture of blood and venom. Clinical enthusiasm for using incision and mouth suction therapy is virtually absent.

The affected body part should be splinted and maintained in a dependent position. The victim should avoid all unnecessary exertion and should be transported immediately to a hospital for antivenin therapy. The victim should not be given alcoholic beverages, and antivenin management should not be attempted in the field because of the risk of anaphylaxis.

Australasian snake envenomations (predominantly elapids) are initially managed by applying a cloth pad (e.g., 8 × 8 × 3 cm) to the bite site under a broad, mildly constrictive bandage that covers the entire extremity to inhibit systemic absorption of venom.[6,17,188] When considering using this technique for North American snake envenomations, the rescuer must bear in mind that pit viper envenomations far outnumber elapid envenomations. It is not known whether local sequestration of pit viper venom worsens local tissue effects.

A constriction bandage should be applied only under these conditions: (1) the victim is a small child or an elderly adult; (2) preliminary tissue signs of envenomation exist (with the exception of the Mojave rattlesnake, in which case a constriction bandage should be used in the absence of signs); (3) the snake is positively identified as venomous; and (4) antivenin therapy will be delayed for more than 2 hours. The purpose of the bandage is to retard proximal spread of venom in an extremity by impeding superficial venous and lymphatic flow. A constriction bandage should be loose enough to admit a fingertip; distal arterial circulation (palpable pulses) should not be compromised. A tourniquet should not be used; taken to the extreme, the decision to apply a tourniquet is to sacrifice a limb to save a life.

Removal of a constriction bandage may be associated with the release of a bolus of venom into the systemic circulation. The physician should be prepared to manage hypotension with antivenin and volume replacement.

Hospital Management

Blood samples are drawn for the following determinations: hemoglobin, hematocrit, red blood cell indices, white blood cell count, whole blood type and crossmatch, platelet count, erythrocyte sedimentation rate, prothrombin time, partial thromboplastin time, arterial blood gases, sodium, potassium, blood urea nitrogen, creatinine, chloride, glucose, creatine phosphokinase, total protein, albumin, and fibrinogen. Urine is obtained for urinalysis, an electrocardiogram is recorded, and a chest radiograph is obtained. If the victim is in respiratory distress, pulmonary function values (forced expiratory volume in 1 second [FEV_1] and forced vital capacity [FVC]) are measured at the bedside.

An intravenous line should be placed for infusion of crystalloid solutions. If antivenin therapy is anticipated or if the patient is hypotensive, a second intravenous line should be placed.

If the bite wound is on an extremity, the circumference of the wound at the advancing edge of the swelling and just proximal to the bite should be measured. The results are recorded every 10 to 15 minutes until no further progression of swelling occurs.

The need to administer antivenin should be determined. If local signs of envenomation (pain, swelling, discoloration) progress rapidly, antivenin is necessary. Antivenin may still be necessary even if there are few or no local signs (e.g., if the bite is from the Mojave rattlesnake). Clearly established systemic signs of envenomation imply a significant venom introduction, and antivenin therapy should proceed without delay.

Antivenin should be administered as described in the following paragraphs.

The severity of envenomation is determined. Although convenient, a numeric grading system (1 to 5) is arbitrary and probably inaccurate.[227] The following system should be used to grade envenomations.

No envenomation. No local or systemic reaction.

Mild envenomation. Local swelling without systemic signs and without abnormal laboratory results. *Close observation is required.*

Moderate envenomation. Progressive swelling or systemic symptoms, any sign of coagulopathy. *Antivenin is necessary.*

Severe envenomation. Severe swelling, severe systemic signs, and/or marked laboratory derangements. *Antivenin is necessary.*

A skin test can be performed for sensitivity to horse serum. This should be done only after the decision to administer antivenin has been made and not to determine whether antivenin should be given. Many manufacturers recommend that a preliminary skin test of diluted antivenin or horse serum be done to attempt to predict whether the product will cause a reaction. However, there are several problems with the skin test. First, it delays actual administration of antivenin, because it takes at least 25 to 30 minutes to administer and read the test. Second, approximately 10% of patients with a negative skin test result still develop an early reaction on infusion of antivenin.[142] Third, a positive skin test result does not prove that the patient will definitely have an early reaction and does not contraindicate giving antivenin in cases of life- or limb-threatening envenomations.[114,226] Fourth, patients occasionally develop anaphylaxis to the skin test itself. Finally, the test in no way predicts who will develop delayed serum sickness.[142,226] For these reasons, it may be wiser just to begin the antivenin infusion at a slow rate with the physician at the bedside, closely monitoring the patient for any sign of reaction.*

If the skin test result is positive, the antivenin should be diluted in sterile water to a 1:100 concentration for administration. Successive vials can be less dilute if the allergic reaction is minimal (controlled by antihistamines and epinephrine).

The effectiveness of antivenin depends on specificity (monovalent, polyvalent), antibody titer, purity, pharmacokinetics of venom versus antivenin, and time and route of administration. The antivenin must neutralize

*References 98, 113, 170, 216, and 258.

the numerous toxic proteins, polypeptides, and peptides in snake venom.

Antivenin is administered. The rational is to provide early and adequate antivenin to neutralize the toxin at the tissue site before it gains a systemic foothold. In the United States, Wyeth Laboratories manufactures two antivenins:

1. Antivenin (Crotalidae) Polyvalent, North and South American antisnakebite serum
2. An antivenin for the venom of the eastern coral snake *(Micrurus fulvius)* (the bite of the western coral snake *[Micruroides euryxanthus]* does not require antivenin because no fatality has ever been reported with this snakebite)

Antivenin should be administered intravenously; care should be taken to provide adequate doses for children and the elderly, who have a decreased volume of distribution and therefore increased sensitivity to the effects of venom.[39] Administering any portion of the antivenin intramuscularly is no longer recommended. The *initial* dose of antivenin should be:

1. *No* envenomation: no antivenin
2. *Mild* envenomation: 0 to 5 vials (50 ml)
3. *Moderate* envenomation: 10 vials (100 ml)
4. *Severe* envenomation: 10 to 15 vials (100 to 150 ml)

The affected extremity should be measured every 15 minutes. Antivenin (5 to 10 vials) should be administered every 1 to 2 hours until there is no further progression of tissue swelling, and major amelioration of systemic symptoms occurs.[42]

A bite from the Mojave rattlesnake *(Crotalus scutulatus)* requires an initial dose of 10 vials, because local signs of envenomation may not adequately represent the potential systemic toxicity of the venom.

Eastern coral snake *(Micrurus fulvius)* bites should be managed initially with 3 to 6 vials of antivenin.[121] A direct correlation exists between the length of this snake and the amount of dried venom elaborated. A large snake (50 to 60 cm) can produce enough venom to require a minimum of 10 vials of antivenin for neutralization.[83]

Although antivenin is most effective if administered within 4 hours of envenomation, any patient who shows progression of the local reaction or any systemic manifestations should be treated in the first 24 hours with antivenin.

If a patient is known to be sensitive to horse serum, has a positive skin test result, or develops signs of an allergic reaction or anaphylaxis during antivenin therapy, aggressive medical management is required.[195] All recipients of antivenin should be pretreated with 50 to 100 mg of intravenous diphenhydramine (1 mg/kg in children). The total dose of antivenin should be reconstituted and mixed in 500 to 1000 ml of saline solution or 5% dextrose in water.[194] If no reaction occurs, the rate of antivenin administration can be increased gradually to get the total dose administered within 1 to 2 hours.[7,229] If signs of anaphylaxis develop, 0.1 to 0.2 ml aliquots of antivenin should be alternated with 0.3 to 1 ml (0.03 to 0.1 mg) intravenous doses of aqueous epinephrine 1:10,000. The patient must be treated in the intensive care unit, using electrocardiographic and blood pressure monitoring. The dose of epinephrine should not exceed that which elevates the pulse rate above 150.

A pregnant woman poses a unique treatment problem. Epinephrine in therapeutic doses may cause alpha-adrenergic constriction of the uterine arteries. Some suggest treating hypotension associated with anaphylaxis in pregnancy with ephedrine (25 to 50 mg slow intravenous push), a noncatecholamine adrenergic drug that preserves uterine blood flow, in combination with an infusion of isoproterenol (2 to 15 μg/minute) to manage bronchospasm.[77]

Tetanus toxoid (0.5 ml) is administered if the patient has not been immunized in the previous 5 years. If the victim has not been immunized in the previous 10 years, hyperimmune tetanus globulin (250 units) is administered in the opposite extremity.

The use of prophylactic antibiotics for the snakebite wound is empiric and controversial. Established infections should be treated on the basis of appropriate culture and antimicrobial sensitivity determinations. The bacteriology of rattlesnake venom has been studied, and isolates of *Pseudomonas aeruginosa, Proteus* species, coagulase-negative *Staphylococcus,* and *Clostridum* species are considered oral flora of the rattlesnake.[105] In view of the propensity of snakebite wounds to develop ischemia and tissue necrosis, it is justifiable to treat the victim of venomous snakebite with moderate intravenous doses of prophylactic penicillin (600,000 units aqueous penicillin G every 4 hours) or a broad-spectrum cephalosporin (cefoxitin, 2 g every 6 hours).

Life support is provided. Snake venom can cause a number of physiologic derangements that may require intense medical management. Hemolysis or coagulopathy may require blood transfusions. Platelet consumption is not uncommon and may require platelet transfusions (corticosteroid administration does not appear to be efficacious). Antivenin treatment must be started before blood products are given to avoid feeding a consumptive coagulopathy. Hypovolemic shock should be treated with crystalloid infusions and fresh frozen plasma. Urine output and renal function should be closely monitored, because hemolysis may cause acute renal failure, and hypotensive nephropathy may cause acute tubular necrosis.

Serum sickness after administration of antivenin is treated with corticosteroids and antihistamines. An initial loading dose of prednisone (40 to 60 mg for adults;

2 to 5 mg/kg, not to exceed 50 mg, for children) should be administered and maintained daily until symptoms are markedly resolved. The corticosteroid should be tapered over a 2- to 3-week course to avoid inducing adrenal insufficiency. Although immune complexes can be measured by various tests, the values may not correlate with the clinical presentation.[96,189]

The site of the wound should be immobilized in a position of function, cushioned, and kept slightly elevated. Devitalized tissue should be surgically debrided. Each day the wound should be gently cleaned with scrubs or brief whirlpool treatments of dilute solutions (no greater than 1:10) of hydrogen peroxide or povidone-iodine, in a manner analogous to burn wound treatment. Skin grafting may be necessary if large surface areas are involved.

Several types of treatment that have been used are controversial and have not been proved effective. These include tourniquets, incision and suction, electric shock, cryotherapy, early excision of the wound, and routine fasciotomy.

The risk of compartment syndrome after such bites is relatively low because most of the venom usually is deposited in subcutaneous tissues.[91,175,226,267] When venom is injected into muscles, the major cause of necrosis is the direct effect of the venom, *not* increases in intracompartmental pressures.[58,89-93,111] Certainly, the possibility of compartment syndrome exists, and because the changes in the bitten extremity may closely mimic a compartment syndrome (pain, swelling, discoloration, numbness), it is important in such cases to monitor intracompartmental pressures using any of the simple, relatively noninvasive techniques available.[89,92] If intracompartmental pressures rise above 30 to 40 mm Hg, fasciotomy and continued administration of antivenin are indicated.[58,89,92,228] Use of routine prophylactic fasciotomies is overly aggressive and only prolongs the patient's hospital stay.[7,33,113,163]

WILD AND DOMESTIC ANIMAL ATTACKS

Animal bites, specifically mammalian (dog) bites, are a common surgical problem, accounting for approximately 1% of emergency department visits in the United States each year.[147,169] The estimated incidence of animal bites ranges from 215 to 809 per 100,000 people each year.[128,200,248] This is probably an underestimate of the true incidence of animal-induced wounds (up to 2 million per year for dog bites alone) because many people do not seek formal medical care.[139,224] The annual cost for animal bite–related medical care may approach $25 million to $50 million.[22,25] In other parts of the world, where humans and undomesticated feral species inhabit common territory, severe attacks, maulings, and deaths are more frequent. Prompt recognition that an injury has resulted from an animal attack, appropriate life-support measures, and meticulous surgical wound care are essential to minimize morbidity and secondary infections from traumatic wounds.[140]

Dog Attacks

More than 100 million dogs and cats are kept as domestic pets in the United States. The number of bites has been estimated to range from 300 to 700 per 100,000 population each year. The incidence of bites probably will increase as the rate of increase in the domestic dog population exceeds that of human population growth. In fact, 1 in 20 dogs will bite a human each year; the average dog bites a human once in its lifetime.[279] Although as many as half of all dog bites may go unreported, nearly 10% of bites require suturing, with an occasional visit to the operating room. Males are more frequently bitten than females, and most victims are under 20 years of age, with preschool and small children at greatest risk.[143,200] Domestic pets and guard dogs, rather than feral renegades, are the most frequent biters.[26] One of three households in the United States owns at least one dog; the family's or neighbor's animal bites most victims.[155] Larger animals—working breeds and guard dogs, such as retrievers, German shepherds, Great Danes, Saint Bernards, and Doberman pinschers—are most commonly implicated in serious attacks.[22,123]

One may say with some justification that for children, no dogs are friendly dogs.[31,155] Dogs bite most adults on the arm, hand, or leg, but they commonly bite small children on the face, scalp, and neck (30% to 80% of bites in children under 5 years of age), presumably because children are willing to bring their faces close to a dog's mouth, will kiss strange animals, may be unintentionally provocative, or will mount an inefficient defense when attacked.* Facial biting may be an extension of the face and mouth biting interaction of dogs with each other. By some estimates, as many as 44,000 children are bitten on the face each year. These bites may lead to scattered multiple skull fractures, dural penetration, cerebral contusions and hematomas, brain abscesses, meningitis, mandibular fracture, nasal fractures, and disfiguring soft tissue injuries, most commonly of the lip, nose and cheek.† Fatalities occur most often in small children, who are physically defenseless against a dog's violent attack.

Although local soft tissue infections are the most common sequelae to dog bites, syndromes resembling generalized Shwartzman phenomenon or thrombotic thrombocytopenic purpura have been reported to follow dog bites.[251]

*References 30, 47, 53, 136, 143, 155, and 156.
†References 34, 156, 197, 206, 209, 237, and 272.

Cat Attacks

Cats are increasingly on the attack, with 5% to 19% of animal bites in the United States attributed to felines, an overall figure of as many as 300,000 bites per year. Women may be more prone than men to cat bites and scratches.[147] Although not as overtly aggressive as dogs, cats have the added weaponry of claws, which are contaminated with saliva from constant preening and in some cases by decaying rodents.[136] A cat bite wound is a puncture wound, with a high propensity for infection, particularly by *Pasteurella multocida*. Some cat bite injuries are deep wounds that may penetrate to bones, tendons, and joint spaces.[66,250,254] In addition to local infection of soft tissue wounds, cat bites and scratches may lead to plague, rabies, tularemia, or cat-scratch disease.[270]

Cat-scratch disease is an ulceroglandular disease transmitted by healthy cats and kittens. The disease may also be transferred by mice, rats, porcupine quills, wood splinters, and fish hooks. The organism *Afipia felis,*[36] which is thought to be an etiologic agent of cat-scratch disease, is a pleomorphic, gram-negative bacillus that stains with Warthin-Starry silver impregnation or modified Brown-Hopp's tissue Gram's stain.[173,268] The organism has been identified in samples of infected lymph nodes and skin from the site of primary inoculation. Seven to 14 days after a cat bite or scratch, which is frequently not recognized, the victim develops a vesicle or pustule at the site of injury. Shortly thereafter, regional lymphadenopathy and lymphadenitis accompany a 2-week illness characterized by nausea, vomiting, malaise, anorexia, fatigue, and fever. In rare cases a victim shows variations of oculoglandular fever, parotitis, erythema nodosum, morbilliform rash, osteolytic lesions, thrombocytopenic purpura, transverse myelitis, or encephalitis.[205,242,256] Cat-scratch disease may mimic diseases of the lymph nodes, such as sarcoidosis, tularemia, Hodgkin's disease, lymphogranuloma venereum, brucellosis, sporotrichosis, and lymphoma. There is no reliable diagnostic test for the disease. The current intradermal skin test is a reaction to an extract of pus taken from the lymph nodes of affected victims.

The disease is self-limited over the course of 2 to 3 months and generally responds to trimethoprim-sulfamethoxazole or rifampin, given for at least 5 to 7 days for an acutely ill child or adolescent.[55] In a severely ill patient, gentamicin is recommended, given every 8 hours for 5 to 10 days, depending upon the clinical response.[29,230] For adults, ciprofloxacin, 500 to 750 mg twice daily given orally, has been effective in 75% to 100% of patients.[133] Tender, fluctuant lymph nodes may be aspirated under sterile conditions to relieve pain.

Rat Bites

Rat bites are predominately a problem of cities, although the wild rodent population in foreign countries carries the risk of rabies virus transmission.[193] Most rats do not attack per se but rather chew on the disadvantaged victim (usually very young, elderly, intoxicated, or infirm) in a feeding activity. Single or multiple bite wounds may be present, but they rarely result in significant tissue loss.

In addition to local soft tissue wound infections, rat bites may lead to rat-bite fever from the gram-negative *Streptobacillus moniliformis* (North America) or *Spirillum minus* (Asia), various forms of plaque *(Yersinia pestis)*, melioidosis, and leptospirosis.[139,171]

Rat-bite fever, including Haverhill fever, which is caused by drinking milk contaminated with *Streptobacillus moniliformis,* develops after a rapidly healing bite, with an incubation period of 1 to 4 days (in rare cases, the onset may be delayed up to 3 weeks). The onset is marked by fever and chills, vomiting, pharyngitis, headaches, myalgia, and weakness. These symptoms are followed in 1 to 7 days by a diffuse, dull red, maculopapular, morbilliform or purpuric rash over the lateral and extensor surfaces of the extremities that may involve the palms and soles with petechiae, accompanied by a polyarticular migratory arthritis. The first episode generally lasts for 10 to 20 days. Untreated, the disease may appear over the course of several months in isolated periods of 4 to 10 days each. Death occasionally follows endocarditis or pneumonia.

The spirochete *Spirillum minus* causes spirillary rat-bite fever. After an average incubation period of 7 to 18 days, the bite wound or primary chancre shows erythema, induration, suppuration, and eschar formation. Lymphangitis and lymphadenitis accompany these tissue signs with relapsing fever, chills, severe myalgia, and a purple or red-brown macular rash that originates at the bite site. Again, although the syndrome usually resolves after a few weeks, it may recur spontaneously at intervals for years. Routine blood tests demonstrate a mild anemia or leukocytosis but generally are not diagnostic. Blood cultures or rising antibody titers are necessary to isolate *S. moniliformis*. *Spirillum minus* may be demonstrated on darkfield microscopy in exudates of the bite wound or in adjacent lymph nodes. Gas-liquid chromatography may permit rapid identification of the streptobacillus.

Both types of rat-bite fever are exquisitely responsive to a 10- to 14-day course of parenteral penicillin (600,000 units procaine penicillin, given intramuscularly every 12 hours), with the exception of rare resistant strains, which should be treated with streptomycin or tetracycline.[139]

Wound Management of Wild Animal Bites

Immediate Management

Management of an animal bite wound or mauling is based on traditional surgical principles, with the caveat that these wounds are often highly contaminated with soil, saliva, animal hair, excrement, and their associated bacteria. In the prehospital setting, attention should be immediately directed to preserving the airway and controlling serious bleeding. Blood loss may be severe, particularly from scalp injuries, and hypovolemic shock should be anticipated. Pressure and compression dressing usually are sufficient to control brisk bleeding. The rescuer should resist the temptation to blindly probe wounds in an effort to clamp bleeding vessels, because this often results in permanent injury to nerves and otherwise uninjured blood vessels. Applying a tourniquet is only appropriate if uncontrollable bleeding from an extremity will lead to exsanguination.

If the victim cannot be carried to a hospital within 12 hours, the wound should be irrigated copiously with clear water, scrubbed gently with soap, and irrigated until clear of all residue. If any chance exists that the bite is from a rabid animal, the wound should be irrigated and then soaked or scrubbed with 1% or 2% benzalkonium chloride, 10% povidone-iodine solution, or hand soap. After a contact period of 5 minutes, the wound should be reirrigated. Unless necessary to allow extrication, neither suturing nor close approximation of the wound edges of an animal bite should be attempted in the field.

Definitive Management

INSPECTION. Regardless of field management, when a victim is brought to an emergency department, the wound should be thoroughly inspected. After a thorough neurovascular examination, the wound should be anesthetized with local infiltration (without epinephrine) or local regional nerve block.[243] If a local anesthetic is used, passing the needle through intact skin rather than through the wound edge often is recommended, although no comparative data exist for infection rates of the different methods. If the animal may have carried the rabies virus, the wound edges should be infiltrated with 1% procaine hydrochloride.

Wounds are explored in a standard fashion, using the operating room and surgical magnification whenever microsurgery will be necessary to repair damaged structures of the hand or face. As previously mentioned, all wounds should be thoroughly irrigated, using a technique that provides sufficient force (10 to 20 pounds/in^2) to dislodge superficial bacteria. One such method is to irrigate the wound thoroughly with a minimum of 250 ml of saline, 1% to 10% povidone-iodine solution in saline, or the surfactant Pluronic F-68, using a commercial irrigation syringe with a 19-gauge steel needle or 18-gauge intravenous plastic catheter to direct the stream.[65,70,221,222,244] Pulsatile wound irrigation has no definite advantage, and commercial irrigation kits are not superior to simple syringe and needle techniques (although they are more convenient). Low-pressure irrigation with a bulb or aseptic syringe (0.05 pounds/in^2) does not remove bacterial contaminants.[244] The size and appearance of the wound determines the volume of irrigant. Jet pressure irrigation (up to 90 pounds/in^2) may actually force bacteria deeper into the wound; irrigation with antibiotic solutions appears to have variable added benefit.[68]

In general, domestic animal bites do not call for routine radiographic studies, with the exception of skull films in infants and small children. Depressed skull fracture, mandibular fracture, dural penetration, meningitis, and brain abscess have been reported to result from animal attacks in which an infant's entire head or a small child's face was clamped in the viselike grip of an animal's mouth.[156,206]

WOUND CLOSURE. Besides the issue of prophylactic administration of antibiotics, the other real controversy in animal wound management involves wound closure. Although many authors decry the use of primary repair, it appears that many animal bite wounds (particularly dog bites) can be sutured if they have been inflicted within 12 hours of repair, are properly irrigated and debrided, do not involve a high-risk area (e.g., the hand), and are not feline, primate, or human in origin.[45,69,223] The risk of infection must be weighed against cosmetic considerations. Fortunately, the face is a highly vascular area with a low inherent risk of wound infection, and most injuries can be closed primarily.

Proper surgical technique is probably the greatest single factor in controlling infection after an animal bite that causes a crush injury rather than a clean laceration.[49,65,66,253] It is not uncommon to underestimate the extent of an animal bite wound when judging by external visual inspection. After a local or regional anesthetic (lidocaine without epinephrine) is administered, all crushed or ragged skin edges should be sharply debrided; macerated subcutaneous tissue and fat should be removed.[279] Hemostasis may be obtained with careful and not overzealous electrical coagulation.[279] If the muscle and bone are involved, they should be conservatively debrided to preserve the normal anatomic appearance. Reapproximation of tissue layers should be achieved using the minimum number of absorbable sutures, because these unavoidably become foreign bodies and a source of infection.[223] If the skin is to be closed, nylon or polypropylene should be used in an interrupted fashion; the running suture technique should be avoided. If additional support is needed to maintain a wound closure that is under tension, adhesive strips may be placed between the interrupted sutures. If skin grafts are required, split-thickness coverage may be preferable to a full-thickness graft.

All wounds closed in the emergency department or outpatient surgicenter should be splinted for 48 to 72 hours.[202] Because dog bite wounds frequently heal initially with indurated, erythematous scars, scar revisions should be delayed for 8 to 12 months, after the scars have softened and faded.[231]

Puncture wounds present unique problems for closure. They have an inherent propensity for infection, primarily because they are difficult to irrigate effectively.[49] Excision of puncture wounds has been suggested for the bites of many animals, but there is no clear-cut advantage to this technique. A puncture wound should never be closed unless provision is made for eliminating dead space with adequate drainage.[231] Application of topical antimicrobial ointments is a two-edged sword. Although these agents clearly decrease the concentration of bacteria on the wound's surface and to a certain extent penetrate the wound's edges, they can create a "grease seal" or plug over a deep puncture wound and prevent adequate drainage. They should be used sparingly and in a nonocclusive fashion.

Extensive tissue damage may require the collaboration of general, plastic, and orthopedic surgeons and neurosurgeons. All scalp wounds and deep facial wounds, particularly in children, should be thoroughly explored to exclude underlying bony injury.[266] Exploration is particularly important when treating the bite of a large animal (e.g., a hunting dog or great cat, such as a lion or tiger). Deep puncture wounds of the neck, caused when a victim is carried by an animal, should be evaluated with cervical spine radiographs. If a fracture is visualized directly by a radiograph or computed tomography (CT) scan, exploration in the operating room is mandatory to inspect the underlying dura and provide complete debridement and irrigation.[156] Wilberger and Pang[272] have recommended that all bone fragments be discarded, and cranioplasty be performed in a delayed fashion as necessary. After surgery, the victim should be given a 7- to 10-day course of oxacillin or cephalothin.

Dog bites. Although the infection rate for most common dog bite wounds is between 5% and 10%, many physicians are not comfortable with primary repair. An acceptable alternative is the technique of delayed primary closure, in which the wound is left open under moist or wet-to-dry dressings for 3 to 4 days. A wound that does not become infected during this period may be closed without detriment to wound cosmetics or rapidity of healing.

Cat bites and hand wounds. Cat bites and wounds of the hand should not be sutured or taped tightly closed, because the infection rate has been reported to approach 50%. They should be irrigated, debrided, and drained around an iodoform gauze wick or left open for delayed primary closure after a minimum of 2 days or after drainage has ceased.

Rat bites. Rat bites do not show an increased propensity for infection, nor do rats in the United States transmit the rabies virus to humans. Rat-bite puncture wounds should be carefully irrigated and left open to heal unless such a method will cause disfigurement.

Splinting. When wound repair involves a joint, a splint should be applied in the position of function for the first few days. The splint should allow frequent inspection of the wound for signs of infection (erythema, swelling, increasing tenderness, purulent drainage, lymphagitic streaking, regional lymphadenopathy, or fever), and the patient should be started on antibiotic therapy. Upper or lower extremity wounds should be kept elevated.

Tetanus immunization. Tetanus immunization is standard and should follow all animal bite wounds or maulings.

Wound Infection and the Bacteriology of Animal Bites

Organisms cultured from animal bite wounds are listed in the box below. Infection can be caused by numerous organisms, and at least one fourth of infected wounds grow out multiple species. *Pasteurella multocida, Staphylococcus aureus,* and *Pseudomonas* and *Streptococcus* species are identified relatively often from infected wounds. Anaerobic species also are commonly present, but because they are mixed with aerobic species, their precise pathogenic role usually is indeterminate.

ORGANISMS CULTURED FROM ANIMAL BITE WOUNDS

Pasteurella multocida
P. mirabilis
P. antipestifer
Pseudomonas sp.
Actinobacillus sp.
Haemophilus sp.
Bacteroides sp.
Peptococcus sp.
Peptostreptococcus sp.
Eubacterium sp.
Veillonella sp.
Propionibacterium acnes
Corynebacterium sp.
Bacillus sp.
Staphylococcus epidermidis
Staphylococcus aureus
Streptococcus viridans
Streptococcus pyogenes
Micrococcus luteus
Neisseria sp.
Moraxella osloensis
CDC alpha-numeric groups M-5, EF-4, IIj, and IIr
Eikenella corrodens
Fusobacterium sp.
Erysipelothrix sp.
Enterobacter aerogenes
Flavobacterium sp.
Chromobacterium sp.*

*References 8, 34, 46, 103-107, and 254.

The flora in animals' mouths is also known to change over the course of the year and to vary according to geographic location and the animal's health and diet. Thus it is difficult to predict what organism is likely to cause a wound infection in any given case.[153]

In addition to local wound cellulitis, the infectious complications of animal bites include osteomyelitis and septic arthritis; meningitis, brain abscess and subdural empyema; endocarditis; pyelonephritis; peritonitis; appendicular abscess; pneumonia and lung abscess; mycotic aneurysm; infection of vascular grafts and prosthetic heart valves; and bacteremia and sepsis. Various species have been identified in these situations. Fatal shock and disseminated intravascular coagulation have been reported following bacteremia caused by both CDC group DF-2 and *Bacteroides* organisms.[153]

Most infections that appear in animal bite wounds during the first 24 hours (in some cases, as rapidly as within 2 hours of inoculation) are likely to involve *P. multocida* and to be accompanied by fever, rapid progression, and marked lymphadenopathy.[35,86,167,255] Wound infections that begin more insidiously, after 24 hours, are more commonly staphylococcal or streptococcal infection.[66]

Recommendations for Drug Therapy

An uncomplicated dog bite wound (less than 24 hours old and not involving the hand, bone, tendon, tendon sheath, joint capsule, or joint space) does not require prophylactic antibiotics.[73] If the wound is complicated, the antibiotics of choice include cephalexin or dicloxacillin (500 mg by mouth four times a day for 5 to 7 days). Erythromycin is a good alternative if the risk of contamination with *P. multocida* is low.

All puncture wounds from a cat bite and significant cat scratches (puncture wound or full-thickness laceration deeper and longer than 2 cm) require prophylactic antibiotic therapy for 7 days. These drugs include penicillin, cephalexin, or dicloxacillin.[74] If the patient is allergic to penicillin, tetracycline may be used (erythromycin is not effective against *P. multocida*).[70,241,269] Given the low cross-reactivity (less than 10%) between the penicillins and cephalosporins, cephalexin may be a better alternative.

All primate bites (and human bites) should be treated with prophylactic antibiotics.[66] These drugs include penicillin and dicloxacillin in combination or a broad-spectrum cephalosporin with anaerobic coverage.[104] In addition, all injured body parts should be splinted in a position of function, and the wounds should be examined daily for signs of infection. If infection occurs after prophylactic therapy, the patient must be hospitalized immediately for intravenous administration of antibiotics, which should include an aminoglycoside.

At the earliest appearance of an infection after an animal bite or mauling, the appropriate cultures should be performed and antibiotics should be administered. If the infection is a minor one, oral agents may be used. Intravenous antibiotics are indicated under these conditions:

1. Cellulitis appears quickly.
2. Signs of lymphangitic spread are present (red streaking, regional lymphadenopathy).
3. The victim is febrile.
4. Swelling is marked.
5. The victim is immunosuppressed.
6. It appears that the victim will not comply with outpatient treatment.

Sepsis has been reported after animal bites and may be caused by unusual and virulent bacterial species. At the earliest sign of systemic infection, cultures for aerobes and anaerobes should be obtained from both wound and blood. Triple antibiotic therapy, pending culture results, may reasonably be initiated with a cephalosporin, aminoglycoside, and penicillin or clindamycin. With regard to the antibiotic susceptibilities of *P. multocida,* the most active drugs appear to be penicillin G, tetracycline, ampicillin, carbenicillin, cephalothin, and chloramphenicol. Penicillin is the drug of choice. Drugs wih relatively low activities include semisynthetic penicillins, clindamycin, erythromycin, and aminoglycosides. Suspected *Pseudomonas* sepsis requires substitution of carbenicillin for penicillin, whereas *Bacteroides* organisms may be treated with clindamycin, metronidazole, cefoxitin, ceftizoxime, or chloramphenicol.

Rabies

The dreaded complication of an animal bite is rabies virus infection. All bites should be reported to the local health department to facilitate the capture and identification of potentially rabid animals. In the United States, rabies has been documented in wild and domestic animals in every state except Hawaii.[51] Abroad, particularly in the Indo-Pacific region and in Asia, Africa, and Latin America, domestic animal immunization practices are haphazard, and dogs are the main source of human exposure.[2] Rabies is a major cause of mortality in India. Australia, New Zealand, Great Britain, Ireland, and Antarctica appear to be human rabies free. As many as 20,000 human deaths related to rabies have been reported to the World Health Organization in a calendar year.

Animals of Risk

Pet vaccination programs in the Untied States have made rabies virus a rare discovery in domestic cats and dogs, including those that have not been vaccinated.[99,260] The greatest reservoir for rabies is found among wild animals, predominately skunks (up to 50%), raccoons, bobcats, foxes, coyotes, and bats (although bats may carry the virus for long asymptomatic periods, recent publications from spelunking agencies suggest that the human rabies risk from bats may be overstated). In the United States, geographic differences exist in the endemic carrier species. For instance, the raccoon is the major reservoir in the mid-Atlantic and southeastern states; the red fox in the eastern states; the spotted skunk in the Plains states; the striped skunk in the Rocky Mountain states and California; and the bat throughout the United States.[275] Other animals that may infrequently carry the rabies virus or secrete it in saliva in low amounts include domestic cows, rodents (rats and mice), squirrels, and lagomorphs (rabbits and hares). In the United States, no case of human rabies has been documented after a rodent bite.

Clinical Infection

Rabies infection is caused by a ribonucleic (RNA) rhabdovirus. The bullet-shaped virus is composed of a coiled RNA-containing core structure (nucleocapsid) that is enveloped by a membrane-derived cover.[275] Surface glycoprotein spikes carry the antigens that elicit an immune response. The virus is synthesized in the cytoplasm and released by budding through the cell membranes, without destroying the host cell.

Transmission of the virus from a rabid animal depends on inoculation of the wound with saliva from the mouth or virus carried on the claws of a preening cat. It may be transmitted by contamination of small lacerations, abrasions, or mucous membranes with saliva or brain tissue from a rabid animal. In rare instances the virus has been reputedly transmitted to spelunkers by inhalation of aerosolized urine from infected cave-dwelling bats. A similar mode of transmission has occurred in the laboratory.[276] Human-to-human transmission has been limited to recipients of corneal transplants from infected donors.[134]

The virus may be secreted in animal saliva before the animal becomes symptomatic. This period ranges from 2 to 3 days in cats and dogs to 15 to 18 days in skunks. A dog infected by the rabies virus becomes ill within 10 days of onset of the carrier state. Rabid animals show clinical signs of excitement, agitation, drooling, frothing at the mouth, and furious and inappropriate behavior.

In humans the rabies virus is deposited in the wound and replicates in striated muscle cells during the early incubation period. After entry into the peripheral nervous system via neuromuscular spindles and perhaps motor end plates, the virus travels centripetally toward the brain within the axons of peripheral nerves at an estimated rate of 3 mm/hour.[275] Wounds on the foot show an average incubation period (until the clinical appearance of rabies) of 60 days, whereas a wound to the face has a 30-day incubation period.[12] Incubation periods may be as short as 10 days or as long as several years.[2]

Overall, approximately 15% of untreated persons bitten by rabid dogs develop clinical rabies infection. The probability of developing clinical rabies infection varies from 0.1% with contamination of a minor wound to 80% following severe wolf bite. Infection of olfactory neuroepithelium in the nares may be the origin of rabies infection following inhalation of aerosolized infected bat urine in caves.[275] The lack of an adequate endogenous immune response in humans infected by the rabies virus has been attributed to the small inoculum of antigen, "shielding" of antigen by muscle tissue of myelin sheaths, survival of cells in the nervous system in which the virus is replicated, and limited release of antigen from the infected central nervous system.[275]

The earliest signs of a rabies virus infection are malaise, fatigue, headaches, anorexia, fever, pain or paresthesia at the bite site, cough, chills, sore throat, abdominal pain, nausea, vomiting, diarrhea, apprehension, anxiety, agitation, irritability, nervousness, insomnia, or depression.[12] The prodromal period may last from 2 to 10 days.

When the virus reaches the central nervous system, the victim shows more serious signs of the disease. This response is related to localization of the infection to the limbic system, with relative sparing of the neocortex.[265] Signs and symptoms include agitation, intermittent hyperactivity, nuchal rigidity, aberrant sexual behavior, hallucinations, seizures, fever, diaphoresis, glossopharyngeal spasm, and copious drooling or frothing at the mouth.[54] Hydrophobia is an aversion to the act of swallowing, which is painful and ultimately impossible for the victim of rabies. Pharyngeal spasm and choking may be induced by exhibiting water to the victim or by blowing air on the face of the patient (aerophobia). (Interestingly, the victim with true rabies often attempts to drink because of thirst, whereas the hysterical victim will not even make the attempt.)

As the disease progresses, "furious" rabies gives way to "dumb" rabies, in which the victim becomes sedated and depressed and ultimately succumbs over a period of days or weeks to paralysis of various configurations (diffuse, symmetric, asymmetric, or ascending), coma, and respiratory arrest.[52]

At the same time that the virus reaches the central nervous system, it is present within the mucus-producing cells of the salivary glands.[275] The infection is initiated from nerves entering the glands and ultimately creates a situation in which the glands may produce up to 1 million virus particles per milliliter. Although the virus may be isolated in postmortem examination from multiple organs (myocardium, muscle, pancreas, lung, liver, kidney, adrenal glands), central nervous system involvement clearly is the major cause of morbidity and mortality.[63,67]

The differential diagnosis of the victim with an unidentified neurologic syndrome is extensive. In a review of diagnoses considered for patients with rabies in the United States and territories for the years 1960 to 1979, the following were recorded: rabies, viral encephalitis, poliomyelitis, postinfectious encephalitis, vaccine reaction, Guillain-Barré syndrome, brain abscess, cerebrovascular accident, brain tumor, tetanus, phenothiazine toxicity, psychosis, rabies phobia, respiratory tract infection, pneumonia, sinusitis, otitis media, viral infection, gastroenteritis, myocardial infarction, hypertension, dissecting aortic aneurysm, arteritis, dehydration, lumbago, and headache.[2]

Identification of Rabies Infection

Any high-risk wild animal that might carry the rabies virus should be captured and killed if it bites a human, particularly if the attack was unprovoked. Care should be taken to avoid extraordinary damage to the head, because the brain must be examined. Any domestic animal that is ill or exhibits inappropriate behavior during the 10-day observation period after a biting episode should be killed immediately. Any stray or unwanted animal that bites a human should be killed immediately. The head and the spinal cord should be double bagged in heavy plastic and transported in a leakproof container under refrigeration to a qualified laboratory for examination of the central nervous tissue by the fluorescent antibody technique.[41] The remainder of the animal should be incinerated. If the transit time to the laboratory will exceed 48 hours, the specimen may be frozen (which delays and complicates testing), or 50% glycol may be used as a preservative. Formalin-fixed tissues may be examined by the fluorescent antibody technique, but specificity may be diminished, with an increase in false negative evaluations. Rabies virus can be found in the saliva of fewer than half of dogs documented as rabid.[275] Rabies virus infection is confirmed by postmortem examination of central nervous system tissue (brain or spinal cord) from the afflicted animal.

Treatment

Unfortunately, no effective treatment exists for an acquired rabies virus infection in humans. Megadose therapy with human rabies immune globulin has been ineffective, as have attempts to use peripheral or intrathecal human leukocyte interferon regimens. The disease is fatal, with scattered reports of survival in isolated cases in all likelihood linked to previous partial immunity or improper documentation of the disease.[127] Clinical care for the victim is supportive. With intensive medical support, a victim infected with rabies virus may survive for 3 weeks or longer. Isolation precautions should be in effect. The issue of postexposure rabies prophylaxis for health care workers in an acute care hospital setting has been addressed, with the following recommendations:

1. All persons who have been in contact with the rabid victim should be identified.
2. The extent and type of contact with the victim should be documented.
3. The risks of human-to-human transmission of rabies should be discussed with each employee who has had contact with the victim.
4. Postexposure prophylaxis should be recommended only to those who have had high-risk contact, defined as percutaneous or mucous membrane contact with saliva, respiratory secretions, corneas (tears), cerebrospinal fluid, or urinary sediment.[217]

Prophylaxis after an Animal Bite (Postexposure Prophylaxis)

First and foremost in postexposure prophylaxis, all bite wounds and scratches from potentially rabid animals should be scrubbed thoroughly with soap and water. The rabies virus is fragile and easily inactivated with disinfectants. Brief irrigation with aqueous benzalkonium chloride 1:750 or 10% povidone-iodine solution may provide virucidal activity. After exposure to a domestic animal suspected to be rabid or a high-risk feral animal (bat, skunk, raccoon, fox, coyote, or bobcat), the victim should be vaccinated against rabies, unless the animal is captured and proven not to be rabid. After exposure to a domestic dog or cat in the United States, vaccination of the victim may be withheld unless the animal appears rabid or is a stray that cannot be captured and is considered at risk by virtue of attack behavior (unprovoked), appearance ("angry, foaming at the mouth"), or if there is a high incidence of rabies in wild animals in the region. Rodents (squirrels, hamsters, guinea pigs, gerbils, chipmunks, rats, and mice) and lagomorphs (rabbits, hares) rarely carry the rabies virus and have not been reported to cause rabies in the United States; therefore, a bite by one of these animals does not generally require rabies prophylaxis, unless it is advised in consultation with the state or local health department.

Wounds at risk for rabies infection include bites that have penetrated the epidermis. Nonbite contacts also may transmit the virus. These exposures include abrasions, open wounds, or mucous membranes contaminated by animal saliva or nervous tissue.

The Immunization Practices Advisory Committee of the U.S. Public Health Service provides recommendations for treatment. Each year, approximately 25,000 people in the United States receive postexposure rabies prophylaxis, although the number of clinical cases per year has dropped since 1960.[127] The greatest number of recipients of postexposure prophylaxis are boys between birth and 14 years of age. This relates to the greater interaction between animals and young children and the lack of a sophisticated medical history. Domestic animals are responsible for a disproportionately large number of immunizations with respect to the actual incidence of rabies in these animals. For instance, in 1981 the percentage of persons who received postexposure prophylaxis because of a domestic animal incident was 66%, whereas only 13% of animals proved to be rabid were domestic, with a frequency of rabies in animals examined of 1.8%. Conversely, the percentage of persons who received postexposure prophylaxis because of wild animal incidents was 28%, whereas 87% of animals proved to be rabid were wild, with a frequency of rabies in animals examined of 16.4%. Possible methods to reduce overtreatment in the United States include (1) expert consultation by the treating physician with the local county or state health department; (2) public education concerning avoiding animals; (3) maintenance of current rabies immunizations for domestic dogs and cats; and (4) elimination of wild animal reservoirs.[128]

The treatment of choice for postexposure prophylaxis is immediate administration of human rabies immune globulin (HRIG) (Hyperab, Cutter Laboratories; Imogam, Merieux Institute) 10 IU/kg infiltrated into the tissue surrounding the bite (if such an injection will not compromise local circulation) and 10 IU/kg intramuscularly at another site (the buttocks have been recommended).[51,129] HRIG is concentrated by cold ethanol fractionation from the plasma of hyperimmunized human donors and has a half-life after administration of 21 days. The rabies-neutralizing antibody content is standardized to contain 150 IU/ml. Anaphylaxis and neuroparalysis have not been reported with HRIG. Postexposure prophylaxis that omits administration of HRIG places the bitten victim at risk of acquiring clinical rabies.[64] However, if HRIG was not given when vaccination with human diploid cell vaccine was initiated, it can be given up to day 8, after which an antibody response will already have occurred.[51]

Simultaneously, the victim should be given an intramuscular 1 ml dose of human diploid cell inactivated virus (HDCV) vaccine (Imovax, Merieux Institute) or rabies vaccine adsorbed (Michigan Department of Public Health) in an extremity (the deltoid region is recommended) other than that used for the HRIG.[3,13,49,51] The intradermal route is not recommended for postexposure prophylaxis. The initial dose of HDCV or rabies vaccine adsorbed should be followed with repeat doses on days 3, 7, 14, and 28.

Persons treated with HRIG and five 1 ml intramuscular doses of HDCV should develop an antibody titer of 1:5 by rapid fluorescent focus inhibition test (RFFIT), as specified by the Centers for Disease Control (CDC). The World Health Organization specifies a titer of 0.5 IU. A person previously immunized with HDCV or with a laboratory-measured adequate antibody response to duck embryo rabies vaccine (DEV) does not need HRIG and requires only booster doses of vaccine on days 1 and 3.[51,81] Because these vaccines are so effective, routinely measuring the antibody titer at the end of HDVC immunization is unnecessary. Patients who suffer from chronic immunosuppression (corticosteroid therapy, acquired immune deficiency syndrome, chronic debilitating diseases) should have the serum rabies antibody titer measured to assess the need for a longer course of immunization.

No contraindication exists to postexposure rabies prophylaxis during pregnancy.[262] Antirabies antibody induced by immunization is passed to the fetus by passive transplacental transfer. In all cases of animal bite, the local public health authorities should be notified.

Pre-Exposure Prophylaxis

Pre-exposure immunization is recommended only for those in high-risk groups, such as veterinarians, laboratory workers, animal handlers, professional hunters, and persons whose travel or avocation (spelunkers, taxidermists) places them in frequent contact with potentially rabid animals. The purpose is to protect against exposure to rabies and to add a margin of safety for those who cannot be rapidly transported to definitive medical care.

HDCV or rabies vaccine adsorbed is administered intramuscularly in three 1 ml doses on days 0, 7, and 28. Because of the excellent antibody response to this regimen, postvaccination serology is not required unless the recipient is known to be immunosuppressed. To maintain an adequate antibody titer (1:5 by RFFIT), a booster dose is required every 2 years unless the RFFIT is measured and adequate.[174]

The Merieux Institute vaccine has been evaluated with intradermal administration for pre-exposure prophylaxis. It is administered intradermally as a 1 ml dose in the lateral aspect of the upper arm over the deltoid area on days 0, 7, and 28. Two to 3 weeks after immunization, routine serologic testing should be performed. If the postimmunization titer is lower than 1:16 (0.16 IU/ml), then an additional dose of the vaccine should be administered and the person retested in 2 to 3 weeks.[50] Serologic testing does not appear to be necessary for persons receiving intramuscular pre-exposure prophylaxis.

A person who has received intramuscular or intradermal (with a rabies titer of 1:16 or above) pre-exposure prophylaxis still requires immediate postexposure prophylaxis after a potential rabies virus inoculation.[50] This is administered as two intramuscular 1 ml doses of HDCV on days 0 and 3. HRIG should not be administered routinely. However, any person who has received intradermal pre-exposure prophylaxis and does not have a documented rabies titer of 1:16 or above should receive a 20 IU/kg dose of HRIG and five intramuscular 1 ml doses of HDCV on days 0, 3, 7, 14, and

28. Up to 6% of persons who receive booster doses of HDCV may suffer from a serum sickness–like syndrome, with urticaria, arthralgia, arthritis, angioedema, nausea, vomiting, fever, and malaise. This has been attributed in part to acquired sensitivity (IgE) to the beta-propiolactone–treated human serum albumin component of the vaccine.[51] The standard treatment of an immune reaction with corticosteroids theoretically could inhibit the development of active immunity to rabies; immunosuppressive therapy therefore should be restricted to the most severe reactions and follow measurement of the serum for rabies antibodies.

Prevaccination and postvaccination rabies prophylaxis is expensive. In countries such as Nigeria where rabies is common, the supply of antirabies vaccines for human use is inadequate. Investigators in these countries currently are exploring the production of less-expensive products, such as suckling mouse brain and fetal bovine kidney cell rabies vaccines.[51,124] These vaccines may carry a higher incidence of morbid side effects.

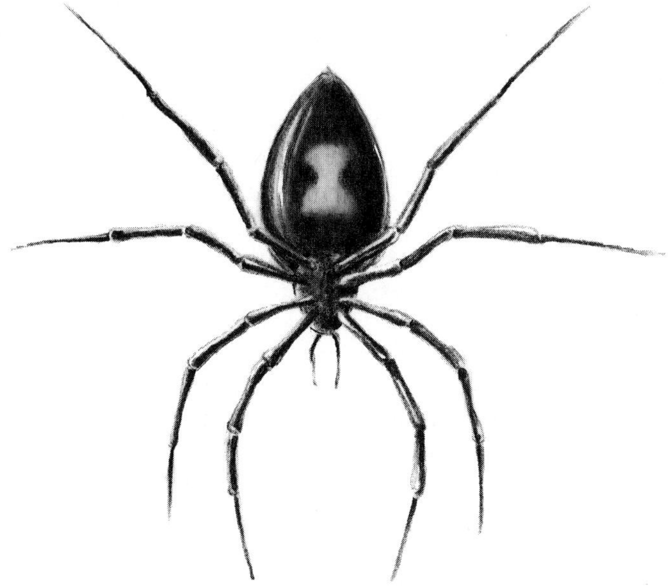

FIGURE 18-2 Female black widow spider *(Latrodectus mactans)* with typical hourglass marking on the abdomen.

SPIDER BITES

Of the 100,000 species of spiders, one fifth can be found in the United States. Spiders are carnivorous creatures, and any specimen with strong fangs can create a human envenomation. Species that have been reported to cause human fatalities include the black widow spider (*Latrodectus* sp.), brown recluse spider (*Loxosceles* sp.), wandering spider (*Phoneutria nigriventer*–South America), and funnel web spider (*Atrax* sp.–Australia). The two common species associated with most serious envenomations in the United States are the black widow and brown recluse spiders.

Black Widow Spider

The black widow spider *(Latrodectus mactans)* is found in both North and South America. Other "widow" *(Latrodectus)* spiders found in the United States are *L. hesperus* (black widow–western states), *L. geometricus* (red widow–Florida), and *L. bishopi* (brown widow–southern states).[162] Adult black widow females are shiny and black, 12 to 18 mm in body length (males are half this size), and have a red or yellow-orange hourglass marking on the underside of the abdomen (Figure 18-2). They are found predominately in fields and forested areas but may also be noted in urban areas associated with sacks of grain or trash collections. The female is aggressive when cornered or provoked and readily bites.

Venom

The venom of the black widow spider is complex and appears to have its greatest effect at the neuromuscular junction.[234] Postulated mechanisms of action include the release of neurotransmitter substances (norepinephrine and acetylcholine) from the presynaptic membrane and inhibition of presynaptic neurotransmitter reuptake, which combine to interrupt normal neurotransmission.[208,210] The role of calcium fluxes at the cellular and mitochondrial membrane is unclear, although it appears that calcium may redistribute in the process.[198]

Clinical Presentation

The initial bite rarely is painful beyond a brief stinging sensation and often is painless. The local reaction usually is limited to a punctate red mark, with minimal swelling or local tenderness. An erythematous halo surrounding the puncture wound or wounds may be noted after the bite of *L. hesperus*. After a 10- to 60-minute interval, the victim begins to complain of local muscle spasm and painful cramps. If the envenomation is significant, particularly if it is on the trunk or proximally located on an extremity, the muscle spasm may become central and severe, with abdominal rigidity and severe thoracolumbar pain. If a spider bite is not suspected, the examiner may misdiagnose the syndrome as an acute condition of the abdomen requiring surgery. Associated systems include paresthesia (diffuse or localized to the soles of the feet), headache, dysphagia, nausea, vomiting, fever, diaphoresis, facial edema, ptosis, conjunctivitis, respiratory distress, and hypertension. The hypertension may be severe enough to necessitate pharmacologic intervention. Priapism has been reported.[246] Infants, small children, and elderly victims are at greatest risk of a severe reaction. The natural course of the envenomation is that most symptom complexes resolve spontaneously over 24 to 36 hours, with 4 days to resolution being the extreme.

Hospital Management

Most victims improve without intervention. However, with a moderate or severe reaction, therapy is indicated. The bite wound should be cleansed, ice packs applied, and tetanus immunization completed. Muscle spasm may be controlled with standard doses of diazepam or with a slow intravenous infusion of 5 to 19 ml (0.1 ml/kg in children) of 10% calcium gluconate, repeated every 2 to 4 hours as needed. Alternatively, adult muscle spasm may be alleviated with a slow intravenous infusion of methocarbamol (1 g or 10 ml, no faster than 100 mg/minute).[144] This may be followed with an intravenous infusion (200 mg/hour) or 500 mg by mouth every 6 hours. In most clinical series, calcium is more efficacious than methocarbamol. Sometimes neither agent is effective, and muscle pain may require administration of narcotics.[194] Severe hypertension that does not resolve with antispasmodic agents may require administration of sodium nitroprusside, hydralazine, or diazoxide. Nausea and vomiting that do not respond to calcium infusions can be controlled with standard antiemetics (prochlorperazine or trimethobenzamide).

Latrodectus antivenin (Merck, Sharp, & Dohme) is prepared from equine serum. To avoid unnecessary sensitization to horse antigens and subsequent anaphylaxis, the antivenin should be used only to treat severe envenomations in those with uncontrolled hypertension or muscle spasm who do not respond adequately to more conservative therapy. Other high-risk groups include pregnant women, young children, and elderly victims in respiratory distress. Skin testing should be performed before intravenous administration of antivenin. The recommended dose of antivenin is 1 ampule (2.5 ml diluted in 10 to 50 ml of normal saline) in a slow (15 minutes) intravenous infusion. A second vial of antivenin is rarely necessary. The risk of delayed serum sickness is moderate. It must be re-emphasized that antivenin administration is rarely indicated and should be done with the expectation of an acute or delayed allergic reaction.

All victims of black widow spider bites should be observed for at least 8 hours, because recurrent symptoms are common. All infants, children, pregnant women, elderly persons, and severely envenomed victims should be admitted to the hospital.

Brown Recluse Spider

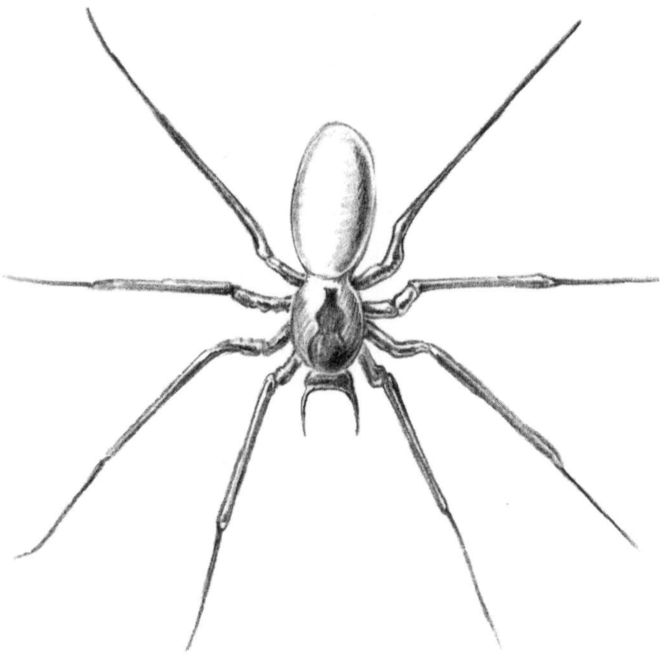

FIGURE 18-3 Brown recluse spider *(Loxosceles reclusa)* with typical dark violin-shaped marking on the cephalothorax.

The brown recluse spider *(Loxosceles reclusa)* and related species are ubiquitous, shy inhabitants of the midwestern and southern United States (Kansas, Oklahoma, Texas, Arkansas, Louisiana, Mississippi, Alabama, Georgia, South Carolina, North Carolina, Tennessee, Kentucky, and Missouri) and increasingly of other regions by virtue of natural migration and transport during interstate commerce.[125,137] Other *Loxosceles* species (*L. unicolor, L. deserta, L. arizonica,* and *L. refescens)* are probably indigenous to the western United States (California, New Mexico, Nevada, and Arizona). The brown recluse spider is 9 to 14 mm in body length and brown or reddish brown, with long, slender legs and three pairs of eyes. A dark, violin-shaped marking may be noted on the dorsum of the cephalothorax (Figure 18-3). Males and females are equal in size and hazard. Although generally not aggressive, the spiders bite when they are trapped in clothing or prodded by the unsuspecting victim. Children are more frequently envenomed than adults. The spiders have relatively weak fangs and tend to cause the most serious envenomations in soft, fatty tissue.

Venom

The venom of the brown recluse spider contains multiple fractions, including hyaluronidase, collagenase, DNase, cholinesterase, RNase, lipase, esterase, and a number of phospholipases (A, C, and D) and proteases.[125] *L. reclusa* venom contains the phospholipase sphingomyelinase D, which binds to cell membranes and likely activates complement, liberates arachidonic acid metabolites, generates leukocyte chemoattractants, and aggregates platelets.* The venom attaches quickly to local tissues, and an active fraction can be detected in the bite wound for up to 5 days. No hemolysin has been found in pure venom.

Clinical Presentation

The initial bite may or may not be painful. After 1 to 4 hours, the victim notices a painful red blister surrounded by a pale or blue-gray ring, occasionally encircled by a hemorrhagic halo (bull's eye lesion) (Figure 18-4). During this early stage, systemic symptoms may include fever, chills, malaise, nausea, and a local scarlatiniform rash. In rare instances a severe reaction of laryngospasm, respiratory distress, and hypotension may develop; whether this represents anaphylaxis or an idiosyncratic hypersensitivity to the venom is unclear.

After 12 to 18 hours the lesion becomes vesiculated, edema worsens, and cellulitis appears. Over the next 2 to 6 days, the local lesion enlarges and becomes necrotic (necrotic arachnidism), with ulceration into the subcutaneous tissue. A central hemorrhagic crater is surrounded by intense inflammation, which represents the response to toxin-mediated arteriolar and venular endothelial damage and subsequent thrombosis. The polymorphonuclear leukocyte response is destructive and severe. Systemic symptoms may persist for 7 to 10 days and include regional lymphadenitis, malaise, fever, and headache. The bite wounds may evolve into indolent ulcers that require months to heal, with large tissue defects. In rare instances failure to heal leads to residual pyoderma gangrenosum.[212]

Severe intravascular hemolytic reactions have been noted in children bitten by *L. reclusa*. Signs and symptoms include spherocytosis, hemoglobinuria, chills, headache, fever, petechiae, jaundice, and hypotension.[71,247] Death may follow pulmonary edema, renal failure, and disseminated intravascular coagulation. The hemolytic crisis is not related to the severity of the local reaction and is putatively linked to alteration of the erythrocyte membrane, which predisposes to complement-mediated destruction of red blood cells.

Hospital Management

Many therapies have been proposed for treatment of the brown recluse spider bite. These include intralesional injection of corticosteroid preparations, early wide excision of the bite wound with primary or delayed closure, systemic corticosteroid administration, and hyperbaric or local oxygen treatment.[80,215]

Surgical wound management is directed at minimizing tissue loss and preventing secondary infection.[9,131] After the necrotic area reaches a diameter of 1 cm, it should be debrided daily using sterile technique.

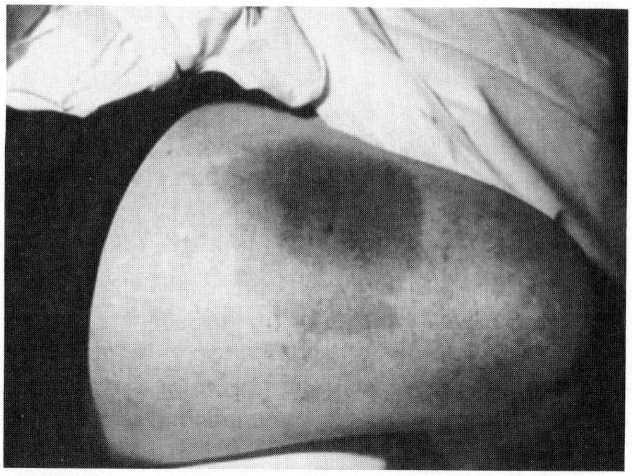

FIGURE 18-4 Typical bull's eye lesion of *Loxosceles* sp. envenomation.

Wet-to-dry dressings, hydrophilic beads, or enzymatic debridement may be used in conjunction with surgical debridement. Split-thickness skin grafts should be applied as soon as no further necrosis is noted and granulation tissue is present, generally after 6 to 8 weeks.

Some exciting new treatment modalities are colchicine and dapsone. In a guinea pig model, dapsone, a polymorphonuclear leukocyte inhibitor, successfully prevented inflammation and necrosis at the site of injection of brown recluse spider venom.[145,233] This effect was subsequently confirmed in clinical reports on human subjects (Figure 18-5). Dapsone therapy is recommended as early as possible after envenomation. The victim should be screened for profound anemia (dapsone can cause bone marrow suppression) and glucose 6-phosphate dehydrogenase deficiency (to avoid hemolysis). The initial dosage is 25 mg by mouth twice a day, up to 100 mg a day. The medicine should be continued for 5 to 10 days, until there is no sign of active local inflammation. Concomitant administration of corticosteroids has not been shown to be beneficial.

FROSTBITE

Frostbite is an injury created when tissue temperature drops below freezing.[182] It is an environmental hazard of all who explore and work in subfreezing temperatures and has figured prominently in injuries to soldiers in ancient and modern times.[201]

Natural History

Tissue temperature in cold environments is a balance between internal heat supply and external heat loss. External cold stress is a function of ambient temperature, windchill, moisture, insulation, and conduction. Internal

*References 85, 94, 213, 214, and 277.

A 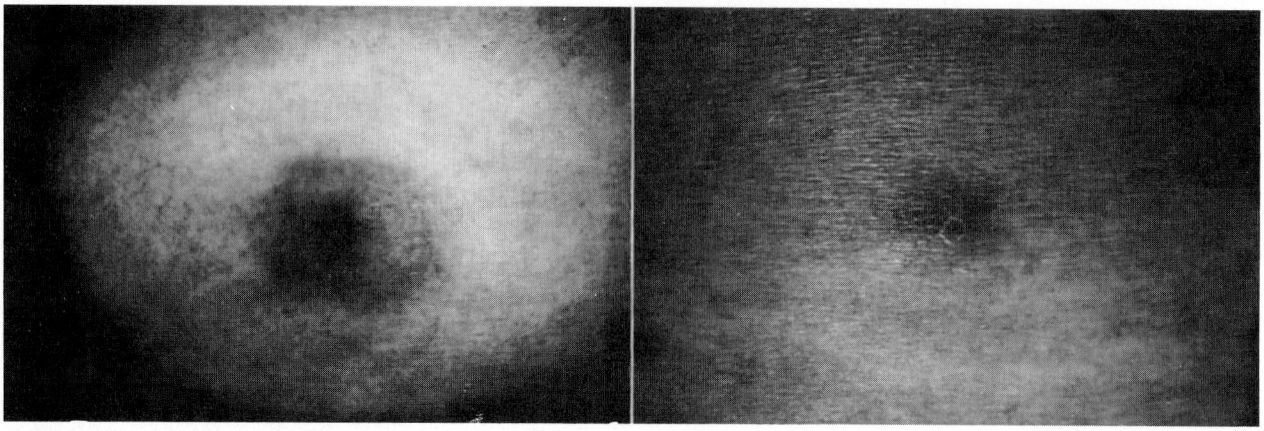 B

FIGURE 18-5 Dapsone therapy of brown recluse spider bite. **A,** Bite wound of the hip after 16 hours and before treatment. The victim complained of malaise, chills, and mild arthralgia. **B,** Twenty-four hours after the initiation of dapsone therapy, the local reaction has nearly resolved; the patient had no systemic complaints.

heat supply is a function of vascularity and blood flow, moderated by vasospasm, shunting, local pressure, drugs, and endogenous alterations in the microcirculation. The lower extremities are most frequently affected by frostbite, followed by the upper extremities, nose, and ears. Less likely tissues, such as the corneas or gingivae, can be involved.[4]

The natural course of a full-thickness frostbite injury varies with the severity of the cold injury but generally falls within the following description. After the frozen tissue is thawed, erythema and warmth develop immediately and last 24 to 72 hours. Darker skin coloration indicates a more severe injury. Sensation initially is intact and diminishes as vesiculation ensues (6 to 24 hours). Edema may or may not be present within the first few hours after thawing and may persist for days.

Cutaneous Response to Cold

As the major thermoregulatory organ, the skin is supplied with a dense system of capillary loops that drain into the subcapillary venous plexus. With extreme cold stress, the cutaneous blood flow can be reduced from a basal level of 200 to 500 ml/minute to 20 to 50 ml/minute, with the greatest variability in the hands, feet, nose, and ears. Both local and systemic cooling influence vasoconstriction. Sympathectomy induces maximum reflex vasodilatation, which can be altered by persistent local temperature–mediated vascular tone.

When a hand or foot is cooled to 15° C (59° F), maximum vasoconstriction occurs. As cooling progresses below 10° C (50° F), periods of vasoconstriction alternate with periods of vasodilatation in 5- to 10-minute cycles (the so-called hunting response). This cold-induced vasodilatation, which varies and can be augmented with acclimatization, is a dominant feature in natives of cold climates and probably contributes to protection from frostbite. When the core temperature is diminished, the circulation to the extremities is diminished to shunt warmed blood to the core. Thus the arms and legs are commonly affected.

Frostbite progresses through four phases, with some degree of overlap.[18] In the *prefreeze phase,* the tissue temperature ranges from 3° to 10° C (38° to 50° F). Cutaneous sensation is abolished at 10° C (50° F). In the chilled state, vasospasm predominates, followed after 24 to 48 hours by leakage of transendothelial red cells and plasma. The putative mechanism is ischemic erosion of capillary endothelium.

In the *freeze-thaw phase,* the tissue temperature drops below the freezing point as the ambient environmental temperature dips below −6° to −15° C (21° to 5° F). Because of the underlying radiation of heat energy, skin must be supercooled to −4° C (24.8° F) to freeze. Because of the windchill factor, moisture and wind increase the rate of cooling. With no circulation, the skin temperature may drop faster than 0.5° C (1° F) per minute. After it is completely frozen, the tissue rapidly shows poikilothermy.

Several factors may cause the damage attributed to freezing of tissues, including intracellular crystallization of ice, intracellular hypernatremia and cellular swelling, and degenerative changes in mitochondria. The susceptibility of tissues to freezing varies, with endothelium, bone marrow, and nerve tissue more sensitive than muscle, bone, and cartilage.

In the *vascular stasis phase,* the tissue temperature returns to normal after thawing. However, vascular stasis predominates secondary to arterial spasm, a hypercoagulable state, endothelial permeability and hemoconcentration, fragmented red blood cells, proteinaceous emboli, and arteriovenous shunting. A period of vasodilatation follows the initial thaw; however, in severe injuries this may not be present, and return to normal vascular patterns may require months.

In the *late ischemic phase,* tissue loss may be attributed to vascular occlusion and tissue hypoxia. Dry gangrene and mummification of soft tissues accompany lesser injuries to bone, nerves, muscle, and cartilage.

Clinical Presentation

Frostbite injuries can be categorized in a manner analogous to burns:

1. *First degree:* erythema, edema, and superficial ice crystal formation (frostnip) without vesiculation.
2. *Second degree:* vesiculation; sensation intact.
3. *Third degree:* vesiculation with extension into the subcutaneous tissue.
4. *Fourth degree:* full-thickness injury, with involvement of bone and muscle; generally results in amputation; less severe bone involvement in children may affect the growth plate and result in developmental digital deformities.[37,47]

The symptoms of frostbite may be categorized as pre-thaw and post-thaw:

1. *Prethaw (frozen tissue).* Numbness, frozen appearance (white, yellow-white, or mottled blue-white); waxy appearance; firmness; absence of blanching or capillary refill—the superficial appearance of a shallow freeze may be identical to that of a solidly frozen part.
2. *Post-thaw (rewarmed tissue).* Pain (burning or throbbing); inflammation; paresthesia (ischemic neuritis); electric current sensation; sensory deficits (touch, pain, and temperature); edema; erythema; vesiculation.

A favorable prognosis can be predicted from the presence of clear vesicles accompanied by normal sensation; hemorrhagic blebs, nonblanching cyanosis, and insensate skin augur a poor outcome. In the first 2 weeks, severely frostbitten skin blackens and hardens, with complete demarcation of nonviable tissue in 3 to 4 weeks (Figure 18-6). Mummification and autoamputation occur from 6 weeks to 6 months. With proper care, superinfection, necrosis, and liquefaction are unusual. No prognostic technique is absolutely accurate in the immediate post-thaw period; a delay of 2 to 3 weeks is necessary to exceed the period of transitory vascular instability.

Treatment

Emergency Field Care

The fundamental principle of prehospital care is that a frostbitten or frozen body part should be thawed only if refreezing can be absolutely prevented. The damage done by a thaw and subsequent refreeze is many times that incurred by nonintervention, thereby prolonging the initial temperature drop. All constricting and wet clothing should be replaced by dry, loose wraps or garments. Alcohol and tobacco should be forbidden. All blisters should be cushioned and left intact. A victim who must walk through snow should do so before thawing frostbitten feet.

If equipment and transportation are available so that a thawed extremity can be kept warm and pliable during the rescue, the tissue may be rewarmed. This should be done in warm water (described later), not with dry heat (difficult to titrate) such as a campfire or automobile exhaust. Vigorous rubbing should be avoided, and topical medications should not be applied. After the thaw, the tissue should be kept warm, dry, and adequately padded, and the victim should be immediately transported to an emergency facility or burn center. Concomitant systemic hypothermia should be anticipated and managed before any attempt at frozen tissue care.

Emergency Department Management

All hypothermic patients should be rewarmed to at least 34° C (93° F) before local frostbite management is begun. Rapid thawing should be done in the emergency department. This is accomplished by placing the frostbitten body parts in a spacious vessel or bath of warm water (41° to 43° C [106° to 110° F]) never to exceed 44° C (112° F). Heated tap water (50° to 60° C [92° to 140° F]) can be too hot and may cause profound discomfort and possible tissue damage. The water should be circulated gently and the temperature monitored constantly to prevent drop-off. Adding antiseptic solutions or inorganic salts to the bath water is not necessary. The thaw is complete when the tissue is pliable and has near-normal color and sensation. This generally requires immersion for 30 minutes. After this time, the application of heat should be promptly discontinued. Pain may be intense immediately after the thaw. The patient should be admitted to a burn care unit for a minimum observation period of 48 hours to allow the extent of the injury to be determined.

Hospital Management

WOUND CARE. In the burn care unit, a minor wound must be placed in moderate sterile isolation. This may be accomplished with loose protective dressings. Serious injuries (e.g., loss of digits expected) should receive total protective isolation, as would a third-degree burn; sterile procedures should be followed whenever tissue is handled. All body parts should be cushioned with sheepskin and blankets to avoid augmenting the injury with pressure-induced ischemia. Elevation is necessary if significant edema persists beyond 7 to 14 days. Pain is frequently severe and requires judicious administration of narcotics.

A B C

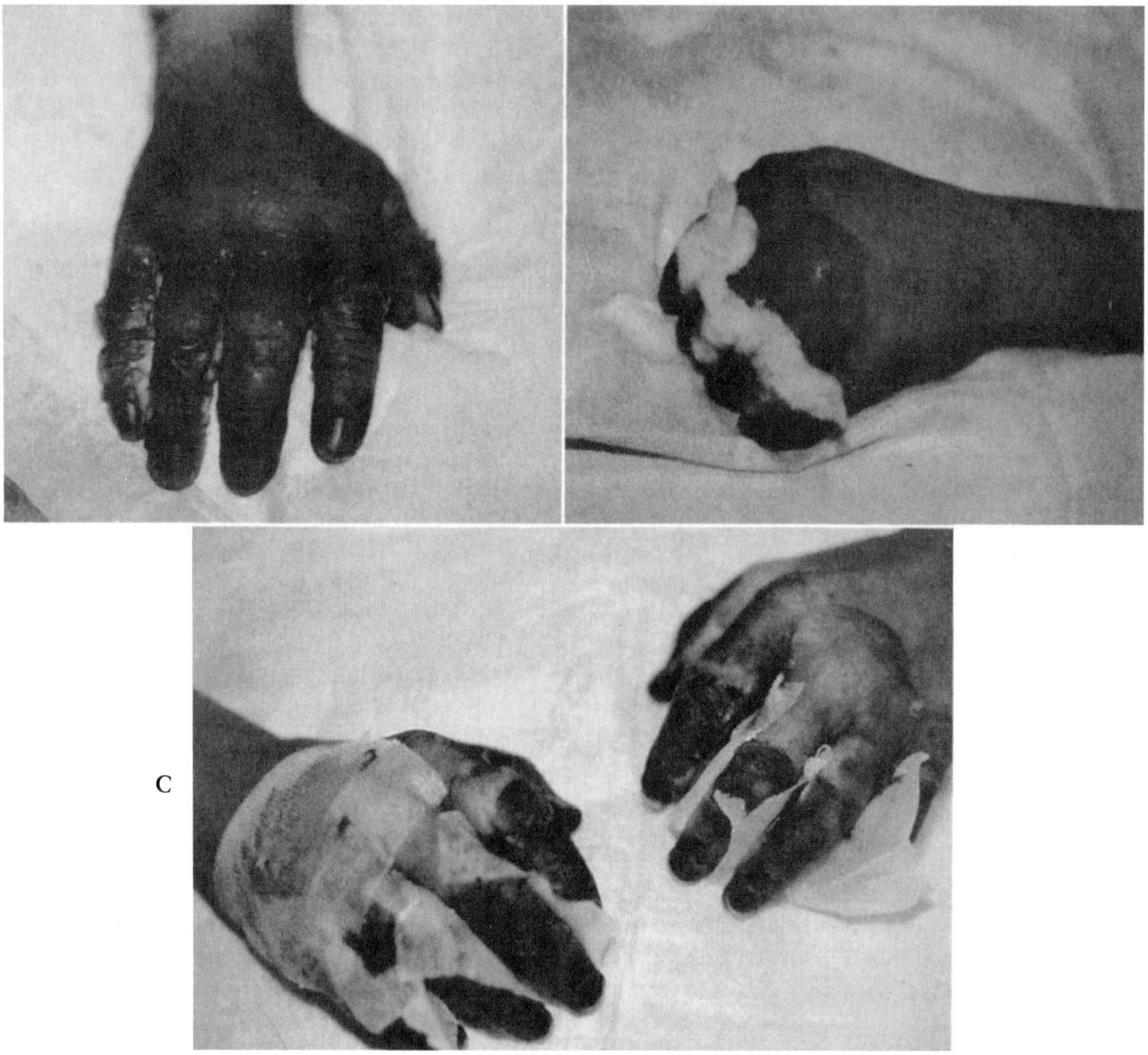

FIGURE 18-6 Frostbite injury. **A,** Over 2 to 6 days, the nonviable tissue becomes hemorrhagic and vesicular; cotton batting cushions are placed between the fingers. **B,** By 2 weeks, early profound necrosis is evident. **C,** Mummification, with clear demarcation of tissue loss, is initiated at 4 to 6 weeks and may evolve over 2 to 4 months. (Courtesy P. Hackett, M.D.)

If the injury is severe, intracompartmental tissue pressures should be monitored. Elevated pressures or distal circulatory compromise or both may necessitate fasciotomies. Whenever possible, the wound should be allowed to self-demarcate (autoamputate) to increase the salvage of viable tissue.

The frostbitten areas should be gently bathed in a whirlpool three times a day for 30 minutes in water 33° to 38° C (90° to 100° F) to which a bacteriostatic agent, such as povidone-iodine, has been added. Obviously devitalized tissue or ruptured vesicles should be cautiously debrided, and early physical therapy with range-of-motion exercise should be undertaken. Use of antibiotics should be limited to established infections (most commonly, group-A beta-hemolytic *Streptococcus*) identified by quantitative tissue culture technique. Areas hardened by eschar can be softened and protected with topical silver sulfadiazine cream.

In most cases the total extent of tissue damage is apparent at the end of 3 to 4 weeks. At that time the decision can be made to allow autoamputation or to complete the process in the operating room.[181] Debridement should be undertaken to shorten the period of disability.[196,204] However, if debridement is done too early, it frequently is necessary to perform additional surgery as further areas of nonviability become apparent. The prognostic value of radionuclide scanning with regard to ultimate outcome is as yet unclear. Patients with small areas of involvement with minimum vesiculation and without potential for tissue loss may be treated as outpatients. All patients who will lose a digit or limb should be hospitalized until the wound has demarcated, surgical debridement is completed, and skin grafting is performed.

Long-term sequelae include phantom limb syndromes, numbness, residual paresthesia, sweating, arthritis, and chronic pain.[28,160,177] Early mobilization and physical therapy are vital to maximum recovery. The victim of previous frostbite suffers from increased susceptibility to cold-stimulated ischemia.

TRENCH FOOT AND CHILBLAINS (PERNIO)

The terms *trench foot, immersion foot,* and *chilblains (pernio)* are used interchangeably to describe cutaneous disorders related to cold exposure without actual freezing of the tissues. These disorders commonly are encountered in wet environments and are attributed to prolonged exposure of unprotected extremities to a cold, humid environment. Frequently noted during wars, trench foot, immersion foot, and chilblains are the sequelae to poor nutrition, inadequate clothing, and constriction of cutaneous blood flow by poorly fitting garments.[19]

The terminology is based on causation rather than pathophysiology. Thus trench foot follows exposure of the foot to cold and moisture, and immersion foot follows exposure to frigid water.[130] In both conditions the immediate symptoms include numbness and painful paresthesia, followed by leg cramping. During the first few hours to days the limb is prehyperemic, with swelling, diffuse discoloration, mottling, and hyposensitivity. After 2 to 7 days the limb becomes hyperemic for a period of up to 6 weeks, during which the condition is marked by paresthesia, regional variation in superficial skin temperature, edema, vesiculation, ulceration, and occasionally gangrene. In the third, or posthyperemic, phase the limb may return to normal temperature but remains exquisitely sensitive to cold.[19] If the injury is severe, liquefaction gangrene may progress.

The chilblain ("cold sore") is a less severe syndrome seen more commonly in women. It is characterized by localized erythema, cyanosis, plaques, nodules and, in rare severe cases, hemorrhage, vesicles, bullae, and ulcerations on the exposed extremities, particularly the lower legs, toes, hands, and ears.[130] The skin lesions appear 12 to 14 hours after exposure to cold and are characterized by intense pruritus and burning paresthesia. Tender blue nodules follow rewarming and may persist for up to 14 days. Chronic pernio may occur in predisposed middle-aged women.

For the purpose of pathophysiologic discussion, all three disorders are referred to as the chilblain syndrome. In general, the dermatologic presentation is related to sympathetic instability and vascular hypersensitivity to cold. Clearly, however, other mechanisms, such as microvascular thrombosis and venous stasis, are contributing factors. One histopathologic study of nine victims of pernio noted a unique lymphocytic vasculitis.[130] Edema of the papillary dermis was a variable feature, as was perivascular lymphocytic infiltration (characteristic of systemic lupus erythematosus, erythema multiforme, or drug eruption).

Treatment of the chilblain syndrome is supportive. The affected skin should be rewarmed in a manner analogous to that used for frostbite, gently washed and dried, and dressed in dry, soft, sterile bandages. Elevation is essential to minimize the swelling that predisposes to bacterial invasion of the compromised tissue. Sympathetic blockade with intra-arterial reserpine has been recommended to ameliorate vasospasm, but the prolonged benefits are unclear. On occasion, healing is followed by local hyperpigmentation. The victim is prone to recurrences on lesser exposure.

LIGHTNING INJURIES

Lightning associated with 50,000 daily thunderstorms strikes the earth more than 100 times each second (8.6 million strikes per day). In the United States, it is directly responsible for three fourths of the forest fires and at least 150 to 300 deaths each year. The natural force with the highest mortality,[57,190,252] lightning traditionally has been the scourge of outdoor laborers, but it is increasingly becoming a hazard to outdoor sports enthusiasts, who account for one fourth of its victims. Although witnessed events are rare, a proper index of suspicion will allow the rescuer to resuscitate the seemingly dead victim.[252] Case reports of multiple victims are not unusual.[38]

Epidemiology

Lightning is a product of thunderstorms and is most likely to strike a person during daylight hours of the summer months. Injuries occur most often in rural territories of the South, the Gulf Coast, the Rocky Mountains, and along the Ohio, Mississippi, and Hudson rivers. Most fatalities (70%) are caused by a single strike (single victim), but clusters of people can be struck by a single strike or multiple strikes. Buildings are struck by lightning based on their height and construction. Relatively few injuries are reported in large cities, where high frameworks and lightning protection devices are numerous.

Types of Lightning

Lightning is created in different forms, including streak lightning (common form), sheet lightning (amorphous, discharged between clouds), ribbon lightning (streak lighting driven by the wind), bead lightning (appears as a "string of beads"), and ball lightning (travels as a softball-sized projectile with unpredictable behavior). Ball lightning has been reported as recently as January 1984, when the Soviet news agency Tass reported that a fireball punctured the forward fuselage of an Ilyushin-18 commercial aircraft, traversed the passenger compartment, and burned through the tail section.

Human Lightning Strike

Pathways

Lightning seeks the most accessible electrical ground through which to discharge. A person can be struck by a bolt of lightning or injured secondarily by a flash discharge from the struck object (such as a tree or building). If the person is electrically grounded, the current passes over or through the victim to reach the ground. *Stride potential* refers to the passage of electricity between the victim's legs, which occurs when the limbs initially carry a different potential. This allows the major current to bypass the thorax and head.

Living tissue, as opposed to a metal rod, is not a pure conductor, because the resistance is not independent of amperage. However, in the same manner that commercial electrical current is carried predominately in the periphery of a metal wire, the lightning current (direct current) frequently travels over the surface of the victim and does not pass internally ("flashover phenomenon").[100] The skin is not appreciably injured, and the presence of lightning is detected when shredded clothing explodes off the victim as a result of vaporization of external skin moisture.[140]

Injuries

TRAUMA. The enormous transfer of current around or through a person causes violent muscle contractions and may cause the victim to be hurled through the air and knocked unconscious (sledgehammer effect). Brief opisthotonic muscle contractions may be severe enough to inhibit respirations. Blunt trauma is common and is similar to that seen after a fall.[184] The sudden discharge of force from lightning produces body tissue shock waves that may cause blast effects in the brain, lungs, bowel, heart, liver, and spleen.[159,203] The amount of damage to clothing or skin cannot be used reliably to estimate the severity of internal injuries.

The electrical current follows preferential pathways of low resistance (and high susceptibility to injury) in the tissues, favoring blood vessels and nerves over muscle and bone. Heat and the dissolution of electrical energy initiate thrombosis and coagulative disruption of the vascular endothelium and often cause muscle damage that resembles a crush injury.

Amperage and temperature are related by Joule's law, which states that heat equals the amperage squared times the resistance ($P = I^2R$). Thus the amplitude of heat energy created by the transmission of electrical energy can be significant in body tissues. Because of the flashover phenomenon and the variability of transmission through the body, a persistent temperature rise is rare. (If a 20 coulomb discharge were to dissipate its energy completely in a 70 kg human body with an average resistance of 5700 ohms, a temperature rise of 14° C [25.2° F] would be induced.) However, significant temperature increases along the pathway of the lightning current in all probability contribute to morphologic changes and organ system dysfunction.

BURNS. Injury patterns in the skin range from a characteristic dermatologic syndrome to more common thermal injuries.[20] Burns occur as sequelae to direct current flow, from ignition of clothing from the superheating of air or metal objects, and from flash-type arc effects. The arc burns resemble welder's injuries and follow exposure to flashes of current from the ground or splashed from nearby objects. Skin exposed to temperatures in the range of 3000° C (5432° F) for microseconds is damaged in a progression from erythema, mottling, and vesiculation to full-thickness eschar formation. Victims who suffer cranial burns or leg burns from lightning injuries have an increased incidence of cardiopulmonary arrest and subsequent death.

Linear burns of first or second degree begin at the head or neck and follow a caudal path delineated by areas of heavy sweat concentration. Punctate burns are unique first-degree (and in rare cases second-degree) injuries that appear in a starburst pattern, composed of tightly spaced, discrete circles that range in diameter from a few millimeters to a centimeter.[176]

The pathognomonic skin sign of a lightning injury is "feathering" or "ferning" (Lichtenberg's flowers, keraunographism), which is created by showers of electrons that penetrate the superficial layer of the skin. A linear, spidery, arborescent, and erythematous skin discoloration follows the pathways of decreased skin resistance of dampness. These markings do not blanch with pressure and may be accompanied by more traditional burn patterns. Because of the flashover effect, the victim is spared the transmission of enormous voltage through the lowered resistance of damaged or wet skin. Classic entrance and exit wounds seen with lower voltage alternating current are absent. The feathery component fades in 24 to 48 hours and leaves no atrophic markings. A seemingly dead victim in the vicinity of a thunderstorm should be rapidly examined for these markings, because prompt resuscitative efforts, even with prolonged down time, can be lifesaving.

NEUROLOGIC INJURY. Most victims struck by lightning are knocked unconscious; recovery ranges from rapid improvement to prolonged disorientation (similar to that seen after electroconvulsive therapy) with anterograde or retrograde amnesia to prolonged coma. The return to consciousness often is accompanied by transient focal motor paralysis and hyporeflexia, which corresponds to spinal cord levels.[14] The lower extremities are most commonly affected. Paralysis of the brainstem respiratory center is followed rapidly by ventricular fibrillation and asystole. Seizures, aphonia and deafness, paresthesia, hypesthesia, and dermatomal sensory deficits spontaneously resolve over 1 to 72 hours. Atrophic spinal paralysis and peripheral nerve ischemia from heat-induced thrombosis in the microcirculation may be permanent. Cerebral edema varies and cannot be predicted by historical features. Ventricular hemorrhage, subdural and epidural hematomas, dural tears, skull fractures, brainstem infarction, and elevated creatine phosphokinase BB measurements have been reported.[56] Survivors suffer from sleep disturbances, storm neuroses, and headaches.

VASCULAR INJURY. Vasomotor spasm is immediate and frequently prolonged, which leads to loss of pulses, mottled and cool extremities, sensory deficits, and peripheral vascular thrombosis. Except for thrombosis, most changes resolve spontaneously over 12 to 36 hours because they result from spasm, not structural thermal injury. In rare instances limb ischemia has necessitated limb amputation. Compartmental syndromes have not been reported, and fasciotomies are rarely necessary.

CARDIAC INJURY. If the heart is in the path of the lightning injury, direct myocardial damage may be reflected in electrocardiogram (ECG) patterns consistent with myocardial infarction, with ST segment elevation and T-wave inversion.[40,138] These findings may accompany coronary artery spasm and subendocardial or epicardial injury, as noted at autopsy. Although rare, transmural myocardial infarction may be confirmed by serial measurement of creatine phosphokinase MB isoenzymes and ECG evolution.[126,157] Increases in serum glutamic oxaloacetic transaminase and lactic dehydrogenase may reflect concurrent injury to other tissues. Coronary artery endothelial injury can lead to delayed endarteritis and thrombosis. Autopsy studies have noted focal cardiac necrosis.

The most common cause of death is cardiopulmonary arrest. Lightning is in effect a massive direct current countershock, which induces asystole.[211] Inherent automaticity regenerates a rhythm, which subsequently deteriorates (ventricular fibrillation) if respirations are inadequate. Other arrhythmias include premature ventricular contractions, ventricular tachycardia, and atrial fibrillation.

MISCELLANEOUS SEQUELAE. Sequelae of lightning strike include personality changes, hypertension, pneumothorax, pneumomediastinum, deafness secondary to rupture of the tympanic membrane and middle ear hemotympanum (serous otitis media), cerebrospinal fluid (CSF) otorrhea, mastoid disruption, basilar skull fracture, cataract, optic nerve atrophy, retinal detachment, retinal burns, hyphema, vitreous hemorrhage, iridocyclitis, vitreous hemorrhage, uveitis, mydriasis, facial nerve palsy, gangrene, and ruptured uterus.*

Emergency Field Care

Successful treatment of lightning injury depends on early, vigorous, and prolonged resuscitative efforts. As with hypothermia, a number of survivors of prolonged resuscitative efforts would have died with less than heroic efforts. An apneic, pulseless victim with dilated pupils who has been recently struck by lightning may be successfully resuscitated. If lightning strikes a group of people, attention should be directed to the seemingly dead first, because those who have a detectable pulse and blood pressure probably will survive.[56]

Lightning victims are not "charged." They can be handled without fear of electrical shock. In the field, rescuers should first stabilize and protect the cervical spine. Because a victim may have fallen or been thrown a distance, fractures should be anticipated. Next, rescuers must manage the airway and support respirations. They should initiate chest compressions if they detect no pulse. Cardiopulmonary resuscitation should not be terminated until the victim reaches a hospital or the rescuers become exhausted.

Hospital Management

The victim should be fully undressed and examined for signs of trauma. All unconscious victims of a lightning injury should have cervical spine radiographs and should be observed on a cardiac monitor. Because gastric hypomotility and dilatation are common, after the airway and cervical spine are secure, a nasogastric tube should be placed to allow intermittent suction to empty the stomach and prevent vomiting and the aspiration of gastric contents. If a serious head injury is suspected, the victim should be started on intermittent antacid or H_2 blocker therapy to normalize gastric pH. A Foley catheter should be placed.

Serial laboratory examinations should include complete blood count, electrolytes, blood urea nitrogen, creatinine, amylase, and glucose. A declining hematocrit should launch an investigation for occult hemorrhage, which may include diagnostic maneuvers such as peritoneal lavage, computed tomography (CT) scan of the abdomen and retroperitoneum, and chest and long-bone (femur, pelvis) radiographs.

CARE OF CEREBROSPINAL INJURIES. Cerebral edema may be treated with hyperventilation to reduce arterial partial pressure of carbon dioxide (P_{CO_2}) and induce

*References 5, 24, 48, 72, 84, 191, and 219.

cerebral vasoconstriction. Mannitol (1 g/kg) should be administered intravenously in life-threatening situations. The efficacy of dexamethasone is a matter of debate; current recommendations do not support its use for cerebral edema caused by trauma, although it may be useful for acute trauma to the spinal cord.

Confusion and antegrade amnesia are not uncommon after lightning injury; however, if the level of consciousness deteriorates, a CT brain scan should be performed promptly to identify remediable intracerebral hemorrhage.

A victim with a ruptured tympanic membrane or cranial burns should be admitted for close observation. Seizures in the immediate period (1 to 4 hours) after the lightning strike may be treated as simple post-traumatic seizures. If seizures prevent return of normal consciousness or persist beyond 4 hours, anticonvulsant therapy should be started.

Dilated pupils do not necessarily indicate brain death in a lightning victim. Diffuse electroencephalographic abnormalities may clear over a period of 24 to 48 hours. Rigorous criteria for brain death should be followed before life support is discontinued.[102,115,264]

CARDIOVASCULAR THERAPY. All victims should be evaluated with an ECG. If direct myocardial damage is suspected, the patient should be monitored for 24 to 48 hours in a coronary care or intensive care unit. Arrhythmias should be managed in standard fashion. A victim without spontaneous respirations should be kept on a ventilator until brain death is formally determined.

RENAL PERFUSION. Close attention should be paid to urinary output, which reflects renal perfusion. Myoglobinuria or hemoglobinuria rarely occurs following lightning strike.[278] If pigments are detected in the urine or serum, urine output should be maintained above 50 ml/hour.

BURN THERAPY. Lightning burns generally are superficial, unlike the injuries associated with high-voltage industrial accidents, and do not cause profound muscle destruction. Still, the urine should be tested for myoglobin. Skin injuries are treated in standard fashion.

DIVING-RELATED ACCIDENTS

The undersea realm has become a highly popular recreational environment. Over 2.5 million sport divers in the United States are joined by an additional 200,000 trained and untrained recruits each year; commercial diving efforts are constantly expanded by the pursuit of offshore petroleum, geologic surveys, and the harvest of marine life.[249] Diving-related medical disorders are noted increasingly by trauma surgeons and emergency physicians who practice in both coastal and inland regions, where modern air travel can return a diver who spent a morning underwater in the tropics.[152]

TABLE 18-1 UNDERWATER DEPTH-PRESSURE RELATIONSHIPS

DEPTH (FSW)*	psig†	psia‡	ATA§	mm Hg (ABSOLUTE)
Sea level	0	14.7	1	760
33	14.7	29.4	2	1520
66	29.4	44.1	3	2280
99	44.1	58.8	4	3040
132	58.8	73.5	5	3800
165	73.5	88.2	6	4560
198	88.2	102.9	7	5320
231	102.9	117.6	8	6080
264	117.6	132.3	9	6840
297	132.3	147	10	7600

From Auerbach PS, Geehr EC, editors: *Management of wilderness and environmental emergencies,* ed 2, St Louis, 1989, Mosby.
*Feet of seawater.
†Pounds per square inch gauge (psig measured by depth gauge).
‡Pounds per square inch absolute (psig plus atmospheric pressure).
§Atmosphere absolute.

COMMONLY USED UNITS OF PRESSURE MEASUREMENT

1 atmosphere absolute = 33 feet salt water (fsw)
= 34 feet fresh water (ffw)
= 5.5 fathoms of seawater
= 14.7 pounds per square inch (psi)
= 760 mm Hg
= 29.9 in Hg
= 1.013 bar

The Underwater Environment

Atmospheric pressure, exerted by air, varies with altitude. At sea level, atmospheric pressure is 760 mm Hg, 14.7 pounds/inch^2 (psi), or 1 atmosphere (atm). Each foot of seawater (depth) exerts a force of 0.445 psi. Therefore, at a depth of 33 feet of seawater (FSW), 1 additional atmosphere of pressure is encountered (see the box above). Underwater, external pressure and depth are related in a linear fashion, as demonstrated in Table 18-1.

As a diver descends, the increasing ambient pressure is transmitted to the entire body. Most body tissues are composed of water and are not compressible, according to Pascal's law, which states that a pressure applied to any part of a fluid is transmitted equally throughout the fluid. However, the air-containing spaces of the body (lungs, middle ears, paranasal sinuses, bowel, tooth and gingival air pockets) respond in accordance with Boyle's law, which states that the volume of a gas at constant temperature varies inversely with pressure (Figure 18-7). The greatest proportionate pressure-volume changes occur near the water's surface.

Depth (feet)	Pressure (ATA)	Relative volume (%)	Relative diameter (%)
0	1	100	100
33	2	50	79.3
66	3	33.3	69.3
90	4	25	63
132	5	20	58.5
165	6	16.6	55

FIGURE 18-7 Pressure-volume relationships underwater.

The sport scuba diver breathes pressurized air from a tank that is either surface-tended or carried on the back. The flow of air is regulated for release at the pressure of the surroundings, to allow the lungs to expand. Thus at greater depths, a greater (potential) volume of air (because it is compressed) is used per breath than is consumed at sea level. A volume of tank-supplied air inspired into the lungs at 33 FSW must expand to two volumes at sea level. Because the greatest pressure-volume changes occur near the surface, shallow depths are exceedingly dangerous for breath-holding ascents.

Arterial Gas Embolism

As the diver ascends, the volume of air contained in the lung expands. The normal release mechanism for this expansion is exhalation. If the diver holds his breath by intention or in panic, if exhalation is prevented by laryngospasm, if air is trapped within an unvented bleb, or if overexpansion occurs in an area of focally increased elastic recoil, a number of the alveoli may rupture, causing the egress of air into the surrounding tissues. Alternatively, a pressure differential of 80 mm Hg is sufficient to force air bubbles across the alveolar capillary membrane without alveolar rupture. If the air tracks along the bronchi into the mediastinum and soft tissues of the neck, pneumomediastinum and subcutaneous emphysema are noted (Figure 18-8). If the visceral pleura is ruptured, pneumothorax, pneumopericardium, and pneumoperitoneum are noted. The dreaded complication is the release of air bubbles into the pulmonary venous circulation, or air embolism.

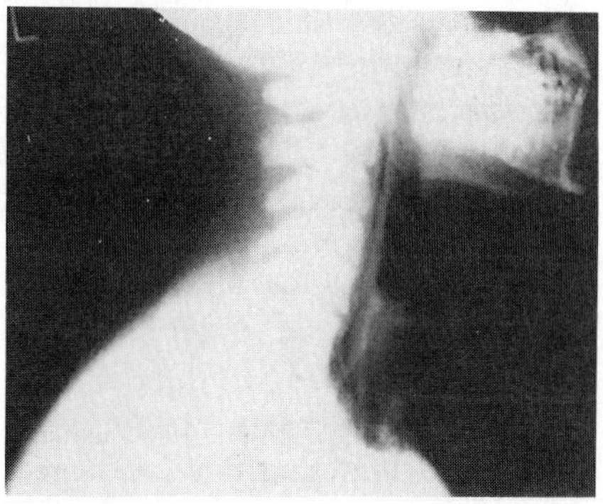

FIGURE 18-8 Retropharyngeal air from pulmonary overpressurization. Air has penetrated the alveolar wall, dissected along the bronchi, and entered the soft tissues of the mediastinum and neck. (Courtesy K. Kizer, M.D.)

The most common type of pulmonary overpressurization is mediastinal emphysema. Symptoms include hoarseness or a brassy voice, substernal chest pain, cough, dyspnea, dysphagia, and subcutaneous air in the supraclavicular fossae or neck. Auscultation of the heart may reveal a crunching sound (Hamman's sign). Radiographs will demonstrate air in the mediastinum, retropharyngeal space, and soft tissues of the neck (Figure 18-9). No immediate therapy is necessary other than admission to the hospital for observation and administration of oxygen based on arterial blood gas measurements. Some authorities believe that oxygen inhalation augments the reabsorption of evolved nitrogen bubbles in the soft tissues. All victims should be examined for a concurrent pneumothorax. In no case should a palpable subcutaneous air collection be aspirated for cosmetic purposes. This action is ineffectual and poses the risk of infection.

Pneumothorax is less common, because it is more difficult for air to rupture through the visceral pleura than to track along the bronchi into the mediastinum. If the pneumothorax develops at depth underwater, it may rapidly proceed to a tension pneumothorax on further ascent. Therapy involves prompt placement of a chest tube to water-seal drainage to allow re-expansion of the lung. A persistent air leak (longer than 72 hours) implies an underlying structural lesion. Recompression therapy is no substitute for tube thoracostomy. If a patient manifests a pneumothorax during recompression therapy, a chest tube frequently is needed to prevent tension pneumothorax.

The pathophysiology of arterial gas embolism (AGE) is that air bubbles released from ruptured alveoli enter the pulmonary venous circulation, traverse the left atrium and ventricle, and are disseminated by the systemic arterial circulation. The bubbles occlude small blood vessels and create an ischemic insult. If the cerebral

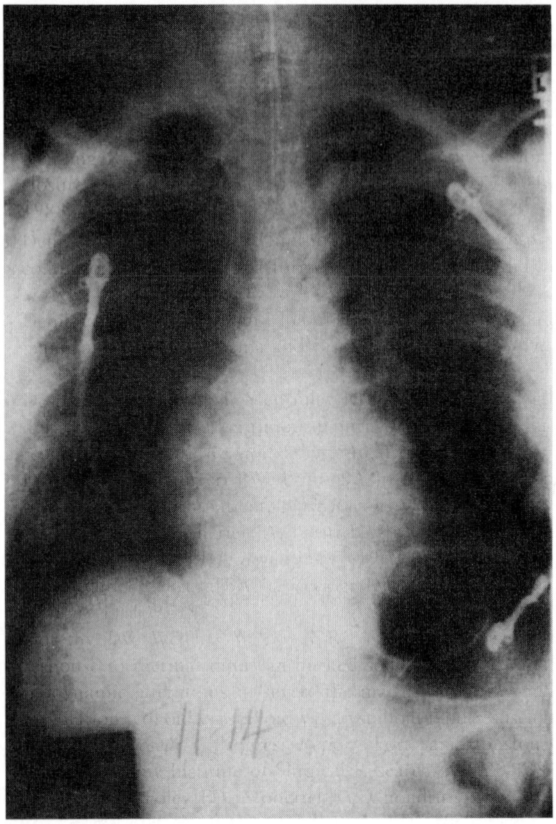

FIGURE 18-9 Radiograph demonstrating air in the mediastinum and soft tissues of the neck. (Courtesy H. Minagi, M.D.)

or coronary circulation, or both, are involved, the result is catastrophic. In an ascending diver, the head-up position seems to predispose to cerebral embolization, perhaps because of the buoyancy of the bubbles.

Symptoms of AGE are often sudden and dramatic, occurring within the first few minutes and no later than 10 minutes after a diver reaches the surface.[95,180] If the coronary arteries are embolized, ischemic chest pain, shortness of breath, hypotension (pump failure), and arrhythmias are noted. Arrhythmias can also be attributed to central nervous system–mediated autonomic stimulation.[44,78] Cardiac arrest without prior apnea has been reported. Most commonly, the cerebral circulation is involved, and multitudinous neurologic deficits are possible, including asymmetric multiplegia, hemiplegia, paraplegia, quadriplegia, paresthesia, blindness, deafness, vertigo, dizziness, headache, seizures, confusion, aphasia, loss of consciousness, and personality changes. Sudden loss of consciousness during ascent or immediately after a dive is pathognomonic for cerebral air embolism. Hemoptysis is rarely reported. Decompression sickness and AGE are frequently seen in combination.

If AGE is suspected, the victim should be placed in the Trendelenburg or the Durant (left lateral, head down) position. If oxygen is available, it should be administered and the victim moved to a hyperbaric chamber facility as quickly as possible. If an unpressurized aircraft is used for transportation, a flight altitude of less than 300 m should be maintained. The pressurized cabin environment should not exceed a 1 atmosphere absolute (ATA) pressure drop if possible. Because the diver is frequently a victim of near-drowning, the rescuer should be prepared to perform cardiopulmonary resuscitation. If consciousness is altered, the airway must be protected from the aspiration of gastric contents.

Hospital Management

The definitive treatment for AGE is recompression and oxygen therapy in a hyperbaric chamber. Delay perpetuates cerebral ischemia and contributes to cerebral edema. However, even if an interval of up to 34 hours has elapsed, recompression therapy should be attempted. Before this therapy, the physician should obtain a chest radiograph, ECG, urinalysis, and a blood sample for a complete blood count, electrolytes, blood glucose, creatinine, and blood urea nitrogen. A CT scan of the brain should be done only if intracranial hemorrhage is suspected; no inordinate delays should be entertained that might postpone recompression therapy. If respiratory distress is severe, as typically is seen with a concurrent near-drowning episode, endotracheal intubation should be performed. Because decompression sickness is a common complication, an intravenous line should be placed and urine output maintained at 1 to 2 ml/kg/hour to encourage capillary perfusion and elimination of inert gas from the tissues.

RECOMPRESSION THERAPY. Clinical and technical recommendations may be obtained 24 hours a day from the National Diving Accident Network (DAN) at Duke University in Durham, North Carolina (Telephone (919) 684-8111). All emergency departments and trauma centers should know the location of the nearest hyperbaric facility. Recompression therapy should be undertaken even if the neurologic manifestations of air embolism have spontaneously resolved by the time the victim reaches the chamber, (as occurs in 10% to 20% of victims). Detailed neurologic examination of such victims often reveals subtle neuropsychiatric or psychomotor impairments that can become permanent without prompt treatment.

Standard therapy for air embolism is recompression in a multiplace (room for multiple patients), double-lock (allows the attendants to enter and exit during therapy) hyperbaric chamber to 6 ATA (165 FSW) on a protocol outlined in the U.S. Air Force modification of U.S. Navy Treatment Table 6A (Figure 18-10). A monoplace chamber (allows one person only) does not allow room for equipment, an attendant, or a resuscitative effort; poses

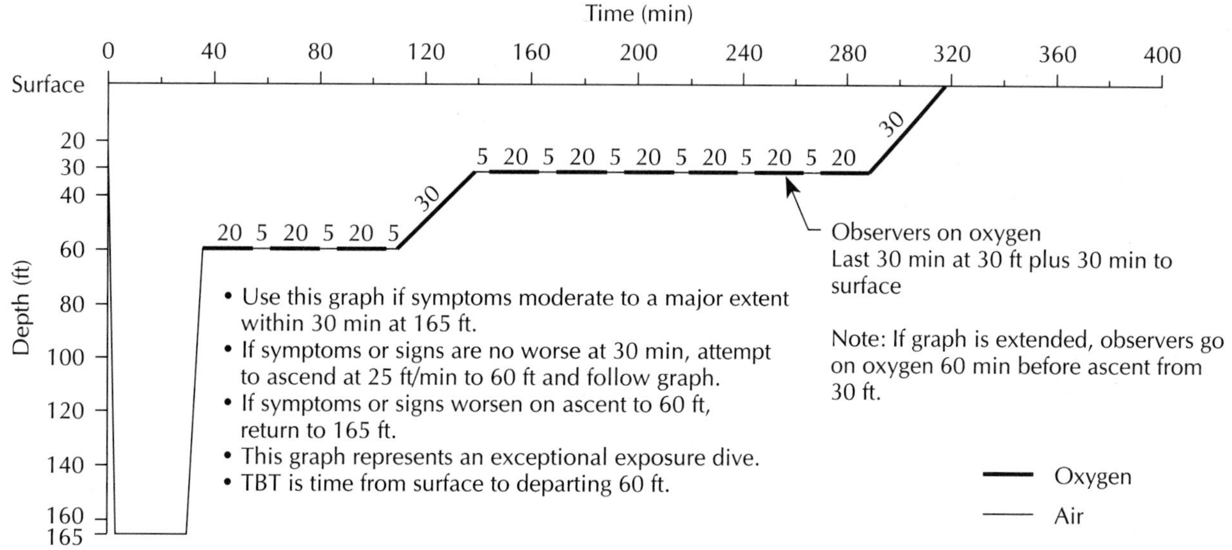

FIGURE 18-10 U.S. Air Force modification of a Navy treatment protocol for the management of arterial gas embolism. (From Auerbach PS, Geehr EC, editors: *Management of wilderness and environmental emergencies,* ed 2, St Louis, 1989, Mosby.)

an increased fire hazard (a pure oxygen atmosphere is used); and cannot be used for recompression below 3 ATA (66 FSW), which may be suboptimal for the management of AGE.

With proper therapy, the victim is rapidly "dived" to a compression depth of 6 ATA, where he breathes air for 30 minutes. After this period, decompression is effected over 4 minutes to 2.8 ATA (60 FSW), where 100% oxygen is administered by face mask in accordance with a 20 minutes on/5 minutes off schedule for at least three cycles. If symptoms improve or show considerable resolution during this period, the victim is decompressed to 1.9 ATA (30 FSW) at a rate of 1 foot/minute; at this depth, six more oxygen-air cycles are completed. To complete the treatment schedule, the victim breathes oxygen and "ascends" to surface pressure over a 30-minute period. An experienced hyperbaric medicine practitioner will modify the treatment table in accordance with the victim's progress.

Intermittent oxygen breathing lengthens the safe time for exposure to hyperbaric oxygen. At 2.8 ATA, where 100% oxygen is used to treat AGE and decompression sickness, pulmonary oxygen toxicity is rarely problematic because oxygen-induced seizures precede pulmonary damage. Central nervous system (CNS) oxygen toxicity is rarely noted and is limited to apprehension, nausea, muscle twitching, auditory changes, tunnel vision, and seizures. In such a case, oxygen breathing is temporarily discontinued without altering the depth of compression, and the patient rapidly returns to his preictal state. Although phenytoin sodium and diazepam may suppress oxygen-induced seizures, anticonvulsants are not generally recommended for this purpose, because elevating the seizure threshold might allow unrecognized CNS toxicity.[60] Anticonvulsants should be used only when recurrent seizures preclude essential hyperbaric therapy.

If the victim is unconscious, cannot cooperate, or is unable to equalize the pressure across the tympanic membrane, a needle tympanotomy is performed to prevent barotitis media and rupture of the tympanic membrane. All inflatable cuffs and balloons should be filled with sterile water or saline, not air. Intravenous fluids should be administered from collapsible plastic bags, not bottles. If a glass bottle must be used, it should be vented.

The benefits of recompression therapy in the management of both AGE and decompression sickness include reduction of bubble size, displacement of tissue nitrogen (replaced by oxygen, which is more rapidly absorbed by the tissues), and overall augmentation of tissue oxygenation. Gradual decompression in the chamber prevents the reformation of gas bubbles. Some hyperbaric medicine practitioners have questioned the necessity of beginning therapy at 6 ATA. In a canine model of cerebral AGE that produced severe cortical dysfunction and cerebral blood flow deficits, the efficacy of treatment was assessed using median nerve somatosensory cortical-evoked potentials, ^{14}C iodoantipyrene autoradiographic cerebral blood flow studies, brain water content measurements, and various physiologic parameters.[165] It appeared that no advantage accrued by preceding oxygen treatments at 18 m with compression to 49.5 m. Application of this study to humans is as yet hypothetical but should be investigated.

Decompression Sickness

Decompression sickness, or "the bends," is a multisystem disorder triggered by liberation of inert gases (predominantly nitrogen) from solution. These bubbles evolve in the bloodstream and tissues of the body as divers ascend and ambient pressure decreases.[97,235,239] The origin of the dissolved gases is the pressurized air that the diver breathes from tanks; if the "no-decompression limit" is exceeded by virtue of excessive time or depth, then more nitrogen is dissolved in the body than can be safely breathed off without staged decompression. According to Henry's law, the amount of a gas that dissolves in a liquid at a constant temperature is related to the partial pressure of that gas in contact with the liquid and the coefficient of solubility of the gas in the liquid. Thus increased absorption of nitrogen and supersaturation of the tissues, particularly those with a high fat content, with inert gas is a prerequisite for decompression sickness. However, the cause is an overly rapid ascent that exceeds the capability of a human to eliminate the gas during decompression. Tissue uptake of nitrogen appears to increase with exercise and obesity. Nitrogen off-loading is diminished in cold water. Predisposition to decompression sickness is noted in the elderly, in a fatigued diver, and in a person who has previously had decompression sickness.

Divers who perform "decompression dives," in which sufficient nitrogen is absorbed to create a situation of risk, practice in-water decompression. In such cases the diver must make "decompression stops" during ascent, pausing at certain depths to eliminate ("off-gas") excess nitrogen and avoid bubble formation. Unfortunately, even with close adherence to the U.S. Navy diving decompression schedules, a diver can develop decompression sickness.

Pathophysiology

Inert gas bubbles in the tissues and bloodstream produce a number of complex mechanical and biophysical effects.[32,62,75,132] Vascular occlusion can occur in numerous vessels, such as the epivertebral venous plexus (Batson's plexus), causing venous stasis and congestive infarction.[116] Bubbles that form in the venous circulation may pass into the arterial circulation via intrapulmonic and intracardiac shunts, causing paradoxic AGE. Lymphatic bubbles may occlude the lymphatics and cause lymphedema. Bubbles that form in the capillary circulation mechanically injure the vascular endothelium and trigger a cascade of inflammation, including activation of factor XII (Hageman factor), which activates the intrinsic clotting, kinin, and complement systems. This promotes platelet activation, microvascular stasis, increased vascular permeability, interstitial edema, and decreased tissue perfusion.[75,116]

Clinical Presentation

Decompression sickness can be divided into type I (joint pain, skin rash) and type II (pulmonary, cardiovascular, central nervous system).[101] The onset of symptoms of decompression sickness usually occurs within 15 minutes to 2 hours after a dive but may be delayed by 24 to 48 hours.[135,148,218] Fatigue out of proportion to the exertion performed often heralds mild decompression sickness. The most common symptom of decompression sickness is periarticular aching joint pain, exacerbated by movement, with associated periarticular numbness or dysesthesia. The knees, shoulder, and elbows are most frequently involved. "Limb bends" also refers to tendinitis or bursitis-like pain attributed to the stretching of tendons or ligaments by nitrogen bubbles. Massage or exercise may exacerbate this pain.

Another frequent manifestation is skin involvement attributed to vasospasm, manifested by itching, serpiginous or scattered scarlatiniform rashes (resembling erysipelas), petechiae on the soles of the feet, and formication. Cutis marmorata marbleization is a darkened mottling that can be noted over the pectoral muscles, shoulders, chest, abdomen, forearms, and thighs. As the rash spreads peripherally, the central area becomes erythematous and warm. Moderate pain at rest and on palpation accompanies the rash. The discoloration blanches with pressure and may persist for 2 to 6 days. Crepitus is absent.

Neurologic decompression sickness may involve the brain, spinal cord, inner ear, or peripheral nerves. Scuba divers frequently have involvement of the lower thoracic, lumbar, and sacral regions of the spinal cord, causing pain, paresthesia, monoparesis, hemiplegia or paraplegia, and bladder and bowel incontinence. If the cerebellum or inner ear is affected, the diver suffers severe vertigo, nausea, vomiting, and ataxia ("the staggers"). Scotomas, visual field defects, migraine-type headaches, hallucinations, alexia, agnosia, dysphasia, seizures, and confusion indicate cerebral involvement.

Pulmonary decompression sickness, "the chokes," implies approximately 10% occlusion of the pulmonary vascular bed by embolic gas bubbles or foam that has originated in the venous system, complicated by induced vasospasm and bronchospasm. Symptoms include chest pain, cough, cyanosis, air hunger, wheezing, tachypnea, and tachycardia. In severe cases of venous air embolism (rarely noted in divers), additional symptoms include increased central venous or pulmonary artery pressure, ECG signs of ischemia or cor pulmonale, decreased end-tidal carbon dioxide fraction, and characteristic precordial Doppler sounds. A chest radiograph does not reveal air in the main pulmonary artery unless the air accumulation is massive (5 to 8 ml/kg).[154] Diffuse systemic venous air emboli can cause hypotension ("decompression shock") and cardiovascular collapse, attributed to increased capillary permeability, rapid leakage of fluid into the interstitial spaces of the body, and functional hypovolemia. In such cases pulmonary and peripheral edema and adult respiratory distress syndrome (ARDS) are noted. These are often complicated by disseminated intravascular coagulopathy.[115] Bradyrhythmias are associated with vasovagal reactions.

Laboratory findings associated with decompression sickness include elevated white blood count, thrombocytopenia, hemoconcentration, and increased prothrombin time.

Emergency Field Care

In the absence of overt symptoms, the diagnosis of decompression sickness can be subtle and easily confused with muscle fatigue or air embolism.[101,151] If symptoms develop several hours after diving, one should note whether the victim exercised vigorously or traveled in an unpressurized aircraft during the interval, because either could initiate the bends. A simple test to diagnose joint bends is to inflate a blood pressure cuff to a pressure of 200 to 300 mm Hg around the affected joint. Pain that is relieved on inflation and returns on deflation is pathognomonic for decompression sickness. The victim should receive oxygen by face mask at a flow rate of 10 L/minute. Transport to a hyperbaric recompression facility should be undertaken immediately. If a nonpressurized aircraft is used, flight altitude should be maintained under 300 m. Pressurized cabin environments should not exceed a 1 ATA pressure drop if possible. Under no circumstances should in-water recompression be attempted.

Hospital Management

At the hospital an intravenous line should be placed and the victim hydrated with crystalloid solution to maintain a urine output of 40 to 50 ml/hour. If the victim has altered mental status or suffers from spinal cord involvement, an indwelling urinary catheter should be placed. A blood sample should be obtained for complete blood count, electrolytes, glucose, creatinine, and blood urea nitrogen. A detailed neurologic examination should be recorded, along with a chest radiograph and ECG. As soon as possible, the victim should be transported to a recompression chamber. Vertigo associated with labyrinthine decompression sickness may be successfully treated with small doses of intravenous or intramuscular diazepam.

Recommendations for adjuncts to therapy have included such modalities as heparin, low-molecular-weight dextran, and corticosteroids. The last has been widely recommended as an adjunct to recompression; however, absolute proof of efficacy awaits controlled clinical trials.[149] Current practice favors initial use of large intravenous doses of a rapid-acting steroid (methylprednisolone sodium succinate, 125 mg), along with a longer-acting maintenance product (dexamethasone, 4 mg every 6 hours). The latter can be continued by mouth for 4 days without prolonged tapering. The putative mechanism of action is related to reduction of capillary permeability, stabilization of lysosomal membranes, activation of prostaglandins, and inhibition of thromboxane that is integral to vascular endothelial platelet aggregation triggered at the blood-bubble interface. Evidence does not yet exist that corticosteroids reduce the cerebral or spinal cord edema associated with decompression sickness, although it is generally accepted that they ameliorate edema of vasogenic rather than traumatic origin.

RECOMPRESSION THERAPY. As stated previously, clinical and technical recommendations may be obtained 24 hours a day from the DAN. Although recompression is most effective if undertaken soon after the onset of symptoms, significant clinical improvement may be noted even after delays in excess of 72 hours. In a review of 50 cases of decompression sickness in which treatment was delayed from 12 to 168 hours after the onset of symptoms, 90% of victims showed complete or substantial resolution, although standard recompression protocols had to be lengthened in many cases.[150]

In the hyperbaric chamber, one popular therapeutic method is to follow the U.S. Navy Treatment Table 6 (see Figure 18-10), in which the victim is rapidly recompressed to 2.8 ATA (60 FSW). At this depth 100% oxygen is administered by face mask in accordance with a 20 minutes on/5 minutes off schedule for at least three cycles. The victim then breathes 100% oxygen during a 30-minute ascent to 1.9 ATA (30 FSW). At this depth the victim completes six additional oxygen-air breathing cycles before ascent to the surface. As with air embolism, the experienced hyperbaric medicine physician may modify the duration at a particular depth in accordance with the victim's clinical response. Some physicians prefer to use U.S. Navy Treatment Table 6A for the management of pulmonary or spinal cord decompression sickness.

If the victim is unconscious, cannot cooperate, or is unable to equalize the pressure across the tympanic membrane, a needle tympanotomy is performed to prevent barotitis media and tympanic membrane rupture.

Barotrauma

Barotrauma is the tissue damage that results from the pressure disequilibrium between the environment and the gas-filled spaces in the body. Barotrauma of descent (volume contraction) is commonly referred to as *squeeze;* barotrauma of ascent is induced by expansion without decompression of gas-filled spaces ("reverse squeeze").

Pulmonary Barotrauma

Lung squeeze is usually encountered by breath-holding (free) divers, who do not breathe pressurized air supplied by scuba tanks. Because the free diver is not breathing compressed air, which would be at the same pressure as the surrounding environment, the air held in the lungs decreases in volume with descent. When the diver attains a depth at which the total lung volume becomes less than the theoretic residual volume, the underventilated air spaces fill with blood and extravasated interstitial lung fluid. This has been attributed to the theoretic decline of intra-alveolar pressure below transpulmonic pressure. Although the world record for free-diving is over 90 m, most people experience lung squeeze at 30 to 40 m. Symptoms appear on ascent and include shortness of breath, coughing, hemoptysis, and respiratory failure. Therapy involves administration of oxygen and, in severe cases, endotracheal intubation and application of positive end-expiratory pressure.

Otolaryngologic Barotrauma

EAR CANAL SQUEEZE. Ear canal squeeze occurs when the external acoustic meatus is occluded by cerumen, bony or cartilaginous exostoses, a wet suit hood, or plugs. Because water cannot enter the external ear to fill the air space, pressure cannot be equalized during descent. A relative negative pressure develops in the blocked ear canal, and the tympanic membrane bulges outward and occasionally ruptures. Edema and bleeding in soft tissue are recognized by petechiae and hemorrhagic blebs.[240] Diving activity should be suspended until healing is complete.

BAROTITIS MEDIA. Middle ear squeeze, or barotitis media, occurs when the pressure in the middle ear cannot be equalized with that of the external environment, generally because of occlusion or malfunction of the eustachian tube.[21] As the diver descends without equalization (via Valsalva's or Frenzel's maneuver), the gas volume in the middle ear contracts and creates a relative vacuum. At a depth of 75 cm below the surface, as the external-to-internal pressure differential across the tympanic membrane reaches 60 mm Hg, the diver senses a feeling of fullness in the ear. At a depth of 1.2 m below the surface, the pressure differential approaches 90 mm Hg, whereupon the medial one third of the eustacian tube collapses and becomes occluded.[250] With further increases in pressure, the mucosa of the middle ear becomes hemorrhagic and edematous, and the tympanic membrane bulges inward (Figure 18-11). Pain is a prominent feature. If descent continues beyond 1.6 to 5.1 m (pressure differential to 100 to 400 mm Hg), the eardrum ruptures, and water rushes into the middle ear, causing severe vertigo, disorientation, and nausea.

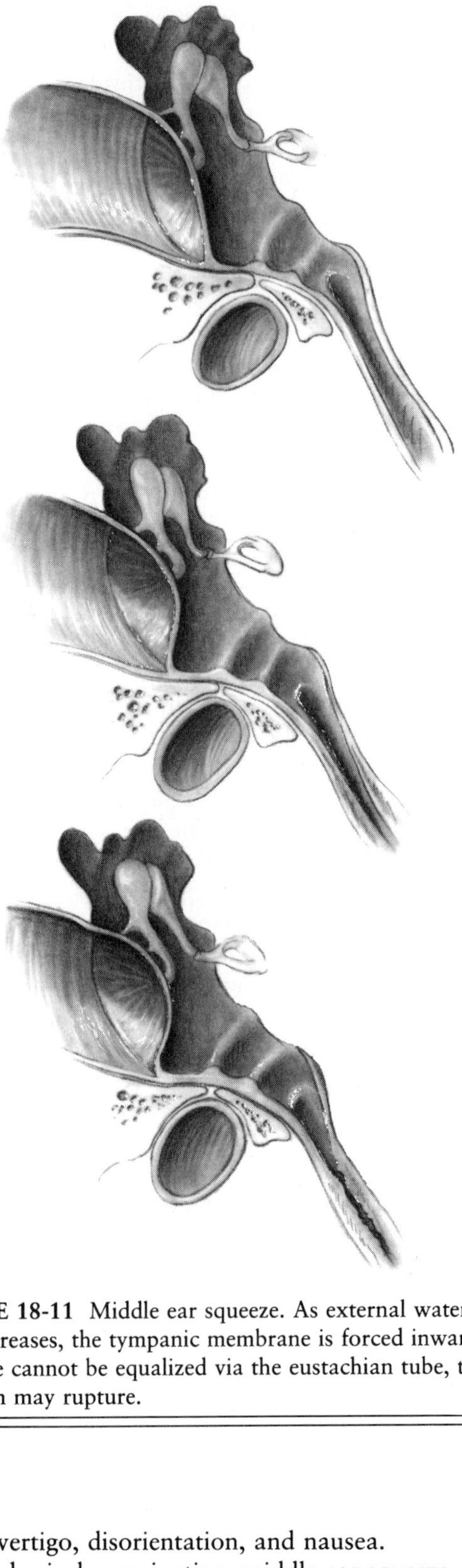

FIGURE 18-11 Middle ear squeeze. As external water pressure increases, the tympanic membrane is forced inward. If pressure cannot be equalized via the eustachian tube, the eardrum may rupture.

On physical examination, middle ear squeeze can be graded on a scale of 0 to 5:

Grade 0 Pain without physical symptoms
Grade 1 Congestion of umbo and pars flaccida
Grade 2 Congestion of entire tympanic membrane

Grade 3 Hemorrhage into the tympanic membrane with or without serous otitis media
Grade 4 Middle ear hemorrhage
Grade 5 Rupture of the tympanic membrane

Most injuries are grade 2 and grade 3, which heal spontaneously within 1 to 2 weeks. Diving activity should be suspended until all symptoms have resolved. If the tympanic membrane has not ruptured, the victim may be treated with a long-acting nasal spray (oxymetazoline hydrochloride, 0.05%, every 12 hours) for 2 to 3 days and an oral decongestant (pseudoephedrine hydrochloride, 60 mg every 8 hours) until the symptoms have resolved. Eardrum pain may be managed with oral analgesics and topical antipyrine-benzocaine-glycerin otic solution. Occasionally, a politzerization procedure using low-pressure air via the eustachian tube is necessary to reinflate the middle ear space.[61]

If the tympanic membrane has ruptured, particularly in polluted waters, the victim should be treated with oral and nasal decongestants and analgesics, started on penicillin or erythromycin therapy, and referred to an otolaryngologist.[23] No solution should be instilled in the ear. Vertigo may be controlled with oral meclizine hydrochloride (25 mg every 8 hours) or intravenous diazepam (5 to 15 mg every 6 to 8 hours).

Alternobaric vertigo is caused by pressure disequilibrium and asymmetric vestibular stimulation between the two middle ears. The condition most commonly occurs on ascent, when expanding air in the middle ear cannot be vented through one of the eustachian tubes.[76,168] This situation frequently occurs if decongestants are used and lose their effectiveness during the dive. An alternate explanation for alternobaric vertigo is that the pressure effect of descent displaces the stapes and oval window inward, causing the round window to bulge outward. Sudden equalization reverses the respective directions of the membranes and increases middle ear and inner ear pressure, which induces vertigo. Regardless of the mechanism, the treatment is identical to that for barotitis media.

LABYRINTHINE WINDOW RUPTURE. The sensory organs of balance and hearing in the inner ear are suspended between endolymph and perilymph. The stapes inserts into the oval window. A membrane that separates the basal turn of the cochlea from the middle ear closes the round window. Barotrauma of the inner ear can cause a rupture of the oval or round window, or both, leading to the formation of a perilymph fistula.[87,88,108,109] The round window is most commonly injured in diving accidents by one of two mechanisms. The first occurs when volume contraction in the middle ear (dysfunction of the eustachian tube) induces spontaneous outward rupture of the round window or causes the tympanic membrane to bulge inward. This forces the ossicles inward and causes subluxation of the stapes footplate through the oval window. The second occurs when the diver performs a vigorous Valsalva maneuver (in an attempt to force air through the eustachian tube to pressurize the middle ear). This increases the cerebrospinal fluid pressure, which is transmitted to the intracochlear perilymph and causes outward rupture of the round window. Alternatively, if the Valsalva maneuver is successful, the sudden rise in middle ear pressure can implode the round window into the inner ear. The labyrinthine fistula can cause permanent damage to the cochlea and hearing loss if not recognized and repaired.

Symptoms include sudden profound tinnitus, vertigo, nausea, vomiting, ataxia, nystagmus, and sensorineural hearing loss. Vertigo is the most common of these symptoms. In some cases only mild tinnitus and a sense of ear fullness may be noted. A fistula test confirms the diagnosis. A pressure change is induced in the middle ear, with positive and negative pressure applied alternately to the external auditory canal. In a positive test, vertigo is reproduced. Interpretation of positive results in a victim with Ménière's disease should be cautiously made. Romberg's sign is frequently normal. A Quix test for body deviation, in which the victim stands with feet together, eyes closed, chin raised, and arms extended, often shows gradual sway in a lateral direction (toward the affected ear when hearing is normal; away from the affected ear when hearing loss exists).

Treatment is controversial. Some otolaryngologists recommend an initial trial of absolute bed rest with the head elevated, and symptomatic treatment for vertigo, whereas others advocate immediate surgical repair of the labyrinthine leak.[207,259] Exploratory tympanotomy accomplishes the latter. To enter the middle ear, the surgeon elevates the tympanic membrane with a skin flap from the wall of the external auditory canal.[164] The patient is placed in Trendelenburg's position to elevate the cerebrospinal fluid pressure, transmitted via the cochlear aqueduct to the perilymphatic fluid. In this way, the round or oval window fistula can be localized by noting the accumulation of leaking fluid. Earlobe fat, perichondrium, or subcutaneous tissue may be used to patch the leaks. If the stapedial footplate is the origin of the leak, a stapedectomy is performed, with insertion of a prosthesis and tissue graft. All grafts are covered with Gelfoam for support.

If the nonsurgical approach is favored, the victim must avoid straining (Valsalva's maneuver), sneezing, or vigorous athletic activity until the ear returns to normal. Recompression in a hyperbaric chamber should not be undertaken unless the symptoms are believed to result from decompression sickness of the inner ear or air embolism, because pressurization will worsen the injury. Obviously, diving should not be attempted until healing is complete.

BAROSINUSITIS. The paranasal sinuses, particularly

the maxillary and frontal sinuses, are subject to "sinus squeeze."[90] This occurs when the diver descends and is unable to force pressurized air into the sinuses. The air within the closed spaces contracts and creates a relative vacuum, producing edema, vascular engorgement, and ultimately hemorrhage of the sinus wall mucosa.[79] Symptoms include intense pain, a feeling of fullness, epistaxis, and bleeding into the throat. Radiography demonstrates a fluid level of opacification of the involved sinuses. Treatment involves administering topical nasal and oral decongestants, analgesics, and antibiotics if fever or purulent discharge is present. A "reverse" sinus squeeze is encountered on ascent if the sinuses cannot vent the expanding air. The major symptom of reverse sinus squeeze is excruciating pain, which may require administration of narcotic analgesics. Over several hours, the air is gradually absorbed without sequelae.

AERODONTALGIA. Dental barotrauma, or aerodontalgia, is encountered if a diver has an enclosed pocket of air within a tooth because of tooth decay or improper repair. If the air pocket undergoes significant contraction during descent, the tooth may implode, causing severe pain. Alternatively, the tooth may fill with blood and gingival tissue, so that expansion of the air space is inhibited on ascent, and the tooth explodes.

HAZARDOUS MARINE LIFE

Encounters with marine animals have increased with the surge in popularity of scuba diving, wind surfing, and other water recreational activities. Such interactions frequently culminate in unique injuries to the participant. The increasing number of saltwater aquaria in private and public collections has created additional risks. Surgeons must be familiar with hazards unique to the marine environment and not rely on therapeutic folklore.

Sharks

Sharks are the most magnificent hazardous marine animals.[11] Surrounded by myth and media attention, these savage animals are under constant biologic and behavioral investigation. Approximately 32 of the 250 species have been implicated in the 100 attacks reported annually worldwide. In U.S. coastal waters (including Hawaii), the most commonly identified man-eaters are the great white, blue, mako, hammerhead, and gray reef sharks. The crescent-shaped jaws of a carnivorous shark contain rows of razor-sharp, rip-saw teeth, so that the leading row can be replaced every few months. With a biting force in larger animals estimated to approach 18 tons psi, shark bites create an unparalleled potential for sudden tissue loss and hemorrhage.

The motivation for shark attacks may be explained by a combination of anomalous behavior, such as violation of courtship patterns, invasion of territorial waters, pursuit of frightened swimmers, and misidentification of victims (such as humans for elephant seals).[16,59] The odds of being attacked by a shark along the North American coastline are roughly 1 in 5 million and are enhanced by swimming in recreational areas, during the afternoon and early evening, and in turbid waters. Most victims are attacked by a single shark without warning, occasionally preceded by a "bumping," in which the shark's rough skin denticles may severely abrade the skin. Victims generally are bitten only once or twice, which precludes feeding as the shark's primary motivation.

Clinical Presentation

Most victims are bitten on an extremity, because they are attacked from below on the leg or bitten on the arm while trying to fend off a frontal assault. In many attacks the laceration patterns indicate open-mouth raking, which yields large slashes without significant tissue loss.[15] However, large sharks can strike with tremendous momentum and can transect a limb or remove a hemithorax (Figure 18-12). The laceration and avulsion of tissue that occur in the ocean create a situation of massive hemorrhage and rapid progression to emotional and hemodynamic shock. In many instances the soft tissue injury is compounded by pneumothorax or hemopneumothorax, evisceration, long-bone or vertebral fractures, or airway obstruction.

Emergency Field Care

If necessary, brisk arterial hemorrhage should be contained with firm pressure. To prevent exsanguination, large disrupted arteries or veins should be ligated if the bleeding cannot be controlled by direct pressure. Injudicious use of tourniquets should be avoided; the decision to apply a tourniquet is one to sacrifice a limb to save a life. If supplies are available, at least two 12- or 14-gauge intravenous lines should be placed in the uninvolved extremities, and vigorous crystalloid infusion (normal saline or lactated Ringer's solution) should be initiated. The patient should be kept well oxygenated and warm while immediate transport to a trauma facility is undertaken.

Hospital Management

The victim should be carefully examined for evidence of cervical, intrathoracic, or intra-abdominal injuries. If blood loss has been severe, cross-matched whole blood or packed red blood cells should be replaced. To temporize, immediate administration of crystalloid appears to be as efficacious as replacement with colloid products such as plasmanate or albumin. Fluorinated hydrocarbon blood substitutes, not yet approved for general use in the United States, have theoretic appeal in this situ-

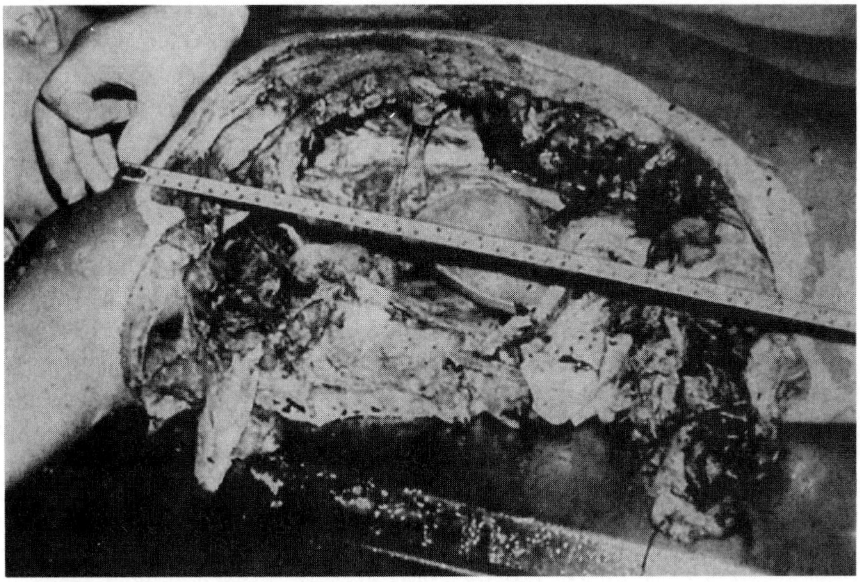

FIGURE 18-12 Massive shark bite. This surfer was attacked by a great white shark estimated to be 16 to 18 feet (4.7 to 5.4 m) long. (Courtesy P. Crossman, Coroner's Division, Salinas, Calif.)

ation. All seriously injured victims should have an indwelling urinary catheter and either a central venous catheter or pulmonary artery catheter to guide administration of fluids and pressor agents.

Debriding any but the simplest abrasion or laceration in the emergency department is inappropriate. Shark bite wounds are a combination of laceration, puncture, and crush injuries. They are frequently more extensive and complicated than they appear and should be explored in the operating room. The wound should be explored to its depths and irrigated vigorously with normal saline. If the wound is very large, a solution of povidone-iodine in saline, not to exceed 10%, may be used for irrigation. It is not uncommon to find shark teeth, pieces of surfboard or wet suit, and copious amounts of sand in the wound. All obviously devitalized tissue should be removed and primary injuries repaired. Although large dead spaces must be closed, the use of absorbable suture material to snugly reapproximate the fat and subcuticular layers is not advised. To minimize the risk of infection, the wounds should be packed open to await delayed primary closure or should be approximated with closed drainage systems.

Tetanus toxoid (0.5 ml intramuscularly) and tetanus immune globulin (250 to 500 units intramuscularly) should be administered. Use of prophylactic antibiotics is controversial and traditionally has been based on the rationale that aquatic debris and shark mouth flora occasionally contain *Vibrio* or *Clostridium* organisms.

Stingrays

Stingrays are the most commonly implicated group of fish involved in human envenomations. Eleven species are found in American coastal waters, and these account for more than 1500 reported injuries each year.[187,225] Rays may grow to more than 3.6 m in length and are identified by their flattened bodies and wide, winglike pectoral fins. The venom apparatus is composed of one to four venomous stings located on the dorsal side of a whiplike, elongated tail. The families Gymnuridae, Myliobatidae, Dasyatidae, and Urolophidae represent an ascending order of risk based on the muscularity and development of the venom organ, which is related to the length and strength of the tail and the location of the sting.[112] The sting is a bilaterally retroserrated dentinal spine attached to the dorsum of the tail by dense collagenous tissue. The sharply toothed spine is encased in an integumentary sheath, overlying symmetric ventrolateral glandular grooves and associated venom glands.

Stingray venom is composed of multifarious toxic compounds, including serotinin, 5′-nucleotidase, and phosphodiesterase. In laboratory animals, the venom effects include peripheral vasoconstriction, cardiac arrhythmias, ischemic ECG changes, respiratory depression, seizures, ataxia, coma, and death.[225]

Clinical Presentation

Most stingrays are encountered as the unwary surf explorer shuffles his feet in shallow water. Stingrays frequently lie partially submerged in the sand, with only the eyes and spiracles exposed. When directly disturbed, they may reflexly lash upward forcefully with the tail, spine erect, inflicting a nasty sting. The integumentary sheath is disrupted, and venom is released into the wound. Thus laceration and envenomation occur simultaneously.

The lower extremities are injured most frequently, followed by the upper extremities, abdomen, and thorax. Because of the retroserrated teeth and powerful strikes, the laceration may be considerable. Fatalities have been reported following intra-abdominal and thoracic trauma.

Envenomation causes immediate, intense local pain, soft tissue edema, and profuse bleeding. The pain radiates centrally and may be severe for 24 to 48 hours and of an intensity to provoke disorientation. The wound initially appears pallorous, dusky, or cyanotic and becomes erythematous, with local hemorrhage within 1 to 2 hours. Delayed necrosis is common; systemic manifestations include weakness, nausea, vomiting, diarrhea, diaphoresis, dyspnea, tachycardia, headache, vertigo, muscle fasciculations, syncope, hypotension, arrhythmias, and death. Paralysis is caused by spastic muscle contraction rather than nerve conduction abnormalties. Puncture of the chest wall can create a pneumothorax or hemopneumothorax.

Emergency Field Care

Treatment is directed at opposing the venom's effects, alleviating pain, and preventing infection.[27] Outside the hospital, emergency measures should include a rapid survey for major traumatic injury, with appropriate stabilization. The wound should be irrigated copiously with saline or fresh water. Hot water irrigation up to 45° C (113° F) may alternate thermolabile protein venom components. Any easily located large pieces of sting or integumentary sheath should be removed from the wound. Local suction (for small puncture wounds) with a rubber suction cup has limited value. When the lower or upper extremity is involved, some authors recommend using a constriction band to occlude superficial venous and lymphatic return, released for 90 seconds every 10 minutes to prevent irreversible limb ischemia. This technique should be considered only if the wound is very large or deep and the time to definitive care will exceed 1 hour.

Hospital Management

As soon as possible, the wound should be soaked in hot water to tolerance (45° to 50° C [115° to 120° F]) for 30 to 90 minutes. This step relieves pain by inactivating some components of the venom. No chemicals (e.g., potassium permanganate, hydrogen peroxide, ammonia, formalin, or magnesium sulfate) should be added to the water, because in this situation such chemicals are tissue toxic or obscure visualization of the wound. Cryotherapy is absolutely contraindicated. Antihistamine, steroid, and proteolytic enzyme (papain) therapies are anecdotal. During the soaking procedure, visible pieces of sting and integumentary sheath should be extracted from the wound.

If no contraindication exists, systemic analgesics should be administered liberally. Narcotics are frequently required. To allow primary debridement of small wounds in the emergency department, the wounds should be infiltrated with 1% lidocaine without epinephrine, or a regional nerve block should be performed. After debridement the wounds should be packed with iodoform gauze or closed loosely and immobilized for 48 to 72 hours. All victims should be observed for systemic effects for 4 hours before they are discharged.

After the soaking procedure, large or complicated wounds should be explored and debrided under sterile conditions in the operating room. The wounds should be closed loosely with drainage or packed open to await delayed primary closure. Tetanus prophylaxis is standard procedure.

The rationale for antibiotic management is the same as for shark bites. If the wound is small and managed in an outpatient (emergency department) setting, the patient should be treated with cephalexin (250 mg four times a day) *and* tetracycline (500 mg four times a day) or trimethoprim/sulfamethoxazole (160/800 mg twice a day).

Urchins

Sea urchins are free-living echinoderms with an egg-shaped, globular, or flattened body. The viscera are surrounded by a hard shell covered with spines and specialized seizing organs (pedicellariae) (Figure 18-13). These predominantly nocturnal animals are most commonly found on rocky bottoms, in coral crevices, or burrowed in the sand.[192]

The venom of sea urchins is delivered by hollow, venom-filled spines or by the triple-jawed pedicellariae. Generally, a single species uses only one of the two mechanisms for envenomation. The spines are either blunt and non-venom-bearing or long, slender, sharp, hollow, and venom laden. The spines of venomous species are brittle and easily broken off in the skin and are keen enough to penetrate rubber gloves, booties, and wet suits. The spines of *Diadema setosum* may exceed 30 cm in length. The pedicellariae are small and are scattered among the spines. A slender stalk attaches the terminal head with its calcareous pincer jaws to the sea urchin's shell plates. The outer surface of each jaw is connected to or covered by a venom gland that contracts and releases venom on stimulation. Pedicellariae will hang onto the victim tenaciously and will be torn from the shell rather than cease biting. Detached pedicellariae

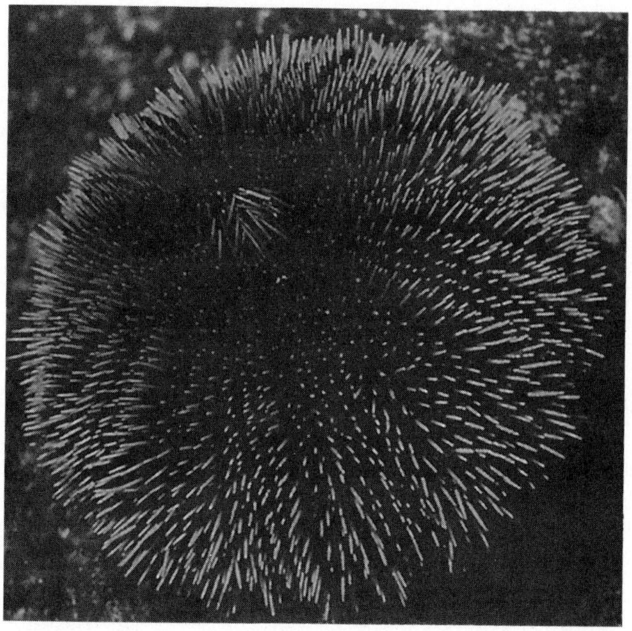

FIGURE 18-13 Sea urchin. The slender, venom-filled spines are sharp, brittle, and easily dislodged or broken after they enter the skin.

may continue to bite and envenom for several hours.[166]

Sea urchin venom contains various toxic fractions, including steroid glycosides, serotonin, and cholinergic substances.[172] The Pacific Ocean urchin, *Tripneustes ventricosus,* carries a potent neurotoxin.

Clinical Presentation

When a venomous spine punctures the skin, the reaction is immediate, characterized by burning pain, and shortly followed by intense aching, erythema, and soft tissue edema.[21] The spines usually break off and remain lodged in the skin. This problem may be confused with purple discoloration left by dye rubbed from the surface of some spines. Spines frequently are lodged in the hand and forearm when the unwary diver brushes up against or handles an urchin. When several spines enter the victim simultaneously, the systemic response may include nausea, vomiting, dyspnea, paralysis, confusion, collapse, and hypotension. The stings of pedicellariae frequently are more intense, causing immediate intense pain with central radiation, severe soft tissue swelling, and local skin hemorrhage. Systemic manifestations include those of spine puncture wounds, as well as syncope, aphonia, respiratory distress, and death. In most cases the pain resolves within 1 to 2 hours; in rare cases focal or generalized muscular paralysis persists for up to 6 hours.

Emergency Field Care

As soon as possible, the wound should be immersed in hot water to tolerance (45° to 50° C [115° to 120° F]), which often substantially relieves the pain. If large spines can be easily grasped, they should be extracted gently, with great care taken to avoid fragmentation in the skin. Blind probing with a surgical instrument in search of spine fragments is fruitless and may exacerbate the injury.

Hospital Management

Visible embedded spines should be removed with the aid of an operating microscope or magnifying loupes. Some spines are radiopaque and can be visualized on plain or soft tissue radiographs. All thick calcium carbonate spines should be removed if possible to prevent infection and the formation of foreign body granulomas. If a spine cannot be easily reached, has entered deeply into the hand or foot, has penetrated a joint, or is closely aligned to a neurovascular structure, the victim should be taken to the operating room for proper visualization (Figure 18-14). Thin, superficially penetrated (subcutaneous) spine fragments may be absorbed in 2 to 21 days and need not be removed unless they cause persistent pain.[110] If left in place, they often are walled off in a granuloma with focal central necrosis and can be removed surgically or injected with intralesional steroids.[146,186,220]

Pedicellariae are removed from the skin most effectively by shaving the skin with a straight razor. Because this procedure can be quite painful, it should be preceded by a hot water soak or topical application of 2% viscous lidocaine, or both.

Scorpionfish

Scorpionfish are second only to stingrays in the number of vertebrate stings recorded in humans.[10] They are found most commonly in tropical waters (and increasingly in private aquaria) and are divided into three groups on the basis of venom organ structure: zebrafish, scorpionfish, and stonefish.[178] Zebrafish are brightly colored, ornate coral reef fish that are found as single or paired swimmers in relatively shallow water. The venom organs are a series of long, delicate dorsal, pelvic, and anal spines, all associated with venom glands. Scorpionfish are more often found on the ocean bottom, where their unique shape and coloration conceal them. Hidden in the rocks, sand, and coral, they are also equipped with stout, venom-laden spines. The sedentary stonefish are found in Indo-Pacific waters, where they conceal themselves in coral crevices or bury themselves in the mud and sand. The spines are heavy and covered with a thick, warty integumentary sheath.

When disturbed, any of these fishes erects the spinous dorsal fin, flares out the armed gill covers, and presents

A
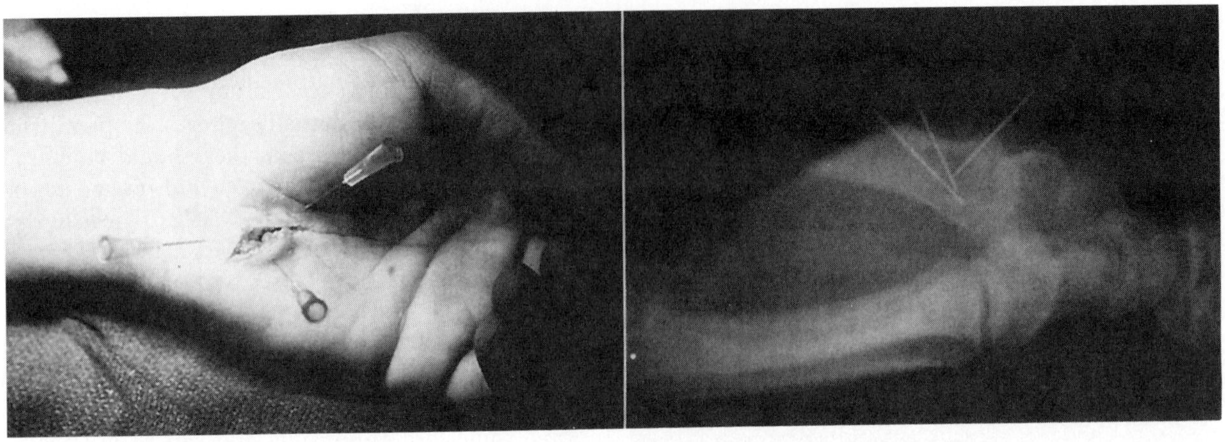
B

FIGURE 18-14 Embedded sea urchin spine. **A,** The spine entered the palm of the victim, who leaned into a tidal pool. Needles were used to locate the spine. **B,** Radiographic film illustrates location of the spine with the needle technique. A 90-minute attempt at surgical removal was unsuccessful. The patient recovered uneventfully.

A
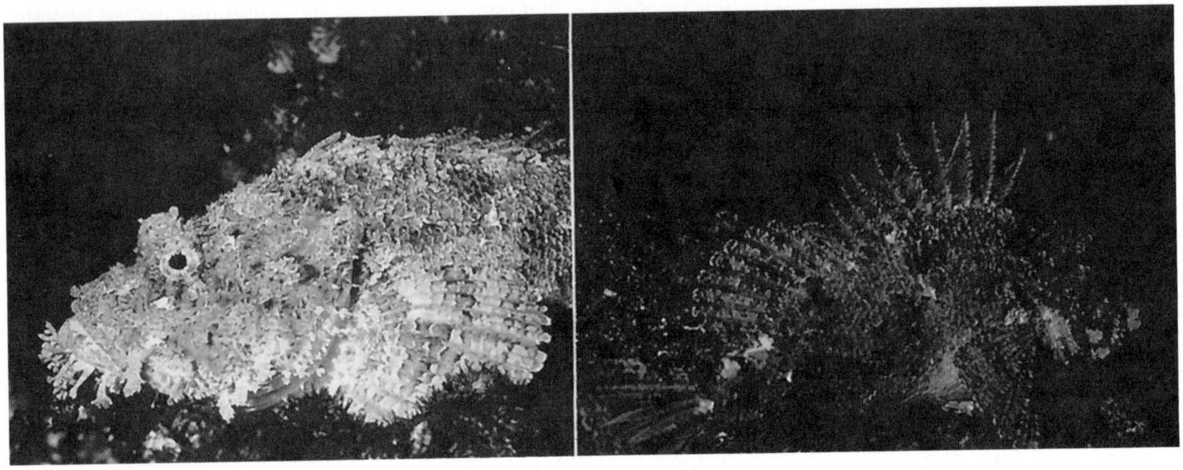
B

FIGURE 18-15 Scorpionfish. **A,** The Galapagos scorpionfish is well camouflaged and blends in completely with the surroundings. **B,** When threatened, the scorpionfish erects its spines; a nasty sting awaits the unwise aggressor.

the anal fins (Figure 18-15). If cornered, they will on rare occasion attack in defense. The venom is carried along the spines underneath the integumentary sheath and is injected into the victim in a manner analogous to that of stingray envenomation. The venom is least potent in the zebrafish, moderately potent in the scorpionfish, and extremely potent in the stonefish.

Clinical Presentation

Most envenomations occur when the unwary fisherman or diver handles or trods on an animal; however, an increasing number of envenomations are noted in owners of saltwater aquaria. The severity of the reaction depends on the amount and potency of venom. Generally, pain is immediate and intense, with central radiation. The pain of a stonefish sting may persist for days at an intensity sufficient to cause delirium. The puncture wound initially becomes ischemic and cyanotic, surrounded by a region of swelling, erythema, and warmth. Over 12 to 24 hours, tissue necrosis and cellulitis develop and may persist in an indolent fashion for weeks to months. In severe envenomations the victim may develop a maculopapular skin rash, nausea, vomiting, diarrhea, sweating, agitation, seizures, focal paralysis, lymphangitis, arthritis, fever, hypertension, respiratory distress, arrhythmias, congestive heart failure, hypotension, and cardiovascular collapse. Death from stings of the dreaded stonefish have been reported.[238]

Emergency Field Care

The field treatment of scorpionfish envenomation is identical to that for stingray envenomation. The wound should be vigorously irrigated; all readily visible spine and integumentary sheath fragments should be removed; and the wound should immediately be soaked in hot water to tolerance (45° to 50° C [115° to 120° F]). Local wound infiltration with lidocaine without epinephrine or regional nerve blocks frequently are needed to control the pain. Cryotherapy is absolutely contraindicated.

Hospital Management

In the hospital the wound should be expeditiously explored to remove all remaining spine and sheath remnants. After the wound has been well irrigated, it should be packed open to await delayed primary closure, or it should be approximated with closed drainage systems. If the sting is from the Australian stonefish and systemic symptoms are severe, a stonefish antivenin is available (Commonwealth Serum Laboratories, Melbourne, Australia). The antivenin is supplied in 2 ml ampules capable of neutralizing 10 mg of dried venom (the equivalent of two significant stings). After appropriate skin tests to establish hypersensitivity to equine sera, the antivenin is administered as a 2 ml intravenous dose slowly. Because absorption varies, intramuscular administration of antivenin is no longer recommended. The administration of antivenin is detailed in the section on snake bites.

REFERENCES

1 Aghababian RV, Conte JE: Mammalian bite wounds, *Ann Emerg Med* 9:79, 1980.
2 Anderson LJ, Nicholson KG, Tauxe RV et al: Human rabies in the United States, 1960 to 1979: epidemiology, diagnosis, and prevention, *Ann Intern Med* 100:728, 1984.
3 Anderson LJ, Winkler WG, Hafkin B et al: Clinical experience with a human diploid cell rabies vaccine, *JAMA* 244:781, 1980.
4 Andors L, Cox DS, Baer PN: Frostbite of the gingiva: a case report, *Periodont Case Rep* 3(1):6, 1981.
5 Apfelberg D, Masters F, Robinson D: Pathophysiology and treatment of lightning injuries, *J Trauma* 14:453, 1974.
6 Anker RL, Straffon WG, Loiselle DS et al: Retarding the uptake of "mock venom" in humans: comparison of three first-aid treatments, *Med J Aust* 1(5):212, 1982.
7 Arnold RE: Controversies and hazards in the treatment of pit viper bites, *South Med J* 72:902, 1979.
8 Arons MS, Fernando L, Polayes IM: *Pasteurella multocida*—the major cause of hand infections following domestic animal bites, *J Hand Surg* 7:47, 1982.
9 Auer AI, Falls BH: Surgery for necrotic bites of the brown spider, *Arch Surg* 108:612, 1974.
10 Auerbach PS: Hazardous marine animals, *Emerg Med Clin North Am* 2(3):531, 1984.
11 Auerbach PS, Halstead BW: Hazardous marine life. In Auerbach PS, Geehr EC, editors: *Management of wilderness and environmental emergencies,* ed 2, St Louis, 1989, Mosby.
12 Baer GM, editor: *The natural history of rabies,* vol 2, New York, 1975, Academic Press.
13 Bahmanyar M, Fayaz A, Nour-Salehi S et al: Successful protection of humans exposed to rabies infection, *JAMA* 236:2751, 1976.
14 Baker R: Paraplegia as a result of lightning injury, *Br Med J* 4:1464, 1978.
15 Baldridge HD: Shark attack: a program of data reduction and analysis, *Contributions from the Mote Marine Laboratory,* vol 1, no 2, 1974.
16 Baldridge HD, Williams J: Shark attack: feeding or fighting? *Mil Med* 134:130, 1969.
17 Balmain R, McClelland K: Pantyhose compression bandage: first aid for snakebite, *Med J Aust* 2:240, 1982.
18 Bangs CC: Hypothermia and frostbite, *Emerg Med Clin North Am* 2(3):475, 1984.
19 Bangs CC, Hamlet MP: Hypothermia and cold injuries. In Auerbach PS, Geehr EC, editors: *Management of wilderness and environmental emergencies,* New York, 1983, Macmillan.
20 Barthlome CW, Jacoby WD, Ramchand SC: Cutaneous manifestations of lightning injury, *Arch Dermatol* 111:1466, 1975.
21 Bayliss GJA: Aural barotrauma in naval divers, *Arch Otolaryngol* 88:141, 1968.
22 Beck AM, Loring H, Lockwood R: The ecology of dog bite injury in St Louis, Missouri, *Public Health Rep* 90:262, 1975.
23 Becker GD, Parell GH: Otolaryngologic aspects of scuba diving, *Arch Otolaryngol Head Neck Surg* 87:569, 1979.
24 Bergstrom L, Neblett L, Sando I et al: The lightning damaged ear, *Arch Otolaryngol* 100:117, 1974.
25 Berzon DR, DeHoff JB: Medical costs and other aspects of dog bites in Baltimore, *Public Health Rep* 89:377, 1974.
26 Berzon DR, Farber RE, Gordon J et al: Animal bites in a large city—a report on Baltimore, Maryland, *Am J Public Health* 62:422, 1972.
27 Bitseff EL, Garoni WJ, Hardison CD et al: The management of stingray injuries of the extremities, *South Med J* 63:417, 1970.
28 Blair JR, Schatzki R, Orr KD: Sequelae to cold injury in one hundred patients: follow-up study 4 years after occurrence of cold injury, *JAMA* 163:1203, 1957.
29 Bogue CW, Wise JD, Gray GF et al: Antibiotic therapy for cat scratch disease? *JAMA* 262:813, 1989.
30 Booker L: Dog bites, *JAMA* 253:1263, 1985.
31 Borchelt PL, Lockwood R, Beck AM et al: Attacks by packs of dogs involving predation on human beings, *Public Health Rep* 98:57, 1983.
32 Bova AA: The basis for drug therapy in decompression sickness, *Undersea Biomed Res* 9:91, 1982.
33 Boyden TW: Snake venom poisoning: diagnosis and treatment, *Ariz Med* 37:639, 1980.
34 Bracis R, Seibers K, Julien RM: Meningitis caused by group II J following a dog bite, *West J Med* 131:438, 1979.
35 Branson D, Bunkfeldt F: *Pasteurella multocida* in animal bites of humans, *Am J Clin Pathol* 48:552, 1967.
36 Brenner DJ, Hollis DG, Moss CW et al: Proposal of *Afipia* gen. nov., with *Afipia felis* sp. nov. (formerly cat scratch disease bacillus), *Afipia clevelandensis* sp. nov. (formerly the Cleveland Clinic Foundation strain), *Afipia broomeae* sp. nov., and three unnamed genospecies, *J Clin Microbiol* 29:2450, 1991.
37 Brown FE, Spiegel PK, Boyle WE Jr: Digital deformity: an effect of frostbite in children, *Pediatrics* 71(6):955, 1983.
38 Buechner HA, Rothbaum JC: Lightning stroke injury—a report of multiple casualties from a single lightning bolt, *Mil Med* 126:755, 1961.
39 Buntain WL: Successful venomous snakebite neutralization with massive antivenin infusion in a child, *J Trauma* 23(11):1012, 1983.
40 Burda CD: Electrocardiographic changes in lightning stroke, *Am Heart J* 72:521, 1966.
41 Burridge MJ: Wildlife rabies in the United States, *Avian/Exotic Practice* 1(1):17, 1984.
42 Butner AN: Rattlesnake bites in Northern California, *West J Med* 139:179, 1983.

43 Cable D, McGehee W, Wingert WA et al: Prolonged defibrination after a bite from a "nonvenomous" snake, *JAMA* 251:925, 1984.
44 Cales RH, Humphreys N, Pilmanis AA et al: Cardiac arrest from gas embolism in scuba diving, *Ann Emerg Med* 10:589, 1981.
45 Callaham ML: Treatment of common dog bites: infection risk factors, *JACEP* 7:83, 1978.
46 Callaham ML: Domestic and feral mammalian bites. In Auerbach PS, Geehr EC, editors: *Management of wilderness and environmental emergencies,* New York, 1983, Macmillan.
47 Carithers HA: Mammalian bites of children, *Am J Dis Child* 95:150, 1958.
48 Castren JA, Kytila J: Eye symptoms caused by lightning, *Acta Ophthalmol* 41:139, 1963.
49 Centers for Disease Control: Rabies postexposure prophylaxis with human diploid cell rabies vaccine: lower neutralizing antibody titers with Wyeth vaccine, *MMWR* 34:90, 1985.
50 Centers for Disease Control: Field evaluations of preexposure use of human diploid cell rabies vaccine, *MMWR* 32:601, 1983.
51 Centers for Disease Control: Rabies prevention—United States, 1984: recommendation of the Immunization Practices Advisory Committee (ACIP), *MMWR* 33:393, 1984.
52 Chopra JS, Banerjee AK, Murthy JMK et al: Paralytic rabies: a clinicopathological study, *Brain* 103:789, 1980.
53 Chun Y, Berkelhamer J, Herold T: Dog bites in children less than 4 years old, *Pediatrics* 69:119, 1982.
54 Clereghino JJ, Mason LC, Sheehan TP: A case of rabies encephalitis, *Northwest Med* 67:258, 1967.
55 Collipp PJ: Cat-scratch disease therapy, *Am J Dis Child* 143: 1261, 1989.
56 Cooper MA: Lightning injuries. In Auerbach PS, Geehr EC, editors: *Management of wilderness and environmental emergencies,* New York, 1983, Macmillan.
57 Cooper MA: Electrical and lightning injuries, *Emerg Med Clin North Am* 2(3):489, 1984.
58 Curry SC, Kraner JC, Kunkel DB et al: Noninvasive vascular studies in management of rattlesnake envenomations to extremities, *Ann Emerg Med* 14:1081, 1985.
59 Davies DH, Campbell GD: The aetiology, clinical pathology, and treatment of shark attack, *J R Nav Med Serv* 3:110, 1962.
60 Davis JC: Diving and barotrauma. In Auerbach PS, Geehr EC, editors: *Management of wilderness and environmental emergencies,* New York, 1983, Macmillan.
61 Davison RA: Ventilation of the normal and blocked middle ear, *Ann Otol Rhinol Laryngol* 74:162, 1965.
62 Dickey LS: Diving injuries, *J Emerg Med* 1:249, 1984.
63 DeHoll D, Rodeheaver G, Edgerton MT et al: Potentiation of infection by suture closure of dead space, *Am J Surg* 127:716, 1974.
64 Devriendt J, Staroukine M, Costy F et al: Fatal encephalitis apparently due to rabies, *JAMA* 248:2304, 1982.
65 Dhingra U, Schauerhamer RR, Wangensteen OH: Peripheral dissemination of bacteria in contaminated wounds: role of devitalized tissue; evaluation of therapeutic measures, *Surgery* 80:535, 1976.
66 Douglas LG: Bite wounds, *Am Fam Physician* 11:93, 1975.
67 Duenas A, Belsey MA, Escobar J et al: Isolation of rabies virus outside the human central nervous system, *J Infect Dis* 127:702, 1973.
68 Edlich RF, Custer J, Madden J et al: Studies in the management of the contaminated wound. III. Assessment of the effectiveness of irrigation with antiseptic agents, *Am J Surg* 118:21, 1969.
69 Edlich RF, Rogers W, Kaufman D et al: Studies in the management of the contaminated wound. I. Optimal time for closure of contaminated wounds. II. Comparison of resistance to infection of open and closed wounds during healing, *Am J Surg* 117:323, 1969.
70 Edlich RF, Schmolka IR, Prusak MP et al: The molecular basis for the toxicity of surfactants in surgical wounds. I. EOI: PO block polymers, *J Surg Res* 14:277, 1973.
71 Edwards JJ, Anderson RL, Wood JR: Loxoscelism of the eyelids, *Arch Ophthalmol* 98(11):1997, 1980.
72 Ehsan M, Waxman J, Finley JM: Delayed gangrene after lightning strike, *Am Fam Physician* 24(5):117, 1981.
73 Elenbaas RM, McNabney WK, Robinson WA: Prophylactic oxacillin in dog bite wounds, *Ann Emerg Med* 11:248, 1982.
74 Elenbaas RM, McNabney WK, Robinson WA: Evaluation of prophylactic oxacillin in cat bite wounds, *Ann Emerg Med* 13:155, 1984.
75 Elliot DH, Mallenbeck JM, Bove AA: Acute decompression sickness, *Lancet* 2:1193, 1974.
76 Enders LJ, Rodriquez-Lopez E: Aeromedical consultation service case report: alternobaric vertigo, *Aerospace Med* 41:200, 1970.
77 Entman SS, Moise KJ Jr: The snake-bitten mother-to-be, *Emerg Med* 16:100, 1984.
78 Evans DE, Korbine AI, Weathersby PK et al: Cardiovascular effects of cerebral air embolism, *Stroke* 12:338, 1981.
79 Fagan P, McKenzie B, Edmonds C: Sinus barotrauma in divers, *Ann Otol Rhinol Laryngol* 85:61, 1976.
80 Fardon DW, Wingo CW, Robinson DW et al: The treatment of the brown spider bite, *Plast Reconstr Surg* 40:482, 1967.
81 Fayaz A, Simani S, Nour-Salehi S et al: Booster effect of human diploid cell antirabies vaccine in previously treated person, *JAMA* 246:2334, 1981.
82 Fitzgibbons JF: Identification of pit vipers of the United States, *Nebr Med J* 65:176, 1980.
83 Fix JD: Venom yield of the North American coral snake and its clinical significance, *South Med J* 73(6):737, 1980.
84 Flannery DB, Wiles H: Follow-up of a survivor of intrauterine lightning exposure, *Am J Obstet Gynecol* 142(2):238, 1982.
85 Forrester LJ, Barrett JT, Campbell BJ: Red blood cell lysis induced by the venom of the brown recluse spider: the role of sphingomyelinase D, *Arch Biochem Biophys* 187:355, 1978.
86 Francis DP, Holmes MA, Brandon G: *Pasteurella multocida* infection after domestic animal bites and scratches, *JAMA* 233:42, 1975.
87 Freeman P, Edmonds C: Inner ear barotrauma, *Arch Otolaryngol* 95:556, 1972.
88 Freeman P, Tonkins J, Edmonds C: Rupture of the round window membrane in inner ear barotrauma, *Arch Otolaryngol* 99:437, 1974.
89 Garfin SR: Rattlesnake bites: current hospital therapy, *West J Med* 137:411, 1982.
90 Garfin SR, Castilonia RR, Mubarak SJ et al: Rattlesnake bites and surgical decompression: results using a laboratory model, *Toxicon* 22(2):177, 1984.
91 Garfin SR, Castilonia RR, Mubarak SJ et al: The effect of antivenin on intramuscular pressure elevations induced by rattlesnake venom, *Toxicon* 23:677, 1985.
92 Garfin SR, Mubarak SJ, Davidson TM: Rattlesnake bites: current concepts, *Clin Orthop* 140:50, 1979.
93 Garfin SR, Castilonia RR, Mubarak SJ et al: Role of surgical decompression in treatment of rattlesnake bites, *Surg Forum* 30:502, 1979.
94 Gebel HM, Campbell BJ, Barrett JT: Chemotactic activity of venom from the brown recluse spider *(Loxosceles reclusa), Toxicon* 17:55, 1979.
95 Gillen HW: Symptomatology of cerebral gas embolism, *Neurology* 18:507, 1968.
96 Gilliland B: Serum sickness and immune complexes, *N Engl J Med* 311:1435, 1984.
97 Gillis MF, Peterson PL, Karagiones MT: In vivo detection of circulating gas emboli associated with decompression sickness

using the Doppler flowmeter, *Nature* 217:965, 1968.
98 Glauser FL: Snakebite treatment: fact and fiction, *Va Med* 114:420, 1987.
99 Glosser JW, Hutchinson LR, Rich AG et al: Rabies in El Paso, Texas, before and after institution of a new rabies control program, *J Am Vet Med Assoc* 157:820, 1970.
100 Golde RH, Lee WR: Death by lightning, *Proc Inst Elec Eng* 123:1163, 1976.
101 Golding FC, Griffiths P, Hempleman HV et al: Decompression sickness during construction of the Dartford tunnel, *Br J Ind Med* 17:167, 1960.
102 Goldowsky SJ: Uniform determination of death, *R I Med J* 66(8):309, 1983.
103 Goldstein EJ, Citron DM, Finegold SM: Dog bite wounds and infection: a prospective clinical study, *Ann Emerg Med* 9:508, 1980.
104 Goldstein EJ, Citron DM, Finegold SM: Role of anaerobic bacteria in bite-wound infections, *Rev Infect Dis* 6:S177, 1984.
105 Goldstein EJ, Citron DM, Gonzalez H et al: Bacteriology of rattlesnake venom and implications for therapy, *J Infect Dis* 140(5):818, 1979.
106 Goldstein EJ, Citron DM, Wield B et al: Bacteriology of human and animal bite wounds, *J Trauma* 13:423, 1973.
107 Goldstein EJ, Citron DM, Wield B et al: Bacteriology of human and animal bite wounds, *J Clin Microbiol* 8:667, 1978.
108 Goodhill V: Leaking labyrinthe lesions, deafness, tinnitus, and dizziness, *Ann Otol Rhinol Laryngol* 90:99, 1981.
109 Goodman P, Morioka WT: Round window membrane rupture, *Laryngoscope* 89:1373, 1978.
110 Gottwald A, Willebrand H: Chronic interphalangeal joint inflammation from intra-articular sea urchin spine, *Handchirurgie* 4:45, 1972.
111 Grace TG, Omer GE: The management of upper extremity pit viper wounds, *J Hand Surg* 5:168, 1980.
112 Grainger CR: Occupational injuries due to sting-rays, *Trans R Soc Trop Med Hyg* 74:408, 1980.
113 Grande CM: *Textbook of trauma anesthesia and critical care,* St Louis, 1994, Mosby.
114 Griffin D, Donovan JW: Significant envenomation from a preserved rattlesnake head (in a patient with a history of immediate hypersensitivity to antivenin), *Ann Emerg Med* 15:955, 1986.
115 Guidelines for the determination of death: report of the medical consultants on the diagnosis of death to the President's Commission for the Study of Ethical Problems in Medicine and Biomedical and Behavioral Research, *Crit Care Med* 10(1):62, 1982.
116 Hallenbeck JM, Bove AA, Elliott DH: Accelerated coagulation of whole blood and cell free plasma by bubbling in vitro, *Aerosp Med* 44:712, 1973.
117 Hallenbeck JM, Bove AA, Elliott DH: Mechanisms underlying spinal cord damage in decompression sickness, *Neurology* 25:308, 1975.
118 Hamby JA, Graybeal GE: Puff adder bite: a case presentation, *Del Med J* 55(10):579, 1983.
119 Hardy DL: Envenomation by the Mojave rattlesnake *(Crotalus scutulatus scutulatus)* in southern Arizona, USA, *Toxicon* 21(1):111, 1983.
120 Hardy DL, Jeter M, Corrigan JJ Jr: Envenomation by the northern blacktail rattlesnake *(Crotalus molossus molossus):* report of two cases and the in vitro effects of the venom on fibrinolysis and platelet aggregation, *Toxicon* 20(2):487, 1982.
121 Hardy DL, Kunkel DB, Russell FE et al: Management of poisonous snakebite, *J Vet Hum Toxicol* 25:135, 1983.
122 Hargens AR, Garfin SR, Mubarak SJ et al: Edema associated with venomous snake bites, *Bibl Anat* 20:267, 1981.
123 Harris D, Imperato PJ, Oken B: Dog bites: an unrecognized epidemic, *Bull NY Acad Med* 50:981, 1974.
124 Harry TO, Adiega A, Anyiwo CE et al: Antirabies treatment of dog-bite victims in Lagos, Nigeria: trial of suckling mouse brain and fetal bovine kidney cell rabies vaccines, *Vaccine* 2:257, 1984.
125 Harves AD, Millikan LE: Current concepts of therapy and pathophysiology in arthropod bites and stings. I. Arthropods, *Int Dermatol* 14:543, 1975.
126 Harwood SJ, Catrov PG, Cole GW: Creatine phosphokinase isoenzyme fraction in the serum of a patient struck by lightning, *Arch Intern Med* 138:645, 1978.
127 Hattwick MAW, Weis TT, Stechschulte CJ et al: Recovery from rabies: a case report, *Ann Intern Med* 76:931, 1976.
128 Helmick CG: The epidemiology of human rabies postexposure prophylaxis: 1980-1981, *JAMA* 250:1990, 1983.
129 Helmick CG, Johnstone C, Sumner J et al: A clinical study of Merieux human rabies immune globulin, *J Biol Stand* 10:357, 1982.
130 Herman EW, Kezis JS, Silvers DN: A distinctive variant of pernio, *Arch Dermatol* 117:26, 1981.
131 Hershey FB, Aulenbacher CE: Surgical treatment of brown spider bites, *Ann Surg* 170(2):300, 1969.
132 Hills BA: Mechanical vs. ischemic mechanisms for decompression sickness, *Aviat Space Environ Med* 50:363, 1979.
133 Holley HP: Successful treatment of cat-scratch disease with oral ciprofloxacin, *JAMA* 265:1563, 1991.
134 Hough SA, Burton RC, Wilson RW et al: Human-to-human transmission of rabies virus by a corneal transplant, *N Engl J Med* 300:603, 1979.
135 How J, West D, Edmonds C: Decompression sickness in diving, *Singapore Med J* 17:92, 1976.
136 Hubbert WT: "Caution: pets may be hazardous to your health," *JAMA* 251:934, 1984.
137 Hufford DC: The brown recluse spider and necrotic arachnidism: a current review, *J Ark Med Soc* 74(3):126, 1977.
138 Jackson SH, Parry DJ: Lightning and the heart, *Br Heart J* 43(4):454, 1980.
139 Jaffe AC: Animal bites, *Pediatr Clin North Am* 30:405, 1983.
140 Jaffe RH: Electropathology: a review of pathologic changes produced by electric currents, *Arch Pathol* 5:839, 1928.
141 Jimenez-Porras JM: Biochemistry of snake venoms, *Clin Toxicol* 3(3):389, 1970.
142 Jurkovich GJ, Luterman A, McCullar K et al: Complications of Crotalidae antivenin therapy, *J Trauma* 28:1032, 1988.
143 Karlson JA: The incidence of facial injuries from dog bites, *JAMA* 251:3265, 1984.
144 Key GF: A comparison of calcium gluconate and methocarbamol (Robaxin) in the treatment of latrodectism (black widow spider envenomation), *Am J Trop Med Hyg* 30:273, 1981.
145 King LE Jr, Rees RS: Dapsone treatment of a brown recluse bite, *JAMA* 250(5):648, 1983.
146 Kinmont PD: Sea urchin sarcoidial granuloma, *Br J Dermatol* 77:335, 1965.
147 Kizer KW: Epidemiologic and clinical aspects of animal bite injuries, *JACEP* 8:134, 1979.
148 Kizer KW: Dysbarism in paradise, *Hawaii Med J* 39:109, 1980.
149 Kizer KW: Corticosteroids in the treatment of serious decompression sickness, *Ann Emerg Med* 10:485, 1981.
150 Kizer KW: Delayed treatment of dysbarism: a retrospective review of 50 cases, *JAMA* 247:2555, 1982.
151 Kizer KW: Management of dysbaric diving casualties, *Emerg Med Clin North Am* 1:659, 1983.
152 Kizer KW: Diving medicine, *Emerg Med Clin North Am* 2(3):513, 1984.
153 Kizer KW: Animal bites. In Gorbach SL, Barlett JG, Blacklow NR, editors: *Infectious diseases,* Philadelphia, 1992, Saunders.
154 Kizer KW, Goodman FG: Radiographic manifestations of venous air embolism, *Radiology* 144:35, 1982.

155 Klein D: Friendly dog syndrome, *N Y State Med J* 66:2306, 1966.
156 Klein DM, Cohen ME: *Pasteurella multocida* brain abscess following perforating cranial dog bite, *J Pediatr* 92:588, 1978.
157 Kleiner JP, Wilkin JH: Cardiac effects of lightning stroke, *JAMA* 240:2757, 1978.
158 Kraner J, Kunkel DB, Ryan P et al: Noninvasive vascular studies in rattlesnake envenomation, *J Vet Hum Toxicol* 25(suppl):68, 1983.
159 Krob MJ, Cram AE: Lightning injuries: a multisystem trauma, *J Iowa Med Soc* 73(6):221, 1983.
160 Kumar VN: Intractable foot pain following frostbite: case report, *Arch Phys Med Rehabil* 63(6):284, 1982.
161 Kunkel DB: Bites of venomous reptiles, *Emerg Med Clin North Am* 2(3):563, 1984.
162 Kunkel DB: Arthropod envenomations, *Emerg Med Clin North Am* 2(3):579, 1984.
163 Ledbetter EO: What's new in the management of snakebite? *Tex Med* 77:41, 1981.
164 Lehrer JF, Rubin RC, Poole DC et al: Perilymphatic fistula—a definitive and curable cause of vertigo following head trauma, *West J Med* 141:57, 1984.
165 Leitch DR, Greenbaum LJ Jr, Hallenbeck JM: Cerebral air embolism. I. Is there benefit in beginning HBO treatment at 6 bar? *Undersea Biomed Res* 11(3):221, 1984.
166 Linaweaver PG: Toxic marine life. *Mil Med* 131:437, 1967.
167 Lucas GL, Bartlett DH: *Pasteurella multocida* infection in the hand, *Plast Reconstr Surg* 67:49, 1981.
168 Lundgren CEG, Tjernstrom O, Ornhagen HL: Alternobaric vertigo and hearing disturbances in connection with diving: an epidemiologic study, *Undersea Biomed Res* 2:153, 1975.
169 Maetz HM: Animal bites: a public health problem in Jefferson County, Alabama, *Public Health Rep* 94:528, 1978.
170 Malasit P, Warrell D, Chanthavanich P et al: Prediction, prevention, and mechanism of early (anaphylactic) antivenom reactions in victims of snakebites, *Br Med J* 292:17, 1986.
171 Mann JM, Schmid GP, Droke WE: Plague and the peripheral smear, *JAMA* 251:953, 1984.
172 Manowitz NR, Rosenthal RR: Cutaneous-systemic reactions to toxins and venoms of common marine organisms, *Cutis* 23:450, 1979.
173 Margileth AW, Wear DJ, Hadfield TI et al: Cat-scratch disease: bacteria in skin at the primary inoculation site, *JAMA* 252:928, 1984.
174 Marwick C: Changes recommended in use of human diploid cell rabies vaccine, *JAMA* 254:13, 1985.
175 McCollough NC, Gennaro JF: Evaluation of venomous snakebite in the southern United States from parallel clinical and laboratory investigations: development of treatment, *J Fla Med Assoc* 49:959, 1963.
176 McCrady-Kahn UL, Kahn AM: Lightning burns, *West J Med* 134:215, 1981.
177 McKendry RJ: Frostbite arthritis, *Can Med Assoc J* 125 (10):1128, 1981.
178 McKinney H, Kizer K, Auerbach P: Scorpaenidae envenomation: a five-year poison center experience, *JAMA* 253:807, 1985.
179 Mebs D, Panholzer F: Isolation of a hemorrhagic principle from *Bitis arietans* (puff adder) snake venom, *Toxicon* 20(2):509, 1982.
180 Menkin M, Schwartzmann RJ: Cerebral air embolism, *Arch Neurol* 34:168, 1977.
181 Miller BJ, Chasmar LR: Frostbite in Saskatoon: a review of 10 winters, *Can J Surg* 23(5):423, 1980.
182 Mills WJ Jr: Summary of treatment of the cold-injured patient: frostbite, *Alaska Med* 25(2):29, 1983.
183 Minton SA: Identification of poisonous snakes, *Clin Toxicol* 3(3):347, 1970.
184 Morgan Z, Heaeley R, Alexander EA et al: Atrial fibrillation and epidural hematoma associated with lightning stroke, *N Engl J Med* 259:956, 1954.
185 Morrison JJ, Pearn JH, Coulter AR: The mass of venom injected by two elapidae: the taipan *(Oxyuranus scutellatus)* and the Australian tiger snake *(Notechis scutatus), Toxicon* 20(4):739,1982.
186 Moynahan EJ, Montgomery PR: Echinoderm granuloma, *Br J Clin Pract* 22:265, 1968.
187 Mullanney PJ: Treatment of stingray wounds, *Clin Toxicol* 3:613, 1970.
188 Murrell G: The effectiveness of the pressure/immobilization first aid technique in the case of a tiger snake bite, *Med J Aust* 2(6):295, 1981.
189 Neale TJ, Theofilopoulos AN, Wilson CB: Methods for the detection of soluble circulating immune complexes and their application, *Pathobiol Annu* 9:113, 1979.
190 NOAA, Weigel EP: Lightning: the underrated killer, *NOAA* 6:2, 1976.
191 Noel LP, Clarke WN, Addison D: Ocular complications of lightning, *J Pediatr Ophthalmol Strabismus* 17(4):245, 1980.
192 O'Neal RL, Halstead BW, Howard LD: Injury to human tissues from sea urchin spines, *Calif Med* 101:199, 1964.
193 Ordog GJ, Balasubramanium S, Wasserberger J: Rat bites: 50 cases, *Ann Emerg Med* 14:126, 1985.
194 Otten EJ: Antivenin therapy in the emergency department, *Am J Emerg Med* 1:83, 1983.
195 Otten EJ, McKimm D: Venomous snakebite in a patient allergic to horse serum, *Ann Emerg Med* 12(10):624, 1983.
196 Page RE, Robertson GA: Management of the frostbitten hand, *Hand* 15(2):185, 1983.
197 Palmer J, Rees M: Dog bites of the face: a 15-year review, *Br J Plast Surg* 36:315, 1983.
198 Pardal JF, Granata AR, Barrio A: Influence of calcium on H-noradrenaline release by *Lactrodectus antheratus* (black widow spider) venom gland extract in arterial tissues of the rat, *Toxicon* 17:455, 1979.
199 Parrish HM: Incidence of treated snakebites in the United States, *Public Health Rep* 81:269, 1966.
200 Parrish HM, Clack FB, Brobst D et al: Epidemiology of dog bites, *Public Health Rep* 74:891, 1959.
201 Pearn JH: Cold injury complicating trauma in subzero environments, *Med J Aust* 1(12):505, 1982.
202 Peeples E, Boswick JA, Scott FA: Wounds of the hand contaminated by human or animal saliva, *J Trauma* 20:383, 1980.
203 Peters WJ: Lightning injury, *Can Med Assoc J* 128(2):148, 1983.
204 Peterson G, Hugar DW: Frostbite: its diagnosis and treatment, *J Foot Surg* 18(1):32, 1979.
205 Pickerill RG, Milder JE: Transverse myelitis associated with cat-scratch disease in an adult, *JAMA* 246:2840, 1981.
206 Pinckney LE, Kennedy LA: Fractures of the infant skull caused by animal bites, *AJNR* 1:264, 1980.
207 Pullen FW, Rosenberg GJ, Cabella CH: Sudden hearing loss in divers and fliers, *Laryngoscope* 89:1373, 1979.
208 Pumplin DW, McClure WO: The release of acetylcholine elicited by extracts of black widow spider glands: studies using superior cervical ganglia and inhibitors of electrically stimulated release, *J Pharmacol Exp Ther* 201(2):312, 1977.
209 Rapuano R, Stratigos GT: Mandibular fracture resulting from a dog bite, *J Oral Surg* 34:359, 1976.
210 Rauber AP: The case of the red widow: a review of latrodectism, *Vet Hum Toxicol* 22(suppl 2):39, 1980.
211 Ravitch MM, Lane R, Safar P et al: Lightning stroke, *N Engl J Med* 264:36, 1961.
212 Rees RS, Fields JP, King LE Jr: Do brown recluse spider bites induce pyoderma gangrenosum? *South Med J* 78:283, 1983.
213 Rees RS, Hawiger J, Des Prez RM et al: Mechanism of platelet

injury associated with dermonecrosis resulting from brown recluse spider venom, *Clin Res* 30:265A, 1982.
214 Rees RS, O'Leary JP, Lynch JB et al: Pathogenesis of systemic loxoscelism following brown recluse spider bite, *Surg Forum* 32:571, 1981.
215 Rees RS, Shack RB, Withers E et al: Management of the brown recluse spider bite, *Plast Reconstr Surg* 68(5):768, 1981.
216 Reid HA, Theakston RDG: The management of snakebite, *Bull WHO* 61:885, 1983.
217 Remington PL, Shope T, Andrews J: A recommended approach to the evaluation of human rabies exposure in an acute care hospital, *JAMA* 254:67, 1985.
218 Rivera JC: Decompression sickness among divers: an analysis of 935 cases, *Mil Med* 17:314, 1964.
219 Robson MC, Heggers JP: Evaluation of hand frostbite blister fluid as a clue to pathogenesis, *J Hand Surg* 6(1):43, 1981.
220 Rocha A, Fraga S: Sea urchin granuloma of the skin, *Arch Dermatol* 85:146, 1962.
221 Rodeheaver GT, Kurtz L, Kircher BJ et al: Pluronic F-68: a promising new skin wound cleanser, *Ann Emerg Med* 9:572, 1980.
222 Rodeheaver GT, Pettry D, Thacker JG et al: Wound cleansing by high pressure irrigation, *Surg Gynecol Obstet* 141:357, 1975.
223 Rosen RA: The use of antibiotics in the initial management of recent dog-bite wounds, *Am J Emerg Med* 3:19, 1985.
224 Roth RM, Gleckman RA: Human infections derived from dogs, *Postgrad Med* 77:169, 1985.
225 Russell FE: Stingray injuries: a review and discussion of their treatment, *Am J Med Sci* 226:611, 1953.
226 Russell FE: *Snake venom poisoning,* ed 2, Great Neck, NY, 1983, Scholium.
227 Russell FE: Treatment of rattlesnake bites, *West J Med* 141:245, 1984.
228 Russell FE, Banner W: *Conn's current therapy,* Philadelphia, 1988, Saunders.
229 Russell FE, Carson RW, Wainschel J et al: Snake venom poisoning in the United States—experience with 550 cases, *JAMA* 233:341, 1975.
230 Schlossberg D, Morad Y, Krause TB et al: Culture-proved disseminated cat-scratch disease in acquired immunodeficiency syndrome, *Arch Intern Med* 149:1437, 1989.
231 Schultz RC, McMaster WC: The treatment of dog bite injuries, especially those of the face, *Plast Reconstr Surg* 49:494, 1972.
232 Simon TL, Grace TG: Envenomation coagulopathy in wounds from pit vipers, *N Engl J Med* 305:443, 1981.
233 Smith CW, Micks DW: The role of the polymorphonuclear leukocytes in the lesion caused by the venom of the brown spider, *Loxosceles reclusa, Lab Invest* 22:90, 1976.
234 Smith JE, Clark AW, Kuster TA: Suppression by elevated calcium of black widow spider venom activity at frog neuromuscular junctions, *J Neurocytol* 6:519, 1977.
235 Smith KH, Spencer MP: Doppler indices of decompression sickness: the evaluation and use, *Aerospace Med* 41:1396, 1970.
236 Smith RL: Venomous animals of Arizona, Tucson, Ariz, 1982, Cooperative Extension Service Bulletin 8245.
237 Sokol AB, Houser RG: Dog bites: prevention and treatment, *Clin Pediatr* 10:336, 1971.
238 Southcott RV: Australian venomous and poisonous fishes, *Clin Toxicol* 10:291, 1977.
239 Spencer MP, Campbell SD: Development of bubbles in venous and arterial blood during hyperbaric decompression, *Bull Mason Clin* 22:26, 1968.
240 Spivak AP: Medical aspects of scuba diving, *Comp Ther* 6:6, 1980.
241 Stevens DL, Higbee JW, Oberhofer TR et al: Antibiotic susceptibilities of human isolates of *Pasteurella multocida, Antimicrob Agents Chemother* 16:322, 1979.
242 Stevens H: Cat-scratch fever encephalitis, *Am J Dis Child* 84:218, 1952.
243 Stevenson TR, Rodeheaver GT, Golden GT et al: Damage to tissue defenses by vasoconstrictors, *JACEP* 4:532, 1976.
244 Stevenson TR, Thacker JG, Rodeheaver GT et al: Cleansing the traumatic wound by high pressure syringe irrigation, *JACEP* 5:17, 1976.
245 Steuven H, Aprahamian C, Thompson B et al: Cobra envenomation: an uncommon emergency, *Ann Emerg Med* 12(10): 636, 1983.
246 Stiles AD: Priapism following a black widow spider bite, *Clin Pediatr* 21(3):174, 1982.
247 Stochosky BA: Necrotic arachnidism, *West J Med* 131:143, 1979.
248 Strassburg MA, Marron JA, Mahoney LE: Animal bites: patterns of treatment, *Ann Emerg Med* 10:193, 1981.
249 Strauss RH: Diving medicine, *Am Rev Respir Dis* 119:1001, 1979.
250 Stucker FJ, Echols WB: Otolaryngologic problems of underwater exploration, *Mil Med* 136:896, 1971.
251 Szalay GC, Sommerstein A: Inoculation osteomyelitis secondary to animal bites, *Clin Pediatr* 11:687, 1972.
252 Taussig H: "Death" from lightning and the possibility of living again, *Ann Intern Med* 68:1345, 1968.
253 Thomson HG, Svitek V: Small animal bites: the role of primary closure, *J Trauma* 13:20, 1973.
254 Tindall J, Harrison C: *Pasteurella multocida* infections following animal injuries, especially cat bites, *Arch Dermatol* 105:412, 1972.
255 Torphy DE, Ray ČG: *Pasteurella multocida* in dog and cat bite infections, *Pediatrics* 43:295, 1969.
256 Torres JR, Sanders CV, Strub RL et al: Cat-scratch disease causing reversible encephalopathy, *JAMA* 240:1628, 1978.
257 Trestrail JH: The "underground zoo"—the problem of exotic venomous snakes in private possession in the United States, *Vet Hum Toxicol* 24(suppl):144, 1982.
258 Trethewie ER: Detection of snake venom in tissue, *Clin Toxicol* 3:445, 1970.
259 Tyler TC: Pressure trauma to the ears and hearing loss, *J Fla Med Assoc* 65:708, 1978.
260 Uhaa IJ, Mandel EJ, Whiteway R et al: Rabies surveillance in the United States during 1990, *J Am Vet Med Assoc* 200(7):920, 1992.
261 Van Mierop LH, Kitchens CS: Defibrination syndrome following bites by the eastern diamondback rattlesnake, *J Fla Med Assoc* 67(1):21, 1980.
262 Varner MW, McGuinness GA, Galask RP: Rabies vaccination in pregnancy, *Am J Obstet Gynecol* 143:717, 1982.
263 Vest DK: Envenomation following the bite of a wandering garter snake *(Thamnophis elegans vagrans), Clin Toxicol* 18:573, 1981.
264 Walker AE: Current concepts of brain death, *J Neurosurg Nurs* 15(5):261, 1983.
265 Warrell DA: The clinical picture of rabies in man, *Trans R Soc Trop Med Hyg* 70:188, 1976.
266 Watson DW: Severe head injury from dog bites, *Ann Emerg Med* 9:28, 1980.
267 Watt CH: Treatment of poisonous snakebite with emphasis on digit dermotomy, *South Med J* 78:694, 1985.
268 Wear DJ, Margileth AM, Hadfield TL et al: Cat-scratch disease: a bacterial infection, *Science* 221:1403, 1983.
269 Weber DJ, Wolfson JS, Swartz MN et al: *Pasteurella multocida* infections: report of 34 cases and review of the literature, *Medicine* 63:133, 1984.
270 Weninger BG, Warren AJ, Forseth V et al: Human bubonic plague transmitted by a domestic cat scratch, *JAMA* 251:927, 1984.
271 White J, Fassett R: Acute renal failure and coagulopathy after snakebite, *Med J Aust* 2(3):142, 1983.

272 Wilberger JE, Pang D: Craniocerebral injuries from dog bites, *JAMA* 249:2685, 1983.
273 Wingert WA: Venomous snake bites. In Auerbach PS, Geehr EC, editors: *Management of wilderness and environmental emergencies,* New York, 1983, Macmillan.
274 Wingert WA, Wainschel J: Diagnosis and management of envenomation by poisonous snakes, *South Med J* 68(8):1015, 1975.
275 Winkler WG, editor: *Rabies concepts for medical professionals,* Miami, Fla, 1984, Merieux Institute.
276 Winkler WG, Fashinell TR, Leffingwell L et al: Airborne rabies transmission in a laboratory worker, *JAMA* 226:1219, 1973.
279 Yales RA, Rees RS, King LE Jr: Inhibition of enzymatic and biological activity of brown recluse spider venom with specific IgG antibody, *Clin Res* 32(2):260A, 1984.
278 Yost JW, Holmes FF: Myoglobinuria following lightning stroke, *JAMA* 228:1147, 1974.
279 Zook EG, Miller M, Van Beek AL et al: Successful treatment protocol for canine fang injuries, *J Trauma* 20:243, 1980.

APPENDIX 18-A
REPRESENTATIVE VENOMOUS SNAKES OF THE UNITED STATES AND CANADA

This listing is selected from a comprehensive directory provided by Jerry Brewer (University of Arizona Health Sciences Center). For the sake of brevity, the snakes noted represent a small fraction of the total number known to carry hazardous venom.

United States

Micruroides euryxanthus euryxanthus (Arizona coral snake)
Micrurus fulvius fulvius (eastern coral snake)
Micrurus fulvius tenere (Texas coral snake)
Agkistrodon contortrix contortrix (southern copperhead)
Agkistrodon contortrix laticinctus (broad-banded copperhead)
Agkistrodon contortrix mokasen (northern copperhead)
Agkistrodon contortrix phaeogaster (Osage copperhead)
Agkistrodon contortrix pictigaster (trans-Pecos copperhead)
Agkistrodon piscivoris piscivoris (eastern cottonmouth)
Agkistrodon piscivoris conanti (Florida cottonmouth)
Agkistrodon piscivorus leucostoma (western cottonmouth)
Crotalus adamanteus (eastern diamondback rattlesnake)
Crotalus atrox (western diamondback rattlesnake)
Crotalus cerastes cerastes (Mojave Desert sidewinder)
Crotalus cerastes cercobombus (Sonoran Desert sidewinder)
Crotalus cerastes laterorepens (Colorado Desert sidewinder)
Crotalus horridus horridus (timber rattlesnake)
Crotalus horridus atricaudatus (canebrake rattlesnake)
Crotalus lepidus lepidus (mottled rock rattlesnake)
Crotalus lepidus klauberi (banded rock rattlesnake)
Crotalus mitchelli pyrrhus (southwestern speckled rattlesnake)
Crotalus mitchelli stephensi (panamint rattlesnake)
Crotalus molossus molossus (northern black-tailed rattlesnake)
Crotalus pricei pricei (western twin-spotted rattlesnake)
Crotalus ruber ruber (red diamond rattlesnake)
Crotalus scutulatus scutulatus (Mojave rattlesnake)
Crotalus tigris (tiger rattlesnake)
Crotalus viridis viridis (prairie rattlesnake)
Crotalus viridis abyssus (Grand Canyon rattlesnake)
Crotalus viridis cerberus (Arizona black rattlesnake)
Crotalus viridis concolor (midget-faced rattlesnake)
Crotalus viridis helleri (southern Pacific rattlesnake)
Crotalus viridis lutosis (great basin rattlesnake)
Crotalus viridis nuntius (Hopi rattlesnake)
Crotalus willardi willardi (Arizona ridge-nosed rattlesnake)
Crotalus willardi silus (west Chihuahua ridge-nosed rattlesnake)
Sistrurus catenatus catenatus (eastern massasauga)
Sistrurus catenatus edwardsi (desert massasauga)
Sistrurus catenatus tergeminus (western massasauga)
Sistrurus miliarius miliarius (Carolina pygmy rattlesnake)
Sistrurus miliarius barbouri (dusky pygmy rattlesnake)
Sistrurus miliarius streckeri (western pygmy rattlesnake)

Canada

Crotalus horridus horridus (timber rattlesnake)
Crotalus viridis viridis (prairie rattlesnake)
Crotalus viridis oreganus (northern Pacific rattlesnake)
Sistrurus catenatus catenatus (eastern massassauga)

CHAPTER

19

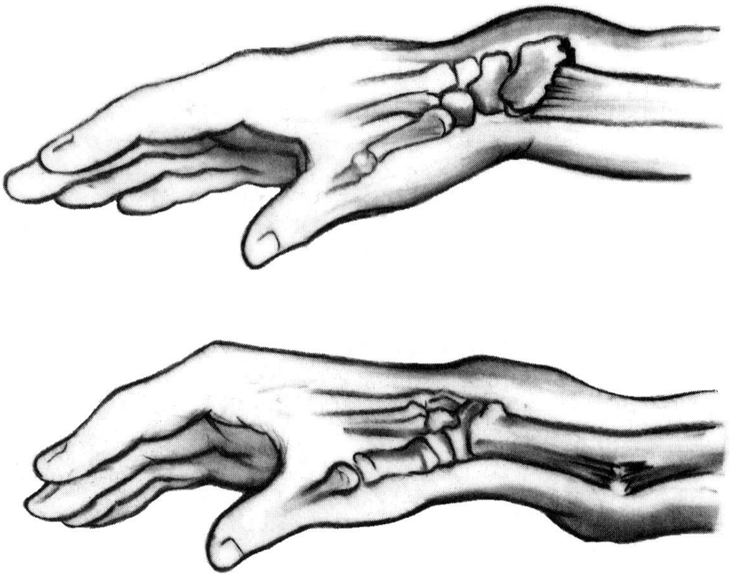

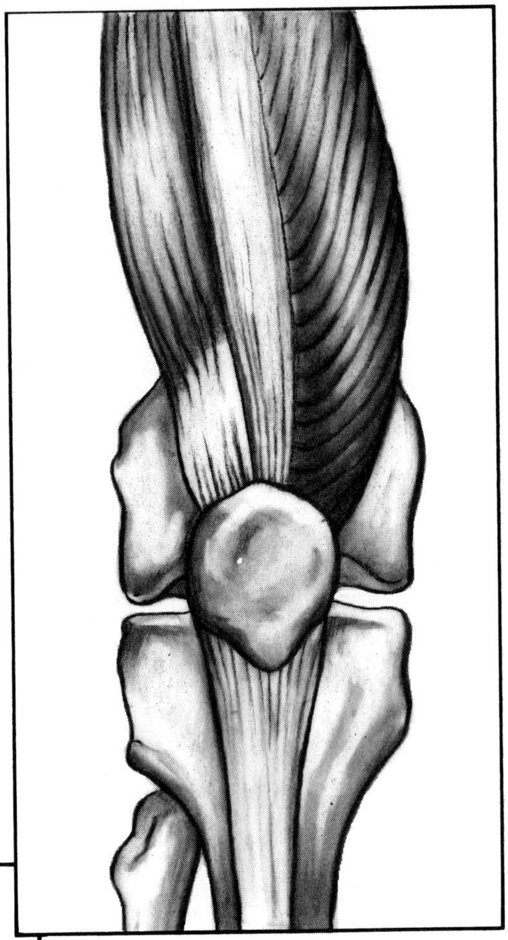

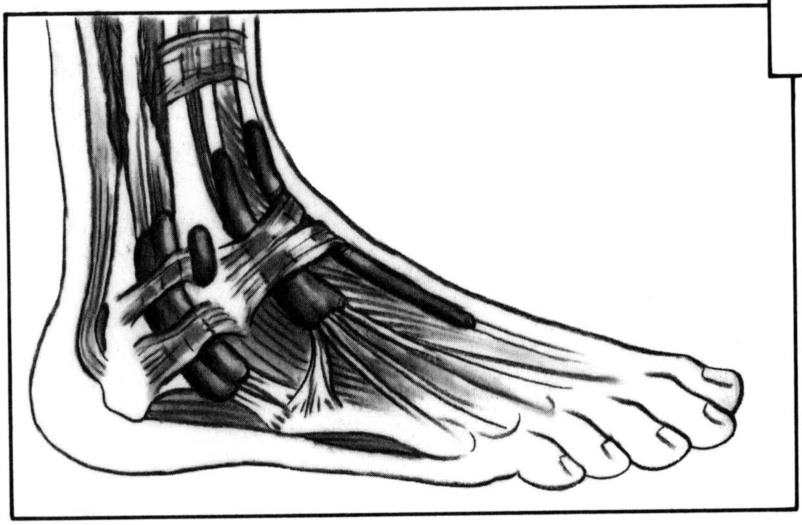

MUSCULOSKELETAL INJURIES AND FRACTURES

Raymond R. White • George M. Babikian

RELATED MATERIAL APPEARS IN CHAPTERS 9, 10, AND 11

We have elected not to try to cover all of orthopedics in a single chapter of a general surgery text. Instead, this chapter outlines for general surgeons what they can and should expect from an orthopedic surgeon who is treating the orthopedic injuries of a patient with multiple injuries.

We have divided the care of such a patient into the following four phases:

1. *Emergency phase.* This phase lasts from the time the patient is injured until the patient is resuscitated (e.g., after all emergency lifesaving procedures have been carried out.)
2. *Acute phase.* After the lifesaving procedures have been carried out (e.g., thoracotomies, abdominal explorations), the orthopedic surgeon must repair the components of the skeletal system that will give the patient an optimal chance of survival. Early surgical stabilization of critical fractures is carried out during this phase.
3. *Reconstructive phase.* This phase covers the same time period as the fourth (rehabilitation) phase.
4. *Rehabilitation phase.* It is during the reconstructive and rehabilitation phases that the patient's care falls more into the hands of the orthopedic surgeon and other subspecialists. During these last two phases, the rest of the patient's skeleton is stabilized, the patient is mobilized, late fracture problems are addressed, and the patient is rehabilitated, both generally and with specific regard to the skeletal system.

We hope you enjoy this chapter.

EMERGENCY PHASE

The first phase of trauma care can be called the emergency phase, and it generally is directed by a general surgical team. The orthopedist plays a secondary but important role in these first few hours of care, when diagnoses are made and resuscitation begun.

Initial management begins at the accident site with transport personnel. They should make careful observations regarding the mechanism of injury, the patient's position, deformities present, and visible blood loss. If possible, a brief neurovascular check of the extremities should be done. Large bits of debris should be removed from open wounds and a sterile dressing applied. Deformities may be splinted in the position in which they lie or gently realigned and splinted. Femur fractures should be placed in traction splints, such as the Hare splint or Thomas splint. Placing gentle traction on the fracture reduces the magnitude of blood loss by decreasing the potential space into which bleeding can occur.

The use of traction splints alone has dramatically reduced the mortality of femur fractures since this type of splint was introduced in the early 1900s. The spine should be completely immobilized with cervical collars and a back board. Splinting should be done expeditiously, because the primary goal is rapid delivery to the hospital.

In the emergency room orthopedic evaluation is begun using the guidelines of the Advanced Trauma Life Support. History is obtained from emergency medical technicians and other attending personnel. The primary survey is carried out, with a preliminary check for bleeding, open wounds, and deformity of the extremities. The secondary survey allows for more detailed examination of the extremities. If the patient is responsive, inquiries should be made regarding the locations of pain. Pelvic stability should be assessed by applying an AP and then a lateral force to the iliac wings of the pelvis, feeling for motion or observing for a pain response. This check can provide preliminary evidence of an unstable pelvic fracture. The appendicular skeleton is examined for evidence of deformity, crepitus, and pain. Careful examination often discloses undiscovered fractures. A meticulous neurovascular examination should be performed and documented so that care can be prioritized and changes assessed. Deformities should be realigned and splinted, and the neurovascular examination repeated. Subjectively decreased pulses after realignment of the fracture should be further investigated with Doppler examination to quantify arterial pressure in the extremity. A mean arterial pressure below 90% of systemic mean arterial pressure indicates possible vascular injury, and further studies are warranted.[14] Dislocations should be noted and promptly reduced. For dislocations of the knee and shoulder, this may be done before radiographic evaluation. With dislocations of the hip and elbow, radiographic films should be taken before relocation.

Radiographic films that should be obtained in the emergency phase include a lateral C-spine view that visualizes from C1 to the C7-T1 disk to allow "clearance" of the C-spine. We also believe that an anteroposterior (AP) view of the pelvis should be obtained at this time to allow characterization of a possible pelvic or acetabular fracture, to obtain clues to sources of bleeding, and to demonstrate the presence of a hip dislocation. Films of all affected extremities should be obtained after the patient's condition has been stabilized. The patient must be carefully monitored while the films are being taken, because during this time much of the patient is lost to examination, and the intensity of care is of necessity decreased. Long-bone fractures should be filmed in both AP and lateral planes from the joint above to the joint below the fracture to rule out concomitant dislocations or second fractures in the areas of the joints.

Computed tomography (CT) scans are helpful for both spine and pelvic fractures but should be performed only if the patient's condition is stable. It is particularly easy to get a CT scan of the pelvis if the general surgical team relies on a CT scan of the abdomen to assess intra-abdominal injuries. Injuries that occur in the plane of the CT scan (transverse spine fracture) are best assessed with tomograms. These are rarely done in the acute period. Vascular studies, such as angiograms, are done in the emergency phase when indicated. They are particularly indicated in all knee dislocations because of the high incidence of clinically occult vascular damage in these injuries.

Initial treatment of orthopedic injuries in the emergency phase includes wound care. Wounds should be examined once, gross debris removed, and a sterile dressing applied. An occlusive wrap may be placed on bleeding wounds; this dressing should not be removed until the patient is in the operating room and ready for debridement. Most fractures can be reduced and aligned with gentle longitudinal traction. They can then be splinted or left in a traction device. The splints and traction device should remain in place until plans for definitive stabilization are underway. Dislocations generally should be reduced in the emergency room. It may be necessary to sedate the patient to relocate major joints such as the hip or shoulder. Local anesthesia generally can be used for dislocations of the knee, elbow, ankle, wrist, and fingers. More peripheral joints should be splinted in neutral position after relocation. After relocation of joints, reduction and splinting of fractures, and dressing of wounds have been accomplished, the patient can be moved for further diagnostic studies or for surgical procedures.

ACUTE PHASE

The major change in orthopedic traumatology over the past two decades has been the general acceptance of an aggressive policy for treating fractures, stressing early complete surgical care of a patient with multiple injuries. Surgical stabilization of long bones ideally should begin immediately after emergency (i.e., lifesaving) intervention is completed and continue until all fractures that would prevent mobilization are fixed. In this scheme orthopedists are correctly considered an extention of the resuscitative team, and only in a very few instances (discussed below) should their efforts be abandoned to "stabilize" the patient's condition. Many studies have demonstrated that the benefits of early complete care far outweigh the risks. Most of the benefits, when viewed simplistically, seem to derive from the ability to mobilize the patient. Because stabilized fractures are less painful, early fixation reduces the need for pain medicine and facilitates nursing care by allowing the patient to be moved. Fracture care with traction enforces the supine position, sometimes called the horizontal crucifixion position. Fixing major weight-bearing bones allows the patient to be moved in and out of bed, which allows an upright chest radiograph, improves ventilatory mechanics, and provides better ventilation-perfusion matching. These benefits reduce the incidence of post-traumatic pulmonary failure, previously the major cause of mortality in these patients. The upright posture also encourages enteral or oral intake of nutrition and allows more normal gastrointestinal (GI) function, which lessens the probability of gut organ sepsis and late septic deaths.[3]

If these general treatment goals are met, the mortality rate for trauma patients with multiple fractures is nearly nil.* The problem is knowing what to fix emergently and how to fix it to allow mobilization. This is our goal in this section.

Pelvic Fractures

Next to skull fracture, pelvic fracture is the skeletal injury that most commonly leads to the death of an injured patient. Pelvic fracture has been described as one of the four "unsolved" areas of trauma.[5] Unrelenting external or extraperitoneal hemorrhage is the major cause of death in patients with a serious pelvic fracture. These patients are subject to massive blood loss, and hemorrhage must be controlled definitively and quickly. This minimizes early mortality from exsanguination and late mortality caused by multiple organ failure, a disorder clearly caused by the prolonged shock/low-flow state. Because a patient with multiple injuries who has a pelvic fracture persists a long list of possible sources of blood loss, the problem remains one of expeditiously defining bleeding sites (intrathoracic, intra-abdominal, retroperitoneal), prioritizing the approach for hemorrhage control (laparotomy or pelvic fracture control first), and choosing the technique for hemostasis for blood loss caused by the pelvic fracture.

An injured patient initially is managed by the ATLS dictum of ABCs: airway management (A); external blood loss control (B); circulatory resuscitation (C); and rapid central nervous system (CNS) evaluation. The secondary survey may reveal physical signs of pelvic fracture such as pain, abnormal position of the leg, pelvic instability on palpation, and groin or flank hematoma; these indicate the possibility of fracture-associated blood loss. A chest radiograph or chest tube placement will rule out intrathoracic hemorrhage. Pelvic radiographs can further clarify any risk of significant bleeding from pelvic fractures. Pelvic views that should be obtained in the emergency room for an adequate appraisal include the AP, inlet, and outlet projections (Figure 19-1).[4] These allow definition of anterior or posterior displacement of the sacroiliac (SI) joint and enable the surgeon to determine whether rotational deviation of the hemipelvis is a factor. These projections also help delineate the relative risk of pelvic fracture bleeding. There are several systems for classifying fractures, but in this situation the crucial decision rests upon whether the posterior pelvic ring injury (the injury around the SI joint) is classified as stable or unstable. With posterior instability, the patient is more likely to hemorrhage.[17] The posterior sacral ligaments are extremely strong; their disruption indicates that a huge amount of force was applied to the pelvis and, by inference, to the neighboring retroperitoneum (Figure 19-2).[4] As such, fractures with posterior element instability have more associated injuries, require more blood products, and have more complications and a higher mortality than stable fractures. A cystogram, which is indicated in almost all pelvic injuries, gives an indirect measure of bleeding by allowing visualization of bladder displacement by the pelvic hematoma.

Even in patients determined to be at high risk for pelvic fracture bleeding, the source of blood loss is not always clear. Pelvic fractures that are likely to bleed are also likely to have associated injuries. As mentioned previously, a chest radiograph or chest tube insertion accurately rules out intrathoracic hemorrhage. If intra-abdominal bleeding is assessed by peritoneal lavage, open supraumbilical placement of the lavage catheter is a superior modification of the technique, because the dissecting retroperitoneal hematoma can be avoided. This minimizes false positive results, which have been reported to be as high as 50% with closed infraumbilical placement. With the open technique, false positive results can be reduced to 8% to 12%, leaving positive results with an 80% to 90% probability of diagnosing intraperitoneal bleeding.[12] This positive lavage data can be further graded according to the degree of positivity. Return of 10 ml of frank blood on insertion of the catheter indicates a high probability of ongoing intraperitoneal bleeding, generally from the liver or spleen. These patients should undergo emergency laparotomy. A patient whose lavage results are positive by red blood cell count alone requires exploration, but often the intra-abdominal lesion is quiescent. Continuous blood loss in these patients and in patients with a negative lavage result should be attributed to the pelvic fracture, and emergency attempts at hemostasis should be directed at this area.[19,20]

Blood loss from pelvic fractures generally stems from multiple lacerations of small and medium-sized arteries and veins, as well as from cancellous bone (Figure 19-3). These vessels bleed freely into the loose areolar tissue of the retroperitoneum, a huge potential space extending from the respiratory diaphragm to mid-thigh and capable of containing 4 L of blood before any tam-

*References 1, 2, 7, 15, 18, 22, 24-26, and 28.

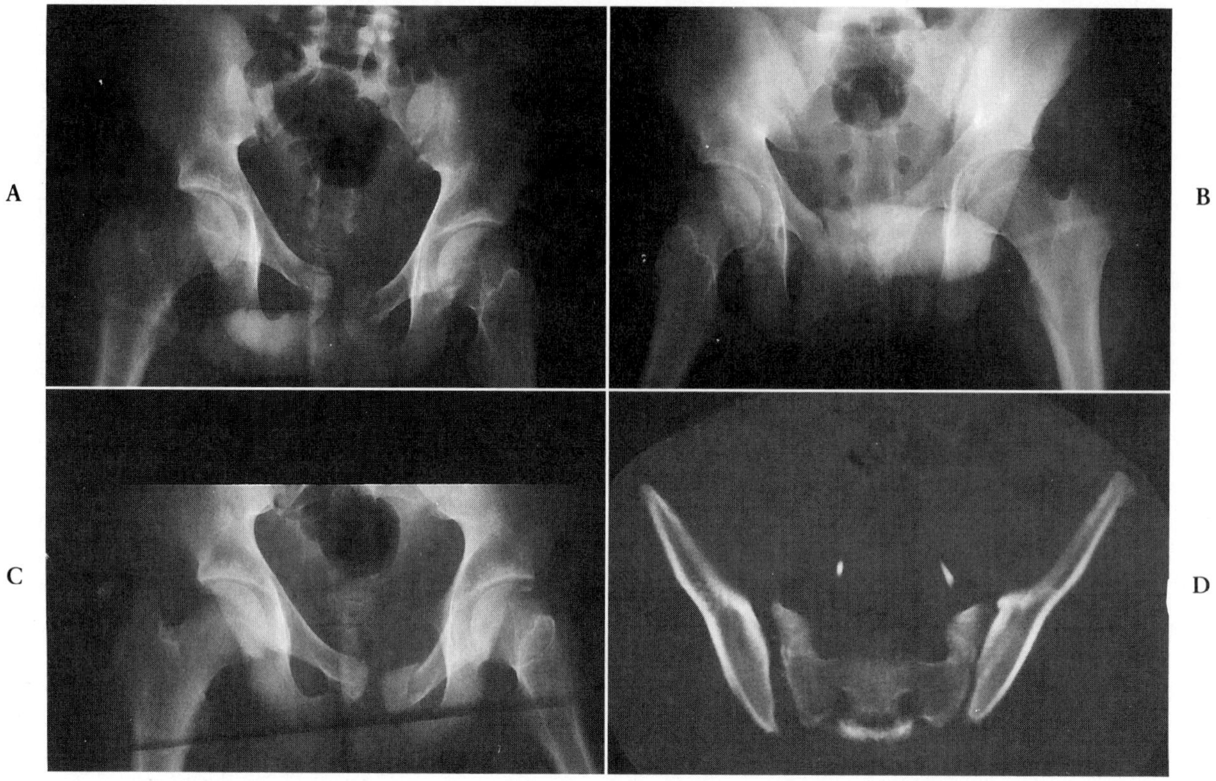

FIGURE 19-1 **A,** AP radiograph, the standard screening view of the pelvis. **B,** Inlet view of the pelvis, showing the fracture's inferior and superior pubic rami. Fractures through the sacral foramen can also be seen in this projection. This view shows vertical displacement of the hemipelvis, if present. **C,** Outlet view of the pelvis, which shows sacral fractures (especially lateral compression fractures) and disruptions of the sacroiliac joint, if present. This view will show asymmetry if a fracture is present. **D,** CT scan, showing subtle changes of the sacroiliac joint.

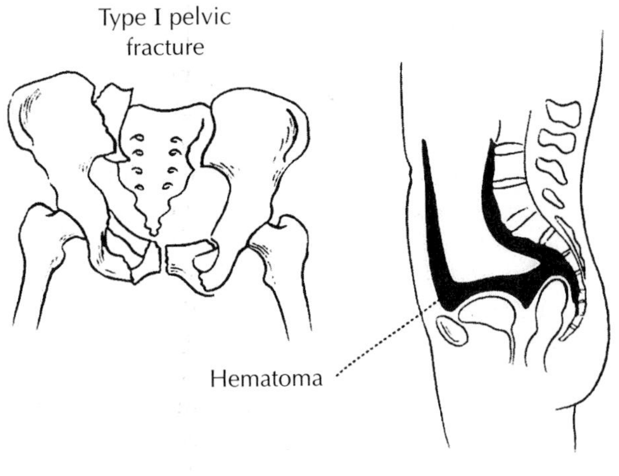

FIGURE 19-2 Unstable fracture caused by posterior pelvic disruption with retroperitoneal hematoma. These fractures cause more associated injuries, blood loss, and mortality than stable fractures. The retroperitoneal hematoma can be large and give a false positive with peritoneal lavage unless an open supraumbilical placement is used.

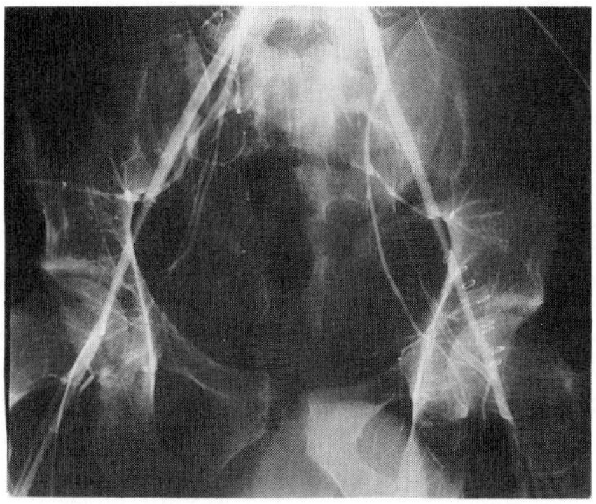

FIGURE 19-3 Pelvic blood supply. The pelvic vasculature has a rich collateral network that makes control of bleeding by direct vessel ligation difficult. This radiograph shows successful constriction of the superior gluteal artery as it passes through to the sciatic notch. Constriction is caused by outward displacement of the ilium.

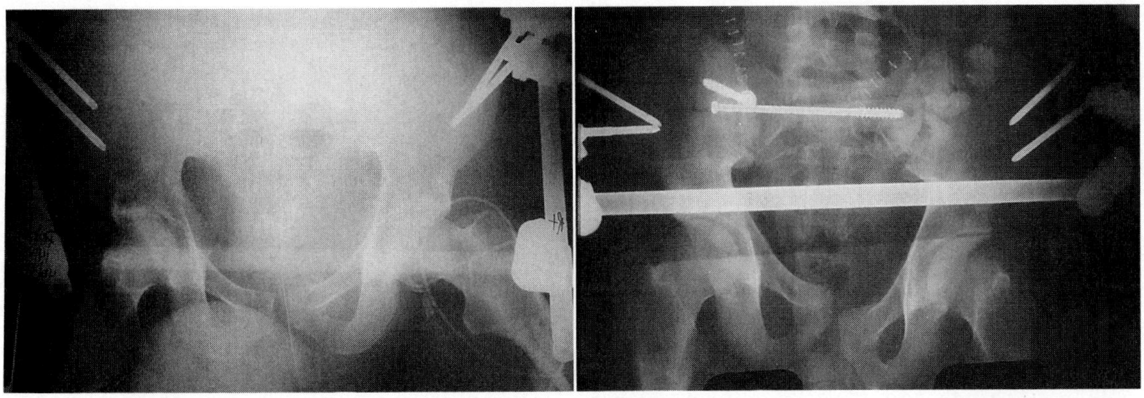

FIGURE 19-4 Pelvic fixation. **A,** The anterior external fixation frame, a simple device that controls bleeding by reducing pelvic volume and stabilizing the soft tissues, was placed during the initial phases of this patient's care. **B,** The posterior screws, which control the posterior ring, were placed during the second surgery.

ponade is realized. Because lacerations of major vessels are the cause of bleeding in only 2% to 10% of cases, most patients do not have surgically accessible bleeding sites that are well defined.[10,11] Attempts have been made to use inflow occlusion (through ligation of the internal iliac artery) to control the numerous bleeding vessels usually encountered, but this technique generally is frustrated by the rich collateral network in the pelvis, which allows for unabated blood loss. Also, approaching the artery requires opening the retroperitoneum and releasing any degree of tamponade that may exist. This allows massive blood loss while control is obtained. Because of the dismal results with this direct approach, it can be recommended only for open pelvic fractures with external bleeding, fractures with angiographically proven injury to major vessels, and patients with extremis. Lacking these indications, an indirect approach to hemorrhage control gives superior results. Military antishock trousers (commonly known as the MAST suit), anterior external fixation, limited internal fixation, and angiography all have a role in patient treatment.

The MAST suit is a three-chambered, external counterpressure device applied circumferentially about both lower extremities and the abdomen. The principal clinical effect with pelvic fractures is hemostatic, with perhaps some element of autotransfusion and increased total peripheral resistance. The device has been used successfully to control hemorrhage with pelvic fractures, but it requires prolonged application (as long as 12 to 24 hours), which has several drawbacks.[5] The MAST suit is ungainly and leaves most of the patient inaccessible to examination. It also enforces the supine position. The pressure required to stabilize a pelvic fracture (40 mm Hg) compromises circulation to the lower extremities and can cause compartment syndromes and skin lesions. Also, hemorrhage control is inferior to that obtained by the external fixator.[9] As such, we believe the MAST suit is best thought of as analogous to the Thomas splint: excellent for transport, minimizes blood loss during this period, but not definitive care.

Anterior external fixation provides a practical approach to indirect control of hemmorhage (Figure 19-4). External fixation controls bleeding by reducing the volume of the disrupted pelvis and producing tamponade. (The pelvis is basically a sphere whose volume is based on the formula $V = 4/3\pi r^3$. Therefore, small increases in the radius lead to large increases in volume.) Also, bone motion, with its attendant continuous damage to soft tissue, is minimized, as is bleeding from cancellous bone if compression can be obtained between fracture fragments. As such, the external frame is a superior tool for controlling acute pelvic fracture hemorrhage. The frame can be placed simply and reduction accomplished quickly, in an average time of 20 minutes. We have placed this device on patients in the emergency room, but it usually is placed in the operating room, using general anesthesia, where 5 mm pins can be inserted after direct visualization of the bony tables of the ilium. This is important, because a disrupted pelvis has abnormally oriented iliac wings, and this orientation must be appreciated to prevent misplacement of the pins. After the pins have been placed, the diastasis can be reduced by medial compression on the pin clusters, and vertical displacement is reduced with traction on the leg. The pin clusters are then connected in the reduced position, using a connecting system in any number of configurations that can even leave the abdomen free, and treatment of the patient is continued. Blood loss stops in up to 95% of patients so managed.[9,19] It is important to realize that this is only provisional fixation for hemodynamic stabilization in patients with posterior sacroiliac disruptions and is not definitive fracture care, because the degree of fracture stability it provides often is inadequate for full patient mobilization. As such, the patient should be stabilized hemodynamically, oxygen delivery ensured, and the fracture fully characterized after the acute period has ended. Definitive fracture care can then be decided on in a nonemergent fashion. If there is an associated posterior disruption, percutaneous or limited open reduction and subsequent internal fixation can be performed from posteriorly using large screws passed from the ilium into the bodies of the sacral vertebrae. This is done under image control, providing definitive fixation and allowing early mobilization. Because posterior exposure is associated with an increase in wound problems, this approach should be used with meticulous technique and careful handling of the soft tissue and skin, and it should be used only for patients in whom it is clearly the superior alternative.

The same goals of acute hemorrhage control can be realized with limited internal fixation. The laparotomy wound created for intraperitoneal exploration provides access to the pubic rami. In the instance of a pubic diastasis, these anterior elements can be reduced and plated, again effectively decreasing intrapelvic volume. This can stand as definitive treatment in open-book-type injuries where the intact posterior SI ligaments keep the pelvis vertically stable.[6]

As mentioned previously, approximately 5% of patients continue to bleed after external fixation. These generally are patients with continuous arterial bleeding, and they are best managed using angiography, with demonstration of bleeding sites and subsequent embolization using Gelfoam or autologous clot.[17,19,21] Major vessel injuries demonstrated angiographically are approached directly. The treatment of the bleeding patient with pelvic fracture requires a multidisciplinary mind set with full cooperation between teams of orthopedists, general surgeons, and radiologists. Priority is given to the injury most likely to be responsible for the greatest blood loss. The external fixator and limited internal fixation are invaluable additions to the treatment of these patients and allow for definitive hemostasis in most. Orthopedic intervention in this setting leads to immediate and dramatic cessation of hemorrhage and impressive improvement in patient mortality and morbidity.

Femur Fractures

The femur is the largest and strongest bone in the appendicular skeleton. It is surrounded by a very large muscle mass and is designed to withstand huge forces, as much as 12 times body weight in the single leg stance and much more than that in active pursuits. The forces required to fracture the femur are large and generally are the result of violent trauma. The surrounding soft tissues are injured both directly by the injuring agent and by the "blast effect" of the shattering bone. These patients often have associated injuries and are at risk both for immediate complications caused by shock from blood loss (which may be as much as 2 units in the thigh) and for late complications related to fracture treatment and associated injuries.

Diagnosis of the femur fracture generally is simple, because most involve both significant deformity and pain. Because the diagnosis often is obvious, subtle findings may be overlooked unless specifically sought. Although rare (less than 1%), vascular injuries do occur and can be disastrous if missed. The pulses in both the popliteal fossa and the foot must be carefully examined, and decreased pulses after alignment of the fracture in a splint should be further investigated with Doppler examination to quantify arterial pressure in the extremity. The neurologic examination is also important and must be meticulous so that any subsequent changes can be appreciated. These changes might herald a compartment syndrome or nerve entrapment from manipulation of the fracture. Also, a nerve injury should alert the surgeon to the increased risk of vascular injury, because these often occur concomitantly.

After examination the fracture should be characterized by AP and lateral radiographs, including the hip and the knee. We discuss here only diaphyseal (shaft) fractures, but an associated hip or distal intra-articular fracture must be ruled out because such an injury would alter therapy. In pure diaphyseal fractures, the radiograph will show the type of fracture, the amount of comminution, and the size of the femur. This information allows intelligent choice of therapeutic options.

Historically, fracture management in patients with multiple injuries and those with isolated fractures was postponed for 7 to 10 days to reduce the nonunion rate and to avoid surgery on patients who were "too sick" for any operation beyond lifesaving and limb-saving intervention. These patients, including those with isolated femur fractures, often had prolonged hospital stays and pulmonary complications, and they occasionally died of respiratory insufficiency, called "fat embolism syndrome." Charts not infrequently read, "traction intact, no complaints" day after day, with a final note describing the patient's death from respiratory failure. This occurred because the major physiologic cost of prolonged immobilization was not recognized. Throughout the 1960s only sporadic reports of immediate fracture care appear, and although late systemic problems seemed dramatically lessened by early surgical fixation, these findings were largely ignored. It wasn't until the 1970s that carefully performed studies began proving the efficacy of early complete care. In several centers, against the surgical authority of the time, policies of early fixation were developed with the reasoning that a trauma patient is never better suited for surgery than at the time of admission. Generally a young trauma victim is in optimum nutritional state and has none of the complications that result from prolonged bed rest. Rüedi and Wolff[25] in 1975, Riska and colleagues in 1976, and Wolff and coworkers in 1978[28] reported large series that showed that immediate internal fixation of fractures following lifesaving interventions dramatically decreased the incidence of post-traumatic pulmonary insufficiency and reduced the complexity of postoperative care. This policy of immediate fixation reduced the incidence of fat embolism syndrome in multiple trauma patients from 22% (observed with conservative fracture management) to 4.5%. Riska and Myllynen[22] followed this up in 1982 with a study that showed that with immediate surgical management of a fracture, the incidence of fat embolism syndrome was only 1.5%. Meek and colleagues[18] (1980) and Goris and coworkers[7] (1982), using Injury Severity Scores (ISS) to quantify the magnitude of trauma, showed that severely injured patients spent many fewer days on a ventilator and had significantly less "septic" mortality if femur fractures were fixed immediately. In 1986 Seibel and associates[26] reported on a group of severely injured patients (ISS of 36 or above) with femur fractures. They demonstrated mathematically that there was no correlation between the magnitude of original injury (as judged by the Hospital Trauma Index/Injury Severity Score) and any measure of the magnitude or duration of the subsequent pulmonary failure septic state. In contrast, all such measures correlated significantly with days of femur traction. The number of positive blood cultures and pulmonary emboli similarly increased with the number of days of femur traction and had no relation to the ISS. Finally, multiple organ failure occurred only in patients with prolonged femoral traction. Results such as this have been reported too often to be ignored. It is now clear that stabilization of a femur fracture is a semi-emergent situation. A final prospective, randomized study by Bone and coworkers[1] in 1988 showed that a delay of 48 hours in fracture fixation significantly increased ICU and ventilator time in a group of patients with moderate injuries. These findings, taken collectively, convinced the American College of Surgeons, which recommended in 1987 that femur fracture care be accomplished within the first 24 hours in patients with multiple injuries.

The reasons a patient benefits so greatly from early fracture care are not completely clear. Certain things are obvious. Conservative fracture care enforces the supine position. Any movement is very painful, and narcotics necessary to control this pain decrease respiratory drive. A prolonged, supine, immobile position is highly abnormal for humans, who even in sleep are normally very active. In the supine position the posterior aspects of the lung are dependent. In this position pulmonary capillary pressure is increased, as is transcapillary fluid loss, and interstitial edema develops, causing a ventilation-perfusion mismatch. Simultaneously, the "activated wound" (the area of the fracture and any other unaddressed problem) is releasing a variety of tissue-destructive agents, and the traumatized zones send embolic materials (fat emboli and platelet and leukocyte aggregates) to the lung. Because of the enforced supine position and the dependent nature of blood flow in the lung, these products are directed to the already edematous posterior aspects of the lungs, further increasing the damage.[2]

The ventilation-perfusion mismatch can be provisionally treated with mechanical ventilation with positive end-expiratory pressure (PEEP), but problems with oxygen transport may persist, depending on the amount of lung damage, necessitating prolonged intubation. This delays enteral nutrition and slows or stops GI function. The penetration pressure of interluminal bacteria increases, and the antibacterial-antitoxin mechanism of the gut mucosum may fail. This leads to gut-origin septic states and late septic–type mortality through activation of the hepatic macrophage.[3]

In contrast, early stable fracture fixation allows patient mobilization in a relatively pain-free manner. The patient may be rolled easily for nursing care and may be upright and out of bed to improve pulmonary mechanics and ventilation-perfusion matching. This prevents prolonged pulmonary failure and resulting intubation. This, coupled with a reduced need for pain medicine, allows normal GI function to resume, thus preventing gut-origin septic states. Problems with decubiti and thrombophlebitis are also virtually eliminated in a mobile patient.

Having established the need for early fixation, the technique must be decided on. Two recent advances have made intramedullary rodding the treatment of choice for virtually all diaphyseal femoral fractures. The first

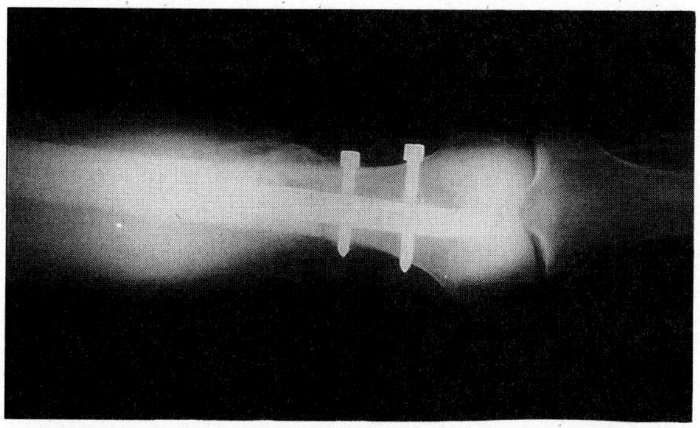

FIGURE 19-5 Femoral fracture fixed with interlocking intramedullary rod. Screws placed proximally and distally "lock" the proximal and distal fragments to the rod, preventing shortening and rotation of the fracture fragments.

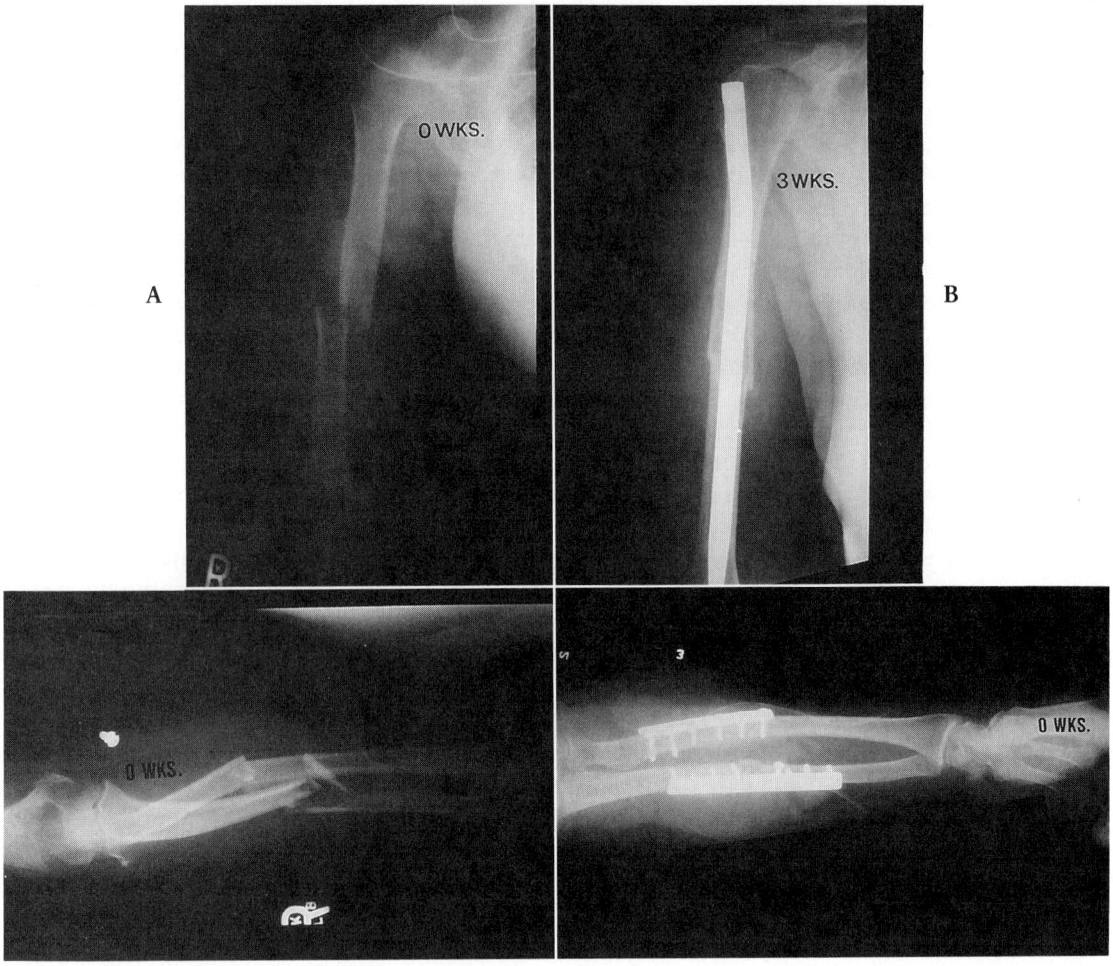

FIGURE 19-6 Floating joint. Ipsilateral humerus (**A**) and forearm fractures (**C**) have been stabilized (**B** and **D**) allowing better initial evaluation of the elbow joint. Fixation also allows the functional rehabilitation of the entire limb.

advance was the realization that placing a reamed rod is safe in open fractures, with little or no increase in infection or the rate of nonunion. The second advance was the development of interlocked rods, which provide axial and rotational stability with cross screws through the proximal and distal aspects of the rod (Figure 19-5). These have expanded the indications for use of the rod to comminuted fractures and to much more proximal and distal fractures. Also, it generally is possible to pass the rod closed without opening the fracture site and disturbing whatever soft tissue connections the fracture fragments have.

Other options for acute care include plating and external fixation. Plating should be considered when other injuries make moving the patient to the fracture table for rodding impossible, or in severe open fractures where extensive soft tissue stripping has already occurred. Technique is critical, with the need to preserve stripping soft tissue connections paramount if union is to be achieved. Union is slower than with rods, and bone defects should be grafted early. An added benefit of plate fixation is that, in the approach to the bone to allow plating, direct access to the fracture zone is realized. This allows debridement of dead muscle and evacuation of hematoma, which decreases the burden of the femur "wound" on the systemic physiology. External fixators have a limited application in the femur but can be used as provisional stabilization. They can be placed very quickly with four pins, two above and two below the fracture. Here they act as outboard, portable traction, which allows early mobilization. However, it is rarely definitive fracture care and should be converted as soon as possible to either intramedullary rod or plating systems.

Floating Joints

Patients with ipsilateral femur and tibia or humerus and forearm fractures have so-called floating joints. All agree that these fractures are indications for immediate fixation both above and below the joint to allow mobilization and proper evaluation of the involved joint. They signify major trauma, and associated injuries, particularly nerve and vascular injuries in the extremity, must be sought. Fixation may involve any combination of techniques as long as stability is achieved, because this, along with repair of intra-articular lesions, gives the best results when done without delay (Figure 19-6).

Contraindications of Early Fixation

Although complete early care is the goal, the risks and benefits must be weighed. In general, major weight-bearing bones must be stabilized immediately so that the patient can be mobilized. This includes the femur and generally the pelvis. The humerus may also be included in patients with multiple injuries. This concept should be abandoned only when further surgery would be detrimental to the patient, such as in the case of hypothermia or coagulopathy. In these situations continued exposure and blood loss only exacerbate the condition, and the procedure should be stopped either to warm the patient or to provide clotting factors.

A less pressing concern is fixation of "minor" weight-bearing joints, where casting can adequately stabilize the fracture to allow pain-free mobilization. Such fractures include the forearm, tibia, ankle, and wrist. Efforts to stabilize these fractures can be safely abandoned if there is concern that an adequate job cannot be done in the acute setting. Factors that come into play include the adequacy of the facility and the surgeon's skill and preparedness. Because morbidity is minimal when these procedures are delayed, it is better to stop operating and "reset the stage" if the surgeon feels that a technically superior job can be done later.

Compartment Syndrome

Compartment syndrome is a condition in which an increase in tissue pressure within a closed space impedes the blood supply and functioning of the tissue within that space. Hence, for compartment syndrome to occur, there must be an envelope that encloses a circumscribed space and increased tissue pressure within that envelope. The envelope may be epimysium, an osseofibrous sheath, as in the anterior and lateral tibial compartments, or fascia alone, as in the femoral or gluteal compartments. Circumferential constricting dressings may also create a "closed compartment." The increase in tissue pressure generally is caused by an increase in the volume of compartment contents (e.g., from bleeding) but can also result from prolonged external compression, as from the MAST suit. Compartment volume can be increased by hemorrhage, interstitial postischemic swelling, or intracompartmental extravascular fluid extravasation or administration. High energy, crush-type injuries associated with fracture, muscle injury, and hemorrhage pose a high risk of compartment syndrome. This situation is most commonly encountered in the tibia but may be present in the thigh, gluteal region, forearm, or upper arm. The presence of shock increases the risk of compartment syndrome for any injury.

The pathophysiology of compartment syndrome is this: Oxygen is delivered across capillaries, and flow across these vessels depends on an arteriovenous pressure gradient. An increase in tissue pressure increases venous pressure by compressing the thin-walled veins. As venous pressure rises, capillary flow ceases, and capillary flow fails. This situation must be reversed quickly or permanent tissue damage results.[27]

The key to treating compartment syndrome is early diagnosis, which requires an alert team with a high index of suspicion. If the patient is awake and responsive, the most important sign is pain out of proportion to that expected from the injury. There is pain on palpation of the compartment, which feels firm. Passive stretching of the muscles of the compartment (e.g., flexion of the toes for the anterior tibial compartment) is very painful. Hyperesthesia may result in the distribution of nerves traversing the compartment, and this may be one of the earliest signs. Paresthesia follows later. Muscle weakness develops as the compartment syndrome becomes established, and it is a late and ominous finding. It is important to note that because this is a failure of capillary flow, pulses distal to the compartment may be intact. Their presence should not decrease the suspicion of compartment syndrome.

In patients in whom the examination is unreliable, or when clinical diagnosis is unsure, tissue pressure can be measured directly. There are many techniques for measurement, all of which involve inserting a needle or catheter into the compartment and obtaining readings of tissue (interstitial) pressure. When these pressures reach a threshold value, fasciotomy should be performed. This threshold is a subject of debate; 30 to 40 mm Hg has been empirically defined as the critical level, although this threshold may be lower in patients in shock who have a low mean arterial pressure.

Compartment syndrome is treated by fasciotomy, which involves releasing skin and enclosing fascia along the entire length of the compartment. When the fascia is opened, the muscle will bulge through the wound as the pressure is released through expansion. Muscle debridement probably should not be done at this time, but rather in a second-look procedure within 24 to 48 hours, because much marginal muscle will remain viable. All compartments affected should be opened completely. This may involve a four-compartment fasciotomy in the lower leg, volar and dorsal fasciotomies in the forearm, and complete fasciotomies of the thigh, buttock, and arm with compartment syndromes in these areas. The surgeon should also be aware of the possibility of foot or hand compartment syndrome. The diagnosis is made as in other areas, and treatment also is fasciotomy of all involved compartments. Wounds should be left open for secondary closure or skin grafting. We provisionally cover these with synthetic material, such as Epiguard.

When compartment syndrome is associated with a fracture, a fasciotomy wound will make it necessary to surgically stabilize the fracture. Releasing the compartments destabilizes the fracture, and the need for open wound care obviates the use of a cast for control. Treatment options include intramedullary nails and plates, and external fixators. Intramedullary nails can be used as an internal splint and can be either unlocked or interlocked, depending on the fracture pattern. In the acute situation it may be preferable to use an unreamed nail; this prevents problems with cortical necrosis and avoids increasing compartment pressures by reaming and pushing intramedullary debris out the fracture site and into the compartment. When direct exposure of the fracture occurs when creating a fasciotomy, it is fairly expeditious to place a plate on the fracture. Again, this should be done with a minimum of soft tissue stripping and maintaining as much periosteum as possible in the area of the fracture. An external fixator can be used, particularly with an open fracture associated with compartment syndrome, for either provisional or definitive stabilization. All of these methods facilitate wound care by allowing access to the soft tissues.

CARE OF OPEN FRACTURES

Open fractures, whether isolated injuries or a component of multiple injuries, are orthopedic emergencies and require special attention. This is because of the obvious inflammation of a bone infection. Bone is a relatively avascular tissue. Once it becomes infected, the infection is extremely difficult to eradicate because of the difficulty involved in delivering white cells and antibiotics to the site of infection. Open fractures are even more challenging in patients with multiple injuries, because fracture care often is delayed while more life-threatening problems are treated.

Open fractures originally were classified as grade I, II, or III, based solely on the size of the wound. A grade I injury had a skin opening less than 1 cm long and was an inside-to-outside injury (the bone itself pierced the skin). Grade II injuries had wounds 1 to 3 cm long and were potentially outside-to-inside injuries (whatever force or object broke the skin also broke the bone). Grade III injuries involved wounds 3 cm or longer and could be either inside to outside or outside to inside, but generally were the latter.

GRADING OF OPEN FRACTURES

Grade I	Wound opening <1 cm. Usually an inside-to-outside injury, i.e., the bone pierces the skin.
Grade II	Wound opening 1-3 cm. Usually an outside-to-inside injury, i.e., the fracture force also causes the skin disruption.
Grade IIIA	Wound opening >3 cm. Minimal bone stripping and muscle contusion. Wound can be closed later by skin closure.
Grade IIIB	Same as grade IIIA but with more contamination or muscle and soft tissue damage. Usually requires muscle transposition or free-tissue transfer for closure.
Grade IIIC	Same as grade IIIB but with vascular injury that requires repair.

This system has been replaced by the Gustilo-Anderson system (see the box above).[8] The new system retains the traditional grade I and grade II classifications, but grade III injuries, which vary considerably, have been subclassified as A, B, or C. In all three subclasses the wound still is 3 cm or longer, but in grade IIIA injuries, soft tissue stripping and contamination are minimal. Grade IIIB injuries have a considerable amount of soft tissue stripping, muscle contusion, and/or comminution; these are also wounds in which the bone itself cannot be primarily covered with soft tissue. A grade IIIC injury is a IIIB injury with vascular damage.[8]

Treatment of open fractures begins at the scene. All noxious materials should be removed from the wound as gently as possible, and the wound should then be covered with a sterile dressing. If the bone is sticking out through the skin, it may return to the skin cavity when the extremity is aligned and splinted. We do not feel that ambulance crews should change the way they normally splint fractures to prevent this. We feel that the receiving orthopedic surgeon is responsible for cleansing the wound thoroughly, and that ambulance crews should not change their overall treatment of the extremity (i.e., splinting) because the fracture is open, especially since failure to align and splint a fracture can lead to vascular compromise and potential loss of the limb. The basic premise for field treatment of an open fracture remains removing noxious contaminants, applying a sterile dressing, splinting the extremity in a normal fashion, and checking neurovascular status before and after such splinting.

In the emergency room the wound should be examined once and once only. All personnel who need to look at the wound should see it at the same time. The wound is then recovered with a sterile dressing. If bone is protruding from the wound, a sterile, moist dressing should be applied to keep the bone from desiccating. The limb should continue to be splinted as appropriate. The wound should not be rechecked until the patient is taken to the operating room. These measures prevent contamination of the wound with hospital-based organisms, which are much more difficult to eradicate if they become established. The orthopedist should attempt to grade the open wound to prepare for surgical care.

In the operating room, the most important aspect of care of an open fracture is debridement, and this is one of the most difficult skills to learn (i.e., what is enough debridement). In our hands, the leg is first prepped with Duraprep and then vigorously irrigated and debrided. The hallmark of this treatment is large amounts of saline delivered via a pulsatile irrigation system. This adheres to the basic tenet, "the solution to pollution is dilution." At this time all devitalized material, skin, muscle, and bone is removed. No piece of bone that is totally devitalized is ever replaced in an open wound, regardless of whether it would add to structural integrity. It is dead. It would take years to incorporate and therefore should not be replaced in the wound regardless of how tempting this may seem. With today's techniques of soft tissue coverage, bone grafting, and bone transportation, there is no need to do anything less than a thorough debridement, removing all devitalized tissue.

After this initial debridement, a formal 10-minute scrub of the extremity is performed. The extremity is draped in the usual fashion, and a second layer of outer drapes is added. A second irrigation and debridement is carried out, this time by extending the wound or making a new incision. The ends of the bone are cleansed of all foreign material, and any further devitalized tissue is removed. The second layer of outer drapes is then removed, leaving a sterile field below, and the surgeon changes gown and gloves. Definitive stabilization of the bone is then carried out. The gold standard for open fractures remains external fixation. These devices have improved in the past 10 years and have gone from very cumbersome devices to simple frames. Most fractures can now be stabilized with four to six pins placed in the bone connected by one or two bars on the outside. In an open tibia fracture, which is by far the most common open fracture, there currently is a move to stabilize grades I through IIIA tibial fractures (see the box on p. 776) with unreamed, locked intramedullary nails. It is felt that by not reaming the medullary canal, there is minimal damage to the already impaired blood supply to the tibia and that locking the nail (i.e., placing screws across the top and bottom of the nail) affords very stable skeletal fixation. Plates can also be used, but only if they can be placed with minimal or no further soft tissue stripping of the bone.

There is always a question of wound closure in open fractures. For us the answer is very simple. We do not close open wounds. As stated earlier, debridement is one of the most difficult things to learn, and even the most experienced surgeons have a difficult time deciding whether a wound should be left open. The simplest thing, therefore, is to leave the wounds open. Any extensions of the wound that the surgeon makes to facilitate debridement can be closed, but the open portion of the wound should be left open, or at least a portion of the wound should be left open. Because the goal of debridement is to eliminate all dead material and dead space, it does not make sense to create dead space by closing the wound. The open wound is kept moist, and the choice of dressings is either moist saline dressings or, in our case, dilute bleach solution, such as Dakin's solution. The dressings are changed three times a day by the nursing staff. This keeps the wound moist and prevents any exposed bony surfaces from desiccating.

Antibiotics are always used in open fractures. Grade I and grade II open fractures with minimal contamination or straightforward road contamination are treated with a first-generation cephalosporin for 48 hours after the first and subsequent procedures. Grade III wounds with more contamination are treated with a first-generation cephalosporin to cover staphylococci, an aminoglycoside to cover the gram-negative organisms, and penicillin to cover the gram-positive rods. This antibiotic regimen is continued for 72 hours after each surgical procedure (i.e., after additional debridements or future fixation or soft tissue procedures).

Before beginning irrigation and debridement, a culture of the wound is obtained. A second culture is obtained after all irrigation and debridement has been completed. Often, by the time of the second look an organism has been isolated from the predebridement cultures, and we can be more selective with our antibiotics. Cultures obtained after completion of the initial debridement are also used to select more type-specific antibiotics at this time.

Most open fractures, especially grade III injuries, require a "second-look" for further debridement. This is carried out 24 to 72 hours after the initial debridement, depending on the status of the wound, the surgeon's assessment of the first debridement, and the patient's general condition. The wound can be closed at this time if it is clean, if minimal further debridement is necessary, and if closure can be obtained without any tension on the skin. If any of these elements is questionable, the wound should be left open and closed at a later date. At this time the wound can be closed by using a split-thickness skin graft or by tissue transfers, either local flap coverage or free tissue transfers. The latter generally are not done in the first 24 to 48 hours, but they are done as early as they safely can be. The surgeon must be certain about the zone of injury before using flaps. If the more proximal vessels have been damaged and used for a free tissue transfer, the transfer may fail. We try to have the bone covered with soft tissue by seven to 10 days with wound closure, local tissue transfers, or with a free tissue transfer. Free tissue transfers have been one of the greatest advances in the care of open fractures. This allows us to do a radical excision of all devitalized tissue at our initial debridement. Even if a large amount of skin has been lost or a large amount of bone is exposed, we will be able to cover this with tissue, which has a rich blood supply.

Primary Amputation

Occasionally, especially in patients with multiple injuries, primary amputation of a severe open fracture must be considered. Vital body systems have been considerably stressed, and it is unjustified to subject these patients to a prolonged operation to try to save an extremity that is unsalvageable. Such surgery can cost the patient's life if the surgeon spends hours trying to replant an essentially dead limb by doing vascular reconstruction, only to have myonecrosis set in and cause renal failure. Deciding when to amputate has always been difficult, but more recently has been well addressed by means of the "mangled extremity severity score" (MESS),[13] which can help the surgeon decide when a lower extremity should be salvaged and when it should be primarily amputated. Table 19-1 gives additional details of this grading system.

The MESS score takes into account the tissue injury, the duration of ischemia, the level of shock, and the patient's age. A score of 7 or higher is 100% positive for eventual amputation. With a score of 6 or less, salvage may be possible. When the warm ischemia time has exceeded 6 hours, the ability to save the limb is dramatically decreased. When deciding whether to salvage the limb, the surgeon should take into account the fact that the patient may be better off in the long run with an adequate below-knee prosthesis than with a limb that clearly will not function normally. Lange and colleagues[16] showed that of patients with grade IIIC injuries whose limbs had been salvaged, not a single person had a normal gait.

TABLE 19-1 MANGLED EXTREMITY SEVERITY SCORE (MESS) VARIABLES FOR LOWER EXTREMITY SALVAGE

	POINTS
Skeletal/Soft Tissue Injury	
• Low energy (stab, simple fracture, civilian gunshot wound)	1
• Medium energy (open or multiple fractures, dislocation)	2
• High energy (close-range shotgun or military gunshot wound, crush injury)	3
• Very high energy (all of the above plus gross contamination, soft tissue avulsion)	4
Limb Ischemia	
• Pulse reduced or absent but perfusion normal	1*
• No pulse, paresthesia, diminished capillary refill	2*
• Cool, paralyzed, insensate, numb	3*
Shock	
• Systolic blood pressure always >90 mm Hg	0
• Transient hypotension	1
• Persistent hypotension	2
Age (yr)	
• <30	0
• 30 to 50	1
• >50	2

*Score doubled for ischemia >6 hours.

RECONSTRUCTIVE PHASE

We have discussed the emergency and acute phases of care of a patient with multiple injuries. In the next two sections we discuss what takes place orthopedically once the patient's condition has been stabilized by the general surgical team. By the time this phase begins, generally after the first 24 hours, the patient has been resuscitated and the major general surgical procedures (e.g., thoracotomy, abdominal exploration, and vascular repairs) have been carried out. The focus of care shifts from these lifesaving measures to those that deal more with the patient's overall ability to function. From an orthopedist's point of view, this means reconstructing the patient's skeletal system.

The reconstructive phase is divided into two parts, an early phase and a late phase. The early phase generally involves the patient's initial hospitalization, during which all necessary fracture stabilization is done. The late phase, which generally covers the time after the patient's initial hospitalization, deals with long-term fracture problems such as delayed union, nonunion, and malunion. This phase may last many years, until the patient's skeletal system is appropriately reconstructed and healed.

Early Reconstructive Phase

In this early phase, it is important to advance the patient from the previous level of function (bed to chair) to the level where the patient is as independent as possible. The major thrust is toward getting the patient ambulatory. Orthopedically, the major goal is to stabilize the patient's skeletal system to allow return to a normal functional life-style. During this phase the skeletal injuries not addressed in the acute phase are addressed in earnest. These procedures include stabilizing weight-bearing extremities, treating periarticular and upper extremity fractures, and continuing open fracture care.

Stabilization of the Weight-Bearing Skeleton

Fractures of the weight-bearing skeleton are stabilized to advance mobilization of the patient. When all of the patient's extremities are weight bearing, even if only

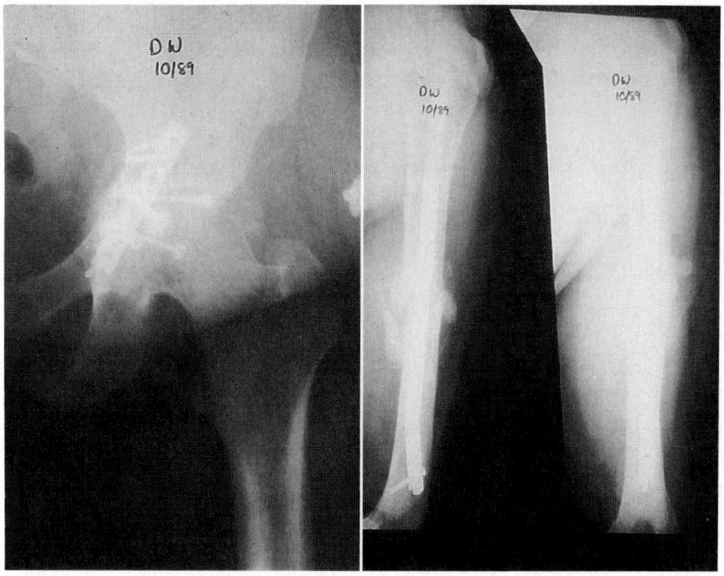

A B

FIGURE 19-7 Upper extremity weight bearing. This patient with upper and lower extremity injuries (**A**) had the humeral fracture fixed with an IM nail, allowing her to bear full weight on the upper extremity (**B**).

partly so, the patient becomes much more mobile. With adequate stabilization, the patient can even ambulate. We feel that ambulation is healthy both physiologically and psychologically.

The optimal situation is to have two weight-bearing lower extremities. Fractures of the lower extremities that were not fixed in the emergency or acute phases are now repaired. The weight-bearing lower extremities generally are stabilized in a way that enables them to bear the maximum amount of weight the fracture pattern will allow. In the tibia and femur, we feel it best to place load-sharing devices, such as intramedullary rods. The rod allows the patient's weight to be transmitted through the bone itself and not through the implant. Intramedullary rods tend to be stronger than plates because of their size and central placement in the bone.

If the posterior aspect of a pelvic fracture is unstable and was not fixed earlier, it is now stabilized. Posterior sacroiliac disruptions and sacral fractures generally are stabilized with screws, which are placed from the outer aspect of the ilium into the body of the sacrum. Occasionally these are augmented by transiliac rods, which go from one iliac crest to the other. This gives the pelvis more stability and often results in nearly full weight bearing through the pelvis.

If fractures of the lower extremity cannot be stabilized so that they are weight bearing (such as an intra-articular fracture), the patient must use the upper extremities to bear weight. The rule of thumb is: Two arms equal one leg. If a patient can use crutches or a walker and has one full weight-bearing lower extremity, the patient can ambulate. If an upper extremity is needed for weight bearing, a fractured humerus is stabilized with intramedullary rods, which allows the humerus to bear full weight. Platform-type adaptive devices for crutches and walkers are also available. These allow the patient to place the weight on the proximal forearm or elbow, so that the patient can bear full weight on the proximal portion of the forearm, even with fractures of the mid-forearm and wrist. In this way, often enough of the weight-bearing long bones can be stabilized to allow the patient to be ambulatory (Figure 19-7).

Spinal Fractures

We generally do not stabilize thoracolumbar spinal fractures during the emergency or acute phase, but others advocate doing this surgery early. Generally, spinal surgery entails a considerable loss of blood and if the patient already has lost blood from other injuries, he could be thrown into disseminated intravascular coagulation (DIC) during spinal surgery. Because spinal surgery is very delicate work that can result in disastrous neurologic complications, we feel it is best undertaken during daylight hours, when the surgeon and the operating room crews are at their best. Spinal fixation is not performed by all orthopedic surgeons, but rather by a limited number, generally at larger hospitals. We feel that this surgery should be done by people trained in it, even if this means a delay of a day or two. Rotating beds can keep the patient supine while rotating from side to side,

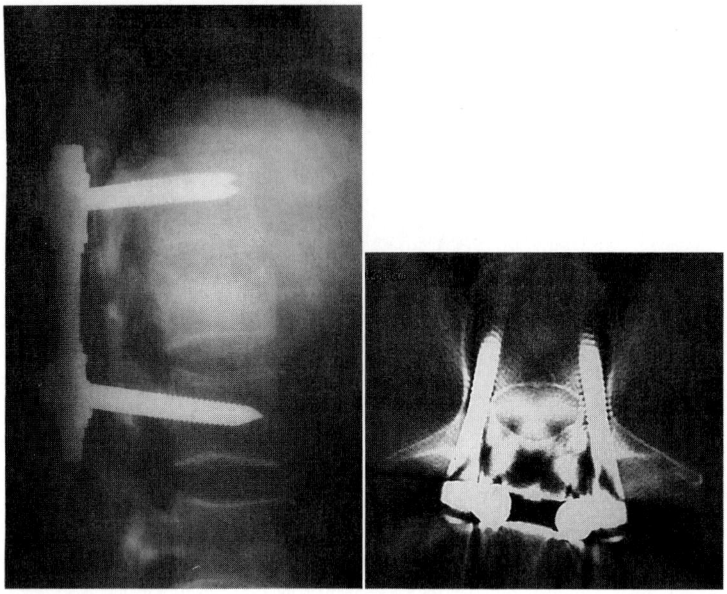

A

B

FIGURE 19-8 Spine fracture fixed with pedicle screws. **A,** The fusion is limited to 3 levels (not 5), 1 above and 1 below the fractured vertebra. **B,** The pedicle screws go through the pedicle into the vertebral body.

thus maintaining adequate pulmonary function until the spinal surgery is done.

Some of the current thinking about spinal surgery may change with the advent of new types of fixation for the spine. The most promising technique appears to be pedicle fixation (Figure 19-1). Placing long screws through the pedicle and into the body of the vertebrae gives very solid fixation without the need for long spans (previously the spine had to be fused over a minimum of five segments, two above and two below the fracture level). With pedicle fixation the same fracture can be fixed with only three levels of fusion, one level above and one level below the fracture (Figure 19-8). Such fixation is simpler and entails less blood loss. The devices used to fuse spines today are stronger and allow patients to be mobilized quickly after surgery, using a removable polyethylene jacket for support.

Periarticular Fractures

Periarticular fractures are fixed during the reconstructive phase, even if they are in the weight-bearing extremities, for three major reasons. First, these fractures often can be stabilized by splinting and still allow the patient to be mobilized (i.e., knee and ankle fractures can be sufficiently stabilized to allow the patient to be mobilized out of bed). Second, these fractures are more difficult and more time consuming to repair than diaphyseal fractures, because the joint surface must be anatomically reconstructed to prevent degenerative arthritis in the future. Third, when fractures in areas such as the acetabulum and distal femur are repaired, blood loss can be considerable. For example, a complex acetabular fracture may take 4 to 8 hours to repair and can involve a blood loss of 1000 to 3000 ml. Subjecting a patient to this lengthy procedure in the emergency phase is unwarranted, and we delay these fractures until the patient's general condition is more stable (i.e., until the reconstructive phase).

When repairing intra-articular fractures, the orthopedist's goal is twofold: first, to obtain anatomic reduction so that the joint surface is perfectly smooth; and second, to achieve stable fracture fixation to allow early motion of the joint. If the surgeon achieves a perfect reduction but is unable to obtain stable fixation, the patient may be unable to move the extremity. If this is the case, the limb quickly becomes stiff and loses function. Weight bearing generally is not a goal with periarticular fractures except in cases such as simple ankle fractures, where weight bearing can be started in an early phase. Most joint fractures are protected from weight bearing until they are sufficiently healed, so that the fracture fragments do not displace. For fractures of the acetabulum, distal femur, or tibial plateau, this can be anywhere from 6 to 16 weeks.

Periarticular fractures generally are stabilized with plates and screws. Whereas intramedullary rods are useful in the shaft portion of the bone, where they can gain purchase above and below the fracture, such is not possible with intra-articular fractures. The devices used to fix intra-articular fractures generally have some way of placing a large amount of fixation in the fragment closest to the joint. Some examples would be an angled blade

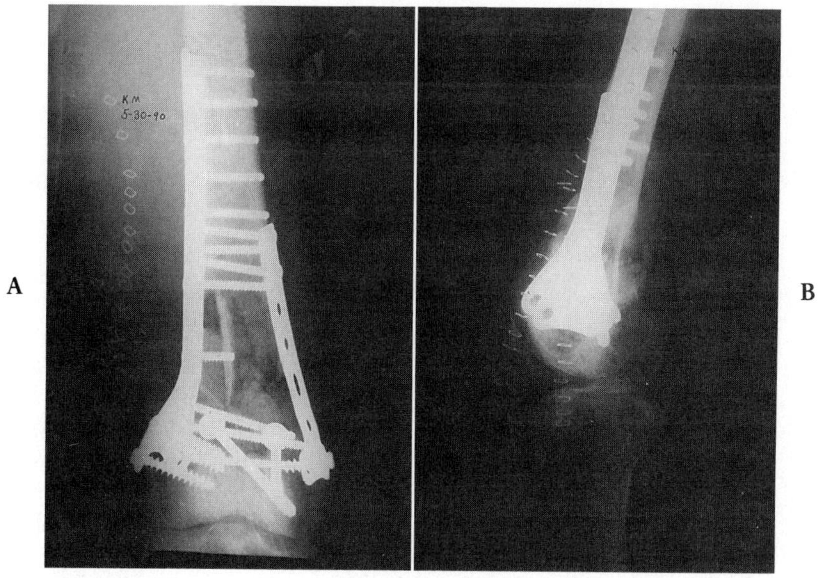

FIGURE 19-9 **A** and **B**, Implants used to stablized joint fractures. The devices have places to insert several screws into the bone near the joint.

plate, a condylar buttress plate, or a T plate. These devices allow a large amount of fixation (as with the blade plate) very close to the joint surface (Figure 19-9). In the upper extremity the devices generally do not need to be as large as in the lower extremity, because the forces acting about the joint are dramatically different in the knee than in the elbow or shoulder. For example, some periarticular fractures (e.g., the proximal humerus) can be stabilized with simple K wire (Kirschner wire) fixation. Also, wrist fractures often can be treated with simple external fixation devices in much the same fashion as they would be as an isolated injury.

In summary, because periarticular fractures are so important to the patient's overall, long-term ability to function, it is critical to repair these injuries as perfectly as possible and to ensure that fixation is not compromised in any way. We feel that these injuries are best treated electively, when the surgeon and ancillary personnel are at their best.

Upper Extremity Fractures

Upper extremity fractures generally are stabilized during the reconstructive phase, because it is not mandatory to fix these fractures to mobilize the patient out of bed. With shoulder immobilizers to stabilize shoulder fractures and splints to stabilize humeral fractures and below, the patient can be mobilized to a chair. To enable these patients to become independently functional, to mobilize themselves out of bed, and also to take care of personal needs such as eating and toileting, at least one and preferably two upper extremities must be stabilized. We try to stabilize these extremities at the second surgical encounter, such as when the lower extremity fractures are being stabilized or when an open wound is being closed.

We fix the fractures of the upper extremity, which traditionally are stabilized regardless of whether the patient has multiple injuries. Fractures involving both bones of the forearm are an excellent example of this. If the forearm shaft fractures are not fixed anatomically and started on early motion, both elbow and wrist motion (flexion/extension and supination/pronation) will be impaired. Forearm fractures are fixed with plates and screws, which are the gold standard for forearm shaft fractures (Figure 19-6). Wrist fractures, as noted previously, often are fixed with external fixation devices and plates. Hand fractures generally are stabilized with either miniplates or K wires; hand fractures rarely require surgical fixation, even in a patient with multiple injuries. Basically we use the same devices as in patients without multiple injuries, except in the humerus, where there is a growing tendency to use intramedullary nailing rather than fracture bracing.

Simple, isolated injuries, such as a simple wrist fracture, often can be treated with closed reduction and a cast. However, if the wrist fracture occurs with an elbow fracture that is stabilized surgically, casting the wrist fracture would impair early motion of the elbow. In these cases we prefer fixation of both fractures to allow complete functional rehabilitation of the entire extremity.

Late Reconstructive Phase

The late reconstructive phase begins after the initial hospitalization. All necessary fractures have been stabilized, and the patient is ambulatory or at least getting about in a wheelchair at home or in a rehabilitation hospital.

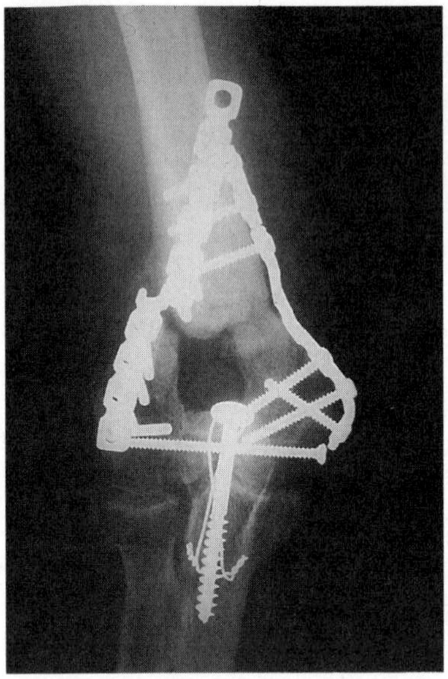

FIGURE 19-10 Broken hardware. Nonunion of a distal humerus fracture has led to plate failure; both plates are broken.

During this phase fracture problems such as delayed union, nonunion, and malunion are dealt with. Also, the normal sequelae of these injuries (e.g., hardware removal) are addressed.

Delayed Union

Fractures often take longer to heal in patients with multiple injuries, partly because of the magnitude of injury the bone and the entire body has sustained. Very simply, small trauma causes small problems, and big trauma causes big problems. Also, patients with severe multiple injuries often are nutritionally depleted, especially protein depleted, and this can delay fracture union. Delayed union generally is defined as delay in the healing of a fracture beyond the expected time frame. For instance, a high-velocity tibia fracture is expected to take up to 6 months to heal. If the fracture is not united after 6 months, it is considered a delayed union, provided it is still progressing toward union.

If a fracture is not progressing toward a timely union, it may be in the patient's best interest to have the healing progress at a faster rate. This is because the patient may be losing ground from a functional point of view (e.g., losing range of motion of an extremity because of casting or prolonged disuse). Also, over the course of a delayed union, especially in periarticular fractures, the fixation could fail, and as a result the reduction could be lost (Figure 19-10).

Delayed unions generally are treated by trying to promote the fracture to unite faster; this usually means bone grafting the fracture to stimulate healing. It is felt that bone graft probably works in two ways: First, it acts as a scaffolding or latticework upon which new bone forms. Second, an autogenous bone graft (generally obtained from the iliac crest) has bone morphogenic protein, which stimulates healing. Research is underway on treating delayed union and nonunion by injecting only bone morphogenic protein into and around the fracture site to promote union.[29]

In cases in which internal fixation has failed because of delayed union, bone grafting is augmented by refixation. Whenever internal fixation is used, a race ensues between union of the fracture and failure of the hardware (e.g., the plate, rod, or screws breaking or the screws loosening in the bone). With delayed union the internal fixation device undergoes excessive stress, and we find it prudent to replace the fixation device at the time of grafting. When delayed union involves a fracture in which an intramedullary rod has been used, treatment is simple: the rod is removed, the medullary canal is reamed, and a larger nail is placed. The reaming provides bone graft and restimulates the fracture, and the larger nail provides greater stability. If there is any component of malunion (e.g., increased angulation or abnormal rotation), this is also corrected at the time of the bone grafting, again involving internal fixation of the fracture.

Nonunion

Nonunion generally is defined as any fracture that has not united after 6 months and that is not progressing toward union (i.e., the fracture healing has in essence stalled). The reasons for nonunion are essentially the same as those for delayed union, except that the progress toward healing has diminished or stopped altogether. There are basically three types of nonunion: atrophic nonunion, oligotrophic nonunion, and hypertrophic nonunion (Figure 19-11).

Atrophic nonunion is nonunion in which minimal healing of the fracture has occurred. There is minimal to no biologic activity toward healing. Clinically the fracture site is of normal temperature and freely mobile. Radiographically virtually no callus formation is present at the fracture site. *Oligotrophic nonunion* is nonunion in which there is modest biologic activity. Clinically the fracture site is warm and has a rubbery feeling. Radiographically callus formation is moderate, and there simply has not been enough callus formation to complete the union of the fracture. *Hypertrophic nonunion* is nonunion in which the body has made a very vigorous effort to heal the fracture. There is considerable biologic activity, and clinically there is a large, warm, palpable mass of callus. The callus often is massive. This type of nonunion often manifests a synovial pseudarthrosis (i.e., in essence the body converts its fracture healing process into the creation of a false joint, to the point where even the ends of the bone are covered with cartilage, the nonunion site is encapsulated, and synovial fluid is present).

Treatment of a nonunion depends on the type. In atro-

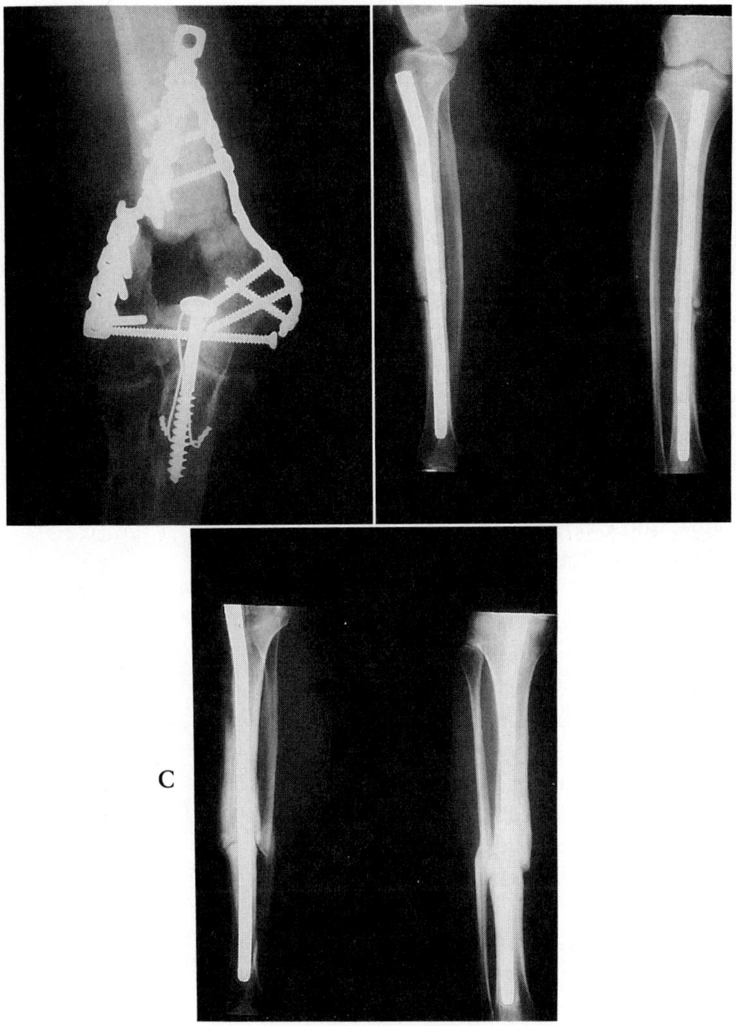

A B C

FIGURE 19-11 A, Atrophic nonunion. Callus (new bone) formation is nearly absent, and bone ends at the fracture site are tapered. **B,** Oligotrophic nonunion. Callus formation is more evident, but the fracture line persists. **C,** Hypertrophic nonunion. Callus formation is extensive, and a large fracture gap is present. This nonunion is also a synovial pseudarthrosis because the nonunion site actually became a false joint. A type of cartilage forms on the ends of the bones, and a synovial fluid is present in the fracture site.

phic nonunion, because the problem is one of poor biology, something must be done to restimulate the fracture to heal. In these cases bone graft must be used to promote the union, and often internal fixation is used as well. In oligotrophic nonunion, the fracture is relatively stable and simply needs additional biologic stimulation (i.e., bone graft or bone morphogenic protein). In hypertrophic nonunion, considerable biologic activity already is present. The body wants to heal this fracture, it simply needs a stable environment to do so. In these cases internal fixation generally is all that is required; once the fracture has been stabilized adequately, it will unite.

There is considerable controversy over whether electrical stimulation should be used to achieve fracture failed to unite, it has not as a result of a process that is union. It is probably best used for oligotrophic nonunion, which needs help in the form of more biologic activity. Electrical stimulation basically promotes calcification of the callus, thereby adding stability at the fracture site. It does not work for gap nonunions (i.e., when the bone ends are more than 1 cm apart), nor does it work for hypertrophic nonunions manifesting a synovial pseudoarthrosis. A major drawback with electrical stimulation is that malalignment is not corrected. Because an oligotrophic nonunion rarely is perfectly aligned, it is most unusual for us to use electrical stimulation to achieve union. We prefer surgical approaches, which improve both biologic activity and alignment.

Infected Nonunion

Infected nonunion presents a most difficult situation for the orthopedic surgeon. Not only has the fracture failed to unite, it has not as a result of a process that is difficult to eradicate. Bone is poorly vascularized tissue, and once it becomes infected, it has a tendency to stay infected. This poor vascularity also presents a challenge in delivering antibiotics to the infection site. Treatment of an infected nonunion basically follows the same lines as that for open fractures. The five treatment basics are (1) irrigation and debridement, with elimination of dead tissue and dead space; (2) soft tissue coverage; (3) bone and wound stabilization; (4) antibiotics; and (5) bony reconstruction.

The first two steps are an effort to obtain a noninfected, closed wound. The first and most important step is radical debridement of all devitalized and infected tissues. This must be done before any infection can be eradicated. It may mean resecting a considerable amount of skin, soft tissue, and bone, and internal fixation devices usually must be removed to allow adequate debridement.

The second step is soft tissue coverage. This often requires use of lôcal tissue transfers, such as a gastrocnemius or soleus muscle transfer in the case of an infected tibia fracture. For more distal fractures, such as in the distal one third of the tibia, this may mean use of a free tissue transfer (i.e., a free rectus or latissimus muscle). This tissue transfer accomplishes three things: It fills dead space; provides a soft tissue envelope; and brings in a new blood supply, through which the needed antibiotics can be delivered.

The third step is bone and wound stabilization. Just as with an open fracture, we feel it is important to stabilize the wound and the bone with some form of internal or external fixation device. Generally this is done with an external fixation device, but occasionally plates are used. Intramedullary rods are rarely used, because rods do not gain the solid fixation possible with an external fixation device and plates. Also, we are hesitant to risk spreading a localized bone infection up and down the entire medullary canal.

The fourth step is antibiotic treatment. These drugs generally are culture-specific antibiotics, and in our cases they usually are administered under the guidance of an infectious disease specialist. Antibiotics generally are necessary for 6 weeks, and we try to gain long-term venous access, usually with a Hickman catheter. Occasionally we use antibiotic-impregnated beads (beads made by adding antibiotic powder to bone cement) to fill the dead space and deliver a high local concentration of antibiotic.

Once a closed, noninfected wound has been achieved, we feel it is safe to begin the fifth step, bony reconstruction. Sometimes this is simple and has already been accomplished at the time of the initial debridement (i.e., if minimal bone is resected, we can often gain direct apposition of the bone ends). If a large amount of bone has been lost, bone grafting can be done to fill this gap, or a newer technique, called bone transportation, can be used. With this technique an osteotomy is made above the gap, and a segment of bone is actually transported slowly (1 mm/day) through the soft tissues to fill the gap. This slow process regenerates bone behind the transported segment. We rarely use this technique, because we have found that bone grafting at the fracture site is an adequate means of filling in gaps and gaining union.

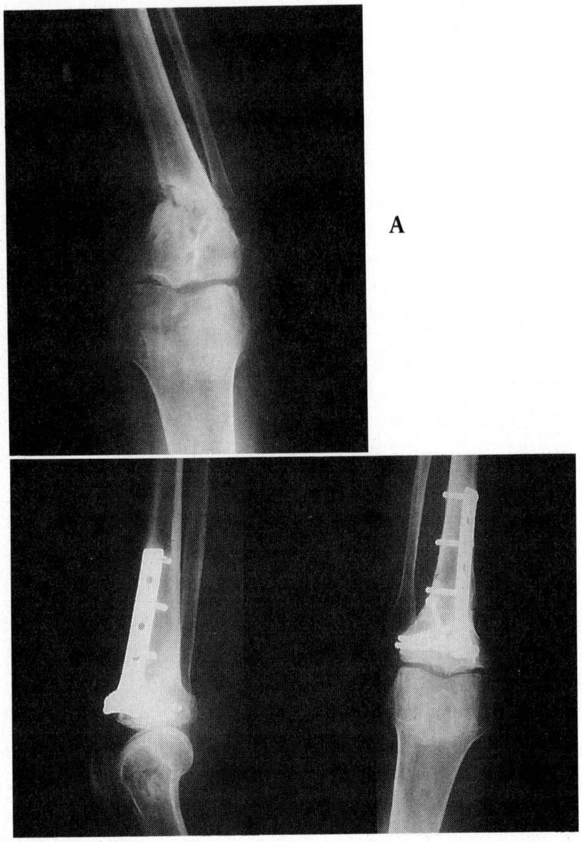
A

B

FIGURE 19-12 **A,** Malunion of a proximal tibia fracture. Varus deformity is severe. This 65-year-old woman, a snow skier, was obviously unable to walk normally. **B,** After corrective osteotomy, the alignment is normal. The patient can walk normally but did not return to skiing.

Our goal for infected nonunion is to have the fracture united within 6 months of the time we begin to tackle the nonunion problem. To date we have been universally successful in treating infected nonunions with the protocol described above.

Malunion

Malunion is a fracture that has healed in a nonanatomic fashion and that causes the patient functional problems. Malunion can be the result of angulation, rotation, or length inequality, which can be caused by loss of position or incorrect reduction (which is rare). Incorrect reduction is more common with intramedullary nailing in which the reduction is not visualized directly but with an image intensifier. Sometimes with considerable bone loss it is impossible to determine the correct length of the extremity and to judge the correct rotation. Generally these problems are not reconstructed until long after the injury, because they often take considerable time to become a problem for the patient. This is partly due to the fact that the patient may not resume normal activities for almost a year after injury.

Malunions can be treated only with surgery, which requires either recreation of the original fracture or a corrective osteotomy (Figure 19-12). Often the deformity is in two or three planes (e.g., angulation in the frontal, lateral, and rotational plane). To correct these problems, a considerable amount of planning is necessary before surgery to ensure that the abnormalities can be corrected and that length can be maintained or corrected if necessary. Osteotomies generally are stabilized, for two reasons: first, to hold the correction that was so painstakingly undertaken and second, to allow the limb to be functionally rehabilitated while healing. The appliances used generally are plates and screws, because these give the most anatomic result. However, for rotational osteotomies, we often use intramedullary nails.

Removal of Hardware

A commonly asked question about internal fixation is, "Should the plate (or rod) be removed, and if so, when?" Before this question can be answered, we must see what the device, the bone, and the patient are doing. Once a fracture has united and the bone has remodeled, the internal fixation does nothing useful for the bone. In fact, it has some negative attributes. It changes the stresses the bone experiences (this is especially true of large plates). Bone reacts to the stresses to which it is subjected, and plates (and, to a lesser degree, rods) shield the bone from normal stresses. Therefore, a plated bone never returns to normal strength until after the hardware is removed. Since the plated segment of bone is relatively stiff compared to normal bone, stresses tend to concentrate at the ends of plates. These stress risers, as they are called, place the bone at higher risk of refracture than normal bone. This risk is higher with rotational injuries. Both these effects are best seen in the shaft portion of weight-bearing bones. Is this reason enough to remove plates and rods? In young, active patients, we feel that all internal fixation devices (rods, plates, and screws) should be removed from the shafts of the femur and tibia. In the upper extremity there is much less concern, because the plates are smaller, the stresses are less, and upper extremity fractures usually are not caused by rotational forces. In fact, in the upper extremity, the risk of refracture is higher after the plates are removed than if they are left in. As a result, we do not recommend routine removal of hardware from upper extremity fractures.

Another indication for hardware removal is pain. This can be the obvious irritation of a tendon passing over a wrist plate or a prominent screw head in the medial malleolus of the ankle, or the very subtle "ache" or stiffness caused by a large screw near a joint. In both such cases patients note an immediate difference when the hardware is removed. In fact, almost all patients are subjectively improved after hardware removal.

Finally, some say hardware should be removed because it may be carcinogenic. Although this has not been proven with internal fixation, stainless steel (by far the most common implant material) contains nickel and chromium, both known carcinogens. This argument for hardware removal is the least pressing, in our opinion.

Why don't we routinely remove hardware in everyone? Because the theoretical risks of fracture and tumor are far outweighed by the very real risks of anesthesia and the complications of removing the implant, including hematoma, infection, nerve damage, and refracture after the implant is removed. The first three are probably due to local scar tissue, which bleeds more and obscures the anatomy. Hardware removal is a very underrated surgery that we do not take lightly. The above considerations are discussed with the patient, who must make the final decision, because hardware removal is not mandatory.

REHABILITATION PHASE

The rehabilitation phase runs concurrently with the reconstructive phase, but we have separated these two phases to illustrate the thought processes of the orthopedist while reconstructing and rehabilitating a patient with multiple injuries. The early rehabilitation phase coincides with the early reconstruction phase and generally is begun during the initial hospitalization. During this time we attempt to achieve two major goals: mobilization and motion. The later portion of the rehabilitation phase generally starts after the patient has left the hospital, and it may last for many years. In the words of baseball great Yogi Berra, "It ain't over until it's over." The late phase continues until the patient and surgeon are satisfied with the final result, which should be union in functional position and a maximally rehabilitated patient.

Our initial goal for a patient with multiple injuries is to achieve the upright head/upright chest position. We feel that this is most important for pulmonary function. The next step is to mobilize these patients out of bed early. We feel it is important for the patient to be mobilized out of bed as early as possible, because this is good for the patient physiologically and psychologically. The orthopedic surgeon should ask the general surgeon, "Where do you want your patient tomorrow?" If the general surgeon wants the patient to be out of bed the next day, it is incumbent upon the orthopedic surgeon to stabilize all fractures necessary to accomplish this goal. A variety of different methods can be used to get the patient out of bed. One is pure muscle power, having the nurses elevate the patient into a chair. Some chairs fold flat like a stretcher; the patient is slid onto the chair, and it is changed to an upright position. Special beds in the intensive care unit can convert directly into a chair position.

A guiding principle of surgical fracture care is "motion is life and life is motion." It is of paramount importance in patients who have undergone internal fixation to have the extremity put into motion. It is especially important to begin early motion in open reduction and internal fixation cases, because reducing and fixing these fractures causes additional trauma to the musculature. This is especially important for articular and periarticular fractures, because these tend to stiffen rapidly if they are not mobilized early. This is because the joint capsule and ligaments will contract and become stiff long before the fracture ever unites. If one waits until the fracture is united to begin motion, the joint will be hopelessly stiffened. Occasionally fixation must be augmented with external support, such as a cast, to allow enough overall stability to hold the reduction. If this is the case, we try to make the cast removable so that the extremity can come out of it periodically for exercise, or we place a hinge in the cast so the joint can remain mobile. An extremity that has been surgically stabilized and then casted without motion has been subjected to the worst of all worlds: stiffness and atrophy resulting from muscle disuse because of the cast, *and* surgical stabilization, with its attendant risks.

Physical therapists play a large role in the mobilization and motion plan. We believe in a vigorous, hands-on physical therapy program in which the therapist does a considerable amount of passive motion of the extremity and then, as the patient can tolerate it, more active exercises. The therapist also is most helpful in mobilizing patients, especially in getting them to the standing and walking positions. We use continuous passive motion machines (CPMs), which automatically move the joint through a predetermined range of motion. At first blush it seems as though the patients would find these uncomfortable; however, the patients tolerate them extremely well. Machines are available that can passively range the hip, knee, ankle, shoulder, elbow, wrist, and fingers. These treatments (continuous passive motion machines and manual physical therapy) are begun as soon as possible. In some cases a continuous passive motion machine is used even while the patient is in the recovery room. When the patient is ready, a walking program is started with a walker or crutches. During this phase we find the physical therapists extremely helpful, because they are quite adept at teaching gait training.

Occupational therapists are particularly helpful with two types of treatment. One is rehabilitating hand and wrist injuries, because occupational therapists are best at dealing with the complexities of these specialized injuries. The second is teaching patients adaptive skills for the activities of daily living. This may range from teaching patients something as simple as using an adaptive device to put on socks, to teaching them new ways to fix a full meal.

Psychiatric Rehabilitation

In our dealings with patients with multiple injuries, especially those with multiple orthopedic injuries, we have found that trauma often is a symptom of an underlying disease, such as alcoholism. These patients often have a life-style that tends to lead to accidents. When we lecture, people always are concerned that they will be our next patient. Obviously, a student sitting at home reading this chapter is at dramatically less risk of becoming one of our patients than a drunk young man speeding down the highway on his motorcycle at 2 AM. Such patients do not tolerate immobility, nor do they tolerate authority figures, such as surgeons and other medical personnel, dictating to them what they need to do. With these patients we find it helpful to have a psychiatrist or psychologist see them and help us with their care. This often also helps us deal with their real or perceived need for pain medication.

We have an unwritten rule on our orthopedic trauma service that patients with two or more fractures should see a psychologist or psychiatrist. This is obviously necessary for patients with underlying alcoholism or self-abusive personalities. A normal, healthy individual with two or more fractures often is devastated by these injuries. One minute he is a normal, healthy person; the next, he is severely impaired, sometimes for life. Patients with multiple fractures or multiple injuries need professional counseling to help them through this traumatic situation. It is actually in these formerly "normal" people that working with a psychologist has been most beneficial. Imagine if you, as the reader of this book, suddenly had both a broken arm and a broken leg. You would need someone to wait on you hand and foot. This would be a very difficult station in life to assume, and you probably would need a professional to help you work through it.

Nutrition

We consider nutrition important to the rehabilitation of patients with multiple injuries. Their bodies have lost a considerable amount of lean muscle mass in an effort to recover from the injuries. In addition, the muscles have become deconditioned. Thus not only have these patients lost lean body mass, the remaining deconditioned lean body mass does not mobilize them as well. This is especially true for older patients, who are not able to regenerate this lost muscle mass as easily as younger patients. We feel that the nutritional rehabilitation phase should start very early on, either with parenteral nutrition or use of feeding tubes. After the patient is eating, we encourage a high protein intake. In overweight patients we do not encourage any weight loss, because these patients continue to lose lean body mass, not adipose tissue. Once their fractures have healed and they have reestablished their lean body mass, we encourage them to lose excess adipose tissue.

Late Rehabilitation Phase

The early rehabilitation phase consists of in-hospital therapy to work on range of motion of the joints and mobilizing the patient into ambulatory status. These are the goals for approximately the first 6 weeks. After 6 weeks the fractures generally are sufficiently united to allow the patient to begin some strength training and, depending on the type of fracture and fixation, to begin weight bearing. We feel that weight bearing is good physiologically, and that once weight bearing is begun, range of motion in the lower extremity improves dramatically and swelling diminishes. Once weight bearing is begun and these muscles begin contracting, especially in the foot and calf, edema fluid is pumped out of the lower extremity.

Generally, sometime between the 6-week and 16-week mark, weight bearing is advanced such that by 16 weeks the patient is full weight bearing or well on the way to full weight bearing. During this time intensive gait training is carried out so that the patient does not limp. As patients advance with weight bearing, they advance from the walker or crutches to a single crutch. This happens when a patient is 60% to 70% weight bearing on the affected extremity. Later the patient goes on to a cane, and then to no support. In the upper extremity, more and more vigorous strengthening exercises are carried out as the fracture union takes place, usually over a similar time frame.

Over the long term, patients are put in a conditioning program to try to increase muscle mass. In severe fractures the muscle mass on the affected side may never quite equal the muscle mass on the uninjured side. However, the strength returns to nearly that of the unaffected side. It is not unusual for a patient to take a year or longer to recover from a devastating orthopedic injury, depending on how long it takes the fracture to unite and whether any residual deformities or neurovascular deficits occur.

The rehabilitation of a patient with multiple injuries is complex because of the severity of generalized damage, including pulmonary function, GI function, musculoskeletal function, and function of the psyche. All these must be integrated into a total rehabilitation program to enable the patient to return to a normal existence.

REFERENCES

1 Bone LB, Johnson KD, Weigelt J: Early versus delayed stabilization of femoral fractures: a prospective randomized study, *J Bone Joint Surg* 71A:336, 1989.

2 Border JR, Allgower M, Hansen ST Jr et al: *Blunt multiple trauma: comprehensive pathophysiology and care,* New York, 1990, Marcel Dekker.

3 Border JR, Hassett J, LaDuca J et al: The gut origin septic states in blunt multiple trauma (ISS = 40) in the ICU, *Ann Surg* 206(4):427, 1987.

4 Burgess AR, Eastridge BJ, Young JWR et al: Pelvic ring disruptions: effective classification system and treatment protocols, *J Trauma* 30(7):848, 1990.

5 Flint LM, Brown A, Richardson JD et al: Definitive control of bleeding from severe pelvic fractures, *Ann Surg* 189(6):709, 1979.

6 Goldstein A, Phillips T, Sclafani SJA et al: Early open reduction and internal fixation of the disrupted pelvic ring, *J Trauma* 26(4):325, 1986.

7 Goris RJA, Gimbrère JSF, van Niekerk JLM et al: Early osteosynthesis and prophylactic mechanical ventilation in the multitrauma patient, *J Trauma* 22(11):895, 1982.

8 Gustilo RB, Mendoza RM, Williams DN: Problems in the management of type III (severe) open fractures: a new classification of type III open fractures, *J Trauma* 24(8):742, 1984.

9 Gylling SF, Ward RE, Holcroft JW et al: Immediate external fixation of unstable pelvic fractures, *Am J Surg* 150:721, 1985.

10 Hawkins L, Pomerantz M, Eiseman B: Laparotomy at the time of pelvic fracture, *J Trauma* 10(8):619, 1970.

11 Huittinen V-M, Slatis P: Postmortem angiography and dissection of the hypogastric artery in pelvic fractures, *Surgery* 73(3):454, 1973.

12 Hubbard SG, Bivins BA, Sachatello CR et al: Diagnostic errors with peritoneal lavage in patients with pelvic fractures, *Arch Surg* 114:844, 1979.

13 Johansen K, Daines M, Howey T et al: Objective criteria accurately predict amputation following lower extremity trauma, *J Trauma* 30(5):568, 1990.

14 Johansen K, Lynch K, Paun M et al: Noninvasive vascular tests reliably exclude occult arterial trauma in injured extremities, *J Trauma* 31:515, 1991.

15 Johnson KD, Cadambi A, Seibert GB: Incidence of adult respiratory distress syndrome in patients with multiple musculoskeletal injuries: effect of early operative stabilization of fractures, *J Trauma* 25(5):375, 1985.

16 Lange R, Bach A, Hansen ST et al: Open tibial fractures with associated vascular injuries: prognosis of limb salvage, *J Trauma* 25:203, 1985.

17 McMurtry R, Walton D, Dickinson D et al: Pelvic disruption in the polytraumatized patient: a management protocol, *Clin Orthop* 151:22, 1980.

18 Meek RN, Vivoda EE, Pirani S: Comparison of mortality of patients with multiple injuries according to type of fracture treatment: a retrospective age- and injury-matched series, *Injury* 17(1):2, 1986.

19 Moreno C, Moore EE, Rosenberger A et al: Hemorrhage associated with major pelvic fracture: a multispecialty challenge, *J Trauma* 26(11):987, 1986.

20 Murr PC, Moore EE, Lipscomb R et al: Abdominal trauma that is associated with pelvic fracture, *J Trauma* 20(11):919, 1980.

21 Panetta T, Sclafani SJA, Goldstein AS et al: Percutaneous transcatheter embolization for massive bleeding from pelvic fractures, *J Trauma* 25(11):1021, 1985.

22 Riska EB, Myllynen P: Fat embolism in patients with multiple injuries, *J Trauma* 22(11):891, 1982.

23 Riska EB, von Bonsdorff H, Hakkinen S et al: Prevention of fat embolism by early internal fixation of fractures in patients with multiple injuries, *Injury* 8(2):110, 1976.
24 Riska EB, von Bonsdorff H, Hakkinen S et al: Primary operative fixation of long bone fractures in patients with multiple injuries, *J Trauma* 17(2):111, 1977.
25 Rüedi T, Wolff G: Vermeidung posttraumatischer Komplikationen durch frühe definitive Versorgung von Polytraumatisierten mit Frakturen des Bewegungsapparats, *Helv Chir Acta* 42:507, 1975.
26 Seibel R, LaDuca J, Hassett JM et al: Blunt multiple trauma (ISS 36), femur traction, and the pulmonary failure–septic state, *Ann Surg* 202:283, 1985.
27 Tscherne H, Gotzen L, editors: *Fractures with soft tissue injuries*, Berlin-Heidelberg, 1984, Springer-Verlag.
28 Wolff G, Dittmann M, Rüedi T et al: Koordination von Chirurgie und Intensivmedizin zur Vermeidung der posttraumatischen respiratorischen Insuffizienz, *Unfallheilkunde* 81:425, 1978.
29 Yasko AW, Lane JM, Fellinger EJ et al: The healing of segmental bone defects, induced by recombinant human bone morphogenetic protein (rhBMP-2), *J Bone Joint Surg* 74A:659, 1992.

The subjects covered in Part Three involve patients who are usually treated by specialists. Nevertheless, the patient's surgeon must be knowledgeable about these areas because the need to provide additional or different care may arise. For example, if a patient has undergone organ transplantation, the surgeon needs to understand the role immunosuppression plays in the diagnosis and management of new surgical problems. Information about our colleagues' capabilities also may bear directly on patients under our care. For example, a general surgeon caring for a trauma patient with a large soft tissue defect needs to know about the kinds of reconstruction his colleagues in plastic surgery have developed and can provide. Furthermore, in some geographic areas, lack of specialists or prohibitive distances may force a general surgeon to provide surgical care usually offered by the pediatric, plastic, or transplant surgeon. Therefore, although these three areas are separate specialties, they are closely associated with general surgery.

PART THREE

SPECIAL AREAS

CHAPTER

20

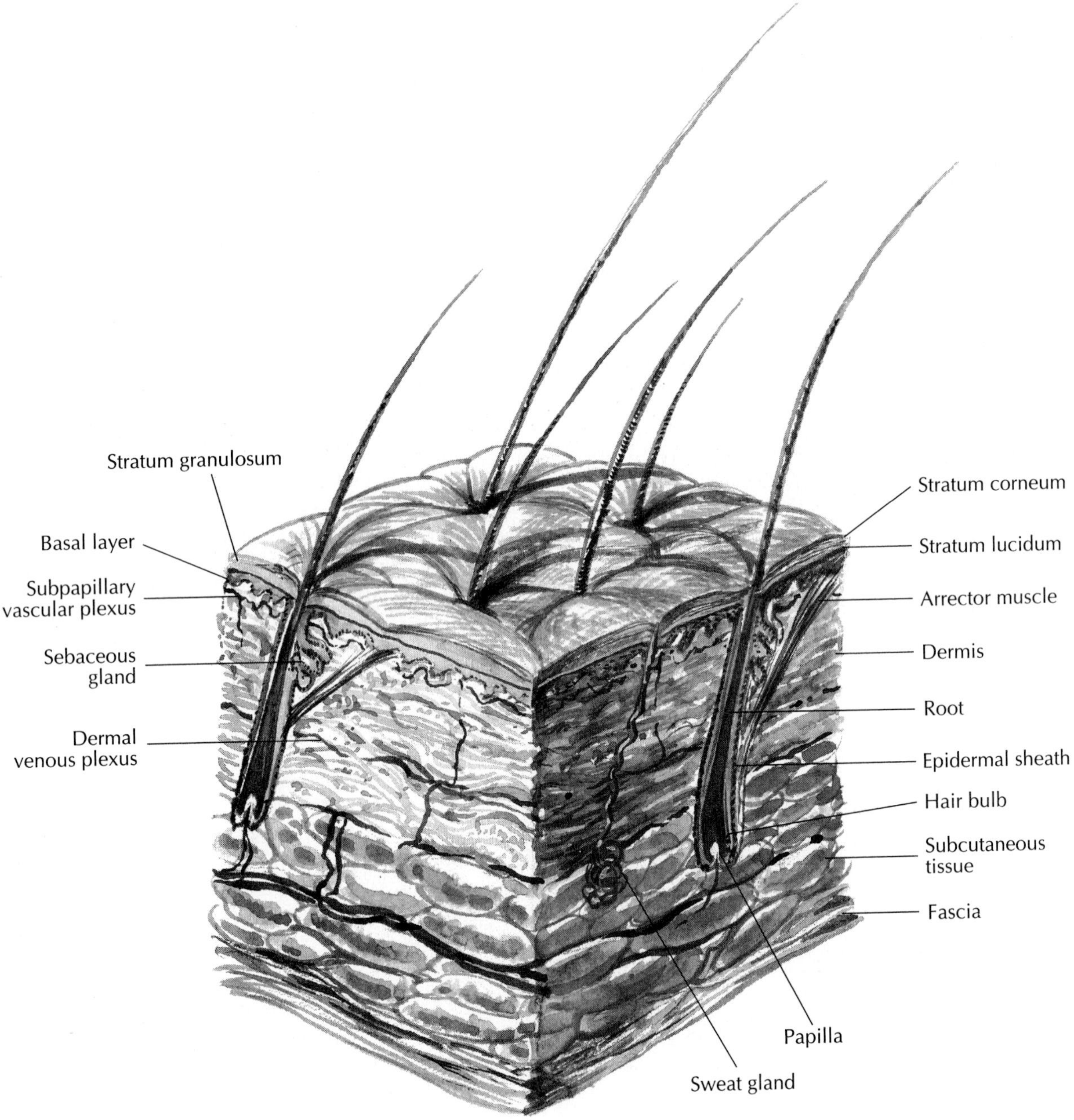

Stratum granulosum
Basal layer
Subpapillary vascular plexus
Sebaceous gland
Dermal venous plexus
Stratum corneum
Stratum lucidum
Arrector muscle
Dermis
Root
Epidermal sheath
Hair bulb
Subcutaneous tissue
Fascia
Papilla
Sweat gland

SKIN AND SOFT TISSUE

Thomas J. Krizek • Roger S. Foster Jr.

RELATED MATERIAL APPEARS IN CHAPTERS 10, 11, and 12

The skin is the largest organ, by size, in the body and second only to muscle in weight. It is the most visible part of us. On occasion blemishes may be "beauty marks" and serve to set us off in a special and attractive way. More often blemishes are matters of at least esthetic and psychologic concern and at worst serious and life-threatening concern.

A *tumor* is defined as any mass of cells that lacks apparently useful function. Particularly for skin and soft tissues, many of these tumors are no more than developmental or acquired cysts. These tumors include birthmarks and other congenital abnormalities, some with no implication other than an unsightly appearance and the distortion of tissue and spirit; others may have real possibilities of becoming malignant and destructive. Tumors of the skin and soft tissues are not respectors of age, sex, race, or even life-style. None of us is immune, and the person without a mole, lump, or bump or two (or more) is most unusual indeed.

Tumors of the skin and soft tissue can arise from any of the various structures that constitute skin: epidermis, dermis, adnexae, its pigment cells, its neurovascular supporting structure, or the mesodermal derived soft tissues that support it. Tumors of the skin and soft tissue are the most common cancers, and more than 600,000 new cases of epidermal carcinomas, 32,000 malignant melanomas, and 5000 soft tissue sarcomas are expected each year.[98,103] Approximately 1 in 80 persons can be expected to require treatment each year, and this may be a low estimate, because these are only cases reported to hospitals and various tumor registries. This figure also does not include benign lesions, which are far more frequent.

Skin and soft tissue tumors are among the most interesting of tumors. More than 200 years ago Sir Percivall Pott noted the apparent induction of cancer in the scrotal area by the repeated exposure to soot, an occupational hazard of chimney sweeps. In the early 1800s Marjolin noted that cancer arose in ulcerated areas, which failed to heal or, when apparently healed, were subject to repeated breakdown from trauma. Shortly after Roentgen's discovery of X rays, the first accidental injuries were followed by the tumor induction from ionizing radiation. Epidemiologic studies confirmed the importance of solar (ultraviolet) radiation in the induction of many forms of skin cancer. The importance of the immune system in these tumors, suspected in many different patient groups, has now been confirmed in the special situations of iatrogenic suppression for purposes of transplantation and of spontaneous suppression in acquired immune deficiency syndrome (AIDS). Thus skin cancers have helped in the identification of chemical agents, traumatic wounds, radiation, and immunodeficiency as predisposing and causative factors in cancer. These observations also form a basis for preventive medicine, and in these problems, more than most, alteration in patient behavior can influence the course and outcome of the disease process.

Certainly the variety of possible tumors in the skin and its contents would defy the efforts of even the most dedicated taxonomist. Presentation of the totality of possibilities would be both exhaustive and exhausting. I have chosen instead to present, as problem situations, clinical situations that the surgeon who treats skin and soft tissue problems might most likely encounter and to include many related problems as part of the differential diagnosis and management concerns. Although this chapter discusses in detail less than 10% of possible skin and soft tissue tumors, it covers more than 99.9% of the problems that surgeons are likely to encounter. The summary table at the end of the chapter provides information on the less common forms.

EMBRYOLOGY

The skin is composed of epidermis, dermis, and an underlying subcutaneous padding; all structures involved are derived from either ectoderm or mesoderm. The epidermis is composed of four different types of cells. The keratinocytes, the most common, are derived from ectoderm. The second most common, the melanocytes, are derived from the neural crest and, like other neural crest–origin tissue, do not readily repopulate themselves. Loss of melanocytes tends to lead to permanent lack of pigmentation in the involved area. The third most common cells, the Langerhans' cells, arise from mesenchymal cells, probably the bone marrow. The least common cell, Merkel's cells, are neural cells that also probably arise from the neural crest. They too will not regenerate.

The supporting dermis, with the exception of the neural supply, is entirely of mesodermal origin with its combination of fibroblasts and vascular supporting structures. Finally, all the soft tissue structures are of mesodermal origin. Malignant tumors of the skin, of ectodermal origin, are usually called *carcinomas;* tumors of the dermis and subcutaneous tissues, of mesodermal origin, are called *sarcomas.*

Much of the primitive embryologic development occurs during the first few weeks of gestation; the complex specialized organs, such as hair follicles and nails, are not completely developed until later; even so, the fetal fingernail in the fifth month is much like that of an adult. The fetal skin is also innervated early, and sensory fibers are identifiable in the dermis by the fifth week.

Some of the premalignant conditions are genetic and developmental. In xeroderma pigmentosa, for instance, the melanocytes are functionally normal but are unable to transfer the pigment to the keratinocytes, and extraordinary sensitivity to ultraviolet radiation is seen.

ANATOMY

Skin

What makes us pretty, much less beautiful, is hard to define; histologically, stratified squamous epithelium covers the movie star as well as the misfit. Wide variations occur in thickness of the skin, from less than 0.05 mm on the eyelids to more than 1.5 mm on the soles of the feet. The skin of the back is much thicker than the skin of the face. Almost all the difference is in the thickness of the dermis rather than the epidermis.

Dermis

The skin is composed of epidermis and dermis (Figure 20-1). The less sophisticated dermis is composed mostly of collagen, which accounts for about 70% of its weight and most of its function—the support of the epidermis.[46] A number of different types of collagen exist. Types I and III are found in the skin; type II is in cartilage. Most skin collagen is type I (80%) and forms the dense network of the deeper portion, the reticular dermis; type III accounts for about 15%, is found in the basement membrane area, and may serve to "anchor" the epidermis onto the dermis. The upper portion of the dermis, between the papillary ridges of epidermis, is the papillary

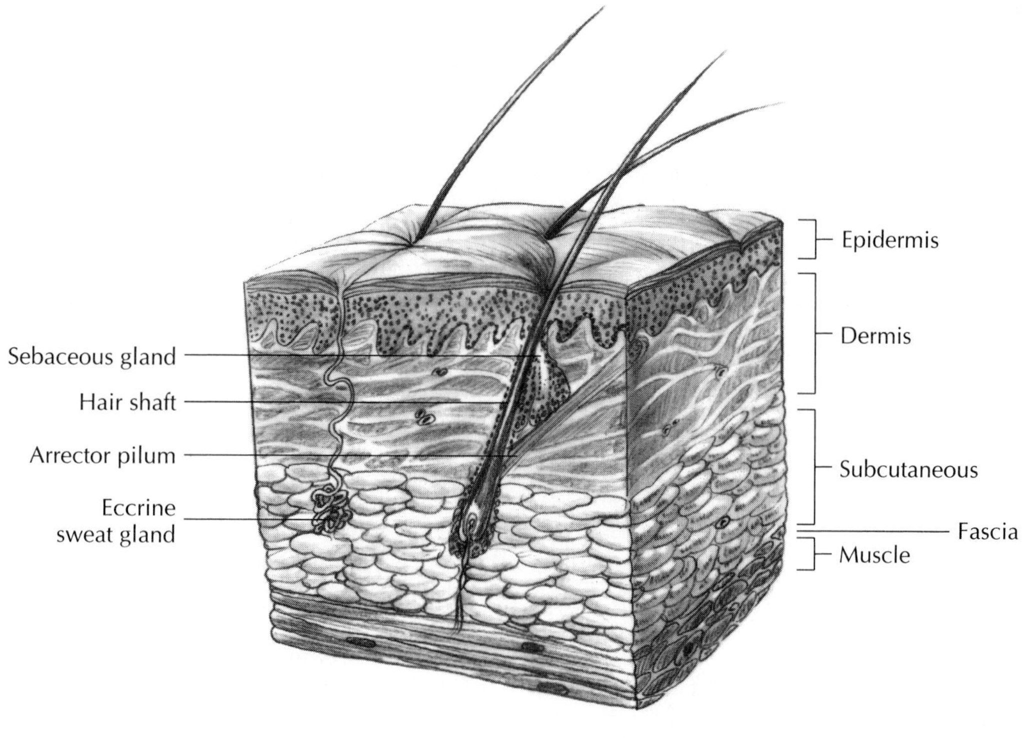

FIGURE 20-1 Epidermis, dermis, and subcutaneous tissue.

dermis; the deeper portion is the reticular dermis. The dermis also contains elastic fibers, which make up less than 1% of its weight but a profound share of its ability to resist deformation and return the skin back to its original position. Finally, the fibers are suspended in a ground substance matrix of mucopolysaccharides, which glue it all together. The nerve and vascular supply to the epidermis courses throughout the dermis; from the epidermis, invaginating down into the dermis, are the hair follicles and glands. Compared with the epidermis, this is primitive material.

Epidermis

The epidermis is among the body's most complex organs. It is critical to life and well-being and yet is so specialized that, when injured or removed, it is not easily replaced. Even its own healing processes leave but a second-rate substitute, a scar. The epidermis contains four cell types.

KERATINOCYTES. The keratinocyte is a basic cell, originating in the basal cell layer or the lining of follicles and glands. Keratinocytes have the capacity to form the cornified, or outer, dead layer of the body, which is our major protection against the world. As they move to the surface, the cells move through basal, spinous, granular, and finally cornified layers. The basal layer cells are almost cuboidal; the spinous layer cells (desmosomes) have intercellular "spines," almost as though they were joining; and the granular layer cells have granules. As the cells reach the surface, the nuclei are gone and the cytoplasm is filled with sulfhydryl-rich filaments; these components are all encased in an insoluble plasma membrane. As the keratinocytes move to the surface, they pick up pigment from the melanocytes, also a major form of protection.

MELANOCYTES. The melanocytes are derived from the neural crest and have as their prime function the production of pigment, which is then transferred to keratinocytes. The melanocytes are found just beneath and intimately attached to the basal cell layer of the epidermis, as well as in the hair follicles, retina, uveal tract, and leptomeninges. Thus some of the pigmented lesions of infancy have connections or are in continuity with skin and meninges. The melanocyte is pale with hematoxylin and eosin stain and black with silver stains, which outline the pigment in the melanosome and also identify the dendritic connection between melanocytes and keratinocytes. Usually melanocytes and keratinocytes are present in a ratio of 1:4 in exposed areas, with as few as 1 melanocyte per 20 to 30 keratinocytes in hidden areas.

Because melanocytes are of neural crest origin, they do not reproduce. When melanocytes have been surgically removed, such as at skin graft donor sites or partial-thickness burn areas, the area may be permanently lighter in color.

LANGERHANS' CELLS. Langerhans' cells are found in the middle of the epidermis and like melanocytes possess dendrites. They are thought to originate from the mesenchyme and function in the immune process. Langerhans' cells possess cell surface antigens and membrane receptors and are thought to play a critical role in recognizing antigens and in interactions with T lymphocytes.

MERKEL'S CELLS. Merkel's cells, also of neural origin, are found at the base of the papillary ridges and look much like melanocytes. They are found particularly on the volar aspect of digits, nail beds, and genitals and have a specialized function in perceiving light touch.

Sensory Cells

The nerves to the skin relay a complex variety of sensibilities (Figure 20-2). Light touch is relayed through Merkel's cells and through the small, branched, shrub-like structures called *Meissner's corpuscles* found in the dermal projections into epidermis between papillary ridges. Not surprisingly, these corpuscles are most concentrated on fingertips. Pressure, a more gross sensation, is transmitted via Pacini's corpuscles found deep in the tissues, even in the subcutaneous tissue. Pain is transmitted through naked nerve endings insinuated between basal cells. Other fibers terminate around follicles and provide sensations such as cold (Krause's end-bulbs), heat, and proprioception. The skin also contains autonomic fibers associated with hair follicles (hair erector muscles), with glands, and with modulate sensations such as "goose bumps," "cold sweat," and the clear watery outflow of the axillary apocrine glands when a person is nervous.

Glands

The skin has three specialized glands with slightly different functions (see Figure 20-1).

Eccrine glands secrete and are referred to as *sweat glands*. Found over the entire body surface, they are in the greatest concentration on the palms of the hand, soles of the feet, and forehead. The hypotonic solution secreted is evaporated on the surface and cools the skin. Anatomically, these glands appear as coiled tubes, which empty directly onto the skin through pores.

Holocrine glands, typified by the sebaceous glands, are found over the entire surface of the skin except the palms of the hands and soles of the feet. Their oily product, sebum, is a function of cell disintegration and is discharged, usually into a hair follicle.

Apocrine glands are found predominantly in the axilla but also the perineum, areola, scrotum, and external ear canal, where they produce cerumen. Their product is discharged into their ducts and then episodically to the surface. The mechanism is by secretion, but because some of the cell also seems to get "pinched off," the mechanism can also be disintegration, as in a holocrine

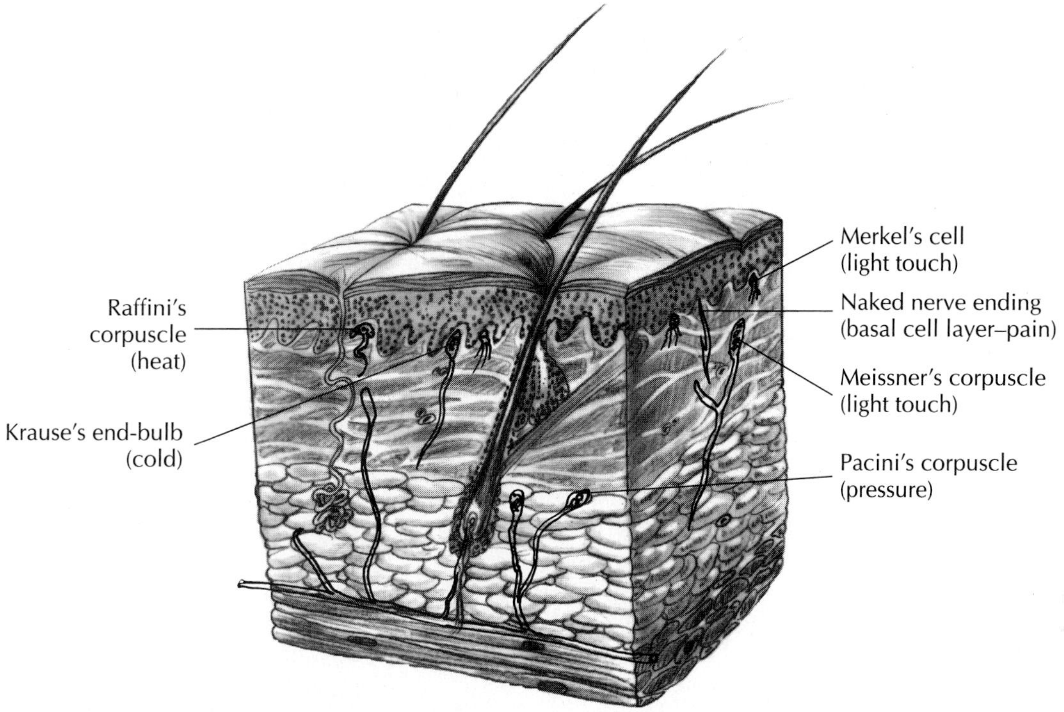

FIGURE 20-2 Nerve supply. A varied and exquisite sensory supply for pain (naked nerve endings in the basal cell layer), light touch in the papillary dermis (Merkel's cells, Meissner's corpuscles), cold (Krause's end-bulbs), heat (Raffini's corpuscles), "goose flesh" (hair erector muscles), "cold sweats" (autonomic to sweat glands), and pressure (Pacini's corpuscles).

gland. Apocrine glands are important sexual glands in other species, and the secretions have the specific identifying and attracting odor.

Hair Follicles

Hair follicles are common to all humans and are distributed over the entire body, except the palms of the hands and soles of the feet. Orientals are the least hairy people and have vertically oriented straight follicles, which lead to straight hair. Blacks have curved follicles, often almost parallel to the skin surface in places, a spiral and therefore curly hair is produced. Whites have combinations of the above and are the hairiest. The hairs, with the exception of the eyebrows and lashes, are related to sex hormones, which accounts for gender differences in facial, pubic, and other body hair.

Adipose Tissue

Fat is derived from mesenchyme and forms the padding on which the skin rests. The mature adipocytes are separated into small compartments called *lobules,* which are located between trabeculae, or partitions, running between the underlying fascia and the overlying skin. This anatomic fact has been of inestimable value to reconstructive surgeons from two perspectives. First, the blood supply to the skin arrives almost entirely from vertically oriented vessels reaching up to the surface. Wide undermining of tissue either by accident or surgically tends to divide the blood supply. Conversely, preservation of this vascularity often enables the surgeon to move large amounts of tissue, including subcutaneous fat and the overlying skin, using the underlying fascia or muscle as a vascular carrier. Similarly, the techniques of suctioning adipose tissue, either to remove tumors or to improve body contour, rely on the vertical trabeculae to preserve the blood supply after the fat has been removed from the compartments.

ROLE OF PHOTOGRAPHY

At the first visit it is important to obtain good photographs. In complicated cases—for instance, when multiple nevi are present—accurate photographs are invaluable for evaluating and documenting perceived changes in the character of individual lesions. The medicolegal value of the accurate photographic documentation of any preoperative and postoperative condition is evident, particularly with conditions that are highly visible and later subject to variations in memory among those involved. Finally, photographs of other patients may be of great value for sharing with the parents and patients examples of the natural history of the disease.

The equipment need not be complicated. An inexpensive 35 mm camera can provide a lasting detailed record. An instant camera can provide an immediate record for the patient's chart. Finally, the hospital photographer is available for elective problems and for hospital records.

PIGMENTED LESIONS

PROBLEM: BENIGN NEVI

Nevocellular nevi are what most people call moles. See the box at right for a listing of types of pigmented lesions.

Clinical Presentation

The patient and family usually cannot state the time nevi appear and rarely notice much change in size. Nevi rarely exceed 3 to 4 mm in diameter. Multiple studies have been done on the incidence of intradermal nevi. The most accurate peak prevalence described was 43 nevi per person for men and 27 for women during the second and third decades of life. As patients age, the nevi seem to disappear spontaneously, and the number of nevi found in elderly patients is relatively small.[100] An average of 15 nevi per adult is probably reasonably accurate.

Pathophysiology

Nevi are derived from nevus cells and are found in cells located entirely in the dermis (intradermal nevi), in the junction between the dermis and the epidermis (junctional nevi), or in both places (compound nevi) (Figure 20-3). The origin of nevus cells is not entirely clear; the

PIGMENTED LESIONS

A. Benign nevi
   1. Intradermal
   2. Compound
   3. Junctional
   4. Letigines
   5. Blue nevus
   6. Nevus of Ota
   7. Nevus of Ito
   8. Mongolian spots
   9. Becker's nevus
   10. Halo nevus
   11. Juvenile nevus (juvenile melanoma)
B. Melanoma precursors
   1. Congenital nevus
   2. Dysplastic nevus syndrome (B-K mole syndrome)
   3. Malignant lentigo
C. Malignant melanoma
   1. Superficial spreading melanoma
   2. Nodular melanoma
   3. Malignant lentigo melanoma
   4. Acral lentiginous malignant melanoma

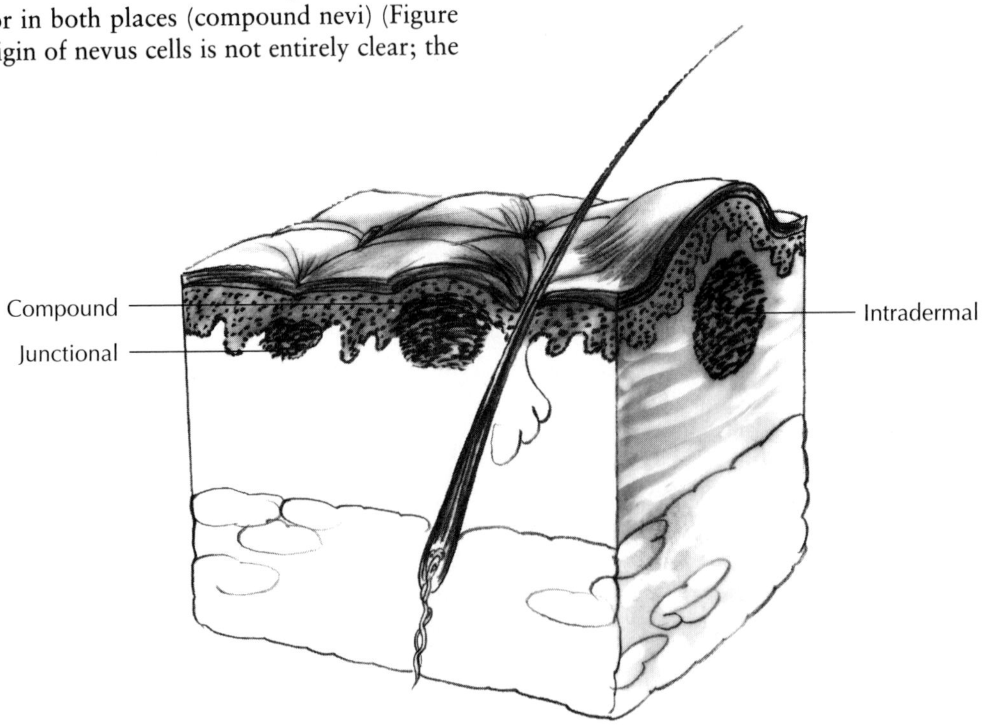

FIGURE 20-3 Comparison of junctional (dermal-epidermal), compound (junction and dermal), and entirely intradermal nevi.

more superficial probably arise in melanocytes, and the deeper cells arise from Schwann cells. Both are obviously of neural origin. Fewer than 1% of persons have any nevi visible at birth. The common differentiation of nevi into congenital and acquired may be artificial. In actuality, acquired nevi are probably present at birth but form no pigment until later, whereas congenital nevi produce pigment in utero and therefore are highly visible at birth.[100]

Classification

Junctional Nevi

Nevi are also classified as junctional, compound, or intradermal. Most of the nevi seen in childhood and adolescence are junctional nevi (Figure 20-4). Junctional nevi are fairly nondescript, small, flat lesions. They are rarely pedunculated. They tend to be smooth, rarely are deeply pigmented, and can be found anywhere on the body but primarily on the face and trunk. These are differentiated from freckles (ephelides), which represent increased activity of melanocytes, by the fact that in junctional nevi an actual mass of tissue is present as opposed to a mere discoloration. Biopsy or excision reveals a lesion with activity of nevus cells at the junction of the dermis and epidermis. The cells' activity increases into adolescence and adulthood and can result in the nevi becoming thicker and elevated.

Compound Nevi

Compound nevi clearly seem to arise from junctional nevi. Components of the junctional nevus, with activity at the dermal-epidermal junction, plus the pushing down of nevus cells into the dermis, may be present in the same lesion (Figure 20-4, *G*).

Intradermal Nevi

Finally, as adulthood approaches, the classic and most common of all nevi, intradermal nevi, are apparent, primarily on the face and the trunk. They are round and elevated from the surface and tend to be smooth because the activity and collection of the nevus cells are primarily in the dermis, pushing the epidermis over the surface of the lesion. Appearances vary widely but growth is basically centrifugal. Therefore the lesions tend to be uniformly round and the elevation increased as the intradermal elements mature. Variations include an irregular border and irregularities in pigmentation (Figure 20-4, *H, I*). They often contain hair, which helps differentiate them from malignant melanomas, which usually do not contain hair.

Natural History

The natural history of the evolution of nevi from junctional to compound to intradermal is usually completed by a change to fibrosis and disappearance in the elderly age group. The chance of nevi becoming malignant is difficult to identify accurately. The number of people who stated that they had a nevus at the site later found to be melanoma has been reported to range from 15% to 85%[90,100]; that is, from as few as one in seven to as many as six in seven patients with melanoma believe that the melanoma began in an area in which a nevus had previously been identified. The wide range in this observation exemplifies how difficult it is to know whether, in fact, such a nevus was actually present. The answer to the rest of the question is even more difficult.

If we assume that each adult in the US population has only 15 nevi at any time, there would be 2.25 billion nevi. Among this population we would expect to identify 32,000 new melanomas per year. If the incidence of melanoma arising in preexisting nevi were low, the one in seven prediction, the statistical chance of any given nevus becoming a melanoma would be one in 500,000. Even if the higher figure were used, that is six in seven melanomas arise in preexisting nevi, the odds of any given nevus becoming a melanoma would be 1 in 83,333. The odds therefore are overwhelming that any given nevus will remain permanently benign, and removal of all nevi as a prophylactic measure is a statistically implausible approach.

Certain characteristics of nevi, however, have been thought to help identify a predilection for malignancy, if not actually which nevi might lead to malignancy. The most common among these would be the congenital or giant nevus. Another characteristic of nevi that has previously been thought to predispose to malignancy is location. Such areas include the belt line, the area a bra rubs, areas other types of clothing might irritate such as shoe tops or sleeves, and other areas predisposed to injury. Unfortunately, none of this can be documented statistically, and there is no evidence that the nevi in these areas are more likely to become malignant than those in any other area. However, nevi that become more deeply pigmented or more easily irritated or bleed from repeated episodes of minor trauma should be removed for biopsy to prove they are not actually melanomas and to relieve apprehension.

Nevi surgery also may be indicated for purely esthetic reasons, again without the need to invoke possible neoplasm as a reason for the surgery. Nevi tend to undergo symptomatic changes during periods of hormonal change, particularly during adolescence and pregnancy, and perhaps during times of stress.

Management

Even though the accuracy of diagnosis is good and statistically favorable for any given lesion diagnosed as benign, all lesions that are removed should be examined microscopically. The technique of lesion removal should be determined by factors such as the esthetic appearance

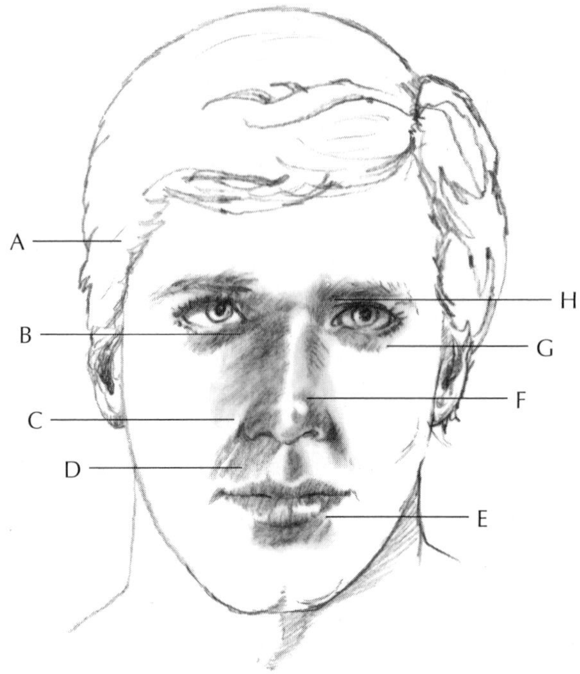

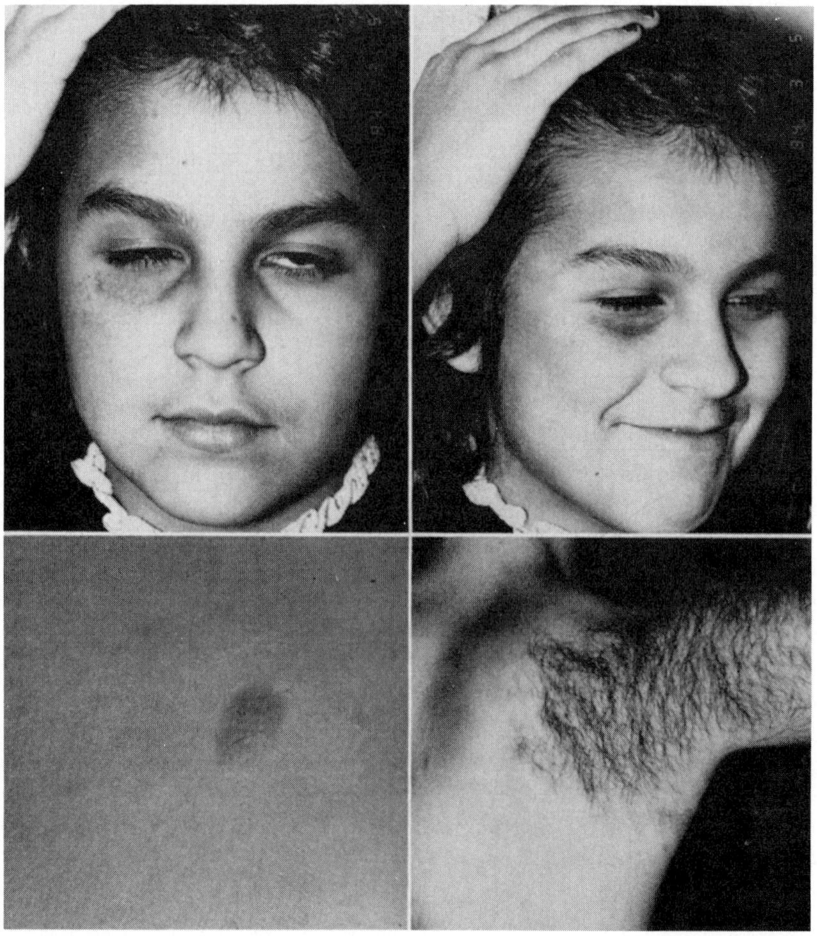

A B C D

FIGURE 20-4 Pigmented lesions. **A** and **B,** Nevus of Ota, melanocytic origin. **C,** Halo nevus with a vague, pale (depigmented) area surrounding the lesion. **D,** Becker's nevus—melanocytic hypertrophy, local hirsutism.

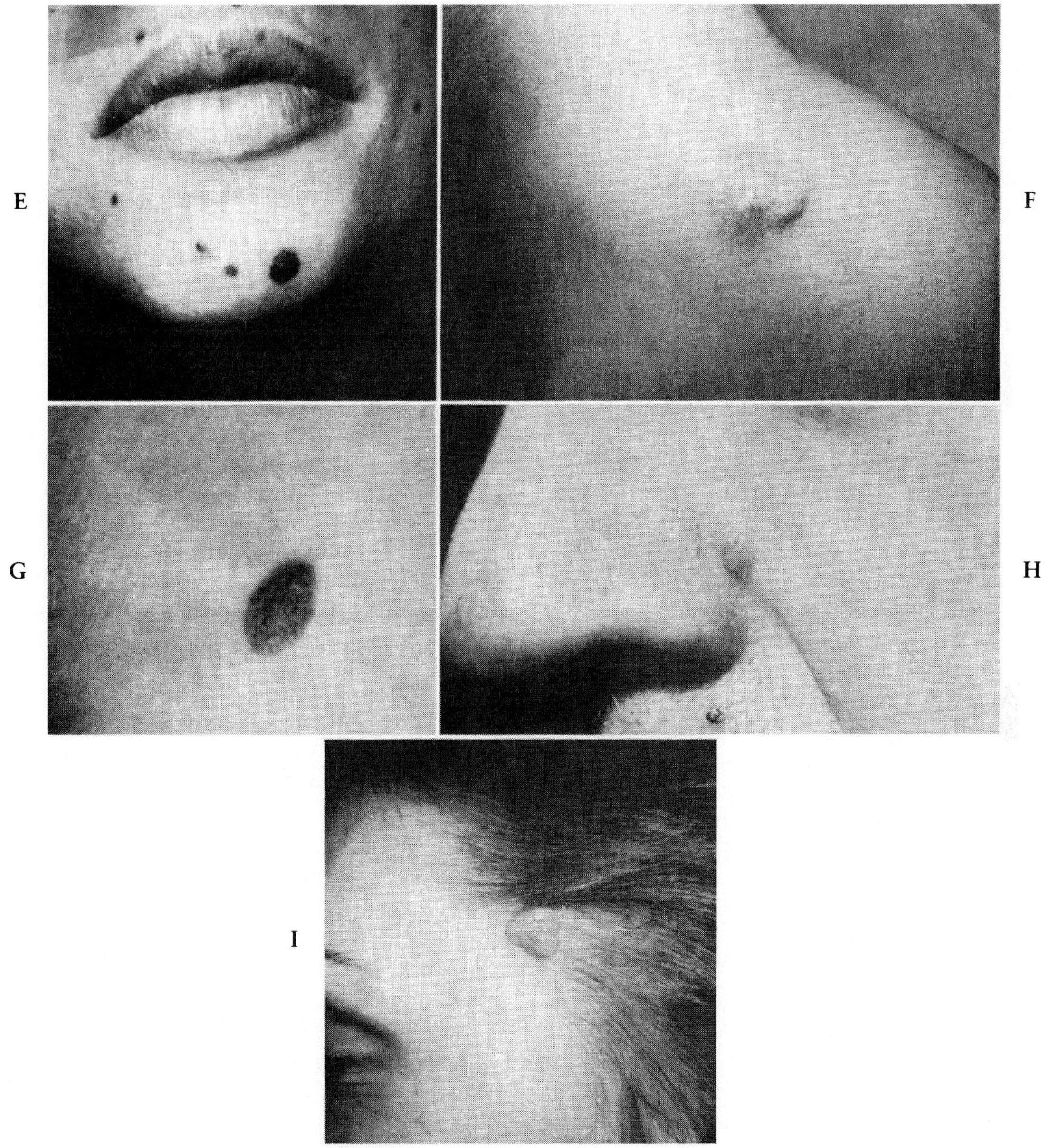

FIGURE 20-4, cont'd **E,** Multiple pigmented intradermal nevi. **F,** Blue nevus. A bluish tinge is distinctly visible in vivo. **G,** Compound nevus in an adolescent. **H,** Intradermal nevus at the nasal/cheek junction. (The lesion on the lip is a cut from shaving.) **I,** Intradermal nevus, almost seborrheic in appearance.

of the healed area, the ease of removal, the skill of the surgeon, and the individual needs of the patient. Excision with a small margin of normal-appearing tissue (1 to 2 mm) with primary closure is the standard approach.

Curetting the lesion and scraping out the base of the nevus cells by curettage and cautery are also theoretically valuable but require secondary healing. Although the healed result is often adequate, the method in some ways is more cumbersome than direct excision. Methods of cautery or other cell destruction that do not provide tissue for biopsy are not recommended. Often patients are seen with melanomas in sites where a lesion previously had been treated by electrocautery without biopsy, and the nature of the original lesion remains forever unknown.

Types

Lentigines

Lentigines are multiple small pigmented lesions that arise from melanocytes rather than new nevus cells.[65] Nevus lentigines are pigmented areas that may appear anywhere on the body, but usually in exposed areas. Although usually pale and light brown, they occasionally become more heavily pigmented, even black. If they can be identified as such, lentigines should be accepted as completely benign and require no specific treatment.

Blue Nevus

The blue nevus is characterized by its clear, blue color. In actuality, the melanin hue is normally somewhat bluish. These blue nevi arise from dermal melanocytes, are usually solitary, may be seen in infancy and early childhood, and have been seen occasionally at birth[22] (Figure 20-4, *F*). They are most frequently found in the head and neck or the dorsum of the hands. They are rarely more than 1 cm in diameter, are moderately firm, and have well-defined borders.

Nevus of Ota

The nevus of Ota is a congenital nevus found most frequently in Asians, especially the Japanese[100] (Figure 20-4, *A-B*). It occurs in the distribution of the first and second branches of the trigeminal nerve on the face, and microscopically it is noted to be a proliferation of dermal melanocytes (Figure 20-3). Almost half of these are present at birth; most others appear in the first decade. They are benign and often disappear spontaneously, although melanoma has been reported arising in a nevus of Ota. The nevus of Ito is identical but appears over the acromioclavicular area.

Mongolian Spots

Mongolian spots are flat, bluish gray or slate gray patches on the lower back and upper buttock area, most commonly found in those of Mongolian descent.[100] The historical migration of people from Mongolia across the mainland and into Korea accounts for an incidence of Mongolian spots of almost 100% in Korea; perhaps because of divergent migration patterns, the incidence among Japanese is approximately 50%. The lesion occurs also among the Chinese and has a varying incidence among blacks, but it is almost never found in whites. In most cases the lesion is present at birth, although occasionally it does not appear until shortly after birth. The most important significance of the Mongolian spot is that it be recognized for what it is. It is a totally benign, self-limited, and self-resolving condition that disappears in early childhood or before adolescence.

Under no circumstances should it be mistaken for something with the potential for malignancy, nor should it require any form of surgical treatment other than a rare confirmatory biopsy. The characteristics of the lesion and its color are somewhat similar to those of bruises, and occasionally these children are reported as being abused.

Becker's Nevus

Becker's nevus is a grayish brown area of pigmentation classically found over the shoulder girdle, anterior aspect of the chest, and scapular region, usually in young men[15] (Figure 20-4, *D*). Heavy hair growth is a characteristic but may not appear until after the pigmentation is first seen. Hyperpigmentation in the basal cell layer is seen. It is not to be confused with a giant congenital nevus. It is benign with no potential for malignancy, and treatment, if any, is for esthetic purposes.

Halo Nevus

Halo nevi are pigmented nevocellular nevi with the hallmark characteristic of a ring of depigmentation surrounding them (Figure 20-4, *C*). They are occasionally accompanied by vitiligo elsewhere in the body. These are particularly fascinating, more for their biologic traits than their clinical significance. The depigmented areas have been identified in several studies as being secondary to an inflammatory infiltrate with T lymphocytes, but without plasma cells or B lymphocytes.[22] The cytolysis of the nevus cell and antibodies against the cytoplasm of melanoma cells have been identified in cell cultures.

The halo of depigmentation seen around the halo nevus and occasionally around actual melanomas may indicate an immune rejection of altered melanocytes or of nevus cells. The halo nevus is not considered premalignant. A decision to perform a biopsy or excision is predicated on the same indications as for other benign-appearing nevi. The need for specific differentiation from the halo that may appear around a melanoma is an additional indication for biopsy. The halo nevus also occasionally dissolves and disappears spontaneously at a much faster rate than that seen with other nevi.

Juvenile Nevus (Spitz Nevus)

Juvenile nevi, also called *benign juvenile melanomas,* were first described by Spitz in 1948.[115] They bear a close histopathologic resemblance to malignant melanoma. They are solitary and occur in preadolescents, although perhaps 15% to 30% may occur in adults.[100] They tend to occur on the face in children and on the trunk and lower extremities in adults. The color is not as deeply pigmented as congenital nevi or melanoma. Telangiectases are also seen. Specific characteristics of the lesion are its histopathology, rather than its clinical appearance or behavior. In favor of the diagnosis is the fact that malignant melanoma is extraordinarily rare in infants and children. Anytime the diagnosis of melanoma is histologically suspected, the surgeon should consider the possibility of a benign juvenile melanoma. Neighboring tissue often contains the characteristics of a compound nevus, which is probably the basic underlying pathophysiologic process involved. The natural history is unclear because removal for complete diagnosis is indicated. There have been reports that incomplete excision has been followed by local recurrence.[99]

PROBLEM: CONGENITAL NEVUS

Congenital nevi deserve a specific category. They are pigmented nevi identifiable at birth. Pigment cells have formed by the time of birth and are laid down in utero, as opposed to other nevi that may appear at birth but fail to pigment until later. The congenital nevi have a higher incidence of melanoma than do any other nevi.[78]

Classification

Small Congenital Nevus

A small congenital nevus is any lesion occupying a surface area of less than 1.5 cm in diameter; medium nevi are 1.5 to 2.0 cm in diameter (Figure 20-5). Most small congenital nevi have an abundance of hair. A handy way of differentiating the small from the large is to label as small those lesions perceived as being easily closed primarily (without the need for a skin graft). More than 90% of congenital nevi fall into the small category. The number of congenital nevi in the population may be more than 1 in every 100 live births.[100]

Even in small nevi, a greater than expected association exists between the nevi and melanoma. The risk for any single person is difficult to determine. The cumulative risk over lifetime is believed to increase approximately 21-fold over normal. Therefore a small congenital nevus in patients who live to age 60 years would have an incidence of melanoma of approximately 1 in 30. This incidence is relatively small, but it is substantially higher in the giant congenital nevi. However, because giant congenital nevi are significantly rarer, those with small lesions may in actuality have a numerically greater risk of developing melanoma. Many believe that *all* small and medium congenital nevi, irrespective of the size and location, should be considered for excision. Once again, the statistics are based only on those patients available for study as the result of biopsy or development of melanoma. The large number of nevi that may be present in the population and are never exised or documented makes statistical studies difficult. Obviously, congenital nevi with pigment and often heavy hair growth present an esthetic problem as well, and elective excision and the subsequent scar offer an appearance superior to the more visible pigmented nevus.

Giant Congenital Nevus

Fewer than 10% of congenital nevi should be termed *large* or *giant.* Their incidence in the population is thought to be 1 in every 20,000 live births.[100] Large nevi are more than 20 cm in diameter, and giant nevi exceed 100 cm^2. These typically occur in the scalp, across the face, particularly around the eyelids, and over the classic "bathing trunk" distribution. These lesions may be only slightly elevated but often are large, verrucous, and indurated. The pigmentation may vary from vaguely pigmented to deep brown or black. The nevi frequently have thick, heavy hair growth with a tendency to increase in density and length with age. Giant nevi may also be associated with other cutaneous lesions, including multiple large nevi. On occasion nevi may cover as much as 85% to 90% of total body surface area (Figure 20-5).

In a study in Denmark, the statistical chance of any given congenital nevus developing melanoma over a lifetime was about 6.3%.[28] For comparison, in the control group of people *without* congenital nevi the chance of developing malignant melanoma was 0.38%. In the United States it is 0.6%, or about 1 in 150. The increased risk therefore is approximately 16-fold.

Giant congenital nevi should be removed as a prophylactic measure against melanoma.[93] The esthetic problems associated with these nevi are further justification for surgery. The basic statistical analysis indicates that the chance of malignancy is approximately the same for each year of life. Including the risks of a general anesthetic in the first year of life and for any year thereafter, the risks of excision are sevenfold better than the risks of leaving the lesion in place.

The depth of surgical excision is also controversial. Histopathology indicates that, except in early infancy (less than 1 year of age), nevus cells are present not only in the dermis but also deep in the reticular dermis, in the subcutaneous tissue, and even deeper. Because the surgeon is operating for prophylaxis against malignancy, it is appropriate to remove all cells with malignant potential. Therefore the excision should be full thickness and probably also include some of the underlying fat.

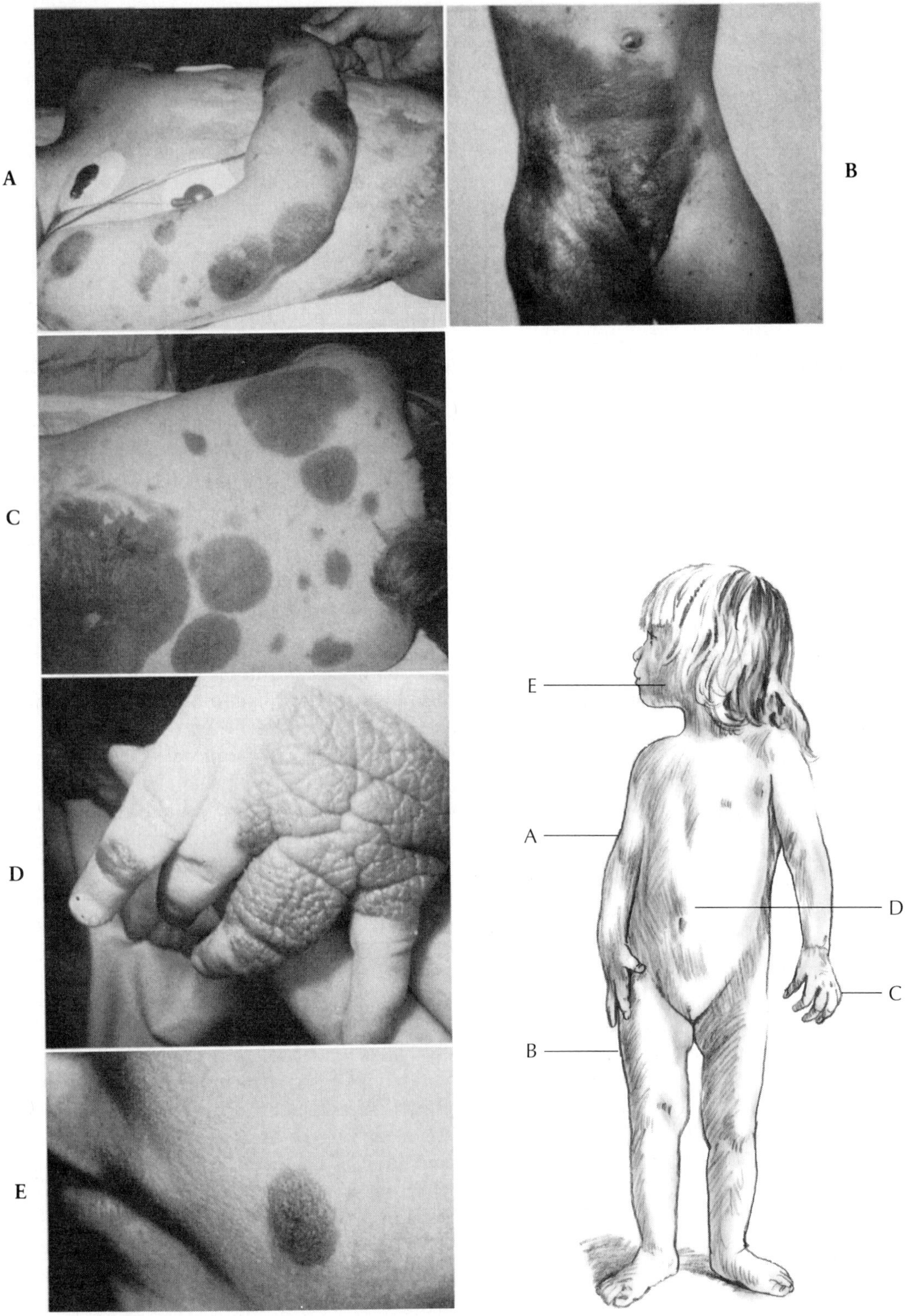

FIGURE 20-5 Congenital nevi. **A,** Multiple nevi—small, medium, and giant—covering 80% to 90% of the body (see also **C**). **B,** Giant congenital nevus—bathing-trunk nevus with multiple nodularities in the pubic area. **C,** Giant nevi with exuberant hair growth. **D,** Congenital nevus in the same patient as shown in **A** and **C.** These are similar to the changes seen in neurofibromatosis. **E,** Small congenital nevus, present at birth.

Clinical Presentation

A multiple number of pigmented lesions can occur.

History (Subjective Findings)

Parents often report that the child was delivered normally; the only abnormal finding at birth was a pigmented lesion. They may bring the child to the surgeon because the lesion has begun to darken, although it has remained the same size. In the first several months and years of life, the patient may develop several other "moles" on the body, trunk, and face. Often no other family member will have unusual moles, and the parents report no family history of malignant melanoma or other malignancy. The child may be normal in every other way.

Physical Examination (Objective Findings)

Physical examination reveals a large pigmented area(s) (Figure 20-6). This area is a raised, multinodular lesion with sparse hair growth and irregular margins. Many other small moles, vaguely pigmented with sparse hair growth, are often present on the trunk and the face.

Diagnostic Studies

Routine diagnostic tests, such as chest radiographs and blood studies, are usually performed. In the absence of other findings, such as suspected involvement of the neural complex or leptomeninges, most special diagnostic measures are unnecessary and excessively costly and provide little, if any, additional information.

A

B

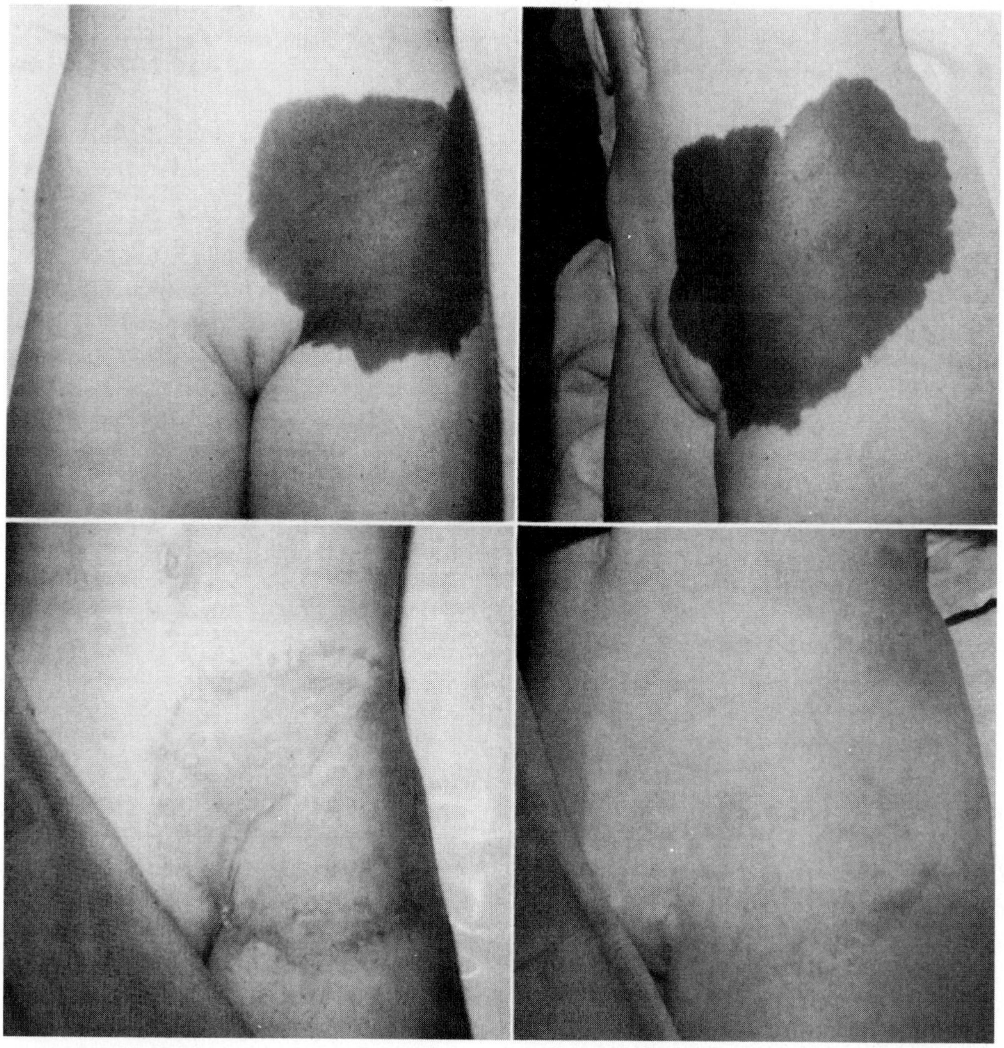

C

D

FIGURE 20-6 Giant congenital nevus of more than 100 cm^2 area in an 8-year-old child. **A** and **B,** Lower abdomen, inguinal region, and buttock. **C,** After excision and split-thickness grafting. **D,** Two years later.

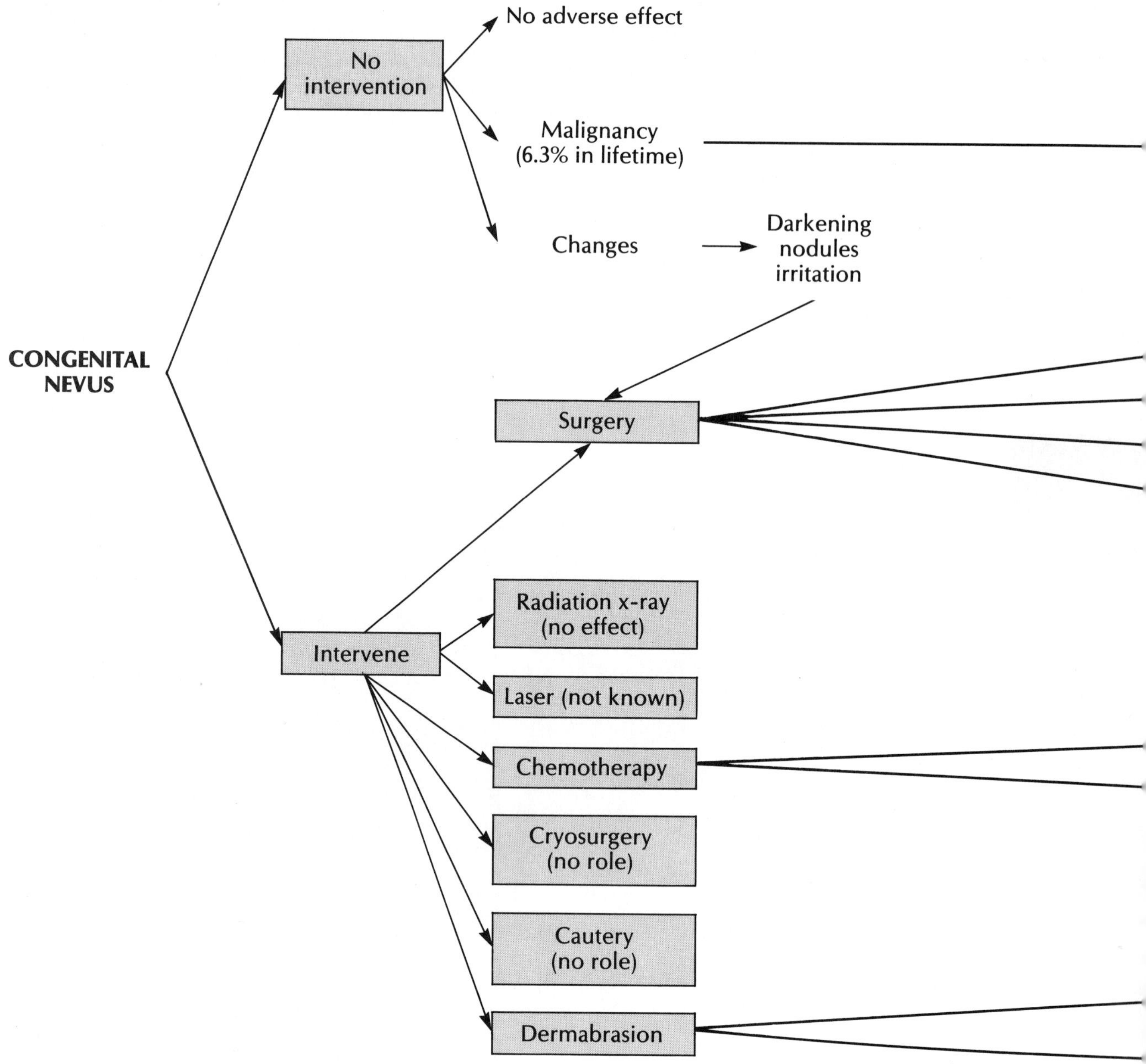

FIGURE 20-7 Algorithm for management of congenital nevus.

Biopsy

Careful clinical evaluation is usually sufficient to identify the nature of the congenital nevus. The critical diagnostic feature is the fact that it was present at birth. Lesions that have changed, primarily by becoming more nodular or darker, or any specific portion of the lesion that is suspected of being malignant should undergo an *incisional* biopsy. However, if the decision is made to perform *total* surgical excision, the preliminary biopsy is not necessary. The excision and the biopsy will be one and the same.

Histology

As opposed to the previously discussed nevi, the congenital nevi have in common nevus cells or clusters of nevus cells in the deep dermis and in the subcutaneous fat, and are oriented along skin appendages. These are often spindle shaped and are thought to resemble Schwann cells. A congenital nevus can histologically and clinically resemble a neurofibroma (Figure 20-5); the more aggressive types have been associated with malignant neurofibromas and other malignancies early in life. These also should be specifically differentiated from ju-

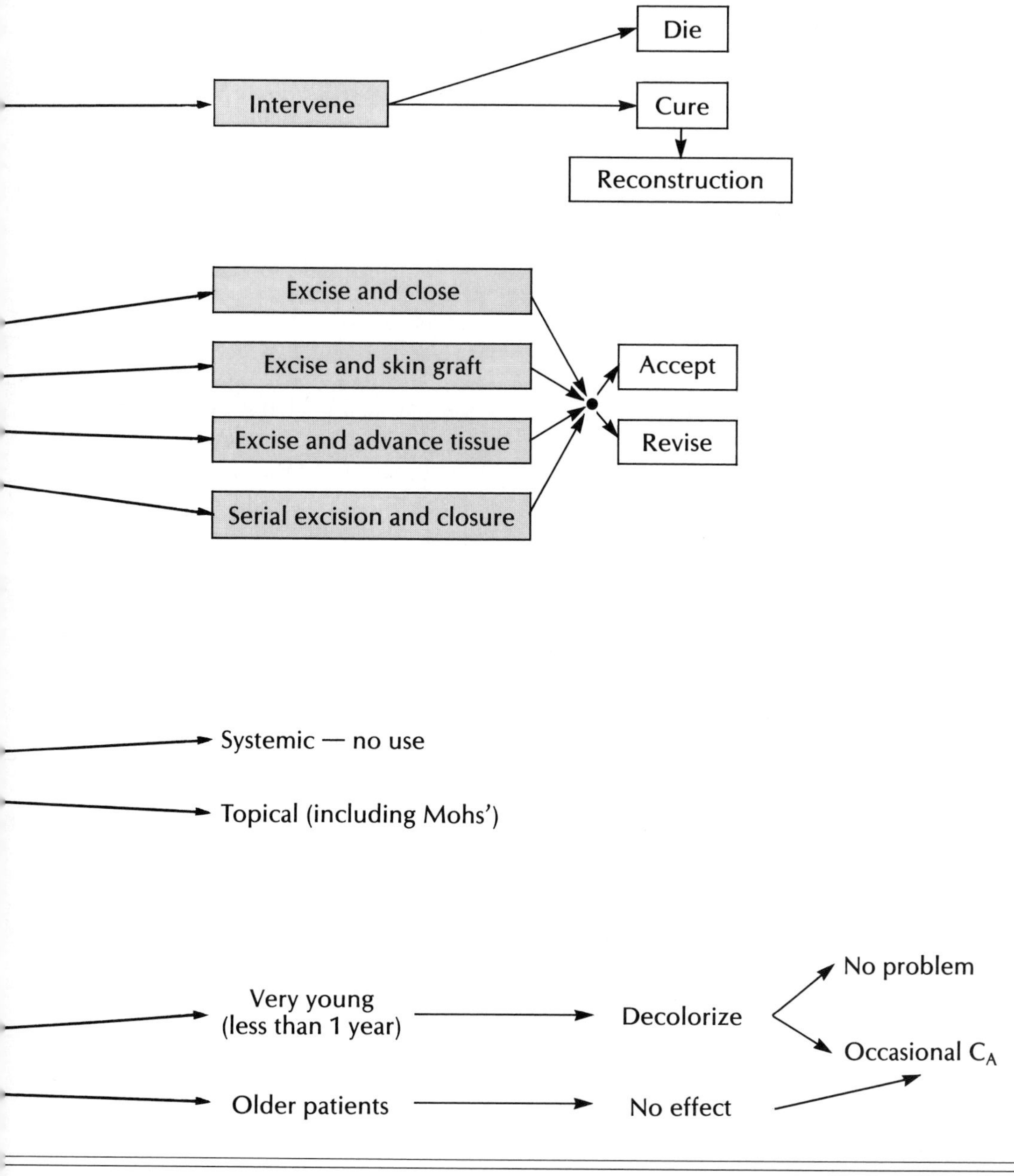

venile melanomas, which are compound in variety, clearly found in the dermis, and clearly benign.

Management

Any therapeutic plan appears clear and nicely outlined when presented as an abstraction in an algorithm (Figure 20-7). Management planning is rarely as clear-cut when the surgeon faces the challenge of removing a large nevus and recognizes the subsequent esthetic and functional deformity that will result and the immediate concerns of the patient and family. The patient and family must decide which therapeutic option to pursue after the surgeon has effectively explained each of the choices available.

Any decision regarding therapeutic intervention, particularly surgical intervention, should begin with the decision on whether to intervene at all (Figure 20-7). To assist the parents in making a decision, the surgeon must outline both the short- and long-term risks of doing nothing compared with the risks of doing something.

No Intervention

The surgeon must explain to the parents that the only reasons for intervening are (1) to make the patient look better; and (2) to prevent the lesion from developing into a malignant melanoma. "Doing nothing" is not an excuse to avoid facing the issue; it should be a positive decision. The chances of a congenital nevus becoming a melanoma are higher than for any other types of nevus and are certainly higher than for normal skin. However, the statistical odds of any given nevus becoming a melanoma in any given year are small. Time devoted to consideration of this and general reflection on the subject with the parents is time well spent. The odds of a congenital nevus that is more than 10 cm in diameter becoming a melanoma are about 6% to 7% in a lifetime and probably no more than 1 in 1000 in any given year.[78] For some parents this might be an attractive statistic; for others it might be entirely unacceptable. No one would suggest, much less accept, bilateral prophylactic mastectomies for female infants even though the chance of malignancy is more than 6% in a lifetime. But the data on nevi are not totally clear; others might suggest the chances of malignancy are as high as 40%.[3,68,100,101]

Intervention

Total surgical removal is the treatment of choice when intervention is chosen. The alternative approaches to surgery are all unacceptable. Radiation has no known efficacy in obliterating nevi and would have permanent and potential harmful effects on a child. Lasers, although of value in some pigmented lesions, are not dependable for lesions of this size. Chemotherapy systemically or topically has no known value. Mohs' chemosurgery, although likely effective, would be an unnecessarily ponderous approach; surgical reconstruction would still be required. Similarly, cryosurgery would destroy the lesion but leave an unacceptable defect.

Dermabrasion has been explored for treating lesions in the very young before the nevus cells descend into the deeper dermal levels. However, dermabrasion always leaves calluses and is not a suitable prophylactic approach. Abrading and perhaps covering with a graft may be aesthetically acceptable if the parents (patient) and surgeon understand and accept the risk.

The entire lesion must be removed. Even large defects can be closed primarily or by rotation of locally available tissue. Larger defects can be closed with skin grafts. Serial partial excision, returning to remove residual tissue after the healing tissue softens, is occasionally used as is "tissue expansion" of the adjacent tissue, which can occasionally be recruited to fill the surgical defect.

Results

The management of any condition with such a statistically unpredictable course as the giant nevus leaves much uncertainty regarding outcome. Certainly those whose nevi are completely excised do not develop melanomas. The control group is almost lacking and we are dependent on the lifetime expectation of melanoma of 6.3% to justify a prophylactic approach.

PROBLEM: DYSPLASTIC NEVUS SYNDROME (B-K MOLE SYNDROME)

Congenital nevi can develop into melanoma and should be thought of as precursors to melanoma. Even more likely to become a melanoma is the dysplastic nevus, as part of the dysplastic nevus syndrome. Clark and associates[25] originally described this syndrome as a precursor of melanoma by identifying two families with atypical nevi and a high incidence of the subsequent development of melanoma. The syndrome was named after the families, whose surnames had the initials *B* and *K* and who were the first two identified as having this; hence the term *B-K mole syndrome,* implying the familial characteristic. The appearance of the melanoma may occur earlier in each of the subsequent generations.

Clinical Presentation

The clinical appearance of the nevus is different enough to be suggestive but not diagnostic. The lesions tend to be irregular, to be larger than other nevi (ranging from 5 to 12 mm in diameter), and to have a multicolored hue of tan and brown, often with a pink border and background. These lesions may appear to be flat, but they are usually raised and are always palpably raised. One of the characteristics of the syndrome is that the lesions are of many different sizes, shapes, and colors, all within the same patient. The dysplastic nevi tend to appear during adolescence and usually are not identified in early childhood.

Those with this syndrome have multiple atypical nevi, although the numbers may range from few to more than 100 (Figure 20-8). They typically occur in the trunk and covered areas and when there are many on the trunk, they are usually also found in the lower extremities.

Diagnostic Studies

The histologic pattern is different enough to give the pathologist a clue, even in the absence of a clinical history or suspicions by the surgeon doing the biopsy. The characteristic changes include atypical basilar melanocytic hyperplasia, elongated rete ridges, mesenchymal changes in the papillary dermis, and a dermal fibroplasia and lymphatic response.

Management

Management of the patient with dysplastic nevus syndrome is difficult and challenging because elimination of all the dysplastic nevi is a formidable undertaking.

A B C

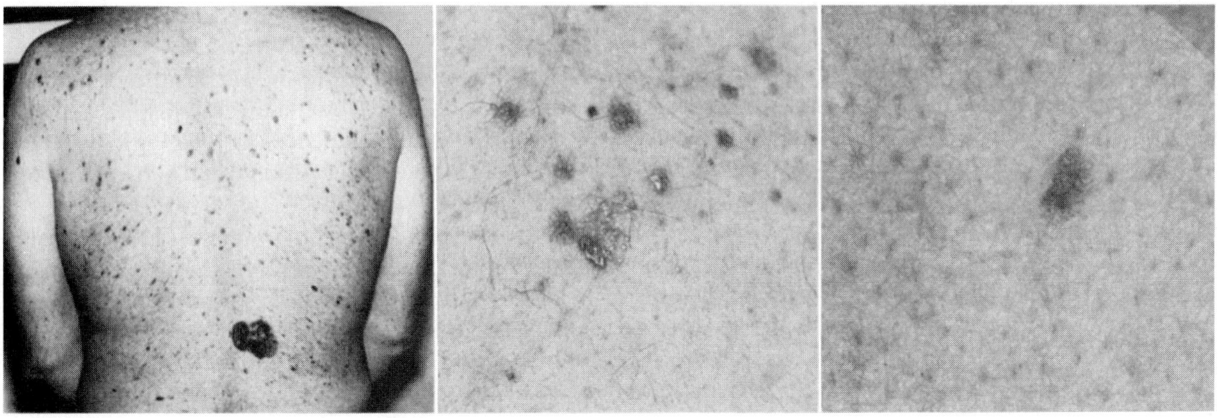

D

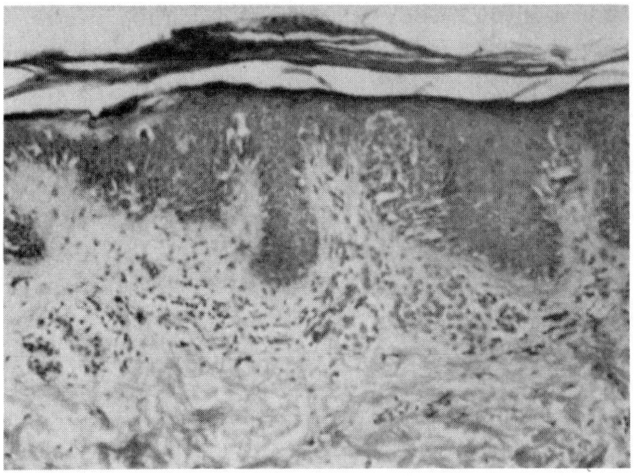

E

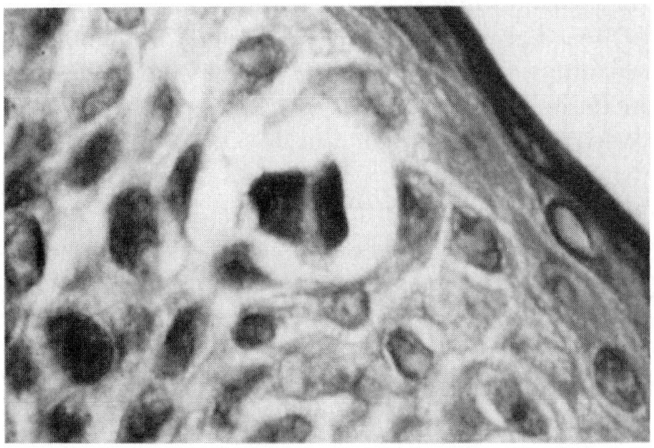

F

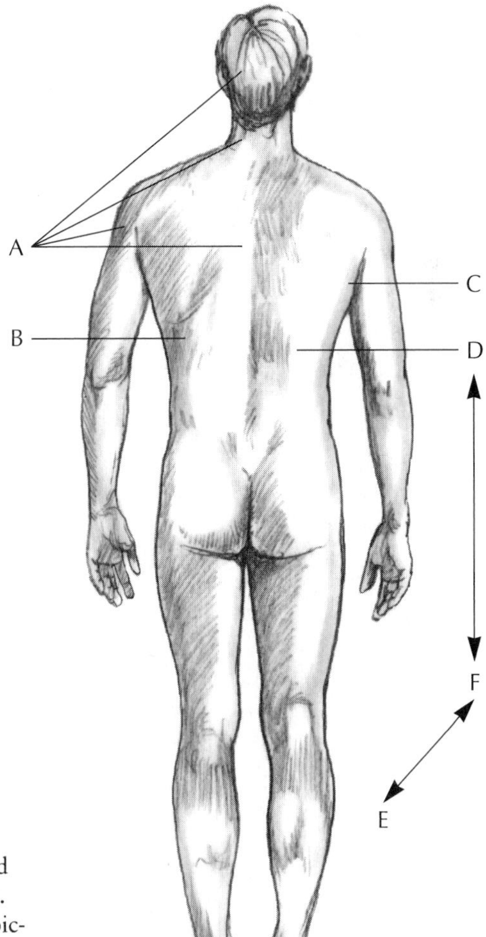

FIGURE 20-8 **A,** Dysplastic nevus syndrome (B-K mole syndrome) and BANS (*B,* Back; *A,* arm; *N,* neck; *S,* scalp). **B,** Multiple dysplastic nevi. **C,** Typical dysplastic nevus—pinkish here at margin. **D,** Microscopic picture of nevus cells. **E,** Vacuolated cell—nevus cell. **F,** Common sites of occurrence. (From Hagstrom WJ Jr, Faibisoff B, Soltani K, Robson MC: *Plast Reconstr Surg* 71:219, 1983.)

Photographs should be taken carefully and used for comparison at the regular follow-up visits every 3 to 6 months.

Lesions that are identified as changing, enlarging, becoming irritated in any way, becoming unusually pruritic, and particularly changing in color should immediately be excised. Once again, destruction by any method that would not provide tissue for histologic examination is condemned. The lesions extend down into the dermis so that superficial scraping and removal are likely to be incomplete.

Patient and Family Education

All first-degree family members should be identified and screened. The incidence of dysplastic nevi among white males in the population ranges from 2% to 8%.[100] This relatively low prevalence of dysplastic nevi in the normal population is in contrast with 134 adults with sporadic melanoma in whom more than one third were found to have dysplastic nevi as well.[42] In true familial melanoma or the B-K mole syndrome (two or more blood relatives with melanoma), more than 90% of the patients with melanoma and 40% of the relatives without melanoma had one or more dysplastic nevi.[25] Convincing evidence of premalignancy has been identified through photographic documentation of invasive melanoma developing from preexisting dysplastic nevi. Similarly, there has been histologic evidence of dysplastic nevus associated with melanoma in the same lesion. It is thought to occur in families as an autosomal dominant trait. An eightfold to twelvefold increase in the risk of melanoma can be estimated for parents, offspring, and siblings of patients with cutaneous melanomas. About 10% of those with dysplastic nevi in the sporadic form will develop melanoma; it may be closer to 100% for melanoma-prone families.[28]

One of the predisposing factors to all melanomas is assumed to be ultraviolet radiation. The effect of sunlight on the dysplastic nevi has not been documented, but all patients and relatives so involved should be advised to avoid sunlight.

PROBLEM: MALIGNANT MELANOMA

Approximately 1 in every 100 white adults will develop a malignant melanoma in his or her lifetime. The overall incidence is relatively small and accounts for somewhere between 1% and 3% of all carcinomas. Approximately 32,000 new cases of malignant melanoma were reported in the United States in 1990. However, the lesion is increasing not only in absolute numbers, but also in the incidence within the population. It is now the second leading cause of death from cancer in males between 15 and 35 years of age.[103] In addition to these increases, there also is evidence that the lesion is appearing earlier rather than at its former peak in the fifth and sixth decades of life. Furthermore, the predominance of melanoma in males is also disappearing, and in 1985 the rates were approximately equal between the sexes.

Malignant melanoma unquestionably seems to be related to radiation, either solar or ionizing radiation, and is most commonly found in those with fair skin, blue eyes, and red or blond hair. In the black patient the incidence of melanoma is low, except on the plantar and palmar surfaces and in the nail beds. Melanoma in the nail beds in whites is almost unheard of. The influence of sun and racial characteristics is important, and Australia and New Zealand have the highest incidence of melanoma in the world, 1 in 60 persons.

In addition to the familial predisposition in the dysplastic nevus syndrome discussed previously, melanoma also trends to arise in family members, and familial melanoma accounts for 1% to 6% of all melanomas.

The traumatic induction of melanoma is difficult to document but should always be considered in any skin cancer or perhaps even in other types of cancer. Melanoma has been found in people with xeroderma pigmentosa, a familial genetic problem with dysplastic skin and a predisposition to many forms of cancer. Melanoma has been reported in vaccination scars and tattoos, but it has not been found with any higher incidence in surgical, burn, or any other traumatic scars.

Some melanomas arise de novo in skin that is thought by patient and physician alike to have been devoid of any blemish or abnormality before appearance of the lesions. However, some clearly do arise in congenital nevi, in dysplastic nevi (B-K mole syndrome), or from nevocellular nevi themselves. The incidence of those arising in preexisting nevi has been estimated to be from 10% to 85%. Conversely, microscopic examination of melanoma shows evidence of benign nevus cells within the melanoma in approximately 40% of cases. The prevalence of nevi is estimated to be 83,333 times the prevalence of melanoma. It is thought that the malignant melanoma arises from the junctional component from the nevus cell—that is, from that area between the dermal epidermal junction—and therefore from junctional and compound nevi rather than from the intradermal component. Thus an intradermal nevus can be considered a benign disease that is not a precursor to melanoma.

Clinical Presentation

History (Subjective Findings)

Patients may report that a lesion is enlarging, has begun to itch intermittently, and clearly is now darker and firmer than in the past. A fair-haired patient may note that, when exposed to the sun, freckles and other moles seem to get darker. Often the patient cannot recall with certainty whether there was a mole where this particular lesion is now located. There may be no family history of malignant melanoma.

Physical Examination (Objective Findings)

The typical lesion has irregular borders. The examiner should record the lesion's greatest diameter (Figure 20-9), its color (often tan to black), and its texture, which may be nodular. Some scaling and evidence of irritation with or without ulceration may be present. Nevi on other areas of the body should be examined carefully.

Regional lymph nodes should also be examined carefully and their presence or absence noted. If the nodes are enlarged, they should be measured and the size recorded accurately in the medical record. Identifying which regional lymph nodes drain an area is often difficult, and lymphoscintigraphy has become a valuable adjunct to determining which node group may drain any given area.

Diagnostic Studies

Biopsy

Obtaining biopsy tissue for examination under the microscope is perhaps more important in melanoma than in any other lesion in the body. There may be a theoretical reason for concern about performing a biopsy on a suspected lesion and the potential danger of either cutting into or not adequately excising the lesion at the first evaluation. Manipulation of a tumor, such as cutting into it, will release tumor cells into the bloodstream. The mere fact that tumor cells are or may be released into the bloodstream should not prevent the biopsy from being performed, and there is no evidence that the biopsy does harm. Before the biopsy the patient should understand that, if the lesion is malignant, more definitive treatment will be necessary.

If the lesion is more than 2 to 3 cm in diameter, has irregular borders, or is located in an area of great functional significance such as the eyelid or lip, an incisional biopsy is appropriate. The biopsy may be accomplished with the patient under local anesthesia as an outpatient. The lesion may be directly incised, much as one would slice a piece of pie, and the portion obtained. The biopsy should extend from the edge of the apparent tumor mass and into normal-appearing tissue in a wedge shape so that the pathologist is given not only the most suspicious area, but the gradations to the margins as well. The biopsy must be generous because it is critical that the pathologist have an adequate amount of tissue to determine the tumor's relative and absolute thickness.

Imaging Studies

Chest radiographs and tomograms are of value in assessing the presence of distant metastases. Among the studies evaluated, tomograms of the lung seem to be more accurate early predictors of distant metastases than routine radiographs and are found to be positive in 40% of patients later found to have distant metastases. Computed tomography (CT) is the method of choice for evaluating distant metastases. The metastatic disease in the lung has a doubling time of approximately 43 days, about three times faster than breast cancer. As part of the follow-up, chest radiographs should be obtained at approximately 6-month intervals. Diagnostic tests, including radionucleotide scans, brain scans, bone scans, and liver and spleen scans, may become positive in the presence of systemic spread.

Lymphoscintigraphy

The description of lymphatic drainage from different parts of the body was described a century ago, and it is not surprising that newer dynamic studies of patterns of

A

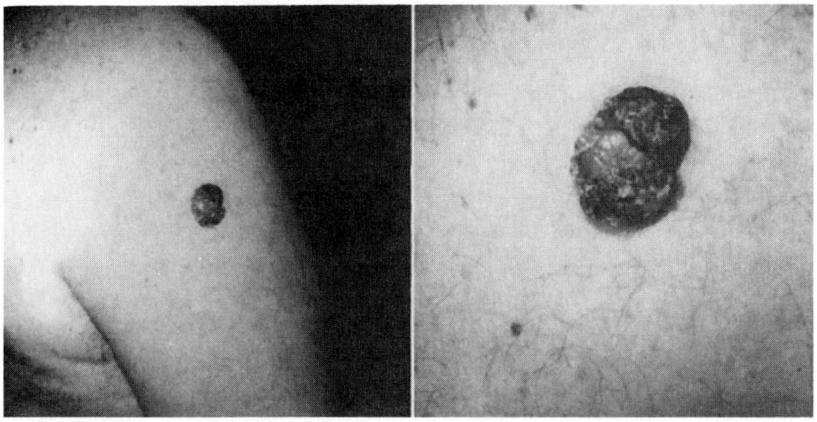

B

FIGURE 20-9 Nodular malignant melanoma. **A,** Nodular melanoma on back of upper arm. **B,** Close-up view of melanoma.

lymphatic spread are somewhat different from classic anatomic descriptions. Radioactive material (technetium-99 antimony sulfur colloid) was injected into the tissue near the primary lesion, particularly for lesions at ambiguous sites on the trunk and head and neck in more than 200 patients at the H. Lee Moffitt Cancer Center at the University of South Florida.[91] When drainage patterns were compared with historical guidelines, the findings were discordant in 63% of patients with tumors on the head and neck and 32% of those with lesions on the trunk. The operative intervention had to be changed because of these findings in 47% of patients with 19% requiring removal of nonclassic lymph node basins. An additional 28% underwent no lymph node dissections because the scintigram failed to demonstrate a predominant drainage basin. Follow-up of up to 3 years failed to show any recurrence in basins not positive on lymphoscintigraphy.

Pathophysiology and Staging

Staging has been a major breakthrough in the understanding of the biology of melanoma and its subsequent contribution to treatment. The observations of Clark and associates,[24] Breslow,[19] Balch and associates,[11] and Day and collegues[33,34,36] indicate that the prognosis of the tumor can be directly correlated with the relative degree of invasion through the skin into the subcutaneous tissue and to the volume of the tumor cells as measured by tumor thickness.

Clark's Classification

Clark's classification is based on the relative degree of invasion of the tumor through different layers of skin.[24] Clark has classified and divided melanomas into five stages (Figure 20-10).

Level I. Level I is the most superficial, and the abnormal cells are confined entirely to the dermal-epidermal junction. There is no evidence of invasion into the dermis.

Level II. In this stage, the earliest stage of the vertical growth phase, melanoma cells are identified as having entered the papillary dermis. They have not totally occupied the papillary dermis and have not extended deeper than the papillary ridges themselves.

Level III. Melanoma cells fill the papillary dermis and extend to the junction of the papillary and reticular dermis.

Level IV. Melanoma cells invade the reticular dermis down to the deepest margin of the dermis but not into the subcutaneous tissue.

Level V. Melanoma cells extend into the subcutaneous tissue.

The profound significance of this classification has been the ability to correlate ultimate survival with this initial degree of invasion observed at biopsy.[10]

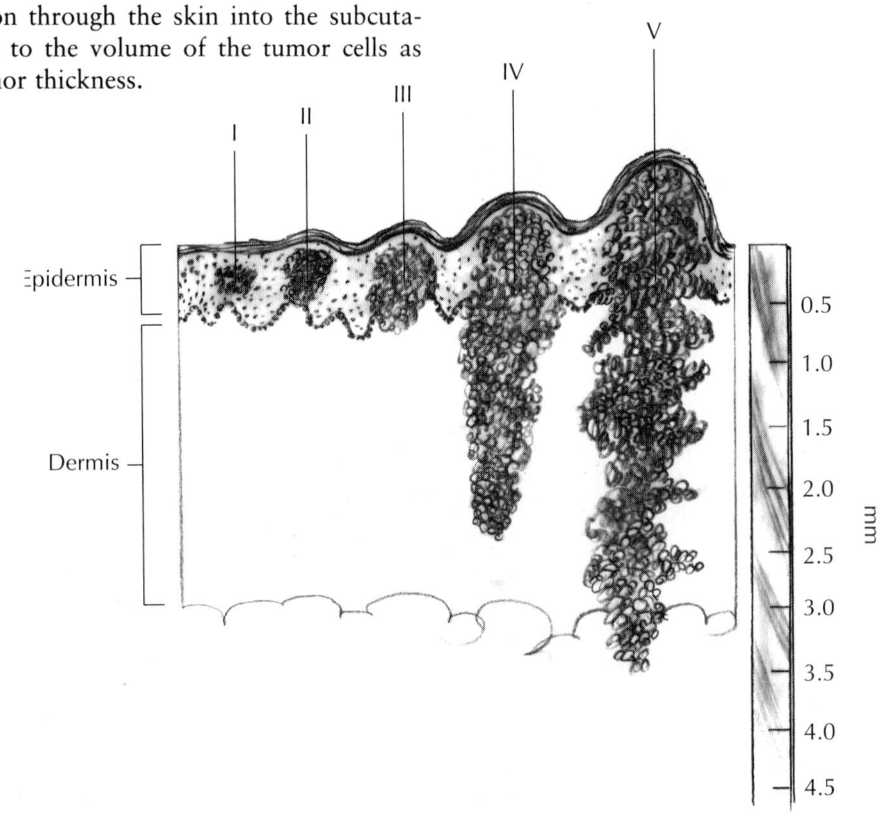

FIGURE 20-10 Clark's classification (levels I to V) is by level of tissue invasion. Breslow's classification is by measurement.

Breslow's Classification

Breslow observed that Clark's classification was relative and was dependent on the thickness of the skin. For instance, the skin of the back is many times thicker than the skin of the eyelid, so a tumor of the back might have a large volume of tumor cells and still be superficial relative to the thickness of the skin. That same absolute thickness and volume of tumor cells found in the cheek or eyelid, where the skin is thinner, might represent a stage when the tumor has actually invaded into the subcutaneous tissue. With that in mind, Breslow reclassified melanoma entirely on the basis of volume, as measured by the absolute thickness of the tumor under the microscope.[19] He placed essentially no importance on its relative degree of invasion through the skin. He emphasized the accuracy of this approach: the degree of invasion may often be difficult to interpret in other lesions, whereas the thickness remains absolute.

Balch compared Clark and Breslow's methods and determined that at 3 years, in a refined measurement of depth, for tumors thinner than 0.75 mm, regional metastasis was 0%.[10] For lesions 0.76 to 1.5 mm, it was 25%; between 1.6 and 3.99 mm, it was 51%; and for those thicker than 4 mm, it was 62%.[10]

Other Classifications

Day refined Breslow's classification to tumors of less than 0.85 mm thick, lesions 0.86 mm to 0.169 mm, those 1.7 to 3.6 mm, and those thicker than 3.6 mm. Day's modification is more specific and can be correlated better with the degree of survival and metastasis[33,34,36] (see the box at right).

STAGING OF MELANOMA

Clark
Level I—dermal-epidermal junction
Level II—papillary dermis
Level III—cells fill papillary dermis and extend to reticular dermis
Level IV—reticular dermis
Level V—subcutaneous

Breslow
Level thinner than 0.75 mm
Level 0.76 to 1.5 mm
Level thicker than 1.5 mm (may be 1.5 to 4.0 mm)
Level thicker than 4.0 mm (modified)

Day
Level thinner than 0.85 mm
Level 0.86 to 1.69 mm
Level 1.70 to 3.6 mm
Level thicker than 3.6 mm

Clinical
Stage I—local only—no regional or distant metastases
Stage II—to regional lymph nodes
Stage III—disseminated

TNM (World Health Organization)
T, Tumor
N, Nodes
M, Metastasis

CLINICAL CLASSIFICATION. For statistical analysis, review, and discussion, an indispensable clinical staging has been added to these histologic observations:

Stage I. Melanoma has either been locally excised or biopsied. There is no evidence of regional lymph node or distant hematogenous metastatic spread. This stage also includes recurrent melanomas found within 4 cm of the primary site and multiple primary melanomas.

Stage II. Melanoma exists with obvious metastatic disease limited to the regional lymph nodes.

Stage III. Disseminated melanoma exists and includes visceral and multiple lymphatic metastases or multiple cutaneous and subcutaneous metastases.

The World Health Organization (WHO) has introduced the TNM classification for the staging for melanoma, in which *T* refers to the characteristics of the tumor itself and follows the Clark and Breslow classifications, *N* is the status of the regional lymph nodes, and *M* represents presence or absence of distant metastasis.

Clinical stagings have proven valuable for stage I melanoma. Balch and associates[15,19] have identified the two dominant pathologic features associated with survival as tumor thickness (which corresponds to the Breslow and Day classification) and the presence of ulceration. They also have identified two clinical factors that influence survival: the initial form of surgical treatment used and the location of the lesion. Tumors found in the BANS area—an acronym for *b*ack, back of *a*rm, *n*eck, and *s*calp (Figure 20-8)—have a particularly poor prognosis.[12] The reason is obvious because each area is hidden to the patient, making early recognition less likely than for areas easily examined.

DESCRIPTIVE CLASSIFICATION. It has been useful over the last years to divide clinical malignant melanoma into four distinct categories for diagnosis and therapeutic planning. The first two of these, superficial spreading melanoma and nodular melanoma, are probably phases of the same process. Malignant lentigo, primarily a variation of melanoma seen in elderly patients, and acral lentiginous melanoma are the most common forms of melanoma found in blacks. The descriptive classification is intimately related to what is believed to be a biologic characteristic of melanoma, namely, its chronologic progression from superficial to deep. Whether the time interval is short or a matter of decades, the basic assumption on which all classification and even management are rationally based is that melanoma will begin as a malignant transformation at the dermal-epidermal junction (where junctional and compound nevi occur). Malignant transformation is then followed by a degree of superficial spreading of the malignancy along the dermal-epidermal junction, which corresponds to the superficial spread of melanoma and is called the *radial phase*. Sometime thereafter, and indeed the interval may be extraordinarily short, the radial converts to a *vertical phase* and begins to invade into the deeper layers of the dermis, through the reticular dermis, and finally into the subcutaneous tissue. This vertical phase is accompanied by a palpable thickening of the lesion and corresponds to the *nodular phase* of melanoma.

Superficial spreading melanoma. Clark and associates[24] first described superficial spreading melanoma in 1969. The term refers more to a phase of melanoma than to a specific entity. It represents a group of approximately 70% to 75% of melanomas at the time they are first seen clinically. The tumor is seen originally as a vaguely pigmented, slightly raised lesion (Figure 20-8). These lesions seem to have a predilection for the back, particularly on women, but they also occur in the lower extremities. The lesions then become increasingly pigmented and more distinctly palpable; as they enlarge in a radial fashion, margins become irregular and the pigmentation becomes blotchy from black to brown, with various areas of deep black pigmentation. Much as in a halo nevus, where the immune system seems to be destroying cells as a response to the nevus cells, various areas of the superficial spreading melanoma may become depigmented (Figure 20-8). The superficial spreading characteristic is thought to be only a phase of melanoma growth; at a certain point the melanoma will become nodular and begin to invade vertically and would no longer be called a superficial spreading melanoma.

Biopsy of the lesion shows variation in cell differentiation but is largely limited to the junctional area between the dermis and epidermis. The superficial spreading type has a relatively more favorable prognosis because of its superficial nature.

Nodular melanoma. Nodular melanoma represents the phase after superficial spreading melanoma when the lesion tends to grow vertically rather than radially. Some 15% to 20% of melanomas will initially be seen as nodular melanomas, often without any evidence of having passed through a superficial spreading phase. They appear more commonly in men than in women and occur some 10 years later in life than the superficial spreading melanoma. These lesions are found more commonly in the head and neck area and on the extremities, compared with superficial spreading melanomas, which are more common on the trunk. The appearance of nodular melanoma is also different from that of the superficial melanoma. Much as the junctional nevus becomes smooth and rounded as it enters its intradermal phase, the nodular melanoma becomes smooth and nodular as it enters its vertical growth phase (Figure 20-9). The color tends to be blue-black and dark brown with occasional variations in hue. The elevated area tends to be smooth; the margins are typically irregular and then develop ulcerations, an uncommon finding in superficial spreading melanomas. Microscopically, the nodular melanoma is distinctly different from the superficial; although evidence of prior spread along the dermal-epidermal junction may be present, the nodular melanoma is invasive into the superficial portions of the dermis, eventually down into the reticular dermis and deeper. These depths of invasion form the basis of Clark's classification; the absolute thickness of the lesion is expressed by Breslow's and Day's classifications.

Malignant lentigo. Malignant lentigo, also known as the *melanotic freckle of Hutchinson,* is a precancerous lesion that arises from abnormal epidermal melanocytes rather than from nevus cells. It falls in the same general category as the lentigines, blue nevi, and nevi of Ota and Ito (Figure 20-11). These lesions may develop malignant characteristics and are then known as malignant lentigo melanomas.

Malignant lentigo melanoma is primarily a melanoma of the elderly, and women are affected more commonly than men. These lesions make up 5% of all presenting malignant melanomas. Almost all melanotic freckles or malignant lentigines occur on the face, typically over the most prominently sun-exposed area and as a patch of flat pigmented area over the malar prominence (Figure 20-11). Lesions enlarge and have an irregular border extending often onto the eyelids, up further on the check toward the temple, down toward the nose, and perhaps occupying the entire cheek. They are almost always deeply pigmented and accompanied by aging skin with wrinkles, actinic changes, and other keratotic and seborrheic changes. As in superficial spreading melanoma, there will often be areas of depigmentation indicating efforts at immune resolution.

The natural history of malignant lentigo melanoma is perhaps better known than that of other forms because surgery is often deferred or treatment not accepted because of the patient's age. Many have remained essentially quiescent for 10 to 20 years. In actuality, the melanoma itself can be monitored for periods of time before distinct evidence of invasive melanoma formation develops. The lesion often appears more malignant by histologic examination than by clinical performance and has all the microscopic characteristics of a true malignant melanoma. In about one third of the patients, however, this malignant lentigo melanoma will develop true nodular traits with thickening and induration (Figure 20-11). The raised areas are characteristic of the nodular melanoma, and it is truly malignant. The distinctive microscopic features of the lentigo melanoma are the pres-

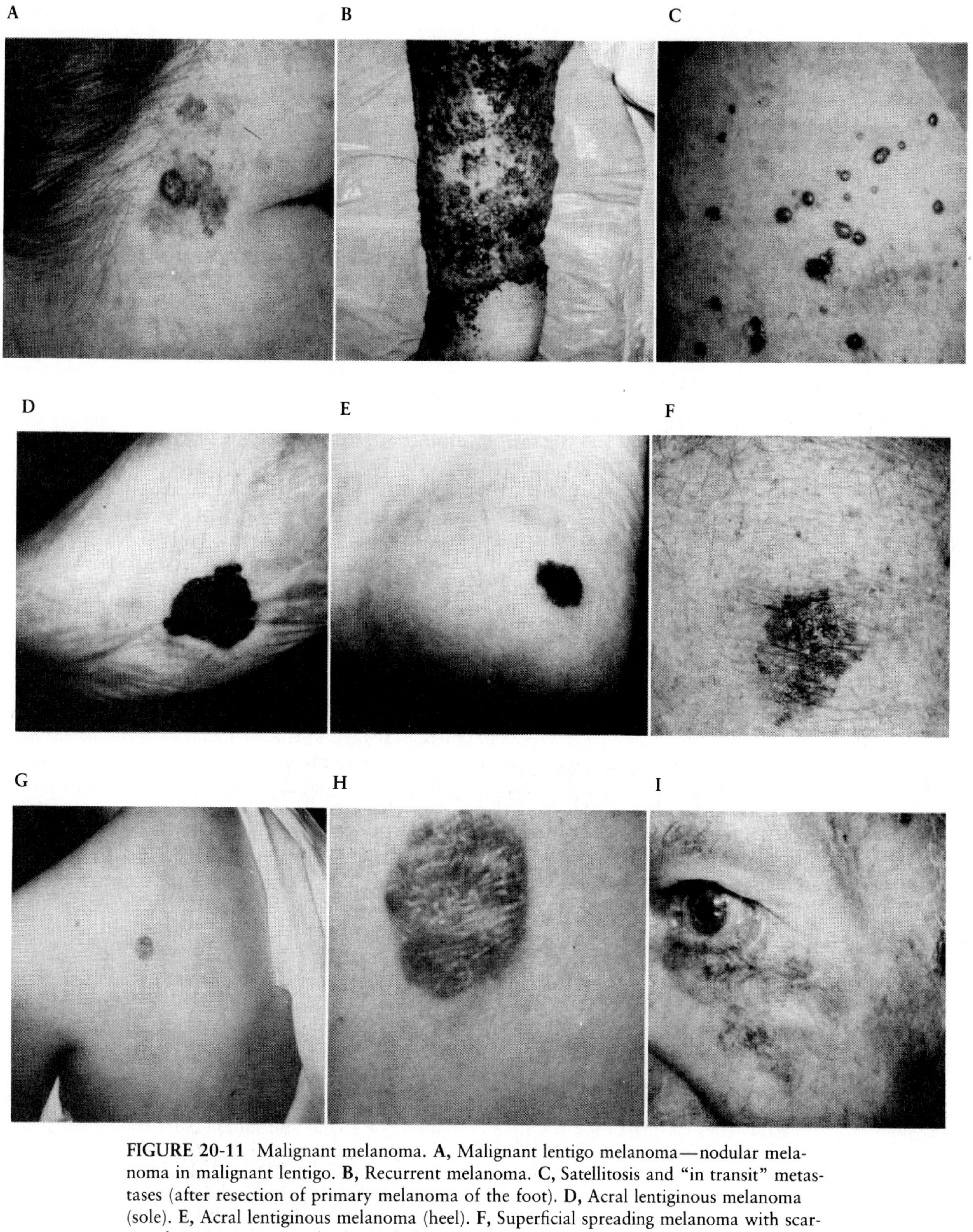

FIGURE 20-11 Malignant melanoma. **A,** Malignant lentigo melanoma—nodular melanoma in malignant lentigo. **B,** Recurrent melanoma. **C,** Satellitosis and "in transit" metastases (after resection of primary melanoma of the foot). **D,** Acral lentiginous melanoma (sole). **E,** Acral lentiginous melanoma (heel). **F,** Superficial spreading melanoma with scarring from spontaneous "healing" (halo). **G,** Superficial spreading melanoma in BANS area. **H,** Closer view of **G. I,** Malignant lentigo.

Continued.

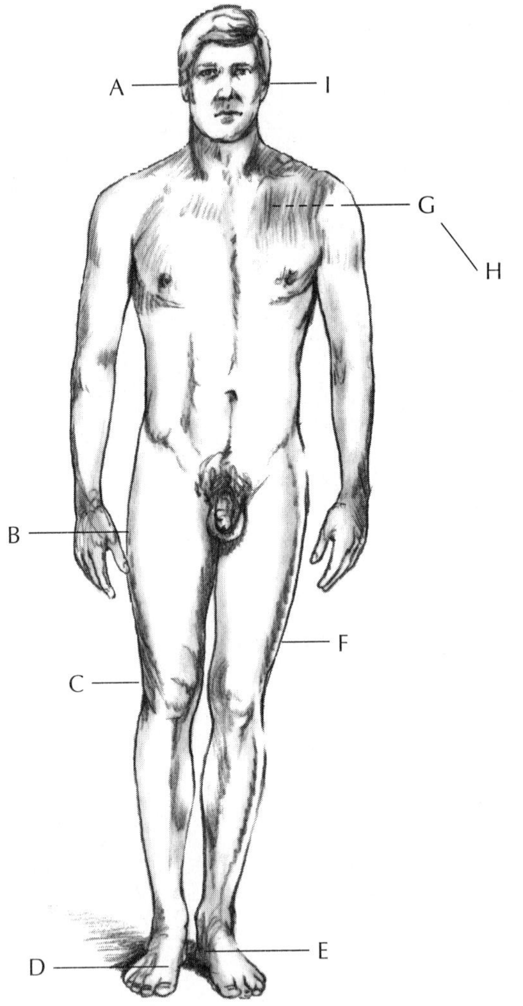

FIGURE 20-11, cont'd For legend see previous page.

ence of the invasive areas of nodular melanoma with adjoining areas of malignant lentigo. These changes begin in the basal cell layer with proliferation of atypical melanocytes.

Acral lentiginous melanoma. Acral lentiginous melanoma has been described only within the last decade. This melanoma tends to occur on the palms, the soles of the feet, and beneath the fingernails (Figure 20-11). Biologically, the melanoma has been thought to be a variation of a malignant lentigo when in fact it is far more aggressive and has a less favorable prognosis. It is not common and in most series accounts for fewer than 10% of primary cutaneous melanomas in white people. However, it is the most common form of melanoma in the black population.

The acral lentiginous melanoma begins and seems to behave at times much like both superficial spreading and malignant lentigo, with a radial growth phase. This behavior is typical, but its duration is often relatively short, and the beginning of the vertical growth phase may be hard to identify. The skin in this area is thick, and any further thickening and nodularity as a result of entry into the vertical growth phase may go unnoticed. Although the superficial and radial growth phases are clearly identified in biopsies of these lesions, most lesions actually have entered into the vertical growth phase by the time they are first examined. Perhaps for this reason, the prognosis is less satisfactory than for other lesions.

Management

The treatment of malignant melanoma is surgical. Any arguments in favor of radiation therapy, chemotherapy, immunotherapy, and other forms of treatment are high in hope but as yet lacking in data.

The basic surgical decisions to be made are how wide and deep the excision should be, how the wound should be closed, and whether the regional lymph nodes should be removed. Each of these decisions should rest on an understanding of the basic biology of the disease.

Surgery

LOCAL EXCISION

Excision width. The width of the excision is based on the assumption that the tumor, at least for a time, spreads radially. If a histologic examination were perfectly accurate, theoretically we should be able to look at the transition of tumor cells in the lesion to normal cells and be able to identify, to within the width of a cell or two, how wide the tumor excision should be. Because light microscopy is not nearly that accurate, there is always a transition zone between where tumor is obviously tumor and normal tissue is obviously normal. In this indefinite area of tissue, tumor cells may well be present but are not sufficiently distinct to be detected by their color, shape, or anatomic distortion, nor are they present in numbers sufficient to displace other tissue. Although their numbers may be biologically significant, they are invisible to the surgeon's eye and even to the eye of the microscopist. What this distance is likely to be underlies the question, "How wide?"

Interestingly, a historical vignette in the evolution of the diagnosis and management of melanoma has seemingly influenced treatment for more than 80 years. Handley,[57] in a Hungarian lecture, described "melanoma" of the foot that he examined at an autopsy. He noted that the tumor mass seemed to spread in a "cone-shaped" fashion such that the tumor mass was smaller at the surface than in the depths of the dermis and in the subcutaneous tissue. He also believed that the tumor had entered into the fascia and would spread along the fascia and muscle through the lymphatics. He therefore recommended that the amount of skin to be removed was approximately 2.5 cm in all directions around the skin lesion, increasing to 5 cm around the tumor mass at the subcutaneous level and then to include the fascia. This decision has been misstated as a principle that the skin margin should be 5 cm, even though Handley never actually suggested this.

Definition of adequate skin margins. No study using primary thickness of the wound as a guide to treatment has demonstrated that even narrow margins of the excision adversely affect survival. In 1983 Day and Lew[32] quoted a number of studies with a total number of patients of more than 1700, and all the data agreed that no adverse effects on survival rates were seen when the margins were narrow, as compared with margins of 5 cm or more. These observations and data again confirm that local recurrence and survival are a function of tumor cell spread beyond any feasible local surgical margin. Therefore the assumption is made that no widening of the excision can possibly help an unfavorable prognosis. Conversely, a very narrow margin excision has no deleterious effects on the most favorable lesions.[2]

With thin melanomas (less than 0.85 mm thick) a number of studies confirm that a narrow margin of excision is more than adequate. Breslow and Macht[20] observed no relapse in lesions less than 0.75 mm thick even though the margins were less than 5 mm. In thin melanomas there seems to be no correlation between narrow margins and recurrence; the cure rate is excellent and the absence of local recurrence is uniform. Therefore an excision should include 1 to 1.5 cm of clinically normal skin around the margins of a melanoma less than 0.85 mm thick. In melanomas 0.85 mm thick or thicker in clincial stage I, the margins should probably be wider.[36] Several studies have indicated that, when the margin for thick melanomas is reduced to less than 2 cm, the recurrence rate increased threefold.[32,35]

The World Health Organization Melanoma Programme randomized a prospective study of 1 cm compared with 3 cm margin excisions for primary melanomas up to 2 mm in thickness; the 1 cm excision margins appeared to be safe for "early" melanomas up to 1 mm thick.[125] Wider margins are indicated for thicker lesions, but margins of greater than 2 cm do not seem warranted for any lesions.

Excision depth. Another question regarding surgical excision is the depth of the excision. The excision depth must encompass the entire tumor mass. The local excision width and depth have no purpose other than to prevent local recurrence. No local treatment has any influence on the development of systemic metastases. In the absence of local recurrence, any distant metastases must be assumed to have occurred before the definitive treatment. The evidence on whether to include fascia in the dissection is anecdotal at best. Kenady and associates[70] found no difference in survival related to removal of fascia, and in Balch and colleagues' survey,[9] 57% of those with stage I and 64% with stage II lesions underwent resection of fascia. It is unclear how much tumor spread through the fascial lymphatics actually occurs. This method of spread also may vary in different parts of the body. A nodular melanoma developing over the cheek, in which the skin is relatively thin, almost immediately comes into continuity with the superficial musculoaponeurotic (fascial) system of the face and the fascia overlying the parotid gland, which also is the first series of lymph nodes. Excision of this lesion might include the fascia; although this excision is technically difficult to perform, it is probably biologically appropriate. On the other hand, for a relatively superficial lesion on the back, with a thick pannus of fat beneath it, removing the underlying fascia hardly seems biologically necessary.

Method of closure. Another basic consideration is the method of closure. It has erroneously been said that any wound that can be closed primarily, without the need for a skin graft, probably represents an inadequate excision. This statement has no sound basis in surgical fact. The width and perhaps depth of the margin influence the prognosis, and the method of closure has no effect on the outcome. The most functional and aesthetically pleasing closure the surgeon can accomplish should be chosen.

REGIONAL LYMPH NODE DISSECTION. Statistically, tumors that are Clark level I and II have essentially no incidence of lymph node metastasis, and routinely removing lymph glands in the regional area of patients with level I and II tumors results in no increase in survival. Whether lymph node dissection is of value in lesions at level V is questionable because the prognosis is poor despite surgery.

Therapeutic regional lymph node dissection(TLND) on theoretic and practical grounds is indicated for patients who are known to have regional lymph node metastases, on the basis of clinically palpable nodes, or for those for whom there is a reasonably high suspicion that the lymph nodes are involved, even though they are not clinically palpable.[87] The pathophysiologic assumption is that some patients have local disease and disease spread to the lymph nodes, but no disease elsewhere. Only for this group would the inclusion of a lymph node dissection be reasonable in an operation designed to be curative. Another group of patients have lymph node involvement and probable spread beyond the nodes to involve visceral organs. A TLND in these patients is, in itself, a biologically unsound operation unless performed to aid diagnosis and to determine whether further therapy is indicated.

Elective regional lymph node dissections (ELNDs) are prophylactic lymph node dissections carried out in the absence of clinical evidence of regional node metastases because of the risk of occult or microscopic metastases existing in these nodes. The theoretic benefit of an ELND is the removal of regional lymph nodes before tumor cells disseminate from the regional lymph nodes to distant sites. Therefore this procedure may increase the survival of these patients over patients treated by delayed therapeutic resection, done only when regional lymph node metastases become evident.

Stage I melanoma. Stage I melanoma, by definition, does not have palpable (and therefore clinically positive) node involvement. The decision to perform an ELND in these patients is predicated on statisically valid suspicion that there may be involvement. In lesions that are thinner than 0.75 mm and are at Clark levels I and II, wide local excision is curative almost all the time, indicating either that the lymph nodes are not involved or that the host defense system is adequate to handle the spread. In either case, the addition of a node dissection would increase morbidity, potential complications with wound healing, infection, and the possibility of lymphedema of the extremity, without adding to the cure rate (Figure 20-12).

In stage I disease, with thicker lesions, the decision to perform an ELND is less clear. The absolute necessity of an adequate biopsy is emphasized by these clinical dilemmas. In lesions of intermediate thickness, ranging from 0.76 to 4.0 mm, or for lesions at Clark levels III, IV, and perhaps V, many persons advocate an ELND particularly when the lesion is in an area where the likely lymph node drainage is obvious. A review by Balch and associates[9] indicated that for lesions of 0.76 to 1.5 mm, 27% of the surgeons surveyed would perform an ELND, and for thicker lesions the percentage increased to 38%. When ELND is performed in these circumstances, the chances of finding positive nodes, when they were not palpable clinically, was 0 for lesions less than 1.0 mm in thickness, 26% to 36% for lesions between 1.0 and 2.0 mm, and more than 50% for lesions thicker than 4.0 mm.

The question of which lymph nodes to remove is pertinent. Lymphoscintigraphy has indicated that the classic described drainage patterns are incorrect in almost half

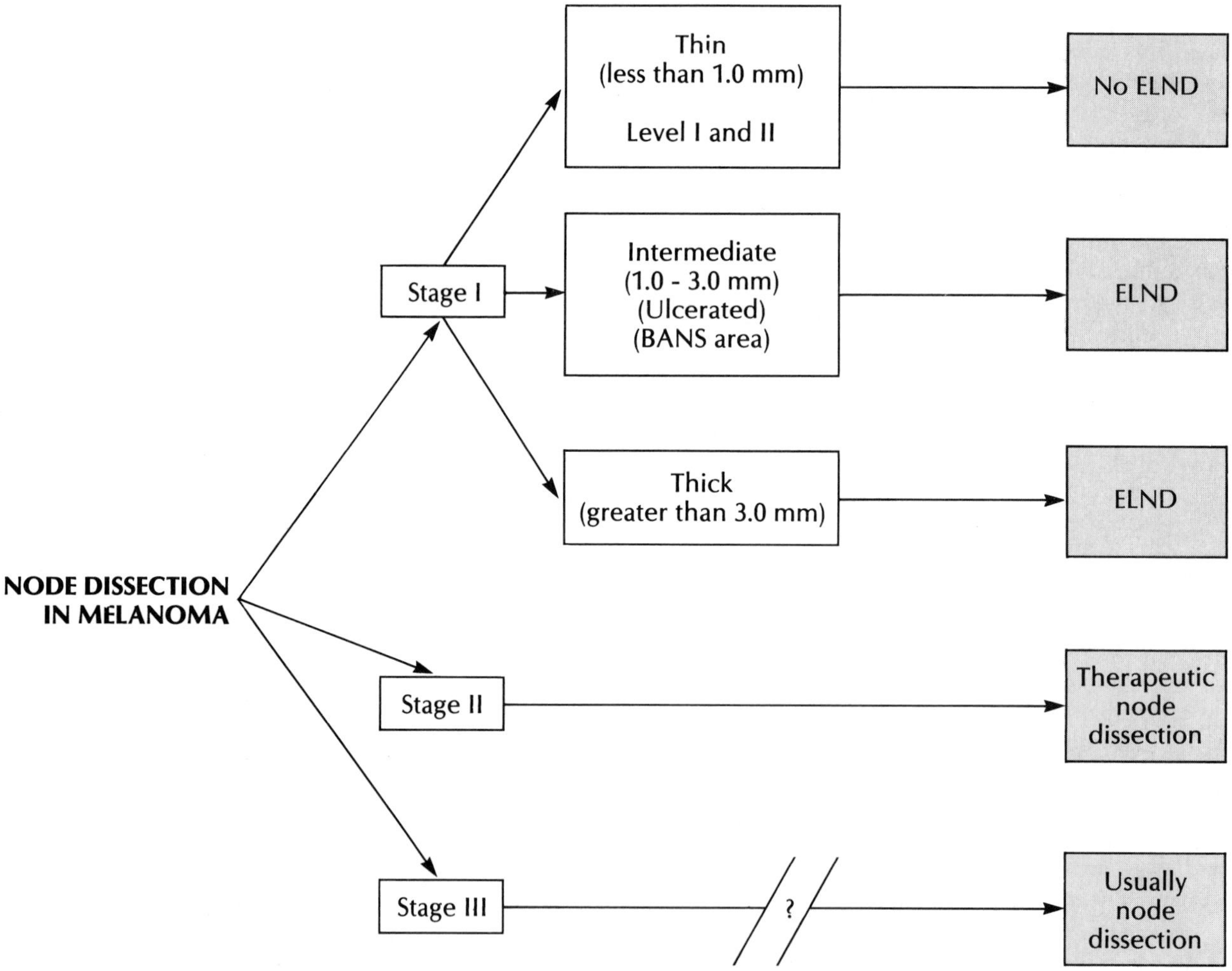

FIGURE 20-12 Algorithm for elective regional lymph node dissection in a melanoma.

of cases of head and neck and trunk lesions. Except for extremity lesions whose drainage is sure, lymphoscintigraphy should be part of the planning.[89]

The *real* question is whether ELND makes any difference, and this is not so clear. Some observers will now refine the indications for ELND to include lesions in which there is or has been ulceration and for lesions in the BANS area.[33] In these circumstances the WHO statistics suggest that the survival of those who have had an ELND is about 22% better over a 10-year period than survival of those in whom the nodes were not removed.[9]

Studies have indicated that, if nodes are to be operated on, they should all be removed because when they are involved, there are almost always several or more nodes involved and the removal of just the enlarged or suspicious nodes is risky.[48] Furthermore, probably it is better, and certainly more practical, for the ELND to be performed, if not in continuity, at least at the same time that the definitive excision is performed. It has been suggested that removing the primary lesion loosens cells into the lymphatics, and the nodes act as a protective filter; their removal several weeks later therefore might be more biologically sound.[99] In practice, this has not been shown to improve survival.

Stage II melanoma. In stage II the lymph nodes are involved clinically. Most agree that this is an indication for regional node dissection. A survey reported that 85% of surgeons would perform a node dissection for clinically positive node involvement, and histologically the nodes are involved about 56% of the time.[9] Therefore it is clear that, even when the nodes are palpable, the findings may be inflammatory or otherwise unrelated to tumor almost half the time. The statistics are always ambiguous and true insight is difficult to achieve. The involvement again is related to thickness. When the primary lesion is between 1.5 and 3.0 mm, the chance of the nodes being involved is 48% and increases to 69% when the lesion is thicker than 3.0 mm.

One approach is outlined in the algorithm in Figure 20-12. For thin stage I lesions (less than 1.0 mm), no ELND is indicated. For lesions in stage I between 1.0 and 3.0 mm, an ELND is probably indicated, particularly if the lesion is or has been ulcerated or is located in the BANS area. For lesions thicker than 3.0 mm and for all stage II lesions, node dissection is indicated.

Stage III melanoma. When distant metastases are present, local removal of tumor and lymph nodes is sometimes appropriate to provide palliation of symptomatic, local, and regional disease.

SENTINEL NODE. The concept of the "sentinel" node evolved from a desire to identify whether a lymphatic drainage basin contains lymph nodes with tumor by some method other than removing all the nodes. When a vital blue dye is injected intradermally at the primary melanoma or biopsy site, the dye will spread lymphatically and stain the most proximal or "sentinel" node of the lymphatic basin. This and perhaps other nearby nodes are excised and subjected to intense histologic examination, perhaps with special melanoma stains. If they are positive, the entire node basin is removed; if they are negative the dissection is stopped. The incidence of tumor "skipping" the sentinel node is less than 1%. Morton and associates[89] identified the sentinel node in 194 of 237 lymphatic basins and detected metastases in 40 (21%) on routine H & E stains. Metastases were present in 47 (18%) of 259 sentinel nodes but in nonsentinel nodes as the only site of metastases in only 2 of 3079 nodes. The false-negative rate was less than 1%.

Adjuvant Therapy

CHEMOTHERAPY. Chemotherapy may be used either as a prophylactic measure or for palliation and may be considered by either the systemic route or perfusion.

Systemic chemotherapy. Systemic chemotherapy has been used primarily for palliation. The drug most used is imidazole carboxamide (dacarbazine, DTIC). The response rate may reach only 20%.[30] Prolonged treatment for at least 6 months after remission seems to be important. Many studies of chemotherapy refer to response rates in which tumor shrinkage is the yardstick. In actuality, a shrinkage of 50% may sound promising, but it makes little difference if it is not accompanied by either improved quality or length of survival.

Regional chemotherapy. Combination chemotherapy is more promising. A combination of DTIC with BCNU (nitrosurea) plus cisplatin plus tamoxifen showed a complete remission rate of 11% and an overall response rate of 46%. Ariyan and associates[5] have studied normothermic regional perfusion of DTIC in 24 patients and have maintained 58% of the patients free from disease for 23 to 70 months. The isolated perfusion technique is only applicable to extremity lesions because the blood supply must be isolated and the drug infused into the extremity in high concentrations and then recovered in venous return to prevent toxic levels from spilling into the circulation. Perfusion also has been used with heat (hyperthermia). Other drugs that have been used include phenylalanine mustard, which has been the standard for 25 years and against which new drugs (dacarbazine, for example) must be measured.[5,85] Many of the studies have involved stage I disease, in which the presence of involved nodes may be unknown; the prognosis for the patients might be good, even without perfusion. Nevertheless, statistics showing survival rates for more than a decade of 78% of patients with stage I, levels IV and V lesions are very impressive.[76]

A combination of cystostatic (melphalan 1-1.5 mg/kg) regional perfusion with hyperthermia (42°C) as an adjunct to definitive surgery has been attempted in high-risk patients. The results showed a recurrence rate of 11% compared with 48% for the control group.

IMMUNE THERAPY. Studies of several decades ago indicated some cross-reactivity between the immune response to melanoma and the response to BCG (bacillus of Calmette and Guérin for tuberculosis) immunization. Melanoma lesions injected with BCG show an almost uniform response; unfortunately it is not a complete response, and only in less than 20% does it have any effect on lesions that were not injected. Gertrude Stein[116] said that "A difference, to be a difference, must make a difference." BCG does not seem to make much of a difference. Humphrey[64] has used an antigen prepared from the melanoma itself, which is clearly more specific, and preliminary data show promising results.

RADIATION THERAPY. Rosenberg and colleagues[108] have recently reported work designed to stimulate the host immune reponse with high-dose interleukin 2 (IL-2).[108] Of the 134 patients with metastatic melanoma treated, 9 (7%) achieved complete regression and 14 (10%) achieved partial regression for a total response rate of 17%. Certain tumors have always been considered "radio resistant," and further clinical trials of new dosage schemes or new methods of delivering the radiation have been slow to appear. However, if the radiation is fractionated differently and the individual treatments are in the range of 400 c-grey, rather than the usual 200 c-grey, the tumors may be responsive.[92]

MOHS' CHEMOSURGERY. Mohs' treatment bascially involves fixing the skin or at least removing the skin, fixing it, and examining it microscopically; this ongoing histologic examination helps determine the margin and depth that are adequate. Since Mohs' chemosurgery involves removing only abnormal-appearing tissue, it theoretically obviates the need to remove normal tissue. Although the data indicate that the cure rate for stage I melanoma treated by Mohs' chemosurgery is identical to that obtained with surgical excision, proof that Mohs' chemosurgery will produce a better functional or esthetic result remains to be seen.[31]

The average melanoma is 2 cm in diameter when first seen. Assuming that Mohs' chemosurgery can remove the entire melanoma, leaving a defect of at most 3 cm in diameter, a depressed circular scar can be the best result hoped for by spontaneous healing after the technique. Secondary surgical reconstruction is often necessary to improve the functional and esthetic appearance. Because the margins around the lesion for melanoma excision are now far less than with previous procedures, the avoidance of surgery and this additional defect would not seem to be a major advantage. The entire diagnosis, staging, prognosis, and need for lymphadenectomy and further adjuvant therapy of melanoma are predicated on an accurate tissue biopsy. An adequate biopsy *must* be obtained before instituting Mohs' treatment as well.

PROGNOSIS FOR MELANOMA

Favorable
Superficial spreading
Malignant lentigo
Thin (less than 1.0 mm)
Levels I and II (papillary dermis or above)
Women before menopause
Younger men
Extremities
Head and neck

Unfavorable
Nodular
Acral lentiginous melanoma
Thick (greater than 3.6 mm)
Levels IV and V (reticular dermis or subcutaneous)
Middle-aged persons
BANS area

Indeterminate or No Effect
Moderate thickness
Level III (upper reticular dermis)
Women during pregnancy

Results

The results of treating melanoma are difficult to present because of the confusing data (see accompanying box). The tumor is terrifying, not because it is necessarily so deadly but because it may be unpredictable and its recurrences may be spread over a decade or so rather than being concentrated, as with many other tumors, in the first year or so after treatment. Most lesions are seen in an early stage of superficial spreading and are relatively thin. Almost all these will be cured, and the overall cure rate is good.

Obviously survival varies depending on the form of therapy. A basic assumption is that all Clark level I melanomas will be cured. With local excision alone, the survival rate for level I melanoma is reported to be 100%. Thus any form of treatment more extensive than simple local excision is of no additional value.

For level II melanomas, even with local excision alone, the cure rates are also over 90%. Conversely, level V melanoma has an extremely poor prognosis, irrespective of the form of treatment used. As will be seen, the major therapeutic controversy and dilemma are in level III and level IV melanomas.

The superficial spreading melanoma is primarily in a radial growth phase; 70% of all lesions are superficial (levels I and II) and less than 0.75 mm thick when first seen. A better prognosis is anticipated for lesions identified in this stage. Similarly, malignant lentigo is usually found in a more superficial phase, and a more benign course is anticipated. When a tumor is identified as being a nodular melanoma with thickening, induration, and the other described characteristics, this corresponds with entry into the vertical growth phase. About 70% of nodular melanomas are in levels IV and V when first identified and have a poor prognosis. The clinical correlation and observations with the histologic staging by Clark have distinct diagnostic and prognostic value.

Modifications of Breslow's classification can also be correlated with survival. Patients with lesions that were less than 0.85 mm thick had an 8-year survival of 99% in the MMCCG* series. Those with lesions of 0.86 to 0.169 mm thick had a cure rate of 93%, those with lesions 1.7 to 3.6 mm thick had a cure rate of 69%, and those with lesions greater than 3.6 mm thick had a 38% survival rate. As expected, the incidence of metastasis increases as the thickness of the tumor mass increases.

PROBLEM: BENIGN SEBORRHEIC KERATOSIS

Keratinocytes and other nonpigmented cells of the skin are also subject to a variety of common benign, potentially malignant, and malignant tumors. Seborrheic keratoses are *not* malignant or premalignant. However, they are lesions that most often must be differentiated from premalignant lesions. Seborrheic keratoses are the most common skin tumors seen in older persons. They occur in men and women equally often and tend to occur centrally (chest, back, and proximal extremities), although they also occur in exposed areas on the face and hands (Figure 20-13, *A*). They begin as small (less than 1 cm), flat, well-defined, pigmented (yellow to brown) spots, often called *age spots*. They then typically enlarge, become raised, and become more pigmented. They often look greasy and scaly, typically appearing "stuck on." Occasionally, they may be rubbed off but will reappear. They sometimes are irritated by friction, particularly by clothing when they are in the groin or axilla. Some, particularly on the face, are pedunculated. The appearance is usually sufficiently characteristic to be diagnostic.

The patient may be reassured of ultimate benignancy. Biopsy is indicated when the differential diagnosis is not clear, such as when the lesions appear suddenly, grow rapidly or extensively, or are repeatedly irritated and inflamed. Biopsy, with the patient under local anesthesia, is indicated in these circumstances. Unless the lesions are small and easily excised, treatment is usually dermatologic by currettage, cautery, or cryosurgery.

PREMALIGNANT LESIONS

Often patients have a variety of benign, premalignant and actually malignant lesions. A combination is not nearly so unusual as might be expected, since the same predisposing factors seem to lead to actinic (solar) keratoses, seborrheic keratoses, basal cell carcinomas, squamous cell carcinomas, malignant lentigo (and malignant lentigo melanoma), and the more unusual keratoacanthoma.

PROBLEM: ACTINIC KERATOSIS

The most common premalignant skin condition is the actinic keratosis. It is the end result of the repeated injury-repair process that not only ages skin but also predisposes the skin to malignant degeneration. This process can result from solar radiation or from the ionizing radiation of roentgen rays used to treat acne or excessive hair growth, usually in women. The solar effect is most likely to take its toll on the areas of the body most exposed over the longest time: the face, back of the hands, shoulders, and back. It tends to occur later in life because it is the function of repeated exposure to the sun. This process can be accelerated and intensified into a shorter period among those whose occupation (farmers or sailors) or avocation (swimming or skiing) increases the exposure (Figure 20-13, *A*). The pigment in the cells is a protective device that evolution and adaptation have provided, but more to some than to others; for example, dark-skinned persons may be almost immune to these changes. Those who have no pigmentation (albinos), lack the ability to transfer pigment to keratinocytes (xeroderma pigmentosa), or are just fair skinned (red-heads, blondes, those of Northern Europe extraction) are the most prone to these changes. Northern Europeans who move to the more intense exposure of Australia develop these changes and the subsequent malignancies in almost epidemic proportions.

Clinical Presentation

Actinic keratoses begin on exposed areas and are initially well-defined, reddened areas with a scaling or papular appearance. There may be a halo of erythema around the lesion. With time they become darker and thicker, and areas of telangiectasia and atrophy can be seen. When malignancy develops, the lesions become firmer and thicker, and the speed of enlargement increases. Ulceration is the hallmark of malignancy. The malignancies developing in actinic keratoses rarely metastasize and are not as serious as those that develop de novo.

Diagnostic Studies

The changes begin in the epidermis with hyperkeratosis, with alternating areas of normal and diseased cells. The dermis begins to thin, and abnormal cells may be found in the upper dermis. There is an accompanying lymphocytic infiltration. The surface changes may be malignant, whereas the adnexal epithelium may preserve the architecture and prevent invasion until frank malignant transformation takes place.

Determining the natural history is difficult because

*Malignant Melanoma Consensus Conference Group

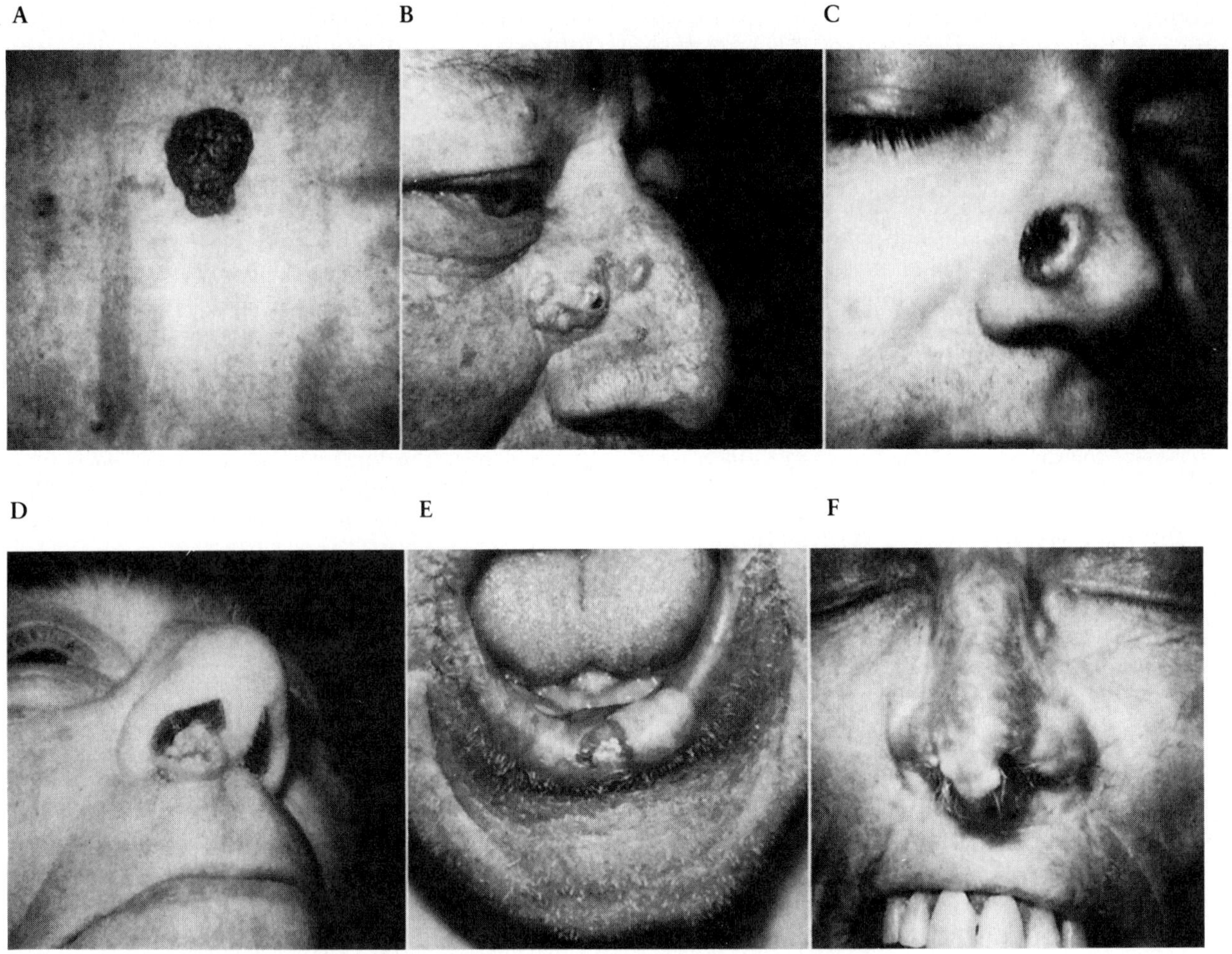

FIGURE 20-13 Common epidermal lesions. **A**, Seborrheic keratosis, with "greasy" stuck-on appearance. Other lesions are actinic keratoses. **B**, Basal cell carcinoma with nodular characteristics. **C**, Keratoacanthoma with a central keratin plug. **D**, Basal cell carinoma with raised, pearly borders and ulcerated craters. **E**, Leukoplakia—a questionable squamous cell carcinoma in the central part of the lip. **F**, Radiation keratoses with atrophy and telangiectasias on cheek 40 years after radiation exposure. **G**, Basal cell carcinoma of lower lid and severe aging changes in both lids. **H**, Squamous cell carcinoma that is highly invasive into the lacrimal apparatus and sinuses.

many lesions remain stable after removal of the offending radiation or other irritant. Others are treated and resolved. It is thought that about 20% to 25% eventually undergo malignant degeneration.

Management

The scope of treatment should be based on the fact that these lesions are superficial and not yet malignant. Destruction of the superficial offending cells is sufficient, and the adnexal epithelium, usually not involved, can repopulate and heal the surface. A variety of dermatologic approaches are effective such as the topical application of 5-fluorouracil or the use of cryosurgery with liquid nitrogen and curettage and cautery. Excision is used for lesions with some question of malignancy.

PROBLEM: LEUKOPLAKIA

The Greeks had a word for the condition leukoplakia: *white patch*. Unfortunately, it is hard to be more specific than the Greeks. Leukoplakia is actually a problem of mucous membrane rather than skin and, pathologically, is the result of irritation. It leads to keratinization, epithelial hyperplasia, and subsequently the development of squamous cell carcinoma. It is instigated by external irritants, particularly smoking.

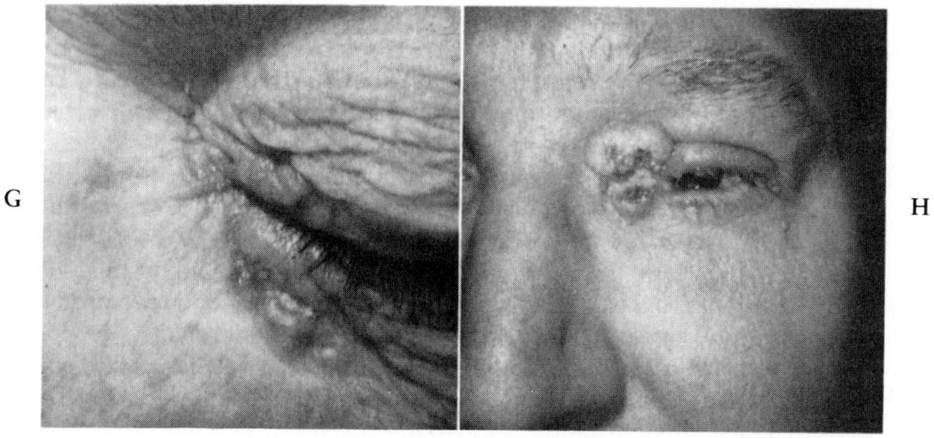

FIGURE 20-13, cont'd For legend see opposite page.

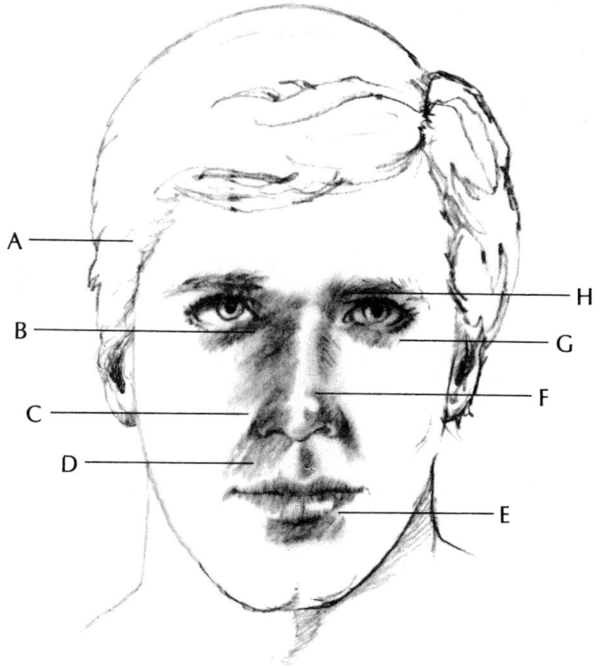

The lesions may be seen early in life in those with congenital skin and mucous membrane diseases, particularly congenital dyskeratosis. More commonly, it is seen as the end result of years of irritation.

About 6% to 10% of cases of leukoplakia are thought to become carcinomas, but this is almost impossible to know because most of these patients probably never seek treatment until malignancy develops. In those lesions seen when ulceration has already occurred, the incidence of malignancy is as high as 25% to 30%. The tumors that arise in areas of leukoplakia are different from those arising in actinic keratosis and should be considered *very* invasive.

Clinical Presentation

Leukoplakia may be found in the vagina, the mucous membrane of the oral cavity, and, pertinently, the lip, particularly the lower lip (Figure 20-13, *E*). The clinical picture is that of whitish, sometimes erythematous patches, which may be indurated, raised, or roughened. They are usually well defined, but as they enlarge, they may become confluent. The development of induration and particularly ulceration should arouse suspicions of malignancy and requires biopsy. Biopsy of leukoplakia shows the hyperkeratosis and acanthosis, as described previously.

MALIGNANT LESIONS

PROBLEM: BASAL CELL CARCINOMA

Basal cell carcinoma is more common in men than women by a 2:1 ratio. Large studies have shown an incidence in the population of 3% to 5% carcinomas of the skin per 1000 persons per year, of which about 60% to 75% are basal cell carcinomas. About 500,000 new cases occur annually.[98]

The most obvious and important predisposing factor is the chronic exposure to wind and probably sun, particularly in fair-skinned persons with less pigment. Certain occupations such as farming obviously aggravate those predisposed. In xeroderma pigmentosa patients the cells are unable to transfer melanin from the melanocyte dendrite to the keratinocytes and are therefore more exposed to solar radiation. Basal cell carcinomas also have been associated with previous injury such as burns, injury from ingestion of arsenicals (usually found in gardening), and years of X-ray exposure, but this is perhaps less true than for squamous cell carcinomas.

Basal cell carcinoma, the most common of malignant skin tumors, outnumbers squamous cell carcinoma by about 5:1. It is the most common skin cancer among whites; among blacks and Orientals, it is unusual. It is most common among the older population (over 50 years) rather than in all ages, even though occasionally it is identified in younger persons and children. It is the most common of tumors found on the face and most other exposed areas, rather than in areas hidden by clothing. It is the most common tumor in those who have xeroderma pigmentosa, a congenital disorder of the skin; it is the most common malignant tumor in children who have the nevoid basal cell carcinoma syndrome; and finally, it is the most common malignancy in patients with the nevus sebaceous of Jadassohn. Therefore, a "most common" description may be a useful statistical maneuver but must be altered and determined for any individual patient.

Basal cell carcinoma is almost always curable if the patient presents the surgeon with the opportunity to treat it at the curable stage and if the tumor is identified and approached thoughtfully with understanding of its pathophysiology and clinical behavior.

Clinical Presentation

History (Subjective Findings)

The lesion may have been present for a long time, perhaps 6 months or so. It tends to become irritated and then may seem to heal with an ointment purchased in the drug store.

Physical Examination (Objective Findings)

The spectrum of lesions that turn out to be basal cell carcinomas range from pink to black, scaling and flat to nodular, and smooth to ulcerated. For descriptive purposes, however, it is useful to divide them into three broad categories.

NODULAR. These are by far the most common. They are to be looked for particularly on the head (86%), most often above a line drawn across the face from the corner of the mouth to the tragus of the ear. They are particularly common along the eyelids (14%), in the nasolabial (16%) and cheek areas, and on the helix of the ear (11%). A fourth occur on the nose and 14% around the eyes, and the remainder of the 86% are distributed about the rest of the face.[112] These are the classic nodules with an umbilicated center and raised, pearly borders (Figure 20-13, *B* and *D*). The epithelial covering is thinned, and the underlying vessels can be seen as telangiectasias. They may be pigmented and confused with melanoma. The center may eventually ulcerate and has been referred to as a "rodent ulcer." Deceptive to patient and physician alike, these ulcerations may even seem to heal for a period.

SUPERFICIAL. These lesions tend to be pinkish, flat, and often scaling and, as opposed to the nodular lesions, occur in the less commonly exposed areas of the back and arms. These lesions may also seem to heal in the center, and there may even be some scarring. These have been described as morphea-like.

SCLEROSING. These slowly growing and ill-defined lesions are usually found on the head and neck. Often yellow and even waxy in appearance, they present the diagnostic problem of lacking a distinct margin. Central sclerosis and the appearance of healing occur with these lesions as well (also called morpheaform).

Diagnostic Studies

Diagnosis is by microscopic examination of tissue obtained by biopsy. In general, the biopsy should include an adequate sampling of the lesion from its center to its margin, including normal-appearing skin. "Shave" biopsies are also diagnostic but lack the precision of determining depth, particularly if the specimen should turn out to be a melanoma and not a basal cell tumor. Certainly the more typical lesions, particularly those smaller than a centimeter in diameter, are most appropriately treated by excisional biopsy in which the diagnosis and treatment are served by the same procedure.

Pathophysiology

Basal cell carcinoma, in its very name, defines itself as being malignant, but it is almost inappropriate to use the term. It is only locally malignant, and it is almost unheard of for a basal cell carcinoma to metastasize to either regional lymph nodes or systemically through the bloodstream; fewer than 200 cases of metastasis have ever been reported. Furthermore, it does not seem to arise from the malignant transformation of preexisting mature epithelial structures and does not possess the true cellular anaplasia usually associated with malignancy.

An interesting, biologically relevant anecdote is the work of Greene,[54,55] who developed a model for growing malignant tumors in the immunologically protected environment of the anterior chamber of the guinea pig's eye. Explants of biopsy tissue from malignant tumors would grow; none of the "benign" tissues tested as a control would grow. There were several exceptions. Benign pleomorphic adenomas of the parotid gland ("mixed tumors") appeared as explants in malignant salivary tumors; and all surgeons are familiar with their tendency to recur, appear in multiple foci, and even invade into normal tissue. On the other hand, the basal cell carcinoma and similar premalignant tissue would not grow.

It is thought that, even though basal cell carcinomas arise from the basal cell layer of the epidermis or from the lining of the hair follicles or sebaceous glands, the damage may begin in the dermis. Repeated solar or chemical injury results in damage to the papillary and subpapillary dermis and probably subsequent changes in the epidermis. Transplantation of normal epidermis onto damaged dermis results in the development of these cancers, whereas transfer of solar or chemically injured epidermis onto normal dermis does not.[123] Cells of similar appearance tend to pile on each other and form palisades at the periphery of the lesion. There is a characteristic fibrous reaction at the periphery, and there is a varying degree of lymphocytic reaction to the tumor.

Basal cell carcinomas usually grow slowly, and doubling times longer than a year have been identified. Even recurrent tumors grow slowly and therefore may not appear for a long time after the initial treatment. This slow, almost indolent behavior provides some latitude in the management choices. The major and critical exception to this description is the basal cell tumor in the immunosuppressed patient. Another exception is the tumor that invades across a mucocutaneous border and into mucous membrane. Whatever growth-retarding characteristics the skin possesses are apparently lacking in mucous membrane, and rapid extension is the rule. The most common areas of concern are in the medial eyelid area, where there is invasion into the lacrimal apparatus and then into the nose and sinuses, into the conjunctiva, and along the orbit and at the junction of the nasal skin and mucous membranes. In these areas growth becomes truly invasive and malignant (Figure 20-14).

Management

Surgical Management

Surgery with a margin of normal tissue, perhaps only 2 to 3 mm, is curative. Unfortunately, normal tissue cannot be identified with perfect accuracy either grossly or even by biopsy and frozen section examination. Nevertheless, a cure rate of 95% should be anticipated. Dellon[37,38] has reviewed patients in whom lesions have recurred in an effort to identify predictive factors. These include squamous differentiation in the cords of tumor cells seen histologically, irregularities in the peripheral palisades, absence of lymphocytic infiltration, and, clinically, the presence of tumor ulceration.

Closure of defects after removal of tumors should be predicated on the plastic* principle of restoring the area to its most satisfactory form, functionally and aesthetically. It makes no biologic difference whether this be by primary closure, by skin graft or flap, or even by leaving the wound open to close by *secondary intention* (granulation, contraction, and epithelialization occurring spontaneously in an open wound) (Figure 20-15).

MARGINS INVOLVED. In some patients, excision and primary closure appear adequate, and the final report some days later will indicate, in the words of the pathologist, that the "tumor is at the margin of resection." In some studies the argument is proposed that, because only about a third or less of these (with "margins involved") actually do recur and those which do can usually be cured by resection of the recurrence, a course of observation is appropriate.[60] Dellon[37,38] has reviewed patients with "positive margins" and determined that those specimens which, on review, showed palisading in more than 75% of the tumor cords had recurrence rates in excess of 95%, compared with no recurrence in those with less than 25% palisading. Tumor ulceration and absence of lymphocyte response were also, but less dramatically, predictive. In areas that are particularly prone

**Plastic,* from the Greek *plastikos,* meaning "shape" or "form." Plastic surgery is the "surgery of form."

A B C

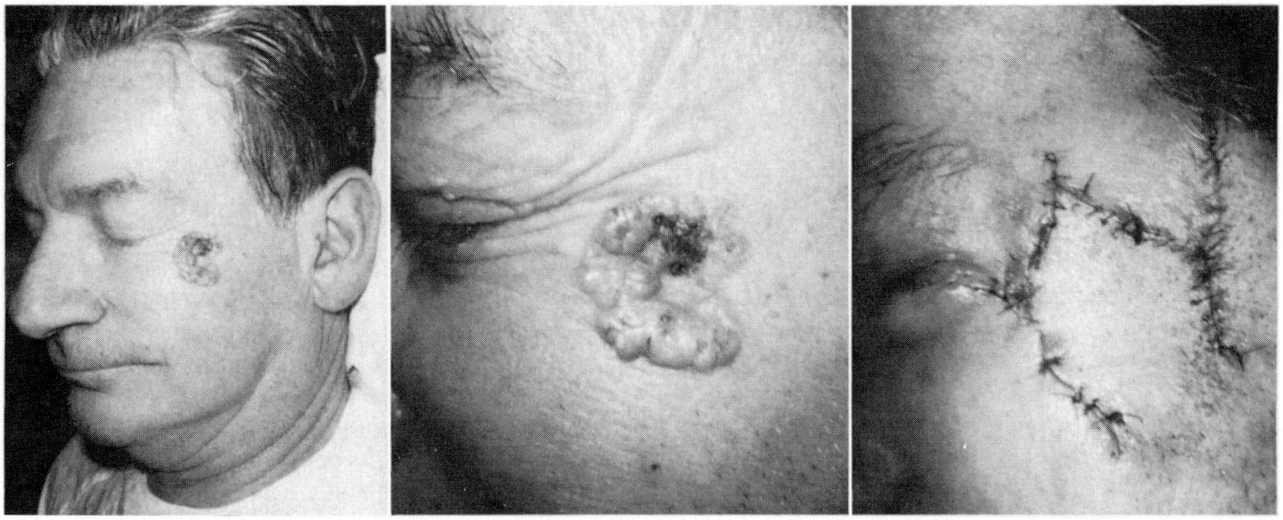

FIGURE 20-14 Basal cell carcinoma. **A,** Basal cell carcinoma of the left cheek. **B,** Close-up view of raised, pearly borders and superficial ulceration. **C,** After excision and closure with a rhomboid flap.

A

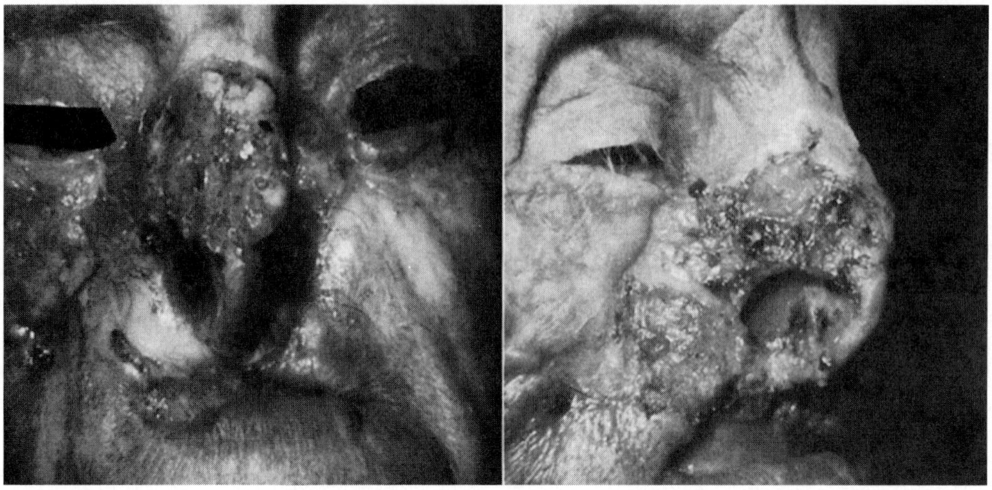

B

FIGURE 20-15 Basal cell carcinoma. **A,** Ulcerating lesion treated for 15 years with ointments in the hope that it would disappear. The lesion was diagnosed as basal cell carcinoma. **B,** Lateral view. There was no metastasis.

to rapid or uncontrolled invasion, such as the medial eyelid and areas near other mucous membranes, reexcision is probably indicated. Conversely, in patients in whom reexcision might be emotionally disturbing, in whom the tumor appeared less aggressive in terms of biology and location, who are readily available and dependable for follow-up, or in whom the reexcision would severely alter the closure problem and require extensive reconstructive procedures, a course of observation might be presented as an alternative.

Curettage

The curettage technique is highly favored by dermatologists and rightfully so, since the cure rate and aesthetic results in well-chosen lesions are excellent. The lesion is basically cored out, the base cauterized, and the wound allowed to close by secondary intention.

Chemosurgery

Mohs' chemosurgery is a highly effective and predictable way of managing basal cell carcinomas and is of most value in those lesions in which margins are difficult to identify grossly and for which removal of adequate margins by standard surgical techniques would be unnecessarily destructive to normal structures.[24] It is also effective for recurrent disease. Serial tissue removal is accomplished and each specimen examined for margins. Mohs' original technique of "fixing" the tissue with zinc chloride has now been modified and simplified, but the principle is valid.[88] The wound, however, remains open. Small areas that close by secondary intention may do so with minimal distortion and produce excellent results. Larger areas, however, may close only with severe distortion, and reconstructive surgery becomes part of the management.

Chemotherapy

Systemic chemotherapy has no role in the management of this disease unless growth becomes uncontrollable, usually via mucous membrane invasion. However, topically applied agents are effective in some superficial lesions. In the nonnodular, nonindurated, superficial, scaling lesions, particularly in areas with mixed premalignant disease such as actinic keratoses, the use of topical 5-fluorouracil may be effective. Its use is probably best reserved for premalignant disease. The patient applies the agent regularly for several weeks, and a highly irritative inflammatory reaction is followed by healing with a smooth, pinkish, normal-appearing epithelial covering. Failure of the treatment can be succeeded by other forms of treatment.

Radiation Therapy

Almost any lesion that can be cured by surgery can be cured by radiation therapy, and vice versa (cure 92%).[40] Therapeutic radiation kills cells by preventing replication; the "kill" occurs only when division and cell-line propagation must occur. Because basal cell tumors divide very slowly, even more slowly than the surrounding normal tissue, the disappearance of the tumor may occur slowly, providing ample time for the normal cells to migrate in and "heal" the defect. This therapy usually leaves a satisfactory aesthetic result. Radiation therapy requires multiple visits, leaves permanent changes in the skin that make further radiation to the same area less safe, and is carcinogenic in itself, a consideration obviously most significant for the younger patient for whom the long lag time between radiation and tumor induction (25 to 30 years) may be a real rather than theoretic problem.

PROBLEM: SQUAMOUS CELL CARCINOMA

As opposed to basal cell carcinoma, squamous cell carcinoma of the skin is a truly malignant tumor, which arises from the keratinizing cells of the skin. The second most common cancer in humans, it occurs in about 1 in 1666 people in the United States per year (100,000 per year). It does, however, account for only about 2000 deaths per year.

Most of the same factors that predispose a person to actinic changes, senile keratoses, and basal cell carcinoma are also likely to lead to squamous cell carcinoma. It too results from exposure to solar radiation, particularly in the fair skinned. It too is related to certain premalignant conditions such as xeroderma pigmentosa, Bowen's disease, and leukoplakia. The exposure to arsenicals is known to be carcinogenic, particularly for squamous cell carcinoma, as is the prior exposure to radiation therapy, whether for the treatment of previous malignant disease or, more commonly, for treatment of benign conditions such as acne or for depilation. Accidental radiation among health workers, particularly dentists, was a striking hazard until the dangers were well recognized and appropriate measures taken to prevent the exposure.

Traumatic induction of cancer has been documented, and any chemical or mechanical injury that can require the tissue to repeatedly heal itself can lead to either premature aging or malignancy. Although the incidence of carcinoma in burn scars is unknown, 2% to 3% of all squamous cell carcinomas do occur in burn scars. Marjolin described this form of malignancy in unhealing

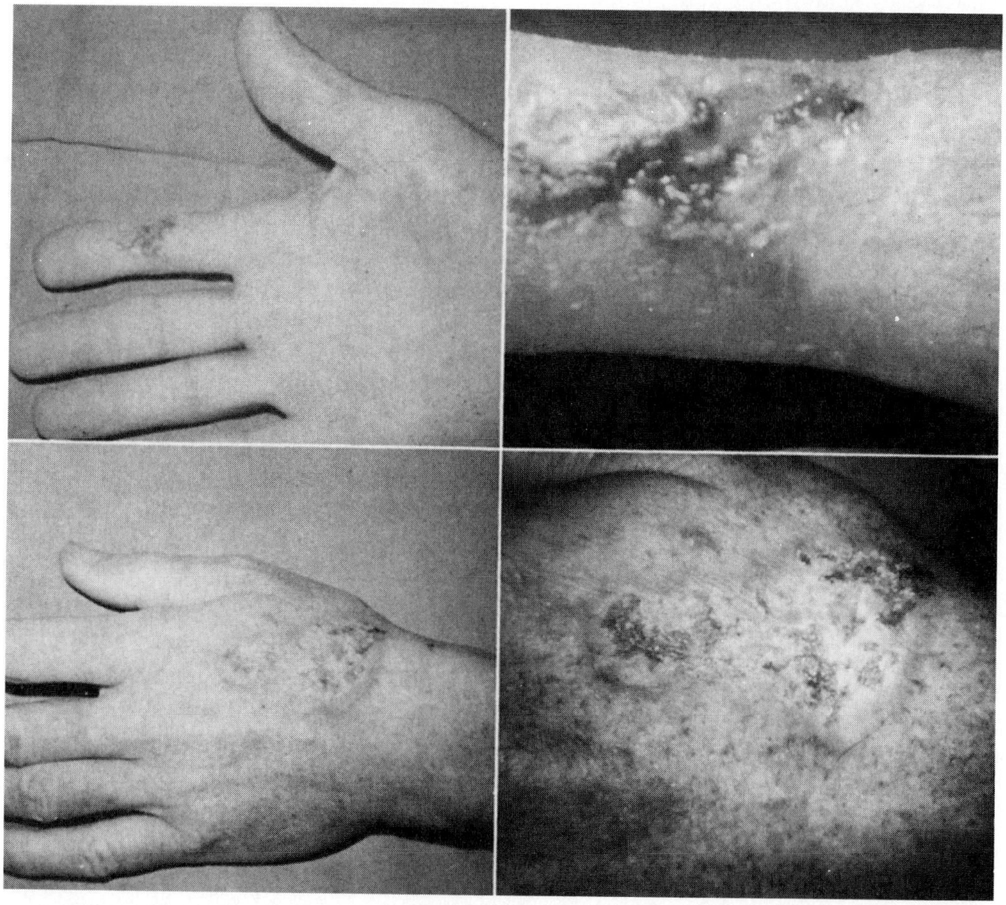

FIGURE 20-16 Squamous cell carcinoma after injury. **A,** Index finger of a dentist who exposed this part to X-ray beams repeatedly for years. **B,** Squamous cell carcinoma. **C,** Back of the hand 15 years after a chemical burn. It never completely healed. **D,** Squamous cell carcinoma.

wounds and includes, in addition to the burns, chronic vascular ulcers, osteomyelitis wounds, and unhealed pressure sores (all are termed *Marjolin's ulcers*)[6,7] (Figure 20-16).

Clinical Presentation

Squamous cell carcinomas tend to occur in the sites most affected by predisposing factors. Because solar exposure and actinic changes are the most important, most of the tumors occur on the face, ears, lips, and hands. Those on the lips tend to affect the lower lip, rather than the upper, and may be associated with leukoplakia. These patients usually have smoking (cigarette, cigar, and pipe) as additional predisposing factors. The lesion often begins within the predisposing lesion, becoming inflamed, then indurated; as it enlarges and becomes raised, it changes its appearance and becomes more ragged and often ulcerated. The course is much more rapid than that of basal cell carcinoma, which may take years to evolve. It must be differentiated from keratoacanthoma, which is also a rapidly growing, raised, smooth lesion but with a characteristic keratin plug in the umbilicated center. Verrucous carcinoma is a variant that can arise in oral papillomas, on the foot, or in preexisting condyloma acuminata around the anal area (Figure 20-17). Marjolin's ulcers are squamous (rarely basal) cell carcinomas arising in areas of chronically unhealed wounds such as burn scars, stasis or other ulcers, and osteomyelitis and tend to occur on the extremities.[6] More than 90% of skin cancers that occur on the hand are squamous cell carcinomas, some of which are associated with prior exposure to radiation (Figure 20-16). Radiation of the face for the removal of hair or to reduce the activity of oil glands in acne causes problems 20 to 25 years after the incident, when the patient is in the late forties and the treating physician is long since gone. The effects are diffuse over the involved area and on occasion may require that areas of the face be resurfaced. Arsenical exposure results in carcinomas on the hand or legs or may be distributed over the trunk, particularly the back.

The presence of lymph node involvement is unusual when the patient is first seen. The presence of larger lesions (more than 2 cm in diameter), poor differentiation, lesions in burn scars, and other Marjolin's ulcer situations has an incidence of nodal involvement of 21% to 35% when first seen.[6,7]

Diagnostic Studies

Early in the course there are often stages of in situ, or noninvasive, carcinomas. Microscopic examination is necessary to confirm the noninvasive nature. It is assumed that these in situ lesions with time will become invasive. The degree of invasion is important, and stages, not dissimilar to Clark's classifications for melanoma, have been applied to squamous cell carcinomas as well. A review of invasive carcinomas showed that the deeper levels of invasion (levels IV and V) had a much higher incidence of recurrence either locally or in regional lymph nodes.

Pathophysiology

Factors that induce a reparative process in tissue may result in the tissue becoming either old or malignant. Hayflick[61] has demonstrated that cells in tissue culture go through approximately 50 cell divisions, at which time they either die of old age or take on the uncontrolled growth characteristics of malignancy. Life experiences

A

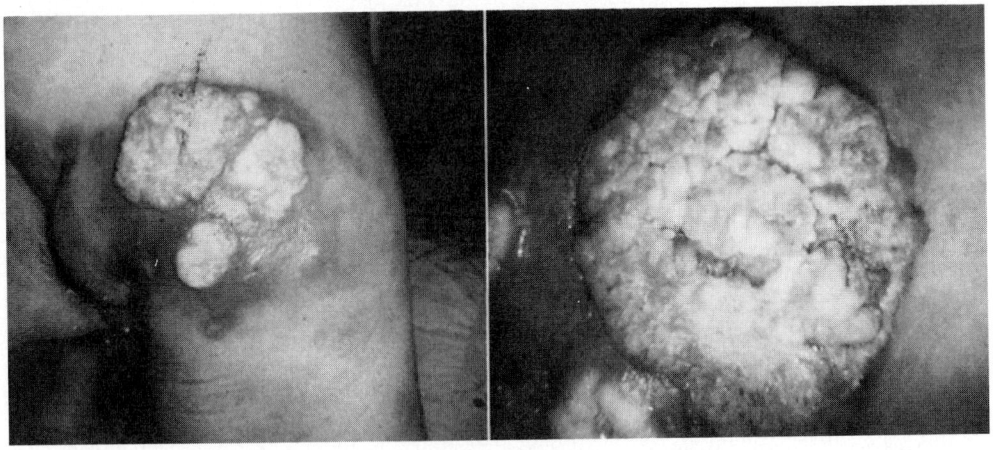

B

FIGURE 20-17 Verrucous squamous cell carcinoma. **A,** This ambulatory patient, who lacks sensation, developed carcinoma in a pressure sore that had failed to heal for 25 years (Marjolin's ulcer). **B,** Close-up view of verrucous carcinoma.

demonstrate that skin exposed to wind, radiation from ultraviolet or X rays, or skin that has been burned loses its elasticity prematurely, looks old because of wrinkles, sags, and has inordinate numbers of "age spots," or keratoses, and a high incidence of skin cancers. Those persons whose skin is least pigmented (the fair skinned and red haired) are far more susceptible to these environmental problems than blacks and more deeply pigmented whites.

Warren[128] has established criteria that should be present before a tumor can be said to have resulted from any specific injury—the "traumatic" induction of cancer. These include evidence that (1) the tissue was normal before the injury; (2) the injury was severe enough to have induced the reparative process and the cell type of the cancer is characteristic of the reparative process; (3) the site of the injury and the site of the subsequent tumor are the same; and (4) there is sufficient time between the injury and the development of cancer.

Burn scar carcinoma is an example. Skin that has been burned and heals by scar epithelium is often unstable, and minor injury may result in repeated efforts at healing. In such areas of repeated breakdown, squamous cell carcinoma may result. Some skin cancer occurs in old burn scars an average of 35 years after the original injury and only in unstable areas. It has never been described in burn areas that have been skin grafted. Arons and associates[7] have reproduced the pathophysiologic process experimentally; animals wounded and then repeatedly wounded as they attempt healing go through stages of reactivity, acanthosis, pseudoepitheliomatous hyperplasia, and finally skin malignancy.

It is the same for humans; each of these stages can be seen sequentially or often at the same time in the same patient. Studies on the induction of squamous cell carcinoma have documented the progression from the inflammation and chronic inflammatory and fibrotic response of the healing process, to hyperkeratosis, and finally to pseudoepitheliomatous hyperplasia as the immediately premalignant phase. In addition there is atrophy (as in aging), telangiectasia, and finally ulceration. Unlike basal cell carcinoma, squamous cell carcinoma, as part of its natural history, can be expected to metastasize. It is assumed that chronologically, after local invasion, the first line of spread is by the lymphatics to the regional lymph nodes and only later by the bloodstream to distant sites.

Another predictive characteristic of tumors is their degree of differentiation on histologic examination. The tumor itself is characterized by irregular squamous epithelium invading into the dermis. Well-differentiated lesions have keratin pearls, and the individual cells are keratinized. Poorly differentiated cells lack these characteristics. Most of the tumors are highly differentiated, which may account for the high degree of success in treatment. Among well-differentiated lesions, the recurrence rate may be less than 10%, compared with 25% to 30% for less differentiated lesions. Furthermore, the presence of a solar change and areas of noninvasive tumor within the specimen is favorable, and an incidence of recurrence of less than 3% has been reported.

Management

The treatment of squamous cell carcinoma uses the same basic modalities as those used in basal cell carcinoma, recognizing further that this is truly an invasive, malignant lesion with the potential for metastasis. The principle involves destroying the local lesion and deciding whether and when to treat regional lymph nodes (Figure 20-18).

Surgical Management

Surgery includes the biopsy. For lesions smaller than 1 cm in diameter, this usually is an excisional biopsy with a 5 to 10 mm margin of normal-appearing tissue. Clear margins and the previously identified prognostic factors help determine whether further excision is indicated. Margins involved with tumor reported by the pathologist require further treatment when the diagnosis is squamous cell carcinoma. Treatment is usually reexcision when feasible because many radiation therapists wish to avoid delivering postoperative radiation to the healing wound. Radiation therapy is better in the more oxygenated preoperative tumor than in the healing wound.

Closure is by the best reconstructive techniques to maintain form and shape and achieve the best aesthetic result possible. There is no scientific benefit in closing a wound in a shabby way or with an unsightly skin graft because the surgeon does not wish to "hide" a recurrence.

Lymph Node Dissection

The indications for ELND are difficult to determine. The best studied situation is for carcinoma of the lower lip, in which prophylactic (when there are no palpable nodes) node dissection has been compared with node dissections performed only when nodes were palpable at the time of treatment of the primary tumor and with nodes that became palpable only after treatment of the primary lesion. The cure rate when treatment is reserved for palpable nodes, even those appearing later, is equal to that when it is done prophylactically. Thus many unnecessary node dissections can be avoided (Figure 20-18). The safest rule of thumb is to strongly consider node dissection for situations in which the lymph nodes are already palpable. The most difficult situation is the patient with no palpable nodes but with a high-risk lesion such as a Marjolin's ulcer or a radiation carcinoma of the hand. There is no easy answer, and multiple other

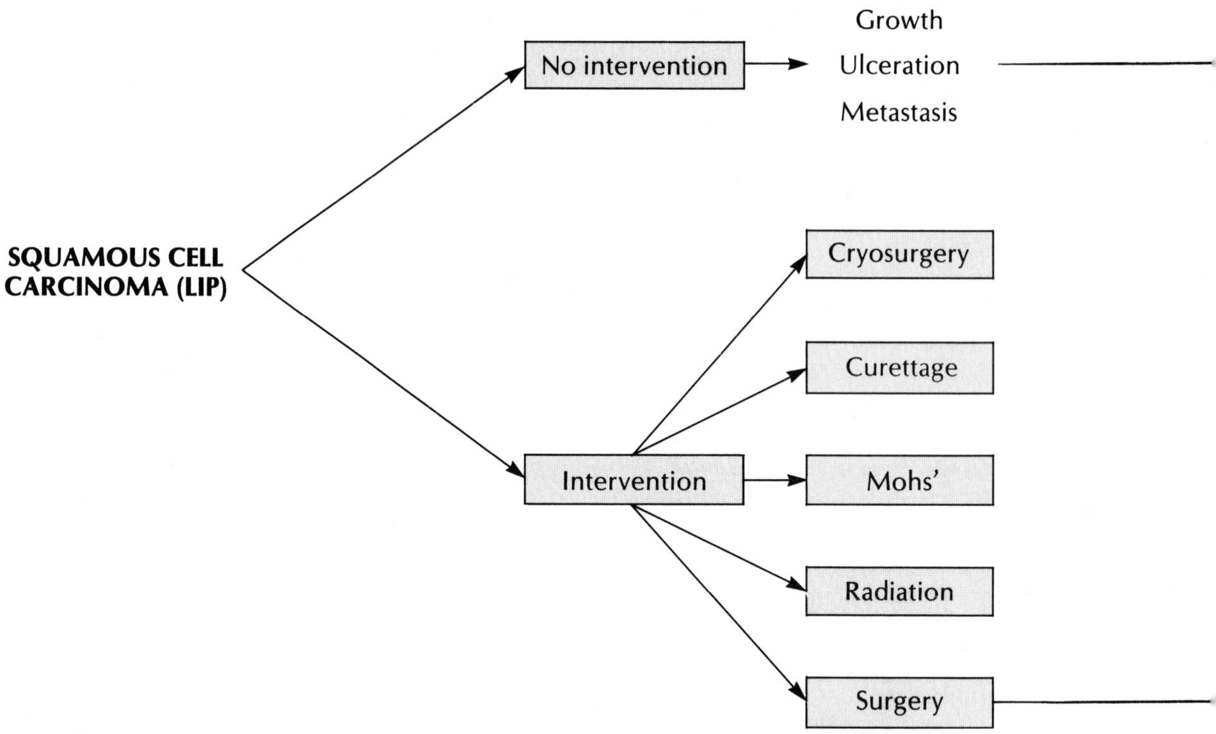

FIGURE 20-18 Algorithm for squamous cell carcinoma. The lip is used as an example.

factors must be taken into account (patient age, location of the lesion, and degree of invasion and differentiation).

Curettage

Curettage and cautery of the base are effective and are usually used by dermatologists rather than surgeons who, in general, are less familiar with and therefore perhaps less comfortable with this technique. Because many lesions are treated by dermatologists, even without biopsy, the vast majority of skin cancers, including squamous cell carcinomas, are never recorded in the tumor registries of hospitals or the states that maintain them. The tumors recorded in hospitals are selected tumors and represent the most difficult in the opinion of those who refer the patients. Furthermore, statistics that are reported by major cancer centers such as the National Cancer Institute are even more selected and may not reflect the true picture in the population.

Radiation Therapy

As in basal cell carcinoma, the cure rate for squamous cell carcinoma from radiation therapy is every bit as good as that from surgery. Certain areas—such as the hands, lower portion of the legs, skin heavily damaged by previous actinic change, and particularly areas of skin previously radiated—tolerate radiation therapy poorly. Good radiation therapy requires careful fractionation of the treatment course over time. Because squamous cell carcinomas have a more rapid turnover rate than basal cell carcinomas, the lesions tend to disappear more rapidly. This rapid disappearance may be only a Pyrrhic victory because the more anaplastic and invasive and the more rapidly a tumor is dividing, the more rapidly it will disappear with radiation; also the more rapidly it will tend to reappear if not cured.

Chemosurgery

Mohs' chemosurgery using either zinc chloride or nonfixation techniques enables the treating physician to remove only tissue that seems to be histologically involved. This selective removal is most important in body areas in which conservation of neighboring tissue is critical, such as the eyelids, the nasolabial area, and around the ears. On the lips, for instance, wedge excision is so effective and the tissue remaining for reconstruction so adequate that the more cumbersome chemosurgery, requiring its special expertise and facility, is less likely to be used. Its cure rate is equal to that of other modalities.

Chemotherapy

Topical chemotherapy with 5-fluorouracil is effective in the early, nonindurated, noninvasive phases of squamous cell carcinoma and in lesions such as Bowen's disease (discussed later). The degree of effectiveness is

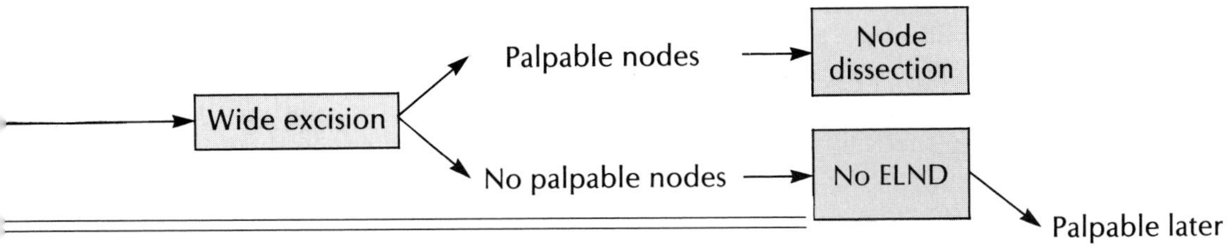

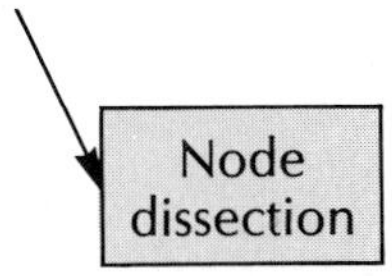

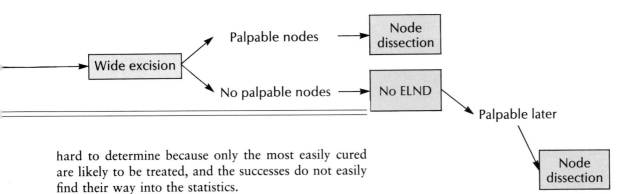

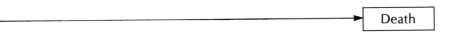

hard to determine because only the most easily cured are likely to be treated, and the successes do not easily find their way into the statistics.

Patient Education and Follow-Up

Almost all skin malignancies and even some premalignant lesions can be statistically and even experimentally linked to the environment. In few areas of patient management is education of such value in preventing recurrence and the development of new malignancies.

Solar Damage

By far the most important of the predisposing factors is the sun. Studies indicate that even a small amount of ultraviolet radiation may be significant, and certainly by the time the patient is seen with clinical lesions, the causative factor has been at play for many years and has involved all the neighboring areas, which may still look essentially normal. After management of the offending lesion the patient should be urged to avoid all unnecessary, unprotected exposure of the skin and, when exposed, to use appropriate sun blockers. Commercial products are rated by their sun protective factor (SPF), and a rating of 15 is adequate protection.

Smoking

Smoking is most assuredly a factor in leukoplakia of the lip and oral cavity, and the need to stop smoking cannot be overemphasized. Studies of oral cancer have indicated that the recurrence rate for those who stop smoking is only a fraction of what it is for those who continue.

Radiation

Currently almost no workers and few patients are ever accidentally exposed to radiation. It is important to continue education of patients and physicians to avoid the use of X rays for management of benign conditions (such as keloids, scars, and hemangiomas) or even trivial aesthetic reasons (such as depilation or acne). The effects of radiation on the skin may not be manifest for 20 to 30 years, but because the radiation is given in childhood or young adulthood, the late effects appear in the prime years.

Arsenicals

The exposure to arsenicals is most unusual and occurs primarily in those involved in serious gardening as a vocation or avocation. Fowler's solution for treating psoriasis also contains arsenic. The association of arsenic and malignancy is not nearly so well documented as the past literature would imply, but avoidance of excessive exposure would be wise.

OTHER LESIONS

PROBLEM: KERATOACANTHOMA

Keratoacanthoma have been described as a "surgeon's dilemma."[22] They are benign and self-limited and yet can be locally destructive and difficult to diagnose. The problem in differentiation from squamous cell carcinoma may be as difficult for the surgical pathologist as for the clinician. Keratoacanthomas may and often do arise from normal skin, in contrast to skin cancers, which tend to arise in solar or otherwise damaged tissue. Their distribution is similar to that of carcinomas—on the face, particularly the nose (Figure 20-13, C), on the cheeks, and around the eyebrows. They also occur on the hands, wrists, and forearms.

The course is one of abrupt onset, with rapid enlargement of a smooth-surfaced, regular, raised, pinkish, nodular lesion; this then usually develops a central umbilication and the classic keratinous central plug. This picture is similar, except in rapidity of growth, to that of nodular basal cell carcinoma. After a quiescent period of weeks to several months the lesions begin to resolve and ultimately disappear, leaving a thin, irregular scar. Unfortunately, this tidy clinical course fails to occur in as many as a third of the cases. An incidence of about 20% to 40% being associated with actual squamous cell carcinoma has been reported.[22]

In some, the lesion size can be impressive, and the local destruction of tissue is hardly benign. In critical areas, such as the medial canthal region of the eyelids, the surgeon cannot afford to allow irreparable damage while anticipating the hoped for resolution.

PROBLEM: NEVOID BASAL CELL EPITHELIOMA

Also known as Gorlin's syndrome or the basal cell nevus syndrome, nevoid basal cell epithelioma is an autosomal dominant condition characterized by the childhood onset of multiple basal cell carcinomas.[52] There are other major problems, including cysts of the jaws, bifid ribs, abnormalities of the vertebrae, and abnormally short metacarpals. Neurologic abnormalities include mental retardation, electroencephalographic abnormalities, and calcification of the dura. Seizures may be encountered. Pits of the hands and feet are almost a characteristic feature of the disease but unfortunately may not appear until later, even into the second decade, well after the other features appear.

The skin lesions are those of basal cell carcinomas but without the classic appearance. Their onset may be as early as the first year or two of life, frequently at adolescence, and they may continue to appear throughout a lifetime. They also lack the predilection for exposed areas, as with other basal cell carcinomas, and actually may be found anywhere on the body. They may be nondescript and look more like seborrheic keratoses or nevi and may occur in crops rather than singly. Despite this ominous sounding combination of problems, the course is benign, and specific treatment of the lesions by standard conservative techniques is complicated primarily by their numbers rather than the malignancy itself.

PROBLEM: NEVUS SEBACEOUS OF JADASSOHN

The nevus sebaceous of Jadassohn is a well-circumscribed, usually solitary, irregularly surfaced, plaquelike or raised lesion, usually found on the scalp, temple, or upper preauricular area. It is seen in children and occasionally is identified at birth[86] (Figure 20-19). It has a waxy appearance, and there is no hair growth. Microscopically there is hypoplasia of hair follicles and sebaceous glands; later the sebaceous glands become hyperplastic. The significance of these lesions is the 10% to 15% incidence of malignancy, usually basal cell carcinoma but also other adnexal carcinomas. These carcinomas also tend to develop early in adolescence, so their potential should be recognized and, where possible, the lesions excised before that time.

PROBLEM: BOWEN'S DISEASE

Bowen's disease is an interesting premalignant phenomenon, more accurately described as carcinoma in situ.[102] About 5% actually become invasive carcinoma (Figure 20-20). Its predisposing factors are the same as for actinic keratoses and carcinoma itself and include age, solar radiation, and a fair complexion. In addition, it is found in perhaps a third of cases in unexposed areas. It has been regularly thought of as part of the arsenical keratosis–carcinoma complex. Most often, however, there are no associated factors. Although there is not much retrospective statistical validation, Bowen's disease is thought to herald the presence of an occult internal malignancy. Because Bowen's disease and internal malignancies of various types are both seen with some frequency, the statistical correlation is difficult to make.

Clinically, Bowen's disease is rather nonspecific, with the most characteristic finding being a substantial degree of keratotic thickening and an underlying erythema. It has regular borders, and in about a third of patients there are multiple lesions. Histologically there are hyperkeratosis and parakeratosis with a distinctive disorganization of the architecture, almost an intraepidermal malignancy. The important feature is that, although the dermis may be inflamed and have a lymphocytic infil-

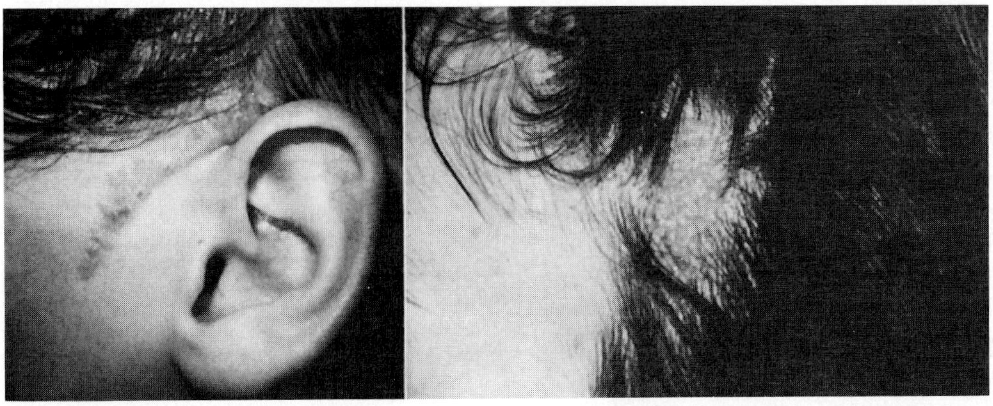

FIGURE 20-19 Nevus sebaceous of Jadassohn. A, Typical lesion—raised, waxy, and hairless. B, Lesion commonly found in the scalp that predisposes the person to basal cell carcinoma.

trate, there is no dermal invasion. When there is dermal invasion, the disease becomes invasive carcinoma and is no longer Bowen's disease.

Treatment includes curettage, cautery, cryosurgery, and topical chemotherapy, but most appropriate is surgical excision for biopsy and therapy.

PROBLEM: ERYTHROPLASIA OF QUEYRAT

Erythroplasia of Queyrat is a disease with a fascinating name that makes it more memorable than its frequency might warrant.[96] In some ways it is equivalent to Bowen's disease, involving mucous membrane, particularly the glans penis and foreskin (when present) and occasionally the vulva. The lesions are plaquelike and painless, with, as the name implies, a reddened surface. It is more likely than Bowen's disease to become malignant; when it does, it tends to be more invasive and aggressive. Local excision for biopsy and therapy is effective, but other topical measures are also appropriate if the superficial and localized nature can be confirmed.

PROBLEM: PAGET'S DISEASE

Paget's disease is its own disease with an eczema-like, crusted appearance developing on the areola of the female breast,[8] although occasionally found in the vulva or the anogenital area and rarely in the male breast.[67] Its major significance in the areolar form is the inevitable presence of underlying breast cancer. This breast cancer usually arises from the underlying ductal tissue and may be intraductal or invasive.

The characteristic findings on biopsy include the presence of Paget's cells within the epidermis. The pathologist can usually identify these characteristic cells on biopsy, which is the initial approach of the suspicious clinician. It is thought that these cells are derived from the underlying ductal tumor; their origin in nonmammary Paget's disease is less clear but probably is from underlying apocrine glands.

The treatment is that of the underlying breast disease and not Paget's disease as such, and the prognosis is related to the underlying disease.

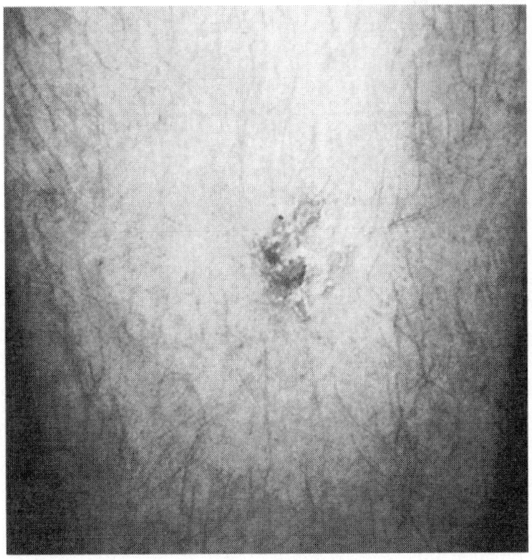

FIGURE 20-20 Bowen's disease (carcinoma in situ). An asymptomatic lesion on the thigh. There is no history of injury. Biopsy confirms the diagnosis.

PROBLEM: TRABECULAR CARCINOMA (MERKEL'S CELL CARCINOMA)

The skin contains epidermal cells with a presumed neural crest origin and a neurosecretory function. Tumors of

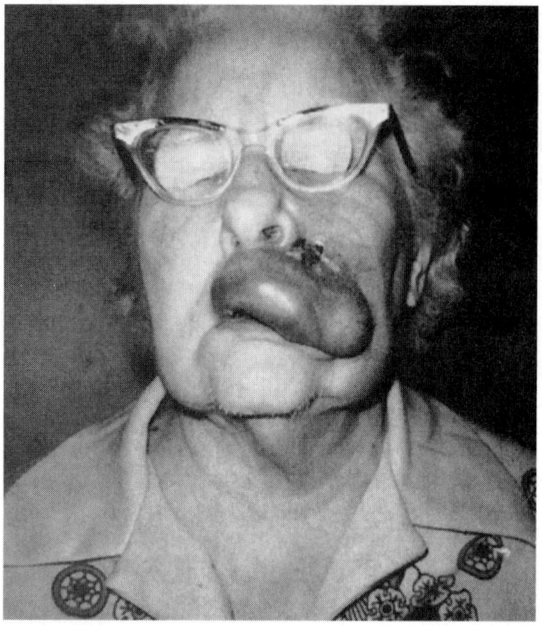

FIGURE 20-21 Merkel's cell carcinoma. Merkel's cells are neurosensory cells in the skin. Tumors are highly malignant and are known as trabecular or Merkel's cell carcinomas.

these cells form an aggressive type of skin cancer, found primarily in an older population[120] (Figure 20-21). Early metastasis to regional lymph nodes is seen, and a series of 54 cases showed that 29 developed local recurrence, 25 developed nodal metastases, and 8 had distal metastases. Although radiation therapy has been palliative for some, the treatment is surgical, with strong consideration given to ELND.

HEMANGIOMAS

Noninvoluting

A. Port-wine stain (small vascular channels) (nevus flammeus)
   1. Present at birth on face (commonly)
   2. Flat, then later raised, nodular
   3. Treatment: makeup, laser, surgery
B. Cavernous hemangioma
   1. Present deeper in tissue
   2. May involve bone (such as the mandible)
   3. May cause gigantism
C. Associated syndromes
   1. Sturge-Weber
      a. Occurs in 85% of port-wine stains with facial nerve distribution involved
      b. Affects cortical leptomeninges
      c. Mental retardation is common
   2. Klippel-Trenaunay-Weber (growth hypertrophy of the extremities)

Involuting

A. Salmon patch, stork bite
   1. Present in half of newborns
   2. Resolves in 4 to 5 months
B. Strawberry hemangioma
   1. Present in first few months of life
   2. Enlarges (proliferative)
   3. Ulceration and bleeding, then resolution and scarring
   4. May obstruct vision and cause amblyopia
C. Associated syndromes
   1. Thrombocytopenia
      a. Platelet trapping
      b. Consumptive coagulopathy
   2. Maffucci's—enchondromas and skeletal abnormalities

CUTANEOUS VASCULAR LESIONS

The vascular cutaneous lesions are among the most common of childhood skin problems and are usually what is meant by the term "birthmark." They have considerable variety in appearance, pathophysiology, prognosis, and management and are not a single disease. They can be divided into two major groupings depending on whether or not they will involute (see box).

PROBLEM: INVOLUTING VASCULAR LESIONS

PROBLEM Strawberry Hemangioma

Clinical Presentation

History (Subjective Findings)

Strawberry hemangioma presents early in infancy. The parents often report the presence of a small pale or pinkish spot on their child at birth. However, at that time no mass is present. The mass appears early in the child's life and may enlarge rapidly. The parents are unable to attribute any specific symptoms or signs to this development.

Physical Examination (Objective Findings)

The mass often is reddish blue and raised (Figure 20-22). The surgeon should measure and record the lesion's widest diameter. The surface epithelium is thinned, and the margins are irregular with areas of roughening. No sign of ulceration or bleeding is present. The mass is soft and compressible, but cannot be completely flattened. No thrill can be palpated, and no bruit can be heard. The physical examination is otherwise normal.

The differential diagnosis in these children is based on a careful review and examination. The box contains an outline of the common hemangiomas found in young

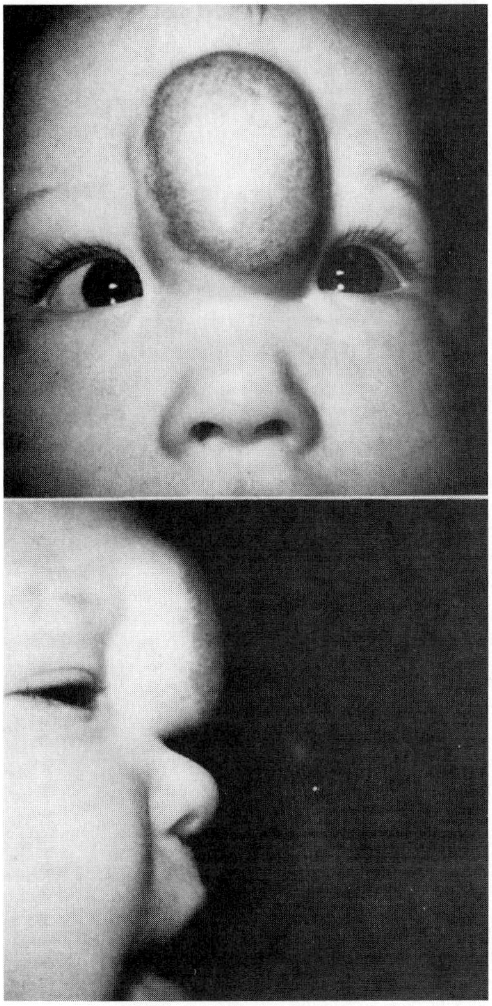

A

B

FIGURE 20-22 Strawberry hemangioma. **A,** Raised lesion, begun as small "herald" spot. It is compressible, with no bruit. **B,** Lateral view.

infants; in general, these may be easily differentiated. The "salmon patches" on the forehead and "stork bites" on the back of the neck are seen as tiny pink lesions present at birth that disappear within months. The port-wine stains, made up primarily of capillary-size vessels, are present at birth and are flat and diffuse, usually over the upper face. Congenital nevi are pigmented, contain hair, and appear to be moles rather than vascular birthmarks.

Diagnostic Studies

Biopsy is usually not indicated in infants because the diagnosis is clear. A blood count may be necessary because certain large vascular lesions can trap platelets, leading to consumptive coagulopathy. A history of bruising or bleeding should alert the physician to this possibility.

Pathophysiology

Strawberry hemangiomas are characterized by the exuberant growth of vascular tissue at a deeper level than found in port-wine stains, which involve capillary proliferation in the dermis. Complex distinctions and classifications based on embryology, histology, and measured cell biology factors (particularly cell dynamics) are useful in large series but unfortunately offer nothing more in terms of prognosis and natural history than is presented in the box. Strawberry hemangioma and pyogenic granulomas are proliferative and have increased tritiated thymidine uptake, tumor angiogenesis factors, and most cell activity. Others, such as port-wine stains and arteriovenous malformations, are adynamic and do not have proliferative and regressive phases. The surface epithelium is thinned, which may lead to ulceration and bleeding. Microscopically there is hyperplasia of endothelial cells and widely dilated vessels.

Management

The therapeutic plan is simple; the choices available are not (Figure 20-23). These lesions predictably involute over a period of years; about 50% resolve by age 5 years, and 75% by 7 years.[114] Further resolution occurs even in adolescence, and more than 90% will resolve. The following factors seem to have no influence on whether, when, or how completely it resolves: the patient's sex, the lesion's size or location, or whether there are multiple or single lesions.

The initial decision should be in favor of observation. The course may be one of essentially no change, followed by a gradual resolution. More likely, lesions will continue to proliferate before beginning to resolve, and in these cases further observation should be chosen. Patients and parents should be seen at regular intervals (every 3 months or so in the beginning, longer intervals later). They are advised about local care—for example, an emollient to avoid drying, scaling, and irritation.

In some cases the lesions may enlarge rapidly and obstruct vision (Figure 20-24). This rapid enlargement is particularly true for deeper, cavernous hemangiomas and it becomes an emergency because even brief obstruction can result in deprivation amblyopia and permanent blindness. Thomson and associates[122] noted visual loss when obstruction was only for a week. Stigmar and Crawford[117] confirmed dangers in patients younger than a year, particularly when obstruction was total. Ulceration and bleeding require immediate care but usually heal without surgery. In some rapidly enlarging lesions, a decision to treat may be made.

Steroids

The first choice is steroids. Zarem and Edgerton[131] noted a response to steroids, and many have confirmed this since. Sasaki and associates[110] demonstrated that

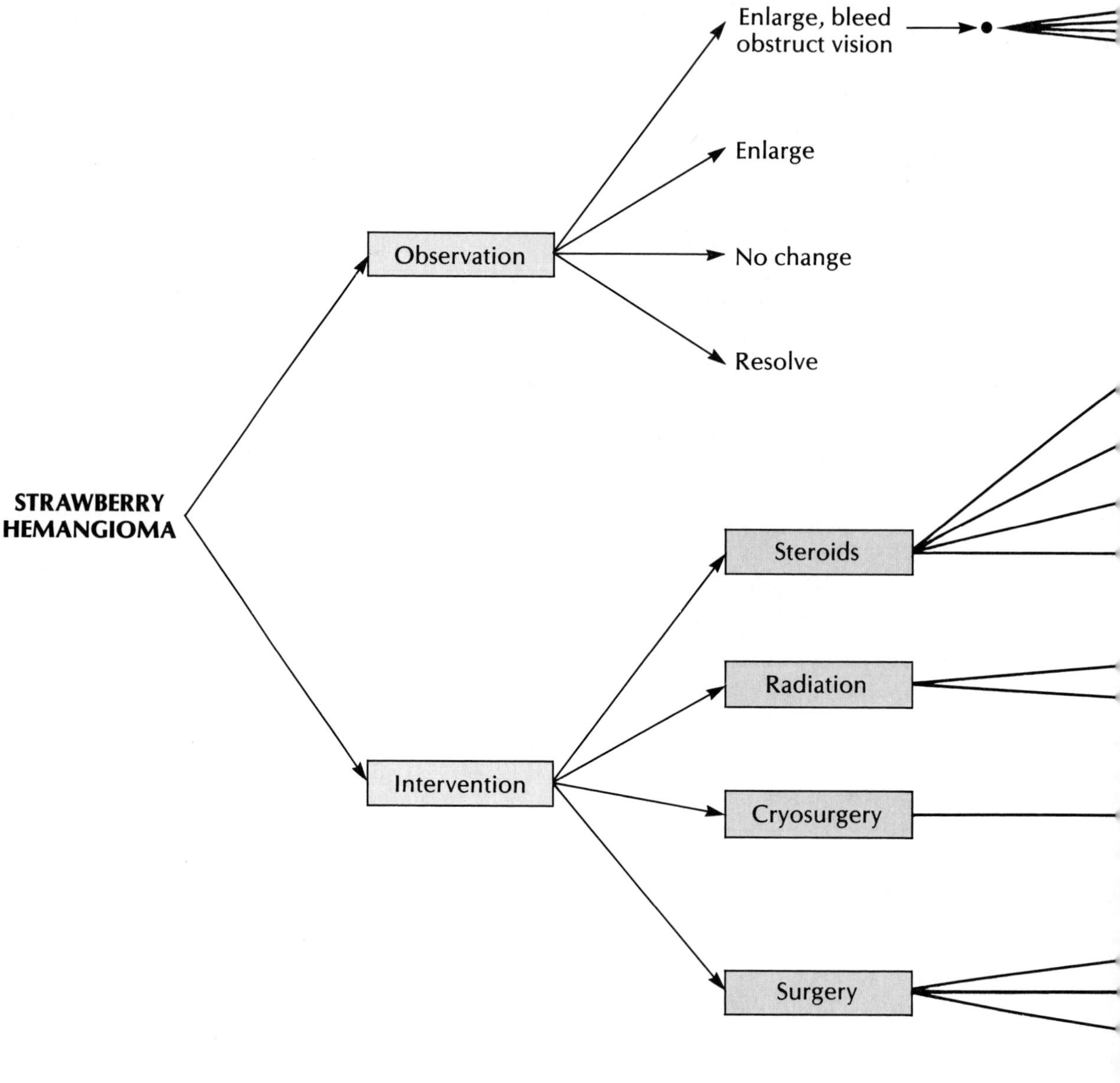

FIGURE 20-23 Algorithm for management of strawberry hemangioma.

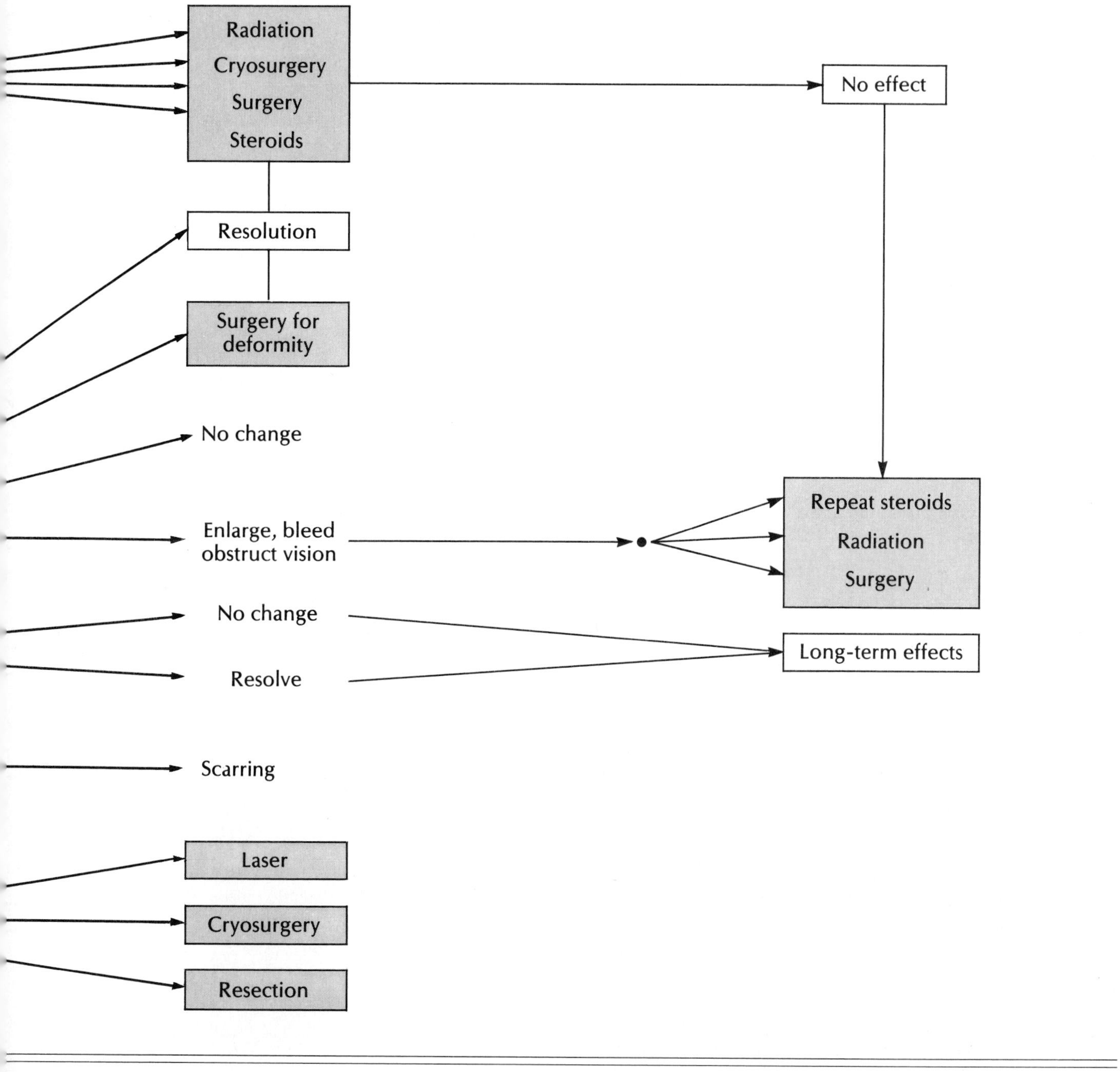
Radiation
Cryosurgery
Surgery
Steroids
No effect
Resolution
Surgery for deformity
No change
Enlarge, bleed obstruct vision
Repeat steroids
Radiation
Surgery
No change
Long-term effects
Resolve
Scarring
Laser
Cryosurgery
Resection

strawberry hemangiomas have estrogen receptors—in particular, serum levels of 17-beta-estradiol (E_2) in levels of 96 pg/ml, compared with 24 to 25 pg/ml in cavernous and port-wine hemangiomas and 18 pg/ml in normal skin. Furthermore, they showed specific 17-beta-estradiol binder activity in biopsy tissue of enlarging strawberry hemangiomas, which subsequently responded to corticosteroid therapy; no such binding capacity (or steroid response) was seen in noninvoluting strawberry hemangiomas, cavernous hemangiomas, port-wine stains, or normal skin. Prednisone, in doses of 2 μm/kg/day for 4 to 6 weeks, results in regression in a high percentage of cases, with few systemic side effects. Complete and permanent resolution, however, does not occur, or we would certainly use this method in all cases.

Surgical Excision

Only in the smallest of lesions should surgical excision be chosen as the initial method of treatment, particularly if there is bleeding, ulceration, or danger to normal neighboring structures. The danger of blindness is the major complication for lesions in the periorbital area, and occasionally an emergency debulking may be required if steroid response is not prompt. For lesions in the oral cavity or hypopharynx, the mass itself or bleeding may be a therapeutic emergency—"Disease desperate grown, by desperate appliance are resolved, or not at all."[111] In these circumstances, radiation therapy may be required.

Radiation Therapy

The lesions have embryonal and undifferentiated cells and often respond to low-dose radiation (400 c-grey) with shrinkage.[126] A response rate of 85% to 90% is at least as effective as doing nothing. It is easy to minimize the long-term effects, which may not manifest themselves for 20 to 25 years, in an effort to effect short-term success. Radiation changes may result in dermatitis, may interfere with normal growth and development of bone and soft tissue, and are carcinogenic; the cancers begin to appear when the patient is in the third decade of life.

Other Options

Other forms of treatment include cryosurgery, which has been a traditional method of destroying smaller lesions. Liquid nitrogen is applied topically, and the frozen area is destroyed; it heals with varying degrees of scarring.

The laser has been used in hemangiomas and has been most effective in treating port-wine stains.[4] The redness in the lesions is attractive particularly to the argon laser beam, and the energy is selectively absorbed and the tissue destroyed. Healing is only by scarring, and the aesthetic result is related to the size, thickness, and configuration of the lesion. The laser may be particularly effective in managing lesions in the hypopharynx because it is a means of hemorrhage control. Injection with sclerosing agents such as hypertonic saline or sodium morrhuate is also occasionally effective but leaves atrophic scarring. The deeper location makes superficial dermaplaning and dermabrasion techniques obviously ineffective. Another investigational drug is interferon, which has had some dramatic effects in the treatment of life-threatening lesions.

A

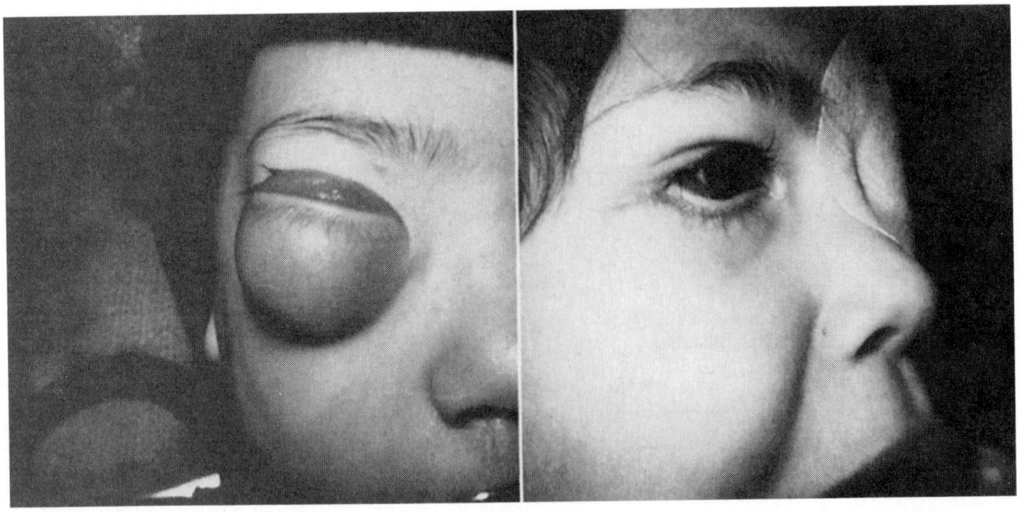

B

FIGURE 20-24 Hemangioma with obstruction of vision. **A,** The hemangioma was followed since infancy. Sudden enlargement obstructed vision, and surgery was performed to avert deprivation amblyopia. **B,** Early postoperative state. The patch on the opposite eye is to encourage use of the involved eye.

Patient Education

It is a marvelous challenge to the surgeon to be the most kind, thoughtful, and understanding of partners with the pediatrician and parents now and with the patient later. The parents are frightened about the immediate implications of this lesion and the potential long-term consequences. No doubt friends and relatives and perhaps even the pediatrician have given the parents information that may be confusing, if not actually terrifying. The surgeon might begin by explaining that these lesions are very common, and perhaps 4% to 5% of all newborns develop this type of hemangioma; of these, 70% are actually born with it.[114] The surgeon should use the term *hemangioma;* the word *birthmark* may carry implications of permanency, and this is often a lesion that involves with time. Because this time may extend over 5 or 6 years, time with the parents now is well spent. These lesions may continue to enlarge over the next months, usually reaching peak growth in about 8 months. Many begin to involute by the end of the first year. They develop a central pallor, begin to discolor, and finally flatten. This involution may be interrupted by growth phases. The surgeon should explain that the surface of these will thin out, but even if they were to be injured or the lesion ulcerate, which occurs in about 10%, severe hemorrhage will not occur and simple pressure will control any bleeding.

The natural history of the disease is one of varying rates of proliferation followed by final involution. The period of management is tortuous and occasionally difficult. A great deal of reassurance is necessary, and the parents' trust is critical lest they seek one who promises a "quick fix." The appearance of the involuted lesion is often better than one might have hoped. The tissue is scar epithelium, thinned and often atrophic. The atrophic area may be excised and revised by one of the reconstructive techniques that will introduce more normal-appearing tissue into the area. The result is never perfect, but it is often inconspicuous and, except for very small lesions, predictably better than early intervention.

PROBLEM Kasabach-Merritt Syndrome

Kasabach-Merritt syndrome is characterized by the association of hemangiomas and thrombocytopenic purpura. The hemangiomas are combinations of the capillary and cavernous varieties. They appear early in life and may involve visceral organs as well. Presumably from the trapping of platelets within the lesion, consumptive coagulopathy and purpura develop with petechiae and ecchymoses. This syndrome has serious portent, and a mortality rate in excess of 30% has been reported.[71]

PROBLEM Maffucci's Syndrome

Maffucci's syndrome is a rare syndrome combining multiple angiomas with enchondromas. The patients develop a complex of vascular problems early in life, including cavernous hemangiomas, phlebectasia, and lymphangiomas. The bony defect is the result of problems with endochondral ossification leading to deformed and shortened bones, particularly of the distal extremity and then to pathologic fractures. Approximately 20% of these patients are thought to develop malignancy either in the bone (chondrosarcomas) or elsewhere (fibrosarcomas and even adenocarcinomas).[74]

PROBLEM: NONINVOLUTING VASCULAR TUMORS—PORT-WINE STAIN (NEVUS FLAMMEUS)

The port-wine stain is present at birth in about 0.3% of newborns; no involution is seen. The lesion is most commonly found on the face, is unilateral, and tends to involve a segment that corresponds loosely to the nerve distribution of the trigeminal nerve. It rarely crosses the midline. The color is initially pink but darkens with age. The lesions tend to thicken with age and in the third and fourth decades may become nodular (Figure 20-25). The lesion involves mature capillaries in the dermis with no evidence of cellular proliferation. Malignant degeneration is not a concern.

The treatment is primarily directed to the aesthetic appearance and in many cases may involve no more than the accurate, skillful application of makeup. Tattooing with flesh-colored dye has been used but is limited by the unsatisfactory distribution and match of the colors. Radiation is again condemned because the results are unsatisfactory and the long-term carcinogenesis of the radiation is an inappropriate risk. Surgical dermaplaning, dermabrasion, and other maneuvers fail to remove the problem, which is in the dermis. Total surgical excision, in general, is unsatisfactory because the skin graft or other tissue replacement is aesthetically disappointing. Treatment with the argon laser is satisfactory in some cases. The argon laser energy is selectively picked up by the red end of the color spectrum and tends to decolorize. The treatment is slow and ponderous and should be preceded by a test area to predict whether the course is worthwhile.

PROBLEM Cavernous Hemangiomas

Some vascular lesions might be classified as massive and include large degrees of arteriovenous shunting. They are usually caused by multiple small shunts rather than any single large one. These large, often plexiform lesions often occur on extremities, but in the head and neck they may involve critical structures.

Figure 20-26 shows a child with a large vascular mass in the left parotid gland. It was a solid tumor without palpable or audible arteriovenous fistulas. Sclerosing agents have been less satisfactory in these large lesions than might have been hoped. Radiation is of doubtful

A B C D

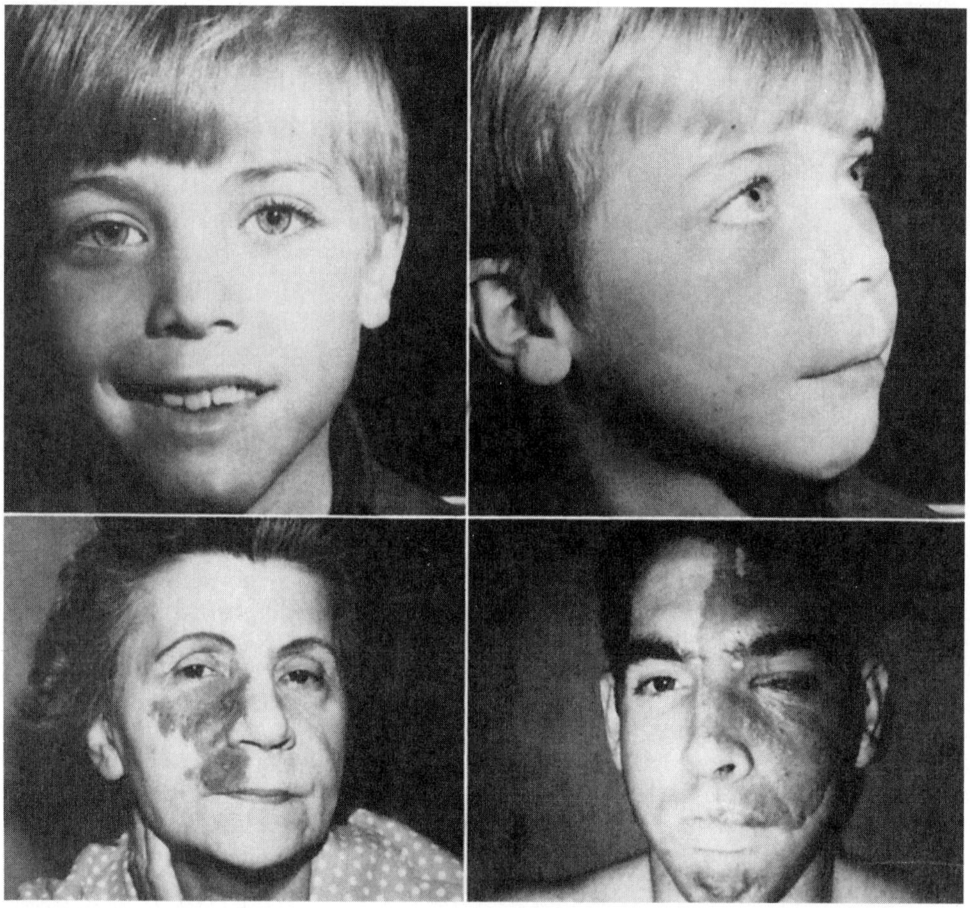

FIGURE 20-25 Hemangioma (nevus flammeus). **A** and **B**, Port-wine stain in a young boy. Although pale, it is unlikely to disappear and may become more nodular with age. **C**, Port-wine stain in an adult, showing more nodularity and degenerative changes. **D**, Sturge-Weber syndrome with port-wine stain. The meninges are also frequently involved, and central nervous system symptoms and retardation may be present.

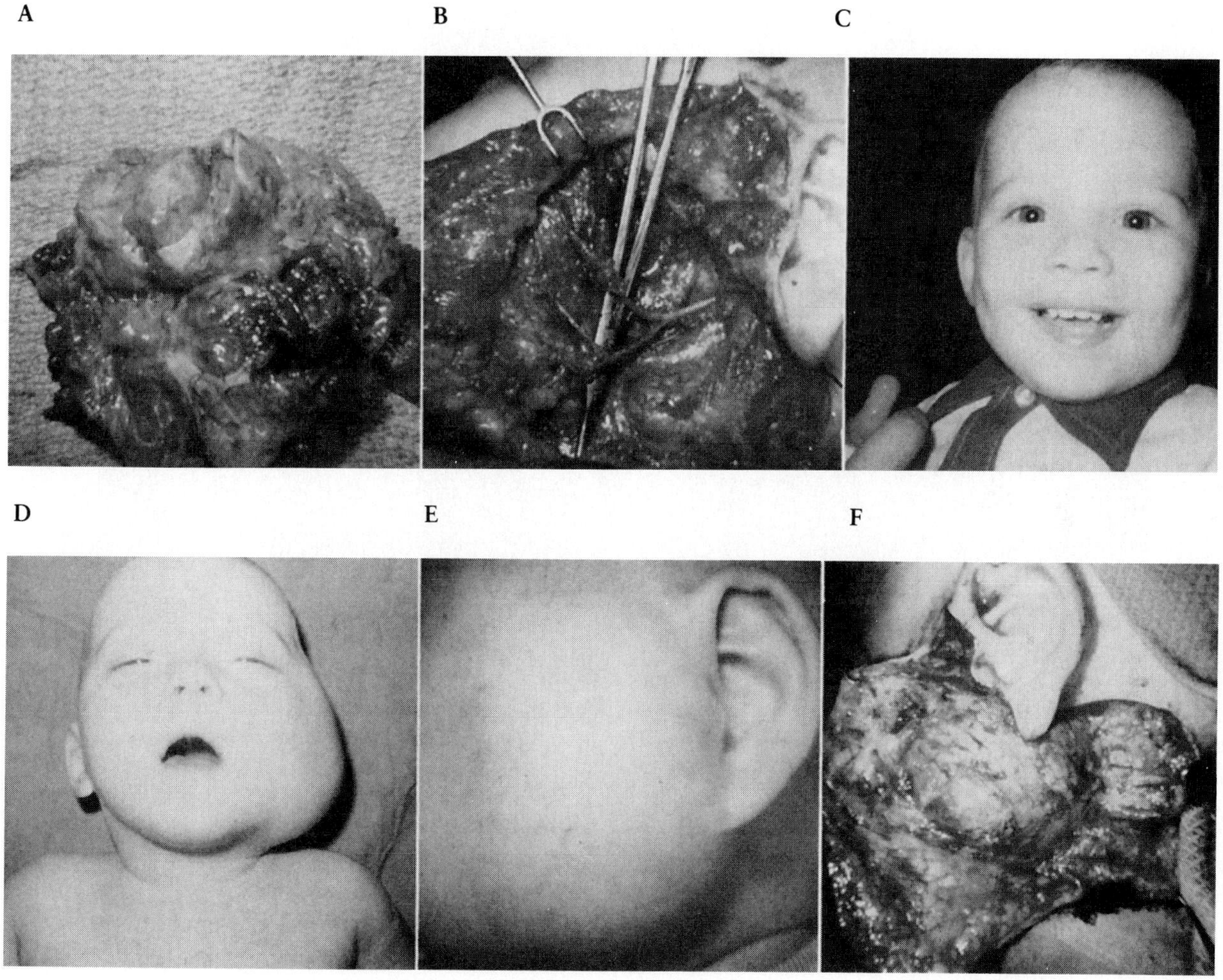

FIGURE 20-26 Massive hemangioma in the parotid gland. **A**, Massive enlargement. Bruit was audible, and multiple feeding vessels were seen on radiography. **B**, Lateral view showing surprisingly little skin involvement. **C**, Mass almost entirely within the parotid gland. **D**, Specimen is solid—a mixed capillary cavernous hemangioma. **E**, Facial nerve is preserved. **F**, A happy result.

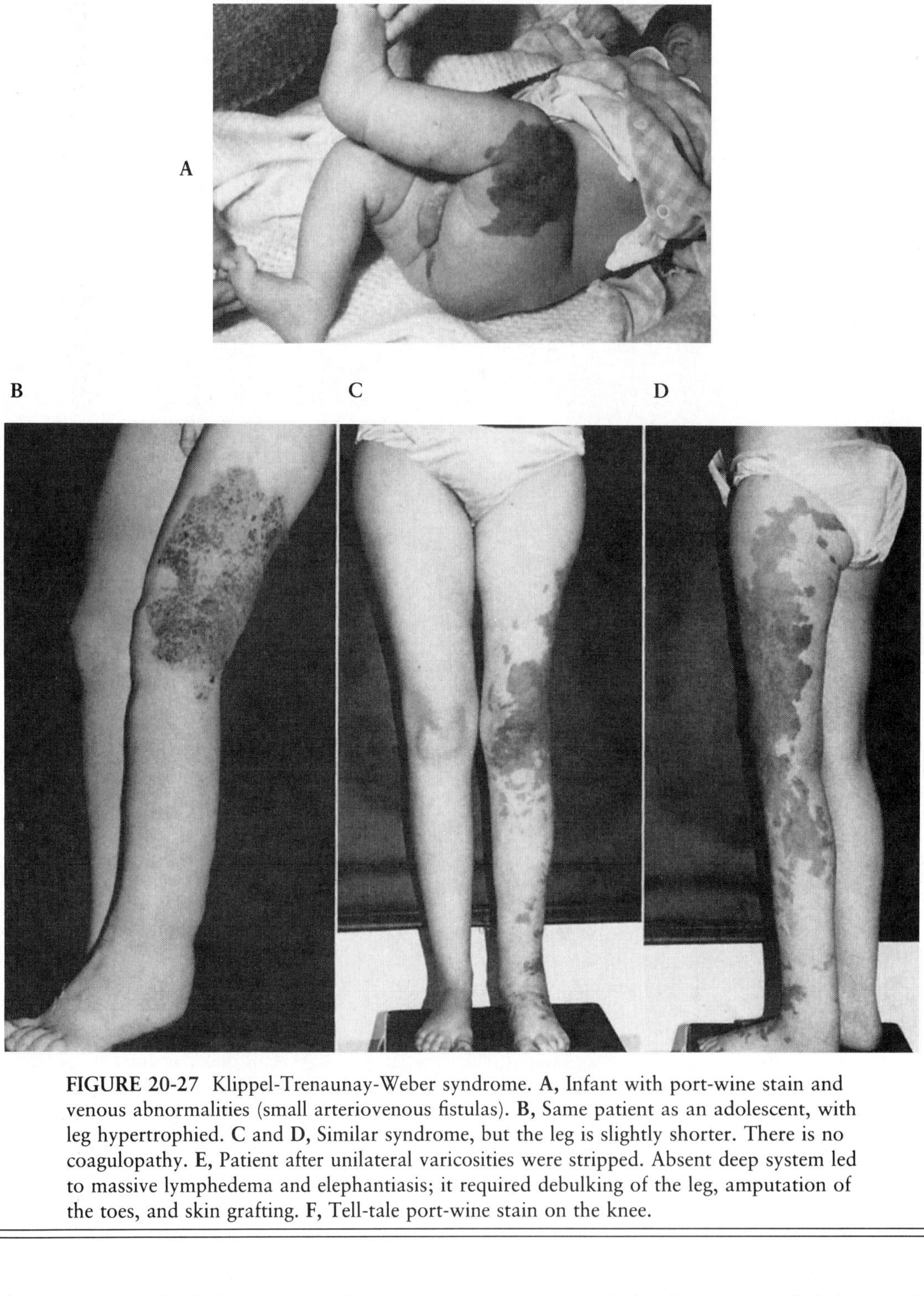

FIGURE 20-27 Klippel-Trenaunay-Weber syndrome. **A,** Infant with port-wine stain and venous abnormalities (small arteriovenous fistulas). **B,** Same patient as an adolescent, with leg hypertrophied. **C** and **D,** Similar syndrome, but the leg is slightly shorter. There is no coagulopathy. **E,** Patient after unilateral varicosities were stripped. Absent deep system led to massive lymphedema and elephantiasis; it required debulking of the leg, amputation of the toes, and skin grafting. **F,** Tell-tale port-wine stain on the knee.

value, and attempts at multiple ligations are disappointing. This lesion was excised, preserving the facial nerve.

PROBLEM Sturge-Weber Syndrome

One special disease in which the port-wine stain forms a hallmark characteristic in more than 85% of cases is Sturge-Weber syndrome.[94] This congenital vascular malformation affects the vessels of the eye, cortical leptomeninges, and the skin in the ophthalmic and maxillary distribution of the trigeminal nerve (Figure 20-25, *D*). Patients develop hemiplegia and seizures, and mental retardation is common. Skull radiographs have a characteristic and almost diagnostic appearance with calcifications in the area of vascular abnormalities. Treatment of the skin lesion is similar to that of other port-wine stains.

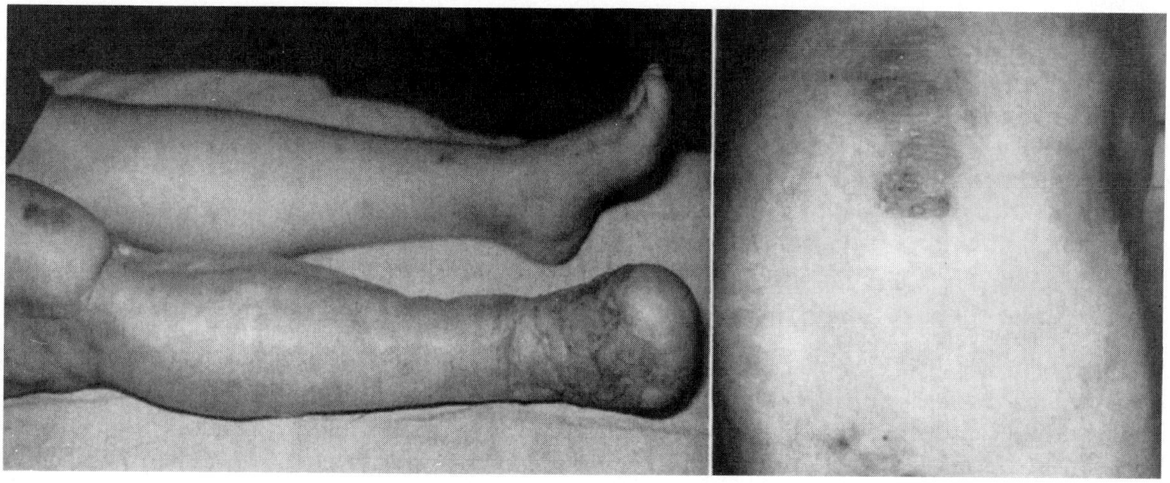

FIGURE 20-27, cont'd For legend see opposite page.

PROBLEM Klippel-Trenaunay-Weber Syndrome

Described initially in 1900, the Klippel-Trenaunay-Weber syndrome is a complex of phenomena that includes the port-wine stain as part of the syndrome.[75] More important, the syndrome usually involves but a single extremity, usually the lower, and often first appears in teenagers with unilateral varicose veins (Figure 20-27). Because of possible small underlying arteriovenous fistulas, it is often accompanied by hypertrophy of soft tissue and bone and leads to a leg length discrepancy. Because the deep venous system is primitive or absent, if the superficial varicosities are removed surgically, inadequate venous return, lymphatic overload, edema, and finally elephantiasis may occur.

PROBLEM Pyogenic Granuloma

Pyogenic granulomas are usually classified as being caused by trauma or infections and are classified as though they were granulation tissue. Rather, they result from a proliferative vascular process of the capillary hemangioma variety, which does arise in an area of trauma.[127] They typically occur on the face and may be related to shaving. They are also found on the digits, particularly around the nails. They begin as red patches, enlarging to reddened, lobulated, and even pedunculated lesions. They do look like the "proud flesh" of granulation tissue. They should be excised or destroyed by curettage and cautery and rarely recur.

PROBLEM Glomus Tumors

Arteriovenous shunting has been invoked as one of the explanations for the vascular changes in pedicle flaps used in reconstructive procedures. These shunts, however, have been difficult to identify anatomically in the human with the exception of arteriovenous malformations and normally in the glomus network, which is found predominantly in the nail beds, but also in the lungs, stomach, bones, and elsewhere.[73] Distinctly arising from smooth muscle cells, the glomus cells invest small canals between arterioles and venules (arteriovenous shunts). The tumors begin as soft reddish and bluish papules and nodules. The characteristic finding is pain, which can be lancinating and radiate up the arm. Occasionally, they occur in multiple digits and are not as painful. They are benign, and surgical excision, when complete, is curative.

PROBLEM Hemangiopericytoma

Unfortunately, hemangiopericytomas are deceptive lesions, with a 20% to 30% incidence of subsequent malignancy, but with few specific identifying characteristics until biopsy.[45] These tumors arise from pericytes, which are primitive perivascular cells whose exact origin and function are unknown. The tumors are present as asymptomatic masses, often subcutaneously with no skin changes. They may enlarge slowly or rapidly and are diagnosed only when removed. Because of the high change of malignancy, they should be widely excised.

LYMPHATIC LESIONS

PROBLEM: LYMPHANGIOMA

Lymphangiomas are congenital malformations of the lymphatic system. There are three major types, two of which have surgical significance.

Lymphangioma circumscriptum is characterized by localized, small, clear cutaneous vesicles. These may become irritated or eroded and leak a clear, almost viscous fluid. The lesions may occur in association with hemangiomas and may eventually develop chronic irritation and require removal.

Cavernous lymphangiomas are larger and deeper confluent channels of lymph vessels, perhaps associated with secondary lymphatic obstruction. When confluent, a single or multiloculated cystic area, known as a *cystic hygroma,* may appear, most commonly in the neck. Surgical excision is curative.

Lymph stasis may lead to edema much as in the lymphedema of congenital absence of lymphatics, the lymphedema precox (Milroy's disease), and lymphedema secondary to tumor, surgery, or infection. The presence of edema in tissue diminishes the local tissue defenses to streptococcal infection and is usually accompanied by some scarring, which increases the edema and also results in thickening of the tissues. The end result is lichenified, thickened tissue with fissures, cracking, new portals for infection, and the clinical picture of elephantiasis.

PROBLEM: LYMPHANGIOSARCOMA

Angiosarcoma occurs in the absence of lymphedema; lymphangiosarcoma occurs in tissue subject to longstanding lymphedema and is seen in the circumstances described previously. Lymphedema does not usually occur from removal of lymph nodes per se nor from merely transecting lymphatic channels. Wound healing problems, which often were seen after radical mastectomy, for instance, lead to infection that, particularly when associated with radiation or the recurrence of tumor, leads to profound lymphedema of the extremity. When the modified radical mastectomy became more popular, the wound healing problems diminished; even though the lymph nodes are also removed, lymphedema is much less common.

Lymphangiosarcoma in the lymphedematous extremity is heralded by the appearance of plaques and nodules, often reddened and purplish in hue. Satellites are often present, and ulcerating lesions confirm the serious nature of the problem. Treatment usually requires amputation, and metastases frequently lead to death.

PROBLEM: ANGIOSARCOMA

There are two major forms of angiosarcoma: those that occur with, after, and in association with lymphedema and those that are unassociated. The lesions that begin in the absence of preexisting lymphedema tend to occur on the face and scalp in the older age group. The lesions begin as reddened and bluish plaques and nodules, which then become "blood blisters" and ulcerate and bleed. They spread by local infiltration through the skin, and the involvement may be diffuse with ill-defined margins, making surgical resection difficult, even with frozen section control, and the cure rate is correspondingly low, with high degree of recurrence and a rate of distant metastasis in excess of 25%.

AIDS-RELATED TUMORS

PROBLEM: KAPOSI'S SARCOMA

Until recently, Kaposi's sarcoma deserved only a small mention as a pathoclinical curiosity. First described in 1872 by Moritz K. Kaposi (who came from Kaposvar in Hungary and adopted the name of his town), this lesion was considered to be a problem of Central Europeans such as Poles and Russians, with a predilection for Jews.[39] It was also found in the Belgian Congo (Zaire) in blacks in an incidence of 9% to 10% of all cancers seen there. It had a peculiar predilection for males, in a ratio as high as 15 : 1. In the 1970s an association of the neoplasm with the immunosuppressed patient was noted among patients undergoing transplantation. Its tendency to be accompanied by a second primary tumor, usually of lymphoreticular origin (for example, lymphoma and leukemia) was noted, and another study reported a high correlation between a primary tumor, a period of immunosuppression, and then the appearance of Kaposi's sarcoma. Others noted an association with autoimmune disease and patients whose immune system might be altered. The link with immunosuppression was then confirmed by its now clear association with AIDS.

Because of clustering, a genetic or infectious origin was suspected and Giraldo and associates[51] identified herpeslike viral particles in tissue culture cell lines from tumor patients. However, a definite link has not been confirmed.

Kaposi's sarcoma is discouraging to manage and not truly a surgical disease in the AIDS patient.[109] Patients with AIDS have symptoms like those of certain varieties of Kaposi's seen in Africa, with diffuse lymphadenopathy, diffuse involvement of the viscera, and the development of additional primary tumors, as in patients with transplants.[80] Kaposi's sarcoma is associated with AIDS (described in 1981) and with opportunistic infections, including *Pneumocystis carinii* pneumonia, candidiasis, cryptococcal meningitis, and central nervous system toxoplasmosis. Appearance of lesions is often first on the upper extremities or trunk. Death is usually from pulmonary or gastrointestinal lesions.[27]

Clinical Presentation

History (Subjective Findings)

In classic forms, the Kaposi's lesions are often preceded by edema and appear on the lower extremities, usually unilaterally initially (Figure 20-28). In AIDS patients the lesions are flat, irregular, and reddish blue (becoming purple and violaceous) and appear on arms

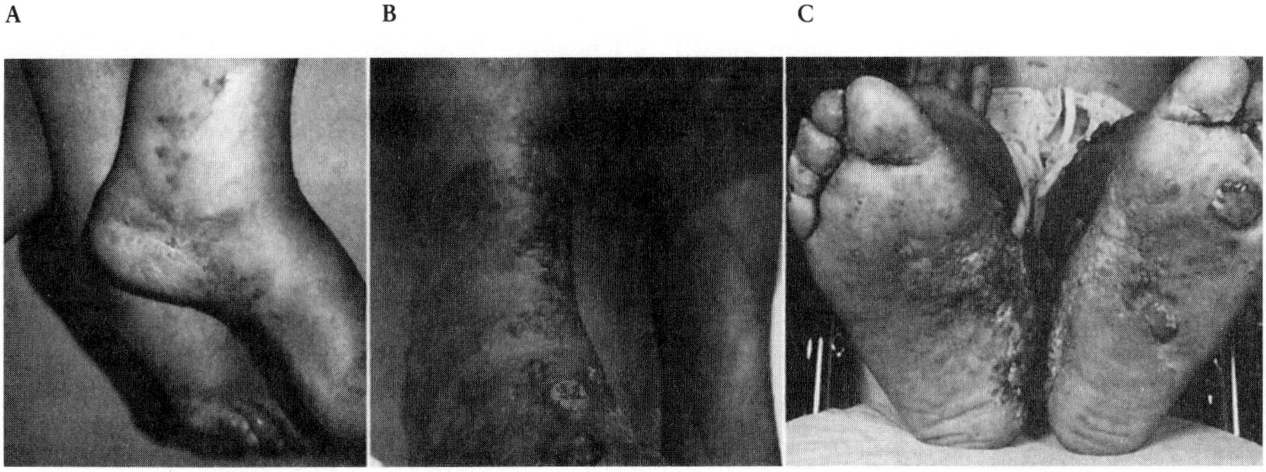

FIGURE 20-28 Classic Kaposi's sarcoma on lower extremities and feet in non-AIDS patients. A, Early lesion—macular, papular. B, Further extension and ulceration. C, Diffuse bilateral involvement.

or the trunk. They may appear several months before the patient seeks medical care. The initially macular lesions become nodular and coalesce to form larger plaques. There may be sudden onset of 5 to 10 new lesions. Pain, pruritus, and burning may be noted. Because the lesions also may be diffuse and involve all internal organs, gastrointestinal symptoms may lead to diarrhea and abdominal symptoms. Whether this diffuse involvement is of multifocal or metastatic origin is unclear.

Physical Examination (Objective Findings)

Examination shows the lesions to be dark purple and nodular, with irregular borders (Figure 20-29). The lymph nodes in the axilla area may be slightly enlarged, soft, and tender bilaterally. Lymph nodes in the neck and inguinal area may also be enlarged and tender. Involvement of lymph nodes is often reactive rather than generated by the tumor itself. Node involvement usually indicates a poor prognosis. The mucous membrane of the oral cavity and hypopharynx is not involved. The rectal examination is usually negative.

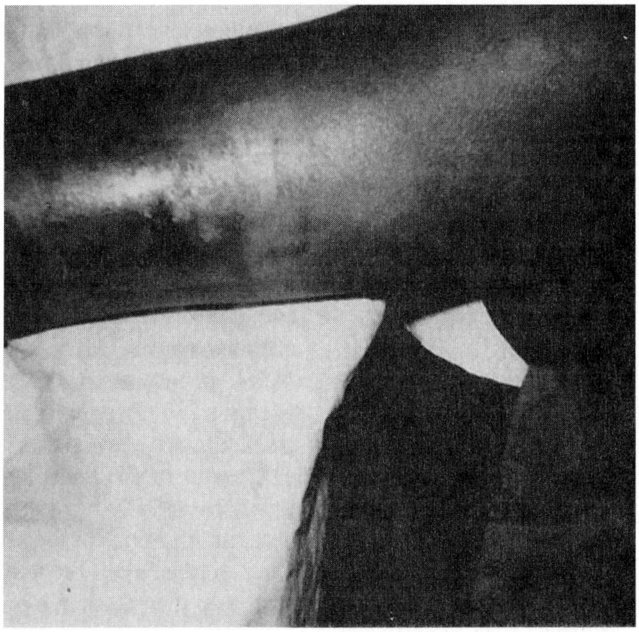

FIGURE 20-29 Kaposi's sarcoma on upper extremities and trunk in a patient with AIDS.

Diagnostic Studies

The prognosis for Kaposi's sarcoma in the non-AIDS patient itself is variable, with some patients surviving for 50 years and longer and others running a progressive course over a decade or so. More commonly the lesions advance rapidly, and a fulminant course over weeks or months may occur.

Management

Kaposi's sarcoma in the absence of AIDS is a challenge; in the presence of AIDS the treatment is symptomatic and palliative. Surgery for localized lesions is effective when they are the only lesions, but the diffuse involvement and the regular appearance of new lesions make this usually a nonsurgical problem.

TUMORS OF ADIPOSE TISSUE–LIPOMAS

Lipomas are the most common of soft tissue tumors and account for about 80% of all benign soft tissue tumors. Although they may occur anywhere on the body, they tend to occur on the neck, back, arms, and thighs. More than 90% occur in women, most commonly those in their thirties and forties, and about 5% are multiple.[1]

Although lipomas may be massive, they are usually but a few centimeters in diameter. They are typically soft, freely movable, and localized in the subcutaneous tissue. Microscopically they appear to be normal fat. No subcutaneous lipomas has ever become malignant. Treatment is surgical and uniformly successful.

Most are removed by excision of the overlying skin and simple enucleation.

Suction-Assisted Lipectomy

The techniques of suction-assisted lipectomy can be successfully used on lipomas. The technique involves the freeing up of fatty deposits by the probing between the subcutaneous fibrous septae and then suctioning the loosened fatty tissue by powerful suction machines. Because the maneuver does not divide the septae, large cavities and dead space are avoided. The suction probes are long, thin, hollow tubes that can be inserted through small incisions often placed in areas where the scar will be hidden by clothing. Small (less than 5 mm long) incisions may be placed in a nearby but hidden area, and the lipomas can be extracted from a distance. They usually do not recur.

PROBLEM: INFILTRATING LIPOMA

Infiltrating lipoma is a term applied to otherwise totally benign lipomas that do not remain subcutaneous but have insinuated themselves between and through tissue planes and into and around the underlying muscles. These are histologically mature adipocytes and show no evidence of atypia or other features suggestive of malignancy. A review of 130 infiltrating lipomas showed that they were found uniformly throughout the body and could be classified into intramuscular and intermuscular categories.[47] The intramuscular lipomas were partially subfascial, completely subfascial, or diffusely distributed throughout the muscle. Those between the muscle were well circumscribed or without any obvious tissue planes. Because these lesions either tend to be fixed to or indistinguishable from the underlying tissue, further studies are required. Radiographic studies usually show the feathery appearance of mature fat, and CT scans may help localize and determine their extent and distribution. In one case the entire gastrocnemius muscle had been replaced by infiltrating lipoma, and only removal of the entire muscle could cure it (Figure 20-30). In other cases biopsy is required to confirm the benign nature of the lesion. In these cases suction technique can help remove lesions in areas that do not lend themselves well to total surgical extirpation.

PROBLEM: HEREDITARY LIPOMATOSIS

Hereditary lipomatosis is characterized by diffuse symmetric lipomas of the extremities and trunk. More than 80% of those affected are men. Madelung's disease is a benign symmetric lipomatosis with deposition of lipomas, particularly around the neck and groin.[26] A "horse collar" appearance has been described. These too are benign and have mature adipocytes on biopsy. Suction techniques offer a more attractive and feasible approach than multiple resections.

PROBLEM: ANGIOLIPOMA

Angiolipomas are a variant of lipomas that have a distinct vascular and fibrous component rather than being purely lipomas. They may be found in large numbers, usually on the upper extremities, and are intimately attached to the undersurface of the dermis, from which they cannot be moved on physical examination and only with great difficulty at surgery.[63] They are characteristically exquisitely tender and symptomatically painful. Adiposis dolorosa, or Dercum's disease, refers to multiple painful lipomas, and the condition may be confused with angiolipoma.

PROBLEM: LIPOSARCOMA

The malignant variety of fatty tumors is relatively rare and there is no evidence that it arises from a previously benign lipoma. Whereas benign lipomas are freely moveable in the subcutaneous tissues, the liposarcoma tends to be fixed to the underlying tissues. Many liposarcomas occur in the retroperitoneum and of those accessible to physical examination, a disproportionate number occur in the medial upper thigh. This, in actuality, is a favorable location for a variety of malignant soft tissue tumors, a factor that should be considered whenever a firm, nonmovable mass is found in this region. The evaluation and management of these sarcomas are discussed later.

TUMORS OF MESODERMAL ELEMENTS

One group of benign and malignant tumors of the skin occurs so frequently that the surgeon should be familiar with their terminology, appearance, and clinical behavior. These are termed *fibrohistiocytic tumors* and arise from fibroblasts, fibrocytes, and histiocytes and defy specific classification. The most common and distinct are discussed here.

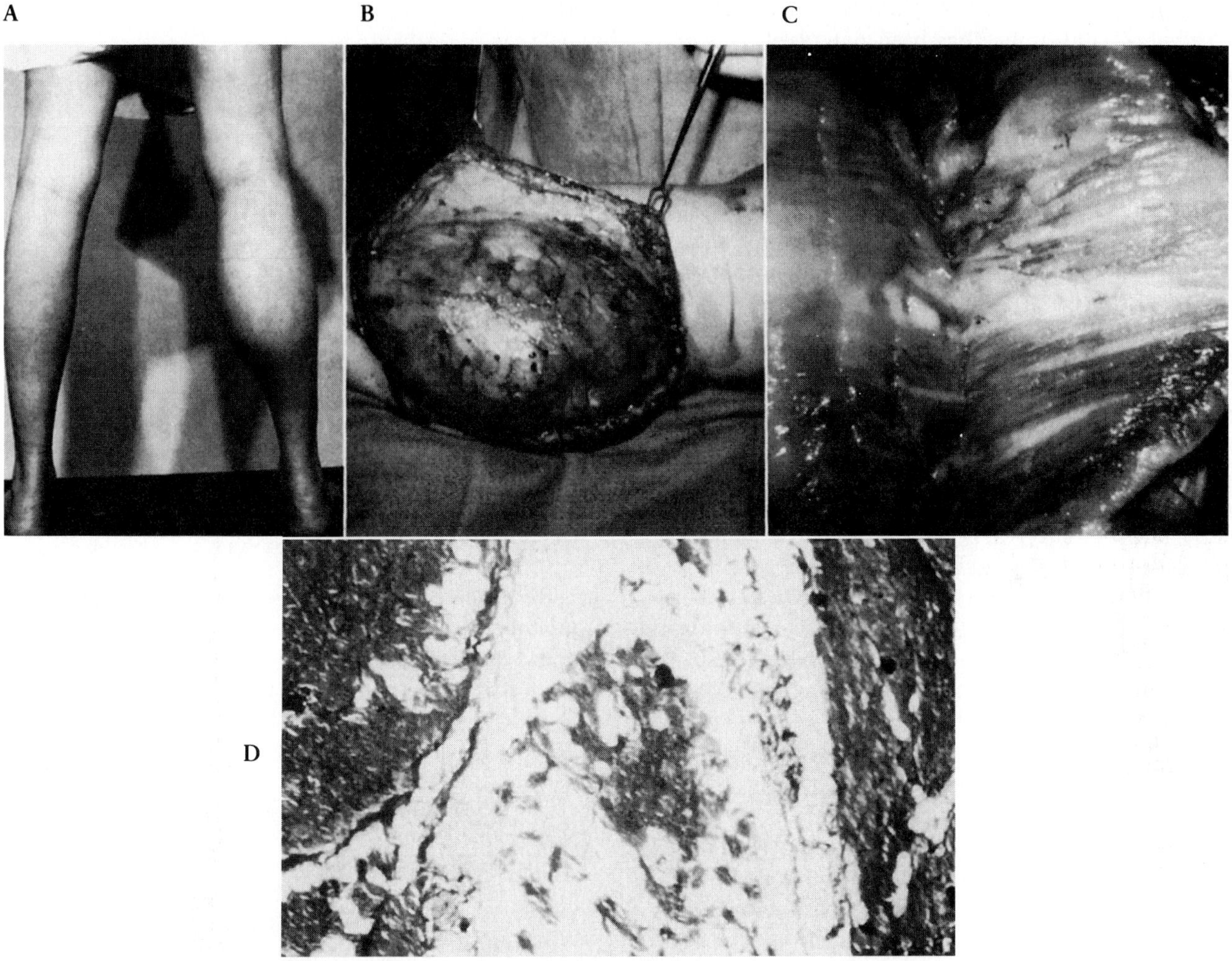

FIGURE 20-30 Infiltrating lipoma. **A,** Painless enlargement of the calf. **B,** Diffuse involvement of the entire gastrocnemius muscle. **C,** Lipoma interdigitating and infiltrating the muscle. **D,** Benign lipoma in muscle.

PROBLEM: FIBROUS HISTIOCYTOMA (DERMATOFIBROMA, SCLEROSING HEMANGIOMA)

Fibrous histiocytomas are common and appear as smooth nodules or papules, usually on the extremities, although any area may be involved. They are usually round or oval, are smooth, and range from yellow to darker brown (Figure 20-31). They are clearly attached to the skin and separate from the underlying tissue. They are usually solitary. Microscopically, there are fibrocytes, bundles of collagen, and whorls of histiocytes. A "cartwheel" appearance has been described, and perivascular hemosiderin deposits are seen. Although an occasional basal cell carcinoma has been found in association, these are to be considered benign, and local excision is accompanied by only a scant recurrence rate.[46]

PROBLEM: DERMATOFIBROSARCOMA PROTUBERANS

Dermatofibrosarcoma protuberans (DFSP) is considered one of the malignant forms of the fibrous histiocytoma, although it is locally invasive into the underlying fat and muscle, is prone to recurrence, and only rarely metastasizes.[121] As opposed to the benign form, which usually is on the extremities, DFSP arises on the trunk, particularly in men. There may be a history of trauma, but the cause-effect relationship between the two is not proven. Early a nodular, firm lesion is attached to the overlying skin. Although there is a long period of slow growth, often a decade or longer, its growth rate increases and multinodularity develops.

Microscopically the tumors are highly vascular and characterized by the cartwheel appearance. There may also be areas of myxoid degeneration.

The treatment is surgical, but unfortunately a recurrence rate in excess of 50% has been reported. Despite this, metastasis is rare. The excision must be wide enough to eliminate this tendency to local recurrence. Although some studies suggest that skin grafting is necessary for closure of the defect, the techniques of tissue transfer make other closures of large defects more satisfactory.

PROBLEM: MALIGNANT FIBROUS HISTIOCYTOMA

Malignant fibrous histiocytomas are the most common of the soft tissue sarcomas in adults. More common in men than women, more than half occur in the skeletal muscle in the lower extremity, particularly the thigh.

These tumors are very malignant; in large series, local recurrence after resection is found in almost half the cases, and metastases are seen in more than 40%. Spread may be hematogenous or to regional lymph nodes.[46] Management is discussed in the Management of Soft Tissue Sarcomas section.

PROBLEM: ANGIOFIBROMA (ADENOMA SEBACEUM)

Angiofibromas are smooth, nodular, flesh-colored lesions that may occur singly or as a conglomerate and are an almost essential characteristic of tuberous sclerosis (90%). Microscopically, these are fibrous and vas-

A

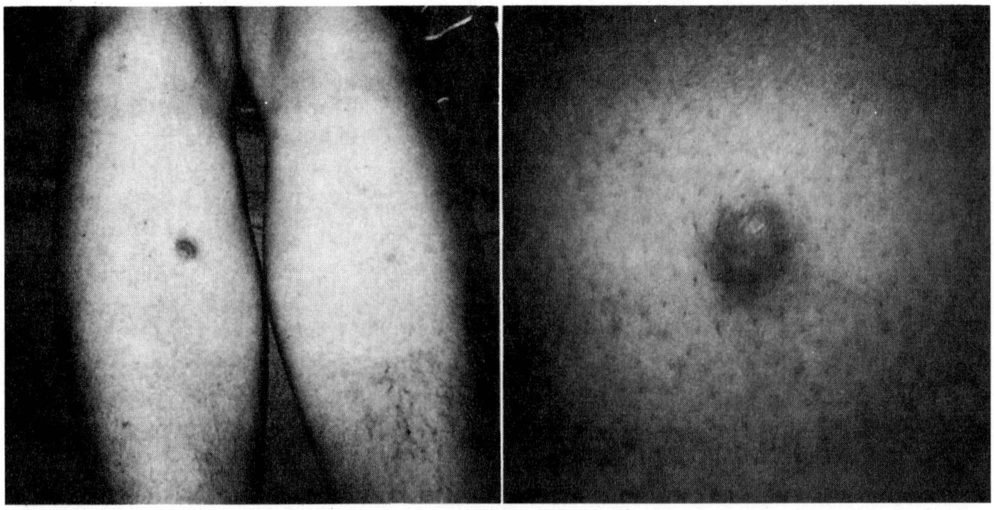

B

FIGURE 20-31 Fibrous histiocytoma (sclerosing hemangioma). **A**, Typical smooth lesion on lower extremity. **B**, Close-up view.

cular in origin. The single lesions can be excised easily, but the more complex collections are a challenge and have been treated with dermabrasion or dermaplaning and skin grafting. They are benign and should be approached as such, reserving the surgery for diagnostic and aesthetic purposes.

PROBLEM: NODULAR FASCIITIS (PSEUDOSARCOMATOUS FASCIITIS)

Nodular fasciitis is a benign, nodular, and proliferative tumor that appears on the upper and lower extremities, particularly in young adults.[23] On examination the lesions are part of neither the skin nor the underlying tissue. They rarely are more than 2 to 3 cm in diameter and are often painful and tender to the touch. The major differential diagnosis is with fibrosarcoma. Nodular fascitis is benign, does not metastasize, and rarely recurs.

PROBLEM: FIBROMATOSES (DESMOIDS)

Fibromatoses are nonspecific and include conditions such as knuckle pads and desmoids. One variety, knuckle pads, arises superficially from the fascia and aponeuroses and rarely invades more deeply. The deeper lesions involving the abdominal wall musculature in particular are the desmoid variety. The microscopic appearance is that of fibrous tissue and collagen bundles. They may be highly cellular and difficult to differentiate from fibrosarcoma. They may arise in old scars and are seen in children and young adults. The extraabdominal desmoids are most often found around the shoulder girdle in adults. These are more aggressive than the abdominal wall variety, and recurrence is seen in as many as 60% of cases.

PROBLEM: DUPUYTREN'S CONTRACTURE

Palmar fasciitis (Dupuytren's contracture) is a disease of the palmar fascia beginning with a chronic, noninfectious inflammatory reaction with nodules developing in the palmar fascia. There is a predilection for the ulnar side of the palm, particularly the ring and little fingers, although all fingers may be involved. It progresses from a phase of nodularity to shortening of the vertical fibers attaching the skin to the fascia, resulting in skin dimpling. Only later does true shortening of the fascia occur, leading to longitudinal contracture along the course of the palmar fascia, particularly the metacarpophalangeal and proximal interphalangeal joints (Figure 20-32). The condition helped in the recognition of the contractile myofibroblasts, which are actively contracting, a process seen as part of normal wound healing.[50]

Dupuytren's contracture is a condition of adults, men and women equally, with no true predisposition to one or the other hand, and is unrelated to handedness. Trauma is always implicated, but this cause is hard to document. The often-implied associations with diabetes, alcoholism, or epilepsy are also difficult to document.

Surgery is directed to release contracture, and intervention may be determined by the course of the disease. Rapid progression over a period of months from nodules to dimples to contracture would suggest earlier surgery is appropriate. In some cases the progression from nod-

A

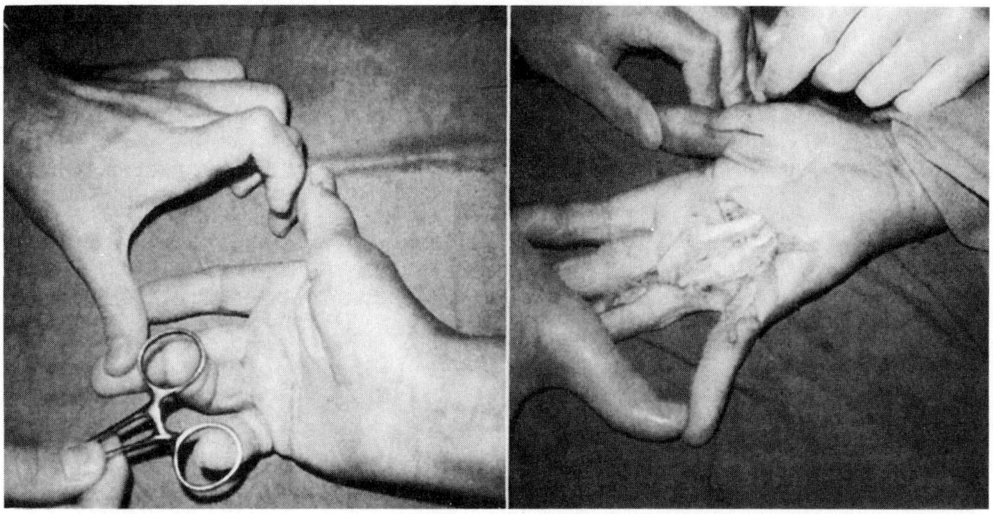

B

FIGURE 20-32 Dupuytren's contracture. **A,** Contracture of longitudinal bands with flexion of ring and little fingers. **B,** Release in the operating room. Closure required skin grafting.

ules to dimpling and early shortening may take years, and surgery may never be required. There is an association between palmar fasciitis and the other fibromatoses.

PROBLEM: PENILE FIBROMATOSIS (PEYRONIE'S DISEASE)

A disease of adult men, penile fibromatosis appears as fibrous plaques on the shaft of the penis, leading to pain and distortion on erection. The pathogenesis is unknown. It is associated with Dupuytren's contracture in 1% to 3% of cases. Surgical excision of the lesions, which are intimately attached to the tunica of the corpora, is best managed by replacement with a dermal graft to prevent distortion and recurrence.

PROBLEM: PLANTAR FASCIITIS (LEDDERHOSE'S DISEASE)

Plantar fasciitis is comparable to Dupuytren's contracture, with which it is occasionally associated. The treatment is the same.

PROBLEM: NEUROFIBROMATOSIS (VON RECKLINGHAUSEN'S DISEASE)

Described by von Recklinghausen in 1882, neurofibromatosis has received widespread lay recognition through the "elephant man," a man publicly displayed as a "freak" at fairs. His grotesque appearance was the result of diffuse tumor involvement, loss of tissue elasticity, and pigmentation (café-au-lait spots), all part of this disease.

The disease is transmitted as an autosomal dominant trait, although it can occur sporadically without a family history.[46] The lesion is heralded in infancy and childhood by the appearance of café-au-lait spots, which are tan macular spots of irregular size and shape. The existence of more than five in children (six in adults) is highly suggestive of neurofibromatosis. Furthermore, a café-au-lait spot found high in the axilla or on the perineum where sun exposure has not occurred is pathognomonic.

Later the tumor masses begin to occur. The classic lesions are soft and pedunculated and have a palpable defect in the skin through which the mass seems to be protruding. They may occur along the course of peripheral nerves (plexiform neuromas) and may accompany loss of elasticity and hypertrophy of the part (elephantiasis) (Figure 20-33). Histologic study shows neurofibromatous elements and is diagnostic. There is no specific site of predilection, but lesions are most obvious around the head and neck. Solitary neurofibromas have been reported. The incidence of malignancy in neurofibromatosis is unknown but is probably about 2% to 5%.

The patient may have severe bony abnormalities or a variety of manifestations, including scoliosis, bowing of bones that may or may not be due to direct involvement in the bone by the neurofibroma itself. Neurologic problems are also common, and the disease may be associated with mental retardation. The acoustic nerve is

A B C

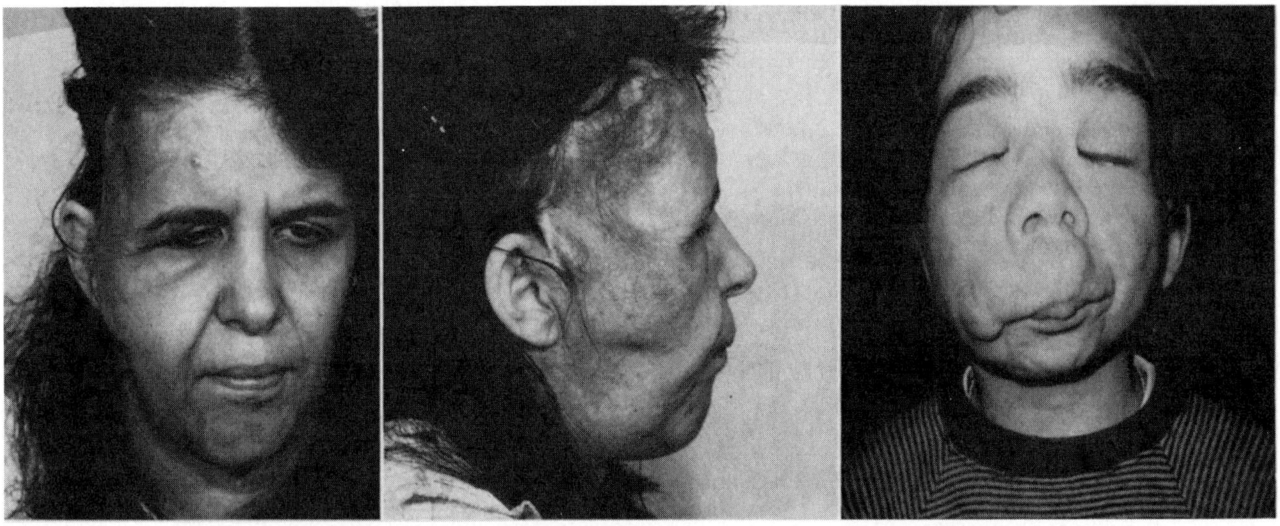

FIGURE 20-33 Neurofibromatosis (von Recklinghausen's disease). **A** and **B**, Neurofibromatosis in an adult, with pigmentation, nodularity, and loss of elastic support. **C**, Neurofibromatosis in a young boy with hemihypertrophy.

particularly likely to be involved, and deafness is common. Gliomas of the optic nerve may produce exophthalmos and decreased visual acuity. There can be intracranial involvement as well, and a few show malignancy. The neurologic symptoms are protean and may include seizures. Finally, there is an association with a variety of endocrine diseases, and a 5% to 10% incidence of neurofibromatosis has been identified in patients with pheochromocytoma.

The etiology remains obscure, although a nerve-stimulating growth factor has been thought to have been found by some investigators.

Treatment is a kindness and not a cure. Debulking and revision of tissue to maintain the best form and function are the challenge for the surgeon. Discouragement by the impossibility of cure should not prevent all efforts to strive toward normalcy through surgery.

SOFT TISSUE SARCOMA

PROBLEM: MANAGEMENT OF SOFT TISSUE SARCOMA • Roger S. Foster Jr.

The preceding sections described some of the various histologic types of soft tissue sarcomas in terms of their presenting characteristics and differentiation from benign soft tissue tumors. This section discusses the management of soft tissue sarcomas as a group because most soft tissue sarcomas have a common biologic behavior, and there is frequently considerable disagreement among pathologists as to the exact histologic type of any given soft tissue sarcoma. The histologic grade of a soft tissue sarcoma is more important than the histologic type. Histologic grade is a very important predictor of biologic behavior and is therefore of major importance in therapeutic decision making, as can be seen in the staging system for soft tissue sarcomas shown in the box below.

Assessment

Because soft tissue sarcomas are composed of relatively compressible tissue, they tend to first appear as soft tissue masses that are large in relation to their anatomic location. Only rarely do soft tissue sarcomas cause pain because of compression or traction on neurologic or vascular structures. The lack of symptoms can be deceiving to the unwary and lead to failure to consider the possibility of a malignancy.

The initial biopsy is an important component of the overall management of soft tissue sarcomas and, except for the smallest tumors, should be an incisional biopsy. As a rule, generous incisional biopsies should be taken

SCHEMA FOR STAGING SOFT TISSUE SARCOMAS BY TNMG

DEFINITION OF TNM

Primary Tumor (T)

TX	Primary tumor cannot be assessed
T0	No evidence of primary tumor
T1	Tumor 5 cm or less in greatest dimension
T2	Tumor more than 5 cm in greatest dimension

Regional Lymph Nodes (N)

NX	Regional lymph nodes cannot be assessed
N0	No regional lymph node metastasis
N1	Regional lymph node metastasis

Distant Metastasis (M)

MX	Presence of distant metastasis cannot be assessed
M0	No distant metastasis
M1	Distant metastasis

HISTOPATHOLOGIC GRADE (G)

GX	Grade cannot be assessed
G1	Well differentiated
G2	Moderately differentiated
G3	Poorly differentiated
G4	Undifferentiated

Stage Grouping

Stage IA	G1, T1, N0, M0, well-differentiated tumor 5 cm or less in diameter; no regional lymph nodal or distant metastases
Stage IB	G1, T2, N0, M0, well-differentiated tumor more than 5 cm in diameter; no regional lymph nodal or distant metastases
Stage IIA	G2, T1, N0, M0, moderately differentiated tumor 5 cm or less in diameter; no regional lymph nodal or distant metastases
Stage IIB	G2, T2, N0, M0, moderately differentiated tumor more than 5 cm in diameter; no regional lymph nodal or distant metastases
Stage IIIA	G3, G4, T1, N0, M0, poorly differentiated or undifferentiated tumor 5 cm or less in diameter; no regional lymph nodal or distant metastases
Stage IIIB	G3, G4, T2, N0, M0, poorly differentiated or undifferentiated tumor more than 5 cm in diameter; no regional lymph nodal or distant metastases
Stage IVA	Any G, T3, N1, M0
Stage IVB	Any G, any T, any N, M1, tumor with distant metastasis

Adapted from American Joint Committee on Cancer: *Manual for staging of cancer,* ed 4, Philadelphia, 1993, JB Lippincott.

before removing soft tissue masses that are larger than 2 to 5 cm to determine if the lesion is malignant and, if so, the histologic grade. Frozen-section reports may be unreliable; therefore decisions should await permanent histologic sections.

The absolute size of a soft tissue tumor that warrants incisional rather than excisional biopsy depends on the anatomic location. Smallest lesions on the hand or foot would warrant preliminary biopsy. In the subcutaneous tissue of the trunk, occasionally somewhat larger lesions may be appropriately removed without preliminary biopsy, but only if the excision will not contaminate tissue planes that would compromise definitive therapy should the lesion prove to be malignant. The problem with excisional biopsies is that soft tissue sarcomas are surrounded by a pseudocapsule that contains elements of invasive tumor that are left behind unless wide excisions are performed. The excisional biopsy of the large soft tissue sarcomas usually opens up and contaminates tissue planes, thus jeopardizing cure, or making the ultimate resection wider than would otherwise have been necessary, or both. Wide excisions are unnecessary and inappropriate for most benign lesions; therefore the preliminary biopsy is important in establishing the appropriate surgical approach.

Needle aspiration biopsy may be of assistance in ruling out a metastatic carcinoma. Needle aspirates are not usually sufficiently definitive to permit a firm diagnosis for primary soft tissue sarcomas, although they may demonstrate sufficient cytologic characteristics to suggest the diagnosis. A large sample of tissue is usually necessary to establish the malignant nature, as well as the histologic grade, of a soft tissue sarcoma. Needle aspirates or core needle biopsies may be of use in establishing the presence of recurrent tumor.

Placement of the open biopsy incision is important in optimizing definitive therapy. Generally, incisions should be placed so they can be completely excised when surgical resection of the tumor occurs and so they do not complicate radiotherapy to the area. Biopsies of tumors on the extremities should be placed longitudinally, and biopsy incisions at other sites should usually be placed parallel to the long axis of the underlying muscle.

Diagnostic Studies

Once the histologic diagnosis has been established, additional studies are carried out to supplement the physical examination, define the clinical stage, and determine resectability. These studies include various imaging tests to establish local and systemic extent of disease. The imaging studies for systemic disease include chest radiographs followed by CT scans of the lung. Liver scans, brain scans, and bone scans are not indicated because they are rarely useful in the asymptomatic patient.

Currently the most useful imaging study for local extent of disease is magnetic resonance imaging (MRI). Soft tissue radiographs have only limited usefulness. Angiography has played a much less important role in the local evaluation of soft tissue sarcomas since the availability of CT and MRI scans. Bone scans have limited usefulness in assessing bone involvement by an adjacent soft tissue sarcoma. A positive bone scan may be caused by a periosteal reaction when no actual erosion by the sarcoma has occurred.

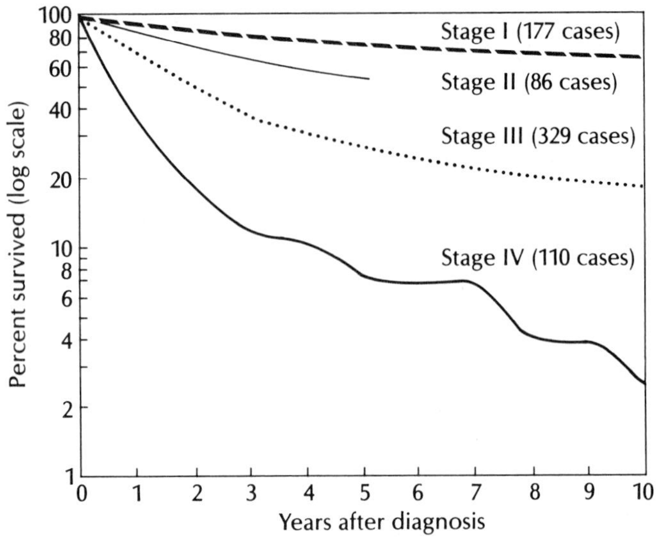

FIGURE 20-34 Survival curves by stage of soft tissue sarcoma patients for 702 cases with complete information for staging; 423 cases with slide review and 279 without. The curve for stage II was not plotted beyond 5 years because at that point the standard error was 5% or higher. (From Russell WO, Cohen J, Enzinger F et al: *Cancer* 40:1562, 1977.)

Staging

Once the histologic grade and anatomic extent of the soft tissue sarcoma have been established, it is possible to establish the stage of disease according to the schema that was presented in the box on page 851. The correlation of this staging system with survival in over 700 patients with soft tissue sarcoma is shown in Figure 20-34.

Pathophysiology

Each of the many histologic types of soft tissue can produce either benign or malignant tumors (sarcomas). Table 20-1 provides a listing of sarcomas with an indication of the usual histologic grade. As previously indicated, the assignment of the various histologic types varies considerably even among highly experienced pathologists. In most series liposarcomas make up about 15% of the total amount of histologic types, but the distribution between the designations of rhabdomyosarcoma, fibrosarcoma, neurofibrosarcoma, and malignant fibrous histiocytoma vary widely in different series.

TABLE 20-1 CELL OF ORIGIN AND USUAL HISTOLOGIC GRADE OF SOFT TISSUE SARCOMA

		GRADE		
NORMAL CELL	SARCOMA	1	2	3
Mesoderm				
Adipose	Well differentiated liposarcoma	×	–	–
	Myxoid liposarcoma	×	–	–
	Round cell liposarcoma	–	×	×
	Pleomorphic liposarcoma	–	–	×
Fibroblast	Fibrosarcoma	–	×	×
	Dermatofibrosarcoma protuberans	×	–	–
Smooth muscle	Leiomyosarcoma	×	×	×
Skeletal muscle	Embryonal rhabdomyosarcoma	–	–	–
	Alveolar rhabdomyosarcoma	–	–	×
	Pleomorphic rhabdomyosarcoma	–	–	×
	Combined rhabdomyosarcoma	–	–	×
Blood vessel	Angiosarcoma	–	×	×
	Lymphangiosarcoma	–	×	×
	Kaposi's sarcoma	–	×	×
Tendosynovial	Synovial cell sarcoma	–	–	×
	Malignant giant cell tumor	–	×	×
Uncertain origin	Epithelioid sarcoma	–	×	×
	Alveolar soft part sarcoma	–	–	×
	Malignant fibrous histiocytoma	–	×	×
	Myxoid malignant fibrous histiocytoma	–	×	×
Ectoderm				
Nerve sheath	Neurofibrosarcoma	×	×	×
	Malignant schwannoma	–	×	×

Modified from Costa J et al: The grading of soft tissue sarcomas. Results of a clinicopathologic correlation in a series of 163 cases, *Cancer* 53:530, 1984.

A group of soft tissue tumors also exists whose members are similar to true sarcomas but rarely metastasize. This latter group, which includes the desmoid tumors and the aggressive fibromatoses, are capable of infiltrating adjacent local tissue just as do true sarcomas. After injury, the proliferative healing response with the presence of mitoses can sometimes mimic the appearance of a soft tissue sarcoma.

Soft tissue sarcomas can arise anywhere in the body. About 40% occur in the lower extremities and 15% in the upper extremities. Approximately 20% originate in the chest and abdominal walls, 15% in the head and neck region, and 10% in the retroperitoneum.

Although most soft tissue sarcomas arise without known predisposing factors, some soft tissue sarcomas have been etiologically related to chemical exposure, radiation injury, and chronic lymphedema.

The factors that influence the prognosis of soft tissue sarcomas include the histologic grade, size of the tumor, site of the primary tumor, location of the tumor, and presence of regional node metastases. Sarcomas located distally on the extremities tend to have a better prognosis than more proximally located tumors. Sarcomas in the mediastinum and retroperitoneum tend to be particularly large at the time of detection and are less likely to be fully resectable, therefore they usually have a poorer prognosis. Soft tissue sarcomas infrequently metastasize to the regional nodes. In the small percentage of cases in which regional node metastases do occur, there is usually evidence of systemic metastases.

The poor prognosis of patients with the higher grades of soft tissue sarcoma is related to the sarcoma's tendency for both invasion into surrounding tissues and hematogenous dissemination. Local invasion tends to be along the fascialplanes that surround muscles, nerves, and blood vessels. After surgery that is done with curative intent, local recurrence rates for high-grade soft tissue sarcomas may be as high as 50%, with over 80% of the local recurrences occurring within 2 years and almost all occurring within 5 years. Sarcomas that recur after the first 2 years are usually of the more differentiated and more slowly growing varieties. A high propensity exists for hematogenous metastases of soft tissue sarcomas to grow in the lungs because the lungs are the most common site of first recurrence of high-grade soft tissue sarcomas.

Despite the general similarity of biologic behavior of the various subtypes of soft tissue sarcomas of equivalent histologic subtypes, more detailed discussions should be sought in other sources.[72,106]

Management in Adults

A variety of approaches have been used in the management of soft tissue sarcomas, including surgery alone, radiotherapy alone, surgery combined with radiotherapy, and surgery combined with radiotherapy and chemotherapy. Multimodality therapy, particularly with radiotherapy, has become increasingly common and has permitted less extensive surgical resections with apparently equally good survival rates when compared with radical surgical resections survival rates.

Surgery

Many soft tissue sarcomas have the misleading appearance of being encapsulated. In fact, this "encapsulation" is almost always a pseudocapsule of compressed fibrous tissue containing sarcoma cells. When soft tissue sarcomas are treated by local surgical resection alone, there is a very high incidence of local recurrence in the range of 60 to 80%.[21] To decrease the chance of local recurrence, proper surgical technique is to remove an envelope of normal tissue around the sarcoma wherever this is technically possible. Some surgeons have strongly promoted the concept of radical compartmental resection in which the entire anatomic compartment involved by the sarcoma is resected.[45,113] Accomplishment of radical compartmental resection implies en bloc removal of skin and subcutaneous tissue surrounding the biopsy site and any involved muscle bundle from origin to insertion, as well as attainment of a wide margin of normal tissue between the tumor and critical tissues such as nerves, blood vessels, and bone. Such wide resection is impossible in many anatomic sites. Amputations formerly were routinely performed to obtain such wide surgical margins for many sarcomas of the extremities. When amputations are performed well above the sarcoma, local recurrence rates have been very low. Local treatment failure after wide radical resection or by amputation well above the tumor, without other adjuvant therapy, is approximately 15%.[106] It is generally believed that prophylactic lymph node dissections are not warranted for most histologic types of soft tissue sarcomas in adults.

Radiotherapy

The experience in the treatment of soft tissue sarcomas with radiotherapy alone is limited. With high doses of radiotherapy (70 to 80 rad delivered over 7 to 8 weeks) relatively small sarcomas (less than 5 cm) may be cured by radiotherapy. The high doses required for sterilization of soft tissue sarcomas are usually followed by radiation fibrosis, which can cause considerable disability.

Surgery and Radiotherapy Combined

The theoretic advantage of combining surgery and radiotherapy is that the combination reduces the morbidity associated with either extreme treatment. It appears that appropriate combinations of conservative surgery and radiotherapy can produce cure rates equivalent to those of radical surgery[97,104,105,107,119], and the amputation rates for extremity sarcomas are greatly reduced. For most patients treated with conservative surgery and radiation, the functional results are very good, but a few have significant functional deficits. The radiotherapy may be given either before or after the surgical resection; there are advantages and disadvantages to each approach. External beam radiotherapy is used most commonly, but good results have been reported with brachytherapy.[18]

When the radiotherapy is administered after surgery, the pattern of extension of the tumor is better defined; the entire unaltered specimen is available for histopathologic study without radiation-induced changes, and no radiation-induced delays in wound healing exist. The advantages of preoperative radiotherapy are that the treatment volume is almost always smaller and the surgical resection usually more conservative. Radiation treatment volumes are usually smaller because it is not necessary to encompass the entire surgical field, which will theoretically have been contaminated by preradiotherapy resections. Surgical resections are usually more conservative because the sarcoma has frequently partially regressed. Whether a preoperative or postoperative approach is used, results are usually better when there is pretreatment planning between the surgeon and the radiotherapist, rather than sequential referral.

When radiotherapy is to be given after surgery, the surgeon can aid the radiotherapist by placing clips at the outer margins of the surgical resection. Usually radiotherapy to doses in the range of 50 rad in 5 to 6 weeks are administered to the entire field involved by the tumor along with all the areas entered in the surgical dissection. The treatment volume is then reduced, and additional treatment to a total dose of 60 to 66 rad is given to the area initially involved by the sarcoma.

The experience with preoperative radiotherapy is less extensive than that with postoperative radiotherapy. When radiotherapy is given preoperatively, an adequate incisional biopsy is first obtained. Doses of radiation in the range of 50 to 60 rad are given in 5 to 6 weeks and are then followed 3 weeks later by conservative surgical resection. Additional radiotherapy is administered to the tumor bed to total doses of 64 to 68 rad using either intraoperative or postoperative techniques.[118,130]

Surgery, Radiotherapy, and Chemotherapy Combined

A number of physicians have used preoperative intraarterial doxorubicin and radiation to treat soft tissue sarcomas of the extremities, followed by conservative en bloc resection, and have reported favorable results.[41,128] The value of adding either infusion or perfusion[46] chemotherapy to the surgery and radiation combination has not yet been established by controlled clinical trials.

A number of trials have been carried out to establish a role for systemic adjuvant chemotherapy in the treatment of high-grade soft tissue sarcomas after complete resection with or without additional radiotherapy. The current consensus is that the efficacy of such adjuvant systemic chemotherapy is not yet established and that further clinical trials are needed.[29]

Management of Metastatic Disease

The treatment of metastatic soft tissue sarcoma involves surgical resection where feasible (including resection of pulmonary metastases) and chemotherapy. Most chemotherapy programs for soft tissue sarcoma are based on using doxorubicin either singly or in combination with other drugs.[53] Intensive chemotherapy programs have shown response rates in the range of 50% with complete remissions in the range of 10% to 15%. Cure appears to occur in 20% to 40% of the patients who obtain complete remissions.[16,106]

Management of Rhabdomyosarcomas in Children

Rhabdomyosarcomas in children seem to respond quite differently from similar tumors in adults. In contrast to its role in adult soft tissue sarcomas, adjuvant chemotherapy is a well-established treatment for nonmetastatic rhabdomyosarcoma in children. Childhood rhabdomyosarcomas respond well to a multimodality approach of surgical resection and chemotherapy with or without radiotherapy. Total excision of the primary lesion is attempted as long as an unacceptable deformity does not result. When satisfactory surgical resections cannot be accomplished, a combination of radiotherapy and chemotherapy is used. Survival of children after treatment of localized rhabdomyosarcoma is over 80%, but it is less than 20% for patients with metastatic disease.[83,84]

CYSTS

PROBLEM: DERMOID CYSTS

Dermoid cysts are among the most common tumors the surgeon is called on to evaluate and treat. They most commonly occur in infancy and are noted by the parents rather than the physician. They may be differentiated usefully by location.

The most common location is in the lateral supraorbital region, in the outer third of the eyebrow (Figure 20-35). Rarely more than a centimeter or two in diameter, they are firm, are nodular rather than cystic, and cannot be compressed. They are often mobile but may be firmly attached to the underlying bony structures. They are not attached to the overlying skin, and there is no pit or pore suggesting such an attachment as in the epidermal or sebaceous cysts seen in adults. They are obviously of great concern to parents, and removal is indicated to alleviate concerns. They also tend to enlarge to worrisome rather than dangerous size and occasionally become infected. They are rarely, if ever, connected to anything other than periosteum. They do not extend to the meninges or brain. The surgeon's ingenuity should be expressed in making the incision and scar as inconspicuous as possible in an infant, such as through the eyebrow itself or through an eyelid fold. The cyst wall is usually nicely circumscribed, without unsuspected extensions, and excision is definitive.

As opposed to the laterally located facial cysts, *any* cyst or other lesion in the midline in an infant or child must be suspected of being developmental and as such connected to any underlying structure with which it may have been associated during development. Dermoid cysts in the upper midline of the nose, for example, often, if not usually, extend between the nasal bones, the leaves of the developing septum, sinuses, and to underlying meninges and brain. The surgeon must be circumspect in identifying this possibility in advance so that a planned simple excision does not become an unplanned craniotomy or disfiguring partial excision. Spreading of the nasal bones, lack of mobility, and telecanthus are some of the clinical signs suggesting deeper extension and indicating a challenging excision.

PROBLEM: EPIDERMOID CYSTS (SEBACEOUS CYSTS, WENS, STEATOMAS)

As opposed to the dermoid cysts, which are congenital, epidermoid cysts are developmental, even in the rarer occasions when they are seen in children. Related to the sebum secretion into the hair follicle, many of these seem to result from a blocked oil gland. This explanation is useful for the patient, who usually is seen with a painless lump (swelling, tumefaction, or cyst) in one of the oilier skin areas on the body such as behind the ear, on the back of the neck, on the cheek, or anywhere on the back (Figure 20-35). They are clearly attached to the skin on examination, and an enlarged pore is often near the surface attachment, which helps in the diagnosis. The cyst is firm and usually not compressible, giving the impression of a solid tumor rather than a cyst. The patient may have previously expressed material from it and might describe it as "cheesy," usually whitish and foul smelling. There may have been previous infection, and frequently patients will come to the surgeon for the first time when they are infected. Removal or at least destruction is indicated because infection occurs in most of the cysts eventually and makes subsequent treatment more difficult. They may be unsightly and, although obviously benign, nevertheless a worry to the patient.

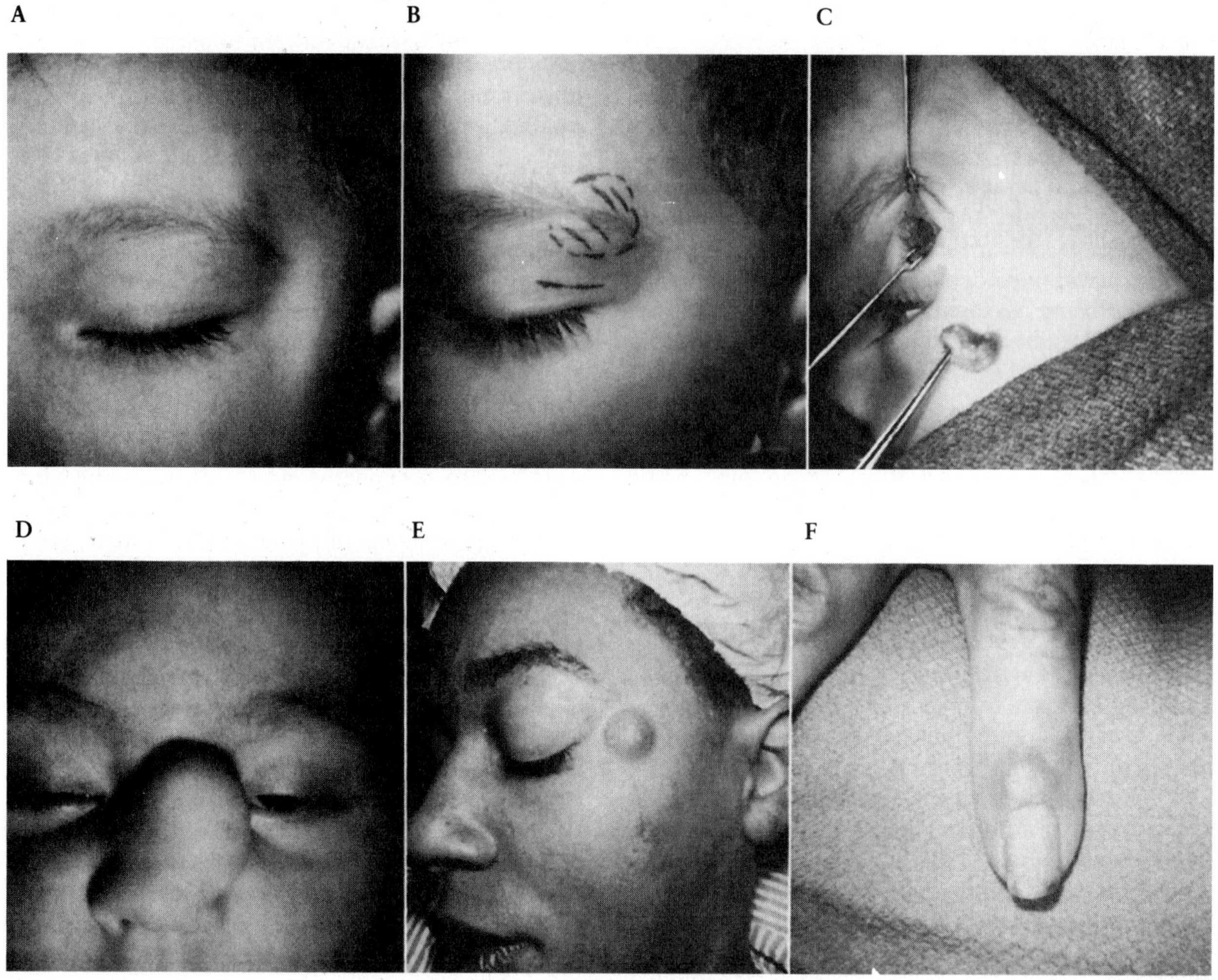

FIGURE 20-35 Cysts. **A,** Dermoid cyst, typical location. **B,** Incision in eyelid. **C,** Cyst removed. **D,** Midline lesion—an encephalocele. **E,** Epidermoid cyst (sebaceous cyst). **F,** Myxoid cyst of the finger.

The pathology of the lesion is that of accumulated sebaceous secretions and keratinaceous material, often under pressure. The wall is that of a pseudocyst, a compressed wall of fibrous tissue and collapsed cells rather than a secreting lining as such. Although incomplete removal may result in reappearance, reappearance in the same or nearby area may occur in situations in which complete removal had been attempted. The acutely inflamed lesion should be incised and drained like any abscess and then removed later when inflammation has subsided. Removal should take into account the benign nature of the condition and the fact that recurrence is more an irritation than a serious consequence. Thus a conservative approach is indicated.

A small incision followed by cautery of the wall is an approach used with considerable success by dermatologists for smaller lesions and should not be ignored by surgeons. Removal of the wall seems desirable; however, a large incision and removal of the cyst intact are unnecessary. Small incisions along expression lines allow the surgeon to evacuate the contents, and then the collapsed wall can be teased out.

Unless clinically infected, the lesions are usually without substantial bacterial growth, and primary wound closure is indicated. Cysts that have been previously ruptured or inflamed may initiate an inflammatory reaction in the tissue, which on occasion has been thought to be neoplastic. The incidence of malignancy in epidermoid cysts is negligible, and they should not be considered premalignant.

PROBLEM: OTHER CYSTS

A variety of other benign cysts are included for completeness. They are as follows:

Pilar cysts from hair follicles, usually the scalp
Mucous cysts: small salivary, inflammatory, usually on lips
Milia: small blocked oil gland on face ("whiteheads")
Myxoid cysts: from trauma, usually on fingers; contain degenerative material (Figure 20-33, *F*)

This chapter includes lesions from the common to unusual and might appropriately conclude with a trivial condition known as a clavus. A clavus is a small painful sinus or cyst found between the toes, usually caused by trauma and an invaginated hair. Identification and removal will gain the gratitude of the patient and the admiration of your colleagues for having known what it was.

PROBLEM: PILONIDAL CYSTS AND SINUSES • Roger S. Foster Jr.

Pilonidal cysts and sinuses occur most commonly in the sacrococcygeal region, but they also occur in other areas such as the beard, the axilla, the umbilicus, and the interdigital web space of the hands or feet. The term *pilonidal* means "hair-nest" (*pilus*-hair and *nidus*-nest). The presence of the hairs in the subcutaneous tissue predisposes the area to infection and abscess formation as may occur with any contaminated foreign body.

Clinical Presentation

History (Subjective Findings)

An uninfected pilonidal sinus tract is usually asymptomatic. The symptoms are related to cellulitis or abscess formation and, during periods of acute infection, consist of pain and swelling. Rarely some spontaneous drainage may occur. Fever and malaise are uncommon. The patient may report previous episodes that have subsided spontaneously. If a previous abscess existed that was simply incised or that drained spontaneously, there may be a history of recurrent episodes of intermittent exacerbation of the infection with periodic drainage from one or more sinuses.

Physical Examination (Objective Findings)

In an acute pilonidal cyst, an area of swelling with tenderness usually exists. Erythema and induration surrounding the abscess are usually minimal. Careful inspection frequently reveals the pit or pits that are the origin of the disease and through which the hairs can gain access to the subcutaneous tissue. The pits in the sacrococcygeal area are typically located in the midline of the natal cleft several centimeters from the anus. If a probe is inserted into the pit, it will usually pass somewhat laterally and cephalad, rather than toward the anus.[77]

Assessment

The surgeon needs to make the distinction between acute pilonidal abscess and chronic pilonidal disease. In the sacrococcygeal area, the skin is relatively thick, and the uninitiated surgeon may not recognize the presence of an abscess. In other areas where the skin is thinner, an infected pilonidal cyst may have the appearance of a small boil or folliculitis, with the cause only being recognized if the surgeon inspects the drainage from the abscess for the presence of the telltale hairs.

Pathophysiology

Many once believed that sacrococcygeal pilonidal disease was a problem of congenital origin. Current evidence strongly indicates an acquired origin for pilonidal disease, with most infections being related to penetration of the skin by hair. Penetration of hair shafts is aided by trapping and alignment of hairs between the buttocks. When hairs are examined under the microscope, it can be seen that they have scales and that the free ends of the scales point towards the hair tip. Rubbing a hair between the fingers in the direction of the long axis of the hair shaft will cause the hair to migrate in the direction of the hair root because of the increased friction of the scales that point toward the tip. When hairs are removed from a pilonidal sinus and examined microscopically, the scales point toward the sinus opening. If hairs are experimentally engaged in the mouth of a pilonidal sinus and the patient instructed to walk about for a period, it can be seen that hairs placed root first will usually migrate into the sinus, whereas hairs placed tip first into the sinus will usually be extruded.[94]

Hirsutism in the buttock and perineal region appears to be associated with development of pilonidal disease, but the shed hairs that are found in sacrococcygeal pilonidal cysts can come from the head and even from other persons. There is some debate as to whether penetration of hair shafts beneath the skin is the single cause of all pilonidal disease because hairs may not always be detected. It has been suggested that the pilonidal sinus may have its origin in distorted midline hair follicles that accumulate desquamated epithelial material, causing enlargement of the follicle. The follicle may then become infected either with or without the presence of penetrating hair.[14] The detection of hairs in pilonidal disease appears to be related in part to the diligence with which the drainage from acute pilonidal cysts and the material in chronic sinuses is searched. Raffman[99] found hair in 115 of 187 specimens examined.[99]

Pilonidal disease usually occurs in young adults and is much more common in men than in women. There is an impression that patients affected with sacrococcygeal pilonidal disease are usually overweight and have a deep sulcus between firm, thick buttocks. The predilection for young adults may be in part related to body habitus and in part to the relatively active and open pores of follicles with sebaceous glands that may provide a port of entry for the hair shaft. Pilonidal disease is not to be confused with the rare, congenital sacrococcygeal dermoid cysts.

Management

Acute Pilonidal Cyst

Because an acute pilonidal cyst abscess is painful and can continue to enlarge quite rapidly, most patients should receive prompt surgical treatment. Antibiotic treatment is rarely indicated, except for patients who are immunosuppressed or for those who have conditions particularly prone to infection, such as valvular heart disease. Acute surgical management consists of either simple incision and drainage of the abscess or careful definitive emergency surgical treatment with drainage of the abscess and opening of all sinus tracts.

Simple incision and drainage has historically been the most commonly performed procedure and is the most appropriate procedure if an experienced surgeon is not available. An incision is made through the skin in the fluctuant area as close as possible to the opening of any visible sinus pit. The wound should be gently probed to make sure that no additional loculations exist, and all collections of hair that can be found are extracted. The patient is promptly relieved of the acute pain by the incision and drainage. Once the inflammatory process has resolved, most patients treated by simple incision require a more definitive procedure to prevent recurrence. The pilonidal cysts occurring in other locations are usually cured by incision and drainage with removal of the foreign body hairs.

When properly performed, definitive emergency treatment of an acute sacrococcygeal pilonidal abscess and sinus can reduce the period of morbidity from the disease. In my experience, and the experience of others,[59] recurrence after such a procedure is uncommon. The procedure needs to be carried out in a minor surgery suite with good lighting and can be carried out under local anesthesia with or without an intravenous analgesia or an ataractic such as diazepam. With the patient prone, the buttocks are shaved and tracted apart with tape to provide wide exposure. An anesthetic such as lidocaine hydrochloride with 1:200,000 epinephrine is used. Injection is begun in uninvolved tissue cephalad to the abscess and is slowly infiltrated subcutaneously around the periphery of the abscess and deep to the abscess. If the local anesthesia is infiltrated slowly and skillfully, there is little pain and most patients will not require intravenous analgesia.

A malleable probe is inserted into the pilonidal sinus pit in the midline and advanced into the abscess cavity, which is usually located cephalad and laterally. An incision is made over the probe to completely expose the abscess cavity, and any secondary sinuses are sought and also incised. No skin is removed except for the epithelial-lined sinus tract leading into the abscess, which is excised along with a minimum of surrounding tissue. The cavity is wiped clean with gauze sponges to remove all hair and granulation tissue; additional local anesthetic with epinephrine is injected to inhibit bleeding and to provide good visualization so that all foreign bodies are removed, and all lateral tracts are identified and opened. Electrocautery may also be used to provide hemostasis. The cavity is loosely packed with a fine mesh gauze moistened with the epinephrine local anesthesia solution. Dressing changes can begin after 2 days, and the dressing may be removed by the patient after a soak in a warm tub. Fresh

SURGICAL DISORDERS OF SKIN AND SOFT TISSUE

DISORDER	INCIDENCE	SIGNS AND SYMPTOMS	DIFFERENTIAL DIAGNOSIS
Nevi			
Junctional nevi		Light brown to black pigmented flat, smooth lesions on feet, hands, face, trunk — arise at dermal-epidermal junction; usually hairless with irregular borders	Other nevi Melanoma
Compound nevi		Combination of junctional and intradermal nevi, elevated and nodular — may be hairy or have a surrounding macular ring	

Compiled by Stephen Payne and Richard L. Gamelli; revised by Thomas J. Krizek fine mesh dressing is best applied once or twice daily by the patient's partner after the patient has soaked in a tub or shower. The wound is examined by the surgeon and carefully probed with a cotton-tipped applicator each week to prevent premature epithelial bridging over the cavity until healed. The patient may return to work or school as soon as the patient is comfortable, which is usually within several days. When skin is not excised in performing this extensive cystotomy (except for a small ellipse around the squamous cell–lined sinus tract) most patients are healed in 2 to 4 weeks. The patient is strongly advised to be meticulous in keeping the area free of hair by using a depilatory cream or by having the area shaved to prevent recurrence.

Chronic Pilonidal Disease

A wide variety of procedures have been described for the management of the chronic pilonidal sinus. These procedures include (1) careful complete cystotomy, opening of all tracts, and removal of epithelialized midline pits; (2) excision and primary closure of the lesion; (3) limited excision without closure, either with or without marsupialization; (4) wide excision; and (5) a wide variety of plastic surgical procedures of tissue transfer and skin grafting.

Many surgeons favor careful, complete cystotomy under local anesthesia as an outpatient procedure. The procedure can be carried out even in the presence of acute infection. Cyst walls are not excised, and care is taken not to excise excessive skin. The disability period is short, usually 1 day or less, and complete healing usually occurs within 4 weeks. Karydakis,[58] Bascom,[13,14] and Lord[77] have described slightly different simple procedures resulting in minimal disability and good long-term control.

Excision and primary closure of the lesion can be carried out when no acute infection exists. Limited but complete excision of all sinuses and foreign bodies is carried out. Most commonly the procedure is performed on admitted patients, but some physicians have reported successful outpatient excision and primary closure.[58,79,131]

Wide excisions lead to delayed healing and long periods of disability. Some surgeons excise the posterior wall of the cyst and then suture the skin to the fascia, marsupializing the cavity. This procedure speeds healing somewhat but still leads to healing periods of 1 to 2 months.

Some authors have reported excisions followed by various plastic surgical procedures that are based in part on the concept of leveling the natal cleft. These procedures seem unnecessary for the majority of patients, but a few patients with complicated and extensive disease may benefit. The types of procedures performed after radical excision include skin grafts, Z-plasties, and other tissue transfers.[17,49,56,62]

ACKNOWLEDGMENT

I wish to express my appreciation for the drawings (in Figures 20-4, 20-5, 20-8, and 20-10) provided by Dr. Kim Olthoff-Van Houten and for patient material graciously provided by Drs. Robert W. Parsons, William J. Hagstrom Jr., Lawrence J. Gottlieb, and Allan Lorincz.

TESTS	RECOMMENDED TREATMENT	MORBIDITY AND MORTALITY	COST CONTAINMENT
Biopsy if suspicious	Excisional biopsy		
Biopsy if suspicious changes occur			

Continued.

SURGICAL DISORDERS OF SKIN AND SOFT TISSUE — cont'd

DISORDER	INCIDENCE	SIGNS AND SYMPTOMS	DIFFERENTIAL DIAGNOSIS
Intradermal nevi ("common moles")	Affects almost entire white population	Very common round, smooth, elevated lesion of dermal origin; may contain hair; usually seen in adulthood Average: 43 lesions per male 27 lesions per female Incidence decreases with age	
Lentigines		Small, medium darkly pigmented flat lesions, usually multiple with no ulceration or hair	Other nevi
Blue nevi		Usually less than 1 cm in diameter, solitary, intensely blue with sharp borders, firm; found on head, neck, dorsum of hand; usually seen in early childhood; may cause pigmentation of draining lymph nodes	
Halo nevi		Depigmentation rings around nevi, may spontaneously disappear more frequently than other nevi	
Congenital nevi	1 in 1000 live births	Darkly pigmented nevi seen at birth; often have hair in them; usually less than 1.5 cm in diameter	Other nevi Melanoma
Giant congenital nevi (10% of all congenital nevi are "giant" type)	1 in 20,000 live births, as large as 20 cm or greater	Scalp, face; large, indurated dark pigmentation; may have thick, hairy growth; high risk of malignancy — up to 20 times that of persons without them	Other nevi Melanoma
Juvenile or "Spitz's" nevi	75% occur in juveniles 25% occur in adults	Solitary childhood lesion; occurs on face most frequently in children Occurs on trunk and lower extremities of adults Differs from congenital nevi or melanoma by having lighter pigmentation; usually has a more regular border and does not undergo suspicious transformations	Compound nevi Junctional nevi Congenital nevi

TESTS	RECOMMENDED TREATMENT	MORBIDITY AND MORTALITY	COST CONTAINMENT
Biopsy if suspicious	Excisional biopsy		
No need to biopsy unless changes occur	None	None	
Biopsy if appearance changes or lesion becomes enlarged or ulcerated	Local excision if biopsy is suspicious		
Biopsy if suspicious	Excisional biopsy		
Biopsy	Full-thickness excision		
Biopsy	Full-thickness excision		
Biopsy	Excisional biopsy		

Continued.

SURGICAL DISORDERS OF SKIN AND SOFT TISSUE — cont'd

DISORDER	INCIDENCE	SIGNS AND SYMPTOMS	DIFFERENTIAL DIAGNOSIS
Keratosis			
Actinic keratosis	Common among older, fair-skinned, sun-exposed persons or those exposed to radiation treatment Considered the most common "premalignant" skin condition	Occurs on skin areas exposed to excessive sunlight — most frequently in older persons with exposed fair skin; lesion consists of a parakeratotic scale in epidermis with resultant cutaneous horn formation. Considered precancerous Well defined, reddened, often scaling areas May have halo of erythema around lesion Skin may be focally thickened or atrophic Malignant change occurs in 20%-25% of lesions — evidenced by rapid enlargement, firmer, thicker lesions that become ulcerated	Squamous cell carcinoma Basal cell carcinoma Keratoacanthoma
Seborrheic keratosis	Most common skin tumor in the elderly (benign); Female to male ratio equal	Wart-like lesion, usually on face or trunk, color varies from gray brown to black and has a greasy surface 1-2 cm, yellow to dark brown, begins flat but becomes raised, greasy, and scaly, appears as if it were "stuck on," may be pedunculated Location: chest, back, neck, proximal extremities, exposed parts of face and hands	Melanoma Actinic keratosis Basal cell carcinoma Keratoacanthoma Actinic keratosis Leukoplakia Ulcers Melanoma
Keratoacanthoma	Usually occurs after age 50 — more often in males, especially with a history of excessive sun exposure Multiple lesions have been associated with immunosuppressed patients	Arises from upper wall of hair follicles, usually arises from previously normal skin, grows rapidly and usually spontaneously regresses; raised, sometimes red lesion Occurs on face — particularly nose, cheeks, around eyebrows, ears, dorsum of hands, sun-exposed skin Marked by rapid growth of pink nodular lesion with classic keratinous plug Often grows rapidly for 4-6 weeks, then often progresses over weeks to months	Commonly confused with well differentiated squamous cell carcinoma Squamous cell carcinoma Basal cell carcinoma

TESTS	RECOMMENDED TREATMENT	MORBIDITY AND MORTALITY	COST CONTAINMENT
Biopsy, incisional or excisional, depending on size	Excision Freezing Topical antineoplastic creams If recognized early, destruction of superficial cells can be accomplished by: Cryosurgery with liquid nitrogen Curettage Cauterization Topical application of 5-fluorouracil If clearly malignant, formal excision is indicated	Approximately 20% undergo malignant change	
Biopsy only if diagnosis unclear or if rapid growth appears or other malignant-type behavior appears	Excision indicated if found to be other than seborrheic keratosis and a premalignant or malignant lesion	Benign; not premalignant	
Excisional biopsy preferred because pathologists must have full cross section to examine If malignant, do wide local excision	Excision Fulgeration Radiation therapy for large lesions	20%-50% may have elements of squamous or basal cell carcinoma	

Continued.

SURGICAL DISORDERS OF SKIN AND SOFT TISSUE—cont'd

DISORDER	INCIDENCE	SIGNS AND SYMPTOMS	DIFFERENTIAL DIAGNOSIS
Hutchinson's melanotic freckle or lentigo maligna	More common in middle age	Slow-growing brown to black macular lesion commonly with interspersed pale areas, found most frequently on face, over 50% develop into melanoma, originates from epidermal melanocytes	Melanoma Blue nevi
B-K mole syndrome or dysplastic mole syndrome	Inherited as autosomal dominant trait	Familial atypical nevi with high incidence of melanoma development Most frequently found on the trunk and lower extremities, usually larger than most nevi (5 mm-12 mm), are multicolored from tan to pink to brown, with irregular borders Slightly raised, characteristically the same affected patient will have several lesions of different sizes, shapes, and colors, usually appear in adolescence	
Melanomas			
Malignant melanoma	1:150 adults will develop one before age 60 1%-3% of all carcinomas Incidence is increasing and affecting younger patients Most common in fair-skinned, blue-eyed patients—rare in blacks		

TESTS	RECOMMENDED TREATMENT	MORBIDITY AND MORTALITY	COST CONTAINMENT
Excisional biopsy of all these lesions	1 – 2 cm wide margin of excision if malignant		
Record lesions by photography every 3-6 months Full-thickness excision and biopsy indicated for any suspicious lesion or lesion undergoing change		10% of dysplastic nevi progress to melanoma	
Full-thickness biopsy	See Treatment Protocol for Malignant Melanoma below		

TREATMENT PROTOCOL FOR MALIGNANT MELANOMA

Stage	Depth of Penetration	Treatment
I	Breslow less than or equal to 0.99 mm thickness Clark level I, II	Local excision with margin of 1 – 2 cm of clinically normal skin; fascial excision not routinely performed
I	Breslow 1.0-3.9 mm thickness Clark level III, IV	Local excision with therapeutic regional lymph node dissection for clinically palpable nodes. With clinically negative nodes, alternative approaches are careful observation versus prophylactic regional node dissection
II	All levels	Regional lymphadenectomy
III		Regional lymphadenectomy indicated only for palliation

Continued.

SURGICAL DISORDERS OF SKIN AND SOFT TISSUE — cont'd

DISORDER	INCIDENCE	SIGNS AND SYMPTOMS	DIFFERENTIAL DIAGNOSIS
Superficial spreading	1%-2% of *all* malignancies	Originates at dermal-epidermal junction, early radial growth phase of melanoma development, 70% of lesions recognized at this stage Variably pigmented, slightly raised lesion, irregular "notched" margins; locations: back, back of arm, neck, and scalp ("BANS") tend to be most malignant areas; the back is the most common site in men, lower legs most common in women	
Nodular melanoma	15%-20% of malignant melanomas present at this stage More frequent in men, occur about 10 years later in life than superficial spreading type	Deeper pigmentation, more raised and nodular secondary to progressive vertical growth, blue to black in color, usually smooth and rounded with very irregular margins — may ulcerate and bleed; most commonly found in "BANS" area, especially head, neck, and extremities; invasive lesion, especially in a vertical direction	Junctional nevi
Lentigo maligna melanoma	More common in elderly women (5% of all malignant melanomas)	Most frequently on sun-exposed face; lesions have irregular borders and can become quite large, and deeply pigmented; often found in association with other seborrheic and keratotic changes; often have depigmented areas within the lesion; very slow growing; one-third develop nodular melanomatous characteristics	
Acral lentiginous melanoma	Most common melanoma of blacks Less than 10% of all melanomas	Occurs on soles of feet, palms of hands, beneath fingernails — tends to develop in areas of thick skin; goes through rapid "radial" phase to a vertical growth phase; firm, slightly raised lesion with irregular borders	Lentigo maligna melanoma Superficial spreading melanoma

TESTS	RECOMMENDED TREATMENT	MORBIDITY AND MORTALITY	COST CONTAINMENT
Full-thickness biopsy	See Treatment Protocol for Malignant Melanoma on page 865		
Full-thickness biopsy	See Treatment Protocol for Malignant Melanoma on page 865 and discussion in text on page 818		
Excisional biopsy	See Treatment Protocol for Malignant Melanoma on page 865 and discussion in text on page 814		
Excisional biopsy	See Treatment Protocol for Malignant Melanoma on page 865 and discussion in text on page 816		

Continued.

SURGICAL DISORDERS OF SKIN AND SOFT TISSUE — cont'd

DISORDER	INCIDENCE	SIGNS AND SYMPTOMS	DIFFERENTIAL DIAGNOSIS
Leukoplakia	Oral lesion more common in smokers	Mucous membrane disease caused by external irritants, particularly smoking when the lower lip is involved Irritation leads to keratinization, epithelial hyperplasia, and subsequent squamous cell carcinoma Found in oral cavity (particularly lower lip) and vagina Characterized by whitish, sometimes erythematous patches Well defined but may become confluent as they enlarge Ulceration heralds malignant change	Squamous cell carcinoma Irritant trauma
Basal cell carcinoma	Male to female ratio 2:1 3:1000 persons/year diagnosed Usually found in persons greater than 50 years old Most common malignant skin tumor in nonblack populations Most common malignant tumor to develop in children with nevooid basal cell carcinoma syndrome and in patients with the nevus sebaceous of Jadassohn	Chronic wind and sun exposure predisposes to development, especially in fair-skinned persons Xeroderma pigmentosa patients at greater risk Appearance: are usually less than or equal to 1 cm Nodular: most common — 85% found on head, especially eyelids, nasolabial fold, cheek, ears; 25% found on the nose — 15% around eyes; classically described as having an umbilicating center with raised pearly borders, usually underlying telangiectasia can be seen; may be pigmented and mimic melanoma; slow growing Superficial: flat, scaly pink appearance in less sun-exposed areas such as back and arms Sclerosing: slow growing, ill-defined borders found on head and neck; usually yellow and waxy with central sclerosis	Melanoma Squamous cell cancer

TESTS	RECOMMENDED TREATMENT	MORBIDITY AND MORTALITY	COST CONTAINMENT
Full-thickness biopsy	Remove irritant: usually smoking, also discontinue dentures and excessive sun exposure Usually only lower lip amenable to surgical resection — the "lip strip" procedure	In general, 6%-10% become carcinomatous Of those lesions already ulcerated, 25%-30% are already carcinomatous	
	Full-thickness biopsy, including normal tissue surrounding lesion Discourage "shave biopsies" Excisional biopsy if possible is preferred: Surgical excision: 2-3 mm "clean" margin adequate, although hard to always accurately identify normal/pathologic interface grossly; closure as appropriate for location and size of tumor excision Curettage: commonly employed by dermatologists — good for carefully selected lesions; wound heals by secondary intention Mohs' chemosurgery: highly effective in skilled hands, especially for lesions where margins are difficult to identify; also useful for some recurrent disease Second intention healing with or without some plastic reconstruction is usual course Radiation therapy: although some believe its use is satisfactory, its own carcinogenicity makes it a less safe and less desirable therapeutic option	Usually curable Almost never metastasize Only locally malignant	

Continued.

SURGICAL DISORDERS OF SKIN AND SOFT TISSUE — cont'd

DISORDER	INCIDENCE	SIGNS AND SYMPTOMS	DIFFERENTIAL DIAGNOSIS
Basal cell carcinoma — cont'd			

DISORDER	INCIDENCE	SIGNS AND SYMPTOMS	DIFFERENTIAL DIAGNOSIS
Squamous cell carcinoma	1.5% of all epithelial tumors, approximately 90% of malignant hand skin carcinomas Most common in elderly males — rare before age 30 2%-3% of all squamous cell carcinoma occurs in burn scars Second most common cancer in man; but accounts for 2000 deaths per year	Occurs in areas of solar or radiation exposure as well as areas of irritation, as with smoking exposure Areas: face, ears, lips, hands; lower lip lesions more common and may be associated with leukoplakia as a predisposing factor Appearance: usually start as red inflamed nodular area, easily confused with lesion of keratoacanthoma Rapidly progressive course, becoming enlarged, indurated, ragged, and ulcerated	Keratoacanthoma Basal cell carcinoma

TESTS	RECOMMENDED TREATMENT	MORBIDITY AND MORTALITY	COST CONTAINMENT
	Note: Although the vast majority of these tumors are slow growing and only locally invasive without significant spread or metastasis, there are important exceptions: These tumors can be much more aggressive in the immunosuppressed patient Basal cell tumors can invade across mucocutaneous borders into mucous membranes, where rapid extension becomes the rule Areas of concern are medial eyelid and edge of nasal skin		
Excisional biopsy — full-thickness depth of invasion important as with melanoma Lymph node involvement unusual unless lesion greater than 2 cm, has poor differentiation, or has arisen from old burn scars or chronically unhealed ulcers (Marjolin's ulcers) Squamous cell carcinoma has potential to metastasize, unlike basal cell carcinoma	Lesions less than 1 cm in diameter: excisional biopsy with .5 to 1 cm margin Lesions greater than 1 cm: excision with 1 cm margin, may require skin grafting Elective regional lymph node (ELND) dissection is controversial but therapeutic node dissection recommended when lymph nodes palpable Some also recommend ELND for higher risk lesions such as Marjolin's ulcers Curettage and cautery Radiation therapy Mohs' chemosurgery: useful in body areas where conserving neighboring tissue is critical, as with eyelids and nasolabial area	Nodal spread found in up to 35% of Marjolin's type lesions Recurrence rates in well-differentiated lesions approximately 10%; can be up to 30% in poorly differentiated lesions	

Continued.

SURGICAL DISORDERS OF SKIN AND SOFT TISSUE—cont'd

DISORDER	INCIDENCE	SIGNS AND SYMPTOMS	DIFFERENTIAL DIAGNOSIS
Nevoid basal cell, epithelious, or "Gorlin's Syndrome," or basal cell nevus syndrome	Not known	Autosomal dominant disorder characterized by childhood multiple basal cell carcinomas associated with cysts of the jaw, bifid ribs, mental retardation and other CNS abnormalities; these often atypical appearing basal cell carcinomas vary from classic nodular or superficial types to appearing more like seborrheic keratoses or nondescript nevi; may occur in "crops" rather than singly; unlike typical basal cell carcinomas, these lesions often lack the predilection for exposed areas of the body	Typical basal cell carcinoma Squamous cell carcinoma Nevi Seborrheic keratosis
Nevus sebaceous of Jadassohn	Rare	Usually solitary, well-circumscribed, irregularly surfaced, plaque-like raised lesion found on scalp, temple, or preauricular areas of children—occasionally at birth; usually has a waxy texture and is hairless; as lesion grows, sebaceous glands become hyperplastic, 10%-15% develop into malignancy, usually of basal cell carcinoma type; this occurs most frequently in early adolescence	
Bowen's disease	Two thirds of patients are same group at risk for actinic keratoses, basal and squamous cell carcinomas; more common after age 50 in patients with history of solar or radiation exposure	Premalignant phenomenon in which keratotic thickening and underlying erythema are found; 5% of cases become invasive carcinoma	Basal cell carcinoma Squamous cell carcinoma Actinic keratosis
Paget's disease		Eczema-like crusted lesions of areolar tissue of female breast; rarely found in vulva, anogenital area, or male breast; in breast, there is inevitably underlying breast cancer of intraductal or invasive type	Eczema Other skin tumors
Merkel's cell carcinoma	More common in elderly white people	Dark red or blue, slowly growing skin nodules; skin of the head, neck, extremities, and buttocks most commonly affected	Other skin carcinomas

TESTS	RECOMMENDED TREATMENT	MORBIDITY AND MORTALITY	COST CONTAINMENT
	Excisional biopsy of suspicious lesions may be complicated by multiplicity of lesions	Rare, have an aggressive malignant course	
Photographic records Biopsy if suspicious change occurs	Excise all lesions that undergo malignant transformation; some advocate excision of *all* of these lesions because of their malignant potential		
Excisional biopsy	Surgical excision for malignancy, curettage and cautery Mohs' technique		
	Treat underlying breast disease after diagnosed by biopsy		
Full-thickness biopsy		Aggressive cancer with early metastasis to regional lymph nodes—frequent distant metastasis and frequent recurrences	

Continued.

SURGICAL DISORDERS OF SKIN AND SOFT TISSUE — cont'd

DISORDER	INCIDENCE	SIGNS AND SYMPTOMS	DIFFERENTIAL DIAGNOSIS
Strawberry hemangioma	5% of all newborns develop this type of lesion — 70% are born with hemangioma	Vascular pink/red, slightly raised lesion in glabellar region; mass is soft and somewhat compressible — no bruit is heard over it; size varies from 1 cm^2 to large lesions (>10 cm^2); usually enlarge and reach peak growth at about 8 months; usually involute over 5-10 years (90%)	
Port-wine stain	Present at birth in 0.3% of newborns; seen in 85% of cases of Sturge-Weber syndrome	Usually found on face on one side over segment loosely corresponding to trigeminal nerve distribution; begins pink but darkens and thickens by third and fourth decades; may become nodular; these lesions *do not* involute	Other hemangiomas
"Salmon patch" or "stork bites"	Very common; up to 50% of newborns have one of these lesions	Tiny flat pink lesions seen at birth that do not grow or ulcerate; seen on forehead or nape of neck	Port-wine stain
Lipoma	Very common	Benign fatty tumor Any body area where fat is present — most often the back, shoulders, neck, head; fat lobules enclosed in a fibrous capsule	Liposarcoma Sebaceous cysts
Dermatofibrosarcoma protuberans	Rare	Protuberant lesion arising from trunk	Other soft tissue sarcomas
Soft tissue sarcoma in adults	0.7% of all cancer	Mass, usually large in relation to anatomic location; symptoms usually minimal	Benign soft tissue tumors
Pilonidal cyst and sinus	Tends to occur in young adults, usually in sacrococcygeal area; can occur in many other areas	Pain, tenderness, and swelling; occurs lateral and cephalad to midline sinus(es) in sacrococcygeal area	Perirectal abscess

TESTS	RECOMMENDED TREATMENT	MORBIDITY AND MORTALITY	COST CONTAINMENT
Serial photographs	Observation Local emollients If lesion enlarges rapidly, obstructs vision, or bleeds badly, must be treated Treatment: Steroids — prednisone daily for 4-6 weeks but not permanent resolution In rare cases low-dose radiation therapy is warranted Argon laser therapy is becoming more widely used, especially for lesions in which bleeding is a problem		Extended cystotomy at time of abscess reduces need for second procedure
Photograph	Treatment: Adequate makeup Tattooing has shown some success Argon laser treatment is gaining popularity		
Photograph	None	Usually fades away during first year of life	
Excisional biopsy	Excision — suction-assisted lipectomy		
Incisional or excisional biopsy	Wide excision with 4-5 cm margin	80% 5-year survival Very low-grade fibrosarcoma, rarely metastasizes	
Incisional biopsy CT scan to establish histologic grade and anatomic extent	Wide surgical resection to include margin of normal tissue Multimodality treatment with radiotherapy and/or chemotherapy should be planned preoperatively (see text)	5-year survival: Stage I, 70% Stage II, 55% Stage III, 25% Stage IV, 10%	
None	Extended cystotomy and limited excision of sinus tract Antibiotics usually not indicated	Wide resections delay healing	Extended cystotomy at time of abscess reduces need for second procedure

REFERENCES

1 Adair FE, Pach GT, Farrior JH: Lipomas, *Am J Cancer* 16:1104, 1932.

2 Aitken DR, Clausen K, Klein JP et al: The extent of primary melanoma excision, a re-evaluation—how wide is wide? *Ann Surg* 198:634, 1983.

3 Alpier JC: Congenital nevi: the controversy rages on, *Arch Dermatol* 121:734, 1985.

4 Apfelberger DB, Maser MR, Lash H: Extended clinical use of the argon laser for cutaneous lesions, *Arch Dermatol* 115:719, 1979.

5 Ariyan S, Mitchell MS, Kirkwood JM: Regional isolated perfusion of high risk melanoma of the extremities with imidazole carboxamide, *Surg Gynecol Obstet* 158:234, 1984.

6 Arons MS, Lynch JB, Lewis SR, Blocker TG Jr: Scar tissue carcinoma. Part I. A clinical study with special reference to burn scar carcinoma, *Ann Surg* 161:170, 1965.

7 Arons MS, Rodin AE, Lynch JB et al: Scar tissue carcinoma. Part II. An experimental study with special reference in burn scar carcinoma, *Ann Surg* 163:445, 1966.

8 Ashikari R, Park K, Huvos AG et al: Paget's disease of the breast, *Cancer* 26:680, 1970.

9 Balch CM, Karakousis C, Mettlin C et al: Management of cutaneous melanoma in the United States, *Surg Gynecol Obstet* 158:311, 1984.

10 Balch CM, Murad TM, Soong SJ et al: A multifactorial analysis of melanoma. Prognostic histopathologic features comparing Clark's and Breslow's staging methods, *Ann Surg* 188:732, 1978.

11 Balch CM, Murad TM, Soong SJ et al: Tumor thickness as a guide to surgical management of clinical stage I melanoma patients, *Cancer* 43:883, 1979.

12 Balch CM, Soong SJ, Murad TM et al: A multifactorial analysis of melanoma, Part II. Prognostic factors in patients with stage I (localized) melanoma, *Surgery* 86:343, 1979.

13 Bascom J: Pilonidal disease: origin from follicles of hairs and results of follicle removal as treatment, *Surgery* 87:567, 1980.

14 Bascom J: Pilonidal disease: long-term results of follicle removal, *Dis Colon Rectum* 26:800, 1983.

15 Becker SW: Concurrent melanosis and hypertrichosis in distribution of nevus unius lateris, *Arch Dermatol Siphilol* 60:115, 1949.

16 Benjamin RS: Soft-tissue sarcomas. In Moosa AR, Robson MC, Schimpff SC, editors: *Comprehensive textbook of oncology*, Baltimore, 1986, Williams & Wilkins.

17 Bose B, Candy J: Radical cure of pilonidal sinus by Z-plasty, *Am J Surgery* 120:783, 1970.

18 Brennan MF, Casper ES, Harrison LB et al: The role of multimodality therapy in soft-tissue sarcoma, *Ann Surg* 214:328, 1991.

19 Breslow A: Thickness, cross-sectional areas and depth of invasion in the prognosis of cutaneous melanoma, *Ann Surg* 172:902, 1970.

20 Breslow A, Macht SD: Optimal size of resection margin for thin cutaneous melanomas, *Surg Gynecol Obstet* 145:691, 1977.

21 Cantin J, McNeer GP, Chu FC et al: The problem of local recurrence after treatment of soft tissue sarcoma, *Ann Surg* 168:47, 1986.

22 Caro WA, Bronstein BR: Tumors of the skin. In Moschella SL, Hurley HJ, editors: *Dermatology*, ed 2, Philadelphia, 1985, WB Saunders.

23 Chung EB, Enzinger FM: Proliferative fasciitis, *Cancer* 36:1450, 1975.

24 Clark WH, From L, Bernardino EA et al: The histogenesis and biologic behavior of primary human malignant melanoma of the skin, *Cancer Res* 29:705, 1969.

25 Clark WH, Reimer RR, Greene MH et al: Origin of familiar melanoma from heritable melanocytic lesion: "B-K mole syndrome," *Arch Dermatol* 114:732, 1978.

26 Comings DE, Glenchur H: Benign symmetric lipomatosis, *JAMA* 203:305, 1968.

27 Conant MA: AIDS and Kaposi's sarcoma, *Curr Probl Dermatol* 13:92, 1985.

28 Consensus Conference: Precursors to malignant melanoma, *JAMA* 251:1864, 1984.

29 Consensus Development Conference Statement: National Institutes of Health consensus development panel on limb-sparing treatment of adult soft tissue sarcomas and osteosarcomas. Introduction and conclusions, *Cancer Treat Symp* 3:1, 1985.

30 Contanza ME: Results with methyl-CCNU and DTIC in metastatic melanoma, *Cancer* 40:1010, 1977.

31 Cottel WI, Proper S: Mohs' surgery, fresh-tissue technique. Our technique with a review, *J Dermatol Surg Oncol* 8:576, 1982.

32 Day CL Jr, Lew RA: Malignant melanoma prognostic factors 3: surgical margins, *J Dermatol Surg Oncol* 9:797, 1983.

33 Day CL Jr, Lew RA, Mihm MC Jr: A multivariate analysis of prognostic factors for melanoma patients with lesions >3.65 mm in thickness, *Ann Surg* 195:44, 1982.

34 Day CL Jr, Mihm MC Jr, Lew RA et al: Prognostic factors for patients with clinical stage I melanoma of intermediate thickness (1.51-3.99 mm): a conceptual model for tumor growth and metastasis, *Ann Surg* 195:35, 1982.

35 Day CL Jr, Mihm MC Jr, Sober AJ et al: Narrower margins for clinical stage I malignant melanoma, *N Engl J Med* 306:479, 1982.

36 Day CL Jr, Mihm MC Jr, Sober AJ et al: Prognostic factors for melanoma patients with lesions 0.76-1.69 mm in thickness, *Ann Surg* 195:30, 1982.

37 Dellon AL: Histologic study of recurrent basal cell carcinoma, *Plast Reconstr Surg* 75:853, 1985.

38 Dellon AL, DeSilva S, Connolly M et al: Prediction of recurrence in incompletely excised basal cell carcinoma, *Plast Reconstr Surg* 75:860, 1985.

39 Dorfman RF: Kaposi's sarcoma revisited, *Hum Pathol* 15:1013, 1984.

40 Dubin N, Kopf AW: Multivariate risk score for recurrence of cutaneous basal cell carcinomas, *Arch Dermatol* 119:373, 1983.

41 Eilber FR, Mirra JJ, Grant TT et al: Is amputation necessary for sarcomas? A seven-year experience with limb salvage, *Ann Surg* 192:431, 1980.

42 Elias PM, Williams ML: Retinoids, cancer and the skin, *Arch Dermatol* 117:160, 1981.

43 Elder DE, Goodman LI, Goldman SC et al: Dysplastic nevus syndrome: a phenotypic association of sporadic cutaneous melanoma, *Cancer* 46:1787, 1980.

44 Enneking WF, Spanier SS, Malawer MM: The effect of the anatomic setting on the results of surgical procedures for soft parts sarcoma of the thigh, *Cancer* 47:1005, 1981.

45 Enzinger FM, Smith BH: Hemangiopericytoma: an analysis of 106 cases, *Hum Pathol* 7:61, 1976.

46 Enzinger FM, Weiss SW: *Soft tissue tumors*, St Louis, 1983, Mosby.

47 Feinstein FR, Krizek TJ: Infiltrating lipomas, Presented at Annual Meeting of American Society of Plastic and Reconstructive Surgeons, Kansas City, October 1985.

48 Finck SJ, Giuliano AE, Morton D: Results of ilioinguinal dissection for stage II melanoma, *Ann Surg* 196:180, 1982.

49 Fishbein RH, Handelsman JC: A method for primary reconstruction following radical excision of sacrococcygeal pilonidal disease, *Ann Surg* 190:231, 1979.

50 Gabbiani G, Ryan GB, Majvo G: Presence of modified fibroblasts

in granulation tissue and their possible role in wound contraction, *Experimentia* 27:549, 1971.
51 Giraldo G, Beth E, Henle W et al: Antibody patterns to herpes bruises in Kaposi's sarcoma. Part II. Serological association of American Kaposi's sarcoma, *Int J Cancer* 22:126, 1978.
52 Gorlin RJ, Goltz RW: Multiple nevoid basal cell epithelioma, jaw cysts and bifid ribs: a syndrome, *N Engl J Med* 262:908, 1960.
53 Greenall MJ, Magill GB, De Cosse JJ, Brennan MF: Chemotherapy for soft tissue sarcoma, *Surg Gynecol Obstet* 162:193, 1986.
54 Greene HSN: The significance of the heterologous transplantability of human cancer, *Cancer* 5:24, 1952.
55 Greene HSN, Lund PK: The heterologous transplantation of human cancers, *Cancer Res* 4:352, 1944.
56 Guyuron B, Dinner MI, Dowden RV: Excision and grafting in treatment of recurrent pilonidal sinus disease, *Surg Gynecol Obstet* 156:201, 1983.
57 Handley WS: The pathology of melanotic growths in relation to their operative treatment, *Lancet* 1:927, 996, 1907.
58 Hanley PH: Symposium: the dilemma of pilonidal disease, *Dis Colon Rectum* 20:278, 1977.
59 Hanley PH: Acute pilonidal abscess, *Surg Gynecol Obstet* 150:9, 1980.
60 Hauben DJ, Zirkin H, Mahler D et al: The biologic behavior of basal cell carcinoma. Part II. Analysis of recurrence in excised basal cell carcinoma, *Plast Reconstr Surg* 69:110, 1982.
61 Hayflick L: The limited in vitro lifetime of human diploid cell strain, *Exp Cell Res* 37:614, 1965.
62 Hirshowitz B, Mahler D, Kaufmann-Friedmann K: Treatment of pilonidal sinus, *Surg Gynecol Obstet* 131:119, 1970.
63 Howard WR, Helwig EB: Angiolipoma, *Arch Dermatol* 82:924, 1960.
64 Humphrey LJ: Adjuvant immunotherapy for melanoma, *J Surg Oncol* 24:303, 1984.
65 Hurwitz S: Epidermal nevi and tumors of epidermal origin, *Pediatr Clin North Am* 30:483, 1983.
66 Jacobs AH: Vascular nevi, *Pediatr Clin North Am* 30:465, 1983.
67 Jones RE Jr, Austin C, Acherman AB: Extramammary Paget's disease. A critical reexamination, *Am J Dermatopathol* 1:101, 1979.
68 Kaplan EN: Incidence of malignancy in small, large, and giant congenital nevi. In *Symposium on vascular malformations and melanotic lesions,* St Louis, 1983, Mosby.
69 Karydakis GE: New approach to the problem of pilonidal sinus, *Lancet* 2:1414, 1973.
70 Kenady DE, Brown BW, McBride CM: Excision of underlying fascia with a primary malignant melanoma: effects on recurrences and survival rates, *Surgery* 92:615, 1982.
71 Lang PG, and Dubin HV: Hemangioma-thrombocytopenia syndrome. A disseminated intravascular coagulopathy, *Arch Dermatol* 111:105, 1975.
72 Lawrence W Jr, Neifeld JP, Terz JJ: *Manual of soft-tissue tumor surgery,* New York, 1983, Springer-Verlag.
73 Laymon CW, Peterson WC Jr: Glomangioma (glomus tumor). A clinicopathologic study with special reference to multiple lesions appearing during pregnancy, *Arch Dermatol* 92:509, 1965.
74 Lewis RJ, Ketchum AS: Maffucci's syndrome: functional and neoplastic significance. Case report and review of the literature, *J Bone Joint Surg* 55:1465, 1973.
75 Lindenauer SM: The Klippel-Trenaunay syndrome. Varicosity, hypertrophy and hemangioma with no arteriovenous fistula, *Ann Surg* 162:303, 1965.
76 Local recurrence and survival in patients with (Clark level IV/V and over 1.5 mm thickness) stage I malignant melanoma of the extremities after regional perfusion, *Cancer* 48:1952, 1981.
77 Lord PH: Anorectal problems: etiology of pilonidal sinus, *Dis Colon Rectum* 18:661, 1975.
78 Lorentzen M, Pers M, Bretterville-Jensen G: The incidence of malignant transformation in giant pigmented nevi, *Scand J Plast Reconstr Surg* 71:163, 1977.
79 Mandel SR, Thomas CC Jr: Management of pilonidal sinus by excision and primary closure, *Surg Gynecol Obstet* 134:448, 1972.
80 Martin J: Acquired immunodeficiency syndrome (AIDS) and Kaposi's sarcoma, *Int J Dermatol* 23:483, 1984.
81 Martin RG, Butler JJ, Albores-Saavedra J: Soft tissue tumors: surgical treatment and results. In *Tumors of bone and soft tissue,* St Louis, 1965, Mosby.
82 Mastrangelo MJ, Berd D, Bellet RE: Aggressive chemotherapy for melanoma. In *Principles and practice of oncology,* Philadelphia, 1991, JB Lippincott.
83 Maurer HM: The Intergroup Rhabdomyosarcoma Study: update, November 1978, *Natl Cancer Inst Monogr* 56:61, 1981.
84 Maurer HM, Moon T, Donaldson M et al: The Intergroup Rhabdomyosarcoma Study. A preliminary report, *Cancer* 40:2015, 1977.
85 McBride CM, Sugarbaker EV, Hichey RC: Prophylactic isolation-perfusion as the primary therapy for invasive malignant melanoma of the limbs, *Ann Surg* 182:316, 1975.
86 Meheegan AH, Pinkus H: Life history of organoid nevi. Special reference to nevus sebaceous of Jadassohn, *Arch Dermatol* 91:574, 1965.
87 Meyer KL, Kenady DE, Childers SJ: The surgical approach to primary malignant melanoma, *Coll Rev Surg Gynecol Obstet* 160:379, 1985.
88 Mohs FE: *Chemosurgery: microscopically controlled surgery for skin cancer,* Springfield, Ill, 1978, Charles C Thomas.
89 Morton DL, Wen D-R, Wong JH et al: Technical details of intraoperative lymphatic mapping for early stage melanoma, *Arch Surg* 127:392, 1992.
90 Moschella SL, Hurley HJ, editors: *Dermatology,* ed 2, Philadelphia, 1985, WB Saunders.
91 Norman J Jr, Cruse CW, Espinosa C et al: Redefinition of cutaneous lymphaic drainage with the use of lymphoscintigraphy for malignant melanoma, *Am J Surg* 162:432, 1991.
92 Overgaard J: Radiation treatment of malignant melanoma, *J Radiol Oncol Biol Phys* 6:41, 1980.
93 Pack GT, Davis J: Nevus giganticus pigmentous with malignant transformation, *Surgery* 49:347, 1961.
94 Page BH: The entry of hair into a pilonidal sinus, *Br J Surg* 56:32, 1969.
95 Peterman AF, Hayles AB, Docherty MB et al: Encephalotrigeminal angiomatosis (Sturge-Weber disease). Clinical study of 35 cases, *JAMA* 167:2169, 1958.
96 Pinkus H, Mehregan AH: Premalignant skin lesions, *Clin Plast Surg* 7:289, 1980.
97 Potter DA, Glenn J, Kinsella T et al: Patterns of recurrence in patients with high-grade soft tissue sarcomas, *Clin Oncol* 3(3):353, 1985.
98 Preston DS, Stern RS: Nonmelanoma cancers of the skin, *N Engl J Med* 327:1949, 1992.
99 Raffman RA: A re-evaluation of the pathogenesis of pilonidal sinus, *Ann Surg* 150:895, 1959.
100 Rhodes AR: Pigmented birthmarks and precursor melanocytic lesions of cutaneous melanoma identifiable in childhood, *Pediatr Clin North Am* 30:435, 1983.
101 Rhodes AR, Wood WC, Sober AJ et al: Nonepidermal origin of malignant melanoma associated with a giant congenital nevocellular nevus, *Plast Reconstr Surg* 67:782, 1981.
102 Richert RR, Brodkin RH, Hutter RVP: Bowen's disease, *Cancer* 27:160, 1977.

103 Rigel DS: Epidemiology and prognostic factors in malignant melanoma, *Ann Plast Surg* 28:7, 1992.
104 Robson MC, Krizek TJ, Wray RC Jr: Care of the thermally injured patient. In Zuidema GD, Rutherford RB, Ballinger WF, editors: *The management of trauma,* ed 3, Philadelphia, 1979, WB Saunders.
105 Romsdahl MM, Lindberg RD, Martin RG: Patterns of failure after treatment of soft tissue sarcoma, *Cancer Treat Symp* 2:251, 1983.
106 Rosenberg SA, Suit HD, Baker LH: Sarcomas of soft tissues. In DeVita VT Jr, Hellman S, Rosenberg SA, editors: *Cancer: principles and practice of oncology,* ed 2, Philadelphia, 1985, JB Lippincott.
107 Rosenberg SA, Tepper J, Glatstein E et al: The treatment of soft-tissue sarcomas of the extremities: prospective randomized evaluations of (1) limb-sparing surgery plus radiation therapy compared with amputation and (2) the role of adjuvant chemotherapy, *Ann Surg* 196:305, 1982.
108 Rosenberg SA, Yang JC, Topalian SL et al: Treatment of 283 consecutive patients with metastatic melanoma or renal cell cancer using high-dose bolus interleukin 2, *JAMA* 271:907, 1994.
109 Safai B, Johnson KG, Myskowski PL et al: The natural history of Kaposi's sarcoma in acquired immunodeficiency syndrome, *Ann Intern Med* 103:744, 1985.
110 Sasaki GH, Pang CY, Witliff JL: Pathogenesis and treatment of infant skin strawberry hemangiomas: clinical and in vitro studies of hormonal effects, *Plast Reconstr Surg* 73:359, 1984.
111 Shakespeare W: *The tragical history of Hamlet, Prince of Denmark,* Act IV, Scene III, London, 1603.
112 Shanoff LB, Spira M, Hardy SB: Basal cell carcinoma: a statistical approach to rational management, *Plast Reconstr Surg* 39:619, 1967.
113 Simon MA, Enneking WF: The management of soft-tissue sarcomas of the extremities, *J Bone Joint Surg* 58A:317, 1976.
114 Spicer TE: Hemangioma, lymphangioma and lymphedema, *Select Read Plast Surg* 3:2, 1984.
115 Spitz S: Melanomas of childhood, *Am J Pathol* 24:591, 1948.
116 Stein G: *Autobiography of Alice B. Toklas,* New York, 1933, Harcourt.
117 Stigmar G, Crawford JS: Ophthalmic sequelae of infantile hemangiomas of the eyelids and orbit, *Am J Ophthalmol* 85:806, 1978.
118 Suit HD, Proppe KH, Mankin HJ, Wood WC: Preoperative radiation therapy for sarcoma of soft tissue, *Cancer* 47:2269, 1981.
119 Suit HD: Patterns of failure after treatment of sarcoma of soft tissue by radical surgery or by conservative surgery and radiation, *Cancer Treat Symp* 2:241, 1983.
120 Tang CK, Toker C: Trabecular carcinoma of the skin, *Cancer* 42:2311, 1978.
121 Taylor HB, Helwig EB: Dermatofibrosarcoma protuberans. A study of 115 cases, *Cancer* 15:717, 1962.
122 Thomson HG, Ward CM, Crawford JS et al: Hemangiomas of the eyelid: visual complications and prophylactic concepts, *Plast Reconstr Surg* 63:641, 1979.
123 Van Scott EJ, Reinertson RP: The modulating influence of stromal environment on epithelial cells studied in human autotransplants, *J Invest Dermatol* 36:109, 1961.
124 Veronesi U, Adamus J, Bandiera DC et al: Delayed regional lymph node dissection in stage I melanoma of the skin of the lower extremities, *Cancer* 49:2420, 1982.
125 Veronesi U, Cascinelli N: Narrow excision (1-cm margin): a safe procedure for thin cutaneous melanoma, *Arch Surg* 126:438, 1991.
126 Walter J: On the treatment of cavernous hemangiomas with special reference to spontaneous regression, *J Fac Radiol* 5:135, 1953.
127 Warner J, Wilson Jones E: Pyogenic granuloma with multiple satellites, *Br J Dermatol* 80:218, 1968.
128 Warren S: Radiation carcinogenesis, *Bull NY Acad Med* 46:131, 1970.
129 Weisenburger TH, Eilber FR, Grant TT: Multidisciplinary "limb salvage" treatment of soft tissue and skeletal sarcomas, *Int J Radiat Oncol Biol Phys* 7:1495, 1981.
130 Wood WC, Suit HD, Mankin HJ et al: Radiation and conservative surgery in the treatment of soft tissue sarcoma, *Am J Surg* 147:537, 1984.
131 Zarem HA, Edgerton MT: Induced resolution of cavernous hemangiomas following prednisolone therapy, *Plast Reconstr Surg* 39:76, 1967.
132 Zimmerman CE: Outpatient excision and primary closure of pilonidal cysts and sinuses, *Am J Surg* 136:640, 1978.

CHAPTER

21

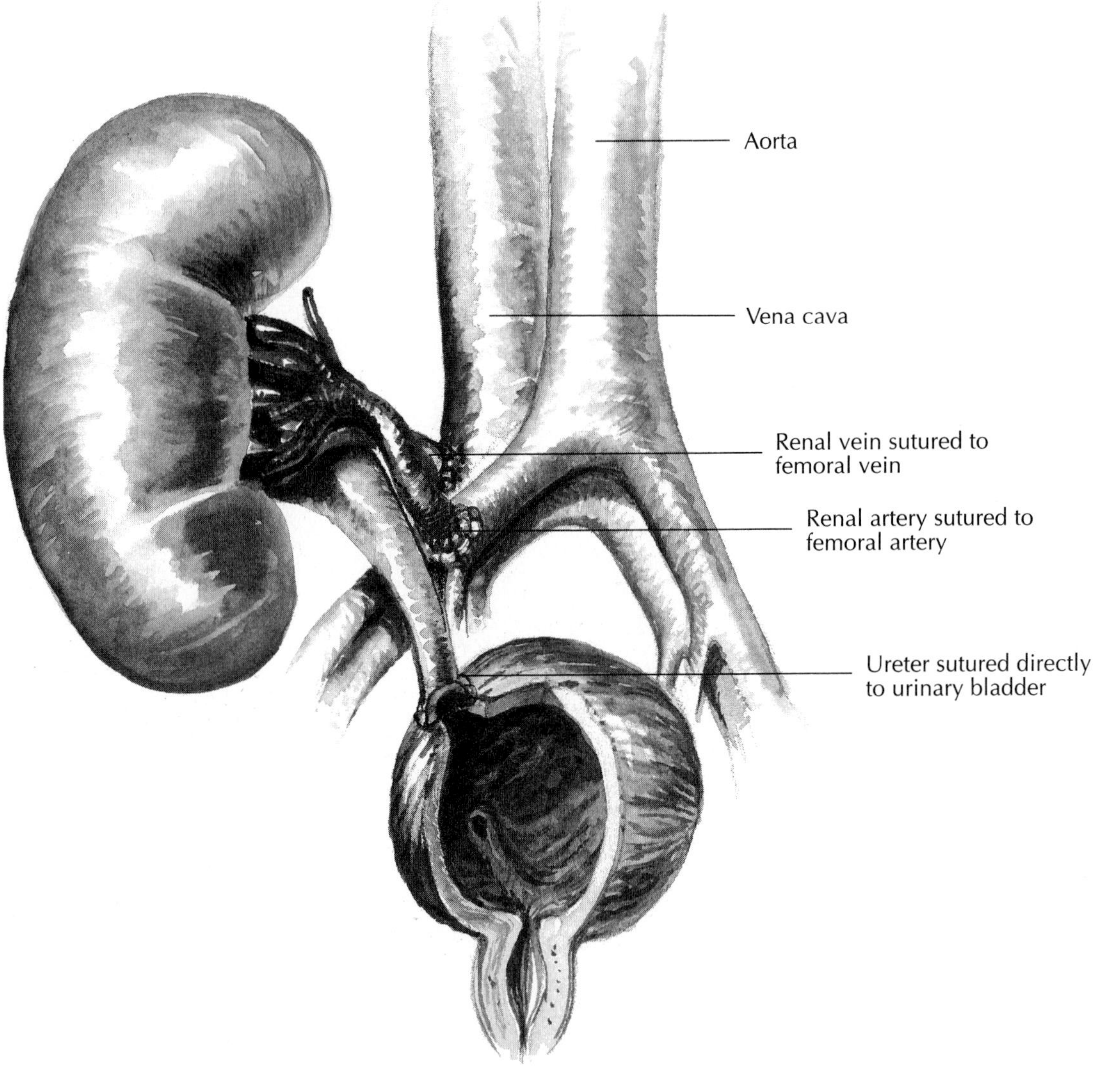

Aorta
Vena cava
Renal vein sutured to femoral vein
Renal artery sutured to femoral artery
Ureter sutured directly to urinary bladder

ORGAN TRANSPLANTATION

Arnold G. Diethelm • Mark H. Deierhoi • W. Henry Barber • Steven C. Poplawski

RELATED MATERIAL APPEARS IN CHAPTERS 13, 14, 34, AND 38

During the last 35 years progress in organ transplantation has far exceeded the expectations of most surgeons, physicians, and immunologists. The spectacular progress achieved in this field is the result of the development of histocompatibility testing, organ preservation, surgical technique, immunology, and especially the pharmacologic development of immunosuppressive agents beginning with azathioprine and corticosteroids in the early 1960s. The recognition that rejection is the result of immune responsiveness to histocompatibility differences in donor antigens has led to the attempt to minimize this genetic disparity by patient selection. This includes ABO matching, the identification of the donor, and recipient antigen profile combined with the exclusion of humoral antibody by a negative crossmatch. The experimental observations in the rodent in the 1960s and 1970s, which documented that the combination of donor antigen and immunosuppressive agents could lead to a form of partial tolerance, have been applied in the clinical setting. It is likely that donor bone marrow combined with new immunosuppressive agents may lead to a form of microchimerism. This in time may not only enhance graft survival but also eliminate the risk of malignancy and other opportunistic infections by decreasing the dosage required for chronic immunosuppression.

The success of clinical transplantation, however, has created a major problem in the shortage of organs that will not be resolved in the foreseeable future. Although the public awareness of organ transplantation has been greatly increased through the media, concurrence with the request for organ donation remains far behind the need. Consequently, organ shortage and rejection are the two paramount obstacles to clinical organ transplantation.

IMMUNOSUPPRESSION

The long-term use of nonspecific immunosuppressive drugs is necessary to prevent recurrent rejection episodes in solid organ transplantation. Although factors such as graft adaptation and the development of decreased host responsiveness to allografted tissue may allow for the reduction in dosage or the elimination of one or more agents, immunosuppression as it is currently used must be continued for the life of an allografted organ. Each drug used over a prolonged time has a unique group of detrimental effects to the host that are associated with its mechanism of action. In general, long-term immunosuppression carries with it the risk of viral and bacterial infections and tumor formation, which in some instances can be fatal to the allograft recipient. The following sections describe the commonly used immunosuppressive medications, their mechanism of action, and their potential complications.

Corticosteroids

Corticosteroids inhibit gene transcription for numerous cytokines, the most important being interleukin-1. These drugs penetrate the cell membrane and bind to specific receptor molecules, which are then transported into the nucleus and inhibit cytokine production at the transcriptional level.[25,32]

The inability of antigen-presenting cells to release interleukin-1 and interleukin-6 produces a greatly diminished inflammatory response. Furthermore, the ability of T cells to develop an interleukin-2 receptor is inhibited; therefore, T cell proliferation is significantly downgraded. In addition to cytokine release, corticosteroids inhibit the release of inflammatory mediators such as leukotrienes, thromboxanes, and anaphylatoxins, thereby decreasing delayed type hypersensitivity responses in tissues. The ability of corticosteroids to halt an ongoing inflammatory response has made them a first line treatment of acute rejection episodes, which although initiated by specific immunologic events, are in large part mediated by nonspecific inflammatory reactions.

The continued long-term use of maintenance corticosteroids is associated with numerous complications, including aseptic necrosis of joints, cataract formation, Cushingoid appearance, and bone demineralization. Therefore, every effort should be made to reduce the dosage to 10 to 15 mg/day or less.

Azathioprine

Azathioprine is an N-methyl-nitromidazole thiopurine synthesized in the early 1950s, which was intended to be a slow-release prodrug of 6 mercaptopurine. It was soon discovered that azathioprine was well absorbed orally, and independent studies performed by Sir Roy Calne in England and Charles Zukoski in the United States demonstrated its immunosuppressive effectiveness in canine renal allografts. Azathioprine was introduced to clinical transplantation in 1963 and along with corticosteroids became the mainstay of immunosuppressive management in human transplantation.

The pharmacologic activity of azathioprine appears to depend on the formation of active intracellular metabolites that inhibit de novo purine synthesis. In addition, a variety of enzymes required for purine interconversion in the salvage pathway are also effectively inhibited.[31] By depleting intracellular purine stores, cellular replication and RNA production are also inhibited. In addition to blocking cellular replication, azathioprine may also block antigen recognition by alkylating thiol groups on T-cell surface membranes.

Although useful as a maintenance immunosuppressive drug, high-dose azathioprine for the treatment of rejection episodes produced bone marrow depression with a righ risk of fatal superinfections in early clinical experience. The primary complication of long-term azathioprine usage is bone marrow suppression due to its effect on rapidly dividing cells. In addition, azathioprine is a direct mutagen, produces rapid dysplastic changes in cervical mucosa, and may facilitate the formation of ultraviolet light induced neoplasms of the skin. This serious side effect increases with the total dose of the drug and is especially severe in patients with prolonged graft survival.

Cyclosporine

Cyclosporine is a lipophilic cyclic endecapeptide isolated in 1970. The subsequent discovery of its potent immunoregulatory activity has not only improved clinical renal allograft survival by 10% to 20% but also has made feasible the transplantation of extrarenal organs such as the heart, liver, lung, and the pancreas, whose success rates before the clinical use of cyclosporine were so low that widespread clinical usefulness was precluded.[15,16]

Cyclosporine does not appear to interact with specific receptors on cellular membranes, and because of its lipophilic nature, crosses the plasma membrane by diffusion. Because of its lack of membrane interaction, it does not affect the binding of antigens to the T-cell receptor complex, signal transduction into immunoreactive cells, or calcium influx. Because cyclosporine does not interfere with the recognition of foreign antigens, the expression of cell surface receptors for a variety of lymphokines, specifically interleukin 2, is not inhibited. Cyclosporine binds to a specific intracytoplasmic binding protein and is carried to the nucleus where it inhibits the transcription of messenger RNA for interleukin 2, other cytokines, and enzymes necessary for the development of effective cytotoxicity. Cyclosporine also inactivates cyclophilin and calmodulin, thus inhibiting cyclic nucleotides, protein kinases, and other activation proteins. The immunosuppressive activity of cyclosporine is thus primarily related to the inhibition of interleukin 2 synthesis and helper T cell function.[40] This inhibition occurs before gene activation and events such as ribosomal translation of messenger RNA are not affected. Because of its mechanism of action, cyclosporine has not proved useful in the treatment of acute rejection episodes and is used exclusively as a maintenance agent. Its primary side effects are renal and hepatic toxicity, which on occasion so limits its use that therapeutic levels cannot be maintained.[62] In addition, cyclosporine may increase the development of lymphoma formation in allograft recipients; however this association has not been conclusively demonstrated. These problems notwithstanding, cyclosporine has become the current cornerstone of immunosuppressive therapy for organ transplantation. A recently developed derivative, cyclosporine G, appears to be significantly less nephrotoxic and possibly equally therapeutic.

Antilymphocyte Antibodies

Polyclonal antilymphocyte antibodies are obtained by the immunization of distantly related species with human lymphocytes or with thymocytes. The most commonly used animals for the production of antihuman lymphocyte antibodies are horses, rabbits, and goats. Immunized animals produce broadly reactive antisera that bind to numerous proteins on human lymphocyte surfaces. Antibodies interacting with platelets and erythrocytes are generally removed by adsorption before use. Polyclonal alloantisera, capable of producing profound short-term immunosuppression, are used primarily as induction agents in the immediate posttransplant course or in the treatment of acute rejection. The mechanism of action of antilymphocyte antibodies has not been altogether clarified; however, it is not entirely related to the bulk elimination of immunoreactive cells. Experimental and clinical evidence suggests that immunomodulation of alloreactive cells by the simultaneous presentation of alloantisera and donor-specific alloantigen is also involved. Long-term use of antilymphocyte agents in almost all cases leads to overimmunosuppression and is a high risk for viral and bacterial infections. Even short-term use for induction therapy or for treatment of acute rejection episodes (14 days or less) is associated with an increased risk of infection, especially from cytomegalovirus.[35] The concomitant administration of intravenous ganciclovir may prevent the risks of cytomegalovirus infection.

Monoclonal antibodies have also been produced that have specificity for T-cell specific surface membrane proteins. Monoclonal antibodies are produced by hybridomas created by fusing murine B cells producing a specific antibody with a malignant plasma cell line. Of the monoclonal antibodies that have been produced, the only one currently in widespread clinical use is directed against the T-lymphocyte cell surface receptor complex (CD3) and is known as OKT3.[19] OKT3 appears to be comparable in its ability to reverse acute rejection with polyclonal alloantisera, and it has also been used in some centers as standard induction therapy.[19,20,22] Like polyclonal sera, its use is associated with an increased risk of infection, especially viral. In addition, the use of OKT3 has been associated with the development of B cell lymphomas. The primary limitation of clinical usefulness with OKT3 is the development of the human antimouse antibodies, which often preclude multiple courses of therapy, as the host antibodies are then capable of rapidly clearing the murine anti-T cell antibodies, thus rendering them ineffective.[18,66]

New Immunosuppressive Agents

In addition to the standard immunosuppressive agents in current clinical use, several recently developed drugs are undergoing clinical trials in transplantation. One or more of these drugs will most likely be incorporated into routine clinical use; however, the precise efficacy and role of the newer agents have not yet been delineated.

FK506

FK506 is a lipophilic macrolide lactone that affects T cell function by inhibiting the production of interleukin 2, interleukin 3, interleukin 4, granulocyte stimulating factor, and interferon alpha in a manner analogous to that of cyclosporine. As with cyclosporine, FK506 has a specific cytoplasmic binding protein that transports it to the nucleus where its immunosuppressive properties are initiated. Because FK506 is almost entirely metabolized in the liver, its elimination is severely impaired in the presence of hepatic dysfunction. FK506 trough levels vary widely with individual patients and with the dose and route of administration. The clinical use of FK506 is rendered somewhat difficult by the poor correlation between blood and serum levels, the degree of immunosuppression, and the occurrence of toxic effects; however, these do not appear to be in reality any more problematic than was the use of cyclosporine shortly after its introduction. Current data would suggest that FK506 is similar in its immunosuppressive efficacy in terms of renal allograft survival to cyclosporine;[75] however, trials are still in progress and its precise role in renal transplantation is not yet clearly defined. The use of FK506 in renal transplantation has been limited by its intrinsic nephrotoxicity; however, one major advantage that has been observed is the lower incidence of posttransplant hypertension in renal transplant recipients. The most serious adverse effects associated with use of FK506 are neurotoxicity and new onset diabetes; these appear to be more severe than with cyclosporine. The most impressive results to date are in recipients of liver and cardiac allografts both as primary immunosuppression and for rescue from rejection.[38,88]

Rapamycin

Rapamycin is a lipophilic macrolide that blocks signal transduction of interleukin 2, interleukin 4, and interleukin 6, which are involved in the triggering of lymphocyte proliferation differentiation.[58] This drug has been effective in prolonging cardiac and renal allografts in experimental animals and early clinical trials have been begun with the use of the drug. The most serious effect of rapamycin is a vasculitis, which may be species specific. The most interesting potential usefulness of rapamycin is the combination with cyclosporine, and in experimental situations, a tenfold reduction in the effective dose of rapamycin dose can be achieved while maintaining adequate immunosuppression.

15-Deoxyspergualin

15-Deoxyspergualin is a guanine derivative that acts primarily on accessory cells involved in immune responsiveness and also reduces the expression of class II alloantigen expression on antigen presenting cells. Currently the drug is available in only an intravenous form, and its long-term usefulness is severely limited by toxic side effects. The drug may find use as an induction agent or to treat selected patients with acute rejection episodes. Early clinical trials indicate that, although the agent is effective in the treatment of acute rejection, profound leukopenia occurs in more than 85% of patients treated.

Mycophenolic Acid

Mycophenolic acid and its analog, mycophenolate mofetil, impair purine-dependent T and B cell functions by inhibiting the enzymes of the purine salvage pathway that catalyze de novo purine synthesis.[3] This property offers unique advantages over many other antimetabolites in that most cells other than immune lymphocytes are able to continue purine synthesis by alternative routes. The avoidance of generalized bone marrow suppression has allowed the use of high-dose therapy to effectively inhibit allograft rejection while maintaining generalized immune competence.[4] In addition the immunosuppressive effect of mycophenolic acid is rapidly reversible, disappearing within 24 hours of the discontinuation of treatment, unlike the prolonged effects seen with other agents. Clinical trials have demonstrated the usefulness of mycophenolate mofetil as both a maintenance agent and in the treatment of acute rejection episodes. This agent may well find a place as a standard immunosuppressive drug in clinical transplantation.

Brequinar

Brequinar sodium, a new immunosuppressive agent still in the experimental stage, has the potential to be an effective adjunctive agent combined with other drugs in preventing acute rejection. It is a 6-fluoro-2-3 methyl-4 quinoline carboxyl acid salt that inhibits the de novo pathway of pyrimidine biosynthesis. The compound interferes with pyrimidine biosynthesis and prevents DNA and RNA synthesis. This interference with DNA synthesis prevents activated cell proliferation and their response to an antigen challenge. The chief immunosuppressive activity occurs when the rejection process is largely mediated by antidonor antibody.[52] Whether this specific feature will be beneficial in preventing humoral antibody responses may be of special importance in preventing allograft rejection in sensitized recipients or in xenografts. The clinical trials of brequinar combined with cyclosporine are still in their infancy and the results are yet to be determined.

ALLOGRAFT REJECTION

Rejection of tumor transplants in mice was noted to be a consistent event when grafts were performed between different strains in experiments performed by Tyzzer and Little[87] more than 70 years ago. These early experiments preceded an era of intense investigation in transplantation biology and immunogenetics. In 1944 Medawar[54] confirmed that immune mechanisms were the cause of allograft rejection by performing a series of skin allograft experiments in rabbits. Medawar described the histologic events of primary rejection and demonstrated the accelerated destruction of secondary skin grafts that occurred via specific immunologic memory. However, in spite of the enormous progress made in the last 40 years in understanding the immune response to allogeneic tissues, the precise series of cellular events that occurs and forms the basis for manipulation of alloresponsiveness is not yet known.

Induction of neonatal tolerance described by Billingham, Brent, and Medawar[9] in 1953 generated new interest in organ transplantation and immunity. The immune reaction was further clarified by the observation that neonatal mice made tolerant would reject allogeneic skin grafts when reconstituted by adoptive transfer of normal lymphoid cells syngeneic to the recipient. Furthermore, in rats skin allograft rejection delayed by irradiation was normalized by adoptive transfer of virgin lymphocytes but not by transfer of lymphocytes from neonatal animals made tolerant. In addition, depletion of T lymphocyte levels by neonatal thymectomy produced prolonged survival of allografts. Mitchison[57] also demonstrated that the rejection process could be adoptively transferred by lymphocytes. It was then noted that congenitally athymic mice were unable to reject skin allografts, with the conclusion that specifically alloreactive T cells, probably cytotoxic T cells, were directly responsible for allograft destruction. In support of a T cell-mediated mechanism was the observation that bursal ablation in chickens had no effect on skin allograft rejection.[13] Although early evidence of antibody involvement was lacking, allospecific antibodies participate in skin and kidney transplant rejection, via either direct complement-mediated cytotoxicity or antibody-dependent cellular cytotoxicity. The interrelationship of cytokine networks is now clearer and most recent work has been directed toward defining the specific cellular elements and soluble factors involved in the host response to allografted tissues.[21]

Pathogenesis

Cellular infiltrates in rejected kidney grafts have a high proportion of graft-specific cytotoxic T cells thought to be responsible for graft rejection. It is also apparent that allograft infiltration is a mixture of T cells, B cells, monocytes, and granulocytes, many of which are nonspecifically trapped in the graft. Thus although graft rejection is probably in part mediated by cytotoxic T cells, the actual damage may be directed by other specifically activated cells that recruit nonspecific effectors of allograft destruction.[50] It has been demonstrated in mice and rats deprived of T cells that skin allograft rejection can be restored by adoptive transfer of T cells with helper phenotype alone, and that the inclusion of specific cytotoxic T cells has no additional effect. Recently it was shown that cloned cytotoxic T cells are capable of skin allograft destruction; however, only minor antigen histoincompatibility was involved, which may involve different effector mechanisms than the rejection of grafts with major histocompatibility complex (MHC) differences.

Some have suggested that mechanisms governing delayed-type hypersensitivity (DTH) reactions may also be responsible for skin allograft rejection. Because DTH reactions involve nonspecific recruitment of effector cells by antigen-specific activating lymphocytes, this type of immune reaction would be consistent with observed patterns of graft rejection. Furthermore, phenotypic DTH T cells have been observed to play a major role in experimental kidney allograft rejection.

The question as to which T cells cause allograft rejection remains controversial. In vivo the process of alloresponsiveness and graft destruction is probably mediated by several T cell subsets that may act alone or in concert to cause rejection.

Histocompatibility Antigens

Tissue antigens that initiate allograft responses have evolved from surface antigens that were present on the earliest multicellular organisms, for example, slime molds, and that primarily functioned in the discrimination of self from nonself. With the appearance of pathogens and the increasing structural complexity of life forms, the original markers of individuality became not only molecules for recognition of self but also recognition and regulation molecules for the various components of the evolving immune system. Base sequence homologies among chromatin materials analyzed from several present-day species, including mice, rats, and humans, indicate a common ancestry for immunoglobulins, antigen receptors on T lymphocytes, and histocompatibility antigens. Thus although the strict differentiation between members of a species no longer represents a major requirement for survival, the involvement of alloantigens in the function of the immune system and their recognition as being foreign, initiate the events leading to rejection of tissue allografts. Although the apparent paradox of the body destroying a nonpathogenic and often life-sustaining transplanted organ remains the greatest obstacle in transplant surgery, other functions of transplantation antigens, such as resistance to diseases, maternal-fetal immunology, and the suppression of neoplastic growth, are dependent in part on differences, rather than similarities, in genotypes.

Gorer[29] first demonstrated the presence in mice of an antigen (H2) that evoked antibody responses and appeared to correlate with tumor allograft acceptance or rejection. The terms histocompatibility genes and histocompatibility antigens, proposed in 1948, denote those genes and antigens involved in tissue compatibility and rejection. As the multiplicity (loci) and polymorphism (alleles) of the genes controlling allograft reactions began to emerge, the term histocompatibility complex was created. Distinctions between antigens causing vigorous skin allograft rejection and those causing more chronic rejection defined the major versus minor histocompatibility antigens, and the MHC designation was used to identify that group of genes coding for major antigens. Thus far, an MHC has been identified in all mammalian species studies, and it is likely to be present in all vertebrates. As mentioned, the biologic importance of the MHC lies not only in its preeminent influence on allograft survival but also in the control of a vast array of biologic phenomena, including immune responsiveness and the development of and susceptibility to diseases.

MHC antigens are glycoproteins and are classified by their biochemical and functional properties. Class 1 molecules consist of a single polypeptide chain with three domains and have a molecular weight in most species of approximately 45,000 daltons. They are noncovalently associated with a small, antigenically invariant chain, beta$_2$-microglobulin. In humans the MHC genes are located on the short arm of chromosome 6, and the A and B loci produce class 1 molecules. Class 1 antigens probably have universal tissue distribution. Incompatibility causes rapid (10 to 15 days) skin graft rejection in the mouse. Class 1 antigens appear to function primarily to guide cytotoxic T lymphocytes in the killing of target cells bearing identical class 1 antigens on their surfaces, which are associated with virus, haptens, or minor histocompatibility antigens.

Class 2 MHC antigens are dimers of noncovalently linked alpha- and beta-chains, which are approximately 25,000 to 33,000 daltons each and are not associated with beta$_2$-microglobulin. The beta-chains tend to exhibit a greater degree of polymorphism. Class 2 antigens are thought to be the products of Ir gene loci, described originally in the mouse as a group of loci (I region) that control immune responsiveness to a variety of antigens. In humans the Ir equivalent is the D/DR area located centromeric to the A-B gene cluster. Thus far, three loci are described biochemically: DP, DQ, and DR. Class 2 antigens have a restricted tissue distribution, being found primarily on B lymphocytes, specialized antigen-presenting cells, vascular endothelium, and other groups of activated lymphoid cells. These antigens have been shown to be the principal determinants that activate lymphocyte proliferation in the allogeneic mixed lymphocyte reaction (MLR) and in initiating graft versus host reactivity. Class 2 antigens appear to function mainly in cell-to-cell interaction regulating immune responses. Anticlass 2 sera also block proliferation responses to synthetic copolymers, and compatibility is necessary for maximum helper T cell support in generation of cytolytic T cell responses.

Class 3 genes code for complement components C4, C2, and factor B. The loci are poorly characterized biochemically and have not been shown to function as alloantigens.

The so-called minor histocompatibility antigens are not associated with MHC and in fact appear to be distributed throughout the genomes of vertebrates. They probably represent the products of loci coding for enzymes and other proteins that have a very limited polymorphism but can act as alloantigens when presented on cell surfaces. However, they evoke no primary antibody response, and skin allografts with minor antigen incompatibilities are usually rejected slowly. Minor antigens are only recognized in association with the original class 1 or class 2 MHC antigen with which the minor antigen was associated in the priming of cytotoxic T cells. Experimental data have suggested that incompatibility for minor antigens can provoke vigorous allograft responses and rejection of skin grafts. However, these same antigenic discrepancies may allow vascularized heart and kidney allografts to survive permanently. By contrast, prior sensitization to minor antigens usually causes accelerated kidney allograft rejection. Minor antigenic incompatibilities appear to be important in stimulating the rejection of vascularized whole pancreas allografts in rats and are probably also important in inducing the graft-versus-host disease in clinical bone marrow grafting.

Immune Responsiveness

The immune system is conveniently divided into two interrelated networks, the humoral (antibody) immune responses and the cell-mediated responses. Lymphocytes that differentiate in the thymus, the T cells, are in large part responsible for the cellular network. T cells have several different subpopulations, which can be generally identified on the basis of their surface antigens and specific function. Helper T cells respond to cell surface antigens on specialized antigen-presenting cells and act as triggering and amplifying components to effector lymphocytes of the cytotoxic and DTH types. Helper cells also appear to augment the activity of suppressor cells, which act to depress immune responses and prevent overstimulation in the absence of antigen. B cells are bone-marrow-derived antibody-producing cells. Most antibody responses are also largely dependent on helper T cells for maximal B cell proliferation, so that the cellular and humoral systems are interdependent. Cell-mediated responses are regulated via both antibody (B cell) and cellular idiotype-antiidiotype networks, which are based on the unique antigen-combining site (idiotype) found on antibodies and T cell receptors, and can themselves act as antigens. Recent work defining the molecular nature of the T cell antigen receptor has been reviewed by Acuto and Reinherz.[1]

Cells of the monocyte-macrophage line are derived from bone marrow and involved with phagocytosis and antigen processing and presentation. One of these, the interstitial dendritic cell, is a highly specialized antigen-presenting cell of this lineage that appears to have an especially strong stimulating capacity in allogeneic responses, as detailed later.

The immune response involves a complex set of reactions on the part of T lymphocytes, B lymphocytes, macrophages, and other antigen presenting cells, and cells of the inflammatory system. In response to antigenic stimulation, helper T cells secrete a set of protein mediators called lymphokines that regulate proliferation, differentiation, and function of other lymphocytes and hematopoietic cells. Many, if not all, of the effects of helper-inducer T cells are mediated by the production of lymphokines. Lymphokines are potent pleiotropic factors that also act on the T cells themselves. Indeed, two T cell-derived lymphokines, interleukin 2 and interleukin 4, function as autocrine growth factors, regulating the growth of the T cells that produce them. Because all or a part of this immune network can be activated in different ways by unique combinations of lymphokines, it is clear that T cells can play a vital role in coordinating the function of different body compartments in the immune inflammatory responses.

The activation of lymphokine genes in T cells by antigen is rapid and temporal; therefore, inflammatory response that involves proliferation and maturation of target cells may be restricted to the site of lymphokine production. Lymphokines or cytokines as they are also known may be involved in either up-regulation or down-regulation of immune responses. Those that are primarily proinflammatory may be further subdivided into those that are primarily growth and differentiation factors and those that are primarily direct functional mediators of inflammation. The clonally characterized growth and differentiation group includes the interleukins 2, 3, 5, 7, 9, 11, and 12.[33] Those that are primarily functional mediators of inflammation include interleukins 1 and 6, granulocyte/monocyte-colony stimulating factor, tumor necrosis factor, interferon alpha, and interferon gamma. Another group of cytokines has been shown to be primarily antiinflammatory or involved in down-regulation of immune responsiveness. These included interleukins 4, 8, and 10 and transforming growth factor β. Studies are currently in progress to characterize the groups of cytokines that are up- or down-regulated during rejection episodes in allograft transplantation and also up- or down-regulated during the process of development of allograft tolerance. A better understanding of cytokine function and the ability to manipulate cytokine regulation may in the future bear clinical importance in the diagnosis of prerejection episodes or in control of the immune response.[21]

The helper T cell appears to be pivotal in the production of cytolytic responses. Cyclosporine, a potent immunosuppressive agent, appears to have its major effect through deactivation of helper T cell function. Experimental evidence suggests that production of IL-1 and IL-2 is markedly depressed by cyclosporine, and that helper T cell and cytotoxic T cell responsiveness to IL-2 is also inhibited. Although the precise molecular mechanism is not known, the abolition of helper T cells effectively eliminates both antibody and cellular cytotoxic responses.

Immune responses to conventional antigens such as viral, bacterial, and haptenic groups follow a characteristic pattern of rise in both humoral (antibody) and cell-mediated responsiveness that wanes as the antigen is processed and cleared from the host. Although B cells and circulating immunoglobulin are capable of free antigen recognition, maximum B cell responsiveness is dependent on helper T cell function. T cells probably do not recognize soluble-free antigen per se but are activated by specialized antigen-presenting cells that process antigen and present it to responding antigen-reactive cells in association with self-class 1 or self-class 2 MHC molecules, depending on the cellular subtype responding. Once primed, these cells or their progeny are capable of recognizing the putative antigen only in association with the original priming self-MHC molecule, a phenomenon known as MHC restriction of immune responsiveness.

Allogeneic recognition of nonself-MHC antigens differs importantly from the response to the previously mentioned conventional antigens and to minor histocompatibility antigens, in that allo-MHC antigens can be recognized by T cells not in association with other class 1 or 2 molecules. Thus no MHC restriction of the responses occurs, and unusually large numbers of precursor cells appear capable of responding to MHC alloantigens.

The presentation of alloantigens to other elements of the immune system appears to be the function of specialized cells of the macrophage/dendritic type. Foreign class 2 antigens on allogeneic antigen-presenting cells represent a usually strong stimulus to helper T cell activation. However, presentation of alloantigens by macrophage/dendritic cells is not an absolute requirement because class 1 disparities alone can stimulate not only development of cytotoxic T cells but also development of anti-class 1 antibodies, which require helper T cell participation. Helper T cells appear to play a central role in the development of allograft responses, in both T cell-B cell cooperation and the maturation of cytotoxic T cells and activated macrophages, via both direct interaction and lymphokine release.

Much current interest in allogeneic sensitization centers on the dendritic cells and their transfer within the organ transplanted, that is, the passenger leukocytes. Early experiments on the effects of elimination of these cells from kidney allografts showed only marginal prolongation of graft survival. However, in selected rat strain combinations, the removal of passenger leukocytes (interstitial dendritic cells) has allowed permanent graft survival. Transplantation antigens per se are not always strongly immunogenic and could be introduced to erythrocytes, platelets, or membrane fragments or in soluble form via the intravenous route to generate a low and sometimes tolerogenic response. Similar results have been obtained in organ culture systems with thyroid or islets of Langerhans in which passenger leukocytes are eliminated during the period of culture, giving permanent allograft survival. The use of anti-class 2 sera to eliminate dendritic-type cells has also proved in some instances effective in islet allografting.

Lafferty and associates[46] proposed a two-signal activation hypothesis to explain the lack of apparent responsiveness seen in cultured allografts. They suggested that allogeneic dendritic cells are capable of directly activating helper T cells via MHC alloantigens on their surface and by the release of costimulating factor (IL-1) in an unrestricted fashion. This event subsequently caused proliferation of immune lymphocytes that directly attack the alloantigens present in the grafted tissues. However, in the absence of allogeneic antigen-presenting cells, foreign MHC antigen must be processed and presented by recipient-derived antigen-presenting cells, and it is proposed that these cytotoxic cells only recognize and destroy cells bearing both host class 2 antigen and donor alloantigens, which would not be present within the graft.

Although there is no doubt that dendritic cell-depleted allografts are less immunogenic and have more readily enhanced survival both with drugs and with enhancing sera, there is no evidence to suggest that cytotoxic responses to MHC alloantigens, when generated by recipient antigen-presenting cells, are in any way MHC restricted, as they are for minor antigens. However, these hypotheses may be applicable to vascularized organ grafts with minor antigen disparities alone, and the depletion of passenger leukocytes appears to be effective in circumventing the rejection of nonvascularized tissues, which depend on recipient capillary ingrowth for their blood supply.

The Rejection Process

The events leading to allograft rejection in nonsensitized patients probably involve numerous facets of the immune system and may be summarized as follows. Graft alloantigens may be presented to the recipient in one of two ways, either directly via dendritic-type passenger leukocytes within the graft or indirectly after antigens are shed from the allograft in soluble or cellular form and processed by the recipient's own antigen-presenting cells of dendritic or macrophage lineage. The initial responding cells are thought to be of the T helper type and require not only antigens but also IL-1, produced by antigen-presenting cells, to become activated and proliferate. T helper cells respond by producing a second lymphokine, IL-2, which drives their own clonal expansion and facilitates the priming and proliferation of effector cells. Activation of the second-order effector lymphocytes again requires the presence of alloantigens. These second-order cells include cytotoxic T cells, T cells mediating delayed-type hypersensitivity (T-DTH), and suppressor T cells. Helper T cells also intensify the humoral antibody response by acting in concert with B lymphocytes, having Ig receptors (idiotypes) for graft alloantigens to produce activated plasma cells. Thus, two arms of the immune system, cellular and humoral, are activated by transplant alloantigens.

Effector T cells of the cytotoxic type attack the transplanted tissues directly and cause damage via direct contact with cells bearing the MHC antigens to which they were primed. Cytotoxic T cells may be the major cause of allograft destruction in transplants having minor incompatibilities alone. Cellular damage by cytotoxic T cells is also caused by the release of intracellular lysosomes, kinins, and vasoactive amines, which potentiate tissue damage by nonspecific lymphoid cells, macrophages, and granulocytes and also cause ischemia via vasospastic responses. Effector cells of the T-DTH type also cause an inflammatory reaction within allograft tissues by activating nonspecific inflammatory cells that have been attracted to the transplant via antigen-specific cellular mechanisms.

Allospecific antibody responses play an important role in the rejection process. Preexisting complement-fixing cytotoxic antibodies are known to mediate hyperacute allograft rejection, and their appearance during an immune response to a transplanted organ is associated with vascular endothelial damage, platelet aggregation, and thrombosis.[44] Antibodies against monocyte/vascular endothelial antigens (non-MHC) have been associated with chronic vascular injury in heart allograft recipients and with rejection of haploidentical living related donor kidney allografts.[68] Other noncomplement-fixing immunoglobulins cause graft damage via cytotoxic cells in the antibody-dependent cell-mediated cytotoxicity system. Cell-mediated mechanisms and antibodies thus act together to cause both direct cytotoxicity and vascular compromise of the allograft. The relative role of each facet is determined by the nature and degree of histoincompatibility and by the state of immunosuppression of the recipient.

Concurrent with the rapid increase in effectors of allograft destruction is the appearance of regulatory mechanisms that dampen the ongoing immune response and that normally occur in the course of any immune reaction to prevent overactivation of host defenses. The decline in the levels of cellular and humoral immunity usually occurs with decreasing amounts of immunogenic antigens and coincides with the destruction of transplanted tissues. Feedback control of both humoral and cell-mediated immunity is thought to occur via the production of antiidiotype antibodies and by the development and maturation of suppressor T lymphocytes. Idiotypes represent the unique antigen-binding receptor on immunoglobulin molecules, and because of this uniqueness they may behave as antigens themselves. Antibodies produced against the receptor portion (idiotype) are termed *antiidiotypic*. The existence of such immunoglobulins and their function in the regulation of immune responses was proposed by N.K. Jerne, and their participation in the suppression (or augmentation, depending on subclass specificity) of allogeneic responsiveness has been shown in numerous systems. The identification of antiidiotypic receptors on T lymphocytes and the identification of suppressor lymphocytes, some bearing antiidiotypes, has prompted interest in their function in transplantation immunology. It is clear that adoptively transferable cells are capable of suppressing allograft responses in experimental animals, and that experimental manipulations of antiidiotype antibodies and suppressor cell populations are capable of producing prolonged allograft survival in the absence of other forms of immunosuppression. The maintenance of organ allografts in nonimmunosuppressed hosts appears to depend on at least three factors, namely, the maturation of antigen-specific suppressor cells; the appearance of humoral factors, probably antiidiotypes; and adaptation of the allograft itself. The concept of graft adaptation, or loss of powerfully immunogenic passenger leukocytes, is recognized clinically by the ever-decreasing requirement for immunosuppressive drugs to maintain function in a nonrejected transplanted organ, seen especially in the first few months after engraftment.

Better understanding of the precise mechanisms of both allograft destruction and the regulation of allogeneic responses will allow the development of donor antigen-specific protocols to enhance the survival of transplanted organs. The current clinical use of nonspecific immunosuppressive drugs will eventually be supplemented by manipulation and administration of donor alloantigens alone and in combination with immunosuppression to augment suppressor function.[28,39,55,65,73] The long-term goal is improved clinical graft survival with lower morbidity and mortality than is currently associated with drug-induced immunosuppression.

Pathologic Classification of Allograft Rejection Responses

The classic description of human kidney allograft rejection comprises three main clinical types: (1) hyperacute and delayed hyperacute (or accelerated) rejection; (2) acute rejection; and (3) chronic rejection.

Hyperacute Rejection

In the presence of preformed cytotoxic antidonor antibodies, the allograft undergoes rapid rejection, with intravascular coagulation and vascular occlusion caused by a direct action of complement-fixing antibodies on the vascular endothelium. These kidneys may produce a minimum amount of urine immediately after transplantation or none at all. They may have a characteristic cyanotic, flaccid appearance soon after restoration of the renal circulation or develop such an appearance in the first few hours. Microscopically, the most striking features are in the small vessels, with clumping of erythrocytes and capillary and arteriolar engorgement. Hemorrhage occurs in the interstitial tissues and is most marked at the corticomedullary junction. There is diffuse polymorphonuclear leukocyte infiltration. A similar pathologic process may occur between the second and fifth postoperative day. Diuresis suddenly stops, the patient's temperature rises, and the graft may enlarge to the point of rupture. Severe thrombocytopenia may occur, and the patient becomes acutely ill. The histologic appearance is similar to early hyperacute rejection; the diagnosis is established by biopsy or radionuclide scanning that demonstrates total or near-total vascular occlusion. Accelerated rejection is a form of hyperacute rejection caused by preformed cytotoxic antidonor antibodies, probably caused by an anamnestic humoral antibody response, in which circulating cytotoxic antibodies immediately before transplantation are present at levels below the sensitivity of standard cytotoxicity assays.[56]

Acute Rejection

Acute cellular rejection of vascularized allografts commonly occurs between the seventh and thirtieth postoperative day but can be seen from a few days to many years after transplantation. The gross appearance of these kidneys may range from moderate edema with normal color to partial or complete cortical necrosis with or without graft rupture. The inflammatory nature of the cellular response was noted by Medawar[54] in skin allografts. Biopsies of kidneys performed during acute rejection episodes demonstrate a prevalence of interstitial lesions, which are characterized by edema with diffuse infiltration of small round cells. There are dense foci of infiltrating lymphocytes that are generally perivascular. Although a variety of lymphoid cells are present, small lymphocytes predominate. There are areas of tubular necrosis, including infiltration of the tubular wall with a mixed cellular infiltration. These changes may be entirely reversible with antirejection therapy of pulsed methylprednisolone or antilymphocyte globulin.[71]

More often there is also a component of fibrinoid necrosis of small arteries and arterioles with platelet aggregates and fibrin thrombi in glomerular and peritubular capillaries. These changes are the consequence of humoral rejection and result in permanent scarring of the involved areas should the overall crisis be reversed. Current protocols for treatment of acute rejection crisis are far more effective at dampening the cellular response, and biopsy specimens showing a predominant vascular injury augur poorly for the long-term prognosis of allograft survival.

Chronic Rejection

Chronic rejection encompasses an ongoing series of events that leads, after a highly variable period, to end-stage fibrosis of the transplanted kidney. The gross appearance of the kidney with chronic rejection reveals a small graft with a pale, granular-appearing cortex. The size of the kidney varies with the duration of the chronic rejection. Renal edema and necrosis are almost never present. A spectrum of histologic change is seen on light microscopy, and all of these changes are related to smoldering vascular damage from humoral antibodies. Immunofluorescent studies show deposits of immunoglobulin, complement components, and fibrinogen in varying patterns. Vascular abnormalities include intimal proliferation, medial necrosis, and other arterial degenerative changes. Glomeruli become progressively sclerotic, and interstitial fibrosis replaces normal parenchyma in ischemic areas. Progressive chronic rejection is an irreversible and currently untreatable process. Attempts to increase immunosuppression do not improve renal function.

HISTOCOMPATIBILITY

Major Histocompatibility Complex

Rejection of an allograft occurs as a result of a complex response of the recipient's immune system to antigens expressed in the donor tissue. The most important group of antigens eliciting the allograft immune response has been termed the major histocompatibility antigens. The genes for the major histocompatibility antigens in mammals are grouped together in a well-defined region on a single chromosome. This region has been termed the major histocompatibility complex (MHC). In humans the MHC is located on the short arm of chromosome 6 and the antigens have been designated the human lymphocyte antigen (HLA).[45]

Gene products of the MHC have been classified into three groups based on their molecular structure. The class I products are MHC antigens expressed on cell surfaces. They are made up of a variable polypeptide chain called an alpha chain noncovalently bonded to an invariant chain termed B_2 microglobulin. The alpha chain is coded by an MHC gene, and B_2 microglobulin is coded on another chromosome. In humans, three class I antigens are expressed on all nucleated cells and are designated HLA A, B, and C. The class II gene products are also MHC antigens and also are made up of two noncovalently bonded polypeptide chains, alpha and beta chains. Both are variable and both are encoded by genes in the MHC. There appear to be three class II antigens in humans, which are expressed as cell surface antigens. These have been designated DP, DQ, and DR and have a limited distribution, being expressed principally on antigen-presenting cells such as B-lymphocytes, monocytes, and vascular endothelial cells. The class III products of the MHC are primarily complement proteins, which are not expressed as cell surface antigens.

The HLA gene products are the most polymorphic in the human genome. Thus there are multiple alleles at each locus and for each expressed antigen. Over 100 HLA antigens have been identified, and with molecular genetic techniques currently available, the list is likely to become much longer.[2,10] The extreme polymorphism of the HLA antigens is central to their function. They are involved in self-nonself discrimination and antigen presentation. Foreign antigens are processed in various ways by antigen-presenting cells such as monocytes, dendritic cells, and B lymphocytes and fragments of these antigens are then presented in intimate association with the individual's HLA antigens to the effector arms of the immune system. Thus the more polymorphic the system, the more likely that an HLA antigen will be available that effectively binds and presents any given foreign antigen. In addition, the HLA antigens are covalently expressed so that each individual has two functional antigens for every locus.

Since foreign antigens are recognized in the context of self-MHC antigens, it should come as no surprise that individuals recognize foreign HLA antigens quite effectively. Although other antigens such as minor histocompatibility antigens and possibly tissue-specific antigens may play a role in allograft rejection, mismatches for the HLA antigens appear to be the most critical for rejection of a transplanted organ.

Histocompatibility Laboratory Tests

The histocompatibility laboratory performs a number of assays that are important in clinical transplantation. These include HLA typing, serum screening for antibodies to HLA antigens, and crossmatch testing of a recipient's serum at the time of transplantation.

HLA typing is one of the principal functions of the histocompatibility laboratory. Currently, most typing is performed using a complement-dependent serologic test. The serum used in clinical HLA typing is obtained primarily from multiparous women who have produced antibodies to one or more HLA antigens. Lymphocytes from the individual being typed are separated into T and B subpopulations and incubated with sera of known specificity in microtiter plates. Complement is then added followed by a supra vital stain that differentiates live and dead cells. The plates are then examined microscopically and the patient's HLA type is determined by identifying the specific sera that react with the individual cells. HLA A, B, and C typing is accomplished using T lymphocytes. DR, DP, and DQ are typed using B lymphocytes.

Although serologic typing is the primary technique used in solid organ transplantation, it has some limitations. Although the majority of known HLA specificities have been identified, occasional patients have unusual antigens for which specific antisera are not available. This is particularly true for minority populations for whom extensive serum screening has not been performed. Thus blanks may be seen in an individual's HLA type. In addition, typing may be technically difficult in leukopenic individuals in whom an adequate number of lymphocytes may not be obtainable. Thus molecular genetic techniques are now being used with greater frequency and provide a second means of obtaining HLA typing.[8] Molecular techniques involve the use of a genomic library of cloned DNA fragments that code for known HLA antigens. An individual's DNA is obtained from lymphocytes, digested using endonucleases, and hybridized to the genomic library. Analysis of the hybridization products allows for identification of the individual's HLA type. Molecular genetic techniques have been particularly useful in typing for class II antigens for which there continue to be difficulties using standard serologic typing.

The crossmatch test is perhaps the most critical assay performed by the histocompatibility laboratory for clinical transplantation. Multiple blood transfusions, pregnancies, or the rejection of a previous allograft may be potent stimuli for a production of anti-HLA antigens by potential transplant recipients. If a patient who has become sensitized to several HLA antigens receives an allograft that expresses those antigens, an immediate reaction termed *hyperacute rejection* may occur.[89] This reaction is essentially the solid organ equivalent of a blood transfusion reaction in which the antibodies from the recipient bind to antigens expressed on the vascular endothelium cell of the donor. These antibodies elicit an immediate reaction with complement fixation, disruption of the vascular endothelium, the position of leukocytes and platelets, and diffuse microvascular thrombosis of the allograft. If a high affinity, high titer antibody is present, this reaction can occur in a few minutes. The crossmatch test is designed to avoid this occurrence.

The standard crossmatch test is a complement-dependent serologic assay performed in the same manner as serologic HLA typing. Serum from the recipient is incubated with donor lymphocytes. Complement is then added and the preparation is examined microscopically for evidence of cell death. A positive crossmatch, particularly if it is directed against HLA A, B, or C antigens, is generally considered a contraindication to proceeding with transplantation, as the likelihood of hyperacute rejection is extremely high.

Recently, several modifications of the standard crossmatch have been introduced to make the test more sensitive. One of these modifications is the antihuman globulin (AHG) crossmatch. In this assay, antibodies to human immunoglobulin that have been produced in another animal species such as goat or rabbit are added after the initial incubation of lymphocytes plus serum. If an anti-HLA antibody is present and has become attached to the donor lymphocytes, this binding will be amplified by attachment of the anti-human immunoglobulin antibodies. Binding of small numbers of anti-HLA antibodies can be detected using this technique.[26]

A second procedure that is gaining popularity is flow cytometry crossmatching. Incubation of donor lymphocytes and recipient serum is performed followed by incubation with a florescence antibody to human immunoglobulin. The binding of this second antibody is then analyzed using flow cytometry for anti-HLA antibody binding, which is currently the most sensitive test available. Although flow cytometry cannot determine whether a specific antibody is complement fixing, extremely small numbers of antibody molecules bound to lymphocytes can be identified.[27]

Screening recipients' sera for anti-HLA antibodies is another important function of the laboratory. Serum samples are obtained at regular intervals from potential transplant recipients who are awaiting a cadaveric transplant. These serum samples are incubated with cells from a panel of lymphocytes that have been selected to represent all of the known HLA antigens. Antibodies to specific antigens can be identified and donors with these antigens can be avoided for those individuals with anti-HLA antibodies of known specificity. Serum screening is not critical for clinical transplantation as antibodies will be identified at the time of the final crossmatch, just before transplantation. However, with long waiting lists, the knowledge that a patient reacts to certain specific antigens can be logistically important by decreasing the chances that an individual who is called for a particular transplant will have a positive final crossmatch.

Another test performed by the histocompatibility laboratory is the mixed lymphocyte culture (MLC), a measure of a recipient's T lymphocyte reactivity to donor antigens. Target lymphocytes are treated with radiation or a similar technique to prevent them from replicating. These cells are then incubated with a responder lymphocyte population in a 5- to 7-day culture. If significant HLA antigenic differences are found between two individuals, the recipient's lymphocytes will identify the donor's foreign HLA antigens and the recipient's cells will undergo proliferation. The recipient's cells are analyzed for a proliferative response to the donor compared to responses to the patient's own cells as well as third-party lymphocytes. T cells respond in an MLC primarily to the class II antigens of the donor, and this test is exquisitely sensitive for HLA class II antigenic incompatibilities. MLC testing was performed originally for living related donor renal transplantation but is used now primarily in bone marrow transplantation.

Clinical Application of Histocompatibility Laboratory Tests

Both HLA typing and crossmatching are currently used in clinical transplantation. They are currently used with greatest benefit in renal transplantation but have some application in the transplantation of extrarenal organs as well.

HLA typing is used extensively in renal transplantation. It is most useful in selecting an appropriate living donor from a family. Because the HLA antigens are found on the same chromosome, they are inherited as a group when passed from one generation to the next. Crossovers within HLA occur, but only rarely. The antigens inherited by an individual from a parent on a single chromosome are designated as a haplotype for the purposes of matching for living related donors. An individual patient who may have potential living related donors will be related to those donors to a varying degree based on shared or nonshared haplotypes. Thus a patient will be a one-haplotype match with his or her parents and offspring. A match with a sibling may be either a zero-, one-, or two-haplotype match. Long-term survival of living related donor transplantations has been shown in multiple studies to be directly related to the degree of the match. Thus two-haplotype matched living related donor transplantation has the best survival, followed by a one-haplotype match sibling, parent or offspring, followed by zero haplotype match sibling. When multiple potential living donors are available, all may be typed, allowing the selection of the best matched individual as the patient's donor.

HLA matching is also beneficial for cadaveric renal transplantation. Because of the complexity of the HLA system, attempts at matching for cadaveric transplantation have been confined to matches for HLA A, B, and DR. There is a stepwise increase in graft survival with increasing matching for HLA antigens in cadaveric transplantation. The most significant benefit from HLA matching comes from a six-antigen match.[86] Further differences in graft survival are seen when HLA DR typing is performed using molecular genetic techniques.[64]

HLA matching is currently not used clinically for extrarenal organs. Because of preservation time constraints and organs size matching criteria, significant logistic difficulties exist in attempting to use HLA matching for these other extrarenal organs, such as heart, lung, and liver. In addition, available evidence on HLA matching indicates significantly less benefit in long-term survival for these organs.

Unquestionably, the most significant histocompatibility test currently used in clinical transplantation is the crossmatch. Crossmatches are currently considered mandatory for renal and pancreas transplantation, and are used increasingly in heart transplantation, particularly for patients who have demonstrated evidence of sensitization to specific HLA antigens.

A serologic lymphocytotoxic crossmatch is currently used most commonly in renal transplantation, although more sensitive techniques are being increasingly utilized. Many centers use the AHG test routinely for all cadaveric and living related donor transplants,[42] whereas others use flow cytometry, particularly for sensitized patients such as those who have lost previous grafts or are sensitized and have detectable cytotoxic antibody levels.[7] Hyperacute rejection has been virtually eliminated by the use of crossmatching. In addition, significant improvements have been demonstrated in the outcome of renal retransplantation with the use of sensitive crossmatching, such as the AHG and flow cytometry.

ORGAN PROCUREMENT AND PRESERVATION

The rapid growth of solid organ transplantation would not be possible without the formulation of brain death legislation and the active efforts of organ procurement agencies and volunteer organizations to promote the donation of organs after brain death. Brain death, formally addressed in the United States by the Harvard Ad Hoc Committee on Irreversible Coma, is a clinical diagnosis made by competent neurologic specialists. Brain death implies irreversible cessation of cerebral and brain stem function and can be arrived at by physical examination. Confirmation can be achieved by electroencephalography, arteriography, or nuclear brain scan.

Establishment of Consent

Failure to acquire consent for organ donation is a major limiting factor in solid organ transplantation. Obtaining consent from the family of a patient who has suffered irreversible brain death requires a patient and compassionate individual who is committed to the concept of organ transplantation. The approval for organ donation may turn a hopeless situation into one that allows the transplantation of hope and life for several other persons.

Donor Evaluation

Once the diagnosis of irreversible brain death has been made and consent for transplantation has been obtained, careful and complete donor evaluation is performed, which requires a complete medical and social history. Organ procurement coordinators play a key role in the accumulation of data and management of potential organ donors. The medical history should include a complete listing of previous illnesses to rule out significant communicable diseases as well as malignancies that may be transmitted with organ transplantation. Careful attention should be paid to social activities associated with a high risk of acquiring transmittable viral infections such as the human immunodeficiency virus and hepatitis B and C, and include alcohol abuse and smoking. The history of the patient's hospitalization should also include the medical management required to maintain hemodynamic stability. Documentation of episodes of cardiac arrest, hypotension, and hypoxia and signs of systemic infection should be sought in the patient's medical record.

Specific laboratory tests are obtained to evaluate organ function and estimate the damage caused by periods of hemodynamic instability. It is important to exclude significant premorbid chronic organ disease such as chronic active hepatitis, chronic renal disease, and previous myocardial disease. The donor's height and weight are required for the transplantation of the liver, heart, and lungs.

Blood typing is necessary and blood and peripheral lymph nodes can be secured for all cross-matching and tissue typing. Serologic examination for transmittable viral infection is carried out routinely. Although the age requirements for organ donation are changing rapidly, individual organ function remains the most important determinant.

Evaluation of cardiac donors often requires examination by local cardiologists. Echocardiography and Swan-Ganz pressure recordings can be helpful in patients with an abnormal history or physical examination. Occasionally, cardiac catheterization is required to evaluate older donors or those donors with risk factors for coronary artery disease.

Medical Management

Medical management of the organ donor is critical for successful organ transplantation. After declaration of brain death, the management is altered from the maintenance of intracranial perfusion pressure to the maintenance of extracranial cellular perfusion. Brain death is often accompanied by diabetes insipidus and ventricular dysfunction that requires fluid resuscitation and vasopressor support. Brain stem herniation may occur at any time and contribute to hemodynamic instability. The majority of organ donors can be maintained in a stable hemodynamic condition with medical management. This condition allows for evaluation and distribution of organs as well as travel time for distant transplant teams. Occasionally, some donors will be hemodynamically unstable in spite of aggressive volume resuscitation and vasopressor support. These donors require expeditious movement to the operating room for emergent cannulation and organ procurement. The decision on organ acceptability for transplantation is best made by the transplanting surgeons. These complex decisions take into account data from the donor as well as the transplanting surgeon's guidelines for organ acceptability and the recipient's medical condition.

After donor identification, distribution is accomplished by the local organ procurement agency in conjunction with the United Network for Organ Sharing (UNOS). This procedure involves a highly structured mechanism for notification and dissemination of donor information to various transplantation centers for organ sharing.

Technique of Organ Procurement

In most cases a midline incision from sternal notch to pubis is made. The thoracic operation involves assessment of cardiac and pulmonary anatomy and the placement of catheters for infusion of cardioplegia and pulmonary preservation solution. The superior vena cava is dissected circumferentially, caudad enough to avoid injury to the sinoatrial node. The point of transection of the inferior vena cava requires adequate distance from the heart to avoid injury to the coronary sinus, and yet provide an adequate suprahepatic caval cuff to be used for transplantation of the liver. The abdominal organ procurement operation requires exposure of the distal infrarenal aorta for cannulation and the placement of a cannula for portal system perfusion with preservation solution. A portal system cannula can be placed either in the superior mesenteric vein, inferior mesenteric vein, the splenic vein, or directly into the transected portal vein. The supraceliac aorta is exposed either in the left chest or through the lesser sac. The ureters are usually identified to facilitate nephrectomy. At this time the patient receives systemic heparinization. The supraceliac aortic cross-clamp is applied, the intrapericardial inferior vena cava and pulmonary veins are transected and the aortic arch cross-clamp is applied. Cardioplegia and abdominal preservation solution cannulas are opened. After the preservation solution has infused, the organs are removed in a sequential fashion. After separation, the organs are packaged and transported back to the transplant center.

As experience accumulates with multiple organ procurement, the abdominal procurement operation has been greatly simplified to allow for rapid en bloc removal of the abdominal viscera, with the organs being separated in a basin of saline slush. This en bloc removal greatly simplifies the procurement of liver, pancreas, and kidneys. The procedure allows for dissection of the vascular pedicles once the organs have been completely cooled in a basin of saline slush. Every effort should be made to procure and match as many organs as possible from each cadaveric organ donor. Each donor has the capacity to donate heart, two lungs, two kidneys, liver, and pancreas as well as tissue such as cardiac valves, cornea, long bones, iliac crests, fascia, and tendons.

Organ Preservation

A key component to transplantation is the ability to preserve the organ ex vivo until reimplantation is feasible. This protection against cell death varies from organ to organ and according to the conditions upon which the organ was procured. The organs are preserved at a

TABLE 21-1 COMPOSITION OF UW SOLUTION

COMPONENT	g/L	mmol/L
Pentastarch (HES)	50	—
Lactobionic acid	35.83	100
KH_2PO_4	3.4	25
$MgSO_4$ $7H_2O$	1.23	5
Raffinose	17.83	30
Adenosine	1.34	5
Glutathione	0.92	3
Allopurinol	0.136	1

Neutralized to pH 7.4 with NaOH : KOH
Na^+ = 20 mmol/L; K^+ = 140 mmol/L
Osmolality, 320 mosm/L

TABLE 21-2 COMPOSITION OF UW MACHINE PERFUSION SOLUTION

COMPONENT	g/L	mmol/L
Na gluconate	17.45	80
KH_2PO_4	3.4	25
Mg gluconate	1.04	5
Adenine	0.68	5
Ribose	0.75	5
Glutathione	0.922	3
$CaCl_2$	0.068	0.5
HEPES	2.38	10
Glucose	1.8	10
Mannitol	5.4	30
Pentastarch	50	—

Na^+ = 100 mmol/L; K^+ = 25 mmol/L
Osmolality, 310 mosm/L; pH = 7.4

temperature of 0°C to 10°C and either by hypothermic storage or pulsatile perfusion. The current perfusate best suited for initial flush and later preservation is the University of Wisconsin (UW) solution developed by Belzer and colleagues.[6,34]

An important limiting factor in organ preservation is the effect of hypothermia on cell swelling. The beneficial effects of hypothermia relate to the decrease in oxygen consumption and a reduction in enzyme activity. An additional benefit of hypothermia is the suppression of bacterial growth during the preservation interval. Prolonged hypothermia eventually induces cell swelling, which in time results in a loss of the cell membrane potential causing Na^+ to enter the cell with water resulting in cell edema and disruption. Thus, hypothermia over time is alone a rate limiting factor in cell preservation.

Renal Preservation

Renal preservation can be effectively achieved by the use of cold (i.e., hypothermic) storage or pulsatile perfusion. The earlier solution developed by Collins was designed to be similar to the intracellular composition of the kidney and contained a high concentration of K^+ and Mg^+ phosphate as a hydrogen ion buffer with the addition of glucose to raise the osmolality of the kidney cells and prevent cell swelling. An alternative to hypothermic storage is pulsatile machine perfusion as developed by Belzer and associates[6] in 1967. Originally Belzer used cryoprecipitate of plasma as a solution for machine perfusion allowing successful preservation of kidneys for up to 72 hours. This solution was later replaced in the 1980s using a synthetic perfusate introduced by Belzer and colleagues. The current UW solution for hypothermic preservation is depicted in Table 21-1. Machine perfusate as noted in Table 21-2 has provided optimal renal preservation.[34] Cold storage is simple and less expensive, but less effective in prolonged renal preservation for more than 30 hours.

Pancreas Preservation

Pancreas preservation is accomplished by cold storage using UW solution with intervals of successful preservation from 6 to 30 hours. However, immediate allograft function is best achieved with preservation times of less than 18 hours. The use of pulsatile perfusion with the pancreas has not been successful due to the development of pancreatic edema.

Liver Preservation

The use of UW solution for hypothermic preservation of the liver has been effective for 24 hours and sometimes longer. However, preservation intervals of 16 hours or less provide better immediate graft function. The advantage of the UW solution for hepatic preservation is obvious in the multiorgan donor where all organs can be procured simultaneously by an en bloc technique with in situ hypothermic perfusion of all organs before removal.

Cardiac Preservation

Cardiac preservation is accomplished by infusion of a liter of hypothermic UW solution into the aortic root. During infusion it is important that the right and left heart chambers are decompressed so that neither chamber becomes distended. Cardiac cooling is supplemented by ice saline in the pericardial cavity. Decompression of the heart is achieved by transecting the vena cava and pulmonary veins. The practical advantage in the logistics of clinical transplantation is readily apparent with the successful prolonged organ preservation of the kidney compared to the heart in terms of the elective nature of the operation.

RENAL TRANSPLANTATION

Successful clinical renal transplantation was introduced by Murray and Merrill at the Peter Bent Brigham Hos-

TABLE 21-3 DEMOGRAPHIC DISTRIBUTION OF 3,359 PATIENTS UNDERGOING RENAL TRANSPLANTATION AT THE UNIVERSITY OF ALABAMA, 1968 TO 1994

SEX		RACE		AGE (YEARS)	
Female	1276 (38%)	Black	1357 (40%)	<10	81 (1%)
Male	2083 (62%)	Other	15 (1%)	10-19	293 (9%)
		White	1987 (59%)	20-29	713 (21%)
				30-39	980 (29%)
				40-49	841 (25%)
				50+	451 (14%)

pital in 1954 following the early experience of Hume and associates.[36] During the next 6 years, functioning allografts were achieved only when the recipient patient with renal failure fortuitously had an identical twin donor.[60] From 1958 through 1962 sporadic efforts at total body irradiation in patients receiving kidneys from a donor who is not an identical twin provided little success and often led to death of the recipient as a result of infection.

The major breakthrough in human renal transplantation began in 1962 with the clinical introduction of azathioprine.[61] Use of this drug was the first successful effort for altering the immune response and allowing foreign tissue to be accepted by the recipient. Azathioprine was soon combined with prednisone, and this combination became the foundation of clinical immunosuppressive therapy until the introduction of cyclosporine in 1983. From 1965 through 1980 a variety of adjunctive procedures were combined with the basic immunosuppressive therapy of azathioprine and prednisone in an effort to improve graft acceptance and diminish rejection. These measures included administration of antithymocyte or antilymphocyte globulin, splenectomy, thoracic duct drainage, and the use of radiographic therapy to the renal allograft during acute rejection. Although many of these adjunctive techniques appeared to provide some improvement of allograft survival, few statistical data provided scientific support for these measures.

In 1979 cyclosporine was introduced in clinical trials and became available for general use in 1983. Cyclosporine combined with azathioprine and prednisone became known as "triple therapy," and when these three drugs were combined with antilymphoid preparations, the protocol was referred to as "quadruple therapy." The use of triple or quadruple therapy has become routine in almost all clinical renal transplant centers. The new immunosuppressive agents, especially rapamycin, FK506, and mycophenolate mofetil will almost certainly replace some of the current drugs.

Clinical Indications

The demographic analysis of the entire University of Alabama transplantation experience is outlined in Table 21-3. The indications for renal transplantation are documented in Table 21-4. The number of patients with diabetes mellitus has nearly doubled in the last 10 years and now is one of the most common reasons for renal transplantation.

TABLE 21-4 CAUSES OF RENAL FAILURE IN PATIENTS AT THE UNIVERSITY OF ALABAMA

CAUSE	NUMBER (%)
Glomerulonephritis	996 (29%)
Hypertension	662 (20%)
Diabetes mellitus	532 (16%)
Unknown	376 (11%)
Polycystic disease	222 (7%)
Other	100 (3%)
Obstructive uropathy	95 (3%)
Other congenital	92 (3%)
Pyelonephritis	88 (3%)
Lupus nephritis	79 (2%)
Alport's syndrome	49 (1%)
Interstitial nephritis	36 (1%)
Hypoplasia/dysplasia	32 (1%)

The current approach to clinical renal transplantation is ideally accomplished by a careful evaluation of the patient before end-stage renal disease and then followed by renal transplantation before dialysis using either a cadaveric or living donor kidney. More commonly, the patient progresses to end-stage disease and requires hemodialysis followed later by transplantation.

The most frequent indication for renal transplantation is glomerulonephritis followed by hypertension, diabetes mellitus, unknown cause, and polycystic renal disease (Table 21-4). Men more often have end-stage disease, and in our institution 40% are black. Most patients undergoing transplantation are between 20 and 50 years of age, although excellent results can be achieved in children and in those over the age of 60.

Technical Considerations

There are many important technical considerations of renal transplantation; only a few are reviewed here. Using the extraperitoneal approach, the recipient kidney is placed in either the right or left lower quadrant. The external iliac artery and vein are dissected free circumferentially. Originally in patients receiving kidneys from related living donors, the vascular anastomosis included ligation of the distal hypogastric artery with placement of a vascular clamp at the takeoff from the common iliac artery and suturing of the divided hypogastric artery end-to-end to the renal artery. This procedure is generally applicable unless the hypogastric artery is less than 2 cm long or there is a major discrepancy between the diameters of the renal and hypogastric arteries. The anastomosis between these two vessels must be performed so that no torsion or angulation occurs that might subsequently lead to renal artery stenosis. If there is advanced atherosclerosis of the hypogastric artery not amenable to endarterectomy, an end-to-side renal artery-external iliac artery anastomosis is indicated. More recently, many transplant surgeons suture the renal artery end-to-side to the external iliac artery thereby avoiding the problems of the hypogastric artery. The renal vein is sutured end-to-side to the external iliac vein. If the kidney is of cadaveric origin, often a donor aortic cuff, including the renal artery, is sutured end-to-side to the external iliac artery. This technique eliminates the need for dissection of the hypogastric artery and decreases the potential risk of renal artery stenosis at the anastomotic site to the external iliac artery. The renal vein anastomosis in the cadaveric recipient is sutured end-to-side to the external iliac vein.

Urologic Reconstruction

The reconstruction of the ureter may be by either a ureteroneocystostomy or an end-to-end ureteroureteric anastomosis of the recipient ureter to that of the donor. The ureteroneocystostomy may be performed using a tunnel technique, placing the ureter posterior to the spermatic cord in men, and entering the bladder through the right or left posterior lateral wall. The ureteroneocystostomy must be performed carefully to avoid torsion or angulation of the ureter in the tunnel. Three posterior sutures are placed firmly through the mucosa and the muscular portion of the bladder, approximating the ureter to the bladder to prevent retraction of the ureter into the tunnel in the postoperative period. It is important to minimize the length of the donor ureter to decrease the risk of ischemic necrosis. The ureteroneocystostomy is accomplished through a midline cystotomy incision closed in three layers.

Anastomosis of the donor ureter to the recipient ureter (ureteroureterostomy) is an alternative approach that is particularly valuable if the bladder is known to have bacterial contamination or has been entered on several occasions for a transplant ureteroneocystostomy or for previous urologic surgery. Recently, the technique of suturing the ureter directly to the bladder without the use of a tunnel has been found to be equally effective. The use of a modified Lich technique has many positive features including simplicity. The importance of reflux in the renal transplant remains unclear. The kidney is placed in the retroperitoneal space. Closure of the wound is accomplished without drainage.

Related Living Donor Nephrectomy

After induction of anesthesia, the donor patient is placed in the lateral position with either the left or right flank anterior, depending on which kidney is to be removed. The skin incision is carried out directly over the twelfth rib, curving caudally along the lateral margin of the rectus muscle. The external and internal oblique muscles are divided. The transversus muscle is split, and the twelfth rib removed. The retroperitonal space is entered directly over the kidney by incising Gerota's fat and fascia. Gerota's fat is dissected away from the renal capsule anteriorly and posteriorly. One must be careful not to enter the renal hilum, and the kidney must not be manually manipulated at this point. Gerota's fat is then dissected free from the cephalad and caudal portions of the kidney. The ureter is identified and dissected caudal to the point where it passes anterior to the iliac artery and vein. Considerable care must be taken to avoid trauma to the ureter, particularly its blood supply. The renal vein is then identified and dissected free circumferentially. On the left side the adrenal and ovarian veins require ligation. The renal artery is then identified slightly cephalad and posterior to the renal vein. This artery is dissected free circumferentially, with the dissection limited to the aortorenal takeoff. The artery is surrounded by sympathetic nerves and ganglia, which can best be identified by observation and palpation. Retraction of the kidney with tension on the renal artery will produce intrarenal spasm and cyanosis of the kidney.

A 10-minute "rest period" is then allowed to relieve intrarenal vascular spasm. Heparin, 2500 units, is administered immediately before clamping of the renal artery. At this point the ureter is divided and ligated, as are the renal artery and vein, and the kidney is removed from the donor. The kidney is then transferred to the recipient surgeon and perfused with EuroCollins solution for 3 minutes at 110 mm Hg nonpulsatile flow at 4° C (39.2° F). This perfusion is performed in the donor operating room on a sterile table. The kidney is then placed into a sterile container with the same solution and taken to the adjacent operating room, where the transplantation procedure is performed.

The donor incision is closed in layers after suture control of the renal artery and vein. Drainage of the operative site is not necessary.

Immunosuppressive Therapy and Allograft Survival

Current immunosuppressive therapy includes cyclosporine, azathioprine, and prednisone (triple therapy) in recipients of one-haplotype match living related donor kidneys with a gradual reduction of prednisone to 10 to 15 mg/day in 21 to 28 days postoperatively. Recipients of two-haplotype match living related donor kidneys may have the prednisone reduced to levels between 0 and 10 mg/day in 3 to 6 months. Cadaveric recipients usually have a 4- to 10-day period of induction therapy with either a monoclonal or polyclonal antilymphocyte antibody. This regimen is combined with azathioprine and prednisone until the serum creatinine reaches a level of less than 3 mg %. Cyclosporine is then initiated, and when a therapeutic level is achieved, the antilymphocyte therapy is discontinued (quadruple therapy). This form of therapy has contributed to a remarkable improvement in renal allograft survival where recipients of a cadaveric allograft have an 80% to 85% function at 1 year, a one-haplotype match allograft of 90% to 95%, and a two-haplotype match of 95% to 97%.

Acute rejection is treated by three bolus injections of Solu-Medrol 500 to 1000 mg/day over 3 days. This regimen may or may not be associated with a concomitant rise in the daily oral dose of prednisone (2 to 5 mg/kg) with a gradual taper over 6 to 10 days. If rejection is not completely reversed, then the use of an antilymphocyte preparation may be indicated. Failure to successfully reverse rejection should be considered as a serious reason to consider transplantation nephrectomy. Multiple attempts to reverse rejection are frequently associated with serious opportunistic infections that are associated with a substantial increase in morbidity and mortality.

There is no successful form of treatment for chronic rejection. The most important consideration is to establish the diagnosis by renal biopsy and accept the fact that in time the graft will undergo complete rejection.

Complications

Early Complications

After renal transplantation the patient may have a completely uneventful course, in which case renal function returns to normal within 3 to 5 days (related living donor kidney) or 7 to 15 days (cadaveric kidney). The most important management aspect after transplantation is the awareness of complications that may impair or alter renal function. Causes for impaired renal function immediately after transplantation include acute and hyperacute rejection, acute tubular necrosis, cyclosporine nephrotoxicity, arterial or venous complications, ureteral complications, pseudorejection because of laboratory error, sudden onset of diabetes, and patient noncompliance in taking medication.

Although cyclosporine is one of the most effective immunosuppressive agents developed thus far, nephrotoxicity occurs frequently and must be considered in every instance in which there is a decline in stable renal function after transplantation. Measurements of blood or serum levels of cyclosporine have been helpful in anticipating drug-induced nephrotoxicity, but by themselves the results do not absolutely confirm or exclude the diagnosis of nephrotoxicity. Some patients are able to tolerate greater dosages of cyclosporine with higher serum or blood levels and maintain satisfactory renal function. Other patients may develop cyclosporine nephrotoxicity in the presence of acceptable blood or serum levels. If cyclosporine nephrotoxicity occurs, a marked reduction in cyclosporine dosage is frequently followed by improvement in renal function in 24 to 48 hours. If there is no improvement in the blood urea nitrogen (BUN) and creatinine levels, other causes of impaired renal function must be considered. Hirsutism, fine tremor of the hands, gum hypertrophy, and hepatotoxicity are all common complications of cyclosporine and in part are related to dosage. The role of renal biopsy in the differentiation of acute rejection from cyclosporine nephrotoxicity remains uncertain. Renal biopsy is most valuable when impaired renal function exists and the biopsy is normal. One can then assume cyclosporine nephrotoxicity is present and reduce the dosage.

Hyperacute and accelerated rejection both result from preformed cytotoxic antibody. Hyperacute rejection occurs within a few hours after transplantation, and accelerated rejection in 48 to 72 hours. In both instances the rejection is irreversible, and immediate transplant nephrectomy is indicated. Fortunately, the serologic crossmatch using donor lymphocytes and the recipient sera has largely eliminated this form of rejection, for which there is no treatment. The radionuclide scan is the procedure of choice to make this diagnosis.

Acute rejection occurred more often with the regimen of azathioprine and prednisone than with the recent experience of triple therapy with cyclosporine. The signs and symptoms include low-grade fever, a tender, enlarged allograft with a decreased urine volume, an increase in weight and blood pressure, and elevated serum creatinine and BUN levels. When patients are treated with azathioprine and prednisone, most acute rejection episodes occur within the first 60 days after transplantation, and approximately 90% of acute rejection episodes occur within the first 90 days after transplantation. Acute rejection after the third posttransplantation month is unusual unless it is preceded by a viral illness, noncompliance, or rapid reduction in the dosage of immunosuppressive therapy.

Patient noncompliance with immunosuppressive therapy must always be considered when sudden deterioration in renal function occurs in the setting of long-term stable function. In patients receiving cyclosporine and prednisone, acute rejection occurs most commonly in the first 6 weeks after transplantation and less frequently after 60 days. Acute rejection may be assumed when both the BUN and creatinine levels increase without other apparent explanation. A renal biopsy may be useful but is subject to sample error. The radionuclide scan is especially valuable because it is noninvasive and can be repeated on a daily basis. The renal image, the estimated renal plasma flow, and the radionuclide uptake by the kidney may separate acute rejection from acute tubular necrosis or renal artery stenosis.[24]

The treatment of acute rejection requires an increase in corticosteroid dosage either orally or with intravenous pulse therapy on a daily or every-other-day basis, using 500 or 1000 mg over 3 to 4 hours. Usually 3 to 4 mg of methylprednisolone will reverse rejection. Rarely should a patient receive more than a total of 6 to 7 g of methylprednisolone. In some patients with acute rejection who do not respond to the use of increased steroid therapy, a short course of antilymphocyte globulin (5 to 10 days) may be beneficial in reversing rejection. Some centers have used antilymphocyte globulin in place of steroids for treatment of acute allograft rejection, thereby decreasing the risks of large-dose steroid therapy.[35] If rejection is not reversed early, transplant nephrectomy will avoid the complications of infection caused by excessive administration of immunosuppressive drugs.

Acute tubular necrosis resulting in impaired renal function and requiring dialysis occurs in less than 1% of patients undergoing related living donor transplantation. This event is uncommon unless technical difficulties were present in procurement of the donor kidney or in the vascular anastomosis of the donor kidney within the recipient patient. However, acute tubular necrosis is almost always present to some degree in patients undergoing cadaveric transplantation regardless of the method of preservation used. Approximately 10% to 30% of patients require dialysis after cadaveric transplantation. The severity of acute tubular necrosis may vary from polyuric renal failure with a slow gradual reduction in serum creatinine level over 5 to 10 days to complete oliguric renal failure, which may persist for a period of days or weeks.

The management of the patient during acute tubular necrosis and oliguric renal failure is accomplished by appropriate diet and fluid restriction with frequent dialysis. The most difficult diagnosis is the differentiation of acute rejection from acute tubular necrosis or recognition of a superimposition of acute rejection on acute tubular necrosis. The separation of these two events can be best determined by a radionuclide scan of the kidney with measurement of the estimated renal plasma flow.[35] The radionuclide studies show that the estimated renal plasma flow improves with subsiding acute tubular necrosis, whereas in patients with acute rejection the renal plasma flow decreases. If impairment of renal function persists for more than 3 to 4 weeks, consideration must be given to renal exploration and transplantation nephrectomy.

Rupture of a renal allograft is an unusual event. Although rupture may occur spontaneously, it usually occurs during an episode of severe acute rejection as a result of renal edema. The incidence is less than 0.5% of patients undergoing transplantation, and rupture usually does not occur unless a graft sustaining severe acute rejection is allowed to remain in situ for a prolonged period rather than being removed early. The indications for prompt exploration include a markedly tender allograft with or without an expanding flank mass, hypotension, and a decreasing hematocrit. The kidney is usually irreversibly rejected at the time of exploration, and a transplant nephrectomy is indicated. On rare occasions the graft is viable, and the site of rupture can be repaired by large absorbable sutures. As a general rule, transplantation nephrectomy is a safe solution to a potentially catastrophic situation.

Vascular complications are uncommon in patients undergoing renal transplantation. Renal artery or vein occlusion occurs in less than 1% of patients. When it does occur, the graft is almost always necrotic, and surgical intevention is of little help. The diagnosis of acute renal artery occlusion is by radionuclide scan, which shows no uptake by the kidney. Prompt surgical exploration combined with immediate transplantation nephrectomy is indicated.

Ureteral complications after transplantation may be serious and require prompt diagnosis and management. These complications include ureteral obstruction caused by periureteral adhesions or improper placement of the ureter through the bladder tunnel with ureteral obstruction. Ultrasonography is the best diagnostic test in the presence of obstruction. If renal function is present, the intravenous pyelogram (IVP) will confirm the diagnosis and demonstrate the site of obstruction. If there is nonfunction of the allograft, with ureteral obstruction, the only suitable diagnostic procedure is ultrasonography. Urine leakage into the retroperitoneal space may occur from ureteral necrosis caused by interruption of the blood supply of the ureter during the ureteroneocystostomy, or by retraction of the ureter from the bladder because of dehiscence of the ureterovesical anastomosis. Proper organ procurement will minimize this complication because the ureteral artery arises from the renal artery where injury will render the ureter ischemic. A urine leak is a serious event that must be diagnosed early if satisfactory surgical repair is to be expected. The diagnostic procedure of choice to confirm extravasation of urine is a radionuclide scan or, in the presence of adequate renal function, an IVP with a cystogram. Disruption of the cystotomy incision is a major problem and requires immediate repair. Most urologic complications occur in the first 6 weeks after transplantation, with the majority in the first 3 weeks.

Pseudorejection may occur in patients undergoing renal transplantation and is often the result of laboratory error or the sudden onset of hyperglycemia associated with volume depletion, causing renal tubular dysfunction and a mild increase in the serum creatinine level. The latter may occur immediately after the transplantation but often occurs several months after transplantation. If it is insidious, it may mimic acute rejection.

Lymphocele, a collection of lymphatic fluid in the perirenal space, may cause compression or angulation of the ureter or both, producing obstruction. In most instances this occurs in the first 3 to 6 months after transplantation and is the result of divided lymphatics along the recipient iliac vein or along the donor renal artery. A lymphocele may be asymptomatic or may cause vague, ill-defined abdominal discomfort. In some instances compression of the iliac vein will cause unilateral edema of the lower extremity. Rarely, the compression on the ureter and renal transplantation is such that acute anuria occurs. If the compression is mild to moderate, impaired renal function may develop, with increased BUN and creatinine levels. The diagnosis is best established by ultrasound or IVP and cystogram. The treatment is internal drainage into the peritoneal cavity. Lymphoceles occur rarely more than 1 year after transplantation.

Late Complications

Late complications of renal transplantation may be related to a variety of factors, including but not limited to chronic rejection, renal artery stenosis, and ureteral obstruction. Long-term cyclosporine use may cause nephrotoxicity several months after transplantation; improved renal function is associated with a reduction in dosage. Chronic rejection, the most common cause of a gradual increase in serum creatinine level during the stable period after transplantation, may occur within the first year after transplantation and progress to ultimate graft failure within 2 to 3 years. In other instances chronic rejection occurs slowly, with a gradually decreasing level of renal function for years and eventual graft loss 10 or more years later. This diagnosis can be established by renal biopsy or by radionuclide studies that show a progressive decline of the estimated renal plasma flow. There is no treatment for chronic rejection.

Renal artery stenosis may mimic chronic rejection by a gradual decrease in renal blood flow with an increase in BUN and serum creatinine levels, and is always associated with progressive hypertension. Renal artery stenosis may occur at the site of the anastomosis as a result of technical errors. An important cause of renal artery stenosis may be torsion of the renal artery when it is anastomosed to the hypogastric artery. This technique of vascular reconstruction is now used much less frequently. However, in some instances intimal injury may occur from trauma by the application of a vascular clamp with subsequent fibrosis and stenosis.

A less common cause may be an atherosclerotic plaque in the hypogastric artery that was incompletely removed by endarterectomy through the divided end of the hypogastric artery at the time of the vascular anastomosis. With vascular stenosis this plaque may increase and cause narrowing of the hypogastric artery. In some instances, for reasons that are not clearly understood, intimal hyperplasia may occur distal to the renal artery-hypogastric artery anastomosis, producing renal artery stenosis of the donor artery. Although this stenosis has been postulated to be secondary to an immunologic injury in the recipient's renal artery, data for this assumption have not been forthcoming.

Treatment of renal artery stenosis is predicated on the assumption that hyperreninemia is present, confirming that anatomic stenosis has physiologic significance. If the stenosis is important, then correction may be achieved by percutaneous transluminal angioplasty or by a direct surgical approach, although the latter is associated with the risk of graft loss. The use of the end-to-side renal artery to external iliac artery has minimized arterial anastomotic problems, especially with the use of a Carrel patch in cadaveric transplantation.

Ureteral obstruction occurring long after transplantation is uncommon. Such occurrence is often caused by adhesions that cause angulation of the ureter. Renal ultrasonography is the simplest diagnostic measure to exclude the presence of hydronephrosis of the transplanted kidney. If hydronephrosis is present, then an IVP is indicated for confirmation of the location of the ureteral obstruction. If the site of obstruction is cephalad to the ureteral tunnel into the bladder, the cause is almost always adhesions. If the stenosis is at the site of the ureteroneocystostomy, then revision of the ureteral implant will be necessary. Patients with mild to moderate hydronephrosis and normal renal function do not require surgical intervention. Renal calculi occur rarely after transplantation.

Avascular necrosis of the femoral head or other bones has been noted to occur in 10% to 20% of patients undergoing renal transplantation, even though not all patients require surgical intervention. The cause of this complication is unclear and probably relates to several physiologic events, including persistent (tertiary) hyperparathyroidism associated with hypophosphatemia and the use of corticosteroids. Although some patients tolerate large dosages of corticosteroids, others will develop avascular necrosis of the femoral head with a minimum amount of steroids. The process rarely becomes symptomatic in the first 3 months after transplantation and seldom occurs more than 4 to 5 years after transplantation. Pain, the most common complaint, is often referred to the knee when the process involves the femoral head. The common physical finding is a decrease in the internal rotation of the hip. The diagnosis of avascular necrosis is then confirmed by radiograph, which reveals early demineralization of the femoral head with or without cortical compression. Surgical intervention for avascular necrosis depends on the patient's tolerance of pain and ability to walk. Total joint replacement, the procedure of choice for avascular necrosis of the hip, has produced excellent results. Partial weight bearing may be beneficial in the management of this condition before the cortex of the femoral head has collapsed. Additional bones involved with aseptic necrosis include the head of the humerus, distal radius, and carpal bones.

Infections are among the most serious life-threatening complications after renal transplantation. Infection in the first 3 months is usually bacterial or viral. Infections that occur more than 3 months after transplantation may be bacterial, viral, fungal, or protozoal. Tuberculosis is relatively uncommon.

Wound infections early after transplantation occur in 1% to 2% of patients and are classified as deep or superficial. A deep wound infection posterior to the external oblique fascia in the perinephric space occurs in less than 1% of patients. When this type of infection is present, prompt surgical drainage is indicated. If the patient has prolonged acute tubular necrosis or impaired renal function of unknown cause and the kidney is cadaveric, transplant nephrectomy in the presence of wound sepsis is often the procedure of choice. However, if the infection is limited in scope and can be adequately drained, then occasionally the graft may be preserved. The most serious complication associated with perinephric infection is the dehiscence of the arterial anastomosis with massive hemorrhage requiring ligation of the external iliac or hypogastric artery. Surprisingly, most patients tolerate ligation of the external iliac artery with little or no difficulty. Superficial wound infections anterior to the external oblique fascia occur in 1% of patients and cause little risk in terms of patient and graft survival.

Nocardia organism infection may initially appear as a low-grade fever and a pulmonary infiltrate or as multiple subcutaneous abscess sites with little or no inflammatory response. Diagnosis may be accomplished by bronchoscopy or needle aspiration. With systemic treatment by sulfa drugs, the prognosis for complete recovery is excellent.

Viral infections caused by herpes simplex, herpes genitalis, and cytomegalovirus are frequently observed in the first 6 to 8 weeks after transplantation. The lesions of herpes simplex, commonly noted in the mucocutaneous membranes of the lips and the soft palate of the mouth, are usually self-limited. Herpetic involvement of the esophagus causes severe dysphagia and usually requires systemic treatment. Herpetic involvement of the genitalia and the anus represents a recurrence of a previous infection and usually occurs within the first 4 to 6 weeks after transplantation. Cytomegalovirus, a common infection in the posttransplantation period, may occur as a primary or recurrent infection.[72] In certain areas of the United States, 90% of patients over 25 years of age will have a history of infection with cytomegalovirus, implying a high risk for recurrence of the disease. If the disease is recurrent, immediate and long-term graft survival is quite good. If the disease manifests as a primary infection, particularly in children, then associated rejection of the graft may occur. Symptoms associated with cytomegalovirus are fever, often with daily temperature elevations to 38.9° C (102° F), malaise, apathy, and anorexia. Leukopenia, an increase in serum creatinine and BUN levels, and abnormal liver function studies are all common occurrences with this infection. The disease generally runs a self-contained course of days or a few weeks. If the disease persists, treatment with intravenous ganciclovir may be beneficial. On occasion acute irreversible graft rejection occurs simultaneously with the onset of acute cytomegalovirus infection.

Fungal infections are a serious problem, usually occurring after 1 or 2 months, and are common in patients requiring large amounts of corticosteroids to manage acute rejection. Pulmonary fungal infections usually manifest as either a low-grade fever with a lung infiltrate or an asymptomatic discrete mass on a routine chest radiograph. Early, prompt, and aggressive diagnostic management is essential. Management includes bronchoscopy and, in the absence of a positive diagnosis, either needle-aspiration or open-lung biopsy. Patients with well-localized pulmonary nodules of fungal origin, with prompt and accurate diagnosis and appropriate treatment, have an excellent prognosis. Patients with vascular invasion of the lung caused by fungi have a poor prognosis and often succumb to widespread infection. Fungal diseases most commonly associated with patients undergoing transplantation include aspergillosis, histoplasmosis, cryptococcosis, blastomycosis, and coccidioidomycosis.

Protozoal infections, most often caused by *Pneumocystis carinii,* are much less frequent when patients are treated postoperatively with sulfa derivatives. Early symptoms of *Pneumocystis* infection include a dry cough and shortness of breath; there is a minimum of findings on chest radiographs. Arterial blood gas determinations reveal a low PO_2. Bronchoscopic examination with washings and lung biopsy often confirms the diagnosis. Treatment must be prompt to avoid rapid spread and death from ventilatory insufficiency. Toxoplasmosis is much less common than *Pneumocystis* infections but is associated with both high mortality and high morbidity.

In general, both diagnosis and treatment of pulmonary infections must be managed aggressively. It is far better to treat with multiple antibiotics, reducing each antibiotic as one approaches an accurate diagnosis, than to observe the patient and allow widespread pneumonia to develop.

Central nervous system infections constitute a small but serious subset of diseases that if not accurately diagnosed and promptly treated will result in patient death. The surgeon should suspect meningitis in any patient who complains of headache, photophobia, stiff neck, nausea, or vomiting. The patient usually describes the headache as the most serious in his or her life. A lumbar puncture with appropriate cultures and spinal fluid analysis is essential and should be performed immediately. It is important to emphasize that a negative cryptococcal antigen in the cerebrospinal fluid does not exclude early infection with *Cryptococcus* organisms, and if the findings are inconclusive, treatment is indicated until a final diagnosis can be established.

Gastrointestinal complications include pancreatitis, gastroduodenal ulceration with bleeding or perforation, and acute diverticulitis. The association of pancreatitis and renal transplantation was recognized in the late 1960s and is an uncommon but serious complication, occurring in 5% to 10% of patients undergoing renal transplantation. The disease may be of sudden onset with rapid progression to acute hemorrhagic pancreatitis and death of the patient. In other instances the disease is chronic, with recurrent episodes and pseudocyst formation. The cause is unknown but may be influenced by the administration of corticosteroids or infection of the pancreas with cytomegalovirus. The treatment is conservative if at all possible, unless drainage of a pseudocyst is indicated.

Acute gastroduodenal ulceration is a serious complication that may be devastating in patients receiving chronic immunosuppressive therapy. Fortunately, the complication occurs much less often than it did 10 years ago, probably as a result of better prophylactic treatment using histamine-blocking drugs and antacids. In the presence of upper gastrointestinal bleeding, immediate endoscopy is indicated, as is prompt surgical intervention if necessary. Patients with serious complaints referable to duodenal ulcer disease should be considered for prophylactic ulcer surgery before transplantation.

Acute diverticulitis is more common in patients over the age of 50 years and should be considered as a cause of generalized lower abdominal pain in these patients after transplantation. The diagnosis and treatment are the same as in the nontransplant patient.

Acute cholecystitis occurs with the same frequency among transplantation recipients as in the general population and does not seem to present a particularly complex problem in management.

Hepatic dysfunction may occur early or late in the posttransplant course. The illness may be mild with recovery or may progress to cirrhosis with a fatal outcome. The outcome of renal transplantation with immunosuppressive therapy in patients who have hepatitis appears less favorable.[67] Patients with hepatitis and impaired hepatic function may be better managed by either complete withdrawal of azathioprine or substitution with cyclophosphamide or a marked reduction of azathioprine.

The most common complication involving patients undergoing renal transplantation is iatrogenic Cushing's syndrome. This syndrome includes the classic findings of truncal and facial obesity, muscle wasting of the extremities, weakness of the quadriceps muscles, and easy bruisability of the legs and arms. Patients with longstanding prednisone dosage greater than 20 mg/day may develop corticosteroid side effects incompatible with a productive life. Certainly most patients with daily prednisone requirements greater than 30 mg/day will have serious complications from the corticosteroid medication; the potential for these complications may justify lowering the prednisone dosage and accepting return to dialysis.

Secondary hyperparathyroidism is a frequent finding in patients undergoing renal transplantation and is more common in patients with a long history of chronic renal failure, especially if transplantation is preceded by chronic dialysis for a number of years. In spite of the high incidence of secondary hyperparathyroidism in patients with chronic dialysis, progression to tertiary hyperparathyroidism requiring surgical intervention is uncommon. The indications for surgical intervention include a persistent calcium level greater than 12 mg/dl, renal calculi, fractures, marked muscle weakness, and severe joint pain. In more than 3359 transplantation operations at the University of Alabama, fewer than 26 patients have required surgery for tertiary hyperparathyroidism.

The risk of malignant disease in recipients of cadaveric and related living donor kidneys is significantly greater than that in an age-matched population. Sheil[77] reviewed recipients of renal allografts who developed malignant disease and noted the incidence of skin carcinoma to increase to 11% in recipients of cadaveric kidneys. Other malignancies were noted to increase six times above the expected level. The risk of carcinoma increases with the duration of graft function and strongly suggests that the immunosuppressive therapy may be a causative factor. The excessive use of azathioprine may be especially deleterious. Therefore reduction of immunosuppressive therapy in recipients of long-term functioning kidneys should be attempted.

Results

Allograft survival has improved dramatically since the introduction of cyclosporine in 1983 with the immunosuppressive protocols combining azathioprine and

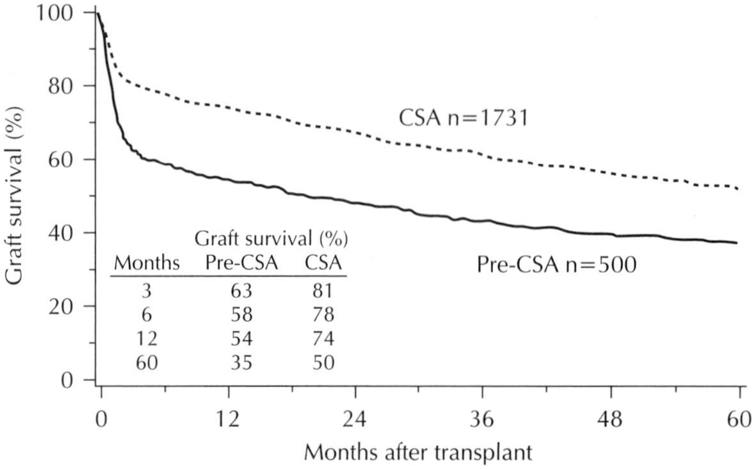

FIGURE 21-1 The substantial improvement in allograft survival after the introduction of cyclosporine in cadaveric renal transplantation is noted above. The prevention of early acute rejection in the first 3 months is apparent.

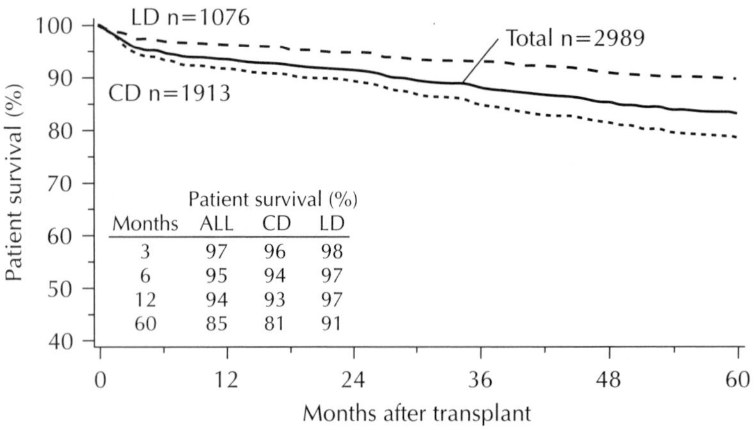

FIGURE 21-2 Patient survival after renal transplantation confirms the excellent early and long-term survival in recipients of both cadaveric and living related donor allografts. *ALL,* Airlifeline; *LD,* living donor; *CD,* cadaveric donor.

prednisone (triple therapy) or the use of antilymphocyte preparation as induction therapy (quadruple therapy) (Figure 21-1). Not only has allograft survival improved but patient survival has increased as well. Recipients of first cadaveric kidneys now have a 1-year graft survival of 80% to 85% and a patient survival of 97% to 98% over the same time interval. Recipients of regrafts experience poorer graft survival. Living donor recipients still have the best patient and graft survival (one-haplotype match 98% and 90%, respectively, two-haplotype match 98% and 95%, respectively) (Figures 21-2 and 21-3). The role of histocompatibility matching in cadaveric transplantation remains controversial and a six-antigen match may provide a 5% overall improvement in graft survival. The use of the cytotoxic crossmatch is still an essential test to exclude those patients with prior sensitization. The sensitivity of this test has been enhanced with the flow cytometer.

Although acute rejection has been reduced in the early posttransplantation months with the use of triple or quadruple therapy, long-term graft survival is best in those individuals free of rejection episodes. Chronic rejection continues to be the most frequent cause of graft loss after 2 years and has no current method of treatment. Interestingly, chronic rejection proceeds at variable rates and may range from less than 1 year to 10 years before complete graft failure.

Renal transplantation in blacks seems to have a

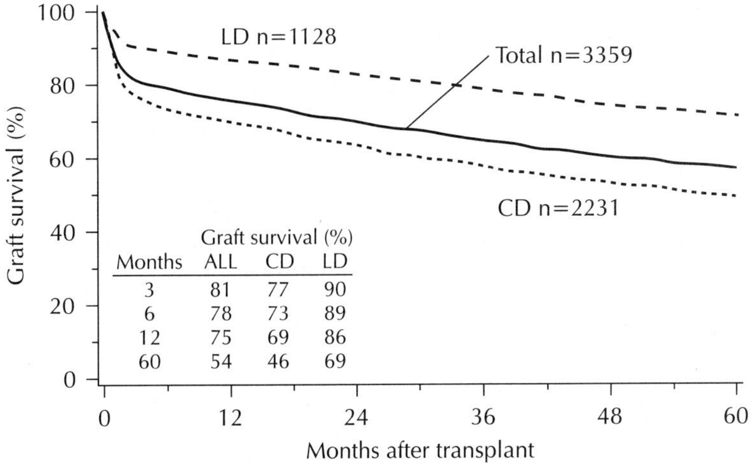

FIGURE 21-3 The total experience at the University of Alabama documents the excellent allograft survival of living related donor transplantation. Early graft loss is largely due to acute rejection, while later graft loss is the result of chronic rejection. *LD*, Living donor; *CD*, cadaveric donor; *ALL*, Airlifeline.

poorer outcome in terms of graft survival for reasons that are unclear. Whether there is a true racial difference in allograft survival is a point of contention and may relate to histocompatibility differences between the two races.

LIVER TRANSPLANTATION

The early clinical experiences in liver transplantation attempted by Starzl and associates[81] in 1963 were met with a very high early mortality rate.[80] Death of the patient was attributed usually to technical or immunosuppressive complications. Survival began to reach acceptable levels after the 1979 clinical trials of cyclosporine and the accumulation of clinical experience primarily by Calne and colleagues[14] and Starzl and associates.[79] Due to the enormous efforts of these pioneers,[78] liver transplantation has become an accepted form of therapy for patients with acute and chronic hepatic failure.[63] Improvements in organ preservation and immunosuppressive technology have resulted in the rapid growth of centers performing liver transplantation, with 2880 liver transplants performed in North America and 2137 performed in Europe in 1990. The most recent 1-year survival rates in many centers exceed 80%.

Clinical Indications

The indications for liver transplantation include acute hepatic failure with progressive encephalopathy, chronic hepatic failure with decompensated cirrhosis, hepatic tumors not resectable by partial hepatectomy, and more rarely, inborn errors of metabolism.

Fulminant hepatic failure is defined as liver failure with the development of hepatic encephalopathy within 2 weeks of the onset of jaundice. Subfulminant hepatic failure describes those cases of hepatic failure where encephalopathy develops between 2 weeks and 3 months after the onset of jaundice. The etiology of fulminant hepatic failure includes viral hepatitis A, hepatitis B, hepatitis delta, hepatitis C, herpes simplex I and II, varicella zoster virus, acute fulminant Wilson's disease, drug-induced disease and Amanita phalloides mushroom poisoning.

Patients with the diagnosis of fulminant hepatic failure require urgent referral to a transplantation center. Encephalopathy can progress to cerebral edema and ischemic brain injury within 24 to 48 hours. Management involves those measures directed against the development of cerebral edema and the maintenance of intracerebral perfusion pressure.[41] Management is facilitated by invasive intracerebral pressure monitoring devices.[49]

Transplantation is indicated in patients with progressive deterioration and stage III or stage IV hepatic coma. In spite of deep coma most patients who receive transplantation before the development of ischemic neurologic injury or herniation can expect a dramatic recovery and good survival. The reduced survival in these patients, compared to those patients electively transplanted, is usually due to the inability to acquire an allograft before the development of neurologic injury.

The causes of chronic liver disease leading to liver transplantation are listed in the box on p. 904. Patients with chronic liver disease are considered for transplantation when the disease has caused the quality of life to deteriorate to an unacceptable level or has placed the patient at risk of dying from complications of liver disease, which is manifested by the development of decom-

DISEASES LEADING TO LIVER TRANSPLANTATION

Chronic Liver Disease
Postnecrotic cirrhosis
- Chronic active hepatitis
  - Hepatitis B
  - Hepatitis C
  - Cryptogenic cirrhosis
- Autoimmune hepatitis
- Alcoholic cirrhosis
- Chronic drug-induced cirrhosis

Cholestatic Liver Disease
Primary biliary cirrhosis
Biliary atresia
Sclerosing cholangitis
Secondary biliary cirrhosis

Metabolic Liver Disease
Alpha-1-antitrypsin deficiency
Wilson's disease
Glycogen storage disease types I & IV
Tyrosinemia
Urea cycle deficiencies
Galactosemia
Hemochromatosis
Polycystic liver

Vascular Disease
Budd-Chiari syndrome

pensated cirrhosis. Signs of decompensated cirrhosis include incapacitating weakness, progressive jaundice, refractory ascites, spontaneous encephalopathy, spontaneous bacterial peritonitis, recurrent gastrointestinal bleeding refractory to sclerotherapy, and the development of the hepatorenal syndrome. Patients with sclerosing cholangitis may present with recurrent biliary tract sepsis in addition to decompensated cirrhosis. Recipients of liver allografts with primary biliary cirrhosis are often referred for transplantation with advanced bone disease, incapacitating weakness, or refractory pruritus before the development of the complications of portal hypertension. Patients with chronic active viral hepatitis face the problem of recurrent viral hepatitis following transplantation.[70] Protocols have been developed to decrease the frequency and severity of recurrent hepatitis B by passive immunization with improved long-term results.[74]

Patients with alcoholic liver disease should demonstrate a period of abstinence and participation in an alcohol rehabilitation program before transplantation. These patients usually undergo a psychiatric evaluation to assess their rehabilitative potential as well as their compliance and social support network.

Transplantation for malignancies of the liver continues to be complicated by disease recurrence despite the lack of apparent extrahepatic disease at the time of transplantation. Survival with conventional resection of hepatocellular carcinoma when compared to that of total hepatectomy and transplantation is similar when stratified by tumor stage.[37] Those patients who cannot undergo lobar resection because of multicentricity or inadequate liver reserve and cirrhosis are considered for organ replacement. These patients are usually enrolled in adjuvant chemotherapy protocols[83] to prevent or delay recurrence. The results of transplantation for cholangiocarcinoma have been extremely disappointing, with a very high rate of early recurrence and death. A combination of preoperative radiotherapy and perioperative chemotherapy is being used in an attempt to improve these dismal results. Total hepatectomy and transplantation for metastatic adenocarcinoma to the liver have been largely unsuccessful due to rapid recurrence of disease. Transplantation for metastatic neuroendocrine tumors has occasionally resulted in good long-term palliation due to the slow growth of these malignancies.

Contraindications to liver transplantation include the presence of extrahepatic malignancy, active substance abuse, extrahepatic infection, irreversible neurologic injury, a history of chronic noncompliance, inadequate psychosocial support network, and concomitant cardiopulmonary disease that makes successful operative intervention unlikely.

Technical Considerations

Successful liver transplantation starts with a carefully procured and preserved organ. Allografts that are subjected to prolonged periods of inadequate oxygen delivery in the donor as well as those with severe fatty change are at an increased risk of primary nonfunction. Vascular abnormalities, including aberrant right and left hepatic arteries, must be recognized in the donor, preserved, and reconstructed during bench preparation of the allograft.

Careful, expert anesthetic management is required for the operative procedure. These patients often have a hyperdynamic cardiovascular system as well as severe coagulopathy and acid-base disturbances on arrival in the operative suite. The anesthesiologist must be prepared for sudden, high volume blood loss as well as the cardiovascular effects seen on reperfusion of the liver.

Recipient Hepatectomy

A bilateral subcostal incision is made. Upper midline extension and xiphoidectomy can facilitate exposure of the suprahepatic vena cava. Often abundant abdominal wall collateral vessels are encountered. Incision and dissection in these patients are greatly facilitated by electrocautery. Sharp dissection is necessarily very limited. The hilar dissection involves exposure and division of the native common hepatic duct, followed by exposure of the hepatic artery and portal vein. Division of the triangular ligaments and gastrohepatic omentum will provide the mobility required for exposure of the supra and infrahepatic portions of the vena cava. Once the cava are dissected circumferentially, the patient is prepared for venovenous bypass if it is to be utilized. Bypass uses inflow from the transected portal vein and a femoral cannula. A nonheparinized pump circulates blood to a large cannula placed either in the neck or upper extremity.

Revascularization of the allograft requires four vascular anastomoses: the suprahepatic and infrahepatic vena cava, the portal vein, and the hepatic artery. The posterior walls of the suprahepatic and infrahepatic vena cava and the portal vein are sutured from the inside of these vessels using an everting technique. Care is taken to avoid constriction of the vessel diameter and consequent stenosis of these venous anastomoses. Various techniques have been developed for hepatic artery reconstruction.[76] Usually the entire allograft celiac axis with an aortic Carrel patch is anastomosed to the native proper or common hepatic artery. If the native hepatic artery is inadequate for reconstruction, a segment of the donor iliac artery can be used to graft to the recipient infrarenal or supraceliac aorta. The presence of portal vein thrombosis requires a graft of the donor iliac vein to the native superior mesenteric vein.[43] After hemostasis is achieved the biliary continuity is reestablished. In adults the biliary reconstruction usually involves a choledochocholedochostomy over a T-tube placed in the native common hepatic duct. If the native common hepatic duct is diseased or unusable, a Roux-en-Y choledochojejunostomy is constructed. In infants and children with biliary atresia a Roux-en-Y choledochojejunostomy is utilized.

At the completion of the operation, immediate graft function is assessed by the production of bile, the rewarming of the patient, the spontaneous correction of acidosis, and the prothrombin time. An allograft with delayed or poor initial function may be salvaged by the infusion of prostaglandin E_1. Primary nonfunction of the graft, while uncommon, should initiate an immediate search for another graft and urgent transplantation. Those patients with primary nonfunction will require intensive care management to support coagulation and acid-base balance while another graft is being sought.

Achieving complete hemostasis before closure of the abdomen greatly facilitates the postoperative course. In the absence of bleeding the coagulopathy often seen at the completion of the transplant does not need to be corrected provided the prothrombin time is less than 25 seconds. Postoperative fluid management is guided by pulmonary artery pressure measurements and urine output.

Posttransplantation immunosuppression is delivered by various protocols, including cyclosporine or FK506, azathioprine, and corticosteroids. Some centers use an antilymphocyte preparation to avoid the use of the nephrotoxic agents cyclosporine and FK506 during the perioperative period. Patients with preoperative renal dysfunction or the hepatorenal syndrome can be managed with azathioprine and steroids for the first 3 or 4 days until the renal function begins to improve. If renal function improves rapidly, cyclosporine or FK506 can be added at that time. If the return of renal function is delayed, immunosuppression can be achieved with the addition of an antilymphocyte preparation for up to 14 days.

Allograft dysfunction in the postoperative period requires specialized investigation. Liver function studies should gradually return toward normal when measured daily. Investigation is required when this improving trend is interrupted or there is a rise in liver enzymes or bilirubin. The usual causes for allograft dysfunction during the first postoperative month are rejection, biliary tract complications, arterial complications, drug toxicity, and sepsis. There is considerable overlap in the presentation of each of these complications, and investigation usually requires the study of each possible complication. The workup for allograft dysfunction requires percutaneous liver biopsy, duplex ultrasonography of the hepatic vessels, and cholangiography. In the early postoperative period, these three systems—parenchymal, vascular, and biliary—are investigated simultaneously with the onset of dysfunction.

The hepatic artery is studied during the first postoperative day with duplex ultrasonography.[59] Failure to locate an adequate Doppler signal in the hepatic artery is an indication for immediate angiography to identify technical problems with the arterial reconstruction.

Rejection is usually noted as laboratory changes of cholestasis. Severe rejection may result in low-grade fever, anorexia, and abdominal pain. However, the usual signs of early rejection are limited to laboratory changes. If there is an external biliary drainage catheter, a change in the color of the bile will be noted. The normal golden-brown color changes first to a dark green and then eventually lightens if left untreated. The diagnosis of rejection is made by microscopic examination of the liver biopsy (Figure 21-4, *B*). Characteristic changes on biopsy show cellular infiltration of the portal tract with activated lymphocytes and eosinophils. Lymphocytes[23] are associated with the bile ductules and can be seen in the subendothelial plane of the portal veins.

The first rejection episode is treated with increasing steroid dose, either as a steroid taper or as bolus therapy with high dose methylprednisolone. Rejection that is resistant to steroid therapy or recurs after a course of increased steroid therapy is treated with monoclonal antibody OKT3. Patients who are receiving cyclosporine and fail antilymphocyte globulin therapy are often rescued with new experimental immunosuppressants or are considered for retransplantation.

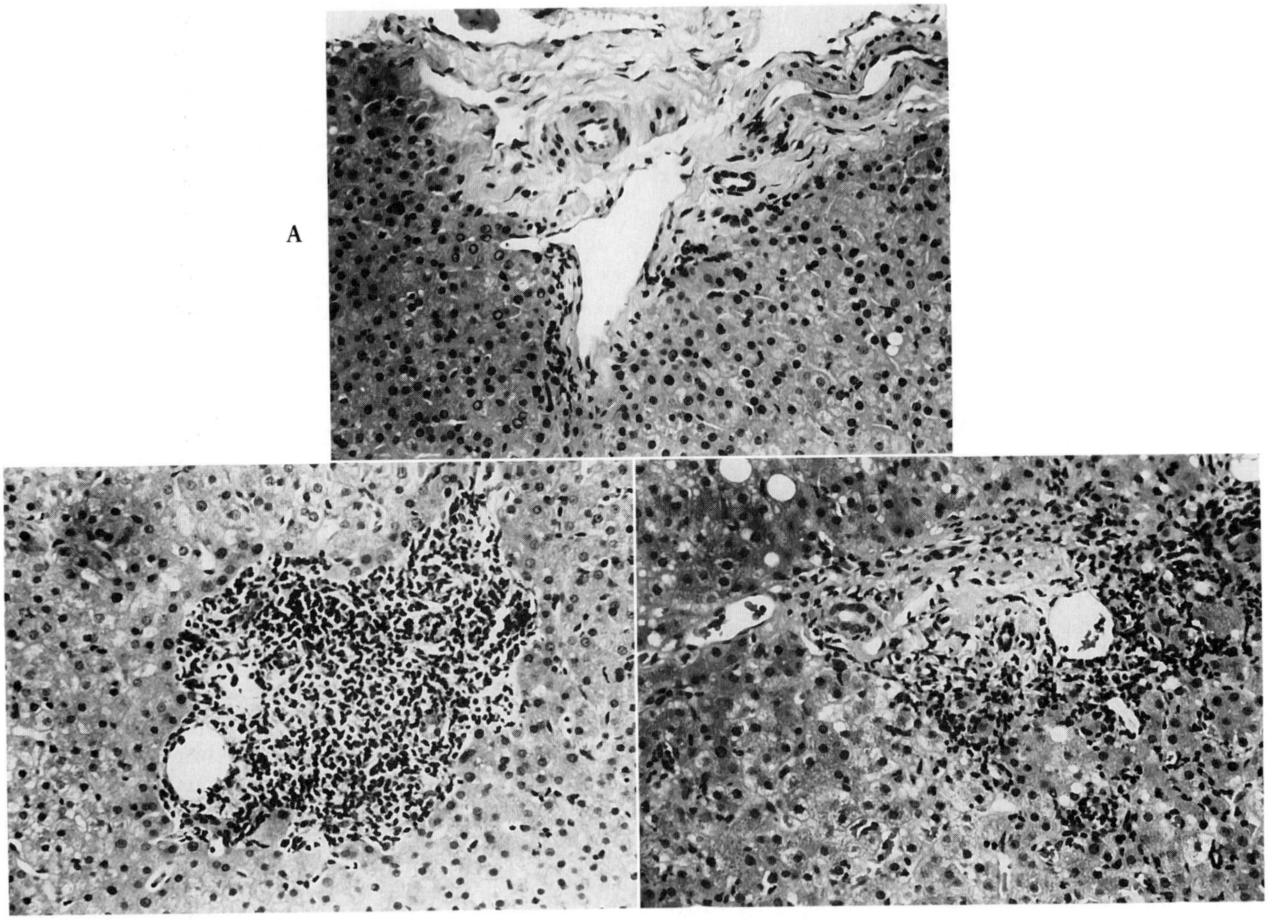

FIGURE 21-4 **A,** An unremarkable portal tract (time zero biopsy). The portal vein *(bottom center)* shows no evidence of subendothelial infiltrates or intravascular lymphocyte adhesion ("endotheliitis" or "endotheliatitis"), the hepatic artery *(upper left,* above portal vein) shows no acute arthrosis or infiltrates, and the bile duct *(lower right)* shows no infiltration by lymphocytes ("ductitis") (400X). **B,** Acute cellular rejection (6 months after transplantation). There is a dense infiltrate of lymphocytes in this portal tract. A portal vein *(lower left)* shows subendothelial infiltration by lymphocytes and intravenous collections of adherent lymphocytes ("endotheliitis"); lymphocytes also infiltrate two bile ducts ("ductitis," one at left center near the portal vein and the other at the lower right edge of the portal tract) (250X). **C,** Recurrent hepatitis C (11 months after transplantation). There are numerous small lymphocytes at the edge of the portal tract and in the adjacent lobular parenchyma, frequently seen in sinusoids. There is focal subendothelial infiltration of the portal vein, without endothelial cell reaction, and the bile duct (at the left edge of the portal tract) shows no evidence of ductitis. Acidophil bodies (not pictured) are also common in recurrent hepatitis (400X).

Cholangiography is utilized to diagnose bile duct leakage or stricture. Unrecognized or delayed recognition of a bile duct anastomotic leak results in intraabdominal sepsis with high mortality. Early bile duct leak usually requires operative repair although experience is increasing in the use of endoscopically placed biliary stents and percutaneous drainage procedures to manage bile duct leaks.[84] Bile duct stricture is usually a technical complication in the immediate postoperative course. These strictures can often be managed with balloon dilatation and stenting. Stricture of the choledochocholedochostomy can be operatively revised to a Roux-en-Y choledochojejunostomy if it is resistant to interventional radiologic procedures.

When arterial problems are suspected by abnormal duplex ultrasound, the patient requires immediate angiography and urgent operative repair if the liver is to be salvaged.[47] Arterial thrombosis may result in hepatic necrosis and abscess formation or may present with dehiscence of the biliary anastomosis. Patients with arterial complications frequently develop intrahepatic bile duct strictures and bile lake formation.[48] Thrombosis of the portal vein is uncommon. Early thrombosis may result in severe portal hypertension and hepatic necrosis. Late portal vein thrombosis usually presents with complications of portal hypertension.[82]

Late Complications

Rejection in liver transplantation continues to be a source of significant morbidity. Although rejection most frequently occurs within the first few months following transplantation, late rejection remains a constant threat. Late rejection episodes are frequently associated with the onset of viral illness or a lapse in compliance with immunosuppressives and histologically appears as vanishing bile duct syndrome and is often unresponsive to conventional therapy and frequently progresses to graft loss.[12] Late bile duct strictures can occur at any time after transplantation. These strictures usually present with laboratory evidence of cholestasis. Occasionally, late bile duct strictures will present with fever and cholangitis. Investigation and intervention can usually be provided by percutaneous cholangiography or endoscopic retrograde cholangiography. Treatment of these strictures can be by balloon dilatation and stenting.

Patients are always at risk of complications due to continued immunosuppression. Later opportunistic infections, such as cytomegalovirus disease, *Pneumocystis* pneumonia, herpes virus infections, and fungal infections are common. Patients on chronic cyclosporine therapy may have a significant decrease in their glomerular filtration rate,[69] although after an initial decline, the glomerular filtration rates tend to be stable in most patients. Some patients, however, develop progressive renal dysfunction. Osteonecrosis from corticosteroids is a frequent complication, especially in patients with primary biliary cirrhosis and in postmenopausal women. Immunosuppression-associated lymphoproliferative disease occurs with varied presentations and is related to Epstein-Barr virus primary infection or reactivation.

The development of lymphoproliferation disease seems to be closely associated with the use of antilymphocyte therapy. The diagnosis of lymphoproliferative disease is made by a biopsy of the affected tissue. Treatment requires reduction in immunosuppression and frequently requires the withholding of cyclosporine until the lymphoproliferative disease resolves.

Recurrence of the original liver disease is occasionally seen. Patients most commonly affected are those with chronic active hepatitis B who remain surface antigen positive and those with chronic active hepatitis C. Protocols using passive immunization for hepatitis B[74] and interferon therapy for hepatitis C have had encouraging results. Diagnosis of recurrence of chronic active hepatitis is made by liver biopsy (Figures 21-4, *A-C*). In these patients, as with patients with rejection, there is lymphocytic infiltration of the portal tract; however, with chronic active hepatitis, there tends to be sparing of the bile ducts. Whether the diseases such as primary biliary cirrhosis, autoimmune hepatitis, or primary sclerosing cholangitis recur following liver transplantation is controversial. It is often difficult to differentiate these diseases from other pathologic changes seen on biopsy of the transplanted liver.

Results

The dramatic achievements leading to the excellent clinical results in hepatic transplantation combine surgical technique, organ preservation, and especially the advances in immunosuppressive therapy. The patient and allograft survival at the Unviersity of Alabama is noted in Figures 21-5 and 21-6. These results include all patients transplanted at this institution and is similar to that reported by others. Long-term graft survival appears to be especially favorable in recipients of liver transplants and may be the result of microchimerism. These impressive results in long-term survival are often associated with a minimal dosage of immunosuppression far less than could be accomplished with other organs. The risk of recurrent disease with hepatitis B is a point of concern in this group of patients and may well limit the use of retransplantation in this select group of patients.

New Developments in Liver Transplantation

Liver transplantation today is severely limited by organ availability. This lack of organ availability is most apparent in children requiring liver transplantation. Because of this shortage, techniques have been developed allowing adult sized organs to undergo reduction to provide a segment or a lobe for transplantation into a smaller child.[11] These techniques require the anatomic division of the graft in a basin of saline slush with meticulous ligation of individual vessels and biliary structures. A logical extension of this technology is development of the living related liver transplant procedure.[12] This elective procedure involves a partial hepatectomy from a relative of the child. Lobectomy in expert hands should be accomplished in a healthy donor with an acceptable morbidity and mortality.

Patients who develop fulminant hepatic failure have the potential to return to normal hepatic function with time. However, because of progressive encephalopathy and intracerebral edema, brain injury occurs before hepatic recovery can occur. A possible solution may be the placement of an auxiliary heterotopic graft. After recovery and healing of the native liver, the immunosuppression may eventually be withdrawn and the aux-

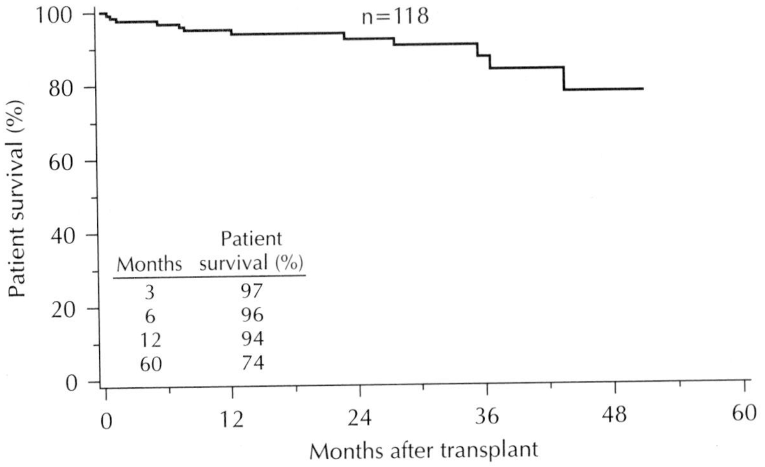

FIGURE 21-5 Patient survival after orthotopic hepatic transplantation at the University of Alabama.

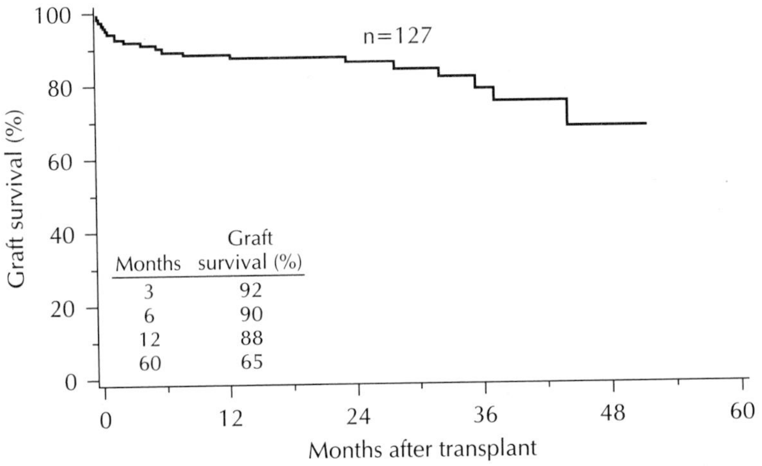

FIGURE 21-6 Allograft survival in all patients, including hepatic regrafts, at the University of Alabama.

iliary graft removed. The ultimate answer to limited organ availability may be the use of xenografts.

PANCREATIC TRANSPLANTATION

Pancreatic transplantation as a treatment for diabetes mellitus includes both islet cell and whole organ transplantation. The application of islet cell transplantation for clinical use remains limited to only a few centers and is largely experimental. Pancreatic transplantation was first attempted in the mid 1960s but failed for immunologic and technical reasons. In 1979 Najarian and associates at the University of Minnesota initiated a carefully constructed trial of segmental pancreatic transplantation between living donor patients.[85] More recently the whole pancreas from cadaveric donors has been utilized and is currently the most common technique.

Clinical Indications

Prime candidates for combined kidney-pancreas transplantation include patients with type I diabetes mellitus of juvenile onset and approaching end-stage renal disease.[30,85] These patients must be carefully selected, usually younger than 40 years of age, not obese, and free of coronary artery disease. Unfortunately these individuals usually have severe retinopathy and gastroparesis in addition to their nephropathy. The ideal time for operation is before end stage and dialysis, which usually is performed with a creatinine between 5.0 and 8.0 mg %. The duration of pancreatic preservation using University of Wisconsin solution is best limited to less than 16 hours. Immediate renal function allows aggressive use of immunosuppression, especially cyclosporine, and provides prompt pancreatic secretion of insulin with correction of hyperglycemia in the first 6 hours after revascularization.

Pancreatic transplantation alone before end-stage renal disease is less successful since rejection of the kidney when combined with the pancreas provides an excellent marker for treatment with antirejection therapy. Usually, but not always, the kidney rejection precedes the pancreas, and treatment seems to prevent the rejection process in the pancreas. The pancreas, however, is surprisingly durable and may continue to function after complete rejection of the kidney. Successful kidney-pancreas transplantation will prevent the progression of retinopathy, but significant improvement of vision is usually not evident. The same appears to be true for peripheral vascular disease.

Technical Considerations

The combined kidney-pancreas operation includes the placement of the whole pancreas in the pelvis, suturing the splenic artery, with an arterial vascular extension graft to the common iliac artery and the portal vein with or without an extension vein graft to the iliac vein. Thus insulin enters the vena cava bypassing the portal vein and liver. Thus far this does not appear to be a major metabolic problem. The most effective management of the exocrine portion of the pancreas has been with duodenocystostomy draining the amylase into the bladder. Urine amylase can be used as a marker for rejection. The kidney may be placed either intraperitoneally or extraperitoneally and the procedure is similar to renal transplantation alone.

Immunosuppressive Therapy

Immunosuppressive therapy is similar to the renal protocol and includes either triple or quadruple drug therapy. Prompt renal function with excellent diuresis allows early administration of cyclosporine and achievement of adequate blood levels. The postoperative reduction of prednisone and long-term immunosuppressive protocol is also similar to that of renal transplantation. Acute rejection usually occurs with an increase in BUN or creatinine before an elevation in blood sugar or a decline in urine amylase. Because the urine amylase concentration is a reflection of the urine volume and amylase secretion, this may be misleading.

Complications

The technical complications of kidney-pancreas transplantation are similar to those of renal transplantation. Pancreas transplantation has the additional risks of splenic artery thrombosis and pancreatic necrosis. The potential for these complications can be determined by either a Doppler flow study or a pancreatic technetium-DPTA perfusion scan. The use of systemic anticoagulation has been advocated by some surgeons to prevent vascular thrombosis; however, we and others have not found it necessary to take this precaution. The occurrence of pancreatitis with an increase in serum amylase is not uncommon and usually not a major problem unless associated with a pseudocyst or disruption of the vascular anastomosis. A duodenal leak or mucosal bleeding may reflect duodenal rejection. Acute irreversible rejection requires pancreatectomy. Peripancreatic fluid levels diagnosed by CT scan or ultrasound need not be treated unless infected.

Results

Combined kidney-pancreas transplantation has a 1-year allograft survival ranging from 65% to 80%, depending on the center with the most common cause of graft loss due to rejection and technical complications.[30,85] If the procedure is successful in the first 3 months, then the long-term outcome is very good for both organs. Unfortunately, patients with long-term graft survival are not free of the progression of complications of diabetes especially peripheral vascular disease. However, the overall quality of life is definitely improved when both organs function well.

CARDIAC TRANSPLANTATION

Heterotopic cardiac transplantation in animals was first reported by Carrel.[17] Subsequently, in 1933, Mann and associates[53] at the Mayo Clinic reported transplantation of the heart into the neck of dogs. The first successful experimental orthotopic cardiac transplantation procedure was reported by Lower and associates[51] in 1961. In spite of these interesting and exciting experimental procedures, it remained for Barnard[5] in 1966 to perform the first cardiac transplantation procedure involving a human donor to human recipient. Because of the frequency of acute and chronic rejection causing the ultimate failure of the transplanted heart, this procedure was pursued in only a few centers until the introduction of cyclosporine. Improved immunosuppressive therapy surveillance techniques for rejection and the development of cardiac procurement and preservation have provided the stimulus for initiating cardiac transplantation programs in a number of centers in the United States.

Clinical Indications

The two most common indications today for cardiac transplantation are end-stage ischemic heart disease and primary cardiomyopathy. Primary cardiomyopathy occurs in three forms: dilated, restrictive, and obliterative, of which the most frequent is the dilated form. End-stage ischemic heart disease is the result of previous myocardial infarction and poor left ventricular function. Congenital malformations thus far represent only a small percentage of patients receiving cardiac allografts. Patients with insulin-dependent diabetes are not ideal candidates because of the predisposition to infection and associated diffuse systemic vascular disease. Patients with active peptic ulcer disease should have appropriate treatment before transplantation. Severe pulmonary vascular disease may be a contraindication for cardiac transplantation. A normal right ventricle will usually fail when the afterload is increased by a pulmonary artery pressure of more than 60 mm Hg.

Donor and recipient must be ABO compatible. Tissue typing has assumed greater importance in renal transplantation than in cardiac transplantation, primarily because of the logistic problems involved between the donor and recipient and the short time interval acceptable for cardiac preservation. In view of these constraints, most centers perform only a preoperative lymphocyte crossmatch to exclude the presence of preformed cytotoxic antibodies in the recipient patient. Thus HLA typing and DR typing have little place in the selection of donor-recipient combinations for cardiac transplantation.

Technical Considerations

Cardiac transplantation requires careful coordination between donor procurement and the transplantation procedure. The transplantation of the donor heart must be performed within 3 to 4 hours of the ischemic interval, although a longer period of preservation appears feasible based on recent experimental studies. The procurement of the donor heart is described in the section, Organ Preservation and Procurement. The size of the donor heart and recipient patient is a critical technical factor in the operation.

The operation is carried out with every attempt to limit the cardiac ischemic time to less than 180 minutes, although preservation of the heart may be extended to 5 or even 6 hours. During procurement of the donor heart, the recipient is simultaneously prepared for transplantation and placed on cardiopulmonary bypass. The donor heart is preserved with UW solution and transported in the same solution at 4° C (39.2° F). Once the donor heart has been delivered to the recipient operating room, recipient cardiectomy is carried out by transsection of the left and right atrium just above the atrioventricular groove and by transsection of the ascending aorta and main pulmonary artery. Thus the pulmonary veins enter a cuff of left atrium and the cavae enter a cuff of right atrium. The suturing of the donor heart to the recipient includes connecting the left atrial cuff of the donor heart to the recipient. The right atrial anastomosis is performed next and the pulmonary artery anastomosis completed in an end-to-end fashion. The aortic anastomosis is then completed.

Immunosuppressive Therapy

During the last 10 years immunosuppressive therapy for cardiac transplantation has been similar to liver and renal transplantation with a few modifications. The immunosuppressive regimen varies from center to center. The regimen at the University of Alabama includes prednisone, azathioprine, and cyclosporine for induction and early maintenance therapy. This includes oral cyclosporine before transplantation, 1 to 4 mg/kg and then posttransplant to maintain 12-hour trough levels at 300 to 400 ng/dl. Methylprednisolone is administered preoperatively, 125 mg, and then postoperatively daily with gradual reduction to 10 mg/day at 3 months and possibly alternate day prednisone therapy if the patient has stable graft function. Azathioprine is administered preoperatively and postoperatively at a dose of 5 mg/kg with gradual reduction to approximately 2 mg/kg. Acute rejection is treated by Solu-Medrol 15 mg/kg/day for 3 days, and if rejection is not reversed, OKT3 monoclonal antibody is administered for 7 to 14 days.

Complications

The diagnosis of cardiac rejection is confirmed by the endomyocardial biopsy. The electrocardiogram and myocardial enzymes are not particularly helpful in identifying rejection in those patients receiving cyclosporine. The endomyocardial biopsy is performed weekly for the first 3 weeks postoperatively and then every 2 weeks for approximately 6 weeks. Biopsy specimens are then obtained every 3 to 4 months. Acute rejection can usually be determined by light microscopy. The treatment for acute rejection is similar to that for renal allografts. Persistence or progression of acute rejection with decreased cardiac performance requires retransplantation.

Cyclosporine in excess of 15 mg/kg/day has been associated with impairment of renal function. Similar experience has been reported by others, with eventual development of chronic renal insufficiency.[62] This renal insufficiency is associated with increased BUN and creatinine levels and responds to a reduction in the dosage of cyclosporine. If the dosage of cyclosporine is not reduced, acute renal failure may develop. In such circumstances, cyclosporine should be discontinued and either antilymphocyte globulin or azathioprine substituted. If hyperkalemia or fluid volume overload occurs during the period of renal dysfunction, hemodialysis may be indicated. Cyclosporine is resumed (3 to 5 mg/kg/day) when urine volume returns to 500 ml/day, and the dosage is gradually increased as the renal function permits. Other complications similar to those noted in renal transplantation include avascular necrosis, cyclosporine

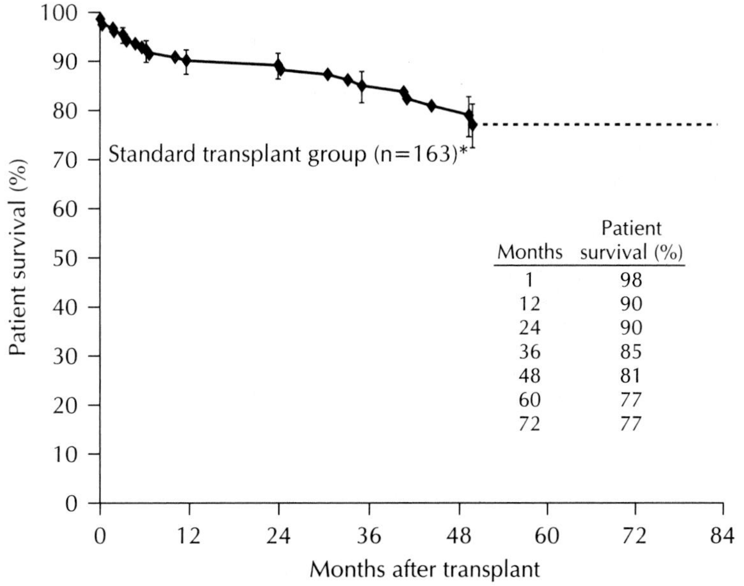

FIGURE 21-7 The clinical outcome after cardiac transplantation is depicted above for a consecutive 7-year experience (Jan 1987—Dec 1993; n = 180) of 160 patients at the University of Alabama; both early and late survival are emphasized.

toxicity, infections, and chronic rejection. In some circumstances patients with cyclosporine-induced nephrotoxicity have had improved renal function after conversion from cyclosporine to azathioprine. The maneuver, however, must be carried out with care to avoid or recognize the risks of acute rejection.

Results

The results of allograft and patient survival following cardiac transplantation have improved tremendously in the last 10 years primarily with the introduction of cyclosporine and the clinical use of the myocardial biopsy technique to confirm the presence of rejection. The results at the University of Alabama are documented in Figure 21-7 and emphasize the impressive control of acute rejection in the first 6 months and the continued persistence of chronic rejection causing graft loss in the next 3 years. The current limitations of cardiac transplantation are the shortage of organs and the present limitation of cardiac preservation requiring the operation to be performed within the first 4 to 6 hours after cardiectomy.

LUNG TRANSPLANTATION

Dr. James Hardy and colleagues in 1963 reported the first human lung transplantation, resulting in patient death 18 days later. Although multiple attempts at transplantation of the lung were attempted from 1963 to 1980, none was successful until 1981 when Retiz and colleagues reported the first heart-lung transplantation. The use of cyclosporine was again the major factor in the success of lung transplantation, combined with improvements in pulmonary preservation and the technical management of the bronchus.

Clinical Indications

Recipients for lung transplantation include patients with end-stage emphysema, pulmonary fibrosis, primary pulmonary hypertension, and Eisenmenger's syndrome. Patients with acute or chronic infection are usually not suitable for lung transplantation and carcinoma. Transplantation may include both lungs and the heart, both lungs, or a single lung. More recently bilateral single lung transplantation has been the procedure of choice.

Donor selection is a key component of lung transplantation and requires clear lung fields, PaO_2 of 300 mm Hg in the presence of a FiO_2 of 100% and 5 cm of positive end expiratory pressure. A bronchoscopy immediately before procurement is necessary to exclude aspiration or purulent secretions. The recipient size is important to be certain the chest can accommodate the donor lung.

Lung Preservation

The heart and lungs are procured together. A pursestring suture is placed in the ascending aorta for UW solution and in the main pulmonary artery above the bifurcation for infusion of the pulmonary flush solution (Euro-

Collins with prostaglandin E1). The trachea is dissected and encircled by an umbilical tape. After cannulation of the ascending aorta and main pulmonary artery, 500 μg of prostaglandin E1 is injected into the superior vena cava. The superior vena cava is then ligated, inferior vena cava transected to decompress the right heart, and the ascending aorta cross-clamped. The UW solution for myocardial preservation is then initiated, as well as the pulmonary flush solution. During procurement the lungs are inflated with 100% O_2. The heart is then excised, the main pulmonary artery divided, and the pericardium anterior to the hilar of each lung excised. The lungs are then removed inflated on 100% O_2, the trachea clamped and divided, and the lungs excised. Further dissection is carried out on a back table where the lungs are separated by stapling the trachea. The lungs are transplanted while inflated.

Immunosuppressive Therapy

The immunosuppressive regimen includes intravenous azathioprine, 2 mg/kg preoperatively. The postoperative course includes antilymphocyte globulin, azathioprine and intravenous cyclosporine infusion of 3 to 4 mg/hr. When the patient can tolerate liquids by mouth, oral cyclosporine is given to achieve blood levels of 300 to 400 ng/ml. The prednisone is decreased orally to a level of 10 mg/day at 3 months with consideration of alternate day prednisone at 1 year. The treatment of acute rejection is with intravenous administration of steroids followed by antilymphocyte globulin if there is no response.

Results

The early and long-term outcome after lung transplantation has improved remarkably in the last 8 years with the current immunosuppressive agents. As noted with other organs, once the surgical technique was established, the primary limitation has become the process of rejection and its control by immunosuppressive drugs.

REFERENCES

1 Acuto O, Reinherz EL: The human T-cell receptor, structure and function, *N Engl J Med* 312(17):1100, 1985.
2 Albert ED, Baur MP, Mayr WR et al: *Histocompatibility testing 1984,* Berlin, 1984, Springer-Verlag.
3 Allison AC, Eugui EM: Immunosuppressive and other effects of mycophenolic acid and an ester prodrug, mycophenolate mofetil, *Immunol Rev* 136:5, 1993.
4 Allison AC, Eugui EM, Sollinger HW: Mycophenolate mofetil (RS-61443): mechanisms of action and effects in transplantation, *Transplantation Reviews* 7(3):129, 1993.
5 Barnard CN: Human cardiac transplantation, *Am J Cardiol* 22:584, 1968.
6 Belzer FO, D'Alessandro AM, Hoffmann RM et al: The use of UW solution in clinical transplantation: a 4-year experience, *Ann Surg* 215(6):579, 1992.
7 Berteli AJ, Daniel V, Mohring K et al: Association of kidney graft failure with a positive flow cytometric crossmatch, *Clin Transpl* 279:611, 1992.
8 Bidwell J: DNA-RFLP analysis and genotyping of HLA-DR and DQ antigens, *Immunol Today* 9(1):18, 1988.
9 Billingham RE, Brent L, Medawar PB: Actively acquired tolerance of foreign cells, *Nature* 172:603, 1953.
10 Bodmer WF, Batchelor JR, Bodmer JG et al: *Histocompatibility testing,* Copenhagen, 1978, Munksgaard.
11 Broelsch CE, Emond JC, Thistlethwaite JR et al: Liver transplantation, including the concept of reduced-size liver transplants in children, *Ann Surg* 208:410, 1988.
12 Broelsch CE, Whitington PF, Emond JC et al: Liver transplantation in children from living related donors, *Ann Surg* 214(4):428, 1991.
13 Burnet FM, Fenner F: *The production of antibodies,* London, 1949, MacMillan Publishers, Ltd.
14 Calne RY, Rolles K, White DJG et al: Cyclosporine A initially as the only immunosuppressant in 34 recipients of cadaveric organs: 32 kidneys, 2 pancreases, and 2 livers, *Lancet* 2:1033, 1979.
15 Calne RY, White DJ: The use of cyclosporin A in clinical organ grafting, *Ann Surg* 196:330, 1982.
16 Canadian Multicentre Transplant Study Group: A randomized clinical trial of cyclosporine in cadaveric renal transplantation, *N Engl J Med* 309:809, 1983.
17 Carrel A: Transplantation in mass of the kidneys, *J Exp Med* 10:98, 1908.
18 Cosimi AB, Burton RC, Colvin RB et al: Treatment of acute renal allograft rejection with OKT3 monoclonal antibody, *Transplantation* 32:535, 1981.
19 Cosimi AB, Colvin RB, Burton RC et al: Use of monoclonal antibodies to T-cell subsets for immunologic monitoring and treatment in recipients of renal allografts, *N Engl J Med* 305:314, 1981.
20 D'Alesandro AM, Pirsch JD, Stratta RJ et al: OKT3 salvage therapy in a quadruple immunosuppressive protocol in cadaveric renal transplantation, *Transplantation* 47:297, 1989.
21 Dallman MJ: The cytokine network and regulations of the immune responses to organ transplants, *Transplant Rev* 6(4):209, 1992.
22 Deierhoi MH, Barber WH, Curtis JJ et al: A comparison of OKT3 monoclonal antibody and corticosteroids in the treatment of acute renal allograft rejection, *Am J Kidney Dis* 11:86, 1988.
23 Demetris AJ, Qian SG, Sun H et al: Liver allograft rejection: an overview of morphologic findings, *Am J Surg Pathol* 14(suppl 1):49, 1990.
24 Diethelm AG, Dubovsky EV, Whelchel JD et al: Diagnosis of impaired renal function after kidney transplantation using renal scintigraphy, renal plasma flow and urinary excretion of hippurate, *Ann Surg* 191:604, 1980.
25 Dupont E, Wybran J, Toussaint C: Glucocorticosteroids and organ transplantation, *Transplantation* 37:331, 1984.
26 Fuller TC, Phelan D, Gebel HM et al: Antigenic specificity of antibody reactive in the antiglobulin-augmented lymphocytotoxicty test, *Transplantation* 32:27, 1982.
27 Garavoy MR, Rheinschmidt MA, Bigos M et al: Flow cytometry analysis: a high technology crossmatch technique facilitating transplantation, *Transplant Proc* 15:1939, 1983.
28 Glass NR, Miller DT, Sollinger HW et al: A four year experience with donor blood transfusion protocols for living donor renal transplantation, *Transplantation* 39:615, 1985.
29 Gorer PA: The genetic and antigenic basis of tumour transplantation, *J Pathol Bacteriol* 44:691, 1937.
30 Groth CG: *Pancreatic transplantation,* Philadelphia, 1988, WB Saunders.
31 Gruber SA, Chan GLC, Canafax DM et al: Immunosuppression in renal transplantation. I. Cyclosporine and azathioprine, *Clin Transpl* 5(2):65, 1991.
32 Gruber SA, Chan GLC, Canafax DM et al: Immunosuppression in renal transplantation. II. Corticosteroids, antilymphocyte globulin, and OKT3, *Clin Transpl* 5(3):219, 1993.
33 Halloran PF, Broski AP, Batiuk TD et al: The molecular immu-

nology of acute rejection: an overview, *Transplant Immunol* 1:3, 1983.

34 Hoffman RM, Stratta RJ, D'Alessandro AM et al: Combined cold storage-perfusion preservation with a new synthetic perfusate, *Transplantation* 47(1):32, 1989.

35 Hoitsma AJ, Van Lier HJJ, Reekers P et al: Improved patient and graft survival after treatment of acute rejections of cadaveric renal allografts with rabbit antithymocyte globulin, *Transplantation* 39:274, 1985.

36 Hume DM, Merrill JP, Miller BF et al: Experience with renal homotransplantation in the human: report of nine cases, *J Clin Invest* 34:327, 1955.

37 Iwatsuki S, Starzl TE, Sheahan DG et al: Hepatic resection versus transplantation for hepatocellular carcinoma, *Ann Surg* 214(3): 221, 1991.

38 Jain AB, Fung JJ, Todo S et al: Incidence and treatment of rejection episodes in primary orthotopic liver transplantation under FK506, *Transplant Proc* 23:928, 1991.

39 Kahan BD: Donor specific transfusions—a balanced view, *Prog Transplant* 1:115, 1984.

40 Kahan BD, Van Buren CT, Flechner SM et al: Clinical and experimental studies with cyclosporine in renal transplantation, *Surgery* 97:125, 1985.

41 Keays R, Potter D, O'Grady J et al: Intracranial and cerebral perfusion pressure changes before, during and immediately after orthotopic liver transplantation for fulminant failure, *Q J Med* 79:425, 1991.

42 Kerman RH, Van Buren CT, Lewis RM et al: Improved graft survival for flow cytometry and antihuman globulin crossmatch-negative retransplant recipients, *Transplantation* 49(1):52, 1990.

43 Kirsch JP, Howard TK, Klintmalm GB et al: Problematic vascular reconstruction in liver transplantation, Part II. Portovenous conduits, *Surgery* 107(5):544, 1990.

44 Kissmeyer-Nielsen F, Olsen S, Peterson VP et al: Hyperacute rejection of kidney allografts associated with preexisting humoral antibodies against donor cells, *Lancet* 2:662, 1966.

45 Klein J: *Natural history of the major histocompatibility complex,* New York, 1986, John Wiley and Sons.

46 Lafferty KJ, Prowse SJ, Simeonovic CJ: Immunobiology of tissue transplantation: a return to the passenger leukocyte concept, *Annu Rev Immunol* 1:143, 1983.

47 Langnas AN, Marujo W, Stratta RJ et al: Hepatic allograft rescue following arterial thrombosis, *Transplantation* 51(1):86, 1991.

48 Langnas AN, Marujo W, Stratta RJ et al: Vascular complications after orthotopic liver transplantation, *Am J Surg* 161:76, 1991.

49 LeRoux PD, Elliott JP, Perkins JD et al: Intracranial pressure monitoring in fulminant hepatic failure and liver transplantation, *Lancet* 335:1291, 1990.

50 Loveland BE, McKenzie IF: Which T cells cause graft rejection? *Transplantation* 33:217, 1982.

51 Lower RR, Stofer RC, Shumway NE: Homovital transplantation of the heart, *J Thorac Cardiovasc Surg* 41:196, 1961.

52 Makowka L, Sher LS, Cramer DV et al: The development of brequinar as an immunosuppressive drug for transplantation, *Immunol Rev* 136:51, 1993.

53 Mann FC, Priestly JT, Markowitz J et al: Transplantation of the intact mammalian heart, *Arch Surg* 26:219, 1933.

54 Medawar PB: The behavior and fate of skin autografts and skin homografts in rabbits, *J Anat* 78:176, 1944.

55 Medawar PB: The use of antigenic tissue extracts to weaken the immunological reaction against skin homografts in mice, *Transplantation* 1:21, 1963.

56 Milgrom F, Litvak VI, Kano K et al: Humoral antibodies in renal homograft, *JAMA* 198:226, 1966.

57 Mitchison NA: Passive transfer of transplantation immunity, *Proc R Soc Lond (Biol)* 142:72, 1954.

58 Morris RE: Rapamycins: antifungal, antitumor, antiproliferative and immunosuppressive macrolides, *Transplant Rev* 6:39, 1992.

59 Morton MJ, James EM, Wiesner RH et al: Applications of duplex ultrasonography in the liver transplant patient, *Mayo Clin Proc* 65:360, 1990.

60 Murray JE, Merrill JP, Harrison JH: Kidney transplantation between seven pairs of identical twins, *Ann Surg* 148:343, 1958.

61 Murray JE, Merrill JP, Harrison JH et al: Prolonged survival of human-kidney homografts by immunosuppressive drug therapy, *N Engl J Med* 268:1315, 1963.

62 Myers BD, Ross J, Newton L et al: Cyclosporine-associated chronic nephropathy, *N Engl J Med* 311:699, 1984.

63 National Institutes of Health Consensus Development Conference: Liver transplantation, *Hepatology* 4(suppl):1s-110s, 1984.

64 Opelz G, Mytilineos J, Scherer S et al: Survival of DNA HLA-DR typed and matched cadaver kidney transplants, *Lancet* 338:461, 1991.

65 Opelz G, Sengar DPS, Mickey MR et al: Effect of blood transfusions on subsequent kidney transplants, *Transplant Proc* 5:253, 1973.

66 Ortho Multicenter Transplant Study Group: A randomized clinical trial of OKT3 monoclonal antibody for acute rejection of cadaveric renal transplants, *N Engl J Med* 313:337, 1985.

67 Parfrey PS, Forbes RDC, Hutchinson TA et al: The impact of renal transplantation on the course of hepatitis B liver disease, *Transplantation* 39:610, 1985.

68 Paul LC, Baldwin WM III, Claas FHJ et al: Significance of monocyte antibodies in renal transplantation, *Dialysis Transplant* 11:119, 1982.

69 Poplawski S, Gonwa T, Goldstein R et al: Long-term nephrotoxicity in liver transplantation, *Transplant Proc* 21(1):2469, 1989.

70 Rossi G, Grendele M, Colledan M et al: Prevention of hepatitis B virus reinfection after liver transplantation, *Transplant Proc* 23(3):1969, 1991.

71 Rowlands DT, Hill GS, Zmijewski CM: The pathology of renal homograft rejection: a review, *Am J Pathol* 85:774, 1976.

72 Rubin RH, Tolkoff-Rubin NE: The problem of cytomegalovirus infection in transplantation, *Prog Transplant* 1:89, 1985.

73 Salvatierra O, Vincenti F, Amend W et al: Deliberate donor-specific blood transfusions prior to living related renal transplantation: a new approach, *Ann Surg* 192:543, 1980.

74 Samuel D, Bismuth A, Mathieu D et al: Passive immunoprophylaxis after liver transplantation in HBsAg-positive patients, *Lancet* 337:813, 1991.

75 Shapiro R, Jordan M, Fung J et al: Kidney transplantation under FK506 immunosuppression, *Transplant Proc* 23:920, 1991.

76 Shaw BW Jr, Iwatsuki S, Starzl TE et al: Alternative methods of arterialization of the hepatic graft, *Surg Gynecol Obstet* 159:491, 1984.

77 Sheil AGR: Transplantation and cancer. In Morris PJ, editor: *Kidney transplantation: principles and practice,* London, 1979, Academic Press.

78 Starzl TE, Iwatsuki S, Van Thiel DH et al: Evolution of liver transplantation, *Hepatology* 2:614, 1982.

79 Starzl TE, Klintmalm GBG, Porter KA et al: Liver transplantation with use of cyclosporine-A and prednisone, *N Engl J Med* 305:266, 1981.

80 Starzl TE, Marchioro TL, Rowlands DT Jr et al: Immunosuppression after experimental and clinical homotransplantation of the liver, *Ann Surg* 160:411, 1964.

81 Starzl TE, Marchioro TL, Von Kaulla KN et al: Homotransplantation of the liver in humans, *Surg Gynecol Obstet* 117:659, 1963.

82 Stieber AC, Zetti G, Todo S et al: The spectrum of portal vein thrombosis in liver transplantation, *Ann Surg* 213(3):199, 1991.

83 Stone MJ, Klintmalm GB et al: Neoadjuvant chemotherapy and liver transplantation for hepatocellular carcinoma: a pilot study in 20 patients, *Gastroenterology* 104:196, 1993.

84 Stratta RJ, Wood RP, Langnas AN et al: Diagnosis and treatment of biliary tract complications after orthotopic liver transplantation, *Surgery* 106:675, 1989.
85 Sutherland DER, Dunn DL, Goetz FC et al: A 10 year experience with 290 pancreas transplants at a single institution, *Ann Surg* 210:274, 1989.
86 Takemoto S, Terasaki PI, Cecka JM et al: Survival of nationally shared, HLA-matched kidney transplants from cadaveric donors, *N Engl J Med* 327:834, 1992.
87 Tyzzer EE, Little CC: Studies on the inheritance of susceptibility to a transplantable sarcoma (J.W.B.) of the Japanese waltzing mouse, *J Cancer Res* 1:387, 1916.
88 Tzakis AG, Reyes J, Todo S et al: Two year experience with FK506 in pediatric patients, *Transplant Proc* 25:619, 1993.
89 Williams GM, Howe DM, Hudson RP et al: Hyperacute renal homograft rejection in man, *N Engl J Med* 279:611, 1968.

CHAPTER

22

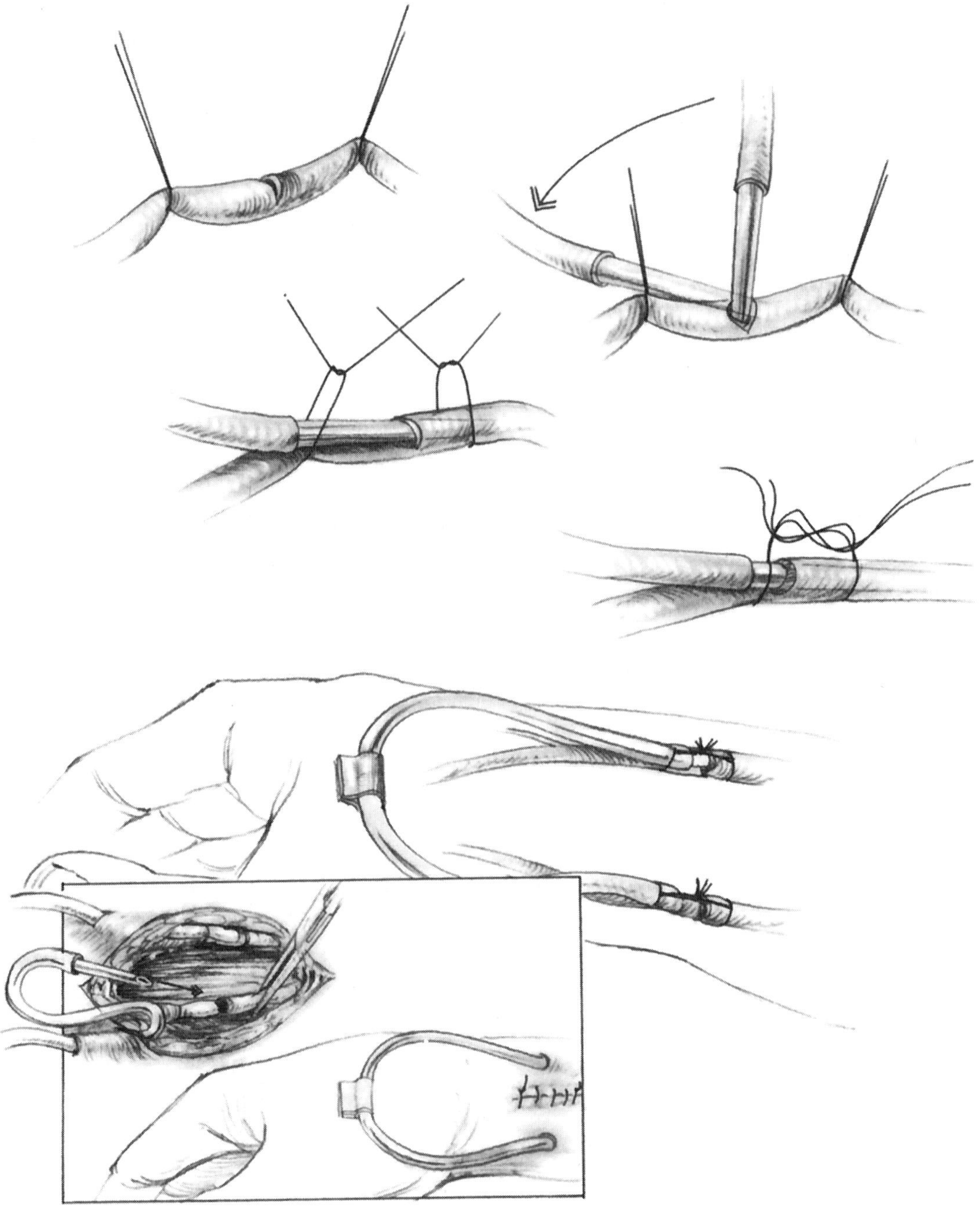

CHRONIC VASCULAR AND PERITONEAL ACCESS

Carl E. Haisch

RELATED MATERIAL APPEARS IN CHAPTERS 7, 14, AND 21

VASCULAR ACCESS

History

Access to the circulation is a major requirement for many forms of therapy today. Frequent access to the blood is necessary for patients undergoing parenteral nutrition, chronic chemotherapy for malignancy, and chronic and acute hemodialysis.

Vascular access is closely related to the development of hemodialysis. Without the need for repeated vascular access into a high-flow system, angioaccess might not have developed. The roots of hemodialysis can be found in the nineteenth century in the laboratory of a chemist, Thomas Graham. George Haas continued Graham's work and attempted the first human dialysis in 1924. He found on subsequent attempts that patients tolerated the procedure, but the dialysis run was too short for therapeutic benefit. In the early 1940s Willem Johan Kolff designed a dialysis machine using cellulose tubing. When heparin became available, Kolff dialyzed his first patient, who had terminal uremia and a blood pressure of 245/150. After each dialysis, the patient improved. However, the patient died on the twenty-sixth day of treatment,[28] when vascular access became unavailable after repeated surgical cutdowns. This case underlined the need for a method of chronic vascular access.

Although a rabbit model of an arteriovenous fistula was constructed using silicon glass conduits, direct application to humans was unsuccessful because of complications of infection and clotting.[28] The next major breakthrough occurred when Quinton and colleagues[75] used a Teflon conduit for constructing arteriovenous fistulas. The major problems were still thrombosis and infection; however, this technique allowed the first long-term dialysis of patients with chronic renal failure. Brescia and associates[13] constructed a natural arteriovenous fistula between the radial artery and the cephalic vein, which minimized thrombosis and infection. However, this approach did not help all patients. For patients without an adequate cephalic vein, May and coworkers[58] tried a saphenous vein jump graft between an artery and a vein. This development has been abandoned, however, because of the high incidence of stenosis and aneurysm formation. The inability to use the saphenous vein led to the use of allografts or synthetic grafts. Bovine grafts were used successfully but have been replaced by polytetrafluoroethylene (PTFE).

The need to give highly irritating solutions to patients and to prevent damage to the blood vessel advanced the developments in vascular access for nutrition and chemotherapy. Aubaniac[6] first described the use of the subclavian vein for vascular access in 1952; later Wilson and associates[105] extensively used the vein for monitoring central venous pressure. Dudrick and Wilmore[30] used it for nutritional support. The subclavian vein was selected because of its easy access and high blood flow. The percutaneous subclavian approach gave central venous access for a limited time. Later the Broviac catheter was developed, which gave long-term vascular access for nutrition[15] but did not allow blood to be drawn through the catheter. The Hickman catheter, with a larger catheter diameter, was developed to meet this need. Currently double- and triple-lumen catheters are available for central venous access. The double-lumen catheter is placed surgically; the triple-lumen catheter is placed percutaneously. Catheters such as the Port-A-Cath and Infus-A-Port allow total skin coverage, thereby decreasing the incidence of infection. These catheters can be used intermittently by puncturing the septum of the access port with a special needle.

Indications

One of the most common clinical settings for chronic or long-term vascular access is acute or chronic renal failure. Other settings include total parenteral nutrition,[110] chemotherapy,[77] repeated blood drawing, and plasmapheresis.

An ideal system or technique for vascular access has not yet been developed. Such a system would feature immediate use after placement, a high blood flow rate, the ability to withstand multiple needle punctures or uses, and no propensity to infection or thrombosis.

External Angioaccess

Dialysis

The first successful vascular access procedure for chronic dialysis was performed using the Scribner shunt[75] (Figure 22-1). The shunt is constructed of Teflon; one tip is placed in the artery, and another in a vein. The portion exiting the skin is made of Silastic, and the two tubes are connected, allowing continuous blood flow. The most common location is between the radial artery and the cephalic vein at the wrist, although a vein more proximal on the arm can be used. The posterior tibial artery and saphenous vein are used for placement in the leg.

Allen's test must be performed before the shunt is placed to ensure adequate blood flow to the hand. The patient is asked to clench the hand tightly, and then the examiner occludes both the ulnar and radial arteries to prevent blood flow to the hand. When the ulnar artery is released, the hand should quickly regain its color. This change ensures adequate collateral circulation via the ulnar artery.

The Scribner shunt is rarely used today. It is indicated for acute dialysis or plasmapheresis in patients with a bleeding diathesis in whom the risk of complications from placement of a percutaneous catheter is prohibitive.[98]

The average life of a shunt is 7 to 10 months, with the range being 2 to 14 months.[49,54] The major complications of shunt failure are thrombosis, infection, bleeding, skin erosion, limitation of activity, and dislodgment of the shunt. Damage to the vessel's intima increases thrombosis. Care must be taken to ensure that the vessel is large enough to accommodate the cannula. The vessel can be gently dilated with coronary dilators, taking care not to tear or injure the intima. The Teflon tip is advanced and tied into place, and the Silastic tubing is brought through a stab wound in the skin. It is wise to tie the Teflon tip in the vessel at two or three points along the vessel, thus making certain that the cannula tip is well secured and will not injure the vessel wall. If thrombosis occurs, a Fogarty catheter can be used to clear the arterial and venous limbs. A small amount of urokinase will lyse clot at the catheter tip.[98] Aspirin (160 mg/day) has been reported to decrease the thrombosis rate from 72% in a placebo group to 32% in the treatment groups over a 5-month period.[42] Coumadin, used to give a prothrombin time 1½ times normal, also decreased the thrombosis rate to one fourth that of a control group.[24]

Infection occurs with a frequency of from 1 in 6.9 patient months to 1 in 35 patient months. *Staphylococcus aureus* is the most common organism. Aggressive local catheter care prevents most infections.[24,78] Placing tubing outside the skin limits the patient's activity, and careless wrapping of the tubing can result in dislodgment, with subsequent exsanguination. Some patients have committed suicide by intentionally disconnecting the tubing, causing exsanguination.

The problem of permanent loss of a potential site for construction of an arteriovenous fistula has led to placement of percutaneous catheters in either the subclavian vein or the femoral vein.[26] Femoral vein catheters, placed using a Seldinger technique, can be used to maintain adequate dialysis for a prolonged time, but patients dislike them because they must be placed and removed before and after each dialysis to prevent infection and thrombosis. The catheters can be placed in a variety of configurations: femoral vein, with a return via a peripheral arm vein; bilateral femoral veins; two cannulas in the same femoral vein; or femoral artery and femoral vein. These configurations allow continuous flow for dialysis. A single catheter may be placed in the vein and an in-and-out dialysis technique used. Another possibility is to place a double-lumen catheter in the femoral vein for continuous dialysis. The complications (less than 1%) include ileofemoral thrombosis, local bleeding, retroperitoneal hematoma, and arterial puncture and injury.[53,85]

Subclavian dialysis catheters are commonly used. They are less subject to infectious complications but have the same complications as placement of any subclavian catheter: arterial puncture, pneumothorax, and malposition (see the section on Complications). Reported additional complications are thrombosis or stenosis of the subclavian vein and perforation of the subclavian vein or superior vena cava, leading to death.[25,34] Subclavian catheters are single or double lumen. Their major advantage is that they can be left in place for a time to allow outpatient dialysis.

A major advance has been the development of a Silastic right atrial catheter. This catheter can have one or two lumens and can be used immediately after place-

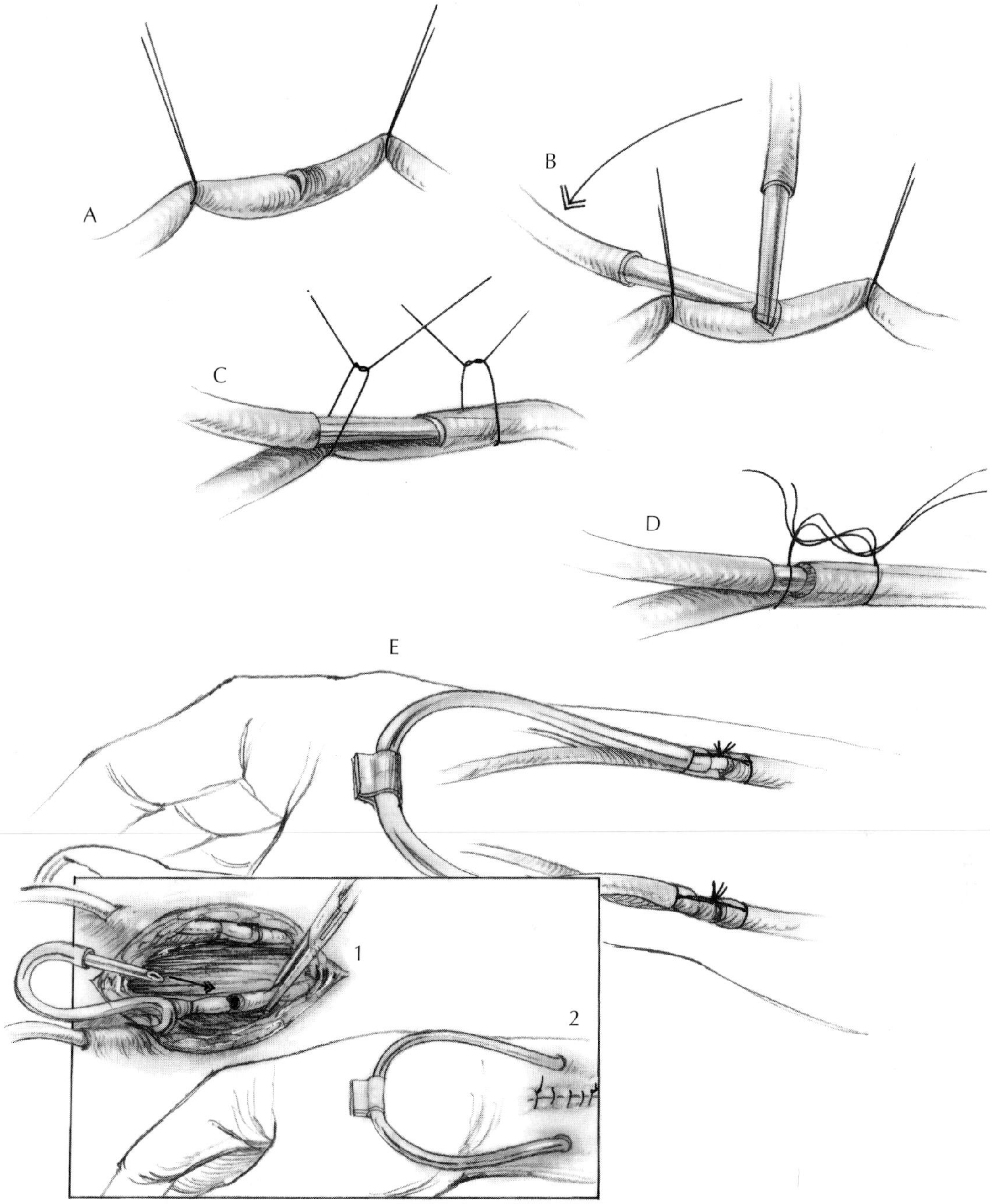

FIGURE 22-1 Placement of a Scribner shunt. **A,** Isolating a blood vessel with an arteriotomy. **B,** Placing the Teflon tip. **C,** Tip being tied into place. **D,** Completing ties. **E,** Finished shunt. Insets: *1,* view of vessels with tip in situ; *2,* completed shunt. (**A** to **D** redrawn from Tilney NL, Lazarus JM, editors: *Surgical care of the patient with renal failure,* Philadelphia, 1982, WB Saunders. **E** redrawn from Rutherford RB, editor: *Vascular surgery,* Philadelphia, 1984, WB Saunders.)

ment. Most commonly a cutdown is performed to the internal jugular vein through the two heads of the sternocleidomastoid muscle. Proximal and distal venous control is obtained, and the catheter is placed into the vein by means of a venotomy. Under fluoroscopic guidance the catheter tip is placed into the superior portion of the right atrium or the superior vena cava. The Dacron cuff is placed at least 3 cm from the skin exit site and deep in the subcutaneous tissues. Between dialysis runs the lumens are filled with heparin (1000 U/ml). Complications with this type of catheter include outflow obstruction, cuff erosion, infection, inflow obstruction, subclavian thrombosis, and perforation of the superior vena cava.[59,88] Forty to 65 percent of Silastic right atrial catheters last about 1 year with revision[64]; percutaneously placed subclavian catheters last 4 to 6 weeks. Moss and colleagues[64] point out that the 1-year survival period for these catheters is approximately the same as the event-free interval for PTFE grafts used for dialysis.

Nutrition or Chemotherapy

Polyethylene catheters commonly have been used in the measurement of central venous pressure and to administer parenteral nutrition. The catheter is placed via the internal jugular vein, subclavian vein, or large veins of the arm. Subclavian placement is the most common method and is described in Chapter 28. The polyethylene catheter is somewhat stiff and can damage the vessel wall, causing bleeding. Care must be taken not to force the catheter, causing it to perforate the vessel wall.

The Broviac catheter, which is made of silicone rubber and has a 1 mm lumen, has been used primarily for parenteral nutrition.[15] The Hickman catheter has a larger lumen than the Broviac catheter and can be used to draw blood or to administer blood products. The Raaf double-lumen catheter is made of similar material but has a round configuration.[76]

The placement techniques for the Broviac, Hickman, and Raaf catheters are limited because of the soft consistency of the silicone rubber. These catheters can be placed through the external jugular vein, the internal jugular vein, the subclavian vein, or the cephalic vein. Placement via the cephalic vein or the internal or external jugular vein calls for a surgical cutdown to the particular vein. The Broviac catheter[43] easily slides through a cephalic vein; however, the Hickman or a double-lumen catheter is too large. If a cephalic vein is not present, another vein must be used. The cardinal guidelines are the same as those for placement of a right atrial catheter for dialysis, outlined previously. A percutaneous technique for placing soft catheters (such as the Broviac catheter) described by Linos and Mucha[55] and Stellato and associates[93] is useful in patients with normal bleeding parameters. However, some double-lumen catheters are too large to place with this technique.

Like the Broviac and Hickman catheters, the Infuse-A-Port and Port-A-Cath catheters provide venous access without having a portion of the catheter exposed. To insert the catheter, venous access is first obtained via the subclavian or internal jugular vein (usually a pacemaker lead introducer is used). The catheter is measured for appropriate length and placed in the vein under fluoroscopic guidance. A subcutaneous pocket is created, with the body (or chamber) of the assembly sutured to the fascia of the pectoralis major muscle. The catheter is used by entering the chamber through the septum with a special needle.[11]

Complications

The complications of external angioaccess can be divided into three basic categories: immediate, malposition, and delayed. Immediate complications are related to placement of the catheter. They are more common with percutaneous placement of catheters via the subclavian vein, which has a complication rate of 4% to 17%.[44,48,82] These complications include pneumothorax, brachial plexus injury, hemothorax, hydromediastinum,[44] cardiac tamponade,[86] air embolus, phrenic nerve injury, thoracic duct injury, bleeding from the puncture site, and puncture of the subclavian artery.[44] Placement of the catheter by experienced surgeons eliminates or reduces the incidence of each of these complications.[44] Immediate complications can also occur when a silicone rubber catheter is placed using a Teflon sheath. Because of the number of complications associated with this technique, one group recommends using a cutdown to place silicone rubber catheters.[74]

Malposition of the catheter tip, which can occur with either polyethylene or silicone rubber catheters, results when the tip of the catheter is placed in the opposite subclavian vein or the internal jugular vein. The location of the silicone rubber catheter should be checked fluoroscopically. Because these are soft catheters, their location can vary considerably.

Delayed complications are mechanical or infectious in nature. Mechanical complications include clotting of the catheter, venous thrombosis, inability to withdraw blood, cuff extrusion, inability of the wound to heal, and defects in the catheter. Clotting of the catheter occurs in 0.7% to 13%[74,97] of those placed. It can be reduced by flushing heparin into the catheter. This flush can be a heparin-saline mix (7 ml, 10 U/ml) or straight heparin (5000 IU/ml) done four times a day.[14,76]

A clotted catheter is treated by injecting urokinase or streptokinase directly into the catheter until patency is restored. In most reports this technique is successful.[23,48] Streptokinase has been associated with allergic reactions when used more than once; therefore urokinase is preferable. Venous thrombosis of the superior vena cava or subclavian vein has also been reported and can prevent the catheter from functioning.[76,99,105] Thrombosis of the vein means access must be found in other locations. A fibrin sheath around the catheter has also been described in these patients. This sheath is found around both polyethylene catheters (14%) and silicone catheters (80%). The sheath could create a nidus for a pulmonary embolus.[102]

Inability to withdraw blood from a catheter placed for chemotherapy or to provide nutrition occurs in approximately 4% of cases.[76] If the catheter cannot be cleared with urokinase or streptokinase, it must be replaced. Cuff extrusion[76] can be prevented by ensuring that the catheter is placed deep in the subcutaneous tissues, at least 3 cm from the skin exit site. Catheter defects can be repaired with a kit from the manufacturer if the catheter break is above skin level.[74]

As more subclavian catheters are being used for short-term dialysis, venous stenosis is being noted more often. This becomes especially evident when an arteriovenous fistula or PTFE graft is subsequently placed in the arm. The patient develops a swollen arm, or the graft clots for no apparent local technical reason. Surratt and colleagues[94] examined 62 extremities and found that a 50% or greater stenosis was present only in patients who had a subclavian catheter in place for a time; they found no stenosis in patients who had not had a subclavian catheter in place. They recommended no preoperative studies for patients who had not had a catheter in place but did recommend a venogram for those who previously had had a subclavian catheter.[94] If temporary access is necessary, a catheter in the internal jugular vein may have fewer long-term sequelae.[20]

Infectious complications can be a major cause of morbidity in patients who use these catheters. Ryan and associates[82] reported a catheter sepsis rate of 7%. They divided catheter sepsis into four categories: bacteriologically confirmed sepsis; clinical catheter sepsis (sepsis that resolved after removal of the catheter without a specific organism being identified); questionable catheter sepsis (sepsis that did not resolve with removal of the catheter; other infections present); and noncatheter sepsis (sepsis that developed secondary to another source). Raaf[76] stated that sepsis occurs in approximately 4% of catheters and that local inflammation of the exit site occurs with 3% of catheters. Inflammation usually can be treated with local therapy, leaving the catheter in place. Dudrick and associates[31] reported catheter sepsis in patients receiving total parenteral nutrition (TPN) at home at a rate of one episode in 2.6 catheter years. Overall sepsis rates are reported from 6% to 27%. The Centers for Disease Control reported an incidence of 7% in 1982, of which cases 54% involved fungal sepsis.[10]

Sepsis is thought to arise from several sources. The main causes include contamination of the infusate, contamination of the hub, contamination from the skin, or endogenous colonization of the catheter. Contamination resulting from poor aseptic technique during insertion or removal is thought to be least common.[7,56]

The source of catheter colonization has been studied. Bjorson and associates[10] showed an association between insertion site and hematogenous catheter tip. They concluded that catheter tip infection stemmed from the subcutaneous portion of the catheter. If this is true, then the value of changing catheters over a guide wire at given time intervals should be questioned.

Rapid identification of an infected catheter is useful in treating a patient suspected of having catheter sepsis. Cooper and Hopkins[21] have reported a technique that allows rapid identification of an infected catheter by direct Gram's stain of catheter segments. This technique can reveal immediately whether a catheter infection is causing sepsis or whether another source should be sought.

Internal Angioaccess

The use of natural tissue in the Brescia-Cimino arteriovenous fistula decreases the incidence of clotting of vascular access. This technique is still considered the "gold standard" against which all other vascular access is compared.[13] Because the Brescia-Cimino fistula, like the Scribner shunt, uses the radial artery, adequate collateral circulation to the hand must be ensured by Allen's test. Numerous anastomotic variations are possible, including side to side (the original description), end of vein to side of artery, end of artery to side of vein, and end of artery to end of vein (Figure 22-2). The side-to-side anastomosis allows great variation in flow and in the length of anastomosis. The usual length of anastomosis is 10 to 12 mm, which results in an average flow rate of 300 to 500 ml/min.[2,18]

Other natural fistulae can be created (Figure 22-3). These include ulnar artery to basilic vein; basilic vein to brachial artery (resulting in retrograde flow into the cephalic vein if the valves are absent or have been destroyed); and cephalic vein to brachial artery at the antecubital fossa or higher in the upper arm.[98]

The patency rates of wrist fistulae vary from 55% to 85% at 2 years.[35,45,73,107] Palder and associates[73] reported a first-month failure rate of 24%. They concluded that the early failure rate is related to the number of patients with poor veins in which the fistula is constructed. Other authors[18,80] have reported an early failure rate of 10% to 15%, and they concluded that the failures are caused by obstruction of venous outflow, excessive dehydration, or hypotension. The brachiocephalic fistula has a patency rate equivalent to that of the wrist fistulae (i.e., 80%).[35]

Complications

Vascular access problems are a major reason for hospital admission of dialysis patients. One study concluded that these problems alone were responsible for 25% of admissions of this group of patients.[47] Complications are less common in patients with natural fistulae than in those with synthetic grafts. The complications are categorized into four major groups: bleeding, occlusion or threatened occlusion, infection, and hemodynamic problems.

Bleeding is quite rare in natural types of fistulae, usually resulting from a broken suture, unrecognized injury

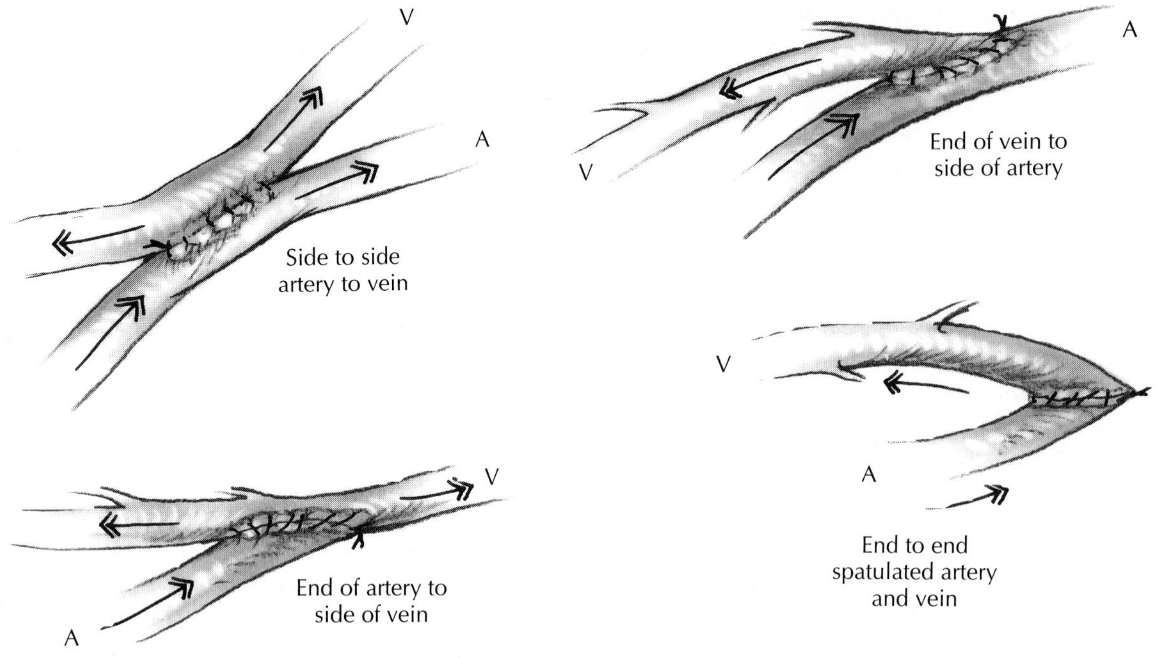

FIGURE 22-2 Four anastomotic possibilities with a Brescia-Cimino fistula. (Redrawn from Fernando ON: Arteriovenous fistulas by direct anastomosis. In Wilson SE, Owens ML, editors: *Vascular access surgery,* St Louis, 1980, Mosby.)

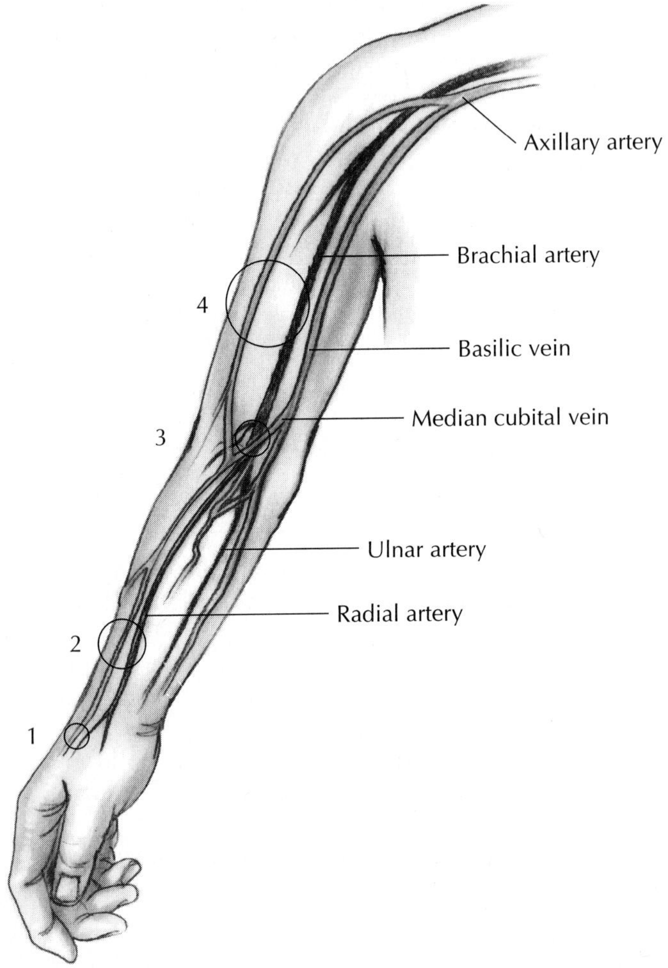

FIGURE 22-3 Four possible anastomotic sites for arteriovenous fistulae in the upper extremity. (Redrawn from Tilney NL, Lazarus JM, editors: *Surgical care of the patient with renal failure,* Philadelphia, 1982, WB Saunders.)

to the vessel, or a poorly ligated branch.

The most common complication is stenosis in the proximal venous limb (48%), followed by thrombosis (9%), and aneurysms (7%).[60] Stenosis in the venous limb can be repaired by excision and reanastomosis or by interposition of a synthetic graft. Thrombosis can be treated by using a Fogarty catheter to remove the clot. If there is no other anatomic reason for failure, these fistulae will last as long as if they had not thrombosed. If an arterial stenosis occurs, the fistula can be reformed at a higher level in the arm. Venous phlebitis makes either of the above options impossible.[98] Thrombosis can be prevented in most instances by careful observation of the dialysis patient. Fistula problems are indicated by an increase in venous resistance, poor flow, difficulty with cannulation, diminished thrill, or a pulsation over the fistula that becomes increasingly prominent.

Aneurysms may thin the skin over a fistula, causing skin breakdown and then infection. These fistulae may be resected and the ends anastomosed, or an interposition graft may be placed. This complication can be prevented by ensuring that access needles are placed in several locations rather than in one area, thus preventing weakening of the vessel.[87]

Infectious complications are much less common in natural fistulae (less than 3%) than in bridge fistulae or external shunts.[46,107] Sterile technique must be used in cannulating these fistulae to prevent infection.

Hemodynamic complications of a fistula can be either systemic or local. The systemic complication is high-output heart failure. It most commonly occurs in patients with borderline cardiac reserve and a fistula flow rate above 500 ml/min. It occurs after a fistula has been present for a period of time (longer than 3 months) and can occur with a 7 mm anastomosis.[1] Treatment involves Teflon banding, closure, or interposition of a narrow segment of PTFE.[1,3,45]

Local hemodynamic complications can have arterial or venous origins. Arterial steal syndrome is uncommon in wrist fistulae (0.25%) but more common in elbow brachiocephalic fistulae (approximately 30%). The steal results because the blood flows into the low-resistance venous system instead of supplying the hand.[41] It is important to remember that approximately one third of the blood flow to a radiocephalic fistula at the wrist comes from the palmar arch.[2] Venous hypertension is seen as a swollen hand, hyperpigmentation, induration of the skin and, eventually, skin ulceration. It is the result of high-pressure venous blood being forced distally. A partial proximal venous stenosis is common in a patient with venous hypertension who has had a side-to-side anastomosis. A study by Wedgewood and associates[103] showed that approximately 25% of patients developed hand hyperemia after a side-to-side anastomosis; no patients in the groups with end-to-side anastomoses developed this complication. The researchers concluded that an end vein-to-side artery anastomosis is preferable. In the case of venous hypertension, the distal venous end can be tied off, which sometimes resolves the problem; however, the fistula may fail after this because of the proximal stenosis that caused the increased distal flow. Neurovascular problems such as pain, weakness, paresthesia, and muscle atrophy may also develop. If not allowed to progress too far, these can be reversed by ligation of the fistula.[57]

Prosthetic Grafts for Vascular Access

Many of the patients who come for dialysis have been chronically ill for a time, or they are older and their superficial veins have been used for intravenous access. There are no veins left for construction of a natural fistula, and a prosthetic material must be used. A prosthetic material allows a vein and an artery not in proximity to be connected using the prosthetic material, and the graft to be used for needle insertion. The ideal material should be nonantigenic, resistant to deterioration in the body, easy to handle and suture, and minimally thrombogenic. It should also be capable of being declotted, able to resist infection and maintain integrity under infected conditions without degeneration or hemorrhage, heal into the body easily, and seal after repeated needle puncture.[83]

Saphenous vein was the first material used as an "artificial" graft. However, extensive dissection was required. Often it was needed for coronary artery bypass or had been used previously, and it had a 50% thrombosis rate at 1 year.[37] Consequently, a number of other materials were tried, including bovine grafts, made from the carotid artery of the cow, and Dacron. Bovine grafts have a tendency to form aneurysms and to become infected, resulting in graft disintegration and subsequent massive life-threatening hemorrhage.[12] Dacron grafts have not been widely used. The Sparks-Mandril graft, made by putting a prosthetic material into the subcutaneous space, has been abandoned because of problems in constructing the graft. The most commonly used prosthetic material is polytetrafluoroethylene (PTFE). This material is incorporated well into body tissues, forms a neointima, and is resistant to degeneration when infected.

Arteriovenous Jump Grafts

As in the construction of a natural fistula, good arterial inflow and good venous outflow are required. One must be sure that numerous needle sticks do not cause a major venous stenosis. While the graft is placed between the artery and vein, care must be taken to avoid rotating the graft or making too sharp a bend in the configuration, because both will compromise blood flow. The graft should be left unused for 2 to 3 weeks to allow tissue ingrowth, preventing a perigraft hematoma when vascular access is started.[45] The plan for placing these grafts is the same as for placing natural fistulae. If possible, the graft should be placed in the nondominant arm as far distal as possible. A straight graft between the radial artery and the cephalic vein can be done in patients with good peripheral arteries or in patients with a previous natural fistula that is unusable because of an aneurysm or high flow. In elderly patients or diabetic patients with poor peripheral circulation, the radial artery-to-cephalic vein graft is not a good configuration. This graft has the lowest patency rate of any of the jump grafts. The best approach in the arm is a loop graft between the brachial or ulnar artery below the elbow and a vein at the elbow. Using the ulnar artery may decrease the incidence of steal syndrome. In the upper arm a graft can be placed between the brachial artery just above the elbow and the axillary vein. Another upper arm configuration is a loop graft between the axillary artery and axillary vein. This latter approach has the disadvantage of causing the patient to externally rotate the arm during dialysis. Both of the upper arm grafts are subject to a greater incidence of steal syndrome because of the size of the vessels used.

The leg also can be used as a site for vascular access. Some dialysis patients prefer this location because of the ease of cannulation. Two approaches have been used: (1) a jump between the popliteal artery and saphenous or femoral vein in the groin; and (2) a loop graft between the femoral artery and the saphenous or femoral vein. Both types of graft are subject to major complications, which have resulted in a 22% amputation rate and an 18% mortality rate.[63]

When all of the above sites have been used, few options are left for hemodialysis. The graft configurations available include axillary artery to axillary vein across the chest, axillary artery to axillary vein with a loop on the chest, or an artery-to-artery graft.[40] All of these configurations are subject to steal syndrome. Tilney and associates[98] have described placing a graft in the upper arm between the brachial artery and the subclavian vein with a course up over the shoulder. This allows easy access to the graft over its long course and the graft is less prone to hemodynamic complications.

COMPLICATIONS. Complications resulting from a jump graft are similar to those of natural fistulae. Bleeding can arise from three sources: the anastomosis, the tunnel, or the graft. The anastomosis can bleed if a suture is broken or the vessel is damaged during surgery. Tunnel bleeding occurs because of damage to superficial blood vessels during placement of the tunnel. Graft hemorrhage is caused by incorrect placement of the needle during cannulation, resulting in a torn graft, or if the graft is used too soon after placement.

Thrombosis of the graft is the leading complication.[33,79] Erythropoietin, by increasing red cell mass, may increase thrombosis. One erythropoietin study showed an increase in graft thrombosis[32]; in contrast, a prospective study showed no increase in graft thrombosis.[8] Thrombosis usually is caused by an inflow or outflow obstruction, with outflow obstruction being more common.[17] The cause of the outflow obstruction is intimal hyperplasia, which can run in the outflow vein for 2 to 4 cm.[51] After declotting with a Fogarty catheter, the involved areas can be repaired with a bypass of the stenotic area, a patch graft, or balloon dilatation.[87] The functional life of the graft after revision is equal to that of a graft that does not require revision.[33,73] Thus an aggressive approach toward graft thrombosis is merited. Thrombolytic therapy with balloon dilatation of stenotic areas has been used with some success.[79,108] There are mixed reports of success in dilating stenotic lesions by means of transluminal angioplasty. The major problem is the stenosis right at the venous anastomosis.[38,89,100] Some attempt has been made to use a venous stent to keep an area of angioplasty open. This has been done in 10 patients on hemodialysis, with patency lasting from 5 to 28 months.[5] In the successful reports it is still difficult to compare the longevity of the graft with those that have been surgically revised, although the data are promising.

Use of an atherectomy device has been attempted in some patients, with patency rates that may be higher than those reported with percutaneous transluminal angioplasty. Use of a Simpson directional atherectomy device was reported in 13 patients. It was successful in 10 patients, with patency from 1 to 13 months. Of the 10 patients with a successful result, three patients underwent the procedure after percutaneous transluminal angioplasty was unsuccessful. This technology is in an infantile stage, and its place has yet to be determined.[109]

Interest has developed recently in the use of color Doppler ultrasound in fistulae and PTFE grafts. Some have suggested Doppler ultrasound examinations at regular follow-up intervals. A recent article by Nonnast-Daniel and coworkers[70] reviewed 51 patients who had either a Brescia-Cimino fistula or a PTFE graft. Doppler ultrasonography was highly accurate in detecting stenoses in these patients. Thrombosis was also easily detected by the Doppler technique. These findings contrast with those of Middleton and colleagues.[61] They showed that the color Doppler procedure correctly identified 20 of 23 stenosed vessels, 3 of 4 occluded vessels, 4 of 4 thrombosed vessels, and 18 of 19 pseudoaneurysms. They concluded that color Doppler ultrasonography may be useful in some patients, but that digital subtraction angiography was the gold standard. Middleton's group did not compare their radiographic or ultrasound results to surgical findings, which Nonnast-Daniel's group did.

Infection is a major problem in jump grafts, with an overall incidence of 19%. A bovine graft, if infected, will disintegrate and cause life-threatening hemorrhage.[12] The use of PTFE has allowed local wound care of an infected graft if the suture line is not involved. An infected, clotted graft and a tunnel infection are both indications for graft removal, because both are likely to involve the suture line. The salvage rate for infected grafts has been estimated at 25% to 50%.[9,73]

A single report has addressed the issue of complications in patients infected with the human immunodeficiency virus (HIV) who need hemodialysis. Most of the patients had PTFE grafts placed. The leading complication, instead of thrombosis, was infection. This occurred in 32% of the patients within 30 days. All the cultures were *Staphylococcus aureus* or other staphylococci, coagulase negative.[66]

Hemodynamic complications of venous hypertension, namely, congestive heart failure and the steal syndrome, can all occur as reported with natural fistulae. Use of the rapid-taper graft (4 to 7 mm) has lowered the incidence of steal syndrome by decreasing blood flow through the graft.[81] Indeed, using theoretic calculations, one can show that the flow through a rapid-taper 4 to 7 mm graft is one fifth that through a straight 6 mm graft.[39] Jendrisak and Anderson[50] have described a technique to reduce the incidence of steal syndrome in patients with vascular insufficiency. They have shown that a branch of the axillary artery can be used for arterial inflow for an upper arm PTFE graft. This has reversed steal syndrome in five patients who developed evidence of upper extremity ischemia after construction of a forearm PTFE graft.[50]

PATENCY. The patency of jump grafts has been thought to be less than that of natural fistulae. PTFE has a 12-month patency rate of 45% to 95%.[80,98] Munda and associates[65] found that the location of the graft influences patency. The best patency was in the forearm loops (78% at 12 months). This compares with a 12-month patency of 60% in the upper arm and 35% patency in the forearm between the radial artery and cephalic vein. Wilson[106] prefers a thigh graft as first choice and reports a 12-month patency rate of 80%. Obviously, patency depends on location and given inflow and outflow rates.

PHYSIOLOGY. The proximal arterial inflow is determined by the size of the fistula. If the fistula is between 20% and 75% of the arterial diameter, the arterial inflow is markedly influenced by the size of the fistula. Because most clinical fistulae are constructed to allow for later stenosis, they are larger than arterial diameter. Other factors of importance are venous outflow resistance, arterial collateral, and peripheral vascular resistance. The fistula may have a diastolic flow of 80% to 90% of the systolic flow, resulting in an increased venous flow.[106]

The classic changes, present primarily in fistulae with large blood flow, include a decrease in both systolic and diastolic blood pressure, an increase in heart rate, an increase in venous pressure, and an increase in blood volume. These are all reversible with closure of the fistula.[27]

Both gross and microscopic changes occur within the blood vessels. The gross changes include vessel enlargement and lengthening of both the arterial and venous segments. Histologic examination initially shows smooth muscle hypertrophy, which will change to smooth muscle atrophy. This atrophy can finally lead to aneurysmal dilatation and vessel tortuosity.

Summary

The development of vascular access was spawned by the need for dialysis, chemotherapy, and nutrition. These three treatments all require high blood flow, either for the dialysis machine to work adequately or to prevent permanent damage to blood vessels. Improvement in the techniques of vascular access and increased understanding of patient needs have decreased complications and improved patency rates.

PERITONEAL DIALYSIS

History

The development of peritoneal dialysis required the demonstration that the peritoneal membrane is semipermeable. Wegner[104] laid the initial groundwork, in 1877, to be followed by the contribution of Starling and Tubby.[90] In 1923 Ganter[36] first used peritoneal dialysis in a patient. Subsequent improvements were made, and the first patient was started on chronic peritoneal dialysis in 1960. Obtaining leak-free access to the peritoneal cavity is the major problem with peritoneal dialysis. Currently most catheters are constructed of Silastic, with Dacron cuffs attached to anchor the catheter and reduce infection. The numerous catheter configurations attempt to keep a good inflow and outflow of dialysate.[29]

Physiology

The precise surface area through which peritoneal dialysis occurs is not known. Of the two peritoneal surface areas, the visceral peritoneum is larger. The blood flow to the peritoneum is estimated at 60 to 100 ml/min.[4] The exchange rates through the peritoneum vary according to molecular size. A middle-sized molecule, such as vitamin B_{12}, is cleared better in chronic ambulatory peritoneal dialysis (CAPD) than in hemodialysis (50 L/week in CAPD compared with 30 L/week in hemodialysis). In a normal kidney, the clearance rate is 1008 L/week. Clearance of small molecules, such as urea, is better in hemodialysis than in CAPD. Normal kidneys give a clearance of 604 L/week, compared with 135 L/week in hemodialysis and 84 L/week in CAPD. Increasing fluid exchange in peritoneal dialysis increases clearance of a molecule; however, practical considerations make this virtually impossible. To obtain a urea clearance of 40 ml/min, 18 L/hour must be exchanged.[69]

The exact role of blood flow is not completely understood. Vasoconstriction decreases peritoneal clearance, and vasodilatation increases clearance. However, in patients in shock, peritoneal dialysis still shows a clearance rate 70% that of normotensive patients. Thus some mechanism other than blood flow is thought to be active.[69]

Indications

Peritoneal dialysis is used in a number of situations: with acute renal failure, while awaiting maturation of vascular access, and for intra-abdominal placement of chemotherapeutic agents. Chronic ambulatory peritoneal dialysis can be used for patients who receive home dialysis, have diabetes mellitus, have cardiovascular instability, have no available vascular access, or are of the Jehovah's Witness faith.[72,96]

CAPD has a number of advantages and disadvantages. The advantages are independence from a machine, steady-state biochemical values and hemodynamic state, control of hypertension and anemia, fewer dietary restrictions, and better rehabilitation potential. The disadvantages include daily dialysis, with exchanges four times a day; peritonitis; and weight gain.[84] Obviously, these factors have to be evaluated for each patient. The only absolute contraindication is lack of diaphragmatic integrity, which allows fluid to move into the chest, causing cardiovascular and pulmonary compromise. Relative contraindications are found in patients with the following: a history of low back pain or disc disease; multiple adhesions, which prevent catheter placement or result in too small an area for dialysate diffusion; a large hernia; a diffuse peritoneal malignancy; a history of respiratory compromise that increasing abdominal volume could worsen; or a history of several previous catheter infections.[69]

Practical Considerations

A number of catheters are available for peritoneal dialysis. These include the curled Tenckhoff, single-cuff Tenckhoff, Toronto-Western, column-disc, Vali, and Gore-Tex catheters. The single-cuff Tenckhoff catheter is the only one that can be placed percutaneously. It is placed aseptically below the umbilicus, with the cuff at the fascial level and the catheter tip directed toward the pelvis. The other catheters must be placed surgically. The incision is paramedian below the umbilicus. After the anterior fascia is opened and the muscles are split, a purse-string suture is placed in the posterior fascia. The catheter is placed through a small incision in the center of the purse string, and then the purse string is tied. The deep cuff is first placed at the posterior fascial level, and then with the purse-string suture, a suture is placed through the Dacron cuff to immobilize the catheter. The anterior fascia is closed, and the catheter is brought out through the skin via a separate stab wound. If used, the second Dacron cuff is placed at least 3 cm from the skin opening. The surgeon must be careful to avoid injuring the bowel and to place the catheter tip in the pelvis. If there is any doubt about the location of the tip, placement and fixation of the catheter under direct vision reduce the incidence of catheter nonfunction.[19,71]

There has been some interest in placing CAPD catheters using a peritoneoscope. One study, a retrospective comparison,[22] used the technique in 150 patients, using local anesthesia. These patients had a much better catheter survival rate at 2 years (84%) than did patients who had had catheters placed by means of an open surgical technique (30%). A second paper also showed excellent results, with 12 complications occurring in 9 of 93 patients. These complications all occurred within the first 4 weeks. The major complication was catheter migration. All procedures were performed using local anesthesia.[16] Despite these encouraging findings, the role of peritoneoscopy in placing catheters and revising complications has yet to be determined.

The electrolyte composition of dialysate is similar to that of serum. The major differences are found in four components: bicarbonate (blood 25 mEq/L, dialysate 0); phosphate (blood 2.5 mEq/L, dialysate 0); lactate (blood 0, dialysate 45 mEq/L); and potassium (blood 4 mEq/L, dialysate 0). The glucose concentration varies, depending on the amount of ultrafiltration needed. A 1.5% glucose concentration causes little ultrafiltration (200 ml for a liter exchange) compared with a 4.5% concentration that is used to remove large amounts of fluid (800) ml for a 2 liter exchange). The most common routine is 2 L exchanged four times a day. The volume and the dialysate glucose concentration can be varied, depending on the patient's needs. The major point to be remembered is that this technique is for a patient who is highly motivated and who will pay careful attention to detail.[52]

Complications

Complications of peritoneal dialysis can be arbitrarily divided into those in the immediate postoperative period and those occurring at a later date. The major perioperative complications include intraperitoneal bleeding, tunnel bleeding, leakage of dialysate fluid, hollow viscus injury, and ileus. Careful attention to technical detail can prevent most of the complications except ileus, which usually resolves within 24 hours.[69]

The most common postoperative complication is peritonitis. Contamination via the catheter lumen is the most common source; however, hematogenous spread from remote sources, transmural spread from the bowel, and contamination by cuffs or catheters also occur.[101] Peritonitis occurs once every 6 to 8 months, or about 1½ episodes per patient per year. Infections are most commonly caused by gram-positive organisms (approximately 75%), with gram-negative organisms being the next most common (approximately 20%). Anaerobes are responsible for about 3% of infections; fungus and tuberculosis are uncommon causes.[69,101] Outpatient treatment of peritonitis is common, with antibiotic therapy dictated by the particular organism and its sensitivity. Tunnel infections can be treated with appropriate antibiotics and local therapy if the Dacron cuff is not involved. If the cuff is involved, the catheter must be removed.[101] Exit site and tunnel infections occur in about 38% of patients followed for 1 year.[99] In patients with a double Dacron cuff, occasionally the superficial cuff becomes extruded and infected. In this instance the cuff can be shaved off and appropriate antibiotics administered.[52]

Mechanical complications result in poor inflow and outflow of dialysis fluid. These complications may be caused by kinking along the catheter track, migration of the catheter out of the pelvis, omental wrapping, or occlusion of the catheter lumen with blood clots or fibrin. Catheter migration can be prevented by using a catheter that will not migrate, such as a Toronto-Western or a curl-tipped catheter, or by tacking the catheter into the pelvis.[19] Careful placement during surgery usually prevents catheter kinking. Omental wrapping can be prevented by a partial omentectomy[95] or by using a catheter that will still function with omentum around it, such as the Toronto-Western or curl-tipped catheter. Urokinase dissolves fibrin and blood clots.

A difficult diagnostic problem in patients receiving peritoneal dialysis is abdominal pain, which can be either peritonitis or another abdominal problem requiring surgical intervention. A study by Moffat and associates[62] reported that 29 of 133 patients with peritoneal catheters required surgical consultation. Of these 29 patients, 10 had catheter sepsis and 19 required abdominal surgery. Eight patients required emergency surgery, and of these four died. A diagnostic test that may be useful in cases of bowel perforation is to look for vegetable fibers in the dialysate. Moffat's study reiterates the difficulty of diagnosing an intra-abdominal surgical problem in patients receiving peritoneal dialysis.

Catheter Longevity

The average catheter survival period is approximately 80% to 85% at 1 year. The figure drops to 60% at 2 years.[92] Survival time for Toronto-Western catheters appears to be slightly longer than that for medically inserted Tenckhoff catheters.[52] Also, catheters placed for the first time have a better survival rate than those placed subsequently.[52]

A discouraging statistic is the percentage of patients who remain on CAPD. Nissenson and associates[67] found that at the end of 42 months, only 40% of patients remained on CAPD (excluding those who had died or who underwent kidney transplantation). Most of the patients transferred to hemodialysis because of infection.

Patients undergoing CAPD have a progressive decline in their ultrafiltration over time, but this has been reversed by switching the patient to solutions containing lactate. After switching these patients to lactate-containing solutions, patients have had stable dialysis for a number of years and additional decreases in ultrafiltration are rarely of clinical significance. These results are promising; however, long-term predictions cannot be made because many of the changes that have been made are less than 5 years old.[68]

The relative benefits of CAPD versus hemodialysis are still not clear. The hematocrit may be higher with CAPD and the cost may be lower, although this information is not yet available.[68]

Summary

Peritoneal dialysis has the advantage of providing adequate dialysis without a machine, thus allowing independence, but mechanical problems and infection still occur. Catheter longevity is equivalent to that with vascular access, but the technique may not be usable for as long a period as hemodialysis.

REFERENCES

1 Anderson CB, Codd JR, Graff RA et al: Cardiac failure and upper extremity arteriovenous dialysis fistulas, *Arch Intern Med* 136:2921, 1976.

2 Anderson CB, Etheredge EE, Harter HR et al: Local blood flow characteristics of arteriovenous fistulas in the forearm for dialysis, *Surg Gynecol Obstet* 144:531, 1977.

3 Anderson CB, Groce MA: Banding of arteriovenous dialysis fistulas to correct high-output cardiac failure, *Surgery* 78:552, 1975.

4 Anne S: Transperitoneal exchange. I. Peritoneal blood flow estimated by hydrogen gas clearance, *Scand J Gastroenterol* 5:99, 1970.

5 Antonucci F, Salomonowitz E, Stuckmann G et al: Placement of venous stents: clinical experience with a self-expanding prosthesis, *Radiology* 183:493, 1992.

6 Aubaniac RL: L'injection intraveineuse sons-claviculaire, *Presse Med* 60:1456, 1952.

7 Bazzetti F: Central venous catheter sepsis, *Surg Gynecol Obstet* 161:293, 1985.

8 Besarab A, Medina F, Musial E et al: Recombinant human erythropoietin does not increase clotting in vascular accesses, *ASAIO Trans* 36:M749, 1990.

9 Bhat DJ, Tellis VA, Kohlberg WI et al: Management of sepsis involving expanded polytetrafluoroethylene grafts for hemodialysis access, *Surgery* 87:445, 1980.

10 Bjornson HS, Colley R, Bower RH et al: Association between microorganism growth at the catheter insertion site and colonization of the catheter in patients receiving total parenteral nutrition, *Surgery* 92:720, 1982.

11 Bland KI, Woodcock T: Totally implantable venous access system for cycle administration of cytotoxic chemotherapy, *Am J Surg* 147:815, 1984.

12 Bone GE, Pomajzl MJ: Prospective comparison of polytetrafluoroethylene and bovine grafts for dialysis, *J Surg Res* 29:223, 1980.

13 Brescia MJ, Cimino JE, Appel D et al: Chronic hemodialysis using venipuncture and a surgically created arteriovenous fistula, *N Engl J Med* 275:1089, 1966.

14 Brismar B, Hardstedt C, Jacobson S et al: Reduction of catheter-associated thrombosis in parenteral nutrition by intravenous heparin therapy, *Arch Surg* 117:1196, 1982.

15 Broviac JW, Cole JJ, Scribner BH: A silicone rubber atrial catheter for prolonged parenteral alimentation, *Surg Gynecol Obstet* 136:602, 1973.

16 Buchner-Beyerlein CH, Albert FW: Endoscopic peritoneal dialysis catheter placement. In LaGreca G, Olivares J, Feriani M et al, editors: CAPD: a decade of experience, *Contrib Nephrol* 89:28, 1991.

17 Butt KMH, Friedman EA, Kounts SL: Angioaccess, *Curr Probl Surg* 13:1, 1976.

18 Cerilli J, Lembert JG: Technique and results of the construction of arteriovenous fistulas for hemodialysis, *Surg Gynecol Obstet* 137:922, 1973.

19 Cerilli J, Walker J, Bay W: A new technique for placement of catheters for peritoneal dialysis, *Surg Gynecol Obstet* 156:663, 1983.

20 Cimochowski GE, Worley E, Rutherford WE et al: Superiority

of the internal jugular over the subclavian access for temporary dialysis, *Nephron* 54:154, 1990.

21 Cooper GL, Hopkins CC: Rapid diagnosis of intravascular catheter-associated infection by direct Gram staining of catheter segments, *N Engl J Med* 312:1142, 1985.

22 Cruz C, Faber MD: Peritoneoscopic implantation of catheters for peritoneal dialysis: effect on functional survival and incidence of tunnel infection. In LaGreca G, Olivares J, Feriani M et al, editors: CAPD: a decade of experience, *Contrib Nephrol* 89:35, 1991.

23 Currow A, Idown J, Behnens E et al: Urokinase therapy for Silastic catheter–induced intravascular thrombi in infants and children, *Arch Surg* 120:1237, 1985.

24 Curtis J, Eastwood J, Smith E et al: Maintenance hemodialysis, *Q J Med* 38:49, 1969.

25 Davis D, Petersen J, Feldman R et al: Subclavian venous stenosis: a complication of subclavian dialysis, *JAMA* 252:3404, 1984.

26 Dorner DB, Stubbs DH, Shader CA et al: Percutaneous subclavian vein catheter hemodialysis: impact on vascular access surgery, *Surgery* 91:712, 1982.

27 Dow P, Hamilton WF: *Handbook of physiology,* vol III, Circulation, Washington, DC, 1965, American Physiology Society.

28 Drukker W: Hemodialysis: a historical review. In Drukker W, Parson EM, Maher JF, editors: *Replacement of renal function by dialysis,* The Hague, 1983, Martinus Nijhoff.

29 Drukker W: Peritoneal dialysis: a historical review. In Drukker W, Parson FM, Maher JF, editors: *Replacement of renal function by dialysis,* The Hague, 1983, Martinus Nijhoff.

30 Dudrick SJ, Wilmore DW: Long-term parenteral feeding, *Hosp Pract* 3:65, 1968.

31 Dudrick SJ, O'Donnell JJ, Englert DM et al: 100 patient years of ambulatory home parenteral nutrition, *Ann Surg* 199:770, 1984.

32 Dy GR, Bloom EJ, Merritts GW et al: Effect of recombinant human erythropoietin on vascular access, *ASAIO Trans* 37:M274, 1991.

33 Etheredge EE, Hard SD, Maeser MN et al: Salvage operations for malfunctioning polytetrafluoroethylene hemodialysis access grafts, *Surgery* 94:464, 1983.

34 Fine A, Churchill D, Gault H et al: Fatality due to subclavian dialysis catheter, *Nephron* 29:99, 1981.

35 Friedman EA, Bett KMH, Pascua LJ et al: Vascular access update, *Trans Am Soc Artif Intern Organs* 25:526, 1979.

36 Ganter G: Über die beseitigung giftiger stoffe aus dem blate durch dialyse (On the elimination of toxic substances from the blood by dialysis), *MMW* 70:1478, 1923 (in German).

37 Girandet RE, Hackett RE, Goodwin NJ et al: Thirteen months' experience with the saphenous vein graft: arteriovenous fistula for maintenance hemodialysis, *Trans Am Soc Artif Intern Organs* 16:285, 1970.

38 Glanz S, Gordon D, Butt KMH et al: Dialysis access fistulas: treatment of stenoses by transluminal angioplasty, *Radiology* 152:637, 1984.

39 Haack D: *Personal communication,* Flagstaff, Ariz, 1985, WL Gore & Associates.

40 Haimov M: Vascular access for hemodialysis: new modifications for the difficult patient, *Surgery* 92:109, 1982.

41 Haimov M, Baez A, Neff M et al: Complications of arteriovenous fistulas for hemodialysis, *Arch Surg* 110:708, 1975.

42 Harten HR, Burch JW, Majerus PW et al: Prevention of thrombosis in patients on hemodialysis by low-dose aspirin, *N Engl J Med* 301:577, 1979.

43 Heimbach DM, Ivey TD: Technique for placement of a permanent home hyperalimentation catheter or prolonged parenteral nutrition at home, *Surg Gynecol Obstet* 143:634, 1976.

44 Herbst CA: Indications, management, and complications of percutaneous subclavian catheters, *Arch Surg* 113:1421, 1978.

cutaneous subclavian catheters, *Arch Surg* 113:1421, 1978.

45 Hertzer NR: Circulatory access for hemodialysis. In Rutherford RB, editor: *Vascular surgery,* Philadelphia, 1984, WB Saunders.

46 Higgins MR, Grace M, Bettcher KB et al: Blood access in hemodialysis, *Clin Nephrol* 6:473, 1976.

47 Hirschman GH, Wolfson M, Mosimann JE et al: Complications of dialysis, *Clin Nephrol* 15:66, 1981.

48 Hurtubise MR, Bottino JC, Lawson M et al: Restoring patency of occluded central venous catheters, *Arch Surg* 115:212, 1980.

49 Ishihara AM, Myers CH: Longevity of arteriovenous shunts for hemodialysis, *Ann Surg* 168:281, 1968.

50 Jendrisak MD, Anderson CB: Vascular access in patients with arterial insufficiency: construction of proximal bridge fistulae based on inflow from axillary branch arteries, *Ann Surg* 212:187, 1990.

51 Jenkins A McL, Buist TA, Glover SD: Medium-term follow-up of forty autogenous vein and forty polytetrafluoroethylene (Gore-Tex) grafts for vascular access, *Surgery* 88:667, 1980.

52 Khanna R, Oreopoulos DG: Complications of peritoneal dialysis other than peritonitis. In Nolph KD, editor: *Peritoneal dialysis,* The Hague, 1983, Martinus Nijhoff.

53 Kjellstrand CM, Merino GE, Mauer SM et al: Complications of percutaneous femoral vein catheterizations for hemodialysis, *Clin Nephrol* 4:37, 1975.

54 Ku G, Moorhead JF: The present status of hemodialysis: *Practitioner* 207:622, 1971.

55 Linos DA, Mucha P: A simplified technique for the placement of permanent central venous catheters, *Surg Gynecol Obstet* 154:248, 1982.

56 Maki DG, Goldman DA, Rhame FS: Infection control in intravenous therapy, *Ann Intern Med* 79:867, 1973.

57 Matolo N, Kostagiv B, Stevens LE et al: Neurovascular complications of brachial arteriovenous fistula, *Am J Surg* 121:716, 1971.

58 May J, Tiller D, Johnson J et al: Saphenous-vein arteriovenous fistula in regular dialysis treatment, *N Engl J Med* 280:770, 1969.

59 McGonigle DJ, Schrock LG, Hickman RO: Experience using central venous access for long-term hemodialysis: a new concept, *Am J Surg* 145:571, 1983.

60 Mennes PA, Gilula LA, Anderson CB et al: Complications associated with arteriovenous fistulas in patients undergoing chronic hemodialysis, *Arch Intern Med* 138:1117, 1978.

61 Middleton WD, Picus DD, Marx MV et al: Color Doppler sonography of hemodialysis vascular access: comparison with angiography, *AJR* 152:633, 1989.

62 Moffat FL, Dietel M, Thompson DH: Abdominal surgery in patients undergoing long-term peritoneal dialysis, *Surgery* 92:598, 1982.

63 Morgan AP, Knight DC, Tilney NL et al: Femoral triangle sepsis in dialysis patients: frequency, management, and outcome, *Ann Surg* 101:460, 1980.

64 Moss AH, Vasilakis C, Holley JL et al: Use of a silicone dual-lumen catheter with a dacron cuff as a long-term vascular access for hemodialysis patients, *Am J Kidney Dis* 16:211, 1990.

65 Munda R, First MR, Alexander JW et al: Polytetrafluoroethylene graft survival in hemodialysis, *JAMA* 249:219, 1983.

66 Nannery WM, Stoldt HS, Fares LG: Hemodialysis access operations performed upon patients with human immunodeficiency virus, *Surg Gynecol Obstet* 173:387, 1991.

67 Nissenson AR, Gentile DE, Soderblow RE et al: Morbidity and mortality of continuous ambulatory peritoneal dialysis: regional experience and long-term prospects, *Am J Kidney Dis* 7:227, 1986.

68 Nolph KD: Current concepts: continuous ambulatory peritoneal dialysis, *N Engl J Med* 318:1595, 1988.

69 Nolph KD: Peritoneal anatomy and transport physiology. In

Drukker W, Parson FM, Maher JF, editors: *Replacement of renal function by dialysis,* The Hague, 1983, Martinus Nijhoff.

70 Nonnast-Daniel B, Martin RP, Linder O et al: Colour Doppler ultrasound assessment of arteriovenous hemodialysis fistulas, *Lancet* 339:143, 1992.

71 Olcott C, Feldman CA, Coplon ND et al: Continuous ambulatory peritoneal dialysis: technique of catheter insertion and management of associated surgical complication, *Am J Surg* 146:98, 1983.

72 Oreopoulos DG: Chronic peritoneal dialysis, *Clin Nephrol* 9:165, 1978.

73 Palder SB, Kirkman RL, Whittlemove AD et al: Vascular access for hemodialysis: patency rates and results of revision, *Ann Surg* 202:235, 1985.

74 Pessa ME, Howard RJ: Complications of Hickman-Broviac catheters, *Surg Gynecol Obstet* 161:25, 1985.

75 Quinton W, Dillard D, Scribner BH: Cannulation of blood vessels for prolonged hemodialysis, *Trans Am Soc Artif Intern Organs* 6:104, 1960.

76 Raaf JH: Results from use of 826 vascular access devices in cancer patients, *Cancer* 55:1312, 1985.

77 Raaf JH: Vascular access grafts for chemotherapy use in forty patients at M.D. Anderson Hospital, *Ann Surg* 182:614, 1975.

78 Ralston AJ, Harlow GR, Jones DM et al: Infections of Scribner and Brescia arteriovenous shunts, *Br Med J* 3:408, 1971.

79 Rodkin RS, Boodstein JJ, Heeney DJ et al: Streptokinase and transluminal angioplasty in the treatment of acutely thrombosed hemodialysis access fistulas, *Radiology* 149:425, 1983.

80 Rohr MS, Browder W, Frentz GD et al: Arteriovenous fistulas for long-term dialysis, *Arch Surg* 113:153, 1978.

81 Rosenthal JJ, Bell DD, Gaspar MR et al: Prevention of high flow problems of arteriovenous grafts, *Am J Surg* 140:231, 1980.

82 Ryan JA, Abel RM, Abbott WM et al: Catheter complications in total parenteral nutrition: a prospective study of 200 consecutive patients, *N Engl J Med* 290:757, 1974.

83 Sabanayagam P, Schwartz AB, Soricelli RR et al: A comparative study of 402 bovine heterografts and 225 reinforced expended PTFE grafts as AVF in the ESRD patient, *Trans Am Soc Artif Intern Organs* 26:88, 1980.

84 Schreiber MJ, Vidt DG, Cunningham RJ: Home therapy for kidney disease: continuous ambulatory peritoneal dialysis and continuous cyclic peritoneal dialysis, *Cleve Clin Q* 52:291, 1985.

85 Sharp KW, Spees EK, Selby LR et al: Diagnosis and management of retroperitoneal hematomas after femoral vein cannulation for hemodialysis, *Surgery* 95:90, 1984.

86 Sheep RE, Guiney WB: Fatal cardiac tamponade: occurrence with other complications after left internal jugular vein catheterization, *JAMA* 248:1632, 1982.

87 So SKS: Complications of vascular access. In Simmons RL, Finch ME, Ascher NL et al, editors: *Manual of vascular access, organ donation and transplantation,* New York, 1984, Springer-Verlag.

88 So SKS: Venous access for hemodialysis in children: right atrial cannulation. In Simmons RL, Finch ME, Ascher NL et al, editors: *Manual of vascular access, organ donation and transplantation,* New York, 1984, Springer-Verlag.

89 Spinowitz BS, Carsen G, Meisell R et al: Percutaneous transluminal dilatation for vascular access, *Nephron* 35:201, 1983.

90 Starling EH, Tubby EH: On absorption from and secretion into the serous cavities, *J Physiol (Lond)* 16:140, 1894.

91 Steinberg SM, Cutler SJ, Nolph KD et al: A comprehensive report on the experience of patients on continuous ambulatory peritoneal dialysis for the treatment of end-stage renal disease, *Am J Kidney Dis* 4:233, 1984.

92 Steinberg SM, Cutler SJ, Novak JW et al: Report of the National CAPD Registry of the National Institutes Health, January 1984.

93 Stellato TA, Ganderer MW, Cohen AM: Direct central vein puncture for silicone rubber catheter insertion: an alternative technique for Broviac catheter placement, *Surgery* 90:896, 1981.

94 Surratt RS, Picus D, Hicks ME et al: The importance of preoperative evaluation of the subclavian vein in dialysis access planning, *AJR* 156:623, 1991.

95 Swartz RD: Chronic peritoneal dialysis: mechanical and infection complications, *Nephron* 40:29, 1985.

96 Tenckhoff H: Home peritoneal dialysis. In Massry SG, Sellers AL, editors: *Clinical aspects of anemia and dialysis,* Springfield, Ill, 1976, Charles C Thomas.

97 Thomas JH, MacArthur RI, Pierce GE et al: Hickman-Broviac catheters: indications and results, *Am J Surg* 140:791, 1980.

98 Tilney NL, Kirkman RL, Whittemore AD et al: Vascular access for dialysis and cancer chemotherapy. In Mannick JA, Cameron JL, Jordan GL Jr, editors: *Advances in surgery,* Chicago, 1986, Year Book Medical Publishers.

99 Torosian MH, Merauze S, McLean G et al: Central venous access with occlusive superior central venous thrombosis, *Ann Surg* 199:770, 1984.

100 Tortolani EC, Tan AHS, Butchart S: Percutaneous transluminal angioplasty: an ineffective approach to the failing vascular access, *Arch Surg* 119:221, 1984.

101 Vas SI: Peritonitis. In Nolph KD, editor: *Peritoneal dialysis,* The Hague, 1983, Martinus Nijhoff.

102 Wagman LD, Kirkemo A, Johnston MR: Venous access: a prospective randomized study of the Hickman catheter, *Surgery* 95:303, 1984.

103 Wedgewood KR, Wiggins PA, Guillon PJ: Prospective study of end-to-side versus side-to-side arteriovenous fistulas for hemodialysis, *Br J Surg* 71:640, 1984.

104 Wegner G: Chirurgische bermerkungen uber die peritonealhohle mit berucksichtigung der ovariotomie (Surgical considerations regarding the peritoneal cavity with special attention to ovariotomy), *Langenbecks Arch Chir* 20:51, 1877 (in German).

105 Wilson JN, Grow JB, DeMay CU et al: Central venous pressure in optimal blood volume and maintenance, *Arch Surg* 85:563, 1952.

106 Wilson WE, Owens MD, editors: *Vascular access surgery,* Chicago, 1980, Mosby.

107 Winsett OE, Wolma FT: Complications of vascular access for hemodialysis, *South Med J* 78:513, 1985.

108 Zeit RM, Cope C: Failed hemodialysis shunts: one year of experience with aggressive treatment, *Radiology* 154:353, 1985.

109 Zemel G, Katzen BT, Dake MD et al: Directional atherectomy in the treatment of stenotic dialysis access fistulas, *JVIR* 1:35, 1990.

110 Zincke H, Hirsche BL, Anomoo DG et al: The use of bovine carotid grafts for hemodialysis and hyperalimentation, *Surg Gynecol Obstet* 130:350, 1974.

CHAPTER

23

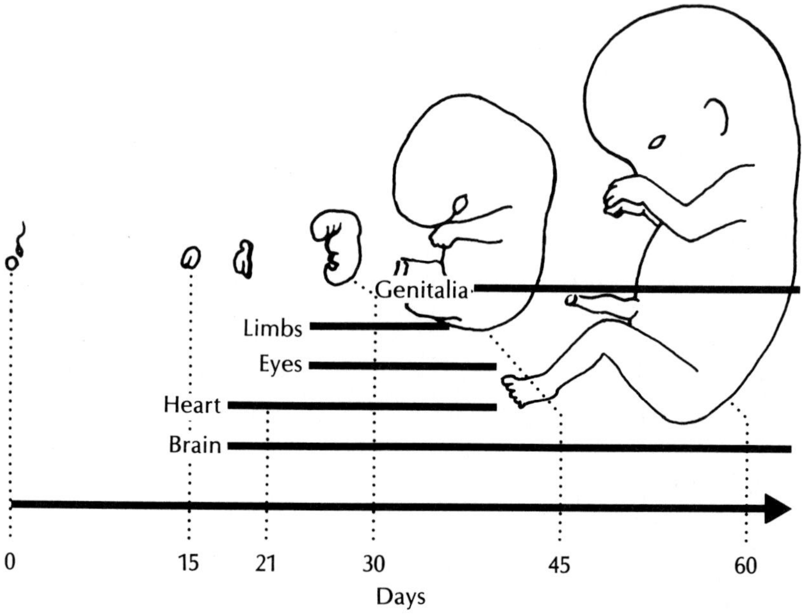
Genitalia
Limbs
Eyes
Heart
Brain
0
15
21
30
45
60
Days

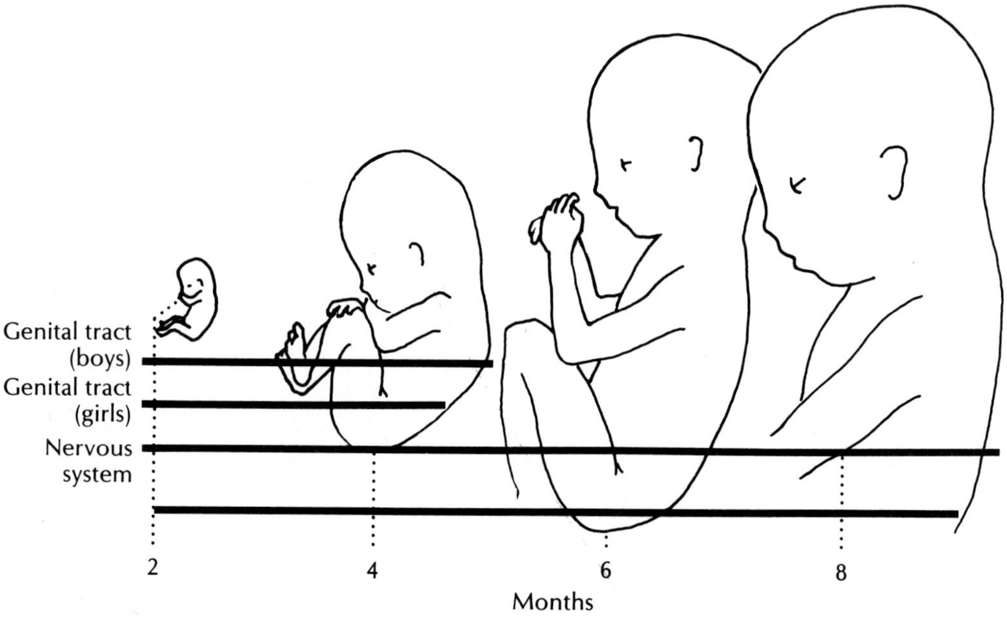
Genital tract
(boys)
Genital tract
(girls)
Nervous
system
2
4
6
8
Months

PEDIATRIC SURGERY

Daniel von Allmen • Moritz M. Ziegler

GENERAL CONSIDERATIONS
Overview
The Newborn

PEDIATRIC CRITICAL CARE
Fluids and Electrolytes
Total Parenteral Nutrition
Physiologic Monitoring
Mechanical Ventilation
Extracorporeal Membrane Oxygenation

PEDIATRIC TRAUMA
Epidemiology
Triage and Management Schemes
Head Injury
Thoracic Injury
Abdominal Injury
Musculoskeletal Injury

AIRWAY, LUNGS, CHEST WALL, AND DIAPHRAGM
Airway Obstruction
Pneumothorax
Congenital Lung Anomalies

PROBLEM: DIAPHRAGMATIC HERNIA

PROBLEM: EVENTRATION OF THE DIAPHRAGM

GASTROINTESTINAL TRACT
Vomiting in Infants and Children

PROBLEM: ESOPHAGEAL ATRESIA

PROBLEM: GASTROESOPHAGEAL REFLUX

PROBLEM: PYLORIC STENOSIS

PROBLEM: DUODENAL OBSTRUCTION—ATRESIA AND MALROTATION

PROBLEM: JEJUNOILEAL ATRESIA

PROBLEM: MECONIUM ILEUS

PROBLEM: MECONIUM PLUG SYNDROME

PROBLEM: HIRSCHSPRUNG'S DISEASE

PROBLEM: IMPERFORATE ANUS

PROBLEM: NECROTIZING ENTEROCOLITIS

PROBLEM: INTUSSUSCEPTION

PROBLEM: INTESTINAL DUPLICATION

PROBLEM: MECKEL'S DIVERTICULUM

PROBLEM: APPENDICITIS

BILIARY SYSTEM

PROBLEM: BILIARY ATRESIA

PROBLEM: CHOLEDOCHAL CYST

PROBLEM: GALLBLADDER DISEASE

PROBLEM: PORTAL HYPERTENSION

ABDOMINAL WALL DEFORMITIES

PROBLEM: OMPHALOCELE AND GASTROSCHISIS

VISIBLE AND PALPABLE LESIONS
Vascular Malformations
Face and Scalp
Neck
Chest Wall
Umbilicus
Extremities
Inguinoscrotal Region

PROBLEM: HYDROCELE

PROBLEM: INGUINAL HERNIA

PROBLEM: UNDESCENDED (CRYPTORCHID) TESTIS

PROBLEM: TESTICULAR TORSION

PEDIATRIC TUMORS

PROBLEM: NEUROBLASTOMA

PROBLEM: NEPHROBLASTOMA (WILMS' TUMOR)

PROBLEM: TERATOMA

PROBLEM: RHABDOMYOSARCOMA

PROBLEM: HEPATOMA

PEDIATRIC TRANSPLANTATION
Overview

RELATED MATERIAL APPEARS IN CHAPTERS 15, 21, AND 40

GENERAL CONSIDERATIONS

Overview

This chapter reviews the common surgical diseases that afflict newborns, infants, and children. In the management of pediatric surgical problems, one must give meticulous attention to the many basic principles peculiar to this age group. Such special considerations include the newborn's increased metabolic rate, inability to maintain body temperature, and an increased susceptibility to infection. In addition care of the infant and child requires continuous attention to optimal nutritional support with the provision of caloric requirements for growth and development. An understanding of fluid and electrolyte requirements as they relate to a child's weight, surface area, and stage of development is essential to avoiding the complications of dehydration and electrolyte abnormalities. A knowledge of normal and abnormal embryologic development helps to accurately diagnose and treat the surgical diseases specific to this patient population. Differences in topographic anatomy, internal organ size, and organ position are all of significance to the surgeon. Treatment of the child must also include consideration of the fears and anxieties of both the patient and their parents.

Congenital abnormalities in newborns are not uncommon. Almost 3% of newborns have a congenital defect noted on initial physical examination, and an additional 4% have anomalies that become evident later. One of every 200 babies requires an emergency operation for congenital anomalies that, unless repaired, are not compatible with life. The skeletal, cardiovascular, gastrointestinal, and central nervous systems are the most common sites of abnormal development.

When approaching the surgical evaluation of a pediatric patient, the family and gestational histories can add important information for appropriate diagnosis and treatment. A family history of previous children with congenital anomalies imparts a 25-fold increased risk of congenital anomalies in subsequent pregnancies. A history of inheritable disorders in the family can tip one off to a specific diagnosis.

The gestational history can also provide important diagnostic information. Abnormal amounts of amniotic fluid (polyhydramnios and oligohydramnios) are frequently associated with congenital anomalies. From the fifth month of gestation on, the fetus normally begins to swallow amniotic fluid, which by late in pregnancy may be as much as 500 ml daily. The fluid is normally absorbed in the small intestine and then is transferred to the mother through the placenta or excreted back into the amniotic sac when the fetus urinates. Thus, gastrointestinal and renal anomalies are often first manifest as abnormal amounts of amniotic fluid.

The newborn physical examination should include inspection of the umbilical cord to see if one or two umbilical arteries are present. A single umbilical artery is associated with an increased possibility of occult anomalies. Small catheters passed through the nares and into the stomach, as well as a thorough inspection of the anus as part of the newborn physical examination, permit very early diagnosis of obstruction at these sites.

The Newborn

The metabolic rate and the rate at which physiologic changes occur in infants are much more rapid than in adults. Relative to body weight, the newborn has about three times the amount of skin exposed to the environment as an adult and has a much thinner layer of subcutaneous fat, both of which make the newborn particularly sensitive to changes in environmental temperature and humidity. In addition to such size differences, there are many physiologic differences between the newborn, the older child, and adults.

The newborn lung is relatively underdeveloped. The alveoli have not matured, and most of the air exchange occurs in the air saccules along the bronchioles. As a result, the newborn has limited pulmonary reserve. Because the ribs are horizontal, the newborn depends almost entirely on the diaphragm for respiration, and any interference with the diaphragmatic excursion limits respiration. The newborn breathes mostly through the nose and not through the mouth; thus any obstruction or narrowing of the nasal passages impairs respiration. Because of the dependent position of the right upper lobe bronchus, the right upper lobe is predisposed to atelectasis. The pulmonary arteries are particularly reactive to stimuli such as hypothermia, hypoxia, acidosis, and hypercarbia, factors which may lead to severe pulmonary vasoconstriction. Pulmonary vasoconstriction may in turn result in limitation of cardiac output or, if the ductus arteriosus remains patent, shunting of the right heart outflow into the systemic circulation.

The normal newborn has a strong heart and is hypervolemic, and the blood has a high oxygen-carrying capacity. The left heart muscle is hypertrophied because during gestation it has been pumping 20% to 30% more blood through the placental circulation. There is normally a relatively high circulating blood volume because of the extra blood from the placenta. The oxygen-carrying capacity of the newborn's blood is frequently 50% higher than that of adults because the normal relative hypoxemia in utero stimulates erythropoiesis.

The newborn has 10% to 15% more total body water relative to weight than does the older child or adult. This excess fluid is lost as urine during the first week of life. Because of this excess total body water, newborns initially need less maintenance fluid during the first few days of life. The normal newborn kidney can handle large volume loads, but it is limited in its concentrating ability. This limitation can lead to a loss of electrolytes and the development of a hypotonic state if fluid replacement is inadequate.

Hepatic function of newborns is deficient in certain enzymes, particularly glucuronyl transferase, which is needed for bilirubin conjugation. Glycogen stores in the neonatal liver are also deficient.

The newborn has certain immunologic deficiencies that place it at increased risk for sepsis. In the absence of antigenic experience, immunoglobulin levels are low. Complement levels are low, and there is deficiency in opsonization and phagocytosis of bacteria. Because the infant can develop septicemia from a minimal bacterial load, the prophylactic use of antibiotics is appropriate if the infant sustains any bacterial contamination.

The premature infant is at particular risk because of the immaturity of many of its organ systems. The lungs are deficient in surfactant, which is needed to prevent atelectasis. Temperature control mechanisms function poorly, and the large surface area relative to size makes hypothermia a particular risk. Central nervous system control mechanisms for breathing and heart rate are immature, placing the premature infant at risk for apnea and bradycardia. Minor stresses of hypovolemia, hypothermia, or hypoxia can result in severe peripheral or splanchnic vasoconstriction that may produce tissue damage.

Providing adequate enteral nutrition is hindered by the premature infant's small gastric capacity and glucose intolerance. Tube feedings may be required to reduce the workload of suckling and to provide feedings at the necessary frequency. Parenteral nutritional support is frequently necessary when enteral feedings are not tolerated.

PEDIATRIC CRITICAL CARE

Fluids and Electrolytes

Fluid therapy in children follows the same general guidelines as fluid therapy in adults except that the margin for error is often smaller. Careful assessment of fluid intake, fluid losses, and electrolyte abnormalities must be made before initiating fluid management and then frequently during the course of therapy to assess the adequacy of treatment.

Several methods are available for calculating maintenance fluid requirements. The formula for fluids based on body weight is as follows:

Body Weight (kg)	Free Water for 24 Hours
0-10	100 ml/kg
11-20	1000 ml + 50 ml/kg for each kg over 10 kg
>20	1500 ml + 20 ml/kg for each kg over 20 kg

For example, a 15 kg child should receive 1000 ml + (5 × 50 ml) = 1250 ml per 24 hours or 52 ml/hr.

TABLE 23-1 REPRESENTATIVE BODY SURFACE AREAS FOR INFANTS OF VARIOUS BODY WEIGHTS

BODY WEIGHT (kg)	BODY SURFACE AREA (m^2)
1.8	0.15
2.7	0.2
4	0.25
5	0.29
8	0.4
10	0.5
20	0.8
30	1.0

Alternatively, fluid may be calculated based on body surface area (Table 23-1). This method requires estimation of body surface area from nomograms using height and weight and then providing 2000 ml/m^2/24 hr as maintenance. Fluids for infants less than 10 kg in weight are more accurately calculated using the body weight formula.

In addition to free water, electrolytes must be included in maintenance fluids. Sodium requirements are 3 to 4 mEq/kg/24 hr. Potassium and calcium requirements are 2 to 3 mEq/kg/24 hr, and these minerals should be included in maintenance fluids once urine output is established.

Abnormal body fluid losses including nasogastric suction, ileostomy output, and diarrhea should be carefully measured and replaced with an appropriate electrolyte solution. Gastric losses are replaced with half normal saline containing 10 mEq/L potassium chloride. Diarrheal, pancreatic, and biliary losses are optimally replaced with equal amounts of lactated Ringer's solution.

Urine output provides an indication of the adequacy of fluid replacement. A volume of 1 ml/kg/hr is generally regarded as the minimally accepted output in infants and small children. Serum electrolyte measurements are used to guide alterations in fluid and electrolyte therapy as the course of treatment progresses.

Acutely hypovolemic children requiring rapid volume expansion should be treated with a bolus of 10 to 20 ml/kg body weight of whole blood, plasma, or 5% albumin. Packed red blood cells are given in 5 to 10 ml/kg increments.

Total Parenteral Nutrition

The advent of total parenteral nutrition (TPN) has dramatically improved the survival of infants and neonates with various surgical problems including necrotizing enterocolitis, intestinal atresia, gastroschisis, and other anatomic and functional causes of the short bowel syndrome. Newborns and premature infants have the highest energy requirements necessary to maintain growth. Nearly 50% of the energy used in term infants less than 2 weeks old and 60% of energy intake in premature infants weighing less than 1200 g is devoted to growth. Paradoxically, deposition of body fat occurs in the later stages of fetal development leaving very premature infants poorly equipped to deal with periods of starvation as short as 2 to 3 days.

The caloric requirement varies with age and concomitant stress factors. In general, infants less than 1 year of age require 90 to 100 kcal/kg/day. Children between 1 and 7 years of age should receive 75 to 90 kcal/kg/day, and those 7 to 12 years old require 60 to 75 kcal/kg/day. Adolescents 12 to 18 years old typically require 35 to 60 kcal/kg/day to maintain normal growth and development. Weight gain and longitudinal growth are good indicators of the adequacy of caloric intake and should be followed closely.

The composition of the TPN should include 30% to 40% of calories provided as fat (0.5 to 3 g/kg/day) and the remainder as carbohydrate. In neonates, glucose administration should be increased slowly beginning with rates less than 6 mg/kg/minute and then advanced slowly to a maximum of 10 to 12 mg/kg/minute. Protein requirements also change with age. Newborns require 2 to 3.5 g/kg/day and have a higher essential amino-acid nitrogen requirement, and older children and adolescents need only 1.5 to 2.0 g/kg/day of protein. Standardized pediatric vitamin and mineral solutions are added to complete the formula.[60]

The pediatric patient receiving TPN must be closely monitored for intolerances of carbohydrate, protein, and fat; for imbalances of fluids and electrolytes; and for deficiencies of vitamins and trace metals. Central line access and maintenance are of greater risk in the pediatric patient; in particular, central line sepsis is the most frequent complication. Cholestatic jaundice, especially in the child who is totally parenterally fed and who has short bowel syndrome, remains a potentially serious problem.

Physiologic Monitoring

Critical care monitoring in older children is similar to that in adults. Neonates and premature infants require several specialized techniques. Arterial lines, placed peripherally or by cannulation of the umbilical artery, provide continuous hemodynamic information and access to blood samples. The limited amount of blood available from these infants and the invasive nature of an arterial puncture have prompted the use of less invasive methods to assess respiratory function. These include the routine use of oxygen saturation monitors and transcutaneous oxygen and carbon dioxide sensors for infants receiving mechanical ventilation. Because pulmonary artery catheters are often not available in sizes appropriate for small infants, assessment of cardiac function relies on physical examination, blood pressure measurements, and echocardiography. Decreased capillary refill, mottling, and metabolic acidosis all suggest impaired perfusion requiring either administration of volume, inotropes, or both.

Mechanical Ventilation

Mechanical ventilation in infants is typically performed with pressure cycle ventilators rather than the volume cycled machines used in adults. Pressure cycled ventilators end their inspiration when a preset peak inspiratory pressure is reached; in contrast, volume cycled ventilators deliver a preset volume of gas. With pressure cycled ventilators, the peak pressure and respiratory rate are varied to adjust ventilation. The fraction of inspired oxygen is altered to provide adequate oxygenation. By limiting the peak inspiratory pressure of a pressure cycled ventilator, the risk of barotrauma in infants can be reduced. However, volume delivery varies depending on the compliance of the lung, and patients must be followed carefully to avoid hypoventilation or hyperventilation as the clinical course progresses.

In infants with severe pulmonary problems, several additional ventilatory techniques can be used. The term *high-frequency ventilation* encompasses a number of ventilatory techniques that use rapid respiratory rates with low tidal volumes. The three basic types of high frequency ventilation are high frequency positive pressure ventilation with rates of 60 to 150 breaths per minute, high frequency jet ventilation with rates of 100 to 900 breaths per minute, and high frequency oscillation with rates of 400 to 2400 breaths per minute. Theoretically, these techniques provide for adequate oxygenation and ventilation while minimizing mean airway pressure and the resultant barotrauma.

Extracorporeal Membrane Oxygenation

Extracorporeal membrane oxygenation (ECMO) is a temporary support technique for infants or children with severe but reversible pulmonary or cardiac disease who would otherwise not survive. When providing ECMO, it is anticipated that the underlying condition will improve. ECMO entails the placement of a large cannula in the internal jugular vein for venovenous bypass[3] or placement of cannulas in the internal jugular vein and carotid artery for venoarterial bypass. Blood is drained from the patient and passed through a membrane lung where carbon dioxide is removed and oxygen is administered. The oxygenated blood is then pumped back to the patient as shown in Figure 23-1.[8,26]

Indications for ECMO in neonates include meconium aspiration, sepsis, persistent pulmonary hypertension, and diaphragmatic hernia. Because of the risk of intra-

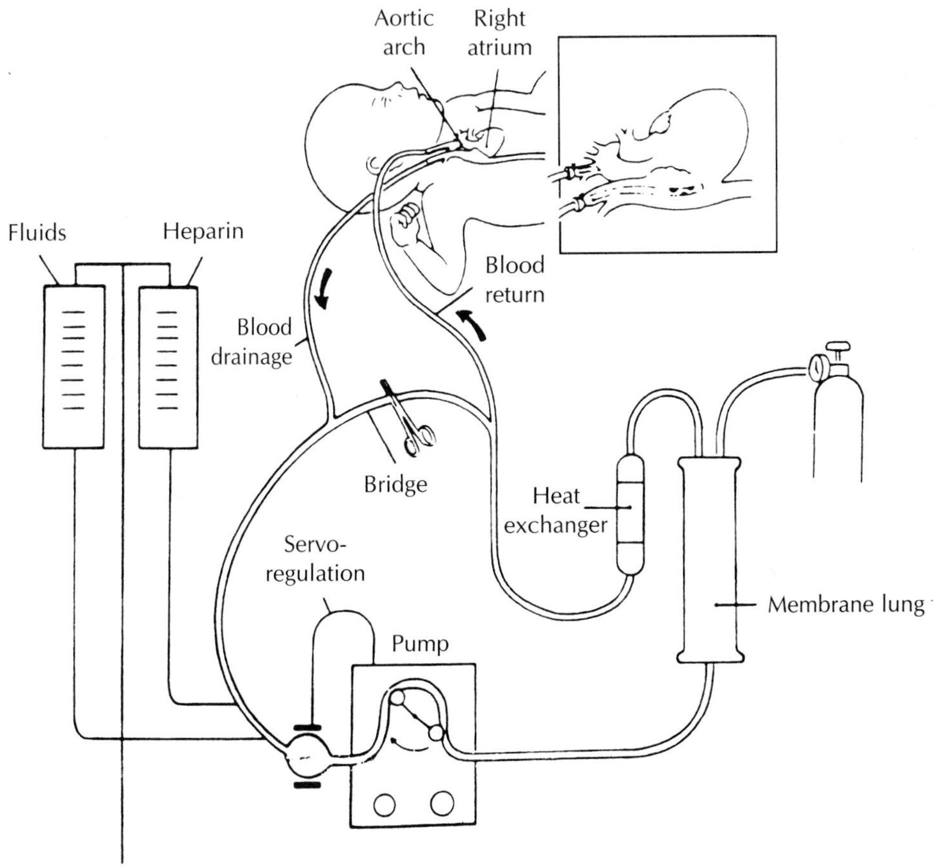

FIGURE 23-1 Diagrammatic representation of an arteriovenous circuit for extracorporeal membrane oxygenation.

cranial hemorrhage associated with the systemic anticoagulation necessary for treatment, premature infants less than 32 weeks' gestation are not candidates for bypass.[8] ECMO is also used in children with severe respiratory failure related to respiratory distress following trauma, smoke inhalation, or reactive airway disease.

Treatment with ECMO extends from 3 days to 3 weeks, depending on the underlying disease. During the time of treatment, the ventilator settings are reduced to "resting" levels. As pulmonary compliance improves, the bypass is weaned and eventually discontinued. The complications of ECMO primarily are related to bleeding resulting from the systemic heparinization. This complication is especially prevalent in neonates who in 10% to 15% of cases develop significant intracranial hemorrhage. Other fortunately uncommon complications are related to mechanical problems such as tubing rupture, oxygenator failure, or air embolism.[33]

The efficacy of ECMO has been well established in near-term, gestational aged neonates.[7,41] Entrance criteria for ECMO therapy are predictive of a 50% to 80% mortality rate without treatment, yet 80% to 85% of patients survive when ECMO support is provided. These outcomes are somewhat dependent on the underlying disease process.[22,55] Patients with diaphragmatic hernia and sepsis have a slightly worse survival rate, whereas those with meconium aspiration and persistent pulmonary hypertension approach 100% survival. The experience with ECMO in pediatric patients beyond the newborn period is limited, but survival rates of 50% to 75% have been reported in this diverse patient population. ECMO remains a drastic but effective method of providing respiratory and hemodynamic support during the worst phases of a potentially reversible illness.

PEDIATRIC TRAUMA

Epidemiology

Trauma is the leading cause of death in pediatric patients and accounts for half of all deaths in children between 1 and 14 years. The peak age range is between 4 and 12 years, with the highest incidence at age 8 years. Thirty percent of infant deaths result from accidental injury. The most frequent mechanism of trauma is blunt injury from motor vehicle related accidents, which account for 30% to 50% of cases. Falls, drownings, and burns account for 25%, 15%, and 10% of cases, respectively. In infancy, deaths are more frequently related to head injury from falls or child abuse, whereas in the 5 to 9-year age group pedestrian injury associated with motor vehicle accidents is the most common mechanism. Penetrating injuries are becoming more prevalent in some urban centers and account for as many as 40% of injuries, especially among adolescents. Blunt trauma often results in multisystem injury, which affects the central nervous system and musculoskeletal systems most frequently. Not surprisingly, these multiply injured children have a higher mortality rate than those with isolated injuries. Of lethal intraabdominal blunt injuries, the liver is most frequently involved.[43,46]

Triage and Management Schemes

The management of pediatric trauma follows many of the same guidelines as used in adults, with several important modifications. The initial assessment and management priorities are listed in the box on the right. During the prehospital phase of treatment, trained Emergency Medical Service personnel may make initial interventions in the care of the trauma patient; but once the child reaches the emergency room, a rapid, reproducible scheme of immediate and subsequent evaluation and intervention should be instituted. The initial assessment involves a primary survey, resuscitation, secondary survey, and eventual triage based on injury severity. In many centers, a trauma team is alerted on arrival of any child with potentially serious injuries, and specific protocols are followed to ensure proper and efficient initial assessment and management.[24]

INITIAL ASSESSMENT AND MANAGEMENT GUIDELINES FOR THE INJURED CHILD

I. Primary survey
   A. Airway maintenance, cervical spine control
   B. Breathing
   C. Circulation
   D. Disability
   E. Exposure
II. Resuscitation
   A. Oxygenation, ventilation
   B. Shock management
   C. Intubations—urinary tract, gastrointestinal tract
III. Secondary survey
   A. Head
   B. Neck
   C. Chest
   D. Abdomen
   E. Extremities
   F. Neurologic
IV. Triage

The first priority in assessment and management is to secure an adequate airway while protecting the cervical spinal cord from a potential cervical spine injury. Cervical spine injuries should be assumed in all patients with major trauma, especially in those with injuries to the face and head. Management of the airway in a child with decreased consciousness or evidence of airway obstruction involves a stepwise sequence of techniques that range from simple jaw thrust to endotracheal intubation. Endotracheal intubation provides the most stable airway but carries a significant risk. It should be performed by the most experienced member of the team using cervical spine immobilization, cricoid pressure, and appropriate sedation. In hemodynamically stable children with head injuries, oral tracheal intubation after sedation with thiopental, intravenous lidocaine, and a nondepolarizing muscle relaxant will avoid increasing the intracranial pressure during the intubation process.[36] A surgical airway is rarely indicated except in cases of severe maxillofacial or laryngeal crush injuries.

Adequate ventilation of the trauma patient occurs only when a patent airway provides sufficient air exchange. In ventilated patients, a tidal volume of 10 to 15 ml/kg is required. The presence of decreased breath sounds, hypotension, and mediastinal shift suggests the possibility of a tension pneumothorax, which should be treated promptly with needle decompression. Tube thoracostomy is the definitive treatment for pneumothorax and hemothorax.[35]

Assessment of circulation involves noting the pulse, skin color, and capillary refill time. Shock is the clinical syndrome that results from inadequate tissue perfusion, and these clinical observations provide an invaluable estimation of peripheral perfusion. Children have very efficient compensatory mechanisms and may maintain a normal blood pressure in the face of significant blood loss. Therefore, it is important to rapidly gain vascular access for potential resuscitation. Since vascular access can be challenging in children, a stepwise sequence of access techniques is mandatory. Initially, percutaneous peripheral access with large-bore catheters is the technique of choice. If access is not rapidly obtained, percutaneous cannulation of the femoral vein or an intraosseous needle should be placed. The intraosseous needle placed in the distal femur or proximal tibia provides a route for rapid administration of fluids including blood products and medications. A venous cutdown on the saphenous vein or antecubital vein provides stable access but is time consuming. Percutaneous cannulation of the internal jugular vein or subclavian vein is rarely indicated in the acute resuscitation phase. Ideally, two large-bore lines should be started on all potentially seriously injured patients.

Resuscitation should be based on the degree of shock

TABLE 23-2 THERAPEUTIC CLASSIFICATION OF HEMORRHAGIC SHOCK IN THE PEDIATRIC PATIENT

	CLASS I	CLASS II	CLASS III	CLASS IV
Blood loss as a percent of blood volume*	Up to 15%	15%–30%	30%–40%	40% or more
Pulse rate	Normal	Mild tachycardia	Moderate tachycardia	Severe tachycardia
Blood pressure	Normal/increased	Decreased	Decreased	Decreased
Capillary blanch test	Normal	Positive	Positive	Positive
Respiratory rate	Normal	Mild tachypnea	Moderate tachypnea	Severe tachypnea
Urine output	1–2 ml/kg/hr	0.5–1.0 ml/kg/hr	0.25–0.5 ml/kg/hr	Negligible
Mental status	Slightly anxious	Mildly anxious	Anxious/confused	Confused/lethargic
Fluid replacement (3:1 rule)	Crystalloid	Crystalloid	Crystalloid + blood	Crystalloid + blood

*Assume blood volume to be 8% to 9% of body weight (80 to 90 ml/kg).

as outlined in Table 23-2. The initial infusion should be given as a push bolus of isotonic crystalloid solution at 20 ml/kg estimated body weight. If no clinical response results from two boluses of crystalloid, resuscitation should be continued with either cross-matched or O negative whole blood. Adequate resuscitation is indicated by stable vital signs, restoration of tissue perfusion parameters, and a urine output exceeding 1 ml/kg/hr.

Once the primary survey is complete, a careful examination of each organ system must be performed. The management and prognosis of specific organ injuries often differ from those in the adult and are described in the following sections.

Head Injury

The head is the most common organ system injured in traumatized children. Infants sustain brain injury from falls and the shaken baby syndrome of child abuse. As children get older, bicycle accidents and pedestrian motor vehicle accidents become the most common etiology. The Glasgow Coma Scale quantifies the severity of head injury based on the best verbal, motor, and eye opening response the patient displays at the time of presentation. In children with evidence of severe head injury, an urgent computerized tomography (CT) scan is the diagnostic test of choice to identify surgically correctable mass lesions such as an epidural, subdural, or intracerebral hematoma. More commonly, diffuse brain swelling is identified and treated by the medical management for intracranial hypertension. Such management includes controlled hyperventilation, diuretics, limitation of positive intrathoracic pressure, and the control of seizures.[52] The outcome of patients with brain injury depends on the degree of injury, but it is generally better than that seen in adults.[20]

Thoracic Injury

Thoracic injuries are relatively uncommon in the pediatric population. The extreme compliance of the chest wall in children can result in significant intrathoracic injury occurring in the absence of rib fractures. Blunt trauma is the most common etiology, and pulmonary contusion is the most common injury. Treatment, as in the adult, is supportive. Pneumothorax and less often hemothorax are treated with tube thoracostomy. In the case of hemothorax, bleeding that continues at a rate exceeding 1 to 2 ml/kg/hr is an indication for exploratory thoracotomy.[35]

The mortality rate associated with thoracic injury is quite high because most such patients also have multiple other injuries. In one series the mortality rate associated with isolated chest injury was 5.3%, and the mortality of combined head and chest injuries was 35%. Thus the presence of thoracic trauma suggests a powerful mechanism of injury and predicts the potential for serious trauma in other organ systems.[17]

Abdominal Injury

Evaluation and management of abdominal trauma in the pediatric age group differs from that in adults. Initial management involves a careful abdominal examination and laboratory studies including liver function tests and a serum amylase. In hemodynamically stable children with abdominal pain or elevated hepatic enzymes, and in patients who cannot be adequately assessed because of neurologic injury, CT is the test of choice to evaluate the abdomen. Elevation of the serum glutamic-oxaloacetic transaminase (SGOT) above 200 and serum glutamate-pyruvate transaminase (SGPT) above 100 IU/dl correlates well with findings of hepatic injury on CT scan. Significant injuries to the spleen and retroperitoneal organs are also accurately diagnosed by CT scan.[51] In the vast majority of cases, these injuries can be managed nonoperatively with bed rest and careful serial assessment for ongoing bleeding.[47] Indications for operation include continued hemodynamic instability despite adequate resuscitation, pneumoperitoneum, a transfusion that totals more than 40% of calculated blood volume, and the presence of large devitalized tissue fragments on CT scan. Injury to the gastrointestinal tract may be missed by CT scan; therefore careful serial abdominal examination becomes an important aspect of the nonoperative management of abdominal trauma.[37,57]

Injuries to the liver and spleen documented on CT scan in hemodynamically stable patients are managed with 7 to 10 days of strict bed rest followed by 1 to 3 months of limited activity. Follow-up CT scans may be performed at that time to document healing. In children who require laparotomy, attempts should be made to salvage the spleen using suture splenorrhaphy, hemostatic agents, partial splenectomy, or splenic wrapping with omentum or absorbable mesh. If total splenectomy is required, the risk of mortality from overwhelming sepsis is 50 times that seen in the normal population. Thus every attempt should be made to salvage the spleen in an otherwise stable patient.

Other organs commonly injured in the abdomen include the pancreas, duodenum, and kidney. Trauma is the leading known cause of pancreatitis in the pediatric population. Treatment is usually conservative because major ductal rupture is uncommon. Parenteral nutrition is initiated and serial examinations performed to identify complications such as pseudocyst formation.

Duodenal hematomas most commonly occur in the third portion of the duodenum from compression of the duodenum against the spinal column. Bilious vomiting in children with an appropriate mechanism of trauma suggests the diagnosis, which is confirmed by the finding of a "coil spring" deformity on barium upper gastrointestinal study. Management is nonoperative; nasogastric decompression and parenteral nutrition is effective in the vast majority of patients. Rarely, operative evacuation of the hematoma is necessary to control hemorrhage or relieve intractable duodenal obstruction.

Injury to the kidneys is suggested by the presence of hematuria. Hematuria is present in 80% to 90% of significant renal injuries, but the degree of hematuria does not correlate well with the degree of injury. Evaluation with an abdominal CT scan demonstrates the severity of injury in most cases. Contusions, superficial parenchymal lacerations, and subcapsular hematomas are managed nonoperatively. Even a contained urinary extravasation in a hemodynamically stable patient can be managed by close observation only. A shattered kidney and vascular pedicle injury require operative intervention.

Musculoskeletal Injury

Long bone fractures are common in pediatric trauma and are often given a lower priority during the initial resuscitation of a multiply injured child. Once the child is stable, however, it is important to assess the vascular status of the extremity distal to the fracture. When the initial physical examination indicates decreased distal perfusion, reduction of the fracture and placement of the limb in traction may restore adequate blood flow to the distal extremity. When vascular injuries do occur, they typically are intimal tears that require operative repair. When a vascular repair is required for an ischemic extremity, fasciotomy should be performed to prevent the development of a compartment syndrome.

AIRWAY, LUNGS, CHEST WALL, AND DIAPHRAGM

Most infants and children with respiratory distress will have problems that require medical rather than surgical treatment. However, certain surgically correctable problems are important to diagnose and treat. In the newborn, surgically correctable problems that can cause respiratory distress include mechanical airway obstruction, pulmonary malformations, pneumothorax, and defects of the diaphragm or chest wall. Mechanical airway problems include choanal atresia, goiter, maldevelopment of the trachea, and cysts and masses in the hypopharynx and neck. Mechanical problems are generally detected by direct inspection. Inability to pass a catheter through the patient's nose into the posterior pharynx suggests choanal atresia. A chest radiograph will usually suggest the diagnosis of cystic adenomatoid malformation, lobar emphysema, pneumothorax, bronchogenic cyst, diaphragmatic hernia, or pulmonary sequestration. Respiratory symptoms exacerbated by feeding suggest the possibility of an esophageal atresia with a tracheoesophageal fistula or a fistula in the presence of an intact esophagus (H-type fistula).

Airway Obstruction

Any child with respiratory distress must be evaluated for airway obstruction. It must never be assumed that respiratory distress is caused by parenchymal lung disease such as hyaline membrane disease or pneumonia until mechanical respiratory problems have been excluded. Evaluation must include inspection of the jaw structure, tongue, nasopharynx, hypopharynx, and larynx. Lateral radiographs of the neck may aid in the demonstration of obstructing lesions of the upper airway, but laryngoscopy and bronchoscopy are frequently required for the definitive evaluation of obstructive airway problems.

If the child's lower jaw structure is underdeveloped (Pierre-Robin syndrome), the tongue will tend to fall back and obstruct the hypopharynx as the child swallows, making ventilation impossible. Sometimes the initial symptoms are mild and become progressive as the infant grows. Infants with mild symptoms may be managed by placing them in the prone position. More severe symptoms may require placement of a decompression tube into the hypopharynx or esophagus or suturing of the tongue to the lip. If these maneuvers are ineffective, a tracheostomy may be necessary.

Choanal atresia is the result of an imperforate nasopharyngeal septal membrane. Infants are obligate nasal breathers, and infants with choanal atresia have difficulty with ventilation. The diagnosis is made by the inability to pass a catheter through the nares into the posterior pharynx and may be confirmed by the injection of a small amount of contrast material. Before correction, the child's ventilation can be maintained with an oral airway, or if necessary, by endotracheal intubation.

Cysts and benign tumors in the hypopharynx, larynx, or trachea may cause airway obstruction and require the placement of a tracheostomy to secure the airway until definitive surgical correction has been completed. Most of these lesions can be resected endoscopically. Mass lesions in the neck, most often secondary to lymphangioma or teratoma, can produce airway obstruction in the neonate. After an airway is assured, a comprehensive treatment plan must be defined.

Pneumothorax

Pneumothorax is the most common respiratory problem requiring surgical correction in the newborn. It is particularly common in hospitals with neonatal intensive care units with large numbers of premature infants. Pneumothorax may occur spontaneously or as a consequence of the ventilatory support of infants with severe respiratory distress syndrome. During ventilation, differential compliance in the neonatal lung can lead to overexpansion of some segments, eventually causing rupture of the alveolar membrane. The air escaping into the pleural space may lead to partial or complete collapse of the lung. Dissecting air can also cause pneumomediastinum, pneumopericardium, or pneumoperitoneum. Evaluation of pneumothorax and other air-block syndromes is through the use of anteroposterior chest radiographs. Equivocal findings can be further evaluated with lateral and decubitus films.

Management of a small pneumothorax producing minimal collapse and minimal respiratory distress is by careful observation and serial chest radiographs. Continued air leakage can lead to a complete collapse of the lung or to the development of a tension pneumothorax in which there may be mediastinal shifting, producing a compromise of expansion of the contralateral lung or a compromise of the venous return to the heart. If complete collapse or a tension pneumothorax is diagnosed, an immediate tube thoracostomy should be performed through the fourth intercostal space in the anterior axillary line. The tube is placed to an underwater seal, and continuous suction may be added if an air leak continues. Temporary emergency decompression of the pneumothorax can be accomplished by aspiration of the pleural space with a small plastic cannula while arrangements for tube thoracostomy are made.

Congenital Lung Anomalies

A variety of congenital malformations of the lung present with nonspecific respiratory distress (tachypnea, cyanosis, and retractions).

Congenital cystic adenoid malformation (also termed bronchiolar malformation) consists of multiple large and small cysts involving a lobe or lobes of either lung. The lesion can be confused with a diaphragmatic hernia, with the cysts resembling loops of bowel in the chest. Unlike in diaphragmatic hernia, however, the abdomen will not be scaphoid, and a barium contrast gastrointestinal series demonstrates the bowel in the abdomen rather than in the chest. Treatment consists of resecting the involved lobe or lobes, the timing of which depends on the severity of the associated signs and symptoms.

Pulmonary sequestration consists of lung tissue that may have no connection with the bronchial tree and that receives its blood supply from a systemic artery (often from below the diaphragm), rather than a branch of the pulmonary artery, and/or drains its venous effluent through a systemic vein. A sequestrum may be extralobar, completely separate from the normal lung (usually located at the left costophrenic angle), or intralobar, most often in the lower lobe. Extralobar sequestrations often are diagnosed early in life, frequently in association with other thoracoabdominal anomalies. Intralobar sequestrations may be first diagnosed during the treatment of an intractable lower lobe pneumonia. After careful definition of the vascular anatomy, the definitive treatment is operative resection.

Congenital lobar emphysema represents a tracheobronchial cartilaginous lesion in which progressive overinflation of one lobe (most commonly the left upper lobe) occurs secondary to airway luminal collapse and distal air trapping. Atelectasis of the adjacent lobes and mediastinal shift may occur with a potential for acute distress. Distinction must be made between lobar emphysema and congenital adenoid malformation of the lung (Figure 23-2), diaphragmatic hernia (Figure 23-3), and pneumothorax. The involved lobe looks like "pink souffle" when viewed at operation and it does not compress. Lobectomy is curative.

PROBLEM: DIAPHRAGMATIC HERNIA

One of the most perplexing problems in pediatric surgery is congenital diaphragmatic hernia. The incidence is between 1 in 2,500 and 1 in 5,000 births, with a wide range of clinical presentation depending on the severity of the defect. Despite early diagnosis by prenatal ultrasound and advanced management techniques, including in utero surgery and ECMO, diaphragmatic hernia continues to have a mortality rate approaching 50%.[10,12]

The most common diaphragmatic hernia is through a defect of the foramen of Bochdalek. These posterolateral defects in the diaphragm result from failure of closure of the pleuroperitoneal canal before the intestine returns to the abdomen during the tenth week of gestation. Eighty percent of the defects are left sided, and only about 10% have a peritoneal lined sac. Herniation of bowel contents through the defect impairs development of the ipsilateral lung by direct compression. The contralateral lung is also compressed by mediastinal shift. In addition to their reduced size, the lungs of these infants are also morphologically and physiologically abnormal. There are decreased numbers of bronchial divisions and increased smooth muscle in the media of the pulmonary arterioles. The vasoconstriction of these abnormal vessels in response to stimuli such as hypoxia and acidosis is exaggerated, leading to pulmonary hypertension and right-to-left shunting through the ductus arteriosus.[11,23,25,28]

Clinical Presentation

The clinical presentation depends on the severity of the diaphragmatic defect and the degree of the pulmonary hypoplasia. Infants usually present within the first few hours of life with increasing respiratory distress. Physical examination reveals a scaphoid abdomen, and occasionally bowel sounds can be auscultated in the chest. The cardiac impulse has shifted away from the site of the hernia. Rarely, such defects are found coincidentally in older children who demonstrate mild respiratory symptomatology.

A

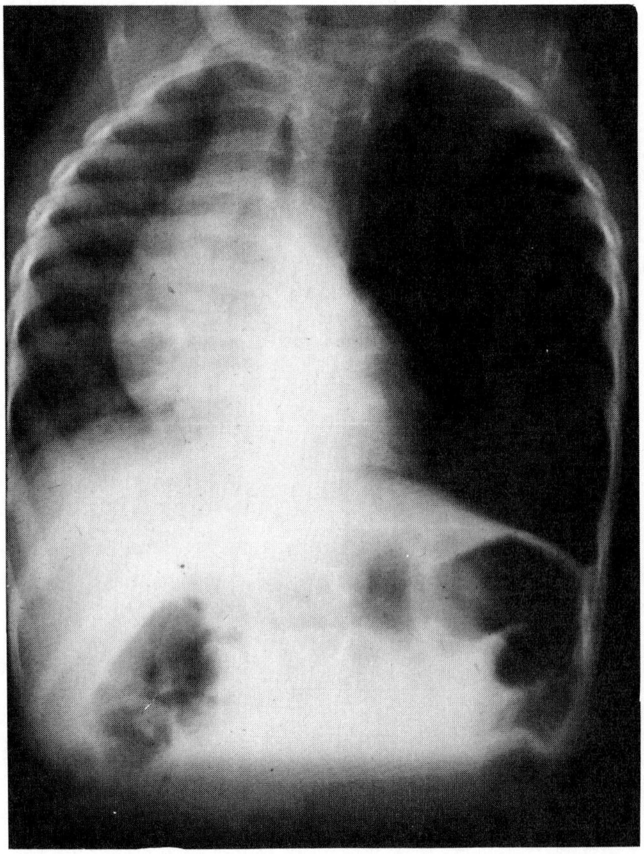

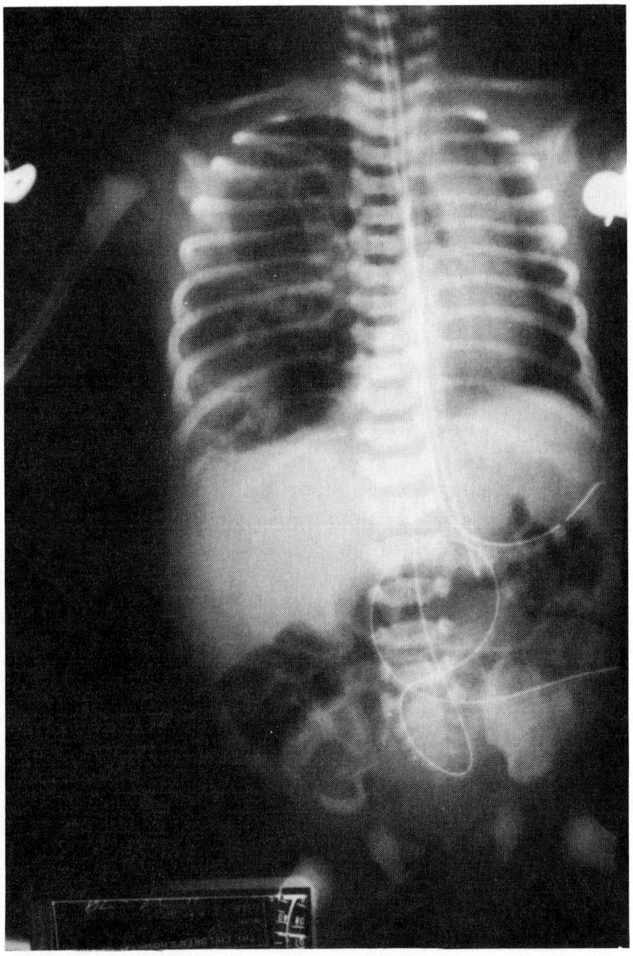

B

FIGURE 23-2 **A,** The left-sided hyperlucent area contains some lung markings, and there is a considerable mediastinal shift to the right. These findings are typical of congenital lobar emphysema. **B,** A cystic and solid right chest lesion in the neonate has produced a mediastinal shift to the left. An intact right hemidiaphragm is most compatible with cystic adenomatoid malformation.

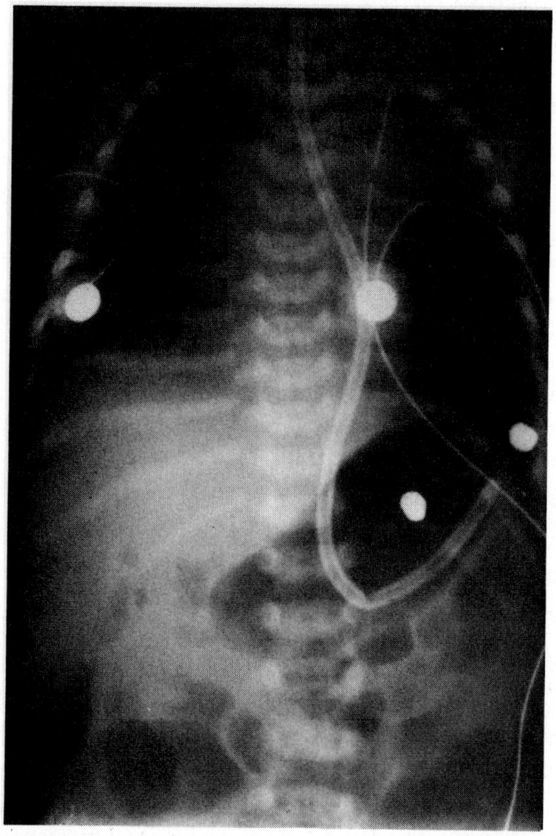

FIGURE 23-3 A radiograph of a left chest lucency compatible with bowel herniating through a defect in the left hemidiaphragm.

Assessment

A chest radiograph may show a marked mediastinal shift with loops of bowel in the chest (Figure 23-4). Placement of a nasogastric tube before obtaining the chest film helps differentiate diaphragmatic hernia from cystic adenoid malformation, which can present with a similar chest radiograph.

Management

The initial management of patients with Bochdalek diaphragmatic hernia is directed towards stabilizing ventilatory function and reversing acidosis. A nasogastric tube is placed to prevent gaseous distention of the stomach and bowel in the chest, which further compromises respiration. Infants with significant respiratory distress should undergo endotracheal intubation and ventilation without delay. Ventilation by face mask and bag is contraindicated because of the risk for further gaseous intestinal distention. Intravenous fluids are initiated and bicarbonate administered to reverse acidosis. Once the child's airway is secured and venous access is established, paralysis with pancuronium may aid ventilation. Major preoperative pitfalls include intubation of the right mainstem bronchus and high ventilatory pressures, which can result in pneumothorax. Rapid clinical deterioration often accompanies contralateral pneumothorax in these infants, and rapid pleural space air evacuation becomes lifesaving.

The surgical treatment of diaphragmatic hernia has evolved with the development of new treatment tech-

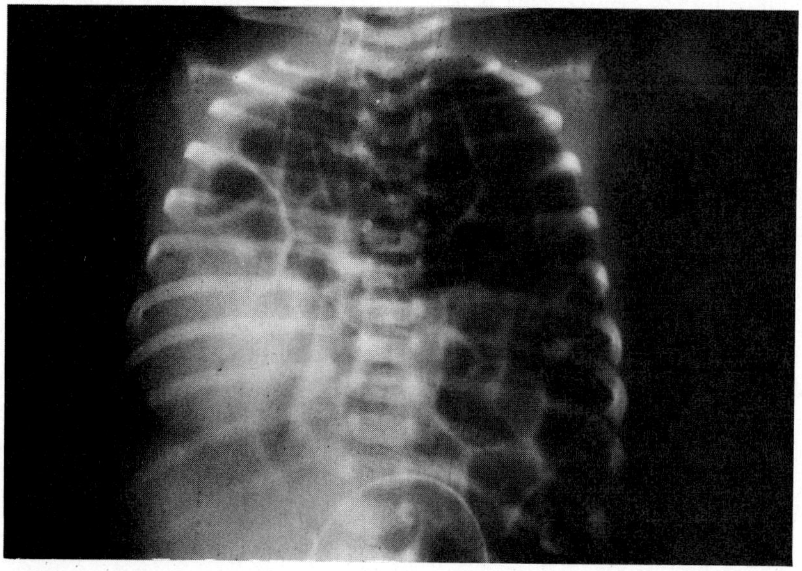

FIGURE 23-4 A multiloculated space-filling lesion of the left chest producing a marked shift of mediastinal structures to the right. This is a classic radiograph of a large left diaphragmatic hernia in a neonate; the respiratory distress is a result of the lung hypoplasia and compression as well as the mediastinal shift.

niques. Classically, these infants underwent emergency operation to reduce the intestine and repair the anatomic defect.[23] Postoperatively, patients were often worse from a respiratory standpoint than before operation. Recent evidence suggests that with the increase in intraabdominal pressure that follows the repair, pulmonary compliance is made worse. As a result many surgeons now advocate delaying the operative repair of the diaphragm until respiratory function is maximized and concomitant medical problems are addressed. ECMO can also play a role in the management of these infants, either before or after repair of the diaphragmatic defect.[30,31,62] The operative repair is usually performed through an abdominal incision. The visceral organs are reduced into the abdomen, and the diaphragmatic defect is closed with nonabsorbable sutures. If the defect is too large for a primary closure, an anterior abdominal wall muscle flap or prosthetic material, such as Goretex, can be used to close the defect. Transthoracic repair is also an option, but this technique is more commonly reserved for rightsided lesions or for repair of diaphragmatic eventration.

The postoperative course in these infants is often complicated by problems related to the pulmonary hypoplasia and vascular smooth muscle hypertrophy. A vicious cycle of hypoxia, hypercarbia, and acidosis resulting in pulmonary hypertension develops, followed by right-to-left shunting and further hypoxia and acidosis. Hyperventilation, creation of a metabolic alkalosis through bicarbonate administration, and adequate oxygenation postoperatively are used to avoid pulmonary hypertension. Some infants demonstrate a "honeymoon period" of relative stability for 24 hours, after which they deteriorate rapidly. Pulmonary hypertension and hypoxia can be treated with pulmonary vasodilators such as tolazoline, nitroglycerin, or nitroprusside. High-frequency ventilation or ECMO may be necessary in severe cases.

Because pulmonary development continues until the age of 8 years, children who survive the initial course following repair of diaphragmatic hernia may recover significant lung function. The number of alveoli per acinus may eventually become normal, but because new airway development is completed by 16 weeks of gestation, the overall number of conducting airways is decreased resulting in a lower total number of alveoli.

Occasionally, the diagnosis of diaphragmatic hernia is not made until several months or even years after birth. These children usually present with gastrointestinal symptoms, do not have significant pulmonary hypoplasia, and generally do very well with operative repair.[45]

Hernias through the retrosternal foramen of Morgagni are unusual lesions often discovered incidentally on chest radiograph. The herniation is beneath the pericardium into the mediastinum. Ventilatory dysfunction is usually mild, and gastrointestinal obstruction or strangulation is uncommon, making repair an elective rather than urgent consideration.

PROBLEM: EVENTRATION OF THE DIAPHRAGM

Congenital eventration of the diaphragm is caused by a failure of formation of the central tendinous portion of the muscular diaphragm. Neurogenic causes of eventration include phrenic nerve injury (acquired eventration) and congenital absence of the anterior horn cells (Werdnig-Hoffman disease). Phrenic nerve damage usually results from a difficult breech vaginal delivery and is accompanied by a brachial plexus injury (Erb's palsy). Acquired eventration secondary to iatrogenic phrenic nerve injury may also be a complication of intrathoracic operative procedures.

Clinical Presentation

The clinical presentation of eventration is a diaphragm that is atonic and moves paradoxically with respiration. The effect is exaggerated in the supine position.

Assessment

The respiratory disturbance caused by eventration of the diaphragm is usually less than that caused by Bochdalek hernia, although the ventilatory dysfunction may lead to atelectasis or pneumonia. The presence of an eventration may be a particular problem for the infant with borderline pulmonary function for some other reason. Diagnostic studies include plain radiographs of the chest but a dynamic fluoroscopy or ultrasound examination of the diaphragm may be necessary to demonstrate paradoxic diaphragmatic motion. The diaphragm on the involved side lies much higher, yet the gas pattern in the abdomen is relatively normal. On the lateral view, the presence of two diaphragmatic leaflets should be visible.

Management

Opinions differ as to whether an eventration of the diaphragm will require operative intervention. Those children having ventilatory difficulty should have plication of the diaphragm. Plication involves either suture imbrication of the diaphragm in a pleat or excision of the central portion of the diaphragm followed by suture closure. The object of these procedures is to eliminate the paradoxic motion on the side of the eventration and to increase intrathoracic space for expansion of the ipsilateral lung. Generally, the prognosis for these infants is good.

GASTROINTESTINAL TRACT

Vomiting in Infants and Children

Vomiting in a newborn or infant is common. Infants who vomit consistently must have a definitive diagnosis made as quickly as possible. Generally, it is preferable to divide neonatal vomiting into two groups, nonbilious and bilious.

The cause of bilious vomiting in a newborn must be assessed as intestinal obstruction and a surgical emergency until proven otherwise. Nonbilious vomiting may also be a surgical emergency, depending on the accompanying signs and symptoms. The amount or frequency of bilious vomiting has little relationship to the type or seriousness of the offending lesion. An infrequent and small amount of bilious emesis is just as significant as frequent and large amounts.

Persistent nonbilious vomiting in the newborn is most often related to feeding technique. It may be associated with respiratory distress in the form of tachypnea, occasional cyanosis, or poor feeding, the latter due either to a poor sucking reflex or early tiring during feeding. Sepsis, meningitis, and noninfectious causes of increased intracranial pressure may be heralded by nonbilious vomiting, early tiring during feeding, hypothermia, and lethargy. Intraabdominal infection, for example necrotizing enterocolitis, may also present in such a way. Cardiac failure associated with tachypnea and hepatomegaly may be manifest initially with nonbilious vomiting. Gastroesophageal reflux is a very common cause of nonbilious vomiting in the newborn, and it must be differentiated in 4- to 6-week-old infants from congenital hypertrophic pyloric stenosis. Projectile nonbilious vomiting, particularly in infants 3 to 8 weeks of age, signals the possibility of pyloric stenosis.

After careful examination of the chest and abdomen, a nasogastric tube should be passed and stomach content aspirated. Plain chest and upright and supine abdominal radiographs should be obtained. A complete blood count, electrolytes, and blood cultures may be indicated. The subsequent work up usually entails contrast studies of the gastrointestinal tract. A barium upper gastrointestinal series is indicated as the initial procedure in infants whose diagnosis is in question to determine the position of the ligament of Treitz and to exclude malrotation of the colon with or without volvulus.

PROBLEM: ESOPHAGEAL ATRESIA

Esophageal atresia occurs in 1 in 3,000 births with an equal sex distribution. One third of the patients are premature, with birth weights less than 2,500 g, and a maternal history of polyhydramnios is common, especially in infants without an associated tracheoesophageal fistula. Although there is no clear evidence for a familial tendency, there are reports of multiple family members and twins with esophageal atresia.

Clinical Presentation

In 85% of esophageal atresia patients with a blind upper pouch and a distal tracheoesophageal fistula, the newborn infant has nonbilious vomiting or regurgitation and an abdomen distended with air. In the 3% to 8% of patients with a blind pouch and no fistula there is regurgitation and the abdomen is flat and airless.

Assessment

When the upper pouch is blind, a nasogastric tube will not pass into the stomach and will be seen coiled in the pouch on radiograph. When there is a distal esophageal fistula, the radiograph will demonstrate the stomach and small intestines filled with air (Figure 23-5). When there is pure esophageal atresia with no distal esophageal fistula, the radiograph may show an air-filled upper esophagus, but there will be no gas whatsoever in the stomach and distal intestines. An isolated tracheoesophageal fistula (H type fistula) with an intact esophagus occurs in 1% to 3% of esophageal anomalies and is usually only

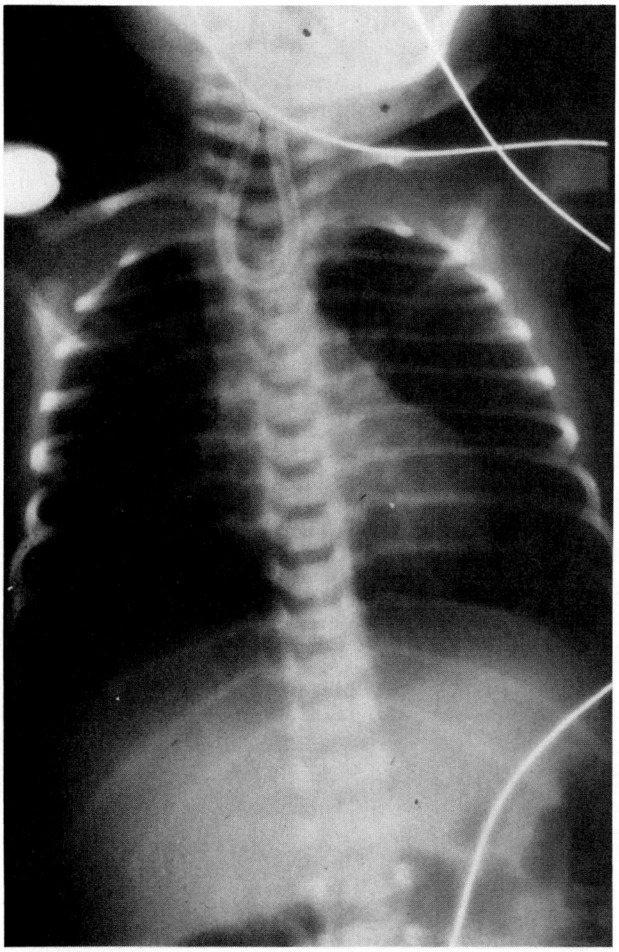

FIGURE 23-5 A radiograph demonstrating a coiled radiopaque catheter in the proximal esophagus along with gas in the gastrointestinal tract. These findings suggest esophageal atresia with a distal tracheoesophageal fistula.

mildly symptomatic. Therefore, the diagnosis of an H type fistula may not be made for days, months, and occasionally for as long as 2 to 3 years after birth. After feeding, such infants will frequently become cyanotic and have episodes of nonbilious vomiting. These cyanotic and vomiting episodes are inconsistent, although coughing with each feeding is usual. A barium swallow is often used to screen for the diagnosis of a tracheoesophageal fistula without atresia, but rigid bronchoscopy is the most sensitive test to not only confirm the diagnosis but to also determine the level of the fistula.[15,18]

Associated anomalies occur commonly with esophageal atresia. Cardiac anomalies are most common, but several types of gastrointestinal and musculoskeletal abnormalities can also occur. Many of these anomalies occur together and are designated as the VACTERL association. These corresponding defects include vertebral, anal, cardiac, tracheal, esophageal, renal, and limb anomalies.[61] The presence of one of these anomalies should prompt a search for others in the association.

Management

Esophageal atresia with tracheoesophageal fistula should be repaired as soon as is feasible by dividing the fistula and doing an end-to-end esophago-esophagostomy. Staged repair with gastrostomy with or without cervical esophagostomy is reserved for severe prematurity or the presence of other life-threatening anomalies.

Preparation for repair requires assessment of associated medical problems such as aspiration pneumonia and evaluation for cardiac anomalies including the position of the aortic arch. Before repair, the patient should be placed in a head-up position with a narrow sump catheter (Replogle tube) placed in the upper pouch attached to constant suction. Maintenance intravenous fluids and administration of prophylactic antibiotics are indicated.

Definitive repair of the usual uncomplicated esophageal atresia and tracheoesophageal fistula is not an emergency procedure. If aspiration pneumonia is present, supportive treatment before repair is justified. Under these circumstances, an initial gastrostomy is indicated, particularly if the fistula is large and is contributing to gastric distention. Emergent division of the tracheoesophageal fistula or balloon occlusion of the fistula may be necessary to maintain high ventilatory pressures in patients requiring mechanical ventilation. In these latter patients the initial gastrostomy should be delayed until after the fistula is controlled.

The definitive operation, an end-to-end esophagoesophagostomy and division of the tracheoesophageal fistula, is performed through a right extrapleural thoracotomy. A small-caliber nasogastric tube is inserted intraoperatively and is left in place postoperatively. An extrapleural thoracostomy tube is left in place for 3 to 7 days as a drain for an esophageal anastomotic leak. An operative gastrostomy is usually not necessary.[48,49]

With pure esophageal atresia, an early gastrostomy is mandatory. Care is taken to place the gastrostomy site away from the greater curvature of the stomach, an anatomic location which subsequently may be used to create a reverse gastric tube as a substitute for the esophagus. A cervical esophagostomy is not initially needed. It is optimal to allow the pressure effects of swallowing to elongate the upper esophagus and to keep the esophagus in its posterior mediastinal position. Infrequently used alternative techniques to bridge a long gap esophageal atresia include preoperative stretching of the upper pouch, operative circular or spiral myotomy, or operatively placing a long suture through both upper and lower pouches along which a fistula forms that can later be dilated. Retrosternal or transthoracic colon replacement and the gastric tube are the preferred alternatives for esophageal substitution in long-gap esophageal atresia. A gastric pull-up is another alternative.

Treatment of the usual proximal esophageal atresia and distal tracheoesophageal fistula should result in a 95% survival. Survival is directly related to a number of factors, the most significant of which is prematurity. The most important additional factors are the association of serious anomalies, particularly congenital heart disease and renal abnormalities. These newborns should always be cared for on a pediatric surgical service in a neonatal intensive care unit.

Three major complications occur after repair of the usual esophageal atresia and tracheoesophageal fistula. Anastomotic leak occurs in 10% to 15% of cases. Without an extrapleural approach (allowing drainage through the extrapleural thoracotomy tube), mediastinitis or empyema might produce a fatality. Stricture at the anastomotic site commonly occurs, especially following an anastomotic leak (25% of leaks); and this may require esophageal dilatation at intervals as frequently as weekly to as infrequently as a single dilatation. Dilatations are most safely accomplished by pulling a dilator through the narrowed site, a technique that requires the establishment of a gastrostomy. The third complication is esophageal obstruction secondary to a foreign body lodging at the anastomotic site. This complication occurs slightly more frequently in patients with a history of stricture formation, but it may occur in any patient after an esophageal atresia repair. Usually the offending substance is a piece of solid food such as a hot dog. Esophagoscopy with foreign body removal and simultaneous dilatations are indicated in these situations especially in the presence of respiratory distress.[13,32]

After esophageal atresia repair, 10% to 20% of patients have serious esophageal dyskinesia resulting in significant gastroesophageal reflux. In these patients when gastroesophageal reflux is refractory to medical and positional management, an antireflux procedure is indicated, even as early as 2 to 4 months of age. This procedure should prevent continuing aspiration, pneumonitis, and esophagitis, the latter contributing to narrowing at the esophageal anastomosis.

Colonic replacement of the esophagus has created several long-term problems including an increased tortuosity of the colonic segment leading to stasis, colitis, polyp formation, and gastroesophageal reflux.

PROBLEM: GASTROESOPHAGEAL REFLUX

Gastroesophageal reflux is a common problem in infants and children. Infants with a history of esophageal atresia, diaphragmatic hernia, or gastrostomy tube placement and children suffering from acquired or congenital mental-motor retardation are particularly susceptible to reflux.[50]

Clinical Presentation

The clinical manifestations are quite protean. Vomiting, failure to thrive, and bronchospastic pulmonary disease are the most common presenting symptoms. Less commonly infants can present with pneumonia, dysphagia, esophageal stricture, or a missed sudden infant death episode. Sandifer's syndrome is a rare manifestation of reflux esophagitis in which the child exhibits dystonic movements of the head and neck simulating seizure activity, a posturing stimulated by the discomfort of esophagitis. Familial dysautonomia (Riley-Day syndrome) is another well-known autonomic nervous system disorder that is associated with intractable vomiting during the autonomic crises.

Assessment

A thorough history and physical examination are followed by radiologic and physiologic testing. A barium swallow, which is often the initial test performed, will demonstrate reflux in severe cases but can have a false-negative rate of up to 85% in mild cases. A hiatal hernia, which is present in 50% to 90% of children with reflux, may be seen. However, the anatomic presence of a hiatal hernia is not pathognomonic for gastroesophageal reflux, and it may be seen in the absence of reflux symptoms in 25% of patients. The barium study also permits an assessment of the gastric outlet to exclude any signs of an obstructive component.

Esophageal pH monitoring is performed for 12 to 24 hours with an esophageal pH probe, and it is the most sensitive method of documenting reflux. A scoring of the frequency, duration, and severity of reflux episodes can then be correlated with symptoms. Esophagoscopy may demonstrate complications of reflux such as esophagitis or stricture. Esophageal manometry may show alterations in lower esophageal motility as well as sphincter pressures, but it is rarely performed. A nuclear medicine gastric emptying scan is most useful to quantify gastric emptying; in the case of delayed emptying a pyloroplasty may warrant consideration.

Management

The management of gastroesophageal reflux involves both medical and surgical therapies. Positional therapy in infants uses gravity to avoid reflux of gastric contents into the esophagus. Infants are maintained in either a 60-degree upright supine position or a 30-degree head-up prone position. Lesser degrees of elevation are not effective, and the position must be diligently maintained. Positional therapy in combination with frequent small, thickened feedings is often effective in relieving symptoms sufficiently so that a child is able to "outgrow" their reflux. Medical therapy in older children consists of treatment with H-2 blockers and metoclopramide.

Indications for operative treatment include a previous resuscitation from sudden infant death syndrome, esophagitis with stricture, recurrent pneumonitis, and treatment failures intractable to medical care. Relative indications include atypical asthma and chronic vomiting.[2,38,65] Several operations are advocated to prevent reflux, but the aim of each is to reestablish a length of intraabdominal esophagus, tighten the esophageal hiatus, increase the esophagogastric angle (angle of His), and create an antirefluxing nipple valve.[14] The Nissen fundoplication, which creates a 360-degree wrap of gastric fundus around the distal esophagus, is traditionally the procedure of choice.[38] A reported higher incidence of complications including gas bloat syndrome and adhesive small bowel obstruction following the 360-degree wrap has lead some surgeons to recommend the Thal procedure, which creates an anterior 180-degree wrap.[65]

In addition to the antireflux procedure, a gastric outlet procedure, i.e., pyloroplasty, is indicated in any patient with evidence of delayed gastric emptying on preoperative gastric emptying scan.

Overall the results of antireflux procedures are very good, a relief of symptoms occurring in over 90% of neurologically normal patients.[4,56] Patients with severe neurologic impairment seem to have a higher recurrence rate despite their treatment program.[19,50,59]

PROBLEM: PYLORIC STENOSIS

Pyloric stenosis occurs in approximately 1 in 400 births and is more common in males.

Clinical Presentation

Patients classically present at 3 to 6 weeks of age with progressive, projectile, nonbilious vomiting. Both younger and older age extremes are possible, the latter especially for the previously premature infant. As vomiting becomes more frequent with most every feeding, the typical picture becomes an infant with a voracious appetite who has stopped gaining weight, whose stool frequency and volume is decreasing, and who is beginning to show stigmata of dehydration.

Assessment

Physical examination may confirm early dehydration. Inspection of the abdomen may reveal a visible peristaltic wave progressing from left to right across the upper abdomen. Careful palpation of the upper abdomen midline to right upper quadrant by the examiner's right hand, with the examiner standing on the infant's left side and cradling the feet and legs in the left hand, will demonstrate a palpable pyloric "olive" or "tumor" in 80% to 90% of infants with pyloric stenosis.

When an irritable infant precludes an accurate abdominal palpation or when the presentation is atypical, ancillary diagnostic studies become useful. A barium upper gastrointestinal series is advantageous when screening for causes of vomiting including gastric outlet anatomic obstruction as well as severe gastroesophageal reflux. Classic findings of pyloric stenosis include indentation on the gastric antrum by the thickened pyloric muscle and a "string" or "railroad track" sign of a narrow column of barium passing through the compressed lumen of the pyloric channel. Ultrasound evaluation of the pylorus depends on size criteria of the pyloric muscle, cross-sectional diameter, length, and channel lumen size.

Management

After the diagnosis is confirmed by either physical examination or ancillary radiographs, the patient is prepared for operation. Often a profound hypokalemic-hypochloremic metabolic alkalosis follows the progressive vomiting, and this aberration must be corrected before the induction of anesthesia. Operative treatment is a Fredet-Ramstedt pyloromyotomy in which a seromuscular incision over the pyloric channel is followed by a gentle separation or splitting of the pyloric muscle (Figure 23-6). This maneuver permits the underlying mucosal tube to bulge out and increase the luminal diameter. This operation is curative and permits the initiation of feeding within 24 hours of the procedure. Only if there is penetration of the pyloric mucosa during pyloromyotomy will complications be more likely.

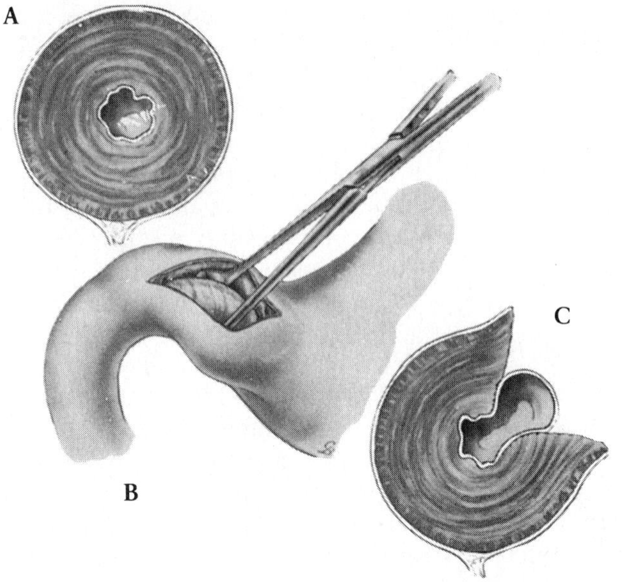

FIGURE 23-6 Hypertrophic pyloric stenosis. **A,** Cross section of thickened pyloric muscle and narrow channel. **B,** Ramstedt pyloromyotomy showing instrument spreading the muscle apart after it has been incised longitudinally, allowing the intact mucosa to bulge outward. C, After muscle spreading, the lumen of the pyloric channel is greatly enlarged and obstruction of the stomach is relieved. (From Liechty RD, Soper RT: *Synopsis of Surgery,* ed 5, St Louis, 1985, Mosby.)

PROBLEM: DUODENAL OBSTRUCTION—ATRESIA AND MALROTATION

Clinical Presentation

Duodenal obstruction in the newborn, due either to stenosis, atresia, or malrotation of large and small bowel, is usually accompanied by bile in the vomitus or nasogastric tube aspirate. Often a distended stomach with a left-to-right peristaltic wave is visible, but additional findings include a scaphoid lower abdomen and little if any stool in the rectum. The baby feeds poorly and is fitful and irritable as if in pain. There may also be coffee ground material in the vomitus. Stigmata of Down syndrome may be present; 20% of patients with duodenal atresia/annular pancreas have Down syndrome.

Assessment

Bilious vomiting in the newborn should be regarded as a surgical emergency until malrotation with volvulus has been ruled out. Plain abdominal radiographs may demonstrate air confined to the stomach and first part of the duodenum, the classic "double-bubble" sign typical of duodenal atresia (Figure 23-7). If air is found distal to the first portion of the duodenum, then malrotation must be excluded. An emergency upper gastrointestinal contrast study is indicated as soon as the newborn is hydrated and decompressed with nasogastric suction. This procedure takes only a few minutes and usually establishes the position of the ligament of Treitz and the type of obstructing lesion (Figure 23-8). Performing this study expeditiously will identify cases of malrotation with volvulus and potential intestinal ischemic injury can be

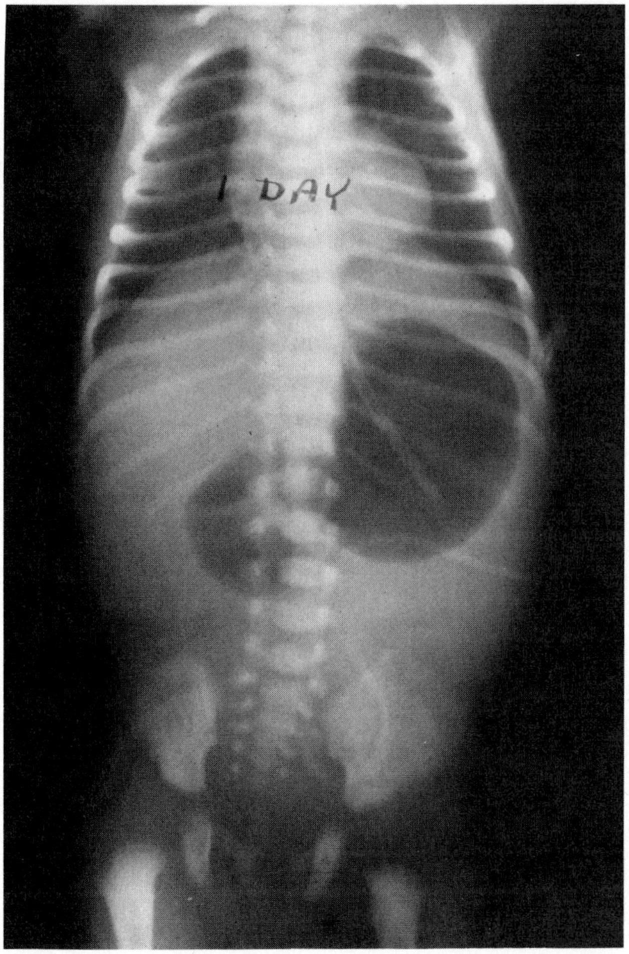

FIGURE 23-7 Radiograph of a 1-day-old neonate with bilious vomiting, demonstrating the classic "double-bubble" sign of duodenal obstruction.

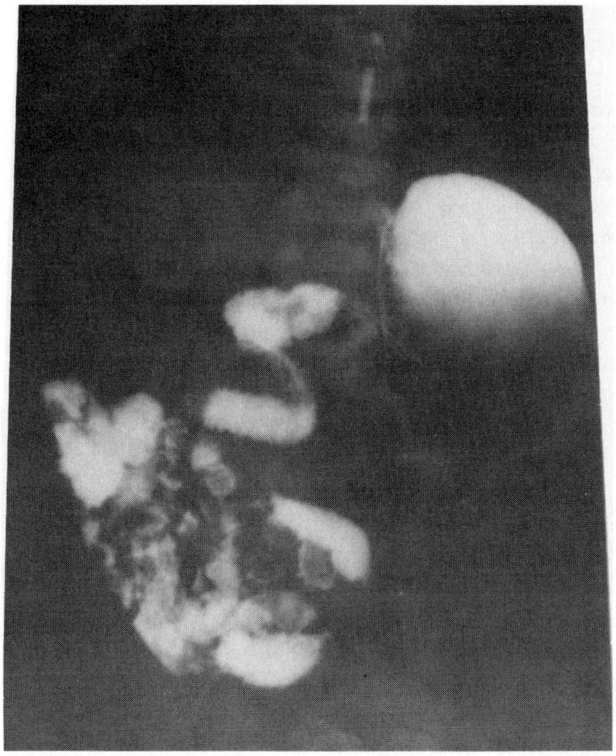

FIGURE 23-8 Upper gastrointestinal contrast radiograph that fails to demonstrate a "C-loop" and the normal position of the ligament of Treitz. This is diagnostic of malrotation.

avoided. A barium enema is less sensitive in ruling in or out a malrotation in a vomiting patient regardless of age.

Management

Electrolyte derangements must be determined promptly and abnormalities corrected rapidly. A nasogastric tube on gravity drainage is mandatory. If the diagnosis of malrotation has been excluded and a duodenal atresia (web, stenosis, or annular pancreas) is identified, operative repair can be performed on a more elective basis. Malrotation, on the other hand, constitutes a true surgical emergency and requires immediate operative intervention.

In patients with evidence of malrotation, the abdomen is entered through an upper abdominal transverse incision. The abdomen is opened widely and the bowel is eviscerated. This allows the inspection of the root of the mesentery and the determination of the degree of volvulus along with assessment of any compromised bowel. The volvulus should be reduced by rotating the bowel in a counterclockwise direction. Ladd's bands, which extend from the cecum across the first and second portion of the duodenum, should be divided to further relieve duodenal obstruction. This maneuver permits the cecum to be placed into the left lower quadrant and the small bowel to be placed along the right side of the abdomen. An appendectomy is performed to avoid confusion in the future with the abnormal cecal placement. If the viability of the bowel is in question at the time of the initial operation, a second-look procedure may be scheduled for 12 to 24 hours after the initial operation to reassess the bowel. A temporary gastrotomy should be made and a balloon-tipped catheter should be passed into the jejunum and withdrawn slowly, with the balloon inflated to rule out any coexisting intrinsic duodenal obstruction.

In patients with duodenal stenosis, duodenal web, or annular pancreas, the abdomen is also explored through a transverse incision. If the obstruction cannot be directly visualized, a temporary gastrotomy is made and a balloon-tipped catheter is passed into the jejunum and withdrawn, with the balloon inflated to determine the level of obstruction. If intrinsic duodenal stenosis in the form of a web or windsock deformity exists, the balloon will be held up at that point. Duodenotomy and correction of the defect can be accomplished directly; however, the surgeon must be extremely careful to identify the ampulla of Vater, which can be involved in the wall of the obstructing duodenal septum. An ampulla proximal to the obstruction would be compatible with a picture of bilious vomiting, while if distal to the obstruction nonbilious vomiting would be more typical. Alternatively a duodenoduodenostomy or duodenojejunostomy may be performed to bypass the area of the intrinsic obstruction.[19,27]

Recovery from intestinal obstruction secondary to malrotation and volvulus is good in cases where there is no evidence of intestinal ischemia. In patients who develop necrosis of their small bowel, the mortality rate increases dramatically. Long-term complications resulting from short bowel syndrome are common in survivors. Intestinal obstruction resulting from adhesions is an established complication following the correction of malrotation.

The survival of isolated duodenal atresia/severe stenosis patients is excellent. Any immediate or long-term mortality is secondary to the severe associated anomalies and is rarely due to the operative correction. Anastomotic leakage and stricture are recognized but rare complications. Occasional problems of failure to thrive and gastroesophageal reflux are recorded postoperatively, but usually are easily corrected by medical management.

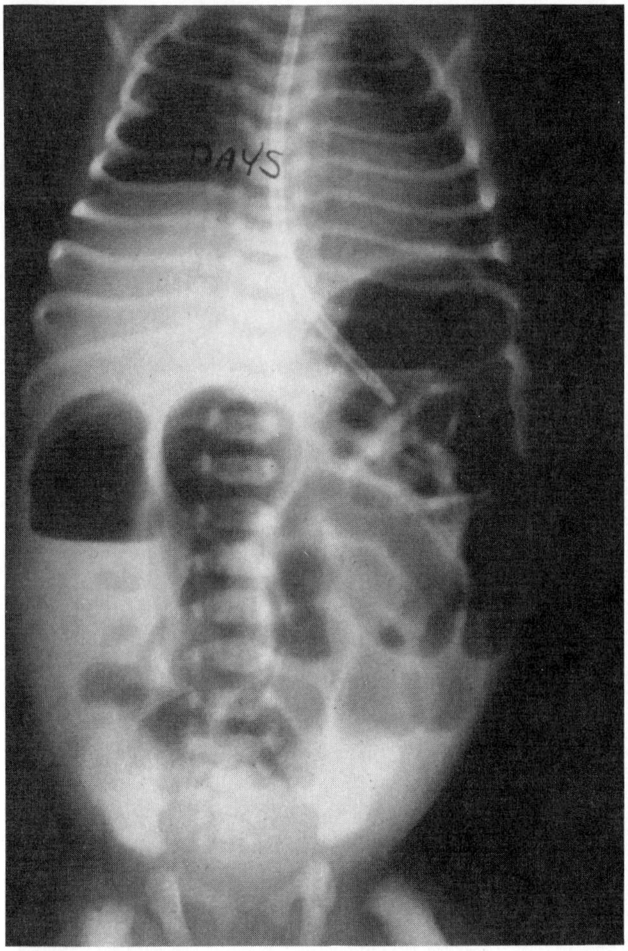

FIGURE 23-9 Plain abdominal radiograph demonstrating multiple dilated bowel loops and air-fluid levels most compatible with a distal bowel obstruction.

PROBLEM: JEJUNOILEAL ATRESIA

Clinical Presentation

Infants with jejunoileal atresia are often born with a soft abdomen but rapidly become markedly distended. Although the infant may pass small amounts of meconium, abdominal distention and bilious nasogastric tube output develop quickly from the complete bowel obstruction.

The most common cause of neonatal intestinal obstruction is intestinal atresia, and jejunoileal atresia follows the duodenum as the most common site for such an obstruction. The etiology of duodenal atresia is thought to be a failure of vacuolization and resorption in formation of a lumen, whereas the most likely explanation of more distal atresia is an in utero mesenteric vascular accident. The resulting obstruction may take the form of an incontinuity obstructing intraluminal membrane to a complete gap between proximal obstructed bowel and the distal segment. Such vascular accidents are usually of unknown etiology, but an in utero volvulus of a loop or an intussusception are possible explanations. The resulting atresias are usually singular, but multiple sites of obstruction may occur. Atresias in the colon are distinctly rare.

Assessment

Neonates with atresia of the small bowel present with bilious vomiting and various degrees of abdominal distention on clinical as well as flat and upright radiographic examination, depending on the site of the obstruction (Figure 23-9). Multiple dilated loops suggest a distal site of the obstruction. To exclude meconium ileus and Hirschsprung's disease as causes of the obstruction and to help localize the site, a contrast enema should be the next diagnostic study (Figure 23-10). If distended loops of bowel remain above the level of a normal caliber or small "unused" colon, then a distal small bowel obstruction is the diagnosis and operative exploration is needed.

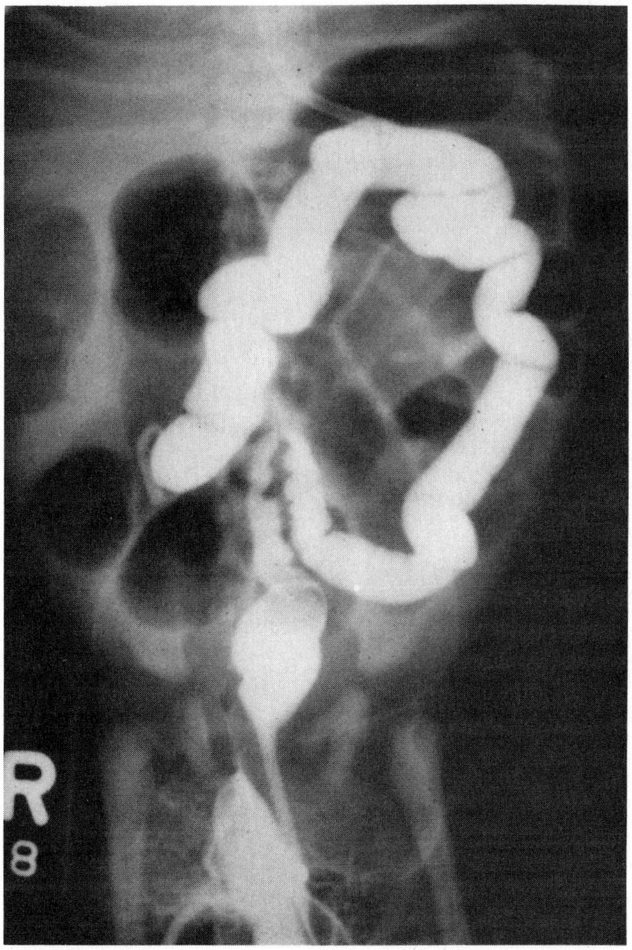

FIGURE 23-10 Contrast enema in the patient depicted in Figure 23-9 with a distal bowel obstruction. The colon is of normal caliber and is patent, and contrast has failed to reach the more proximal dilated small bowel. Operative exploration is indicated for what most likely will be a distal small bowel atresia.

Management

After appropriate nasogastric decompression and fluid rehydration, the baby should undergo operative exploration. The bowel is thoroughly explored and the atretic segments identified; the preferred management is segmental resection with primary anastomosis. At times an obstructing intraluminal membrane, especially when distal to a more proximal obstruction, is identified by insertion of a catheter into the bowel and infusing saline to assure luminal patency. Surgery should preserve as much intestinal length as possible, but if necessary the proximal dilated segment may be partially resected, or tapered, to improve on the proximal to distal anastomotic size discrepancy. A longitudinal enterotomy with excision of the membrane and transverse closure of the intestine is preferred for the treatment of obstructing intraluminal membranes. Because of the typically prolonged anastomotic dysfunction postoperatively, the use of a concomitant gastrostomy and a parenteral nutritional access line may be prudent. Such prolonged but temporary anastomotic dysfunction is a much more likely complication than would be anastomotic leakage or actual stenosis.

The rare colon atresia may also be amenable to primary anastomosis. At times a neonatal colostomy is preferred followed by a delayed restoration of intestinal continuity after recovery and several months of systemic growth have been achieved.

When intestinal length is adequate, recovery is complete and uncomplicated in the majority of patients.

PROBLEM: MECONIUM ILEUS

Meconium ileus represents an intrinsic distal small bowel obstruction secondary to the intraluminal accumulation of an abnormal meconium.

Clinical Presentation

Infants with meconium ileus are born with abdominal distention, the only type of bowel obstruction that does not require the swallowing of gas to produce this distention. The abnormal meconium is the product of a lack of normally secreted pancreatic and intestinal exocrine juices in utero, the abnormality being secondary to cystic fibrosis. Infants with meconium ileus have cystic fibrosis; with a known family kindred for this disease plus chorionic villus sampling and genetic analysis, the in utero diagnosis of cystic fibrosis can be confirmed. Cystic fibrosis occurs once in every 1,000 to 2,500 live births, and meconium ileus occurs in approximately 15% of this population. If in addition fetal bowel distention is seen by in utero ultrasound, the antenatal diagnosis of meconium ileus can be suspected.

Assessment

At birth the distention is visualized, and plain supine and upright radiographs of the abdomen demonstrate classic findings: large and small disparate sized distended bowel loops, a bubbly picture of air admixed with stool (meconium) in the right lower quadrant, and no significant air-fluid levels (Figure 23-11). The history, physical examination, and plain radiographs are collectively diagnostic; but further evidence is the finding of an unused or microcolon seen at contrast enema radiograph (Figure 23-12). At times inspissated pellets of meconium can also be seen in the right colon and distal ileum, and proximal to this are the distended loops of bowel.

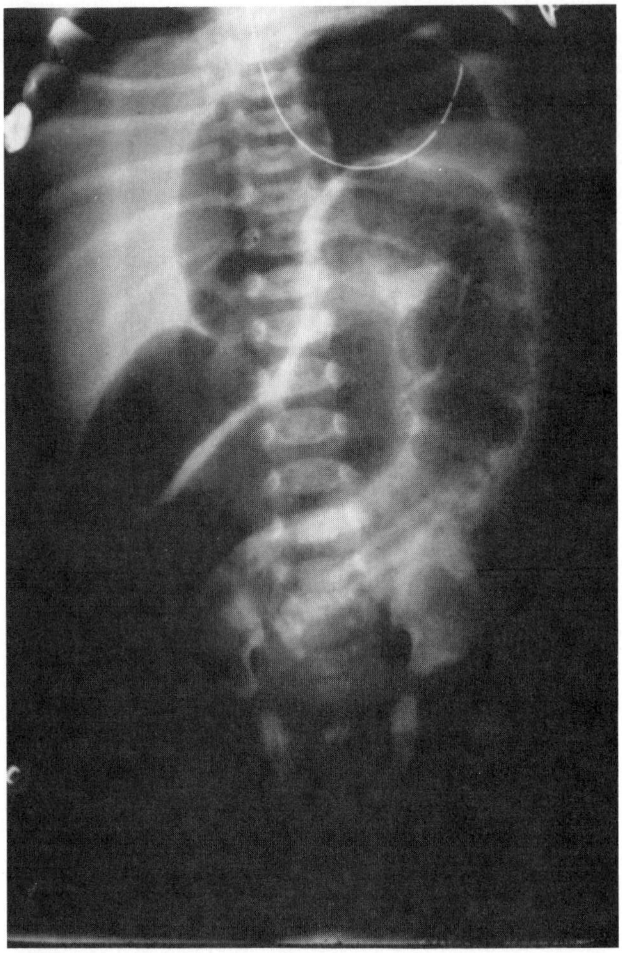

FIGURE 23-11 Classic plain film radiograph of a patient with meconium ileus, showing large and small distended loops, a bubbly picture of air admixed with the meconium stool in the right lower quadrant, and few air-fluid levels.

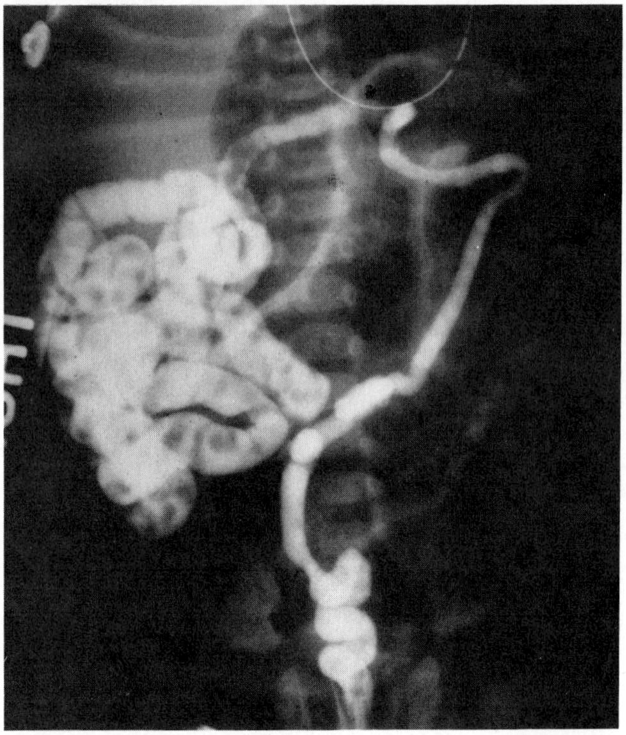

FIGURE 23-12 Contrast enema radiograph in the patient depicted in Figure 23-11. An unused microcolon is demonstrated, and contrast has refluxed into the dilated terminal ileum, which is filled with "pellets" of inspissated meconium. This is an ideal patient for administering hyperosmolar solubilizing agents to relieve the intraluminal obstruction.

Management

In almost two thirds of cases the nonoperative management of meconium ileus may be effective. After nasogastric tube decompression and fluid resuscitation at one to two times maintenance, a contrast enema using hyperosmolar meglumine diatrizoate (Gastrografin), which contains a solubilizing agent, is administered. The goal is to reflux Gastrografin through the colon proximally into the meconium-laden dilated bowel loops. Fluid is pulled by the hyperosmolar agent into the bowel lumen, and the meconium is liquefied and begins to pass as the enema is expelled. The sequence may need to be repeated to assure complete evacuation of the obstructing inspissated meconium.

If the therapeutic enema proves unsuccessful, or if there is evidence of meconium peritonitis or a meconium cyst suggesting an in utero bowel perforation, then operative intervention is needed. At operation the first goal is to confirm the diagnosis of a meconium obstruction not complicated by either atresia secondary to a twist of a heavy bowel loop or a meconium perforation. Atresia or a perforation with cyst formation would best be managed by resection and primary anastomosis if no distal intraluminal meconium exists. With extensive bowel involvement, short bowel syndrome may be a practical postoperative problem.

Several options are available for managing an obstruction secondary to inspissated meconium alone. An intraoperative intraluminal injection, either through a needle or via a catheter enterotomy, of a meconium solubilizing agent such as Gastrografin, a 4% solution of n-acetyl-cysteine (Mucomyst), or a pancreatic enzyme solution (Viokase) may be effective in liquefying the meconium, which facilitates its distal passage. If this proves ineffective then segmental resection of the dilated ileal segment may be advisable, after which several added options may be entertained: primary anastomosis, double barrel side-by-side ileostomies (Mikulicz stoma), end- (proximal) to-side (distal) ileostomy (Bishop-Koop procedure), or end- (distal) to-side (proximal) ileostomy (Santulli procedure). The postoperative administration of pancreatic enzymes via the distal limb of the ostomy further facilitates dissolution of meconium in the more distal ileum and colon. When infants have recovered, their stomas can be closed either formally in the operating room or at times by bedside ligature of the defunctionalized ileal chimney (Bishop-Koop).

The prognosis for infants with meconium ileus is largely dictated by the pulmonary and pancreatic severity of their cystic fibrosis. In complicated meconium ileus where an in utero perforation has produced a meconium cyst or where a volvulus of a meconium-laden loop has produced an atresia, the outcome will be related to the extent of the short bowel syndrome secondary to intestinal loss and to nutrient malabsorption because of cystic fibrosis.

PROBLEM: MECONIUM PLUG SYNDROME

Occasionally, newborns will present with a distal bowel obstruction with mild abdominal distention with or without bilious vomiting. Such babies have not passed meconium. On contrast enema radiograph a "plug" or "cast" of meconium is identified in the transverse or descending colon and at times a size disparity exists, with the descending or left colon being of smaller caliber. After the enema is complete the baby will pass the "plug", and thereafter the obstruction will be relieved. A small fraction of such infants may in fact have either Hirschsprung's disease or a form of meconium ileus with underlying cystic fibrosis. Depending on the clinical progress of the patient it may be prudent to evaluate the patient further with a rectal biopsy and/or sweat test.

PROBLEM: HIRSCHSPRUNG'S DISEASE

The most common functional congenital obstruction of the colon is Hirschsprung's disease or congenital aganglionosis. The cause of the obstruction is the congenital absence of intramuscular (Auerbach's) and submucosal (Meissner's) autonomic ganglion cells in a segment of the rectum or colon. In contrast, cholinergic nerve fibers are increased in size and density in the diseased segment. As a result of the absence of these ganglion cells, peristalsis does not occur in the affected section. The term *megacolon* describes the dilatation and hypertrophy of the normally innervated colon proximal to the aganglionic section. The length of aganglionic bowel is quite variable and ranges from ultrashort segments of distal rectum to total bowel aganglionosis. The most common transition zone is in the rectosigmoid or sigmoid colon.

Neonates: Clinical Presentation

In the neonate, Hirschsprung's disease may produce early intestinal obstruction characterized by abdominal distention, the rectal passage of little or no meconium, and bilious vomiting. Occasionally, the occurrence of paradoxical diarrhea, which may herald enterocolitis, may confuse the diagnosis.

Assessment

A presumptive diagnosis of short segment Hirschsprung's disease may be made by physical examination of the rectum. The examiner notes a normal anal orifice, a narrow rectal ampulla, and withdrawal of the finger often results in the explosive passage of gas and meconium. In addition, anorectal manometry demonstrates the failure of the internal anal sphincter to relax when the rectum is distended. The diagnosis is made definitively by rectal biopsy, which reveals the absence of ganglia in the autonomic nerve plexus in the submucosal and intramuscular plexi. Because these ganglion cells are scattered throughout the myenteric and submucosal plexus and every section may not contain a ganglion cell, the pathologist makes several "steps" through the tissue and several sections of each step (Figure 23-13). An alternate technique is to apply histochemical stains for acetylcholinesterase to the tissue, an increased concentration of the enzyme being diagnostic for Hirschsprung's disease.

Management

The goal of initial management is to relieve the intestinal obstruction. At operation, biopsies are performed to identify the transition zone from distal aganglionic to proximal normally innervated bowel, and a colostomy is created proximal to this transition level. Rarely, a good risk infant can undergo primary definitive corrective surgery. However, in a small or otherwise compromised infant, the preference is to delay such definitive operation until later in infancy or young childhood.

After Infancy: Clinical Presentation

Less symptomatic children may not be diagnosed in infancy but during the first year of life suffer episodes of distention, vomiting, and paradoxical diarrhea between periods of constipation. Bacterial overgrowth can predispose children to an acute enterocolitis, which carries a mortality rate of approximately 20%. Because the dominant complaint of the older child becomes chronic constipation, the risk of life-threatening complications of bowel perforation, enterocolitis, and sepsis increases with age.

Parents of older infants and children with Hirschsprung's disease will give varied reports. Abnormal bowel function will have been present since the day of birth. The rectal passage of meconium after birth may

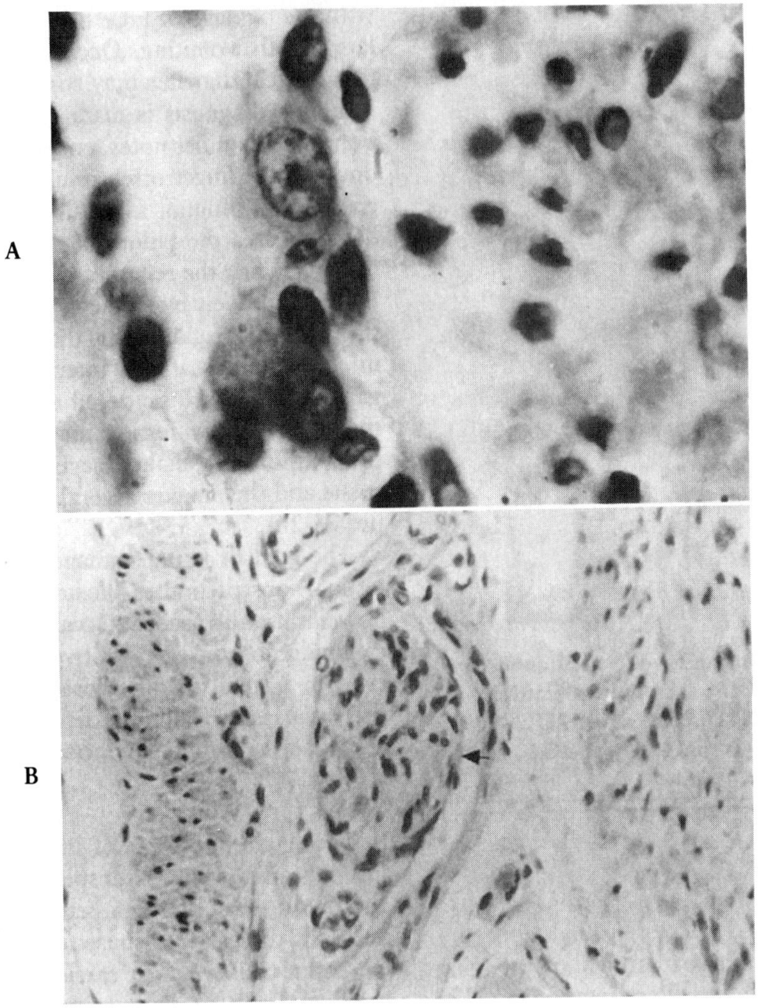

FIGURE 23-13 A, Typical ganglion cells in the myenteric plexus of a normal bowel. Note their "kite" shape and their large nuclei with distinct nuclear material and prominent stippled cytoplasm. B, Myenteric plexus of a child with Hirschsprung's disease, with absence of ganglion cells and a hypertrophied nerve bundle *(arrow)*. (From Filston HC: *Surgical problems in children*, St Louis, 1982, Mosby.)

have been delayed from 24 to 48 hours. They will report degrees of explosive diarrhea followed by constipation. Common signs include abdominal distention, poor weight gain, and vomiting of feedings. Medical measures taken for control of symptoms (laxatives, enemas, suppositories) produce no results.

Assessment

On physical examination, the surgeon finds a pale and malnourished child with soft abdominal distention. The examiner often can feel loops of colon distended by gas and hard feces. As with the infant, digital examination reveals a small rectal ampulla. Withdrawal of the examining finger may produce an explosive escape of liquid stool and gas.

A barium enema study on an unprepared bowel will aid the diagnosis by revealing the characteristically narrow or normal-sized rectum that flairs through a funnel-shaped transition zone into a megacolon above the point of obstruction (Figure 23-14). The examiner should use only small amounts of barium and not attempt to fill the entire colon. Delay in the expulsion of the barium (over 24 hours) is a second diagnostic element of the study. As with infants, rectal wall biopsy definitively confirms the diagnosis.

Management

The definitive management of Hirschsprung's disease is operative. Initial efforts are aimed at relieving the obstruction, usually by a colostomy, which must be

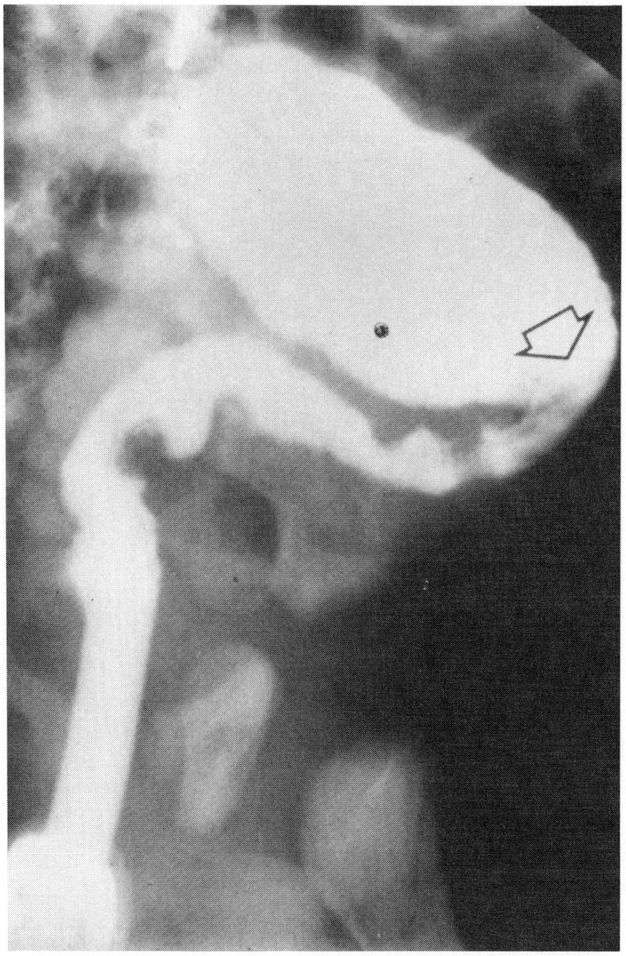

FIGURE 23-14 Barium enema radiograph depicting classic rectosigmoid Hirschsprung's disease. There is proximal colon dilatation, a funnel-shaped transition zone, and a collapsed distal aganglionic segment.

placed within an area of normal ganglionated bowel. Seromuscular biopsies of the colon are again performed to identify the appropriate level.

Definitive treatment is achieved by using one of several abdominal perineal pull-through techniques in which the surgeon anastomoses the ganglionated proximal colon to the aganglionic anorectal pouch. A Duhamel procedure involves pulling the normally innervated colon down to the anus behind the aganglionic rectum and anastomosing the bowel segments "side to side." This maneuver provides peristaltic movement without sacrificing the sensation of stool in the rectal vault. In cases of long segment aganglionosis, the side-to-side anastomosis between normal and aganglionic bowel can be extended proximally to avoid sacrificing large segments of colon. Alternatively, a Soave procedure may be performed in which the rectal mucosa is stripped down to the anorectal level of the transitional epithelium, and the normal ganglionated bowel is pulled through the muscular sleeve of the rectum and anastomosed to this site, thus bypassing the aganglionic bowel completely.

The outcome for children with aganglionosis confined to the distal colon is excellent. Children with aganglionosis involving the total colon and portions of small bowel fare less well and may suffer from short gut syndrome.[53,58]

PROBLEM: IMPERFORATE ANUS

Imperforate anus occurs in one of every 4,000 to 5,000 newborns and is slightly more common in males. The spectrum of the entity is complex, but practically lesions can be separated into low- or high-type imperforate anus based on the position of the end of the rectum in relationship to the puborectalis muscle sling (Figure 23-15).

Clinical Presentation

Generally, the rectum in low-type imperforate anus will have penetrated the muscle sling and will exit on the perineum as a fistula anterior to the proper anatomic position of the anus. In a female this fistula may be located on the perineum from the vaginal forchette anteriorly to the perineal body posteriorly. In the male the fistula will open on the perineum at any position anterior to the position of the true anus all the way to the base of the scrotum. Rarely the low ending rectal pouch will end not in a fistula but will end blindly.

The rectum in high-type imperforate anus will not penetrate the puborectalis muscle. In a male the rectum will uniformly end in a fistula into the urinary tract, most commonly as a rectourethral fistula into the bulbus or prostatic urethra. In a female the variations are greater. When imperforate anus is present but two perineal orifices are seen, the rectum usually ends as a rectovaginal fistula along the upper portion of the posterior vaginal wall. If only one perineal orifice is seen, a cloacal deformity exists in which a common channel exiting to the outside connects on the inside to the bladder-urethra, vagina, and rectum.

Assessment

The diagnosis of imperforate anus is made by neonatal physical examination and close perineal inspection. Distinguishing low- from high-type imperforate anus is often more difficult. Though mostly of historic significance, the Rice-Wagensteen "invertogram" permits visualization of the distalmost air in the rectal pouch relative to a line drawn from the pubis to the ischium to the coccyx (Figure 23-16). A pouch ending above that line suggests a high lesion. A pelvic-perineal ultrasound examination may be a useful technique to visualize the

A C B D

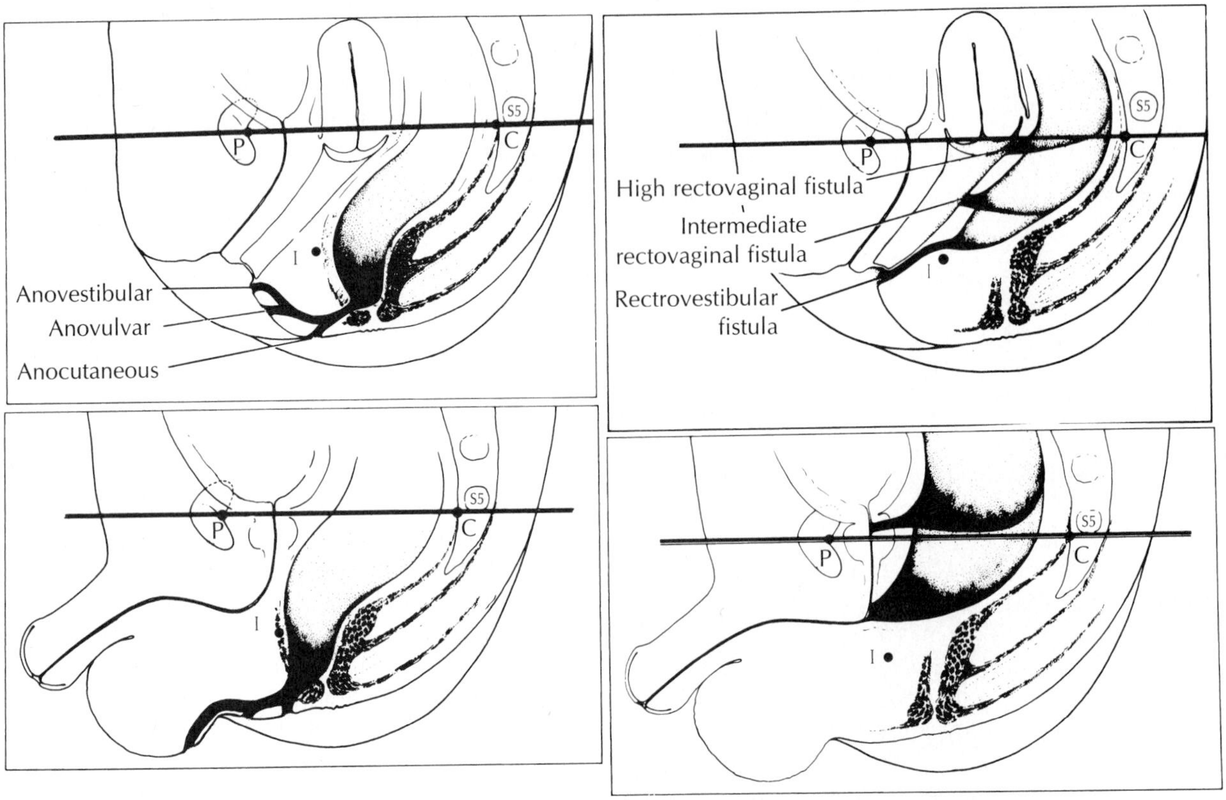

FIGURE 23-15 Imperforate anus, levels of the rectal pouch, and location of fistulae. **A,** Low imperforate anus anomalies in the female almost always have an external fistulous tract. **B,** Low imperforate anus anomalies in the male usually have an external fistulous tract. **C,** Intermediate and high imperforate anus lesions in the female are usually associated with a fistula to the posterior vagina. **D,** Intermediate and high imperforate anus in the male is usually associated with a fistula to the urinary tract. *P,* Pubis; *C,* coccyx; *I,* ischium. (From Templeton JM, O'Neill JA Jr: Anorectal malformations. In Welch KW, Randolph JC, Ravitch MM et al, editors: *Pediatric surgery,* ed 4, St Louis, 1986, Mosby.)

same distal extent of the pouch relative to the same line or to the perineal skin. The rectourinary fistula in a high male imperforate anus can often be demonstrated by a retrograde voiding cystourethrogram. The evaluation of a complex cloacal anomaly will require careful endoscopic inspection complementing contrast radiography.[21]

Evaluation of the neonate with imperforate anus needs to be expeditious, but ideally it should include a careful reinspection of the perineum at 24 hours of age when there is evidence of a perineal fistula, indicating a low lesion. Additionally, the passage of air or meconium in the urine of a boy will confirm a rectourinary fistula of a high lesion. During this interval the infant can be more thoroughly evaluated. Inspection of the perineum for a projected anal orifice that responds to local stimulation suggests an intact external component of the muscle complex. Radiographic evaluation of the sacral spine may demonstrate anomalies, which may imply impaired innervation of the pelvic musculature. Genitourinary evaluation by ultrasound is especially important in high-type imperforate anus where 35% to 50% of babies will have associated urinary tract findings that may be life-threatening.

Management

The general principles of management depend on accurate neonatal diagnosis: primary immediate or early perineal anoplasty without colostomy for low-type imperforate anus and neonatal colostomy followed by a delayed pull-through with colostomy closure at a third operation for high or intermediate imperforate anus. Either a loop colostomy or a colostomy whose ends are purposefully divided to separate fecal from urinary streams in the presence of a rectourinary fistula and renal anomalies is preferred.

The definitive reconstruction of high-type imperforate anus can be accomplished by a variety of pull-through

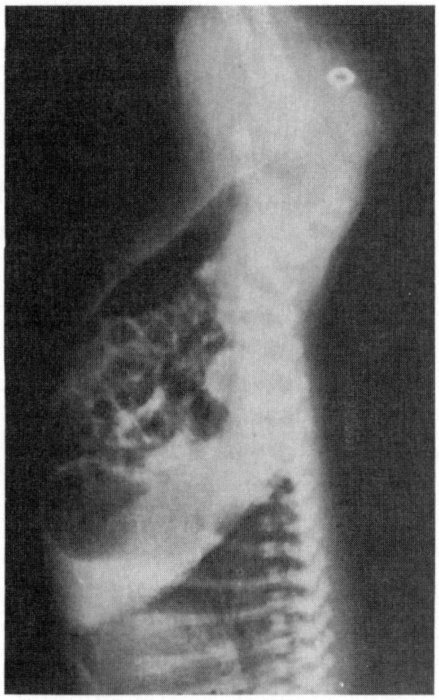

FIGURE 23-16 Lateral radiograph of a baby taken after the infant was inverted for several minutes, showing distance from the perineum (radiopaque marker) to end of atretic, air-filled rectum. (From Liechty RD, Soper RT: *Synopsis of surgery,* ed 5, St Louis, 1985, Mosby.)

procedures.[16] In cloacal anomalies the midline sagittal anorectoplasty has the advantage of meticulously identifying all aspects of the pelvic muscle complex, separation of the rectum from any aberrant connections, sizing or tapering the rectum to fit the available muscle complex, and reconstruction of a urethra and vagina under direct anatomic visualization.[44]

The measured results of imperforate anus repair include reconstruction of a "normal anatomy" for urinary, genital, and rectal tracts as seen at operation relative to the musculature and as visualized by perineal inspection and electrical stimulation. Patients with low anomalies should both appear normal and have normal continence. However, patients with intermediate or high lesions fare less well in relation to voluntary bowel control, soiling, constipation, and diarrhea[34]; and classically they have followed a one-third rule: one third have normal stool control, one third have occasional soiling, and one third are incontinent. With careful attention to operative detail, the results can be expected to be somewhat better, but a significant volitional-maturity factor is involved because continence usually improves with age. Rarely, patients will require permanent colostomy or have a limited life expectancy secondary to associated anomalies, usually of the urinary tract.[42]

PROBLEM: NECROTIZING ENTEROCOLITIS

Necrotizing enterocolitis (NEC) is a common gastrointestinal disorder that affects 2% to 8% of premature neonates in critical care units. Most of these infants are premature, with birth weights less than 2,500 g, but approximately 10% are term infants with normal birth weights. The age at onset of the disease ranges from 1 day to 3 months, with term infants usually developing symptoms earlier in life than premature infants.[29]

The etiology of NEC remains unknown. Many risk factors have been suggested including umbilical vessel catheters, asphyxia, hypothermia, and congenital heart disease, but controlled studies do not definitively implicate any of these. There is a strong association of NEC with feeding, and 90% to 95% of patients have been fed either formula, breast milk, or a combination of both before developing symptoms. Hyperosmolar formulas are thought to be more damaging than isosmolar feedings and they should be avoided. Breast milk may have some immunoprotective properties due to passively transmitted factors such as IgA.

NEC may occur in epidemics, suggesting that an infectious agent may be etiologic; however, no specific agent has been consistently cultured in NEC patients and blood cultures are positive in only 30% of infants. Bacteria must play some role in the development of NEC, likely in combination with some of the other factors noted earlier.[6,39,40]

Clinical Presentation

In mild forms of the disease, infant stools become seedy and flecked with blood while post-feeding residuals and mild abdominal distention develop. In more severe cases the stool may be frankly bloody and abdominal distention is obvious and may be accompanied by bilious vomiting. As the disease progresses, peritonitis may develop with abdominal wall erythema, edema, and palpable fixed loops of bowel. Shock and multisystem organ failure may follow with or without perforation.

Assessment

Laboratory findings are nonspecific and suggest an evolving pattern of sepsis. The white blood cell count may be either elevated or decreased. Thrombocytopenia is common and should be closely followed. Progressive acidosis also suggests severe disease.

Plain radiographs of the abdomen reveal pneumatosis intestinalis (gas within the bowel wall) and an ileus pattern in the majority of cases; it is the pneumatosis which makes the diagnosis definitive (Figure 23-17). Gas may also be present in the portal vein, a finding which is not itself an indication for operative intervention. Free intraperitoneal air signifies intestinal perforation and is an absolute indication for operation.

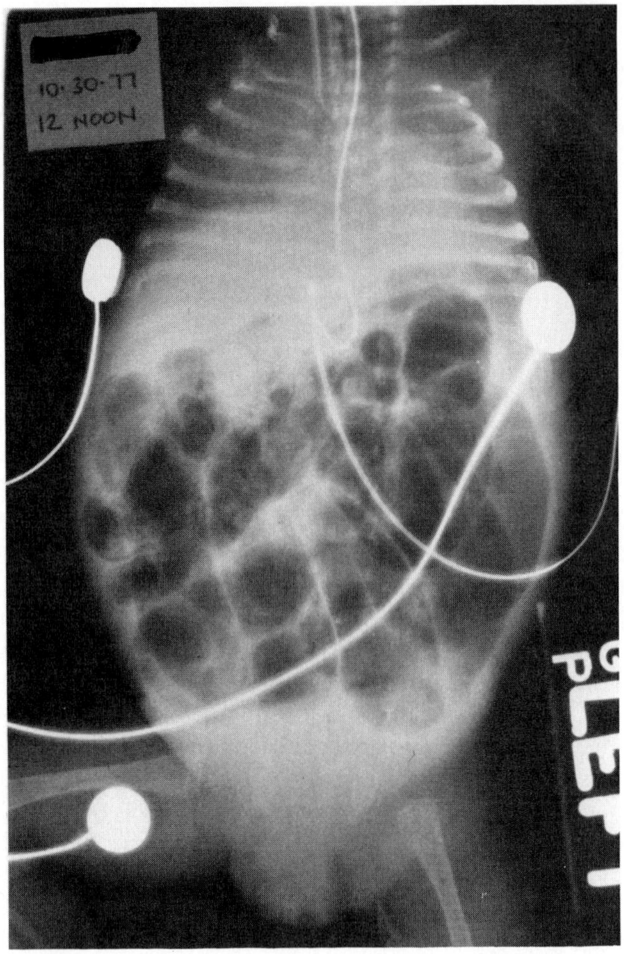

FIGURE 23-17 Abdominal radiograph of a patient with advanced necrotizing enterocolitis. There is a pattern consistent with ileus, and pneumatosis intestinalis (intramural intestinal air) is present in several areas, most easily seen in the right lower quadrant.

Management

Most patients with neonatal necrotizing enterocolitis respond successfully to medical management if begun early. Treatment includes bowel rest, suction decompression of the stomach, broad-spectrum antibiotics to cover both aerobic and anaerobic organisms, intravenous fluids to expand intravascular volume, and respiratory support as needed.

Operative intervention is required when signs of parietal peritonitis develop or for perforation. The clinical evidence of peritonitis may be any or all of the following: (1) physical signs of peritonitis, such as increasing abdominal tenderness, abdominal rigidity, and erythema and edema of the abdominal wall; (2) progressive deterioration despite treatment for sepsis; and (3) progressive or persistent metabolic acidosis despite treatment for sepsis. Operative therapy consists of resection of necrotic bowel with conservation of as much bowel as possible. All necrotic bowel should be resected with exteriorization of all marginally viable ends. Resection with primary anastomosis has been reported, but is not commonly performed. If clinical improvement ensues, the child should be returned to the operating room in 3 to 4 days for the placement of a central line for parenteral nutrition. After 10 to 14 days of antibiotics and parenteral nutrition, refeeding is started and slowly advanced using an elemental diet. Before the take down of any stomas all distal bowel must be studied for the presence of NEC ischemia-induced strictures.[9,29]

The overall survival of patients undergoing operation for NEC is 60% to 70%. The major early morbidity is related to complications of prematurity; the morbidity in long-term survivors is short gut syndrome, especially in infants requiring extensive resection.[1,53,54,63,64] These patients experience growth retardation and the hepatotoxic effects of prolonged parenteral alimentation.

PROBLEM: INTUSSUSCEPTION

Intussusception most commonly occurs between 2 months and 2 years of age. The pathophysiology involves telescoping of one segment of bowel, the intussusceptum, into another segment of bowel, the intussuscipiens, most commonly the terminal ileum into the right colon. Ninety-five percent of intussusceptions are idiopathic and do not have a pathologic lead point such as a polyp, hemangioma, Meckel's diverticulum, or even a lymphoma. Most idiopathic intussusceptions are ileocolic intussusceptions and are frequently associated with a preceding viral illness, often caused by an adenovirus.

Clinical Presentation

Classically, a child in the appropriate age range will exhibit sudden onset of crampy abdominal pain. Between episodes of drawing up legs and fussing, the child looks well and behaves normally. As the disease progresses, bilious vomiting and currant jelly stools develop. Not infrequently after several hours such children become quiet, have reduced responsiveness, and stare into space. On physical examination a mass may be palpable in the abdomen. Overt signs of peritonitis may not develop even in cases where the intussusceptum has become gangrenous because it is surrounded by the distal bowel segment.

Assessment

A high index of suspicion in children with an appropriate history is necessary. Plain abdominal films are often nonspecific, but they may demonstrate a mass effect in the

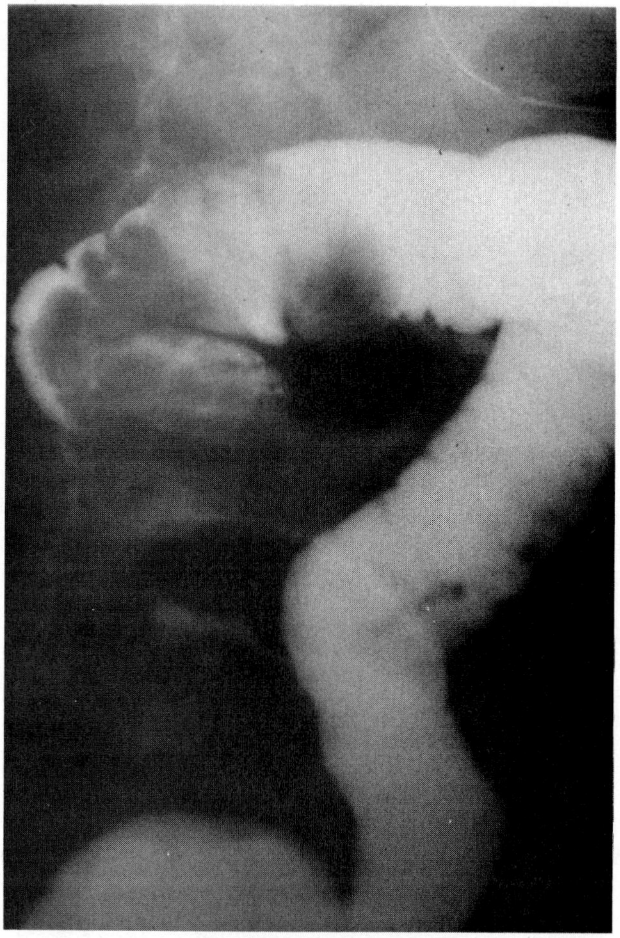

FIGURE 23-18 Barium enema radiograph demonstrating the "spring-coil" sign of an intussusception located near the hepatic flexure of the colon.

right abdomen. A contrast enema, either air or radiopaque material, is diagnostic and, in about two thirds of cases, therapeutic, resulting in pneumatic or hydrostatic reduction of the intussusception (Figure 23-18). A barium enema must be performed with careful technique with the column of barium being raised no more than 3 feet above the patient to avoid the risk of perforation. The more recently devised air enema has proven equally, if not more, effective, and theoretically the air decreases the risk of peritoneal contamination if perforation occurs. In the presence of peritonitis, no therapeutic enema should be performed, and the child should be taken directly to the operating room.

Management

The child with intussusception should be treated like any other child with an intestinal obstruction, that is, admitted to the hospital and hydrated with intravenous fluids. If the enema is not successful in reducing the intussusception, immediate operative reduction is indicated. At operation the intussusception is reduced by applying pressure along the distal segment rather than traction on the proximal segment. If the reduced bowel does not appear viable, it should be resected. A primary anastomosis can be performed with antibiotic coverage. The recurrence rate of any idiopathic intussusception is about 8% to 10% following enema reduction and 2% to 3% when reduced by operation. The overall prognosis in these children is good.

Lead points occur in 5% to 8% of all cases of intussusception. Although a Meckel's diverticulum is the most common lead point, other potential lead points include polyps and even small bowel lymphomas. The latter are more common in the older patient.

PROBLEM: INTESTINAL DUPLICATION

Duplications of the intestinal tract may occur anywhere from the pharynx to the rectum. About three fourths of all duplications occur in the small intestine, particularly in the ileum. Duplications appear on the mesenteric side of the gastrointestinal tract and are usually closely adherent to the parent bowel. They may be cystic or tubular, communicating or noncommunicating (Figure 23-19). They have a complete muscle coat of both the inner circular and outer longitudinal muscle and have an alimentary mucous membrane lining.

Clinical Presentation

Duplications may be entirely asymptomatic or they may obstruct the bowel, become inflamed, or perforate. Both intussusception and segmental bowel volvulus may be caused by duplications.

Management

The treatment of duplications is operative. Usually duplications involve only a short segment of bowel, and the simplest treatment is resection of the duplication with the adjacent segment of bowel followed by reanastomosis. Duplications may involve long segments of bowel, even rarely the entire small intestine. When resection of the duplication and the adjacent normal bowel in continuity would result in short bowel syndrome, the appropriate surgical approach is an endointestinal stripping of the mucosa of the duplication. This approach allows the normal bowel to be left in place, preserving normal bowel length.

PROBLEM: MECKEL'S DIVERTICULUM

A Meckel's diverticulum occurs in 2% of the population approximately 2 feet proximal to the ileocecal valve as a partial persistence of a portion of the embryonic omphalomesenteric duct. Most are asymptomatic, but in a diverticulum containing ectopic tissue—stomach or pancreas—a diverticulitis may occur, or gastric acid output may produce an adjacent ileal ulcer with gastrointestinal bleeding. Such ectopic gastric tissue may be visualized by a technetium pertechnetate scan. Operative resection is indicated for such a symptomatic diverticulum.

PROBLEM: APPENDICITIS

Appendicitis must be considered in the differential diagnosis of any child with abdominal pain. Acute appendicitis is the most common surgical emergency in childhood, and the diagnosis challenges even the most astute and experienced clinician.

A

B

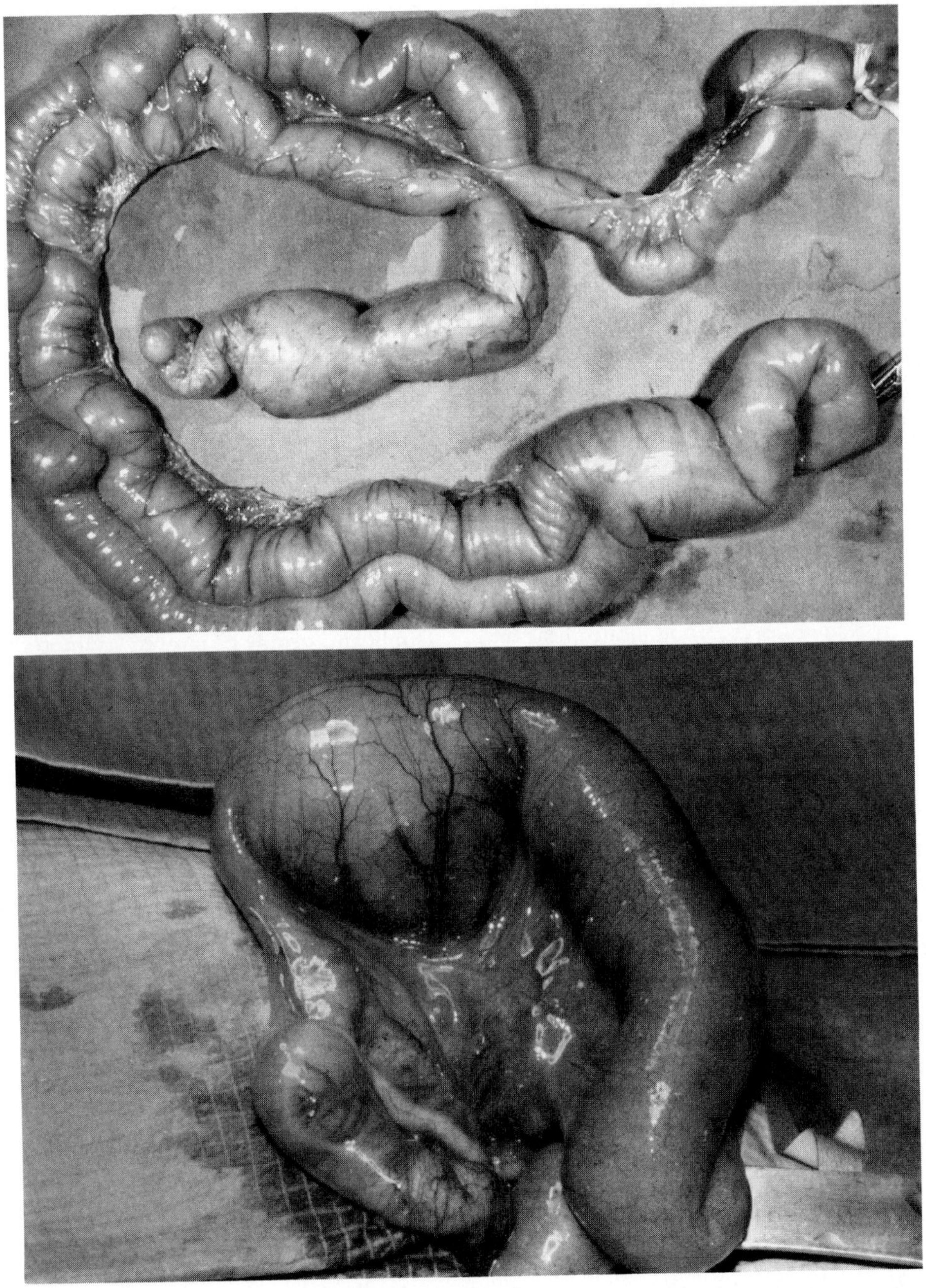

FIGURE 23-19 **A,** Small bowel tubular duplication. **B,** Small bowel cystic duplication demonstrating its mesenteric-side location.

Clinical Presentation

The clinical presentation of appendicitis may be quite protean, and the diagnosis is especially difficult in younger children. In children under 4 years of age, perforation is a common finding at the time of diagnosis. The peak incidence of appendicitis in the pediatric population is 6 to 10 years of age.

The classic patient with appendicitis presents with a several hour history of vague periumbilical pain, which shifts to the right lower quadrant and becomes a steady aching pain. Anorexia and vomiting follow shortly after the onset of pain. A low-grade fever of 38 to 38.5°C is common.

On physical examination the child will have tenderness to percussion and to palpation localized to the right lower quadrant. This finding is frequently accompanied by involuntary guarding of the muscles in the right lower quadrant. The child must be relaxed and cooperative for an optimal examination to be made, and the examiner should be gentle and attempt to distract the child with conversation. Other findings include tenderness on rectal examination, along with discomfort elicited by various leg movements (psoas sign, obturator sign).

Assessment

Although the diagnosis is primarily a clinical one based on history and physical examination, laboratory studies may also be helpful. Mild elevation of the white blood cell count and a left shift frequently are present, and a urinalysis should be normal. Abdominal plain films are helpful if the diagnosis is not clinically obvious, a calcified fecalith being found in 12% of patients with appendicitis. Other less specific signs of right lower quadrant inflammation may also be seen. Ultrasound examination may be helpful in making the diagnosis of simple acute appendicitis, but its value is greater when excluding pathology in adjacent organs, such as an ovarian cyst in the female. It may also demonstrate a right lower quadrant mass or abscess in a patient with a ruptured appendix. Selected use of a barium enema study may reveal evidence of cecal deformity and inflammation. Any child in whom appendicitis is suspected should be admitted to the hospital for observation, and serial abdominal examinations should be performed until the diagnosis can be confirmed or excluded.

The patient with a ruptured appendix may present with a high fever, a markedly elevated white blood cell count, and peritonitis, sometimes with diffuse and poorly localizing abdominal tenderness. The history of the illness is very helpful in making the diagnosis. Abdominal films may show a mass effect or localized ileus in the right lower quadrant or a small bowel obstruction (see Chapter 32).

Management

Patients with acute appendicitis are treated by appendectomy. Patients with a ruptured appendix and diffuse peritonitis require extensive fluid resuscitation including bolus infusions of 10 to 30 ml/kg of intravenous fluids to establish adequate urine output before operation.

Occasionally, patients with a perforated appendix present with a localized abscess in the right lower quadrant. This abscess may be treated conservatively with antibiotics or antibiotics with percutaneous drainage. A subsequent interval appendectomy is then performed approximately 6 to 8 weeks after initial presentation.

The most frequent complications of appendicitis are recurrent abscess, most commonly in the pelvis, and adhesive intestinal obstruction. There is a slightly higher incidence of infertility in the female who has had either simple appendicitis or a ruptured appendix as compared with the general population.

BILIARY SYSTEM

PROBLEM: BILIARY ATRESIA

The most common type of neonatal jaundice is either physiologic or infectious in etiology, and surgical causes are rare. Biliary atresia, a progressive intrahepatic and extrahepatic bile duct obliterative disease occurs rarely in but 1 in 15,000 newborns, an incidence which may be higher in Asian countries.

Biliary atresia classically has been described as correctable or uncorrectable depending on whether or not a portion of the proximal extrahepatic bile ducts was patent—a finding which would permit operative diversion of the "obstructive jaundice" into the gastrointestinal tract. In contrast, uncorrectable biliary atresia represents a completely obliterated extrahepatic biliary tree treatable only by diversion at the hepatic porta, by the so-called portoenterostomy or Kasai operation. Additionally, Alagilles syndrome represents a biliary hypoplasia, an entity characterized by an association with pulmonary valvular stenosis and elfin faces, but not typified by a severe hepatopathy in the neonatal period. The typical liver pathologic picture of biliary atresia is a background of fibrosis in a green and contracted liver which demonstrates cholestasis and bile duct proliferation.

Clinical Presentation

When neonatal jaundice persists beyond the first 2 weeks of life or if a direct fraction conjugated hyperbilirubinemia is present, a thorough and rapid evaluation must be performed.

Assessment

Cholestasis secondary to biliary atresia is not associated with bile excretion into the duodenum; therefore an analysis of duodenal content by tube aspiration or nuclear medicine hepatobiliary imaging with technitium iminodiacetic acid will usually distinguish obstructive from hepatic parenchymal jaundice. Ultrasound images of the liver in biliary atresia will demonstrate a contracted or even absent gallbladder. Most diagnoses, however, depend on liver biopsy and the specific findings noted earlier. It is necessary at times to proceed to laparotomy with operative cholangiography to finally determine whether the extrahepatic bile duct is patent and amenable to operative correction.

Management

With the confirmation of the diagnosis of biliary atresia, early operative intervention is warranted; if operative exploration confirms the diagnosis of biliary atresia, then a portoenterostomy is indicated. Only in the patient with end-stage liver disease whose diagnosis of biliary atresia was delayed beyond 6 months of age should portoenterostomy not be performed. In such a case a primary liver transplant would be the preferred procedure. At portoenterostomy, originally described by Kasai in Japan in the 1950s, the scarred remnant of the extrahepatic biliary tree is identified and traced proximally to the porta hepatis just lateral to the hepatic artery and anterior to the portal vein. At that point the obliterated and fibrotic duct system is excised in hopes that the portal plate will contain microscopic-sized ducts capable of serving as excretory channels. A limb of jejunum fashioned into a Roux-en-Y configuration is most often chosen for the neoduct excretory channel, and a nonrefluxing intussusception valve may be constructed in it. Postoperatively, antibiotics may play a role in minimizing cholangitis, and corticosteroid administration may minimize scar obliteration of the biliary ductules at the portal plate. Cholegogues may be useful in enhancing bile flow, and appropriate nutrients are required to minimize fat malabsorption.

The cessation of bile flow and recurrent cholangitis are the most common complications after portoenterostomy. In patients undergoing operation before 3 months of age, it can be expected that from one third to one half will have prolonged excretion through their conduit, although a slowly evolving picture of biliary cirrhosis may follow. Older children do less well and early liver transplanation becomes a life-sustaining therapy.

PROBLEM: CHOLEDOCHAL CYST

Cystic dilatation of the biliary tree, predominantly extrahepatic but also intrahepatic, is classified into a number of variations, the most common of which are cystic dilatation of the common bile duct with or without dilatation of intrahepatic ducts (Figure 23-20). Presentation of a choledochal cyst will occur on in utero ultrasound as a cystic mass; as a coincidental finding when evaluating the neonate with obstructive jaundice; or in the older child as the classic triad of right upper quadrant pain, jaundice, and a palpable mass.

A choledochal cyst is a pseudocyst characterized by a fibrotic inflammatory wall and an ulcerated or absent mucosal lining. When located in intrahepatic ducts, such cysts are referred to as Caroli's disease. In this location or when repeated episodes of infection and biliary obstruction have occurred, cholangitis and adjacent liver parenchymal injury is the rule. Because of the cystic nature of this disease, ultrasonography is the diagnostic procedure of choice.

Classically, choledochal cysts were treated by cyst enterostomy. However, recurrent cholangitis was common, and in the face of a 20-fold greater incidence of biliary carcinoma in a choledochal cyst, the preferred treatment has become cyst excision with biliary reconstruction by choledochojejunostomy of the Roux-en-Y type. Careful identification and protection of the orifice of the pancreatic ducts are mandatory.

The result of treatment of an extrahepatic choledochal cyst is excellent. Cyst excision minimizes the incidence of cholangitis, pancreatitis, biliary cancer, and bile duct obstruction. In contrast, Caroli's disease may be characterized by recurring bouts of cholangitis, eventually progressing to end-stage liver disease, and such patients may require liver transplantation.

PROBLEM: GALLBLADDER DISEASE

Though uncommon, acalculous cholecystitis and hydrops of the gallbladder occur in critically ill children. The evaluation of jaundice in such acutely ill patients requires an abdominal ultrasound for diagnosis, and if signs of progressive gallbladder distention or inflammation develop then cholecystostomy or cholecystectomy is warranted.

Calculous cholecystitis with or without choledocholithiasis is uncommon in children, but is more likely to be problematic in children with an underlying propensity for hemolysis, namely, sickle cell disease, spherocytosis, and thalassemia. In the face of documented cholecystitis, cholecystectomy, either by laparoscopic or open technique, is warranted. In patients with known stones and a propensity for hemolysis, cholecystectomy is also indicated. However, if gallstones are found coincidentally in a child and have not produced symptoms, then sequential serial follow-up is the only therapy needed.

PROBLEM: PORTAL HYPERTENSION

Portal hypertension is discussed in detail elsewhere in this text (see Chapter 34). The most important distinc-

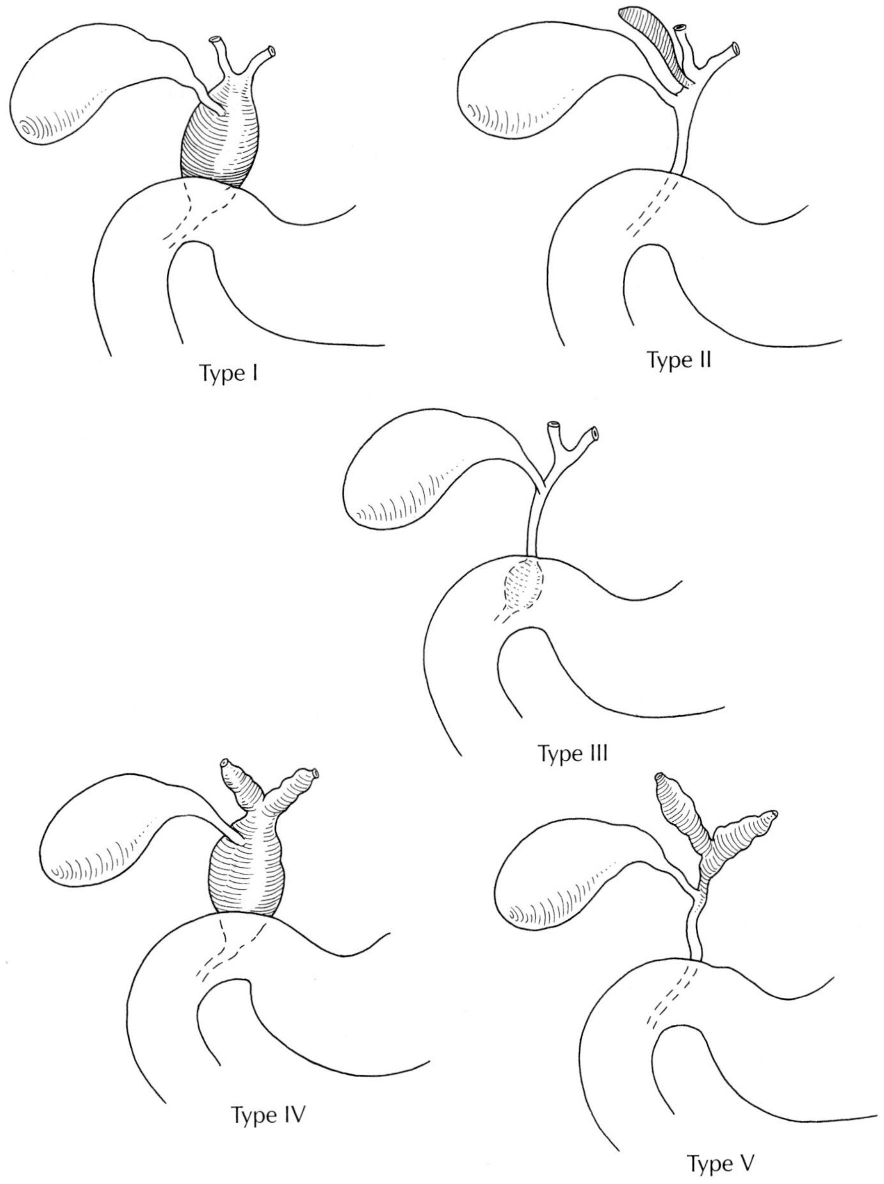

FIGURE 23-20 The five most commonly seen and identified varieties of choledochal cysts. The type I cystic dilatation of the common duct, with either complete or incomplete duct obstruction, is the most frequently encountered anatomy. (From O'Neill JA Jr, Templeton JM Jr, Schnaufer L et al: Recent experience with choledochal cyst, *Ann Surg* 205:533, 1987.)

tion to make about pediatric portal hypertension is that almost half of all pediatric cases are a result of portal vein obstruction in infancy secondary to omphalitis or umbilical vein catheterization. The resulting vein thrombosis creates portal hypertension; but over time the resulting cavernous transformation of the portal vein, collateral channel formation, and recanalization lowers portal pressures. In most cases, spontaneous improvement occurs as the child ages. In those cases in which such improvement does not occur, the cavernous change precludes portocaval shunting. In such patients the preferred decompressing operation is either a distal splenorenal shunt, a mesocaval shunt, or an esophagogastric variceal ligation procedure. Because of the slow but continued spontaneous improvement in portal hypertension in children with extrahepatic portal vein obstruction, variceal sclerotherapy has received broad application.

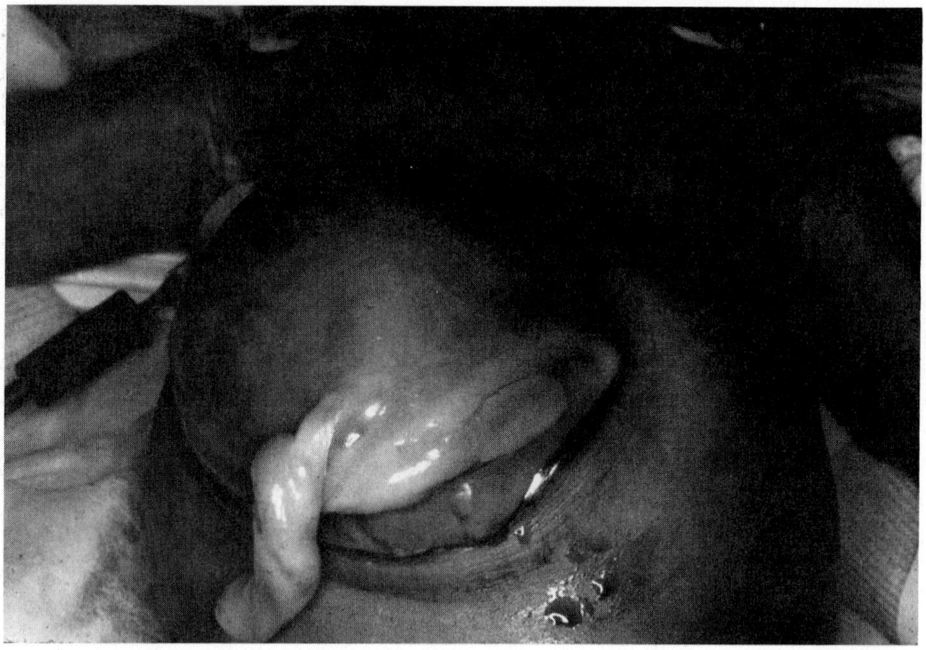

FIGURE 23-21 A patient with an omphalocele abdominal wall defect. The membrane-covered midline defect may be variable in size. The contents beneath the sac included the liver in this patient.

ABDOMINAL WALL DEFORMITIES

PROBLEM: OMPHALOCELE AND GASTROSCHISIS

Omphalocele ("hollow navel") and gastroschisis ("belly separation") occur at an incidence of 1 per 10,000 to 20,000 live births. Although there is a suggestion that these two entities represent variations of a single process, they have unique and distinctive features.

An omphalocele is a midline, membrane-covered defect of variable size (Figure 23-21). Small lesions less than 4 cm in diameter are often called hernias of the umbilical cord. Moderate or large omphaloceles in addition to representing a variable deficiency of skin, subcutaneous tissue, muscle, and fascia may also be associated with a smaller abdominal cavity. Omphaloceles may be isolated or they may be associated with chromosomal anomalies (trisomy 13 or trisomy 18), systemic syndromes (Beckwith-Wiedemann, prune-belly), or regional upper midline defects including ectopia cordis anomalies of the chest wall, pericardium, diaphragm and heart, or regional lower midline defects including vesicointestinal fissure and cloacal exstrophy.

In contrast, gastroschisis is a right paramedian uncovered defect of 2 to 4 cm in diameter with a skin bridge at times separating the defect from the umbilical cord (Figure 23-22). The amniotic-fluid bathed bowel has a typical thickened and foreshortened appearance with covering by a thickened peel. Associated anomalies are infrequent in contrast to omphalocele (10% versus 35% to 40%) and consist largely of intestinal atresia and the posttreatment hypoperistalsis syndrome.

The embryologic origin of these abdominal wall defects occurs between the fifth and twelfth gestational week at a time when the somatopleure folds and joins to form the abdominal wall, the myotomes grow and fuse to form abdominal wall musculature, and the body stalk remains enlarged to receive and hold an elongating midgut, which eventually will retract back into the abdominal cavity, rotate, and fix as development is complete. An omphalocele develops when the body stalk persists or has not been replaced by a lateral mesodermal ingrowth. Gastroschisis may represent a local abdominal wall vascular injury with a secondary mesenchymal damage.

An alternate explanation is that gastroschisis may be the result of an in-utero rupture of the membrane covering of a hernia of the umbilical cord. Genetic and teratogenic influences have been implicated in these abdominal wall deformities. Gastroschisis more likely occurs in the first-born baby of a younger mother. The baby is more likely to be premature, and omphaloceles are significantly more likely to be found in the presence of associated anomalies.

Clinical Presentation

It is commonplace that both omphalocele and gastroschisis are diagnosed by in-utero ultrasound. If other

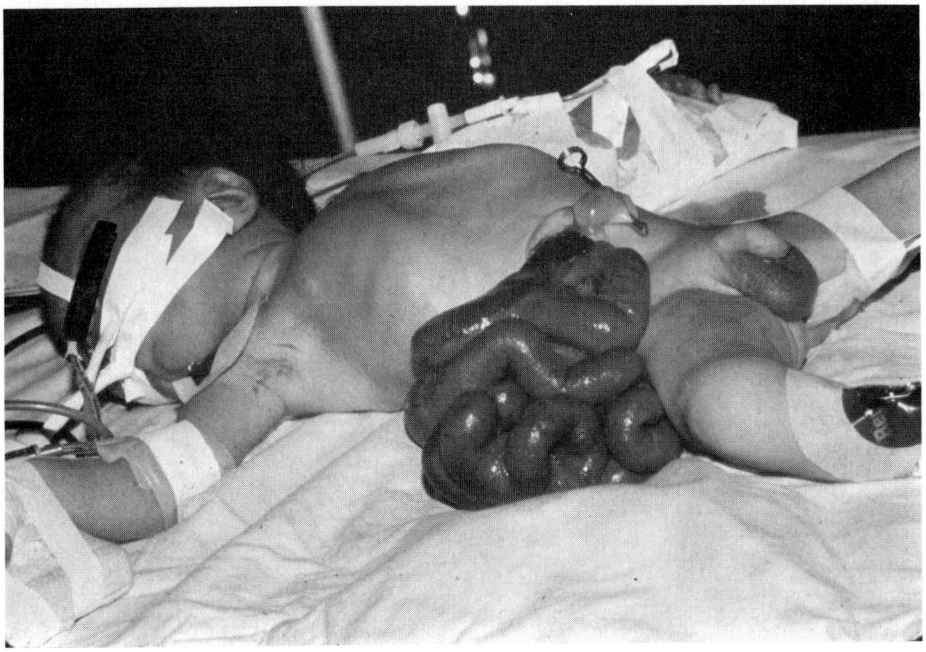

FIGURE 23-22 A patient with a gastroschisis abdominal wall deformity. The right paramedian defect is 2 to 4 cm in diameter, and through it herniates varied lengths of uncovered intestine.

anomalies are not detected and if fetal growth is appropriate, then there is advantage to carry the pregnancy to as close to term as is possible.

Management

At birth the newborn with an abdominal wall defect should be kept warm, the omphalocele membrane or the uncovered gastroschisis bowel should be kept moistened with saline, and the gastroschisis bowel must be supported in a position that will not permit a kink or twist of the mesentery, which in turn could impair mesenteric circulation. Prompt operative treatment of the defect should follow.

Treatment options for omphalocele may be categorized into one of four choices: primary fascial closure of small defects usually after excision of the membrane, skin closure only over an intact omphalocele membrane, application of a topical antiseptic agent to the membrane to produce a surface that will either secondarily epithelialize or serve as a bed to accept a skin graft, or application of a Silastic silo that can be used to slowly reduce the protruding viscera into the abdominal cavity followed by a delayed closure of abdominal wall fascia (Figure 23-23).

Gastroschisis may be treated by abdominal wall stretching, visceral reduction and fascial edge closure, or application of a temporary Silastic silo. The prolonged postoperative ileus also makes insertion of a gastrostomy tube desirable. After the bowel is inspected for the presence of an associated atresia and after excessive air and meconium are evacuated from the stomach, small bowel, and large bowel, mechanical abdominal wall stretching increases the cavity space lost with "domain loss" by the protruding viscera. As the viscera—usually stomach, small bowel, and large bowel—are reduced, the appropriate intraabdominal pressure may be gauged by measuring intragastric, intravesical, or intracaval pressures. Rarely, a small prosthetic patch will effectively fill a fascial defect before approximating skin. Usually, if the viscera cannot be safely reduced, a temporary "silo" should be applied and thereafter the viscera gradually reduced.

Postoperatively, patients with a primarily closed omphalocele will begin enteral feeds early because bowel functional recovery is rapid. In contrast, patients with a primarily closed gastroschisis characteristically have prolonged intestinal nonfunction for several weeks. Both patient groups after a staged repair have a prolonged interval of recovery before feeding can resume.

The outcome of patients with small- to medium-sized omphalocele deformities is uniformly good, limited only by associated anomalies that occur in about one third of patients. Patients with large hepatomphaloceles and the need for a staged repair offer a real challenge. In addition to associated anomalies, other factors that contribute to morbidity include infection secondary to the prosthetic silo, intraabdominal organ compression potentially producing ischemic injury, and respiratory fail-

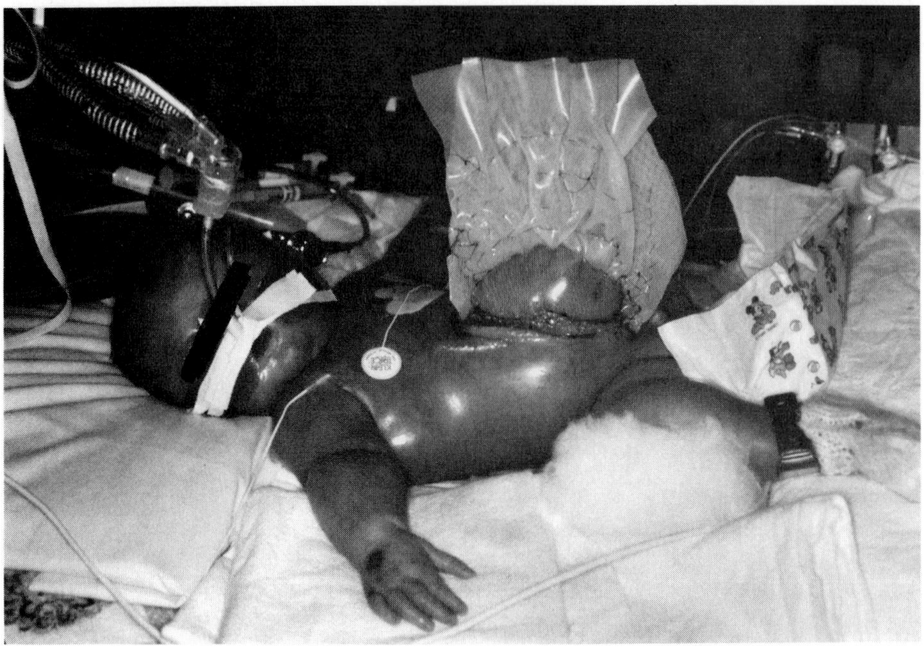

FIGURE 23-23 A patient with "Silastic-silo" in place for the staged management of an abdominal wall defect. The suture lines across the Silastic indicate the several reductions of herniated contents back into their intraabdominal location.

ure secondary to the elevation of the diaphragm due to increased intraabdominal pressure. At times reduction of a protruding liver may produce angulation of the suprahepatic inferior vena cava, which adversely influences cardiac output. In contrast to these problems are practical issues related to obstetrical recognition of a small omphalocele-hernia of the umbilical cord, where improper placement of the umbilical cord clamp may produce injury to the contents of the sac.

The results of the treatment of gastroschisis depend on the degree of intestinal injury-dysfunction, as well as on the ability to achieve primary abdominal wall closure. Patients undergoing staged repair have a more prolonged pattern of ileus, but those undergoing either primary or staged repair have an enhanced outcome by the early and aggressive use of total parenteral nutrition. If atresia complicates gastroschisis, an initial diverting stoma followed by a delayed reanastomosis is prudent. Except in the profoundly growth retarded baby, survival should exceed 90%.

VISIBLE AND PALPABLE LESIONS

A large portion of any pediatric surgeon's clinical practice is the diagnosis and management of visible and palpable lesions, the "lumps and bumps" of childhood. Generally it is easiest to consider these relative to the body region in which they occur.

Vascular Malformations

These "birthmarks" are abnormal collections of vascular channels either in or beneath the skin surface. They vary from flat, reddened discolorations at the base of the posterior neck, the "stork bite," to raised deeply reddened capillary hemangiomas, the so-called strawberry lesions (Figure 23-24). Both of these malformations are characterized by early progression followed by eventual fading; the residual after regression is minimally noticeable. Other hemangiomas may be formed of larger cystic channels (cavernous hemangiomas) or may be located largely beneath the dermis (hemangioendotheliomas). These lesions are not characterized by spontaneous regression. The port wine stain, purplish in hue and often found on the face, also does not spontaneously regress. Watchful waiting is the most acceptable approach to hemangiomas, although some progressing lesions are amenable to intralesional or systemic corticosteroid therapy, laser ablation, or conventional operative excision.

A lymphangioma is an abnormal collection of lymph channels and cysts and is most commonly found in the neck, chest wall, or axilla, but potentially found anywhere in the body. These lesions when composed of huge cystic components and when localized to the neck are also called a cystic hygroma (Figure 23-25). Lymphangiomas are spongy, irregular soft tissue masses, which when they involve the skin produce small punctate lym-

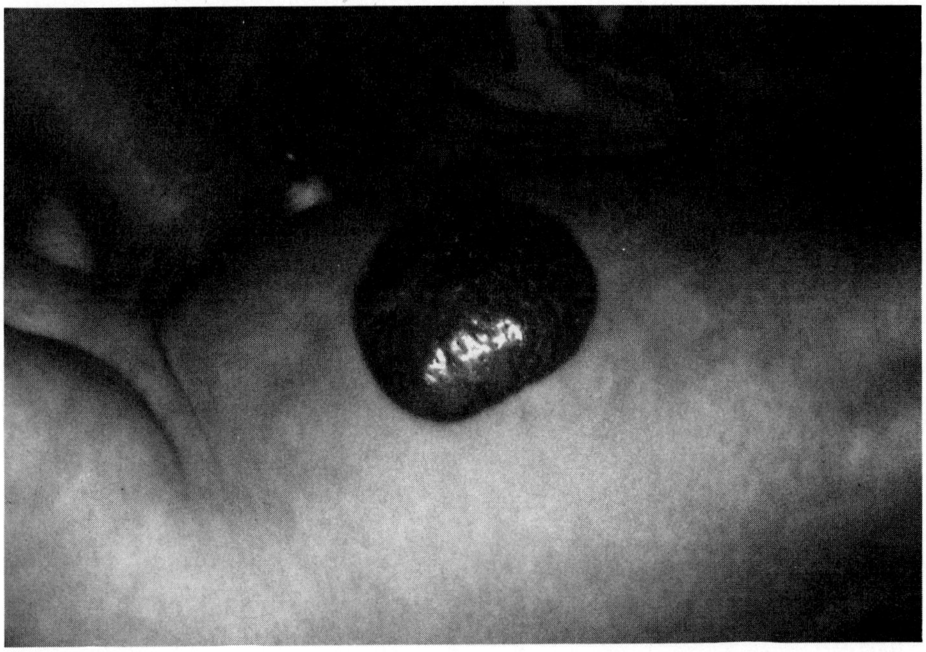

FIGURE 23-24 A patient with a capillary hemangioma of the abdominal wall. It is anticipated that this large lesion will undergo a pattern of spontaneous regression, leaving the patient with a flattened area of redundant skin in which the coloration will have nearly completely faded.

A

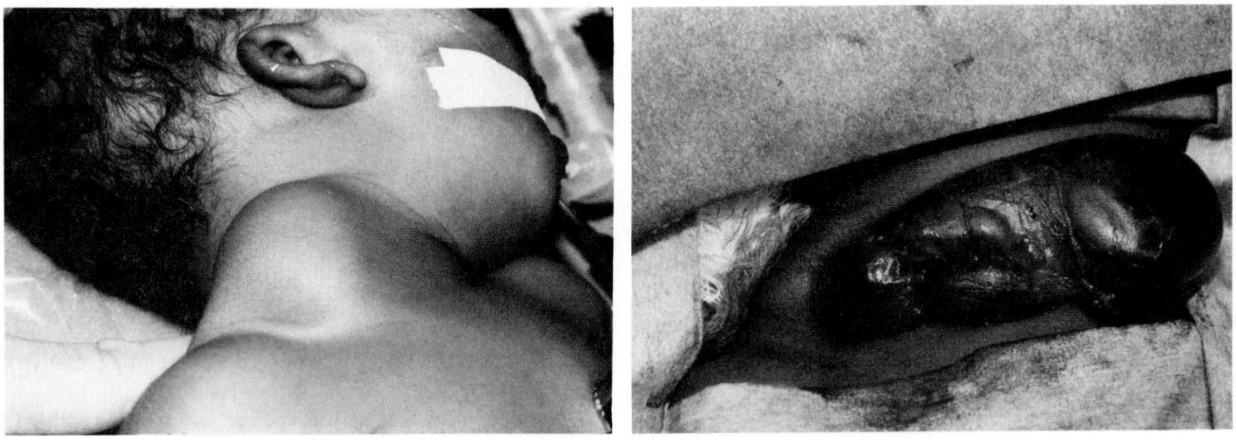

B

FIGURE 23-25 **A,** A young patient with a large cystic mass filling the right neck. **B,** The mass being excised; it is a multilocular cystic hygroma.

phectasias. They tend to grow into or enwrap adjacent normal structures. The gross appearance varies from a fine honeycomb to large clusters of grapes, and they are filled with a thin, yellow proteinaceous fluid. They are prone to secondary infection becoming firm, reddened, and tender; but most important they do not spontaneously regress. Lymphangiomas are optimally treated by nondestructive operative excision for prevention of infection and for relief of symptoms related to their position. Intralesional injection of sclerosing agents—chemical or bacterial products—may be selectively useful.

Mixed vascular lesions at times involve the extremities. The concomitant presence of arteriovenous malformations, hemangiomas, and lymphangiomas in an

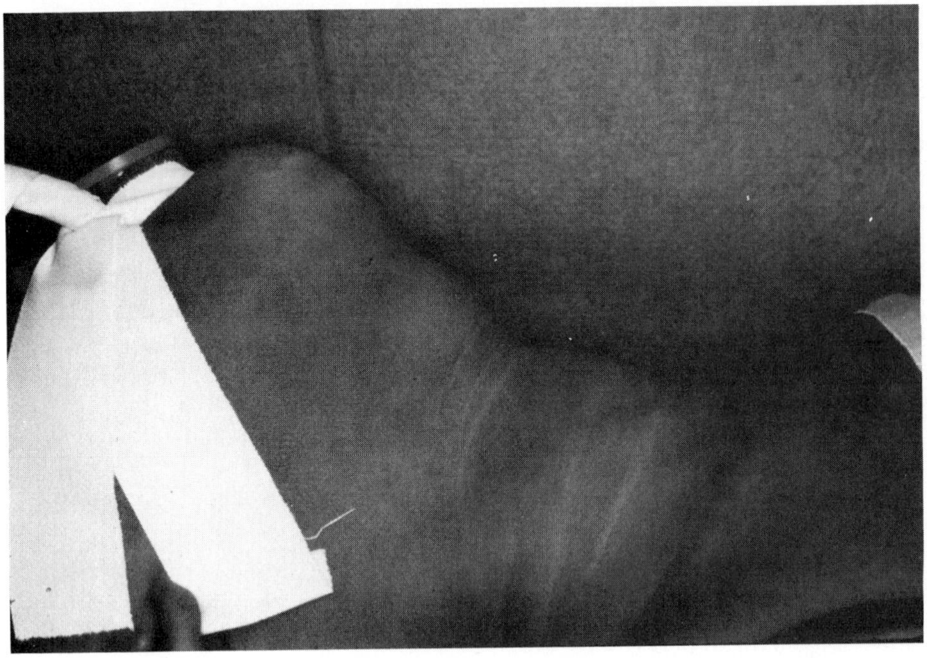

FIGURE 23-26 A child awaiting operation for a midline neck nodule located in the upper one third of the neck. This lesion is a thyroglossal duct cyst, a diagnosis proved at operation.

extremity may produce hyperemia and extremity overgrowth or pain and recurrent infections. Management of such problems must be individualized.

Face and Scalp

The most common lesion on the face and scalp in addition to a hemangioma is the soft tissue dermoid or epidermoid cyst. Discrete, circumscribed, and close to the skin, these lesions most commonly are found beneath the lateral aspect of the eyebrow or on the scalp. Because of their propensity for progressive growth and erosion of the underlying skull, excision is recommended. Preauricular sinuses are common, but unless associated with an underlying cyst that has been infected, they do not require excision.

Tongue-tie, a tight anterior frenulum of the tongue, may bind down the tongue tip, producing problems of mandibular dentition. Rarely does tongue-tie contribute to speech pathology. When the tongue-tie contributes to maldevelopment of the teeth, frenulotomy is indicated.

Neck

Lesions of the neck are best defined as midline or lateral. Classic midline neck lesions are an enlarged submental lymph node, dermoid cyst, and thyroglossal duct cyst. A thyroglossal duct cyst is a developmental remnant from the descent of the thyroid from its origin at the posterior third of the tongue to its typical neck site. Such lesions move with swallowing and protrusion of the tongue and lie at or above the notch of the thyroid cartilage (Figure 23-26). Their apparent deep fixation is secondary to an extension through the body of the hyoid bone to the base of the tongue. These cysts require excision for diagnosis and prevention of secondary infection. To prevent recurrence the resection must include the cyst and its proximally extending tract through the center of the hyoid bone (Sistrunk procedure).

The most common lateral neck lesion is an enlarged cervical lymph node (lymphadenopathy), which may be enlarged secondary to bacteriologic infection (suppurative lymphadenitis) most often due to a staphylococcal organism. Antibiotic therapy and occasionally aspiration or incision and drainage are needed for treatment. Lymphadenopathy may have protean additional causes including infections such as cat-scratch fever or tuberculosis as well as lymphoma. As a result an asymmetrically enlarged node may require excisional biopsy for diagnosis.

A soft tissue nodule along the anterior border of the sternocleidomastoid muscle often associated with a skin sinus represents a second branchial arch anomaly. If a sinus is present it will extend proximally and end in the tonsillar fossa coursing deeply in the neck between the external and internal carotid artery bifurcation (Figure 23-27). A first branchial arch anomaly usually lies in the submandibular triangle or over the angle of the mandible

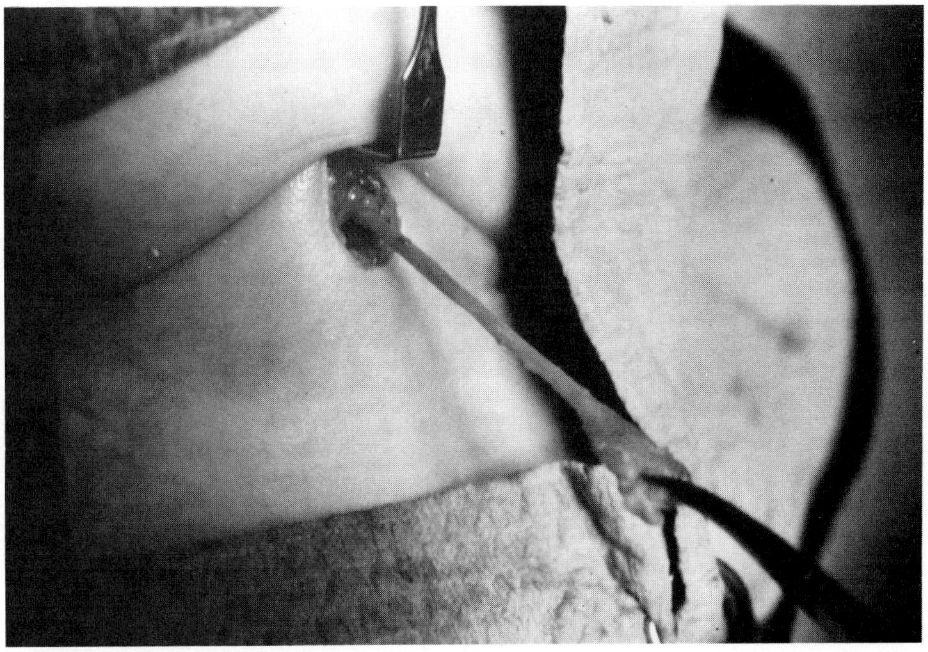

FIGURE 23-27 Excision of a second branchial arch cyst and sinus whose proximal tract extends between the branches of the carotid artery to end in the tonsillar fossa.

and a tract if present will lead to the external auditory canal. Branchial remnants may contain cartilage, there may be a cyst alone, or there may be a cyst and sinus. Excision is required to confirm the diagnosis, to prevent infection from the communicating sinus, and to prevent a carcinoma in situ in adulthood.

In the neonatal period a firm mass palpable in the body of the sternocleidomastoid muscle associated with a head-tilt toward the side of the lesion most typically represents torticollis (wry neck) (Figure 23-28). This mass is due to hemorrhage in the muscle secondary either to in utero positioning or to the delivery process. Incisional release of the scarred muscle was the historic treatment of choice, but passive and active range-of-motion exercises are almost uniformly effective in softening the contracture and restoring full head and neck range of motion, thus normalizing facial development.

Chest Wall

Breast enlargement in a neonate is common and is usually due to simple hypertrophy. This self-limited problem is likely secondary to the baby's exposure to transplacental or breast milk maternal estrogen, and no specific treatment is indicated. When a neonatal breast mass is associated with redness and tenderness, a staphylococcal breast abscess is the likely diagnosis, and incision and drainage coupled with antibiotic therapy is the preferred treatment. Gynecomastia, enlargement of the male breast, may be unilateral or bilateral. These lesions have no signs of overlying inflammation but they often are tender. Careful physical examination, which includes a testicular examination to screen for tumors, is mandatory. Observation is most often successful for this self-limited problem, but in selected patients a subcutaneous mastectomy is indicated for pain control and for psychologic support.

The most common breast tumor in a pediatric patient is a benign fibroadenoma. These firm, discrete masses vary from pea-sized to a tumor that replaces or distorts the entire breast. If they do not stabilize or get smaller, excision is indicated.

Pectus excavatum or funnel chest occurs secondary to an irregular overgrowth of costal cartilages between the ribs posteriorly and the sternum anteriorly (Figure 23-29). An apparent inner retraction of the sternum develops, which can compress the substernal heart and encroach on intrathoracic volume. It is difficult to document, but selected patients with pectus excavatum may develop a cardiorespiratory disability that can be relieved or prevented by pectus excavatum repair. In other patients supportive therapy only is needed.

In contrast pectus carinatum, pigeon chest, is a cosmetic deformity. It is amenable to cosmetic repair, ideally when longitudinal growth has been completed. Usually no functional disability results from this lesion. Other more rare chest wall lesions include Poland's syn-

A

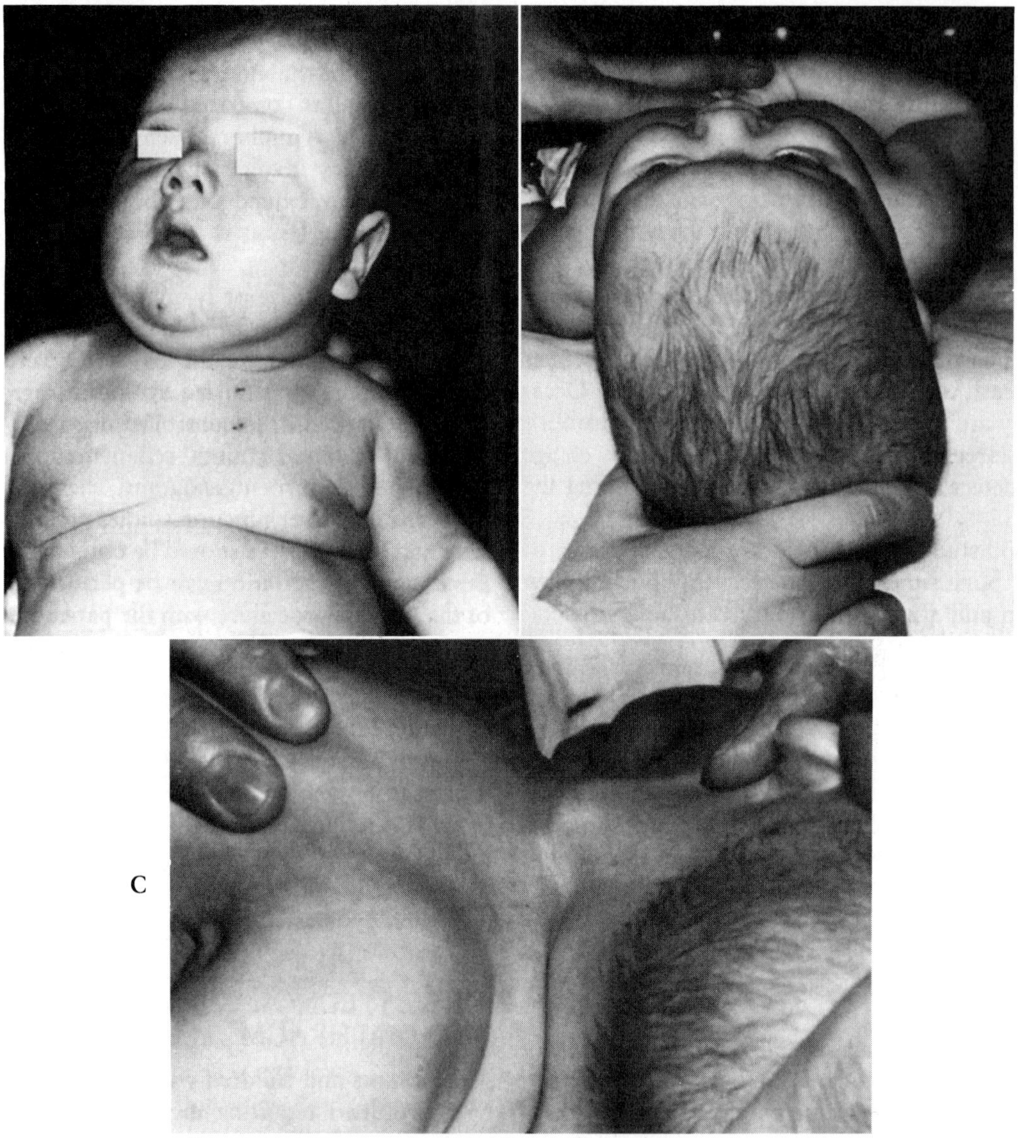

B

C

FIGURE 23-28 A, Marked facial asymmetry and skull molding secondary to a torticollis tumor of the left sternocleidomastoid muscle. B, The molding and obliquity of the anteroposterior diameter of the skull are seen when the face is placed in the straightforward position. C, The tight sternocleidomastoid "tumor" is both visible and palpable. (From Filston HC: *Surgical problems in children*, St Louis, 1982, Mosby.)

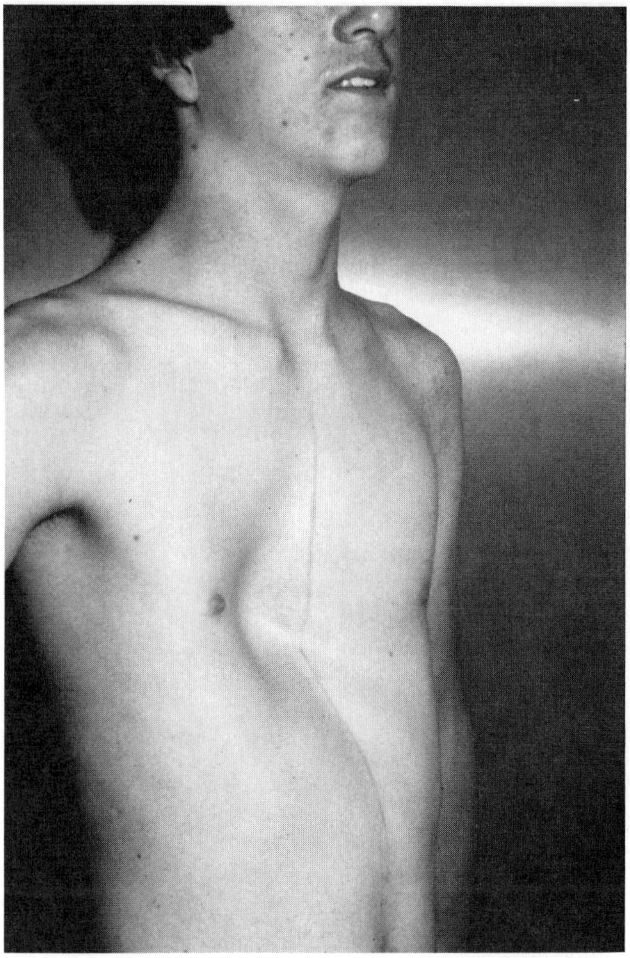

FIGURE 23-29 Patient with pectus excavatum. This funnel-chest deformity is typically asymmetric, with the depth of the defect to the right of the patient's midline.

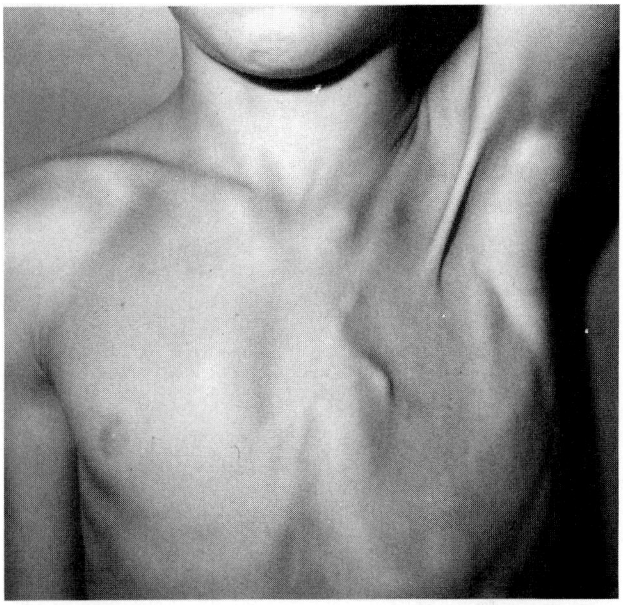

FIGURE 23-30 A patient with a left-sided Poland's syndrome characterized by deficiencies of the second, third, and fourth ribs as well as the overlying pectoralis major and minor muscles.

drome, a deficiency or absence of the pectoralis major and minor muscle and ribs 2, 3, and 4 (Figure 23-30). Ectopia cordis, the uncovered heart, is a still more rare problem for the neonate.

Umbilicus

Weeping lesions of the umbilicus may represent a granuloma, a patent urachus, or a patent omphalomesenteric remnant. An umbilical granuloma is a reddened protruding mass occurring at the site of separation of the umbilical cord clamp. They vary in size from 2 to 3 mm to 20 to 30 mm in diameter, and they are best treated by silver nitrate cauterization when small or cauterization and excision when large. A patent urachal remnant is more common in males and may be due to bladder outlet obstruction. An abdominal wall ultrasound may prove diagnostic, but a voiding cystourethrogram demonstrates not only the lesion in continuity with the dome of the bladder, but also the presence or absence of posterior urethral valves (Figure 23-31). A patent omphalomesenteric duct communicating with the terminal ileum at the site of a Meckel's diverticulum often drains a feculent material (Figure 23-32). Both of the latter umbilical lesions require excision at the time of operative umbilical exploration.

An umbilical hernia is secondary to a persistence of the umbilical ring. These lesions are more common in black children. In more than 80% of cases, the ring continues to contract after birth until it has closed. If closure has not occurred in boys by age 4 years and in girls by age 3 years, or if the ring exceeds 2 cm in diameter, operative closure is indicated. Umbilical herniorrhaphy prevents the unusual complications of incarceration, strangulation, and evisceration.

Midline fascial defects of several millimeter diameter through which preperitoneal fat may protrude are termed epiploceles. When symptomatic or enlarging, these defects should be closed. A true epigastric hernia is rare and is usually located in the immediate supraumbilical region. Repair is indicated. Separation of the bodies of the rectus abdominus muscles with resulting tubular protrusion of the widened midline is diastasis recti. No treatment is needed.

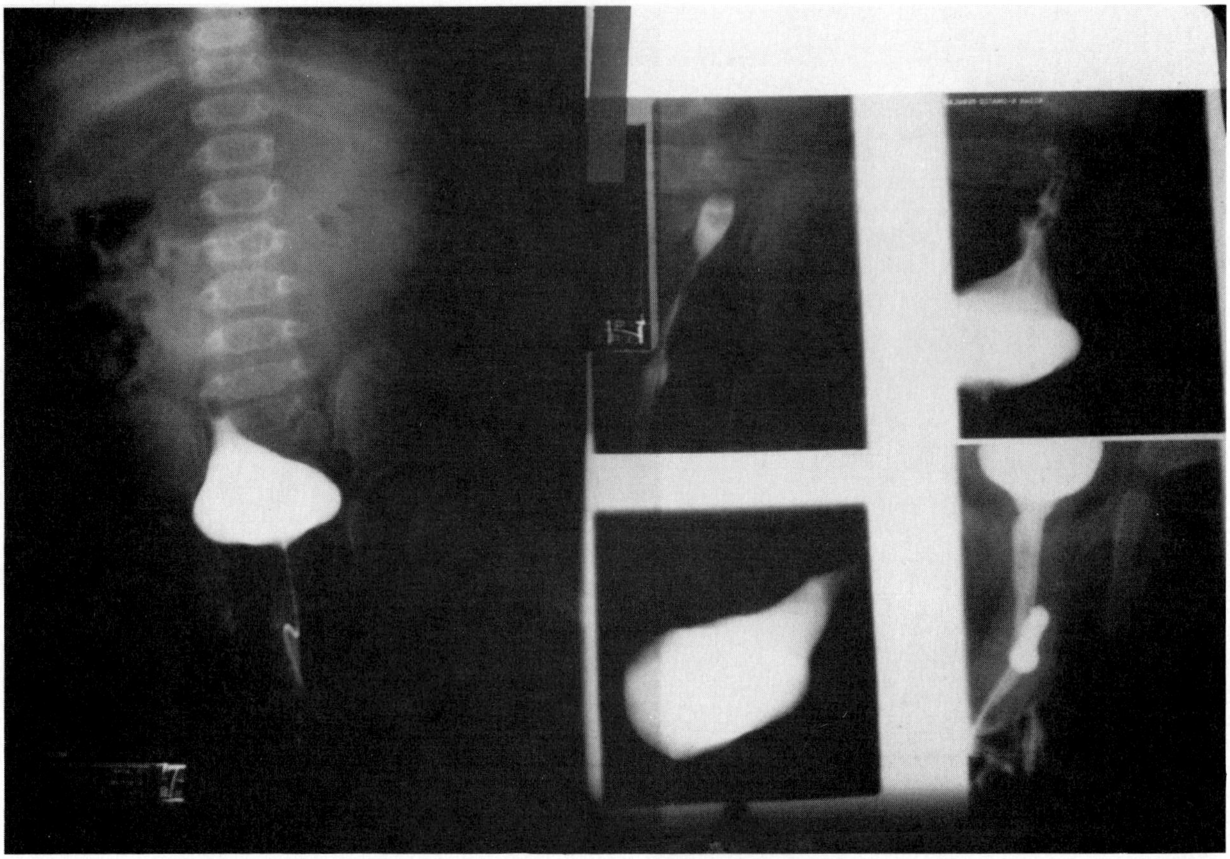

FIGURE 23-31 Voiding cystourethrogram demonstrating a urachal remnant extending from the dome of the urinary bladder.

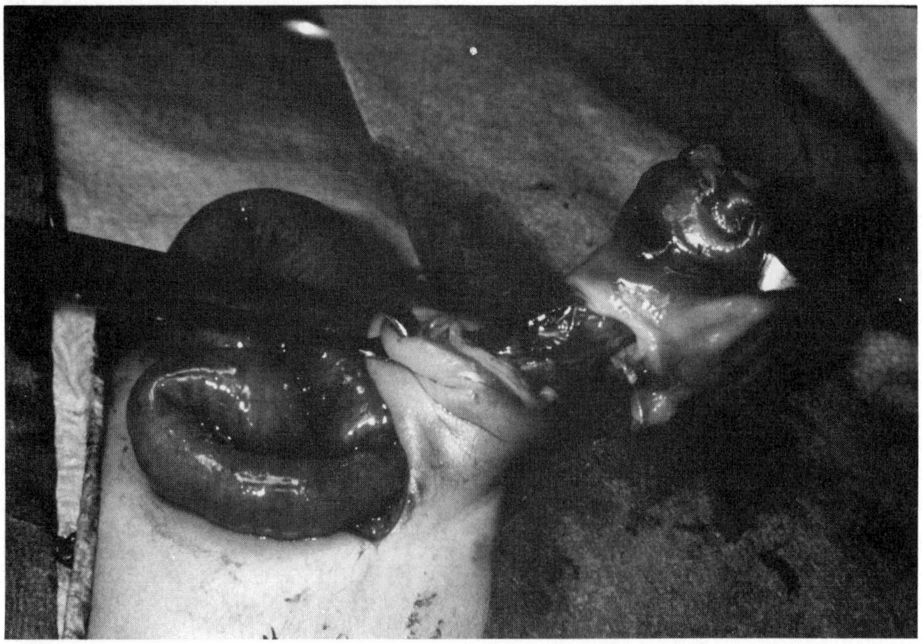

FIGURE 23-32 A patient with an omphalomesenteric duct connecting the terminal ileum with the umbilicus. Intestinal contents draining from the umbilicus suggests the presence of this anomaly.

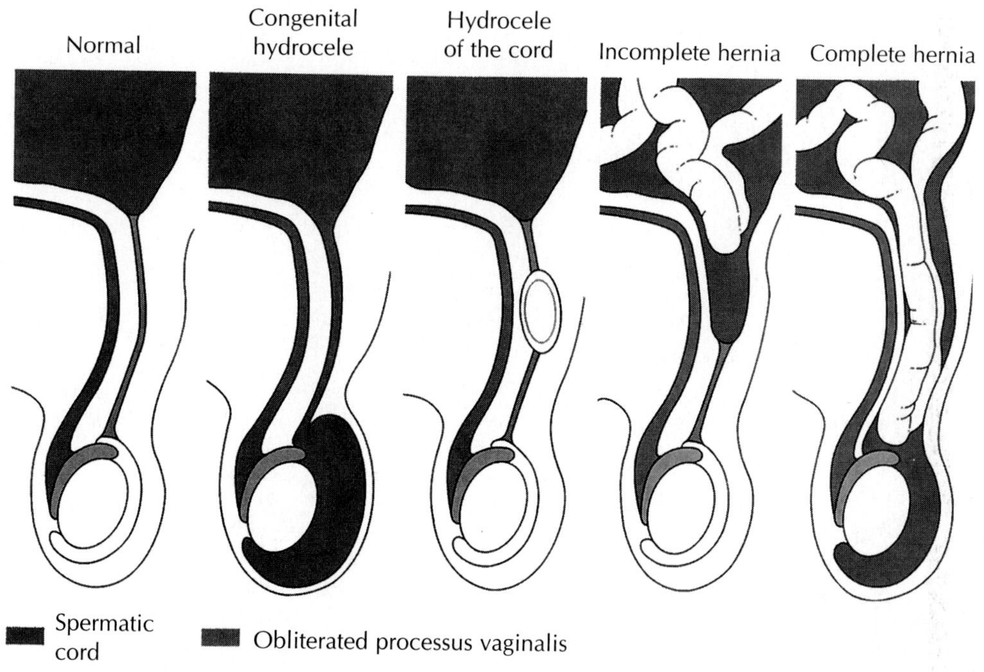

FIGURE 23-33 Diagrammatic representation of the spectrum of developmental defects of the processus vaginalis and its obliteration. From left to right is depicted normal anatomy, a congenital hydrocele with fluid accumulating in the scrotum, a hydrocele of the cord, an incomplete hernia protruding into the inguinal canal, and a complete hernia protruding into the scrotum. (From Nakayama DK: *Pediatric surgery: a color atlas,* Philadelphia, 1992, JB Lippincott.)

Extremities

Pigmented skin lesions may occur on the trunk or on the extremities. Congenital nevi have a significant incidence of malignant degeneration into a melanoma, and if possible such lesions should be excised. Acquired nevi require monitoring only, and the risk of malignancy is not enhanced by a palmar, plantar, or genital location.

Soft tissue subcutaneous nodules are common. Synovial cysts of joint or tendon sheath lining occur on the dorsum of the wrist (ganglion cyst) or in the popliteal fossa (Baker's cyst). Asymptomatic lesions can be followed, but enlarging or painful cysts require excision. Firm, irregular, mobile lesions at times attached to the skin are likely to be pilomatrixomas (calcified epithelioma). They slowly enlarge and should be excised.

Infections of the extremities require aggressive management. Acute suppurative infections around finger or toenails produce paronychia, which require drainage and possible partial nail excision. Infection of the distal palmar space of the digits produces a felon, which also requires drainage in addition to antibiotics. A plantar puncture wound is best treated by local debridement, survey for a retained foreign body, and systemic antibiotics for aerobic and anaerobic organisms. Local extremity cellulitis may be treated with oral antibiotics as can the reddened streaking of lymphangitis. However, when the patient exhibits lymphadenitis proximal to an extremity infection, local care plus parenteral antibiotics become necessary.

Inguinoscrotal Region

Testicular descent is accompanied by extension of a sac of parietal peritoneum into the scrotum, the processus vaginalis. The lumen of this structure normally obliterates by the seventh month of fetal life, a process that occurs later on the right side than on the left (Figure 23-33).

PROBLEM: HYDROCELE

Proximal obliteration of the processus with entrapment of a distal fluid collection in the scrotum produces a physiologic hydrocele that will resorb spontaneously, usually by 6 months of age. A communicating hydrocele or hernia-hydrocele occurs when the processus is patent but the neck is too narrow to permit anything but fluid to enter the scrotum. Intermittent size change of the hydrocele and its failure to spontaneously disappear both confirm its diagnosis. A communicating hydrocele is treated electively by inguinal hernia repair.

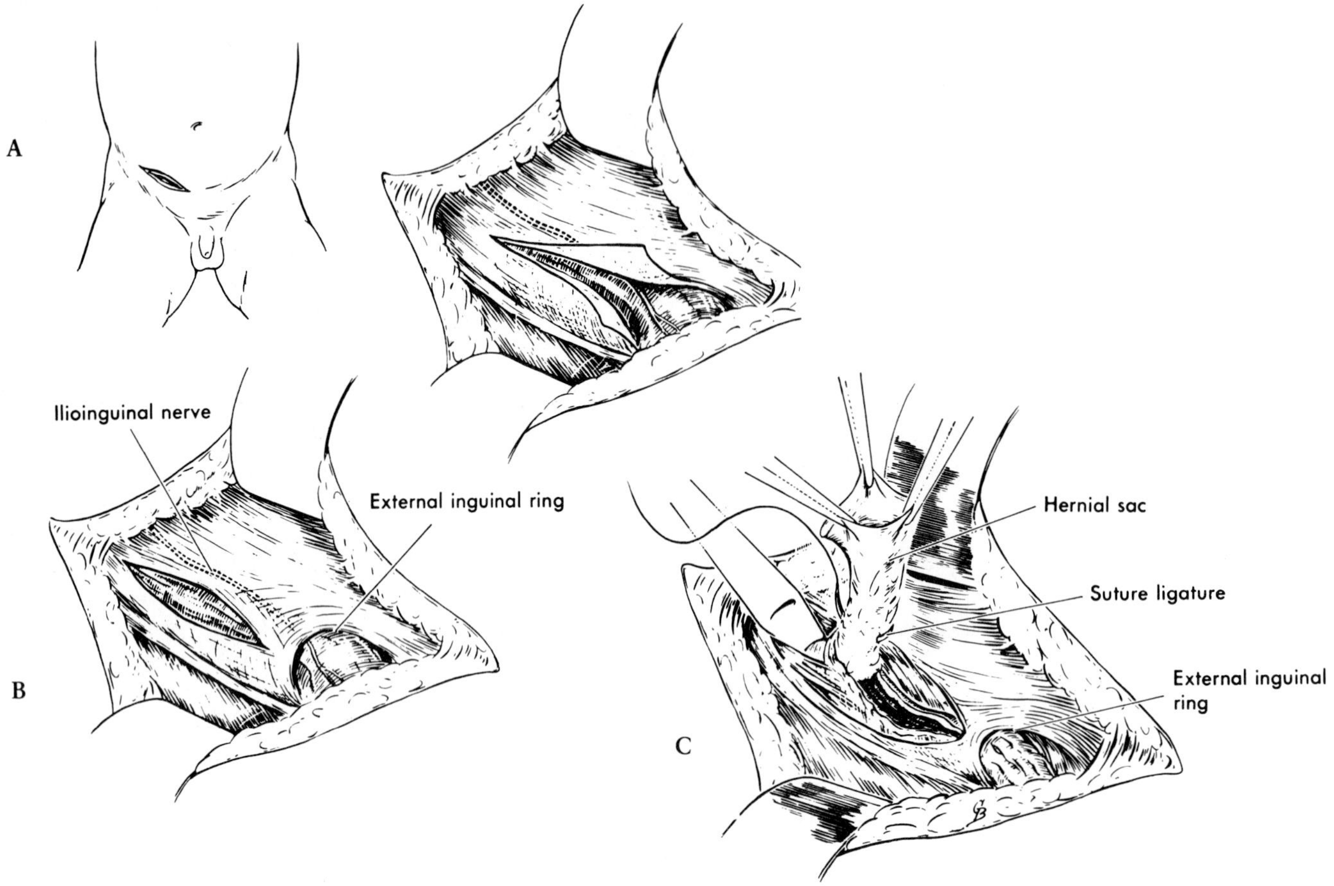

FIGURE 23-34 Repair of right indirect inguinal hernia in an infant. **A,** Groin skin-crease incision. **B,** Incision in external oblique aponeurosis exposes hernia and cord structures; the ilioinguinal nerve should be protected. **C,** Hernial sac has been separated from cord structures and divided, and contents have been reduced; suture ligature is closing the neck of the sac. (From Liechty RD, Soper RT: *Synopsis of surgery,* ed 5, St Louis, 1985, Mosby.)

PROBLEM: INGUINAL HERNIA

An inguinal hernia is defined as a protrusion of intraabdominal contents through the deep inguinal ring into the wider-neck patent processus.

Clinical Presentation

In addition to the inguinal canal bulge that comes and goes, a hernia may extend down into the scrotum. A hernia entrapped in the inguinal canal is incarcerated; a diagnosis is made when the hernia is painful, tender, and nonreducible. Signs and symptoms of small bowel obstruction may follow. The incarcerated hernia progresses to a strangulated hernia when the blood supply to the entrapped viscera is compromised.

Management

A communicating hydrocele or hernia-hydrocele or inguinal hernia should be repaired electively when diagnosed to prevent the 5% per year incidence of incarceration. Treatment is high ligation of or obliteration of the hernia sac (Figure 23-34). Urgent inguinal exploration is indicated for a nonreducible inguinal hernia; reduction of an incarcerated hernia should be followed by repair within 24 to 72 hours. Inguinal hernias are more common in boys and in premature babies and are more often located on the right side. They often are familial. Both direct inguinal hernias and femoral hernias are rare in children.

PROBLEM: UNDESCENDED (CRYPTORCHID) TESTIS

Approximately 50% of undescended testes occur on the right side, 25% on the left side, and 25% are bilateral. This incidence coincides with the order of testicular descent, which occurs earlier on the left than the right.

Clinical Presentation

The parents of a child with an undescended testis will relate that they have never seen the involved testis in the boy's scrotum.

Assessment

Careful physical examination with a relaxed patient will often yield identification of a palpable testis in the inguinal canal that cannot be brought into the scrotum. The true undescended testis must be differentiated from the retractile testis, a normal testis intermittently pulled out of the scrotum by the cremasteric reflex. A testis sometimes in the scrotum and sometimes not is a retractile testis and does not require surgical repair. The retractile testis can be detected by parental observation and repeated physical examinations. At puberty these testes will assume their normal intrascrotal location and require no other treatment.

Management

The rationale for treatment of cryptorchid testes is twofold. First, cryptorchid testes are exposed to higher body temperatures, which result in decreased spermatogenesis. The degree of testicular damage may be related to the length of exposure to the increased temperatures, and the operative return of the testis to the scrotum may be associated with the preservation of fertility. The exact timing of repair is the subject of some debate. However, recent studies using electron microscopy have shown that changes in the testes occur as early as 2 years of age, suggesting that operative repair should be undertaken at or before this time.

The second rationale for repair of the undescended testis is the issue of malignant change. The overall incidence of testicular malignancy is quite low, but there is a 40-fold increase in the risk of malignancy in patients with cryptorchid testes. Interestingly, in patients with a unilateral cryptorchid testis, the incidence of malignant change is increased in both the descended and undescended testicle. Although return of the testis to the scrotum does not decrease the risk of malignant change, it does provide the opportunity for earlier diagnosis.

Embryologically, testicular descent occurs at approximately the twenty-eighth week of gestation. Proper descent of the testis through the inguinal canal into the scrotum requires adequate amounts of male hormones. Medical treatment of undescended testes consisting of the administration of hormonal therapy, androgens, or pituitary hormones has been proposed; however, controlled studies fail to demonstrate a reproducibly significant efficacy. Only 6% to 19% of children with cryptorchid testes responded to human chorionic gonadotropin or gonadotropin-releasing hormone in a randomized study.

Ninety percent of undescended testes are located in the inguinal canal. The operative treatment of simple cryptorchidism when the testis is palpable in the inguinal canal is relatively straightforward. An inguinal skin crease incision is made as for an inguinal herniorrhaphy, the accompanying hernia sac is ligated, and dissection is performed along the spermatic vessels dividing the cremasteric muscle and internal spermatic fascia until enough length is attained to position the testis in a scrotal dartos pouch. If necessary, additional length can be gained by dividing or tunnelling the testicle under the inferior epigastric vessels or by continuing the dissection along the spermatic vessels into the retroperitoneum.

The intraabdominal testis poses a more difficult problem. Preoperative studies such as an abdominal ultrasound may be performed to attempt to locate the intraabdominal testis. Intraoperatively, laparoscopy has also been used to attempt to identify the location of the testis, which can lie anywhere from the renal hilum to the inguinal canal. If simple mobilization of the vessels does not provide sufficient length for placement of the testicle within the scrotum, a number of staged procedures and microvascular techniques have been described to position the testis in the scrotum.

PROBLEM: TESTICULAR TORSION

Any male with the acute onset of severe scrotal pain must be considered to have testicular torsion until proven otherwise. Torsion most commonly occurs in patients with a "bell clapper" suspension of the testis and cord within the tunica vaginalis. The stabilizing normal posterior attachment of the epididymis to the tunica vaginalis is lacking, which allows the cremasteric muscles to apply a rotational force to the testicle, potentially resulting in twisting of the blood supply and ischemia.

Clinical Presentation

Classically, in testicular torsion a sudden onset of exquisite scrotal pain occurs. Pain may also be referred to the lower abdomen, back, and thigh. Although torsion is the most common cause of acute scrotal pain and occurs in all age groups, the most common age at diagnosis is early adolescence.

On physical examination, the scrotum is red or bluish and exquisitely tender. The involved testis is pulled higher than the one on the contralateral side and may lie in a transverse rather than vertical plane. The epididymis is rotated anteriorly.

Assessment

The differential diagnosis includes torsion of an appendix testis, epididymitis, infectious orchitis, or an incarcerated inguinal hernia. Torsion of an appendix testis presents with well-localized tenderness and a visible "blue dot" sign near the upper pole of the testis or epididymis.

When the diagnosis can be made clinically, immediate

operation is required. If the diagnosis is in question, several other tests may be useful. Ultrasound Doppler flow studies may be helpful, but a technetium 99 testicular scan is the study of choice in cases where the diagnosis is unclear. This study is unreliable in smaller children, and regardless of the results of such studies they should not dissuade the surgeon from operating based on clinical suspicion.

Management

At operation, the torsion should be untwisted and bilateral orchidopexies should be performed. Orchidopexy can be accomplished through either bilateral transverse scrotal incisions or a single incision along the median scrotal raphe. Repair involves simply exposing the testis and fixing it to the tunica vaginalis with sutures. If at the time of operation a torsion of the testicular appendage is diagnosed, it should be treated by excision. In cases of testicular torsion, long-term results depend on the duration of ischemia. Patients with symptoms lasting less than 6 hours have an 85% to 95% testicular salvage rate. Those whose symptoms have lasted longer than 24 hours have a less than 10% testicular salvage rate. Aggressive surgical therapy therefore is indicated to avoid the potential loss of a testicle from prolonged ischemia.

PEDIATRIC TUMORS

Cancer is second only to trauma as the leading cause of death in childhood. Although leukemias and lymphomas account for most of these cancers, solid tumors that fall into the realm of pediatric surgery include neuroblastoma, Wilms' tumor, rhabdomyosarcoma, hepatoma, and teratoma. The improved outcomes in childhood cancer are a product of national cooperative groups and multimodal therapies, operative resection being but one part of this treatment strategy.

PROBLEM: NEUROBLASTOMA

Neuroblastoma develops from sympathogonia at the site of neural crest tissue anywhere in the body. These tumors have several unique features. They metabolize catecholamines, which produce metabolically active products that may serve as a tumor marker (vanillylmandelic acid, VMA). They have the ability to mature from a highly malignant to a totally benign ganglioneuroma cell type. They are the most common human tumor to undergo spontaneous regression. Finally, there is a tumor-associated oncogene, n-*myc*.

Neuroblastomas occur at a frequency of 1 per 12,000 live births. The tumor is diagnosed most commonly in early childhood: 50% are under age 2 years, 75% under age 4 years. As a part of the neuralcristopathies, neuroblastoma may be familial and may be associated with other similar entities, for example, Hirschsprung's disease.

Neuroblastomas are small, round cell tumors whose typical histology is rosette formation. The tumor most commonly arises in the retroperitoneum (75%), either in the adrenal medulla or the paraspinal ganglia (Figure 23-35). An additional 20% of tumors occur in the posterior mediastinum, and less than 5% occur in either the neck or the pelvis.

Clinical Presentation

Patients characteristically present with a palpable abdominal mass, but other features include potential spinal cord compression, the black eyes of retroorbital metastases, and signs and symptoms of excessive catecholamine secretion including hypertension, diarrhea, and nutritional wasting. There is also the peculiar opsoclonus myoclonus syndrome characterized by an acute cerebellar ataxia, a remote effect of usually a mediastinal primary tumor.

Assessment

The radiographic diagnosis of neuroblastoma is facilitated by the fact that 50% to 80% of tumors demonstrate finely stippled tumor calcification. Body imaging is useful for staging tumors as well as for defining encroachment on adjacent normal structures such as the kidney, celiac axis blood vessels, and the spinal cord when dumb-bell tumors invade through the intervertebral foramina. I-meta-iodobenzylguanidine (I-MIBG) is taken up by chromaffin cells much the same way as is noradrenaline, and it has been used as a sensitive tumor marker for longitudinal follow-up before and after treatment.

Neuroblastoma is staged based on extent of disease, from I (local disease) to II (tumor extending beyond the organ of origin but not crossing the midline) to III (disease crossing the midline) to IV (systemic metastases to lymph nodes, bone, bone marrow, liver and other organs). There also is a unique stage, IV-S, defined as a local tumor with dissemination limited to liver, skin, and bone marrow; this disease stage is limited to the infant under age 1 year and carries a favorable prognosis.

Management

The treatment of neuroblastoma is multimodal and is dictated by tumor stage as well as prognostic risk factors. Stage I and II local tumors are treated operatively by resection. In poor prognosis stage II tumors demonstrating n-*myc* oncogene amplification, adjuvant chemotherapy and radiotherapy are considered. In stage III tumors primary resection or cytoreduction is performed if possible followed by adjuvant therapy. In stage IV metastatic neuroblastoma, the role of operative resection of the primary tumor is less clear; but if the patient ad-

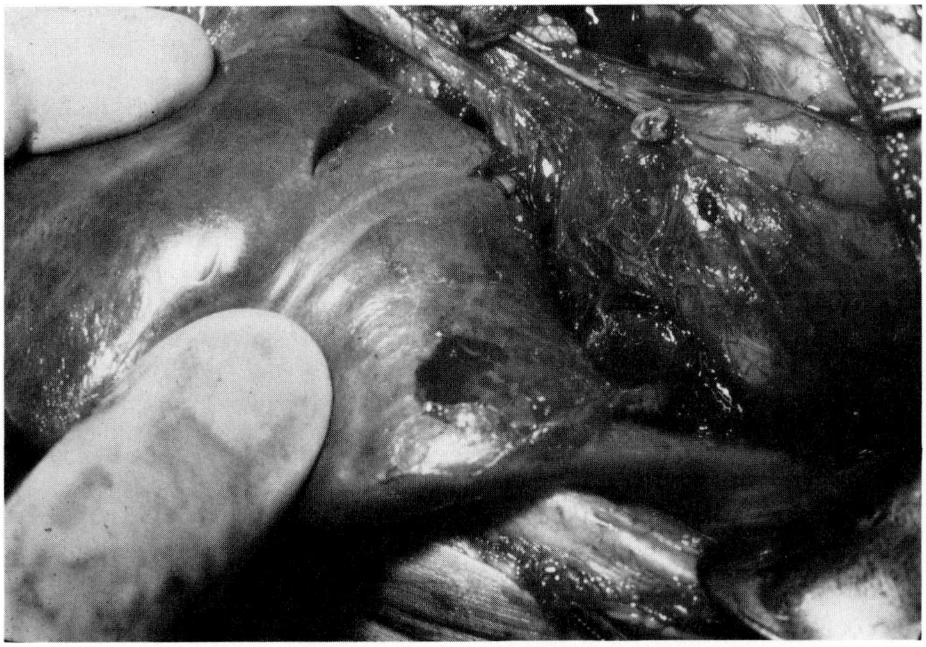

FIGURE 23-35 A patient with an infrahepatic suprarenal right upper quadrant neuroblastoma.

vances to kill and rescue chemotherapy, total body irradiation, and bone marrow transplant, then delayed or second look operative removal of the original tumor becomes imperative. Stage IV-S primary tumors may or may not be removed. Waiting for spontaneous regression rather than intensive chemotherapy/radiotherapy is the preferred mode of treatment of this disseminated disease form.

The outcome for neuroblastoma patients has not changed dramatically over the last 40 years. Survival is best in low stage, young patients; it is also better for cervical and thoracic locations than for retroperitoneal/pelvic tumors. Additional features associated with a favorable outcome include less than 10 copies of n-*myc* oncogene, low neuron-specific enolase, a normal serum ferritin, and a favorable histologic pattern. Stage related 3-year survival when these features are optimal are the following: Stage I, 90%; Stage III, 70%; IV-S, 91%. However, high stage tumors often have unfavorable prognostic features, which has a profoundly adverse influence on outcome: Stage II, 20%; Stage III, 20%, Stage IV, 10%.

PROBLEM: NEPHROBLASTOMA (WILMS' TUMOR)

Wilms' tumor is a malignant tumor originating from the metanephric blastema. Along with neuroblastoma it represents the most common solid abdominal tumor of childhood; nevertheless it is rare. It tends to present between 1 and 5 years at a mean age slightly older than that for neuroblastoma. The occurrence of Wilms' tumor may be related to a loss of a tumor suppressor gene located on chromosome 11; 10% to 15% of patients with Wilms' tumor also have additional congenital anomalies such as aniridia, genitourinary malformations, hemihypertrophy, and Beckwith-Wiedemann syndrome.

This tumor of the metanephric blastema may histologically contain elements of mesenchymal and epithelial differentiation. In contrast, adverse histologic features include cellular pleomorphism (anaplasia) and clear cell or rhabdoid sarcomatous change.

Clinical Presentation

Most patients with Wilms' tumor present with the sudden onset of a painless abdominal mass. Such lateral flank masses may be associated with hypertension as well as with microscopic hematuria.

Assessment

Historically, intravenous pyelography was the study of choice for Wilms' tumor, a test that would demonstrate intrarenal calyceal distortion by a mass while simultaneously providing a functional assessment of the status of the opposite kidney (Figure 23-36). Today abdominal ultrasound is more commonly used as a diagnostic screening study, and a contrast CT scan provides a tumor

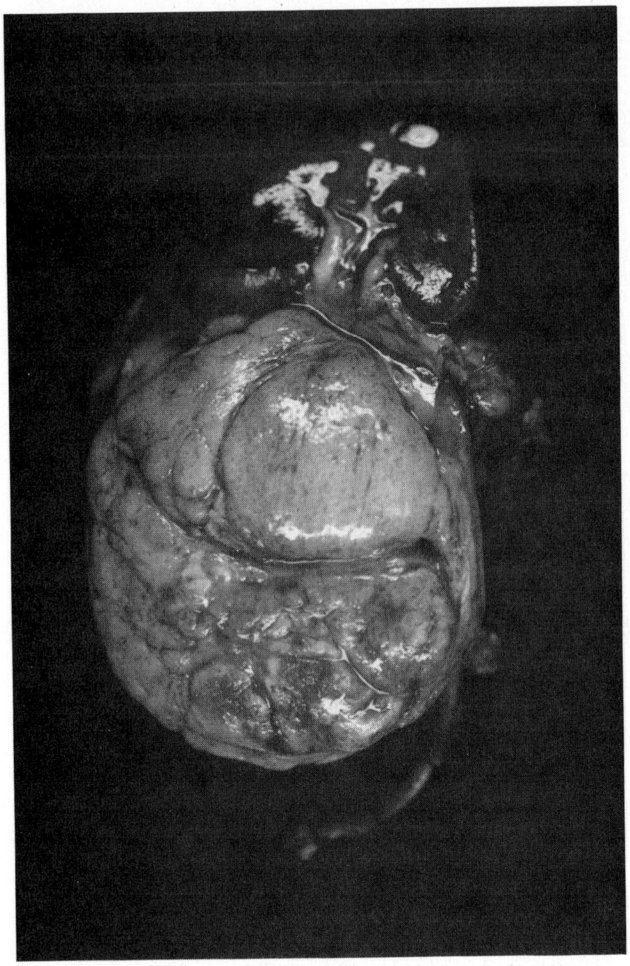

FIGURE 23-36 Large intrarenal tumor distorting the normal architecture of the kidney. This pattern is typical of a Wilms' tumor.

road map as well as a functional assessment of the opposite kidney. In addition to local and intravenous vascular extension, Wilms' tumor metastasizes most frequently to the lung. Therefore chest radiography is also imperative in the initial diagnostic evaluation of these patients.

Wilms' tumor also is staged from I to IV, indicating local disease, regional disease, and metastatic systemic disease respectively. The tumor may also occur bilaterally, stage V tumor.

Management

Wilms' tumor represents the pinnacle of success in multimodal therapy, which includes operation, chemotherapy, and radiotherapy as administered in national cooperative trials. To date the following results have been demonstrated: (1) Lymph node disease and unfavorable histology adversely influence the prognosis; (2) stage I and II tumors are best treated by adjuvant actinomycin D and vincristine, and additional radiotherapy is not needed; (3) actinomycin D and vincristine together as adjuvants are better than either drug alone; and (4) the addition of a third adjuvant, doxorubicin, improves the results for stage II, III and IV disease; in contrast the use of four drug therapy with the addition of cyclophosphamide only improves outcome for patients with anaplastic tumors.

Nephrectomy remains the operative procedure of choice for Wilms' tumor for all stages, although it may be delayed in stage IV patients. In addition, in stage V disease renal preservation is the goal; therefore primary or delayed operation should spare renal mass rather than considering the patient for bilateral nephrectomy and eventual renal transplantation. A transabdominal approach is made to the tumor, and the procedure must include a careful inspection and palpation of the contralateral kidney. Any suspicious area should be biopsied to exclude Wilms' tumor as well as nephroblastomatosis, a potential tumor precursor. Hilar control of the vascular pedicle is advised when performing the nephrectomy, and the renal vein must be closely observed for evidence of potential intravascular extension.

Multimodal therapies for stage I through III favorable histology Wilms' tumor have produced 4-year disease-free survival rates of 97% and 85%, respectively. In contrast survival rates for all stage IV tumors and unfavorable histology stage I through III tumors vary from 52% to 86%.

PROBLEM: TERATOMA

These rare embryonic tumors are defined as a tumor composed of multiple tissue or cell types foreign to their site of origin. Their location varies from the brain, mouth, neck, thorax, retroperitoneum, testes, ovaries, and presacral areas; the latter two are most common in childhood. Almost two thirds of teratomas are benign and are composed of well-differentiated mature tissue. Malignancy is heralded by immature, undifferentiated tissue, a feature more common in older patients who have sacrococcygeal teratomas. Teratomas occur more frequently in girls.

The diagnosis of teratomas depends on their site of origin. Sacrococcygeal exophytic tumors are commonly noted on in utero ultrasound or by inspection at delivery (Figure 23-37). Intrapelvic lesions are readily palpated by rectal examination. Gonadal teratomas produce mass-effect symptoms, and either the masses are palpable or are defined by imaging studies. Tumor markers are useful in defining the presence of malignant elements in teratomas. Elevated human chorionic gonadotropin (HCG) suggests a choriocarcinoma, whereas an elevated

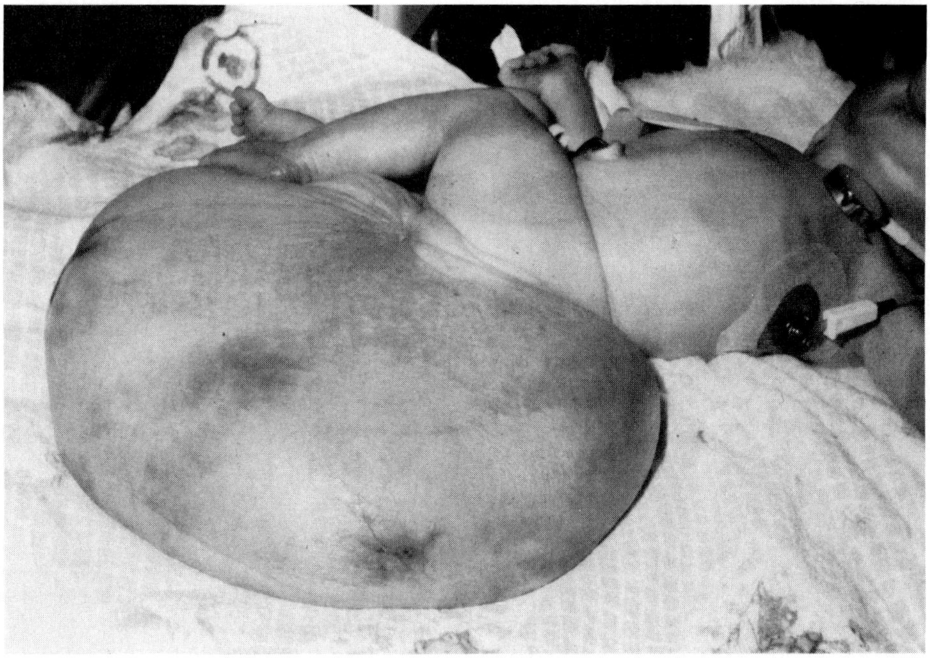

FIGURE 23-37 Gigantic cystic and solid sacrococcygeal mass in a newborn. This exophytic mass also had an intrapelvic extension and proved histologically to be a mature teratoma.

alpha fetoprotein (AFP) is indicative of a teratoma containing an entodermal sinus or yolk sac tumor.

Resection is the preferred treatment for both mature and immature teratomas. Resection of sacrococcygeal teratomas may require a simultaneous transabdominal and transperineal approach in which the coccyx is also removed. Adjuvant multiagent chemotherapy has proved useful in immature teratomas, but if the tumor is not amenable to a curative resection, ultimate cure will be difficult to achieve.

PROBLEM: RHABDOMYOSARCOMA

These small, round-cell tumors originate from embryonic muscle cells. They account for 5% to 15% of malignant solid tumors of childhood, but in older adolescents they are more common than neuroblastoma and Wilms' tumor. In infancy and early childhood the most common tumor location is the bladder, prostate, vagina, and head and neck; in older children and young adults paratesticular, trunk, and abdominal organ sites are more common. Orbital and limb tumors are found at any age.

The diagnosis of a rhabdomyosarcoma depends on a tissue analysis after presentation as a mass. The most common tumor sites include the head and neck (40%), genitourinary tract (20%), extremities (20%), trunk (10%), and other sites (10%). Tumor histology is variable and prognosis varies from least to most favorable as follows: botryoid, embryonal, alveolar, and small round-cell sarcomas. Embryonal tumors are most common and alveolar types quite rare. Alveolar subtypes are rarely found in the favorable sites—the orbit, bladder, prostate, vagina, or paratesticular areas—and are more common on the trunk and perineum.

Rhabdomyosarcomas spread locally, to regional lymph nodes, and via the bloodstream to the lungs, bone marrow, and soft tissues. Staging is classified I through IV based on the presence of residual disease and metastatic spread.

Treatment of these tumors has changed to the predominant scheme of primary chemotherapy-radiotherapy protocols, with delayed, conservatively limited, or even no operative treatment. This approach is the predominant treatment for tumors of the orbit, nasopharynx, paranasal sinuses, middle ear, bladder, prostate, and vagina. However, primary tumor resection with wide tumor-free margins remains the therapeutic goal as long as tumor removal does not cause long-term disability.

The outcome of rhabdomyosarcoma is related to histologic type, primary tumor location, and extent (or stage) of disease. Embryonal tumors have the best outcome, alveolar tumors the worst (69% versus 52%, respectively). Orbital (86%) and head and neck (78%) primaries have the best outcome, whereas extremity tumors have the worst (54%). Survival ranges from 81% for stage I rhabdomyosarcoma to 27% for metastatic stage IV disease.

PROBLEM: HEPATOMA

Malignant liver tumors fall into one of two types: the embryonic tumor form hepatoblastoma and the tumor more typically associated with cirrhosis, hepatocellular carcinoma. Although hemangiomas are the most common liver tumors in childhood, hepatoblastoma and hepatocellular carcinoma are the most common malignant liver tumors. Hepatoblastoma typically occurs in the child younger than 4 years of age, whereas the peak age of incidence for hepatocellular carcinoma is between 10 and 15 years.

Hepatoblastoma contains hepatic epithelial cells that resemble embryonal fetal tissue. The tumor has several histologic variants, the pure fetal histology being associated with an improved survival. Patients usually present with a visible or palpable abdominal mass, and an elevated AFP level is a useful tumor marker. The hepatocellular carcinomas are composed of large cells and broad cellular trabeculae, considerable nuclear pleomorphism, and frequent tumor giant cells. A characteristic cell type with a more favorable outcome is the fibrolamellar variety. When metastatic, both tumors tend to spread to lung, lymph nodes, and adjacent viscera.

Tumor imaging is particularly important for liver tumors because operative resection for cure plays a vital role in patient management. Angiography or contrast MRI provides a safe road map for anatomic lobectomy in tumor management. Adjuvant chemotherapy is usually administered after resection using combinations of vincristine, cyclophosphamide, doxorubicin, and 5-fluouracil. Bilobar or multicentric malignant liver tumors may be treated by total hepatectomy and liver allotransplantation.

The survival of patients with malignant liver tumors depends on stage (resectability) and histology. Overall survival rate of patients with hepatoblastoma is 35% to 40%, but for patients with pure fetal history it may approach 90%. Overall survival in patients with hepatocellular carcinoma is 30% to 35%, but it may be as high as 40% to 45% for the fibrolamellar histologic variant. Two-year survival after transplantation for hepatoblastoma approaches 58%, whereas the same survival rate for transplantation for hepatocellular carcinoma is only 20% to 30%.

PEDIATRIC TRANSPLANTATION

Overview

Transplantation is discussed elsewhere (Chapter 21) in this book. The unique features of pediatric transplantation relate to the etiology of end-stage disease: obstructive uropathy for renal failure; biliary atresia and metabolic errors for hepatic failure; the technical challenges of the small-sized recipients; the impact of the pediatric physiology in preoperative and postoperative care; and the intensity of the allograft reaction in the human species born immunocompetent. Although the results of pediatric renal transplantation may not be as good as in the adult population, the results for whole organ and segmental liver transplantation are superior to those seen in adults.

Pediatric heart, heart lung, and single lung transplantations have also been performed with some success; and the next frontier awaiting good results is pediatric bowel and pancreatic transplantation.

REFERENCES

1 Adzick NS, Harrison MR, Glick PL: Diaphragmatic hernia in the fetus: prenatal diagnosis and outcome in 94 cases, *J Pediatr Surg* 20:357, 1985.
2 Alison PR: Reflux esophagitis, sliding hernia and the anatomy of repair, *Surg Gynecol Obstet* 92:149, 1951.
3 Anderson HL, Otsu T, Chapman RA: Venovenous extracorporeal life support in neonates using a double lumen catheter, *Trans Am Soc Artif Intern Organs* 35:650, 1989.
4 Ashcraft KW, Holder TM, Amoury RA et al: The Thal fundoplication for gastroesophageal reflux, *J Pediatr Surg* 19:480, 1984.
5 Ashcraft KW: Gastroesophageal reflux. In Ashcraft KW, Holder TM editors: *Pediatric Surgery,* Philadelphia, 1993, WB Saunders.
6 Ballance WA, Dahms BB, Shenker N: Pathology of neonatal necrotizing enterocolitis: a ten-year experience, *J Pediatr* 117:56, 1990.
7 Bartlett RH, Roloff DW, Cornell RG: Extracorporeal circulation in neonatal respiratory failure, a prospective randomized study, *Pediatrics* 76:479, 1985.
8 Bartlett RH, Gazzaniga AB, Toomasian J: Extracorporeal circulation in neonatal respiratory failure: 100 cases, *Ann Surg* 204:236, 1986.
9 Bell MJ, Ternberg JL, Feagin RD: Neonatal necrotizing enterocolitis, *Ann Surg* 187:1, 1978.
10 Bianchi A: Intestinal loop lengthening—a technique for increasing small intestinal length, *J Pediatr Surg* 15:145, 1980.
11 Bohn DJ, Tamura M, Perrin D: Ventilatory predictors of pulmonary hypoplasia in congenital diaphragmatic hernia, confirmed by morphologic assessment, *J Pediatr* 111:423, 1987.
12 Cullen ML, Klein MD, Philippart AI: Congenital diaphragmatic hernia, *Surg Clin North Am* 65:1115, 1985.
13 Delins RE, Wheatley MJ, Coran AG: Etiology and management of respiratory complications after repair of esophageal atresia with tracheoesophageal fistula, *Surgery* 112:527, 1992.
14 DeMeester TR, Wernly JA, Bryant GH: Clinical and in vitro analysis of determinants of gastroesophageal competence, *Am J Surg* 137:39, 1979.
15 Depaepe A, Dolk H, Lechart MF: The epidemiology of tracheo-esophageal fistula and oesophageal atresia in Europe, *Arch Dis Child* 68:743, 1993.
16 De Vries PA: The surgery of anorectal anomalies: its evolution with evaluations of procedures, *Curr Probl Surg* 21:5, 1984.
17 Eichelberger M: Thoracic trauma. In Ashcraft KW, Holder TM, editors: *Pediatric Surgery,* Philadelphia, 1993, WB Saunders.
18 Ein SH, Shandling B, Wesson D: Esophageal atresia with distal tracheoesophageal fistula: associated anomalies and prognosis in the 1980s, *J Pediatr Surg* 24:1055, 1989.

19 Fonkalsrud EW, DeLorimer AA, Hayes DM: Congenital atresia and stenosis of the duodenum, *Pediatrics* 43:79, 1969.
20 Gennarelli TA, Champion HR, Sacco WJ: Mortality of patients with head injury and extracranial injury treated in trauma centers, *J Trauma* 29:1193, 1989.
21 Glasier CM, Seibert JJ, Golladay ES: Intermediate imperforate anus: clinical and radiographic implications, *J Pediatr Surg* 22:351, 1987.
22 Glass P, Miller M, Short B: Morbidity for survivors of extracorporeal membrane oxygenation: neurodevelopmental outcome at 1 year of age, *Pediatrics* 83:72, 1989.
23 Gross RE: Congenital hernia of the diaphragm, *Am J Dis Child* 71:580, 1946.
24 Harris BM, Barlow BA, Ballantine TV: American Pediatric Surgical Association principles of pediatric trauma, *J Pediatr Surg* 27:423, 1992.
25 Harrison MR, DeLorimer AA: Congenital diaphragmatic hernia, *Surg Clin North Am* 61:1023, 1981.
26 Hill JD, DeLeval MR, Fallat RJ: Acute respiratory insufficiency. Treatment with prolonged extracorporeal membrane oxygenation, *J Thorac Cardiovasc Surg* 64:551, 1972.
27 Kiernan PD, ReMine SG, Kiernan PC: Annular pancreas, *Arch Surg* 115:46, 1980.
28 Klell D, Petersen C, Zimmerman HJ: The developmental anatomy of congenital diaphragmatic hernia, *Pediatr Surg Intern* 2:322, 1987.
29 Kliegman RM, Fanaroff AA: Neonatal necrotizing enterocolitis, *N Engl J Med* 310:1093, 1985.
30 Lally KP, Paranka MS, Roden J: Congenital diaphragmatic hernia—stabilization and repair on ECMO, *Ann Surg* 216:569, 1992.
31 Langer JC, Filler RM, Bohn DJ: Timing surgery for congenital diaphragmatic hernia. Is emergency operation necessary? *J Pediatr Surg* 23:731, 1988.
32 McKinnon LJ, Kosloske AM: Prediction and prevention of anastomotic complications of esophageal atresia and tracheoesophageal fistula, *J Pediatr Surg* 25:778, 1990.
33 Nagaraj HS, Mitchell KA, Fallat ME: Surgical complications and procedures in neonates on extracorporeal membrane oxygenation, *J Pediatr Surg* 27:1106, 1992.
34 Nakayama DK, Templeton JM, Ziegler MM: Complications of posterior sagittal anorectoplasty, *J Pediatr Surg* 21:488, 1986.
35 Nakayama DK, Ramenofsky ML, Rowe MI: Chest injuries in childhood, *Ann Surg* 210:770, 1989.
36 Nakayama DK, Waggoner T, Venkataraman ST: The use of drugs in emergency airway management in pediatric trauma, *Ann Surg* 216:205, 1992.
37 Newman KO, Bowman LM, Eichelberger MR: The lap belt complex: intestinal injuries in childhood, *J Trauma* 31:1169, 1991.
38 Nissen R: Gastropexy and fundoplication in surgical treatment of hiatal hernia, *Am J Dig Dis* 6:954, 1961.
39 Novicki P: Intestinal ischemia and necrotizing enterocolitis, *J Pediatr* 117:514, 1990.
40 O'Neill JA: Necrotizing enterocolitis, *Surg Clin North Am* 61:1013, 1981.
41 O'Rourke PP, Crone RK, Vacanti JP: Extracorporeal membrane oxygenation and conventional medical therapy in neonates with persistent pulmonary hypertension of the newborn: a prospective randomized study, *Pediatrics* 84:957, 1989.
42 Parrott TS: Urologic implications of anorectal malformations, *Urol Clin North Am* 12:13, 1985.
43 Peclet MH, Newman KD, Eichelberger MR: Patterns of injury in children, *J Pediatr Surg* 25:85, 1990.
44 Pena A: Surgical treatment of high imperforate anus, *World J Surg* 9:236, 1985.
45 Reid IS, Hutcherson RJ: Long term follow up of patients with congenital diaphragmatic hernia, *J Pediatr Surg* 11:939, 1976.
46 Rouse TM, Eichelberger MR: Trends in pediatric trauma management, *Surg Clin North Am* 72:1347, 1992.
47 Schiffman MA: Non-operative management of blunt abdominal trauma in pediatrics, *Emerg Med Clin North Am* 7:519, 1989.
48 Shaul DB, Schwartz MZ, Marr CC: Primary repair without routine gastrostomy is the treatment of choice for neonates with esophageal atresia and tracheoesophageal fistula, *Arch Surg* 124:1188, 1989.
49 Spitz L, Kiely E, Brereton RJ: Management of esophageal atresia, *World J Surg* 17:296, 1993.
50 Stringel G, Delgado M, Guestin L: Gastrostomy and Nissen fundoplication in neurologically impaired children, *J Pediatr Surg* 24:1044, 1989.
51 Taylor GA, Eichelberger MR, O'Donnell R: Indications for computed tomography in children with blunt abdominal trauma, *Ann Surg* 213:121, 1991.
52 Tepas JJ, DiScala C, Ramenofsky ML: Mortality and head injury. The pediatric perspective, *J Pediatr Surg* 25:92, 1990.
53 Thompson JS, Pinch LW, Murray N: Experience with intestinal lengthening for the short bowel syndrome, *J Pediatr Surg* 26:721, 1991.
54 Touloukian RJ, Smith GJW: Neonatal intestinal length in preterm infants, *J Pediatr Surg* 18:720, 1983.
55 Towne BH, Lott IT, Hicks DA: Long-term follow up of infants and children treated with extracorporeal membrane oxygenation (ECMO), *J Pediatr Surg* 20:410, 1985.
56 Turnage RH, Oldham KT, Coran AG: Late results of fundoplication for gastroesophageal reflux in infants and children, *Surgery* 105:457, 1989.
57 Umali E, Andrews HG, White JJ: A critical analysis of blood transfusion requirements in children with blunt abdominal trauma, *Am Surg* 58:736, 1992.
58 Vanderhoff JA, Langnas AN, Pinch LW: Short bowel syndrome: a review, *J Pediatr Gastroenterol Nutr* 14:359, 1992.
59 Vane DW, Harmel RP, King DR: The effectiveness of Nissen fundoplication in neurologically impaired children with gastroesophageal reflux, *Surgery* 98:662, 1985.
60 Warner BW: Parenteral nutrition in the pediatric patient. In Fischer JE, editor: *Total parenteral nutrition,* Boston, 1991, Little, Brown.
61 Weaver DD, Mapstone CL, Yu P: The VATER association, *Am J Dis Child* 140:225, 1986.
62 West KW, Bengston K, Rescorla FJ: Delayed surgical repair and ECMO improves survival in congenital diaphragmatic hernia, *Ann Surg* 216:454, 1992.
63 Williamson RC: Intestinal adaptation: structural, funtional, and cytokinetic changes, *N Engl J Med* 298:1393, 1978.
64 Wilmore DW: Factors correlating with a successful outcome following extensive resection in newborn infants, *J Pediatr* 80:88, 1972.
65 Ziegler MM, Bishop HC: Reflux peptic esophagitis in children. In Nylus L, Baker R, editors: *Mastery of surgery,* Boston, 1984, Little, Brown.

CHAPTER

24

LARYNGOSCOPIC VIEW OF LARYNX
WITH PATIENT SUPINE

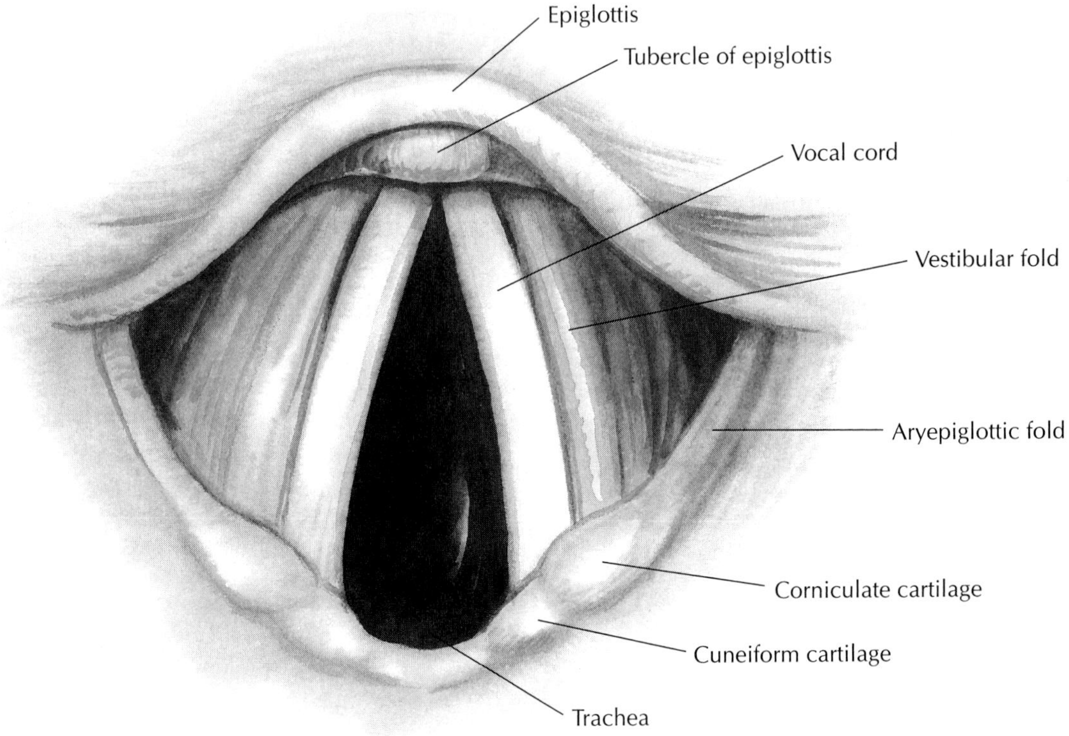

PERIOPERATIVE ANESTHESIA

David H. Stern

This chapter presents an overview of the anesthetic considerations germane to the preoperative, intraoperative, and postoperative care of surgical patients. It is designed to present to the surgeon and student of surgery the thought processes of the anesthesiologist when assessing the patient, planning and implementing the anesthetic, and participating in the patient's postoperative care.

Anesthetic considerations are organized around organ systems for two purposes. The first is to focus on the various physiologic and pathophysiologic aspects of each organ system that contribute to the planning and implementation of *all anesthetic procedures;* for example, assessment of the potential impact of recent myocardial infarction (cardiovascular), choice of anesthesia for the pregnant patient (reproductive), and management of the patient with bowel obstruction (gastrointestinal). The second purpose is to evaluate the anesthetic considerations associated with *surgical procedures on specific organ systems;* for example, use of the double-lumen endotracheal tube for certain thoracic operations (respiratory), anesthetic management of patients undergoing transurethral prostate resection (genitourinary), and anesthetic management of patients undergoing craniotomy in the sitting position (nervous).

This chapter is not intended to teach anesthesiology to surgeons but rather to explain how anesthesiologists think. The goal is to help surgeons better understand some of the problems anesthesiologists encounter and how the management of these problems might interact with surgical care during the perioperative period.

PATIENT ASSESSMENT AND PREPARATION

Interview, Evaluation, and Discussion

The goals of the preanesthetic consultation are (1) to identify medical conditions of concern during the course of anesthesia; (2) with informed consent of the patient or guardian, to decide on an appropriate anesthetic plan; and (3) to allay anxiety by discussion and premedication as needed.

After review of the patient's chart, a directed history and physical examination is performed, with emphasis on cardiovascular, respiratory, hepatic, renal, and neurologic areas. Also covered are previous anesthetic problems, drug allergies, bleeding disorders, diabetes, hypertension, current medications, and abuse of alcohol, tobacco, or drugs. Particular attention is devoted to evaluation of the airway. The anesthesiologist must then decide whether additional studies or consultations are necessary.

Discussion varies with the needs of each patient, but most should be informed about fasting before surgery, preoperative sedation to be ordered, any uncomfortable procedures to be performed before surgery (such as intravenous or arterial cannulation or awake intubation), method of induction of anesthesia, aftereffects, and risks. Choice of anesthetic technique is based primarily on surgical needs (anatomic region, duration, and patient positioning) and preexisting disease, but must also take into account the skills of the anesthesiologist and the patient's preference.

Patients scheduled for Monitored Anesthesia Care with local anesthesia and sedation require a comprehensive evaluation like that for general anesthesia. These patients are frequently elderly and have numerous medical problems that may be troublesome intraoperatively. Furthermore, alternate techniques must be planned in the event of unsatisfactory tolerance of local anesthesia or an untoward drug reaction or other event.

Preoperative Sedation

A reassuring preoperative visit can dramatically reduce the need for sedative drugs, but most patients benefit from anxiolytic medications. Narcotics are most useful in patients who are in pain, but are often combined with other sedatives. Benzodiazepines, such as diazepam, lorazepam, and midazolam, are the most effective anxiolytics and are frequently given alone. Barbiturates and related drugs (secobarbital, pentobarbital, chloral hydrate) potentiate the effects of other sedatives and are often used alone in children. Droperidol was at one time frequently given in combination with fentanyl (Innovar), but because it can cause extrapyramidal symptoms, dysphoria and severe psychologic distress despite an outwardly calm appearance,[83] it is now rarely used except in small doses as an antiemetic.[66] Promethazine and hydroxyzine are antihistamines that also have useful sedative properties in combination with narcotics.

Oral medications are preferred in children who can swallow them reliably, but even in adults, oral diazepam and lorazepam are effective when given 1 to 2 hours in advance.

Anticholinergic drugs such as atropine, scopolamine, and glycopyrrolate, when given intramuscularly in advance, offer little protection against bradycardia, but can be useful antisialagogues in patients with excessive secretions or before performing flexible fiberoptic laryngoscopy. Scopolamine is rarely used today but can be combined with morphine as a long-acting sedative and amnesic.

CARDIOVASCULAR SYSTEM

Acquired Cardiovascular Disease

The patient with coronary artery disease must be evaluated from two standpoints: (1) ischemia, in which oxygen delivery cannot meet myocardial oxygen demand; and (2) ventricular dysfunction resulting from ischemia, loss of muscle fibers, or both. Anesthetics that minimize ischemia may cause intolerable myocardial depression, whereas those preserving or enhancing contractility may precipitate or worsen ischemia.

Risk Factors

Numerous risk factors for perioperative infarction have been identified; the most significant is recent myocardial infarction. A classic 1977 study found that patients undergoing surgery during the first 3 months after myocardial infarction had a 37% risk of reinfarction.[45] The risk fell to 16% between 3 and 6 months and to 5% after 6 months. Because average mortality for reinfarction was 54%, elective surgery should probably be postponed for at least 6 months after acute myocardial infarction. However, Rao and El-Etr[90] more recently suggested that aggressive treatment based on invasive monitoring of systemic arterial and pulmonary arterial and wedge pressures may reduce the risk of reinfarction during the first 6 months after myocardial infarction.

Congestive heart failure and dysrhythmias were also

found to be major risk factors for perioperative myocardial infarction, as were the following: extremes of age (more than 70 years); intraabdominal, intrathoracic, or major vascular surgery; emergency status; hemodynamically important mitral or aortic stenosis; and poor general medical condition. All these factors increased perioperative mortality. In addition, a positive correlation was found between postoperative mortality and length of procedure.

Besides evaluation of these risk factors, preoperative assessment should note the presence of hypertension, anemia, abnormal pulmonary function, impaired exercise tolerance, current cardiac and other medications, and any recent anginal episodes, along with their precipitating circumstances and the response to medications.

Laboratory Studies of Cardiovascular Importance

Laboratory studies of value in guiding anesthetic management of patients with cardiac risk factors include the electrocardiogram (ECG) to identify preexisting ischemic changes, conduction abnormalities, rhythm abnormalities, and prior infarction; echocardiogram to reveal ventricular wall motion abnormalities, valvular defects, and pericardial effusion; ECG stress testing to identify ischemia related to rate-pressure product; cardiac enzymes to confirm suspected recent damage; electrolytes, particularly potassium; arterial blood gases (acidosis may indicate tissue hypoperfusion, whereas hypoxemia warrants corrective measures to prevent myocardial hypoxia); and chest roentgenograms to evaluate effusion, coexisting pulmonary disease, cardiomegaly, and congestive heart failure. Data from cardiac catheterization and angiography are also useful to the anesthesiologist because they may substantiate the need for monitoring intraoperative cardiovascular status with a pulmonary artery catheter. Elevated wedge pressure and low ejection fraction indicate that central venous pressure will be an inadequate correlate of left ventricular filling pressure.[112] Baseline pressures indicate intraoperative goals, and the location of stenotic coronary lesions may dictate the best ECG lead for intraoperative monitoring.

Important Cardiovascular Considerations in Choosing an Anesthetic

Valvular lesions may be stenotic, regurgitant, or combined. Anesthetic management depends on the severity and type of valvular lesion. Contractility depressants are usually avoided because myocardial function is already impaired. In mitral stenosis, preservation of sinus rhythm and prevention of tachycardia are important to maximize ventricular filling. The anesthesiologist, therefore, would usually avoid deep levels of volatile anesthetics, which could cause junctional rhythm or bigeminy. Likewise, heart rate could be increased by either inadequate depth of anesthesia or by certain agents such as pancuronium, a neuromuscular blocker. In patients with mitral regurgitation, cardiac output is best maintained using intravenous fluid to maintain adequate left ventricular filling pressure, along with vasodilators and positive chronotropes. Heavy preoperative sedation is avoided because it can cause bradycardia as well as hypoxemia. Similar therapeutic goals apply to aortic insufficiency. Mitral valve prolapse, which is found in about 5% of otherwise normal patients,[30] may result in potentially fatal arrhythmias.[107] Aortic stenosis is associated with myocardial ischemia because of concentric hypertrophy and high ventricular wall tension coupled with low coronary perfusion pressure. Vasodilation resulting from either high volatile anesthetics, or certain intravenous anesthetics such as thiopental and propofol, can cause hypotension and further ischemia. Patients with severe heart disease have poor tolerance for the adverse changes in sympathetic tone, body position, and fluid balance that commonly occur during surgery. Although intraoperative monitoring is helpful, it is important that these patients are stable and receiving optimal therapy preoperatively.

Prophylactic antibiotics for patients with valvular lesions are most valuable when given intravenously at least 1 hour before events that cause bacteremia.[62] Although nasotracheal intubation can produce significant bacteremia, orotracheal intubation usually does not.[7]

In patients with idiopathic hypertrophic subaortic stenosis, anesthetic agents that depress contractility are beneficial because they lessen the muscular outflow tract obstruction, whereas arterial vasodilation alone can further worsen coronary perfusion pressure. Cardiomyopathy, whether caused by drugs, toxins, or disease, is managed much the same as other lesions that damage heart muscle and impair contractility.

Patients with congestive heart failure should be treated aggressively preoperatively, in many cases using a pulmonary artery catheter to optimize fluid balance and adjust drug therapy. Unfortunately, this approach may not be possible with emergency procedures, when anesthetic hazards associated with a "full stomach" are usually present as well. This combination presents serious problems for the anesthesiologist. Hemodynamic stability is difficult to maintain in patients with congestive heart failure during the "rapid-sequence" induction and intubation aimed at preventing aspiration of gastric contents. Regional block or local infiltration anesthesia for these procedures is not always safer than general anesthesia. Anesthesiology consultation should be sought as early as possible. Most important, the urgency of the surgery should be carefully weighed against the substantial risks.

Antihypertensive medications must be continued through the morning of surgery. Although hypertensive patients at rest in their hospital beds often remain normotensive despite discontinuation of therapy, they are likely to exhibit large swings in blood pressure when exposed to anesthetic drugs, tracheal intubation, and surgical manipulation. Serial blood pressures recorded preoperatively can help the anesthesiologist anticipate hemodynamic lability and set safe limits for intraoperative blood pressures.

In victims of major trauma, the anesthesiologist's approach to establishing cardiovascular stability has three facets; in order of priority they are: (1) support of tissue oxygenation and perfusion (airway management, ventilation, restoration of blood volume and circulation to correct shock); (2) identification and treatment of specific organ system compromise and allowance for altered drug response and clearance; and (3) administration of anesthetic drugs to blunt sympathetic response, prevent movement, reduce muscle tone, and depress consciousness. Included in point 2 are pneumothorax, hemothorax, fat embolus, cardiac contusion or pericardial tamponade, kidney injury, and intracranial hemorrhage or contusion causing intracranial hypertension. Undiagnosed problems may worsen while masked by general anesthesia.

Cardiovascular Drugs

Through the day of surgery, any drug regimen on which the patient is stable preoperatively must be maintained. Sudden discontinuation of antihypertensive medication at best may lead to lability under anesthesia, making it difficult to keep the arterial pressure within reasonable limits.[89] At worst, dangerous postoperative hypertension may result. Clonidine must be gradually tapered and replaced with another agent preoperatively if oral medications are not feasible postoperatively. Propranolol and other beta-adrenergic blocking drugs are safe to continue up to surgery[63]; rebound angina may occur if they are suddenly discontinued.

Diuretics are of anesthetic concern for two reasons: (1) hypertensive patients may require fluid loading before anesthesia because they have a contracted intravascular volume[108]; and (2) potassium loss may lead to chronic depletion of total body potassium. Except in urgent cases, surgery should be delayed until hypokalemia can be gradually corrected. Rapid intravenous replacement may temporarily raise the serum potassium level without correcting an underlying deficit of hundreds of milliequivalents; it may also result in intraoperative hypokalemia with serious ventricular arrhythmias resistant to antiarrhythmic therapy.[23,118]

Digitalis preparations are best continued. Serum level measurement is indicated if any suspicion of toxicity exists, particularly if potassium is low.

Anticholinergics, such as atropine and glycopyrrolate, are used principally to reduce oral secretions when necessary. They are of little value in preventing reflex bradycardia when given intramuscularly an hour before induction; intravenous atropine is the therapy of choice.[77] Atropine-induced tachycardia can precipitate ischemia in patients with coronary disease and decrease cardiac output in those with aortic or mitral stenosis.

Intraoperative Considerations

Cardiovascular Implications of Anesthetic Technique

Regional anesthesia is not necessarily better than general anesthesia for patients with cardiovascular disease. The ultimate effect of anesthesia on the patient depends not only on the technique but also on the anesthesiologist's skill and judgment; timing, dose, and rate of drug administration; preoperative preparation and medication; coexisting disease; and postoperative management.

Tracheal intubation is an intense stimulus that often results in sympathetic response. Agents used to block this response cause variable degrees of myocardial depression. Thus cardiovascular stability is difficult to maintain during tracheal intubation, making it particularly hazardous to patients with cardiac disease.

Spinal anesthesia lowers blood pressure by venodilation. This effect is minimal if the level of blockade is kept low; hypotension can be treated with fluids and vasopressors. High levels of spinal anesthesia may also cause cardiac sympathetic blockade. Epidural anesthesia causes less precipitous but similar changes.

Local infiltration is often thought to be safest for patients with severe cardiac disease. Nevertheless some anxious patients may develop ischemia from tachycardia and hypertension. Anxiety-related increases in preload and afterload may also worsen congestive heart failure. Attempts to alleviate anxiety with heavy sedation may cause hypoxemia and hypercarbia with further sympathetic outflow. Furthermore, if excessive doses of a local anesthetic are used, or if systemic absorption of the local anesthetic is more rapid than anticipated, a toxic reaction may ensue. Although lidocaine toxicity is usually heralded by neurologic signs and symptoms, bupivacaine toxicity may rapidly progress to cardiac arrest without early neurologic signs. Anesthesiologists are frequently called on to monitor patients undergoing local infiltration anesthesia. These patients require the same evaluation and preparation as those undergoing general anesthesia. Early consultation with the anesthesiologist aids in choosing the safest technique.

Cardiovascular Effects of Anesthetic Agents and Adjuncts

General anesthetics may have profound effects on the cardiovascular system. For example, halothane at 0.8% concentration (a typical anesthetic dose) causes a 30% depression of myocardial contractility.[11] This depression may be beneficial in ischemic disease because it reduces oxygen consumption, but it may lead to heart failure when ventricular function is marginal. Thiopental, a common intravenous induction agent, also causes cardiac depression. Propofol appears to have a greater hypotensive effect than thiopental. Other anesthetic agents such as ketamine have sympathomimetic properties with effects opposite to those just listed and may be contraindicated when myocardial oxygen supply is marginal. Many anesthetic drugs, such as some neuromuscular blocking agents, release histamine or block sympathetic ganglia, causing vasodilation.

Some anesthetic drugs are arrhythmogenic. Halothane sensitizes the heart to catecholamines. Epinephrine used for hemostasis during halothane anesthesia should be limited in a 70 kg patient to 10 ml of 1:100,000 epinephrine solution/10 minutes, and 30 ml/hour.[64] Pancuronium and aminophylline interact with halothane to increase ventricular irritability. This increase may be exacerbated by light levels of anesthesia or hypercarbia, which cause catecholamine release. Junctional rhythms are common, particularly with halothane, which causes sinus node depression. Enflurane and isoflurane, both newer inhalation agents, tend to cause tachycardia.

Monitoring Cardiovascular Function

Noninvasive monitors used routinely by the anesthesiologist include observation (skin color, salivation, lacrimation, pupil size, sweating), auscultation (continuous monitoring of breath and heart sounds), indirect blood pressure measurement (by Korotkoff sounds or oscillometric automatic cuff), ECG, and body temperature. Doppler ultrasound is often used at the wrist to detect radial artery blood flow when Korotkoff sounds are inaudible or on the precordium to detect central venous air embolism.

Invasive monitors include systemic arterial, central venous, and pulmonary arterial catheters. Other devices, such as left atrial catheters, may be inserted surgically. Invasive monitoring may be indispensable for safe anesthetic management, even in the absence of surgical indications. For example, in patients with ventricular dysfunction, a pulmonary artery catheter is helpful in determining whether intravenous fluid or inotropic drugs are needed during intraabdominal procedures that may involve major fluid shifts or blood loss.

Other Intraoperative Cardiovascular Considerations

Inhalation anesthetics are potent vasodilators. Without surgical stimulation, the combination of venous pooling and arterial dilatation will result in hypotension. Mechanical means (elevation of the legs), fluid loading, vasoconstrictors, or reduction of the anesthetic concentration can compensate for this tendency. Reducing concentration is only a temporary solution, because anesthetic depth may then be inadequate for the incision.

Cardiac and Aortic Surgery

Anesthesia for open heart surgery is a subspecialty. Extensive monitoring is used to follow and treat moment-to-moment changes in hemodynamics, because disturbances that are inconsequential in healthy patients can be catastrophic in these patients. Although sympathetic responses must be adequately suppressed, myocardial depression or vasodilatation may be poorly tolerated. These requirements can be met by using high-dose narcotic anesthesia at the expense of prolonged respiratory depression requiring postoperative ventilation and increased risk of awareness of events under anesthesia.

Patients with aortic disease often have concurrent coronary disease, making anesthetic management a challenge. During surgery on the aorta, avoiding left ventricular ischemia or failure may be difficult if cross-clamping is too abrupt; pharmacologic corrections take much longer than mechanical changes. Likewise, advance warning and slow execution of aortic declamping allow the anesthesiologist to infuse enough fluid to raise preload and prevent hypotension.

Continuous epidural anesthesia for abdominal aortic surgery offers the advantages of vasodilatation from sympathetic blockade and postoperative pain relief without excessive sedation or respiratory depression. Pain relief with epidural narcotics can improve postoperative gas exchange. Disadvantages include the need for close patient monitoring by trained nurses and the risk of epidural hematoma in anticoagulated patients.

Using an arterial cannula for continuous monitoring of blood pressure and periodic measurement of arterial blood gases and pH, the anesthesiologist can carefully control arterial oxygen and carbon dioxide partial pressure (Pa_{O_2}; Pa_{CO_2}) as well as blood pressure.

RESPIRATORY SYSTEM

Preoperative Assessment and Preparation

Only with adequate preoperative assessment of respiratory status can the anesthesiologist anticipate intraoperative requirements for tissue oxygenation and carbon dioxide elimination. Knowledge of baseline status is essential to providing optimal intraoperative management and ensuring a prompt return to preoperative pulmonary status.

Patients with bronchospastic disease should have therapy optimized preoperatively. If this measure is not taken, uptake and elimination of anesthetic gases will be prolonged; at worst, surgical stimulation and tracheal instrumentation will precipitate life-threatening bronchospasm.

Upper respiratory infections are not benign in surgical patients. General anesthesia carries the risks of increased tracheobronchial secretions, laryngospasm, and spread of the infection to laryngotracheitis or pneumonia. Normal airway mucociliary clearance is depressed with general anesthesia, increasing the risk of lung contamination and obstruction of small airways by secretions.

Preoperative preparation of patients with pulmonary disease has been shown to reduce respiratory morbidity and mortality.[46] This preparation may include bronchodilators, antibiotics, oxygen, chest percussion, and treatment of cor pulmonale. In patients with chronic respiratory muscle weakness or with restrictive or obstructive disease for which no specific pharmacologic therapy exists, preoperative training for postoperative coughing, deep breathing, and incentive spirometry can help minimize postoperative atelectasis.

Short-term preoperative cessation of smoking will increase the margin of safety by reducing blood carbon monoxide levels, leaving more hemoglobin available for oxygen transport.[24] Beneficial recovery of mucociliary transport, which tobacco smoking paralyzes, may also occur.

Upper abdominal and thoracic incisions markedly reduce vital capacity after surgical procedures, resulting in increased pulmonary complications.[109] When baseline vital capacity and forced expiratory volume are poor (less than half normal), postoperative mechanical ventilation may be necessary to prevent respiratory failure.

Pharmacologic Respiratory Considerations

Drugs used to treat respiratory disorders may benefit anesthetic management by improving physiologic status. However, they may also interact with anesthetic drugs.

Patients whose disease is under pharmacologic control, particularly asthmatic patients, should continue to receive their medications preoperatively. Methylxanthines (theophylline, aminophylline) should be continued through the perioperative period to maintain effective plasma levels, even though the intraoperative tachycardia they sometimes cause can be troublesome. Beta-sympathomimetic drugs have the potential for increasing ventricular irritability, which may require avoidance of certain drugs such as halothane and pancuronium.

Depending on dose and duration of therapy, patients receiving corticosteroid drugs for bronchospastic disease may have enough adrenocortical dysfunction to require preoperative steroid prophylaxis against stress-related adrenal insufficiency. It is controversial, however, whether "stress" doses should be given unless indicated intraoperatively.

Laboratory and Radiologic Studies

One of the most valuable means to evaluate respiratory function is to measure arterial blood gases. Elevated preoperative $Pa{CO_2}$ is an important finding because it may indicate that ventilation is stimulated by hypoxia rather than hypercarbia, rendering such patients susceptible to respiratory arrest during spontaneous breathing of high inspired oxygen tensions. Postoperative criteria for extubation depend on preoperative ventilatory status, making preanesthetic baseline blood gas analysis invaluable in patients with severe disease.

Pulmonary function testing at the simplest level includes forced vital capacity and forced expiratory volume in 1 second. These basic tests constitute a good preoperative screening for restrictive disease and small airway obstruction and help determine the need for postoperative mechanical ventilation.

Routine preoperative chest radiographs yield little in healthy patients,[93] but are valuable in patients with known or suspected pulmonary disease.

Intraoperative Considerations

Respiratory Implications of Anesthetic Technique

In selecting anesthetic technique, the anesthesiologist must consider operative positioning and the surgical site, both of which can seriously compromise respiration.

Clinicians sometimes incorrectly assume that regional anesthesia is preferable for patients with lung disease. Certain regional anesthetic techniques, such as brachial plexus block and low spinal or epidural block, allow surgery on the extremities without instrumentation of the airway or interference with respiration, which is an advantage as long as the patient can tolerate the necessary positioning. If anesthesia must include the abdomen or chest or if the positioning and its duration are intolerable to the patient, a general anesthetic with endotracheal intubation and control of ventilation may be safer than regional anesthesia. High spinal or epidural anesthesia can interfere with the accessory muscles of respiration. Furthermore, heavy sedation can lead to respiratory depression and poor clearance of secretions. Because much depends on individual skills and experience, the anesthesiologist should determine which technique will be best.

Respiratory Effects of Anesthetic Agents and Adjuncts

In selecting agents for general anesthesia, the anesthesiologist considers the agent's benefits versus its effect on respiratory function. Inhalation agents can suppress ventilatory drive and, therefore, delay their own uptake and elimination in the spontaneously breathing patient. Halothane causes bronchodilatation and depresses airway reflexes. Other inhalation agents, such as isoflurane and enflurane, are also bronchodilators but can irritate the upper airway, increasing the incidence of coughing and laryngospasm. All inhalation agents, as well as thiopental and the narcotics, suppress hypoxic drive to ventilation. This suppression occurs at subanesthetic levels of the commonly used volatile agents and has dangerous implications for patients who retain carbon dioxide and depend on hypoxemia for respiratory drive.

Mucociliary function is depressed by volatile agents and by dry, inspired gas mixtures.[41,42] Humidification of anesthetic gases, therefore, can be helpful. Deep breathing and coughing also help mobilize secretions postoperatively.

The effects of residual neuromuscular blockade range from impairment of deep breathing, coughing, and the ability to protect and maintain the airway to impairment of even normal tidal ventilation with resulting hypercarbia and hypoxia. Attainment of high motor blockade with regional anesthesia (i.e., subarachnoid or epidural block) has similar adverse effects.

Monitoring Respiratory Function

The simplest but least accurate indicator of arterial oxygenation is color of the skin or nail beds. Likewise, blood in the operative field may give some indication of hemoglobin saturation, but depends on lighting and background colors and is notoriously deceptive. When the question of hypoxemia arises, more direct means of assessing oxygenation are indicated.

The pulse oximeter is now a standard of care for general anesthesia. This noninvasive device uses a clip-on or adhesive sensor applied to the finger, ear, nose, or other tissue. Beat-to-beat determination of oxygen saturation is achieved by measuring two wavelengths of light that have different transmission curves as a function of hemoglobin saturation. This device, though sometimes subject to interference from external light, low local blood flow, and abnormal hemoglobin, has reduced the need for frequent blood gas sampling and dramatically increased safety and the ability to use lower oxygen concentrations during anesthesia, because changes in saturation can be detected immediately. The transcutaneous oxygen sensor is another device that offers continuous noninvasive monitoring, but it requires careful application, must be heated, and is unreliable when skin blood flow is reduced. It has not found wide acceptance in anesthesia.

Changes in airway pressure can be detected using a gauge on the anesthetic circuit. Increases in peak airway pressure may reflect bronchospasm or endobronchial location or obstruction of the endotracheal tube. Decreases in airway pressure may result from leaks or disconnections. High pressures may cause barotrauma and pneumothorax, particularly in patients with emphysema.

Bronchoconstriction and airway secretions, as well as the adequacy of ventilation, can be assessed by continuous auscultation through a precordial or esophageal stethoscope.

An arterial cannula allows serial blood gas measurements, useful for adjusting ventilation and detecting ventilation/perfusion mismatch requiring increased inspired oxygen fraction (FiO_2) or changes in ventilator settings. When there is severe ventilation/perfusion mismatch, therapy can be guided by calculating shunt fraction, which requires measurement of oxygen partial pressure in venous blood (P_VO_2) sampled from a pulmonary artery catheter.

Continuous measurement of expired carbon dioxide tension can be performed by capnograph based on infrared light transmission; Raman scattering device (RASCAL™), which uses laser light; or mass spectrometer. Although originally used to detect air embolism, these devices are becoming routine for noninvasive approximation of $PaCO_2$. The capnograph has reduced the need for frequent blood gas measurement and is also the most reliable means of rapidly identifying unintentional esophageal intubation and other ventilation problems.

Intraoperative Respiratory Problems

Ventilation and gas exchange have highest priority during anesthesia. Mechanical problems range from disconnections or a malfunctioning anesthesia machine to soft tissue obstruction of the airway and malposition or obstruction of an endotracheal tube. Intraoperative positioning, especially head down, may lead to ventilation/perfusion mismatch and restriction of lung expansion.

Major intraoperative derangements of respiratory function include bronchospasm, pneumothorax, and pulmonary embolism. Bronchospasm, which is more easily prevented than treated, is prevented by ensuring adequate levels of anesthesia before airway instrumentation or surgical stimulation and by establishing therapeutic levels of bronchodilators preoperatively in the susceptible patient. Intraoperative bronchospasm can be a life-threatening emergency when ventilation becomes nearly impossible. Treatment options include parenteral bronchodilators as well as aerosols delivered through the breathing circuit. Although an effective bronchodilator, halothane sensitizes the heart to sympathomimetic drugs (i.e., those used to treat bronchospasm) and may cause or exacerbate ventricular dysrhythmias.

Pneumothorax can occur spontaneously but is more often related to excessive intrathoracic pressure, surgical disruption of the pleura, or rupture of emphysematous blebs. The likelihood of barotrauma, leading to either pulmonary interstitial emphysema or pneumothorax, is minimized by limiting peak airway pressure to 50 cm H_2O); however, the pressure at which barotrauma occurs ranges from 25 to 80 cm H_2O.[81] Tension pneumothorax during general anesthesia is heralded by tachycardia, hypotension, rising airway pressure, a decrease or loss of breath sounds unilaterally, and tracheal deviation. This emergency warrants immediate pleural decompression by needle or chest tube. Nitrous oxide continued in the presence of pneumothorax will rapidly diffuse into and enlarge the pleural gas collection.

The chronically immobilized patient is at risk for venous thrombosis, which can lead to pulmonary embolism with as little provocation as transfer to the operating table. In patients predisposed to venous thrombosis, support stockings and preoperative anticoagulation are indicated.[60] Intraoperative detection is often possible only for very large emboli; transient tachycardia may be the only sign.

Thoracic Surgery

Most patients undergoing thoracic procedures are positioned in lateral or anterolateral positions, which can adversely affect cardiopulmonary function and increase chances for peripheral nerve injury. Ventilatory impairment results from restriction of chest motion and lung expansion, which can be minimized by placing rolls under the axilla and hip to better inflate the dependent, well-perfused lung. The lateral position can also impair venous return, causing a decrease in cardiac output. Peripheral nerve injuries may result from stretching or compression of the brachial plexus, radial, ulnar, or peroneal nerves. The dependent eye must be free of pressure to avoid retinal artery occlusion with postoperative blindness.

Opening the chest cavity during thoracic surgery causes physiologic derangements, which add to the already impaired lung function in most of these patients. Exposure of the nondependent lung creates severe ventilation/perfusion mismatch because the less-perfused upper lung is under little restriction and receives greater ventilation. Surgical retraction of the lung collapses the airways, markedly increasing the shunt. PaO_2 usually falls, requiring higher FiO_2 to prevent hypoxemia.

Some procedures such as pneumonectomy and control of pulmonary hemorrhage are facilitated by the placement of a double-lumen endotracheal tube, such as the Carlens, White, or Robertshaw, so that one lung may be selectively ventilated while the other is collapsed and isolated. Although this placement benefits the surgical procedure, it causes a large shunt with potential for hypoxemia unless careful monitoring is carried out and appropriate actions are taken. Continuous or intermittent insufflation of oxygen or continuous positive airway pressure to the collapsed lung can minimize hypoxia. The value of positive end-expiratory pressure to the dependent lung is not well proved. Proper endobronchial placement of the double-lumen tube has a very small margin for error; improper placement will compromise ventilation. Double-lumen tubes are more likely than standard tubes to traumatize the larynx, trachea, or bronchi. The surgeon must be aware of position of the tube, which has occasionally been sutured into the bronchial stump closure.

On completion of one-lung anesthesia, reexpansion of the collapsed lung will help prevent postoperative atelectasis and will improve venous return by bringing the mediastinum back to the midline. To avoid coughing that could disrupt fresh bronchial stump closures, anesthetic depth is coordinated with the degree of surgical stimulation, particularly airway manipulation. Double-lumen tubes must be removed or replaced with conventional endotracheal tubes following completion of the procedure.

Postoperative Respiratory Considerations

Postanesthetic management after thoracic procedures includes several major considerations. Positioning may be critical because cardiac herniation and collapse can occur after pneumonectomy and pericardiectomy if the operated side is dependent. Coughing can disrupt the bronchial stump closure. Inadequate analgesia limits tidal volume, whereas excessive narcotic analgesia causes respiratory depression. Intercostal nerve blocks are helpful, at the risk of local anesthetic toxicity and pneumothorax. Thoracic epidural or subarachnoid narcotics are effective for long-term pain control with early ambulation but pose the hazards of delayed respiratory depression, pruritus, nausea, and urinary retention.[59,73] Small doses of naloxone appear to be effective in treating these symptoms without reversing the analgesia.

Criteria for extubation are based on preoperative baseline function. Typical criteria might include sustained (4 to 5 seconds) headlift or adequate nerve stimulator response, indicating adequate reversal of neuromuscular blockade; inspiratory force of at least -25 cm H_2O and vital capacity of at least 15 ml/kg body weight; $PaCO_2$ within 5 mm Hg of baseline; alveolar-arterial oxygen difference less than 300 mm Hg with FiO_2 of 100%; and the patient's ability to protect the airway.

When aminoglycoside and certain other antibiotics have been given, neuromuscular blockade may be potentiated to the extent that it cannot be reversed with the usual agents.[14] In such cases mechanical ventilation is necessary until neuromuscular function is adequate.

GASTROINTESTINAL SYSTEM

Aspiration of Gastric Contents

One of the most feared complications of anesthesia is the pulmonary aspiration of gastric contents. Thus the anesthesiologist is concerned with factors contributing to the risk of aspiration pneumonia,[61] including the following:

1. *Gastric volume.* A volume of more than 25 ml is considered a major risk factor.[17] Fasting for 6 to 8 hours after solid food intake is usually allowed for the stomach to empty, although anxiety, trauma, late pregnancy, and drug therapy can delay gastric emptying.[15,52] Anxious patients may

have preoperative aerophagia and an inflated stomach.[3,22] A recent review suggests that in nonpregnant, nonemergency patients, 150 ml of clear liquids may be administered up to 3 hours preoperatively, with no adverse effect on gastric volume in adults.[25]

2. *Gastric pH.* Pulmonary aspiration syndrome (Mendelson's syndrome) is more severe when the aspirated material has a pH of less than 2.5. Several drugs can be used to elevate the pH of gastric contents. To be effective, histamine receptor blockers such as cimetidine or ranitidine should be given orally or intravenously at least 2 hours before induction of anesthesia.[19] The pH of gastric contents can be buffered by oral antacids.[53] Clear, nonparticulate antacids such as sodium citrate are preferred because they provoke less tissue reaction if aspirated.[114,119,128,135]
3. *Esophageal sphincter tone.* Tone of the lower esophageal sphincter, which is the anatomic barrier to regurgitation,[20] may be reduced by many commonly used drugs, such as narcotic analgesics and anticholinergics.[94]

Patients with the following conditions are at increased risk for aspiration: bowel obstruction, long-standing diabetes, advanced age, pregnancy, hiatal hernia, acute abdomen, and history of vomiting during previous induction of anesthesia.

Anesthetic management of the patient with a full stomach focuses on protecting the airway. If general anesthesia is used, the trachea is intubated either with the patient "awake" (moderate sedation can be used as long as protective airway responses are intact) or by means of the "rapid-sequence" induction technique, sometimes referred to as "crash induction." Two major goals of rapid-sequence induction are (1) to produce sudden loss of consciousness; and (2) to prevent an increase in intraabdominal pressure favoring silent regurgitation of gastric contents.

Intraabdominal pressure can be increased by retching, coughing, or succinylcholine-induced muscle fasciculations.[80] Rapid-sequence induction involves preoxygenation (or more correctly, denitrogenation) to prevent hypoxemia during the subsequent period of apnea, pretreatment with a small dose of a nondepolarizing neuromuscular blocking drug to prevent muscle fasciculations, and injection of intravenous anesthetic and rapid-acting neuromuscular blocking drug in quick succession. An assistant applies firm pressure over the cricoid cartilage, compressing the esophagus between the cricoid ring and the anterior body of the sixth cervical vertebra, thus minimizing the likelihood of passive regurgitation of gastric contents.[38] As soon as the muscles are relaxed, the trachea is intubated as quickly as possible with a cuffed endotracheal tube. The cuff is inflated and tube position checked by auscultation before cricoid pressure is released. As the patient emerges from anesthesia, the endotracheal tube should be left in place until protective airway reflexes have returned.[92,97,105]

Patients with Gastrointestinal Disease

Esophagus

Patients with a history of anatomic or physiologic abnormalities of the esophagus, particularly those with a history of motility problems, should be treated with the precautions against regurgitation and aspiration just listed. Included are patients with a history of achalasia, Zenker's diverticula, or hiatal hernia, particularly with symptoms of gastroesophageal reflux.[18,84]

The patient with esophageal varices often has portal hypertension, hepatosplenomegaly, ascites that may be severe enough to cause respiratory compromise, thrombocytopenia and coagulopathy, and various degrees of liver dysfunction. The passage of a nasogastric tube may lacerate a varix and cause substantial hemorrhage.

Stomach

Patients undergoing surgery for herniation, obstruction, tumor, or hemorrhage in the stomach should be considered at risk for regurgitation. The patient with a perforated gastric ulcer presents special problems. Besides having a full stomach, these patients are usually in severe pain, which is worsened by inspiration; thus they are often tachypneic and hypercarbic. Atelectasis and sympathetic pleural effusions are common.[102]

Gallbladder

In patients with biliary obstruction, narcotics typically used in anesthesia (morphine, fentanyl) may cause increased intrabiliary pressure by increasing the tone of the sphincter of Oddi. This pressure can be attenuated by pretreatment with traditional anticholinergics, such as atropine, glycopyrrolate, or scopolamine,[54] or antagonized by the narcotic antagonist naloxone.

Subcostal retraction may interfere with ventilation. The painful right subcostal incision may cause postoperative "splinting" and hypoventilation.[102]

Liver

Impairment of liver function must be advanced before it significantly affects the metabolism of anesthetic agents. More important, certain factors, such as hypoxia and hypotension, can further compromise a failing liver. In addition to reduced drug metabolism, patients with liver disease may have ascites, which when severe, can restrict ventilation. Serious metabolic derangements and high serum ammonia levels with hepatic encephalopathy may also exist. These patients may have delayed return of both consciousness and protective airway reflexes. Coagulopathy, portal hypertension, and esophageal varices may be present; and the anesthesiologist considers all these when planning the anesthetic.

The issue of "halothane hepatitis" has been of concern for many years.[10,12,13,87] This disorder, marked by postoperative liver necrosis, is exceedingly rare. The mechanism of toxicity, when it occurs, does not appear to be dose-related but rather associated with autoimmunity or hypersensitivity. Halothane hepatitis is an overused diagnosis; many other, more likely causes of postoperative jaundice exist. In one large study, one patient in 700 had elective surgery cancelled because of liver chemistry abnormalities; of these, one third developed jaundice. Many of these abnormalities would have been attributed to halothane if it had been used.[95] No specific tests are available to diagnose halothane hepatitis, although work continues in this area.[39] It is fortunate that children do not appear to be susceptible, because halothane is still the most satisfactory halogenated agent for inhalation induction. Although no evidence indicates that preexisting liver disease is exacerbated by halothane, risk seems to be greater with obesity, hypoxia, recent exposure to halothane, and chronic exposure to polychlorinated biphenyls.[100,120] Today anesthesiologists use halothane freely in children but limit its use in adults to cases when its properties are advantageous, as in bronchospasm and mask induction.

Bowel

Bowel obstruction carries a high risk of pulmonary aspiration of gastric contents. Thus rapid-sequence induction or awake intubation is chosen in these patients.

Patients with lower intestinal obstruction often have abnormalities in fluid and electrolyte balance that should be recognized and treated preoperatively.[93] However, the anesthesiologist must be aware that these patients often require large volumes of intravenous electrolyte solution intraoperatively.

Lower gastrointestinal perforation is more common in elderly patients and at first may be unrecognized. These patients typically have peritonitis and are severely dehydrated from loss of fluid into the "third space." Thus they may benefit from invasive hemodynamic monitoring.

The patient with toxic megacolon presents a particular anesthetic challenge. Preoperative abdominal films indicate the degree of colon dilatation. Some commonly used drugs, such as narcotics and anticholinergics, should be avoided, because they can predispose to further dilatation and even colon rupture. During emergency colectomy for toxic megacolon, however, narcotics and anticholinergics may be safely used as adjuncts to the anesthetic agents.

The nitrous oxide concentration in gas-filled spaces of the body increases toward the concentration in the blood. Therefore, if 50% nitrous oxide is administered, the volume of closed, gas-filled spaces can nearly double. With bowel obstruction, nitrous oxide diffuses into gas trapped in the bowel and increases intraenteric pressures.[35] Under these circumstances nitrous oxide can be used during the induction of anesthesia but then is usually discontinued.

RENAL, GENITOURINARY, AND REPRODUCTIVE SYSTEMS

Renal Function

The anesthesiologist is interested in the patient's renal function because general anesthesia affects renal function and because the patient's renal function can influence general anesthesia.

General anesthetics temporarily decrease renal function.[22,67] Because of myocardial depression and vasodilation, anesthetics decrease renal function by decreasing renal flow.[79] Mechanical ventilation may further decrease renal flow by decreasing cardiac output.[21,55]

The metabolism of methoxyflurane leads to the formation of free inorganic fluoride ion,[110] high serum levels of which can produce high-output nephropathy (azotemia, increased serum osmolality, increased serum sodium). Methoxyflurane is now seldom used in general anesthesia but may occasionally be used in obstetrics for labor analgesia. Enflurane, another volatile anesthetic, is also metabolized to inorganic fluoride ion, but to a much lesser extent than methoxyflurane. Some cases of fluoride nephropathy caused by enflurane have been reported.[71] In controlled studies, temporary, mild decreases in ability to concentrate urine were seen in healthy volunteers exposed to prolonged, deep levels of enflurane anesthesia.[16,75] Nephrotoxicity has not been reported with isoflurane, an isomer of enflurane that is metabolized to a lesser extent.

Patients with Renal Failure

The kidney is the principal means of excretion of many commonly used drugs, such as nondepolarizing neuromuscular blockers. The anesthesiologist, therefore, must be alert for increased duration of action of these agents in patients with renal failure. A peripheral nerve stimulator is one means of measuring residual neuromuscular blockade, which may necessitate prolonged ventilation if reversal with agents such as neostigmine or edrophonium is inadequate.

Patients with chronic renal failure tend to have a lower hematocrit level than healthy patients, but because compensatory mechanisms allow these patients to maintain adequate oxygen transport, preoperative transfusion to increase the hematocrit to "normal levels" is rarely indicated. Anesthetic technique, however, must be modified to maintain adequate oxygen transport.

The patient undergoing chronic hemodialysis may be

hypovolemic after dialysis. Predialysis and postdialysis body weights may assist in assessing the state of hydration. Monitoring central venous pressure, or in some cases pulmonary arterial pressure, helps to quantify volume depletion and avoid unintentional fluid overload. Serum potassium level should be no higher than 5.5 mEq/L following dialysis if general anesthesia is planned. Succinylcholine, a muscle relaxant used for intubation, leads to a transient rise in serum potassium concentration during muscle fasciculations, and is best avoided in the presence of hyperkalemia. A recently dialyzed patient should also undergo coagulation studies (prothrombin and partial thromboplastin times) to rule out residual anticoagulation, which may contraindicate spinal or epidural anesthesia and may lead to excessive intraoperative bleeding.

Patients receiving chronic hemodialysis usually have peripheral arterial fistulae, typically in the nondominant forearm. Blood pressure measurements, venipuncture, and intravenous infusions are avoided in that arm. By monitoring the bruit or thrill generated by the fistula, the anesthesiologist can detect whether fistula flow becomes inadequate, posing the risk of thrombosis. If the bruit disappears, hydration with a bolus of intravenous fluid may reestablish blood flow. Although intravenous fluid should be administered judiciously, the risk of loss of the fistula due to volume depletion and a drop in cardiac output is more serious than the risk of overhydration, which can be treated postoperatively by dialysis.

Nephrotoxic drugs, including enflurane, methoxyflurane, and aminoglycoside antibiotics, are avoided in patients with impaired renal function.

Genitourinary Surgery

Transurethral Resection of Prostate

During this procedure, water intoxication, blood loss, and bladder perforation are key problems confronting the anesthesiologist.[28] Glycine solution is usually used for irrigation because it is clear, nonconductive, and isosmotic. Large volumes of this fluid may enter transected venous sinuses during transurethral resection of the prostate, resulting in circulatory volume expansion, hemodilution, and sometimes hyperkalemia due to hemolysis.[106] Circulatory overload leads to hypertension and eventually pulmonary edema. The most pressing concern with hemodilution is hyponatremia (serum sodium level below 120 to 125 mEq/L), which manifests in the awake patient as restlessness, confusion, headache, and nausea. The condition progresses to lethargy, convulsions, and coma. Water intoxication can be confirmed by measurement of serum sodium concentration. Hyponatremia is safely treated with diuretics, along with isotonic saline solution to maintain intravascular volume. In severe cases the serum sodium concentration can be increased with intravenous hypertonic saline, although this technique is potentially hazardous and controversial.

Spinal anesthesia is often chosen over general anesthesia for transurethral resection of the prostate because it allows early diagnosis of hemodilution and hyponatremia. Additional advantages of spinal anesthesia are early recognition of bladder perforation, reduced intraoperative blood loss, and postoperative relief of bladder spasm and pain from traction on the urethral catheter. On the other hand, uncooperative patients and those with pulmonary disease can be poor candidates for regional anesthesia because a poorly timed cough could result in bladder perforation.

Patient Positioning in Urologic Surgery

The lithotomy position reduces pulmonary vital capacity and drains blood from the legs. These effects are even more pronounced if the operating table is adjusted so that the shoulders are lower than the hips. The awake patient experiences increased work of breathing. During general anesthesia, ventilation/perfusion mismatch worsens, and the endotracheal tube can migrate into a bronchus as the hilum of the lung moves cephalad, resulting in shunting and hypoxemia. Autotransfusion from the elevated legs can precipitate pulmonary edema or mask hypovolemia; as the legs are lowered at the end of a procedure performed in the lithotomy position, a reduction in preload can cause hypotension.

The kidney position, in which the patient is in a lateral decubitus position with hips elevated and head and feet dependent, causes substantial cardiorespiratory impairment. Blood pools in the upper body and legs. If the kidney rest is positioned incorrectly under the flank, respiration and venous return are compromised even more; the kidney rest should be located under the iliac crest, where it most effectively stretches the opposite flank to facilitate surgical exposure.

Gynecologic Surgery

Laparoscopy is a common procedure that most gynecologists regard as preferable to laparotomy for diagnosis and for tubal ligation. However, the procedure presents several areas of concern to the anesthesiologist:

1. Abdominal insufflation with gas to facilitate exposure, combined with a head-down position, impairs diaphragmatic excursion. Intubation of the trachea with mechanical ventilation is nearly always indicated.
2. Insufflation is usually accomplished with carbon dioxide because it is physiologic and rapidly absorbed. Absorption of carbon dioxide into the circulation can produce respiratory acidosis, which causes release of catecholamines, resulting in hypertension and tachycardia. This problem is easily avoided if the anesthesiologist augments ventila-

tion to accommodate the exogenous carbon dioxide load. Halothane is well known to sensitize the myocardium to the arrhythmogenic effects of catecholamines and is usually avoided in laparoscopy.

3. Carbon dioxide embolism with acute cardiovascular collapse can occur when vascular integrity is disrupted or during unintentional extraperitoneal insufflation.
4. During insertion the laparoscope can puncture bowel, inflated stomach, distended bladder, or even the vena cava or aorta. A nasogastric tube is sometimes inserted to decompress the stomach.

Pregnant Patients

Because of concern about the effects of surgery and anesthesia during the first trimester of pregnancy, when organogenesis is in progress, elective surgery is postponed in the pregnant patient. The teratogenic effects of anesthetic drugs in human beings are still poorly defined.[37,85]

If surgery is necessary, regional anesthesia is used in the pregnant patient, when possible. When general anesthesia is required, barbiturates and nitrous oxide have been used without evidence of increased fetal mortality. After about the twelfth week of pregnancy, patients have increased gastric volumes and delayed gastric emptying time. They should be considered, therefore, to have full stomachs and warrant rapid-sequence induction and intubation if general anesthesia is chosen.[91]

In late pregnancy a large uterus can compress the vena cava and decrease venous return, leading to decreased cardiac output and blood pressure. Called the *supine hypotension syndrome,* it is manifested by a falling blood pressure associated with tachycardia and sweating. Seen as early as the thirtieth week of pregnancy, the syndrome is more severe when the uterus is abnormally large, as in polyhydramnios or multiple gestation. Placing a pillow under the right hip or tilting the table to the left helps shift the uterus away from the aorta and vena cava and can ameliorate this syndrome. Vasopressors may occasionally be required.

When a pregnant patient undergoes surgery after the first trimester of pregnancy, fetal heart rate should be monitored, either by Doppler pulse meter or fetal ECG.

NERVOUS SYSTEM

Concerns of the anesthesiologist regarding the surgical patient with neurologic disease include intracranial pressure (ICP) and brain perfusion, air embolism, and neurologic deficit.

These concerns dictate the emphasis of the preoperative evaluation. Preoperative blood pressure values help determine the safe range of intraoperative values in patients with cerebrovascular disease. Patients with intracranial aneurysms require careful preoperative sedation and precise control of hemodynamics intraoperatively. Elevated ICP warrants important changes in anesthetic technique.

Concomitant disease is often more important than the neurologic problem. A comatose patient requires thorough pulmonary evaluation because of possible atelectasis, aspiration, or rarely neurogenic pulmonary edema. Coronary disease frequently accompanies cerebrovascular lesions. Differential diagnosis of coma includes diabetes, liver dysfunction, kidney failure, and electrolyte imbalance, which all have major anesthetic implications.

Preoperative sedation should be mild or omitted entirely in patients with central nervous system depression. State of consciousness is often a valuable guide to rising ICP or vascular compromise. In addition, narcotics and sedatives depress respiration; the resulting elevation of Pa_{CO_2} causes a further rise in ICP. Small doses of diazepam have anticonvulsant properties that may be advantageous.[72]

Neurosurgical procedures limit the anesthesiologist's access to the airway, which necessitates careful positioning and fixation of the endotracheal tube. Extreme neck flexion may kink standard endotracheal tubes; kink-resistant, wire-reinforced tubes are available. In patients with cervical fracture or vertebrobasilar insufficiency, improper head positioning can do irreparable damage. In any patient, head manipulation may advance the tube down one bronchus, resulting in atelectasis of one lung. The prone position requires that the tube be securely fixed to the face; rapid reintubation in this position in the event of unexpected extubation is very difficult.

Intracranial Pressure

Elevated ICP is important not only because certain anesthetic agents worsen it, but also because the anesthetic technique must minimize coughing and elevation of central venous pressure. Predisposing factors to increased ICP include head trauma with cerebral edema, space-occupying intracranial lesions, intracranial hemorrhage, and hydrocephalus. When ICP increases sufficiently to cause medullary ischemia, the patient will demonstrate the Cushing triad of systemic hypertension, bradycardia, and irregular respiration.

Preoperative sedation is usually mild or omitted altogether in patients with elevated ICP and in those with central nervous system depression. In addition to the risk of respiratory arrest, there is risk of further elevation of ICP due to hypoventilation leading to an elevated Pa_{CO_2}, which in turn increases cerebral blood flow. In addition, sedation may mask progression of symptoms.

With elevated ICP, the goal of anesthesia induction

is adequate depression of sympathetic reflexes and muscle activity to avoid further increases in ICP, without significant cardiovascular depression. Hyperventilation is the most important mechanism for reducing ICP on induction of anesthesia. Nondepolarizing neuromuscular blocking agents are often used in place of succinylcholine, which can cause some increase in ICP. Intravenous lidocaine lessens the sympathetic response to tracheal intubation, whereas intravenous propranolol helps block sympathetically mediated tachycardia and hypertension.

Preoperative control of ICP is typically aided by decreasing intravascular volume. This decrease can result in hypotension when anesthesia is induced because many anesthetics are vasodilators.

Nitrous oxide and oxygen with a narcotic and muscle relaxant are frequently chosen to avoid the cerebral vasodilatation effect of volatile anesthetic agents. However, hyperventilation to establish hypocarbia before the use of volatile agents has been found to prevent the rise in ICP, making this technique acceptable as well.[68,115] Optimal Pa_{CO_2} is about 30 mm Hg; further decreases do not appreciably reduce ICP but may cause deleterious cerebral vasoconstriction.[99] In some situations, such as air entrapment in the ventricles or venous air embolism, nitrous oxide must be discontinued to avoid its diffusion into and consequent enlargement of air spaces. Ketamine is generally contraindicated in the presence of elevated ICP.

Despite precautionary measures, ICP occasionally rises to dangerous levels. Reduction of ICP before induction of anesthesia may be achieved by one or more of the following methods:

1. Removal of cerebrospinal fluid.
2. Hyperosmolar agents (mannitol, urea, or glycerol). Rebound rise of ICP is marked with urea, less with mannitol, and rare with glycerol. Large doses of these agents can produce marked brain shrinkage and tearing of cortical veins and dural sinuses.[74]
3. Systemic diuretics. Furosemide and ethacrynic acid reduce ICP by both reduction of intravascular volume and decreased formation of cerebrospinal fluid.
4. Steroids, such as dexamethasone.
5. Barbiturates, such as thiopental in large doses (30 mg/kg). This reduces cerebral blood flow. Because of the myocardial depression and prolonged unconsciousness produced by these large doses, the use of barbiturates to control ICP is limited.

Positioning and Air Embolism

Surgical considerations determine patient positioning. Careful positioning can avoid obstruction of the jugular veins, which increases ICP, and pressure on bony areas or peripheral nerves, which can lead to pressure necrosis and nerve injury.

The sitting position offers better surgical exposure and wound drainage for certain procedures, such as posterior fossa craniotomy and cervical laminectomy. However, surgery in the sitting position carries the risk of venous air embolism, a potentially fatal complication that can occur whenever the surgical wound is above the level of the right atrium.[78]

The anesthesiologist has several means of detecting and treating venous air embolism. A precordial Doppler probe placed over the right side of the heart is the most sensitive detector but is sometimes difficult to use and interpret reliably. Pulmonary blood flow obstruction is reflected by a fall in end-tidal Pa_{CO_2}, which can be detected with a capnograph. Precordial or esophageal heart sounds change with significant amounts of air, eventually becoming a continuous "mill wheel murmur"; however, this sign usually occurs too late to be useful. Additional signs include tachycardia, hypotension, cardiac arrhythmias, and elevation of central venous pressure. With air embolism, a right atrial catheter is often helpful in evacuating air and confirming the diagnosis. Rapid repositioning of the patient may be necessary if flooding or packing of the wound does not stop air entry.

Neurologic Deficits

Iatrogenic lesions include nerve injury resulting from improper positioning, as well as neuropathy caused by nerve trauma or hematoma during regional anesthesia. Documenting preoperative deficits is essential.

Spinal cord lesions require special anesthetic considerations. For many weeks after the onset of paraplegia, degenerating muscles release large amounts of potassium when succinylcholine is given, which can lead to cardiac arrest.[111] When a spinal cord lesion is above the seventh thoracic dermatome, autonomic hyperreflexia can occur; 85% of patients with lesions above the fifth thoracic level exhibit this syndrome. Initiated by a cutaneous, proprioceptive, or visceral stimulus below the lesion, the syndrome may consist of flushing of the head and neck, caused by cutaneous vasodilatation above the lesion, and paroxysmal hypertension, with increased vagal tone leading to bradycardia, premature ventricular beats, and heart block.[96] Ganglionic blocking agents such as pentolinium can block this reflex in nonanesthetized patients.[5]

Other Neurologic Diseases

Regional anesthesia is rarely contraindicated for medical reasons in patients with myopathy, peripheral neuropathy, or multiple sclerosis; however, because the patient may attribute worsening of the disease to a regional anesthetic, anesthesiologists are reluctant to use this technique.

Enflurane can precipitate seizures in patients with a seizure history, particularly in the presence of hypocarbia. Halothane and isoflurane, which do not significantly lower seizure threshold, can be used instead. Phenobarbital and phenytoin should usually be continued through the preoperative period to maintain control of seizures.

Patients with intracranial aneurysms require special treatment. They are often more heavily sedated in an effort to minimize stress and hypertension, are best kept hydrated during the procedure, and require precise control of blood pressure. Deliberate hypotension by various methods, a potentially hazardous technique, can help control bleeding and provide optimal surgical conditions.[33,69]

Although general anesthesia is usually preferred for optimal surgical conditions, one should remember that local infiltration of the scalp and periosteum is adequate for burr holes and other minor procedures, including stereotactic ablation in the awake patient.

Postoperative Care of Neurosurgical Patients

Neurosurgical patients are at risk for intracranial hemorrhage, particularly if hypertension occurs. Hemorrhage usually appears as increasing ICP in the recovery room, which may be manifested by reduced level of consciousness, change in respiratory pattern, bradycardia, or hypertension. Cerebral edema is minimized by elevating the head, provided blood pressure is adequate in this position. ICP can be measured continuously with an intraventricular or epidural cannula.

When the return to consciousness is slow, a cuffed endotracheal tube is left in place to protect the airway, although ventilatory assistance may also be necessary. If neck motion is restricted, extubation may also be delayed until the patient is alert, because reintubation may be difficult. Level of consciousness is checked frequently and classified using any of several criteria, such as the Glasgow Coma Scale (see Chapter 26).[57]

Pain is usually treated with mild analgesics to avoid respiratory depression and the attendant risks of hypercarbia and intracranial hypertension.

SKELETAL MUSCLE AND THE MYONEURAL JUNCTION

Patients with primary disorders of skeletal muscle and the neuromuscular junction may exhibit diminished motor reserve and increased sensitivity to neuromuscular blockade. Musculoskeletal disorders of primary concern to the anesthesiologist include rheumatoid arthritis, scoliosis, muscular dystrophies, and myasthenia gravis, as well as malignant hyperthermia, a dreaded anesthetic complication.

Rheumatoid Arthritis

Patients with rheumatoid arthritis present the anesthesiologist with many systemic manifestations and side effects of pharmacologic management.[56] All joints may be affected, including those involved with the upper airway (cervical spine, temporomandibular joints, cricoarytenoid joints).[43] Immobility of these joints can make direct visualization of the glottis during endotracheal intubation very difficult. Furthermore, atlantoaxial subluxation can cause compression of the cervical spinal cord or vertebral artery during neck extension.[35,103] Thorough airway assessment before anesthesia induction is vital in these patients. In difficult cases the best method may be "awake" intubation, either by inserting the endotracheal tube "blindly" into the larynx via the nasopharynx or by threading the endotracheal tube over a flexible fiberoptic laryngoscope under topical anesthesia of the posterior pharynx. Elective tracheostomy may be necessary, although regional anesthesia is often a valuable alternative.

Malignant Hyperthermia

Malignant hyperthermia (MH) is perhaps the most dreaded of anesthetic complications. Because it is often recognized too late or not at all, resulting mortality is high.

MH is a primary disorder of the sarcoplasmic reticulum. When the disease is triggered, a calcium excess in the myoplasm results in a hypercatabolic emergency. Known triggering agents include many drugs used during anesthesia, such as halothane and succinylcholine. Although certain anesthetic drugs are considered "safe," no anesthetic is absolutely safe, because stress alone can precipitate the syndrome.

The earliest signs of MH are variable and nonspecific but may include tachycardia, hypertension, arrhythmias, and muscle rigidity.[48] Hypercarbia and metabolic acidosis are early findings. Rise in body temperature can occur late in the course. Myoglobinuria and renal failure may follow. Measurement of serial serum creatine phosphokinase (CPK) and urine myoglobin is helpful in patients suspected of having an episode of MH because the diagnosis is mainly clinical. Although special muscle biopsy tests for MH are available, none is fully reliable without clinical supporting evidence. Dantrolene is an effective treatment if used promptly but is expensive and time consuming to prepare.[49]

Patients at risk for MH are usually identified by family history or a prior suspected episode of MH. Dantrolene may be given prophylactically. Special precautions must be taken to avoid exposure to trace amounts of halogenated agents; this approach may be difficult or impossible on short notice. The need to avoid succinylcholine and halogenated agents complicates anesthetic management, especially when a halogenated agent is indicated in a patient with asthma or hypertension. Because no anesthetic is absolutely safe, regional techniques in a properly sedated patient may be safest, when feasible. Ester local anesthetics are safe, whereas amides such as lidocaine are theoretically a risk. Most authorities on MH believe local infiltration with amide anesthetics for biopsies and dental procedures poses little risk, but this hypothesis has not been proven.[50]

Myasthenia Gravis

Myasthenia gravis, an autoimmune disorder of the muscle acetylcholine receptor, is most often characterized by ocular and oropharyngeal weakness. Respiratory weakness is less common than in the muscular dystrophies and is most often seen in severe myasthenia; however, aspiration resulting from dysfunction of the swallowing mechanism remains a hazard.

Surgical stress alone can precipitate a myasthenic crisis. Myasthenic patients are extremely sensitive to neuromuscular blocking drugs; postoperative ventilatory support may be necessary even when these agents have not been used. Although some clinicians advocate that muscle relaxants never be used, they are sometimes clearly necessary, but in minuscule doses. According to some studies, regional anesthesia is less troublesome, but ester local anesthetics should be avoided because anticholinesterase therapy may interfere with their metabolism.[31] Patients with dysphagia and respiratory impairment should continue to receive anticholinesterase therapy throughout the perioperative period.

Before extubation of the trachea, patients should be capable of maintaining adequate ventilation and clearing secretions. Suitable criteria might include adequate arterial blood gases, inspiratory force greater than -30 cm H_2O, and vital capacity of 15 ml/kg after a 1- to 2-hour trial of spontaneous ventilation.[70]

HEMATOLOGIC SYSTEM

Hematologic disorders concern the anesthesiologist when they interfere with oxygen transport, blood flow, or clotting. In addition, some hematologic diseases damage other organ systems. For example, leukemia may result in tissue infiltration affecting the heart, brain, liver, and kidney; it is occasionally associated with a myasthenic syndrome; and it increases susceptibility to infection. Anemia is frequently a sign of another disease, such as renal failure, which affects anesthetic management.

Blood Cell Disease

Anemia limits oxygen transport to the tissues. In the past, it was thought that a hemoglobin concentration of 10 g/dl, or about 30% hematocrit with normal erythrocytes, was a reasonable minimum to allow adequate oxygen delivery.[44] More recently, studies have demonstrated that there is no increase in perioperative morbidity in otherwise healthy patients with preoperative hematocrits as low as 7 g/dl, or about 21% hematocrit.[47] Therefore, preoperative transfusion is no longer thought to be indicated in patients with hemoglobin levels greater than 7 g/dl, in the absence of significant cardiorespiratory or other disease impairing oxygen delivery to vital organs. Patients with long-standing anemia, such as those with chronic renal failure, have increased cardiac output and other compensatory mechanisms and generally need not be transfused preoperatively unless hematocrit has dropped below their baseline. In fact, an optimal balance between reduced oxygen-carrying capacity and improved flow characteristics resulting from reduction in blood viscosity occurs at about a 30% hematocrit. This balance can be demonstrated following cardiopulmonary bypass, when hemodilution has reduced blood viscosity and cardiac output is maintained at reduced stroke work and myocardial oxygen consumption.[82] Patients with hemoglobin levels chronically as low as 7.2 g/dl have shown treadmill exercise tolerance comparable to that of nonanemic patients.[104] Polycythemia is itself a risk; patients with hemoglobin concentration greater than 16 g/dl have demonstrated increased perioperative mortality that can be reduced by preoperative phlebotomy.[116]

Some types of anemia pose hazards beyond a reduction in oxygen transport; these hazards include sickle cell disease, thalassemia, and autoimmune hemolytic anemia. Sickle cell anemia occurs in patients with the abnormal hemoglobin (Hb) S. Sickle cell disease, the homozygous form (Hb SS), is found in about 0.2% of the black population in the United States, but it is the most serious type of anemia in the surgical patient. Sickling of red cells results in obstruction of small blood vessels, followed by tissue infarction, hemolysis, and bone marrow exhaustion with aplastic crisis and severe anemia. Sickling can be prevented by administering high inspired oxygen concentrations to prevent hypoxemia and by avoiding acidosis and hypothermia. The patient should be well hydrated to maintain peripheral blood flow and positioned to avoid peripheral venous stasis. During sickle cell crisis, the concentration of normal adult Hb A is sometimes therapeutically increased by exchange transfusion.

Autoimmune hemolytic anemias are troublesome when transfusion is necessary. If cold antibody is present, the patient must be kept warm and all administered fluids must be warmed. Cross-matching blood may be difficult, and hematology consultation is advisable. Patients are sometimes asked to donate blood preoperatively for intraoperative administration.

The patient with a history of acute intermittent porphyria is rare but at high anesthetic risk. Frequently used anesthetic drugs such as barbiturates (thiopental) and benzodiazepines (diazepam), as well as phenytoin, sulfonamides, ergot preparations, chlordiazepoxide, meprobamate, and pentazocine, can precipitate an attack, which may progress to lower motor neuron lesions, psychiatric disorders, and bulbar paralysis. Because an acute attack may mimic the acute abdomen, the anesthesiologist must be aware of possible porphyria when preoperatively assessing the patient with an acute abdomen.

Hemostatic Disorders

Clotting disorders can lead to uncontrollable hemorrhage. In addition, regional anesthesia may be contraindicated because of the risk of neurovascular deficit from a hematoma compressing a blood vessel, nerve, or spinal cord.

Routine preoperative evaluation should include inquiry about bleeding problems and the use of drugs that impair platelet function, such as aspirin. Bleeding time is the most useful test for evaluating platelet function, whereas prothrombin time, partial thromboplastin time, and platelet count constitute the rest of a coagulation screening profile. Additional studies such as fibrinogen level can be reserved for more specific evaluation.

The most common platelet disorders in surgical patients are dilutional thrombocytopenia and platelet dysfunction. Thrombocytopenia results from large volumes of transfused blood or other fluid, whereas platelet disorders are usually caused by drugs. A single dose of aspirin irreversibly acetylates platelet cyclo-oxygenase; platelet function requires more than a week to return to normal. Other drugs, such as indomethacin and furosemide, have reversible effects, and platelet function returns to normal in 1 to 2 days. If emergency surgery is required, 2 to 5 units of platelets/70 kg body weight will restore normal platelet function.[101]

Hemophilia, von Willebrand's disease, and other specific clotting factor deficiencies are managed preoperatively with replacement of the appropriate factors to approximately 40% of normal.[8] Vitamin K or fresh frozen plasma is typically used to reverse the effects of coumadin, whereas protamine rapidly reverses heparin.

Intraoperatively, the replacement of large blood losses with whole blood and packed red blood cells results in dilutional thrombocytopenia. Platelet counts below 100,000/mm^3, occurring at about 5000 ml blood loss in an average adult, have been shown to exacerbate surgical bleeding, whereas counts below 50,000/mm^3 are nearly always associated with bleeding.[79] One unit of platelets will increase platelet count about 10,000/mm^3 in an average 70 kg adult.[93]

Transfusion of packed cells results in dilution of coagulation factors V and VIII. By contrast, whole blood has adequate levels of these factors, so deficiency is unusual when whole blood is given. Minimum levels of 20% factor V and 30% factor VIII are needed for surgical hemostasis. About 2 units of fresh frozen plasma per 10 units of packed erythrocytes transfused are required.

Heparin given during vascular surgery can be reversed by using about 1 mg protamine/mg heparin. Because heparin has a half-life in the blood of only 1 to 3 hours, the dose of protamine can be reduced according to the interval since the last administration of heparin. Protamine is not a benign drug; a dose exceeding the amount required to neutralize heparin molecules (an acid-base reaction) decreases platelet aggregation and interferes with thromboplastin generation, compounding a coagulopathy. Protamine does not reverse the impairment of platelet aggregation caused by large doses of heparin; if activated clotting time is normal, excessive additional protamine doses should not be given. Furthermore, rapid injection of protamine is associated with hypotension. Finally, protamine has been reported to cause severe anaphylactoid reactions in some patients, particularly those taking protamine zinc insulin or those who have had vasectomies and have formed antibodies to sperm.[51]

Less common causes of intraoperative coagulopathy include disseminated intravascular coagulation resulting from transfusion reaction, sepsis, or other disease. The treatment of disseminated intravascular coagulation with heparin is controversial. Fibrinogen is administered if levels are less than 100 mg/dl. Aminocaproic acid (Amicar) is indicated only in primary fibrinolysis; its use in disseminated intravascular coagulation may lead to intravascular thrombosis.

Blood Transfusion

Because blood transfusion is not without risk, minimizing the transfusion of blood and blood products is best. When blood loss is not excessive, blood volume can be maintained with crystalloid solutions until the hematocrit decreases to 25%. Target hematocrit may be lower in the patient with chronic anemia and higher in patients with disease affecting oxygen delivery, such as coronary disease or cerebrovascular disease. A formula for the *allowable blood loss* to meet this criterion can be derived in a straightforward way to yield:

$$\text{Allowable blood loss} = \text{Estimated blood volume} \times \frac{[\text{Initial hematocrit} - \text{Target hematocrit}]}{\text{Hematocrit of lost blood}}$$

In most cases, crystalloids are given during the initial phase of blood loss to maintain blood volume, so that the hematocrit of lost blood decreases with time. However, it is safest to use the initial hematocrit value for the hematocrit of lost blood, to compensate for the drop in preoperative hematocrit with hydration. In nonanemic patients the allowable blood loss usually exceeds 20% of blood volume. With rapid and continuing blood loss, earlier transfusion may facilitate maintenance of blood volume and compensate for surgical blood loss often being underestimated because of loss into drapes and gowns and onto the floor and because of the delay in measuring it.

Component blood therapy in many cases is preferable to whole blood administration. Packed erythrocytes are less likely to result in volume overload than whole blood, have a lower risk of antibody reaction, and conserve other components that are often in short supply. Packed red cells, therefore, are the initial choice for intraoperative blood replacement in adults. With greater amounts of blood loss, whole blood can be more rapidly administered without need for dilution with saline solution and avoids the need to replace factors V and VIII with fresh-frozen plasma from additional donors, thereby reducing the patient's risk of hepatitis. Functional platelets are not present in significant numbers in either whole blood or packed cells and must be given when losses exceed 10 to 20 units of blood.

Recognition of a transfusion reaction is more difficult in the anesthetized than in the awake patient. The earliest sign is often oozing at venous puncture sites and increased blood loss in the incision. Early recognition is crucial; treatment after discontinuance of blood transfusion is standard and is discussed in Chapter 6.

ENDOCRINE AND METABOLIC SYSTEMS

Thyroid

Hyperthyroidism

Patients with hyperthyroidism tend to have a higher than normal anesthetic drug requirement. Plasma catecholamine levels are usually elevated, and hyperthyroid patients are prone to hypertension, tachycardia, and hyperthermia. The choice of anesthetic drugs and adjuvants, therefore, requires great care. Drugs known to increase heart rate, such as anticholinergics, gallamine, and pancuronium, are avoided. Halothane, which sensitizes the myocardium to the arrhythmogenic effects of catecholamines, is also usually avoided. Pulse rate should be well controlled preoperatively, preferably to below 80 beats/minute.

The most severe form of hyperthyroidism is thyrotoxicosis, or thyroid storm, which can be life threatening, particularly in a patient with preexisting cardiovascular disease. Surgical manipulation of the thyroid can also precipitate thyroid crisis. Beta-adrenergic blocking drugs should be immediately available.

Hyperthyroid patients have increased oxygen consumption and carbon dioxide production, which can lead to respiratory and metabolic acidosis. Frequent arterial blood gas determinations, therefore, are helpful in managing these patients.

Intravenous fluids are infused at more rapid rates in the hyperthyroid patient to compensate for the greater insensible fluid loss. Hyperthermia may occur; atropine should be avoided because it inhibits heat loss.

Hypothyroidism

Hypothyroid patients have low metabolic rates and sluggish circulation. Anesthetic requirement is reduced, consciousness is more rapidly lost, and emergence is prolonged. Hypothyroid patients are unusually sensitive to sedatives and often require no preoperative sedation. Their anxiety level is usually low. Hypothyroid patients are more prone to narcotic-induced respiratory depression than the euthyroid patient. Cardiac reserve is often limited, and even mild hypovolemia is poorly tolerated. If hypotension fails to respond to cautious volume replacement, intravenous hydrocortisone may be useful. In severe cases monitoring of central venous or pulmonary artery pressure helps guide fluid therapy and prevent circulatory overload.

Hypothyroid patients have decreased heat production. Intraoperative hypothermia, with increased risk for arrhythmias, should be anticipated. A warming blanket may help. Intravenous fluids should be warmed, and inspired gases can be warmed and humidified to minimize loss of body heat.

Parathyroid

Hyperparathyroidism

Patients with hyperparathyroidism have hypercalcemia; the serum calcium level should be brought below 14 mg/dl before induction of anesthesia. After the removal of the parathyroid glands, profound hypocalcemia can occur, with symptoms ranging from neuromuscular irritability to frank tetany and convulsions. Intravenous calcium gluconate should be available and attention paid to serum magnesium and potassium levels, because hypomagnesemia and hypokalemia aggravate the symptoms of hypocalcemia.

Adrenal Gland

Adrenal Cortex

Decreased secretion of cortisol is seen in surgical patients for various reasons, including autoimmune disease of the adrenal cortex, granulomatous disease, and metastatic invasion of the adrenals. The patient with chronic adrenocortical hyposecretion shows the symptoms of Addison's disease, including hyponatremia, hyperkalemia, hypovolemia, and abnormal skin pigmentation. Acute adrenal insufficiency in patients with overwhelming sepsis is a very serious condition characterized by marked hypotension.

Probably the most common cause of adrenocortical

hyposecretion is the use of pharmacologic doses of steroids to treat other diseases. No criterion for preoperative steroid treatment in patients with a history of corticosteroid treatment is universally accepted. When therapy has been recent and of sufficient duration that pituitary suppression or adrenocortical atrophy likely has occurred, a dose equal to the maximum adrenal output may be given preoperatively (about 300 mg/70 kg/day hydrocortisone in divided doses).[86] This dose typically is given as 100 mg intramuscular hydrocortisone acetate the night before and morning of surgery; intravenous hydrocortisone sodium succinate has a more rapid onset of action. Intravenous corticosteroids may be needed intraoperatively to treat hypotension in patients with adrenal insufficiency, but before resorting to this therapy, the anesthesiologist must rule out other more likely causes.[113]

Adrenocortical excess (Cushing's syndrome) occurs both as a primary disease and as a result of steroid therapy. Significant problems influencing anesthetic management include hypertension, obesity, hyperglycemia (which is quite sensitive to insulin), hypokalemia, and polycythemia.[86]

Pheochromocytoma

Patients with pheochromocytoma have either sustained or episodic arterial hypertension, which can be life-threatening; subarachnoid hemorrhage is one consequence. Acute, malignant hypertension can be treated with an intravenous vasodilator such as phentolamine. The patient is typically prepared for surgery with several days of oral phenoxybenzamine. As the hypertension responds to therapy, blood volume increases because of decreased filtration pressure in the kidneys, and the hematocrit falls. If possible, a minimum drop in hematocrit of 4% should be achieved before surgery.

Relatively heavy preoperative sedation helps to minimize the stress response. The potential need for rapid blood volume expansion dictates the insertion of several large-bore intravenous cannulas. Direct intraarterial blood pressure monitoring is indicated to follow potentially rapid and large swings in vascular tone and blood pressure. Central venous or pulmonary arterial pressure monitoring allows optimal volume replacement.

Before subjecting the patient to noxious stimuli such as endotracheal intubation or surgical incision, alpha-adrenergic blockade should be adequate and time must be allowed to establish a deep level of anesthesia. Surgical manipulation of the tumor, even under deep anesthesia, may cause rapid and severe hypertension. Intravenous vasodilators such as phentolamine or nitroprusside must be immediately at hand.

As venous drainage of the tumor is interrupted, a rapid drop in blood pressure usually occurs because of vasodilatation; vasoconstrictors then may be urgently needed to support the circulation until adequate amounts of fluid can be infused. If the blood pressure does not drop at this time, the anesthesiologist should alert the surgical team, because additional tumor may be present in another focus. Ten percent of pheochromocytomas lie along the sympathetic chain and occasionally occur simultaneously in the contralateral adrenal gland.[26,29,88]

Diabetes Mellitus

The patient with diabetes mellitus for more than 5 years is subject to multisystem diseases that must be considered before anesthesia. Markedly decreased gastric motility poses a risk of regurgitation and pulmonary aspiration of stomach contents. Peripheral vascular disease and neuropathy often bring these patients to the operating room for amputations or debridements; coexisting coronary artery disease, often asymptomatic in diabetic persons, and autonomic neuropathy with hypertension make anesthetic management more difficult. One must assume that any patient with diabetic retinopathy is likely to have diabetic nephropathy. Hypotension and nephrotoxic drugs may further impair renal function, which should be followed closely in the perioperative period even if the preoperative blood urea nitrogen and serum creatinine levels are normal.

The most feared complication in the diabetic surgical patient is intraoperative hypoglycemia, the signs of which anesthesia can mask. Insulin needs fluctuate widely with changing oral intake and perioperative stress. Long-acting hypoglycemic drugs, both insulin and oral hypoglycemic agents, therefore, are difficult to use, particularly if a long period without oral intake is anticipated. During lengthy procedures, the best control is achieved with doses of regular insulin guided by frequent blood glucose determinations. The development of chemical reagent strips and the portable apparatus to read them has greatly simplified this approach. Slightly higher blood glucose levels are preferable in the interest of avoiding hypoglycemia. The stress of anesthesia and surgery may cause some hyperglycemia. A rigorous, tightly controlled regimen is unnecessary for short procedures if the patient is expected to resume oral intake soon. In this case a maintenance intravenous glucose infusion should be started the morning of surgery and a reduced insulin dose (one-third to one-half normal) given. Alternatively, but less common, insulin is withheld until after oral intake has resumed. Scheduling surgery early in the day greatly simplifies perioperative management of the diabetic patient.[98,117]

Alcoholism

Excessive ethanol consumption presents the anesthesiologist with two possible situations. First, the acutely intoxicated patient, who must be treated as having a "full stomach," may not cooperate with the insertion of vascular catheters or with the necessary preoxygenation. Anesthetic needs may be significantly reduced; protective airway reflexes may be depressed. Alcohol withdrawal syndrome may develop in the postoperative period.

Second, the chronic alcoholic has an increased anesthetic requirement. Possible associated disorders, such as liver dysfunction, cirrhosis, renal dysfunction, malnutrition, and metabolic derangement, all affect anesthetic management.[58,65]

POSTOPERATIVE CARE

The Postanesthesia care unit is staffed by specially trained nurses skilled in managing postanesthetic problems. They usually work under the supervision of an anesthesiologist.

Problems in the immediate postoperative period include airway obstruction, hypoventilation, and hypoxemia; nausea and vomiting, pain, and agitation (emergence delirium); aberrations in body temperature; circulatory instability and arrhythmias; hemorrhage; and drug interactions and allergic reactions.

Respiratory Problems

Airway obstruction may be caused by residual neuromuscular blockade, excessive sedation, laryngeal edema, or hemorrhage into or around the airway. Acute management consists of airway support, reversal of muscle relaxants (not always possible), and aerosol treatment for laryngeal edema. Endotracheal intubation may be necessary. Additional problems include bronchospasm and excessive secretions stimulated by anticholinesterase drugs given to reverse relaxants. The threat of pulmonary aspiration is present, particularly in the elderly, whose airway reflexes are depressed.

Hypoventilation can result from the causes of airway obstruction just listed. In addition, ventilation can be depressed directly by anesthetic drugs and indirectly by depression of hypoxic drive. Atelectasis, secretions, and foreign body aspiration can cause intrapulmonary shunting and resulting hypoxemia. Attention is directed toward correcting the primary disorder, but mechanical ventilation remains a useful temporizing measure.

Cardiovascular Problems

Hypotension in the recovery room is most often caused by hypovolemia but may also result from myocardial infarction, cardiac tamponade, anaphylaxis, pulmonary embolus, or sympathetic blockage following major regional anesthesia. Hypertension typically follows carotid endarterectomy and intracranial surgery and is common in patients with preexisting hypertension. Any patient may develop hypertension and tachycardia in response to pain.

Postoperative arrhythmias are common. Although often caused by cardiac disease, arrhythmias seen in the absence of such disease include sinus tachycardia resulting from pain, fever, or hypovolemia; premature atrial and ventricular contractions caused by catecholamine release, hypoxia, or hypercarbia; and sinus bradycardia resulting from vasovagal reflex.

Emergence: Pain and Delirium

Agitation and confusion are common in elderly patients, but may occur in anyone under the influence of residual anesthetics and adjuncts, especially ketamine and scopolamine.[34] Physostigmine is effective in reversing scopolamine delirium and may also counteract other centrally depressant drugs.[9,32] Flumazenil is a benzodiazepine antagonist that will reverse the effects of diazepam or midazolam. Hypoxia should always be considered in the differential diagnosis of agitation and confusion and must be ruled out before other measures are undertaken.

Postoperative pain must be judiciously treated to avoid excessive sedation and respiratory depression. Local anesthetic infiltration and intraoperative nerve block are alternatives to parenteral narcotics.

Many anesthesia departments now run acute pain management services. In contrast to clinics devoted to chronic pain management in a multidisciplinary setting, the acute pain service is concerned with postsurgical pain. Whereas PCA (patient-controlled analgesia) pumps delivering IV narcotics can generally be run by the nursing service, epidural infusions are likely to be managed by the acute pain service.

Lumbar or thoracic epidural infusions of narcotics and/or local anesthetics can minimize sedation and other side effects of systemic narcotics, allowing patients to be more active and alert while offering highly effective pain relief for several days. Still, these patients must be monitored for pruritus, urinary retention, nausea, and most important, delayed respiratory depression. The latter can be life-threatening and may require monitoring for 12 to 24 hours after narcotic infusion is discontinued.

Nausea and Vomiting

Nausea and vomiting are frequent postoperative problems and range in severity from mild discomfort to serious fluid and electrolyte imbalance. Retching may also strain a surgical closure. Although no anesthetic technique can guarantee absence of postoperative nausea, the following steps can be taken to minimize it:

1. Avoid narcotic premedication in patients without preoperative pain.
2. Avoid gastric inflation during positive-pressure ventilation by mask.
3. Administer prophylactic antiemetic drugs.

Patients often give a history of prolonged postoperative nausea following previous surgery and mistakenly attribute it to the anesthetic rather than to the analgesics used postoperatively. In addition, nausea may be caused by ancillary drugs, anxiety, aerophagia, surgery involving the eye or ear, or other factors causing gastric distention.

If an antiemetic drug of the phenothiazine group (chlorpromazine, prochlorperazine, promethazine) or butyrophenone group (droperidol) is given, the dose of narcotic analgesics should be decreased because the drugs are synergistic. Metoclopramide (0.15 mg/kg) is an alternative, particularly after tonsillectomy in children.[40] Ondansetron is a new antiemetic drug that is effective but extremely expensive and is generally reserved for patients receiving chemotherapy who have been unresponsive to other less costly agents.

Allergic Reactions

Allergic reactions are often not recognized until the patient leaves the operating room because (1) early dermatologic manifestations of such reactions may be hidden by the surgical drapes; and (2) anesthetic drugs attenuate the allergic reaction. Although many drugs given by the anesthesiologist cause transient histamine release without anaphylaxis, blood and antibiotics are the most common causes of true anaphylaxis.

Transfer from the Postanesthesia Care Unit (PACU)

Patients are discharged from the PACU when cardiovascular and respiratory conditions are stable enough that close monitoring is no longer needed. The anesthesiologist is expected to make a postoperative visit after discharge from the recovery room, typically the day after surgery, to identify any anesthetic sequelae and to discuss any concerns with the patient. Although most complications are apparent within the first 24 hours, some are not. In such cases the anesthesiologist will appreciate prompt consultation by the person who discovers a late complication. The anesthesiologist not only might bring additional expertise to assist in managing the complication, but the information may also be useful in preventing future similar complications.

▪This chapter is a revision of Stern DH, Watson WJ, Faaberg JE, Marshall SLH, Sheth NN: Perioperative anesthesia. In Davis JH: *Clinical Surgery*, St Louis, 1987, Mosby.

REFERENCES

1 Alberti KGMM, Thomas DJB: The management of diabetes during surgery, *Br J Anaesth* 51:693, 1979.
2 Anderson WH, Dossett BE Jr, Hamilton GE: Prevention of postoperative pulmonary complications, *JAMA* 186:763, 1963.
3 Awe WC, Fletcher WS, Jacob SW: The pathophysiology of aspiration pneumonitis, *Surgery* 60:232, 1966.
4 Bannister WK, Sattilaro AJ: Vomiting and aspiration during anesthesia, *Anesthesiology* 23:251, 1962.
5 Basta JW, Niejadlik K, Pallares V: Autonomic hyperreflexia: intraoperative control with pentolinium tartrate, *Br J Anaesth* 49:1087, 1977.
6 Bell H, Stubbs D, Pugh D: Reliability of central venous pressure as an indicator of left atrial pressure, *Chest* 59:169, 1971.
7 Berry FA, Blankenbaker WL, Ball CG: A comparison of bacteremia occurring with nasotracheal and orotracheal intubation, *Anesth Analg* 52:873, 1973.
8 Blatt PM, Brinkhous KM, Culp HR et al: Anti-hemophilic factor concentrate therapy in von Willebrand's disease, *JAMA* 236:2770, 1976.
9 Brebner J, Hadley L: Experiences with physostigmine in the reversal of adverse post-anesthetic effects, *Can Anaesth Soc J* 23:574, 1976.
10 Brown BR: Halothane hepatitis revisited, *N Engl J Med* 313:1347, 1985.
11 Brown BR, Crout JR: A comparative study of the effects of five general anesthetics on myocardial contractility. I. Isometric conditions, *Anesthesiology* 34:236, 1971.
12 Bunker JP, Blumenfeld CM: Liver necrosis after halothane anesthesia: cause or coincidence? *N Engl J Med* 268:531, 1963.
13 Bunker JP, Forrest WIT, Mosteller F et al: A study of the possible association between halothane anesthesia and postoperative hepatic necrosis, National Halothane Study, Washington, DC, 1969, US Government Printing Office.
14 Burkett L, Bikhazi GB, Thomas KC Jr et al: Mutual potentiation of the neuromuscular effects of antibiotics and relaxants, *Anesth Analg* 58:107, 1979.
15 Cannon WB: The passage of different food-stuffs from the stomach and through the small intestine, *Am J Physiol* 12:387, 1904-1905.
16 Carter R, Heerdt M, Acchiardo S: Fluoride kinetics after enflurane anesthesia in healthy and anephric patients and in patients with poor renal function, *Clin Pharmacol Ther* 20:565, 1976.
17 Chase HF: The role of delayed gastric emptying time in the etiology of aspiration pneumonia, *Am J Obstet Gynecol* 56:673, 1948.
18 Cohen S, Harris LD: Does hiatus hernia affect competence of the gastroesophageal sphincter? *N Engl J Med* 284:1053, 1971.
19 Coombs DW, Hooper D, Colton T: Pre-anesthetic cimetidine alteration of gastric fluid volume and pH, *Anesth Analg* 58:183, 1979.
20 Cotton BR, Smith G: The lower esophageal sphincter and anaesthesia, *Br J Anaesth* 56:37, 1984.
21 Cournand A, Motley HL, Werko L et al: Physiologic studies of the effects of intermittent positive pressure breathing on cardiac output in man, *Am J Physiol* 152:162, 1948.
22 Cousins MJ, Mazze RL: Anesthesia, surgery and renal function: immediate and delayed effects, *Anesth Int Care* 1:355, 1973.
23 Daniell HW: Arrhythmia in hypokalemia, *N Engl J Med* 284:1385, 1971.
24 Davies JM, Latto IP, Jones JG et al: Effects of stopping smoking for 48 hours on oxygen availability from the blood: a study on pregnant women, *Br Med J* 2:355, 1979.
25 Davies JM (chairman), Davison JS, Nimmo WS et al: The stomach: factors of importance to the anaesthetist, Symposium Report, *Can J Anaesth* 37:896, 1990.
26 De Blasi S: The management of the patient with phaeochromocytoma, *Br J Anaesth* 38:740, 1966.
27 Del Guercio LRM, Cohn JD: Monitoring operative risk in the elderly, *JAMA* 243:1350, 1980.
28 Desmond J: Complications of transurethral prostatic surgery, *Can Anaesth Soc J* 17:25, 1970.
29 Desmonts JM, le Houelleur J, Redmond P et al: Anaesthetic management of patients with phaeochromocytoma, *Br J Anaesth* 49:991, 1977.

30 Devereux RB, Perloff JK, Reichek N et al: Mitral valve prolapse, *Circulation* 54:3, 1976.

31 Drachman DB: Myasthenia gravis, *N Engl J Med* 298:136, 1978.

32 Duvoisin RC, Katz R: Reversal of central anticholinergic syndrome in man by physostigmine, *JAMA* 206:1963, 1968.

33 Eckenhoff JE: Deliberate hypotension, *Anesthesiology* 48:87, 1978.

34 Eckenhoff JE, Kneale DH, Dripps RD: The incidence and etiology of postanesthetic excitement, a clinical survey, *Anesthesiology* 22:667, 1961.

35 Edelist G: Principles of anesthetic management in rheumatoid arthritic patients, *Anesth Analg* 43:227, 1964.

36 Eger EI II, Saidman LJ: Hazards of nitrous oxide anesthesia in bowel obstruction and pneumothorax, *Anesthesiology* 26:61, 1965.

37 Eriksson M, Catz CS, Yaffe SJ: Drugs and pregnancy, *Clin Obstet Gynecol* 16:199, 1973.

38 Fanning GL: The efficacy of cricoid pressure in preventing regurgitation of gastric contents, *Anesthesiology* 32:553, 1970.

39 Farrell G, Prendergast D, Murray M: Halothane hepatitis: detection of a constitutional susceptibility factor, *N Engl J Med* 313:1310, 1985.

40 Ferrari LR, Donlon JV: Metoclopramide reduces the incidence of vomiting after tonsillectomy in children, *Anesth Analg* 75:351, 1992.

41 Forbes AR: Humidification and mucous flow in the intubated trachea, *Br J Anesth* 45:874, 1973.

42 Forbes AR: Halothane depresses mucociliary flow in the trachea, *Anesthesiology* 45:59, 1976.

43 Funk D, Raymon F: Rheumatoid arthritis of the cricoarytenoid joints: an airway hazard, *Anesth Analg* 54:742, 1975.

44 Gillies IDS: Anaemia and anaesthesia, *Br J Anaesth* 46:589, 1974.

45 Goldman L, Caldera DL, Nussbaum SR et al: Multifactorial index of cardiac risk in noncardiac surgical procedures, *N Engl J Med* 297:845, 1977.

46 Gracey DR, Divertie MB, Didier EP: Preoperative pulmonary preparation of patients with chronic obstructive pulmonary disease, *Chest* 76:123, 1979.

47 Greenwalt TJ (chairman) et al: Perioperative Red Blood Cell Transfusion, Consensus Conference, *JAMA* 260:2700, 1988.

48 Gronert GA: Malignant hyperthermia, *Anesthesiology* 53:395, 1980.

49 Gronert GA, Thompson RL, Onofrio BM: Human malignant hyperthermia: awake episodes and correction by dantrolene, *Anesth Analg* 59:377, 1980.

50 Hermens JM, Bennett MJ, Hirshman CA: Anesthesia for laser surgery, *Anesth Analg* 62:218, 1983.

51 Horrow JC: Protamine: a review of its toxicity, *Anesth Analg* 64:348, 1985.

52 Horton RE, Ross FGM, Darling GH: Determination of the emptying-time of the stomach by use of enteric-coated barium granules, *Br Med J* 1:1537, 1965.

53 Husemeyer RP, Davenport HT, Rajasekaran T: Cimetidine as a single oral dose for prophylaxis against Mendelson's syndrome, *Anaesthesia* 33:775, 1978.

54 Innes IR, Nickerson M: Atropine, scopolamine, and related antimuscarinic drugs. In Goodman LS and Gilman A, editors: *The pharmacologic basis of therapeutics,* ed 5, New York, 1975, MacMillan.

55 Järnberg PO, de Villota ED, Eklund J et al: Effects of positive and end-expiratory pressure on renal function, *Acta Anaesth Scand* 22:508, 1978.

56 Jenkins LC, McGraw RW: Anesthetic management of the patient with rheumatoid arthritis, *Can Anaesth Soc J* 16:407, 1969.

57 Jennett B, Teasdale G: Aspects of coma after severe head injury, *Lancet* 1:878,1977.

58 Johnstone RE, Kulp RA, Smith TC: Effects of acute and chronic ethanol administration on isoflurane requirement of mice, *Anesth Analg* 54:277, 1975.

59 Kafer ER, Brown JT, Scott D et al: Biphasic depression of ventilatory responses to CO_2 following epidural morphine, *Anesthesiology* 58:418, 1983.

60 Kakkar VV, Corrigan TP, Fossard DP et al: Prevention of fatal postoperative pulmonary embolism by low doses of heparin: an international multicentre trial, *Lancet* 1(8011):567, 1977.

61 Kallos T, Lampe KF, Orkin FK: Pulmonary aspiration of gastric contents. In Orkin FK, Cooperman LH, editors: *Complications in anesthesiology,* Philadelphia, 1983, JB Lippincott.

62 Kaplan EL, Anthony BF, Bisno A et al: Committee on prevention of rheumatic fever and bacterial endocarditis of the American Heart Association, prevention of bacterial endocarditis, *Circulation* 56:139A, 1977.

63 Kaplan JA, Dunbar RW: Propranolol and surgical anesthesia, *Anesth Analg* 55:1, 1976.

64 Katz RL, Bigger JT Jr: Cardiac arrhythmias during anesthesia and operation, *Anesthesiology* 33:193, 1970.

65 Keilty SR: Anesthesia for the alcoholic patient, *Anesth Analg* 48:659, 1969.

66 Korttila K, Kauste A, Auvinen J: Comparison of domperidone, droperidol, and metoclopramide in the prevention and treatment of nausea and vomiting after balanced general anesthesia, *Anesth Analg* 58:396, 1979.

67 Larson CP, Mazze RL, Cooperman LH et al: Effects of anesthetics on cerebral, renal and splanchnic circulation, recent developments, *Anesthesiology* 41:169, 1974.

68 Lassen NA, Christensen MS: Physiology of cerebral blood flow, *Br J Anaesth* 48:719, 1976.

69 Leigh JM: The history of controlled hypotension, *Br J Anaesth* 47:745, 1975.

70 Leventhal SR, Orkin FK, Hirsh RA: Prediction of the need for postoperative mechanical ventilation in myasthenia gravis, *Anesthesiology* 53:26, 1980.

71 Loehning RW, Mazze RI: Possible nephrotoxicity from enflurane in a patient with severe renal disease, *Anesthesiology* 40:203, 1974.

72 Maekawa T, Sakabe T, Takeshita H: Diazepam blocks cerebral metabolic and circulatory responses to local anesthetic-induced seizures, *Anesthesiology* 41:389, 1974.

73 Magora F, Olshwang D, Eimerl D et al: Observations on extradural morphine analgesia in various pain conditions, *Br J Anaesth* 52:247, 1980.

74 Marshall S, Hinman F: Subdural hematoma following an administration of urea for diagnosis of hypertension, *JAMA* 182:813, 1962.

75 Mazze RI, Calverley RK, Smith NT: Inorganic fluoride nephrotoxicity: prolonged enflurane and halothane anesthesia in volunteers, *Anesthesiology* 46:265, 1977.

76 Mazze RI, Schwartz FD, Slocum HC et al: Renal function during anesthesia and surgery. 1. The effects of halothane anesthesia, *Anesthesiology* 24:279, 1963.

77 Meyers EF, Tomeldan SA: Glycopyrrolate compared with atropine in prevention of the oculocardiac reflex during eye-muscle surgery, *Anesthesiology* 51:350, 1979.

78 Michenfelder JD, Martin JT, Altenburg GM et al: Air embolism during neurosurgery, *JAMA* 208:1353, 1969.

79 Miller RD, Brzica SM: Blood, blood component, colloid, and autotransfusion therapy. In Miller RD, editor: *Anesthesia,* New York, 1981, Churchill Livingstone.

80 Miller RD, Way WL: Inhibition of succinylcholineinduced increased intragastric pressure by nondepolarizing muscle relaxants and lidocaine, *Anesthesiology* 34:185, 1971.

81 Nennhaus HP, Javid H, Jullian OC: Alveolar and pleural rupture, *Arch Surg* 94:136, 1967.

82 Nicolaides AN, Bowers R, Horbourne T et al: Blood viscosity, red-cell flexibility, haematocrit, and plasma-fibrinogen in patients with angina, *Lancet* 2:943, 1977.
83 Patton CM: Rapid induction of acute dyskinesia by droperidol, *Anesthesiology* 43:126, 1975.
84 Payne WS, Ellis FH: Esophagus and diaphragmatic hernias. In Schwartz SI, editor: *Principles of surgery,* New York, 1969, McGraw-Hill.
85 Pederson H, Finster M: Anesthetic risk in the pregnant surgical patient, *Anesthesiology* 51:439, 1979.
86 Pender JW, Basso LV: Diseases of the endocrine system. In Katz J, Benumof J, Kadis LB, editors: *Anesthesia and uncommon diseases,* ed 2, Philadelphia, 1981, WB Saunders.
87 Pohl LR, Gillette JR: A perspective on halothane-induced heptotoxicity, *Anesth Analg* 61:809, 1982.
88 Pratilas V, Pratila MG: Anaesthetic management of phaeochromocytoma, *Can Anaesth Soc J* 26:253, 1979.
89 Prys-Roberts C, Meloche R, Foex P: Studies of anaesthesia in relation to hypertension. I. Cardiovascular responses of treated and untreated patients, *Br J Anaesth* 43:122, 1971.
90 Rao TLK, El-Etr AA: Myocardial reinfarction following anesthesia in patients with recent infarction, *Anesth Analg* 60:271, 1981.
91 Roberts RB, Shirley MA: Reducing the risk of acid aspiration during Cesarean section, *Anesth Analg* 53:859, 1974.
92 Roe RB: The effect of suxamethonium on intragastric pressure, *Anaesthesia* 17:179, 1962.
93 Roizen MF: Preoperative evaluation of patients with diseases that require special preoperative evaluation and intraoperative management. In Miller RD, editor: *Anesthesia,* vol 1, New York, 1981, Churchill Livingstone.
94 Sanchez GC, Kramer P, Ingelfinger FJ: Motor mechanisms of the esophagus, particularly of its distal portion, *Gastroenterology* 25:321, 1953.
95 Schemel WH: Unexpected hepatic dysfunction found by multiple laboratory screening, *Anesth Analg* 55:810,1976.
96 Schonwald G, Fish KJ, Perkash I: Cardiovascular complications during anesthesia in chronic spinal cord injured patients, *Anesthesiology* 55:550, 1981.
97 Sellick BA: Cricoid pressure to control regurgitation of stomach contents during induction of anaesthesia, *Lancet* 2:404, 1961.
98 Shapiro FL, Kjellstrand CM, Goetz FC: End-stage diabetic nephropathy, Kidney International Meeting #6, suppl 1, 1974.
99 Shapiro HM: Neurosurgical anesthesia and intracranial hypertension. In Miller RD, editor: *Anesthesia,* New York, 1981, Churchill Livingstone.
100 Shingu K, Eger EI II, Johnson BH: Hypoxia may be more important than reductive metabolism in halothane-induced hepatic injury, *Anesth Analg* 61:824, 1982.
101 Simpson MB: Platelet function and transfusion therapy in the surgical patient. In Schiffer CJ, editor: *Platelet physiology and transfusion,* Washington DC, 1978, American Association of Blood Banks.
102 Skillman JJ, Bushnell LS, Hedley-Whyte J: Peritonitis and respiratory failure after abdominal operations, *Ann Surg* 170:122, 1969.
103 Smith P, Benn RT, Sharp J: Natural history of rheumatoid cervical subluxations, *Ann Rheum Dis* 31:431, 1972.
104 Sproule BJ, Mitchell JH, Miller WF: Cardiopulmonary physiological responses to heavy exercise in patients with anemia, *J Clin Invest* 39:378, 1960.
105 Stept WJ, Safar P: Rapid induction/intubation for prevention of gastric-content aspiration, *Anesth Analg* 49:633, 1970.
106 Still JA, Modell JH: Acute water intoxication during transurethral resection of the prostrate, using glycine solution for irrigation, *Anesthesiology* 38:98, 1973.
107 Swartz MH, Teichholz LE, Donoso E: Mitral valve prolapse: a review of associated arrhythmias, *Am J Med* 62:377, 1977.
108 Tarazi RC, Frohlich ED, Dustan HP: Plasma volume in man with essential hypertension, *N Engl J Med* 278:762, 1968.
109 Tarhan S, Moffitt EA, Sessler AD et al: Risk of anesthesia and surgery in patients with chronic bronchitis and chronic obstructive disease, *Surgery* 74:720, 1973.
110 Taves DR, Fry BW, Freeman RB et al: Toxicity following methoxyflurane anesthesia. II. Fluoride concentrations in nephrotoxicity, *JAMA* 214:91, 1970.
111 Tobey RE, Jacobsen PM, Kahle CT et al: The serum potassium response to muscle relaxants in neural injury, *Anesthesiology* 37:332, 1972.
112 Toussaint GPM, Burgess JH, Hampson LG: Central venous pressure and pulmonary wedge pressure in critical surgical illness, *Arch Surg* 109:265, 1974.
113 Vandam LD, Moore FD: Adrenocortical mechanisms related to anesthesia, *Anesthesiology* 21:531, 1960.
114 Viegas OJ, Ravindran RS, Shumacker CA: Gastric fluid pH in patients receiving sodium citrate, *Anesth Analg* 60:521, 1981.
115 Wahl M, Deetjen P, Thurau K et al: Micropuncture evaluation of the importance of perivascular pH for the arteriolar diameter on the brain surface, *Pflugers Arch* 316:152, 1970.
116 Wasserman LR, Gilbert HS: Surgical bleeding in polycythemia vera, *Ann NY Acad Sci* 115:122, 1964.
117 Williamson JR, Kilo C: Current status of capillary basement-membrane disease and diabetes and diabetes mellitus, *Diabetes* 26:65, 1977.
118 Wright BD, DiGiovanni AJ: Respiratory alkalosis, hypokalemia, and repeated ventricular fibrillation associated with mechanical ventilation, *Anesth Analg* 48:467, 1969.
119 Wrobel J, Koh TC, Saunders JM: Sodium citrate, an alternative antacid for prophylaxis against aspiration pneumonitis, *Anaesth Int Care* 10:166, 1982.
120 Zauder HL: A possible interaction of PCB and halothane in man, *Anesthesiology* 51:96, 1979.

SUGGESTED READINGS

Cousins MJ, Bridenbaugh PO, editors: *Neural blockade in clinical anesthesia and management of pain,* ed 2, Philadelphia, 1988, JB Lippincott.

Covino BG, Vassallo HG: *Local anesthesia: mechanisms of action and clinical use,* New York, 1976, Grune & Stratton.

Dripps RD, Vandam LD: *Introduction to anesthesia: the principles of safe practice,* ed 7, Philadelphia, 1988, WB Saunders.

Eger EI II: *Anesthetic uptake and action,* Baltimore, 1974, Williams & Wilkins.

Goodman LS, Gilman A, editors: *The pharmacological basis of therapeutics,* ed 7, New York, 1985, Macmillan.

Lebowitz PW, Newberg LA, Gillette MT, editors: *Clinical anesthesia procedures of the Massachusetts General Hospital,* Boston, 1982, Little, Brown.

Miller RD, editor: *Anesthesia,* ed 3, New York, 1988, Churchill Livingstone.

Motoyama EK, Davis PJ, editors: *Smith's anesthesia for infants and children,* ed 5, St Louis, 1990, Mosby.

Mueller RA, Lundberg DBA: *Manual of drug interactions for anesthesiology,* New York, 1988, Churchill Livingstone.

Shnider SM, Levinson G: *Anesthesia for obstetrics,* ed 2, Baltimore, 1987, Williams & Wilkins.

Smith NT, Corbascio AN: *Drug interactions in anesthesia,* ed 2, Philadelphia, 1986, Lea and Febiger.

Stoelting RK, Dierdorf SF, McCammon RL: *Anesthesia and co-existing disease,* ed 2, New York, 1988, Churchill Livingstone.

Stoelting RK, Miller RD: *Basics of anesthesia,* ed 2, New York, 1989, Churchill Livingstone.

APPENDIX 24-A
AMERICAN SOCIETY OF ANESTHESIOLOGISTS (ASA) RISK CLASSIFICATION

A simple system of classifying the overall medical risk of patients about to undergo anesthesia is still used. The following physical status classification was adopted by the ASA in 1962:

1. Normal, healthy patient
2. Patient with a mild systemic disease
3. Patient with a severe disease that limits activity but is not incapacitating
4. Patient with an incapacitating disease that is a constant threat to life
5. Moribund patient not expected to survive 24 hours with or without surgery

In the event of emergency surgery, an E precedes the number. The anesthesiologist assigns physical status following the preoperative assessment. This risk classification system is useful because it corresponds with perioperative mortality.[27] As a group, emergency patients also have a greater risk than nonemergency patients within each physical status class.

APPENDIX 24-B
ANESTHESIA EQUIPMENT

Although the anesthesia machine has undergone vast changes in appearance and features, such as the addition of alarms, safety devices, and integral physiologic monitors, its function has changed little in the last few decades.

The primary function of this apparatus is to provide precise concentrations and flow rates of oxygen, nitrous oxide, air, and volatile agents. This function is accomplished by hoses and pipes that connect to hospital pipelines, backup gas tanks, needle valves with accurate gas flowmeters, and vaporizers for volatile liquid agents such as halothane, enflurane, and isoflurane. A separate "flush" valve routes high flows of oxygen directly to the patient breathing circuit. Most modern machines incorporate one or more safety mechanisms; the most basic cuts off all other gas flows if oxygen pressure drops. More sophisticated designs attempt to prevent administration of hypoxic concentrations of oxygen. Despite various safety designs, the literature is replete with case reports of serious malfunctions with the potential for patient injury. In short, nothing substitutes for the anesthetist's vigilance.

The gas mixture is delivered to a breathing circuit, which is connected in turn to the patient's airway via an endotracheal tube, mask, bronchoscope, or other attachment. Breathing circuits have numerous designs. In the "circle" system, one-way valves constrain gases to follow a unidirectional path through the circuit, which also incorporates a chemical carbon dioxide absorber. A reservoir bag or ventilator bellows allows spontaneous or controlled respiration. Anesthetic gases flow continuously into the circuit, and a pressure-set "pop-off valve" allows gas to exit the system. A gauge monitors airway pressure; some systems also incorporate gas flowmeters to monitor tidal or minute volume.

Although the circle system can be used in most pediatric patients, some anesthesiologists prefer a different type of circuit, which has no carbon dioxide absorber but depends on adequate fresh gas inflow to prevent rebreathing and carbon dioxide retention. This type of system (some variations are known as *Bain, Mapleson D, Jackson-Rees,* and *Ayers*) is compact and lightweight and offers little resistance to breathing; but its conservation of anesthetic gas, heat, and humidity is poor. A humidifier may be added to this or a circle system to help maintain body heat and minimize drying of the airway.

In the past, excess anesthetic-laden gases were discharged into the operating room. Most modern systems use a "scavenging" adapter to trap these gases and route them outside.

In addition to the anesthesia machine, much other equipment is kept available in the operating room. Airway equipment consists of laryngoscopes, oral and nasal airways, endotracheal tubes, and other specialized devices used in securing and maintaining a patent airway. Suction is kept ready to clear the airway rapidly. An oxygen analyzer continuously monitors inspired oxygen concentraton. A multitude of intravenous drugs, fluids, and associated equipment for their administration is kept at hand. Automatic oscillometric blood pressure devices that connect to a standard blood pressure cuff are common, and direct arterial pressure monitors are used frequently.

Electrocardiographic monitors are routine, but some will perform sophisticated arrhythmia and ST segment

APPENDIX 24-B cont'd
ANESTHESIA EQUIPMENT

analysis, trending, and hemodynamic calculations. Many monitors now include a pulse oximeter, capnograph, interfaces for pressure transducers, and other functions that previously required freestanding devices. Mass spectrometers can monitor expired gases for an entire suite of operating rooms, although there is a trend toward individual gas monitors in each room. Other devices finding increased use by anesthesiologists include monitors for evoked potentials and processed EEG and transesophageal echocardiography machines.

APPENDIX 24-C
ANESTHETIC AGENTS AND TECHNIQUES

The following tables provide a summary of three major regional anesthetic techniques and the most important general features of the inhaled and intravenous anesthetics, narcotics, anticholinesterase and neuromuscular blocking drugs, and local anesthetics used by the anesthesiologist. The tables are not intended to provide adequately detailed or complete information for the use of these agents and techniques, but rather to introduce the reader to the relative effects of these agents and their uses.

INHALED ANESTHETICS

AGENT:	NITROUS OXIDE	HALOTHANE	ENFLURANE	ISOFLURANE
MAC%*	105†	0.75	1.68	1.15
Myocardial depression‡	+	+ + +	+ + + +	+ +
Arrhythmias§	±	+ + + +	+ +	+
Vasodilation	±	+ +	+ + +	+ + + +
Pungency	0	+	+ + +	+ + + +
Respiratory depression	±	+	+ + +	+ +
Muscle relaxation	0	+	+ + +	+ + + +
Comments	Low potency, diffusion into gas-filled spaces	20% metabolized, rare hepatotoxicity	5% metabolized, possible fluoride nephrotoxicity, lowers seizure threshold	Minimally metabolized

* *MAC*, minimum alveolar concentration, is a measure of anesthetic potency. It is the alveolar concentration of anesthetic gas at which 50% of a sample population will not move after surgical incision.
†Nitrous oxide is not a "complete" anesthetic; when used alone, partial pressure greater than 1 atm would be required in most patients to prevent response to incision.
‡Decrease in myocardial contractility and stroke volume.
§Potentiation of the arrhythmogenic effects of either endogenous or injected catecholamines.

INTRAVENOUS ANESTHETIC INDUCTION AGENTS*

AGENT:	THIOPENTAL	KETAMINE	DIAZEPAM	MIDAZOLAM	PROPOFOL
Hypnotic dose (mg/kg)	1-5 (IV)	1-5 (IV) 6-10 (IM)	0.1-0.5 (IV)†	0.1-0.3 (IV)	1-2.5 (IV)
Onset of loss of consciousness (min)	0.5-1	1-3 (IV) 3-5 (IM)	1-4 (IV)	1-3 (IV)	0.5-1 (IV)
Duration (min)	10-15 (3)	5-10 (IV) 10-20 (IM)	5-15‡	5-15 (3)	8 (IV)
Respiratory depression	+ + + +	±	+ (variable)	+ +	+ + + +
Cardiovascular effects	Hypotension	Hypertension, tachycardia	Occasional hypotension	Occasional hypotension	Hypotension
Comments	Releases histamine, decreases cerebral blood flow and intracranial pressure	Psychotomimetic, emergence hallucinations, increases cerebral blood flow and intracranial pressure, causes salivation and increased intraocular pressure; increases airway reactivity	Pain, phlebitis at IV site, amnesia	Water soluble, less irritation to vein than diazepam	Fat emulsion, shorter half life than thiopental, may cause local pain on injection

* Doses and times are approximations for comparative purposes. Wide variations are found.
† Intramuscular injection not typically used for induction of anesthesia because of unpredictable absorption.
‡ Short duration is caused by redistribution rather than metabolism. Large doses have a long elimination half-life (10-12 hours for thiopental, 24 hours for diazepam, 1-4 hours for midazolam; active metabolites of diazepam have 2-8 day elimination half-lives).

NARCOTIC ANALGESICS AS ANESTHETIC ADJUNCTS*

AGENT:	MORPHINE	MEPERIDINE	FENTANYL	SUFENTANIL	ALFENTANIL	BUTORPHANOL
Dose†	0.1-0.3 mg/kg	0.5-1 mg/kg	1-100 μg/kg	0.1-20 μg/kg	8-245 μg/kg	0.5-2 mg/70 kg
Onset (min)	5-10	5-10	1-3	1-3	1	1-3
Duration (hr)‡	2-4	1-4	0.5+	0.3-0.5+	0.5+	3-4
Comments§	Vasodilatation, euphoria	Tachycardia,‖ mild anticholinergic effect, mild negative inotropic effect	Marked truncal rigidity may occur, impairing ventilation	Similar to fentanyl but 5-10 times as potent	Similar to fentanyl but very short acting, often given by continuous infusion	Agonist-antagonist**

* Doses and times are approximations for comparative purposes. Wide variations are found. Upper dosages for fentanyl, sufentanil, and alfentanil reflect their use as a sole anesthetic agent.
† Dose is individualized for each patient. Doses listed are by intravenous route, for typical young, healthy patients. For fentanyl, sufentanil, and alfentanil, lower dose ranges are for supplementation of other anesthetics, whereas the highest doses provide a complete anesthetic with a long duration.
‡ Durations listed are for small doses only and vary widely among individuals.
§ The narcotics can cause respiratory depression, nausea and vomiting, and constipation. With the possible exception of meperidine, narcotics can increase intrabiliary pressure, an effect that can be antagonized by anticholinergics.
‖ Most narcotics cause bradycardia.
** Butorphanol may precipitate withdrawal symptoms in narcotic-addicted patients. Nalbuphine, another agonist/antagonist, in small doses has been advocated for reversal of fentanyl-induced respiratory depression.

NEUROMUSCULAR BLOCKING DRUGS ("MUSCLE RELAXANTS")

AGENT:	SUCCINYLCHOLINE	d-TUBOCURARINE	METOCURINE	PANCURONIUM
Dose (mg/kg)*	1-2	0.6	0.3-0.4	0.08-0.10
Onset (min)†	1	5-8	5-8	2-3
Duration (min)‡	10-15	30-90	30-90	30-90
Metabolism	Plasma hydrolysis (pseudocholinesterase)	60% kidney, 40% liver	Almost exclusively kidney	Mostly kidney
Comments	Depolarizing type of blockade, muscle fasciculations, postoperative myalgia, hyperkalemia§ occasionally, prolonged action caused by abnormal pseudocholinesterase	Histamine release and ganglionic blockade may cause hypotension‖	Little cardiovascular effect‖	Tachycardia, hypertension‖

* Intravenous dosage required for profound muscle relaxation, as during tracheal intubation. In practice, much smaller doses may be given, guided by peripheral nerve stimulator response, to achieve only 75% to 95% receptor occupancy.

† Time to achieve satisfactory intubating conditions. Onset of weakness occurs much sooner.

‡ Time until additional dose is needed. This depends on the size of the previous dose. Metocurine has a somewhat longer duration of action than curare or pancuronium.

§ Succinylcholine typically causes a 0.5 to 1 Eq/L transient rise in serum potassium. This may be dangerous in patients with serum potassium above 5.5 mEq/L preoperatively. Also, the rise in potassium is much greater in patients with massive trauma, burns, or denervated muscle.

‖ Many drugs potentiate the effect of the nondepolarizing neuromuscular blockers, including the volatile anesthetics, aminoglycoside and polymyxin antibiotics, lithium, magnesium, procainamide, and quinidine.

** Hofmann elimination is a nonenzymatic process that occurs at physiologic temperature and pH; ester hydrolysis is catalyzed by nonspecific esterases. Atracurium is therefore metabolized even in the presence of severe liver and kidney disease.

ANTICHOLINESTERASE DRUGS FOR REVERSAL OF NEUROMUSCULAR BLOCKADE*

AGENT:	NEOSTIGMINE	PYRIDOSTIGMINE	EDROPHONIUM
Dose (mg/kg)	0.5-0.8	0.1-0.3	0.5-1
Onset (min)	2-5	3-7	1-3
Peak effect (min)	7-10	12-15	3-5
Comments			Muscarinic effects less than other agents

* If these agents are not preceded with an anticholinergic agent such as atropine or glycopyrrolate, all have similar side effects caused by parasympathetic action: bradycardia, salivation, bronchorrhea, and gastrointestinal cramping.

COMMONLY USED LOCAL ANESTHETICS

AGENT:	LIDOCAINE	BUPIVACAINE	MEPIVACAINE	TETRACAINE	CHLOROPROCAINE
Structure	Amide	Amide	Amide	Ester	Ester
Duration*	Medium	Long	Medium	Long	Short
Max. dose (mg/kg)	3-7	2-3	3-7	2-3	10-12
Common use	Infiltration, nerve block, spinal, epidural, or topical administration	Infiltration, nerve block, spinal, or epidural administration	Infiltration or nerve block	Spinal or topical administration	Epidural administration
Comments		Cardiac toxicity occurs sooner than with other agents		Occasional anaphylaxis	Occasional anaphylaxis, can cause paralysis if injected into the subarachnoid space

* The addition of epinephrine in a ratio of 1:200,000 (0.1 mg/20 ml) prolongs the duration of local anesthetics by most routes but may cause vasospasm if used in hands or feet.

VECURONIUM	ATRACURIUM	MIVACURIUM	PIPECURONIUM	DOXACURIUM
0.08-0.10	0.4-0.5	0.08	0.07	0.25-0.40
2-3	2-3	2.5-4	3-5	4-6
20-40	20-40	12-20	50-80	60-80 (variable)
Liver	Ester hydrolysis and Hofmann elimination in plasma**	Not dependent on renal elimination	Mostly renal	Mostly renal
Little cardiovascular effect‖	Histamine release‖	Metabolized by plasma cholinesterase, slight histamine release	Minimal cardiovascular effect	Minimal cardiovascular effect

COMMON MAJOR REGIONAL ANESTHETIC TECHNIQUES

TECHNIQUE:	SPINAL	EPIDURAL	BRACHIAL PLEXUS NERVE BLOCK*
Description	Small-bore needle inserted through dura, usually below the second lumbar interspace. Small doses of anesthetic are used (e.g., 50-100 mg lidocaine).	Large-bore needle inserted through yellow ligament (ligamentum flavum) into epidural space, identified by sudden loss of resistance to injection or "hanging drop" technique. Catheter often passed for subsequent injections. Typical volume, 5-25 ml (1.5%-2% lidocaine).	Proximity of needle to nerve identified by paresthesia, electrical stimulation, arterial puncture, or tactile sensation of needle passing through tissue structures. Usually requires 20-60 ml injected volume.
Uses	Short procedures (less than 3 hours) on lower extremities, perineum, lower abdomen, and sometimes upper abdomen.†	Long procedures, same regions as spinal but sometimes used for thoracic operations if injection is made at thoracic level.	Operations on the upper extremities, usually below the shoulder; catheter may be passed for subsequent injections during long procedures.
Onset of surgical anesthesia (min)‡	5-10 min	10-30 min	15-40 min
Characteristics	Profound sensory and motor blockade below level of block, which depends on dose, speed of injection, and other factors difficult to control.	Segmental blockade controlled by location of catheter and volume injected.	Difficult to block reliably all plexus nerves, resulting occasionally in inadequate anesthesia.
Hazards	Rapid onset hypotension, postural headache caused by dural puncture, nausea with high levels.	Slow-onset hypotension, occasional unintentional dural puncture, epidural hematoma, intravascular or subarachnoid injection.	Hematoma, pneumothorax, intravascular injection, local anesthetic toxicity, neuropathy.

*The several approaches to brachial plexus blockade include interscalene, supraclavicular, infraclavicular, subclavian perivascular, and axillary. The axillary approach is safest and used most often but is usually inadequate for surgical procedures above the elbow.

†Suitable for longer procedures if a catheter is passed into the subarachnoid space ("continuous spinal"); however, this is associated with a high incidence of postlumbar puncture headache.

‡Onset depends on local anesthetic agent used.

Note: Intravenous regional nerve block, or "Bier Block," provides complete anesthesia below a tourniquet placed on the upper arm. Typically, up to 3 mg/kg of 0.5% plain lidocaine is injected into the exsanguinated arm with tourniquet inflated. Onset of anesthesia is about 5 minutes; duration is limited to about 2 hours because of tourniquet ischemia. Anesthesia disappears rapidly when the tourniquet is deflated. Deflation within 15 minutes of initial injection may release large amounts of anesthetic into the circulation, causing symptoms of toxicity.

CHAPTER

25

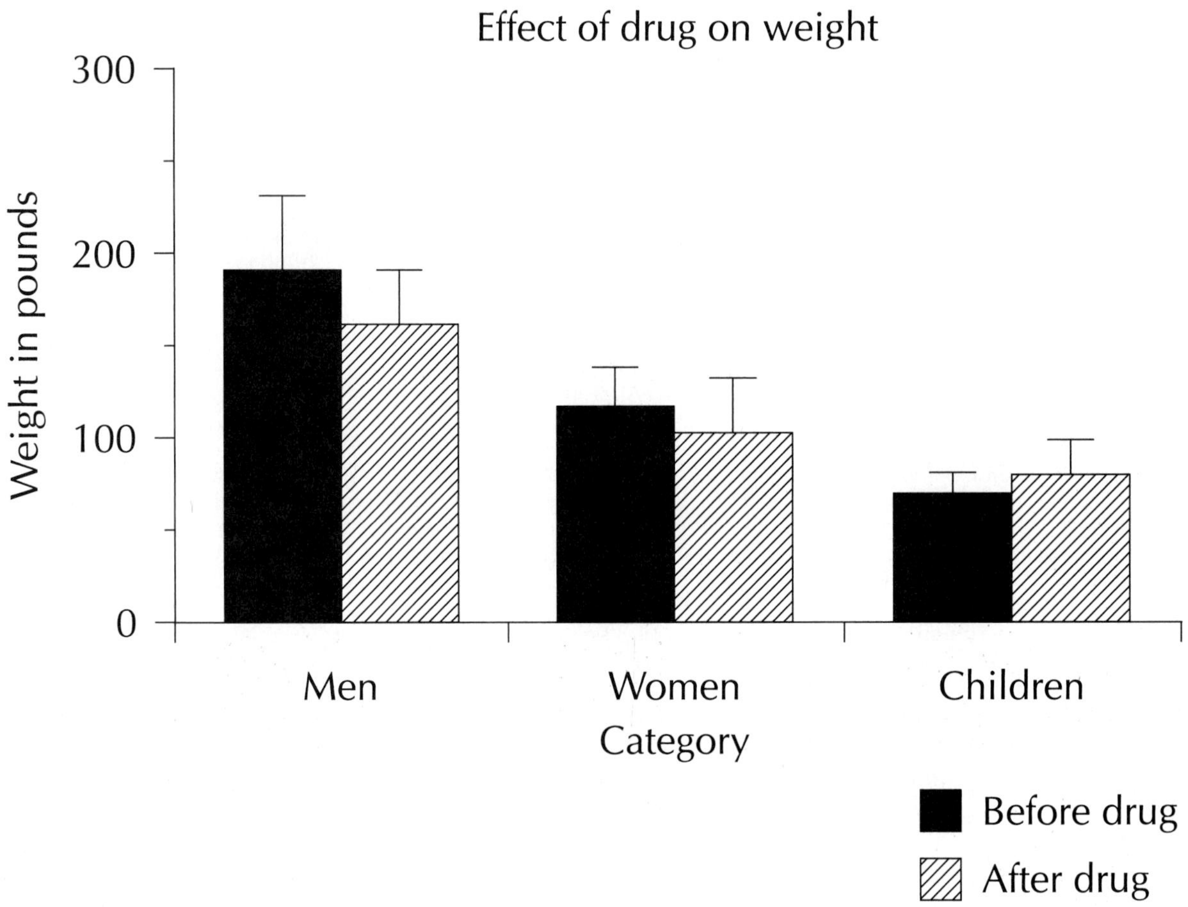
Effect of drug on weight
300
200
100
0
Weight in pounds
Men
Women
Children
Category
Before drug
After drug

CRITICAL EVALUATION OF DATA

Blair A. Keagy • George J. Palmer

With the availabililty of the microcomputer and its accompanying statistical analysis software, the medical scientist can be less concerned with the mechanics of statistical testing and can concentrate instead on proper application of these techniques and the interpretation of the resultant analysis. In addition to data analysis, the microcomputer may be used as a word processor to generate reports, grant applications, abstracts, and articles. Graphics programs are available that allow construction of clear and useful graphs and slides. The computer can also be used in conjunction with a telephone modem to perform medical topic searches through low-cost bibliography services. It is not necessary to develop computer programming skills to use the available software because these programs are quite user friendly; indeed, failure to make use of these inexpensive computer-based techniques results in a large amount of unnecessary "busy work." This chapter provides (1) a basic understanding of testing techniques; and (2) guidelines of how and when they should be used. Rather than including the mathematics behind these various statistical tests, appropriate references are listed at the conclusion of the chapter.

For purposes of this discussion, it is useful to review several commonly used terms. A *population* refers to an entire group of events, organisms, or objects. A *sample* indicates a subset of a population that is composed of a group of *subjects*. The term *raw data* refers to the basic information collected in its original form before being altered by various mathematic manipulations.

Most statistical software programs require the raw data to be tabulated in a spreadsheet format. By convention, the data are arranged to occupy rows, and variables are listed in columns. An example of a spreadsheet that can easily be used by almost all statistics programs is shown in Figure 25-1.

The first step in data analysis is the establishment of a clearly stated hypothesis to be tested. A *hypothesis* refers to a supposition or working theorem used to explain a series of observations. Secondly, a *probability level (P)* must be established, which estimates the probability that the observed events occured by chance rather than being the result of an intervention or an actual difference in measured parameters. The probability level is an arbitrary number designated by the investigator, but by convention a 5% ($P < .05$) level is usually chosen. Most often the working theorem is stated as a *null hypothesis*, which holds that there is *no* difference between observations from a group of subjects under examination. If the probability obtained from a statistical test is sufficiently small (generally less than .05), the null hypothesis is rejected. Thus because the thesis that there is no difference in the observations is rejected, one may reasonably accept the proposition that there is a differ-

SUB	CO	AOP	HR	HCT
1	5.5	120	70	45
2	4.0	130	80	40
3	3.9	90	100	30
4	5.1	120	90	38
5	4.2	110	70	42
6	2.0	80	120	28
7	2.1	85	130	26
8	3.0	100	70	35
9	6.0	130	60	40
10	1.9	70	140	25

FIGURE 25-1 Sample spreadsheet. *SUB,* Subject number; *CO,* cardiac output; *AOP,* systolic aortic pressure; *HR,* heart rate; *HCT,* hematocrit.

ence in the observations and that these differences are not the result of chance occurrence.

The following sections describe some of the statistical tests available for the analysis of raw data. The mathematics behind these tests are not given in great detail, but the information provided elucidates the indications for using the technique in question.

SENSITIVITY AND SPECIFICITY

Popular statistical methods used in data analysis are sensitivity and specificity. These parameters are often used to describe the success of predictive tests such as the duplex scan, which is a newly developed noninvasive technique used to detect the presence and degree of carotid artery stenosis. The *sensitivity* of a test is its ability to correctly identify those patients who truly have the disease in question, whereas the *specificity* is the ability of a test to classify as negative those patients who do not have the disease. Stated in mathematic terms, the sensitivity is :

Number with a positive test/Total number with disease

The result is generally expressed as a percentage and reflects the ability of the test to correctly predict the disease. The specificity is:

Number with a negative test/Total number without disease

Again this test is expressed as a percentage and reflects the ability of the test to indicate the absence of the disease. The easiest way to set up the raw data for analysis with these techniques is in the form of a row-and-column table. For example, what are the sensitivity and the specificity of oculoplethysmography in the detection of hemodynamically significant carotid artery disease? In the example shown in Figure 25-2, the specificity of the test is good, and there is a low incidence of false-positive examinations. However, the lower sensitivity (65%) indicates that a fair number of persons with hemodynamically significant carotid lesions are not detected with this test.

Bayes' Rule

Many low-risk noninvasive diagnostic tests that are developed and described in the literature have a high sensitivity and specificity. As a result, the creators of these tests suggest that they should be used as general screening tests for the detection of a certain type of disease in

Result of OPG	Tight carotid stenosis: Present	Tight carotid stenosis: Absent	
Positive	130	60	190
Negative	70	740	810
	200	800	1000

Sensitivity = 130/200 × 100 = 65%

Specificity = 740/800 × 100 = 92%

FIGURE 25-2 Sample row-and-column table.

the general population. However, one additional factor must be taken into account before citing a certain test as a good screening device—the incidence of the disease in the general population. For example, suppose a new test for the detection of severe carotid artery disease has been developed that has a 90% specificity and a 90% sensitivity. In this example it is further assumed that the frequency of carotid stenosis in the general population is 2%. Bayes' rule states that the probability of the patient having the disease when the screening test is positive is:

$$\frac{\text{Prev} \times \text{Sens}}{(\text{Prev} \times \text{Sens}) + (\text{Abs} \times \text{Fpr})^*}$$

In our example the formula becomes:

$$\frac{0.2 \times .90}{(0.2 \times .90) + (.98 \times .10)} = .155$$

In other words, with the test described, only 15% of all patients with a positive screening test would be found to have a significant carotid disease. Thus although a new technique may have a high sensitivity and specificity, its usefulness as a screening device is limited in a population with a low prevalence of the disease in question.

DESCRIPTIVE STATISTICS

Descriptive statistics give the scientist some idea of the nature of the raw data and are commonly used to summarize a set of observations by reporting measures of central tendency. The most commonly used parameters include the mode, median, and mean. The *mode* is the most commonly recorded observation; the *median* is the middle-ranked observation that has the same number of observations above and below it; and the *mean* is the arithmetic average, or the sum of the observations divided by the number of data points. The example in Table 25-1 demonstrates these parameters with reference to the ages of a group of 11 subjects.

Another example demonstrates the use of *categories* in examining data for central tendency: After 2 years of general surgical training, residents were tested for the acquisition of new operating skills. Table 25-2 shows the tabulated results. The mode of new operating room skills is 19 to 21, with a frequency of 10. The median of new operating room skills, or the number at which there is an equal frequency above and below that value, is 21.5 (note that there are 15 observations above and 15 observations below the median). The mean of this sample is calculated by using the midpoint of the range as the representative number of new skills. From the data shown in Table 25-3, the arithmetic mean then formulates to:

$$([29 \times 3] + [26 \times 7] + [23 \times 5] + [20 \times 10] + [17 \times 5])/30^* = 20.6$$

The median and the mode should be similar to the value of the mean in the case of a normal distribution. When the data do not conform to a normal distribution, special

**Sens,* Sensitivity (90%); *Fpr,* false-positive rate (1 − Spec) (10%); *Prev,* prevalence of carotid disease in general population (2%); *Abs,* absence of disease (1 − Prev) (98%).

*30 represents the number of observations.

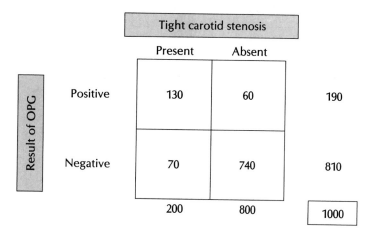

TABLE 25-1 THE COMMON PARAMETERS OF CENTRAL TENDENCY: MODE, MEDIAN, AND MEAN

SUBJECT	AGE
A	22
B	30
C	32
D	32
E	36
F	38
G	40
H	40
I	40
J	40
K	52

Mode, 40; median, 38; mean, 40.2.

TABLE 25-2 USE OF CATEGORIES IN EXAMINING CENTRAL TENDENCY IN STUDY OF NEWLY ACQUIRED OPERATING SKILLS

NUMBER OF NEW SKILLS	FREQUENCY
28-30	3
25-27	7
22-24	5
19-21	10
16-18	5

TABLE 25-3 THE MEAN OF NEWLY ACQUIRED OPERATING SKILLS

NUMBER OF NEW SKILLS	FREQUENCY
29	3
26	7
23	5
20	10
17	5

TABLE 25-4 SAMPLE RANGE OF THE ARTERIAL OXYGEN PRESSURE IN DOGS THAT HAD UNDERGONE LUNG TRANSPLANTATION

PRESSURES	
DOG	TORR
1	80
2	65
3	40
4	100
5	75

techniques, known as nonparametric tests (discussed in later sections), are used to analyze the data.

Measures of Variability

It is desirable to have some idea of the variability of the data around the calculated mean. The simplest measure of variability is the *range,* or difference between the highest and lowest observation in the sample. For example, measurements of the arterial oxygen pressure in dogs that had undergone unilateral lung transplantation are shown in Table 25-4. The range uses only two data points—the maximum and the minimum values. In the example the range is 60 torr (100 − 40).

The *variance* uses all the scores in a sample and represents the sum of the squared deviations of individual values from the mean, divided by one less than the sample size. The formula† for calculating the variance is:

$$\text{Variance} = \frac{\text{Sum of all } (X - \overline{X})^2}{n - 1}$$

The square root of the variance is the *standard deviation* of the sample. The standard deviation is a useful tool in describing characteristics of curves of known distribution, specifically the bell-shaped curve. It provides some indication of the variability of the data around the mean. Thus the data set is generally presented with a mean value plus or minus one standard deviation. If the data follow a normal or dumbbell-shaped distribution, 68% of the data points will be included within one standard deviation above or below the mean value. Two standard deviations above or below the mean value encompass 95% of the data, and 99% of the data are included in three standard deviations above or below the mean. The example in Table 25-5 shows calculation of these measures of central tendency in a group of patients with essential hypertension.

T Tests

In many cases, the medical scientist finds it necessary to look for possible differences in the mean values of a variable between disparate patient groups or between observations recorded before and after some treatment intervention was applied to the same group of subjects. This type of analysis examines continuous or numeric data, such as age, height, or blood glucose levels. The two types of t tests that may be used for these analyses are Student's t test and the paired t test. Student's t test is used when comparisons are made between the means of two different patient populations, such as a comparison of mean blood glucose levels between a group of diabetics and a group of nondiabetics. The paired t test,

†*X*, Each individual measurement; $\overline{X}$, mean of all measurements; *n*, number of observations.

on the other hand, is used when comparing values in a single patient group before and after some form of treatment intervention, such as a comparison of diastolic blood pressures before and after treatment with an antihypertensive medication (a more detailed explanation of these tests is given in the following paragraphs).

Student's (Unpaired) T Test

Student's t test is used to compare continuous (numeric) data in two different populations. This is a widely used statistic in medical research because comparison of variable values from patient groups is important in determining an optimal form of treatment.

The example in Table 25-6 shows a simple use of Student's, or unpaired, t test. In this example the weights of a group of boys are compared with the weights of a group of girls to see whether boys, in general, weigh more. There is no requirement in this test that the two groups be of equal size. The test will generate a t statistic, and in most cases, microcomputer programs will provide the *P* value as part of the printout, thus avoiding the necessity for the researcher to refer to statistical tables. If the *P* value is .05 or less, the observer may reject the null hypothesis and conclude with 95% or greater certainty that there is a real difference between the two groups.

This test provides a means of comparing only two variables (note that the mean values for more than two variables can be examined using analysis of variance). It is important for the researcher to eliminate (as much as possible) other variables that may affect the results. For instance, if the girls in the study are much older than the boys, it may be erroneously concluded that girls on the average weigh more. The age factor was not taken into account. It is up to the researcher to eliminate all the other variables that might affect the results.

In the example given in Table 25-6, the *P* value is .002; thus there is greater than a 99% chance that there is indeed a difference in the average weights, and that boys weigh more than girls.

Paired T Test

The paired t test provides the same t statistic as the unpaired t test and allows the observer to obtain a *P* value either directly from the computer program or from a book of statistical tables. The difference between the paired and unpaired statistics is that the paired t test mandates that the same study population be examined.

For example, the data in Table 25-7 compare the diastolic blood pressures in a group of patients before and after administration of an antihypertensive drug. The study was undertaken to see whether the drug in question lowered the blood pressure in the study group. Because the measurements in a paired t test are taken

TABLE 25-5 SAMPLE MEASURES OF CENTRAL TENDENCY IN STUDY OF PATIENTS WITH ESSENTIAL HYPERTENSION

AGES OF HYPERTENSIVE PATIENTS		
X_i	$(X_i - \bar{X})$	$(X_i - \bar{X})^2$
58	−5.3	28.1
47	−16.3	265.7
70	6.7	44.9
60	−3.3	10.9
45	−18.3	334.9
80	16.7	278.9
52	−11.3	127.7
73	9.7	94.1
69	5.7	32.5
79	15.7	246.5
		1464.2

Mean, 63.3 years; variance, 1464.2/9 (162.7); standard deviation, 12.8.

TABLE 25-6 SAMPLE OF STUDENT'S OR UNPAIRED T TEST IN STUDY COMPARING WEIGHTS OF BOYS AND GIRLS

WEIGHT (Lb)	
BOYS	GIRLS
95	80
90	77
86	68
77	59
100	72
92	60
73	59
68	
85	
90	

T value, 3.747; degrees of freedom, 15; *P* value, .002.

TABLE 25-7 SAMPLE OF PAIRED T TEST USED TO COMPARE DIASTOLIC BLOOD PRESSURE IN PATIENTS BEFORE AND AFTER MEDICATION

DIASTOLIC BLOOD PRESSURE (mm Hg)	
BEFORE DRUG	AFTER DRUG
100	90
90	85
80	70
110	100
95	90
80	70
120	100
85	70

T statistic, 6.065; degrees of freedom, 7; *P* value, .001.

TABLE 25-8 APPLICATION OF PEARSON'S PRODUCT MOMENT FORMULA IN CARDIAC OUTPUT STUDY

CARDIAC OUTPUT (L/Min)			
EMF* PROBE	SWAN-GANZ CATHETER	ULTRASOUND PROBE	DYE DILUTION
5.4	4.8	5.3	5.0
4.8	5.1	4.7	4.5
2.9	1.5	3.0	2.5
3.7	3.6	3.5	4.0
4.1	4.8	3.9	3.3
6.0	5.2	5.8	5.9
2.5	3.0	2.7	2.2
3.3	3.3	3.0	3.0
4.4	4.1	4.2	4.1

r Values

	EMF	Swan	Ultrasound	Dye
EMF	1	.71	.98	.94
Swan		1	.67	.62
Ultrasound			1	.92
Dye				1

* *EMF*, Electromagnetic flow.

TABLE 25-9 DATA GENERATED IN STUDY OF THE DEPENDENCE OF HEIGHT ON WEIGHT

HEIGHT (In)	WEIGHT (Lb)
60	140
50	80
68	160
72	180
78	190
65	142
80	220
45	60
65	120
40	62

before and after some form of intervention, the number of sample points in the comparison groups must be the same. In the example, the low *P* value indicates that the null hypothesis can be rejected and that the investigator can say with greater than 95% certainty that the drug is effective in lowering the diastolic blood pressure. Again, it is up to the investigator to be certain that no variables other than the drug might have influenced the results.

Correlation Coefficient

The correlation coefficient is a measure of association between variables. In medical research this statistic is often used to determine whether one parameter is a good predictor of another.

For example, is the amount of internal carotid artery stenosis, as measured with a noninvasive device such as the duplex scanner, similar to the amount of stenosis determined with a conventional arteriogram? The measure of association between variables is expressed as an r value. The highest r value is one, indicating that one variable is an exact predictor of another. An r value of zero would indicate that there is absolutely no association between the two variables. The Pearson's product moment formula may be used to determine these r values, and in the case of more than one variable, the association between all the variables is expressed in tabular form. The columns of data representing the different variables may be entered into a computerized statistics program, and r values may be generated without any knowledge of the mathematics involved in their calculation. In addition to the r values, a *P* value is given that indicates whether the r value represents a significant degree of association.

In the example in Table 25-8, the correlations (r values) between four different methods of determining cardiac output at nine different points in time are demonstrated. The highest association is between the values observed with the electromagnetic flow probe and the values obtained with the ultrasound probe (r, .98). The lowest association is between the Swan-Ganz catheter and the dye dilution methods (r, .62).

Regression Analysis

Regression analysis gives a more detailed analysis of the association between two variables. Generally this would be used to determine whether one variable can predict the other. For example, is a patient's height an accurate predictor of weight (Table 25-9)? This question can be examined visually by using a scattergram that plots one point against the other (Figure 25-3). By viewing the scattergram, one can see how close the association is between the dependent variable (usually displayed on the y axis) and the independent variable (usually displayed on the x axis). A computer-generated line can be drawn between these points, based on the sum of the least squares. The line is based on an equation that draws a line in which the square of the distance of each point from the line is at its minimum.

The correlation coefficient, or r value, is a measure of association between the two variables. As with Pearson's product moment formula, a perfect correlation would be indicated by an r value of one, whereas absolutely no predictive value or association between variables would be indicated by an r value of zero. In addition to evaluating the strength of the association, regression analysis also generates an equation that shows

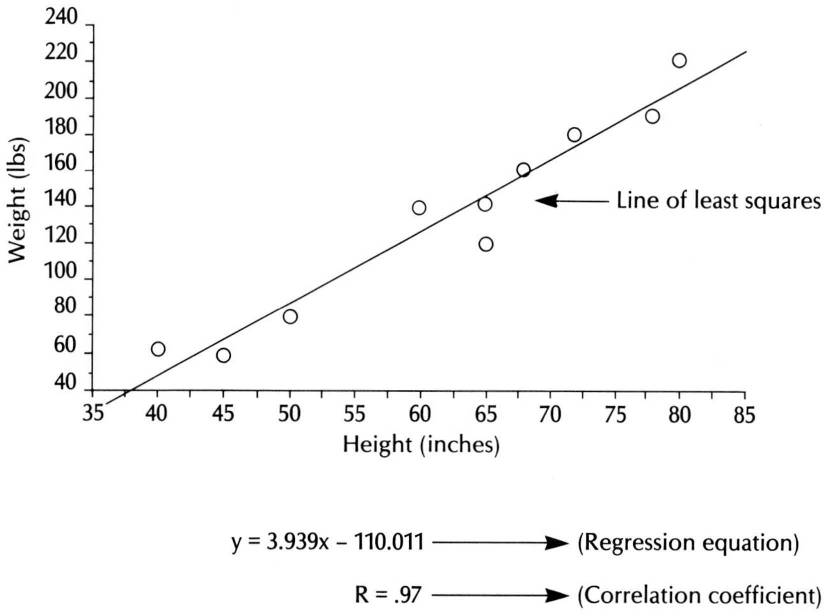

FIGURE 25-3 Sample scattergram plotting data from a study of the dependence of height on weight.

the nature of the relationship between the two variables.

The most common relationship is linear. The linear regression equation indicates the slope, or steepness, of the linear regression line and the point at which the line crosses the y axis (the y intercept). This linear regression equation can then be used to predict other points on the linear regression line.

In some instances the relationship may be parabolic rather than linear. In these cases the regression line would be curved, and the equation might be second order, that is, a nonlinear association. Regression equations can be higher than second order; however, when values are much above the second order level, the proposed relationship is of questionable value.

In some cases the dependent variable may relate to more than one independent variable. For example, a knowledge of both hematocrit and fibrinogen level would provide a better means of predicting viscosity than knowing one variable alone. This program is best approached with *stepwise regression analysis*, in which each variable is sequentially added to the equation to determine whether the predictive ability is increased with the addition of this variable. If the addition of a variable does not improve the predictive ability of the equation, that variable will not be included.

Chi-Square Test

When comparing discrete variables, such as the number of patients in different categories or subgroups, chi-square analysis is the appropriate test to use. It is a method commonly encountered by general medical readers because it is easy to use and has wide applicability. The raw data should be set up in the form of a contingency table, which involves counting the number of persons or subjects in each specifically defined group. In its simplest form, this test can be set up as a two-by-two table, and χ^2 equals the sum of the squares of the observed values (O) minus the expected values (E), divided by the expected value:

$$\chi^2 = (\text{Sum of all})\frac{(O - E)^2}{E}$$

For example, is there a difference in the incidence of hypertension between black patients and white patients? To examine this problem, a two-by-two table is set up, classifying blacks and whites as hypertensive or not hypertensive (Figure 25-4).

The counted values are entered into a computer program and a chi-square statistic is generated. In addition, a *P* value will be given by most computer programs and represents the probability that the difference in frequency of the values in the various cells was not the result of chance. The *P* value can also be easily obtained by referring to standard tables in a statistical textbook. If a table is used, it is necessary to know the degrees of freedom (DOF) in addition to the chi-square value. The DOF is calculated by subtracting 1 from the total number of cells.

	Black	White	
Hypertensive	15	4	(19)
Not hypertensive	30	41	(71)
	(45)	(45)	(Total = 90)

$X^2 = 8.073$

$p = .004$

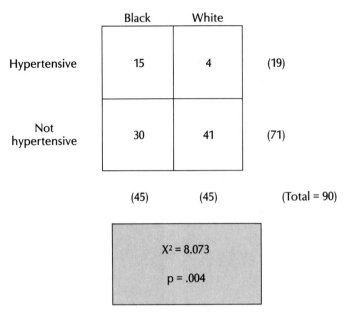

FIGURE 25-4 Sample two-by-two table classifying blacks and whites as hypertensive or not hypertensive.

The *P* value indicates the confidence with which one can reject the null hypothesis. In the example given above, the chi-square value is 8.073, and the probability that the observed values were different from an expected normal distribution of equal numbers in all cells is 0.004. Thus the null hypothesis is rejected, and it is assumed that blacks have a higher incidence of hypertension than whites.

The two-by-two table used in the above example represents one of the simplest applications of the chi-square test. Larger tables (three-by-three, four-by-three, etc.) may also be constructed, and the chi-square statistic can be used to see if there is any difference among the cells. It must be kept in mind that, for example, in a three-by-three table, a statistical difference may be demonstrated, but to localize the variables responsible for this difference, individual chi-square analyses must be performed. (The chi-square test is inappropriate for small sample sizes because the distribution of data is often skewed. A nonparametric test, the Fischer exact test, is a special modification of the chi-square test used when the sample size is small.)

ACTUARIAL ANALYSIS

Although surgical therapy may be initially successful, the long-term success of some procedures may be less than anticipated. Therefore some statistical technique is necessary to assess the survival of various groups of patients. Actuarial techniques have been in existence since the sixteenth century but were only introduced into the surgical literature in the 1950s. The statistical treatment of time-related events in a given group (often referred to as survival curves) is frequently used to compare mortality among groups, although any event, such as prosthetic valve infection, colonic leak rate, or postoperative heart block, could be measured with these techniques.

There are two fundamental ways of determining the event rate among groups: The life-table method and the Kaplan-Meier method. Both of these techniques are based on several basic assumptions:

1. The interval before the event has a unique starting time (that is, the beginning of therapy or the operation).
2. A discrete endpoint or event can be defined (for example, death, thrombosis, or infection).
3. The length of follow-up can be variable after the begininning of the study.

With the actuarial or life-table method, observations are grouped into fixed time periods, such as minutes, days, or years, to estimate an event curve. The probability of "surviving" or having an event-free interval is estimated by using the following formula:

$$Px = \frac{Nx - Ex - Lx/2}{Nx - Lx/2}$$

Nx represents the number of patients without event in xth interval. Ex is the number of events in the xth interval, Lx is the number lost to follow-up in the xth interval. Px is the probability of an event-free xth interval.

The probability of an event-free interval is then determined by multiplying the probability of each succeeding interval:

$$Vx = P_1 \times P_2 \times - \times Px$$

Vx represents the probability of an event-free interval beginning at time zero to interval x. The event-free curve is then estimated by connecting the Vx points generated.

As an example, 15 patients who had undergone "curative" gastric resection for carcinoma were followed for up to 5 years. The results are shown in Table 25-10. If these data are examined at 12-month intervals, then for the first Px it is noted that in the first 12 months, 2 patients died and none were lost to follow-up. This then fits into the equation as:

$$P_1 = \frac{15 - 2 - 0/2}{15 - 0/2} = .87$$

TABLE 25-10 DATA FROM STUDY OF PATIENTS WHO HAD UNDERGONE "CURATIVE" GASTRIC RESECTION FOR CARCINOMA 5 YEARS PREVIOUSLY

PATIENTS	DEATH (MONTHS)	LOST TO FOLLOW-UP (MONTHS)
1	8	—
2	10	—
3	20	—
4	—	22
5	—	25
6	—	28
7	30	—
8	32	—
9	—	34
10	34	—
11	37	—
12	—	38
13	40	—
14	42	—
15	43	—

In the next year, one patient died, and one was lost to follow-up. This then fits into the equation as:

$$P_2 = \frac{13 - 1 - 1/2}{13 - 1/2} = .92$$

The probability of a patient surviving resection for gastric carcinoma for 24 months is $E_x = P_1 \times P_2$, or in this case, $.87 \times .92 = .804$. By carrying out the appropriate calculations, one generates the life table shown in Table 25-11. Thus the probability of surviving gastric resection up to 4 years in this series was 15.5%; there were no survivors after this.

The Kaplan-Meier method estimates the event curve by using the exact time of death. It differs from the life table in that a patient who was lost to follow-up is assumed to be alive and is not corrected for in the equation. This method assumes that the probability of an event occurring is zero until that event happens; thus the generated curve is steplike and not a curve at all. Although each method is applicable to grouped or individual data, the life-table method is commonly used for groups and the Kaplan-Meier method is used for individuals. The above data are reexamined here using the Kaplan-Meier method. The formula for the Kaplan-Meier method is:

$$Px = \frac{\text{No. of patients without event at time x}}{\text{No. of event-free patients at time x + No. of events at time x}}$$

In these data, the first death occurred at 8 months. This transforms the equation to:

$$P8 = \frac{14}{14 + 1} = 0.93$$

The next patient died at 10 months:

$$P10 = \frac{13}{13 + 1} = 0.93$$

At 34 months 5 patients are still surviving or lost to follow-up. This converts the equation to:

$$P34 = \frac{5}{5 + 1} = 0.83$$

Note that the patients lost to follow-up before the event

TABLE 25-11 LIFE TABLE GENERATED FROM DATA IN TABLE 25-10

MONTHS AFTER OPERATION	NO. OF PATIENTS ALIVE	NO. OF EVENTS	PATIENTS LOST TO FOLLOW-UP	Px	Vx
0-11	15	2	0	.87	.87
12-23	13	1	1	.92	.80
24-35	12	3	3	.71	.57
36-47	06	4	1	.27	.15

TABLE 25-12 TABLE DERIVED BY APPLYING KAPLAN-MEIER METHOD TO DATA IN TABLE 25-10

MONTHS	NO. OF PATIENTS ALIVE	NO. OF PATIENTS DEAD	Px	Vx
6	14	1	.93	.93
10	13	1	.93	.86
20	12	1	.92	.79
30	8	1	.88	.70
32	7	1	.87	.61
34	5	1	.83	.51
37	4	1	.80	.41
40	2	1	.66	.27
42	1	1	.50	.13

at 34 months were ignored in this calculation. The patients lost to follow-up after the 34-month event are assumed to be alive. By carrying out the calculations, Table 25-12 is generated by the Kaplan-Meier method.

One-Way Analysis of Variance

Student's t test has been used to compare the difference between the means of two variables, but this test is limited in that it can compare only *two* means. Analysis of variance (ANOVA), on the other hand, is used for the comparison of the means of three or more independent groups. It is a requirement for the use of this test that the variances are equal; if they are not, a nonparametric test should be used (discussed in the latter part of this chapter). The null hypothesis states that there is no significant difference between the groups. The alternative hypothesis (if the null hypothesis is rejected) is that there is a significant difference between at least two of the population means.

An F ratio is calculated with the ANOVA test, which places the variance between the groups in the numerator and the variance within the groups in the denominator. Stated another way, the numerator is the average of the squared differences between the group means and the mean of all the scores, and the denominator is the variance of all scores. The test is used to see if the variability in the data is caused by variability within groups or variability between groups.

Values for the F distribution can be calculated and tabulated for known degrees of freedom, and the F ratio can be compared with this table for determination of sufficient smallness for acceptance of the null hypothesis. In theory, the variance estimate should equal 1 if the null hypothesis is correct. If the observed F value is greater than the *P* value that has been selected by the investigator, then the null hypothesis is rejected and the groups are assumed to be unequal. In most microcomputer programs, the user is asked to pick three or more variables and then choose ANOVA from the menu of tests. The F statistic is given along with a probability value, allowing the user to accept or reject the null hypothesis. It is important to note that the analysis of variance does not predict any relationship among or within the variables once the null hypothesis is rejected.

TABLE 25-13 DATA GENERATED FROM STUDY OF MEAN VISCOSITY LEVELS

VISCOSITY LEVELS (SECONDS)		
DRUG A	DRUG B	DRUG C
32.1	28.5	38.5
38.6	22.8	40.2
20.6	20.4	50.9
34.9	18.6	48.7
22.6	17.5	42.3
41.2	30.8	39.8
35.9	25.6	42.5
26.4	21.7	41.6
	24.4	37.7
		44.4

Mean: A, 31.5; B, 23.4; C, 42.6.
Standard deviation: A, 7.6; B, 4.4; C, 4.3.

In the example in Table 25-13, the mean viscosity levels were measured using a new Merrill porous bed viscometer (which registers in seconds) in three groups of patients, each of which had been treated with a different drug. The null hypothesis assumes that there is no difference in viscosity levels among the three groups.

On first inspection of the raw data it would appear that there is a difference among the means of the three groups. A one-way analysis of variance as shown below is used to see if this difference is significant.

ANALYSIS OF VARIANCE

	DOF	Sum Squares	Mean Square
Between groups	2	1785.357	892.679
Within groups	24	721.323	30.055
TOTAL	26	2506.68	
F test = 29.701			$P \leq .0001$

The F ratio is high in this example, and the probability that the differences in the means occurred by chance is less than 0.05. Therefore the null hypothesis is rejected, and it is assumed that a difference in group means exists. T tests may be used to identify the difference(s) in more detail.

Two-Way Analysis of Variance

Two-way analysis of variance (ANOVA) accomplishes essentially the same thing as the previous test except that the data may be influenced by two independent variables. As an example, assume that viscosity was again measured after administration of drugs A, B, and C. This time, however, the investigator was also interested in whether the sex of the patient contributed to variance between the groups. The data would be set up as in Table 25-14.

The two-way ANOVA would examine each of the individual factors, as well as the interaction of the two factors (Table 25-15). The data suggest that the two variables together do influence the viscosity; furthermore, the drug seems to exert a greater effect than does sex.

TABLE 25-14 DATA GENERATED IN STUDY OF EFFECT OF SEX ON VISCOSITY LEVELS

	DRUG A	DRUG B	DRUG C
Males	46	29	35
	42	27	38
	45	24	34
	40	30	40
	38	22	45
Females	35	21	47
	33	24	38
	34	18	42
	29	17	45
	37	20	49
		23	39

Nonparametric Testing Techniques

Many nonparametric testing techniques are available. Their unusual names create confusion for the majority of medical personnel attempting to make sense from data analyses in various journal articles. The most important thing to remember is that the purpose behind these examinations is the same as in those presented in previous sections of this chapter. However, the other tests (t tests, chi-square, correlation coefficient, etc.) presume that the data being analyzed have a normal distribution about the mean. Nonparametric tests are distribution independent and may be used with data that do not have a normal distribution. In many cases this indicates a small number of patients. The calculations from these tests are easily made with microcomputer software. In the following discussion the corresponding nonparametric test is related to its counterpart that depends on a normal distribution of data.

The Mann-Whitney U test is used to compare two independent samples of continuous data. The sample sizes do not have to be equal, and this test corresponds to Student's t test, which is used when there is a normal distribution of data. The other nonparametric test that may also be used in this situation is the Wilcoxon ranked sum test.

In examining the effect of a certain drug, a parameter is examined before and after the treatment is administered to see if the drug makes a difference to the condition of the patients. In the parametric world the paired t test is used; the nonparametric equivalent is the Wilcoxon signed rank test.

When comparing the means of more than two independent populations to see if any differences are present, the nonparametric Kruskal-Wallis test may be used. It is based on the ranks of the data rather than on the actual values. The Kruskal-Wallis test compares with the one-way ANOVA technique described earlier. The corresponding nonparametric test for the two-way ANOVA is the Friedman test.

Contingency tables are set up in the form of cells when discrete data or a number of patients with a certain

TABLE 25-15 TABLE GENERATED BY APPLICATION OF ANOVA TO DATA IN TABLE 25-14

SOURCE	SUM OF SQUARES	DEGREE OF FREEDOM	MEAN SQUARES	F RATIO	P>F
Sex	84.424	1	84.424	6.509	0.126
Drug	1981.242	2	990.621	76.375	0.001
Interaction	272.975	2	136.488	10.523	0.001
Error	337.233	26	12.971		
TOTAL	2675.875	31			

a	b
c	d

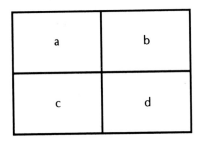

$$\text{Probability} = \frac{(a+b)!\ (c+d)!\ (a+c)!\ (b+d)!}{N!\ a!\ b!\ c!\ d!}$$

FIGURE 25-5 Formula used for computing the Fisher exact test.

	Alive	Dead	
No heparin	1	5	6
Heparin	3	3	6
	4	8	12

FIGURE 25-6 Two-by-two contingency table for study of the effect of intraoperative heparin on mortality.

	Alive	Dead	
No heparin	0	6	6
Heparin	4	2	6
	4	8	12

FIGURE 25-7 Reducing the smallest cell by one and keeping the marginal totals constant yields the more extreme or less likely probability. (See Figures 25-5 and 25-6.)

condition are analyzed. Significant differences between the observed numbers and the expected numbers (based on chance) are detected by the chi-square test. When the sample sizes are small or there is not a normal distribution of data, the Fisher exact test is the procedure of choice.

The Spearman-Rho test is a nonparametric test used to detect a significant relationship between continuous variables. This test is useful when the data are not intervally numeric but ranked, such as medical student grades that might be honors, high pass, pass, marginal, and fail. It is similar to the techniques described to obtain a correlation coefficient. The Kendall-Tau test is another nonparametric test used to detect an association between variables. It is based on the ranks of data rather than their actual values.

Two examples of nonparametric testing techniques are given below to help familiarize the reader with these types of statistical methods.

Fisher Exact Test

The two-by-two contingency table has been discussed. The null hypothesis for the Fisher exact test is the same as for the chi-square test (i.e., that the variables are independent). It assumes that the marginal totals of the contingency table will be constant; thus by manipulating the individual cells of the table yet maintaining the marginal totals constant, several P values can be generated, and the sum of these is the probability according to the Fisher exact test. The formula used in computing the Fisher exact test is shown in Figure 25-5 in which *(!)* indicates the factorial value:

$$4! = 4 \times 3 \times 2 \times 1 = 24$$

For example, 12 patients with mesenteric venous thrombosis were examined to see if intraoperative heparinization changed mortality. The two-by-two contingency table constructed is shown in Figure 25-6. The contingency table is examined as follows:

$$P = \frac{(1 + 5)! \times (3 + 3)! \times (1 + 3)! \times (5 + 3)!}{12! \times 1! \times 3! \times 3! \times 5!} = .24$$

The smallest cell is reduced by one, whereas the marginal totals are kept constant to obtain the more extreme or less likely probability. This process now converts the table to that shown in Figure 25-7, and the probability is calculated again:

$$P = \frac{(0 + 6)!\ (4 + 2)!\ (0 + 2)!\ (6 + 4)!}{12!\ 6!\ 4!\ 2!\ 0!} = .22$$

This process of reducing by one is continued until zero is reached. To obtain the probability for the Fisher exact test, the computed probabilities are added:

$$0.24 + 0.22 = 0.46$$

TABLE 25-16 DATA GENERATED FROM STUDY MEASURING ARTERIAL PRESSURE OF OXYGEN OF DOGS BEFORE AND AFTER UNILATERAL LUNG TRANSPLANTATION

DOG NO.	BEFORE OPERATION	AFTER OPERATION	DIFFERENCE	RANK	SIGNED RANK
1	100	80	20	7	7
2	80	80	0	—	—
3	94	96	−2	1	−1
4	60	85	−25	8	−8
5	75	62	13	4	4
6	65	80	−15	5	−5
7	85	90	−5	3	−3
8	80	62	18	6	6
9	92	45	47	9	9
10	89	93	−4	2	−2

Thus the null hypothesis that survival is independent of heparin effects is rejected. As the numbers in each cell get larger, this test becomes cumbersome, and the chi-square becomes appropriate. Note that this is the result of a one-tailed test. A two-tailed test value is obtained by multiplying the probability by two.

Wilcoxon Signed Rank Test

The Wilcoxon signed rank test itself ranks the raw data relative to other data points. By knowing the sum of the positive ranks, the sum of the negative ranks, and the number of samples, a table of critical values can be consulted for the level of significance. For example, the arterial pressure of oxygen of dogs was measured before and after unilateral lung transplantation. The results are shown in Table 25-16. To rank the samples, the signs are initially ignored, and the rank is obtained from lowest to highest with any zero values detected from the population. This generates the rank column in Table 25-16. The signed rank then assigns positive or negative as in the difference column. The sum of the positive ranks is 26; the sum of the negative ranks is 19; and the n of this group is 9. After comparison with a signed rank table, we obtain a *P* value that allows us to reject the null hypothesis.

DATA PRESENTATION

The basic tenet to be used when preparing data for presentation to a group of people is to *keep it simple.* When faced with a large row-and-column table filled with numbers, the average listener loses interest and gains little from the presentation.

It is often better to present data in graphic form rather than as numbers on a slide, and three basic types of charts can be used to represent data to an audience: the bar graph, the pie chart, and the line graph.

Bar Graph

An example of a bar graph is shown in Figure 25-8. This illustration was constructed to show the effect of a certain drug on weight in different groups of people. The graph is simple and self-explanatory. While the audience is examining the slide the presenter can elaborate on different aspects of the data, such as how the groups were defined and how long the drug was administered. The y axis of the graph should be constructed so that the data fit on the graph in a pleasing manner but are not so compressed that differences in the data will not be appreciated.

In general more than four categories on a graph become confusing and a line chart should be considered. It is important that a legend accompany the illustration so that the meaning of the different colored bars can be readily appreciated. In Figure 25-8 two time periods are represented—before and after administration of the drug. Three bar shades or situations are about all that should be used in one graph; the data tend to get confusing if more than this number is used.

The labels for the x and y axes should be simple but should accurately express the meaning of the categories or classifications. Abbreviations are acceptable if they are easily understood by the audience.

The Ts on top of the bars represent either one standard deviation or one standard error of the data. Which of these two parameters is in use should be made clear to the audience because the standard error is usually much smaller than the standard deviation.

This type of graph is ideal for presenting comparisons done with the paired t test. In Figure 25-8, a paired t test could be done before and after administration of the drug in each of the three categories (men, women, and children). A P value could then be placed over the two corresponding bars for each of the comparisons.

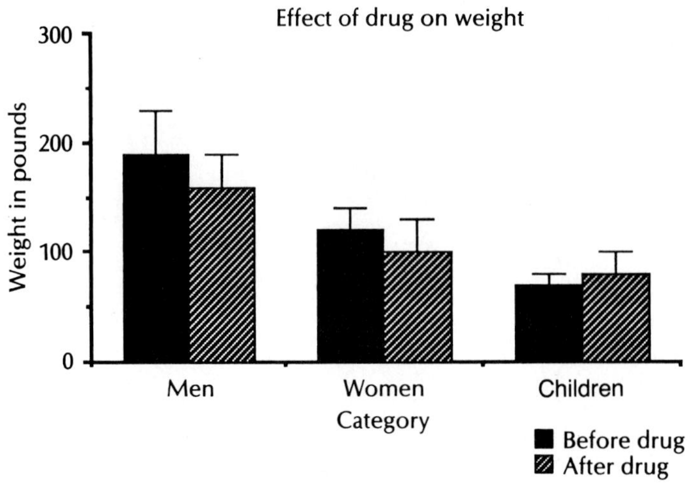

FIGURE 25-8 Bar graph showing the effect of a drug on weight in different groups of people.

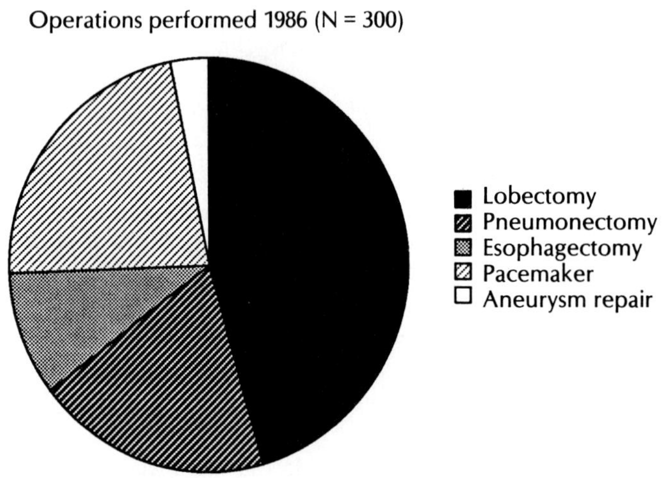

FIGURE 25-9 Pie chart presenting the number and types of operations performed during a given time period by a general thoracic surgery service.

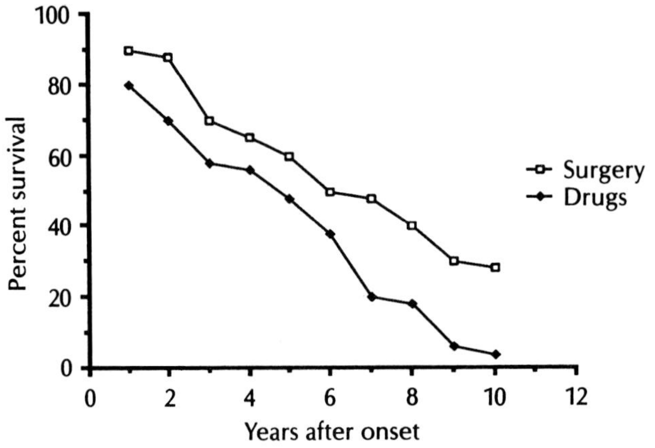

FIGURE 25-10 Line graph comparing surgery and drug therapy in the treatment of disease *X*.

Pie Chart

The pie chart is particularly helpful when the presenter is trying to emphasize the percentage that each of the categories contributes to the population as a whole. The example in Figure 25-9 graphically presents the number and types of operations performed by a general thoracic surgery service during a certain time period. The audience can easily appreciate which were the most and least frequent types of operations. These types of charts can be quite simple but effective in displaying various kinds of demographic data. Because this is basically a percentage type of graph where elements are presented as a part of the whole, it is important to indicate somewhere on the graph the number of patients under examination. In this example the number (n = 300) is displayed in the graph title.

Line Graph

When a number of data points are to be plotted on the same graph, the data may be plotted on a line chart (Figure 25-10). This type of chart is particularly useful for displaying actuarial data. The observer can readily see the percentage of patients surviving a certain disease each year after its diagnosis. In addition, this medium provides a way of visually displaying the results of two different kinds of treatment. As with all other graphs and situations, it is important to keep the amount of information displayed on the graph simple.

SUGGESTED READINGS

Daniel WW: *Biostatistics: a foundation for analysis in the health sciences,* New York, 1983, John Wiley & Sons.

Remington RD, Schork MA: *Statistics with applications to the biological and health sciences,* Englewood Cliffs, NJ, 1970, Prentice-Hall.

Rimm AA, Hartz AJ, Kalbfleisch JH et al: *Basic biostatistics in medicine and epidemiology,* New York, 1980, Appleton-Century-Crofts.

Rosner B: *Fundamentals of biostatistics,* Boston, 1982, Duxbury Press.

Sharp VF: *Statistics for the social sciences,* Boston, 1979, Little, Brown.

Sincich T: *Statistics by example,* San Francisco, 1982, Dellen Publishing.

INDEX

G

H

I

J

P

W

X

Y

Z